SETHI'S
Quantitative Analysis *of* Pharmaceutical Formulations

SETHI'S

Quantitative Analysis *of* Pharmaceutical Formulations

Methods With Reaction Mechanism

Fourth Edition

Volume 1

Dr. P.D. Sethi
M.Pharm., Ph.D.

CBS

CBS PUBLISHERS & DISTRIBUTORS PVT. LTD.

NEW DELHI • BENGALURU • PUNE • KOCHI • CHENNAI

ISBN : 978-81-239-2187-7

Third Edition : 1997
Reprint : 2003, 2004, 2005, 2008, 2010, 2011
Fourth Edition : 2012

Published by:
Satish K. Jain and produced by Vinod K. Jain for CBS Publishers & Distributors Pvt. Ltd.,
4819/XI Prahlad Street, 24 Ansari Road, Daryaganj, New Delhi - 110002 (India)
E-mail: cbspubs@airtelmail.com, delhi@cbspd.com • www.cbspd.com

Branches:
- ***Bengaluru:*** 2975, 17th Cross, K.R. Road,
  Bansankari 2nd Stage, Bengaluru - 560070
  Ph.: +91-80-26771678/79
  E-mail: cbsbng@gmail.com, bangalore@cbspd.com
- ***Pune:*** Bhuruk Prestige, Sr. No. 52/12/2+1+3/2,
  Narhe, Haveli (Near Katraj-Dehu Road By-pass), Pune - 411051
  Ph.: +91-20-64704058/59, 32342277 • E-mail: pune@cbspd.com
- ***Kochi:*** 36/14, Kalluvilakam, Lissie Hospital Road, Kochi - 682018, Kerala
  Ph.: +91-484-4059061-65 • Fax: +91-484-4059065
  E-mail: cochin@cbspd.com
- ***Chennai:*** 20, West Park Road, Shenoy Nagar, Chennai - 600030
  Ph.: +91-44-26260666, 26208620 E-mail: chennai@cbspd.com

Printed at :
Aegean Offset Printers, Greater Noida (UP)

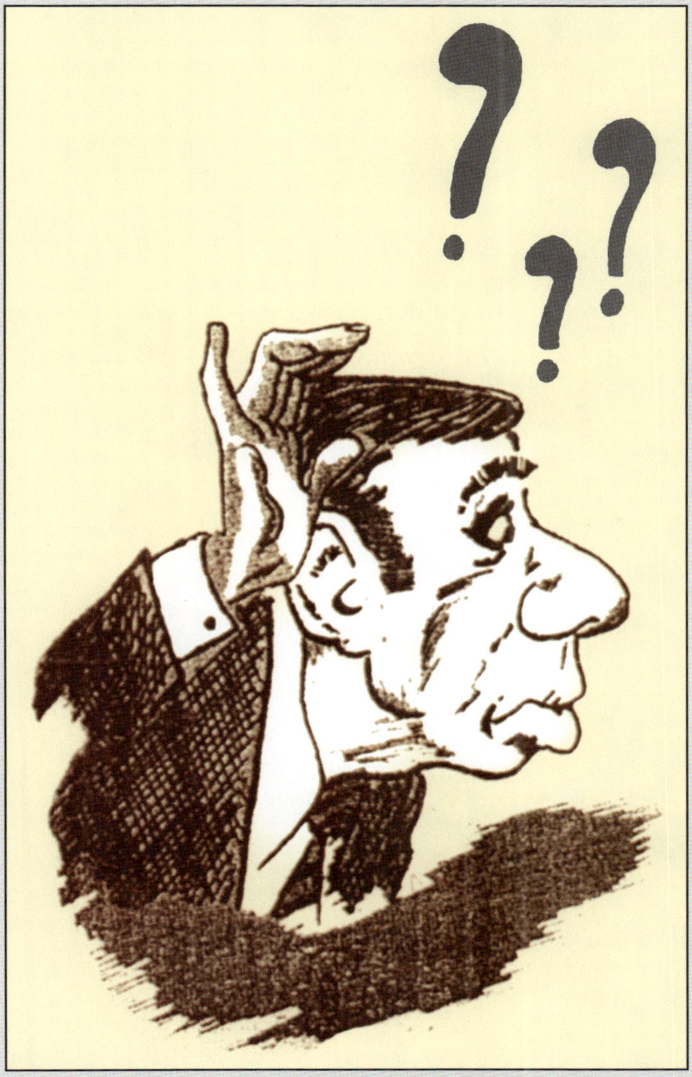

What technology may not solve, the idea may!

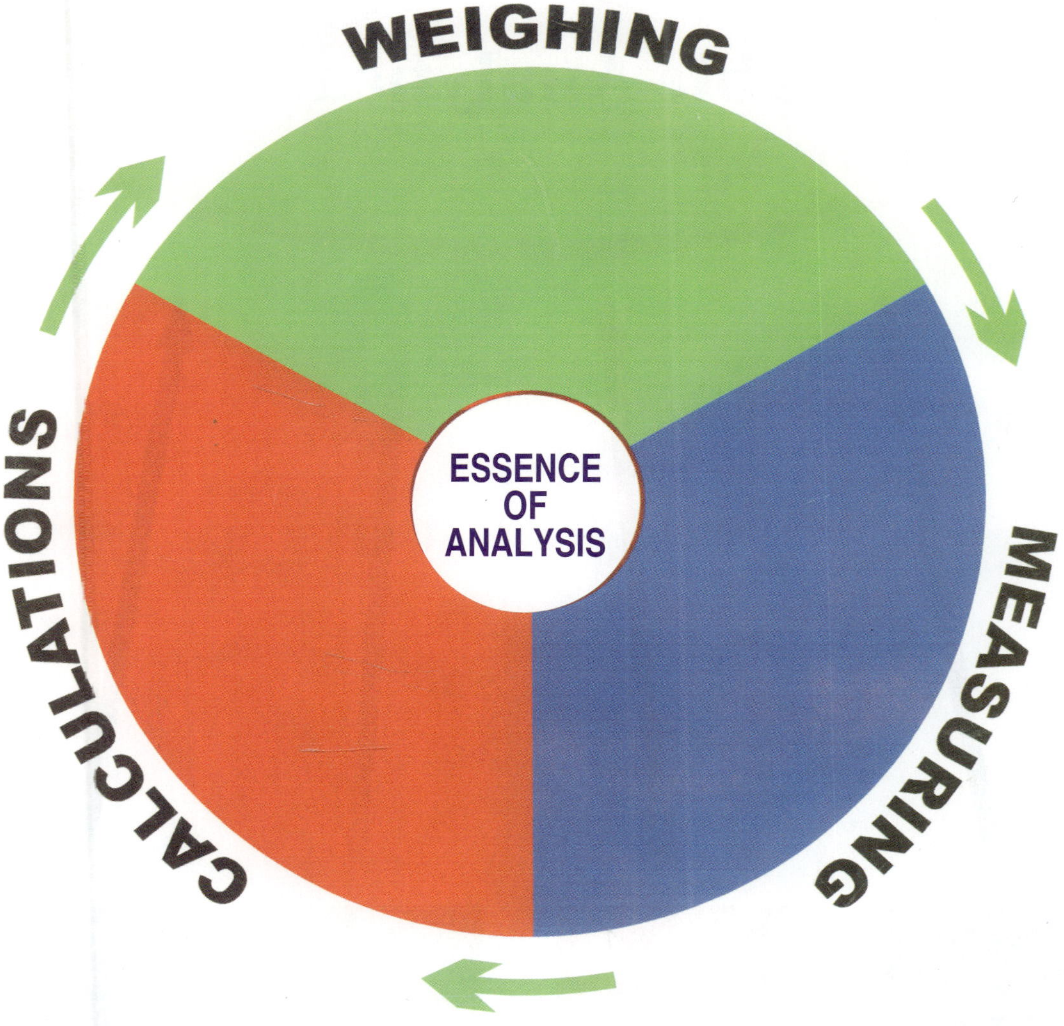

"If from any art, you take away which concerns weighing measuring and arithmetic, how little is left of that art."

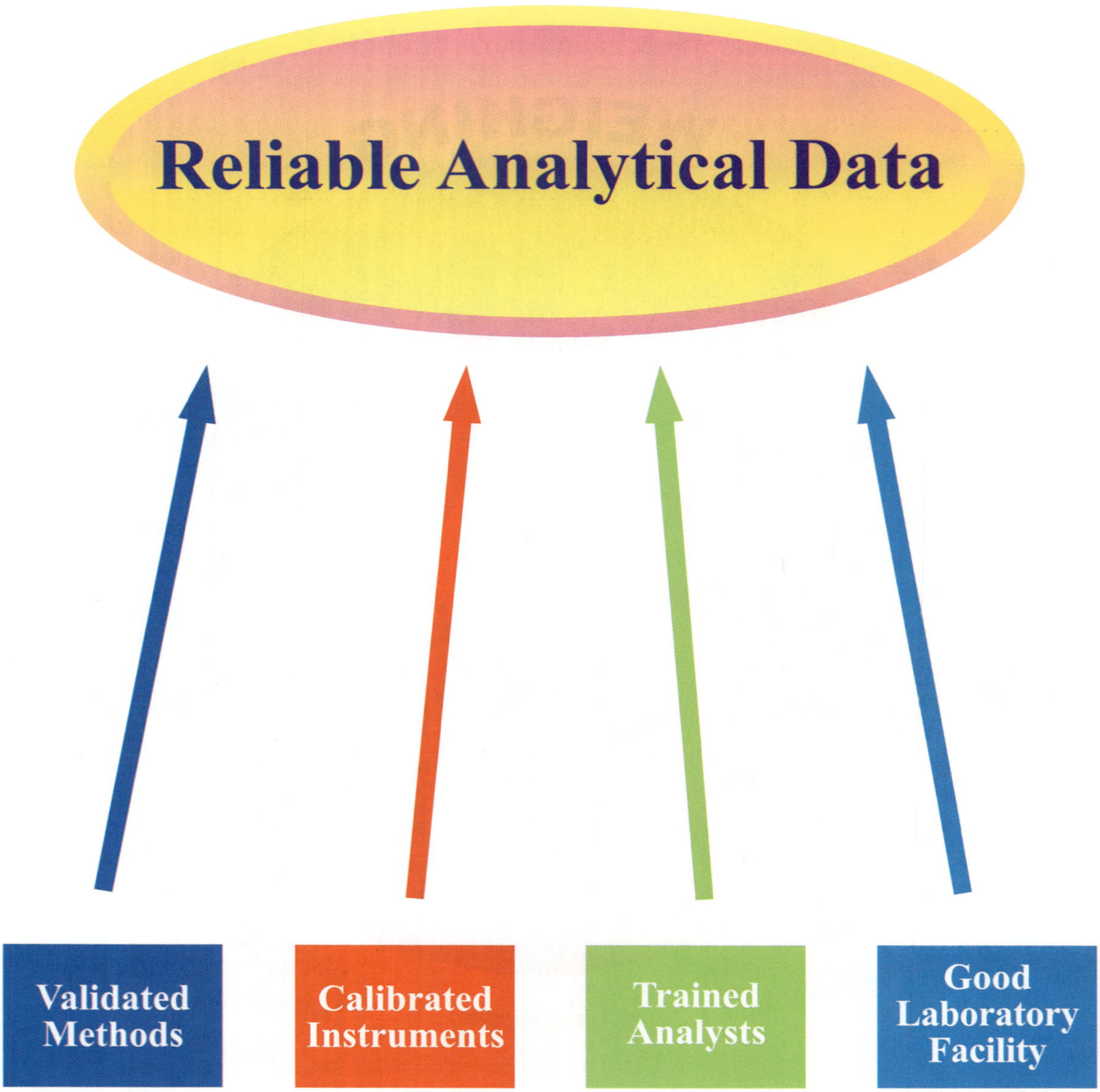

Talent, Attitude and Practical Experience Have No Subtitute

To

Usha, my wife

Although no one is ever born talented nor talent obtained
as a gift or lucky coincidence, it is a resource acquired
through one's own endeavour,
but without her active support and inspiration,
I would never have been an author.

Dedicated to Fellow Analysts, Students, Teachers, Professionals and Mentors

I am quite aware that this compilation may not be flawless, but if I would have waited till it could be done without any error, probably this would never have been possible considering the fact that incompleteness is inevitable feature of any book. I do hope that this compilation will provide adequate stimulus for you to be a sound professional. I would like to appeal the fellow analysts, students, teaching fraternity and professionals to evaluate my efforts in proper perspective. It took me almost 15 years to scan most of the old analytical journals from 1950 onward, the period when analytical methods based on chromogenic reactions were most prevalent. I would like to express my gratitude to fellow analysts, teachers and the mentors in the profession who helped me to shape my ideas for compiling this text. The wide popularity of my books on spectrophotometric analysis, TLC, HPTLC and HPLC among pharmaceutical analysts, students and teachers has been gratifying and encouraging. My aim has never been to use my knowledge as a vehicle but only as a means of sharing my experience with prefessional fraternity.

P.D. Sethi
Pharmaceutical Analyst

"There is no barrier to acquisition of knowledge. Nobody owns it, everybody partakes it and the world becomes richer."

Preface to the Fourth Edition

After the first edition this book appeared in 1985, analytical and teaching fraternity have been of the considered opinion that for professional competency the knowledge of the chemistry involved in the analytical methods i.e. "Reaction Mechanism" needs to be provided, even though not legally mandated, to enable the analysts to perceive the methodology in proper perspective since all aspects of different methods are ultimately founded on chemistry. This is how the idea for contents of this book originated.

Although I had conceptualized the project in 1992 but being busy in compiling books on other subjects of current importance i.e. TLC, HPTLC, HPLC including revision of this title, I could not take up this project due to paucity of time and resources. Further, in view of complexity of the project, I did harbour serious doubts regarding its ultimate completion if and when taken up. If anyone feels that the books can be written by setting an author on his or her way and then waiting for the manuscript to appear, they are delusioned. It needs constant adaptation, definite level of discipline and hunger to keep going. I had been exploring the possibility of associating some teachers with sound knowledge of basic organic chemistry, but met with no success. It has been my ultimate **desire** to complete the project before I close my shop forever.

Knowing fully well that nothing can be achieved without enthusiasm and dedication, being **SCORPIO** decided to accept the challenge with the **SELF BELIEF** and complete the project by myself. I sincerely hope that this series shall find permanent place in every analytical laboratory and teaching institutions with the assurance that such an exhaustive compilation on the subject may never be available.

"Desire is perhaps the starting point of achieving something."

"Belief is the knowledge that we can do something. It is the inner feeling that what we undertake, we can accomplish."

"Scorpio have creative mind with sharp memory, truly explorer of new intelligent horizon, have great stamina and never shy away from challenges, extremely introspective with analytical mind, highly intuitive, determined in pursuit of their goal, passionate about every thing they do, have strong sense of purpose in life with determination to do nothing half-heartedly."

For practical consideration, in addition to introductory chapters, the book has been arranged in 13 principal chapters each containing different multi-component formulations. Analytical methods for each ingredient in a formulation have been described on the pattern similar to 3rd edition using mainly UV-Vis spectroscopy as principal analytical tool. However, as clear from the title, uniqueness of 4th edition is that with each method "probable reaction mechanism" has been described for proper understanding of the methodology as describing methods while ignoring chemistry was considered to be an incomplete endeavour. This should help analysts to integrate fully the analytical methods with the chemistry involved and enable them to transmit the knowledge to others who want to learn. Majority of the reactions included in the text are of the type – addition, elimination, substitution, condensation, rearrangement or oxidation-reduction invariably resulting in the formation of a coloured end product, which could easily be quantified spectrophotometrically in visible region (400-800 nm). This once again established the importance of UV-Vis spectroscopy as an indispensable, reliable and well established analytical tool in spite of steep increase in the use of other physical methods of analysis (HPLC, HPLC/MS, GC, GC/MS, HPTLC, etc.). Analytical methods based on chromogenic reactions have stood the test of time and are still recommended for the fledgling analysts.

Understanding the reaction mechanism allows us to know its specificity and the reaction with the drug being analysed. For drugs having more than one functional group, the methods have been designed depending on the specificity of a particular functional group. With selective chemical reactions, the analyst can manipulate the sample to reveal the desired information and increase the selectivity of the analyte eliminating the possible interference due to other substances present in the formulation while analyzing. It is not

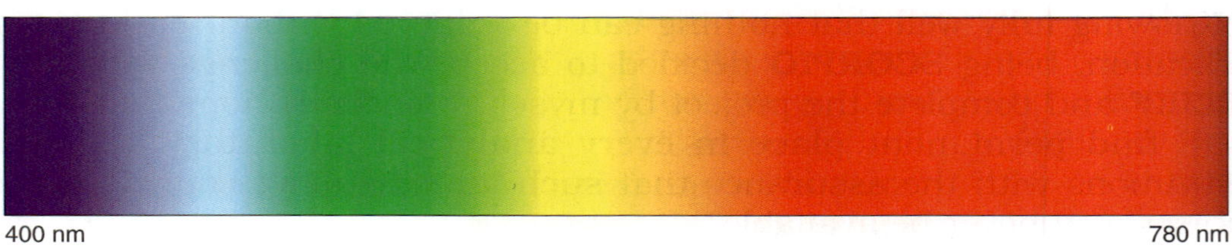

The light that human eye can perceive ranges from deep-violet (short wavelength) through blue, green, yellow and orange to deep red (long wavelength).

"One who never made a mistake never learnt anything."

necessary to learn thousands of individual reactions, instead we can learn few common reactions really well and apply the knowledge to similar cases.

Based on the functional group present in a molecule, the following reagents have been most commonly employed for quantification of the drug molecule: Gibbs' reagent, Bratton-Marshall reagent, Emerson's reagent, Ehrlich's reagent, Pauly's reagent, INH reagent, MBTH reagent, Besthorn's reagent, Folin's reagent, Van Urk's reagent, Wurster's Red reagent, Sanger's reagent, Chromotropic acid reagent, N-Bromosuccinimide reagent and DNPH reagent.

Most of the reaction mechanisms described in the text are as reported by the authors for which relative references have been cited under each reaction. However, the book "Pharmaceutical Chemistry, Vol. 2" by H.J. Roth et al. has been extensively referred to and has been extremely helpful in visualizing the reaction mechanism of several drug substances. Other textbooks of organic chemistry and analytical chemistry invariably consulted have been added under references at the end of introduction.

I am confident that 'Reaction Mechanism' described in this book along with method of analysis shall provide the most stimulating learning experience and will enable you to appreciate the excitement of this fascinating field.

Since newer molecules are invariably chemical modifications of existing drug substances, this compilation should be of help to the analysts in developing suitable method of analysis for newer drug molecules and also understand the chemistry involved and the confidence to tackle newer situations.

Over the years it was observed that at postgraduate level several practical exercises in pharmaceutical analysis were based on the methods described in 1st, 2nd and 3rd editions of this book. The students were invariably keen to know the detailed chemistry involved in methods. I do hope, my attempt in this direction will help students to perform practicals with better understanding. I expect this four-volume book on pharmaceutical analysis with reaction mechanism should make analytical science easier to understand for students, analysts and educators.

The icon representing structure of codeine with "Reaction Mechanism" reflects the underlying concept of this book.

Although I have exerted all my efforts to ensure that the text is free from errors, but it is quite possible that methodology details, certain structures and reaction mechanism may be inaccurate. I hope my efforts shall be evaluated in proper perspective.

It is the analyst who is consistently if not constantly involved with all the aspects of analysis. His/her interest necessarily is not of a curious bystander. This book does not purport to make analysts out of its readers, although it is hoped that some will be "turned on" to such a pursuit.

New Delhi, India

P.D. Sethi, M.Pharm., Ph.D.
Pharmaceutical Analyst

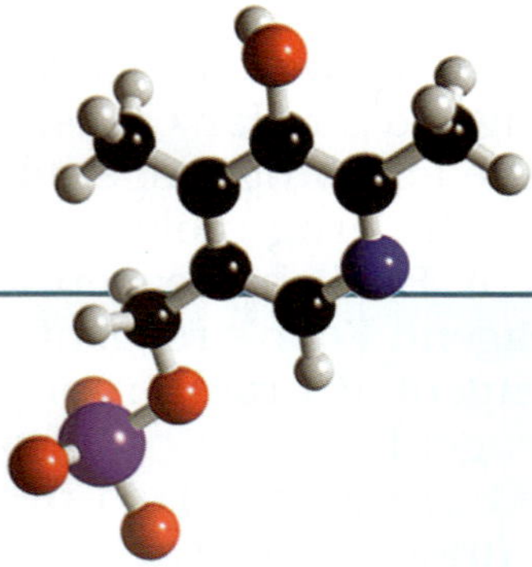

Acknowledgement

I would like to express my most sincere gratitude to analysts, students, teachers and professionals for their continuous support and encouragement and shaping my analytical career and ideas for compiling this book. The support extended by Professor Vijay K. Kapoor, University Institute of Pharmaceutical Sciences, Panjab University, Chandigarh in explaining and correcting several reactions included in the text is sincerely acknowledged. I am deeply indebted to Mr. Dilip Charegaonkar, Managing Director, M/s Anchrom Enterprises (I) Pvt. Ltd., Mumbai for supporting my scientific activities. I would like to convey my appreciation to the management of M/s Anchrom Enterprises (I) Pvt. Ltd., Mumbai and Kongposh Publications Pvt. Ltd., New Delhi for independently establishing life-time annual awards for Best Research Papers in "HPTLC Analysis" and "Pharmaceutical Analysis" respectively in recognition of my contribution in the field of Pharmaceutical Analysis. I am confident, their gesture shall provide impetus to young analysts for their interest in pharmaceutical analysis, currently the most creative and challenging field.

Without the support and untiring efforts of Mr. Dharmvir of 'CBS' my hand-written text particularly the reactions would never have been converted into book, thanks for his dedication and commitment for completing the assignment meticulously. I am thankful to Mr. Satish K. Jain, Managing Director, CBS, for accepting the hand-written manuscript of most challenging project and providing all the required facilities to bring this series to fruition.

New Delhi, India

P.D. Sethi, M.Pharm., Ph.D.
Pharmaceutical Analyst

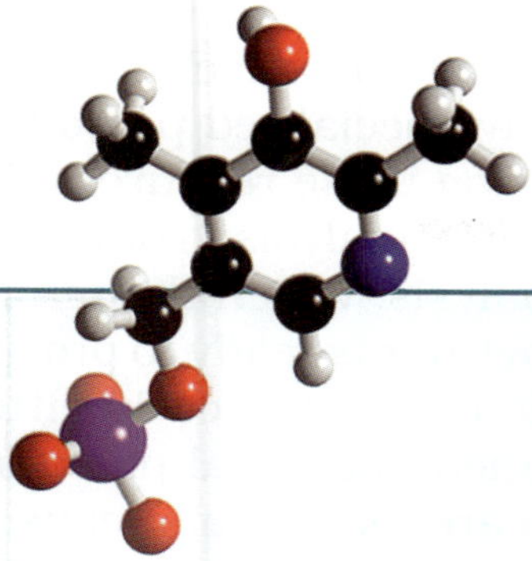

Preface to the First Edition

Devising accurate assay procedures for each ingredient of complex dosage formulations containing several therapeutically and chemically compatible drugs with very similar chemical nature is a monumental undertaking. The very idea of separation, identification and estimation of each ingredient in such complex formulations would make the analyst's hair stand on end. Not only are the multiple active constituents present but they are usually there in widely divergent concentrations depending upon their relative potency and therapeutic need of the patient. The presence of additives, excipients and decomposition products further complicates the development of analytical procedures. Many of the classical tests long regarded as specific for certain substances are now answered by many more compounds. Nevertheless, the therapeutic advantage of such complex drug combinations should take precedence over any potential analytical problem which is ultimately the concern of the analyst. The increasing complexities of pharmaceutical preparations and the marked emphasis on quality control by the ethical manufacturers have placed greater load on the ingenuity of the quality control chemist.

An analyst who is in the need of an analytical method may be obliged to survey tremendous amount of literature in order to select one procedure which may appear to suit his need and facilities available, but when he subjects the selected procedure to actual test, he may find that he cannot reproduce the method. It is, therefore, essential that the practising analyst should have access to analytical procedures which are simple, reliable and workable under routine laboratory conditions.

"No one is ever born talented nor talent obtained as a gift or lucky coincidence. It is a resource acquired through one's own endeavour. In this process, others may provide some help and inspiration, but it is a quality earned by one's own hard endeavour."

Modern analytical techniques rely increasingly on complex techniques of analysis that require expensive equipments and highly specialized personnel. Such methods are not of much help in countries lacking these resources. For the most part, modern analytical techniques merely permit analysis to be carried out more rapidly than the conventional method of analysis, which though not bad are tedious and time-consuming. Even if a manufacturer is ready to procure and install modern instruments/equipments, their maintenance in fittest condition is a herculean task. Non-availability of trained analytical personnel and precise, simple and suitable methods of analysis are major handicaps for pharmaceutical manufacturers in developing countries.

Taking into consideration the technical and economic constraints, it is necessary that the recommended methods should permit their use by drug laboratories located in developing countries. It is significant to stress that even simple instruments like colorimeter and spectrophotometer result in sensitive and accurate measurements with clear advantage of speed, simplicity and easy maintenance. The large volume of literature devoted to their application in almost every field of scientific research constitutes irrefutable evidence of their utility. It is, therefore, reasonable to assume that the analytical procedures involving the use of such simple instruments will find greater application. Selection of analytical method is a very critical point. The method must be accurate, sensitive, selective, reproducible and convenient.

In view of rapid advance during the last several years in the field of pharmaceutical analysis and marketing of ever increasing multi-component formulations, the available texts dealing in pharmaceutical analysis that have been written so far do not in general deal with the analysis of each component in wide range of complex pharmaceutical dosage formulations, particularly in presence of interfering substances. The official compendias are rarely of help in such formulations. To fill the existing gap in literature and keeping in view the economic and technical limitations of drug manufacturers, particularly in medium and small scale sector, it was felt that there exists a need to have a compilation of a simple, suitable and reliable methods for analysis of each ingredient of multi-component drug formulations.

This text, a maiden attempt, is meant to fulfill these needs. Analytical procedures for more than 200 drug formulations of divergent combinations have been compiled to serve as a convenient source of information for analysts and scientists engaged in the field. The focal point for this compilation is the presentation of practical aspect of the methodology using colorimeter and spectrophotometer as the main analytical tools.

For practical considerations, the drug formulations have been classified into 23 different categories based upon their common therapeutic uses as under:

1. Analgesics and antipyretics
2. Antacids and other ulcer healing drugs
3. Antacids, sedatives, antispasmodics
4. Anthelmintics
5. Anti-allergic drugs
6. Antibiotics
7. Anti-diarrhoeals
8. Anti-inflammatory drugs
9. Antimalarials
10. Anti-tuberculous drugs
11. Bronchospasm relaxants (anti-asthma)
12. Enzymes and digestives
13. Expectorants and cough suppressants
14. Eye, ear preparations
15. Keratolytics and cleansers
16. Laxatives, purgatives and lubricants
17. Nasal preparations
18. Oral rehydration salts
19. Rubefacients
20. Sedatives and tranquillisers
21. Topical antifungal, anti-infective preparations
22. Urinary anti-infective preparations
23. Vitamins, minerals and other nutritional additives.

For most of the formulations, several alternative methods have been described for a particular substance so that the analyst can intelligently select and apply the method to suit his need and the laboratory facilities available. Preliminary treatment of the sample for analysis utilizing conventional isolation and extraction procedures have been applied wherever necessary to eliminate the presence of potentially interfering substances. In other cases, the methods are sufficiently specific to permit the analysis of individual ingredients without pre-treatment. The procedures have been described in sufficient details highlighting the important steps in methodology so that these can be reproduced without much difficulty. Merits and demerits of each method and possibility of its application to other formulations have been discussed. To help the analyst and to enhance the book's usefulness, several worked out examples based on actual experimental data have been included. For drug manufacturers, who are interested to set up their independent quality control division, chapter on the profile of a quality control laboratory has been included giving brief outline of different sections.

Its importance for pharmaceutical teachers, students and institutions imparting special course in drug analysis cannot be overestimated. Science graduates interested in pursuing career as analytical chemist will find this compilation invaluable for daily use which will provide ready answers to most of their analytical problems. It is earnest feeling of the author that knowledge of the basic inorganic and organic chemistry tempered by judicious changes and the special skill needed in pharmaceutical analysis and the information included in this text will enable the analyst to overcome most specific problems and he will be able to analyse any viable combination of drug formulations he may encounter in future. It is pertinent to mention that analyst should cautiously choose the method and interpret the results carefully before certifying the product. It is hoped that this text will enable the analyst to take their rightful place in the pharmaceutical industry and in government laboratories concerned with the quality control of medicinal preparations.

The author is indebted to his wife, Usha for her moral support throughout his career.

The author wishes to express his sincere appreciation to Dr. O.P. Ghai, Professor and Head, Department of Pediatrics, All India Institute of Medical Sciences, New Delhi, for his helpful suggestions and guidance.

How far I have succeeded in my attempt, the decision is left to my fellow pharmacists and analysts.

New Delhi, India **P.D. Sethi**
1985

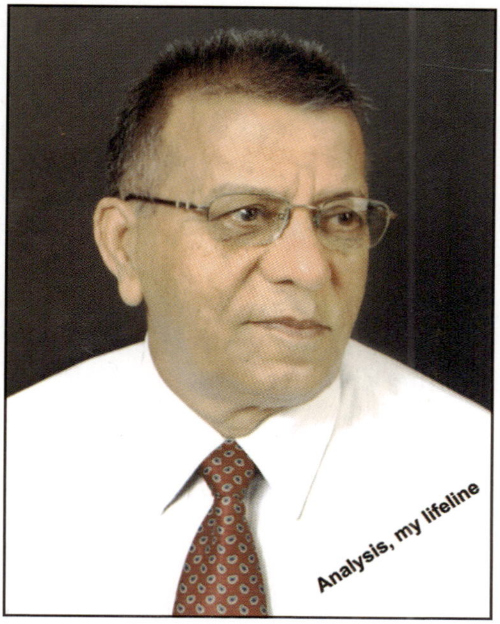

Dr. P.D. Sethi
(1936 -)

Making of An Analyst & The Author (My Story)

"Practical experience is mastered in the laboratory; scientific knowledge is mastered in the library."

Dr. C.K. Atal, my guide for M. Pharm at Punjab University, Chandigarh, now residing at Delhi often asks me, in spite of majoring in pharmacognosy both in M. Pharm. & Ph.D. programmes, how I became a pharmaceutical analyst. This prompted me to pen down my journey towards being an analyst & the author. This is what my story is all about.

I obtained my M. Pharm. (1962) and Ph.D. (1973), both in Pharmacognosy. During my Ph.D. programme, I worked on isolation and characterization of withanolides and physalins from Solanaceous plants. After a short stint at

"No one is ever born talented nor talent obtained as a gift or lucky coincidence. It is a resource acquired through ones own endeavour, in this process, others may provide some help, inspiration and guidance".

BHU, Varanasi, I joined Central Indian Pharmacopoeia Laboratory (CIPL), Ghaziabad in Sept. 1975 as Senior Scientific Officer (Gr-I). The main function of the laboratory was to update Indian Pharmacopoeia (IP) in addition to analysis of drug samples received from CDSCO and drugs control departments of some States. Being next to the Director, I was entrusted with overall charge of the chemistry division, the major division of the laboratory. The chemistry division had two officers (SSO-II) and few SSA's in addition to about 30 bench analysts.

Before joining CIPL, I had practically no experience in analysis of drugs, thus interacting with analysts during routine rounds of the laboratory was quite embarrassing. I stopped taking rounds of the laboratory and decided first to update my scientific knowledge in the field.

Mr. N.C. Dhawan, then SSA, was the immediate supervising officer responsible for assigning samples to different analysts for testing and guiding them in routine analytical work. During lunch hours, I started discussing with him common analytical methods being followed in the laboratory. However it was felt that both scientific knowledge of the methods and practical experience are very much essential.

Fortunately, the laboratory had a good collection of Indian and foreign analytical journals and books. I started spending most of my free time in the library collecting references and cataloguing them. Occasionally, I visited National Medical Library (NML) New Delhi for the purpose This helped me to a great extent in knowing the scientific as well as practical aspect of different methods. For practical experience, I set up a separate bench-space in the laboratory and started parallel analysis of samples, comparing the assay results with that of the analysts who had been initially assigned the samples for analysis. Limited practical experience along with scientific knowledge of the methods gave me adequate confidence. After about three months, I started taking rounds of the laboratory and interacting with bench-analysts. Whenever draft test reports were submitted to me for scrutiny, I started calling the concerned analyst in my room and discussed the nitty-gritty of each step involved in the analysis, difficulties encountered and how they were solved. These practical tips were regularly recorded and were incorporated as foot notes in my first book "Quantitative Analysis of Pharmaceutical Formulations" published in 1985. I continued the practice of interacting with bench analysts at their working benches and having a separate bench-space for experimental work till my retirement.

Dr. P.R. Pabrai, the director gave me a free hand in organising the laboratory. I constituted a separate R&D group and started working on development of analytical methods on problems often encountered by the industries. Our work was published in important journals and presented at annual Indian

Pharmaceutical Congress and much appreciated. Soon our laboratory became the leading centre for R&D work in pharmaceutical analysis with excellent standing among analytical fraternity.

In 1976, during my visit to State Drugs Laboratory, Baroda, Gujarat, I had a chance to study working of their repository for working/reference standards and protocols for analysis of patent and proprietary formulations. I set up a separate section at CIPL for maintaining working/reference standards and analytical protocols and started obtaining protocols for different formulations from the manufacturers. Soon the section developed into a full-fledged division (Repository) with good collection of protocols and working/reference standards. While analysing samples as per protocols received, practical difficulties encountered and changes made were recorded.

In view of contradictory test reports often emanating from different laboratories mainly due to different protocols being followed, to bring uniformity, Drugs Controller of India (DCI) constituted a committee with Director CDL, Calcutta as its chairman, government analysts of Maharashtra, Karnataka and Gujarat as its members and myself as convenor. The methods being followed in different laboratories in respect of certain common formulations were obtained and after comparative evaluation, final methods to be followed were circulated to all laboratories. This exercise gave me several alternate methods for significant number of formulations.

While analysing samples, compendial identification tests, usually based on test tube tests, were being followed. Analysts had then very limited experience in application of thin layer chromatography (TLC). Realizing the practical importance of this technique, I encouraged analysts in the use of this technique, trained them in preparation of laboratory hand-made TLC plates. We locally got fabricated the entire plate-coating assembly suitable for 20×10, 10×10, 5×10 and 2.5×10 cm plates and soon TLC was routinely used as an alternative analytical technique for identification. Later on, we could develop semi-quantitative assay method by TLC "Quick Assessment System" for several dosage forms and an analyst could analyze 40-50 samples of such formulations everyday. The use of TLC was further extended to identification of individual component in multi-component formulations. Each densitogram so obtained was traced on paper and attached with analytical data along with detailed chromatographic conditions as a permanent record. Salient feature of this study was that we could work out a single solvent system, so called "Universal Solvent System", which could separate different ingredients for identification in more than 80 formulations of divergent combinations. TLC data based on actual laboratory experiments was later on compiled and published as a book "Identification of Drugs in Pharmaceutical Formulations by TLC" in 1992.

In 1977, our laboratory was approved by Meerut University as a R&D centre and my name was only approved as guide for the Ph.D program. Probably due to my increasing popularity as an analyst because of my professional competency and the university not approving the name of Dr. P.R. Pabrai as guide due to his fewer research publications, created a wedge between us and our relations started drifting. Though there were some administrative reasons, but it will not be appropriate to discuss them. He divested me of all my official responsibilities and withdrew all the facilities including my office room, telephone, peon etc. I was made to sit in the laboratory alone with no staff member allowed to interact with me. All possible efforts were made on daily basis to humiliate and demoralize me. Initially I was quite depressed but with confidence in my professional knowledge and being a **Scorpio** (hindrance and obstacles bring out the best), I decided to accept the situation and make best use of adversity to my advantage. Now when I look back I realize that adversity had in fact been the major driving force for me to be an analyst & the author, for this I am extremely obliged to Dr. P.R. Pabrai. I started spending most of my time in the library, collecting published literature on analytical methods. It was observed that some of the most popular books in pharmaceutical analysis were quite old and not of much use for analysis of currently available formulations, except the book by Hashmi, "Assay of Vitamins". Considering the challenge being faced by analysts for analysis of fixed-dose multi-component formulations due to mutual interference of different ingredients present in the formulations, I decided to explore the possibility of compiling available analytical methods and sharing my practical experience with fellow analysts.

Since I was not allowed to use any of the office facility, I hired a typewriter and requested Mr. V.K. Arora, P.A. to the director to type the draft manuscript of the book at his home. As the subject was very new, no publisher was prepared to take the risk of publishing the book. Ultimately with the help of a friend dealing with sale of scientific books, I decided to get the book published at my own level. In December 1984, during IPC at Bangalore, I circulated a brief synopsis of the proposed book. I was rather thrilled and surprised with the response. Orders for more than 200 copies were received within a week with advance payments.

Believe me, not even a single page of the final manuscript of the proposed book was ready at that stage. I took two months leave and worked for 12-14 hrs a day to complete the manuscript. In those days hand composing was done for final printing. My publisher was based in East Delhi. Daily I used to visit him every evening on my way back home from Ghaziabad to hand over fresh manuscript and collect proof of the earlier part and reach home after 10 pm. The efforts put in by my wife, Usha in managing the home and education of the children is hard to ignore, in fact nothing would have been possible without her full support. When the book ultimately appeared in mid-1985, the entire stock (1000 copies) was sold out in few weeks. The book ultimately established me as an analyst & the author. Although this book was revised in 1992 (2nd ed.), & 1997 (3rd ed.), the first edition (1985) even today is prized possession of analysts and is considered the most popular practical compilation ever published in the field.

After Dr. Pabrai retired in August 1983, in spite of being senior most officer in the laboratory, I was not promoted as director due to some adverse remarks recorded in my ACR by Dr. P.R. Pabrai. Dr. S.C. Sharma was transferred from CDL, Calcutta to CIPL as director on ad hoc basis. After my repeated representation to the authorities of the fact that as per ruling of SC, adverse remarks in the ACR are to be communicated to the officer concerned, which was never done in my case. The authorities, taking a view that sudden sharp fall in the skill of the officer being suggestive of bias, stroke off the adverse remarks and I was promoted as director CIPL in February 1986.

On the special request of Ministry of Health and Family Welfare, the laboratory started the testing of oral contraceptive pills. The analysis of ethinyl estradiol, the minor component required 5 cm glass cell for colorimetric analysis. Most of the laboratories in the country were not equipped with this facility, hence unable to analyse such samples. Although our laboratory was testing the samples the method being tedious and lengthy, only 4-5 samples could be analyzed in a day. Having adequate experience in application of TLC/HPTLC and the laboratory having HPTLC system (Camag), we validated HPTLC method for simultaneous estimation of both ethinyl estradiol and norgestrel and could analyse 20-25 samples each day. The credit for this entire work goes to Dr. Murugesan, then JSA at CIPL and now Director RDTL, Chennai.

In February 1992, I was transferred to Bombay as director CDL. In fact there was no functional laboratory and I was not provided even a chair to sit which had to be borrowed from CDSCO (WZ). Ministry of Health had just taken over possession of part of 4th floor of ESI hospital at Thane. There was hardly any work done on alteration of different wards into the laboratory. Though my office was situated at Antop Hills along with the office of the CDSCO but I was spending most of my time at site coordinating with CPWD who was entrusted with completion of entire project. As the work on the project started progressing satisfactorily, I initiated the process of procurement of laboratory equipments and instruments and recruitment of sanctioned staff. By September 1992, the laboratory was handed over to us and by that time most of the technical and administrative staff was in position. I shifted my office to the laboratory at Thane. All equipments such as IR, HPLC, UV, balances were in position.

Microbiology and Pharmacology divisions along with animal house were fully functional. In mid November 1992 the functioning of the laboratory was inaugurated. Within a period of 6-8 months I could establish a well equipped laboratory from scratch with excellent facilities. Leading analysts from the Industries and institutions frequently visited the newly established laboratory to see the set-up and discuss their analytical problems.

Since the analysts were not having adequate work and with past experience in the application of HPTLC, I decided to extend R&D work on the application of HPTLC in analysis of fixed-dose multi-component formulations. Since, CDL was not equipped with HPTLC system, Mr. Charegaonkar, MD, Anchrom Enterprises (I) Pvt. Ltd., Bombay was kind enough to extend all the facilities available at his analytical laboratory in Mulund. Within 2 years, we could develop and standardize HPTLC methods for more than 150 divergent fixed-dose formulations. This project would not have been completed without the support of Ms. Virinda, then JSA, CDL and Sujata of Anchrom. Entire analytical data as obtained in the laboratory and information retrieved from published literature was compiled and published as a book "Quantitative Analysis of Drugs in Pharmaceutical Formulations by HPTLC" in 1999. This book proved to be the ultimate guide for all HPTLC practitioners and even today is cited as reference almost in every publication related to application of HPTLC in pharmaceutical analysis. Chromatographers started associating me with TLC/HPTLC technique.

HPLC, then another up-coming analytical technique, was gaining popularity. Dr. Vaibhav working as JSA in the laboratory had earlier worked for his Ph.D under Dr. R.T. Sane on application of HPLC in pharmaceutical analysis, I assigned him the job of screening published literature on application of HPLC in analysis of fixed-dose formulations. After getting permission from libraries of IIT, BARC and Bombay college of pharmacy, Dr. Vaibhav regularly visited these libraries and collected copies of published papers. By the time I retired in 1994, I had fairly good collection of published literature on the subject which I continued to update. After I was free from revision of other titles I started work on the compilation of all available data on HPLC and finally volume 1 was published in 2001. In sequence to volume 1, volume 2 appeared in 2006 and volume 3 & 4 in 2010. I intend to continue the series if health and life permits.

During one of my visit to the office of my publisher at Delhi in 1992, I purchased one book Pharmaceutical Analysis (volume 2) by H.J. Roth for our CDL Library. This book contained detailed chemical reactions of drugs based on their functional groups. Since analytical methods described in 1st & 2nd editions of my book "Quantitative Analysis of Pharmaceutical Formulation" were primarily based on colour reactions of the functional groups with specific reagents, I realized that for proper understanding of the methods, chemistry involved i.e. "Reaction Mechanism" need be provided along with the methods. It is how the idea of this project was conceptualized. I discussed this subject with Ms. Padma, one of the JSA in the laboratory who had just obtained her M.Sc. in organic chemistry. She readily agreed to take up the project and could write down reaction mechanism for almost all the methods included in 1st & 2nd edition of my book as well as in respect of published methods. When I retired, the literature on HPLC collected by Dr. Vaibhav and reaction mechanism compiled by Ms. Padma was the only treasure I carried home and left behind a fully equipped functional laboratory with well trained analysts.

During the first APA convention held at Bombay in 1997, I presented "Reaction Mechanism" of some important pharmacopoeial identification tests. The presentation being unique was well appreciated. I made up my mind to revise the 3rd edition of my book giving reaction mechanism for each method included in 1st, 2nd, 3rd, editions of the book. In view of complexity of the subject, I initially did harbour some doubts about its ultimate completion. Since it was my **DESIRE** to complete the project before I close my shop, knowing fully well that nothing can be achieved without dedication, and it shall need constant adaptation, definite level of discipline and above all hunger to keep going, I decided to accept the challenge with **SELF BELIEF**.

It gives me pride to state that the final manuscript of the book (4th ed.) "Quantitative Analysis of Drugs in Pharmaceutical Formulations" complete with "Reaction Mechanism" for each method (4 volumes series) is in press.

The books authored by me so far in the field of pharmaceutical analysis using different analytical techniques (UV-Vis spectrophotometry, TLC, HPTLC, HPLC) continue to have excellent response and have proved to be a cradle for my success. How useful these books have been to analysts in discharging their analytical functions; I leave the decision to them. Although I can claim being an analyst by virtue of my professional contribution, but what standing I enjoy among pharmaceutical analysts of the country, let the present and future generation of analytical fraternity take a view. However today whatever I possess i.e. name, fame and money, it is simply because of my being an analyst & the author.

"DESIRE is perhaps the starting point of achieving something"

"Belief is the knowledge that we can do some thing. It is the inner feeling that what we undertake, we can accomplish"

I am deeply indebted to Mr. Dilip Charegaonkar, M.D. Anchrom Enterprises (I) Pvt. Ltd. Mumbai for extending every possible support for me to be a sound HPTLC practitioner. I express my gratitude to Anchrom Enterprises (I) Pvt. Ltd., Mumbai and KONGPOSH Publication Pvt. Ltd. New Delhi for independently establishing lifetime annual awards for Best Research Papers in HPTLC Analysis & Pharmaceutical Analysis respectably in recognition of my contribution in the field.

I humbly bow my head before the temple (Central Indian Pharmacopoeia laboratory), where I started my analytical career and which provided me all the facilities and inspiration to be an analyst. I express my gratitude to all the bench analysts of CIPL particularly N. C. Dhawan and Ms. Savita Devi from whom I learnt basics of analysis. In my becoming an analyst & the author, Dr. Y.K.S. Rathore, Dr. N. Murugesan and Dr. S.C. Mathur had played major role, thanks to them for giving practical shape to my ideas.

Before I close my story I would like to share one important aspect of my being an author. I had no access to any of the modern gadgets i.e. Computer, Internet, E-mail, etc. All the published literature on different subjects was surveyed by frequent personal visits to different libraries. The manuscript of all books authored by me had been handwritten and given to the publisher for publication. It was only the **passion** to achieve something that kept me performing.

At the end I would like to express my sincere gratitude to fellow analysts, students, researchers, teachers, professionals and mentors for their continuous support and inspiration in shaping my analytical career spanning about four decades.

With a pledge to dedicate my knowledge and experience to the fellow analysts, I end my story with the hope that it will inspire some to be analyst.

P.D. Sethi

"Nothing dies faster than the idea kept in closed mind, so share your knowledge and experience and let the world be richer."

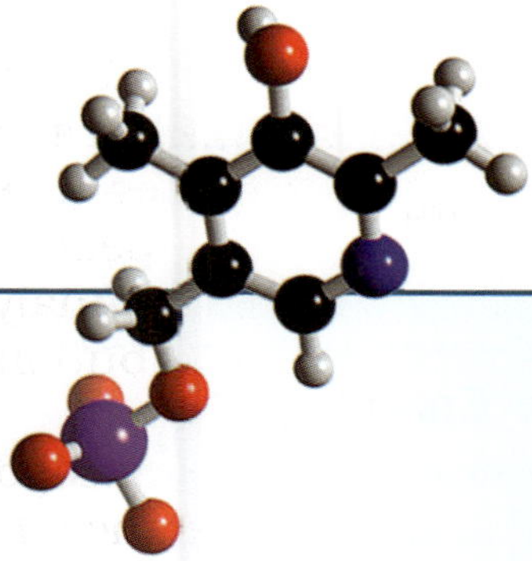

Brief Contents
Volumes I – IV

VOLUME 1

VOLUME 2

VOLUME 3

VOLUME 4

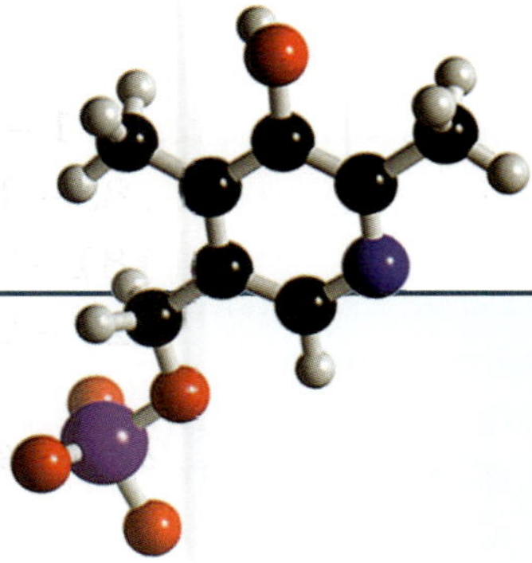

Contents

CHAPTER 3
Calibration of Analytical Instruments 153–177

CHAPTER 4
Method Development – Optimization – Validation – Transfer – Revalidation 179–206

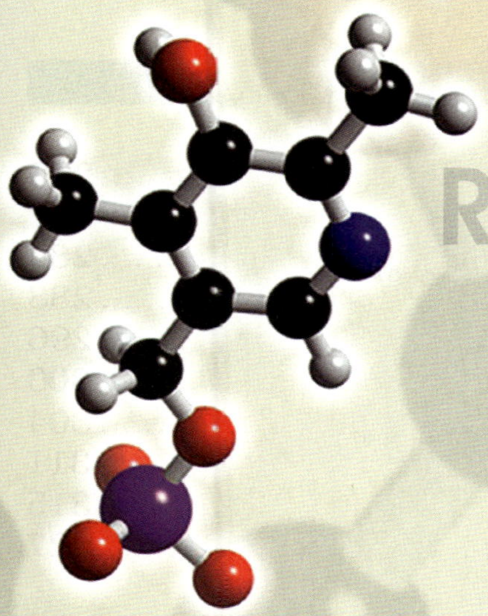

Reaction Mechanism

1

Introduction

Quality is important in every product or service but it is vital in medicine as it involves life. Unlike ordinary consumer goods there can be and there is no "second" quality in drugs. Quality control is a concept which strives to produce a perfect product by series of measures designed to prevent and eliminate errors at different stages of production. As a matter of fact, it is built in from the time of inception of the thought to make a product, to the time, it is finally made and sent out with an 'OK' quality report. In popular practice, the quality of medicines or pharmaceutical products is assured through quality control. It is, therefore, essential that quality assurance department must adopt "Good Laboratory Practice" to ensure reliability and accuracy of results given out by them. The assurance of the quality and the reliability of pharmaceuticals, together with their careful control are our moral obligations arising from the humanism towards the sick human beings. Consequently, the manufacture and the control of drugs are very responsible tasks and they need substantial knowledge of the science.

The decision to release or reject a product is based upon one or two types of control actions or combination of both. If the product is a single entity of high purity, the analytical data is the basis for decision but most of the time, the formulation is a physical mixture of several potent drugs. With the growth of pharmaceutical industry during the last several years, there has been rapid progress in the field of pharmaceutical analysis involving complex instrumentations. Providing simple analytical procedures for complex formulations is a matter of foremost importance.

Generally Acceptable Specifications for Different Dosage Forms

(a) **Tablets:** Appearance, friability, hardness, colour, odour, moisture, strength, disintegration and dissolution.

(b) **Capsules:** Strength, moisture, colour, appearance, shape, brittleness and dissolution. For soft gelatin capsules, the fill medium should be examined for precipitate, cloudiness and pH.

(c) **Emulsions:** Appearance (such as phase separation), colour, odour, pH, viscosity and strength. Storage on the side or inverted is suggested for assessment of the closure systems. It is recommended that a heating/cooling cycle be employed (e.g. between 4°C and 45°C) to test physical stability.

(d) **Oral solutions and suspensions:** Appearance (precipitate, cloudiness), strength, pH, colour, odour, redispersibility, dissolution (suspensions), and clarity (solutions). Liquids and suspensions should be stored on their side or inverted in order to determine whether contact of the drug product with the closure system affects product integrity.

After storage, samples of suspensions should be prepared for assay according to the recommended labelling.

(e) **Oral powders:** Most oral powders are marketed for reconstitution prior to administration. The following characteristics of the powder should be examined: appearance, strength, colour, odour and moisture. The reconstituted product should be prepared according to the recommended labelling. Specific characteristics to be examined on the reconstituted material should include: appearance, pH, dispersibility and strength throughout the recommended storage period.

(f) **Metered-dose inhalation aerosols:** Strength, delivered dose per actuation, number of (metered) doses, colour, clarity (solutions), particle size distribution (suspensions), loss of propellant, pressure, valve corrosion, and spray pattern. Because the container contents are under pressure, filled containers must be checked for weight loss over the expiration dating period. For suspensions, aggregate (or solvate) formation may lead to clogged valves or to the delivery of a pharmacologically inactive dose. Corrosion of the metering valve or gasket deterioration may adversely affect the delivery of the correct amount of drug substance. If the drug product is intended for use in respiratory system, it is important to confirm that the initial release specifications are maintained to assure the absence of pathogenic organisms (e.g., *Staphylococcus aureus*, *Pseudomonas aeruginosa*, *Escherichia coli*, and *Salmonella* species) and the total microbial limit per canister.

(g) **Topical and ophthalmic preparations (ointments, creams, lotions, pastes, gels, solutions):** Appearance, clarity, colour, homogeneity, odour, pH, resuspendibility (lotions), consistency, particle size distribution, strength and weight loss (plastic containers). The ophthalmic preparation needs test for sterility. Ointments, pastes and creams in containers larger than 3.5 grams should be assayed by sampling at the surface, middle, and bottom of the container. In addition, tubes should be sampled near the crimp.

Evaluation of nonmetered aerosols should include appearance, odour, strength, pressure, weight loss, net weight dispensed, delivery rate and spray pattern.

(h) **Small-volume parenterals (SVPs):** SVPs include an extremely wide range of preparations. Evaluation of these drug products should include strength, appearance, colour, particulate matter, pH, sterility, and pyrogenicity (at reasonable intervals). Stability studies on powder products should demonstrate that the residual moisture content remains within acceptable limits and that the product is stable throughout the recommended storage period.

The stability of reconstituted products should also be determined after they are constituted according to the recommended labeling. Specific parameters to be examined at appropriate intervals throughout the maximum intended use period of the constituted drug product, stored under condition(s) recommended in labeling, should include appearance, odour, colour, pH, strength, dispersibility and particulate matter.

Continued assurance of sterility for all sterile products may be assessed by a variety of means, including evaluation of the container-closure integrity by appropriate challenge test(s), testing for preservatives (if present), and/or sterility testing.

For terminally sterilized drug products, a specification for maximum process parameters should be provided. Stability studies should evaluate and support the adequacy of the maximum release specification for process lethality.

Parenterals (except ampules) should be stored inverted or on their sides in order to determine, by comparison, whether contact of the drug product or solvent with the closure system affects product integrity or results in leaching of chemical substances from the closure material.

(i) **Large-volume parenterals (LVPs):** Similar to those for SVPs, a minimum evaluation should include strength, appearance, colour, clarity, particulate matter, pH, volume (plastic containers), extractables (plastic containers), sterility and pyrogenicity (at reasonable intervals). Continued assurance of sterility for all sterile products may be assessed by a variety of means, including evaluation of the container-closure integrity by appropriate challenge test(s), by testing for preservatives (if present), or by sterility testing.

These products should be stored some inverted and some on their sides in order to determine whether contact of the drug product or solvent with the container-closure system affects product integrity, or results in leaching of chemical substances from the container-closure material.

(j) **Suppositories:** Suppositories should be evaluated for strength, softening range, appearance and dissolution. The effect of aging may also be observed from a hardening of the suppository and a polymorphic transformation of the drug substance; therefore, control and stability testing should include dissolution time at 37°C.

(k) **Drug additive:** For any drug product that is intended for use as an additive to another drug product, the possibility of incompatibilities exists. In such cases, the drug product labelled to be administered by addition to another drug product (e.g. parenterals, aerosols) should be studied for stability and compatibility in admixture with the other drug product.

The Art & Science of Pharmaceutical Analysis

Analysis of so-called drugs is based on sound scientific principles. The chemistry and mathematics are subtly combined for accurate measurements. Even the highly trained and experienced analyst may have little mastery over common laboratory procedures. The analyst has the necessary tools and the techniques of his profession and is able to exercise judgement and transcribe indefinable state of mind into action while working in the laboratory.

The Pharmacopoeias permit maximum 5-10% deviations from the labelled claim. This deviation is permitted for various reasons: (a) no drug can be put into dosage form without compounding errors; (b) some drugs are unstable and gradually deteriorate on storage; (c) no method of analysis is so precise as to provide recovery values free of error. Although analyst has no control over first two reasons but can definitely ensure that error in analytical procedure is as small as possible by performing all the analytical steps carefully and quantitatively, remembering that the art of analysis is always mastered in the laboratory and science of analysis in the library. He is, therefore, ought to be careful in choosing common tools as flasks, separating funnels, pipettes, burettes to be used in analysis. For example, for measuring 10 ml of a solution, using 100 ml of graduated cyclinder is not suitable. For micro-titration the use of microburette is desirable. For conical flasks, often used for titration, the total volume of the sample and the titrant must be considered. It shall be analytically wrong to use 250 ml conical flask when total volume shall be less than 50 ml. The apparatus and tools should be chosen on the basis of experience and common sense.

In case of suspension in liquid either the solid has to be recovered quantitatively for further analysis or the suspended particles to be removed/discarded before continuing with analysis. In both cases, filtration is called for.

The simplest approach shall be to pass the suspension through small plug of cotton wool packed into neck/filtering funnel, thus removing coarse particles and permit the passage of finer particles into filtrate. This procedure is mostly not recommended provided small amount of particles in the filtrate have very little effect on analytical results. Most common approaches to filtration in the use of filter paper, which differ in size, porosity, wet strength and ash contents, for example Whatman No. 1 filter paper or its equivalent retains particles of average size and allow the fluid to pass rapidly and is not suitable for quantitative gravimetric analysis. In contrast, if solid is to be removed by filtration, ignited and analysed gravimetrically, low ash filter paper is recommended such as Whatman No. 40, 41 and 42 for recovery of fine crystals, No. 41 for coarse and gelatinous and No. 42 for very fine crystals. The size of the filter paper shall depend on the size of filtering funnel. The paper folded into quarters and seated into the funnel and wetted with the solvent, until tight seal between the paper and glass is obtained. The top of the filter paper should never extend above the edge of the funnel and be rather within 2-3 cm of the rim. However, some analysts are of the opinion that paper should not form seal with the funnel as space between the paper and glass makes the filtration faster. However, it should be ensured that there is tight seal between paper and the glass near rim.

For gravimetric assay, the precipitates are collected in ashless filter paper and transferred to a porcelain crucible. The crucible will glow at 500°C, becomes red at 600°C, appears orange at 1000°C.

The objects are never cooled in closer desiccator as during cooling partial vacuum is created and on opening the desiccator air rushes in and tends to blow the sample out of the container resting on the porcelain plate.

Particularly attention should be paid to recording on analytical results. It is the analyst who gives his/her stamp of approval for release of a particular product. Hence the analyst cannot be excused for not keeping detailed laboratory record book as he/she proceeds step by step through analytical procedure. Proper recording of analytical data needs no over-emphasis. "Whatever is not written is not done."

Analytical Techniques

Some of the medicinal products are still being assayed by the time-tested procedures of gravimetric and titrimetric technique, though use of electronic balances and recording titrators have improved these classical procedures considerably. A wide diversity in the type of analytical technique has been characteristic of assay method for pharmaceuticals. Simple distillation is useful for determining alcohol contents of the glanicals, or other substances being volatile in current of steam such as menthol, thymol and even certain alkaloids such as ephedrine. Moisture contents have been determined by drying in a desiccator or in a heated oven. Use of moisture balance in which sample pan is directly heated by infrared lamp without removing the sample from the balance has been an innovation, though the most specific and convenient procedure being Karl-Fischer titration method, end point being detected manually or by electrometric with automatic titration. Separation techniques, particularly chromatographic method are valuable in analysis of pharmaceuticals. Modern spectrophotometer which incorporates features such as microprocessor control, diode array detector have become essential tools for analysis. Assay methods based on absorption in the ultraviolet and visible portion of electromagnetic spectra are used extensively. Some colourless substances required to be analysed are converted to a derivative having colour, the intensity of colour measured at suitable wavelength and compared with known amount of reference substance of known purity. The fluorometer measures fluorescence that may be present in the sample such as riboflavin or may be developed into the sample such as thiamine hydrochloride.

Solvents used for dilution for UV spectrophotometric assay require special purification which is often exacting and different from the requirement for other uses. It is preferable that blanks are run on the solvent and reagents used to obtain a correction for their inherent absorbances.

The following analytical techniques have been employed for estimation of different components in formulations included in the text.

1. Titrimetric and gravimetric
2. Spectrophotometric
3. Paper chromatography
4. Preparative thin-layer chromatography
5. Column chromatography
6. Ion-exchange chromatography
7. Flame photometry and atomic absorption spectrometry (AAS).

1. Titrimetric methods

A. Acid-base titration
   1. Direct titration
      (a) Titration of an acid by a base
         (i) Titration of a liberated acid.
         (ii) Sorenson-Formol titration (free amino group present is first treated with formaldehyde to form a derivative methylamine, resulting in reduction in the basicity of amino group, to enable titration of free carboxylic group of the amino acid.
         (iii) Non-aqueous titration (Table 1.1): Non-aqueous solvents have greater coefficient of expansion than water; even small difference in temperature during standardization and actual sample analysis can result in significant error. Further for non-aqueous titrations sample must be finely powdered and passed through sieve 100 before suspending it in glacial acetic acid. The coarse sample powder usually gives inconsistent end point and lower assay values as coarse particles do not disintegrate fully in non-aqueous medium to liberate the active drug for titration, hence leading to inconsistent end point.

Preparation of 0.1 N perchloric acid: Add slowly, keeping temperature below 20°C, 8.7 ml of perchloric acid to 1000 ml of glacial acetic acid. Allow the mixture to stand for about 1 hr. Determine quickly the moisture contents (% w/v) and designate this as 'A'. To the above solution add slowly [(A – 0.03) × 52.2] ml of acetic anhydride with shaking. Allow the solution to stand for 24 hrs and standardize with potassium hydrogen phthalate.

Table 1.1. Experimental conditions for non-aqueous titration

Type of titration	*Titration of bases and their salts*	*Titration of acids*
Solvent	Glacial acetic acid Acetic anhydride Formic acid Propionic acid	DMF Pyridine n-Butylamine Ethylenediamine
Indicators	Crystal violet Quinaldine red p-Naphtholbenzein Malachite green	Thymol blue Thymolphthalein Azo violet O-Nitroaniline
Electrodes	Glass—Calomel Glass—Silver-silver chloride	Antimony-calomel Glass-calomel Platinum-calomel

(b) Titration of a base by an acid
(i) Titration of metal salts
(ii) Non-aqueous titration.

2. Residual titrations
Titration of excess acid by a base
(i) After distillation of a volatile base
(ii) After addition to carbonate residue
(iii) Alkaloidal assay.

B. Precipitation reactions

C. Redox titration
(i) Cerric sulphate or cerric ammonium nitrate.
(ii) Potassium permanganate.
(iii) Dichlorophenol indophenol
(iv) Potassium dichromate.
(v) Ferrous ammonium sulphate.
(vi) Potassium ferricyanide.
(vii) Sodium nitrite.
(viii) Iodometric and iodimetric.

D. Complexation titration
(i) EDTA
(ii) Other miscellaneous titrants such as sodium lauryl sulphate.

2. Gravimetric method

(i) Weigh drug after extraction.
(ii) Weigh a derivative after separation.
(iii) Weighing residue after ignition.

3. Spectrophotometric method

(i) Dye complex method
(ii) Colorimetric involving a chromogenic reagent
(iii) Ultraviolet (UV) absorption
(iv) Fluorimetry.
(v) Flame photometry.
(vi) Atomic absorption spectrometry

4. Electrochemical method

(i) Potentiometry

5. Chromatographic method

(i) Thin layer chromatography
(ii) Paper chromatography
(iii) Column chromatography

6. Miscellaneous

(i) Optical
(ii) Enzyme assay
(iii) Differential solubility

Spectrophotometric Methods

In most of the spectrophotometric methods use of reference/working standard in conjunction with the sample under assay is recommended to avoid any error due to wavelength, or slit-width variations among various brands of spectrophotometers as well as to avoid error arising from differences in transmittance and placement of cells.

(i) Dye-Complex Method (Ion-Pair Complex Formation)

Most of the procedures for extractive spectroscopic determination of basic drugs are based on formation of ion-associates between onium compounds and dye anions. The anionic dyes which are frequently used are of two categories:

(a) Monoprotic drugs - Picric acid, 2,6-dichlorophenol indophenol and tetrabromophenolphthalein ethyl ester (TBPE).
(b) Diprotic drugs: Bromophenol blue (BPB), Bromocresol green (BCG) and bromothymol blue (BTB).

Diprotic dyes show narrow optimum pH range and poor extractability of the ion-associate whereas monoprotic dyes show higher sensitivity and best extractability (T. Sakai, *Analyst*, 107, 640-646, 1982).

Amines in their protonated state form a complex with an anionic species (acidic dye) to form natural ion-pair complexes which are distinguished by their solubility in organic solvents such as chloroform, benzene, dichloromethane. Thus by using a pairing agent, a coloured complex is produced and the amines can thus be measured colorimetrically. The equilibrium expression for ion-pair formation can be expressed as:

$$A^{+}_{aq} + D^{-}_{aq} \rightleftharpoons AD_{org}$$

A_{aq}^{+} is the protonated amine in aqueous phase, D_{aq}^{-} is the anionic pairing dye in aqueous phase and AD_{org} is the final ion-pair complex extractable into organic phase. These complexes are readily decomposed by extracting the complex with aqueous acid or alkali depending on the anion pairing dye.

The formation of ion-pair complex method has been extensively used in this text for estimation of several basic nitrogenous substances employing several anionic pairing ions (dyes). The relevant experimental conditions (pH of the buffer, extracting solvent and absorption maxima) for several compounds are given in Table 1.2.

Table 1.2. pH of the buffer, extracting solvent and absorption maxima for different compounds

Drug	*Dye*	*Buffer* (pH)	*Extracting solvent*	λ_{max} (nm)
Astemizole	BCG	2.5 (phosphate)	$CHCl_3$	424
	Tropeolin OOO	0.1 M HCl	$CHCl_3$	500
	Superchem violet 3B	1.3 (Glycine-HCl)	$CHCl_3$	590
Amitriptyline HCl	BTB	—	$CHCl_3$	620
Atropine SO_4	BTB	7.5 (phosphate buffer)	$CHCl_3$	450
Antazoline	MO	6.0 (phosphate buffer)	$CHCl_3$	420
	BCG	3.4 }		
	BPB	2.5 }	$CHCl_3$	420
	BTB	2.8-4.0 }		
Acebutalol	Orange-II	0.1 M HCl	$CHCl_3$	480
Amolodipine	Orange-II	—	$CHCl_3$	470
	BCG	—	$CHCl_3$	410
Amodiaquine	BPB	2.5	$CHCl_3$	420
	BCP	6.0		415
Buspirone HCl	BCG	2.4 } phthalate buffer		415
	BPB	3.4 } phthalate buffer	$CHCl_3$	410
	BTB	2.6 } phthalate buffer		415
	BCP	3.4 } phthalate buffer		405
	MO	4.2	$CHCl_3$	450
Benzalkonium chloride	BTB	7.5 (phosphate)	H_2O	610
	MO	10 (KCl + NaOH)	$CHCl_3$ + HCl	510
Bromhexine HCl	BCP	Acidic	H_2O	410

(*Contd.*)

Drug	*Dye*	*Buffer* (pH)	*Extracting solvent*	λ_{max} (nm)
Clidinium bromide	BCP	7.00	$CHCl_3$	420
Chlorhexidine gluconate	BCG	5.7 (citrate phosphate)	$CHCl_3$	410
	Alizarin yellow G	PO_4 buffer pH 7.6	CH_2Cl_2	405
	BTB	7.5 (phosphate)	H_2O	610
Cyclomate Na^+	Azure-A	5.8 (borate-PO_4)	$CHCl_3$	652
Chlordiazepoxide	Fast red-A	(acidic)	$CHCl_3$	515
	Orange-II	5.0 phthalate	$CHCl_3$	495
	Fast green FCF	5.0 phthalate	$CHCl_3$	630
Cimetidine	BTB	5.5 (citrate PO_4)	$CHCl_3$	420
Chloroquine PO_4	BTB	5.6 (citrate PO_4)	$CHCl_3$	410
Ciprofloxacin	BCP	4.5 (phthalate) }		
	BPB	2.5	$CHCl_3$	420
Clotrimazole	BPB	3.4 (phthalate)	$CHCl_3$	410
	CI and orange 4S	0.1 M citric acid	$CHCl_3$	422
Codeine PO_4	BPB/BTB	3.0	$CHCl_3$	420
	MO	3.5	$CHCl_3$	410
	BCG	3.8 (citrate-PO_4)	$CHCl_3$	418
Cisapride	Ergioglaucine A (EG-A)	—	$CHCl_3$	640
Celerazine HCl	MO	3.6	$CHCl_3$	423
Chlorpromazine HCl	SBT	2.0		
	SDB	3.0 }	$CHCl_3$	520
	FSB FF	4.0		
Cyclizine HCl	SBT	2.0		
	SDB	3.0 }	$CHCl_3$	520
	FSB FF	4.0		
Cyproheptadine HCl	SBT	2.0		
	SDB	3.0 }	$CHCl_3$	520
	FSB FF	4.0		
Clonidine HCl	BTB	7.6 (citrate-PO_4)		420
	Metanil yellow	Dilute acetic acid	$CHCl_3$ + HCl	530
Domperidone	Suprachem violet 3B	1.3	$CHCl_3$	565
Diltiazem	Orange-II }	0.1 N HCl	$CHCl_3$	490
	Alizarin red	0.1 N HCl	$CHCl_3$	440
Diazepam	Alizarin violet 3B	Glycine + HCl	$CHCl_3$	560
	Orange-II	0.1 N HCl	$CHCl_3$	515
Diphenhydramine HCl	BCG	3.0 (phthalate)	$CHCl_3$	415
	BCG/BPB	4.4 (citrate-PO_4)	$CHCl_3$	412
	MO	5.0 (citrate-PO_4)	$CHCl_3$ + acidified CH_3OH	525
Doxepen HCl	MTB	4.0 (citrate-PO_4)	$CHCl_3$	413
Diclofenac Na^+	Methylene blue	6.8	$CHCl_3$	640
Dicyclomine HCl	Methylene blue	—	H_2O	590
Dextropropoxyphene HCl	BCG	4.0 (phthalate)	$CHCl_3$	420

(*Contd.*)

Drug	*Dye*	*Buffer* (pH)	*Extracting solvent*	λ_{max} (nm)
Dextromethorphan HBr	BCP	4.0 } citrate-PO_4	$CHCl_3$	415
		5.3 }		420
	BTB	7.5 (phosphate)	$CHCl_3$	405
Ephedrine HCl	BTB	7.0 (phosphate)	$CHCl_3$	425
Ethambutol HCl	Alizarin violet 3B	2.0	$CHCl_3$	415
Emetine HCl	MO	5.0 (citrate-PO_4)	$CHCl_3$ + acidified CH_3OH	460
Enalapril	BCG	3.1	$CHCl_3$	413
Erythromycin	SBT	2.0 }		
	SDB	3.0 }	$CHCl_3$	520
	FSB FF	4.0 }		
Etoricoxib	BCG	3.5	$CHCl_3$	416
	BCP	2.5	$CHCl_3$	408
Fluphenazine	Light green	5.0 (phthalate)	$CHCl_3$	635
	Orange G	0.1 M HCl	$CHCl_3$	560
Flunarizine	BCG	3.0 }		
	BCP	2.0 }		
	BPB	3.0 }	$CHCl_3$	415
	BTB	2.0 }		
Glycyrrhizin	Methylene blue	9.2 (citrate-PO_4-borate)	$CHCl_3$	640
Glibenclamide	BTB	5.6 (citrate-PO_4)	$CHCl_3$	410
Homatropine methyl bromide	BTB	10.5 (borate)	$CHCl_3$	420
	BTB	7.5 (citrate-PO_4)	$CHCl_3$ + ammoniacal CH_3OH	420
Hydroxyzine HCl	BPB	2.6	$CHCl_3$	420
	BCG	3.5		
	MO	4.5		
	SBT	2.0 }	$CHCl_3$	520
	SDB	3.0 }		
	FSB FF	4.0 }		
Hyoscyamine	BCP	2.5 (phosphate)	$CHCl_3$	440
Isopropamide	MO	10.2 (phosphate-bicarbonate)	$CHCl_3$ + HCl	510
Imipramine HCl	SBT	2.0 }		
	SDB	3.0 }	$CHCl_3$	520
	FSB FF	4.0 }		
	BCG	3.4 } phthalate	$CHCl_3$	418
	BPB	3.2 }		416
Ketotifen	BTB	2.6 } phthalate	$CHCl_3$	411
	BCP	2.8 }		407
Ketoconazole	BCG	2.5 }		420
	BCP	2.5 }		420
	BPB	1.5 }	$CHCl_3$	415
	MO	2.75 }		430

(*Contd.*)

Drug	*Dye*	*Buffer* (pH)	*Extracting solvent*	λ_{max} (nm)
Loperamide	Tropeolin OO	3.0 (citrate-PO_4)	$CHCl_3$ + acidified CH_3OH	540
	BCG	5.3 (citrate-PO_4)	$CHCl_3$	408
Lignocaine HCl	BCG	4.2 (phthalate)	CH_2Cl_2	420
Lidocaine HCl	BCG	4.2 (phthalate)	CH_2Cl_2	420
	SBT	2.0	$CHCl_3$	520
	SDB	3.0		
	FSB FF	4.0		
Lomofloxacin	BTB	4.0	$CHCl_3$	410
	BCG	3.0		415
	BCP	3.0		405
	BPB	3.0		400
Miconazole NO_3	BCG	3.0 (citrate-PO_4)	$CHCl_3$	420
	Solochrome dark blue	4.0 (phthalate)	$CHCl_3$	530
Melclopamide	BTB	7.5 (citrate-PO_4)	$CHCl_3$	425
	BTB	5.7 (citrate-PO_4)		420
Metronidazole benzoate	BTB	4.4 (citrate-PO_4)	$CHCl_3$	430
Mebeverine HCl	BTB	—	$CHCl_3$	405
	Fast green FCF	—	$CHCl_3$	625
	Eriochrome black	0.1 N HCl	$CHCl_3$	500
	Alizarin red		$CHCl_3$	410
Methdilazine HCl	Brilliant blue	—	$CHCl_3$	420
Nifopam HCl	BCG	3.0		
	BPB	3.0 phosphate	$CHCl_3$	410
	BTB	2.6		
	BCP	2.6		
Norfloxacin	BTB	—	$CHCl_3$	422
Nortriptyline HCl	Orange-II	2.0	$CHCl_3$	495
	Light green FCF	5.0	$CHCl_3$	630
Naphazoline NO_3	BCG	3.4		
	BPB	2.5/4.0	$CHCl_3$	420
	BTB	6.0		
	MO	6.0		
	SBT	2.0	$CHCl_3$	520
	SDB	3.0		
Noscapine	BCP	1.0 (NaCl + HCl)	Toluene	410
Oxymetazoline	BPB	2.5	$CHCl_3$	420
	BCG	3.4	CH_2Cl_2	
Orphenadrine	BCG	—	$CHCl_3$	430
	BPB			
	MO			
Oxyfedrine HCl	BCG	3.5		
	BPB	2.5	$CHCl_3$	420
	MO	4.5		
	Eriochrome black T	2.0	$CHCl_3$	520
	Solochrome dark blue	4.0		

(*Contd.*)

Drug	*Dye*	*Buffer* (pH)	*Extracting solvent*	λ_{max} (nm)
Pentazocine HCl	Cobalt thiocyanate	2 N HCl	CH_2Cl_2	625
Pilocarpine NO_3^-	BCG	6.0 (citrate-PO_4)	$CHCl_3$ + 0.1 N NaOH	580
	BCP	6.0		
Piperazine citrate	BTB	5.7 (phosphate)	$CHCl_3$	420
Procylidine HCl	BCG	3.5		
	BPB	2.5		
	BTB	2.8	$CHCl_3$	410
	MO	4.5		
	Solochrome black T	2.0	$CHCl_3$	520
	Solochrome dark blue	4.0		
Phenylbutazone	Basic fuchsin	7.8 (citrate-PO_4)	$CHCl_3$	545
Prazosin HCl	Orange-II	—	$CHCl_3$	490
	Alizarin violet 3B	—	$CHCl_3$	570
Promethazine HCl	BCG	2.8 (citrate-PO_4)	$CHCl_3$	415
	Sunset yellow	1.0		480
	SBT	2.0		
	SDB	3.0	$CHCl_3$	520
	FSB FF4	4.0		
Pyrimethamine	BPB	2.5		
	BCP	3.5 phthalate	$CHCl_3$	420
	BTB	3.8		
	MO	4.5		
Probenecid	Basic fuchsin	7.0	$CHCl_3$	415
Quarternary ammonium salts	BCG	1.3	CH_2Cl_2	415
	MO	10.0 (KCl + HCl)	CH_2Cl_2	415
	BTB	7.5 (phosphate)	H_2O	610
Reserpine	Alizarin violet 3B			
	Alizarin brilliant violet B	1.2 (glycine + HCl)	$CHCl_3$	560
Sparteine	BCG	4.0	$CHCl_3$	420
Timolol	BCG	2.2	$CHCl_3$	410
	Solochrome black T	2.8		515
Tamoxifen	Alizarin	1.5 (glycine + HCl)	$CHCl_3$	440
Ticlopidine HCl	BCG	3.6		
	BPB	3.2 phthalate	$CHCl_3$	415
	BTB	2.8		
	BCP	3.0		
Trimethoprim	BTB			
	BCG	4-6 (citrate-PO_4)	CH_2Cl_2	430
	BCP			
	BPB	3.2 (citrate-PO_4)	$CHCl_3$	418
Trihexyphenidyl	BCP	5.3 (PO_4)	$CHCl_3$	410
Tolazoline HCl	SBT	2.0		
	SDB	3.0	$CHCl_3$	520
	FSB FF	4.0		

(*Contd.*)

Drug	*Dye*	*Buffer* (pH)	*Extracting solvent*	λ_{max} (nm)
Triprolidine HCl	SBT	2.0		
	SDB	3.0	$CHCl_3$	520
	FSB F	4.0		
Xylometazoline HCl	SBT	2.0		
	SDB	3.0	$CHCl_3$	520
	FSB F	4.0		
	BCG	3.4		
	BPB	2.5		
	BTB	3.8	$CHCl_3$	415
	MO	6.0		
Albendazole	Tropaeolin OOO	1.3	$CHCl_3$	590
Albendazole	Suprachen violet	1.0	$CHCl_3$	495
Mebendazole	Tropaeolin OOO	1.3	$CHCl_3$	590
Mebendazole	Suprachen violet	1.0	$CHCl_3$	495
Fenbendazole	Tropaeolin OOO	1.3	$CHCl_3$	590
Fenbendazole	Suprachen violet	1.0	$CHCl_3$	495
Astemizole	Saprachen violet	1.0	$CHCl_3$	490
Astemizole	Tropaeolin OOO	1.3	$CHCl_3$	590
Lomofloxacin	BPB	3.0	$CHCl_3$	412
	BTB	3.4	$CHCl_3$	422
	BCP	2.8	$CHCl_3$	416
	BCG	2.4	$CHCl_3$	416
Sildenafil	Orange-II	0.1 N HCl	$CHCl_3$	495
	Eriochrome black-T	0.1 N HCl	$CHCl_3$	520
Secnidazole	BTB	4.4	$CHCl_3$	431
Ceterizine	TB	3.6	$CHCl_3$	413
Lignocaine	BTB	4.6	$CHCl_3$	420
Tetracaine	BTB	4.6	$CHCl_3$	420
Bupivacaine	BTB	4.6	$CHCl_3$	420
Ketamine	BTB	4.6	$CHCl_3$	420
Oxiconazole	MO	2.3	CH_2Cl_2	427
Loratadine	BPB	0.1 N HCl	$CHCl_3$	625
Clarithromycin	BCG	0.1 N HCl	$CHCl_3$	615
Rimapril	BPB	2.6	$CHCl_3$	414
Quinine	Tropaeolin 00	4.6	CH_2Cl_2 + HCl	545
Repglinide	BTB	2.4	$CHCl_3$	438
Amlodipine	MO	4.0	$CHCl_3$	417
Reserpine	MO	4.6	$CHCl_3$ + HCl	530
Desloratadine	BCP	0.1 N HCl	$CHCl_3$	416
Fexofenadine	BTB	2.6	$CHCl_3$	412
Linezolid	BCG	2.6	$CHCl_3$	420
Verapamil	Alizarin red-S	—	$CHCl_3$	428
Azelastine HCl	BCG	3.6	$CHCl_3$	420
	BTB	3.2	$CHCl_3$	420
	BPB	3.6	$CHCl_3$	420

(*Contd.*)

Drug	*Dye*	*Buffer* (pH)	*Extracting solvent*	λ_{max} (nm)
Pefloxacin	BTB	3.0	$CHCl_3$	415
	BCG	2.4	$CHCl_3$	420
	BPB	2.4	$CHCl_3$	422
	BCP	2.0	$CHCl_3$	415
Losartan	BCG	3.5	$CHCl_3$	420
	Wool fat blue	1.5	$CHCl_3$	595
	Safranine	9.8	$CHCl_3$	530
	Methylene blue	9.8	$CHCl_3$	655
Ibuprofen	Safranine	7.4	$CHCl_3$	520
Disopyramide	Alizarin red-S	0.1 N HCl	$CHCl_3$	440
	Tropaeolin 000	0.1 N HCl	$CHCl_3$	495
Chondroitin sulphate (decrease in absorption value)	Victory blue B	4.0	—	614
Lacidipine	Tropaeolin 000	3.5	$CHCl_3$	420
	BCG	3.5	$CHCl_3$ + acid	500
	Azocarmine	1.5	$CHCl_3$	540
Lomofloxacin	BCG	4.0	$CHCl_3$	420
	Eriochrome black-T	4.0	$CHCl_3$	490
Sildenafil	BTB	3.0	$CHCl_3$	420
	BCG	2.2	$CHCl_3$	435
	BPB	3.0	$CHCl_3$	415
Amlodipine	Orange-II	1.2	$CHCl_3$	487
Tizanidine	Metanil yellow	2.4	$CHCl_3$	410
Propranolol	BPB	3.0	$CHCl_3$	420
	BCP	5.0	$CHCl_3$	410
	BCG	5.0	$CHCl_3$	420
Metoprolol	BPB	3.0	$CHCl_3$	420
	BCP	3.0	$CHCl_3$	415
	BCG	5.0	$CHCl_3$	415
Clarithromycin	Tropaeolin OOO	0.1 N citric acid	$CHCl_3$	500
Cisapride	Metanil yellow	2.4	$CHCl_3$	408
Domperidone	BTB	2.4-4.0	$CHCl_3$	420
	BCG		$CHCl_3$	410
	BPB		$CHCl_3$	418
	Tropaeolin OOO		$CHCl_3$	420
Sibutramine	BTB	3.4	$CHCl_3$	420
	BCG	3.2	$CHCl_3$	420
Lomefloxacin	BTB	3.0	$CHCl_3$	410
	BCG	1.5	$CHCl_3$	415
	BCP	1.5	$CHCl_3$	405
	BPB	1.0	$CHCl_3$	400
Chlorhexidine gluconate	Alizarin yellow G	7.6	CH_2Cl_2	405
Mebeverine	Eriochrome black-T	0.1 N HCl	$CHCl_3$	500
	Alizarin red-S	0.1 N HCl	$CHCl_3$	410

(*Contd.*)

Drug	*Dye*	*Buffer* (pH)	*Extracting solvent*	λ_{max} (nm)
Donepezil HCl	Orange-G	0.1 N HCl	$CHCl_3$	480
Cetalopram	Orange-G	0.1 N HCl	$CHCl_3$	476
Rabeprazole	Orange-G	0.1 N HCl	$CHCl_3$	477
Labetalol, Cisapride, Roxythromycin, Econazole, Levamisole, Tamoxifen	Wool fast blue BL	1.5	$CHCl_3$	600
Gentamycin, Tobramycin	Aniline blue (acidic medium)	Water (decrease in absorption)		606
Atenolol, Timolol, Nandolol	BPB, BTB, BCP	1.2	$CHCl_3$	415
Carvedilol	BCG	0.1 N HCl	$CHCl_3$	415
Tegaserod maleate	BCG	2.5	$CHCl_3$	415
Rabeprazole	BTB, BCG, BPB, BCP	2.0	$CHCl_3$	454
Amoxycillin	Methylene blue (MB)	3.3	CH_2Cl_2	657
Sibutramine HCl	Congo-red	Weak acidic medium	CH_2Cl_2	490

BCG – Bromocresol green; BTB – Bromothymol blue; MO – Methyl orange; BPB – Bromophenol blue; BCP – Bromocresol purple; SBT – Solochrome black T; SDB – Solochrome dark blue; FSB FF – Fast sulphone black FF.

Theoretical conditions which help in choosing a rational system for a particular determination involves the knowledge of the dissociation constant of acidic dye and the basic compound and the pH dependence of the partition characteristics of the two substances and their addition product between aqueous and organic solvent. Since dyes are used in excess one of the basic requirements of this technique is that unreacted dye must be wholly retained in aqueous phase at the pH employed. If the initial partition coefficient of the dye (in acid form) is high, the pH of the buffer must be above the pKa of the dye. However, if acid form of the dye is insoluble in the organic phase, pH of the buffer may not have much role. As pH has no significant influence on partition characteristics of the dye above its pT; it is always advisable to explore the area between pK and pT (Table 1.3) to find out the most critical pH for a system i.e. the lowest pH at which the dye is wholly retained in the aqueous phase on shaking with an organic solvent.

Table 1.3. The lowest pH values at which the dye is wholly retained in the aqueous phase on shaking with an organic solvent

Dye	*pK*	*pT*	*pH*	*Organic solvent*
Bromocresol purple	6.3	6.8	5.4	Benzene
Bromothymol blue	7.0	7.6	5.0	Toluene
Bromocresol green	4.7	5.4	6.6	Chloroform
Bromophenol blue	4.0	4.6	5.6	Chloroform
Bromochlorophenol blue	4.2	4.8	4.0	Benzene
Chlorophenol red	6.0	6.6	6.5	Benzene
Methyl orange	3.8	4.4	5.0	Ethylene dichloride/chloroform, benzene
Thymol blue	2.0	2.8	5.0	Chloroform
Tropaeolin	2.2	2.6	3.2	Chloroform

Most nitrogenous bases of pharmaceutical interest have pK between 4 and 8. Thus at a particular pH, the extent to which any base will exist in its free form will depend on its pKa value. The condition required is that the medium may not be too acidic so as to retain the base in the aqueous phase. It is sometimes necessary to operate at a pH somewhat higher than the pT of the indicator (dye). General guideline is that pH of the buffer chosen should be somewhat above the pKa of the base to be estimated and then select the dye for which this pH is optimum. For example, for methyl orange-chloroform system at pH 5.0, pKa of the base must be below 7.0.

The sensitivity of this method depends primarily on molar extinction coefficient of the dye in the medium in which the absorbance is measured. To increase the sensitivity of the method, the ion-pair complex so formed and extracted into organic layer, is brought back to aqueous layer (acidic or basic) by shaking the organic layer with 0.1 N HCl or 0.1 N NaOH depending on the dye initially used for complex formation. The dye used in the complex formation is quantitatively extracted with aqueous layer and the absorbance of the resultant aqueous solution is measured as is the case with clonidine and pilocarpine.

*Note:*1. Most of these complexes being yellow in colour absorb in far ultraviolet region in the range of 360-420 nm, the maxima is not sharp and difficult to locate.

2. Reagent blank usually is very high.
3. As formation of complexes is pH-specific, presence of other substances can effect the pH. For estimation of codeine in presence of aspirin, usually pH of higher value is required for formation of complex with methyl orange.

(ii) Colorimetry involving chromogenic reagents

The instrument (colorimeter) employs tungsten radiation source and broad band (~ 300 nm) optical filters of nominal wavelength. It is usually difficult to establish linearity range in a colorimeter due to relatively broad spectral band-width employed. While employing colorimetric methods comparison with the standard is absolutely essential.

Colorimetric methods involving chemical reactions confer certain degree of specificity, thus other components present in the formulation do not interfere in the analysis, however the analyst should consider the following practical aspects while using colorimeter methods.

1. Colour reagent should be selective for drug substance of interest to discriminate it from its degradation products, impurities and other excipients/matrix present in the formulation.
2. Effect of other parameters such as solvent, pH, reagent volume, order of adding reagent, age of reagent, reaction temperature, which may have bearing on the colour reaction should be identified and established.
3. Time required for optimum colour intensity.
4. Stability of chromophore formed.

(iii) Ultraviolet and visible spectroscopy

(a) Single beam spectrophotometer: Uses prism or high quality diffraction grading monochromator and intense source of ultraviolet radiation—deuterium (hydrogen) lamp. As the sample and reference cells are manually moved in and out of radiation beam at each wavelength of interest, scanning of spectrum is not possible.

(b) Double beam spectrophotometer: Contains high quality optical components as in the case of single beam spectrophotometer but radiation in the monochromator splits into two identical beams, one passing through the sample and other through the reference cell, thus making scanning of spectra possible.

Analytical absorption spectroscopy in ultraviolet and visible region of electromagnetic spectrum is widely used for quantitative analysis in the field of pharmaceutical and biomedical analysis. Since, this technique has been extensively used in this text while describing analytical procedures, it is appropriate that analyst is made conversant with some important and practical aspects of this technique.

The scope of absorption spectroscopy is further extended by use of colour reactions often with concomitant increase in sensitivity and/or selectivity. Such reactions are used to modify the spectrum of an absorbing molecule, so that it could be detected in visible region well separated from other interfering

Table 1.4. Complimentary colours*

Wavelength (nm)	*Colour absorbed*	*Colour observed (complimentary colour)*
400-435	Violet	Yellowish-green
435-480	Blue	Yellowish
480-490	Greenish-blue	Orange
490-500	Bluish-green	Red
500-560	Green	Purple
560-580	Yellowish-green	Violet
580-595	Yellow	Blue
595-610	Orange	Greenish-blue
610-750	Red	Bluish-green

* If white light is deprived of one of its colours by absorption, the resulting light will appear as complimentary colour.

components. Chemical modification is also useful for transforming non-absorbing molecule to a stable derivative possessing significant absorption spectral behaviour. Selectivity can further be enhanced by number of chemical or instrumental techniques such as difference spectroscopy, derivative spectroscopy, derivative-difference spectroscopy and dual wavelength spectroscopy, however, such methods should be validated.

The prescribed unit used in UV-visible spectroscopy is wavelength expressed as nanometres (nm). The position of maximum absorbance of a peak is designated λ_{max}. The wavelength in this region is divided into two ranges, i.e., 200-400 nm (ultraviolet region) and about 400-800 nm (visible region). Outside these limits are designated as far ultraviolet (vacuum ultraviolet) and near infrared. The group in the molecule which is responsible for absorption is described as chromophore whereas group having little or no intrinsic absorption of its own, but modifies the absorption spectrum of the molecule is called auxochrome.

Measurement of chromophore in visible region has been extensively used. Most of the time, chemical species do not possess suitable chromogenic properties and are made to react with a suitable reagent giving rise to coloured species. Compounds having phenolic functional group with ortho or para position yield spectrophotometrically useful chromogens through nitrosation. The stability of nitroso-derivative is increased by addition of alcohol or alkalinization of the medium. Coordination of a transition metal with polydentate-ligand (ortho-nitroso-derivative) results in the formation of a stable water soluble metal chelate. Most of the drug substances with phenolic functions included in this text have been estimated either through their nitroso-derivative or metal chelate or both such as paracetamol, oxyphenbutazone, amoxycillin, salbutamol sulphate.

Ortho-nitroso-derivative (having para position occupied) are usually unstable in acidic medium, whereas para-nitroso-derivatives are stable in both the acidic and alkaline medium. Ortho-nitroso phenol derivations are capable of forming chelates with cobalt (II) ion, whereas para-nitroso derivatives do not form cobalt chelates. The cobalt chelate is sparingly soluble in water but easily extractable with organic solvents such as chloroform (yellow chromogen). Copper chelates are usually purple in colour.

The extent of absorption of radiation by a given absorbing system at a specific monochromatic wavelength is governed by two classical laws of absorptiometry.

Lambert's (Bougner's) law: At a given concentration (C) of a homogeneous absorbing system, the intensity of transmitted light decreases exponentially with increase in path light.

The complimentary Beer's law concerned with concentration (C) states that for a layer of defined path length, the intensity of transmitted light decreases exponentially with increase in concentration (C) of a homogeneous absorbing system. The combination of both these laws gives the popular law i.e. Beer-Lambert law i.e.

$$\log \frac{I_o}{I} = kcb \qquad \text{where } k = \text{absorptivity of the system}$$

When concentration is expressed in g/100 ml, k is described as specific absorption and is designated by the symbol $A_{1\text{cm}}^{1\%}$ or A (1%, 1 cm) i.e. absorbance of a 1% w/v solution of a substance in a cell of 1 cm path length. The term is also expressed as A_1^1 and is widely used in analytical chemistry. $A_{1\text{cm}}^{1\%}$ values have been used in the text for calculating assay values, however, because of instrumental differences and possible effect of solvents, these values are subject to considerable variations. It is therefore advisable not to use these values where accurate assay is required or in case of dispute, use of reference substance is called for.

Molar absorptivity: Absorbance of a one molar solution in a cell of 1 cm path length. As per American convention absorptivity (a) is defined as absorption of 1 g/L solution of a substance in a cell of 1 cm path length.

$$\text{Absorptivity (a)} = \frac{A_1^1}{10} = \frac{\text{Value of A1\%,1cm}}{10}$$

i.e. Absorptivity (a) is $\frac{1}{10}$th of specific absorption (A_1^1).

Example: Aspirin (Acetyl salicylic acid)

λ_{max} (acid) = 230 nm

A_1^1 (230 nm) = 466

Absorptivity (a) = 46.6

Molar absorptivity = 8397.32 ...(46.6 × 180.2)

Red or bathochromic shift: Shift in the peak position (λ_{max}) to a higher wavelength due to effect of substituents, solvents or molecular re-arrangement. This is often large (> 100 nm). This effect is exploited for quantitative and qualitative purpose.

Blue or hypsochromic shift: Shift in the peak position (λ_{max}) to a lower wavelength sometime as much as 30 nm.

Hyperchromic and hypochromic shift: Increase or decrease in the absorptivity value.

Bathochromic/hypsochromic shifts are usually accompanied with hyper- or hypochromic effects.

Isobestic (iso-absorption) point: The point (wavelength) at which molar absorptivity of different ionic species is identical. To determine this point, UV absorption spectra of different ionic species is scanned under identical conditions and concentrations. This property has been extensively used to develop analytical techniques for bi-component drug formulations. Certain methods described in the text are based on this technique.

Note:

1. Quantitative spectrophotometric analysis should preferably be carried out above 235 nm as in the range of 190-210 nm, special precautions are required to be observed.
2. Spectrophotometric measurements should be carried out at the peak of spectral absorption of the substance under estimation. It is always desirable to actually determine the peak wavelength of the compound in the instrument under use as minor variations in the apparent wavelength of the peak are observed from instrument to instrument.
3. Spectrophotometric measurements should usually be made first with the standard solution.
4. The concentration of sample and standard should be so chosen that the absorption value of final solution is in the range of 0.40 to 0.75 for least error.
5. When an assay is carried out with routine frequency, use of reference substance can be omitted and instead a suitable standard curve prepared with reference substance may be used.
6. When a new apparatus or new lot of reagents are used, standard curve needs confirmation.
7. In the event of uncertainty or dispute, direct comparison with the reference substance is necessary.

Validity of Beer-Lambert law

The validity of the Beer-Lambert law is affected by number of factors. If the radiation is non-monochromatic the observed absorbance usually is lower than for monochromatic radiation. Thus sharp bands are more susceptible than broad bands to absorbance error on this account. Further if absorbing species undergoes association, dissociation, photodegradation, solvation, complexation or adsorption or emits fluorescence, then positive or negative derivations from the Beer's law may be observed. Stray light effects and the type of solvent used can also lead to non-compliance with the Beer's law.

For single-beam instruments the absorbance range for precise measurement should be below 0.3-0.6 absorbance units, the optimum range being 0.45 absorbance units. For double-beam spectrophotometry, the optimum range lies between 0.6 and 1.2 absorbance units. Five or more standard solutions whose absorbances are within working range should be measured in duplicate in a matched pair of cells against solvent as reference. The cell constant should be substituted for each individual measurement and needs to be checked regularly. If a graph absorbance (A) versus concentration (C) indicates any systematic (positive or negative) deviation, then additional points be inserted and working range estimated.

Practical application of absorbance values A_1^1 depends on various factors such as purity of substance, solvent used and precise conditions employed in the reference instrument and the type of instrument available. It is therefore desirable to ascertain the reported absorptivity data in one's own laboratory. It is advisable not to depend on reported absorptivity values when accurate assay values are required or in matter of dispute the use of reference substance for comparison is called for. The absorptivity values should be periodically determined if sufficient quantity of drug in pure form is available.

The validity of Beer-Lambert law should be established for each drug under the measurement conditions prevailing in the laboratory over the concentration range of interest. The reported range more than often is required to be re-established.

Absorption cells

For visible region (400-700 nm) matched pair of glass cell is used. For ultraviolet region, fused silica or quartz cells having high transmittance in the range of 190-1000 nm are employed (glass has poor transmission property in the ultraviolet region). In routine analytical work, cells with 1 cm path length are used; however, cells of longer path length (up to 10 cm) are available and employed in case where the concentration of the substance to be determined is too low or the substance has low absorbance values. For estimation of ethinyloestradiol by colorimetric method employ glass cell of 5 cm path length whereas glass cell of 2 cm path length is used for assay of promethazine hydrochloride in elixir promethazine. Flow cells now available primarily to minimise the turbulent flow through the cell are used for monitoring changes in the absorbance during a reaction dissolution studies or for HPLC. For enzymatic or temperature controlled studies, cells are provided with thermostatic control. Cells to be used for spectrophotometric analysis have optical surface opposite to each other whereas optical surface is at right angle to each other in case of fluorometric analysis.

Careful handling and care of cells is pre-requisite for precise and accurate measurements. The cells should be matched for absorbance of less than 1%. For correct identification, each pair of matched cells should be similarly marked i.e. more strongly absorbing cell as sample cell and other being coded as reference cell and this orientation should be maintained during actual analysis. This will ensure that cell constant is always possible and there is no oscillating error due to change in orientation (cell constant should be checked at wavelength of measurement or by scanning the baseline over the range of measurement).

Cleaning of cells: If the cell contained aqueous solutions, it can be rapidly cleaned by repeated rinsing with distilled water and then with methanol or ethanol. After day use, cell should be preferably soaked overnight in very dilute solution of detergents. Periodically the cells and stopper should be soaked in fresh solution of chromic acid followed by thorough rinsing with distilled water to restore their matched performance. Use of strong alkali or acid is not recommended and test solutions should be left in the cell for least possible time. Sharp glass or metal objects should not be introduced in the cell. Optical side of the cells should not be touched, preferably cleaned with soft muslin cloth or photographic lens tissue. Cells should be stored in pair in a closed protective container usually supplied by the manufacturer.

Solvents

Quality of spectral measurement is directly affected by the type and purity of solvent used. Each solvent has a cut-off wavelength (Table 1.5) and should not be used below its cut-off wavelength even if reference cell is used for compensation as there is greater risk of stray light effect.

Distilled water, alcohol (methanol, ethanol), chloroform and dilute solutions of acid and alkali are most commonly used solvent for spectrophotometric analysis. The solvent should be free from UV absorbing contaminants and should not interact with the substance to be analysed. Analytical grade of solvents are usually suitable except in spectrophotofluorometric analysis.

It is preferable to use distilled water as deionised water may be contaminated with absorptive fragment of ion-exchange resin, or may contain bacterial metabolites contributing to non-specific absorbance. 95% alcohol should be used

Table 1.5. UV cut-off points for commonly used solvents (corresponding to about 10% transmittance)

Solvents	*Wavelength (nm)*	*Solvents*	*Wavelength (nm)*
Water (distilled)	190	Chloroform (stabilized)	245
Dilute inorganic acid	190	Carbon tetrachloride	265
Cyclohexane	210	Acetic acid glacial	250
Cyclopentane	210	n-Butyl alcohol	215
Ethanol (96% v/v)	210	1,4-Dioxan	220
n-Heplane	210	Ethyl acetate	253
n-Hexane	210	Methyl ethyl ketone	330
Isopropyl alcohol	210	Iso-octane	210
Methanol	210	N,N-Dimethyl formamide	270
Ether	220	Benzene	280
Sodium hydroxide (0.2 M)	225	Pyridine	305
Ethylene dichloride	230	Acetone	330
Methylene chloride	235		

as dehydrated alcohol is likely to be contaminated with traces of benzene used to form azeotropic mixture for distillation. Acetone, usually used to clean the cell is highly absorptive and difficult to remove. Chloroform and carbon tetrachloride absorb around 250 nm and should be used above 280 nm. Ether, though transparent even down to 220 nm, has problem of volatility (inconsistent standard solution) and inflammability. Use of strong acids and alkalies should be avoided. Solvent so chosen should not interact with the substance to be analysed.

Filtration

In methods involving colour development, it is preferable to centrifuge the final coloured solution as use of filter paper or passing through layer of anhydrous sodium sulphate results in loss of colour intensity. In certain methods, use of glass sintered funnel is indicated, it must be adhered to.

Phase separation filter (Whatman No. 1 PS)

It is a filter impregnated with water repellent (stable silicone) for effecting rapid separation of immisible mixture of aqueous and organic liquid on a laboratory scale. Since these filters are hydrophobic in character, organic liquids readily pass through the paper whereas aqueous liquid and solid are retained, thus rapid separation of two liquids is attained.

- Fold the paper in normal way and keep it in conical filter funnel.
- Pour mixed phases directly into the paper. It is not necessary to allow the phases to separate clearly before pouring.

- Allow the organic phase to filter completely through the paper, retained aqueous phase may be if required washed with small volume of solvent. This is necessary particularly when separating phase which is lighter than water in order to clean the meniscus of aqueous phase.
- Do not allow the aqueous phase to remain on the filter paper for long time after phase separation as it will start seeping through because of evaporation of organic solvent from pores of filter paper, creating a local vacuum which in turn draws the water through—seeping process.

Variables in quantitative analysis

- Inhomogeneity of the medicament
- Sampling error
- Preparation of sample such as extraction
- Precision, accuracy and ruggedness of the method
- Random error including that of the operator

It is, therefore, essential that the analytical procedure must reasonably assess quality of the sample and should be capable of revealing inhomogeneity, suitability of the sampling procedure, precision and accuracy of the method and the extent of possible errors at different stages of the procedure.

Common Units of Measurement

Units of Mass

Symbol	*Prefix*	*Power of Ten*	*Ordinary Notation*
g	gram		
m	milli	10^{-3}	0.001
μ	micro	10^{-6}	0.000 001
n	nano	10^{-9}	0.000 000 001
p	pico	10^{-12}	0.000 000 000 001
f	femto	10^{-15}	0.000 000 000 000 001
a	atto	10^{-18}	0.000 000 000 000 000 001
z	zepto	10^{-21}	0.000 000 000 000 000 000 001
y	yocto	10^{-24}	0.000 000 000 000 000 000 000 001

Units of Length	**Units of Volume**		**Units of Time**	**Units of Temperature**
Metre (m)	Litre (L)		Day (d)	Degree Celsius (°C)
Centimetre (cm)	Millilitre (ml)	10^{-3} L	Hour (h)	
Millimetre (mm)	Microlitre (μl)	10^{-6} L	Minute (min)	
Micrometre (μm)			Second (s)	
Nanometre (nm)				

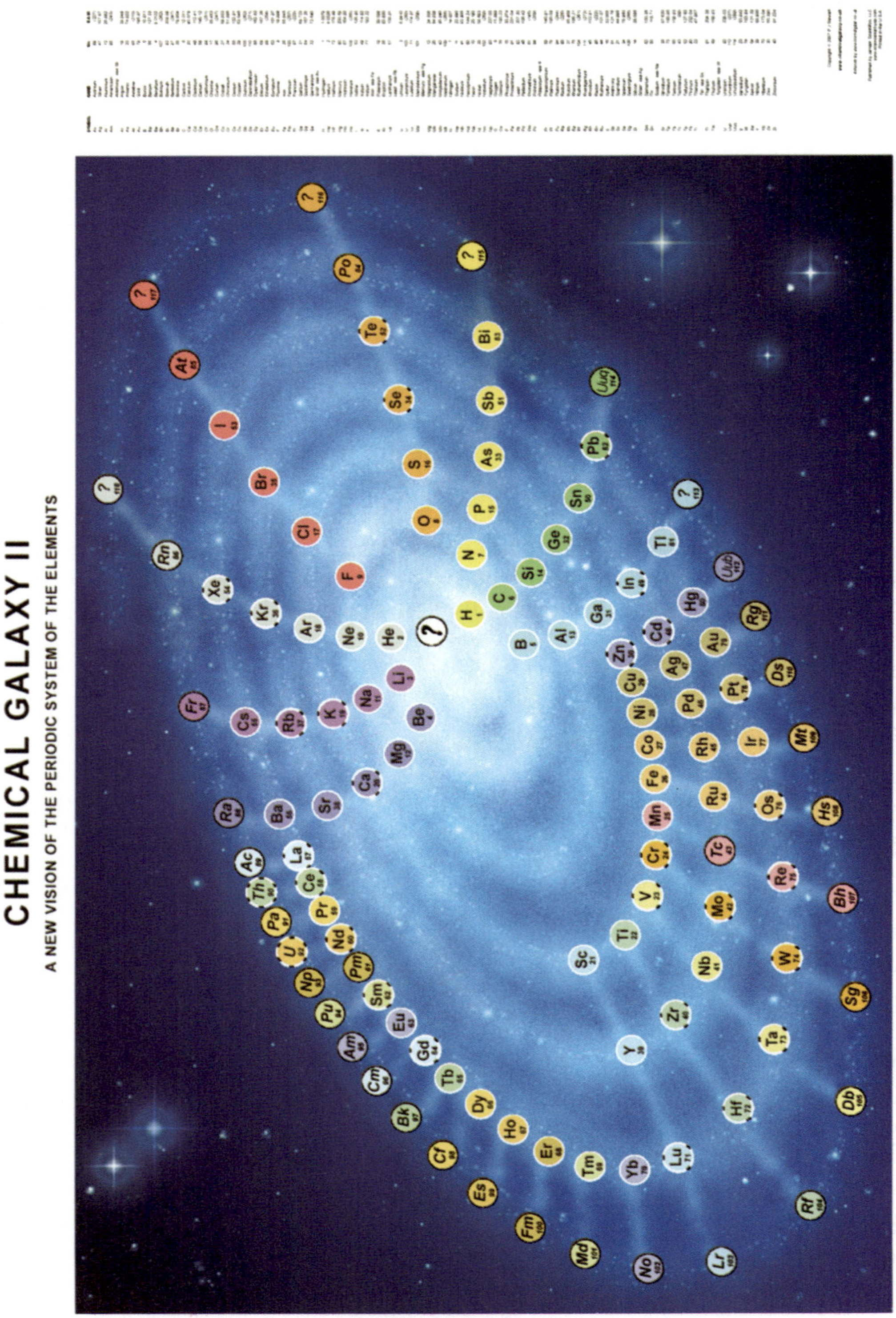
CHEMICAL GALAXY II
A NEW VISION OF THE PERIODIC SYSTEM OF THE ELEMENTS

List of Common Reagents and Drugs Reacting to Produce Coloured Species (Chromogens)

Reagent

- Emerson Reagent (4-aminoantipyrin, potassium ferricyanide reagent)

Drugs

- Amoxycillin, Salbutamol, Piroxicam, Thymol, Eugenol, Phenylbutazone, Guaiacol sulphonate, DIHQ, Niclosamide, Nylidrin, Labetalol, Triamcinolone, Orciprenaline, Phenylephrine HCl, Nelfinavir, Nitrendipine (after reduction), Doxycycline, Chlorocresol, Dopamine

Reagent

- Bratton-Marshall Reagent

Drugs

- Primary aromatic amines, Sulphonamides, Benzodiazepine, Benzocaine, Thiacetazone, Bromhexine, Metoclopramide, Folic acid, Nimesulide, Phenylbutazone, Urea, Chloramphenicol (after reduction), Mosapride, Ambroxol, Paracetamol, Phenoazopyridine, Nimodipine, Metronidazole, Captopril, Eugenol, Isosorbide dinitrate, Pyridoxine, Piperazine, Ethinylestradiol, Salbutamol, Isoxsuprine, Amoxycillin, Niclosamide, Amodiaquin, Terbutaline, Pentazocine, Phenylephrine, Acebutolol

Reagent

- Gibbs' Reagent (2,6-Dibromoquinone-4-chloroimide or 2,6-Dichloroquinone-4-chloroimide)

Drugs

- Salicylamide, Amoxycillin, Piperazine, Oxyphenbutazone, Salbutamol, Primaquine, Resorcinol, Thymol, Rifampicin, Cloxacillin, Piroxicam, Barbiturates, Guaiacol sulphonate, Stanazalol, 8-OH-quinolins, Pyridoxine, Anti-epileptic drugs, Thiamine, Cimetidine, Isoxsuprine, Nylidrine, Labetalol, Aminophylline

Reagent

- Wurster's Red Reagent (N,N-Dimethyl-1,4-phenylene diamine reagent)

Drugs

- Paracetamol, Salbutamol, Terbutaline, Thiamine, Vitamin E, Triamcinolone, Isoxsuprine, Thiouracil, Nylidrin.

Reagent

- Iodine Reagent

Drugs

- Aspirin, Ascorbic acid, Benzocaine, Isoniazid, Analgin, Papaverine, Paracetamol, Resorcinol, Phenol, Piperazine, Salicylic acid, Thymol, Barbiturates, Quinine, Vitamin D, Morphine, Codeine, Phenylbutazone, Theophylline, Caffeine, Penicillin, Diazepam, Captopril, Emetine, Cephaeline, Imidazole derivatives, Propoxyphene, Antipyrin, Ethambutol, Sulphaguinidine, Glycin, Hydrocortisone, Salicylamide, Thiamine, Phenothiazines

Reagent

- Marquis Reagent (Formaldehyde-sulphuric acid reagent)

Drugs

- Morphine, Codeine, Promethazine, Propranolol, Nadolol, Chlorpromazine, Atropine, Amtriptylene, Chlordiazepoxide, Chlorphenaramine maleate, Cyclizine, Dextropropoxyphene, Diazepam, Diphenhydramine, Diphenoxylate, Ephedrine, Imipramine, Lignocaine, Mephenesin, Guaiphenesin, Mepyramine, Naphazoline, Phenylpropanolamine

Reagent

- MBTH Reagent, Besthorn's Reagent (3-Methyl-2-benzothiazolinone-hydrazine reagent)

Drugs

- Paracetamol, Analgin, Mephenesin, Ethambutol, Omeprazole, Sulphadoxine, Methyldopa, Pyridoxine, Sparfloxacin, Gatifloxacin, Pefloxacin, Enrofloxacin, Tobramycin, Cefpirome, Rofecoxib, Oxyclozanide, Nimesulide, Lansoprazole, Bisacodyl, Nelfinavir, Finasteride, Lacidipine, Benzthiazide, Hydrochlorothiazide, Hydroflumethiazide, Nabumelone, Trimelazidine, Lamivudine, Stavudine, Ketosteroids, Carbonyl compounds, Penicillin and Cefdinir

Reagent

- Emmerie-Engel Reagent (2,2′-Bispyridine-Iron (III) chloride reagent)

Drugs

- Salbutamol, Terbutaline, Captopril, Vitamin E, Vitamin C, Nylidrine, Isoxsuprine

Reagent

- Para-Aminophenol Reagent (PAP reagent)

Drugs

- Thiamine, Oxyphenbutazone, Thymol, Sulphadoxine, Methyl dopa, Diloxanide furoate

Reagent

- Folin's Reagent (1,2-Naphthoquinone-4-sulphonic acid reagent)

Drugs

- Amino acids, Chlorthalidone, Hydrochlorthiazide, Pyrimethamine, Analgin, Folic acid, Primaquine, Dapsone, Piroxicam, Metoclopramide, Cimetidine, Tranexamic acid, Rofecoxib, Sparfloxacin, Baclofen, Nateglinide, Dequalinium chloride, Ergot alkaloids, Dapsone, Prochlorperazine

Reagent

- Ninhydrin Reagent

Drugs

- Amoxycillin, Lysine, Cimetidine, Ephedrine, Methyldopa, Pantothenic acid, Neomycin, Diloxanide, Diazepam, Naphazoline, Lisinopril, Pyrazinamide, Primaquine, Promethazine, Gentamycin, Hydralazine, Phenytoin, Phenylpropanolamine, Naleglinide, Folic acid, Paracetamol

Reagent

- DNPH Reagent (2,4-Dinitrophenylhydrazine reagent)

Drugs

- Corticosteroids, Nitrofurantoin, Norfloxacin, Ciprofloxacin, Allantoin, Rifampicin, Methyltestosterone, Paraformaldehyde, Menadione, Dihydroascorbic acid, Buspirone, Dexamethasone, Triamcinolone

Reagent

- Pauly's Reagent (Diazotized sulphanilic acid reagent)

Drugs

- Histamine, Clotrimazole, Tinidazole, Metronidazole, Flavonoids, Salbutamol, Primaquine, Pyramethamine, Alendronate, Cimetidine, Isoxsuprine, Terbutaline, Nylidrin, Pioglitazone

Reagent

- Iron (III) chloride reagent

Drugs

- Salicylic acid, Phenothiazines, Paracetamol, Morphine, Ergotamine, Diclofenac, Norfloxacin, Galifloxacin, Ciprofloxacin, Ofloxacin, PAS, Meloxicam, Metoprolol, Lisinopril, Iodochlorhydroxyquinoline, Phenolic drugs, Gallic acid, Flavonoids, Catechols, Cholesterol

Reagent

- Sanger's Reagent (2,4-Dinitrofluorobenzene reagent)

Drugs

- Amoxycillin, Metoprolol, Ampicillin, Propanolol, Nitrazepam

Reagent

- Barton's Reagent [Iron (III) chloride - Potassium ferricyanide reagent]

Drugs

- Ibuprofen, Ketoprofen, Diclofenac, Clopidogrel, Sildenafil, Terazosin, Meloxicam, Lacidipine, Tobramycin, Cefpodoxime, Proxetil, Aromatic amines, Tubocurarine, Estradiol, 4-Aminoantipyrin

Reagent

- p-Chloranil Reagent

Drugs

- Sulphonamides, Ephedrine, Piperazine, Emetine, Reserpine, Berberine, Morphine, Papaverine, Lidocaine, Procaine, Phenothiazine, Ampicillin, Amoxycillin, Cloxacillin, Furosemide, Tolbutamide, Gliclazide, Metoprolol, Propranolol, Albendazole, Oxprenolol, Captopril, Pyrimethamine, Fluoroquinolone, Fenfluramine, Benzthiazide

Reagent

- INH Reagent (Isonicotinic acid hydrazide reagent)

Drugs

- Diloxanide, Nitrofurantoin, Spironolactone, Ketosteroids, Dichloroquinolines

Reagent

- Ehrlich's Reagent (4-Dimethylaminobenzaldehyde - Hydrochloric acid), Van Urk's Reagent (4-Dimethylaminobenzaldehyde - Sulphuric acid Reagent) Note: Instead of 'PDAB', 'PDAC' can be used.

Drugs

- Sulphonamides, Paracetamol, Bromhexine, Benzocaine, Chlordiazepoxide, Thiacetazone, Isoniazid, Oxyphenbutazone, Amoxycillin, Indomethazine, Ergotamine, Ergometrine, Urea, Atropine, Scopolamine, Carvone, Chlorthalidone, Metoclopramide, Biotin, Ranitidine, Frusemide, Phenothiazine, Barbiturates, Analgin, Terbutaline, Nitazoxanide, Satranidazole, Cisapride, Metronidazole, Nateglinide, Primary aromatic amines, Flutamide, Meprobamate, Promethazine, Aminophylline, Tinidazole

Reagent

- Blue Tetrazolium Reagent

Drugs

- Corticosteroids, Isosorbide, Spironolactone, Pyraquantel

Reagent

- Sodium nitrite Reagent

Drugs

- Paracetamol, Pentazocine, Chloroxazone, Terbutaline, Amodiaquine, Piperazine, Dithranol, Mefenamic acid, Indomethazine

Reagent

- N-Bromosuccinimide Reagent

Drugs

- Paracetamol, Amodiaquine, Amoxycillin, Quercetin

Reagent

- Chromotropic acid Reagent

Drugs

- Analgin, Pilocarpine, Formaldehyde, Paraformaldehyde

Structures of Some Drug Substances Whose Methods of Analysis Are Described in the Text

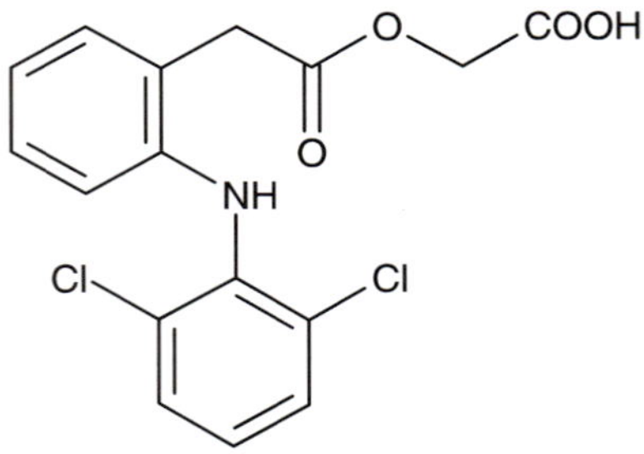

Aceclofenac

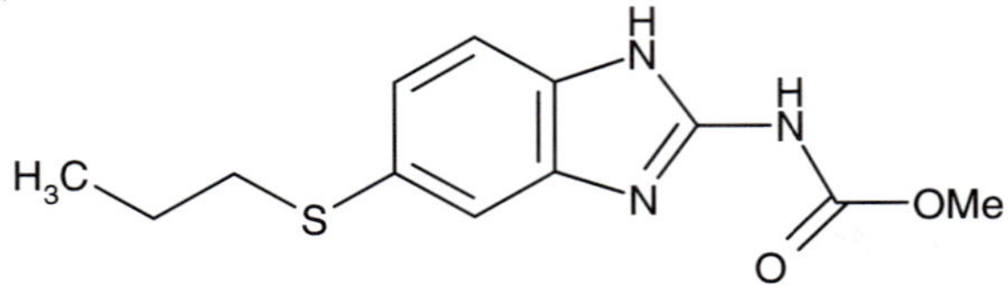

Albendazole

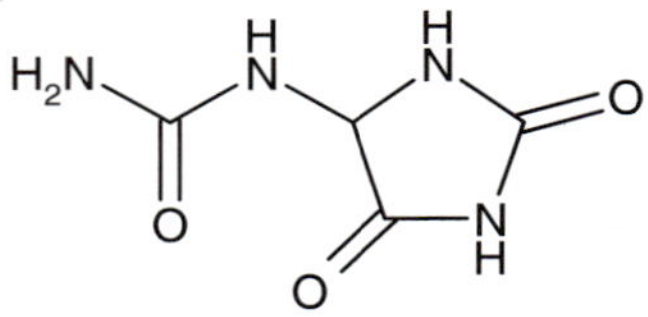

Allantoin

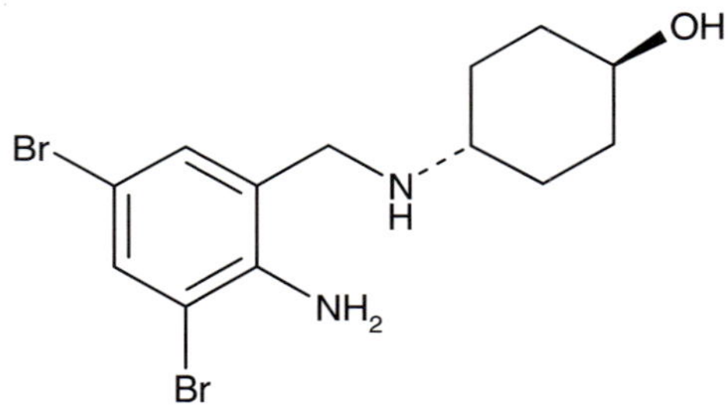

Ambroxol

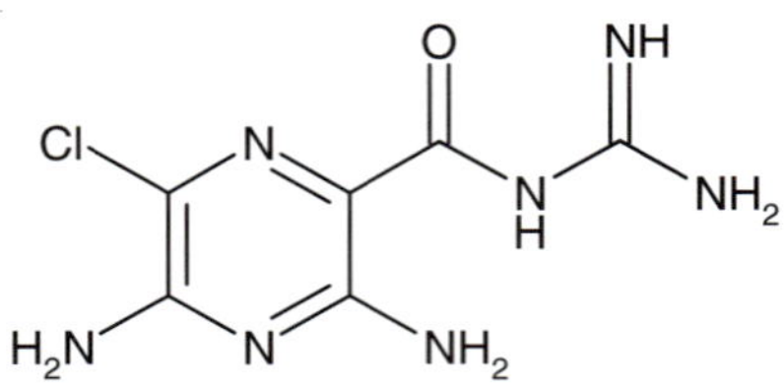

Amiloride

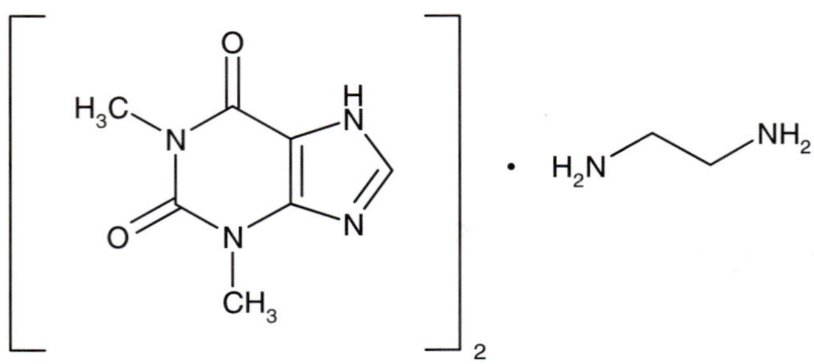

Aminophylline

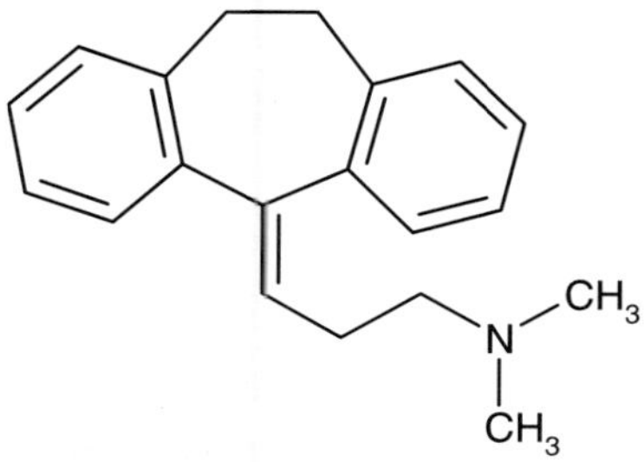

Amitriptyline

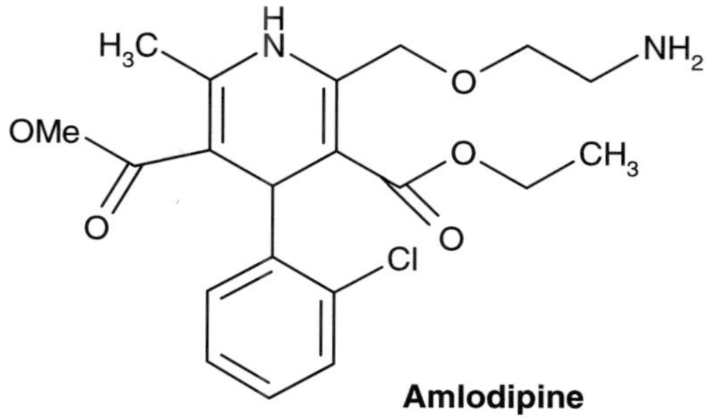

Amlodipine

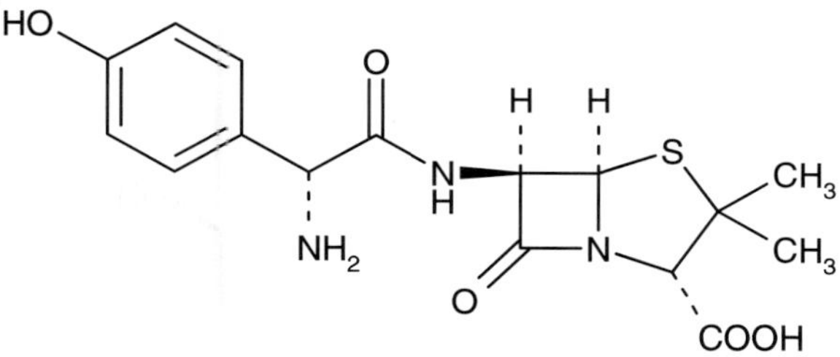

Amoxycillin

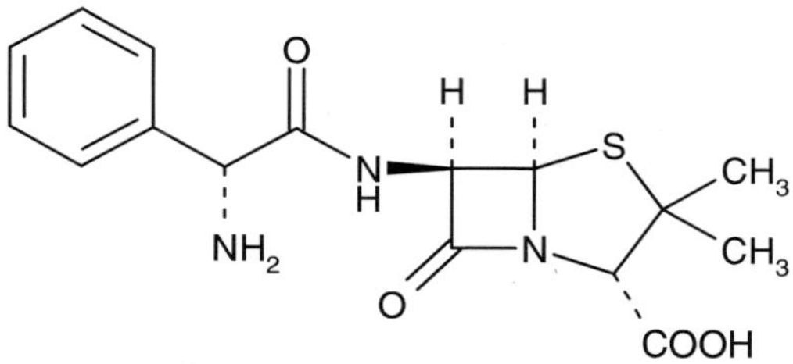

Ampicillin

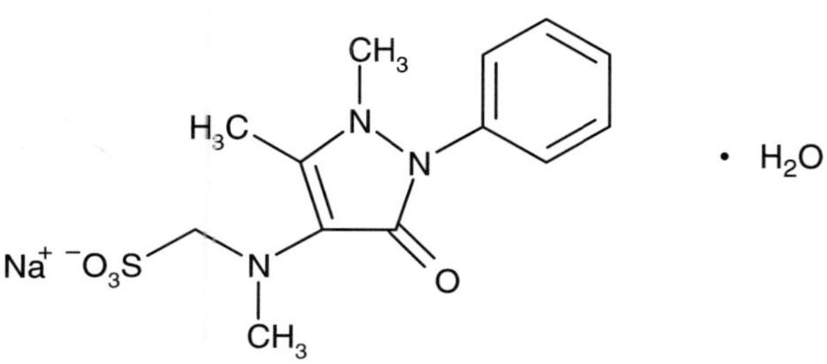

Analgin (Dipyrone)

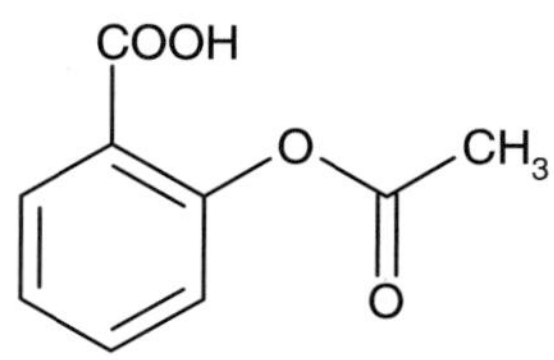

Aspirin

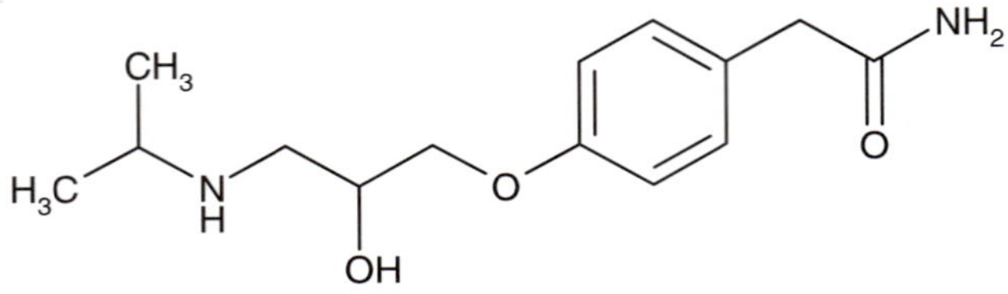

Atenolol

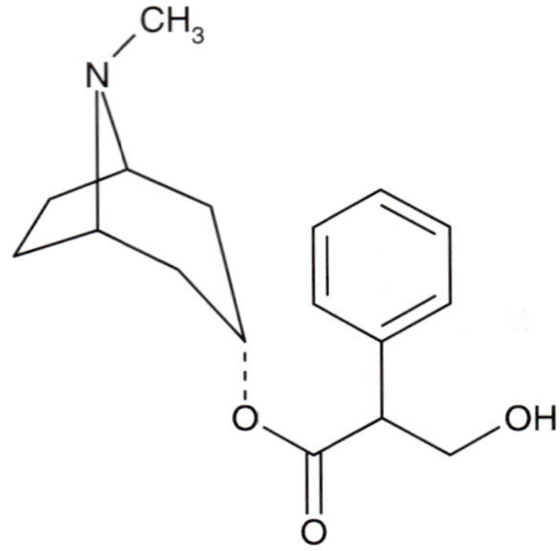

Atropine

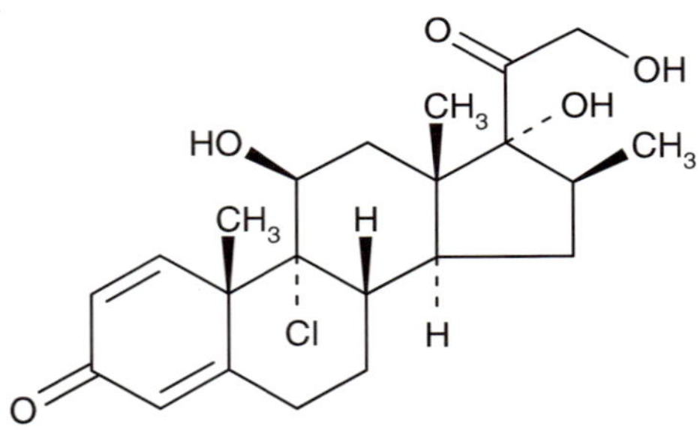

Beclomethasone

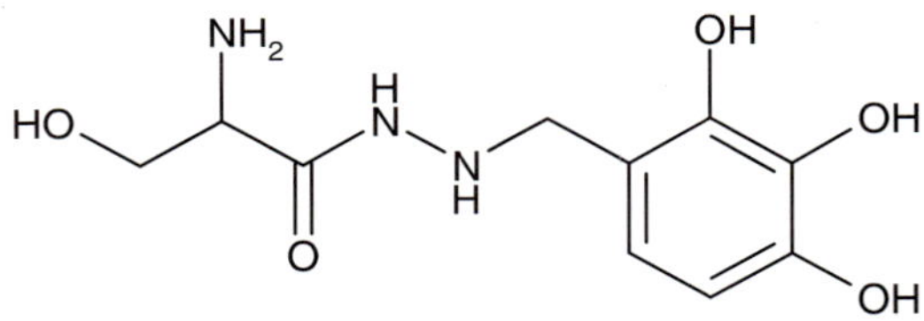

Benserazide

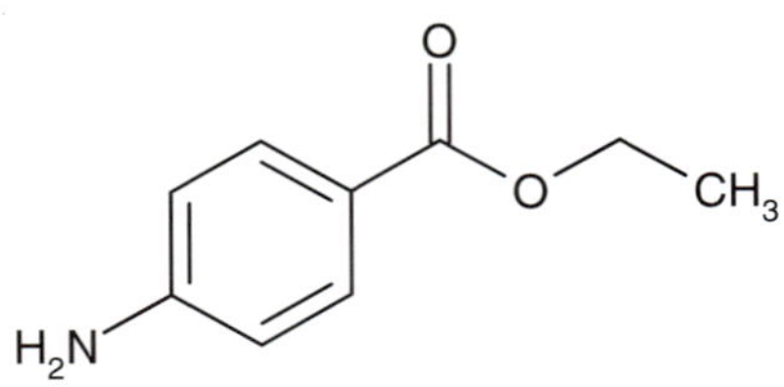

Benzocaine

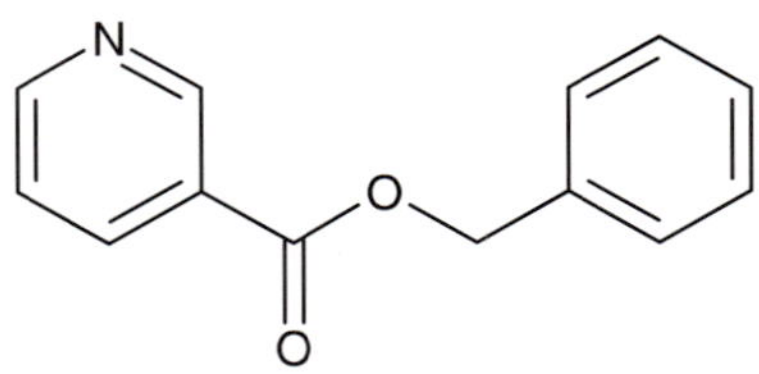

Benzyl nicotinate

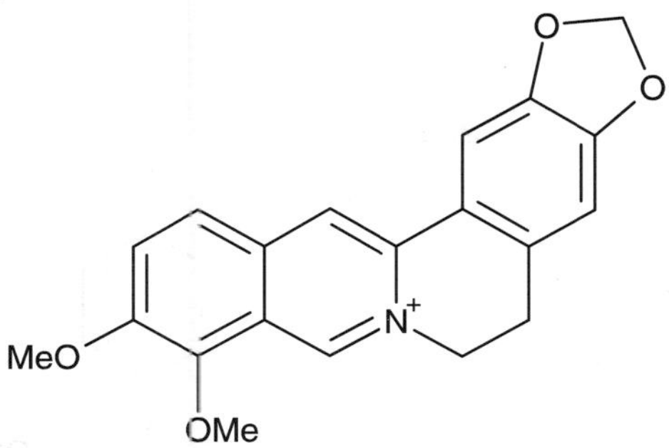

Berberine

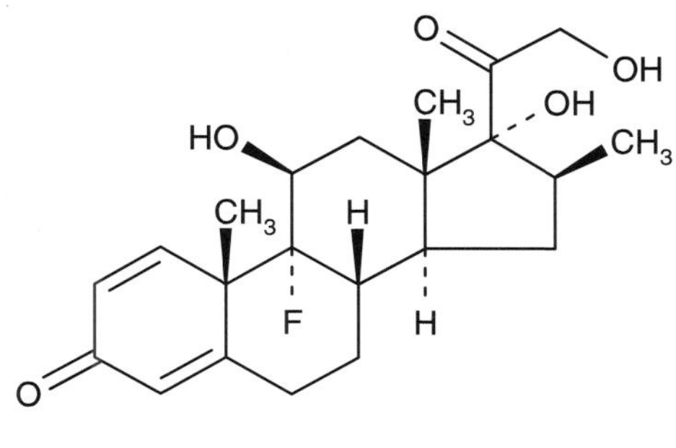

Betamethasone

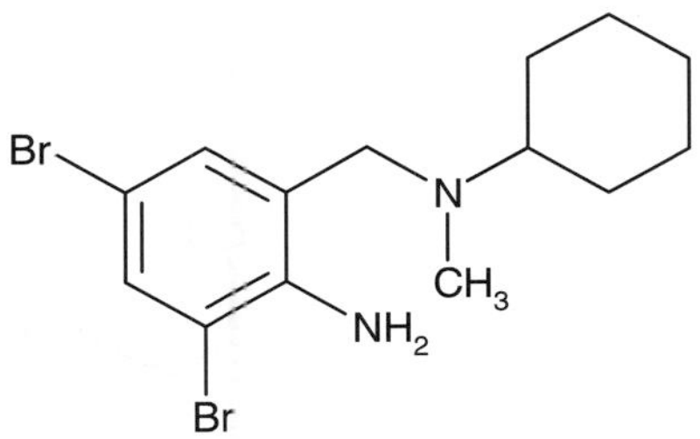

Bromhexine

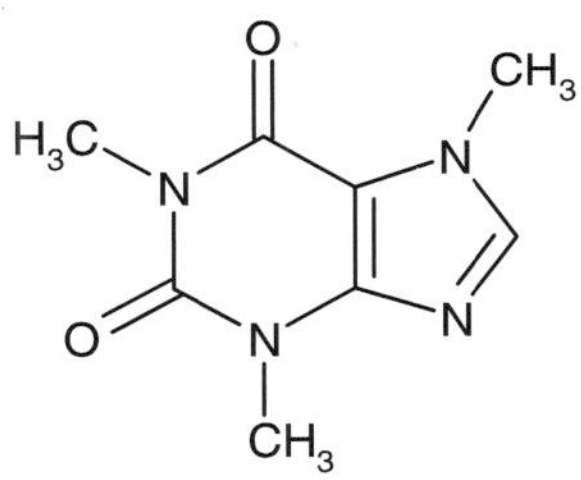

Caffeine

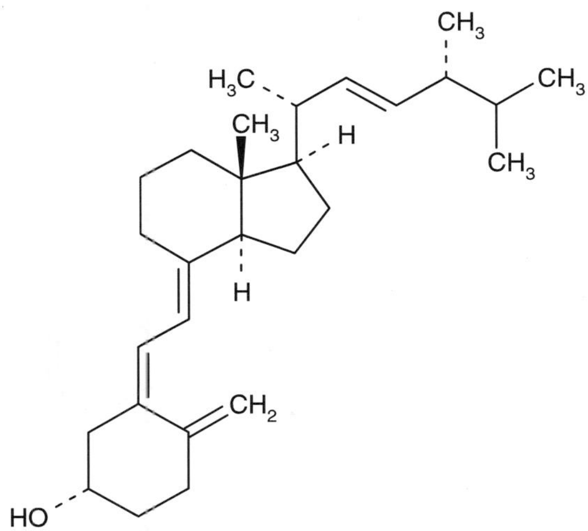

Calciferol (Vitamin D_2)

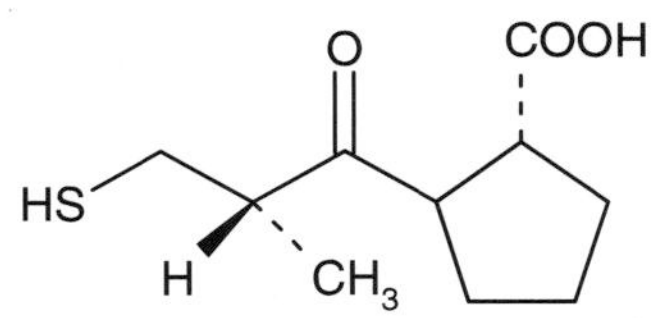

Captopril

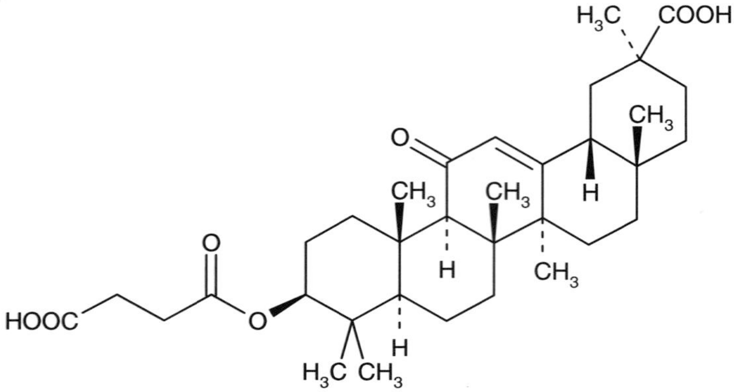

Carbenoxolone

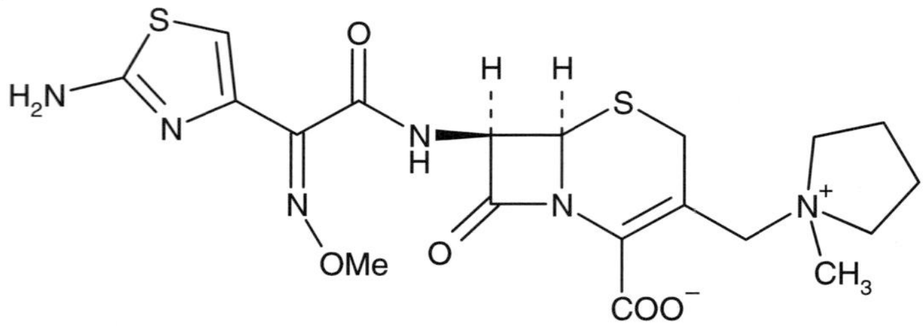

Cefepime

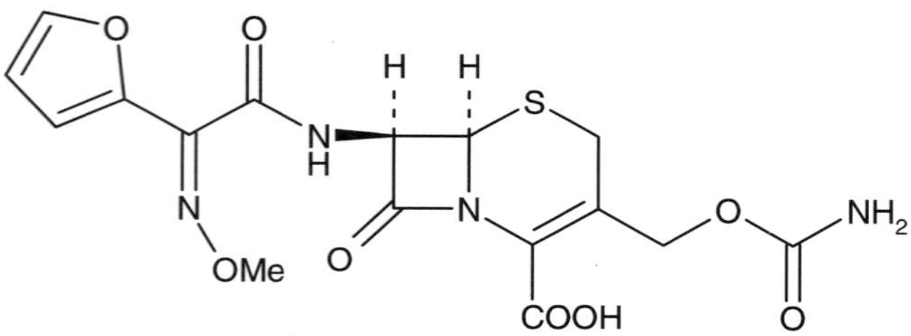

Cefuroxime

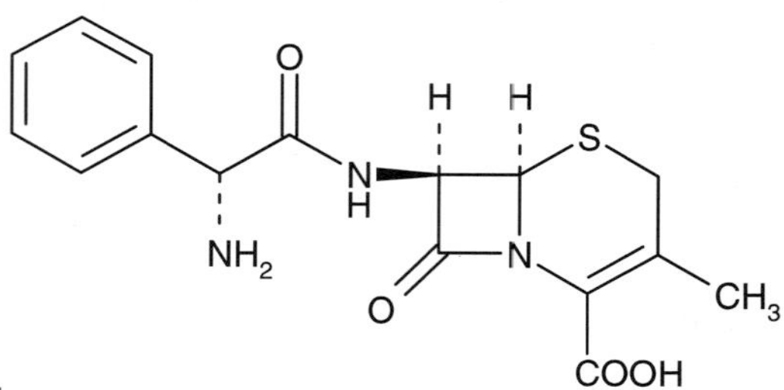

Cephalexin

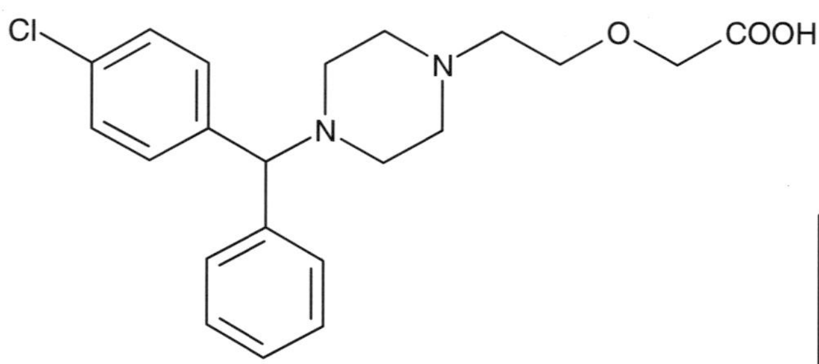

Cetirizine

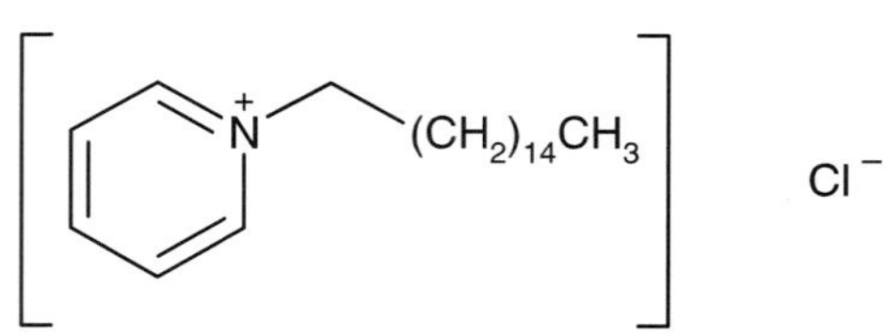

Cetylpyridinium chloride

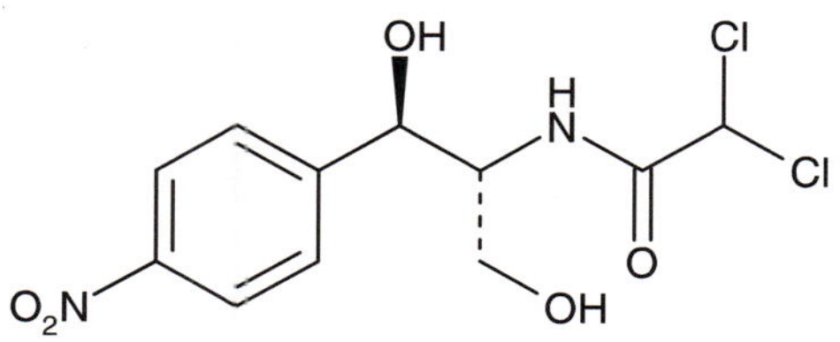

Chloramphenicol

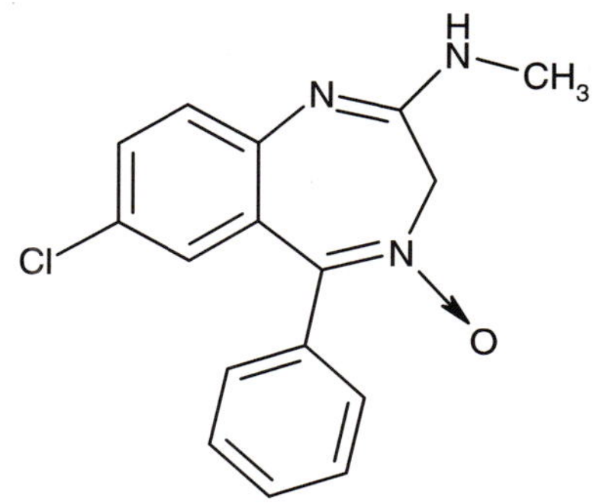

Chlordiazepoxide

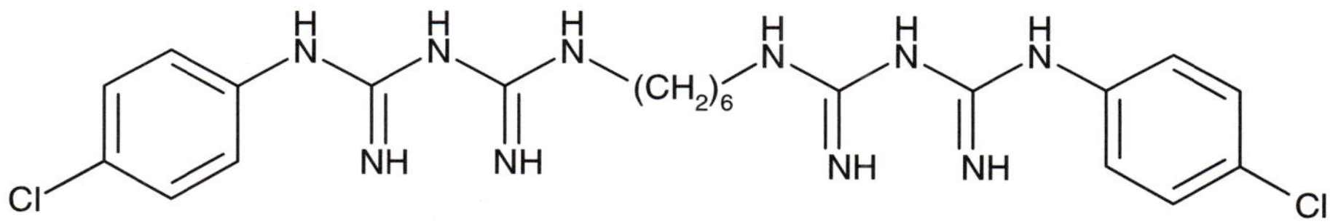

Chlorhexidine

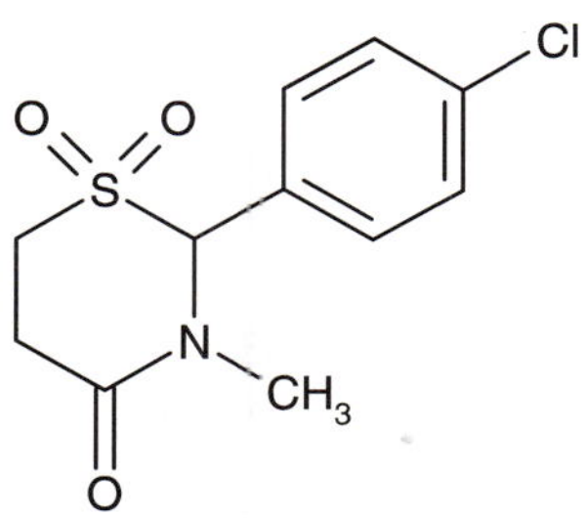

Chlormezanone

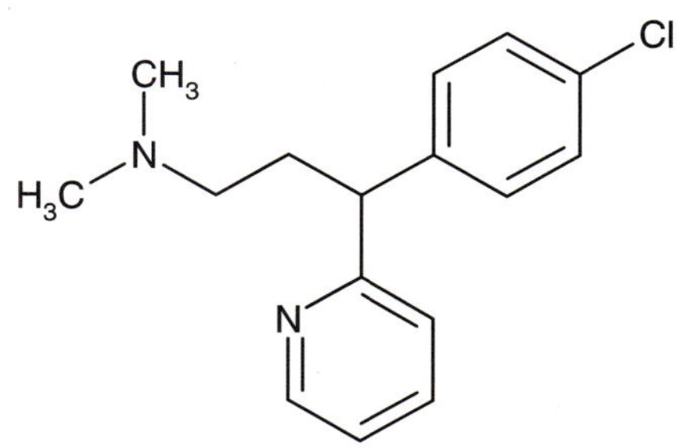

Chlorpheniramine

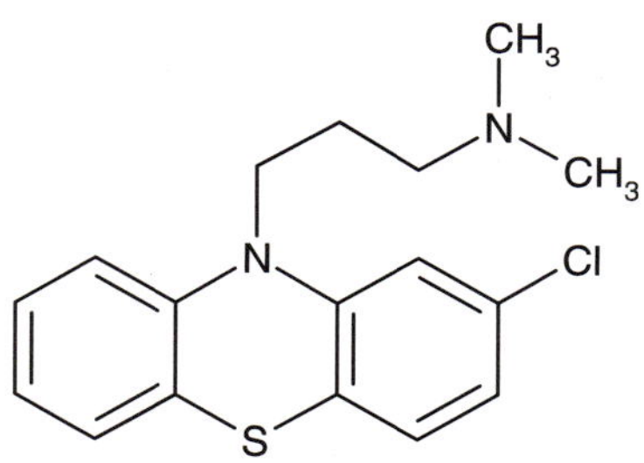

Chlorpromazine

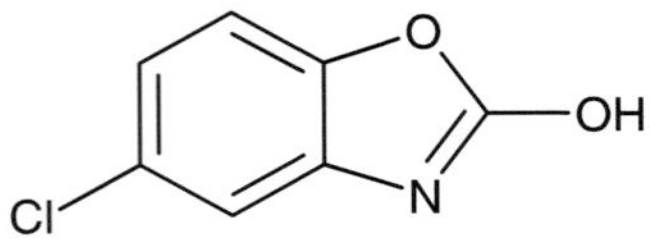

Chlorzoxazone

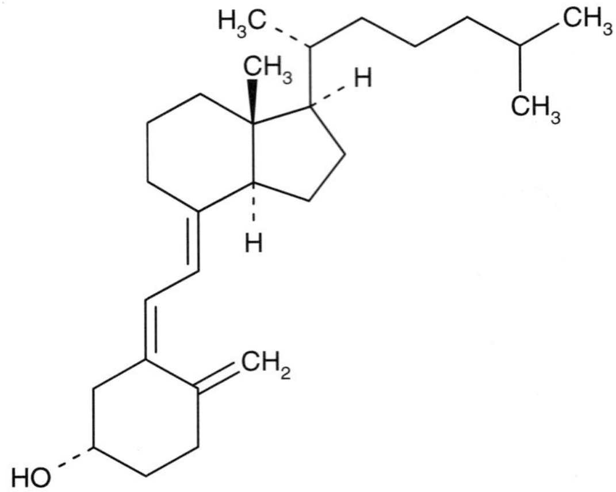

Cholecalciferol (Vitamin D$_3$)

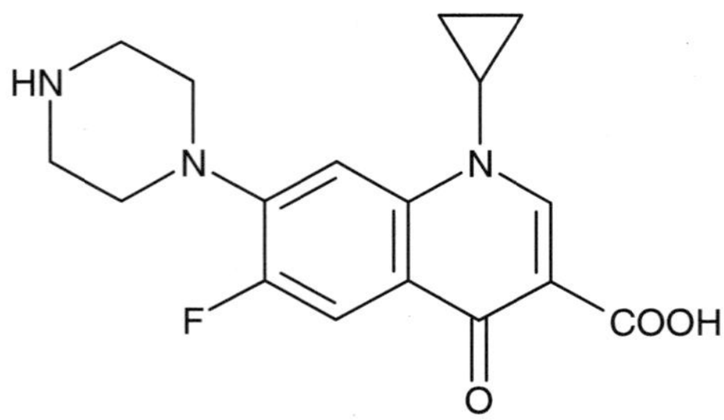

Ciprofloxacin

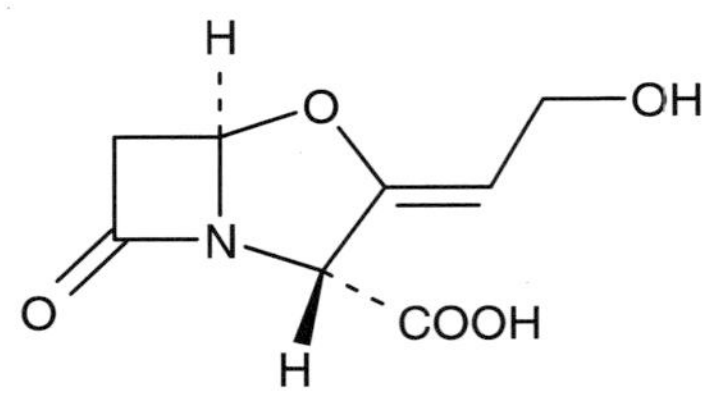

Clavulanic acid

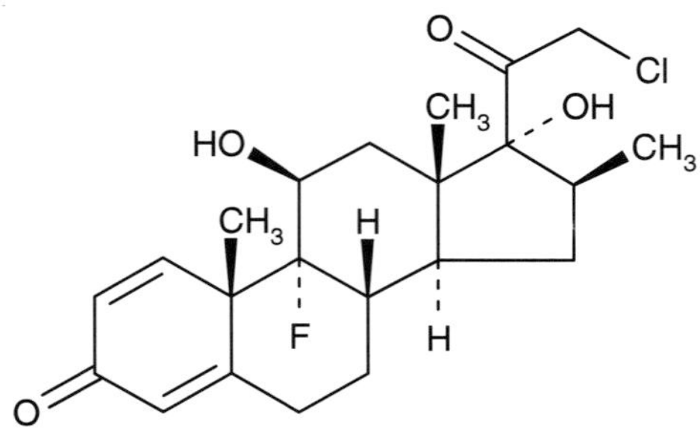

Clobetasol

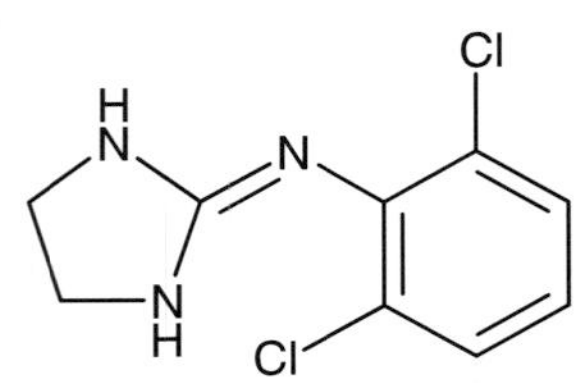

Clonidine

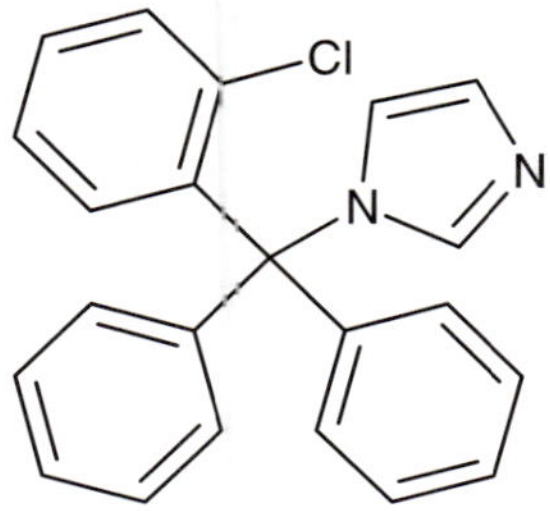

Clotrimazole

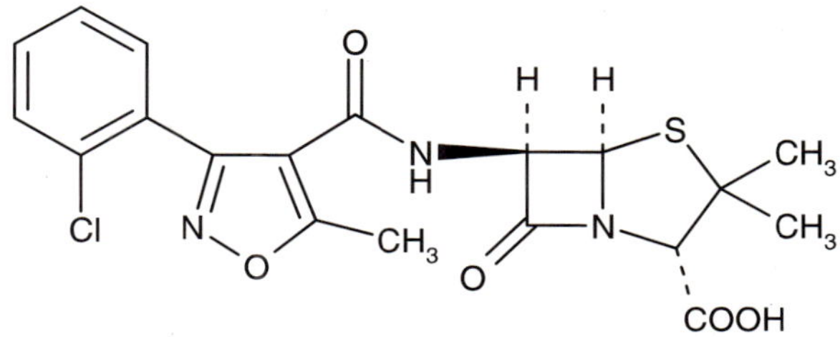

Cloxacillin

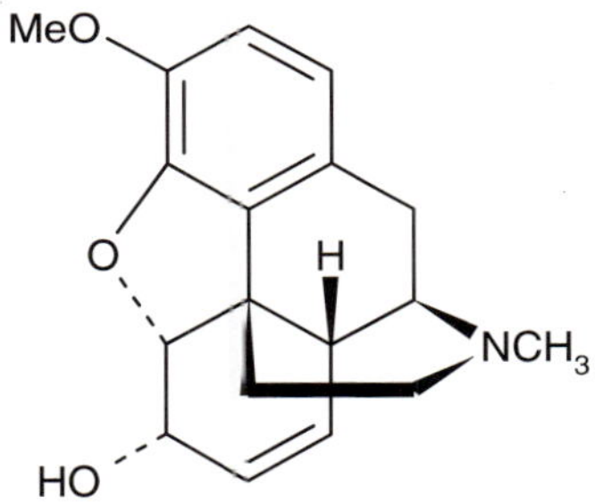

Codeine

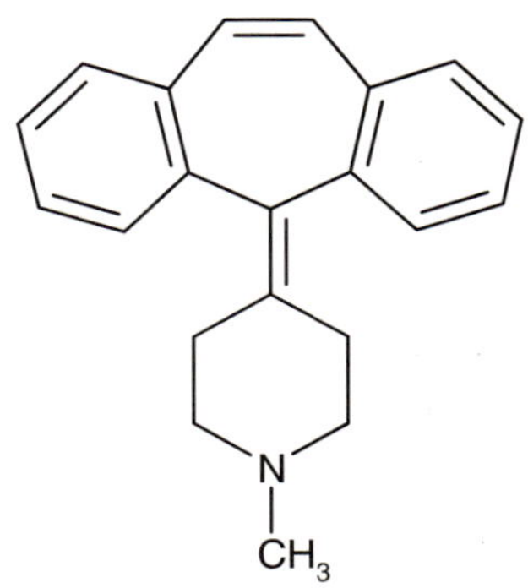

Cyproheptadine

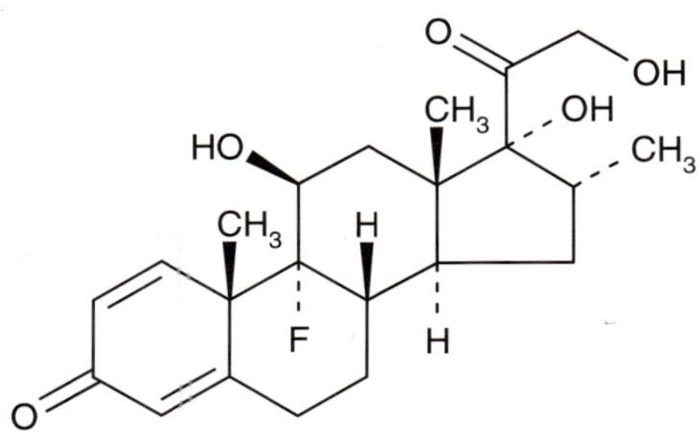

Dexamethasone

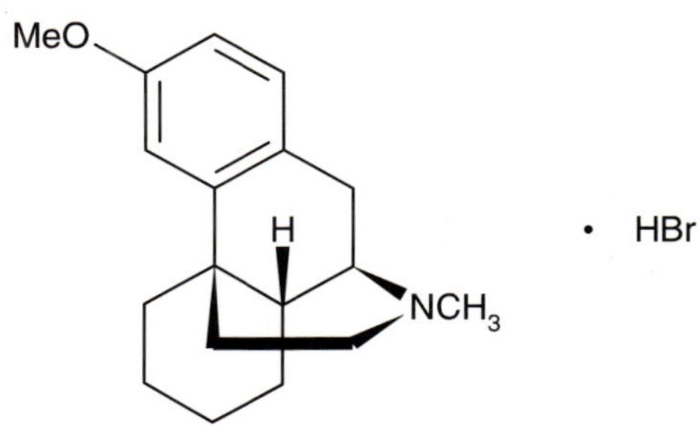

Dextromethorphan hydrobromide (Racemethorphan)

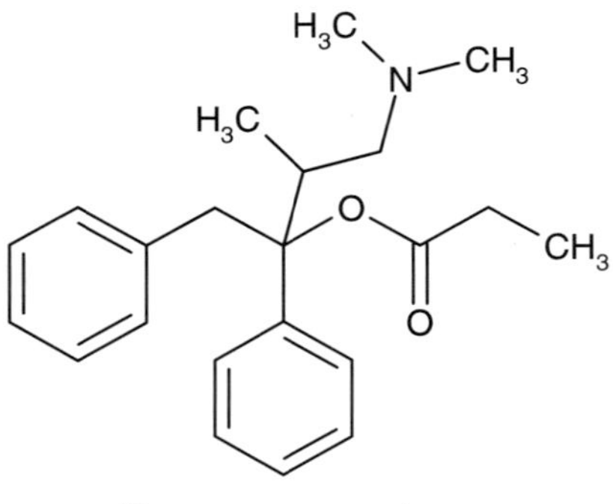

Dextropropoxyphene (Propoxyphene)

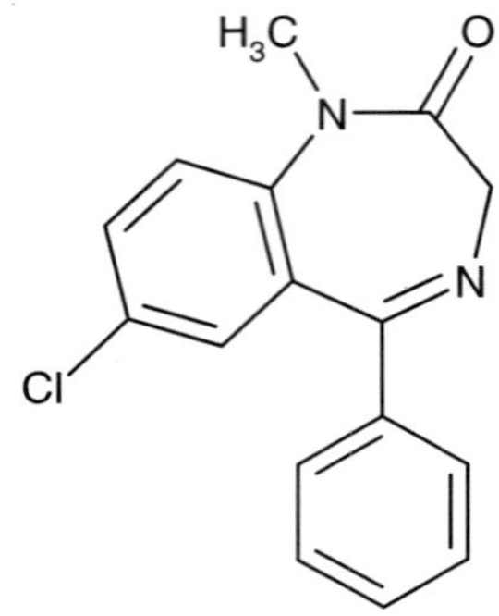

Diazepam

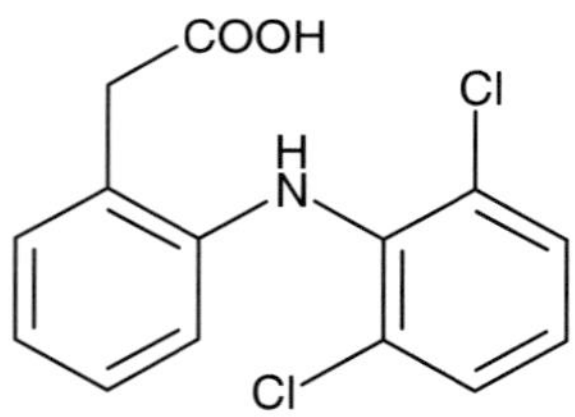

Diclofenac

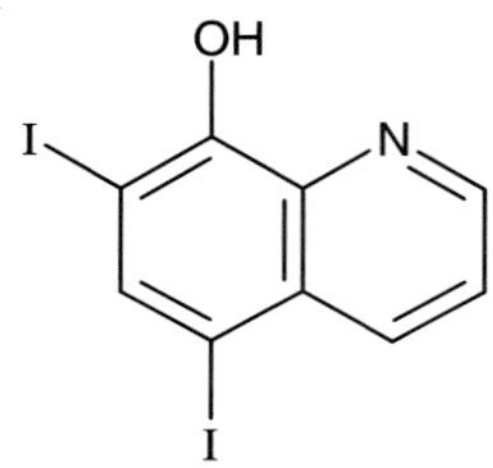

Diiodohydroxyquinoline

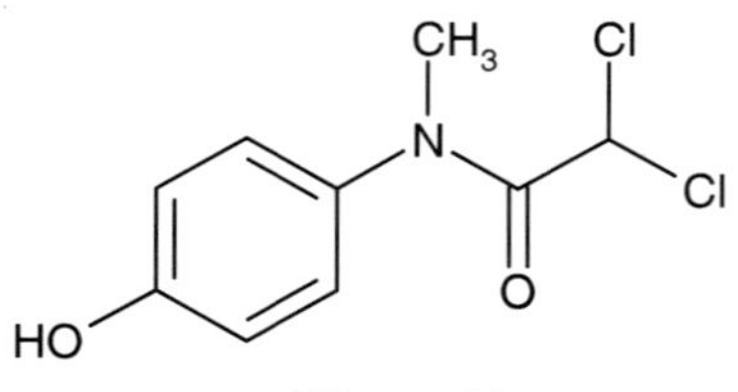

Diloxanide

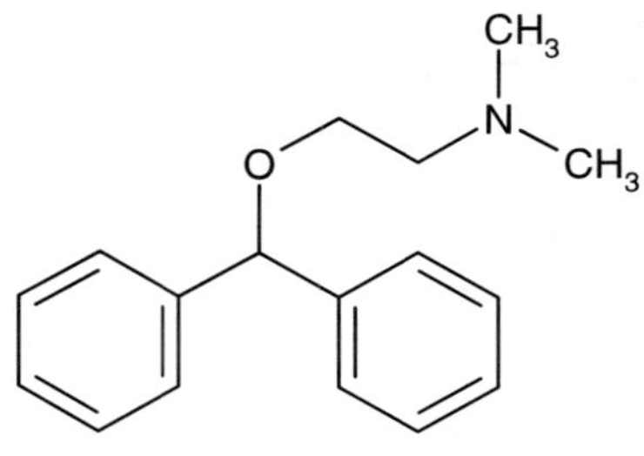

Diphenhydramine

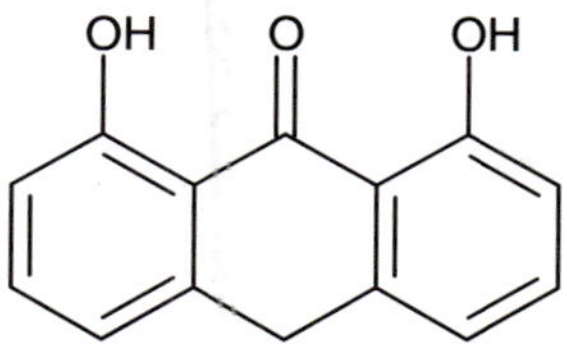

Dithranol (Anthralin)

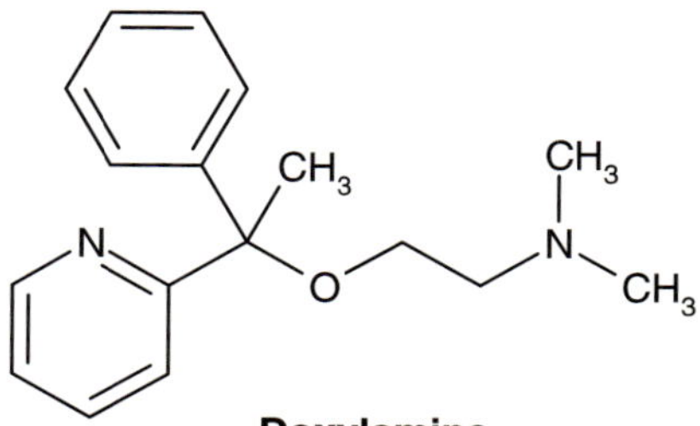

Doxylamine

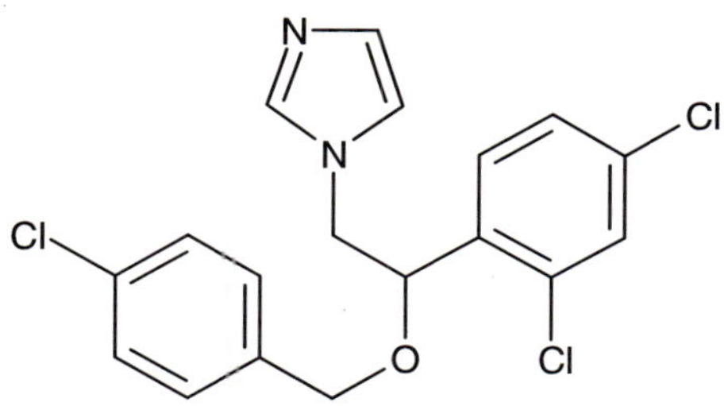

Econazole

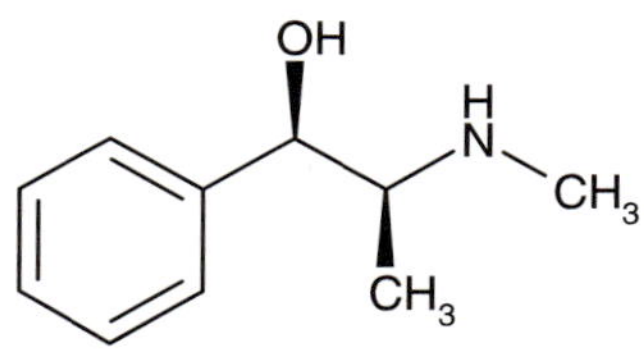

Ephedrine

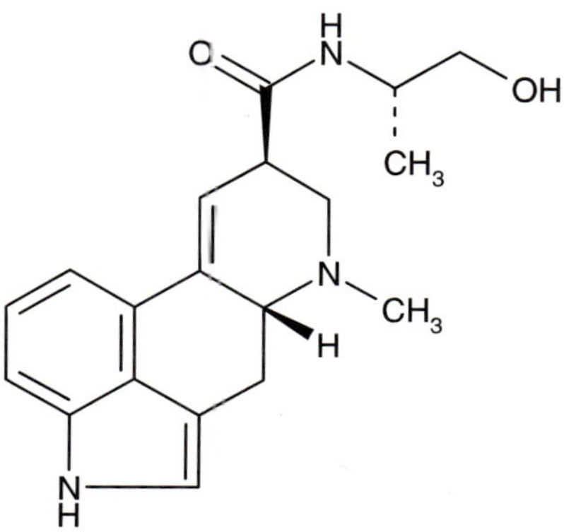

Ergometrine (Ergonovine)

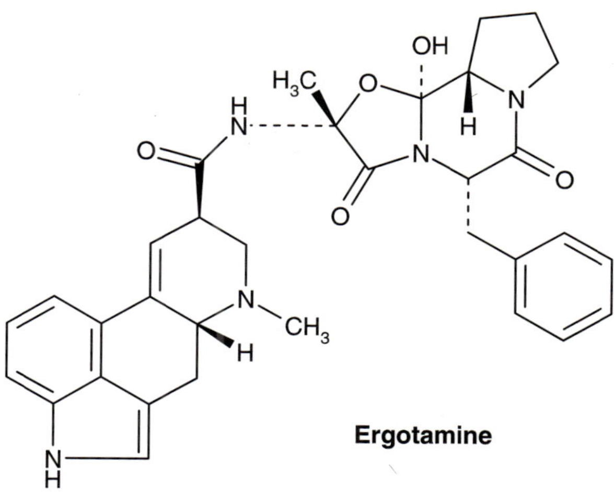

Ergotamine

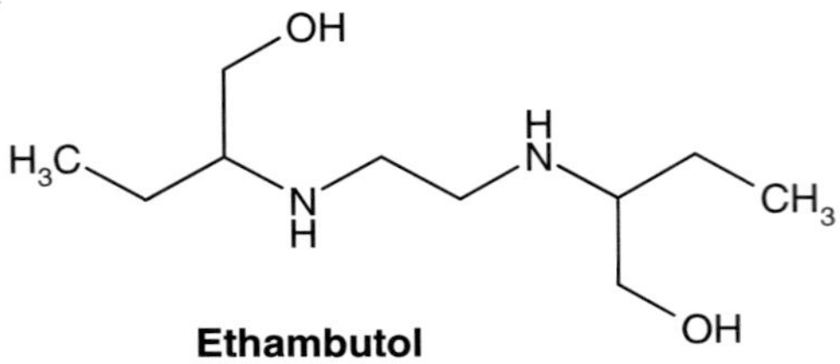

Ethambutol

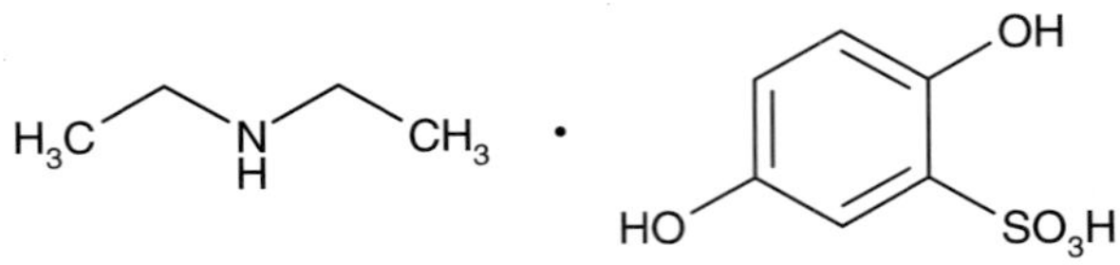

Ethamsylate

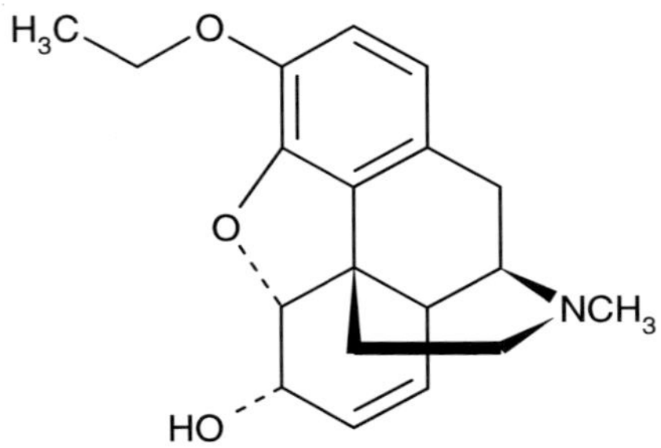

Ethylmorphine

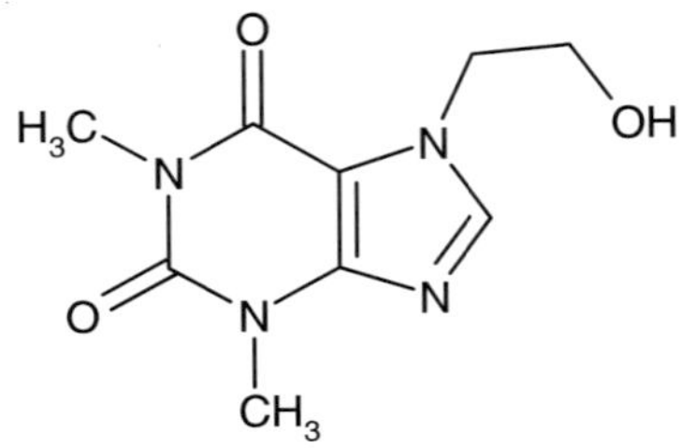

Etofylline (Hydroxyethyltheophylline)

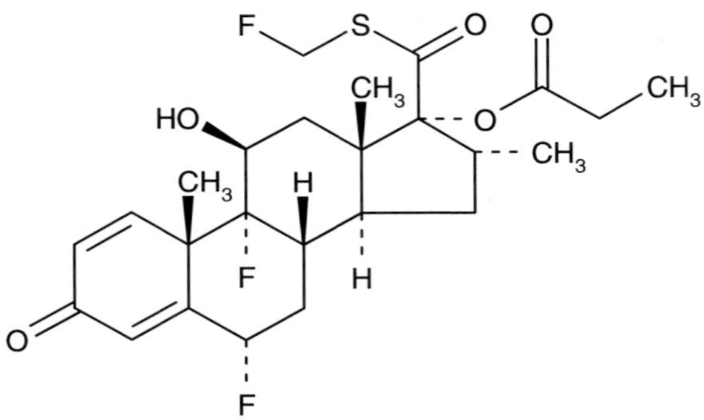

Fluticasone propionate

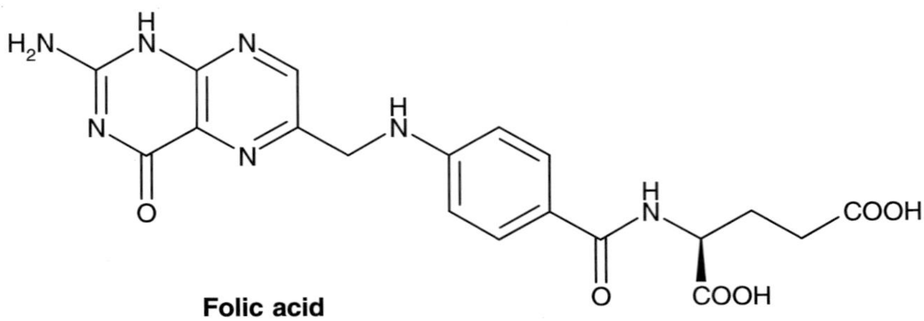

Folic acid

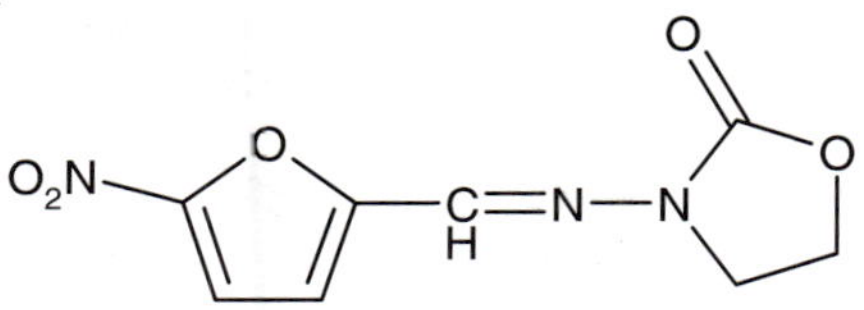

Furazolidone

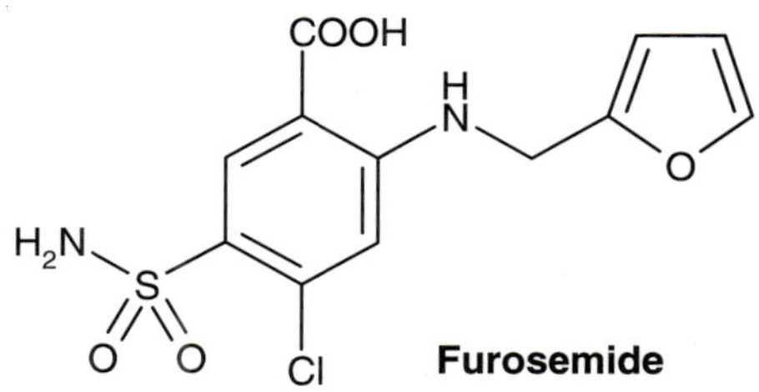

Furosemide

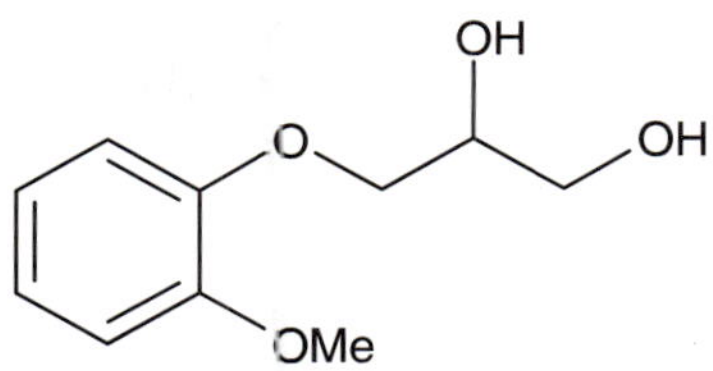

Guaiphenesin (Guaiacol glyceryl ether)

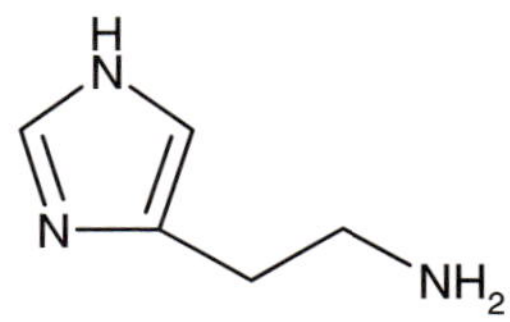

Histamine

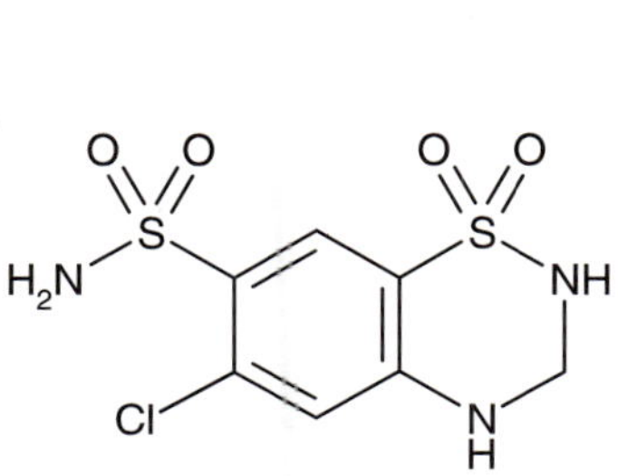

Hydrochlorothiazide

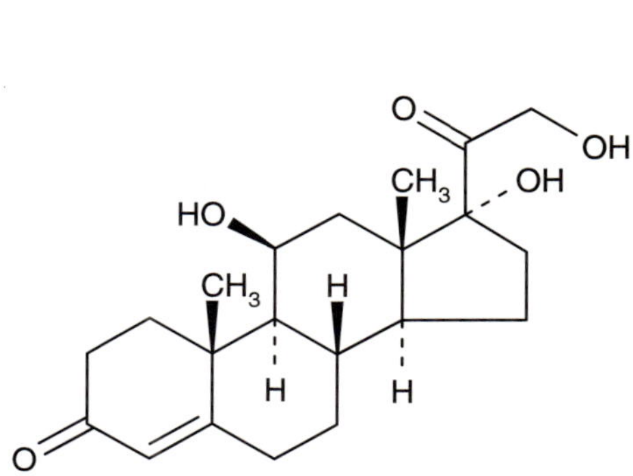

Hydrocortisone

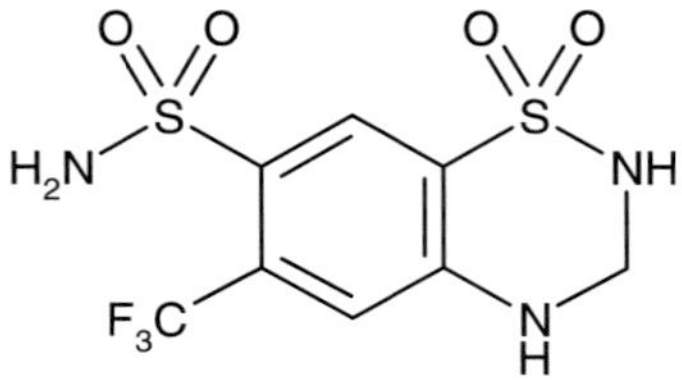

Hydroflumethiazide

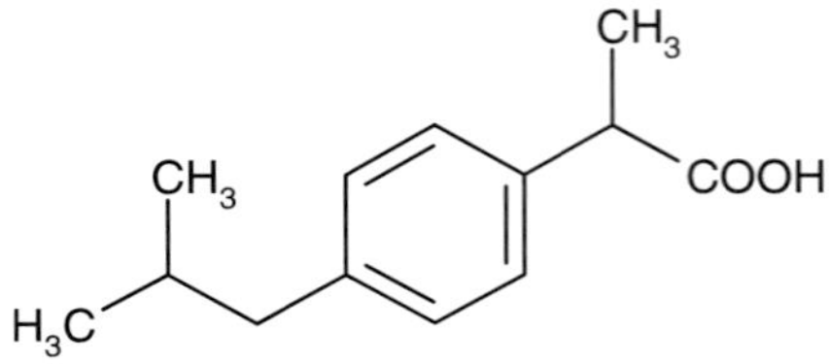

Ibuprofen

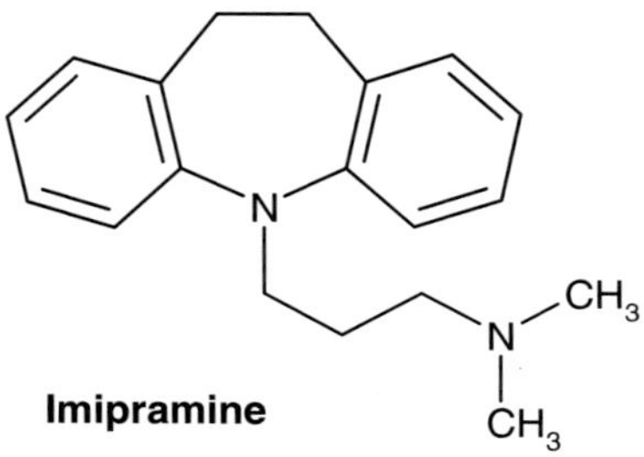

Imipramine

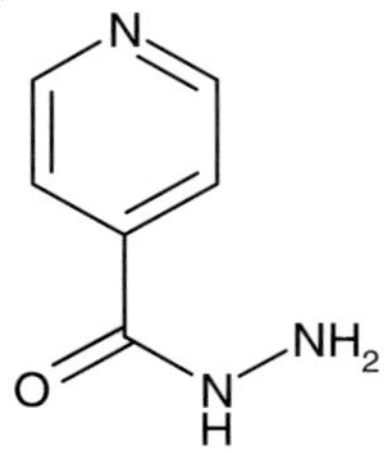

Isoniazid

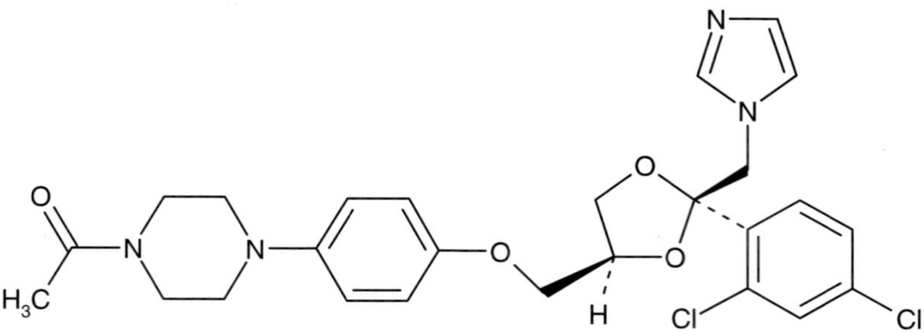

Ketoconazole

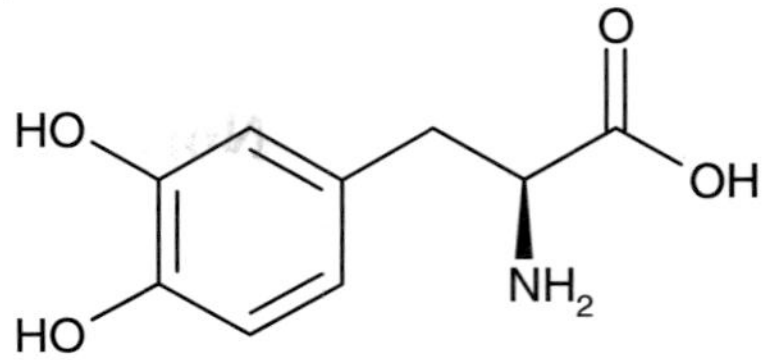

Levodopa

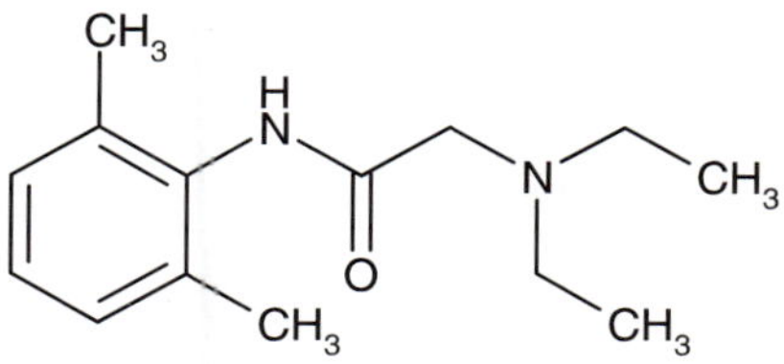

Lidocaine (Lignocaine)

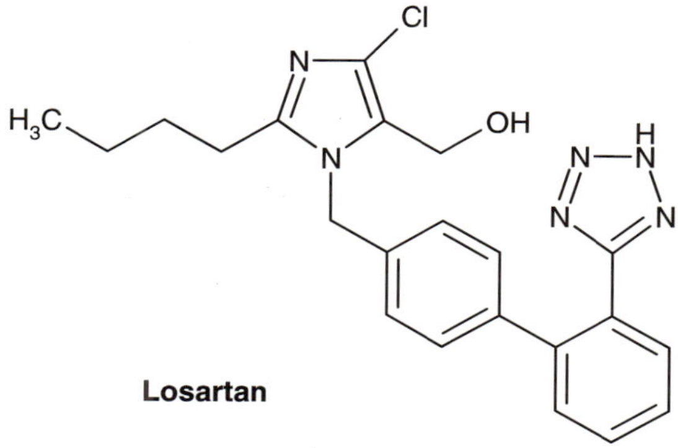

Losartan

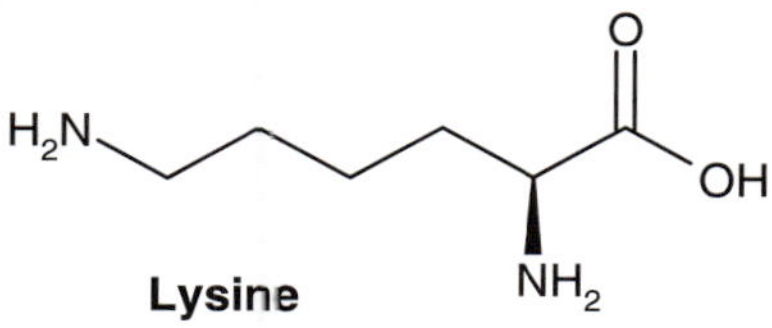

Lysine

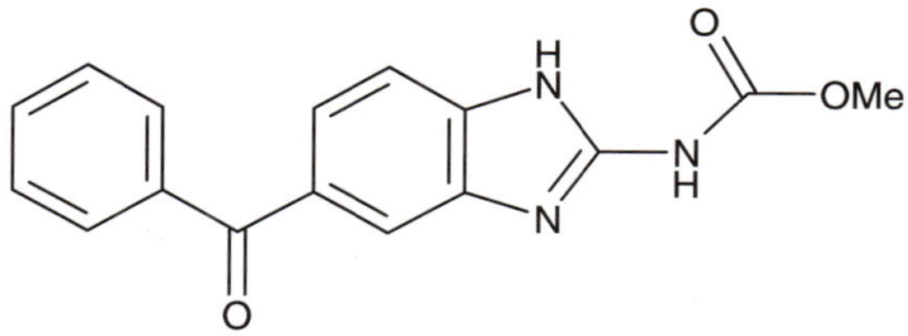

Mebendazole

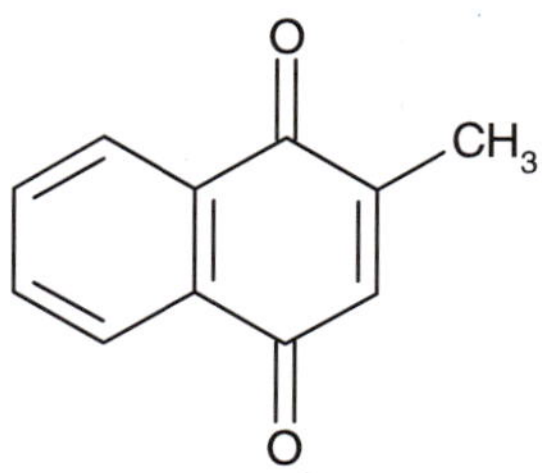

Menadione (Vitamin K_3)

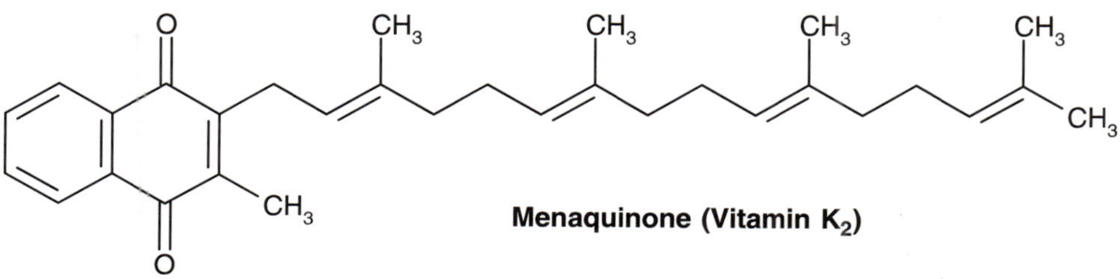

Menaquinone (Vitamin K_2)

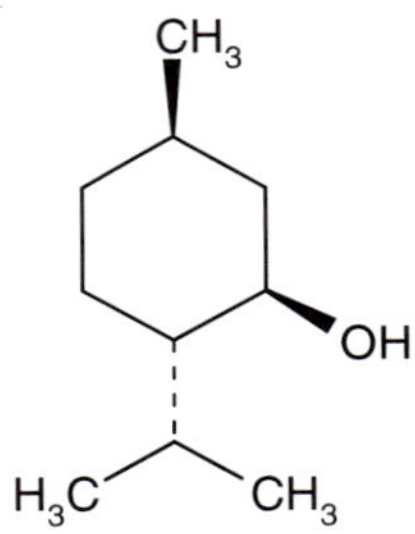

Menthol

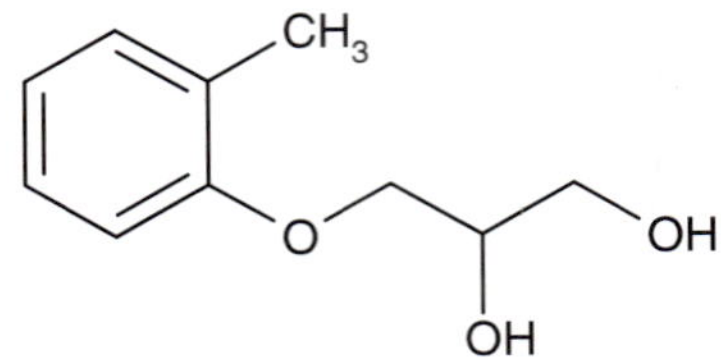

Mephenesin

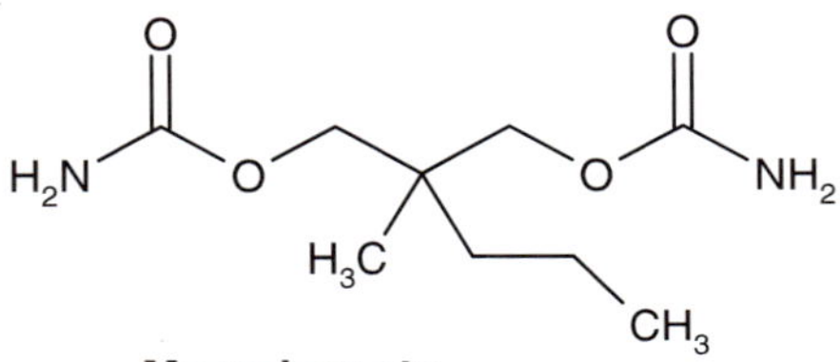

Meprobamate

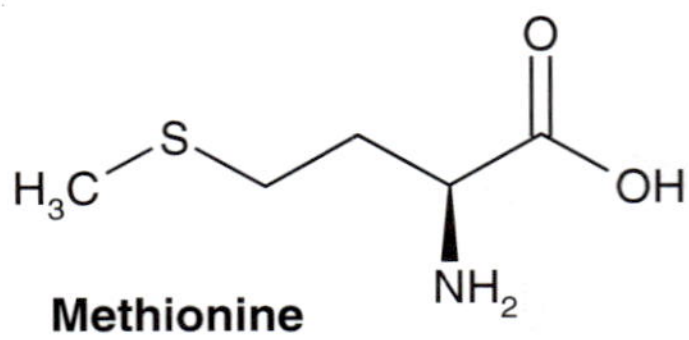

Methionine

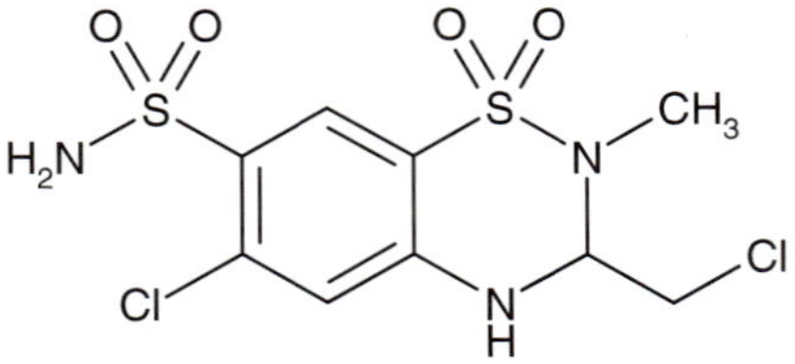

Methyclothiazide

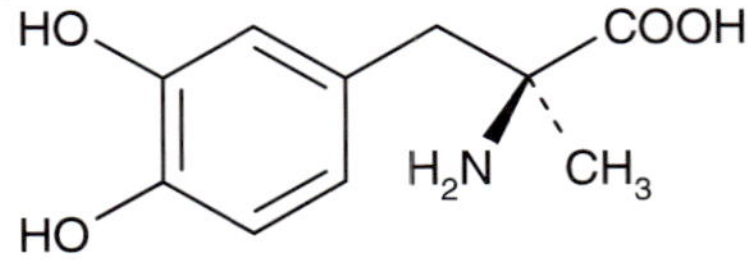

Methyldopa

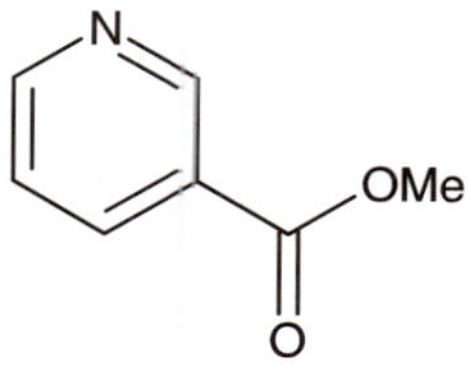

Methyl nicotinate

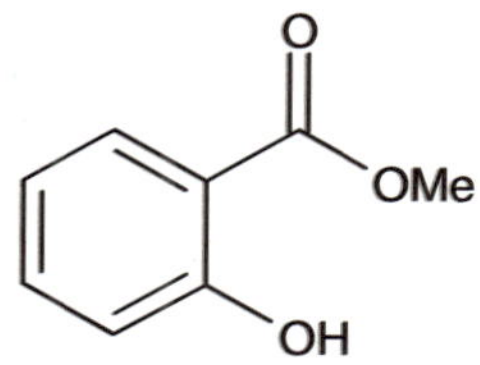

Methyl salicylate

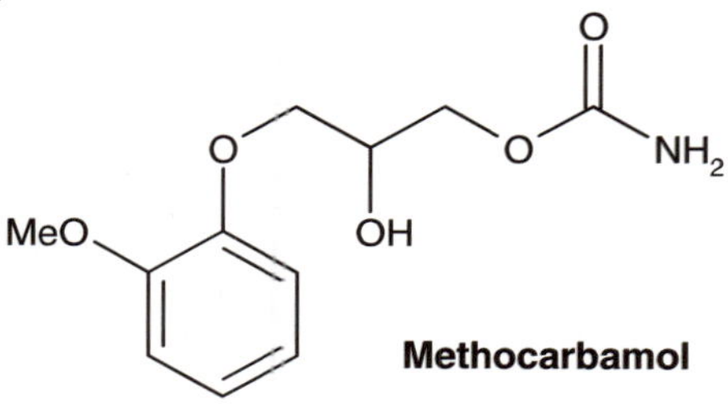

Methocarbamol

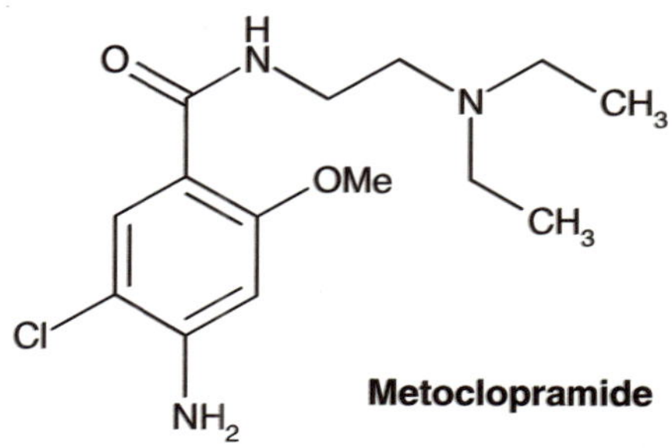

Metoclopramide

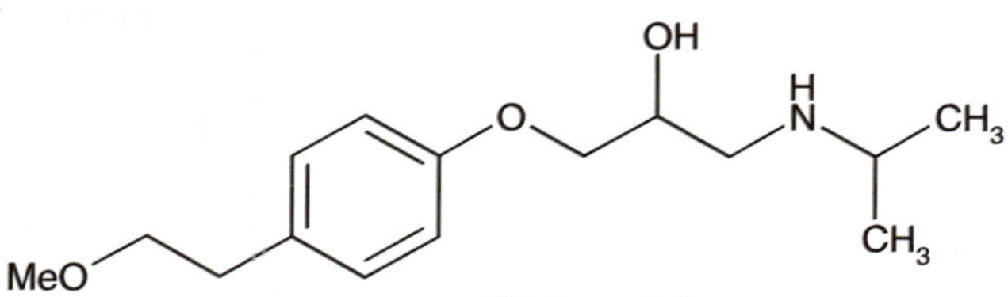

Metoprolol

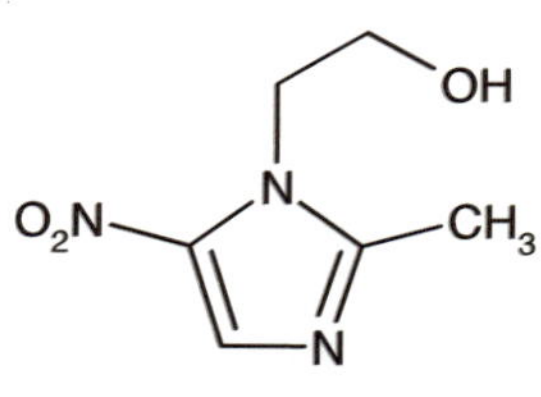

Metronidazole

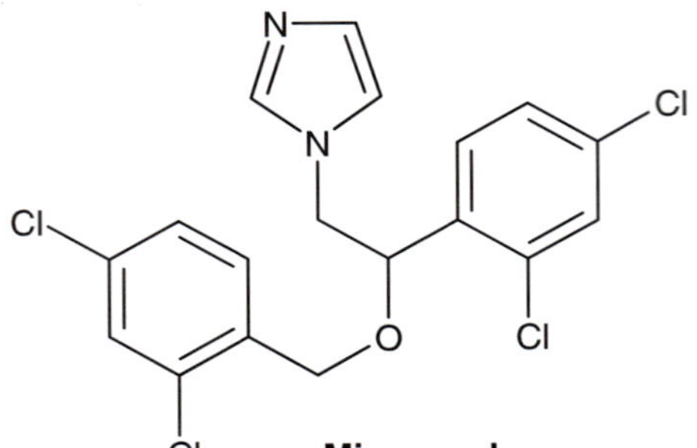

Miconazole

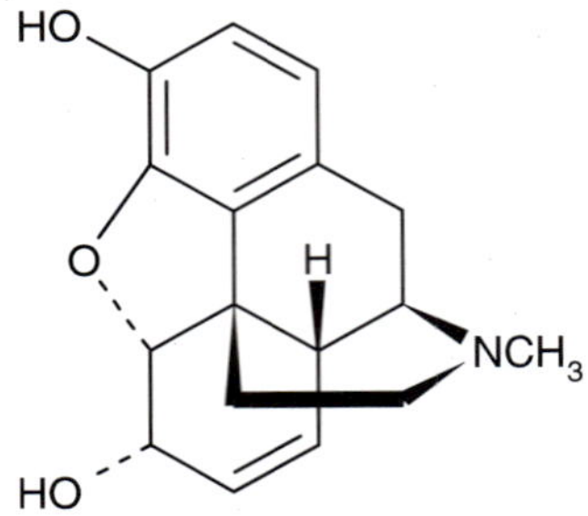

Morphine

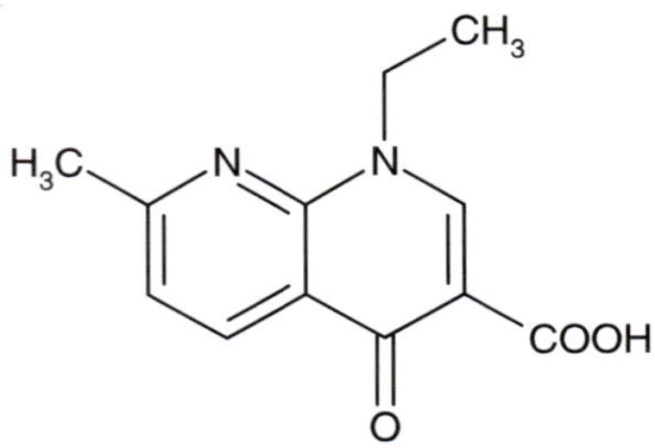

Nalidixic acid

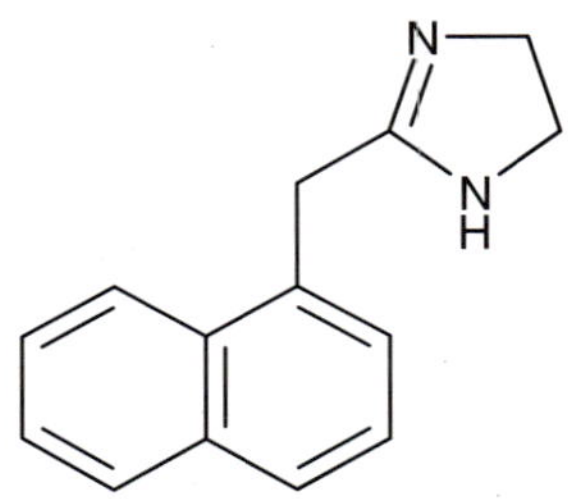

Naphazoline

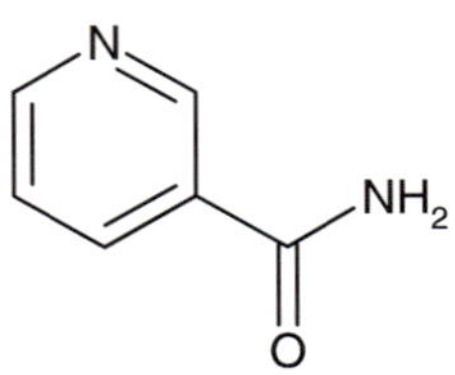

Nicotinamide

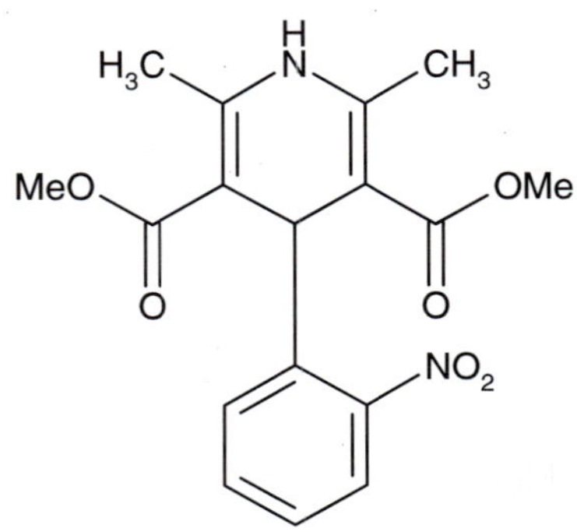

Nifedipine

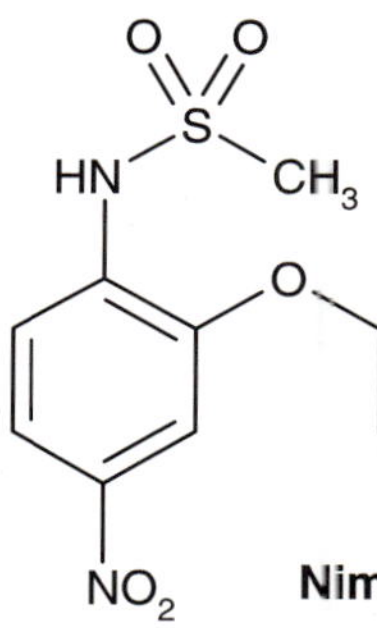

Nimesulide

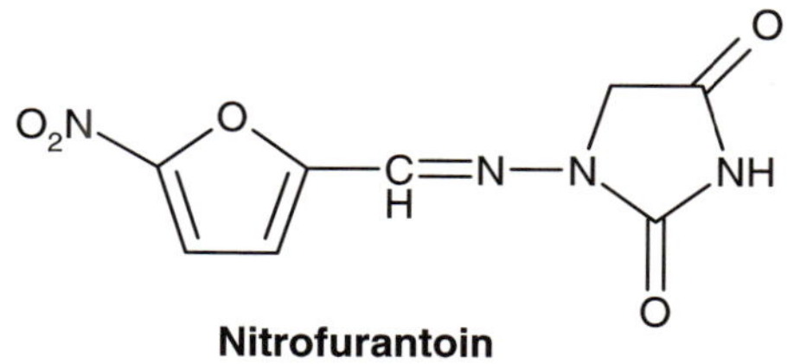

Nitrofurantoin

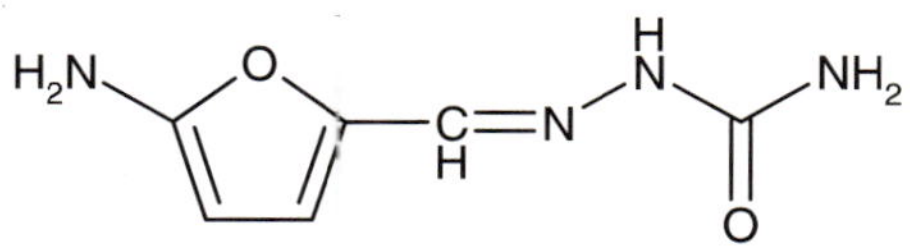

Nitrofurazone

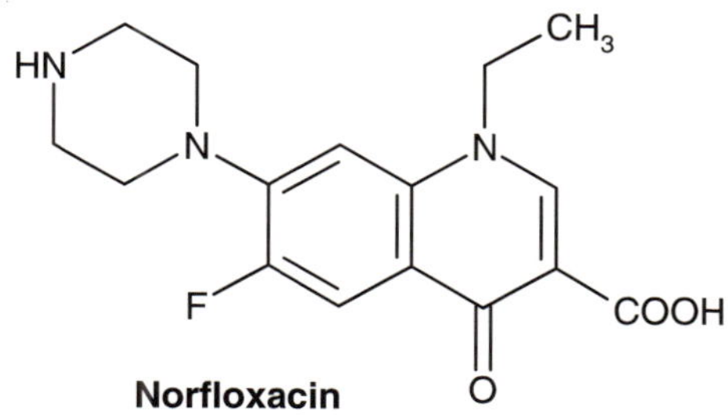

Norfloxacin

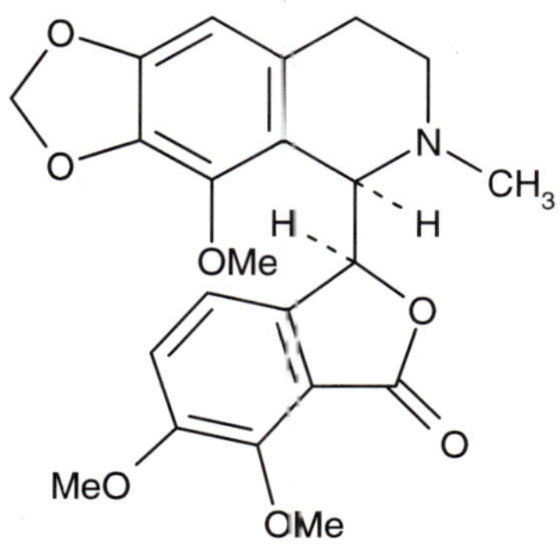

Noscapine

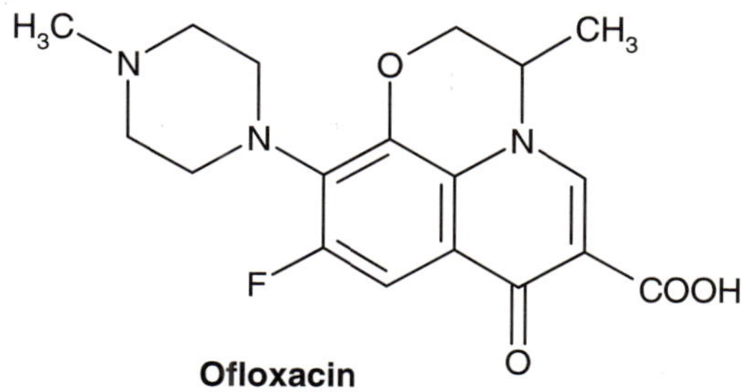

Ofloxacin

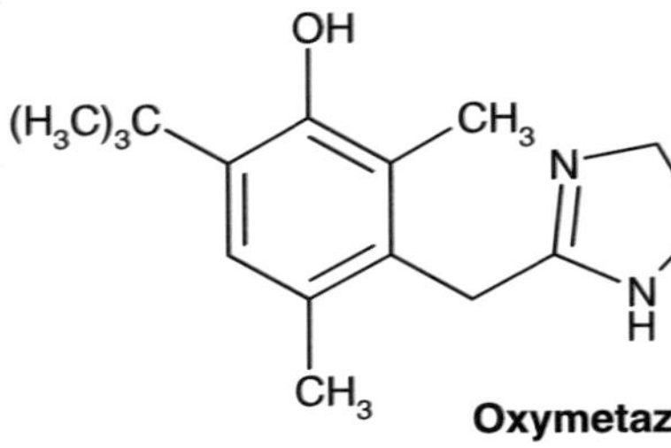

Oxymetazoline

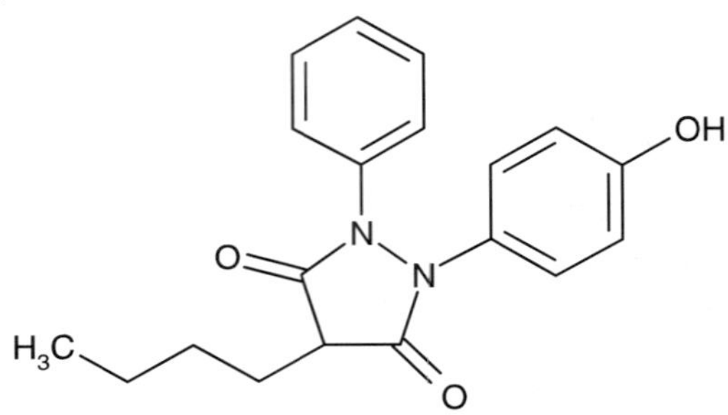

Oxyphenbutazone

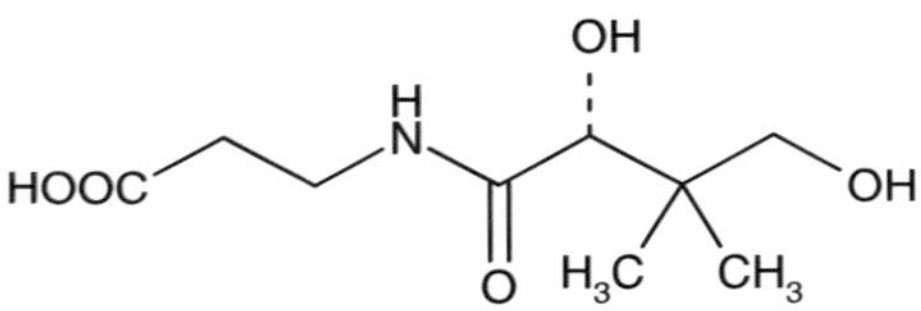

Pantothenic acid (Vitamin B_5)

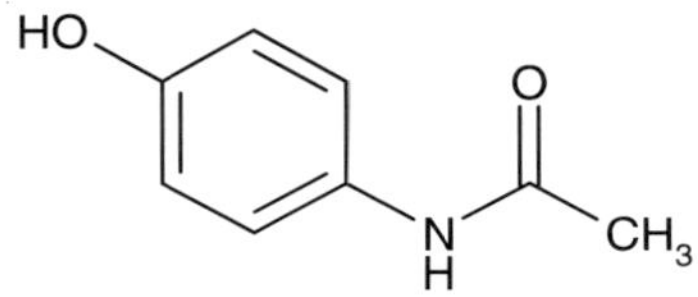

Paracetamol (Acetaminophen)

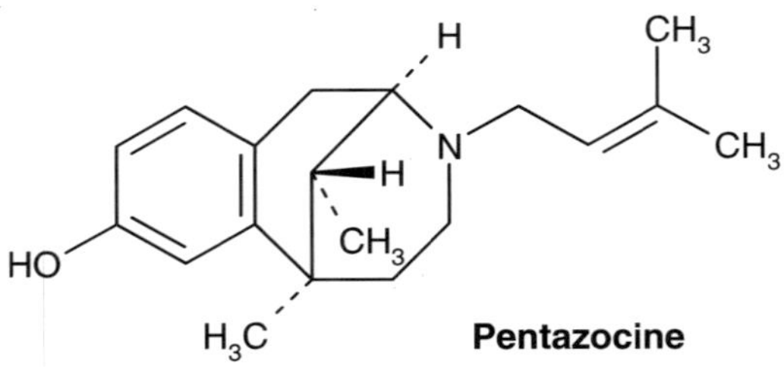

Pentazocine

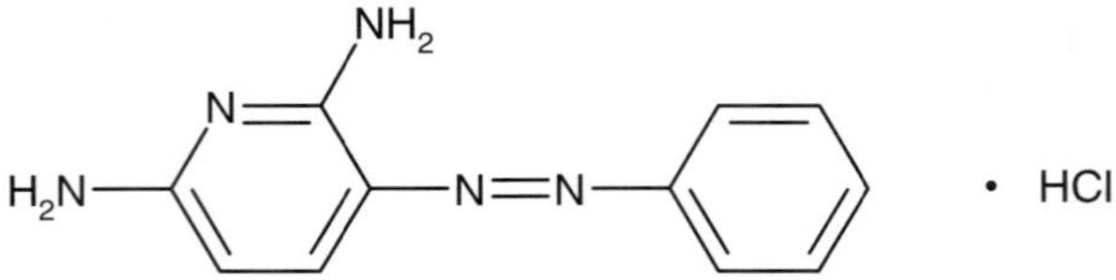

Phenazopyridine hydrochloride

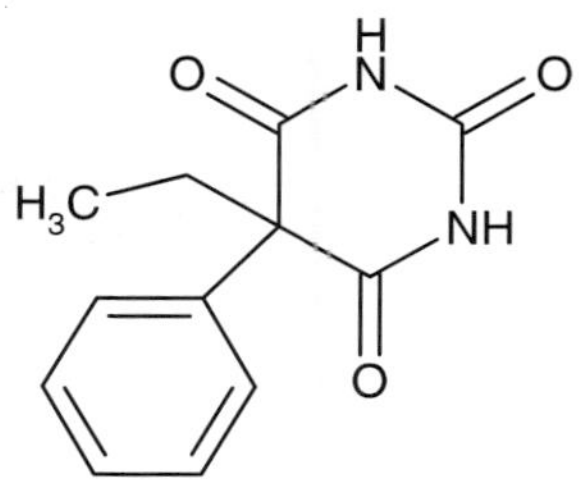

Phenobarbitone

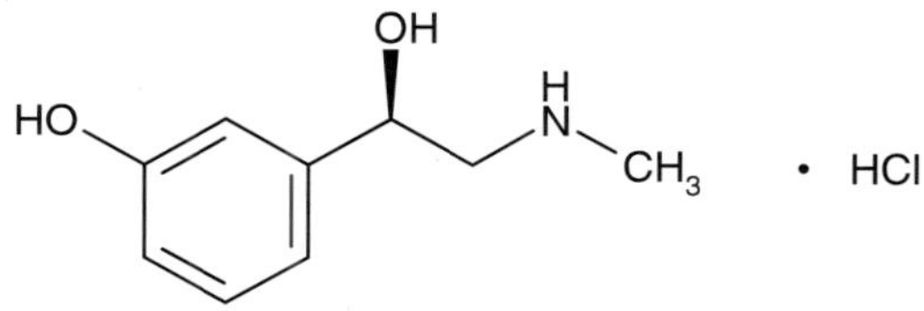

Phenylephrine hydrochloride

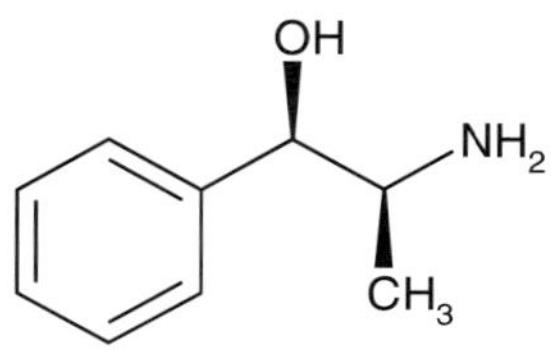

(+)-Form

Phenylpropanolamine

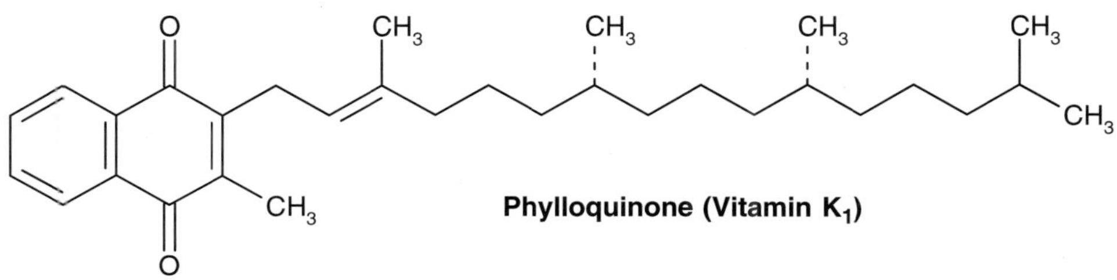

Phylloquinone (Vitamin K_1)

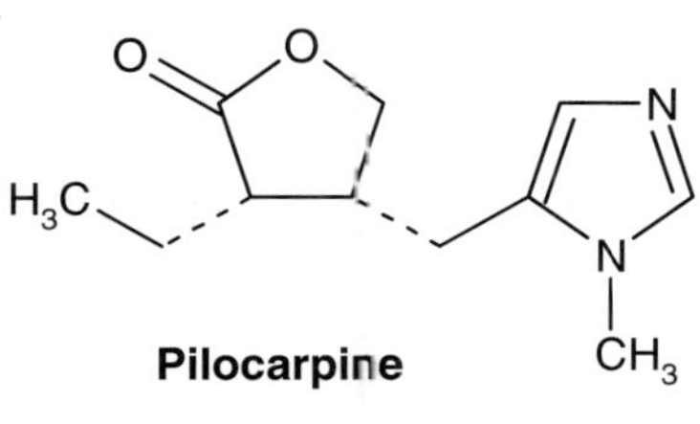

Pilocarpine

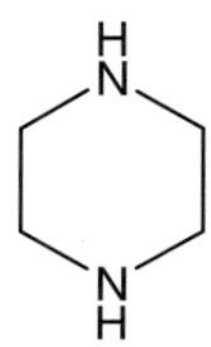

Piperazine

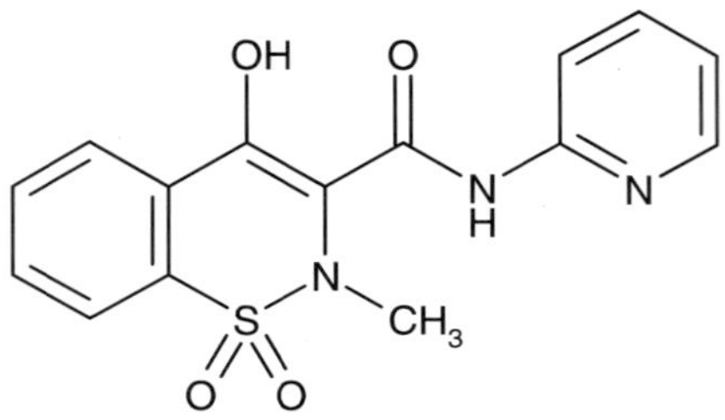

Piroxicam

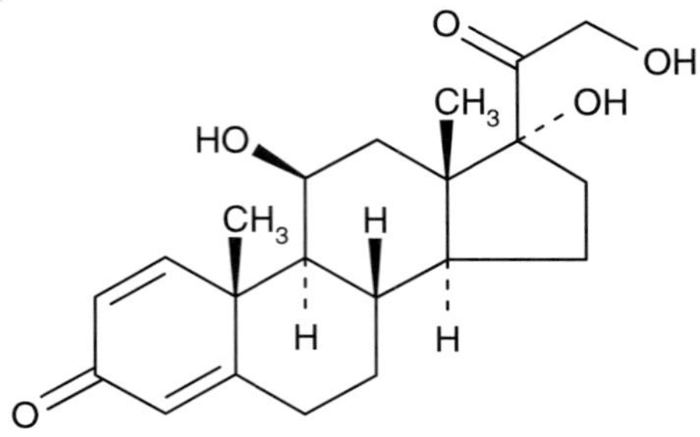

Prednisolone

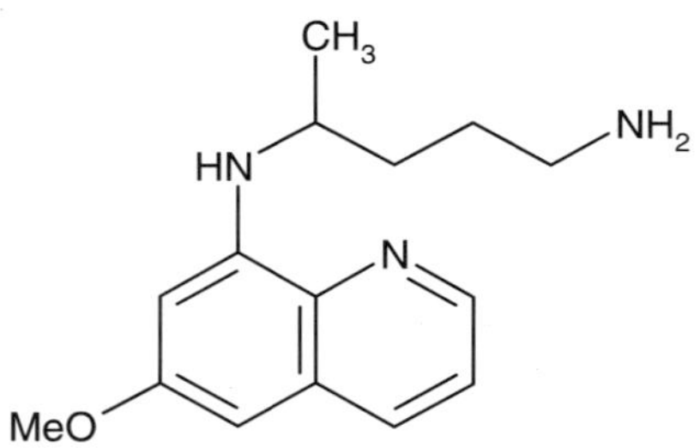

Primaquine

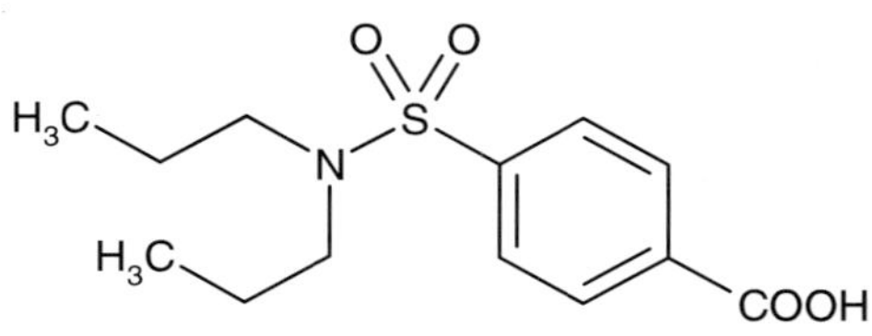

Probenecid

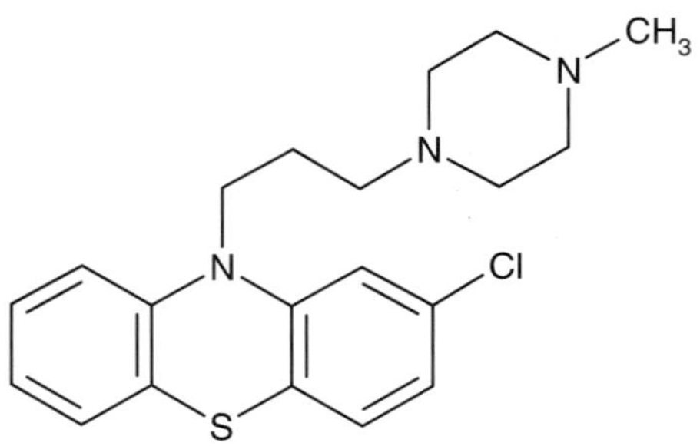

Prochlorperazine

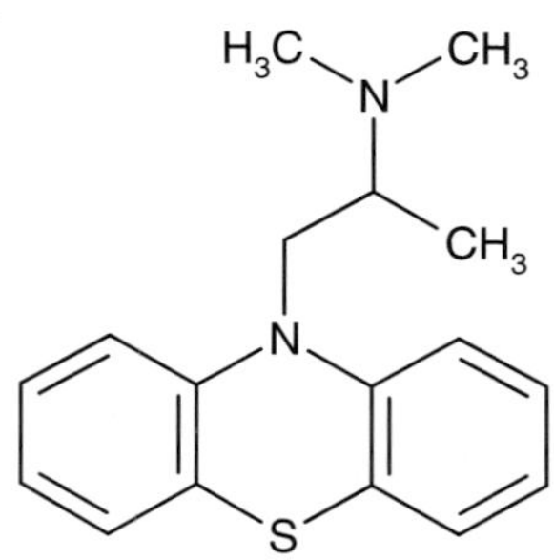

Promethazine

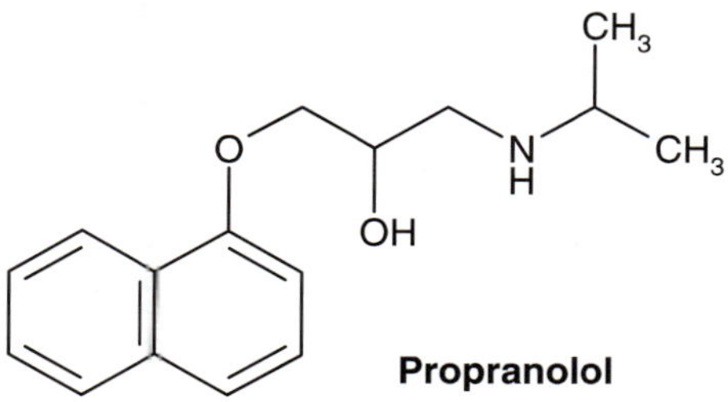

Propranolol

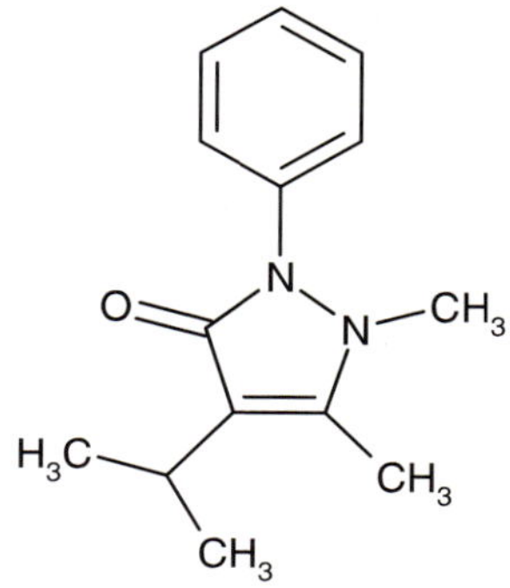

Propyphenazone

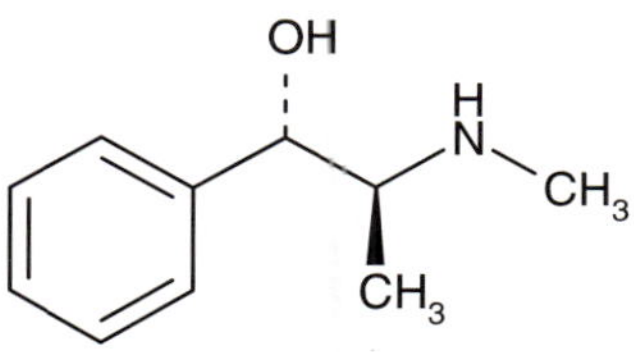

Pseudoephedrine

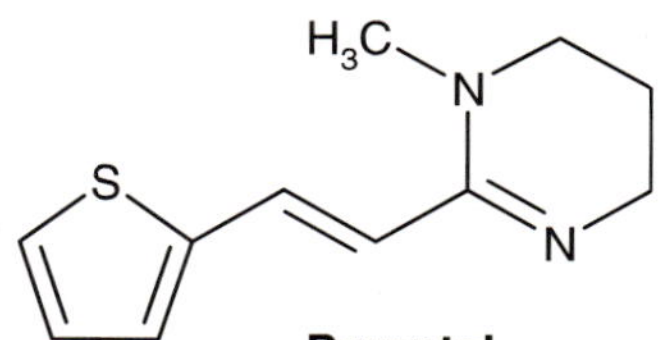

Pyrantel

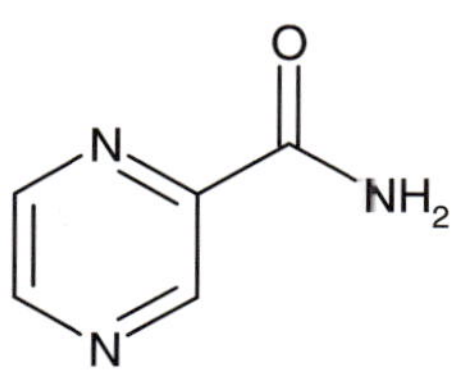

Pyrazinamide

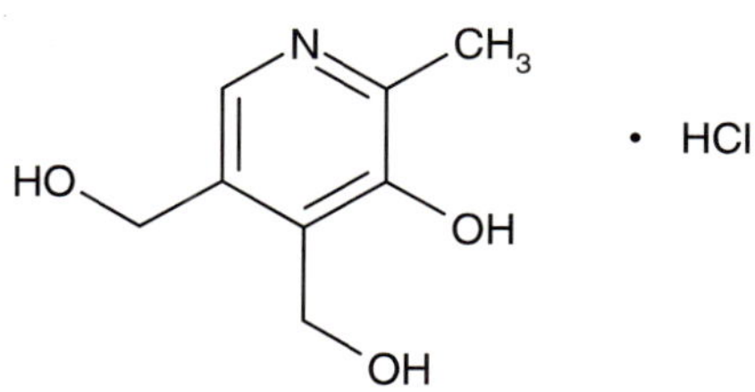

Pyridoxine hydrochloride (Vitamin B_6 hydrochloride)

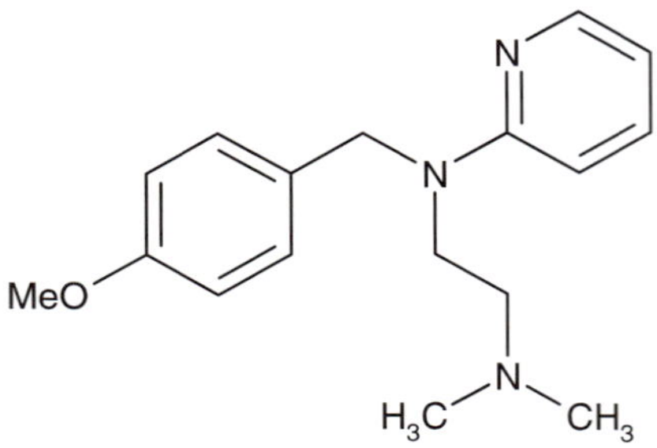

Pyrilamine (Mepyramine)

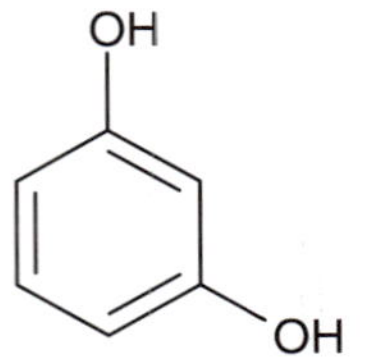

Resorcinol

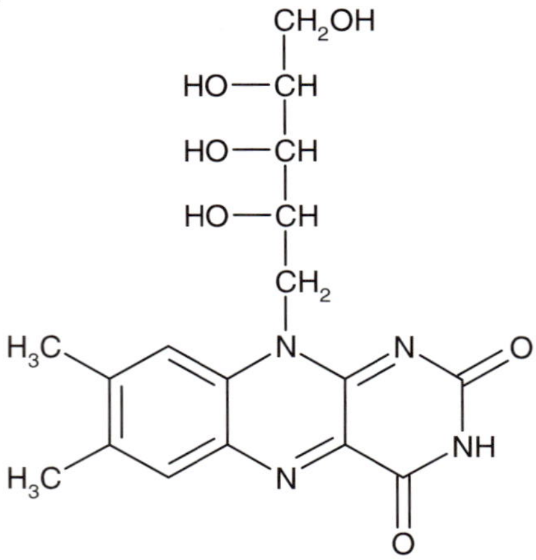

Riboflavin (Vitamin B_2)

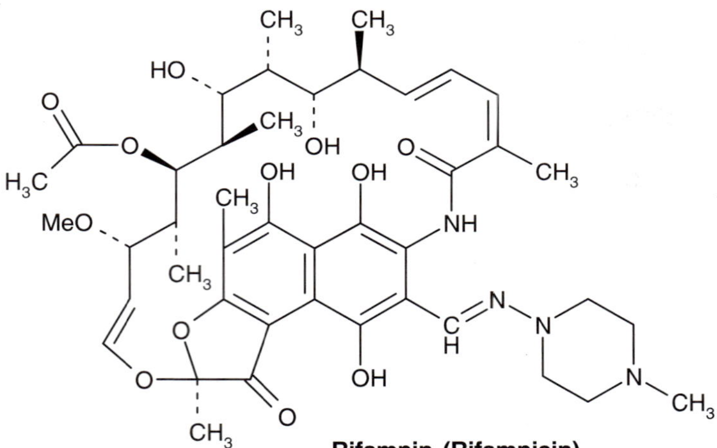

Rifampin (Rifampicin)

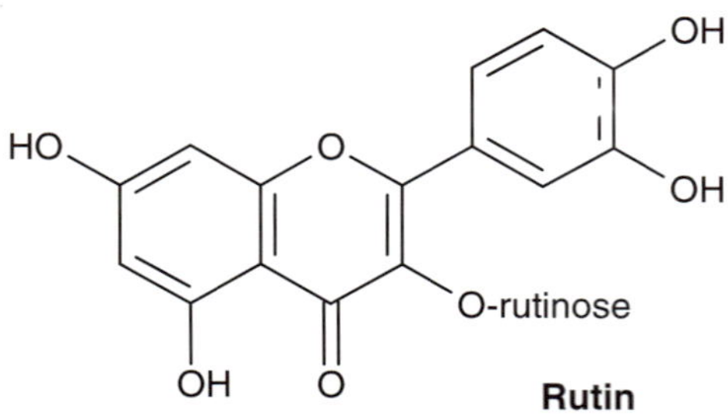

Rutin

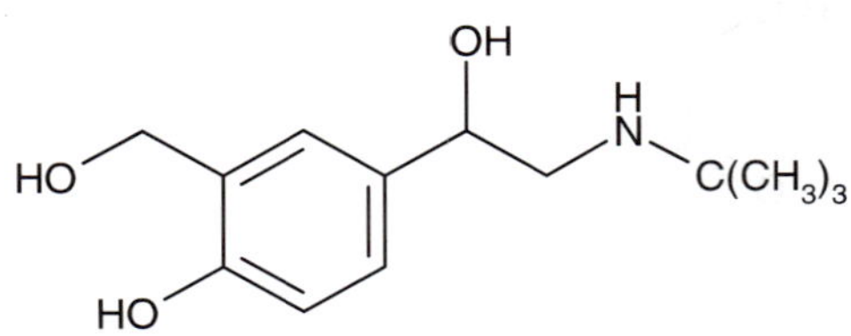

Salbutamol (Albuterol)

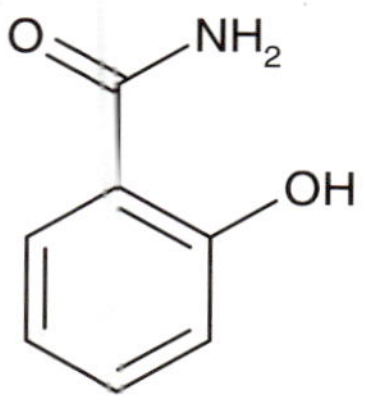

Salicylamide

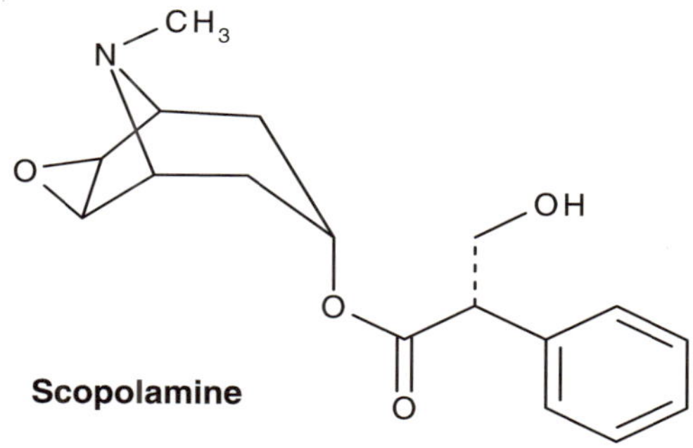

Scopolamine

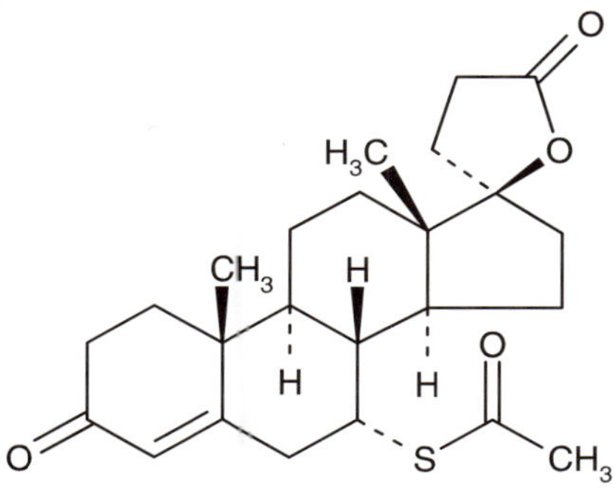

Spironolactone

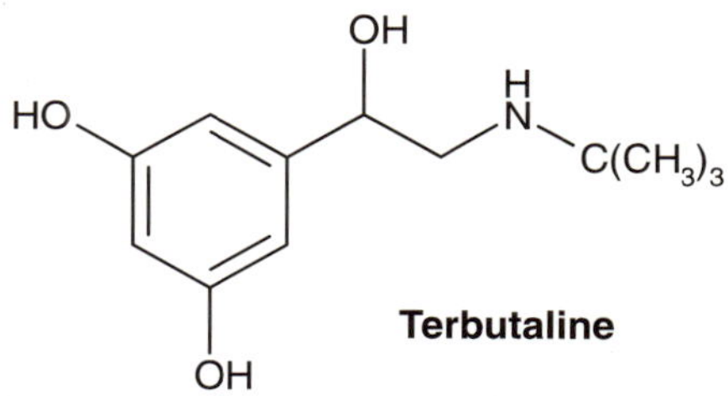

Terbutaline

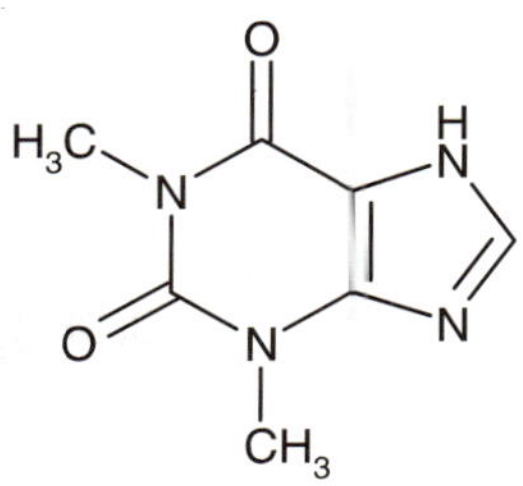

Theophylline

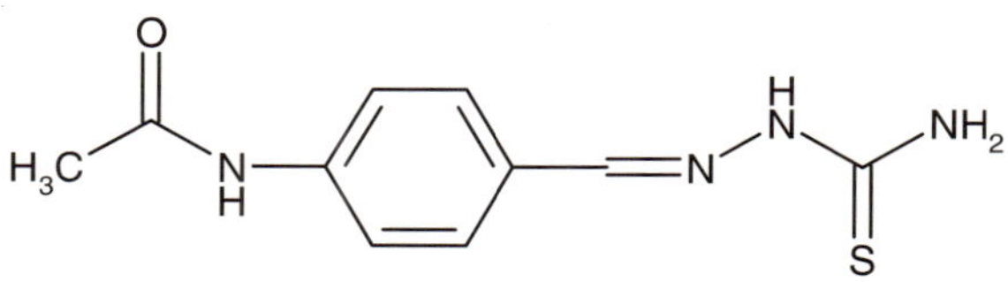

Thiacetazone

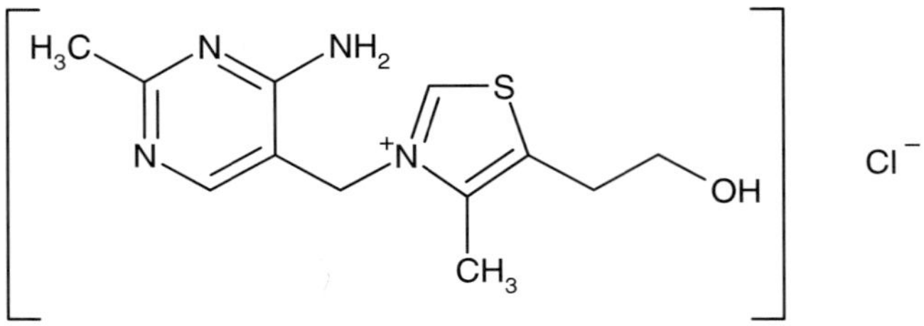

Thiamine (Vitamin B_1)

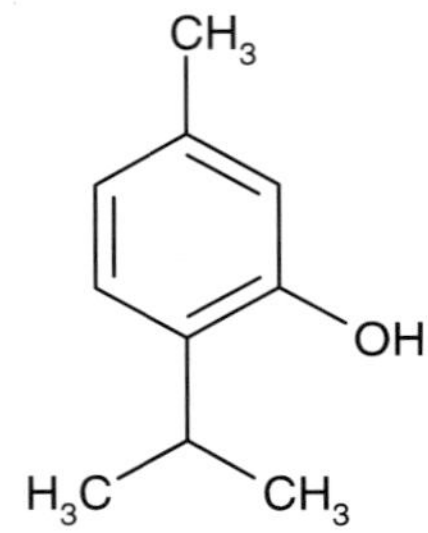

Thymol

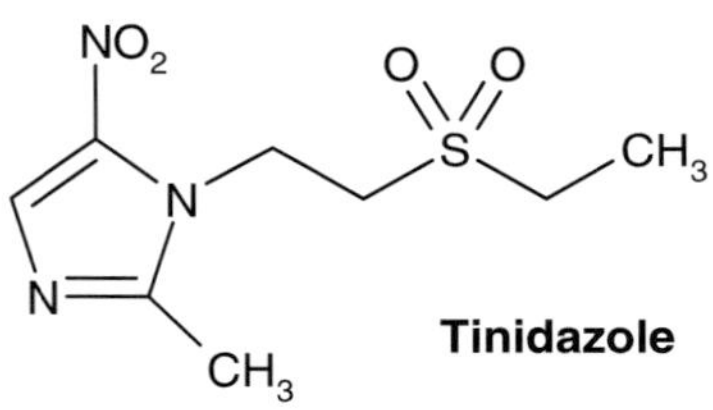

Tinidazole

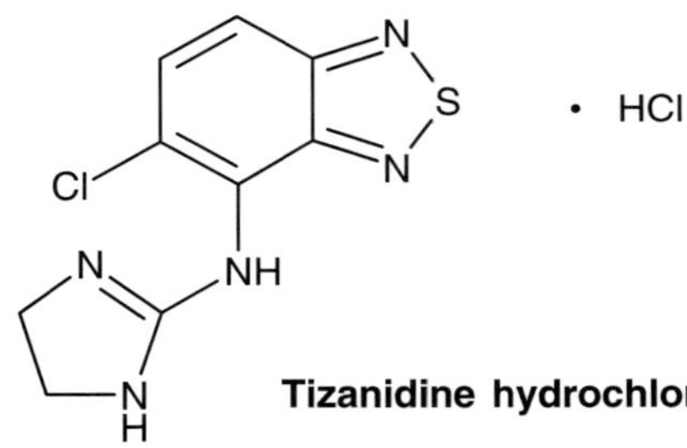

Tizanidine hydrochloride

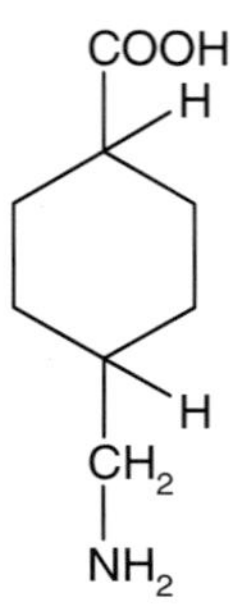

Tranexamic acid

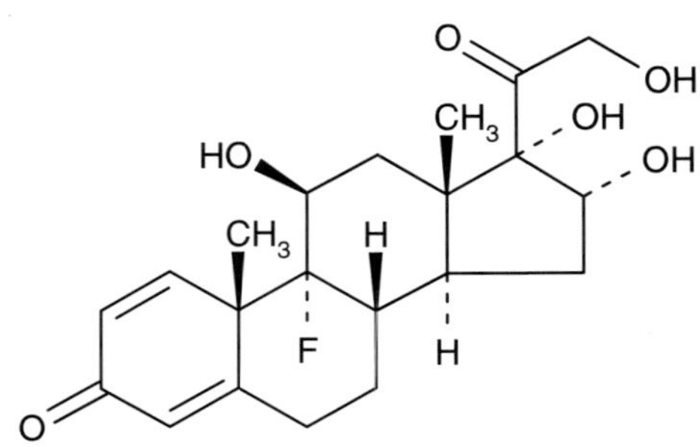

Triamcinolone

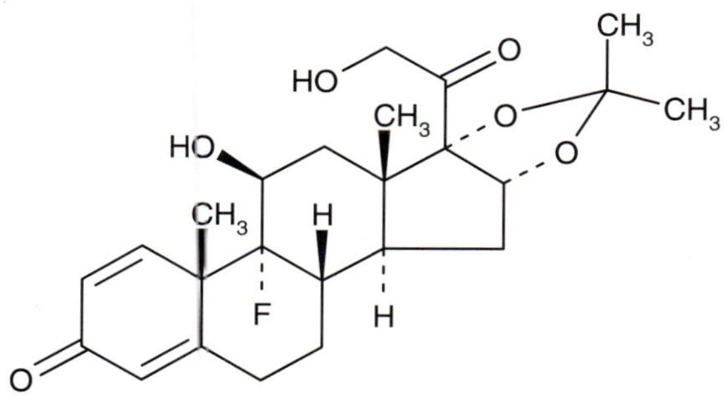

Triamcinolone acetonide

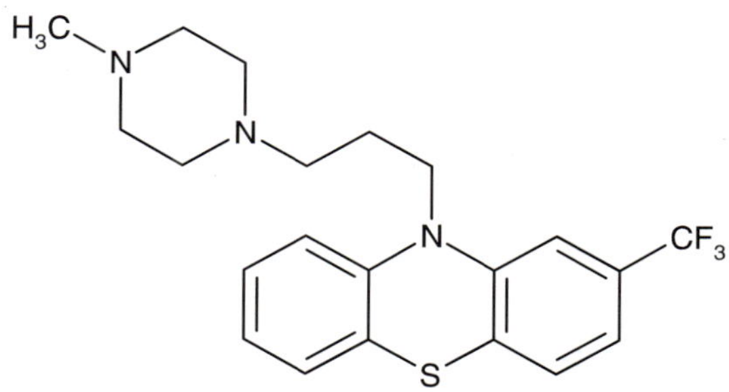

Trifluoperazine

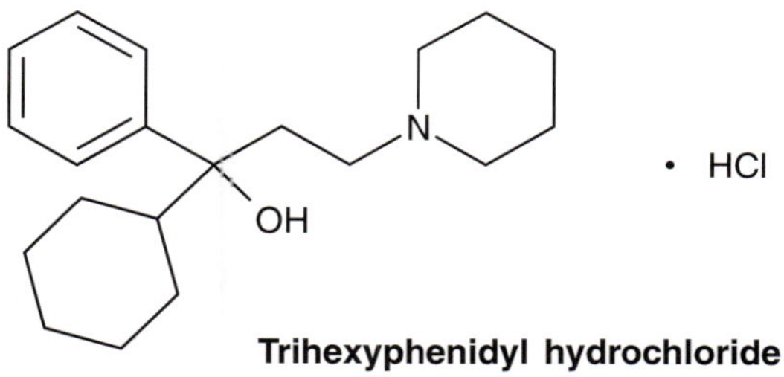

Trihexyphenidyl hydrochloride

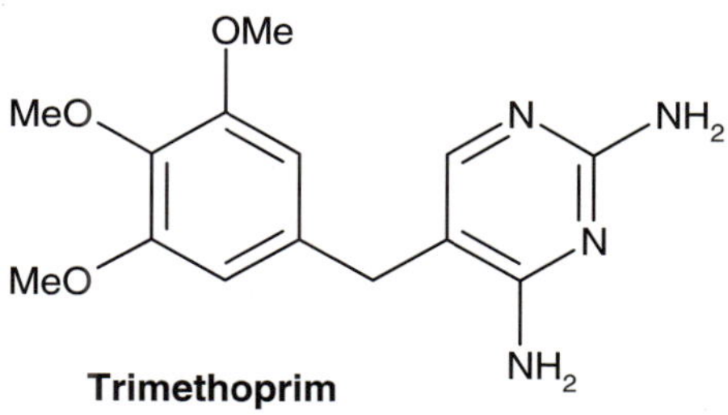

Trimethoprim

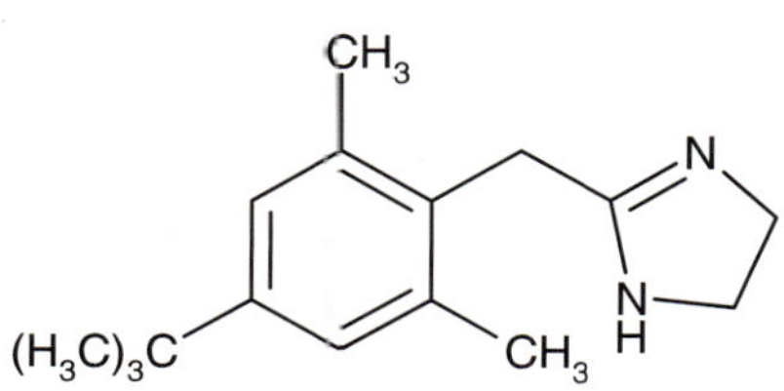

Xylometazoline

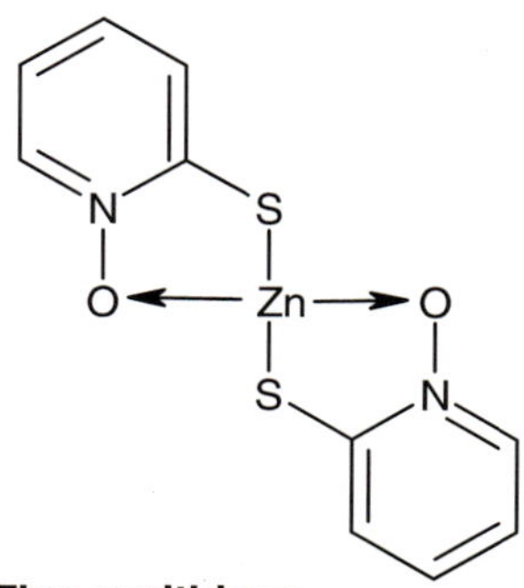

Zinc pyrithione

References
(Books Consulted)

1. H.J. Roth, Kurt Eger, Reinhard Troschütz, *Pharmaceutical Chemistry*, Vol. 2 (1991), Drug Analysis, Ellis Horwoodsens, New York.
2. Kenneth A. Connors. *A Textbook of Pharmaceutical Analysis*, 3rd ed. (1999), John Wiley & Sons, New York.
3. R.M. Verma, *Analytical Chemistry*, 3rd ed. (1994), CBS Publishers & Distributors, New Delhi, India.
4. *Vogel's Textbook of Quantitative Chemical Analysis*, 6th ed. (2000), Pearson Education Limited.
5. *Vogel's Textbook of Practical Organic Chemistry*, 4th ed. (1978), Longman Groups Ltd., London.
6. I.L. Finar (1973), *Organic Chemistry* (Vol. 1), 9th Indian Reprint (2004), Pearson Education Ltd.
7. Norman L. Allinger et al., *Organic Chemistry* (1971), Worth Publishers Inc., New York.
8. Marye Anne Fox et al., *Organic Chemistry*, 2nd ed. (1997), John & Bartlett Publishers, USA.
9. George Lunn & Louise C. Hellwig, *Handbook of Derivatization Reactions for HPLC* (1998), John Wiley & Sons Inc.
10. T. Higuchi et al. (1962), *Pharmaceutical Analysis*, 1st Indian ed. (1997), CBS Publishers & Distributors, New Delhi, India.
11. H. York et al. (1994), *Thin Layer Chromatography: Reagents and Detection Methods* (Vol. 1a and 1b), VCH Verlags GmbH, Germany.
12. Christian, *Analytical Chemistry*, 6th ed. (2005).
13. R. Kellner, *Analytical Chemistry: A Modern Approach to Analytical Science*, 2nd ed. (2004).
14. David C. Lee & M. Webb, *Pharmaceutical Analysis*.
15. A.H. Becket & J.B. Stenlake, *Practical Pharmaceutical Chemistry*, 4th ed. (Vols. 1 & 2).
16. S. Ahuja, *Handbook of Pharmaceutical Analysis* (2005).
17. D.C. Garett, *Quantitative Analysis of Drugs*.
18. Higson, *Analytical Chemistry*, 2005.
19. Rouessac, *Chemical Analysis: Modern Instrumentation Methods*, 2005.
20. Chung Chow Chan & Y.C. Lee, *Analytical Method Validation and Instrument Performance*, 2004.
21. Jie Jack Li, *Named Reactions*, 2nd ed., 2004.
22. Jerry March, *Advanced Organic Chemistry*, 4th ed., 1992.

23. M.H. Willard, *Instrumental Method of Analysis*, 7th ed.
24. Hashmi, *Assay of Vitamins in Pharmaceutical Preparations*, 1973.
25. Gunzler, *Handbook of Analytical Techniques.*
26. Schirmer, *Modern Methods of Pharmaceutical Analysis*, 2nd ed. (Vols. 1 & 2).
27. V. Alexeyev, *Quantitative Analysis* (1994).
28. Ohannesian, *Handbook of Pharmaceutical Analysis.*
29. J.W. Enke, *Art and Science of Chemical Analysis.*
30. Solomons, *Organic Chemistry*, 8th ed.
31. K. Florey, *Analytical Profile of Drug Substances* (Vols. 1-30).
32. L.G. Chatten, *Pharmaceutical Chemistry, Vol. 1: Theory & Application*, 1966.
33. Hans Thacher Clarke, *A Handbook of Organic Analysis* (*Qualitative & Quantitative*), 4th ed., 2007.

Reaction Mechanism

2

Good Laboratory Practices

Good lab
and condi
monitored
of GLP en
means to
their full
the studie
quality an
of the drug
Comm

(a) Tec
acc
con

(b) Imp

(c) Pro

(d) Imp

Under
of the d
achieve
imagen
instrum
control
the mo
photom
enterpr
the tech
commerc
is comm
must ha
sophistic
perform
The
procedu
in such
Control
sound a
that the
strength
in help
quality

Good laboratory practices (GLP) is concerned with the organisational processes and conditions with which the laboratory studies are planned, performed, monitored, recorded and reported. Adherence by laboratories to the principle of GLP ensures the proper planning of studies and the provision of adequate means to carry them out. It facilitate the proper planning of studies, promotes their full and accurate reporting and provides means whereby the integrity of the studies can be verified. The application of GLP to analysis assures the quality and integrity of data in taking accountable decision regarding quality of the drug.

Common lapses and defaults relating to GLP are:

(a) Technical personnel being unaware of the importance of protocols, accurate observations, proper performance of the test procedures and accurate record-keeping.
(b) Improper laboratory procedures.
(c) Failure to critically review the data.
(d) Improper supervision of the personnel.

Undoubtedly, the Quality Control Laboratory is the most essential component of the drug industry. The trust and consistency of a laboratory's results are achieved by developing attitudes and environments that are based on proper management of human resources, ongoing controls (validation of materials, instruments and techniques) and successful communication. Of course, quality control may be easy for a well equipped and staffed enterprise, which has all the necessary facilities including sophisticated instruments like spectrophotometer, chromatographic apparatus etc., at their command, but the small enterprises may have some problems mainly due to financial constraints and the technical manpower. Such companies can engage the services of approved commercial testing laboratories to augment their testing capabilities. This policy is commonly being followed by many organisations. However the company must have a laboratory capable of performing in process controls not requiring sophisticated instruments such as infrared spectrophotometer, high-performance liquid chromatography.

The establishment of any specifications, standards, sampling plan, test procedures or any other laboratory control procedures, including any change in such specifications should be finally reviewed and approved by the Quality Control Laboratory. The laboratory controls shall include the establishment of sound and appropriate specifications, standards and test procedures to assure that the final drug product conforms to the required standards of identity, strength, quality and purity. The Drug Control Authorities do have the interest in helping the industry to improve its quality control facilities to raise the quality assurance level of their products. The authorities should provide training and technical expertise to the industry in establishing their quality control laboratories. There exists some disagreement between the Regulated and the Regulators in this respect, but both the Drug Control Authorities and the Drug Industry are in agreement that consumer's interest is in everyone's best interest, because it is its mission and assignment both as a matter of conscience and business outlook.

For any discussion regarding Drug Control Laboratory, it is necessary to consider the specific functions of different kind of Laboratories. The Industrial Quality Control Laboratory is essentially concerned with routine examination of a limited range of raw material, intermediates and finished products. In a drug control laboratory owned by a company, the entire manufacturing history can be made available to the analyst. In contrast, the laboratory of a regulatory authority has to examine a much wider range of finished products about which very little background information is available. Other laboratories may be concerned solely with the developments of newer methods of analysis and analytical profile of new medicinal substances. The quality control laboratory has an important role to play in providing technical service leading to decisions as to the use or release for sale of material or to decision of legal nature. For such service to be efficient and effective, essential requirements are:

- Technical competence.
- Well equipped.
- Good internal organisation and co-ordination of the activities of the various sections of the laboratory.
- Co-ordination with other departments.

To inspire the confidence and respect that is so necessary for functioning of a laboratory, the above conditions are required to be fulfilled.

The laboratory is usually required to carry out the following type of testing: Chemical, instrumental, general microbiological, sterility, microbiological assay (potency testing of antibiotics and vitamins), routine pharmacological. The division of the laboratory into sections may be based either on the main techniques used or on the type of products to be tested. However, care should be taken that the work load is evenly distributed among various sections and it should not restrict communication between the staff involved in testing of same sample.

The organisational setup of a laboratory usually depends on the work load, the nature and variety of the work, availability of trained personnel and equipments. The head of such organisation may be designated as Quality Assurance Manager who has the overall responsibility for all aspects of quality in the organisation. He must be satisfied that all key members of the laboratory staff have the requisite competence and matching responsibilities i.e. depending on the assignment, then, through a proportionate combination of education and experience, each person must have demonstrated competency for the responsibilities of that assignment.

Technical competence: The selection of the staff for this work is of prime importance. Not all graduates/post-graduates in pharmacy, chemistry or other allied sciences possess the aptitude and attitude of mind to become competent analysts. Patience, enthusiasm, determination, mental acuity and a critical approach to problems are most desirable characteristics for an analyst (see Desirable qualities of an analyst). The new graduates may acquire necessary knowledge and experience from training organised within the laboratory or by working under the directions of senior colleagues (see Grading of analysts). The training should not overlook the more basic procedures, the basic training should include exercises such as determination of moisture, sulphated ash, weight per millilitre, refractive index, total solids, alcohol contents, alkaloidal contents, melting point, boiling range, limit tests for heavy metals and specific rotation. The trainees should be encouraged to understand fully all calculation procedures and should avoid the application of arithmetical formulae without first understanding them. The more experienced staff should have an opportunity for specialised training in topics such as GLC, HPLC, HPTLC and IR spectrophotometry.

According to their qualifications and experience, the analysts fit into three general categories: Trainee/probationary, Experienced and Seniors. There can be overlap between these groups as senior analyst can be trainee in some new technique. However the skill attained and intended functions can help in grading the analysts. New analyst will require extensive training for procedures in use in the laboratory. The amount of time spent on training will vary depending on the background and previous experience of the individual analyst. With the increasing complexicity of analytical procedures and instrumentation, individual specialization cannot be avoided. Analyst at all levels should have the following minimum skill before he is allowed to handle the analysis of samples:

1. Knowledge of basic chemical principles, theories and laboratory techniques as gained through completion of degree course in pharmacy, chemistry or other allied sciences.
2. Use of common instruments like balance, UV, pH meter, polarimeter, melting point apparatus, refractometer required in compendial procedures.
3. Adequate knowledge of CGMP and CGLP.
4. Established laboratory safety procedures.
5. Communication of laboratory results in written reports.

Development of analytical procedures is an important function of the laboratory in which all analysts should be involved to some extent. It promotes job satisfaction and stimulates the critical attitude that is so necessary for an analyst.

Note: Head of the laboratory must be of high professional standing with adequate experience in drug analysis and laboratory management and shall be responsible for:

(a) ensuring maintenance of documents including that of quality system as per legal requirements;
(b) planning and organizing audit of quality system;
(c) investigation of technical complaints;
(d) recommending any regulatory action in case of non-compliance of analysed samples;
(e) assigning duties to the analysts according to their technical competence.

GRADING OF ANALYSTS

This is primarily based on skill and functions, though there may be some overlapping.

Grade 1

1. Knowledge of basic chemical principles, theories and laboratory techniques as would be acquired through the successful completion of 4 year college course in Pharmacy, Chemistry.
2. Use of common instruments such as balances, pH meter, melting point apparatus, refractometer, colorimeter, polarimeter, moisture balance, required to be used in compendial methods in conformance with SOP.
3. Application of required quality assurance procedures.
4. Adherence to established laboratory safety procedures.
5. Communication of results in writing.

- Can analyse samples of pharmaceuticals (bulk and finished products) under guidance from supervisor or senior analyst.
- His work and analytical data needs to be discussed while in progress.

Grade 2

In addition to that of Grade 1, he should have attained:

1. Knowledge of use of more advanced instruments such as computer controlled HPLC/GC/IR, automated dissolution rate apparatus etc.
2. Knowledge of application of special techniques such as HPTLC/TA/Microscopy.
3. Knowledge of CGMP/CGLP.

- Can independently analyse samples using established and validated analytical procedures.
- His work is reviewed and discussed while in progress.

Grade 3

In addition to that of Grade 2, he should have:

1. Knowledge of agency's regulatory programme and objectives.
2. Experience in analysis of samples using compendial and manufacturer's method.
3. Previous experience or hands-on training with the instruments or techniques required by the method to be studied.
4. Knowledge of validation techniques and criteria for method acceptance.
5. Can select and apply the appropriate analytical method.
6. Can develop new methods or revise existing methods and validate the method so developed.
7. Participate in collaborative studies at inter- or intra-laboratory level.

- His work is discussed, if needed, otherwise be accepted.

Grade 4

In addition to Grade 1-3, the analyst should have:

1. Knowledge for use of advanced instruments such as FTIR, GC, Mass spectrometer and AA/MS.
2. Knowledge about validation of analytical procedures.
3. Planning of work for most efficient use of the resources.
4. Knowledge of statistical methods for data evaluation.
5. Leadership of a small group of analysts.

- He should be able to analyse samples (very difficult, complex, unusual and controversial), in addition to carry out check analysis or samples with doubtful results.
- Can evaluate methods submitted with NDA or ANDA.
- Can serve as a team leader for a project or study.
- Can supervise the proficiency testing of the analysts.
- His work is accepted as valid.

Grade 5

1. Expertise in operation and calibration of analytical instruments.

- Acts as a team leader.
- Conducts collaboration studies.
- Evaluates new laboratory methods.
- His work is considered as authoritative.

Scientists have given drugs to the people, the analyst guarantees quality of these drugs now and in future.

Validation of analysts

In addition to in-house audit programme, there should be a proven basis of evidence for reviewing the performance of an analyst called "proficiency testing".

1. Analysis of pre-analysed samples in respect of potency/assay/impurities.
2. Analysis of standard samples prepared for validation purpose.
3. Analysis of samples in replicate and measure of SD/RSD.
4. Analysis of samples for recovery studies after spiking the pre-analysed samples.

DESIRABLE QUALITIES OF AN ANALYST

1. Possesses aptitude and attitude of mind to become competent analyst.
2. Enjoys his assignment with pride.
3. Punctual and disciplined.
4. Has pleasant personality, is humane and modest.
5. Well organised and methodological.
6. Has initiative, drive, creative urge and ability to interact.
7. Flexible and appreciates other's view-point.
8. Imbibes confidence in his colleagues.
9. Able to work independently and as member of a team.
10. Plans his work for efficient use of time and resources.
11. Can complete his assignment (practical and written) in a given time frame.
12. Pays full attention to details (theoretical and practical).
13. Can identify the cause and solve the problem.
14. Able to think and evaluate scientifically and critically.
15. Questions what he is doing and why.
16. Always more than willing to improve upon quality of his work.
17. Possesses experimental skill.
18. Has sound knowledge of basic chemical principles and theory of laboratory techniques.
19. Able to follow oral and written instructions.
20. Good presentation and communication skill.
21. Sound knowledge of CGLP and CGMP.
22. Knowledge of method validation techniques as criteria for method acceptance.
23. Knowledge of basic statistical method for data evaluation.
24. Sound knowledge of common compendial procedures.
25. Knowledge in operation, calibration and maintenance of common analytical instruments.
26. Adheres to established laboratory safety procedures, while performing his analytical functions.

ANALYST AND ANALYTICAL DATA

Excellent laboratory facilities + Advance validated analytical instruments + Validated methods + Validated analysts	**Most reliable data**
Average laboratory facilities + Advance validated analytical instruments + Validated methods + Validated analysts	**Reliable data**
Average laboratory facilities + Routine validated analytical instruments + Validated methods + Validated analysts	**Data likely to be reliable**
Excellent laboratory facilities + Advance validated analytical instruments + Validated methods + Non-validated analysts	**Unreliable data**

"While dealing with the man and the laboratory the analyst has definite place in the sun. Analysts are not merely the measuring-tape wielders but equal partners and often troublesome as their results cost money. Let the analysts be on guard against any analytical non-sense."

The function of the analyst is to obtain results as close to true value as possible by the correct application of analytical procedure employed. The level of confidence the analysts may enjoy in their analytical results will be very small unless they have the knowledge of the accuracy and precision of the method as well as being aware of the errors which may get introduced. Quantitative analysis is not simply taking a sample, carrying out single determination and then claiming that the values so obtained are irrefutable. It requires sound knowledge of chemistry involved and the possibility of interference from other possible sources.

TRAINING OF ANALYST

Why analyst should be trained

1. To enable him/her to perform analytical functions correctly.
2. To reduce time and cost of analysis.
3. To avoid frequent false positive/negative results.
4. To comply with statutory requirements.
5. To do analysis right every time.
6. To improve confidence level.
7. To improve competence.
8. To enable him/her to better his/her career.

When to train analyst

A. On induction.
B. Before receiving any new instrument.
C. Before introducing a new product.
D. Before using a new API.
E. Before implementing new SOP.
F. Before introducing any new statutory changes concerning quality control.
G. Before implementing new method of analysis.
H. Before assigning any new/additional responsibility.
I. Before making any changes in CGMP.
J. On observing that analyst is making repeated errors (chronic offender).
K. On receiving any adverse report from FDA.
L. On encountering an accident.

Adapted from presentation made by Gidy Asrani (Vice-Chairman, Quality Management Sub-Committee, IDMA) on 12th Pharmaceutical Analysts Convention, 2009.

How to train the analyst

B. Before receiving a new instrument

- Obtain advance copy of instruction manual of the instrument.
- Let the analyst read the manual.
- Analyst be deputed to manufacturer of the instrument for training and demonstration.
- Already trained individual in the organization make presentation on the said technique.
- Depute the analyst to training seminars.
- Let the analyst interact with other analysts using same instrument.
- Familiarize the analyst with regulatory requirements of the instrument.
- Evolve a sound procedure to evaluate the performance of the analyst for the assignment.

C. Before introducing a new product

- Explain the importance of new product.
- Allow the analyst to be familiar with new technology.
- Explain him different equipments needed and their functioning.
- Explain detailed role of each ingredient in the new product.

D. Before using a new API

- Let the analyst first read all the relevant literature.
- Explain him the purpose of new API.
- He should know the properties and characteristics of new API.
- Highlight the hazards in handling and storage of new API.
- Explain rationale of different specifications of new API.
- Explain stability profile of new API.
- The analyst should know the vendor.

E. Before implementing SOP

- Explain the purpose of SOP.
- Describe the benefits and consequences of not following the SOP.
- Elaborate each step of SOP.
- Provide any clarification, if needed.
- Allow the analyst to perform as per proposed SOP.
- Correct/compliment the performance of analyst.
- Authorize the analyst implementation of SOP – the same may be appropriately recorded.

F. Statutory changes

- Explain the purpose and rationale of required changes.
- Allow the analyst to study the required changes correctly.
- Explain the importance of such changes.
- Explain the consequences of non-conformation.
- Inform the date when required changes shall be effective.
- Let the analyst draw up a schedule for implementing the changes.

G. Before introducing new method of analysis

- Explain the reason/rationale for change of the existing method.
- Explain the benefit of new method.
- Explain the consequences of the change.
- Explain different steps of methodology and technique involved.
- Highlight the most important steps in methodology which are likely to affect the analytical results.
- Explain the chemistry of the new method if involved.
- Demonstrate the working of new instrument involved in performing the new method.
- Caution on the handling of new chemicals and reagents.
- Explain recording system of analytical results.
- Inform the effective date of change.

H. Assigning new/additional responsibilities

- Explain the new responsibility being assigned.
- Explain its benefits.
- Amend the list of responsibilities.
- List the skill required to carry out new responsibilities.
- Guide the analyst on how to perform the new functions.
- Authorize the individual to perform new responsibility.
- Establish the mechanism to verify how the analyst is performing new responsibility.
- Carry out the occasional appraisal of how the new/additional responsibilities are being performed.
- Obtain the feedback about the performance of individual from reliable source.
- Record the implementation of new responsibilities.

I. Making changes in CGMP

- Explain the changes being made.
- Explain the reasons for the change.
- Explain the benefits of change.

- Explain other associated changes being made in documents and records.
- Guide the analyst to implement the changes.
- Guide the analyst to maintain the record in effective manner.

J. When the analyst is making repeated errors (chronic offender)

- Investigate the cause of repeated errors.
- Explain the consequences of such errors.
- Find out why and how the errors are being made repeatedly.
- Demonstrate the corrections.
- Highlight the benefits from prevention of errors.
- Train the analyst to carry out the procedure correctly to avoid errors.
- Carefully observe correct performance.
- Counsel/reprimand/reward the analyst.

K. Adverse FDA report

- Allow the analyst to study the adverse report and determine the possible causes.
- Allow the analyst to verify the adverse report.
- Let the analyst evaluate the ultimate consequences of adverse report.
- Let the analyst suggest changes required.
- Let the analyst suggest action to prevent recurrence.
- Let the analyst initiate the draft reply to FDA report.
- The draft reply be evaluated by competent personnel.
- Let the analyst evaluate possibility of such adverse report in other areas of his functions.

L. On encountering an accident

- Train the analyst for an immediate course of action.
- Analyst should study and outline the possible causes of accident.
- Analyst should recommend necessary changes to avoid such incidents in future.
- Explain the method of recording the accident.
- Explain details of regulatory requirements.
- Explain how to evaluate the consequences.
- Explain the possibility of recurrence.
- Counsel/reprimand the individual responsible for the accident.

Common Issues Confronting the Analysts

1. Lack of understanding of theoretical background of the method.
2. Unfamiliarity with the instrument and the technique.
3. Not following the correct procedure while conducting the tests.

4. Lack of patience while conducting the test.
5. Does not have adequate experience to carry out a particular test.
6. Not adequately trained to interpret/evaluate the analytical results.
7. Lack of adequate professional training including GLP.
8. No up-grading of analytical knowledge.
9. Lack of interaction with fellow analysts.
10. Lack of reading habits.
11. Lack of inquiring mind.
12. Frequent change of jobs.

Even though the laboratory may have several specialised divisions or sections under the direction of competent staff, the ultimate responsibility rests with the quality assurance manager. It is, therefore, absolutely essential that he should have high professional standing and have had extensive experience in drug analysis and laboratory management in a quality control laboratory in the regulatory department or in industry and be conversant with the methods used in different sections of the laboratory and be aware of their capabilities and limitations. Head of the quality control who is ultimately responsible for final decision relating to the acceptability of the finished product should report to some higher level of authority other than the one directly responsible for producing the product. This will ensure independent function of both the divisions while taking ultimate decision on the acceptability or rejection of the products. It can be argued that a quality control unit might not have all the expertise required to carry out its responsibilities which include anything that may or may not have impact on drug quality. But the discipline of quality assurance includes the ability to ask proper questions about the functioning of various aspects of drug production in order to ensure quality. However judgement by a quality control unit must be based on facts and opinion which can be relied upon in reaching the conclusion.

It is important that instruments and other apparatus be regularly calibrated and maintained in working order. It is convenient to allocate responsibility to individual analyst and to fix a card to the instrument stating who is responsible so that all problems related to the instrument may be referred to that person.

In the entire analytical sequence, the personnel accountability should be documented and record should be maintained for each laboratory employee which should include:

1. Name
2. Academic qualification
3. Relevant experience with detail
4. Refresher courses and training undergone
5. Scientific publications

6. Responsibilities in the laboratory and the list of tests and assays the personnel is qualified to perform
7. Periodic validation of personnel.

It is preferable to segregate the work based on type of analysis with periodic change over to expose the analysts to different types of analysis.

When a person is being qualified to perform a particular assay method, there should be no access to verbal guidance from other laboratory staff, that is, the person being qualified must carry out the procedure as per written instructions only. If the written directions are not adequate, the individual will not be able to perform the test without additional instructions, reflecting the measure of method's transferability.

Internal quality control procedures facilitate correct operations. The use of control charts to record the analytical results for consecutive batches of a single product provide the means of detecting non-random variations and undesirable trends either in production or in the laboratory. Previously analysed samples and standard samples should be periodically submitted for re-analysis to check the accuracy of analytical procedures and performance of the quality control personnel. The services of a referral laboratory, if available, may be utilized where pre-analysed samples can be referred for post-testing auditing. This procedure should not be considered to have been simply designed to check the integrity of the analyst but in overall interest of the laboratory. Based on audit report, adequacy of existing staff, management and training programme of the analysts can be reviewed. It has been observed that errors mostly occur during preparatory work such as weighing, dilutions, quality of reagents (unsuitable or deteriorated), purity of reference drug substances, inappropriate methods (method which are difficult to reproduce) and variations in laboratory environments. The main cause of such errors is carelessness, fatigue, inadequate training and lack of aptitude and attitude in analytical work. The staff being assigned work beyond their level of competence should normally be avoided. The possibility of in-service training programmes should be explored to update professional competence and keep staff abreast of advances in analytical methods and instrumentation. For continuous automated analysis, standard should be assayed at regular intervals to correct for drift and to assure the accuracy of the results. Analytical method development units must develop and qualify and the quality control units must review and approve drug testing specifications for each component and raw material to be utilised in the product and its production. A representative sample from each assigned control number must meet the requirements of its protocols before the material can be released for use. The testing specifications established for each item should include the following data:

1. Product's name and number.
2. Required tests:
   (a) Refer to pharmacopoeial requirements or in-house specifications and should include amount of sample required for testing and retention for future analysis.
   (b) An amount of each reagent, buffer etc. necessary for various tests.
   (c) Equipment required.
   (d) Instrument required.
   (e) Personnel qualified for test.
   (f) Exact details of the testing procedures.
   (g) Procedure for computation of the results.
3. Tolerance allowable for each test: This should reflect pharmacopoeial requirements or in-house variance limits. It is preferable if the in-house tolerance limits are more stringent than the compendial limits to ensure that released product meets official requirements when subjected to regulatory inspection and testing.
4. Frequency for re-assaying each item.
5. A procedure for sampling protocols should be established and should include the following information:
   (i) Who has the responsibility and authority to draw sample from received goods.
   (ii) Number of units to be sampled based on the number of in-coming containers per control number.
   (iii) Method of selecting containers to be sampled.
   (iv) Size and distribution of sample from each container.
   (v) Entering sample information in the continuous log book maintained in the control laboratory.

The analyst must then determine what specification is to be used to assess the quality of the sample. If no suitable pharmacopoeial monograph exists, the analytical specifications and methods of analysis may be obtained from the manufacturer or drafted in the laboratory on the basis of published information or personal experience. Whatever may be the case, detailed note on the specifications adopted and method of analysis used must be recorded in the work sheet.

The testing specifications and sampling protocols are official master records and must be maintained in a secure storage area with limited access. The master record should be placed under the control of a single competent person with appropriate academic training and experience to make necessary and appropriate corrections, additions or deletions. The specifications of work in-process and finished products must meet the same stringent requirements as imposed on raw material. Calibration of instruments, apparatus, gauges and other recording devices at suitable intervals should be done in accordance with an established written programme containing specific directions, schedules, limits for accuracy and precision and provision for remedial action, in case accuracy and/or precision limits are not met. Instruments, apparatus, gauges and other recording devices not meeting the established specifications shall not be used. Even if the calibration of equipments has been contracted to outside agencies, the responsibility for the same must still rest with the analyst of the quality control department. The calibration procedures, acceptance criteria and the frequency must have his approval. It is not adequate to report that the equipment is acceptable, but calibration result must be recorded. Frequency of calibration is usually decided on the basis of experience and past performance of the equipment. It is always desirable that the analyst should always record the specific instrument and reference standard used in any analysis. This will narrow down the field of rechecking the analytical results in case of controversy. One can resort to mini calibration until and unless one has reasons to suspect about the satisfactory performance of the equipment. However, if a sample has been found not conforming to the prescribed specifications, the analysis should be repeated by another analyst using fresh lot of reference standard, chemicals and reagents.

Pharmacopoeial monographs describe tests for identity, limits for certain impurities, strength (per cent of active substance or biological potency) and also perhaps tests for stability or physical properties relevant to biopharmaceutical activity of the substance. The monographs generally include several tests for identity. Each individual test is not necessarily specific for the substance but may identify a certain chemical group or ion. A particular Rf value being selective is not a characteristic of one substance only. The intention of the monograph is that the qualitative and quantitative tests considered as a whole should provide adequate evidence as to identify. Pharmaceutical limits for impurities refer particularly to those substances whose presence might be expected from knowledge of the manufacturing process or decomposition route. However, the pharmacopoeia for example states in its general notices, "The requirements are not framed to provide against all possible impurities, it is not to be presumed, for example, that an unusual impurity is tolerated which is not precluded by the prescribed tests should rational consideration require that it be absent."

A problem arises when new routes are developed for the synthesis of a medicinal substance. The alternative routes may lead to impurities other than those limited by pharmacopoeial tests. For the licensing of a pharmaceutical formulation of a new medicinal substance, regulatory authorities normally require full details to be disclosed regarding the synthesis of that substance, likely impurities and control methods used to limit those impurities. However, for the manufacture of formulations of established drugs, there is generally no restriction on the source or method of manufacture of the ingredients. It appears that application of pharmacopoeial limit tests for impurities alone may sometimes be insufficient. As the suppliers of raw materials may be unwilling or unable to divulge the manufacturing process and the potential impurities, the problem is not easily resolvable. The pharmacopoeial requirement for potency or per cent purity is in some cases intended to allow for some deterioration on storage. Clearly then, when deterioration under normal storage conditions is to be expected, the raw material as purchased and the finished pharmaceutical product leaving the factory must be well above the minimum pharmacopoeial requirement. The pharmacopoeial limits are intended for application by the regulatory authority and make allowance for some decomposition during the shelf life of the product. The lower limit does, nevertheless seem very generous and the upper limit seems unnecessarily high. It is therefore, necessary for the company to set its own minimum standards.

It is a good general policy to examine representative samples submitted by potential suppliers of materials before deciding from which source to purchase.

Compendial monographs for sterility, dissolution test and content uniformity are quite specific. Achieving compliance with compendial requirements is considered as meeting a minimal quality criteria. The product manufacturers are required to ensure that quality of the product not only meets the labelled claim but also retains its potency throughout the shelf life within prescribed limits. The specifications for each product as developed and recorded is an official document and normally include the following data:

1. Product's name and number.
2. Required tests (compendial or in-house specifications) which include:
   - (a) Potency test.
   - (b) Identity test for ingredients, known contaminants and degradation products.
   - (c) Hardness friability.
   - (d) Dimension.
   - (e) Colour determination.
   - (f) Moisture determination.
   - (g) pH determination.
   - (h) Weight variation/content uniformity.
   - (i) Disintegration time/dissolution time.
   - (j) Visual defects (chipping, mottling, coating defects).

(k) Abrasiveness or foreign material present in ophthalmic products.
(l) Sterility.
(m) Pyrogen.

3. Amount of drug and reagents required for each test.
4. Equipments and instruments required for each test.
5. Personnel qualified for the test.
6. Details of the exact test or assay procedures.
7. Permissible tolerance or variation for each test.
8. Recording of the analytical data.

SYSTEMS AND PROCEDURES IN A QUALITY CONTROL LABORATORY

1. Good laboratory practices.
2. General procedures for analysis abstracted from IP/BP/USP.
3. Current approved and authorized specifications and standard test procedures.
4. Authorised documents for analysis.
5. Retention of analysed samples.
6. Reference substances and certified working standards and their periodic update.
7. Volumetric solutions and reagents and their standardization schedule.
8. Reporting system for each sample.
9. Analytical reference number.
10. Calibration of instrument, maintenance of log book and calibration schedule of each instrument.
11. Handling of product complaints.
12. Cleaning of laboratory glassware.
13. Records of temperature and humidity of critical areas of the laboratory.
14. Laboratory safety guidelines.
15. Opening and closing of the laboratory.
16. Validation (instruments, personnel and analytical procedures).
17. Regular job-based training and evaluation of quality control personnel.
18. Possible evidence that the systems continue to perform reliably and reproducibly.
19. Analyst data validation.
20. Periodic validation of analytical methods in use.
21. Periodic validation of analyst.
22. No dispatches without approval of quality control department.
23. Continuous upgrading of quality system.
24. Continuous upgrading of quality standards.

STEPS FOR SUCCESSFUL ANALYSIS

1. Working bench and apparatus should always be kept clean.
2. If glassware are to be kept in hot air oven, these should be rinsed with distilled or demineralized water. Inside of the glass should never be cleaned with cloth. Usually soap or detergent solution such as teepol is satisfactory for cleaning. If cleaning mixture (sodium dichromate in concentrated sulphuric acid) is employed, large volume of water shall be required for rinsing the wares. Glass apparatus (flasks, beakers etc.) should be kept in the hot air oven in inverted position to avoid deposit of any residue after evaporation of water.
3. Do not use broken or chipped glassware.
4. Graduated apparatus should neither be heated nor any hot liquid poured into it, because the apparatus will expand and may not contract to its initial volume on cooling to room temperature.
5. All reagent bottles must be returned to their correct position—reagent shelf—immediately after use.
6. Stopper of the reagent bottle must not be kept on bench, preferably held in left hand and replaced in the bottle as soon as the reagent has been used.
7. All reagent solutions should be labelled indicating identify, titre value or concentration and special storage condition, if any. If water bottle contains liquid other than water, it should be labelled appropriately (often for rinsing of cuvettes, methanol is introduced into water bottle).
8. In case of non-aqueous titrations, both standardization and sample analysis should be carried out at the same temperature as far as possible as non-aqueous solvents have greater coefficient of expansion than water so even small difference in temperature can result in significant error.
9. While taking out reagents, the position of the label on bottle should be on the top to avoid getting label spoiled.

Essential requirements of analytical measurements

1. Analytical measurements should be made to satisfy the desired and agreed parameters.
2. Analytical measurements should be made using methods, protocols and equipments which have been tested and validated to ensure that they are fit for intended measurements.
3. Personnel making analytical measurements should be professionally qualified and competent to undertake the analysis.
4. Technical performance of the laboratory should be regularly assessed by an independent authority.

5. Analytical data obtained in one location should be consistent with those elsewhere—reproducibility.
6. The laboratory should have well-defined quality control and quality assurance procedures.
7. Proper selection of the method taking into consideration the nature and purpose of analysis and facilities available and to decide whether accuracy and precision are really important in given situation.
8. When a particular procedure fails, when should the analysis be terminated to try another method.
9. The samples may be grouped for analysis such as samples containing vitamins for high throughput.
10. Possible use of "Quick Assessment System" by which approximate idea about the quality of the drug (90-110% of claim) can be assessed.

RESPONSIBILITIES OF KEY PERSONNEL IN QUALITY CONTROL LABORATORY

As part of good laboratory practices, it should always be possible to trace who was responsible for certain results. Responsibility should be taken by people who should not only be trained to bear such responsibility but should have personality to cope with the responsibility in term of emotion, experience and knowledge. For this, the individual needs to have appropriate character, education, commitment, leadership and empowerment.

1. Approval or rejection of all raw materials, packaging materials, intermediate, bulk and finished products.
2. Evaluation of batch records.
3. Approval of sampling instructions, specification, test methods and other quality control procedures.
4. Checking the maintenance of laboratory premises and equipment including all instruments.
5. Ensuring initial and continuing training of quality control personnel relevant to their needs.
6. Ensuring validation/proficiency testing of analysts.
7. Ensuring validation of quality control procedures and calibration of equipments and maintenance of their records.
8. Setting up a system of quality assurance.
9. Preparing a quality control manual giving all details about the systems to be followed.

STANDARDS OF TOTAL QUALITY MANAGEMENT

1. Commitment: Believe in the philosophy of quality and show constancy of purpose towards improvement of product and service if one wants to stay in the business for the foreseeable future.
2. Leadership: Show quality of leadership by example. Leadership is not the domain of managers only, but for everyone.
3. Customer orientation: It is entirely because of customers that you are here. Determine their needs and educate them for better understanding of their needs.
4. Team work: We are all in this together. Build yourself and the organisation on each other's ideas and strengths.
5. Communication: Always appreciate others' viewpoints. Communication is vital to business – national or international.
6. Empowerment: As a boss, take the blame and pass on the credit. Give people power, responsibility, pride of workmanship and recognition to the one who deserves; remove barriers to achieve this goal.
7. Training: Continuing education is important for continuous improvement. Build awareness of the need and opportunity for improvement.
8. Style: Believe in your own quality system. Learn from pioneers in the field, taking best from each to suit your system.
9. Pride of workmanship: Enjoy your work. You can hold your head high if you did the job right way and the quality way.
10. Drive out fear so that every one may work effectively for the organisation. Do not be revengeful.
11. As we are in new economic age, one can no longer succeed with mistakes, defective material and defective workmanship.
12. Do you depend on mass inspection, build in the quality through evidence.
13. The characteristics that indicate quality and measurement of its success must be well defined. Critical quality problem be defined and the management must take the lead in solving them.
14. Quality is to be achieved by understanding and improving the system rather than reducing the defects through inspection and corrections.
15. Create a structure in the top management that should push everyone to improve.

Those who ignore "Total Quality Management Concept", do so at the peril of their future business. Charles Darwin's law of survival of the fittest, though a cruel law, and unrelenting, holds in the free enterprise. The only survivors will be the companies with constancy of purpose for quality, productivity and service.

SAFE LABORATORY PRACTICES

Do's and Don'ts

Most of them are of common sense.

1. To protect clothing from chemical damage, wear a lab apron or lab coat. Long hair should be tied back to keep it from coming into contact with lab chemicals or flames.
2. An open flame may be ignited only when no flammable solvents are in the vicinity. The person lighting the flame must check with analyst in the vicinity to see if they are working with flammable solvents.
3. Exercise great caution in handling volatile, flammable solvents such as ether, acetone and methanol. Never evaporate these solvents on a hot plate in an open system. An efficient condenser system must be used.
4. In case of injury (cut, burn, fire, etc.) notify the instructor immediately.
5. In case of a fire or imminently dangerous situation, notify everyone who may be affected immediately; be sure the lab instructor is also notified.
6. If chemicals splash into someone's eyes, act quickly and get them into the eyewash station; do not wait for the instructor.
7. In case of a serious cut, stop blood flow using direct pressure using a clean towel; notify the lab instructor immediately.
8. Know the location and operation of:
    - Fire extinguishers
    - Safety showers and eyewash stations (near chemical section)
    - Fire alarm boxes
    - First-aid box
    - Exit doors
    - Telephones
9. Eating, drinking and smoking are prohibited in the laboratory at all times.
10. Never work in the laboratory without proper supervision by an instructor.
11. Never carry out unauthorized experiments. Come to the laboratory prepared. If you are unsure about what to do, please ask the instructor.
12. Never pipette using mouth suction. Avoid inhaling and never taste any chemical in the lab.
13. Never force glass tubing through a rubber stopper. If glass tubing must be inserted into a rubber stopper, be sure to lubricate both the stopper and the tubing (glycerol or soapy water). Protect your hands, wrap the glass tubing in a towel while inserting.
14. Always remember, **HOT** glassware looks exactly the same as **COLD** glassware, be careful what you touch. 100°C = 212°F (boiling point of water).

Other safety aspects

1. Adequate ventilation.
2. Gas cylinders should be kept outside the laboratory in upright position.
3. Off & on switch of the fuming hood should be outside the panel.
4. Laboratory coat should be made of cotton with snap fasteners.
5. Nylon and polyester clothes should be avoided.
6. Poisons and toxic substances should be kept under lock & key.
7. Be aware of the methods for safe disposal of corrosive or dangerous chemicals by neutralization or deactivation.

TEN COMMANDMENTS OF GLP*

Follow CGLP (Current Good Laboratory Practices) for ensuring that the analysis of (releasing/rejecting) a product is dependable and correct.

- ⇨ Thou shalt write procedures!
- ⇨ Thou shalt follow thy written procedures!
- ⇨ Thou shalt correctly document thy work!
- ⇨ Thou shalt review and retain thy work!
- ⇨ Thou shalt validate thy work!
- ⇨ Thou shalt plan and build and procure proper systems facilities and instruments!
- ⇨ Thou shalt audit to control systems, facilities and instruments for assessing quality of products!
- ⇨ Thou shalt maintain and improve thy systems, facilities and instruments!
- ⇨ Thou shalt be competent! (As result of education, training and experience)
- ⇨ Thou shalt be clean and neat in thy work!

Thou shalt write procedures!

- Each and every step involved in the analysis shall be written down. These procedures are termed as standard operating procedures (SOPs).

Thou shalt follow thy written procedures!

- Written procedures shall be followed without any deviation, otherwise it shall amount to violation.

---

* Adapted from article by Dr. (Mrs.) S.K. Gehani, IDMA PAC-99.

Thou shalt document thy work!

- Any thing left to memory is a rumour. Any thing recorded is valid and dispels all doubts. Having followed the written procedures, documentary evidence is necessary for audit and using for further reporting.
- Raw data documentation should be done in a numbered bound registers.

Thou shalt review and retain thy work!

- The data shall be preserved as per regulatory requirement. The preservation of documents both manufacturing and analytical should be under the control of quality assurance department.

Thou shalt validate thy work!

- GLP expects that every analytical result of a product is almost mirror image of the previous analytical results. This can only be achieved if one follows written procedures without deviation. For this analyst, instruments and procedures are validated to give reproducible results.

Thou shalt plan and build and procure proper systems facilities and instruments!

- Quality of analysis has to be built-in from initial stages for reproducibility of the results. For this, we need proper facilities, rugged validated methods and instruments qualified for IQ, OQ and PQ.

Thou shalt audit to control systems, facilities and instruments for assessing quality of products!

- It is essential to audit the systems to control them for giving only quality results in quality line which are right the first time.

Thou shalt maintain and improve thy systems, facilities and instruments!

- It is necessary to have a "Master Validation Plan" which encompasses the periodic validation of procedures, instruments, facilities and systems.
- "Master Calibration Schedule" for performance of instruments as well as have a calendar for training of personnel.

Thou shalt be competent!

- The people have to be competent in their specific area.
- This competency is achievable by their education in the field, followed by training in specific job and thereafter by the experience and familiarity of work.

- Competent people are expected to do their job right the first time and every time, thereby cutting down cost of the analysis incurred due to repeat analysis.

Thou shalt be clean and neat in thy work!

- If anything unclean comes in contact with the sample under analysis it shall contaminate the sample.
- Use all glassware certified to be clean before starting analysis.
- Ensure environmental cleanliness usually wherever required by chemical, microbial evaluation and particle count of air.
- Personnel in contact be clean; wearing clean uniform. Hands to be cleaned after eating, visiting toilet and after handling different chemicals and products.
- No eating, smoking, chewing, spitting shall be allowed in laboratory.
- Wear masks to control coughing, sneezing directly on any product.
- The working in the department shall be systematic and orderly to control untidiness in area.
- All the material shall be in their proper slot, instead of its lying about disorderly.
- All the rubbish shall be thrown only in dustbins and not just anywhere.
- Any material spillage shall be cleaned up immediately and disposed of suitably.
- All incoming material and its container shall be checked for its cleanliness.
- Samples to be analysed in clean surroundings with clean glassware by clean personnel.

SOP ON OUT OF SPECIFICATION (OOS) LABORATORY RESULTS

Objective

To establish procedural guidelines for investigation and evaluation of Out of Specification Laboratory Results.

Scope

This procedure is applicable to all test results including routine, non-routine analysis and those generated as a part of the commercial stability programme of chemical and instrumental analysis for Drug Products (formulations), and Bulk Pharmaceutical Chemicals.

Responsibilities

1. MQC/MQA/Production incharge shall be responsible for carrying out investigations on out of specification laboratory result.
2. The out of specification laboratory results are caused by laboratory error or operator error or manufacturing process error. This operating procedure provides system to investigate and evaluate laboratory test failure, laboratory error, manufacturing process error and operator error.
3. These investigations represent a key issue in deciding whether a product may be released or rejected or reprocessed and shall form the basis for retesting and resampling. The laboratory errors occur when analysts make mistakes in following method of analysis or use incorrect standards or make errors in the calculations and interpretation of the results, etc.
4. The manufacturing process errors occur when manufacturing process is not followed as per the Master Batch Records, faulty and non-validated equipments are used, processes are not validated or standardised process parameters are not maintained, etc. Operator errors occur when there is a lack of training on the job or operator's negligence.

Procedure

Following procedure shall be adopted as guidelines for failure investigation to identify the cause of Out of Specification Laboratory Results (OOS) and its evaluation:

(a) Retesting from same solution of the original sample shall be carried out by the same analyst as per guidelines provided for laboratory failure investigation.

(b) When the laboratory investigation is conclusive and indicates identifiable laboratory error, the results shall be recalculated or original laboratory sample shall be retested once. The retest data shall replace the original data. However, the original data shall be retained.

(c) When the laboratory investigation is inconclusive and reason for the error is not identified, then the following retesting procedure shall be followed for further investigation.

Retesting shall be carried out minimum in order to establish whether the OOS result was due to an undetermined laboratory error. Retesting shall be carried out from the original sample and from fresh sample in the absence of any appropriate scientific data. However, number of retests shall be reduced depending upon the nature of material, the precision of analytical method (historical) trend analysis data of process and quality parameters of product and other scientific data. A detailed retest protocol shall be written and approved by Q.C. Manager/Q.C. Incharge. This protocol shall contain details of retesting, analyst and acceptance criteria for retest results.

After completion of retesting, the Q.C. Manager/Q.C. Incharge shall evaluate the data in order to decide whether or not the initial OOS result was erroneous and therefore can be considered invalid. This decision shall be based upon the variability of the data, the quality trend of the product, the precision of analytical method employed and other relevant scientific data.

Resampling and testing

- Resampling shall be treated as a part of failure investigation and only as a supportive data.
- Resampling and testing the material of batch under question shall be permitted, provided, it shall be proved from the laboratory investigations that the OOS laboratory result is due to incorrect/faulty sampling procedure adopted OR if the residual quantity of the original laboratory sample is insufficient for retesting.
- Results of testing after resampling shall be documented in failure investigation report and the analyst's protocol notebook.
- No averaging of variable results which also include "Out of Specification Results" is allowed.

Documentation

Investigation documentation shall include the following:

- A detailed report on the failure investigation carried out shall include purpose, identification and reasons of failure investigation (Annexure IV).

Findings on cause of OOS laboratory results shall be classified into three categories, namely:

1. Laboratory error (analysts, sampling)
2. Non-process related or operator error.
3. Process related or process error (instruments, procedure).

The report shall have recommendation of Q.A. for further action.

Have inquiring mind and try to understand and evaluate unexpected laboratory results.

GUIDELINES FOR INVESTIGATION REPORT ON OOS LABORATORIES RESULTS

(Laboratory Failure Investigation)

1. Name of the product under investigation:
2. Stage of Mfg.
3. Batch No. Mfg. Date: Exp. Date:
4. Investigation started on: Completed on:
5. Details of OOS laboratory results:
6. Name of the analyst who has reported OOS laboratory results:
7. Results of retesting from the same solution of original sample ....

   Analyst ....
8. Checklist for failure investigation: (To be tick marked appropriately)

	Yes / No
(a) Method of analysis followed is approved and current.	/
(b) Specifications are approved/current/relevant.	/
(c) There is no deviation in every step of method of analysis followed by analyst.	/
(d) Correct standard solution/reagents/glasswares used while performing the analysis.	/
(e) Correct working standards (approved/current) used wherever applicable.	/
(f) The analytical instrument used is calibrated and in working condition (instrument performance).	/
(g) The analyst is trained and certified for the test to be carried out (supporting records).	/
(h) The analytical findings and results are correctly entered in the analyst's notebook of protocols.	/
(i) The calculation formula and the method of calculation and interpretation of the results are correct/approved (chromatograms to be attached).	/
(j) Any other observations/findings which may affect the system followed (validation of analytical method/system suitability requirements, etc.).	/
(k) Correct/approved sampling procedure is followed.	/
(l) The sample drawn is representative of the batch (homogenity of the batch).	/

Conclusion:

Q.C. Manager/Incharge

SCHEMATIC CHART OF ACTIVITIES FOR OUT OF SPECIFICATION LABORATORY RESULT AND FAILURE INVESTIGATION

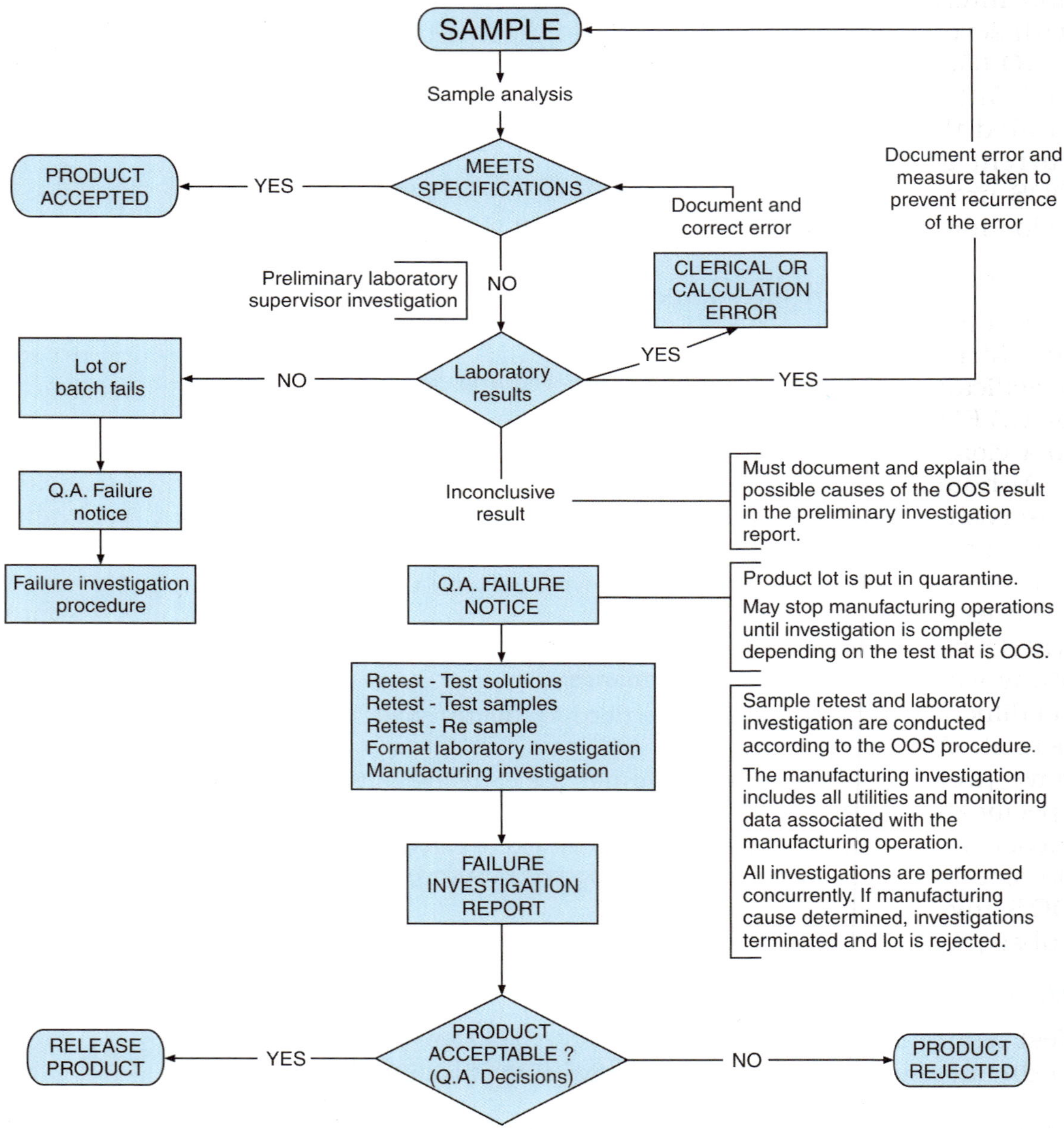

INVESTIGATION OF OUT OF SPECIFICATION RESULTS*

About the Article

During my working span of nearly 35 years with various highly reputed national and international pharmaceutical companies, I had the privilege to interact with several inspectors from US FDA, MHRA (UK), MCC (SA), ANVISA (Brazil), WHO (Geneva) and many others. Every regulatory inspection that I attended had Out of Specification (OOS) as a mandatory part in their checklist. I have drafted this article based on my discussions/interactions/presentations and current guidelines, with an objective to develop clear understanding about OOS procedures. I honestly feel such a clear understanding will immensely help Indian Pharmaceutical Industry to minimize non-compliances in this area.

Background

Out of Specification (OOS) has become a buzz word today in Pharmaceutical Industries across the globe. Reason being the fact that improper out-of-specification investigation is a leading cause of warning letters and 483's issued by US FDA. Form 483 contains those observations that can be directly linked to a violation of regulations, not suggestions, guidance, or other comments.

Although the 483 does not contain references to the regulations, each observation is directly traceable to a section of the applicable regulations. Items placed on a form 483 are the opinion of the FDA investigator on the scene, and may be subject to review by others within FDA.

Other regulatory agencies like MHRA of UK have also come out strongly with OOS as one of the weak links through their inspections conducted globally. Many workshops, seminars, consultants, and guidances are available today, yet difficulties and inconsistent approaches to out-of-specification investigations persist. Varying degrees of understanding of current expectations in this area have probably led to different approaches towards investigation of out-of-specification results. Look at the following chart which gives us an idea about most common cGMP deficiencies noted by US FDA during inspections conducted outside US. Maximum deficiencies are noticed in the area related to Failure/ OOS investigations. Though the exact statistics is not available for the subsequent years, areas of concern have remained almost same.

What is OOS?

Test results lying outside the final specifications are classified as OOS Results and confirmed OOS results are classified as failures. Failure is a departure

* Vijay U. Kshirsagar, Executive Vice President, Corporate Quality & Regulatory, Unichem Laboratories Limited, Mumbai, India

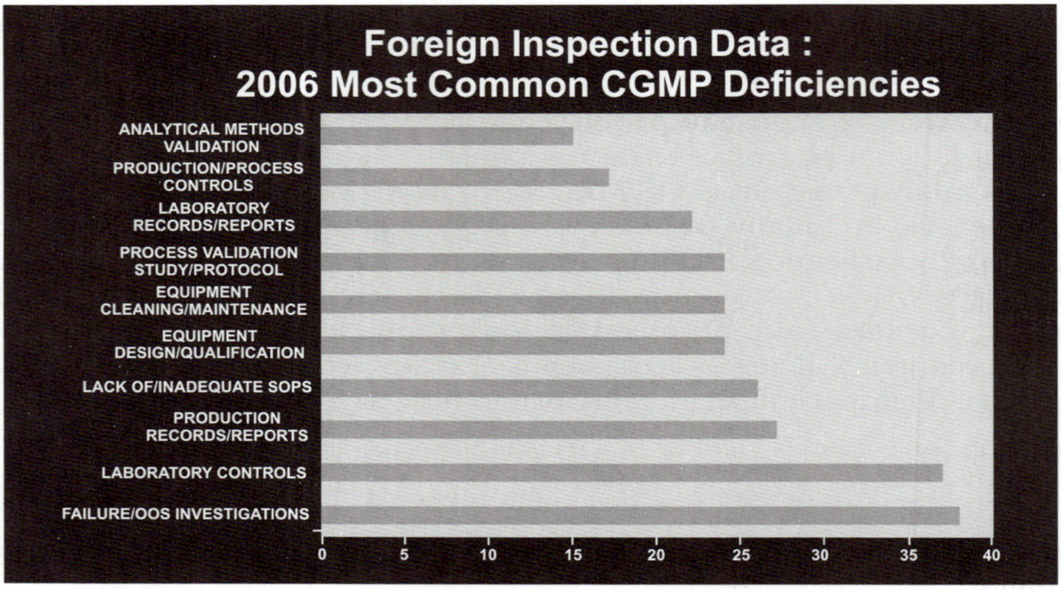

from a set standard or the specification. Failures also include unplanned deviations and system failures. OOS or Failure does not include Out of Trend (OOT) observations which are still within the limits or the finding where only alert limits are crossed but not the action limits.

Historical Court Case in US

It was Judge Wolin from US court who first coined the word Out of Specification (OOS). He preferred to use the term OOS rather than failure. The guiding principles for out-of-specification investigations are based on a historical legal ruling by Judge Wolin in 1993. US FDAÆs final guidance published in 2006 after a debate which ran for almost 8 years has its genesis in the landmark judgment passed by Judge Wolin while presiding over a case brought by FDA enforcement action against a generic-drug manufacturer namely Barr Laboratories in US. Among the issues that FDA cited were averaging out-of-specification values with in specification values to get a passing result; discarding raw data; conducting multiple retests with no defined end point.

FDA had also commented that failure investigations were carried out in a nonscientific manner and analytical methods were lacking in validation. Judge Wolin's responsibility was to listen to experts from both sides and craft an opinion that was based on the testimony and the law. In addition, he had to interpret the current regulations about good manufacturing practices. The trial itself generated 2300 pages of testimony, 400 exhibits and declarations. So now let us look at the important elements of this historical ruling.

Judge Wolin came down very heavily against indiscriminate retesting which was considered as 'Testing to Compliance' which means test and retest the product till it passes. He did allow retests, but only when the laboratory investigations were completed and an analyst error or sampling error was established.

An identified lab error can overcome the OOS result. Judge Wolin further directed that retests were to be done on the same sample and not a different sample, but retests might be conducted on a second aliquot from the same portion of sample or on a portion of the same larger sample previously collected for laboratory tests. Judge Wolin put several restrictions on 'Outlier Tests' which could be an attempt to disqualify a genuine OOS results. Whenever you have a result which is significantly different than other results for the same sample, general tendency is to term it as 'Outlier' and disregard it. Judge remarked that it cannot be used frequently by the firm and further added that it is not applicable for chemical results. General understanding is that in microbiological testing at times it is possible to get 'Outlier Results' due to inherent variability. OOS investigation needs to be completed in 30 days time.

Regulatory Expectations

It is first necessary to understand the minimum expectations of the Regulatory Bodies. I am quoting below from the respective guidelines as it appears:

EU Commission Directive 2003/94EC
"... All process deviations and product defects shall be documented and thoroughly investigated ..."

US 21CFR 211.192 & Other Provisions in 211
"Any unexplained discrepancy ... shall be thoroughly investigated ... The investigation shall extend to other batches ... that can have been associated with the Specific failure or discrepancy. A written record of the investigation shall be made and shall include the conclusions and follow-up."

ICHQ7, GMP for API's
"Any deviation from established procedures should be documented and explained. Critical deviations should be investigated, and the investigation and its conclusions should be documented.", "All deviation, investigation and OOS reports should be reviewed as part of the batch record review before the batch is released."

Case Study

Now let us take a case study for discussion. A firm has been manufacturing a particular API for years together without any problem. Suddenly a batch (blended) came with pink shade and failed in description as it is supposed to be white to off-white in appearance. Primary investigation revealed that there is no lab error or sampling error. No possibility of cross contamination was noticed. Similarly there was no manufacturing or packing (container/closure) error. There was no deviation or change done w.r.t. routine procedure.

Subsequently the team listed various possible causes for this problem e.g. coloured impurity formation during reaction, contamination coming from un-cleaned reactors , blenders, unidentified impurity in the starting materials, significant processing time difference for a stage/s etc. Each cause was thoroughly verified. Finally it was found that the root cause was 'use of unclean blender'. Blender though dedicated for a product was used 28 days before and it was cleaned partially (dry cleaning) after its previous use. Invisible residue was left behind which got discoloured over a period of time due to reaction with the metal/aerial oxidation. The pink colour could only be seen in IPA which was used for flushing the reactor.

Firm had not done any dirty equipment and clean equipment hold time studies. On previous occasions, blender did not remain unused for such a long time of 28 days. So, as a corrective action, batch in question was rejected and immediate previous 10 batches control samples were checked for description. As a part of preventive study, concerned impurity was separated on preparatory HPLC and identified. Dirty equipment and clean equipment hold time studies were done for each type of cleaning i.e. partial cleaning and complete cleaning.

Investigation Tools

Investigation is a science. In many instances, information about the last event and the starting event is reasonably well known. Information about what occurred between these endpoints, however, is often unclear, confusing, and perhaps contradictory. Hence it calls for good subject knowledge, sound analytical experience, lot of probing/questioning, data search, objective analysis of the data gathered and finally arriving at the root cause of the problem. Somebody who has hands on experience of HPLC analysis can only effectively investigate the OOS result obtained in Assay by HPLC. There are lots of techniques which are available today like Fault Tree Analysis (FTA), Failure Mode Effect Analysis (FMEA), Fish Bone Analysis, Hazard analysis of critical control points, etc.

The FTA method can diagnose the reliability and security of processes, mainly those that can be a potential source of hazardous and catastrophic events. It follows a top down approach where analysis starts from a top unwanted negative event and then developing all causal intermediate events in a descending way until reaching the final independent events of origin. From this analysis, a representative logical information flow diagram is obtained. FTA is useful for qualitative analysis because it reveals the various combinations of failures and cause-and-effect relationships that provoke the unwanted top event, as for quantitative analysis in case of calculating the top event occurrence probability from those to which the basic independent event can arise.

FMEA can be used to discover and analyze all potential failure modes conceivable for a process or system and the effects they can cause as well as to determine how to correct or mitigate those. Correction is based on the evaluation of the degree of severity and criticality as well as their occurrence and cause detection levels. From there, the actions to be taken are determined.

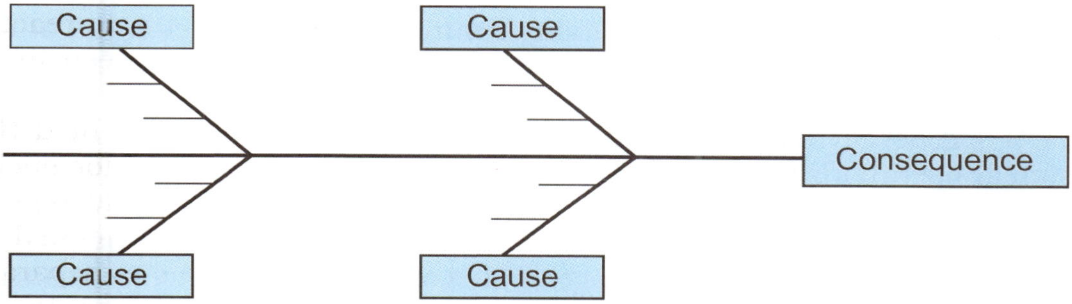

Fish bone figure shown above is self explanatory as to how various causes are aligned and can finally lead to a consequence which could be an OOS result. By sequencing them properly and doing the impact analysis of each, one can arrive at a root cause/s.

First Step: Develop a SMART SOP

It is a well known convention that Standard Operating Procedure (SOP) should be SMART in the sense it should be Specific to the purpose, parameters described in the SOP should be Measurable, Achievable. SOP should be Relevant to the job actually carried by the firm and it should be Traceable i.e. it should be properly numbered, controlled and it must be possible to track the changes made in the SOP.

Additionally the SOP that governs OOS investigations should give checklist to know the assignable cause of OOS and help the analyst and the supervisor uncover laboratory error. The SOP also should define the options for what to do in the event that no assignable cause is discovered. SOP should describe finite reporting times for the various phases of the investigation, and describe requirements of the internal documentation that will demonstrate that the SOP was indeed followed. The SOP should emphasize how essential it is that all data generated during testing and during the subsequent investigations be retained.

SOP must clearly define role and responsibilities of Analyst, Supervisor and Manager as applicable. The SOP should distinguish between out-of-specification investigations and out-of-trend investigations The SOP should include careful consideration of measurements that may be exempt from out-of-specification investigations.

Scope of the SOP

SOP on OOS is expected to address all the OOS results obtained during Chemical, Physical & Microbiological testing of Active Pharmaceutical Ingredients (API), Raw Materials, Packing Materials, Various Intermediates of API & Finished Drug Products, Stability testing of drug product & API at own lab as well as contract lab. It is applicable to products manufactured on contract basis too.

OOS is generally not applicable to results obtained during machine setting or similar operations where variability could be there. Similarly data generated during training or generated under a technology transfer protocol may be excluded if the suspect data were generated by a person not yet qualified to perform the method. Similarly, data generated on intentionally stressed samples (part of forced degradation study) need not have to be investigated as out of specification.

OOS Investigation: Phase I

Phase I deals with a laboratory investigation. A checklist of possible sources of error may aid this part of the investigation. Checklist items to use in reviewing the analyst's notebook can include points like:

- Was the correct amount of sample taken?
- Were the sample dilutions correctly performed?
- Were other reagents and solutions correctly prepared and used?
- Are the calculations correct?
- Were the correct volumetric flasks and pipettes used?
- Whether the analyst was trained to do the activity?
- Whether all instruments/glassware used for the analysis were calibrated?
- Whether atmospheric conditions were proper which could have led to absorption of moisture etc.
- Was there any deviation from the prescribed standard testing procedure?

Similar checklists can be developed to identify sources of error in sample integrity and handling, instrument performance, method parameters, analyst's technique, the test procedure, standards and instrument output.

Laboratory error should be relatively rare. Frequent errors suggest a problem that might be due to inadequate training of analysts, poorly maintained or improperly calibrated equipment, or careless work.

Whenever laboratory error is identified, the firm should determine the source of that error and take corrective action to prevent recurrence. When clear evidence of laboratory error exists, laboratory testing results should be invalidated and retesting should be carried out by two analysts including the original analyst who is equally trained and qualified. Reanalysis should be done on the same solution which was used earlier (e.g. injected in HPLC) or on remaining part of the same sample. If all results are found OK within a permissible variation, batch can be released.

When evidence of laboratory error remains unclear, a Full-scale OOS investigation (Phase II) should be conducted to determine what caused the unexpected results.

OOS Investigation: Phase II

Phase II includes sampling investigation, manufacturing investigation and retesting if justified.

Sampling Investigation

When all data have been evaluated, an investigation might conclude that the original sample was prepared/stored/handled improperly and was therefore not representative of the batch quality. Improper sample preparation might be indicated, for example, by widely varied results obtained from several aliquots of an original composite (after determining there was no error in the performance of the analysis). Resampling should be performed by the same qualified, validated methods that were used for the initial sample. However, if the investigation determines that the initial sampling method was inherently inadequate, a new accurate sampling method must be developed, documented, and reviewed and approved by QA.

Reporting Testing Results

General practice is to average out the results obtained. However the guideline demands that one has to exercise utmost precaution while doing so. There are both appropriate and inappropriate uses of averaging test data during original testing and during an OOS investigation. Averaging data can be a valid approach, but its use depends upon the sample and its purpose. For example, in an optical rotation test, several discrete measurements are averaged to determine the optical rotation for a sample, and this average is reported as the test result. If the sample can be assumed to be homogeneous, using averages can provide a more accurate result. In the case of microbiological assays, it is customary to report the average result because of the inherent error observed in microbiological analysis. However in all these cases the firm has to define allowed relative standard deviation for each type of test. This must be based on method validation studies.

Averaging test data should be used during an OOS investigation only if they were used during the original testing too that produced the OOS result.

However reliance on averaging has the disadvantage of hiding variability among individual test results. For this reason, all individual test results should normally be reported as separate values along with the average and relative standard deviation. Averaging can also conceal variations in different portions of a batch, or within a sample. For example, the use of averages is inappropriate when performing powder blend/mixture uniformity or dosage form content uniformity determinations. In these cases, testing is intended to measure variability within the product, and individual results provide the information for such an evaluation. In such cases each individual result has to fall within the acceptable limit along with RSD and the average result.

US Guideline gives an example of an assay of a finished drug with a specification of 90 to 110 percent, an initial OOS result of 89 percent followed by additional retest results of 90 percent and 91 percent would produce an average of 90 percent.

While this average would meet specifications, actually additional test results also tend to confirm the original OOS result. However, in another situation with the same specifications, an initial OOS result of 80 percent followed by additional test results of 85 percent and 105 percent would also produce an average of 90 percent, but present a much different picture. These results do not confirm the original OOS result but show high variability and may not be reliable. In both examples, the individual results, not the average, should be used to evaluate the quality of the product.

It is difficult to put the whole process in words. Easiest way to learn about the actions to be taken at different stages is to have a flowchart in your SOP. Please find attached herewith two OOS Decision Trees. One of them is for investigation of OOS result obtained for Finished Product/API and another one is for Raw Materials and Finished Products.

Time Cycle for Various Activities

Though there is no fixed period but generally laboratory investigation should take maximum about 7 days, sampling investigation needs to be completed in 2-7 days, production investigation can take from 2 to 21 days. Thus the final report can be prepared and decision can be taken within 30 days from the date of occurrence of the event. Above time lines are only indicative in nature; actual time taken shall depend on the nature of OOS result. US FDA requires that if an OOS result is confirmed for the commercial batch which is already into the market (e.g. stability failure), Field Alert Notification has to be submitted to US FDA within 3 days.

Investigation Report

It must describe what happened exactly, where it happened and when it happened. Root cause/s must be stated in the report to the extent possible. Investigation must not be limited to only to the batch/s in question but it must be extended to all other batches where there is a reason to believe that similar error could have happened . It must state the final disposition like 'OOS result confirmed, batch rejected' or 'OOS result not confirmed, error identified, batch rechecked, found OK, hence released', etc. Immediate corrective action for the batch/s in question must be stated along with preventive actions to avoid similar problem in future. Actions taken thereof must be reviewed subsequently for their effectiveness.

SUMMARY

In reality a firm can get an OOS result which needs to be reported in a transparent manner and investigated scientifically. Unless OOS is confirmed it is not a failure. Fortunately today we have clear US guideline on OOS. The article describes essentials for conducting an investigation of an out-of-specification result in a compliant, reliable, and timely manner. However, no guideline can describe every possible scenario that can exist in a practical life. Hence every firm has to make use of scientific logic and take the decision based on Decision has to be guided by the interest of customer i.e. customer.

The best practice is to minimize the generation of OOS results through a corrective and preventive mechanism. Careful description of methods and reportable values and having appropriate system suitability parameters can help to avoid out-of-specification results. Qualification of equipment and analysts and rigorous transfer of analytical technology will help to ensure that a laboratory is fully capable of performing an analytical method.

REFERENCES

1. "FDA's Summary of Judge Wolin's Interpretation of GMP Issues Contained in the Court's Ruling in USA vs. Barr Laboratories", (GMP Institute), www.gmp1st.com/barrsum.htm
2. "Guidance for Industry, Investigating Out of Specification (OOS) Test Results for Pharmaceutical Production", Food and Drug Administration, October 2006, http://www.fda.gov/cder/guidance/index.htm

3. J.D. Hofer and E.C. Rickard, "A Guide to Determining Sample Sizes and Outlier Criteria in Analytical Investigations", Pharm. Technol. 25 (3), 52–66 (2001). PT
4. ICH Q9, Quality Risk Management, Nov 2005 http://www.ich.org/LOB/media/MEDIA1957.pdf

Note: Whatever is written in this article is in my personal capacity. It should not be considered as regulatory opinion or the opinion of my company.

OOS INVESTIGATION FLOW CHART FOR APIs, DRUG PRODUCTS AND THEIR INTERMEDIATES

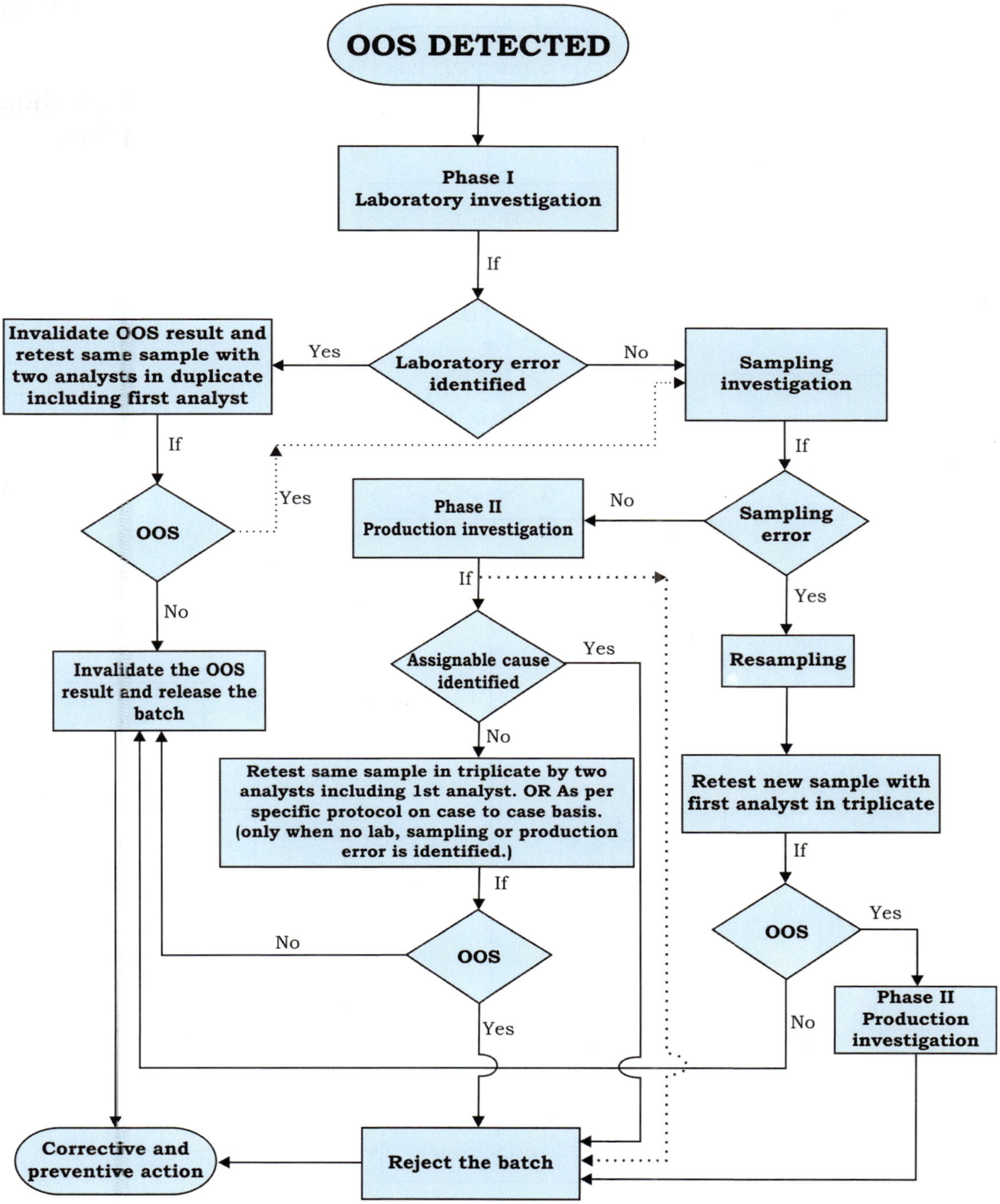

OOS INVESTIGATION FLOW CHART FOR RAW MATERIAL AND PACKAGING MATERIAL

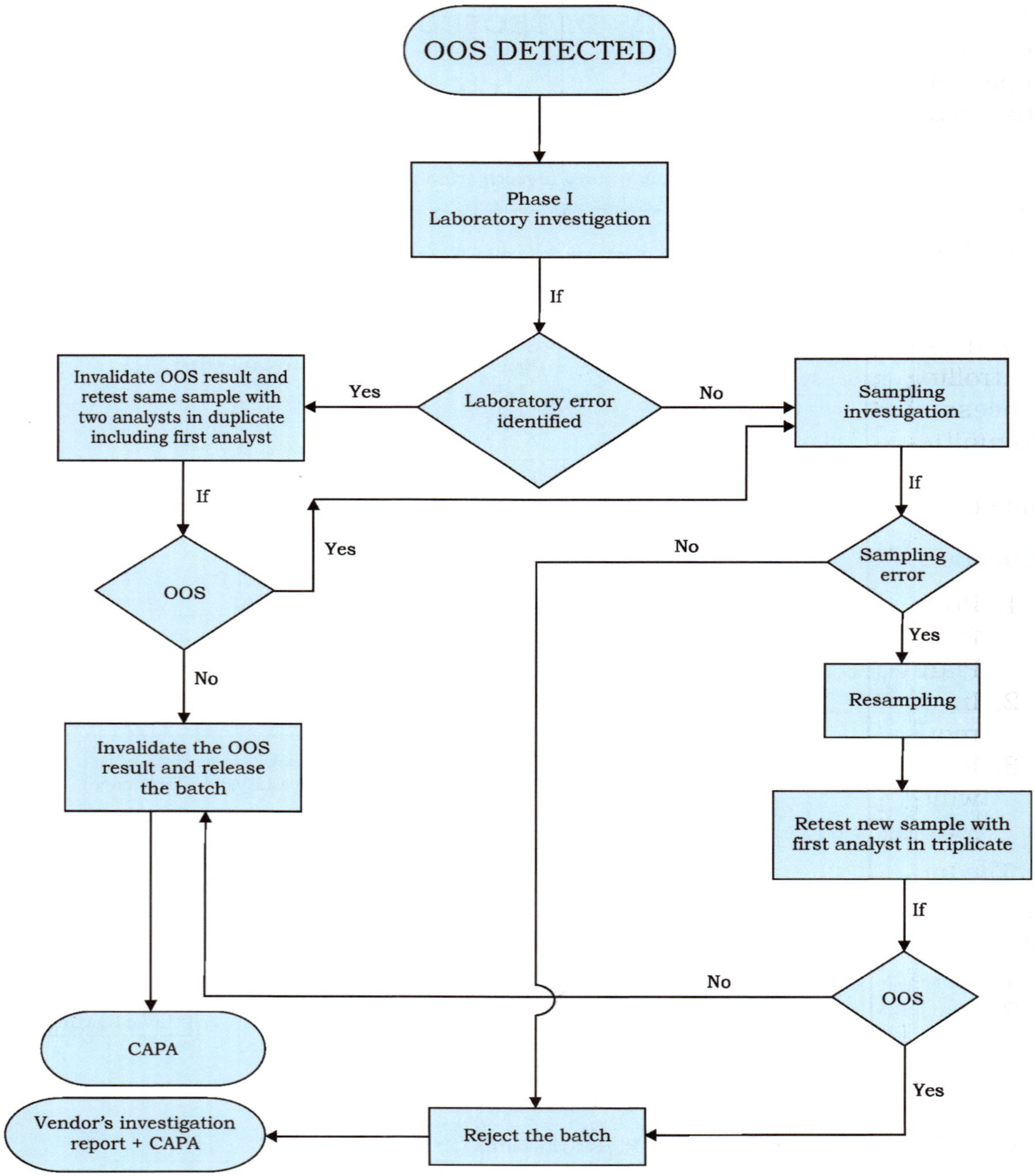

SOP ON CHANGE IN SPECIFICATIONS
(Instrument, Analytical Method or Analytical Environment)

Objective

To establish a systematic approach for notification, evaluation and implementation of technical changes in specifications, instruments, chemicals, analytical methods and analytical environment.

Scope

This change shall apply for the technical changes pertaining to analysis of Drug Products, Bulk Pharmaceutical Chemicals and Intermediates.

Responsibility

Members of change control committee shall be responsible for evaluating, controlling and approving the changes made in the procedures for analysis, process specifications and related areas. In all cases, Change Control Committee, which includes Q.A. head as one of the essential management team members, who shall have the final authority to approve and implement the changes.

Procedure

1. Proposal for change may be initiated by the concerned R&D (Drug Products) and (Chemicals), Regulatory Dept., Projects Dept., Corporate Planning Dept. or concerned locational Quality Control laboratory.
2. In case of technical changes pertaining to deviation from compendial requirement, the intimation shall include comparative data.
3. Request for change pertaining to the following aspects but not limited to which are likely to influence quality shall be prepared by the concerned Manager/Department Head/Section.

The Incharge in the prescribed format shall forward to Coordinator Manager, Q.A. at location for proposals raised at location and in case of proposal raised at Corporate, shall forward to the Divisional Head of Quality:

1. General procedures for laboratory working.
2. Material specifications.
3. Packaging material specification.
4. In-process/intermediate specifications.
5. Finished product's specifications.
6. Test procedures (methods of analysis)
7. Laboratory equipment/instrument.

8. SOPs pertaining to laboratory procedures.
9. Any other procedure pertaining to Quality Control.
10. Analytical laboratory site.

Plan of Action and Implementation

1. Change Control Committee shall review the proposal received.
2. After evaluation of the proposal, the Change Control Committee shall approve or reject the proposal for change. The decision shall be conveyed to Manager Q.A.
3. The change shall be implemented at location through Manager Q.A.
4. The implementation of change, after approval from Change Control Committee, shall be conveyed by the originator of the proposal to the Manager Q.A. at location.
5. After implementation of the change, the necessary data, when required by Change Control Committee, shall be forwarded by Q.A. Manager.

Documentation

1. Documents undergoing such changes/revisions shall have revision cards attached to it and "controlled" copy holder shall update the change.
2. Such revised written procedures/pages/sections/part of the document shall be forwarded to the "controlled" copy holder concerned for replacement of the obsolete pages/sections/part of the document.
3. Obsolete pages/sections/part of the document shall be destroyed after their replacement with revised copy/copies.
4. One set of such obsolete pages/sections/part of the document shall be maintained at location Manager Quality Assurance with "Obsolete/Void" stamp in red ink marked on it.
5. A set of "Master copies" of such "OBSOLETE" document shall be maintained at Corporate Quality Division with "OBSOLETE/VOID" stamp in red ink marked on pages.

FORMAT FOR CHANGE IN SPECIFICATIONS

01. Location: Department: Proposal No. and Date:
02. Proposed change(s):
03. Scientific rationale/justification:
04. Supporting data (if required): Enclosed/Not required
05. Probable date of implementation:
06. Date forwarded to *C.C.C.: (a) Initial
    (b) After first review by Corporate
07. Proposal requested by: *C.C.C. (Location)

(To be signed by concerned Section Heads)

Analyst	M.Q.C.	M.Q.A.

Conclusion: Approved/Rejected/Comments

Evaluation - *C.C.C. (Corporate) Approval			
M.Q.C.	M.Q.A.	M R&D	Divisional Head Quality

*** C.C.C. = Change Control Committee**

GUIDELINES FOR SETTING UP A PHARMACEUTICAL CONTROL LABORATORY

As per schedule-M to the Drugs and Cosmetic Act, for each manufacturing unit it is mandatory to have a quality control laboratory equipped with professionally experienced staff and laboratory equipments to carry out tests for potency, efficacy and safety of drugs and to establish that the subject sample complies with appropriate specifications. The reliability and consistency of the test results primarily depend on overall attitude of the analyst in addition to instrument and analytical technique employed for analysis. A typical pharmaceutical control laboratory is composed of several divisions/sections for carrying out various tests requiring different analytical techniques.

Various Divisions/Sections

1. Chemical and Physico-chemical.
2. Instrumental
3. Microbiology
   (a) General microbiology testing
   (b) Antibiotic assay
   (c) Vitamins assay
   (d) Sterility testing
4. Pharmacognosy
5. Pharmacology
   (a) Pyrogen testing (using rabbits and BET)
   (b) Bioassay
   (c) Animal house
6. Reference/working standards/Protocols repository

List of Common Instruments for Central Instrument Laboratory

- Double beam UV-visible spectrophotometer.
- FTIR spectrophotometer (may require controlled humidity).
- High performance liquid chromatograph (HPLC), isocratic/gradient system with different detectors.
- High performance thin-layer chromatographic (HPTLC) system with different accessories.
- Gas liquid chromatograph (GLC) with different detectors.
- GC-MS system.
- Spectrophotoflourimeter.
- Atomic absorption spectrometer (AAS); with various lamps.
- Polarimeter, digital.

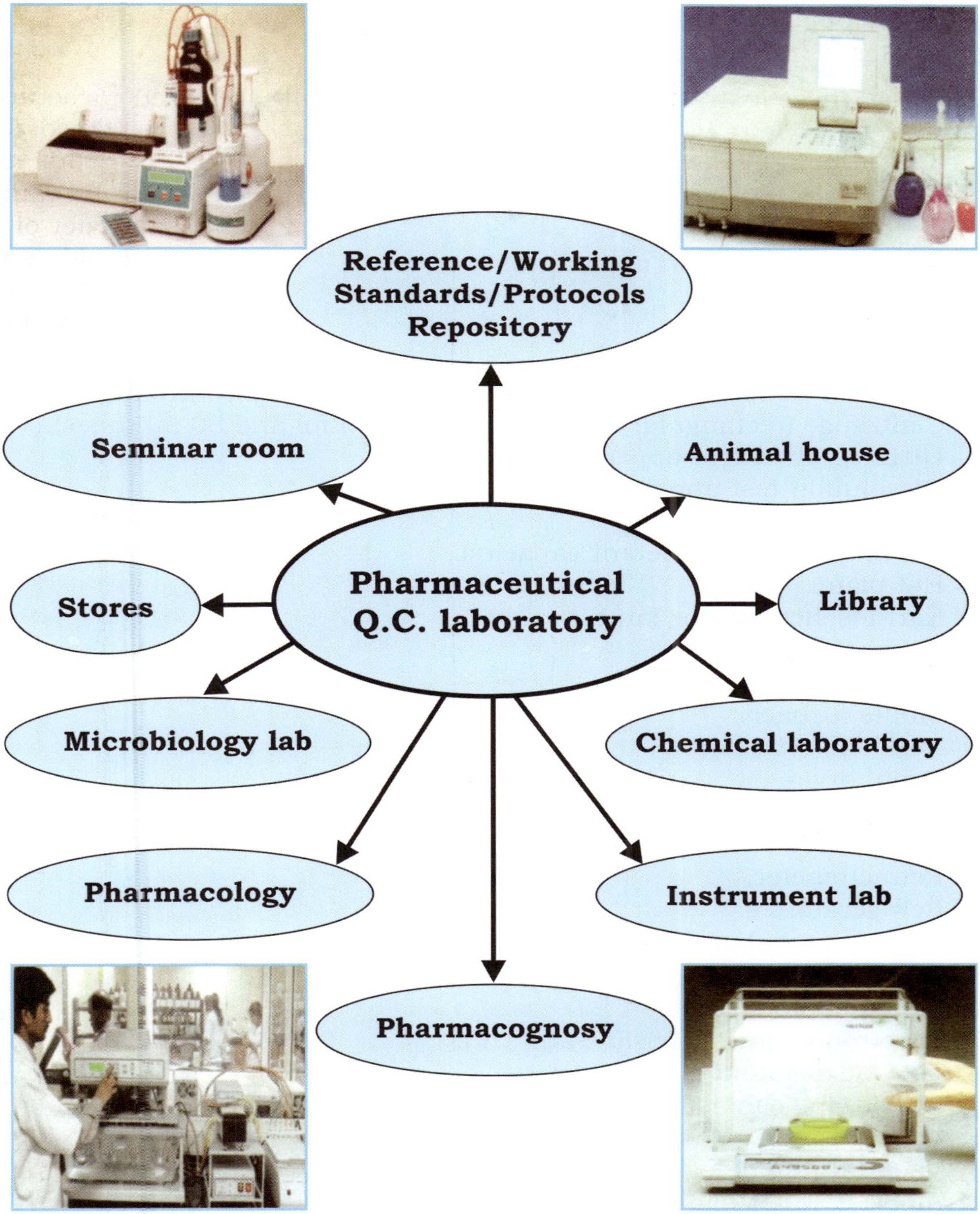

Different divisions/Sections of a Quality Control Laboratory

- Analytical balance with printer.
- pH meter.

Note: All these instruments should be provided fully stabilized current and housed in air conditioned room.

Common Instruments/Equipments for Chemical and Physico-chemical Analysis

1. Ammonia distillation apparatus.
2. Balance, analytical.
3. Top-pan balance.
4. Boiling-range apparatus.
5. Constant temperature water-bath (thermostatically controlled).
6. Centrifuge (rectangular with head to hold 15 ml and 50 ml tubes).
7. Disintegration test apparatus.
8. Dissolution test apparatus.
9. Flourimeter.
10. Heating mantles (different capacity).
11. Hot plate.
12. Karl-Fischer titrator (auto-tirator).
13. Magnetic stirrer.
14. Melting-range apparatus.
15. Muffle furnace.
16. Nesslers' cylinders.
17. Oven, drying.
18. pH meter.
19. Polarimeter.
20. Refractometer.
21. Refrigerator.
22. Semi-microbalance.
23. Sieves (set).
24. Flame photometer.
25. Spectrophotometer (visible and UV).
26. TLC kit including accessories.
27. UV viewing cabinet (short and long wavelength).
28. Vacuum oven.
29. Vacuum pump.
30. All glass water distillation assembly (single, double or triple).
31. Hot-air oven.
32. Vortex mixer.
33. Sonicator with heating assembly.

34. Deep freezer.
35. Potentiometric titrator.
36. Oxygen flask combustion apparatus.
37. Fuming chamber.
38. Infrared moisture balance.
39. Bulk density apparatus.
40. Refrigerated centrifuge.
41. Particle size analyser.
42. Columns for GLC and HPLC analysis. TLC/HPTLC pre-coated plates.
43. Viscometer.
44. Magnetic stirrer with hot plate.
45. Vacuum (rotary) evaporator (film flash evaporator).
46. Hot and cold air blower.
47. Rotary shaking machine.
48. Grinder mixer.
49. Soxhet extraction apparatus.
50. Dessicator (plain and vacuum type).

Note: Specific equipments shall be required to undertake the testing of any specific material such as sutures, surgical, condoms, disposable/non-disposable syringes, needles, blood bags, etc.

No listing of chemicals, reagents, glassware and general laboratory implements is given, as such lists can easily be compiled at the laboratory. Specific equipments will depend on the number and types of various units and sample to be analysed. However, it has to be stressed that sufficient glassware be kept in stock in the laboratory to allow for possible breakage in use, especially in situation where long lead times are needed to get replacements. This should pertain to items of everyday use like burettes, pipettes, separating funnels, conical and volumetric flasks and graduated cylinders.

List of common instruments/equipments for microbiology testing

1. Antibiotic zone reader.
2. Autoclave (horizontal).
3. Colony counter with magnifier (table model).
4. UV-visible spectrophotometer.
5. Deep freezer.
6. B.O.D. incubator.
7. Laminar flow, bench type.
8. Membrane filtration assembly (both single and three stages).
9. Microbalance/analytical balance.
10. Microscope (binocular).

11. Hot air sterilizer/oven.
12. pH meter.
13. Refrigerator.
14. Water-bath (thermostatically controlled).
15. Sonicator.
16. Centrifuge.
17. Hot plate.
18. Magnetic stirrer with hot plate.
19. Vacuum pump.
20. Vacuum oven.
21. Top-pan loading balance.
22. Vial decapping machine.
23. All glass double water distillation assembly.
24. Fluorescence microscope.

General chemicals, reagents and glassware may be compiled in the laboratory itself.

Note:

(a) Facility for 'AHU' with positive pressure.
(b) Walls, floors and ceiling should be non-shedding, non-cracking.
(c) Flooring should be unbroken both at the junction between the walls and the floor as well as and the ceiling.
(d) No sink and drain.
(e) Doors and windows shall be made of non-shedding materials like aluminium, stainless steel or glass.
(f) Doors and windows shall be of double panes.
(g) All entrances fitted with air-lock system.
(h) Use of wood should be avoided.

List of equipments for pharmacological testing

Pharmacological analysis primarily involves:

1. Pyogen testing.
   (a) Using rabbits.
   (b) LAL (Bacterial Endotoxin Test - BET)
2. Toxicity tests.
3. Bio-assays.

Equipment

1. Isolated organ bath.
2. Kymograph complete with operation table, respiration pump.

3. Manometer.
4. Hot air oven/sterilizer.
5. Oxygen cylinder.
6. Pyrothermometer with 6 probes.
7. Self-indicating balance to weigh animals.
8. Analytical balance.
9. Rabbit restraint boxes.
10. Animal cages as per requirement.
11. BOD incubator.
12. pH meter.
13. Dessicator (plain and vacuum type).
14. Top-pan loading balance.
15. Refrigerator.
16. Centrifuge.
17. Vial decapping machine.
18. Microscope.
19. UV-visible spectrophotometer.
20. Water-bath.
21. Water-bath thermostatically controlled.
22. Magnetic stirrer with hot plate.
23. Shadowless lamp.
24. Facilities for conducting LAL/bacterial endotoxin test.
25. Hot plate.
26. All glass double water distillation assembly.

List of chemicals, glassware, syringes, surgical, equipments and other accessories may be compiled.

Manufacturing unit output in finished product, laboratory output in analytical data

Environmental requirements

Light	≥ 600 Lux
Noise level	NMT 45 decibels
Humidity (RH)	35–55%
Temperature	25 ± 2 °C
Electricity	Constant, use of UPS recommended
Fume hoods	Fitted with heavy duty exhaust fans
Furniture	Movable module type

Note: The laboratory should preferably be centrally airconditioned.

Protocols/Specifications Repository

1. Every drug testing laboratory must have the correct edition of all the Pharmacopoeia official in the country including latest supplements, addendums.
2. All updates, corrections must be noted in the principle volumes of the pharmacopoea to prevent any possibility of obsolete portion being used.
3. A separate repository should be compiled for patent and proprietary medicines. The test methods or specifications be validated by the respective manufacturer or the laboratory itself. The validated methods so developed either by the manufacturer or in the laboratory must comply with the requirements of pharmacopoeia in respect of accuracy, precision, linearity, reproducibility, specificity and ruggedness.

GOOD LABORATORY PRACTICES (An Update)*

"Object of analysis is to obtain information that offers the greatest possibility of translation into a useful and satisfying statement of the properties of material system."

– Chirnside 1961

Any laboratory environment consists of people, facility, instrumentation, chemicals supplies and samples submitted for analysis. There has to be a logical and scientific manner of organization and management which drive the laboratory system. Since each laboratory works in individual manner, it requires customised approach and attitude. Every laboratory depends on consistency and development of system which ensure consistency. The consistency in laboratory depends upon well managed and adequately trained people well maintained facilities calibrated instrumentation, high quality chemicals, adequate supplies and proper handling of samples. All these combined in a system are termed as good laboratory practices or GLPs. Good laboratory practices are applicable to all types of laboratories which undertake testing of samples of drug substances or drug products and are attached to a manufacturing unit (private), test samples on behalf of other manufacturers (commercial) and set up by government organizations, e.g., various FDA's laboratories, custom's laboratories or central drugs laboratory.

Quality control has been worded (ASQC, 1983) as "the operational techniques and activities which sustain quality of a product or service which will satisfy a given need." Quality assurance also bears a closely worded explanation "as planned or systematic actions necessary to provide adequate confidence that a product will satisfy given needs" (here the product is to be treated as analytical report).

Both quality control and quality assurance attain greater importance as all pharmaceutical operations depend heavily upon sample testing. (Techniques such as PAT, i.e., process analytical technologies and process-simulation techniques through six-sigma are emerging science and may become popular in times to come.)

Pharmaceutical quality control testing of a manufacturer is usually a matter of repetitive testing of samples of active pharmaceutical ingredients or of a limited number of pharmaceutical products, whereas other quality control laboratories such as public testing laboratories or government department laboratories deal with a much wider range of pharmaceutical substances and products. Public testing laboratories or government department laboratories

---

* Kapil Bhargava, Ex. Dy. Drugs Controller (India)

therefore, have to apply a wider variety of test methods. All these quality control laboratories may perform some or all quality control activities, e.g. sampling and testing of APIs (drug substances), excipients and pharmaceutical finished formulations (drug products), stability testing, testing against specifications (part analysis) and investigative testing (testing of complaint samples), etc. Whereas bigger laboratories may develop their own code for good practices for various activities in their laboratory, special consideration for set-up and methodology of testing is to be given to laboratories attached to small or medium scale pharmaceutical firms having limited resources.

There are mainly two types of activities in pharmaceutical quality control laboratories:

- Compliance testing of APIs, pharmaceutical excipients and pharmaceutical products employing "official" methods/pharmacopoeial methods, validated analytical procedures developed by the laboratory or validated analytical procedures provided by another manufacturer and verified by the laboratory or
- Investigative testing of sub-standard quality medicine, suspicious or counterfeit products, received by the laboratory for examination and comments.

Good Laboratory Practices are to be applied to both these type of activities as result of both these type of testing bear a very significant after-effect.

For the quality of a drug/medicine sample to be correctly reported, the laboratory should be in position to draw sample by its own personnel according to SOPs or should be able to correctly assess the sample submitted to it so that the analysis is correctly planned and meticulously executed. Analytical results must be competently evaluated to determine whether the sample complies with the specifications or other relevant criteria. Thus in order to attain these objectives, proper persons should be employed by the laboratory and it is to be properly set-up in respect of its premises and must possess necessary instruments/equipment needed.

Various GLP codes are available and these are quite close to one another. The Codes from WHO, PIC (pharmaceutical inspection convention) and Schedule L1 of Drugs and Cosmetics Rules of India are popular ones. Most GLP codes are presented in form of "guidelines", it may be mentioned that usage of word "should" in the codes makes the requirement as essential and is expected to be followed at all the times. Whereas conditions in Schedule L1 of Drugs & Cosmetics Rules, are mandatory and "requirements" are to be followed by all drug testing laboratories in India. The key aspects of GLPs are mentioned below.

Personnel

The laboratory must have sufficient personnel with the necessary education, training, technical knowledge and experience for their assigned functions. The technical management should ensure the competence of all persons who operate specific equipment, instruments or other devices, who are performing tests and/or calibrations, validations or verifications. This can be done through training of staff. Their training should be appropriately supervised and should be assessed on completion. In case of receipt on a new instrument in the laboratory, particular staff member should undergo additional training and this should be documented.

The laboratory should maintain current job duties and responsibilities for all personnel involved in testing and/or calibration, validation/verifications. The laboratory should also maintain records of all technical personnel, describing their qualifications, training, and experience.

Head of laboratory (supervisor) should have qualifications appropriate to the position, with good experience in analysis of pharmaceuticals and laboratory management of a pharmaceutical quality control laboratory either in the regulatory sector or in industry. He/she is responsible for issue of COAs or and analytical testing reports. This person also ensures that procedures for performing calibration, verification and re-qualification of instruments, monitoring of environmental and storage conditions are in place and are conducted as required and person trained according to their job functions. This person is also responsible for ensuring various regulations applicable to laboratory. It may be pointed out in case samples of narcotic substances are handled by the laboratory, the laboratory in-charge will ensure that all provisions are met. Other levels of personnel may be depicted in an organisation chart and their reporting hierarchy.

Analysts are normally graduates in pharmacy, analytical chemistry, microbiology or other relevant subjects with the requisite knowledge, skills and ability to adequately perform the tasks assigned to them by management and to supervise other technical staff. Adequate number of persons are to be employed for testing and other activities in the laboratory. Indian regulation does not clarify adequacy of staff in the laboratory Schedule L1, however mention that "staff in the laboratory shall possess necessary qualification, proper training and shall have adequate, experience for the assigned duties"; the adequacy depends upon type of samples received and analysis conducted. As a thumb-rule close to two samples per analyst per day are usually treated as adequate in case of chemical and instrumental analysis in a laboratory attached to a manufacturing site as the samples are known. This statistics generally reduces for commercial laboratories and further reduce in government laboratories.

Premises

The laboratory facilities are to be suitably located, of adequate size and be of sound construction. The facilities in the lab are to be designed to suit the functions and operations to be conducted. Rest and refreshment rooms should be separate from laboratory areas. Changing areas and toilets should be easily accessible and appropriately provided for number of users.

The laboratory facilities must have adequate safety equipment located appropriately and measures must be in place to ensure good housekeeping. Each laboratory is to be equipped with adequate work benches, work stations, fume hoods, etc. and required instrumentation/equipment are to be provided.

The environmental conditions, including lighting, energy sources, temperature, humidity, air pressure, etc., are to be appropriate to the functions and operations to be performed. The laboratory shall ensure that the environmental conditions are monitored, controlled and documented and do not invalidate the results or adversely affect the quality of the measurements. The laboratory therefore can be partitioned into analytical sections for Chemical Analysis (wet lab), Instrumental Analysis, Microbiology Analysis and Biological analysis (if required). It is good to provide a separate "hot area" for experiments or supplies (distilled water preparation) requiring heat and a glassware washing and drying area. As now-a-days experiments of wet analysis are reduced and most analysis is done through liquid chromatography, this lab, therefore, may be accordingly sized. (For adequacy and working benches here and for comfortable working, I recommend minimum 5 linear feet to be provided for one chemist – internationally it is 15 feet.) While making or re-designing the laboratory, provision is to be made for one room for routine instruments UV and IR spectrophotometers, the other for HPLC, and third for GLC (in case that is installed). Air-conditioning for temperature control and dehumidifier for humidity control are to be provided as required for instrument and samples under analysis. All considerations are to be given for providing these conditions for stability of analyte in solution. In case experiment requires monochromatic light or dark room these are to be provided. Microbiology lab is to be divided at least into media preparation room, washing and sterilization room, experiment room (with LAF work-station) and incubation room. All clean room conditions such as provision of "class-conditions" in testing room (class 10,000), two air locks for proper gowning and pass box for sample and supplies to be taken to testing area, are to be provided. In case sterility testing is undertaken the set-up and conditions are to be the same that are provided for manufacture of sterile provided to ensure that an inadequately set-up lab atmosphere does not compromise sterility test results.

Schedule L1 of Drugs and Cosmetics Rules was published in Gazette of Govt. of India. Requirements of premises are depicted below:

(a) (i) The laboratories shall be designed, constructed and maintained so as to prevent entry of insects and rodents besides cross contamination;
(ii) interior surface (walls, floor, and ceilings) shall be smooth and free from cracks, and permit easy cleaning and disinfection;
(iii) adequate provision is made not only for space and equipment for carrying out necessary test but also for utilities like water, power and gas;
(iv) air ventilation system shall ensure dust free environment.

(b) The laboratories shall be provided with adequate lighting and ventilation and if necessary, air-conditioning to maintain satisfactory temperature and relative humidity that will not adversely affect the testing and storage of drugs or the accuracy of the functioning of the laboratory equipments or instruments.

(c) The drainage system facilities shall be such as to facilitate proper maintenance and prevent water logging in the laboratory.

(d) Tabletops shall be constructed with acid, alkali and solvent resistant material and shall be smooth and free from crevices as far as possible.

(e) All bio-medical laboratory waste shall be destroyed as per the provisions of the Bio-Medical Waste (Management and Handling) Rules, 1996.

(f) Adequate space with proper storage conditions in the laboratory shall be provided for keeping reference and working standards and be maintained by the quality control department. Standard Operating Procedure (SOP) for the maintenance of reference standards and evaluation of Working and Secondary standards shall be prepared by the laboratory.

(g) The air circulation is maintained in the area where sterility test is carried out as per Schedule 'M'.

(h) Bio-burden shall be routinely maintained in the controlled and uncontrolled area (e.g., air locks).

These requirements are to be followed by all testing laboratories of a manufacturing site.

In case the laboratory is handling highly potent or toxic substances, special precautions must be taken and, if necessary, there should be separate and dedicated unit/equipment (e.g. isolator, laminar flow work bench) to handle, weigh and prepare (for analysis) these substances.

Archiving (record room) facilities should be provided to ensure the secure (preferably fire-proof) storage and retrieval of all documents. The design and condition of the archives should be such as to protect the contents from deterioration. Access to the archives must be restricted to designated personnel.

Procedures must be in place for the safe removal of different types of waste including toxic waste (chemical and biological), reagents, samples, solvents and air filters.

If in-vivo biological testing (e.g., rabbit pyrogen test) is included in the scope of the laboratory then the animal houses must be isolated from the other laboratory areas with separate entrance and air-conditioning system. The rooms required to be provided are animal quarantine, animal quarters, pre-conditioning room, testing room, cage washing room, feed storage room, feed preparation room and room for sick animals. Air conditioning and air displacement system (for fowl smell removal) are to be provided. There is other relevant literature available for maintenance of animal house and Schedule L1 has to mention as under:

(i) Animal House shall have the approval of the Committee for the Purpose of Control and Supervision on Experiments on Animals (CPCSEA).
(ii) Designed in such a way that there is an arrangement to quarantine the new animals procured or purchased and have a provision for clean corridor and dirty corridor.
(iii) In case of a diseased animal proper diagnosis shall be done and proper record of treatment shall be maintained.
(iv) Different types of animals shall be housed separately with proper identification.
(v) A Standard Operating Procedure shall be prepared for breeding and care of animals, maintenance, cleaning or sanitation with suitable schedule for cleaning of animal cages, racks, floor and other equipments.
(vi) The animal house shall have proper air-conditioning (temperature and humidity) with proper lighting and be monitored regularly and documented periodically.

Laboratory Storage Facilities

The storage facilities should be well organized for the correct storage of samples, reagents and equipment.

Separate storage facilities must be maintained for the secure storage of samples, retained samples, reagents and laboratory accessories, reference substances and reference materials. Storage facilities must be equipped to store material, if necessary, under cold temperature (2°C to 8°C).

Appropriate safety procedures should be designed and strictly followed for flammable reagents are stored or used. The laboratory must provide separate rooms or areas for storing flammable substances, fuming and concentrated acids and bases, volatile amines and other reagents, such as hydrochloric acid, nitric acid, ammonia and bromine. Self-igniting materials, such as metallic sodium, must also be stored separately. Small stocks of acids, bases and solvents may be kept in the laboratory store but the main stocks of these items should be retained preferably in a store separate from the laboratory building. Gases used for GLC also should be stored in a dedicated and secured place outside the testing laboratory and placement of cylinders should be such that gas pipes be not of excessive length.

Quality Management System

The laboratory management should establish, implement and maintain a quality management system in accordance with the laboratory activities. While designing this system, it should be kept in mind the type of analysis being conducted there, quantum of samples for testing, and calibration, validation and verification activities the laboratory undertakes. The laboratory management must ensure that systems, programmes, procedures and instructions are clearly spelt out for assuring the quality of the test results laboratory generates. A copy of this system must be communicated and be made available to all concerned personnel for implementation. It is clarified here that QC laboratories attached to a manufacturing unit may have these aspect spelt out in main quality policy document of the site and a separate document is not to be made.

The quality manual should contain as a minimum:

- A quality policy statement, including at least the following:
  - a statement of the laboratory management's intentions with respect to the standard of service it will provide;
  - a commitment to establishing, implementing and maintaining an effective quality management system;
  - the laboratory management's commitment to good professional practice and quality of testing, calibration, validation and verification;
  - a requirement that all personnel concerned with testing and calibration activities within the laboratory familiarize themselves with the documentation concerning quality and the implementation of the policies and procedures in their work.
- Structure of the laboratory (organizational chart).
- Procedures to be followed for retaining quality and the persons responsible for implementation of these.
- References to specific quality assurance procedures for each test e.g. (validated/verified methods are being followed).
- Information on the appropriate qualifications, experience and competencies that personnel are required to possess.

- Information on initial and in-service training of staff.
- Policy for internal/external audit (or both) and management review.
- Policy and procedure to inform staff of corrective and preventive actions introduced as a consequence of discrepancies detected.
- Policy for dealing with complaints.
- Policy for selecting, establishing and approving analytical procedures.
- Policy for handling of out-of-specifications results.
- Policy for usage of reference/working substances and reference materials.
- Policy for participation in appropriate proficiency testing scheme (analyst's validation) and evaluation of the performance.
- Policy to select suppliers of materials and services.

Besides standard test procedures (STPs) the laboratory must establish, implement and maintain authorized written standard operating procedures (SOPs) at least for:

- Matters relating to personnel, including qualifications, training, clothing and hygiene.
- Change control.
- Receipt of consignments of materials (e.g., samples, reagents).
- Procurement, preparation and control of reference substances and reference materials.
- Internal labelling, quarantine and storage of samples (and materials).
- Qualification of equipment (e.g. KBr press, Autoclaves, LAF workstations etc.).
- Calibration of instruments (general policy).
- Preventive maintenance and verification of instruments and equipment.
- Sampling of starting materials and intermediate products (if performed by the laboratory).
- Handling of atypical and out-of-specification results.
- Validation of analytical procedures.
- Verification of pharmacopoeial or validated analytical procedures.
- Cleaning of laboratory facilities including bench tops, equipment, work stations, clean rooms (aseptic areas for sterility testing and other microbiological testing), laboratory glassware.
- Monitoring of environmental conditions, e.g., temperature and humidity (wherever it is controlled say in some of the instrument rooms and in microbiology laboratory).
- Monitoring temperature of storage conditions.
- Disposal of reagents, solvents, samples, other laboratory waste.
- Safety measures.

The effectiveness of the quality management system should be reviewed periodically to ensure the continued compliance with the requirements of the system and to apply any necessary corrective and preventive measures.

The quality manager is responsible for planning and organizing internal audits addressing all elements of the quality management system. Such reviews must be recorded, together with details of any corrective and preventive action (CAPA) taken (a specimen check-list is annexed towards the end of this chapter).

Management review of quality issues should be regularly undertaken at least once a year. The review generally includes:

- reports on internal and, if conducted, external audits or inspections and any follow-up required to correct deficiencies pointed out in that inspection
- outcome of investigations carried out as a result of complaints received, atypical results reported in collaborative trials and/or proficiency tests
- corrective actions applied and preventive actions introduced as a result of these investigations

Documentation

Documentation is an essential part of the quality management system. Laboratory must establish and maintain procedures to control the documents. System to control documents here in laboratory also is similar document control system related to manufacturing operations. Here in laboratory too all documents are to be reviewed at a prescribed interval and review report is made. The review can be done by QA persons from the laboratory or any designated person by the management (in case of other big laboratories who undergo different types of quality audits, viz. ISO or NABL, may have this activity performed through outside expert persons). During periodic review, in case there is no change in any of the document, "no-change" remark can be made on copies of the document and this can be revalidated.

Documentation procedure is to ensure that:

- each document has a unique identification number (SOP number or STP number), version number and date of implementation;
- all SOPs are available at the relevant locations, e.g. near instruments;
- documents are kept up-to-date and reviewed as required;
- invalid document is removed and replaced with the authorized, revised document with immediate effect;
- any revised document includes references to the previous document;
- old, invalid SOPs are retained in the archive to ensure traceability of the evolution of the procedures (their copies are to be destroyed); and
- all the relevant staff is trained for the new and revised SOPs.

Change Control System

A system of change control must be in place to inform staff of new and revised procedures. No experiment or analysis should be undertaken with following change control procedures. System must ensure that:

- revised documents are prepared by the initiator, or a person who performs the same function, reviewed and approved at the same level as the original document and subsequently released by the quality manager; and
- staff acknowledges by a signature that they are aware of applicable changes and their date of implementation.

Materials, Equipment, Instruments and Other Devices

Reagents

All reagents and chemicals, including solvents and materials used in tests and assays, must be of appropriate quality.

Reagents should be purchased from reputable, approved suppliers and should be accompanied by a certificate that specifies its date of manufacture / packing and if possible a date it will retain its desired quality and the material safety data sheet, if required.

In the preparation of reagent solutions in the laboratory:

- responsibility for this task must be clearly specified in the job description of the person assigned to carry it out; and
- prescribed procedures must be used which are in accordance with published pharmacopoeial or other standards, where available. Records should be kept of the preparation and standardization of volumetric solutions.

The labels of all reagents must clearly specify:

- content;
- manufacturer;
- date received and date of opening of the container;
- concentration, if applicable;
- storage conditions; and
- expiry date or re-test date, as justified.

The labels of reagent solutions prepared in the laboratory must clearly specify:

- name;
- date of preparation and initials of technician/analyst; and
- expiry date or re-test date, as justified.

The labels for volumetric solutions prepared in the laboratory must clearly specify:

for use by the appropriate laboratory personnel together with a schedule of the dates on which it is due for qualifications verification and/or calibration.

Instrument/Equipment Logs: Records must be kept of each item of equipment, instrument or other device used to perform testing, verification and/or calibration. The records must include at least the following:

- the identity of the equipment, instrument or other device;
- the manufacturer's name, model, serial number or other unique identification;
- the qualification, verification and/or calibration required;
- the current location, where appropriate;
- the equipment manufacturer's instructions, if available, or an indication of their location;
- the dates, results and copies of reports, verifications and certificates of all calibrations, adjustments, acceptance criteria and the due date of the next qualification, verification and/or calibration;
- the maintenance carried out to date and the maintenance plan;
- a history of any damage, malfunction, modification or repair.

Usage Logs: It is also recommended that records should be kept and additional observations made of the time for which the equipment, instruments or devices were used.

Procedures should include instructions for the safe handling, transport and storage of measuring equipment. On re-installation, re-qualification of the equipment is required to ensure that it functions properly on installation.

Maintenance procedures should be established, e.g. regular servicing must be performed by a team of maintenance specialists, whether internal or external, followed by verification of performance.

Equipment, instruments and other devices, either subjected to overloading or mishandling, giving suspect results, shown to be defective or outside specified limits, must be taken out of service and clearly labelled or marked. Wherever possible they must not be used until they have been repaired and re-qualified.

When the equipment, instruments and other devices are outside the direct control of the laboratory for a certain period of time or have undergone a major repair, the laboratory must re-qualify the equipment to ensure its suitability for use.

For preparation of SOPs on calibration, verification of performance and qualification of equipment requirements in various pharmacopoeia, these official books can be referred. USP and EP in their general chapter have made references.

Traceability

I. The result of an analysis should be traceable, when appropriate, ultimately to a primary reference substance.

II. Calibrations or qualification of instruments should be traceable to Certified Reference Materials and so to SI units (metrological traceability).

Working procedures

Incoming samples

Sample in the laboratory may be of starting materials (active and excepients both), intermediate products, finished formulations and also packing materials and these samples are received by the laboratory for purpose of release (or rejection). Sample is to be collected according to sampling plan and SOP. Samples should be representative of the batches of material from which they are taken and sampling should be carried out so as to avoid contamination and other adverse effects on quality or mix-up of, or by, the material being sampled. The quantity of sample in all cases to be such that it is sufficient enough for conducting complete analysis and also repeat analysis if this to be performed (re-sampling is not a good practice). In case of starting materials, where more than one containers are sampled, pooling is to be done in the sampling area itself. Such samples are prepared in duplicate (or triplicate) i.e. one for immediate testing; the second for confirmation of testing if required; and the third for retention, in case of dispute (sample is rejected and starting material is to be returned to manufacturer – more so if the item is not manufactured locally and is imported. For further reference, WHO expert committee has published a document for sampling and that could be referred for finalizing different SOPs related to sampling activity.

Test request

A standard test request form should be filled out and accompany each sample submitted to the laboratory. In case of a pharmaceutical manufacturer's laboratory the requirements may be given in the master production instructions.

The test request form must provide or leave space for the following information:

- the source of the material;
- a full description of the drug (medicine), including its composition (in case of formulations), Generic Name & brand name;
- dosage form and concentration or strength, the manufacturer and the batch number;
- the size of the sample;

- the type of analysis (complete or partial);
- the date on which the sample was collected;
- the size of the consignment from which it was taken, when appropriate;
- the expiry date (for pharmaceutical products) or re-test date (for APIs and pharmaceutical excipients);
- the specification to be used for testing;
- the required storage conditions;
- remarks, if any.

At times complaint samples are received by the laboratory for investigation. The laboratory must review the test request to ensure that:

- the requirements are adequately defined and the laboratory has the capability and resources to meet them;
- the appropriate tests and/or methods are selected and capable of meeting customer's requirements.

Any issue must be resolved with the originator of the request for analysis before testing starts and record of review must be kept.

Inward of samples and labelling

All newly delivered samples and accompanying documents (e.g. the test request) must be assigned an inward/unique id (in case LIMS is in place) number. Separate inward numbers must be assigned to each of the sample received for analysis even though two or more medicines, different dosage forms, or different batches of the same medicine or different sources of the same batch are received in one receipt-memo. A unique id number must also be assigned to incoming retained sample and samples received for stability testing.

A label bearing the inward number must be affixed to each container of the sample. Care must be taken to avoid obliterating any other markings or inscriptions.

A sample inward register must be kept, which may be a record book, a card file or data-processing equipment, where the following information is recorded:

- the inward number of the sample;
- the date of receipt;
- the specific unit to which the sample was forwarded (if mentioned e.g. sample for bulk sterility is generally forwarded directly to microbiology department).

Inspection/checking of the submitted sample and testing

The sample received must be inspected/checked by laboratory staff to ensure that the labelling is in conformity with the information contained in the test request. The findings must be recorded, dated and signed. If discrepancies are found, or if the sample is damaged, the observation must be recorded on the test request form and information is brought to the notice of the head of laboratory for further decision.

The specific unit to which the sample is sent for testing is determined by the person responsible. The examination of a sample must not be started before the relevant test request has been received. The sample must be properly stored until all relevant documentation has been received. A request for analysis may be accepted verbally only in case of emergencies. All details must immediately be placed on record pending the receipt of written confirmation. Copies or duplicates of all documentation must accompany each numbered sample when sent to the specific unit.

Analytical worksheet

The analytical worksheet is an internal document for recording information by the analyst about the sample, the test procedure, calculations and the results of testing. It is to be complemented by the raw data obtained in the analysis.

The analytical worksheet contains documentary evidence either to confirm that the sample being examined is in accordance with the requirements; or this supports an out-of-specification result.

The analytical worksheet must provide the information – the inward number of the sample and the sample number, the date of the test request; the date on which the analysis was started and completed, the name and signature of the analyst, a description of the sample received, references to the specifications and a full description of test methods to which the sample was tested, including the limits, (if possible the identity of the test equipment used û this information is already there on chromatography graphs and may be recorded in case of an IR spectrophotometer), the identification number of reference substance used, the results obtained, the interpretation of the results and the final conclusions (whether or not the sample was found to comply with the specifications). The analytical work sheet is to be signed by each of the analysts involved and approved and signed by the supervisors. Any further comments, for example, for internal information or detailed notes on the specifications selected and the methods of assessment used or any deviation from the prescribed procedure, which must be approved and reported, or whether and when portions of the sample were forwarded to other units for special tests, and the date when the results were received may be a part of worksheet.

All values obtained from each test, including blank results, must immediately be entered on the analytical worksheet and all graphical data, whether obtained from recording instruments or plotted by hand/software, must be attached or be traceable to an electronic record file or document where the data is available.

The completed analytical worksheet must be signed by the responsible analyst(s) and approved and signed by the supervisor.

When a mistake is made in analytical worksheets or when data or text needs to be amended, the old information should be deleted by means of a line (not erased or made illegible using white ink) and the new information added alongside. All such alterations should be signed by the person making the correction and the date of the change inserted. The reason for the change should also be given on the worksheet.

The completed analytical worksheet must be kept safely, together with all attachments, including calculations and recordings of instrumental analyses.

Validation of analytical procedures

The laboratory should have the documented evidence that any analytical procedure used for testing is suitable under actual conditions for the intended use. This evidence is obtained through validation. Validation also serves to establish acceptance criteria for system suitability test. Validation should be performed according to a validation protocol, which includes analytical performance characteristics to be verified for various types of analytical procedure. The results should be documented in the validation report.

It may be clarified here that a pharmacopoeial method or externally validated analytical method, which is being performed for the first time utilizing the equipment and reagents available, should be verified under actual conditions of use in order to demonstrate that is suitable for the substance or product to be tested. The extent of verification should be justified on the basis of risk management principles. Further guidance on validation of analytical procedures the texts such as guideline elaborated by the International Conference on Harmonisation of Technical Requirements for Registration of Pharmaceuticals for Human Use (ICH) and General chapters of the U.S. Pharmacopeia on Validation and Verification of compendial procedures may be referred.

Testing

The sample must be tested in accordance with the work-plan of the laboratory after completion of the preliminary procedures. If testing of sample is not feasible the reasons must be noted in the analytical worksheet and the sample must be stored in a secure place pending analysis.

In case some specific tests required to be carried out by another unit or by a specialized external laboratory (R&D laboratory of a company), the responsible person should handle this procedure. Test procedures should be described in detail and should provide sufficient information to allow properly trained analysts to perform the analysis in a reliable manner. Where system suitability criteria are defined in the method they should be fulfilled. Any deviation from the test procedure must be approved and documented.

In case sample fails to meet the specifications with the approved standards it should be investigated. Since the consignment, from which the sample has been taken, is in quarantine stage, that status of quarantine should be maintained. The possibility of any re-testing is to be evaluated, only if this is defined in SOP and if this aspect is not defined, the sample should be rejected.

Retesting

If SOP permits re-testing of a doubtful or suspected out-of-specification (OOS) result, a review of procedures applied during testing process is to be undertaken by the supervisor with the analyst/technician/lab assistant (if involved in any process of testing) before re-testing is permitted. The following should be addressed:

- confirm with the analyst/technician/lab assistant that the appropriate procedure(s) was applied and followed correctly;
- examine the raw data to identify possible discrepancies;
- check all calculations for their correctness;
- check that equipment employed was qualified, calibrated and that system suitability tests were performed and were acceptable;
- ensure that the appropriate reagents, solvents and reference substances were used.

I would like to quote here an important judgement in one of the district courts in USA in a case where re-testing to pass a sample was being argued. The relevant line of the judgement reads: "*the firm should have a pre-determined testing procedure and it should consider a point at which testing ends*". It is not known if the judge had a scientific background, he/she, however made a scientifically very sound statement.

While finalizing SOP the aim of re-testing is to isolate an out-of-specification result and re-testing should not continue infinite number of times (till sample passes!). In case of quality control laboratories of a manufacturing site, the cause of failure is to be investigated (process related or process not related); if findings are true and determination is made about the defect in product, out-of-specification results should not be repeated. The judgement further reads: "*additional re-testing for the purpose of testing a product into compliance is not acceptable*" and the judgement continues to state: that re-testing:

- must be done on the same, not a different sample;
- may be done on a second aliquot from the same portion of the sample that was the source of the first aliquot;

- may be done of the same larger sample previously collected for laboratory purpose.

It is mentioned earlier in this chapter that re-sampling is not GMP and any successful re-sampling should not invalidate earlier out-of-specification results unless it is proved that original sample was improperly prepared or is not a representative sample.

Evaluation of test results

Test results must be reviewed and evaluated statistically after completion of all the tests to determine whether they are mutually consistent and meet the specifications used. The evaluation should take into consideration the results of all the tests (all test data).

Whenever doubtful (atypical) results are obtained they should be investigated. The complete testing procedure needs to be checked according to the internal quality management system.

An SOP must be in place for the conduct of an investigation of an out-of-specification test result. The SOP should give clear guidance on a number of re-tests allowed (based on sound statistical principles). All investigations and their conclusions must be recorded. In the event of an error any corrective action taken and any preventive action introduced must be recorded and implemented. A decision path for sample analysis may appear as under:

Sample by analyst A

Passes – consider release

Does not pass –

- Results are to be reported to supervisor and cause is to be investigated, batch deviations could be possible – investigation needed for finding out production defects – sample is to be rejected.
- No production defects – sample to be reanalysed by the analyst A – Passes – sample can be released.
- Reanalysis by analyst A – Sample fails in one or more tests the testing is to be repeated by two analysts – both pass the samples – sample can be released, in case both fail the sample – it should be rejected.
- If only one analyst passes the sample and the other fails – it is to be analysed by another senior analyst – sample passes – released and if sample does not pass – sample is to be rejected.

All individual results (all test data) with acceptance criteria should be reported. All conclusions must be entered on the analytical worksheet.

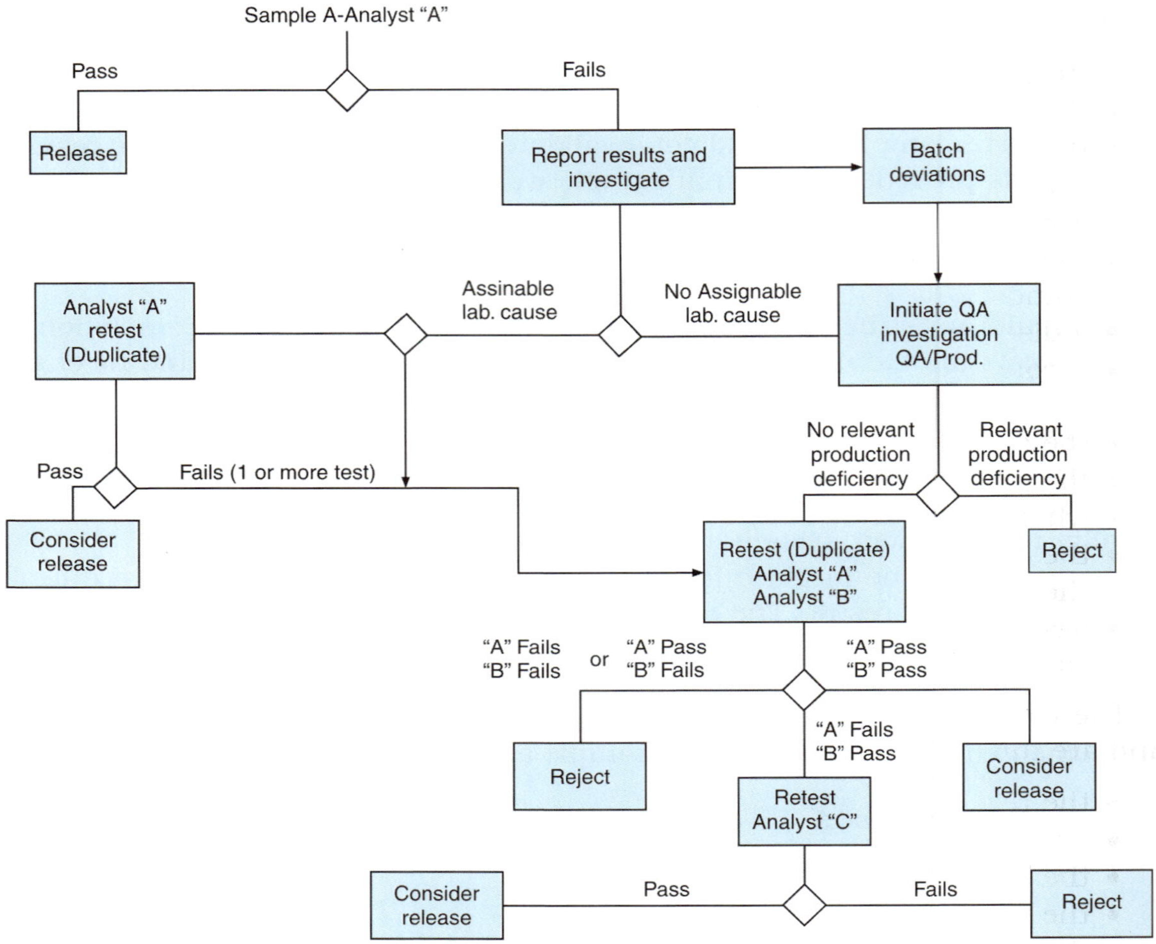

Analytical test report

The analytical test report is a compilation of the results and states the conclusions of the examination of a sample. It must be issued by the laboratory, based on analytical worksheet. Any amendments to the original analytical test report will require the issue of a new corrected document.

Uncertainty of measurement: It is evident that pharmacopoeial assay limits are set, taking into account the uncertainty of measurement, and the production capability and therefore acceptance criteria for an analytical result should be predefined. This measurement uncertainty can be estimated either from validation data or from the data obtained from proficiency tests of analysts. These limits will assist in taking decision to release a product.

The analytical test report should provide the following information:

- the laboratory registration number of the sample;
- the laboratory test report number;
- the name and address of the original manufacturer;
- the name and description and batch number of the sample, where appropriate;
- the results of all the tests performed or the numerical results with the standard deviation of all the tests performed (if applicable);
- a discussion of the results obtained;
- a conclusion whether or not the sample(s) was found to be within the limits of the specifications used;
- the date on which the test(s) was completed;
- the signature of the head of the laboratory or authorized person;
- whether or not the sample(s) complies with the requirements;
- the date on which the sample was received;
- the expiry date or re-test date, if applicable;
- a statement indicating that the analytical test report, or any portion thereof, cannot be reproduced without the authorization of the laboratory.

The contents of Certificate of Analysis (COA) are mentioned in drug rules and are to be followed. These contents are to have following information:

- the registration number of the sample;
- date of receipt;
- the name and address of the laboratory testing the sample;
- the name and description and batch number of the sample;
- the name and address of the original manufacturer;
- the reference to the specification used for testing the sample;
- the results of all tests performed;
- a conclusion whether or not the sample was found to be within the limits of the specification;
- expiry date or re-test date, if applicable;
- date on which the test(s) was completed;
- the signature of the head of laboratory or other authorized person.

Retained samples

Samples should be retained as required by the legislation. There should be sufficient retained sample to allow at least two re-analyses. Retained sample should be kept in its final pack.

Safety

General rules for safe working are in accordance with national regulations and several SOPs where safety has been mentioned. Safe working in a laboratory is closely connected to laboratory design, chemicals used and other safety measures employed. These may include following requirements:

- MSDS must be available to staff before testing is carried out;
- smoking, eating and drinking in the laboratory must be prohibited;
- staff must be familiar with the use of fire-fighting equipment, including fire extinguishers, fire blankets and gas masks;
- staff must wear laboratory coats or other protective clothing, including eye protection;
- special care must be taken, as appropriate, in handling, for example, highly potent, infectious or volatile substances;
- highly toxic samples should be handled in a specially designed facility to avoid the risk of contamination;
- all containers of chemicals must be fully labelled and include prominent warnings (e.g. "Poison", "Flammable", etc.) whenever appropriate;
- safety rules in handling cylinders of compressed gases must be observed and staff must be familiar with the relevant colour identification codes;
- staff must be aware of the need to avoid working alone in the laboratory;
- first-aid materials must be provided and staff instructed in first-aid techniques, emergency care and the use of antidotes.

Protective clothing must be available, including eye protection, masks and gloves. Water showers should be installed. Rubber suction bulbs must be used on manual pipettes and siphons. Staff must be instructed in the safe handling of glassware, corrosive reagents and solvents and particularly in the use of safety containers or baskets to avoid spillage from containers.

Warnings, precautions and instructions must be given for work with uncontrollable or dangerous reactions when handling specific reagents (e.g. mixing water and acids, or acetoneûchloroform and ammonia), flammable products and highly oxidizing agents.

Poisonous or hazardous products must be labelled appropriately and stored separately, but it must not be taken for granted that all other chemicals are safe. Unnecessary contact with reagents, especially solvents and their vapours, must be avoided. The use of known carcinogens and mutagens as reagents must be limited or totally excluded if required by local regulations. Replacement of toxic solvents and reagents by less toxic materials or reduction of their use must always be the aim, particularly when new techniques are developed.

"Purpose of analysis is to obtain information that has the greatest chance of providing a meaningful solution not only to a problem, but for the business."

– Lucchesi 1995

Few Bullet Points for Laboratory

General criteria for a lab design

- Functionality
- Safety
- Flexibility
- Communication/interaction
- Cost-effectiveness
- Possibilities of enhancement
- Synergism with other parts of laboratory

Synergistic effects of a good design may impart

- Greater creativity
- More informal interaction
- More team-work
- Better performance
- Greater productivity

Special design needs

- Incorporation into a larger unit
- Specific expansion
- General growth
- Proximity to a certain unit
- Location
- Regulatory sample receiving
- Storage spaces
- Factors judging QC lab vs. R&D lab
- Openness (more open)
- Appearance (different from QC laboratory)
- Exit from each area
- Location for interaction/or no interaction
- Traffic (more traffic as number of departments visit this area)
- Design for each area
- Lighting
- Safety
- Other spaces (archiving library conference, etc.)
- Cost per sq. foot

Traits of a person promoted to a manager

- Works without supervision
- Well organised
- Good at details
- Resourceful in tough situations
- Need to see things "done right"
- Makes decision quickly
- Pushes personal problems aside
- Concentrates on Job at Hand
- Driven toward perfection
- Self critical
- Constantly wants to improve

Five important leadership skills are ability to:

- Communicate
- Focus
- Coach
- Provide relevant feedback
- Build commitment

People with these skills can

- Communicate expectations
- Listen before talking
- Catch people doing right
- Find face saving when people do wrong
- Tolerate well intended mistakes
- Seek group inputs and decisions
- Trust their intuition
- Delegate

In case you are in a situation to retire old equipment/instrument

- Sell to a re-conditioning company
- Donate to a college/university
- Sell to a client/company
- Send to company/plant lab
- Rent or lease to a temporary projects
- Lease with an option to buy
- Send to a consulting/testing lab

REFERENCES

1. Quality assurance of pharmaceuticals. A compendium of guidelines and related materials. Volume 2, Second updated edition. Good manufacturing practices and inspection. Geneva, World Health Organization, 2007.
2. ISO/IEC 17025:2005.
3. WHO TRS, No. 885, 902, 929, 937, 953.
4. Uncertainty of measurement - Part 3: Guide to the expression of uncertainty in measurement (GUM1995) 2008, ISO/IEC Guide 98-3.
5. The U.S. Pharmacopoeia, 32nd edition. General chapters: <1058> Analytical Instrument Qualification, 2009.
6. ICH Q2 (R1): Validation of Analytical Procedures.
7. EU QA Documents Validation of Analytical Procedures.
8. The U.S. Pharmacopoeia, 32nd edition. General chapters: <1225> Validation of compendial procedures, and <1226> Verification of compendial procedures, 2009.
9. Schedule L1 of Drugs & Cosmetics Rules (India).
10. Several other WHO texts referring good laboratories practices.

Questions for Preparation of A Self-Inspection Checklist of the Laboratory

(Reference: PIC guidance document for inspection of laboratories)

The checklist has a regulatory inspection ad-memoire colour; this however will help laboratories in preparing their own checklist and conduct self-inspection accordingly. The laboratories attached to a manufacturing site may combine relevant questions to self-inspection/internal audit format.

QUALITY ASSURANCE

QA system

- Is document available for QA system Or If quality manual prepared.
- Are names of key personnel, their reporting lines and responsibilities clearly defined.
- What is review period (procedures, processes) for this system.
- Vendor's approval system for ensuring quality of supplies:
  - If vendor approval system defined and followed
  - Is there a policy for supplier's quality assessment
  - Is approval supported by site visits/qualification/evaluation

Self inspection

- Is any self inspection performed, if yes, mention names of self inspection team member.

- What is the frequency of self inspection.
  (mention date of last inspection carried out.)
- What is the reporting style
  (check-list, written report, only non-compliance etc.)
- Mentioned the procedure of corrective measures taken

Trending of Results/OOS-results

- Are analysis trends assessed, if yes, by whom.
- Is SOP available for this

Change control system, responsibilities, follow up actions

- Who is responsible for change control procedures
- What follow-up actions are taken and if these changes documented, managed,

Risk management

- Is any risk management method/approach incorporated in the methods
- Are all critical parameters included
- Is this related to validation process, if yes, how

DOCUMENTATION

General information

- Is there a system exist for preparation, revision. distribution, archiving of documentation, change control and handling of copies of controlled documents.
- What is syntax of documents – electronic/paper or both.
- Is procedure in writing available for document format, numbering system, approval criteria, distribution, return, interval for revision etc.
- How is the process of archiving managed for their location and protection.
- Has SOP mention the authorisation for copying and identification of copies (e.g., controlled copy, uncontrolled copy, etc.) from official and controlled documents.

Laboratory documentation

- Are specifications for materials and products; consistent with in-house/ pharmacopoeial requirements.

Standard Operating Procedures (SOPs)

- Do SOPs exist for sampling, testing, equipment handling and other laboratory processes.

- Is there a standard form used for preparing all SOPs.
- Are these prepared for
  - test instructions
  - analytical procedures
  - methods of using specific equipment.
- Have working details been described.
- If SOPs are in conformity with the approved method of testing.
- Are batch testing records/testing protocols data comply with instructions.
- Are all alterations signed and commented

Log books

- What is the form and content of the analyst's analytical notebooks, worksheets and general lab notebooks.
- Do log books exist for equipment, calibration, maintenance, standards, sample receipt etc. Mention if the data is recorded elsewhere.
- Does standard form include complete data (including raw data) e.g. chromatograms, spectra, results and printouts or any other data that you consider as raw data.
- Are all the note-books page numbered or if loose sheet in form of formats are used do these formats have document number.
- Are sheets of raw data recorded/attached directly into relevant laboratory report/notebooks. There should not be any scrap or loose paper.

Data traceability

- How data traceability is ensured e.g. if procedures are available for record on receipt and usage of materials or standards.
- Is all analytical raw data easily traceable – mention if separate analyst's books are used for noting weights, etc.
- How is traceability ensured? For example, how is traceability of working standards to primary standards ensured.
- How is the "history" of sample recorded, e.g., receipt log, storage conditions, handling, security, safety data, etc.

Personnel

- Is laboratory organogram available, attach if available. Mention QC manager and deputy (other key personnel).
- Are personnel (including analysts) adequate in number specified to positions and different testing. Mention total number of employees (total).
- What is the annual average staff turnover?
- Is there a document specifying qualifications, experiences, duties, responsibilities and staff presence on site?

Training - Training system, programme / plan and training on special reasons

- Is training schedule or calendar prepared. If prepared, is it followed and persons trained accordingly.
- Are training program documented and SOP is available for training. Does training system describe as who is responsible for training, who imparts training and the trainer's qualifications.
- How evaluation of training effectiveness is done. Orally, through written tests or through blinding of samples for analysis.
- Are all persons evaluated and re-evaluated on a periodic basis for the training imparted.
- If any specific training is given to other personnel e.g. maintenance, cleaning staff, etc.

Premises

- Is laboratory suitably located and laid according to approved lay-out plan.
- Is Quality Control laboratory separate from production areas?
- If the facility design has considered separation of rooms for different activities e.g. clean (instrument room) and dirty (washing of glassware etc.) hot room and other rooms. Mention these provided for chemical, microbiological and biological testing with respective areas.
- Are all rooms identified, clearly labelled and their status indicated.
- Is the laboratory instrument/equipment located in appropriate area (e.g. clean equipment in clean room).
- How are sensitive instruments protected.
- Is separate storage area provided for defective equipment/instrument storage.
- If temperature, humidity and ventilation, etc. adequate, maintained and monitored constantly (during working).
- Is any recording system or alarms provided in case of malfunctioning/failure of these system.
- If system of alarm available for critical equipment (e.g., LAF work station), when these do not work.
- Does laboratory has separate areas for storage of reagents, chemicals, samples, control samples and documents.
- Are storage conditions monitored (only in case where special storage conditions provided).
- How are the documents protected e.g. stored in fire proof almirah/cabinets.
- Is there clearly indicated dedication of rooms, areas (directions), status?

Equipment, Instruments

- Brief description of major equipment available – List is to be provided.

- Is there as approved URS (user requirement specification) and person authorised to approve this. It is expected to have a document including names of suppliers and/or may be procured from third party.
- Is there a procedure for assembly of equipments, instruments and services and their qualifications such as design qualification (DQ), installation qualification (IQ), operational qualification (OQ) and performance qualification (PQ), Calibration, status labelling, log books (maintenance and usage) and cleaning.
- Mention the status of qualification. Are these performed prior to first use.
- If details on specifications and acceptance criteria provided and operators have been trained or if this is done through contracted services (generally done for sophisticated instruments such as liquid particle counters or solid particle counters).
- Are relevant qualification documents, SOP available for all possible assembling configurations of instruments and equipments in the laboratory.
- Is appropriate environmental conditions clearly mentioned for housing the instruments and equipments.
- If procedures using these equipment are validated e.g. when autoclaves are used for sterilization of media, accessories and dresses etc. sterilization cycle is to be validated.

Calibration

- Are calibration procedures defined in writing.
- If documentation/records are available.
- Have interval for calibration mentioned and calibration status indicated for all instruments and equipments.
- Does SOP for instrument/equipment mention calibration procedure and frequency.
- If sufficient detail of procedures, materials/certified reference materials are available for performing calibration.

Cleaning & sanitation

- If cleaning and sanitation procedures are validated according to requirements and if the process has been documented.

Maintenance system

- How is preventive maintenance procedures programmed, performed and documented?
- Is preventive maintenance program conducted in-house or contracted out.
  - If part of maintenance is contracted out, mention which is contacted out.
  - Are responsibilities of contact giver and contract acceptor mentioned and followed.

- Are all critical systems, areas and equipment included in maintenance program.
- After break-down maintenance who "releases" equipment for laboratory's use.
- Is there system available for the formal acceptance of equipment back into service.

Materials and supplies

Laboratory reagents, standards reference substances and reference materials (reference cultures, etc.)

- Is handling procedure and MSDS of highly toxic, hazardous and sensitising materials, poisons etc. available.
- Is list of such materials available along with names of suppliers.
- Is there a procedure available for handling, labelling, storing and expiry dating of chemicals and reagents in the laboratory.
- Is there any requirement for identity testing (especially for titrimetry indicators)?
- Please list out primary standards available in the laboratory.
- List out official reference standards available in the laboratory.
- If traceability to official standards assessed (through proper procurement document and also information of current lot in circulation from internet!).
- Is there a procedure available for preparation of working standards.
- Is there a procedure/SOP for in-house calibration of working standards and reference material used for preparation of these standards.
- How expiry date, potency value and LOD, etc. are assigned to each in ûhouse reference material.
- What is the procedure for handling and storing of these materials.
- Is there any procedure for ensuring the security of these materials.
- What are measures introduced to avoid cross contamination of reference materials.
- Is SOP for waste disposal available.

Water, water systems, water sampling and water testing

- Has laboratory water system been described – mention what types of water(s) are used for analysis – PW, DW, RO, UHQ, etc. and how laboratory water is prepared.
- Is any special quality of water used for microbiological testing.
- What is the sampling procedure of laboratory water and how is laboratory water sampled. Mention if manufacturing area's PW water sampling SOP also covers sampling of water from laboratory.
- What kind of quality testing is done for water used in different types of analysis.

Sampling and Samples

- Mention SOP number for sampling of various materials. Does it mention the type of sampling plan e.g. *n-plan*, *p-plan* or *r-plan*.
- In case reduced sampling is done (in case of APIs) does SOP mention reasons for reduced sampling.
- Does SOP mention name of person responsible for sampling, place of sample and pooling (preparation of composite sample) of starting materials sample.
- What is the representative quantity of sample as defined in the SOP – 5 gm, 10 gm, etc.
- Does SOP include the details of container (in which sample will be placed), labelling, cleaning process (in case re-usable bottles are used) and cleaning of equipment, etc.
- Is there separate sampling area in stores or materials are sampled at the point of receipt? How is the risk of cross contamination/bacterial contamination prevented during sampling.
- In case in-process sampling is done by QC laboratory, does the procedure mention IPC's sampling or intermediate item's sampling.
- In case QC is involved in environment monitoring, does SOP mention procedure of air sampling for viable and non-viable counts.
- Does SOP exist for sampling of water at various user points, including laboratory user points.
- What is the procedure for keeping retain samples.
- What is the procedure for disposal of analysis left-over quantity of the items analysed.
- How and for how much time retain-samples of starting materials are kept? Mention storage area and conditions.
- How long are samples stored prior testing and if this is mentioned in STPs.
- Is re-sampling done in case of OOS results. If yes, is there a procedure for re-sampling and if a decision tree for this activity available.
- Air sampling
  - What type of air sampler is used. Mention type of air sampler
  - Does SOP mention the sample volume of air (100 L/200 L or more) its testing time, and media used for testing.
  - Is air sampling equipment calibrated
- Which methods are used for testing: standardised (e.g., Pharmacopoeial), modified or developed "in house"?
- If methods developed in house or modified validated.
- If any analysis is done on contract basis and if yes, a formal contact for such analysis has been made.
- Are specifications and STPs for testing of all the starting materials available. Is identity test done on sample from each container and if yes, which method is used.

- If any procedure is there for releasing the materials based on supplier's certificate.
- Is SOP available for preparation of reagents and standards.
- Who controls the testing equipment quality and is the person trained for this activity.
- In testing of intermediates if the person(s) identified for sampling.
- If all test methods are validated.
- Which policy of test method validation is followed – ICH or any other.
- Is method validation is part of Validation Master Plan (VMP).
- Is there a general SOP on method validation with details of reporting and final approval of method.
- Tick if all these parameters of method validation are covered — precision (System and method), intermediate precision, Accuracy, Specificity, Reproducibility, Linearity (range), Limit of detection, Limit of quantitation, Robustness (including solution stability and filter compatibility).
- Mention if these are documented in each SOP or protocol and acceptance criteria for each parameter defined and met.
- System suitability test procedure has been developed and acceptance criteria for each system suitability parameter defined and met.
- How is raw data stored.
- In case any LIMS installed how raw data is transferred to this system.
- Mention in brief the procedure for evaluation of test results and if analytical data reviewed by responsible person.
- What is change control system in the laboratory and its operations.
- Mention who is responsible for writing the final protocol and who is responsible for comments and evaluation of the results (QC manager or any other person).
- In case of failures/OOS test results what system is followed.
- Are laboratory errors (operator, equipment), Process/Procedure related errors evaluated for OOS results and test results rendered invalidated.
- Mention who is authorised to invalidate the test results.
- Is there a SOP for OOS result investigation?
- OOS are reported to whom – QA or QC in-charge.
- What is the procedure on decision related to OOS.
- On failures if retesting and re-sampling performed.

Chemical testing

- Is procedures in place for reagents preparation, handling volumetric glassware and volumetric solutions, indicators for titration.
- How often volumetric glassware (e.g., pipettes and volumetric flasks) calibrated.

- How are primary standard solutions labelled and if date of preparation, normality/molarity, stability and validity and storage conditions mentioned in SOP.
- What is the procedure for general housekeeping of indicators and at what interval titration indicators are changed.
- How often thermometers are calibrated and if calibration corresponds to the parameters specified in relevant methods.
- If conductometer/pH measurements, Refractometry, Relative density testing unit, Polarimetry, Viscometer, KF titration unit, MP apparatus, DT apparatus, Dissolution testing units, etc. are calibrated; if yes, mention frequency.
- Are all balances calibrated prior to use and if standard weights available for this purpose.
- Which certified materials/device is used for calibration (e.g. dissolution calibrator tablets from USP). The documentation on physical calibration (shaft wobble, level, spindle speed, vibration, vessel temperature) is to be checked and commented upon.
- In-house calibration register is to be maintained and entries filled. If calibration buffers are relevant for pH range measured in laboratory.
- If following parameters are covered:
  - UV VIS spectrophotometers: Absorbance accuracy, accuracy, resolution, limit of stray light controlled for UV equipment?
  - IR spectrophotometer: Verification of wave number scale has been carried out and accuracy, resolution, base line flatness controlled for the instrument.
  - Atomic Absorption Spectrophotometer (AAS): If performance monitored, linearity and trends assessed, by choosing frequently analysed elements or another element such as copper.
  - HPLC/GC: Is there well defined system suitability tests and acceptance criteria defined.
  - TOC Analyser: Which material is used for calibration.

Microbiology Laboratory including sterility testing

Premises

- Comment on areas provided for micro assays, other micro work e.g. culture manipulation and sterility testing (there should be at least three separate testing areas and other ancillary areas).
- What is HVAC (Heating Ventilation and Air Conditioning) system in microbiological laboratory. Are there any visual alarms provided and design has incorporated proper pressure differentials between different areas.
- Is there any re-qualification program for HVAC and HEPA filters.

- Are area of preparation and washing room provided.
- Are interior surfaces smooth in this area and no un-cleanable recesses are created – mention type of interior surfaces e.g. epoxy coating/PU coating/ Epoxy painting, smoothly polished floorings, etc.
- If logical number of air-locks provided for entering and exit from clean rooms.
- If appropriate gowning instructions for access into the critical areas exist.
- If logical number and type (static or dynamic) pass boxes provided for material transfer.
- If enough LAF work stations or bio-safety cabinets provided for all micro-biological manipulations
- Mention "cleanliness class" (grade A/B or A/C) in sterility testing area and air-locks.
- What measures are taken for protection against microbiological contamination during aseptic operations.
- Is "house-culture" prepared for various positive controls.
- Is there separate area and procedure for decontamination of materials from microbiological testing.
- Is there effective segregation of washing area to the clean and non-clean part?
- Equipment
  - Are equipment such as autoclaves, incubators, LAF work stations, HEPA filters etc qualified (IQ, OQ & PQ) before use and respective processes validated.
  - Is main autoclave double ended.
  - For sterilisation process validation if cold points and load pattern etc. have been identified.
  - What type of steam is used for sterilisation process.
  - Is there a procedure for recording sterilisation details in respect of equipment and other accessories.
  - Are equipment such as colony counter, air ampler and particle counter etc. qualified for use.
- Mention if testing materials settle plates, culture media etc are prepared in-house or procured from outside as readymade.
- If all reference cultures available. What is procedure of maintaining purity of assay cultures. If these are traceable to official source and identified on receipt.
- Mention if any validity is mentioned on label of thee cultures.
- Is SOP available for maintenance of these cultures (slants/stabs). If maintained in stabs if culture revival procedure is available.
- What are the arrangements for maintaining powder media and if all required media available.

- Is SOP mention for testing each lot/batch for growth promotion, selectivity, and purity.
- What protective garments are used in laboratory for microbiology work and for sterility testing.
- How are gowns washed and sterilised. Facilities are to be in-house.
- Which protective garments are used by operators at sterility testing. If these are suitable for intended use.
- Are the laboratory coats kept and located in appropriate manner.
- Are instructions available for use.
- Testing
  - If STP in respect of microbiological testing of product has mention details for Incubation, Growth promotion, Positive controls, Negative controls and Bioburden, etc.
  - If incubation period justified. What is the incubation time and temperature.
  - What is the frequency of observation of sample during incubation – daily or at the end of incubation time.
  - If the procedure for sub-culturing available.
  - How often positive and negative controls performed – with each test or with each lot of media prepared.
- In microbiological testing if procedure is available for Environmental Testing (monitoring).
- If procedure mention sampling location, swabs to be used, settle plates and contact plates to be exposed.
- Mention if environment monitoring is performed at rest/in operation condition.
- Mention which media is used, what is the method, time exposure and surface area covered/limits and recovery rate?
- Is there a procedure for recovery in EM, if yes what is the procedure, specially in sterility testing area.
- Mention if sampling procedure available for MLT for various types of waters for pharmaceutical use.
- If location/sampling sites identified and adhered to. If worst case determined in case of Water system and clean area.
- What are action and alert limits and if there a procedure if the limits exceed the parameters.

Reaction Mechanism

3

Calibration of Analytical Instruments

A key to maintain consistent and reliable results within laboratory remains strongly attached to the validation and calibration of analytical detection systems used in daily analysis. Instrument calibration record is most frequently sought after and among the most cited observations during regulatory inspections. It is vital for the laboratories to maintain a rigorous regime of instrument qualifications and calibration. It must be realized that the users (not the instrument supplier) are responsible for the maintenance of the instrument in the laboratory.

Calibration is the process of establishing how the response of measurement varies with respect to the parameter being measured. It is often regarded as adjusting the output of an instrument to agree with the value of applied standard with reasonable accuracy. The usual way to perform calibration is to subject the reference material to the measurement process to prepare a calibration curve i.e. graphical plot of a signal as a function of analyte quantity/ concentration. Analytical measurements in different laboratories must be comparable independent of their location/site or the time of measurement. Thus, it is important to establish traceability to common standards. Calibration of instrument is essential in determining the performance attributes of a method. It is thus important that analytical instruments are suitably calibrated with reference standards before the sample is actually analysed.

Every laboratory instrument should comply with:

(a) **Installation qualifications (IQ):** Checking of instrument against standard of operating environments, physical connections, safety parameters and functional parameters prior to the initial utilisation of the system. It will confirm that the system is correctly installed.

(b) **Operational qualifications (OQ):** It is the process to ensure that the instrument performs consistently as specified over all the intended operating ranges.

(c) **Performance qualifications (PQ):** It is the process of testing normal operations and requires continuing evidence that the system is in control such as by generating control charts with calibrating data.

Common Laboratory Instruments, Equipment and Apparatus Need to be Calibrated

1. Karl Fischer apparatus and auto-titrator
2. Analytical balance
3. UV-visible spectrophotometer
4. Infrared spectrophotometer

5. pH meter
6. Thermometer
7. Refractometer
8. Polarimeter
9. B.O.D. incubator
10. Laboratory oven
11. Disintegration test apparatus
12. Dissolution test apparatus
13. Gas chromatograph (GLC)
14. HPLC/LC-MS
15. HPTLC
16. AAS/ICP-MS
17. Glass apparatus (used for measurement)

Objectives of Calibration

- To ensure the accuracy/reliability of the reading obtained from an instruments/equipments, laboratory glassware with authentic reference standard having traceability.
- To track the measurement results back to national and international standards.
- To maintain the quality control and quality assurance in the production to comply with requirements.
- To promote national/international recognition like NABL, GLP, ISO 9000, HACPP, ISO/IEC 17025, etc.

Frequency of Calibration

- Varies from instrument to instrument.
- As recommended by the manufacturer.
- Laboratory experience.
- Accuracy and precision required for the analytical method.
- Extent of use.
- However, the calibration must be done at the time of:
  (a) Installation
  (b) Service/repair
  (c) Relocation (change of site)
- Spectrophotometer — 3 to 6 months
- Chromatographic systems (6-12 months)
- Glassware — One time if not exposed to high temperature
- pH meter — Every time before use

Basic Requirements for Calibration

- Standard reference material/calibrator
- Controlled environmental condition
- Competence and responsibilities of laboratory personnel performing calibration
- SOP for calibration
- Traceability of standard
- Documentation/records of calibration:
  1. Procedure for issuing calibration sticker to track the status of the instrument.
  2. Remedial measures taken in case of calibration failure.
  3. Procedure to inform the actual user.

  Suggested environmental conditions are:

  (a) Temperature: 25 ± 1°C
  (b) Relative humidity: 45-60%
  (c) Light: 400-500 lux
  (d) Acoustic level (sound): 60 dBA (max)
  (e) Power supply: 250 V ± 1%
  (f) Vibration: Almost nil

Typical Calibration Data Sheet

1. Name of the instrument.
2. Manufacturer's name.
3. Instrument identification number: Description, Model No., Serial No., Range/Scale.
4. SOP procedure number.
5. Calibration date and time.
6. Calibration site/location.
7. Environmental conditions (temperature, humidity, pressure).
8. Calibration completion date and calibration record.
9. Calibration status: Accepted/Rejected.
10. Calibration frequency.
11. Next calibration due date
12. Name and signature of calibrating technician/analyst.
13. Maintenance of log-book.
14. Analyst responsible for monitoring calibration and maintenance status.

Methods of Calibration

External standards: Different concentrations of the known standards are prepared and response measured by the analytical system. The sample parameters are determined with respect to that of standard.

Internal standards: A known amount of standard whose physicochemical property is close to that of the analyte is added to the sample. The analyte concentration can be obtained by comparing the value from the standard with the value from the analyte.

Standard addition: The sample is first measured in analytical instrument. Then known amount of the analyte is added to the sample and the sample is measured again. By comparing of the values before and after addition of the analyte, concentration of the analyte in the sample can be calculated.

Type of standards used for calibration

(a) **Primary standards:** These are the instruments/equipments which are available with approved national calibration laboratories. These are about 4 times more accurate than secondary standards.

(b) **Secondary standards:** These instruments are available with the manufacturers. These instruments are normally used to calibrate, measuring standard equipment and are normally 4 times more accurate than measuring standards.

(c) **Measuring standards:** These are the instruments which are used in analytical laboratories and are used to measure process parameters.

CALIBRATION OF ANALYTICAL BALANCE

Since analytical balance is the most important instrument employed in any analytical laboratory and may contribute significantly to any analytical error, the detailed procedure for its use, maintenance and calibration is described for guidance of analysts particularly the newer ones.

Factors influencing the accuracy of a weighing balance

It is presumed that the analysts are well acquainted with the principles of weighing and its use in weighing. Weighing accuracy is usually not indicated in the protocols of an analytical procedure. Accuracy (agreement between weighing results and actual mass of the sample) largely depends on the analyst who weighs the sample and the environment rather than the BALANCE. Validity of any analytical work depends on how accurately the sample has been weighed and if the weighing is not accurate, the validity of analytical result will always remain questionable.

Following points are intended to draw attention to certain important practical aspects to ensure accuracy of the balance and consequent weighing:

- Sample must not be weighed directly on the balance pans.
- Hot objects must be cooled to room temperature before introducing into the balance. If the sample is warm relative to the balance, convection currents cause the pan to be buoyed up; weighing results will be unstable and non-reproducible, hence weigh the sample at ambient temperature neither cold nor hot.
- Some samples may take up water or carbon dioxide from the air during weighing or lose weight even at room temperature due to volatile nature. For meaningful results, the sample must be handled and weighed in a sealed, capped bottle.
- Liquid samples should always be weighed in a suitable stoppered container—weighing bottle—to avoid spilling of material on the balance pan or inside the case of balance.
- A sample carrying a charge of static electricity is attracted to various parts of the balance or has tendency to jump when handled with a spatula tip, leading to erratic, non-repeatable weighing results. This can easily be overcome by controlling the humidity to constant level, i.e., above 30% RH or static electricity may be discharged with anti-static gun, if available.
- As a rule, finer the reliability of a balance, the more critical is the choice of location. Preferably analytical balance should be kept away from air current such as windows, doors, heat, air-conditioning outlets. Exposure to strong radiant heat source such as direct sunlight, ovens, hot water baths should be avoided.
- Never locate the electronic balance in the main chemical laboratory or near water taps, wash basin.
- Instrument room housing electronic equipments should have no water connection; any waste may be collected in a suitable container and disposed of outside.
- The balance should preferably be installed on a vibration proof table, stone tables are preferred (balances are affected by vibrations—from rotating machines, elevators, slamming doors, nearby road traffic). Electronic balances are less prone to the effect of vibrations than the mechanical balances.
- Balance should not share the same powerline circuit with another equipment as it may cause interference. A powerline filter is usually recommended.
- Zero point and calibration of the balance are affected by variations in temperature. Normal indoor laboratory conditions are adequate. Since electronic balances produce heat (10-20 W), it is desirable that the balance is left constantly under power in order to avoid warming off drift at the beginning of any weighing. It is for these reasons that in most of the electronic

balances "ON-OFF" is for turning off the display, but keeps power "ON" for rest of the system.

- Allow the balance to stabilize before making any weighing, preferably leave the balance turned on permanently.
- Keep the balance chamber closed at all times except when adding or removing the objects to be weighed as changes in temperature, humidity, air current, vibrations will alter the readings.
- Handle all the containers or objects with either tweezers or tongs. Handling with fingers can change the temperature or leave grease smudge that will obviously alter the weight; to handle tared apparatus, make use of finger cots or gloves.
- Make readings without delay, allow enough time for sample to come to an equilibrium and the display to stabilize.

  Note: It may not be necessary to weigh the sample to a degree of accuracy if same level of accuracy cannot be achieved in subsequent steps of analysis. In volumetric work, the accuracy of the apparatus (volumetric flasks, pipettes) is about ± 0.2%, therefore for weighing 1 g of the sample up to ± 0.0001 g is not necessary as it will give an error of only ± 0.01% in weighing.
- Since electronic balances read the weight directly, the analyst is likely to become complacent and may assume that all readings are correct at all times—it is not so. Balances need frequent calibration—for this a calibrated 100 mg weight can serve as a useful daily check on balance and gives confidence in balance reading.
- To clean the weighing pan and housing, a soft cloth with a mild detergent is sufficient. Do not use any strong solvent for the purpose. To remove solid residue use of nylon brush is suggested.
- Small bags containing dried silica gel (indicating type) should be kept inside the chamber of the balance. When silica gel turns pink, it may be regenerated by heating in an oven at 105°C till it acquires uniform blue colour.
- In balances having built-in calibration facility, manufacturing tolerance is usually 100 ± 0.0002 g. This small uncertainty is of no significant value in practical applications. However, serious problem often confronted is that due to surface contamination, the built-in weight may change. It is therefore desirable that occasionally calibration must be checked with a reliable standard mass—a certified weight.
- There are deviations in weighing results when the sample is kept in the middle and then in other position on weighing pan. This kind of error is usually small, however, weighing load should never be kept off centre.
- Balance doors must be closed when final weighing is done. Balances with facility for auto opening-closing of doors are now available.

Note: Minimum sample weight should be at least 3000 times the standard deviation of the balance.

General Precautions For Weighing the Sample

- In case of samples being hygroscopic, or deliquescent, the exposure to atmosphere be reduced to minimum.
- If the sample is to be transferred to a vessel with narrow aperture, make use of funnel.
- Ensure that mouth of the vessel to which sample is being transferred is absolutely dry.
- Do not return any sample to weighing bottle after it has been transferred to receiving vessel.
- Weighing vessel should not be too large to avoid any changes due to absorption of moisture and also avoid exceeding the capacity of the balance.

Standard Operating Procedure and Calibration of Analytical Balances

Weighing is the single most used step in all analytical procedures. Most common problem encountered during weighing is the balance drift, the primary causes for the same are:

1. Improper leveling of balance.
2. Balance doors not closed while weighing.
3. Vibration from other operations in the laboratory.
4. Balance not located in suitable laboratory area.
5. Temperature variations in balance housing and the sample.

Before weighing any sample these causes should be eliminated. All direct reading electronic balances should be left with power 'ON' as electricity consumption is negligible. This will ensure that balance has temperature equilibrium while weighing. Alternatively, at least 1 hour is recommended for equilibrium (microbalances even may need 24 hours to reach equilibrium).

Note: Balance drift, if any, can be determined by weighing a fixed weight on daily basis.

The following guidelines are intended to ensure that the weighing, the most common source of error, is correct and reliable.

1. Check power and position of the level bubble.
2. Calibrate with internal 20 g weight for analytical balance and with 100 mg as a microbalance before making any weighing.
3. Do not depend on any prior calibration.
4. Each day, a fixed weight stored in the balance housing should be weighed and any deviation of more than one in the place indicated below for the particular balance should be reported.

(a) Analytical balance: Use 20 g weight; there should be no variation in the observed weight in the first four places to the right of decimal.

(b) Microbalance: Use 100 mg weight; there should be no variation in the first three places to the right of decimal.

Note: Accuracy of weight (20 g or 100 mg) is not important, aim of above check is to find out if any drift has been there. Weighing of fixed weights will determine whether the knife edge is defective or not. If there is no drift, there will be no variation in the observed weight in the first four or three places as the case may be.

5. Weigh the samples when they are at the same temperature as the balance.
6. Record the weight after the reading is stable for at least few seconds. Do not allow the sample to remain on the balance for longer period as there can be change in weight due to humidity.
7. If the sample has been stored in refrigerator allow sufficient time for the sample and the container to attain temperature as that of balance.
8. Do not open the container until sample and container are at equilibrium to prevent condensation of moisture in the sample.
9. Weights or samples should be just placed (not dropped) on the pan to avoid damage to the balance.

Note: The above procedure will eliminate or reduce the errors. The extra time required for checking will be compensated by improved accuracy of the results.

Calibration of pH Meter

Requirements

- Reference buffer solutions of pH 4.0, 7.0 and 9.0
- Calibrated voltmeter (multimeter)

Procedure

- As per SOP set the instrument at pH 4.0, 7.0 and 9.0 using reference buffer solutions.
- Check the electrode for its millivolts output and compare with initial one.

Calibration frequency

- Every time for pH performance.
- Six months for electrode performance.

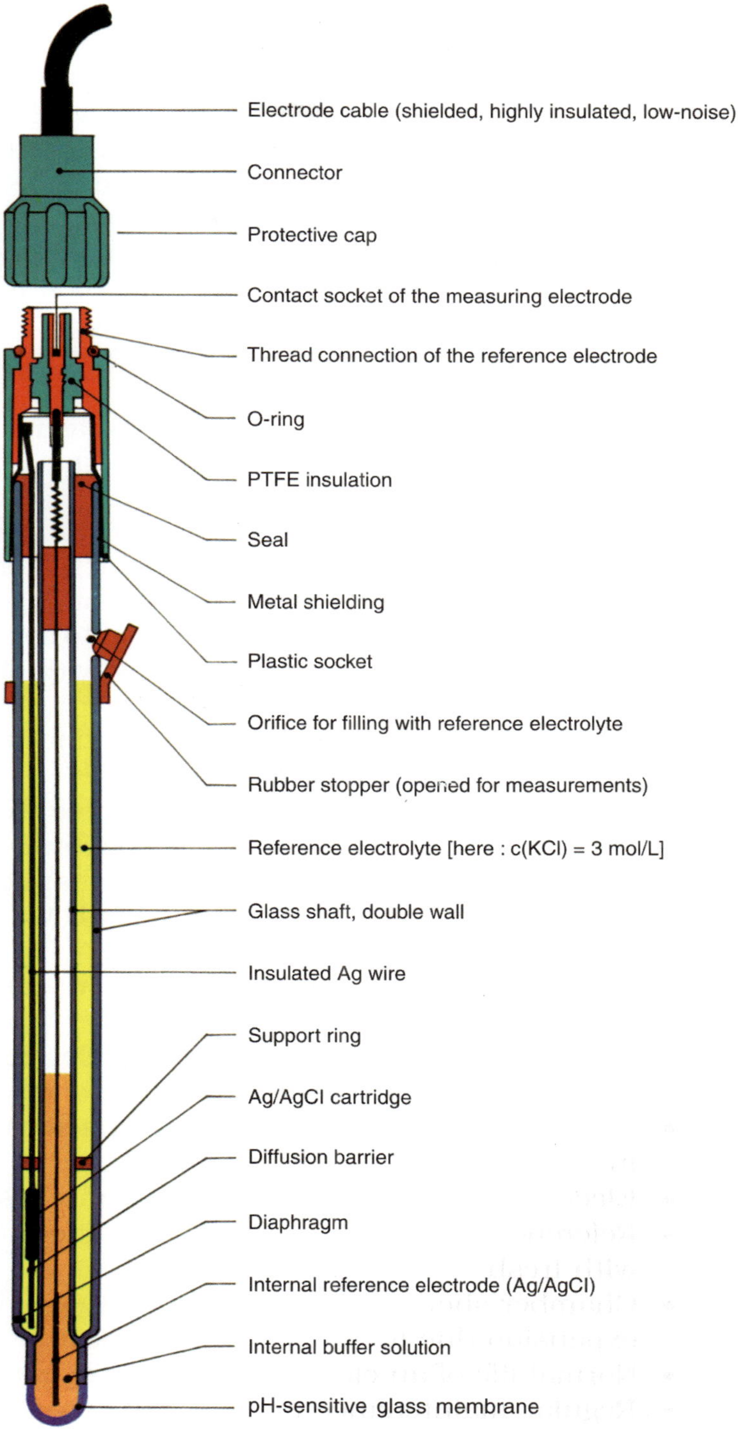

Metrosensor long life (LL) combined pH electrode with Ag/AgCl cartridge; quicker response to temperature and more reliable pH measurements. (*Courtesy:* Metrohm, Switzerland through M/s Micro-Devices & Computers, Chennai, India)

Note:
- pH meter can only correct the temperature behaviour of the electrodes and never that of the solution to be measured.
- If electrodes stored in dry condition, there is likelihood of zero point drift; can be corrected by storing in water.
- If the solution components react with electrodes, one may observe slow response, zero-point drift; can be corrected by treating with etching salt/HCl.
- On deposition of solid on electrode membrane, there is slow response and zero-point drift; store the electrode in storing acid or heat with etching salt/HCl. Deposition of protein on electrode membrane leads to zero-point drift; can be corrected by heating with 5% pepsin in 0.1 M HCl.
- Measurement of pH of water-organic solvent involves risk of precipitation of KCl electrolyte at the junction between reference electrode and measuring electrode.
- For measuring pH of mixed solvents (water-organic), electrodes require frequent rehydration, i.e., soaking in water or acidic buffer.
- While measuring pH of semisolids (ointment, cream and syrup), the diaphragm of the electrode is subject to contamination; after measurement it should be cleaned properly with ethanol followed by purified water.
- Electrodes should not be left in solution with high sugar contents as dehydration of the gel may occur.
- Water used as medium should be free from CO_2 as this can cause problem in case of samples with low buffering capacity.
- Electrodes must be frequently cleaned as per manufacturer's instructions, however, soaking in 0.1 M HCl or HNO_3, 0.1 M NaOH and finally with acid.
- In case of silicone contamination (from grease), soaking in nitric acid (5 hours) will dissolve the silicone.
- Long storage in storage solution accelerates aging process. Store, dry and soak in buffer before use.
- Bulb of the electrodes should be cleaned with soft tissue paper soaked in n-propanol.
- Electrodes must be inspected for scratches, cracks and deposits, etc.
- Reference electrode of refillable electrode should be drained and refilled with fresh solution frequently.
- Chamber should be filled upto 70-80% of its capacity to take care of expansion due to temperature changes.
- Normal life of an electrode is about 2 years if maintained properly.
- Regular maintenance and proper storage of electrodes shall ensure proper performance and extended life.

Calibration of UV-Visible Spectrophotometer

UV-visible (UV-Vis) spectrophotometer is the most commonly used instrument in any analytical laboratory. Its popularity is primarily due to the fact that it is easy to use particularly at the hands of fledgling analysts and the speed of analysis.

One of the most important part of any validation plan is the procedures put in place to ensure that the instrument systems are in calibration as calibration is one of the fundamental building blocks that ensure compliance. For calibration of UV-visible spectrophotometer many methods have been suggested each having its problems and limitations. Various parameters to be validated are absorbance, accuracy, wavelength accuracy, stray light (220 nm and 340 nm), drift and noise.

Most commonly recommended method for checking absorbance accuracy is to use solution of potassium dichromate (6.006 mg/100 ml in 0.005 N sulphuric acid). It exhibits characteristic spectral graph having minima (valley) at 235 and 313 nm and maxima at 257 and 350 nm. In addition to resulting process errors that arise from making up the solutions, potassium dichromate is a notorious oxidizing agent resulting in very poor stability of the solution. Off-the-shelf made up solutions have their merits but their stability cannot be guaranteed once the bottle has been opened. Many customers use filters those having calibration traceable to international standards. Filter tolerances have to be taken into account but these errors are consistent for a given set of conditions. Usually, a set of four neutral density filters are available. Holmium filler for absorbance accuracy, Didymium filter for wavelength accuracy and two filters designed to assess stray light at 220 nm and 340 nm. One can use 1.2% solution of potassium chloride to check the level of stray light. It should be less than 1% transmittance. Figure shows the typical spectral graph with Holmium oxide glass filter with characteristic maxima at 241.5, 287.5, 360.9 or 536.2 nm.

Note: 1. For calibration of wavelength, tolerance of ±1 nm in the range of 200-400 nm and ±3 nm in visible range (400-600 nm) is usually recommended.

2. Level of stray light increases with the age of instrument.

Indian Pharmacopoeia recommends the use of holmium perchloride solution, the emission lines of deuterium lamp or the lines of mercury vapour lamp. Using the emission lines from deuterium lamp has the benefit as the source is present in an instrument. However, this source has only two useful wavelengths i.e. 656.1 nm and 486.0 nm, hence the complete wavelength range especially the UV region cannot be checked. Incidentally, most of the drug substances absorb in UV region. Recently, new models of UV-visible spectrophotometer having mercury vapour lamp have been introduced. The emission lines of mercury vapour lamp covers the entire wavelength range.

Parameters to be Validated

- Absorbance accuracy
- Wavelength accuracy
- Linearity check
- Drift
- Noise (0A/2A)
- Stray light (220/340 nm)

Absorbance accuracy of UV-visible spectrophotometers using 60.0 mg/litre of potassium dichromate solution in 0.005 M sulphuric acid

Wavelength (nm)	*A 1%, 1 cm*	*Absorbance*
235 nm (minima/valley)	124.54 (122.9-126.2)	0.748 (0.740-0.756)
257 (maxima)	144.02 (142.4-145.5)	0.865 (0.856-0.894)
313 nm (minima/valley)	48.62 (47.0-50.3)	0.292 (0.289-0.295)
350 (maxima)	106.56 (104.9-108.2)	0.640 (0.634-0.646)

Note: For absorbance accuracy, potassium nitrate solutions (1.065%, 0.710% and 0.355% w/v) can be used. The absorption of these solutions is measured at 302 nm. The calculated absorbance values (A 1%, 1 cm) should not differ by more than 0.010 of the values 0.75, 0.50 and 0.25.

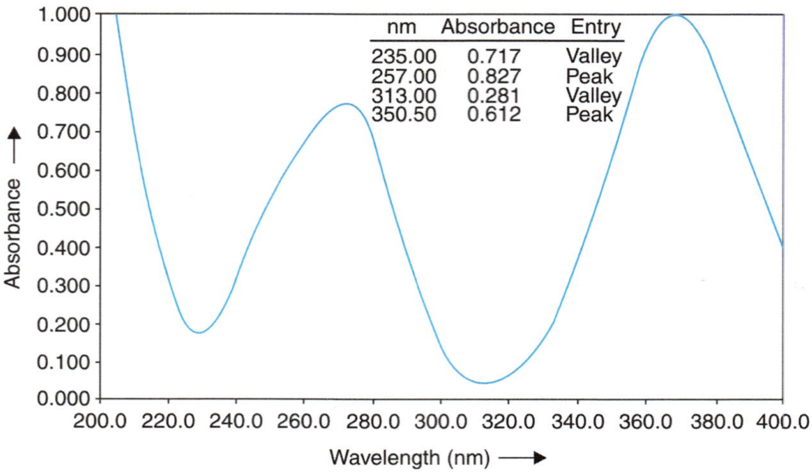

Typical spectrum of potassium chromate solution in 0.01 N sulphuric acid for checking absorbance accuracy of UV-visible spectrophotometer.

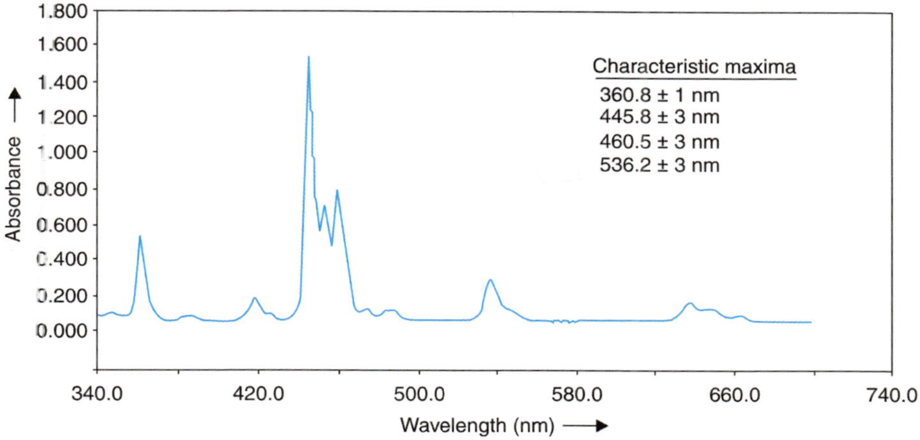

Typical spectrum using calibrated holmium oxide glass filter for checking wavelength accuracy of a UV-visible spectrophotometer.

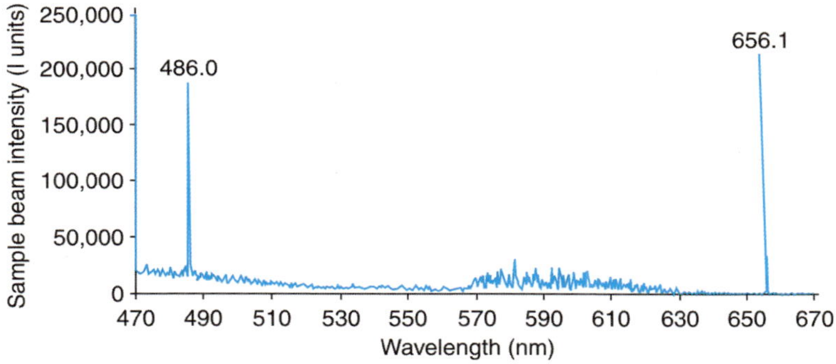

Deuterium lamp emission spectrum for checking wavelength accuracy of a UV-visible spectrophotometer.

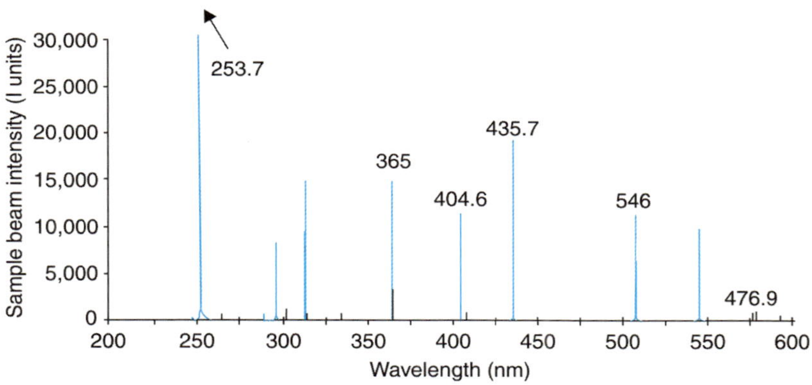

Typical mercury lamp emission spectrum for checking wavelength accuracy of a UV-visible spectrophotometer.

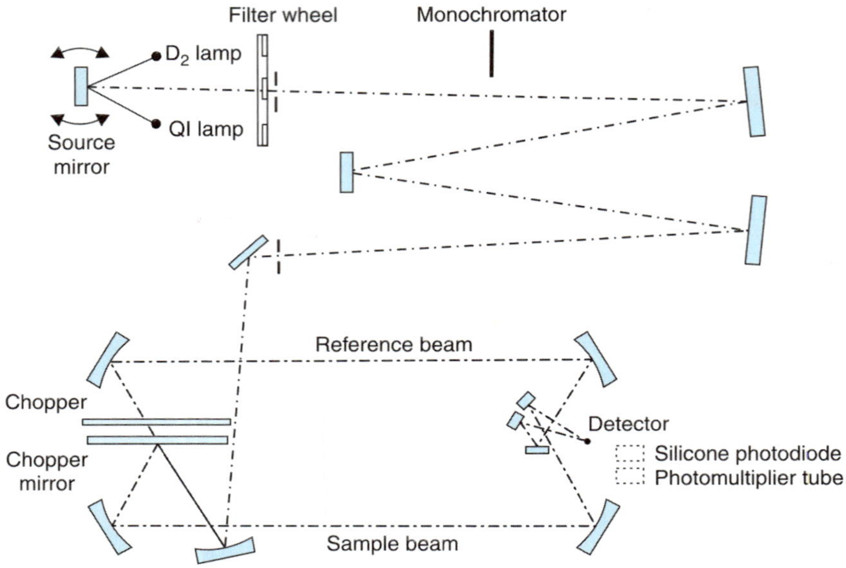

Optical system of a double beam, monochromator UV-visible spectrophotometer.

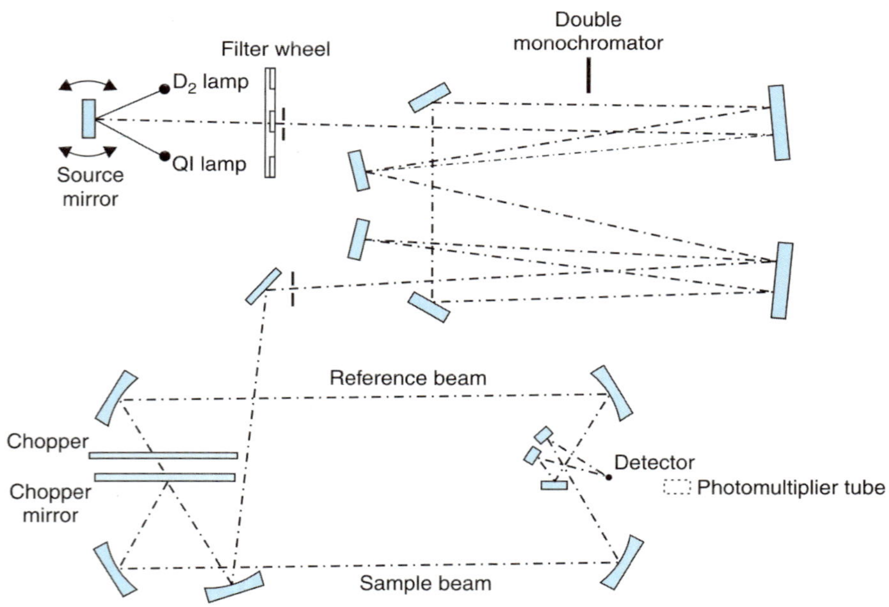

Optical system of a double beam, double chromator UV-visible spectrophotometer.

TYPICAL CALIBRATION/VALIDATION RECORD OF AN INSTRUMENT (CALIBRATION CERTIFICATE)

Name of the instrument:	UV-visible spectrophotometer
Name of the manufacturer:	Perkin-Elmer
Model No. and year of manufacture:	LAMBDA-25 (λ_{25})
Date of installation:	May 2008
Laboratory division/section where instrument is installed:	Instrumental Division
Environmental temperature:	25 ± 2 °C
Range of calibration:	190-1100 nm
Date of previous calibration:	May 2009
Date of calibration:	29.8.2009
Calibration standard and its tracibility:	$K_2Cr_2O_7$ solution in 0.005 M H_2SO_4
Calibration results:	Described
Date of re-calibration (next date of calibration):	28.11.2009

Name and signature of
calibrating analyst

(Authorised signatory)

CALIBRATION OF UV-VISIBLE SPECTROPHOTOMETER

(a) Absorbance accuracy

S. No.	Wavelength (nm)	Absorbance (1%, 1 cm) observed	Specified value of absorbance	Maximum tolerance
1.	235	125.68	124.5	122.9 to 126.2
2.	257	144.50	144.5	112.4 to 145.7
3.	313	47.69	48.6	47.0 to 50.3
4.	350	105.74	106.6	104.9 to 108.2

(b) Resolution power (Toluene & N-hexane)

S. No.	Absorbance at 266 nm	Absorbance at 269 nm	Observed value of ratio of ABS at 269/ABS at 266	IP requirement for ratio of ABS at 269/ABS at 266
1.	1.382	2.375	1.71	NLT 1.5
2.	1.384	2.376	1.71	NLT 1.5
3.	1.384	2.377	1.71	NLT 1.5
4.	1.388	2.374	1.71	NLT 1.5
5.	1.401	2.373	1.71	NLT 1.5
6.	1.408	2.366	1.71	NLT 1.5
7.	1.386	2.372	1.71	NLT 1.5
8.	1.379	2.376	1.71	NLT 1.5
9.	1.381	2.373	1.71	NLT 1.5
10.	1.375	2.372	1.71	NLT 1.5

Decrease in resolution shall cause decrease in extinction coefficients at the measurement wavelengths leading to inaccurate analytical results. Thus, sensitivity of the measurement is compromised and finer features of the spectrum are likely to be lost. The resolution of UV-Vis spectrophotometer is directly related to its spectral band width (SBW). Obviously, smaller the SBW, finer the resolution. SBW is dependent on the slit width and dispersion power of the monochromator. For higher resolution, spectrophotometer with variable slit width are required whereas for routine analytical work, spectrophotometer with fixed slit width will be suitable. In spectrophotometer equipped with diode array detector, the resolution is also dependent on the number of diodes in array.

(c) Stray light (Potassium chloride solution)

S. No.	Absorbance at 200 nm	IP requirement	S. No.	Absorbance at 200 nm	IP requirement
1.	2.366	>2	6.	2.326	>2
2.	2.357	>2	7.	2.315	>2
3.	2.340	>2	8.	2.344	>2
4.	2.345	>2	9.	2.336	>2
5.	2.325	>2	10.	2.316	>2

Stray light is defined as the detected light of any wavelength that is outside the band width of the wavelengths selected for measurement. Stray light causes decrease in absorbance and reduces the linearity range of the instrument. High absorbance measurements are likely to be affected more severely by stray light. It is reported that at 1% transmittance, stray light at 1% of the incident light may cause 15% drop in absorbance. Further, stray light is likely to cause deviation from linearity particularly at high absorbance. At the same time, noise is likely to cause deviation in linearity at low absorbance range. Interestingly absorbance values in the range of 0.3-1 AU is most preferred range in UV-Vis analysis, being less susceptible to deviation by stray light and noise.

(d) Linearity

Linearity of the instrument was checked with caffeine (λ_{max} 271.66 nm). See enclosed linearity curve.

(e) Baseline check (Noise level)

See enclosed spectra from 200–1100 nm.

Note: The calibration results reported in this certificate are valid at the time of calibration and under the stated conditions of measurement for particular sample identified.

Practical Tips

1. Check the intensity and age of the lamp before starting the analysis as the lamp which has been used for long period usually gives high baseline noise and unstable energy output.
2. Check the cells; make sure they are clean and free from contamination. Optical characteristics of any pair of cells should match closely.
3. Only certified reference material should be used for performance check of the instrument.
4. While using potassium dichromate solution, ambient temperature should be between 21-25°C. For temperatures outside this range, data need to be corrected as per instructions given along with reference standard material.

Commonly Commercially Available Reference Materials

1. Potassium dichromate solution
2. Toluene-hexane solution
3. Potassium chloride solution
4. Neutral density fillers
5. Holmium oxide solution

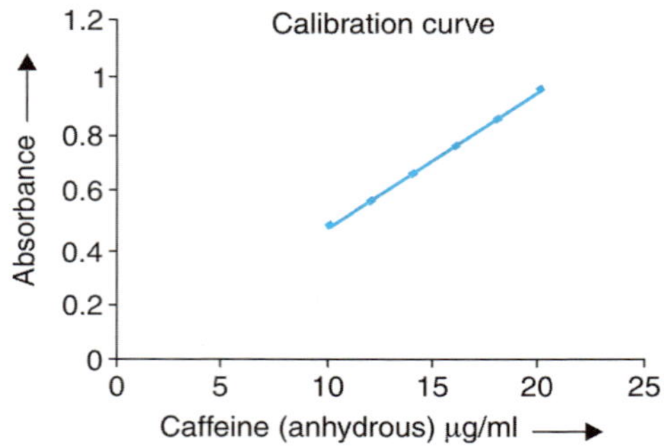

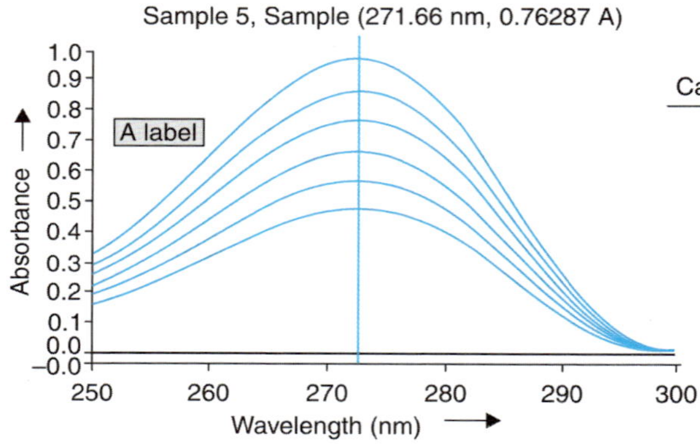

Solution of Caffeine in water (10-20 µg/ml)

Caffeine	Conc. (µg/ml)	Abs.
1	10	0.4795
2	12	0.5689
3	14	0.6646
4	16	0.7649
5	18	0.8579
6	20	0.964

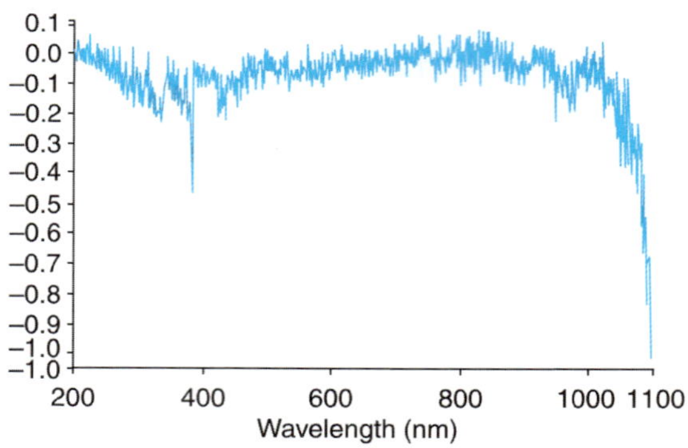

Base-line check (Noise level)

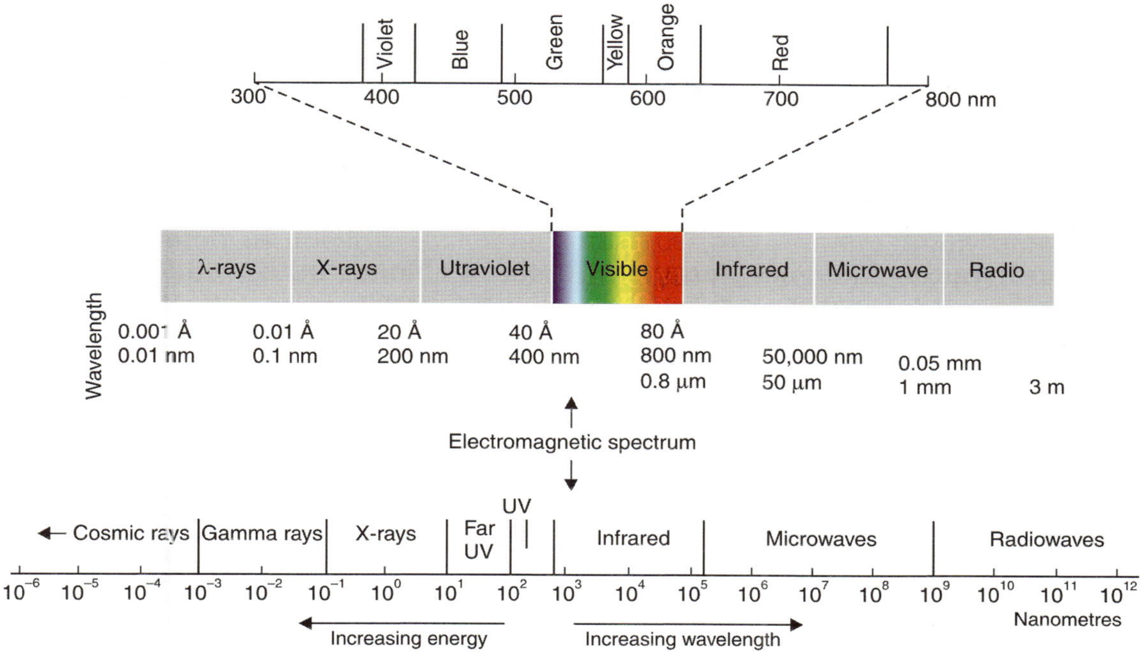

Region	*Wavelength (nm)*
Far ultraviolet	10-200
Near ultraviolet	200-380
Visible	380-780
Near infrared	780-3,000
Middle infrared	3,000-30,000
Far infrared	30,000-300,000
Microwave	300,000-1,000,000,000

Note: The human eye is only sensitive to a tiny proportion of the total electromagnetic spectrum between approximately 380 and 780 nm (visible region) and within this area we perceive the colours of the rainbow from violet through to red. If the full electromagnetic spectrum shown in the figure was redrawn on a linear scale and the visible region was represented by the length of one centimetre, then the boundary between radio and microwaves would have to be drawn approximately 25 kilometres away!

PROCUREMENT OF ANALYTICAL INSTRUMENTS

Requirement

Before planning purchase of an instrument, one should have sound rationale for purchasing the required instrument. It should justify the expenses. The purpose of acquiring an instrument may be:

(a) Increasing productivity
(b) To meet specific need
(c) To meet regulatory requirement
(d) To enhance the capability of the laboratory

Preparation of Specifications of Analytical Instruments

1. Nature of analytical work (quality control, R & D, in-process control).
2. Is the analysis required qualitative, semi-quantitative or quantitative?
3. Are the reference standards available for comparison?
4. What is the degree of analytical precision and accuracy required?
5. What is the expected range of analyte concentration?
6. What is the quantity of sample usually available for each analysis?
7. What is the probable sample matrix and which component of the matrix is likely to interfere in the analysis?
8. Are you required to follow only compendial (USP/BP/IP/EP/JP) methods or alternative methods of analysis can also be employed?
9. Pre-installation requirements.
10. What safety practices are required?
11. Number of samples to be analysed per day (throughput per day).
12. How quickly the results are required?
13. Is automation required? If so, to what extent?
14. Do you plan to upgrade the instrument at later date to meet future requirements?
15. What type of instruments are being used in other laboratories engaged in similar analytical work?
16. Spares and consumables.
17. Are there any economic constraints? Strike balance between the cost and the performance of the instrument. Remember, least expensive instrument may not be the best investment and most expensive instrument may not be the best investment for a particular purpose.
18. Academic qualifications and training level of the personnel who will handle the instruments in your laboratory.

Note: 1. Some degree of compromise may sometimes be necessary. One must assign priorities to various factors considering the ultimate objective of analysis and future planning.

2. All the users (analysts) may not be ready to tackle complicated operations due to lack of professional competency.

3. For routine assay of main active ingredients in dosage form for product release, isocratic HPLC system with variable wavelength detector may be adequate, however, if laboratory is involved in stability indicating assay or to study impurity profile, gradient HPLC system with more sensitive detector may be needed.

SELECTION OF VENDORS (SCIENTIFIC EQUIPMENT SUPPLIERS)

"Certification and qualification of vendors/suppliers of raw material, instruments and other inventories should be the responsibility of quality control department and be part of pre-approval programme of all potential vendors/ suppliers."

One of the most difficult task in choosing an instrument is selecting a vendor because human interaction, personalities and emotions come into the picture. It is advisable to make several contacts with one or more vendors' representatives before selecting an instrument as people will be your main source of information about the product and the manufacturer. You should feel comfortable while speaking with them, asking them questions and hearing their advice. Try calling the technical support line and see how quickly and accurately they answer your questions. The best measure of a vendor is the satisfaction of the current users of the product you are planning to purchase. Most vendors will supply you the names, addresses and telephone numbers of only selected users, who are almost always happy with the product and after-sale service. To get less biased evaluation of a vendor, it is preferable if you can find users through other channels such as professional societies, scientific seminars/conferences and other professional contacts. However, it is preferable that the vendor (SES) should have greater expertise than the customer on the technique and the instrument being offered.

To help the analysts to select the vendors for procurement of instrument with required specifications, some important guidelines have been compiled.

1. Is the vendor specialized in the analytical field or is just a trader?
2. Is the vendor dedicated to selling analytical instruments only or is just a small part of a big organisation?

3. What is the financial status of the vendor? Purchasing an instrument from a financially unsound vendor can be risky.
4. For how long the vendor has been in the field of selling analytical instruments (vendor's previous experience)?
5. Vendor's familiarity with CGMP and CGLP?
6. Does the vendor have the list of customers particularly in your region to whom he has supplied the instruments in the recent past?
7. Can the vendor establish that the instruments under consideration are proven to operate satisfactorily in Indian laboratory conditions?
8. Will the vendor carry out after-sale service of the instrument? Has he the facilities for annual service contract? If so, what will be the charges? Reliability of the vendor needs to be established; find out from current users.
9. Before finalising the purchase, can the vendor arrange practical demonstration of the instrument with actual sample analysis of your field?
10. Is the vendor equipped with application laboratory and has trained technical personnel?
11. Will the vendor provide necessary help and guidance in developing and validating method of analysis?
12. Does the vendor support the customer for training including the level of training in his application laboratory? If so, are there any financial effects?
13. Does the vendor usually stock substantial amount of consumables required for maintenance and after-sale service of the instrument?
14. Does the vendor has the facilities for updating the knowledge of your analysts from time to time with application notes?
15. Will the vendor be arranging workshop/seminars from time to time? If so, what shall be the charges for participating in them?
16. Has he informed you the additional facilities required in your laboratory for installation and operation of the said instrument and has your laboratory been adequately equipped as suggested by the vendor?
17. Have you any previous experience with the vendor either directly or through knowledge gained from other laboratories? If so, how do you assess his general performance particularly in respect of after-sale service and technical expertise?
18. Have you prepared the detailed specifications of the instrument you are looking for, considering the requirements of your laboratory before making trade enquiries?
19. Have you consulted your fellow analysts in the field known to you before making final choice of the instrument?
20. Are you satisfied that the instrument to be procured shall meet your present requirements and can be updated to meet future requirements?

21. If you are duplicating the instrument, take into consideration the past performance of the existing one.
22. While making budgetary provisions for the purchase of an instrument, consider procurement of consumable spares at least for 2-3 years.
23. Carry out comparative evaluation of technical and financial aspects of various marketed brands of the instrument meeting your specifications before making the final choice.
24. Has any of your technical personnel been trained in the operation and maintenance of different analytical instruments including the one under consideration for purchase?

*Note:*1. Although technical and economic factors have significant bearing on the selection of vendor, however final decision should be made after properly assessing each prospective vendor's capabilities in respect of above factors. This will help you in short-listing the vendors.

2. Strong relationship with fewer but better suppliers is mutually beneficial to facilitate improvement in quality, cost and overall responsiveness.
3. Once the vendor is chosen, he should be considered important player of your team. The vendor should provide all the possible assistance in establishing the equipment validation. The vendor will carry out normal operations checks for its pre-qualification acceptability criteria.
4. Once the vendor has demonstrated the equipment validation, optimal limitation of the instrument should clearly be understood by the analytical chemist.

"For wrong selection, you will probably be reminded every day."

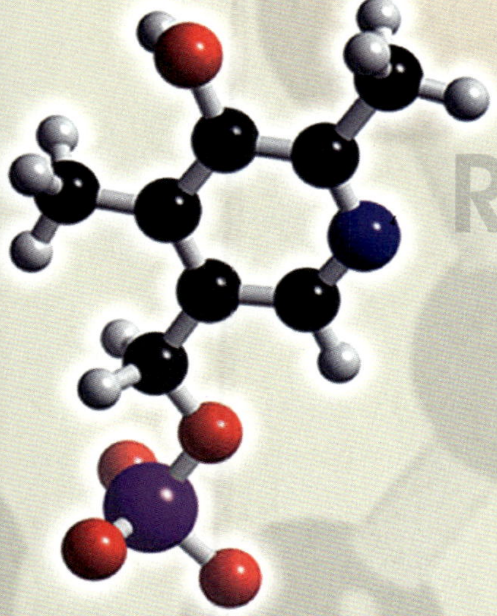

4

Method Development
Optimization
Validation
Transfer
Revalidation

METHOD DEVELOPMENT

Developing a method of analysis is usually based on existing literature using quite similar instrumentation. In fact, it is rare that a method is developed that does not in some way relate or compare to existing literature-based approach. The development of any new or improved method usually tailors existing approach and instrumentation. Method development usually requires selecting the method requirements and type of instruments to use and why.

Reasons for Developing A New Method

- There may not be a suitable method for a particular analyte.
- Existing methods may be too error-, artifact, and/or contamination-prone, or may have poor accuracy or precision.
- Existing methods may be too expensive and time consuming.
- Existing methods may not provide adequate sensitivity or analyte selectivity in samples of interest.
- Newer instrumentation and techniques may be available that provide improved analyte identification or detection limits, greater accuracy or precision.
- There may be need for an alternative method to confirm analytical data for legal reasons.
- There may be scientific reason.

Type of Analytical Problems

1. It may be essentially a problem already solved and the earlier validated analytical procedure may be directly applied such as compendial procedures.
2. It may be related to earlier problem and the existing validation procedure may be applicable with some judicious changes/modifications.
3. It may altogether be a new problem, one might not have encountered or solved before. It is here that the experience/skill/expertise of the analyst is called for and the options are:
   (a) Use personal experience and knowledge of analytical chemistry.
   (b) Try out well-established procedures.
   (c) Survey the literature; unfortunately in most of the reported methods, the knowledge/information about various parameters of the method (LOD, LOQ, precision, accuracy, range, interference) is often inadequate, and some degree of optimization is always required.

"Errors are troublesome opponents of accurate and precise analytical results."

Selection of Analytical Method

One of the most difficult situations that an analyst may be confronted with is to select most suitable procedure for a particular problem. With ever increasing number of analytical methods being reported, it is impossible to familiarize with all the available methods. We are mostly relying on knowledge, experience, scanning of literature, dependent on habits/fashion. One is usually tempted to apply those methods which are well established or the analyst may have personal experience, though the choice is often limited because of laboratory facilities in term of instruments/personnel. In view of variables in quantitative analysis such as inhomogeneity, sampling error, random error (instruments/ operator), the selected method must reveal all these variables. First stage in the selection or development of method is to establish what is to be measured and how accurately it should be measured. Unless one has series of methods at hand to assess quality of the product, validation programme may have limited validity. The selected method must have the following parameters:

1. As simple as possible.
2. Most specific.
3. Most productive, economical and convenient.
4. As accurate and precise as required.
5. Multiple source of key components (reagents, columns, TLC plates) should be avoided.
6. To be fully optimised before transfer for validation of its characteristics such as accuracy, precision, sensitivity, ruggedness etc.

Note: (a) Method validation for a particular analytical problem may not always be applicable in other situations due to interference of other ingredients present in the formulation.

(b) The method so developed must discriminate between the available for which it is designed, process contamination, decomposition products, related substances.

(c) Before finally selecting a method for application in a given case, trial run of the proposed method is advisable.

Data for Analytical Procedures

(Before finalising the method, it is preferable to enlist the proposed analytical specifications to be applied to a particular substance or its dosage form.)

1. Justification for proposing an analytical procedure with comparison to other possible alternatives should be described.
2. Scientific basis i.e. the principle involved in the proposed procedure should be elaborated. If the proposed method is intended to replace the existing procedure comparative laboratory data including merits/demerits should

be made available. Understand customer expectations (analysis time, ease of use, analysis cost, available instrumentation).

3. List of all necessary reagents, test solutions with directions for their preparation. Unstable reagents be identified, their storage conditions and usable shelf life be specified.
4. List of instruments required along with their parameters such as instrument type, cell dimensions, GLC/HPLC columns, TLC plates and sensitivity required.
5. Detailed step by step procedure along with equilibration, extraction and centrifugation time, system suitability parameters if required, preparation of sample, standard, use of blank and other procedural details as required.
6. Detailed complete formulae for calculation of analytical results with all terms/symbols defined along with representative calculations for each parameter.
7. Precautions or any other unusual hazards in carrying out the method be indicated.
8. It must be specified whether the method is capable of detecting decomposition products/impurities/related substances or not.
9. Whether the proposed method is stability indicating or not.
10. Understand customer expectations (analysis time, ease of use, analysis cost, available instrument).

Note: The proposed method must provide comprehensive details as deemed necessary to allow reasonably trained analyst to perform it in a reliable and reproducible manner.

OPTIMIZATION

During optimization, the analytical conditions that have been worked out during initial stage of development are further improved/maximized in term of LOD, LOQ and overall ability to quantify the analyte of interest. While attempting optimization of the method, one must provide analytical figures of merit which are required to meet the assay requirements, i.e. accuracy, precision, LOD, LOQ, linearity must be clearly defined, otherwise, it may be difficult to optimize any analytical method.

Results obtained during optimization should be evaluated against the limits set forth by the figures of merit. At this stage, the analyst should evaluate how does the newly developed and optimized method compares with the currently accepted method of analysis for the analyte of interest. If the new method offers any significant advantage, only then one should put in additional time, efforts and resources; if there is no apparent advantage, additional efforts may not be justified. Further, the analyst should evaluate the scope of the new method; whether it is applicable only to the main analyte of interest or other related analytes such as impurities, degradation products/related substances, since the method for a specific analyte has far less utility.

Optimization of method can follow either manual or computer-driven approach. Manual approach involves varying only one experimental variable at a time while keeping other constant and recording the changes in response. This univariable approach is slow, time-consuming and quite expensive; however, it provides better understanding of the principle and theory involved. Most of the analytical methods are expected ultimately to be used in quality control laboratory; they require an additional degree of optimization compared to research papers.

HAS THE METHOD BEEN ADEQUATELY OPTIMIZED

General criteria

1. LOD is at least one order lower than needed.
2. Calibration curves are linear over wider range starting with LOQ.
3. Sample throughput is increased.
4. Sample preparation prior to analysis is minimized.
5. Interference is identifiable and minimum.
6. Analytical data can be easily acquired.
7. Reproducibility of analytical figures of merit is demonstrated with acceptable level of accuracy and precision.
8. Cost of analysis per sample is minimized.

Note: 1. The end user should plan on verifying method performance prior to making it as SOP.
2. Properly developed and fully optimized method is readily validated.

Since optimization of the method is one of the most time-consuming parts of the overall method development procedure requiring acquision of large amount of quantitative data, the analyst should ensure that the method so optimized has broader practical utility instead of just meeting immediate requirements.

Validation of analytical method

Since validation is a time-consuming exercise, the method should not be taken up for validation until and unless fully developed and optimized.

To communicate effectively and purposefully on the subject like validation it helps if all can communicate from similar concept. Attitude, proper management of human resources and communication skill are few inputs for validation of product/instruments/personnel/analytical methods.

VALIDATION

It may be defined in many ways, but most important point to emphasize is its practical application, concept, its significance and impact.

- A process involving confirmation or establishing by laboratory studies that a method/procedure/system/analyst give accurate and reproducible result for intended analytical application in a proven and established range.
- To establish that performance characteristics of the method (accuracy, precision, sensitivity, ruggedness, etc.) meet the requirements of intended analytical application.
- Process of providing documented evidence that the system/procedure does what it is intended to do precisely and reliably.
- Systematic approaches to identify, measure, evaluate, document, re-evaluate all the critical steps responsible to ensure qualitative/quantitative detection of analytes accurately and precisely before establishing the validation of the method under evaluation.
- Collection and evaluation in a documented form of repetitive evidence collected according to agreed protocols to provide high degree of assurance that the procedure under consideration will consistently produce a product meeting its pre-determined specifications or quality attributes.

A validated transferable analytical method that will serve its end-users for an extended period of time with minimal complications. Method validation is partly science, partly art and remaining major part being book-keeping and accounting. To be very honest, very few laboratories do satisfactory job while executing different components. Methods are often developed and validated by R&D scientists who are not end-users of the method. Obviously, the requirements of end-users are often ignored leading to a complex but scientifically elegant method getting developed. Though QC chemists are well educated and technically sound, often they have to work under great pressure and complexity of the method may make their life difficult. Therefore, methods should be as simple and robust as possible keeping in mind the requirements of the end-users.

Types of Validation

(a) Prospective validation: This is employed when historical data of the product is not available or is not sufficient and in-process and finished product testing are not adequate to ensure reproducibility or high degree of compliance to product likely attributes. Such validation is conducted prior to release of either new product or product made under revised/new manufacturing process where revision may effect the product characters.

(b) Retrospective: This provides trend of comparative result i.e. review and evaluation of existing information for comparison when historical data is sufficient and readily available. Retrospective validation is acceptable provided specific test results generated by reliable analytical method on number of samples are available to allow statistical analysis. Simply pass/fail test results would not be accepted as part of retrospective validation—useful for trend setting.

(c) Concurrent: Based on information generated during implementation of a system. For this extensive testing and monitoring are performed as part of initial run of the method. Concurrent validation verifies the quality characteristics of a particular batch and provide assurance that the same quality would be attained again when subsequent batches are manufactured and analysed under similar conditions.

Analytical Validation

Analytical monitoring of a pharmaceutical product or of specific ingredients within the product is necessary to ensure its safety/efficacy throughout all phases of its shelf life (storage, distribution and use). Such monitoring is in accordance with the specifications elaborated/validated during the product development. Analytical validation ensures that the selective analytical method will give reproducible and reliable results adequate for intended purpose. It is therefore necessary to define precisely both the conditions in which the procedure is to be used and the purpose for which it is intended. These principles are applicable both for pharmacopoeial and non-pharmacopoeial procedures being used. These guidelines are also applicable for examining physicochemical as well as biological procedures.

Reasons/Purpose for Validation

1. Enables scientists to communicate scientifically and effectively on technical matters.
2. Setting standards of evaluation procedures for checking compliance and taking remedial measures.
3. Economic: Reduction in cost associated with process sampling and testing. The consistency and reliability of validated analytical procedure is to produce a quality product with all the quality attributes, thus providing indirect cost saving from reduced testing or re-testing and elimination of product rejection.
4. As quality of the product cannot always be assured by routine quality control because of testing of statistically insignificant number of samples, the validation thus shall provide adequacy and reliability of a system or a procedure to meet the pre-determined criteria/attributes providing high

degree of confidence that the same level of quality is consistently built into each unit of finished product from batch to batch.

5. Retrospective validation is useful for trend comparison of results compliance to CGMP/CGLP.
6. Closer interaction with pharmacopoeial forum to address analytical problems.
7. International pharmacopoeial harmonisation particularly in respect of impurities determination and their limits.
8. For taking appropriate action in case of non-compliance.

As quality control process is not static, some form of validation/verification should continue till the validated process is in use. It should not be the concept that once the procedure has been initially developed/validated and then forgotten. Pharmacopoeial methods are usually considered validated.

In validation studies, suitability of the final method for a given analyte in a selected matrix is demonstrated using specific instrumentation including different experimental steps so that the method can be transferred from one laboratory to another laboratory suitably equipped and staffed.

Although, there are well-established guidelines for validation of a method, but there may be several approaches that can be employed. However, the primary concern of the analyst should be to select an approach that will prove to be true validation. Thus, finally, it is the responsibility of the analyst to select correct validation approach.

Validation approaches may include zero, single and double blind spiking method, inter-laboratory collaborative studies and comparison with currently available compendium methods.

(a) Zero-blind method

Single analyst using the method to demonstrate accuracy, precision and recovery of the method. Though this approach is fast, simple and quite useful, but it is very much biased and may lead to subjective results creating doubts for unbiased reviewer or final user of the method. However, this approach requires minimum time, manpower and cost and may be good to start validation process. If this approach fails, one may not proceed with the validation of the method.

(b) Single-blind approach

In this case, one analyst prepares the sample at varying concentration and passes on to the second analyst who actually carries out the analysis of the sample. The results so obtained are compiled and returned to the first analyst for comparison. This approach appears to be unbiased but may invite biased approach on part of the first analyst who compares the data in that he may try to bring two sets of data into better agreement. However, if single-blind approach has proved successful one can think of including additional analysis.

(c) Double-blind approach

This involves three analysts, one who actually prepares the sample at varying concentration, second does the actual analysis and third compares both sets of analytical data received separately from first two analysts. Both first and second analysts have absolutely no access to the data. This is most objective approach provided third analyst has no bias.

(d) Inter-laboratory collaborative study

This is probably the most widely and accepted procedure to validate any analytical method; however, it has several serious drawbacks. This is costly and time-consuming and difficult to organize. This approach is rarely employed when the method is being described in the literature for the first time.

It provides unbiased information on the performance of the analytical method. These are usually indicated when variability in analyst to analyst, instrument to instrument is high. Regulatory authorities invariably require the use of validated methods. The validation process produces performance data which is then evaluated by analysts to determine "fitness of purpose" before use in the laboratory. The candidate methods are first evaluated in a single laboratory to ascertain satisfactory repeatability data and robustness. Replication experiments also serve to highlight problems caused by heterogeneous distribution of analyte in the sample matrix. The method should then be tested in a properly organised collaborative study indicating a minimum of eight participating laboratories. Careful thought will need to be given to the material to be tested and the level of analyte present. Mode of incorporating analyte into the matrix is critical. Usually the mean of all acceptable results obtained in the collaborative study is acceptable. Confirmation of these values could be achieved by analysis using other analytical techniques. Recovery studies can help in confirming the results. However, the possibility of matrix-analyte interaction in real sample which could effect the applicability and performance of the method must be considered.

The data received from laboratories participating in the collaborative studies should be scrutinised for obvious discrepancies. Any such result should be referred back to the originator for checking or remedial purpose on technical grounds. The remaining results are then subjected to statistical evaluation and in particular, the removal of outliner using Cochran and Grubbs tests. IUPAC recommendations permit the removal of up to 22 of the participants in this way—it obviously implies that more than 78% of the participants ought to be able to obtain satisfactory results with a properly validated method as participating laboratories are normally at their "best behaviour" while taking part in such collaborative studies. On the other hand it may indicate that these laboratories were unfamiliar with the method or technique involved.

Analysis today is so complex that few workers would guarantee obtaining a correct result first time. This highlights the need to ensure that the method is indeed written up in sufficient details that the analysts who had not been involved in its development can obtain satisfactory results.

The analyst must be careful not to use such a method outside its tested range and field of application without checking that the data obtained are equally valid.

Procedural Details for Collaborative Studies

1. The method should be clearly and precisely written (no ambiguity).
2. The method so chosen must be demonstrated to apply to concentration of analyte of interest in presence of matrices.
3. All the critical variables and their effect on the results must have been determined and the need and the way for their control must be emphasized.
4. The method should provide full written details by the leader of the team and preferably tested by junior analyst or an analyst who does not have background of the method.
5. All the reagents, equipments including unusual ones should be located and available from common supplier to make collaborating laboratories to procure the same. Alternatively sufficient quantity should be procured and supplied to the collaborating laboratories.
6. The samples must be identical and homogeneous to keep sampling error to minimum.
7. For inter-laboratory collaborative studies, at least 8 laboratories should participate to analyse sufficient samples to generate minimum of 40 point data.
8. Samples must be stable to withstand stress and strain of transport/ storage.
9. Reserve samples (to replace lost sample or for re-analysis of sample—to evaluate the cause in case of abnormal results).
10. Instructions for carrying out collaborative studies should be clear and reviewed by personnel not associated with study.
11. If the analyte is not very stable, all participants should start analysis at the same time.
12. Practice samples to be provided for establishing recovery, repeatability of the methodology.

Design of Collaborative Studies

1. Triplicate sample
2. Six replicates
3. Single analyst
4. Single day
5. Analyst to analyst
6. Day to day
7. Lot to lot

Advantages

1. Regulatory credibility for method validation.
2. Best estimate for reproducibility.
3. Best way to test that the method works as written.
4. Well-defined guidelines.

Disadvantages

1. Time and resources required for conducting the study.
2. Employment of highly qualified and experienced personnel.
3. Usually large number (8-12) of laboratories are required to participate to obtain a good reproducibility estimate.

(e) Comparison with a currently accepted method or compedium method

Comparison with a currently accepted or compendium analytical method is yet another validation approach. This is usually done by a single analyst, but it can be done by two analysts using a split sample. This approach uses results from the currently accepted method as verification of the new method's results. Agreement between results initially suggests validation. Disagreement is a serious cause for concern of future acceptability of the new method. However, disagreement could also suggest that the currently accepted method is invalid, creating additional problems. If the analyst can prove that the currently accepted method is indeed invalid, the analyst must then initiate an alternative approach to validate the new method. The question will eventually arise as to how many samples should be analyzed in any validation approach — 1, 2, 6, 12? In general, the more the better, and the greater the variety of samples and variation in the concentration range the better. Ideally, the method should be validated for the analyte using several different sample types, with several of each type determined separately for statistical and validation purposes. A single, zero-blind or a single, single-blind study is obviously less meaningful and less acceptable than an inter-laboratory collaborative true double-blind study of several sample matrices at widely different concentration levels. Initial validation approaches are generally less rigorous and demanding than ones performed for standard reference material (SRM) development.

Strategy for Validation of Methods

The validity of a specific method should be demonstrated in laboratory experiments using samples or standards that are similar to the unknown samples analyzed in the routine. The preparation and execution should follow a validation protocol, preferably written in a step-by-step instruction format. Possible steps for complete method validation are listed.

Steps in Method Validation

1. Develop a validation protocol or operating procedure (SOP) for the validation.
2. Define the application, purpose and scope of the method.
3. Define the performance parameters and acceptance criteria.
4. Define validation experiments.
5. Verify relevant performance characteristics of equipment (IQ, OQ, PQ).
6. Qualify materials, e.g., standards and reagents.
7. Perform pre-validation experiments.
8. Adjust method parameters and/or acceptance criteria if necessary.
9. Perform full internal (and external) validation experiments.
10. Develop SOPs for executing the method in the routine.
11. Define criteria for revalidation.
12. Define type and frequency of system suitability tests and/or analytical quality control (AQC) checks for the routine.
13. Document validation experiments and results in the validation report.

A Validation Report Should be Prepared That Includes

1. Objective and scope of the method (applicability, type).
2. Type of compounds and matrix.
3. Detailed description of chemicals, reagents, reference standards and control sample preparations.
4. Procedures for quality checks of standards and chemicals used.
5. Safety considerations.
6. Method parameters.
7. Critical parameters indicated from robustness testing.
8. Listing of equipment and its functional and performance requirements.
9. Detailed description of conditions on how the experiments were conducted, including sample preparation.
10. Statistical procedures and representative calculations.

11. Procedures for quality control in the routine (e.g. system suitability tests).
12. Representative plots, e.g. chromatograms, spectra and calibration curves.
13. Method acceptance limit performance data.
14. The expected uncertainty of measurement results.
15. Criteria for revalidation.
16. Person who developed and initially validated the method.
17. Summary and conclusions.

Scope for application of validation

1. Manufacturing process control (raw material).
2. Pre-formulation evaluation of dosage forms.
3. Stability studies.
4. Environmental control/check.
5. Cleaning controls (contamination).

Common Problems for Successful Validation

1. Failure to include sample of critical impurity, degradation product or internal standard necessary to assess the adequacy of the method.
2. Failure to list complete specifications of the method.
3. Selection of unsuitable specifications such as those which do not account for assay building.
4. Failure to provide sufficient details of reagent preparation or equipment parameters.
5. Use of arbitrary arithmetic correction.
6. Use of single source of equipment or reagent without full specifications.
7. Use of specialized tools, equipments not commercially available.
8. Use of internal standard or any other reagent which is not commercially available.
9. Failure to provide fully characterized reference standard.
10. Failure to submit complete, legible data and labelled chromatographs and spectra.

Future of validation

In spite of the advances in analytical technology offering newer methods of analysis which are more accurate and precise, the need for validation shall always remain.

It is better to do modest amount of validation work on as many assays/ products as possible rather than do an exhaustive job for few and no work on others.

As quality control process is not static, some form of validation/verification should continue till the validated procedure is in use. It should not be a concept that once the method is initially developed and validated, it is forgotten.

Responsibility

For validation work, one may require personnel with specialized training/ qualifications beyond that usually required for routine quality control. Such personnel should not only bear the responsibility but should have personally to cope with the responsibility in terms of emotion, experience and knowledge for which individual needs to have appropriate character i.e. education, commitment, leadership and empowerment.

It is advisable to get this work done from consultants under contractual obligations instead of hiring specialized personnel and facilities.

Consultant

Consultants are individuals or a group of persons hired by a company or organisation on a contractual basis. The advantages and disadvantages of having a work performed by consultants are the same in any given situation.

Consultants are able to review the present protocols and are in a position to apply experience gained in other organisations and field to problems that the personnel within the hiring company might not have anticipated. This has definite advantages as the hiring company need not go through potentially time-consuming and arduous task of recruiting technical personnel with specialized talent for particular job. This is more economically viable as work is taken up under contractual agreement with pre-determined cost and completion schedule.

Precaution: Since such works are time and cost bound, the initial contract must clearly spell completion schedule of the project and the overall cost.

Summary of validation procedure

Type of validation	*Test for*
Specificity	Interference
Accuracy	Recovery; Linearity
Sensitivity	Limit of detection; Limit of quantitation
Precision	Repeatability; Reproducibility; Ruggedness
Personnel	Qualifications; Experience; Responsibility; Proficiency
Equipment	Specifications; Vendor; Calibration; Maintenance
Service	Sanitation; Water, Waste disposal

Analytical Parameters/Analytical Performance Characteristics to be Validated

- Accuracy
- Precision
  - Repeatability
  - Intermediate precision
  - Reproducibility
- Specificity
- Limit of detection (LOD/DL)
- Limit of quantitation (LOQ/QL)
- Linearity
- Range
- Robustness
- Extraction efficiency
- Filter retention
- Stability study

Additional data

1. Representative instrument output
2. Representative calculations

Accuracy

Accuracy is the closeness of the test results to the true or accepted value i.e. measure of exactness of the analytical method. It provides an indication of any systematic error or bias in the method. In pharmaceutical industry, this is typically a straight line with a given slope and zero intercept. It is usually expressed as % recovery by assay of known or added amount of analyte within linearity range. For this, one can design experiment for recovery of known or spiked samples (usually ±10% of the claim in presence of drug product placebo matrix). The spiking may be done either by adding standard solution or dry spiking of API into matrix followed by thorough mixing, keeping the amount of matrix constant. One can also determine accuracy of a method by comparing the results with those obtained by an alternate validated method.

Precision

It expresses the degree of agreement among individual test results when the method is applied to an homogeneous sample under given conditions. Precision consists of different components i.e. repeatability and intermediate precision and reproducibility.

Repeatability (under same conditions)

It reflects the variation in the results experienced by same analyst, single day, same method, same set of reagents, same instrument within a short interval of time, only difference being the sample. Repeatibility does not distinguish between variation from the instrument or system along but also from sample preparation process. During validation, repeatibility is performed by analysing multiple replicates of the sample by the proposed method and recovery (%) values calculated for each assay value. This parameter is the main criteria for compendial assay procedure, often called method precision.

Intermediate precision (formerly known as ruggedness)

Degree of reproducibility of test results obtained by analysing the same sample under variety of test conditions such as different:

- Analysts
- Instruments
- Days
- Reagents
- Columns and TLC plates

i.e., lack of influence of environmental variables on the method. Comparison of reproducibility of test results to the precision of assay is the direct measure of ruggedness of the method.

Reproducibility (under different conditions)

When the subject method is carried out by different analysts in different laboratories, using different equipments, reagents and laboratory settings and on different days — variability of analytical results as function of analyst, day-to-day, laboratory-to-laboratory, equipment-to-equipment, etc. using the samples from same homogeneous batch. Problems connected with reproducibility of the test results are naturally compounded when tests are performed in different countries. When discussing confidence in test results, a major concern is assuring a sufficient degree of producibility. Ideally all test methods should produce accurate results with high degree of precision and be described in such a way as to ensure high levels of repeatability and reproducibility. Unfortunately, test methods processing all these characteristics are rare and considerable efforts are required in this direction.

In terms of international trade, problems with reproducibility often lead to serious disputes.

Reproducibility of test results requires:

(a) Inter-laboratory trials (proficiency tests) are required on a continuing basis to ensure that laboratories are maintaining satisfactory level of performance and may be used to generate reliable reproducibility data.

(b) The tests must be based on test methods which do not allow different procedures or interpretation.

(c) The accuracy and/or precision of the test methods must be known in advance. This requires the adoption of test methods which have been properly validated.

(d) Technical competence of the laboratory must be demonstrated which requires some kind of evaluation.

It is not part of routine validation process. It is important for method transfer to different sites.

Specificity/selectivity

Ability of the method to measure accurately and specifically the analyte of interest in presence of matrix and other components likely to be present in the sample matrix and impurities, degradation products and other related substances. For this, one may compare the test results of analysis of samples containing other ingredients/impurities/degradation products/related substances/placebo ingredients with those obtained from analysis of sample without these, i.e., the method must allow distinct analytical measurement of analyte of interest and exclusion of all other relevant interferences. If the impurities/degradation products or potential contaminants are not available, one can apply a proposed method to the strained and stressed (heat, light, himidity) samples. Degree of agreement among results will explain specificity of the method.

If the impurities/degradation products are not available, one may carry out additional purity tests by chromatography — HPLC/HPTLC.

The term selectivity is often interchangeable with specificity, however, there is distinct difference. Selectivity of the method is defined as its ability to separate analyte of interest from other components that may be present in the sample including impurities. Thus, for a method to be selective, it has to show every component in the sample i.e. a method may be specific but not necessarily be selective as well. This terminology is often used in chromatography methods i.e. HPTLC, HPLC, GC, but is not feasible in spectroscopic methods of analysis.

Limit of detection (LOD or DL)

Lowest concentration of the analyte in the sample that the method can detect but not necessarily quantify under the stated experimental conditions simply indicates that the sample is below or above certain level. Limit test prescribed as percentage or as parts per million (ppm—mcg/ml). The LOD will not only depend on the procedure of analysis but also on the type of instrument.

A. Instrumental:
   (a) S/N 2 : 1 or 2 : 1
   (b) 2-3 times of SD of blank response.
B. Non-instrumental: One has to establish the minimum level at which analyte can be reliably detected – usually LOD is 2-3 times lower than LOQ.

Obviously LOD is influenced by absolute value of the blank and SD of the method of analysis.

Limit of quantitation (LOQ or QL)

LOQ of an analytical procedure is the lowest amount of analyte in a sample that can be quantitatively estimated with acceptable accuracy and precision. It is a parameter of quantitative assay for low concentration of compounds in sample matrices and is used particularly for determination of impurities and degradation products and expressed as concentration (% or ppm).

The procedure usually followed is to analyse samples containing decreasing known quantity of the analyte and determine the lowest level at which acceptable level of accuracy/precision is attained. However, it is preferable to validate the method at or near LOQ.

- Instrumental: Usually 10 times of standard deviation of blank response; 2-3 times higher than LOD.
- Non-instrumental: One has to establish the level experimentally depending on the method of analysis employed.

Linearity

It is the ability of the analytical procedure to elicit test results that are directly proportional to the concentration of analyte present in the given sample. In a linear method the test results are directly, or by well-defined mathematical transformation, proportional to the concentration of analyte within a given range. During validation, linearity is established for all active compounds, preservatives and impurities and performed using standard.

- Analysis in duplicate.
- Determination by least square method/regression line, slope of curve will provide rsd.
- Response-concentration curve on graph paper to establish Beer's law—response to be linear on at least 5-6 points.

Note:

- Extrapolation of the curve at either end is not desirable.
- Three-point linearity curve in the concentration range of 80-120% of the claim gives an error of ±1.0% and may be resorted to.
- Slope of regression line—measure of linearity.
- Y intercept—measure of potential assay bias.

Range

This is defined as the interval between the lowest and highest levels of analyte in the sample for which the method has been demonstrated to give test results with suitable level of precision, accuracy and linearity in the range of 80/100/120 % of the claim. The range, often referred to as linearity of the method, is evaluated by spiking a placebo.

Robustness

It is the measure of the capacity of the analytical method to remain unaffected by small but deliberate variations in procedure such as pH, temperature, instrument. It provides indications for reliability of the test procedure during normal application of the method in normal laboratory conditions. It is most important parameter for transferring the method after its validation.

Extraction efficiency

It reflects the effectiveness of the extraction of the active substance from the sample matrix. The extraction efficiency can be checked by varying shaking/sonication time, temperature, the amount of extraction solvent, etc.

Filter retention

It is reasonable to expect that some components may be retained on filter paper or filtration assembly may contribute some unknown components. This parameter needs to be evaluated. Ibuprofen is significantly adsorbed on filter paper during filtration of the sample.

Analytical data required for assay validation

	Type of analysis			
	1	2		3
Parameter	*Assay*	*QT*	*QL*	*Assay*
Accuracy	Yes	Yes	—	—
Precision	Yes	Yes	No	Yes
Specificity	Yes	Yes	Yes	—
LOD	No	No	Yes	—
LOQ	No	Yes	No	—
Linearity	Yes	Yes	No	—
Range	Yes	Yes	—	—

Validation/Proficiency of Analysts

In addition to in-house audit programme, there should be a proven basis of evidence for reviewing the performance — "Proficiency testing" of the analyst:

1. Analysis of pre-analysed samples in respect of potency/assay/impurities.
2. Analysis of standard samples prepared for validation purpose.
3. Analysis of samples in replicate and measure of SD/RSD.
4. Analysis of samples for recovery studies after spiking the pre-analysed samples.
5. Services of a referral laboratory may be obtained for post-testing audit.
6. Corrective action based on validation report.

Note: By approaching method development, optimization and validation in a logical, stepwise manner, laboratory resources can be used in more efficient and productive manner.

Information Supporting the Suitability of Analytical Method for Dosage Form

1. Data demonstrating accuracy, precision and linearity of the method over 80-120% of the labelled claim.
2. Data demonstrating the specificity of the method and its suitability for determining the limits of known/unknown impurities, degradation products, related substances and other drug substances likely to be present in the finished product (multiple component formulations).
3. Data demonstrating recoveries from sample matrix.
4. Data demonstrating that neither the fresh nor degraded placebo interferes with the proposed method.
5. Data demonstrating the stability of the analyte during purification, extraction, assay.
6. LOD and LOQ to be established and documented.
7. Degradation scheme (acid/base hydrolysis, temperature degradation, photolysis and oxidation) of active ingredients.
8. If the method is not stability indicating, then limit test for degradation product must be included for assessing quality of the product.
9. System suitability test (for chromatographic assays) and standardization of dissolution test apparatus may be carried out and documented.
10. While analysing samples often overages are required to be added due to stability problem, data about repeatability parameter should be available.
11. Ruggedness data (reproducibility of results by analysis of same sample i.e. day-to-day, lab-to-lab, analyst-to-analyst, instruments-to-instrument, different time, different lots of reagents) to confirm lack of operational variables should be documented.
12. Legible reproduction of representative instrumental records/chromatogram.

Summary of Tests Required for Validation

Test	*Definition*	*Determination*
Accuracy (Recovery)	Closeness between the actual and found values, often expressed as recovery by assaying the known added amount of analyte.	Placebo spiked with analyte covering 50% to 150% of the sample concentration and analysed recoveries of each calculated.
Precision repeatability (Method precision)	Variation observed by a single analyst on single day and on single instrument.	Multiple replicates of a homogenous sample are analysed using the proposed analytical method and recovery (%) values of each calculated.
Intermediate precision (Ruggedness)	Variation observed within a laboratory on different days with different instrument and with different analysts.	A second analyst repeats the analysis of sample analysed under repeatability; recovery (%) values found and compared with the results of first analyst.
Specificity	It measures only the desired component without interference from other components that might be present (impurities, degradation products, excipients). Separation is not required (difference from selectivity).	Sample blank sample matrix known related impurities to be evaluated to find interference, if any.
Detection limit (DL/LOD)	Lowest concentration of analyte that can be detected, just to determine if the analyte concentration is above or below a specific limit.	The LOD is based on signal to noise ratio (3 : 1) and expressed as % or ppm or ppb.
Quantification limit (QL/LOQ)	Lowest amount of analyte in a sample that can be quantified with acceptable accuracy and precision; used for determination of impurities and degradation products.	Estimated from determination of signal to noise ratio (10 : 1).
Linearity	Evaluates the ability of analytical procedure to obtain a response that is directly proportional to the concentration of analyte in the sample.	Linearity is usually established for active substances. Evaluation is done on standards.
Range (Linearity of the method)	The interval between lower and upper concentration of analyte in the sample for which the method has been demonstrated to have acceptable level of precision and accuracy.	Evaluated by spiking the placebo with analyte in the range of 50-100% of the labelled claim.
Robustness	Ability of the method to remain unaffected by small but delibrate changes in different parameters of the method.	By varying the parameters and measuring the effect on the method by analysis of the sample.
Filter retention	Comparison of test results between filtered and the ııltered sample to determine whether the sample has been retained on filter.	Blank sample and standard solutions are analysed with and without filtration and recovery values compared.
Extraction efficiency	It ia a measure of the effectiveness of the extraction of the drug from sample matrix.	Investigated by varying the shaking time, sonication time or temperature.

General Information

1. The documents should be designed, prepared, rechecked and distributed with care. They should comply with relevant part of the manufacturing process.
2. Documents should be approved, signed and dated by appropriate authorized persons. No document should be changed without authorization.
3. Documents should have unambiguous contents i.e. title, nature and purpose should be clearly stated.
4. Documents should be regularly reviewed and kept up-to-date. When a document is revised, a system should be available to prevent inadvertent use of the superseded version of the method.
5. Any alteration made in a document should be signed and dated. The alteration should permit the reading of original information. Where appropriate, the reason for alteration should be recorded.
6. Records should be made or completed when any action is taken, so that all significant activities are traceable.
7. Data may be recorded by electronic data-processing system/photographic or other reliable means. If documentation is handled by electronic data-processing method, only authorized persons should be able to enter/modify/delete the data.

Stability studies

1. Quality control (QC) department should evaluate the quality and stability of the finished pharmaceutical product, if necessary, of starting material/intermediate product.
2. QC department should establish expiry dates and shelf life specifications on the basis of stability tests related to storage conditions.
3. A written programme for ongoing stability determination should be developed and implemented. Elements are:
   (a) Complete description of the drug involved in the study.
   (b) Complete testing protocols/parameters and method describing all tests to check potency, purity, physical characteristics with documented evidence that these protocols will indicate stability.
   (c) Provision for inclusion of adequate number of batches.
   (d) Testing schedule for each drug.
   (e) Provision of special storage conditions.
   (f) Provision for sample retention.
   (g) Summary of all experimental data generated, its evaluation and conclusion of the study.

Stability of the product should be determined prior to marketing following any significant changes in process, equipment or packing material.

Criteria for stability indicating method

The proposed method must be capable of discriminating between principal compound and other:

1. Known impurities
2. Active degradation products oxidation/hydrolysis
3. Placebo degradation products
4. Excipients, preservatives

Methods usually employed are TLC/HPTLC/HPLC.

METHOD TRANSFER

Most of the pharmaceutical houses usually have two independent laboratories

A. This laboratory (designated as R&D lab or AMD lab) is assigned the function of developing analytical procedure and its validation.

- This is well-equipped (instruments/personnel skill and experience and numbers) with sophisticated analytical instruments, high level of technical expertise required.
- Not working under pressure for batch release.

B. QCL: Where the methods so developed and validated are routinely used.

- It is this transfer of analytical methodologies which presents a formidable challenge for obtaining validated results during routine use.

AMD laboratory should take care of major problem area which might have caused difficulties while developing the method before transfer to QCL.

1. Should discuss all practical aspects with authorized personnel from QCL before transfer.
2. Should provide written protocols with all details which defines the basis of acceptance of an analytical method.
3. Background information on the method.
4. Should set up method transfer protocols and performance of testing.
5. Difficulties encountered.
6. Suggested precautions.
7. All critical steps in methodology that may require special attention.
8. Training to the analysts working in QCL (receiving laboratory).
9. Ability of the receiving laboratory to carry out the method.

Note: Review the data for conformance and arrange follow-up with AMD laboratory if needed. Before transfer it is preferable that an analyst from QCL is sent to AMDL to observe the more experienced analyst of AMDL run the actual test or may be allowed to run the test under close supervision of experienced analyst. This creates mutual faith.

Note: 1. If the analytical method is found not to be optimum or if any deficiency and difficulty are observed during application, the method should be returned to the originating chemist for re-evaluation.

2. It is absolutely essential that AMD laboratory is aware of the facilities and conditions to which the method is to be sent for actual quality control use.
3. Validation procedures usually consist of exhaustive comparative study between QCL and AMD laboratory. This study consists of both laboratories arranging three different lots of drug products with 10 samples being assay from each lot.

Method Transfer Documents

- Detailed method: The procedure should be unambiguous.
- Method development report: Linearity, precision, recovery and representative batch testing.
- Validation summary: Should include validation activities and the results.

Method Transfer Protocols

A qualified person from the transferring laboratory should write the transfer protocols. The quality assurance (QA) representative of both transferring and receiving laboratory should approve the transfer plan which may contain the following:

- Clear understanding of the analytical procedure by participating laboratories
- Scope
- Material (chemicals, instruments and standards) required. The standard should accompany certificate of analysis.
- Acceptance criteria for different parameters (linearity, accuracy, precision).
- Method transfer documents.
- Copies of the validated method.
- Form of final report.

Method transfer study design

1. Analyst to analyst
2. Day-to-day
3. Lab to lab

Minimum requirements are:
(a) Triplicate samples of distinct lots
(b) Six replicates
(c) Single analyst
(d) Single day

Acceptance criteria for method transfer

- Compare accuracy (bias) and precision.
- Have pass/fail limits agreed by AMD and QC laboratories.
- Carry out statistical tests.

RE-VALIDATION

As the method under validation is required to be used as written, any modification (given below) requires revalidation. The degree of revalidation shall depend on the changes made.

- One may be required to quantify additional components or new impurity/ degradation product.
- Method simplification or improvement (outdated technology).
- Safety concern (such as use of benzene is no more recommended).
- Changes in manufacturing process/product change.
- Economic consideration.
- Sample throughput.
- Complexity of the method (method simplification/improvement).
- Change of column/TLC plates due to manufacturer.
- Regulatory agency guidelines/requirements (issue of new requirement).

Note: There has to be a formal monitoring system by which qualified representatives of the AMD or QCL review the proposed or actual changes that may affect the validated status of the method and cause corrective measures/ actions to be taken to ensure that the analytical method retains its validated status during use.

Note: Analytical methods have finite life time; should be reviewed periodically and then revised or changed if required.

Following examples call for revalidation:

1. Change of sample preparation.
2. Change in dilution steps.
3. Change of chromatographic column.
4. Change in impurity profile.
5. Change in degradation profile.

1. Sample preparation (whole tablets vs. powdered composite)
   Recovery, Linearity, Precision } To be revalidated
2. Dilution steps
   A. Same analyte concentration and identical solvent ratio. Precision to be revalidated.
   B. Different solvent ratio. Linearity and precision to be revalidated.
   C. Different analyte concentration. Linearity, precision, specificity to be revalidated.
3. Change of chromatographic column or brand of TLC plates
   Precision, Specificity, Resolution, Recovery } To be revalidated

Essential Requirements of Analytical Measurements

1. Analytical measurements should be made to satisfy the desired and agreed parameters.
2. Analytical measurements should be made using methods, protocols and equipments which have been tested and validated to ensure that they are fit for intended measurements.
3. Personnel making analytical measurements should be professionally qualified and competent to undertake the analysis.
4. Technical performance of the laboratory should be regularly assessed by an independent authority.
5. Analytical data obtained in one location should be consistent with those elsewhere—reproducibility.
6. The laboratory should have well-defined quality control and quality assurance procedures.

Quality control and quality assurance (QA)

One question often asked is why the quality control function cannot also be responsible for quality assurance. Quite apart from the responsibilities of QA cutting across various functions, assurance also covers the review of QC procedures and records. How can this review be unbiased if the head of QC were to don the QA hat as well? When bias comes in, out goes quality assurance!

Unfortunately, often unhealthy tension is noticed among the QA and QC. Efforts should be made to reduce such tension during the methods validation programme. It must be remembered that validation work done by QC department has to be exhaustively reviewed by the reviewers. You have to present accurate account of your work which may raise some questions. Obviously 'QA' should be treated as you first line of defence. If you cannot make QA understand your work, how will the reviewer understand. So treat QA as your friend.

	Quality control	**Quality assurance**
1. Activity	Functional	Multi-functional
2. Relationship	Part of GMP	Product design + GMP
3. Responsible to	The head of the manufacturing unit (for administrative matters) and to the head of QA (for functional matters)	Responsible to top management (Chief Executive Officer of the company)
4. Main responsibilities	1. Laying down specifications for input materials, intermediates and finished products and testing methods. 2. Sampling, inspecting and testing. 3. Maintenance and calibration of testing equipment. 4. Validation of test methods. 5. Test records. 6. Stability testing and quality review. 7. Laboratory personnel training.	1. Review and approval of product design and development. 2. Review and approval of production and quality control documentation for compliance with GMP and GLP requirements. 3. Product labelling. 4. Review of the controls on the quality of starting materials, intermediate and finished products. 5. Review of batch production and quality control records and release of batches. 6. Handling product complaints. 7. Review of stability data and shelf-lives of products. 8. Process and equipment cleaning validations. 9. Technical audits. 10. GMP training. 11. Regulatory affairs.

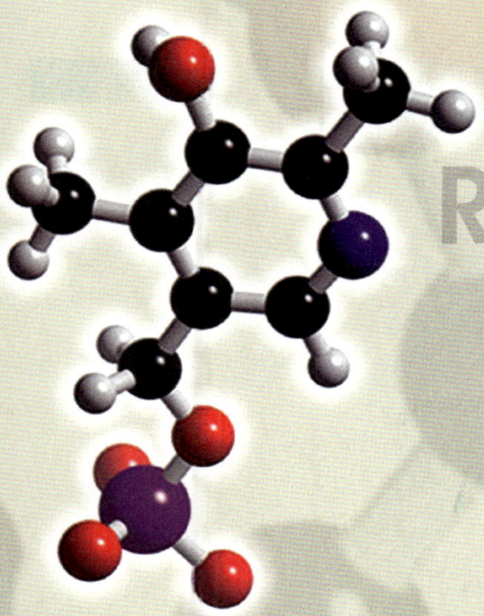

Reaction Mechanism

5

SOP on Reference and Working Standards

Any person engaged in the quality assurance of drugs and pharmaceuticals must be fully aware of the need of reference material with which the test material is to be compared before deciding about its quality. Various tests like identification by UV absorption spectrophotometry or determining the presence and/or absence of impurities/decomposition products/related substances or determination of potency/strength, one would need the use of reference material of known purity or potency. The use of such reference standards during determination of individual ingredient of multi-drug formulations needs no emphasis with respect to accuracy and ease of such determinations.

In India Central Drug Laboratory (CDL)*, Calcutta has been responsible for making available only IP reference standards to the drugs manufacturers as well as to approved drug testing laboratories, but all the required reference standards may not be available. Further, most of the related substances/ decomposition products for which pharmacopoeial limits are prescribed are usually not available thus jeopardising the very purity of drug substances.

Indian Foundation for Pharmaceutical Reference Standard Substances (IFPRESS), Mumbai has been supporting the activities of CDL to limited extent in respect of API reference substances and their impurities.

Since primary reference standards are available in small quantities and are very expensive, it is desirable that working reference standards should be prepared and used for day to day analysis. The bulk drug substances may be obtained from the manufacturers of basic drugs and then standardized.

In this direction, Drug Control Authorities of certain States such as "Delhi" have taken the initiative of allowing certain approved Drug Testing Laboratories (M/s Arbro Pharmaceutical Ltd., New Delhi) in their jurisdiction to prepare, standardize and distribute working standards reasonably priced for use by the pharmaceutical manufacturers in the state. If drug authorities of other states take similar initiative, the problem can be solved to a great extent.

Objective

The SOP on "Reference and Working Standards" is to establish a system for procurement, storage and usage of reference standards and preparation, usage, storage of working standards.

Scope

The scope of SOP is procurement, distribution, preparation, usage and storage of reference standards and working standards for analysis as required by compendial requirement.

* Since "Indian Pharmacopoeia Commission" has been established, this responsibility has been taken over by the commission.

Responsibility

Personnel responsible for the activity will be mainly from analytical laboratory who have to provide details and specifications to the purchase department for procurement of material.

Procedure

Activities involved in procurement, preservation, usage, preparation of working standards, storage can be as per guidelines indicated.

1. Procurement

Quality Control department has to raise a purchase requirement for a new compendial Reference Standard or in case of any change in Lot/Batch No. of existing Reference Standard or if the existing Reference Standard is exhausted.

2. Storage

The Reference Standards are to be stored as per the instructions given in respective pharmacopoeia or as per label.

3. Usage

The usage of the Reference Standards has to be recorded which shall also include the quantity used for generation of Working Standards.

4. Preparation of Working Standards

- Samples from latest manufactured and released batch shall be selected for preparation of Working Standard.
- The analytical profile of selected batch shall be nearest to that of Reference Standard.
- The Working Standard shall be dispensed like Reference Standard and stored similarly.
- Total quantity of Working Standard shall be recorded and its usage indicated.
- The label of Working Standard bottle, vial as well as the Certificate of Analysis generated for it shall bear the relevant batch details identifying the source.
- The Certificate of Analysis shall also have all the enclosures like chromatograms (UV, IR, GLC/HPLC).

Storage of Working Standards

The unit/container in use shall be stored at 25°C, protected from light, humidity and environment contamination:

- Room temperature: 25-30°C (< 50% RH)
- Room temperature/Dessicator:
- Refrigerator (2-8°C)
- Freezer: –25°C to +10°C
- Dessicator
- Deep freezer (< –50°C)
- Nitrogen or any other inert gas blanket.

Usage

Usage of the reference/working standard has to be recorded along with the quantity.

A TYPICAL SCHEMATIC CHART OF ACTIVITIES FOR REFERENCE AND WORKING STANDARDS

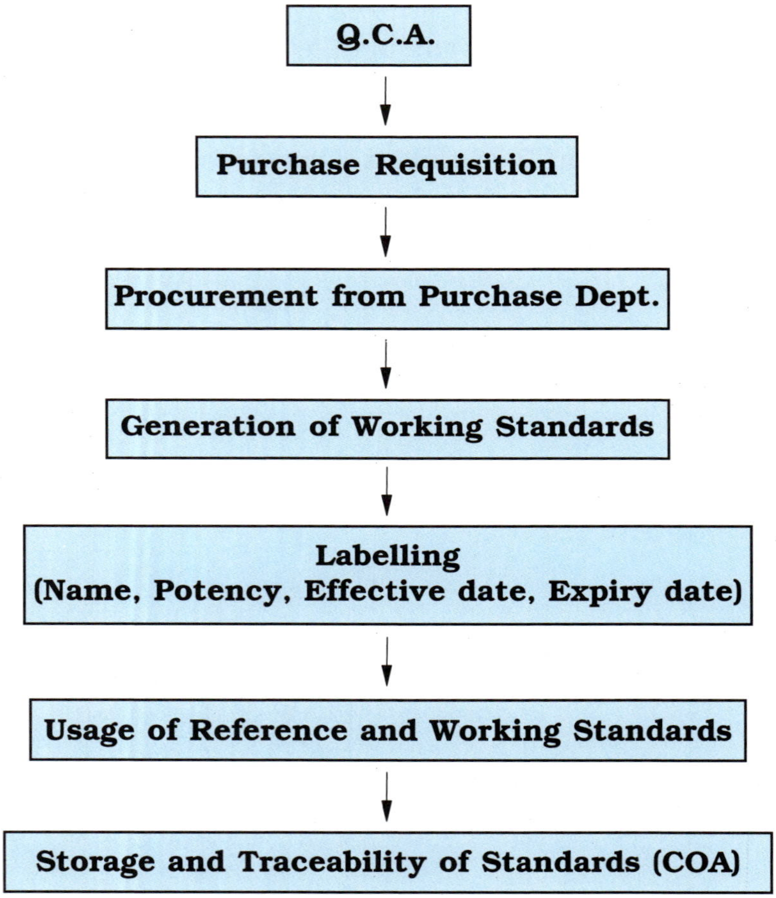

DEVELOPMENT PROCESS FOR PHARMACOPEIAL REFERENCE STANDARDS

(i) New monograph

or

(ii) New request for an existing reference standard

or

(iii) Present stock depletion

↓

The bulk material is sourced preferably from leading manufacturer

↓

The material is tested and characterized through collaborative testing involving a minimum of 3 laboratories, industry and FDA (CIPL, CDL, CDTL).

↓

Data from the collaborative study are reviewed by Pharmacopeial scientist.

↓

Compilation of collaborative study is sent to the Pharmacopeial Reference Standards Committee for evaluation along with all the test procedures used to generate the data, copy or original of all raw data, copy of method validation and finalized characterization report.

↓

Pharmacopeial reference standard committee accepts, recommends further testing, or rejects the material.

↓

The approved material is subdivided and suitably labelled.

↓

The material is released into Pharmacopeial inventory for distribution.

TYPICAL CHARACTERIZATION FLOWCHART

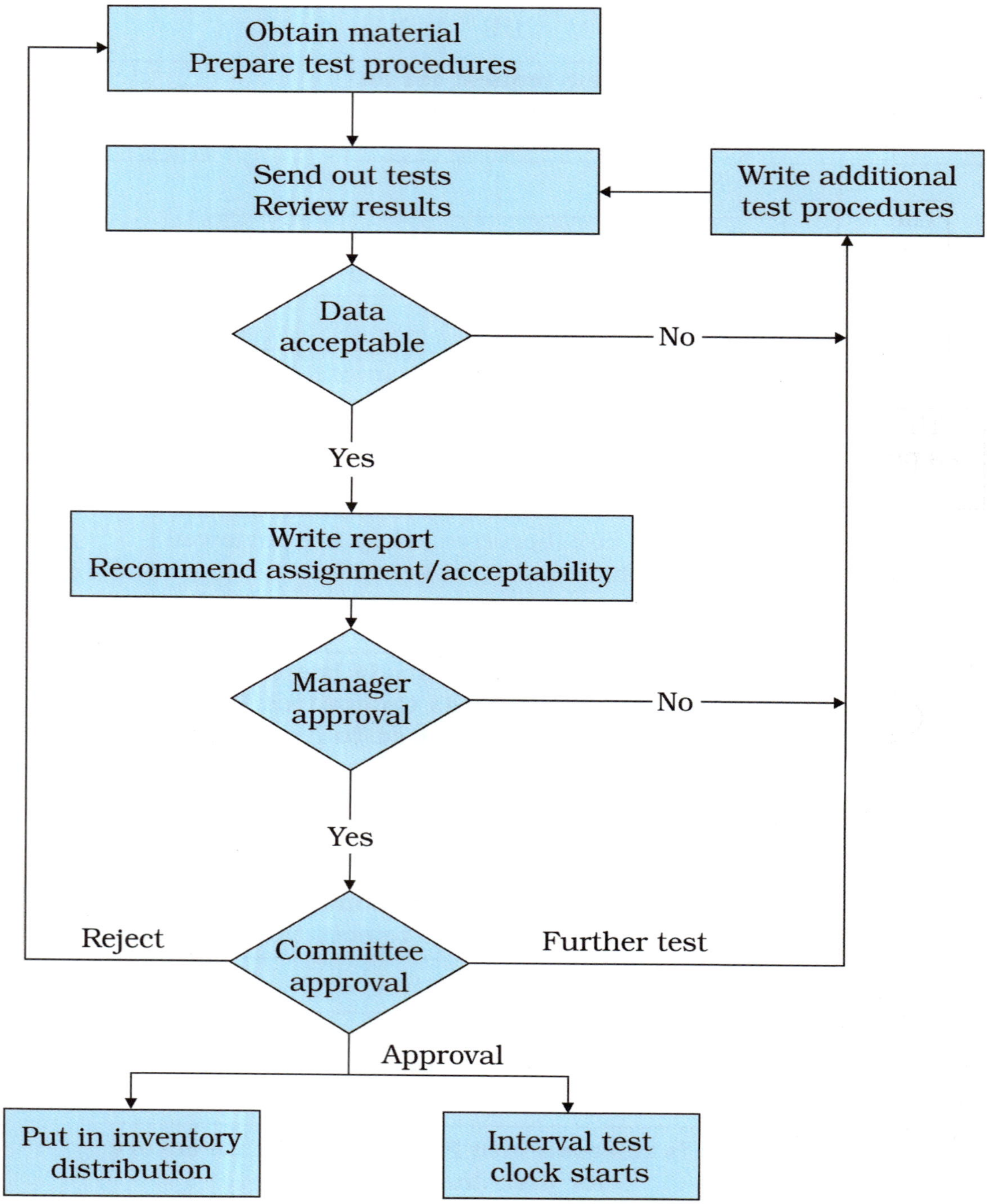

FLOWCHART FOR PREPARATION OF WORKING STANDARDS

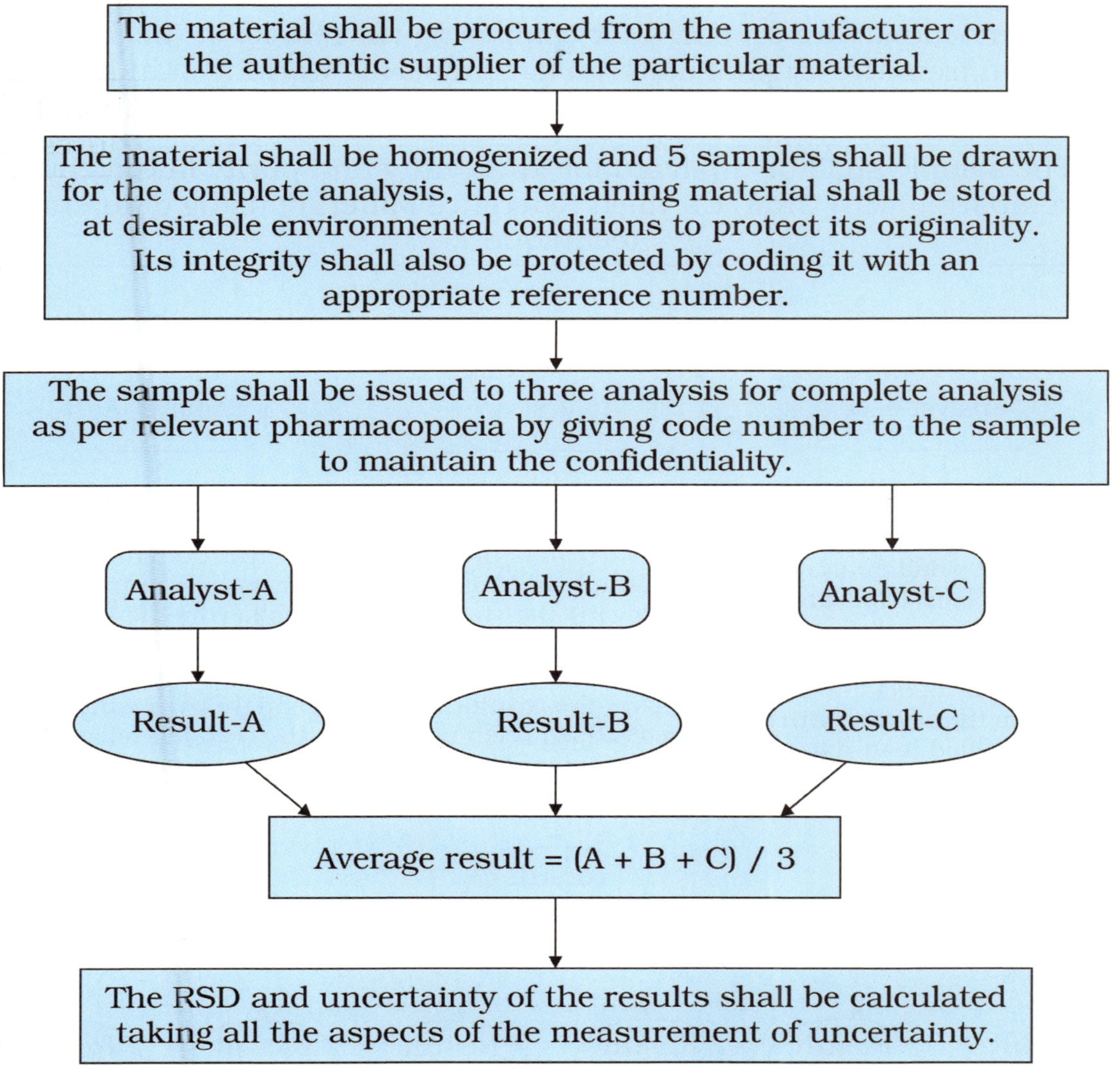

Average results of complete analysis compiled and compared with pharmacopoeial requirements to take final decision about its acceptance or rejection as working standard.

VERIFICATION WITH CERTIFIED REFERENCE MATERIAL

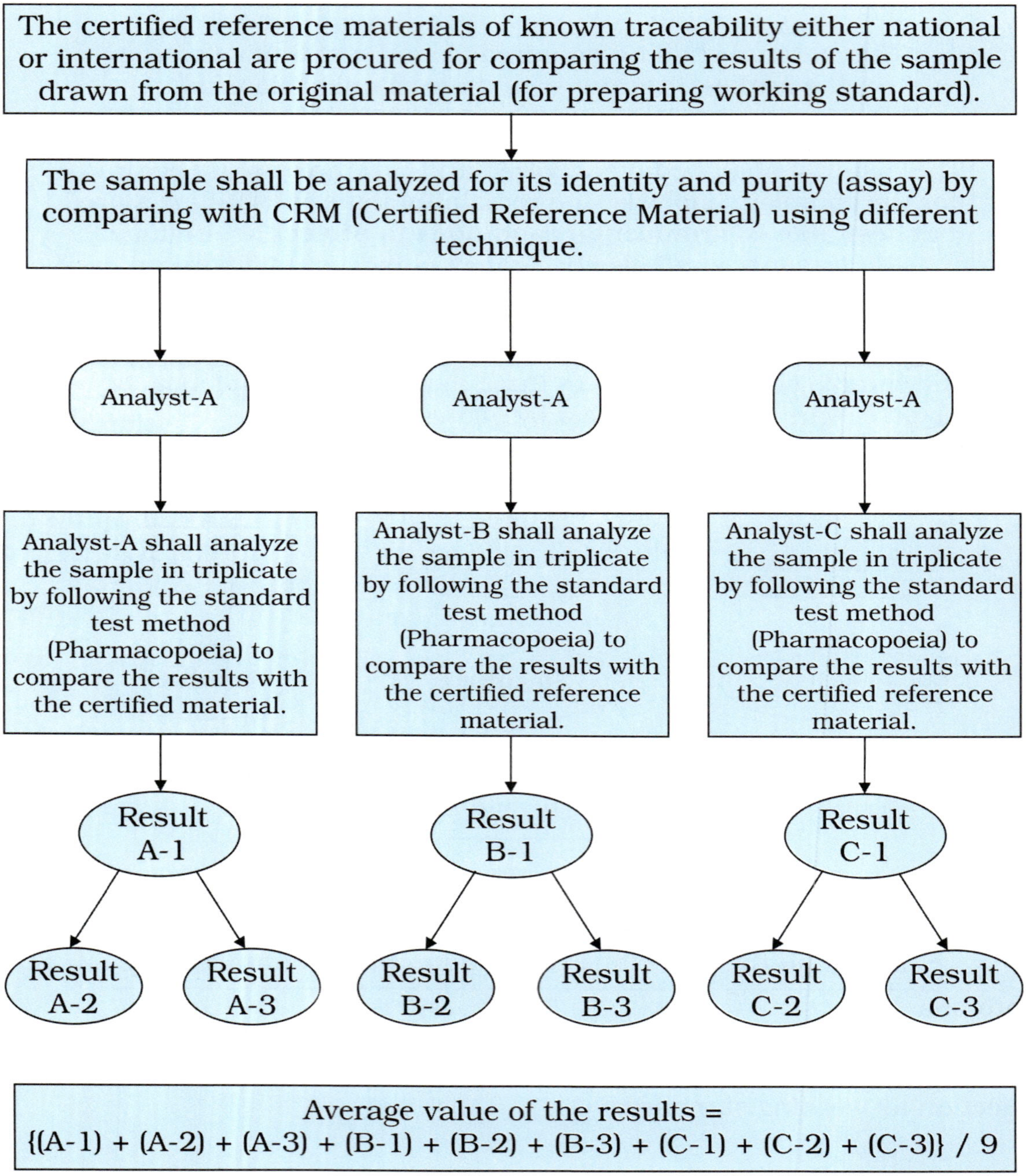

COLLABORATIVE TESTING

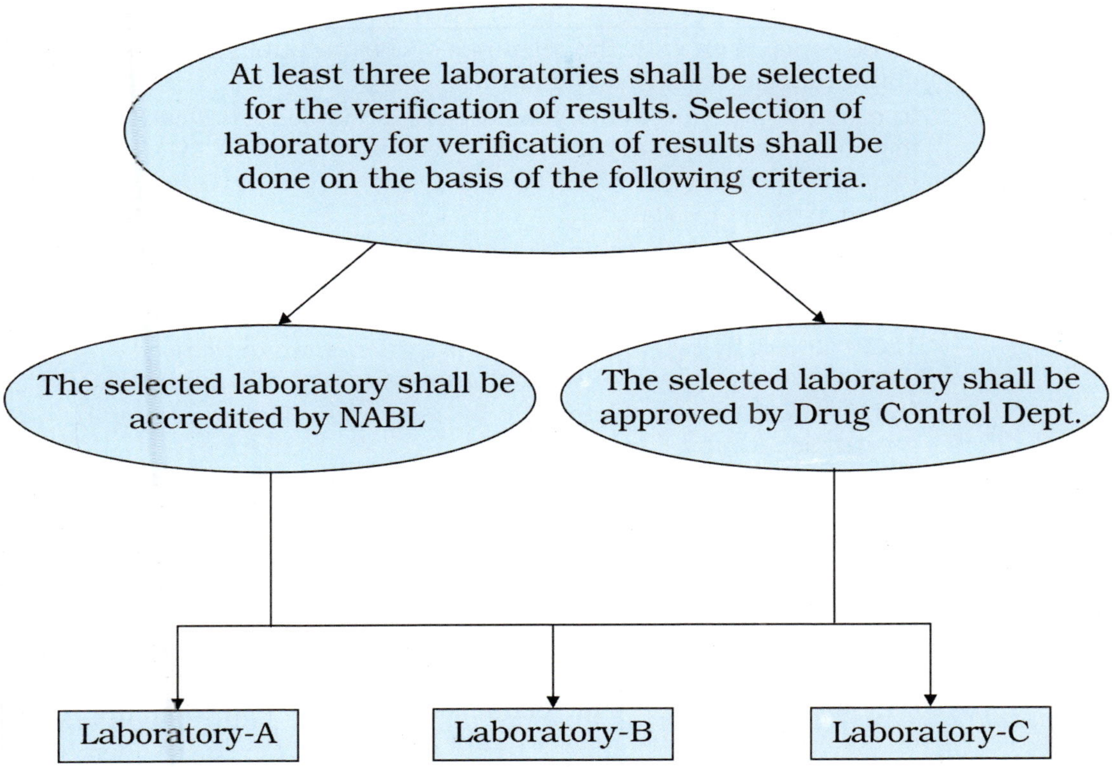

Data from collaborative testing reviewed and decision taken for acceptance/ rejection.

Note: The approved material is subdivided and suitably labelled for release into pharmacopoeial inventory for distribution.

Analytical data required for working standard

In addition to pharmacopoeial tests, the following tests should be carried out to obtain an elaborate analytical data on th working standard.

Infrared spectrum	To be concordant with the reference spectrum published or spectrum obtained from reference standard.
Selective test	In case IR spectrum is not considered a suitable identification method, complementary methods such as TLC and HPLC are recommended for identification.
UV spectrum	Maximas to be indicated.
Assay	Chemical assay data, microbiological assay data, if any, the data obtained from manufacture of substance and laboratory findings compared.
Purity	TLC – Generally two different solvent systems are to be used and spots identified and compared for total impurities/specific impurities. HPLC – Two different systems to be used and selection depending on a greater separation efficiency.
Other characteristics	LOD, water (KF), Specific Optional Rotation, any specific limit test characteristic to the product.
Stability of known hygroscopic substance	In case the information is available about the hygroscopic nature of the substance to be accepted as working standard, the percentage of water (H_2O) preferably by Karl-Fischer is to be tested by exposing the substance for 24 hours to uncontrolled room temperature, controlled conditions (desiccate) and 70-80% Rh and readings noted.
Storage	Conditions of storage to be mentioned. (Quantity in a container should be as little as possible to avoid unnecessary exposure and contamination of the standard by repeated opening of the container.)

Note: A material conforming to various tests and showing results within acceptable limits should be accepted as working standard.

CERTIFICATE OF ANALYSIS - COA
(Working Standards)

Material:	Evaluated against:	Traceability of CRM
Batch No.:	B. No./Lot No.:	
Mfg. date:	Validity/Expiry date:	
Make:	Analysis Report No.:	
Date of evaluation:	Effective date:	

Protocol of Test	Specifications	Results
Description		
Identification		
Related substances		
Loss on drying/water		
Assay		

Remarks: The above substance conforms with Reference Standard/Batch No./ Lot No. and is qualified for Working Standard No. ....

Storage:

Analyst
Date

Manager Quality Assurance
Date

LABEL OF WORKING STANDARD

WORKING STANDARD
(Not for medicinal use)

Name of working standard:
Laboratory reference of working standard (Batch No.):
Traceability of Working Standard (COA) No.:
Assay/Potency:
Loss on drying/water:
Quantity of working standard:
Date of preparation:
Date of expiry:
Storage condition*:

(Authorized signatory)

* Room temperature (25-30°C, <50% RH)
Room temperature/Desiccator
Refrigerator (2-8°C)
Freezer (–25°C to +10°C)
Desiccator
Deep freezer (< –50°C)
Nitrogen or any other inert gas blanket

LIST OF REFERENCE / WORKING STANDARDS

Sr. No.	Name of reference/ working standard	Compendial IP/BP/USP/EP	Dt. of receipt	Qty. recd.	Lot No./ B. No.	Storage condition	Assay	To be used for

USAGE / DISPENSING RECORDS

Sr. No.	Name of reference/ working standard	Date of use	Batch No./ Lot No.	Qty. used	Opening stock	Closing stock	Initial of the person who dispensed

Note: 1. The log book dealing with the inventory of the standards should indicate who, when and how much quantity of the standard was removed.

2. Exercise care while handling to avoid contamination of the reference substance.

READY RECKONER FORMAT
LIST OF WORKING STANDARDS

S. No.	Name of the standard	Batch No.	A.R. No.	LOD/ water	Potency	Date effective	Retesting date	Sign

CHANGE IN LOT OR BATCH NO. OF REFERENCE STANDARD

S. No.	Name of reference standard	Current lot No.	Change lot No.	Pharmacopoeia	Effective from	Applicable to

Detailed Addresses of Agencies for Procurement of Certified Reference Materials (CRM) for Pharmaceutical Analysis

INDIAN SOURCE

- **LGC Promochem India Private Ltd.**
  P.O. Box 8061, No. 142, 3rd Floor, 5th Cross,
  Rajamahal Villas Extension, Bangalore - 560080 (India)
  Tel: (+91) 80-23611256 or (+91) 80-23611257
  Fax: (+91) 80-23613859, E-mail: in@promochem.com
- **LGC Promochem India Private Ltd.**
  No. 408, B Wing, Galleria
  Hiranandani Gardens, Powai, Mumbai-400076 (India)
  Tel: (+91) 022-25700244, 25706044
  Fax: (+91) 022-25703741, E-mail: promochem@vsnl
- **LGC Promochem India Private Ltd.**
  No. 7-1-213/B, 1st Floor, Opp. Govt. Hospital
  Ameerpet, Hyderabad-500016 (India)
  Tel: (+91) 040-23736378, Fax: (+91) 040-23736379,
  E-mail: promochem@vsnl.net
- **LabIndia**
  372, Udyog Vihar, Phase-II
  Gurgaon-122016, Haryana (India)
  Tel: (+91) 124 2843200, Fax: (+91) 124 2843299
  E-mail: lipldelhi@vsnl.net
- **Indian Pharmacopoeia Commission**
  CIPL Campus, Rajnagar, Ghaziabad - 201001
  Tel: 95-120-2783392
- **National Physical Laboratory (NPL)**
  Indian Reference Materials Section
  Dr. K.S. Krishnan Marg, New Delhi-110012
  Tel: 91-011-25734649, E-mail: aka@nplindia.ernet.in
- **IFPRESS - Indian Foundation for Pharmaceutical Reference Standard Substances**
  A-21, MIDC, Street 3, Andheri (E), Mumbai-400093 (India)
  Tel: 91-22-28218921, Fax: 91-22-28377927, M - 09820490494
  E-mail: klenzaids@mtnl.net.in, i@vsnl.net

- **Sigma-Aldrich Chemicals Private Ltd.**
  A-2, The Qutab Hotel Complex
  Shaheed Jeet Singh Marg, New Delhi-110016
  Tel: 91-11-41654255, Fax: 91-11-41654266

INTERNATIONAL SOURCE

- **ICRS** – (International Chemical Reference Substances)
  WHO Collaborating Centre for Chemical Reference Substances,
  Apoteket AB, Production and Laboratories, Central Laboratories, ACL,
  Prismavagen 2, SE-14175 Kungens Kurva, Sweden
  Tel.: +46 8 466 1799, Fax: +46 8 740 6040
- **BPCRS** – (British Pharmacopoeia Chemical Reference Substances)
  Medicines Control Agency Laboratory
  Government Buildings (Block 2), Honeypot Lane,
  Stanmore HA71AY, England
  Tel: +44 (0) 171-972 3608, Fax: +44 (0) 181-951 3069
- **USP** – U.S. Pharmacopoeial Convention, Inc., Reference Standards Order Department, 12601 Twinbrook Parkway, Rockville, Maryland 20852, USA
  Tel: (800) 227-8772, Fax: 1-301-816-81-48,
  Website: www.usp.org/dsd/refstd
- **EPCRS** – European Pharmacoeia Commission Secretariat, Council of Europe, BP 907, F 67029 Strasbourg Cedex 1, France
  Tel: (88) 41 28 52, Fax: (88) 41 27 71
- **NIST** – National Institute for Standards and Technology, Office of Standard Reference Materials, Room B311, Chemistry Building, Gathersburg, MD 20899, USA
- **ORM** – Office of Reference Materials, Laboratory of the Government Chemist, Teddington, TW 110LW, UK
- **UKBS** – National Institute for Biological Standards and Control, P.O. Box 1193, Blanche Lane, South Mimms, Potters Bar, Hertfordshire, EN6 3QH UK
  Tel: +44 (1707) 646399, Fax: +33 (1707) 646977
- **JPRS** – Japanese Pharmacopoeia Reference Substances
  1. National Institute of Hygienic Sciences, Osaka Branch, 1-1-43, Hoensaka, Chou-ku, Osaka 540, Japan
     Tel: +81-6-941-1533, Fax: +6-942-0716
  2. The Society of Japanese Pharmacopoeia, 2-12-15, Shibuya-ku, Tokyo 150, Japan
     Tel: +81-3-3400-5634, Fax: +81-3-3400-3158

- **ARS** – ASEAN Reference Substances issued under ASEAN TCDC Programme on Pharmaceuticals. Available at individual participating laboratories:
  1. National Quality Control Laboratory of Drug and Food, JI. Percetaken Negara No. 23, Jakarta, Indonesia
     Tel: (021) 41507, Fax: (021) 4201427
  2. National Pharmaceutical Control Bureau, Ministry of Health, Jalan University, P.O. Box 319, 46730 Petaling Jaya, Malaysia
     Tel: (603) 7573611, Fax: (603) 7562924
  3. Bureau of Food and Drugs, D.O.H. Compound, Alabang, Muntinlupa, Metro Manila, Philippines
     Tel: (632) 8422213, Fax: (632) 8424603
  4. Institute of Science and Forensic Medicine, Outram Road, Singapore 0316
     Tel: (065) 2216800, Fax: (065) 2290749
  5. Drug Analysis Division, Department of Medical Science, Ministry of Public Health, Tiwanon Road, Nonthaburi 11000, Thailand
     Tel: (662) 5915233, Fax: (662) 5910203
- **FPRS** – (French Pharmacopoeia Reference Substances) Agency du Medicament, 14, rue Ecole de Pharmacie, 34000 Montpellier, France
  Tel: 67 02 31 31, Fax: 67 60 78 84
- **MXPRS** – (Mexican Pharmacopoeia Reference Substances) Laboratorio Nacional de Salud Publica, Secretaria de Salud, Mexico D.F., Mexico X
- **NIH** – Laboratory of Antibiotic Drugs, Dept. of Biological and Blood Products, 2 Titan Tan Xi
  Tel: (0425) 61-0771
- **SR-FNA** – Sustancia de Referencia – Farmacopea National Argentina, Instituto Nacional de Medicamentos, Servicio de Materials de Referencia, AV Caseros 2161 (1264) Buenos Aires, Argentina
  Tel: (541) 340-0800 ext 2600, Fax: 340-0853
- **SPCR** – (Swiss Pharmacopoeia Reference Substances) Office federal de la sante publique, Laboratoire federal de pharmacopel, Case postal 3001, Beme, Switzerland
- Laboratory of Antibiotic Drugs, Department of Biological and Blood Products, The National Intitute of Health, 4-7-1 Gakuen, Musahimurayama City, Tokyo 208, Japan

There are certain other materials which may not be required in the anlysis of drugs; pharmaceutical manufacturers may require them for associated testing like test for pesticides, aflatoxins, metals in herbal medicines, test for environmental pollution control. For such testing, Certified Reference Materials (CRM) are available from some well-established institutions.

Sources for other certified reference materials

1. Institute for Reference Materials and Measurements (IRMM), Retieseweg, B-2440 Geel, Belgium
2. Reidel-de Ha'en Aktiengesellschaft Wunstorfer Straße 40, P.O. Box D-30918, Seelze (Outside Germany represented by Hoechst AG)
3. Institute for Environmental Research and Technology, National Research Council of Canada, Montreal Road, Ottawa, Ontario, Canada K1A0R6
4. Bureau of Analysed Samples Ltd. (BAS), Newham Hall, Newby Middlesbrough Cleaveland, England TS8 9EA
5. The Office of Reference Materials, Laboratory of the Govt. Chemist, Queens Road, Teddington, Middlesex TW 11 OLY, UK

REFERENCE STANDARDS FOR MICROBIOLOGY

- **IMTECH (Institute of Microbial Technology)**
  Sector-39A, Chandigarh
  0172-2690562, 2695215-216, Fax: 0172-2690632, 2690585
  E-mail: curator@imtech.res.in
- **Kitten Enterprises Pvt. Ltd.**
  203, Malwa, Patanwala Industrial Estate
  L.B.S. Marg, Ghatkopar (W)
  Mumbai-400086
  91-22-25007007
  E-mail: info@kitten.co.in

Note:

- All activities pertaining to microbiology testing shall be carried out in an aseptic area by an authorized person.
- If any culture has become non-viable or mutant, it may be destroyed by autoclaving under supervision of an authorized person.
- Viability of a culture may be ensured before starting an analysis.

6

Cardiovascular System

Reaction Mechanism

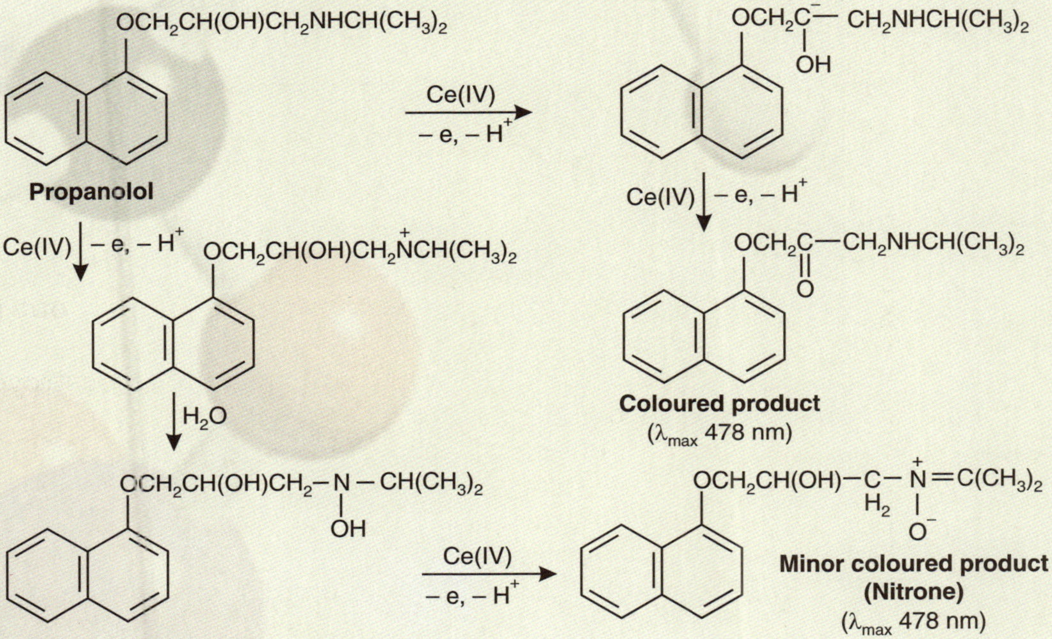

Formulation 1

Dihydralazine sulphate, Hydrochlorothiazide, Reserpine

ESTIMATION

Dihydralazine sulphate

METHOD 1

Reagents

1. 1 M hydrochloric acid.
2. 2 M hydrochloric acid.
3. Methanol.
4. 2% w/v solution of 4-dimethylaminobenzaldehyde (PDAB) in methanol.

Standard solution

100 mcg/ml of dihydrallazine sulphate in 1 M hydrochloric acid.

Sample solution

Suspend accurately weighed quantity of the sample in 50 ml of 2 M hydrochloric acid and shake mechanically for 60 min, dilute to 100 ml with water (100 mcg/ml).

Procedure

To 4 ml each of sample and standard solutions, add 10 ml of methanol and 5 ml of 'PDAB' reagent. Keep at room temperature for 30 min and dilute to 100 ml with methanol.

Measure the extinction of both sample and standard solutions at 405 nm against reagent blank and calculate the contents of dihydralazine sulphate by comparison.

Probable Reaction Mechanism

This colour reaction is based on the condensation of primary amine with 4-dimethylaminobenzaldehyde (PDAB) in acidic medium to give yellow-coloured Schiff's base—bishydrazone (λ_{max} 405 nm).

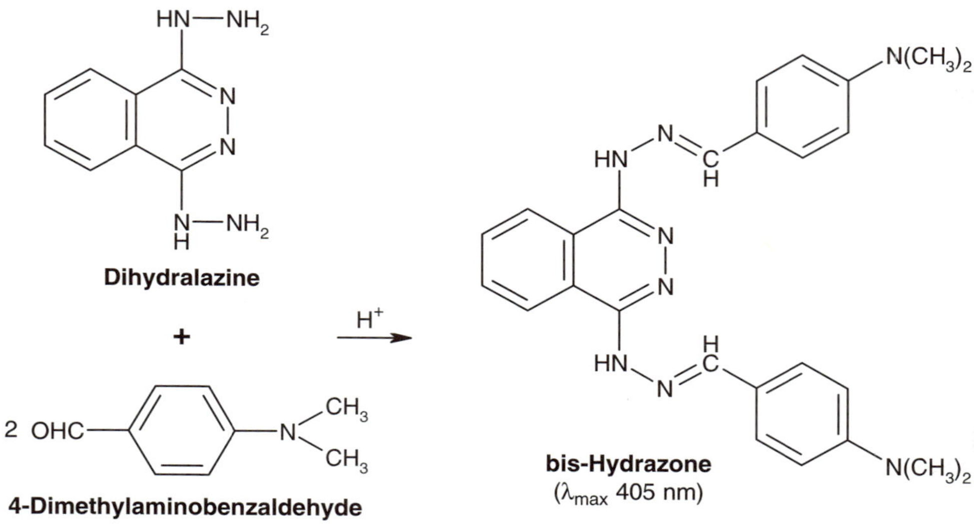

Reference

Pharm. Chem. (Vol. 2) by H.J. Roth, p. 644.

METHOD 2

Reagents

1. 0.1 M hydrochloric acid.
2. Methanol.
3. 1% w/v solution of O-phenanthroline in 0.1 N hydrochloric acid (dye).
4. Methanol – 0.1 M hydrochloric acid (1 : 1) mixture (solvent).
5. 0.20 w/v solution of ferric nitrate in 0.1 M hydrochloric acid.

Standard solution

50 mcg/ml of dihydralazine sulphate in the solvent.

Sample solution

Weigh accurately powdered sample equivalent to 10 mg of the substance, add 10 ml of 0.1 M hydrochloric acid and shake for 30 min, dilute to 25 ml with methanol. Filter and dilute appropriately with solvent to get solution of 50 mcg/ml.

Procedure

To 5 ml each of sample and standard solutions, add 10 ml of ferric nitrate solution and 10 ml of dye solution. Swirl the flask and warm at 60°C in water-bath for 30 min. Cool and adjust to 100 ml with water.

Measure the absorbance of both sample and standard solutions at 508 nm against solvent blank and calculate the contents of dihydralazine sulphate by comparison.

Probable Reaction Mechanism

On acid hydrolysis and oxidation with Fe (III), p-quinone is formed and Fe (III) is reduced to Fe (II) which forms chelate with o-phenanthroline to form tri-phenanthroline-Fe (II) complex of orange-red colour (λ_{max} 508 nm).

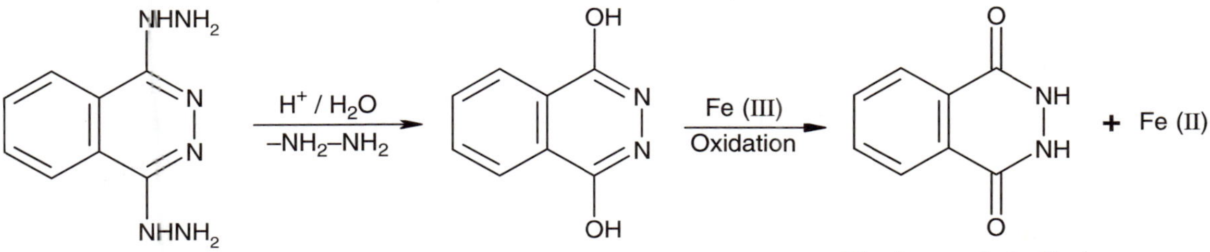

Diquinone derivative

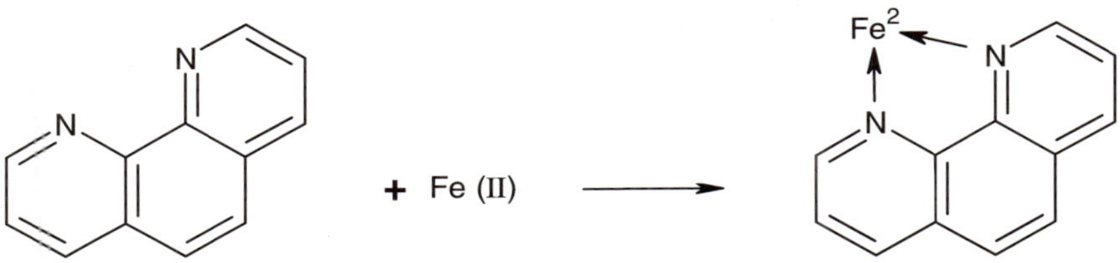

1,10-Phenanthroline

Fe (II) – o-Phenanthroline chelate (Ferroin)
(λ_{max} 508 nm)

METHOD 3

Weigh accurately powdered sample equivalent to 100 mg of substance, add 50 ml of water, stir for 15 min, add 50 ml 2 M hydrochloric acid and titrate with 0.1 M sodium nitrite till blue colour is produced when a glass rod dipped into the titrated solution is streaked on the smear of starch-potassium iodide paste. Each ml of 0.1 M sodium nitrite is equivalent to 14.415 mg of dihydralazine sulphate.

Probable Reaction Mechanism

This method is based on titration of primary amine with $NaNO_2$ based on diazotization reaction. The excess of HNO_2 reacts with KI to liberate I_2 which in turn reacts with starch to give blue colour, the end point. Since 2 mols of HNO_2 react with 1 mol of dihydralazine, the equivalent factor shall be 1/2 of the molecular weight of the compound.

$NaNO_2 + HCl \longrightarrow NaCl + HNO_2$

$2HNO_2 + 2KI \longrightarrow I_2 + 2KNO_2 + H_2O$

I_2 + Starch ⟶ Blue-coloured starch—Inclusion complex—End point

Diazotization Reaction

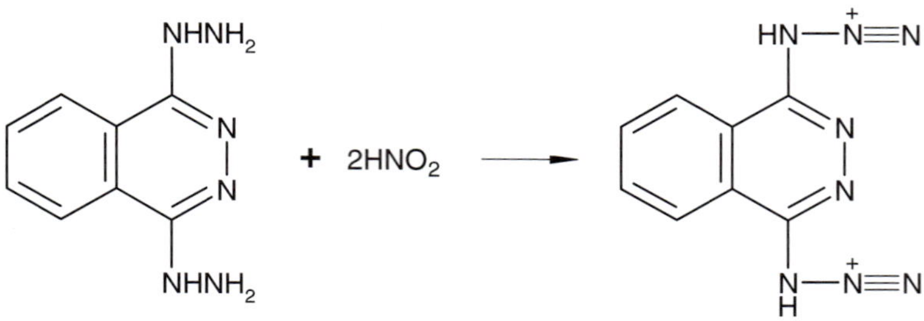

Diazide

Like any other hydrazine derivative, such as isoniazide, its reaction with 1-chloro-2,4-dinitrobenzene (2) in alkaline solution gives bis-2,4-dinitrophenyl hydrazide derivative which has red colour. This reaction can be used for quantitative estimation.

Dihydralazine has 2 nucleophilic nitrogen atoms of which hybridized hydrazide nitrogen is the more nucleophilic under these conditions. It attacks nucleophilically at the chlorine-bearing C-atom of 1-chloro-2,4-dinitrobenzene to form bis-dinitrophenyl hydrazide, having red colour.

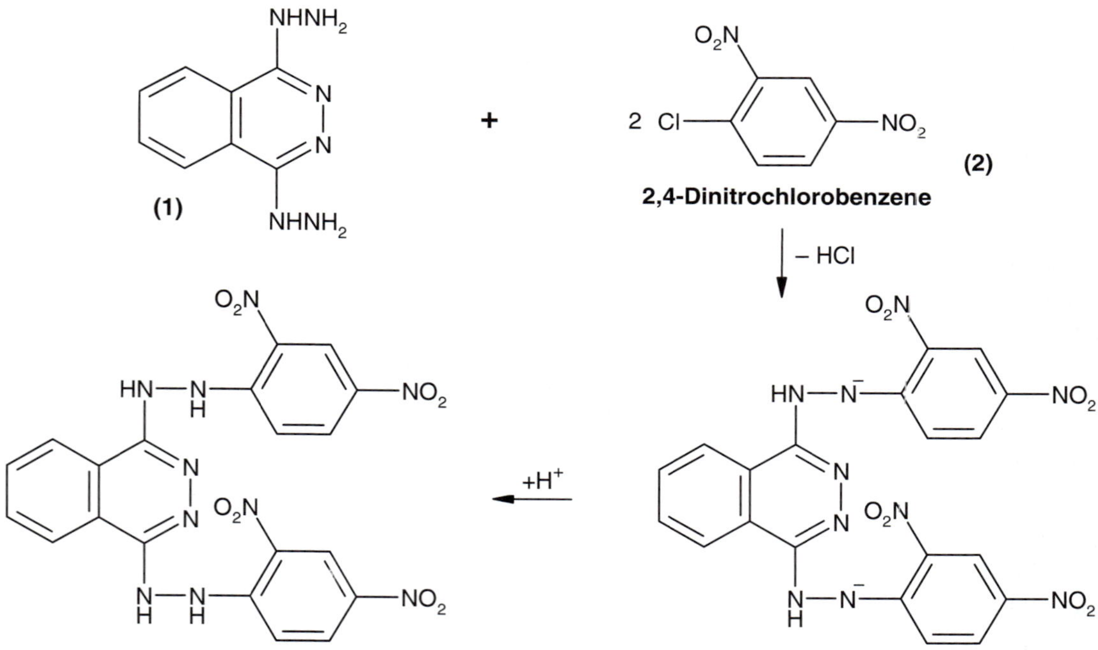

bis-Dinitrophenylhydrazide
(λ_{max} 490 nm)

Reference

Pharmaceutical Chemistry (Vol. 2) by H.J. Roth, p. 645.

Hydrochlorothiazide

METHOD 1

Reagents

1. 2 M ammonium hydroxide.
2. 2 M sodium hydroxide.
3. 2 M hydrochloric acid.
4. 0.2 M sodium nitrite.
5. 2% w/v solution of ammonium sulphamate in water.
6. 1% solution of N-(1-naphthyl)-ethylene diamine dihydrochloride (NED).

Standard solution

To 25 mg of the substance, accurately weighed, add 50 ml of 2 M ammonia and dilute to 500 ml with water (50 mcg/ml).

Sample solution

Suspend accurately weighed sample equivalent to 25 mg of the substance in 50 ml of 2 M ammonia, shake for 30 min and dilute to 500 ml with water.

Hydrolysis of sample and standard

To 20 ml each of sample and standard solutions, add 20 ml of 2 M sodium hydroxide and heat to boiling under reflux for 90 min. Cool and add 25 ml of 2 M hydrochloric acid, cool to 20-25°C, add further 25 ml of 2 M hydrochloric acid, add 1 ml of 0.2 M sodium nitrite. Mix, after 3 min add 2 ml of ammonium sulphamate solution, stir and allow to stand for 10 min, add 2 ml of 'NED' reagent and dilute to 100 ml with water.

Measure the absorption of both sample and standard solutions at 515 nm against reagent blank and calculate the contents of hydrochlorothiazide by comparison.

Probable Reaction Mechanism

On hydrolysis, the heterocyclic ring is opened to yield disulphonamide as aniline derivative with primary amino group and formaldehyde. The amino group is diazotized and coupled with N(1-naphthyl)-ethylenediamino to yield azo dye (λ_{max} 515 nm). The compound can also be quantitatively determined by reaction of chromotropic acid with formaldehyde (see under analgin).

Note

1. The extended conjugation in the end product is responsible for the strong absorption of the light in visible region of the spectrum.
2. The method is based on reaction with "Bratton-Marshall reagent". Other common compounds reacting with this reagent are bromhexine, benzocaine, sulphonamides, phenylbutazone, urea, folic acid and metoclopramide.

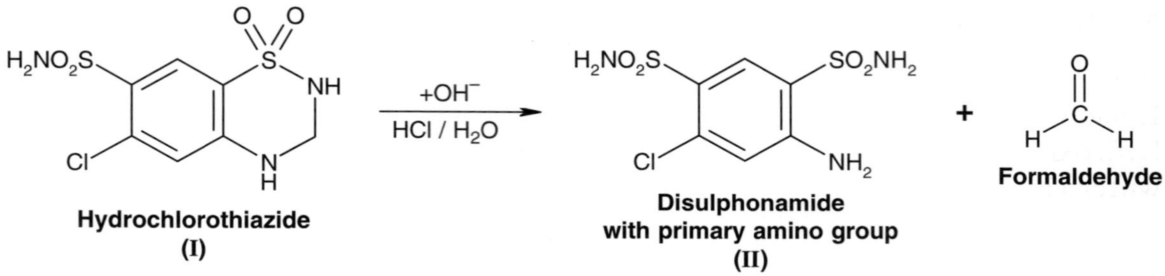

$$NaNO_2 + HCl \longrightarrow HNO_2 + NaCl$$

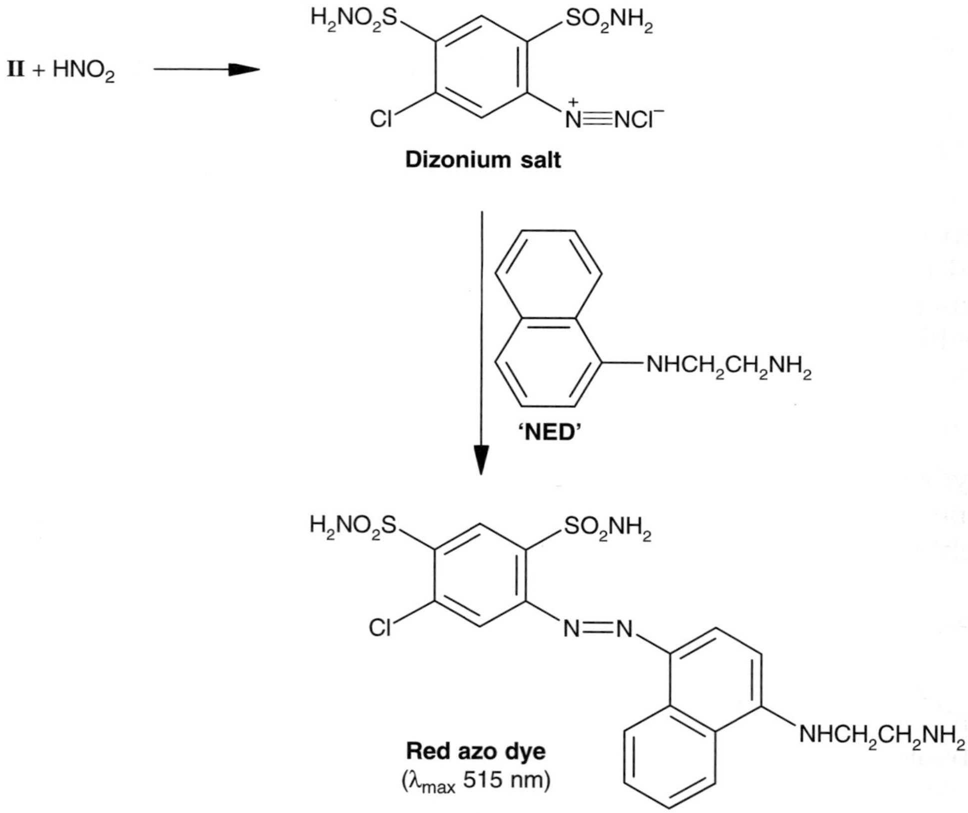

Ammonium sulphamate is added to remove excess of HNO_2 as it will react with the dye and thus interfere.

$$\underset{}{HNO_2} + \underset{\text{Ammonium sulphamate}}{NH_4SO_3NH_2} \longrightarrow N_2\uparrow + \underset{\text{Ammonium hydrogen sulphate}}{NH_4HSO_4} + H_2O$$

METHOD 2

Standard solution

Dissolve 10 mg of the substance, accurately weighed, in 10 ml of 2 M sodium hydroxide and dilute to 100 ml with water. Further dilute 5 ml to 50 ml with water (10 mcg/ml).

Sample solution

Accurately weighed quantity of the sample equivalent to 10 mg of the substance is suspended in 20 ml of water and extracted with 4 × 15 portions of chloroform. To the aqueous layer, add 10 ml of 1 M sodium hydroxide and further extract with 4 × 15 ml portions of chloroform. Aqueous alkaline extract is diluted with water to get final concentration of 10 mcg/ml.

Concomitantly measure the absorption of both sample and standard solutions at 273 nm against reagent blank and calculate the contents of hydrochlorothiazide.

Explanatory Note

On extracting the sample suspended in water with chloroform, reserpine gets passed on to chloroform layer. On basifying the aqueous layer, followed by extraction with chloroform, dihydralazine gets extracted with chloroform, leaving hydrochlorothiazide in alkaline aqueous layer which is estimated by measuring its absorption at 273 nm.

METHOD 3

The hydrolytic product (disulphonamide) of the compound forms a dye complex with methylene blue in pH 7.0 phosphate buffer. The complex can be extracted with chloroform and has λ_{max} 540 nm.

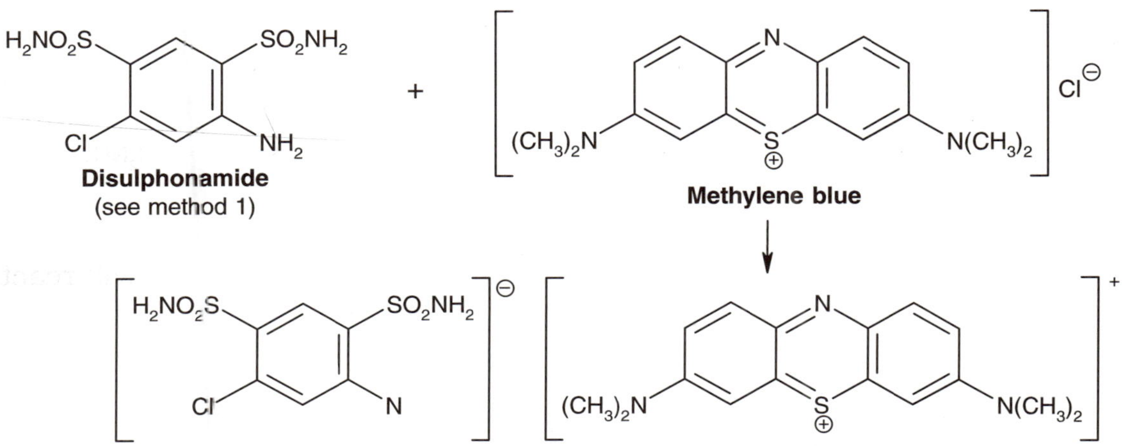

Drug-dye complex - ion-pair complex
(λ_{max} 540 nm)

METHOD 4

A spectrophotometric method has been reported by F. Belal et al. (1986) for determination of several benzothiadiazines, i.e., hydrochlorothiazide, methylclothiazide, bendroflumethiazide, benzthiazide and chlorothiazide. This method is based on coupling reaction of diazotized amine, being an electrophilic substitution, with carbanions associated with an active hydrogen atom. Carbanionic compounds such as ethyl acetoacetate with an active methylene group is used as reagent for coupling with diazotized primary aromatic amines.

Reagents

1. 5% ethanolic solution of ethylacetoacetate.
2. 0.5% sodium nitrite solution.
3. 2% urea solution.
4. 20% and 50% solution of sodium hydroxide.
5. 1 M HCl.
6. Conc. HCl.

Standard solution

Dissolve 50 mg of the substance in 10 ml of 20% sodium hydroxide solution by boiling under reflux for 30 min, cool, add 15 ml of conc. HCl and dilute to 100 ml with water. Further dilute 10 ml to 100 ml with 1 M HCl (50 μg/ml).

Sample solution

Extract powdered sample equivalent to 50 mg of the substance under analysis with 3 × 25 ml of 0.8% sodium hydroxide solution, filter, dilute to 100 ml with water. Boil 10 ml of this solution with 10 ml of 20% sodium hydroxide solution and proceed further as under standard solution.

Procedure

To 5 ml each of sample and standard solutions add 10 ml of sodium nitrite solution, cool the flask in ice, add 2 ml of urea (to destroy excess of HNO_2) and after 3 min add 1 ml of ethyl acetoacetate solution, followed by 6 ml of 50% NaOH solution. Measure the absorbance at about 430 nm against reagent blank.

Probable Reaction Mechanism

Benzothiadiazines on alkaline hydrolysis yield 2,4-disulphamoylanilines which are diazotized and coupled with the reagent i.e. ethyl acetoacetate in strong alkaline solution.

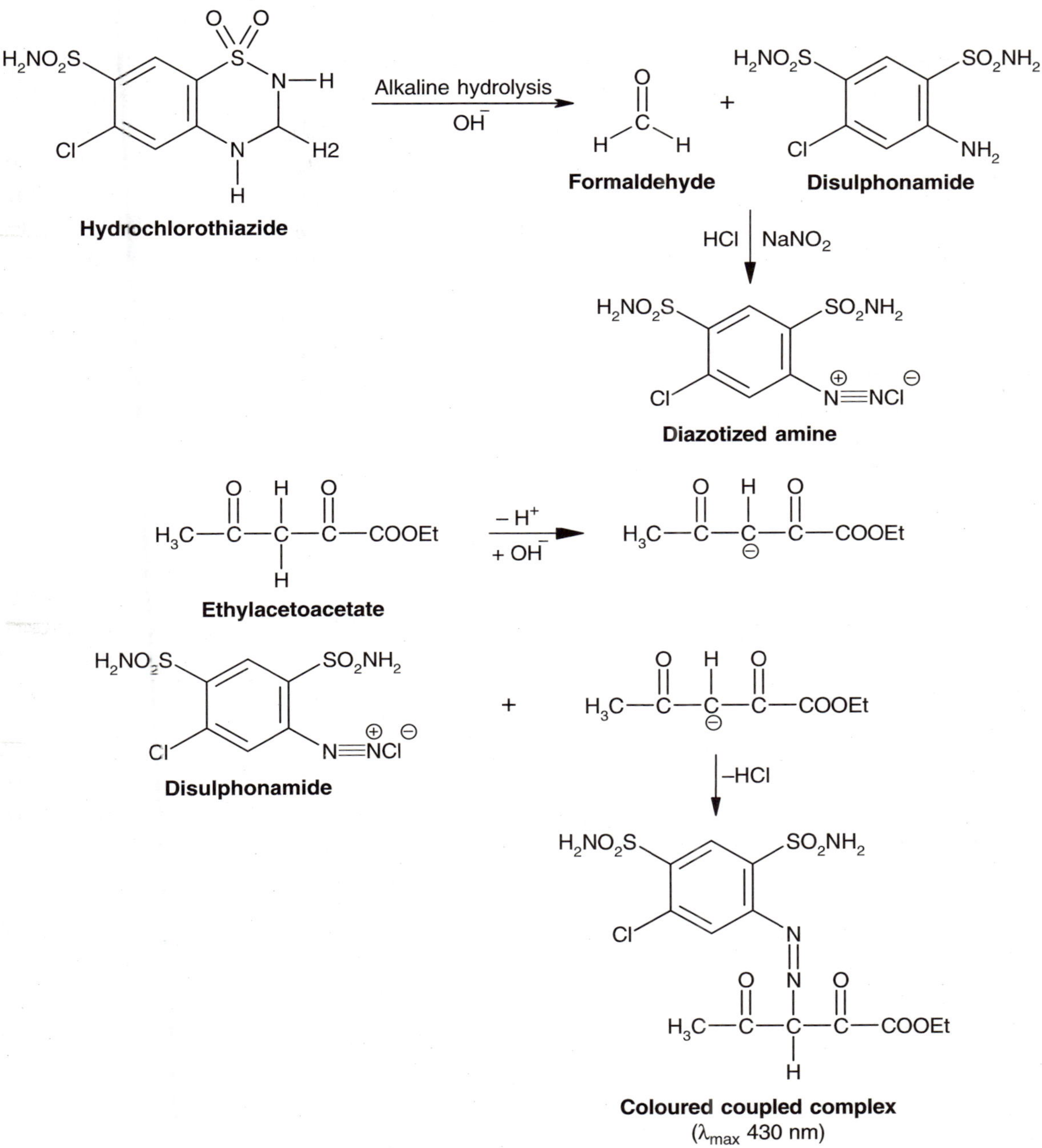

Note

1. The coupling reaction is instantaneous and colour is stable for 24 hours.
2. Hydralazine and reserpine which are co-formulated do not interfere.
3. Molar absorptivities of product with different benzothiazides is the same.

Reference

1. S. Belal, E.A. El-Neanacy and S. Soliman. *Talanta*, **25**, 290, 1978.
2. F. Belal, M. Rizk, F. Ibrahiem and M. Sharaf El-Din. *Talanta*, **33** (2), 170-172, 1986.

A method has been described for the estimation of several diuretics by Sastry et al. (1989) based on reaction of p-N,N-dimethylphenyldiamine hydrochloride (DMPDH) and chloramine T. Several diuretics studied were amiloride (AML), frusemide (FRU), acetazolamide (AZ), benzothiazide (BZT), hydrochlorothiazide (HCT), hydroflumethiazide (HFT), polythiazide (PT), trichlormethiazide(TCM). All drugs except amiloride were first hydrolysed with 5 M sodium hydroxide and then analysed by the proposed method. The hydrolysed sample was treated with 'DMPDH' reagent and chloramine T. The absorbance of the end reaction product in all the compounds except amiloride was measured at 540 nm except 660 nm for amiloride.

Probable General Reaction Mechanism

In the presence of chloramine T, 'DMPDH' undergoes a 2-electron oxidation to yield a less stable but highly reactive species, p-N,N,-dimethylbenzoquinone-imine (DMBQDi). This species reacts with amino compounds by electrophilic attack at para or ortho position to the amino group to give a dye which is finally oxidized to indo-dye. However, in the case of acetazolamide and amiloride, the reaction takes place by expulsion of electron withdrawing groups such as —Cl in case of amiloride and SO_3H in case of acetazolamide.

Drugs Analysed

Drugs	R_1	R_2	R_3	R_4
1. Hydrolysed BZT, TCM, HCZ	SO_2NH_2	Cl	SO_2NH_2	—
2. Hydrolysed PT	SO_2NH_2	Cl	SO_2NHCH_3	—
3. Hydrolysed HFT	SO_2NH_2	CF_3	SO_2NH_2	—
4. Hydrolysed FRU	SO_2NH_2	Cl	COOH	—
5. AML	—	—	—	$CONH—C(=\overset{+}{N}H_2Cl^-)—NH_2$

Reference

1. D.N. Kramer and L.U. Tolentino. *Anal.Chem.*, **43**, 834, 1971.
2. C.S.P. Sastry, M.V. Suryanarayana and A.S.R.P. Tipirneni. *Talanta*, **36(4)**, 491-494, 1989.

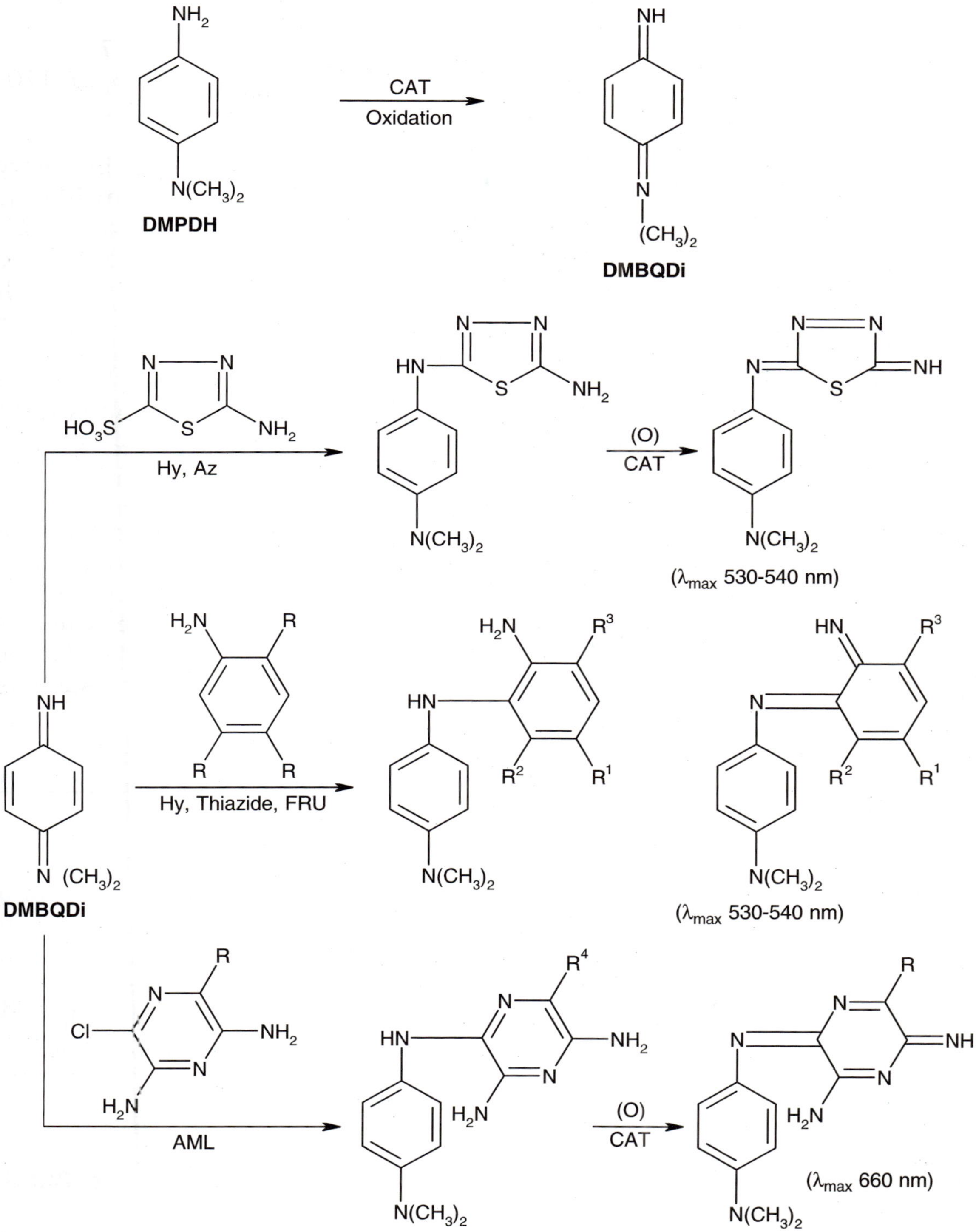

NH2
N(CH3)2
DMPDH
CAT
Oxidation
NH
N
(CH3)2
DMBQDi
HO3S
NH2
Hy, Az
HN
(O)
CAT
(λmax 530-540 nm)
H2N
R
Hy, Thiazide, FRU
R3
R2
R1
HN
(λmax 530-540 nm)
NH
N (CH3)2
DMBQDi
Cl
AML
R4
(O)
CAT
(λmax 660 nm)

Reserpine

METHOD 1

Reagents

1. 2% w/v solution of citric acid in water.
2. 1% w/v solution of sodium bicarbonate in water.
3. 0.3% w/v solution of sodium nitrite in 50% methanol.
4. 5% w/v solution of ammonium sulphamate in water.
5. Methanol.
6. Hydrochloric acid.
7. Chloroform.

Standard solution

Dissolve 25 mg of accurately weighed substance in 1-2 drops of chloroform, mix about 30 ml of methanol (previously warmed to 50°C). Cool and dilute to 250 ml with methanol (protect this solution from light—use amber coloured glass apparatus). (Just before start of estimation, take 10 ml of the solution, add 35 ml of chloroform and dilute to 50 ml with methanol).

Sample solution

Extract accurately weighed quantity of the sample equivalent to 1 mg of the substance with 10 ml of chloroform by shaking for 5 min. Add 10 ml of citric acid and shake for 2 min, collect chloroform layer, wash citric acid layer with further 10 ml of chloroform. To the combined chloroform layer, add 10 ml of sodium bicarbonate solution, shake for 2 min. Collect chloroform layer into 50 ml flask through pre-moistened cotton plug. Extract the aqueous layer with 2×5 ml portions of chloroform, combine chloroform layer and dilute to 50 ml with methanol.

Procedure

To 5 ml each of sample and standard solutions, add 2 ml methanol, 1 ml of sodium nitrite solution and 5 drops of hydrochloric acid. Mix and allow to stand for 30 min. Add 0.5 ml of ammonium sulphamate solution and dilute to 10 ml with methanol. Allow to stand for 10 min. Determine the absorbance of both the solutions at 390 nm against solvent blank (chloroform-methanol-water, 3.6 + 5.4 + 1.0 v/v) and calculate the contents of reserpine.

Explanatory Note

Reserpine is freely soluble in chloroform, successive extraction with citric acid and sodium bicarbonate removes other interfering substance. Treatment with HNO_2 brings about oxidative breakdown of reserpine leading to yellow colour (λ_{max} 390 nm) due to 3-dehydroreserpine.

Probable Reaction Mechanism

$$NaNO_2 + HCl \longrightarrow NaCl + HNO_2$$

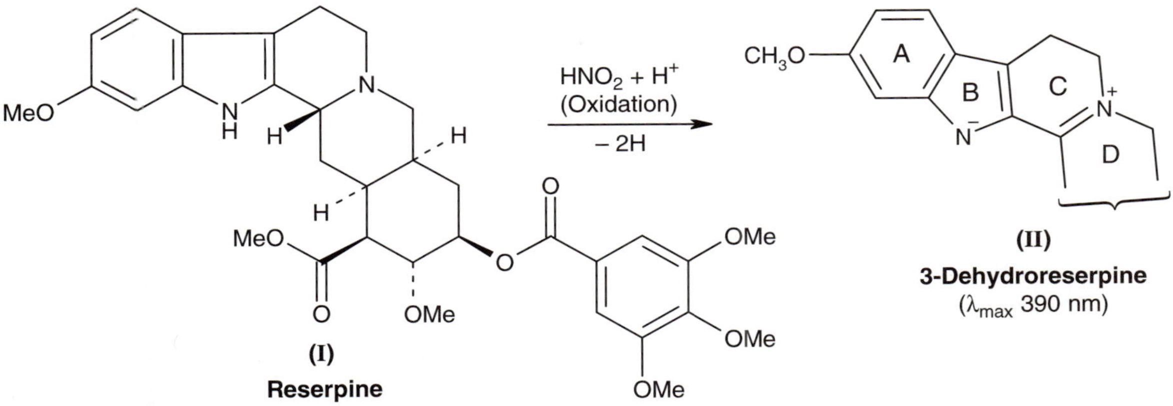

(I)
Reserpine

(II)
3-Dehydroreserpine
(λ_{max} 390 nm)

Note

Ammonium sulphamate is added to remove excess of HNO_2.

METHOD 2

Reagents

1. To about 200 mg of vanadium pentoxide, add 20 ml of water and 200 ml of orthophosphoric acid, shake vigorously and dilute to 1000 ml with absolute alcohol. Allow to stand at room temperature for 60 min and filter.
2. Methanol – 0.1 M hydrochloric acid mixture (1 : 1), solvent.

Standard solution

200 mcg/ml of reserpine in methylene chloride. Dilute 5 ml to 100 ml with solvent.

Sample solution

Suspend accurately weighed quantity of the sample equivalent to 2 mg of substance in 100 ml of 0.1 M hydrochloric acid, stir for 30 min and heat in ultrasonic water-bath for 1 min, cool and dilute to 200 ml with methanol.

Procedure

Dilute 3 ml each of sample and standard solutions to 50 ml with vanadium pentoxide reagent. Determine the contents by fluorimetry using solvent as blank.

Excitation wavelength : 400 nm
Emission wavelength : 496 nm
Calculate the contents of reserpine in the sample by comparison.

Explanatory Note

Reserpine on oxidation with vanadium pentoxide in acidic medium gives tetrahydroreserpine which has yellow-green colour with intense fluorescence with ex: 400 nm, em: 496 nm.

Probable Reaction Mechanism

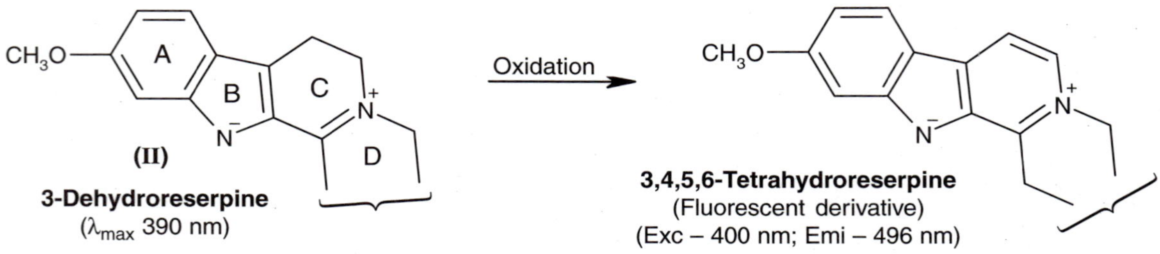

On acid or alkaline hydrolysis which occurs at C-18 forming trimethoxy-benzoic acid which can form the bases of titrimetric assay.

Probable Reaction Mechanism

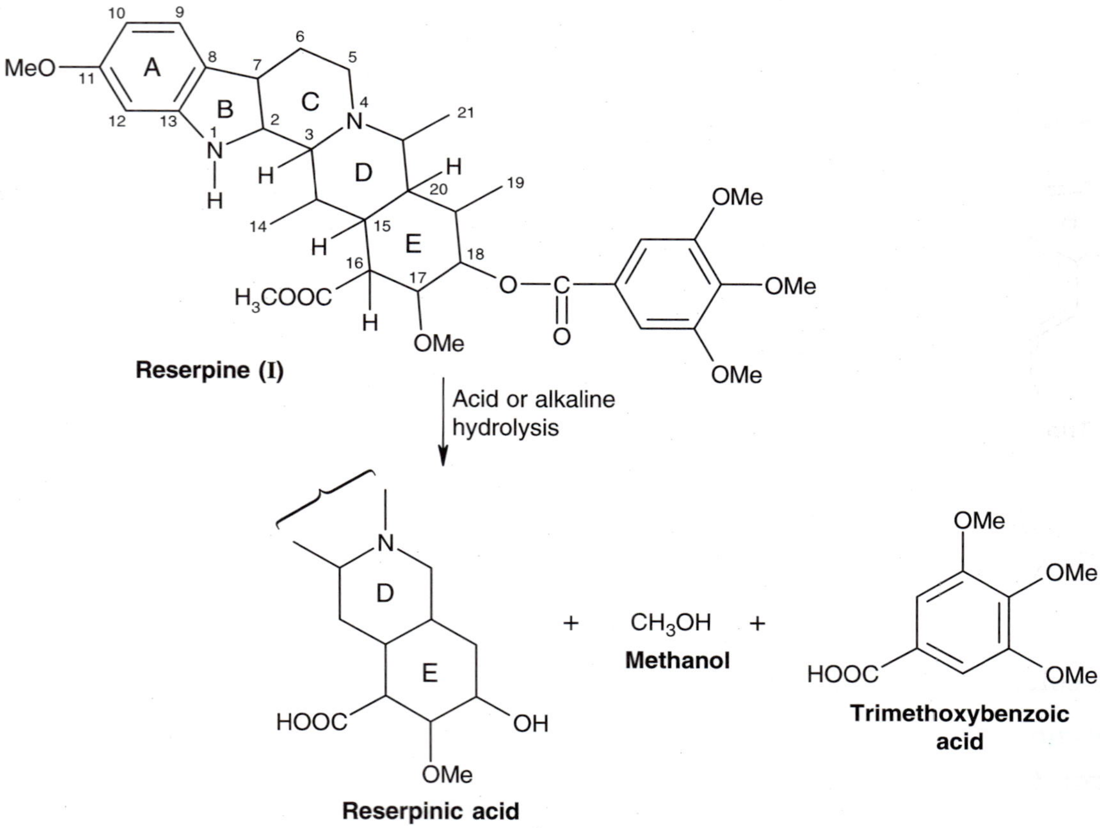

The compound reacts with vanillin or 4-dimethylaminobenzaldehyde (PDAB) in acidic medium. The aldehyde attacks at C-10 of the intact molecule. The position C-10 is activated by the methoxy (OCH_3) group present at C-11 giving a red-coloured complex which forms the basis of spectrophotometric analysis.

Probable Reaction Mechanism

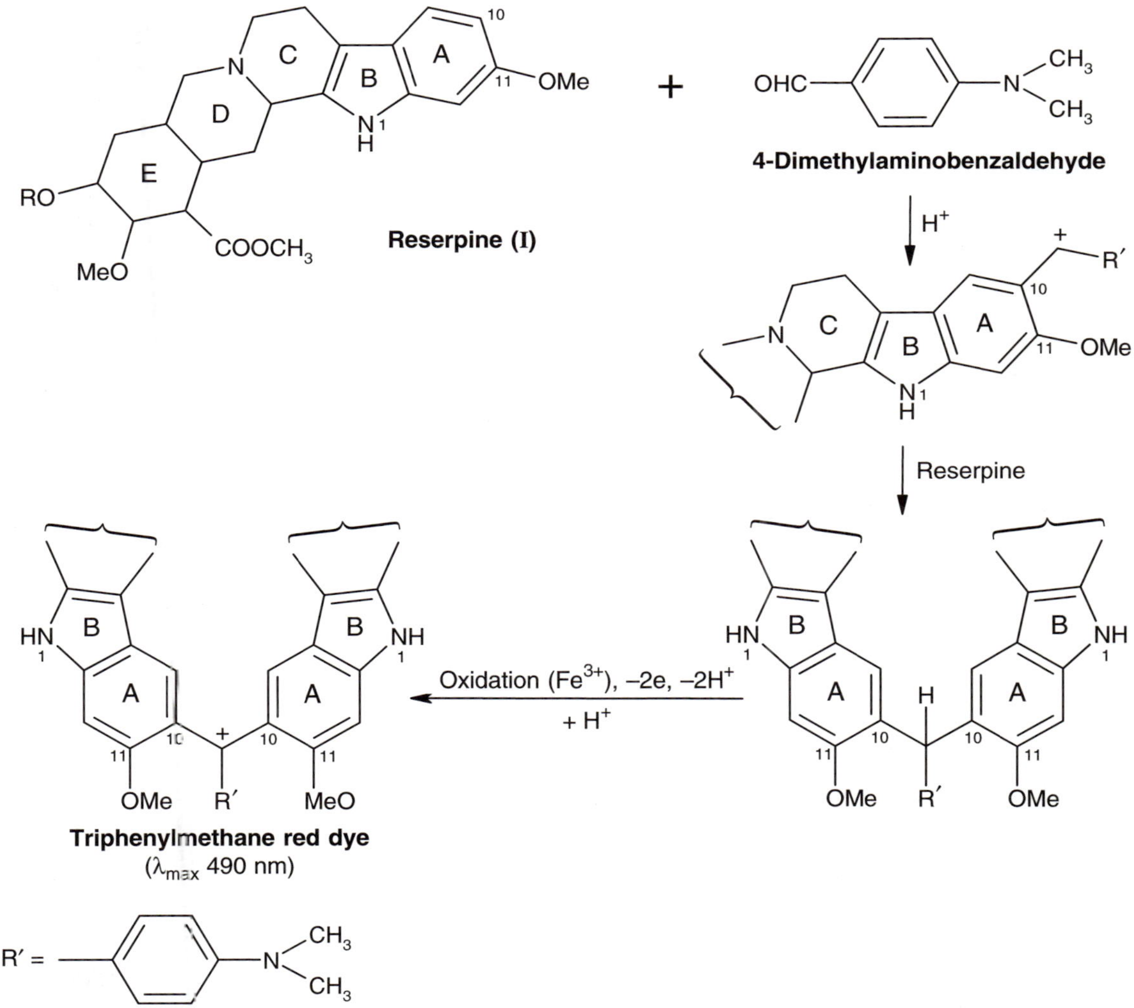

Note

Pink-coloured dye is formed when vanillin is used as aldehyde.

Reference

Pharm. Chem. (Vol. 2) by H.J. Roth, p. 576-578.

Formulation 2

Hydrochlorothiazide, Propranolol hydrochloride

ESTIMATION

METHOD 1

Both these substances in acidic medium have isoabsorption point at 284 nm; thus could be used for total contents of hydrochlorothiazide and propranolol, whereas propranolol has no absorption at 326 nm, absorption being solely due to hydrochlorothiazide. Hence at 326 nm there will be no interference from propranolol.

Standard solution

1. 2 mcg/ml of propranolol hydrochloride in 0.1 N hydrochloric acid.
2. 1 mg/ml of hydrochlorothiazide in 0.1 N hydrochloric acid.

Sample solution

Accurately weighed quantity of the sample equivalent to 40 mg of propranolol was extracted with 50 ml of methanol in ultrasonic bath and diluted to 100 ml with 0.1 N hydrochloric acid.

Both the sample and standard solutions were further diluted appropriately and absorption measured at isoabsorption point (284 nm) for total contents of both the substances and at 326 nm for hydrochlorothiazide. Thus the contents of propranolol could be obtained by difference. The method observed Beer's law with range of 10-80 mcg/ml at 284 nm for both the substances and 10-250 mcg/ml at 326 nm for hydrochlorothiazide. The method is suitable for dissolution studies.

Explanatory Note

At isoabsorption point (284 nm) both the substances have same absorption, thus absorption value obtained at this wavelength will give total amount of both the substances, whereas the amount of hydrochlorothiazide found by measuring its absorption at 326 nm can be subtracted from the total found at 284 nm will give amount of propranolol hydrochloride.

METHOD 2

Standard solution

1. 80 mcg/ml of propranolol hydrochloride in water.
2. 50 mcg/ml of hydrochlorothiazide in 0.04 M sodium hydroxide.

Sample solution

Accurately weighed quantity of powdered sample equivalent to 40 mg of the propranolol hydrochloride was extracted with 50 ml of 0.1 N hydrochloric acid by shaking for 30 min (80 mcg/ml).

Procedure

To 6 ml each of sample and standard solutions, add 1 ml of 5 N sodium hydroxide and 25 ml of n-heptane, shake for 5 min and allow the layers to separate (reserve alkaline aqueous layer for estimation of hydrochlorothiazide).

Concomitantly measure the absorbance of n-heptane layer (test and standard-2) at 293 nm against n-heptane blank extract and calculate the contents of propranolol hydrochloride in the sample. The absorbance of aqueous extracts (test and standard-2) is measured at 273 nm against aqueous blank extract and calculate the contents of hydrochlorothiazide in the sample.

Probable Reaction Mechanism

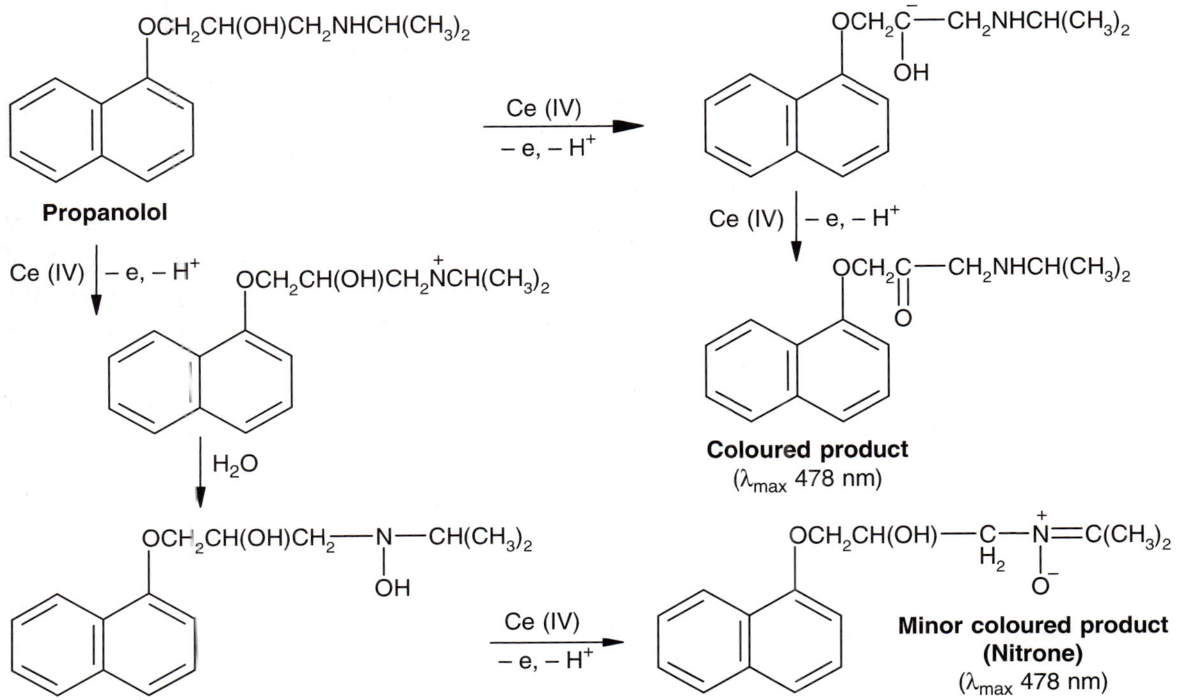

Explanatory Note

On basification with sodium hydroxide, propranolol is extracted into n-heptane layer whereas hydrochlorothiazide remains in aqueous alkaline layer. Absorbance of n-heptane layer is measured at 293 nm (propranolol) and alkaline aqueous layer at 273 nm (hydrochlorothiazide).

n-Heptane layer containing propranolol is evaporated and residue taken up in water can be subjected to quantitative analysis by oxidation with ceric (IV) giving an orange-coloured product (λ_{max} 478 nm). Oxidation of the molecule takes place at N-alkyl ethanolamine site as usual. As Ce (IV) is a strong oxidizing agent, number of other side reaction products are formed in small amount. The authors have confirmed the formation of nitrone by IR and NMR studies which is probably due to oxidation of secondary amine site.

Reference

Sajid Husain, A.S.R. Krishnamurthy, R. Sekar and P. Ravi Prasad. *Indian Drugs*, **32(12)**, 574-577, 1995.

Sanghavi et al. (1980) have reported spectrophotometric method based on nitration of naphthalene ring with potassium nitrate/sulphuric acid.

Reagents

1. 5% w/v solution of urea in water.
2. 2% w/v solution of potassium nitrate in water.
3. Conc. sulphuric acid.

Sample and standard solutions

250 μg/ml solution in 1 M hydrochloric acid.

Procedure

To 2.5 ml each of sample and standard solutions, add 1.5 ml of potassium nitrate solution, followed by 0.5 ml of conc. sulphuric acid. Keep aside for 10 min, then add 2 ml of urea solution (to remove any HNO_2 formed), keep aside for for 5 min, dilute to 50 ml and measure the absorbance of yellow colour at 360 nm against reagent blank.

Note

1. Hydrochlorothiazide/hydroflumethiazide, if present, did not interfere.
2. Alprazolam/diazepam, usually present, did not interfere.

Probable Reaction Mechanism

Since propanolol is substituted at α-position, the electrophilic group (NO_2^+) will attack at position-2 or position-4 or both depending on the reaction temperature (at room temperature – mono; and at higher temperature – dinitro derivatives shall be formed).

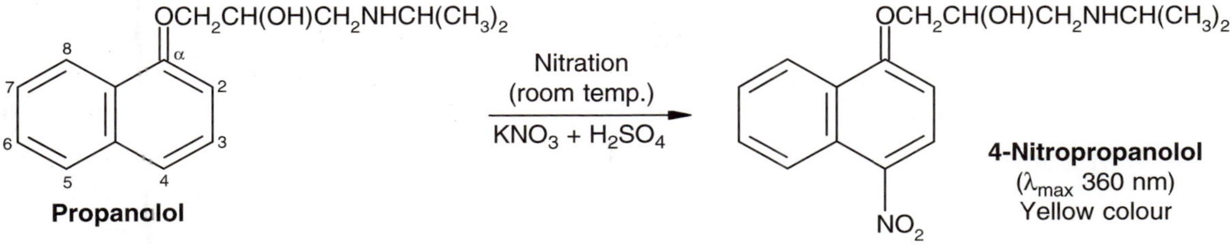

Sulphuric acid, being a strong acid, protonates nitrate to give $H_2NO_3^+$ which on losing water gives nitronium ions (NO_2^+). Sulphuric acid helps in this reaction by taking up water molecule, being anhydrous. Nitronium ion (NO_2^+) then attacks the naphthalene ring to give nitro derivative.

$$KNO_3 + H_2SO_4 \rightleftharpoons KSO_4^- + H-\overset{+}{\underset{H}{O}}-NO_2 \rightleftharpoons H_2O + NO_2^+ \text{ (taken up by } H_2SO_4\text{)}$$

$$(H_2NO_3^+ \text{ or } H_2ONO_2^+)$$

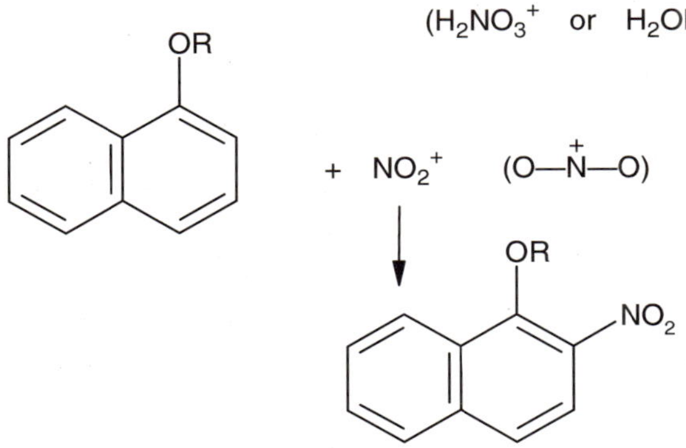

Reference

1. N.M. Sanghavi and N.G. Jivani. *Talanta*, **27**, 591-592, 1980.
2. Organic Chemistry by Norman L. Allinger, Worth Publishers, 1971, p. 353.

Basavaiah et al. have proposed titrimetric and spectrophotometric methods.

(a) Titrimetric method

Suspend adequate quantity of the sample in water to get 1 mg/ml solution, add 2 ml of 1 M HCl, 2 ml of 10% KBr solution and titrate with 0.02 M chloramine T (CAT) solution using methyl orange as indicator. From the volume of 0.02 M CAT solution consumed, calculate the amount of propanolol (PPL) in the sample under analysis. The molar ratio PPL : CAT being 1 : 3.

(b) Spectrophotometric method

Reagents

1. 1 M hydrochloric acid.
2. 500 µg/ml solution of 'CAT' in water.
3. 0.2% w/v solution of metol.
4. 0.1% w/v solution of sulphanilic acid.
5. 1 M sodium acetate solution.

Sample and standard solutions

50 µg/ml of the substance in water.

Procedure

In each flask, separately mix 1 ml each of 1 M HCl and 1 ml of 'CAT' solution, then to each flask add 2 ml of sample/standard solutions, dilute to 5 ml with water, keep aside for 10 min with occasional shaking. Then, to each flask, add 1.5 ml of sodium acetate solution, followed by 1 ml each of metol and sulphanilic acid solutions, dilute to 10 ml with water and measure the absorbance of both sample and standard at 520 nm against reagent blank within 20 min.

Probable Reaction Mechanism

p-N-Methylbenzoquinone formed in situ from metol-CAT interaction is a good electron acceptor to form charge-transfer (C-T) complex with aromatic amine (sulphanilic acid) as the electron donor.

Initially, propanolol is oxidized by 'CAT'. Excess of the reagent reacts with metol to give benzoquinone monoimine which forms C-T complex with aromatic amine.

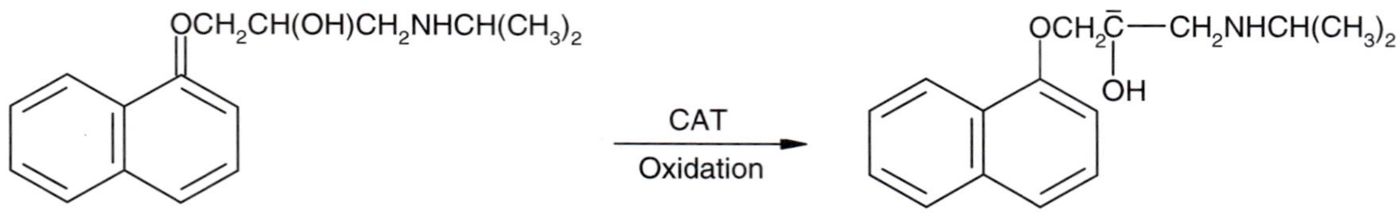

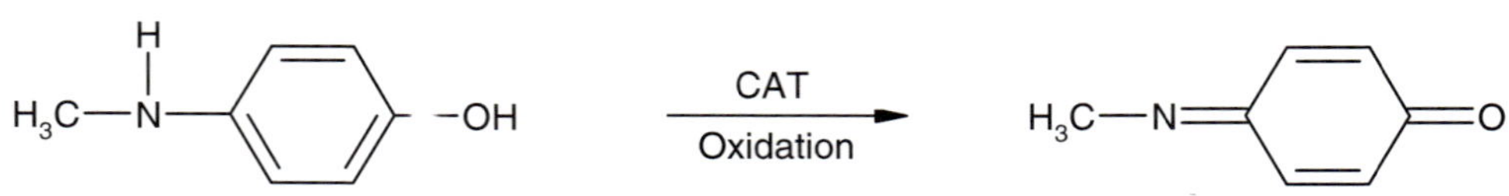

Metol
(p-N-methyl aminophenol)

p-N-methyl benzoquinone monoimine

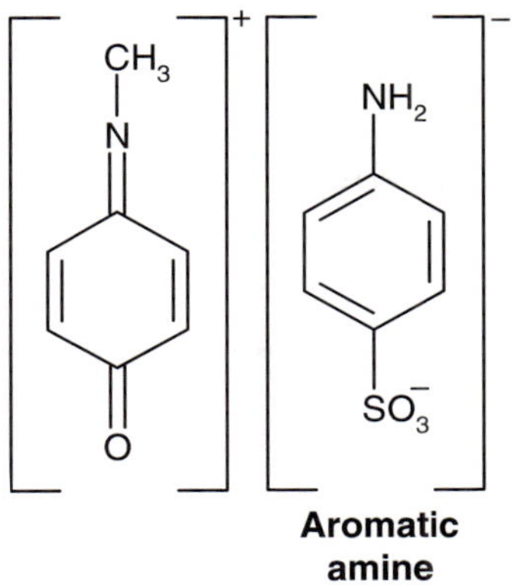

Charge-transfer complex
(λ_{max} 520 nm)

Note

This reaction is similar to the one described for adrenaline and noradrenaline (Indian Drugs, **28(6)**, 272, March 1991).

Reference

K. Basavaiah, U. Chandersekar, H.C. Prameela and P. Nagegowda. *Indian Drugs*, **41(5)**, 303-305, 2004.

An alternative method using 'NBS' as oxidizing agent and coupling with 'INH' was earlier described by C.S.P. Sastry et al. for this drug.

Reference

C.S.P. Sastry, A. Sailaja and T. Thirupathi. *Indian Drugs*, **29(3)**, 132-133, 1992.

Formulation 3

Propranolol hydrochloride, Hydroflumethazide

ESTIMATION

Propranolol hydrochloric and Hydroflumethazide

Standard solution

1. 20 mcg/ml of propranolol in 0.1 N hydrochloric acid.
2. 10 mcg/ml of hydroflumethazide in 0.1 N sodium hydroxide.

Sample solution

Suspend accurately weighed quantity of the sample in 10 ml of water, add 25 ml of 0.1 N sodium hydroxide and extract with 3 × 50 ml portions of water-washed anaesthetic ether. Combine the ether extract and wash with 20 ml of water. Retain the main aqueous alkaline layer and the washing for estimation of hydroflumethazide.

Extract the ether layer with 3 × 50 ml portions of 0.1 N hydrochloric acid, dilute the acid layer to 200 ml with acid and mix. Dilute further 10 ml of the resultant solution to 100 ml with 0.1 N hydrochloric acid and measure the extinction of both the solutions at 290 nm using 0.1 N hydrochloric acid as blank and the contents of propranolol are calculated by comparison.

Transfer the aqueous alkaline layer to 250 ml volumetric flask and dilute to mark with 0.1 N sodium hydroxide. Further dilute 10 ml of this solution to 100 ml with 0.1 N sodium hydroxide. Measure the absorption at 275 nm and of contents of hydroflumethazide are calculated by comparison.

Explanatory Note

Ether layer containing propranolol is extracted back into acid layer to get propranolol hydrochloride. Its absorbance measured at 290 nm for quantitative estimation; whereas alkaline layer contains hydroflumethazide (λ_{max} 275 nm).

Alternatively, propranolol can be estimated by its reaction with 1-fluoro-2,4-dinitrobenzene in alkaline medium (2.5% borax).

This reagent is known as Sanger's reagent (developed by Frederick Sanger – awarded Nobel Prize in 1958 for establishing the sequence of amino acids in proteins) and reacts with secondary amino group present in alkylamine group with loss of one molecule of hydrofluoric acid (HF).

Probable Reaction Mechanism

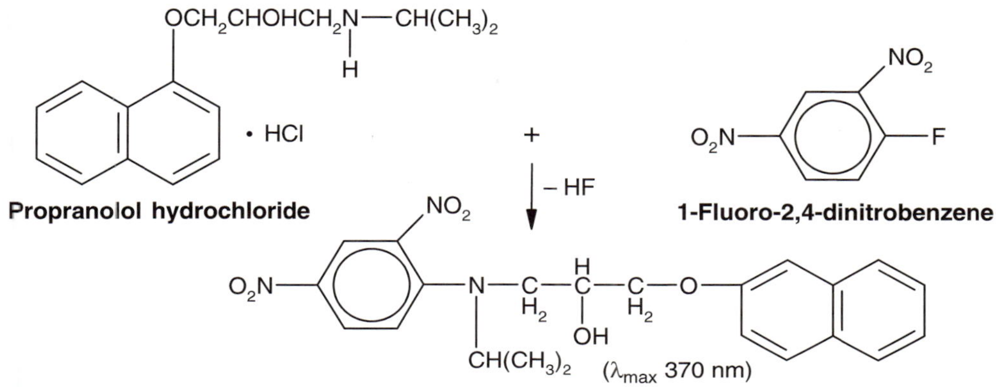

Reference

D.M. Shingbal and J.S. Prabhu Desai, *Indian Drugs*, **21(7)**, 304-305, 1984.

Note

Metoprolol is reported to react with 'DNFB' reagent and p-chloranil in similar way.

Reference

D.M. Shingbal et al., *Indian Drugs*, **24(5)**, 270-273, 1986; **24(7)**, 373-374, 1986.

The secondary amino group of propranolol, which is nucleophilic, will attack the benzene skeleton of chloranil, resulting in Michael addition like product. The reaction proceeds with the loss of a molecule of HCl.

Probable Reaction Mechanism

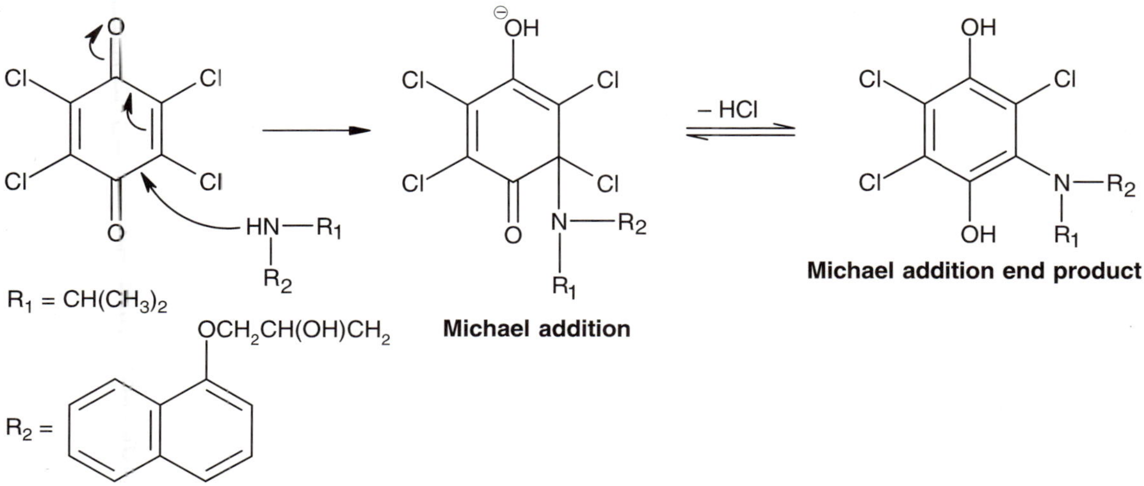

The final product shall have the following structural representation.

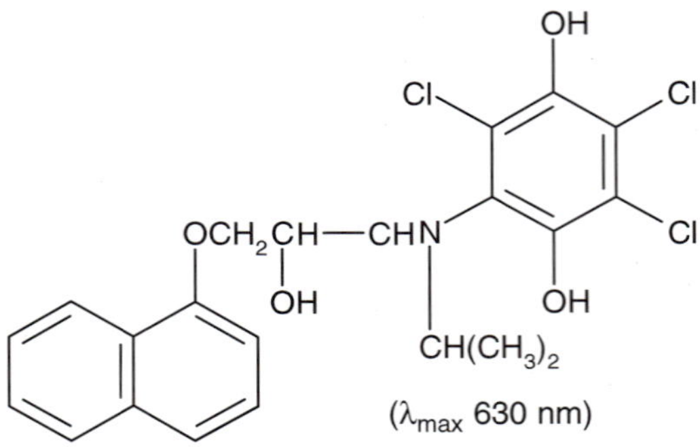

(λ_{max} 630 nm)

Reference

1. D.M. Shingbal and A.B. Khandeparkar, *Indian Drugs*, **24(7)**, 365-366, 1987.
2. Pharmaceutical Chemistry (Vol. 2) by H.J. Roth, p. 107.

Chloranil and dichlorodicyano-1,4-benzoquinone (DCQ) show typical addition and redox reactions and can be used as reagents for the estimation of several common drugs: ephedrine, emetine, berberine, reserpine, papaverine, morphine, piperazine (alkaloids), procaine, lidocaine (local anaesthetics), promethazine, benzodiazepine (phenothiazines), ampicillin, amoxycillin, cloxacillin, ofloxacin (antibiotics), furosemide, benzothiazide (diuretics), sulphonamide, piperazine and pyrimethamine.

Hydroflumethazide

The compound shall answer all the reactions of hydrochlorothiazide. The analytical methods described for hydrochlorothiazide can be used for this compound.

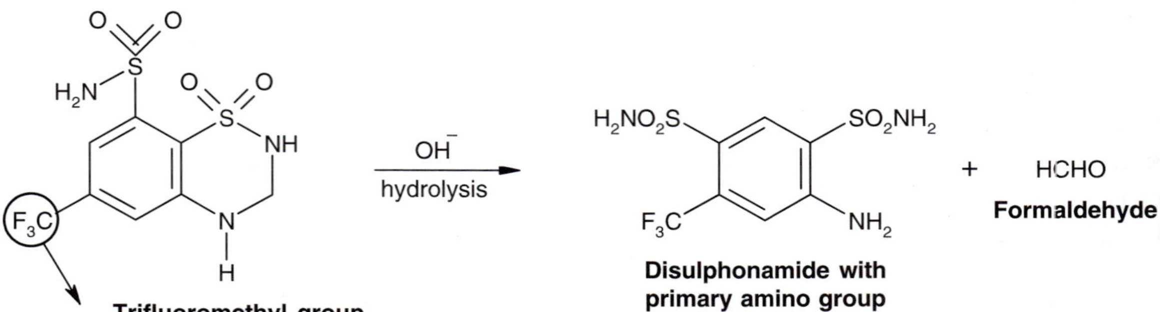

The primary amino group can be diazotized and coupled with N-(1-naphthyl)ethylene diamine to give azo dye. For details refer to formulation 1 of this chapter under hydrochlorothiazide.

Formulation 4

Propranolol hydrochloride, Hydralazine hydrochloride

ESTIMATION

Propranolol hydrochloride and Hydralazine hydrochloride

Standard solution

1. 20 mcg/ml of propranolol hydrochloride in methanol.
2. 10 mcg/ml of hydralazine hydrochloride in water.

Sample solution

Extract accurately weighed quantity of powdered sample equivalent to 200 mg of propranolol with 10 ml of methanol by shaking for 10 min. Filter, use the filtrate for estimation of propranolol and preserve the residue for estimation of hydralazine. Dilute 2 ml of filtrate obtained above to 100 ml with methanol, mix and further dilute 5 ml to 100 ml with methanol (20 mcg/ml) and measure the absorbance of both the solutions at 290 nm using methanol as blank and contents of propranolol calculated by comparison.

Transfer the residue obtained above to 500 ml volumetric flask and dissolve in water. 5 ml of the resultant solution is further diluted to 250 ml with water.

Absorbance of both sample and standard solutions is measured at 260 nm using water as blank and contents of hydralazine calculated by comparison.

Explanatory Note

This method is based on differential solubility; propranolol hydrochloride being soluble in methanol and hydralazine being insoluble. This procedure has to be carried out on finely powdered sample (dry) and the filtration should preferably be done through G4 sintered funnel.

Hydralazine can also be estimated by its reaction with ninhydrin.

Reagents

1. 10% w/v solution of ninhydrin in methanol.
2. 0.2 M phthalate buffer pH 3.0.

Sample and standard solutions

20 μg/ml in 0.2 M phthalate pH 3.0 buffer.

Procedure

To 4 ml of sample/standard solution add 4 ml of pH 3 buffer and 2 ml of ninhydrin solution. Allow the solution to stand in dark for 1 hour at room temperature, dilute to 50 ml with water and measure the absorbance at 442 nm of both sample/standard solutions for estimation.

Probable Reaction Mechanism

Condensation reaction occurs between hydralazine and ninhydrin resulting in the formation of the product as shown below:

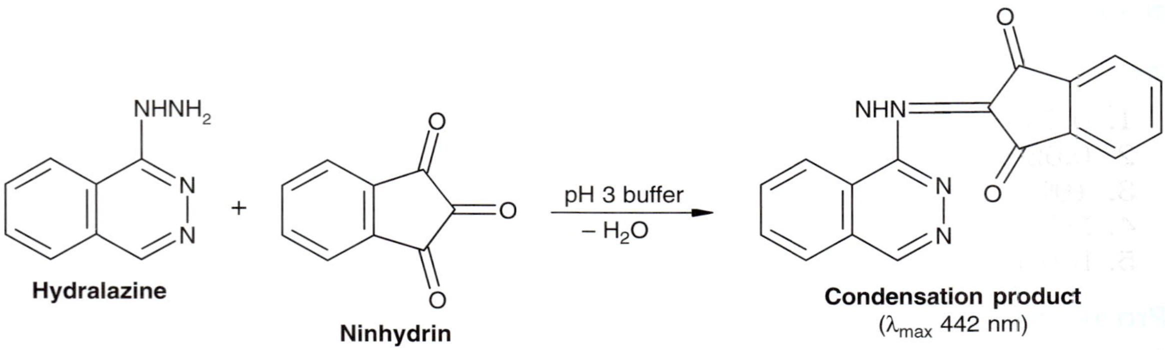

Reference

Manesh C. Dutt et al. *J. AOAC.*, **66(6)**, 1455-1457, 1983.

Formulation 5

Propranolol hydrochloride, Dihydralazine sulphate, Hydrochlorothiazide

ESTIMATION

Propranolol hydrochloride

Reagents

1. 0.05 N silver nitrate.
2. 0.05 ammonium thiocyanate.
3. 10% w/v solution of ferric ammonium sulphate.
4. Dilute nitric acid.
5. Nitrobenzene.

Procedure

Accurately weighed quantity of the powdered sample equivalent to 200 mg of propranolol was suspended in 25 ml of water, shake in mechanical shaker for 30 min and dilute to 50 ml with water. To 25 ml of filtrate, add 10 ml of dilute nitric acid and 25 ml of 0.05 N silver nitrate. Titrate excess of silver nitrate with 0.05 N ammonium thiocyanate using ferric ammonium sulphate as indicator. Carry out a blank titration. Each ml of 0.05 N silver nitrate consumed is equivalent to 14.79 mg of propranolol hydrochloride.

Note

This is non-specific assay method involving estimation of chloride moiety.

Both propanolol hydrochloride and metoprolol hydrochloride form ion-pair complex with acidic dyes such as bromophenol blue, bromocresol purple and bromocresol green in potassium phthalate buffer pH 3. All complexes are extractable into chloroform and have λ_{max} in the range of 410-420 nm.

Reference

Somashekara, P.G. Ramappa and H.D. Rovanasiddappa, *Indian Drugs*, **38(2)**, 98-99, 2001.

Both these drugs also form ion-pair complex with different food colours such as carmosine-S, indigo-carmine, sunset yellow, Evan's blue, fast red-E and other acidic dyes such as solochrom black-T, fast sulphone black-FF, solochrome cyanine-R in acidic buffer. These have been used for quantitative estimation of the drugs.

Reference

R.T. Sane, M.L. Kural, V.G. Nayak, V.B. Malkar and R.S. Sawant, *Ind. J. Pharm. Sci.*, **46(4)**, 151-154, 1984.

Sajjan et al. (2002) have reported two methods based on nitration of the drug with uranyl nitrate or thorium nitrate in acidic medium yielding coloured nitro derivatives (λ_{max} 377 nm).

Probable Reaction Mechanism

Since propanolol is a mono-substituted naphthalene i.e. substituted at α(1) position, electrophilic substitution shall take place preferably at position-4 or 2, preferably at position-4. In case of dinitro derivative, we will get 2,4-dinitro analogous to the dye Martin's yellow.

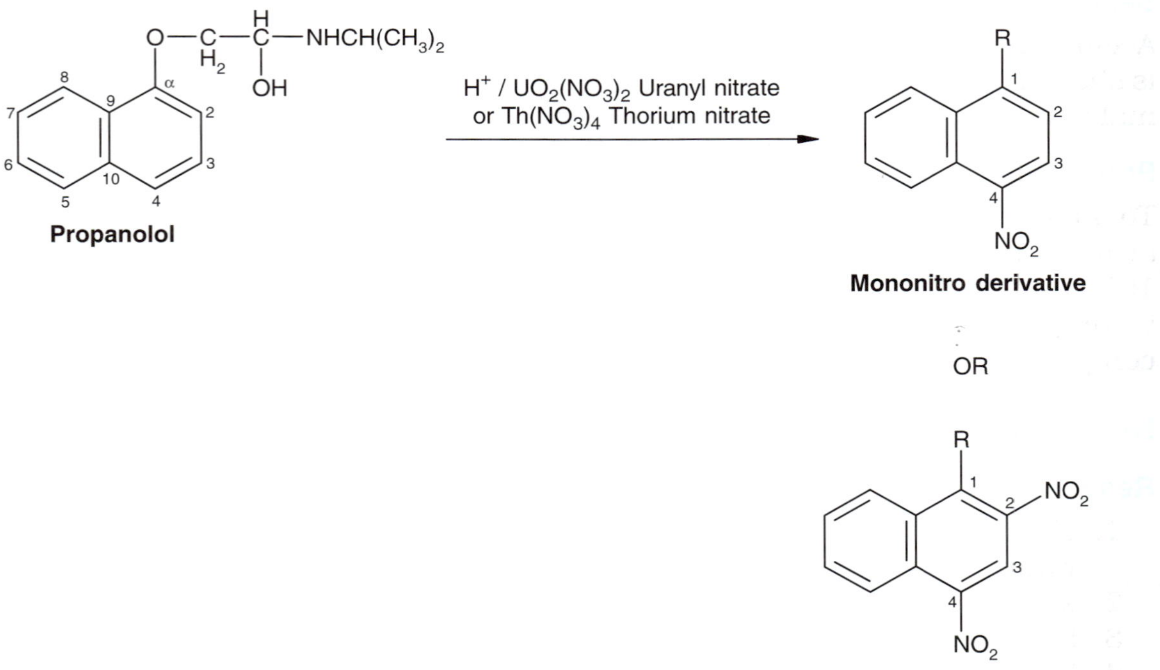

Yellow-coloured 2,4-dinitro derivative
(λ_{max} 377 nm)

Note

1. For reaction to proceed, the reaction mixture is required to be heated in water-bath (70–80°C) for 2 min.
2. Colour is stable for 2 hrs.
3. Excipients do not interfere.

Reference

Aparna G. Sajjan, J. Seetharamappa and Sarswati P. Masti, *Ind. J. Pharm. Sci.*, **64(6)**, 68-70, 2002.

Dihydralazine sulphate

Reagents

1. 0.05 M sulphuric acid.
2. 1 M sodium hydroxide.
3. FC phenol reagent (1 : 1).

Standard solution

250 mcg/ml of the substance in 0.05 M sulphuric acid.

Sample solution

Accurately weighed quantity of the sample equivalent to 25 mg of the substance is shaken with 50 ml of 0.05 M sulphuric acid for 50 min in mechanical shaker, make up to 100 ml.

Procedure

To 4 ml each of sample and standard solutions, add 2 ml of 0.05 M sulphuric acid, 1 ml of FC phenol reagent and 1 ml of 1 M sodium hydroxide, dilute to 100 ml with water and measure the absorbance of both sample and standard solutions at 610 nm against reagent blank and calculate the contents by comparison.

Hydrochlorothiazide

Reagents

1. 1% w/v solution of n-(1-naphthyl)-ethylene diamine dihydrochloride in water.
2. 2 M hydrochloric acid.
3. Dimethyl sulphoxide.
4. 2% w/v solution of sulphamic acid in water.
5. 0.02 M sodium nitrite.
6. 2 M sodium acetate.

Standard solution

25 mg of a substance is suspended in 10 ml of sodium hydroxide solution and heated under reflux for 60 min, cool, add 80-100 ml of water and 20 ml of 2 M hydrochloric acid and dilute to 200 ml with water.

Sample solution

Extract the sample with 100 ml of acetone. 5 ml of acetone extract is evaporated and residue hydrolysed with 10 ml of sodium hydroxide and further proceeded as with standard solution.

Procedure

To 10 ml each of sample and standard solutions, add 1 ml of sodium nitrite solution and allow to stand for 10 min, then add 2 ml of sulphamic acid solution and after further 10 min, add 5 ml of dimethyl sulphoxide and 2 ml of 'NED' solution and make up the volume to 100 ml with sodium acetate solution and measure the absorption of both sample and standard solutions at 513 nm against reagent blank and calculate the contents by comparison.

Explanatory Note

The method is based on alkaline hydrolysis, acidification, diazotization and coupling with n-(1-naphthyl)-ethylene diamine. For detailed reaction mechanism, see Formulation No. 1 of this chapter.

Formulation 6

Metoprolol tartrate, Hydrochlorothiazide

ESTIMATION

METHOD 1

Reagents

1. Carbonate buffer solution, pH 11.0 : Mix 2.5 ml of 1 M sodium bicarbonate and 65 ml of sodium carbonate and dilute to 1000 ml with water.
2. Dichloromethane, saturated with water.
3. 1 M hydrochloric acid.
4. 1 M sodium hydroxide.

Metoprolol standard solution

4 mg/ml of metoprolol tartrate in dichloromethane.

Hydrochlorothiazide standard solution

Dissolve 100 mg of the substance in 2-3 ml of 1 M sodium hydroxide and dilute to 100 ml with buffer solution, pH 11.0.

Sample solution

Accurately weighed quantity of the powdered sample is suspended in 25 ml of buffer solution, add 25 ml of dichloromethane. Shake vigorously for 30 min, centrifuge to separate to layer. Aqueous phase (upper layer) is used for estimation of hydrochlorothiazide whereas organic phase is used for estimation of metoprolol.

Metoprolol tartrate

Dilute 5 ml of organic layer to 200 ml with dichloromethane and measure the absorbance of the solution at 277 nm.

Hydrochlorothiazide

Dilute 10 ml of aqueous phase to 50 ml with water and finally 5 ml is diluted to 50 ml with 0.1 M hydrochloric acid. Measure the absorbance at 272 nm.

Note

Treat 25 ml of each standard solution with buffer and dichloromethane and treat organic layer and aqueous layer as above.

METHOD 2

Metoprolol tartrate

Standard solution

100 mcg/ml of metoprolol tartrate in 0.1 M hydrochloric acid.

Sample solution

Extract accurately weighed quantity of the sample with 0.1 M hydrochloric acid by shaking for 30 min and filtering.

Procedure

To 10 ml each of sample and standard solutions, add 2 ml of 2.5 M sodium hydroxide and extract with 3 × 25 ml portions of chloroform, passing each extract from pre-rinsed glass wool, dilute to 100 ml with chloroform and measure the absorbance of both the solutions at 276 nm using chloroform as blank.

METHOD 3

Reagent

0.2% w/v solution of $FeCl_3$ in 0.05 M HCl.

Sample and standard solution

100 μg/ml in 0.05 M HCl.

Procedure

To 1 ml each of sample and standard solutions, add 2 ml of the reagent, keep aside for 5 min and measure at 380 nm.

Probable Reaction Mechanism

Fe(3) forms complex with the drug in acidic medium resulting in formation of coloured complex (λ_{max} 380 nm).

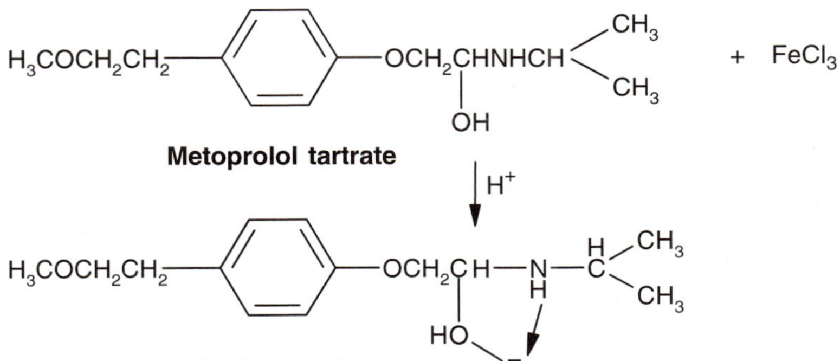

Ferric complex
(λ_{max} 380 nm)

Reference

Indian Drugs, **25(10)**, 424, 1988.

Metoprolol reacts with 2,4-dinitrofluorobenzene "Sanger's" reagent. In this reaction, secondary amino group present in the molecule is involved. The reaction proceeds with loss of HF. The reaction product is yellow in colour with λ_{max} 380 nm. The compound also reacts with chloranil in alkaline medium. Here the secondary amino group adds to the enone system of the reagent with loss of HCl. Both reactions are reproduced.

Probable Reaction Mechanism

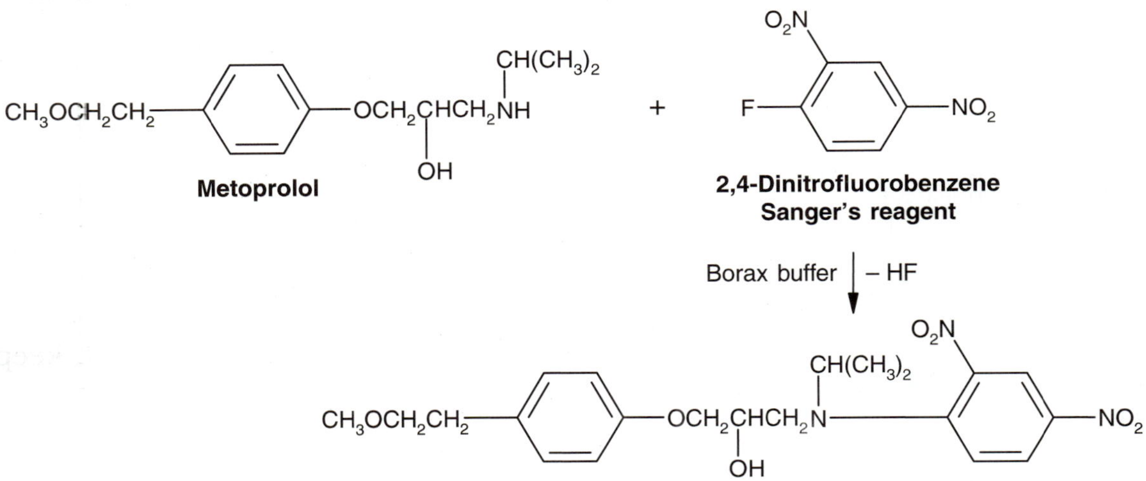

End reaction product
(λ_{max} 380 nm)

Reference

Indian Drugs, **24(5)**, 270, 1987.

Probable Reaction Mechanism

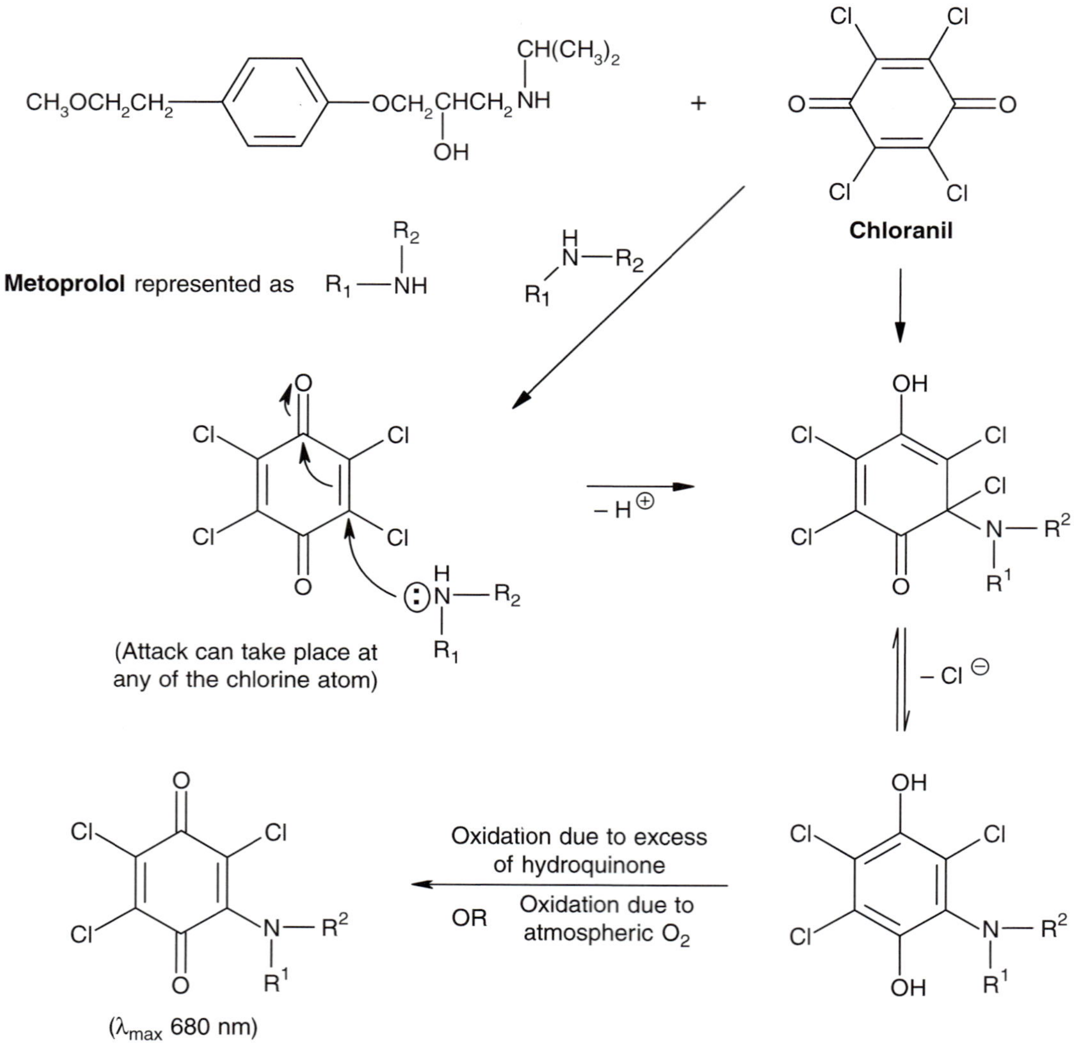

Reference

Indian Drugs, **24(7)**, 373, 1987.

Hydrochlorothiazide

Standard solution

50 mcg/ml of hydrochlorothiazide in methanol.

Sample solution

Accurately weighed quantity of the sample is suspended in 15 ml of water, add 60 ml of methanol and sonicate for 5 min and dilute to 100 ml with methanol. Further dilute 10 ml to 50 ml with menthol.

Concomitantly measure the absorption of both the solutions at about 316 nm using methanol as blank, and calculate the contents of hydrochlorothiazide by comparison.

Formulation 7

Frusemide, Amiloride hydrochloride

ESTIMATION

METHOD 1

Both frusemide and amiloride have iso-absorption point at 260 nm in acidic solution, whereas frusemide has no absorption at 395 nm. This property has been used for quantitative estimation of both the substances. The absorption values at iso-absorption point (260 nm) gave total concentration of both the substances, whereas at 315 nm the absorption is solely due to amiloride. Thus frusemide could be calculated by difference.

Standard solutions

1. 8 mg/ml of frusemide in 0.1 M hydrochloric acid.
2. 1 mg/ml of amiloride in 0.1 M hydrochloric acid.

Sample solution

Accurately weighed quantity of the powdered sample equivalent to 40 mg of frusemide was separately extracted with 50 ml of 0.1 M hydrochloric acid in ultrasonic bath and diluted to 100 ml with 0.1 M hydrochloric acid. Both sample and standard solutions were further diluted appropriately and absorbance measured at 260 nm and 395 nm, and results calculated by comparison. At 260 nm, total quantity of both the substances in the sample was obtained. The amount of amiloride present in the sample is calculated from absorption values at 395 nm and subtracted to get the quantity of frusemide.

The method obeyed Beer's law in the range of 5-30 mcg/ml for both the substances at 260 nm and 5-75 mg for amiloride at 395 nm. The method is suitable for dissolution studies as well.

METHOD 2

The method is based on the physical property of the components. Amiloride hydrochloride is soluble in water, whereas frusemide being insoluble could thus be separated by simple extraction with water.

Accurately weighed quantity of the sample equivalent to 4 mg of amiloride (AMD) was suspended in 20 ml of water, shaken for 5 min and filtered through G_3 sintered glass funnel. The filtrate was diluted to 50 ml with water. Further dilutions were done with water to get a final solution of 10 mcg/ml in respect of AMD.

The residue thus retained on the funnel was extracted with 0.1 M methanolic sodium hydroxide and further diluted to get a solution of 10 mcg/ml in respect of frusemide (FRS). Standard solution of both the substances were prepared in water (AMD) and in methanolic sodium hydroxide (FRS).

Absorbance of both sample and standard solutions were measured at 281 nm (AMD) and 274 nm (FRS) and results calculated by comparison.

METHOD 3

Frusemide

Accurately weighed quantity of the powdered sample is extracted with 0.1 M sodium hydroxide to get solution of 10 mcg/ml. The absorbance is measured without delay at 271 nm and the results are calculated taking 580 as value of A 1%, 1 cm at 271 nm.

Note

Frusemide may be dissolved in DMF and the carboxylic group present can be titrated with sodium hydroxide using bromothymol blue as indicator. Alternatively, on boiling with hydrochloric acid under reflux, hydrolysis takes place and an aniline derivative is produced which is diazotized and coupled with NED to give violet dye.

Probable Reaction Mechanism

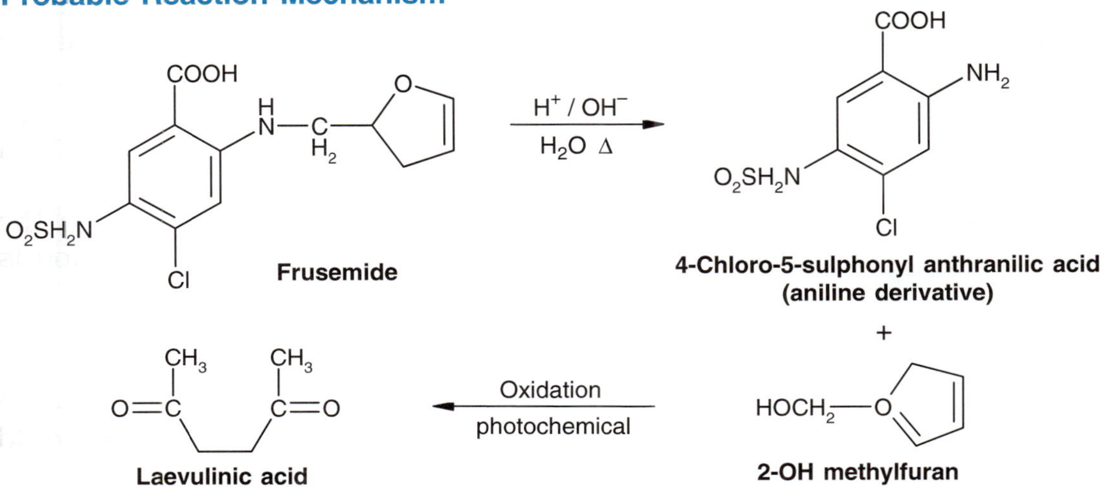

Note

Aniline derivative so formed on acid hydrolysis can be diazotized and coupled with 'NED' to give violet-red complex (λ_{max} 545 nm).

Reference

Pharmaceutical Chemistry (Vol. 2) by H.J. Roth, p. 447.

Alternatively, aniline derivative obtained above as a result of acid hydrolysis can be condensed with p-dimethylaminobenzaldehyde (PDAB) to form Schiff's base. Further, amino group of the sulphonamide moiety present in the molecule being non-substitute can directly condense with 'PDAB' to form Schiff's base.

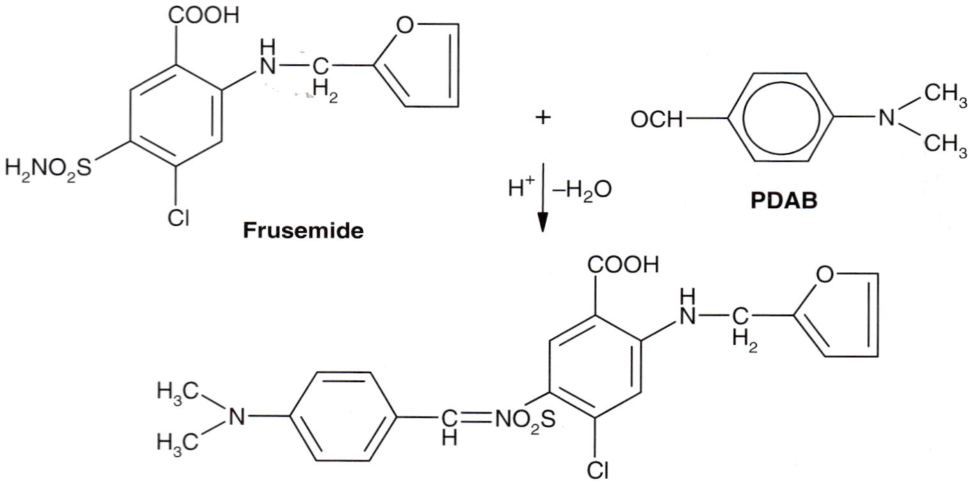

Schiff's base
(λ_{max} 484 nm)

Reference

P.T. Sudharashan, L.N. Subash & K.R. Dutt, *Indian Drugs*, **42(2)**, 113-115, 2005.

Furan part of the molecule couples with diazonium salt to yield azo dye (λ_{max} 540 nm).

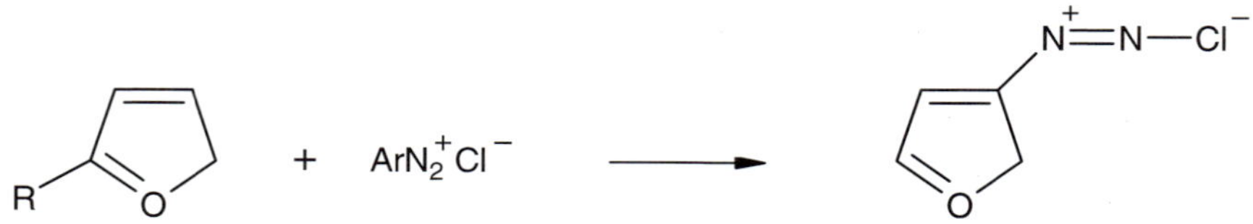

Azo dye
(λ_{max} 540 nm)

Reference

Pharmaceutical Organic Chemistry (Part 1) by Rama Nadenla, 2005.

Note

Frusemide having carboxylic group (COO^-) can be dissolved in DMF and titrated with sodium hydroxide using bromothymol blue as indicator.

Amiloride hydrochloride

To accurately weighed quantity of powdered sample equivalent to 10 mg of amiloride hydrochloride, add 10 ml of methanol and dilute to 100 ml with 0.1 N sodium hydroxide. Transfer 4 ml of the resulting solution to a 50 ml stoppered centrifuge tube, add 10 ml of methanol and 20 ml of tributyl orthophosphate (previously washed with water) and shake vigorously for 2 min and centrifuge for 5 min. Collect the upper layer and repeat the extraction with further 20 ml of tributyl orthophosphate (water-washed). Combine the extracts, add 2 ml of methanol and dilute to 50 ml with water-washed tributyl orthophosphate. Measure the absorbance of resulting solution at 363 nm against blank (24 ml of water-washed tributyl orthophosphate and 1 ml of methanol) and calculate the results taking 692 as value of A 1%, 1 cm at 363 nm.

Formulation 8

Spironolactone, Frusemide

ESTIMATION

METHOD 1

Accurately weighed quantity of powdered sample equivalent to 50 mg of spironolactone (SPT) was suspended in 15 mg of chloroform and filtered through G_3 sintered glass funnel. The filtrate was diluted to 50 ml with chloroform. Further dilutions were made to get concentration of 10 mcg/ml of SPT.

The residue retained on the funnel was extracted with 0.1 M methanolic sodium hydroxide and diluted to get concentration of 10 mcg/ml in respect of frusemide (FRS).

Extinction of both sample and standard solutions was measured at 244 nm for SPT and at 274 nm for FRS and results calculated by comparison.

Explanatory Note

SPT being freely soluble in chloroform whereas the residue left on sintered funnel pertains to FRS. For acceptable analytical results, the sample powder should be very fine and dry.

METHOD 2

Spironolactone

Reagent

1. Isonicotonic acid hydrazide (INH) reagent.

Standard solution

40 mcg/ml of spironolactone in methanol.

Sample solution

Extract appropriate quantity of powdered sample with methanol to get concentration of 40 mcg/ml.

Procedure

Evaporate 2 ml each of sample and standard solutions to dryness, add 5 ml of INH reagent. Close the tubes and heat for 60 min at 50°C. Cool and measure the absorbance of both the solutions at 405 nm against reagent blank and calculate the results by comparison.

Explanatory Note

The α-β unsaturated carbonyl group (C==O) at C-3 reacts with INH reagent to give yellow-coloured hydrazone derivative (λ_{max} 405 nm) which forms the basis for quantitative estimation.

Probable Reaction Mechanism

The reaction mechanism is based on Umberger reaction.

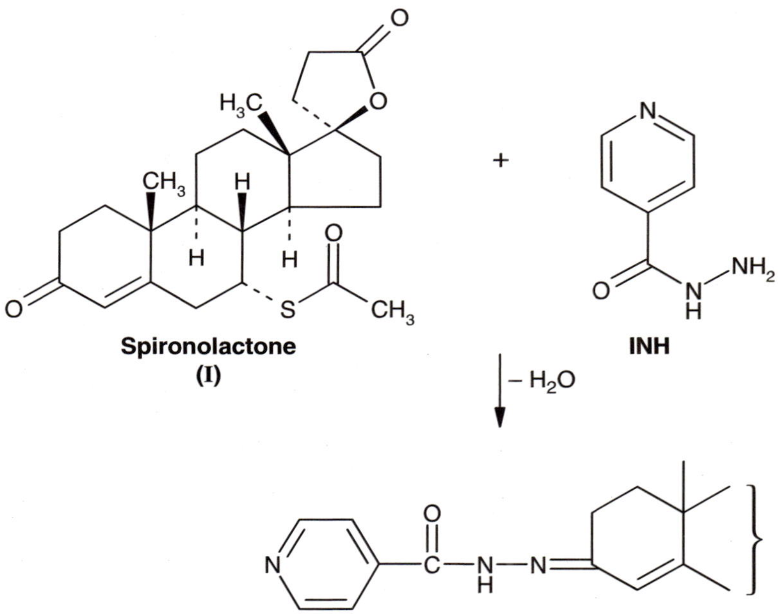

Hydrazone derivative
(λ_{max} 405 nm)

Reference

D.M. Shingbal & J.S. Prabhu Desai, *Indian Drugs*, **21(7)**, 306-307, 1984.

Spironolactone reacts with tetrazolium salt, the thiol group present in the molecule reduces tetrazolium salt in alkaline medium (tetramethylammonium hydroxide) to form coloured formazone.

Probable Reaction Mechanism

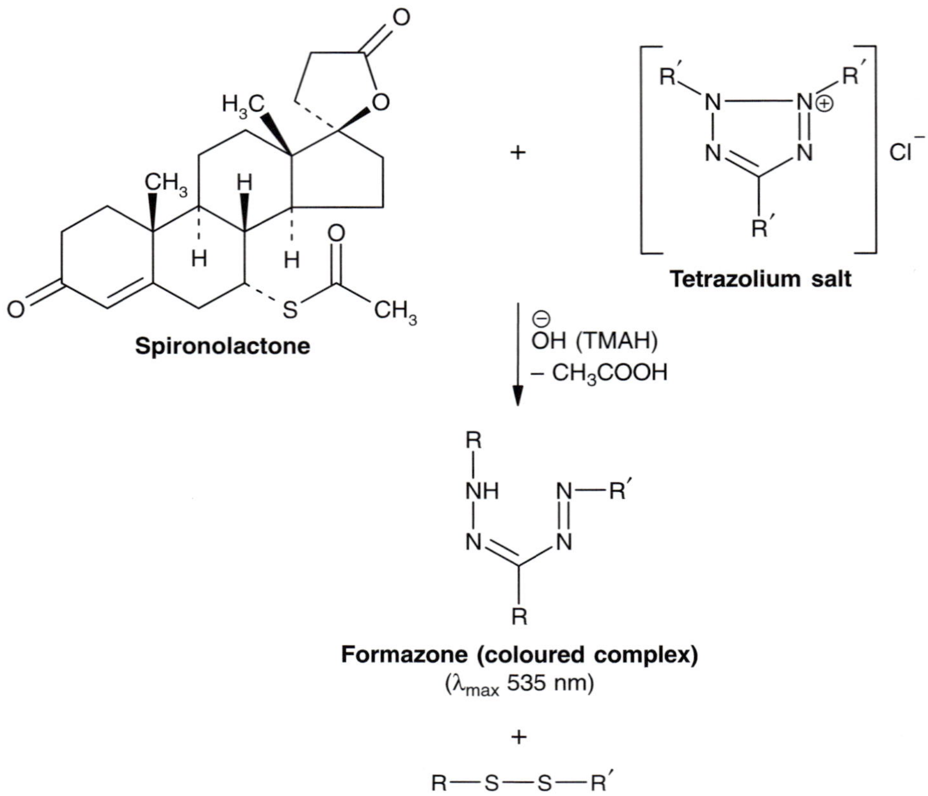

where R =

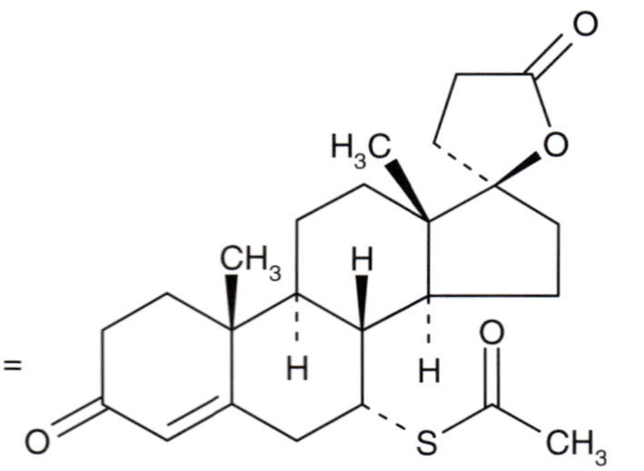

Reference

R.G. Sharma et al., *Eastern Pharmacist*, p. 121, 1992.

Alternate reaction mechanism is explained below:

The compound reduces triphenyltetrazolium compound in alkaline medium to give coloured formazone (λ_{max} 480 nm).

Probable Reaction Mechanism

The lactone ring of the drug opens up under alkaline conditions, i.e., under tetramethylammonium hydroxide employed resulting in the formation of the following species.

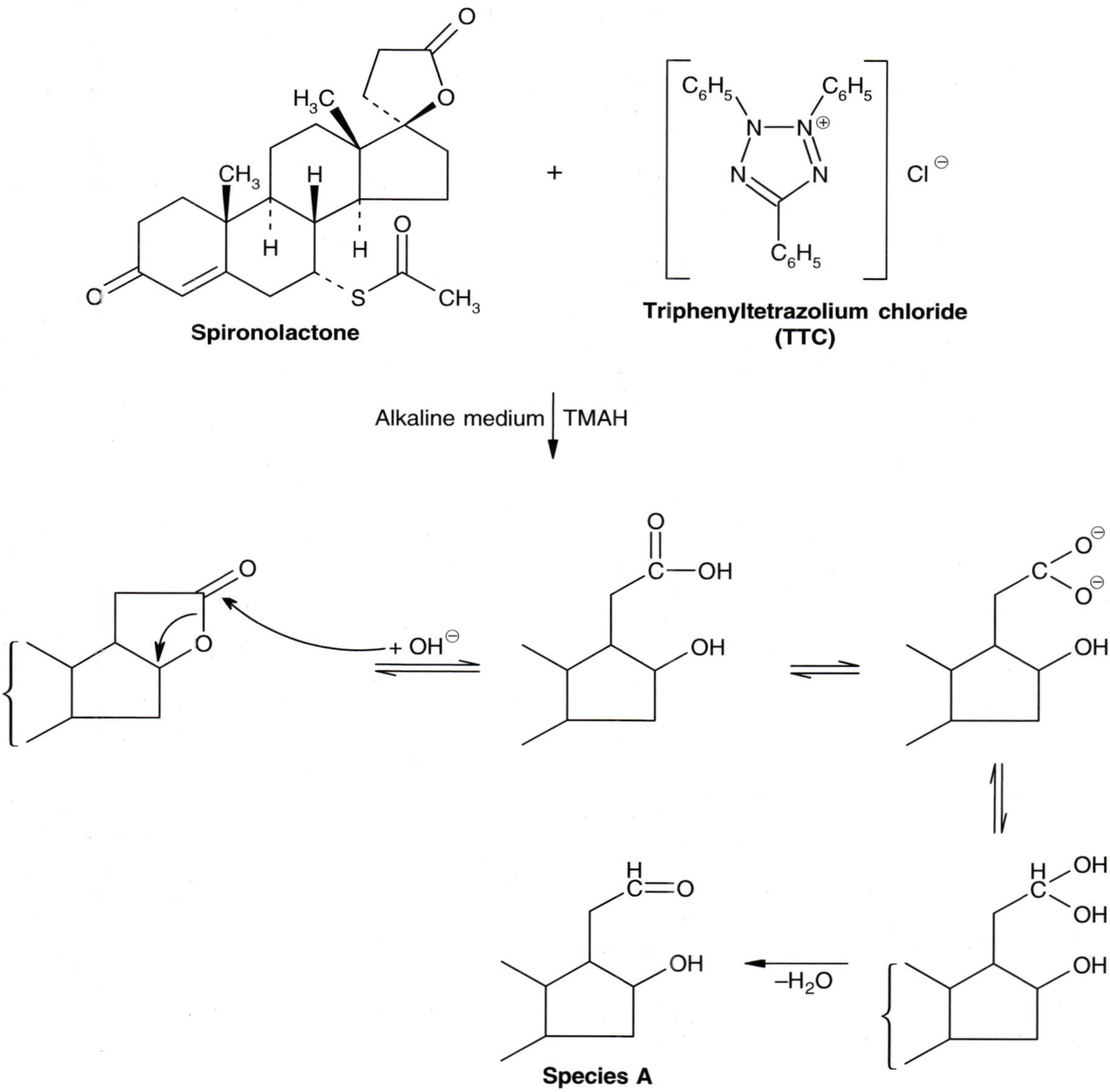

The alcoholic-OH group of species A is then oxidized by triphenyltetrazolium chloride in alkaline solution, where the reagent itself undergoes reductive opening of the heterocyclic ring to give the red-coloured triphenyl formazone.

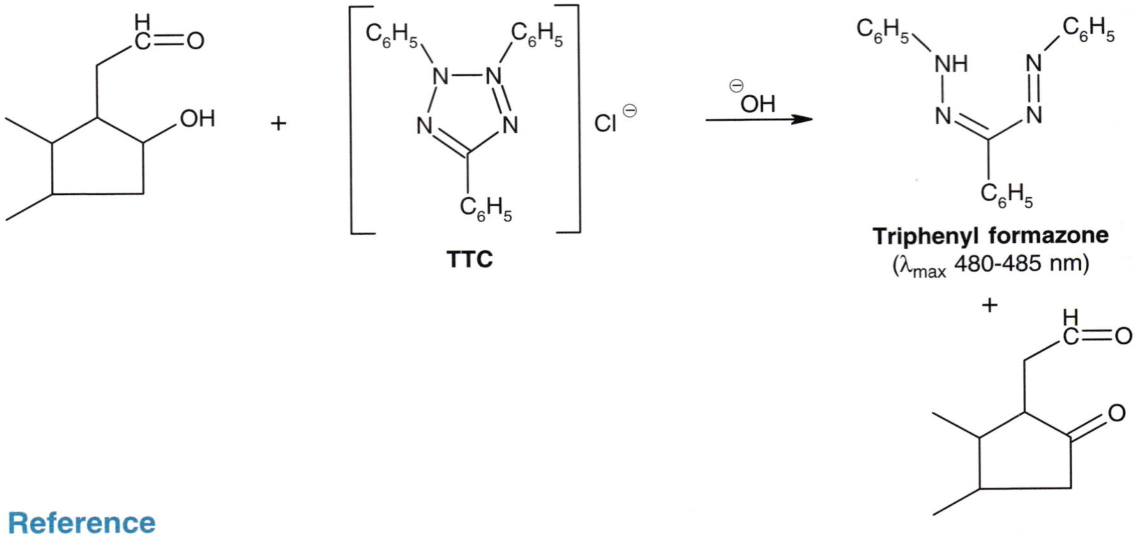

Reference

1. Pharmaceutical Chemistry (Vol. 2) by H.J. Roth, p. 470.
2. Vinay Nevrekar, *Indian Drugs*, **21(8)**, 347-350, 1984.

Spironolactone reacts with dinitrobenzene in the presence of alkali to give Meisenheimer salt.

Alkali removes the acidic proton next to carbonyl group in ring A of the molecule resulting in the formation of carbonium ion. Carbonium ion so formed interacts with dinitrobenzene resulting in the formation of a yellow-coloured complex.

Probable Reaction Mechanism

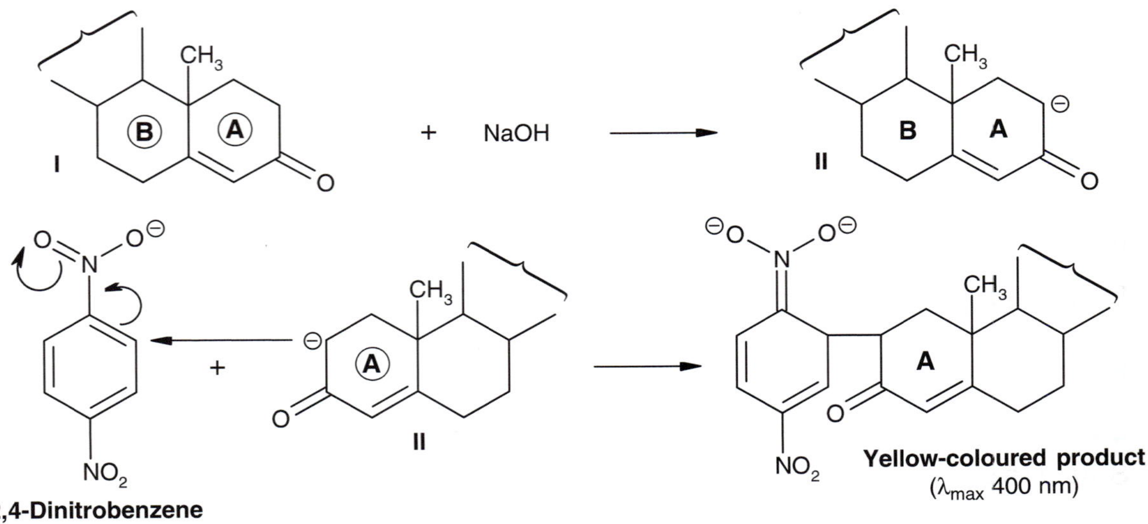

Reference

D.M. Shingbal & V.R. Rao, *Indian Drugs*, **23(4)**, 232, 1986.

Spironolactone (I) reacts with thiosemicarbazide/semicarbazide resulting in formation of thiosemicarbazone or semicarbazide (λ_{max} 430 nm). The reaction of thiosemicarbazide or semicarbazide is at carbonyl function in ring (A) as according to Woodward Fieser's law, product formed should have extended conjugation, the product formed due to reaction in ring E will not have extended conjugation, hence no conjugation at 430 nm.

Probable Reaction Mechanism

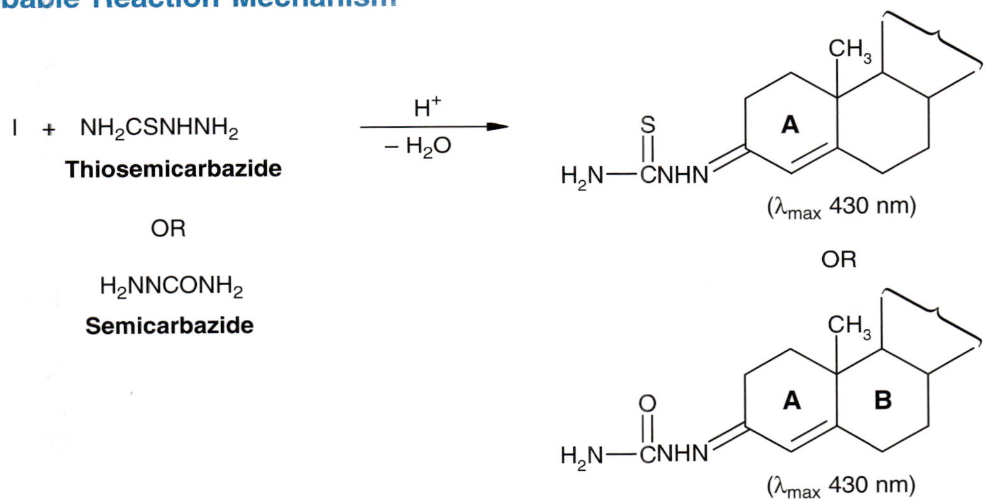

Reaction product with ring (E)

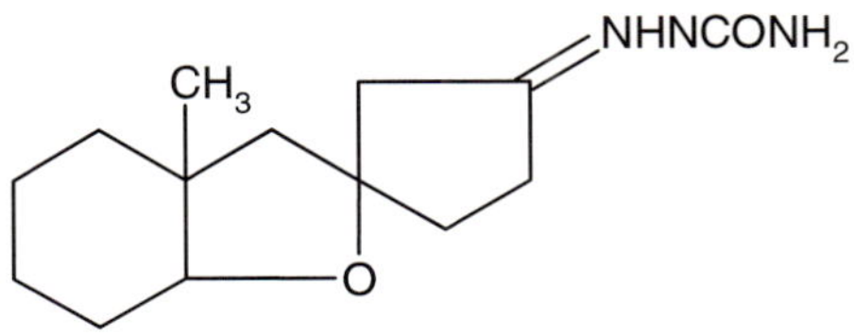

No extended conjugation, hence no absorption at 430 nm

Reference

D.M. Shingbal et al., *Indian Drugs*, **24(9)**, 450-451, 1987.

Frusemide

Standard solution

8 mcg/ml of frusemide in 0.1 M sodium hydroxide.

Sample solution

Accurately weighed quantity of the sample equivalent to 20 mg of the sample is extracted with three 10 portions of ethyl acetate. The combined ethyl acetate extract is shaken with five 20 ml portions of 0.1 M sodium hydroxide and finally diluted to 250 ml. 5 ml of the resultant solution is diluted to 50 ml with 0.1 M sodium hydroxide (8 mcg/ml).

Measure the absorbance of both sample and standard solutions at 272 nm using 0.1 N sodium hydroxide as blank and calculate the results by comparison.

Explanatory Note

Ethyl acetate extract containing both SPT and FRS is shaken with sodium hydroxide to get FRS in aqueous alkaline layer (λ_{max} 272 nm).

Formulation 9

Spironolactone, Hydroflumethazide

ESTIMATION

METHOD 1

Spironolactone

Follow the method 3 described in formulation 8 of this chapter.

Hydroflumethazide

The aqueous extract obtained during estimation of spironolactone is appropriately diluted and extinction measured at 274 nm. For details see method 3 in formulation 8 of this chapter under frusemide.

METHOD 2

Standard solution

10 mcg/ml each of spironolactone (SPN) and hydroflumethazide (HFT) in methanol.

Sample solution

Accurately weighed quantity of the powdered sample was extracted with methanol by vigorously shaking for 10 min and diluting appropriately to get final concentration of 10 mcg/ml. Absorption of the sample and standard solutions was measured at 238 nm, being the absorption maximum of SPN and at 273, the absorption maximum of HFT. The results were calculated by comparing with the standard. Spectral measurements at respective maxima did not show any interference. The method is suitable for routine quality control.

METHOD 3

Reagents

1. 0.2% w/v solution of hematoxylin.
2. 0.4% w/v solution of chloramine T (CAT).
3. Phosphate buffer pH 7.0.

Standard and standard solutions

20 µg/ml in methanol.

Procedure

To 1 ml of the reagent (1) add 1 ml of reagent (2) and 15 ml of buffer. Keep aside for 30 min and then add 1 ml each of sample/standard solution. Heat on water bath (70°C) for 15 min, dilute to 25 ml with water and measure the absorbance of sample and standard at 550 nm against reagent blank.

Probable Reaction Mechanism

First hematoxylin is oxidized by 'CAT' reagent. The drug is hydrolysed to disulphonamide and then sulphonamide reacts with oxidized hematoxylin to form the resulting product.

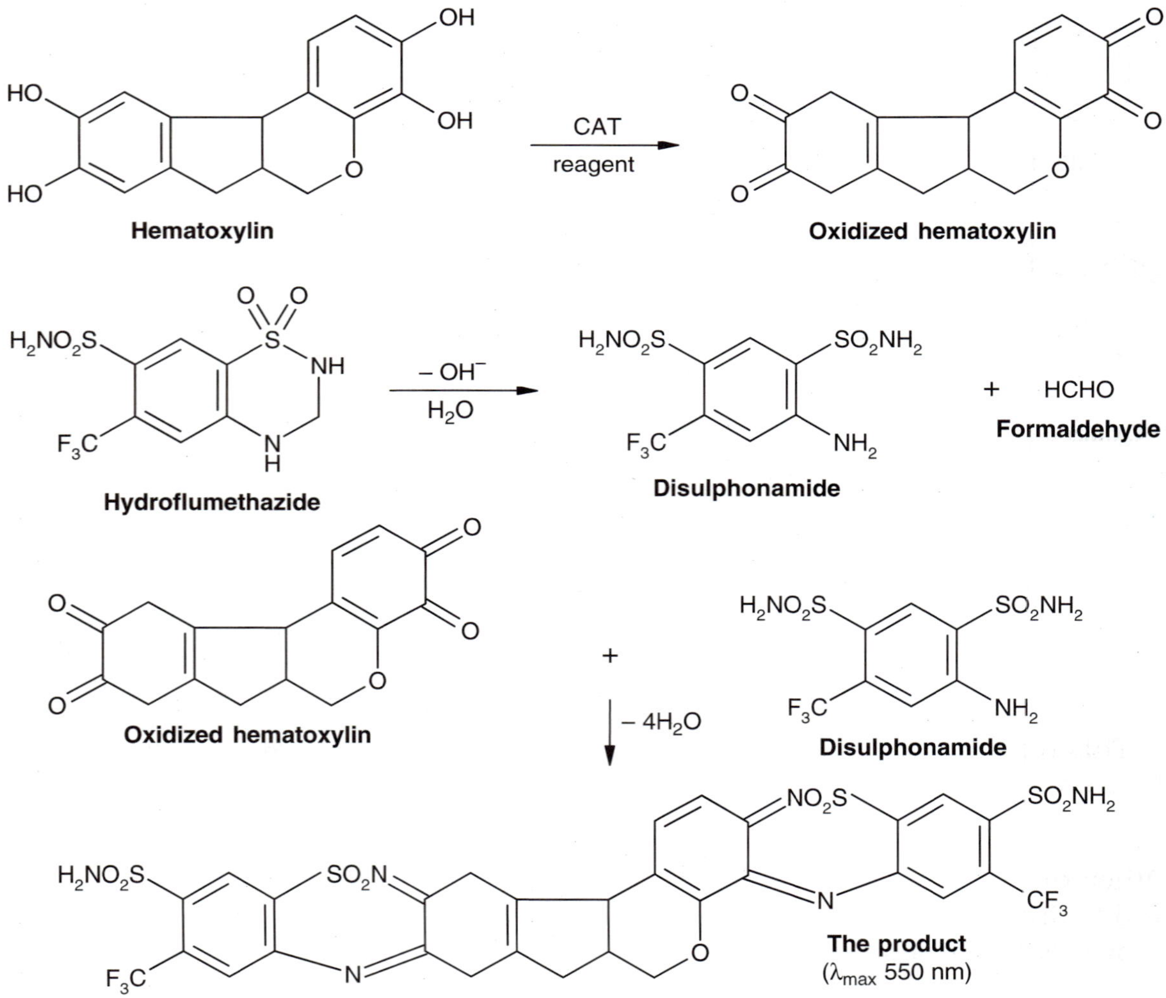

Reference

Indian Drugs, **26(6)**, 304, March 1989.

METHOD 4

The hydrolysed product (disulphonamide) is allowed to react with MBTH reagent (3-methyl benzthiazolin-2-one-hydrazone in the presence of oxidizing agent Ce (IV), Fe (III) or IO_4.

Probable Reaction Mechanism

Initially 'MBTH' reagent loses 2 electrons and a proton and then reacts with disulphonamide to give desired coloured product. Since para position to the amine group in sulphonamide is blocked, the coupling takes place at ortho position as shown.

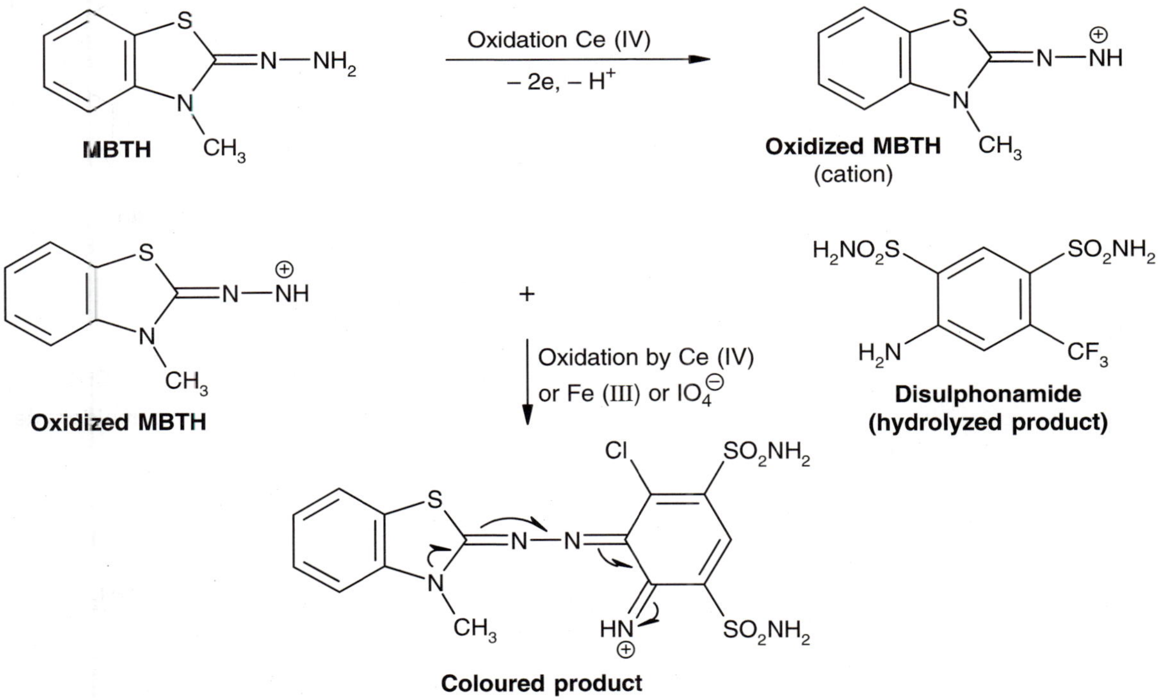

This resonance is possible due to the availability of lone pair of electrons on 'N' atom.

Note

Other diuretics which couple with 'MBTH' reagent are amiloride, frusemide and hydrochlorothiazide. General formula for coloured products obtained with above reagents is:

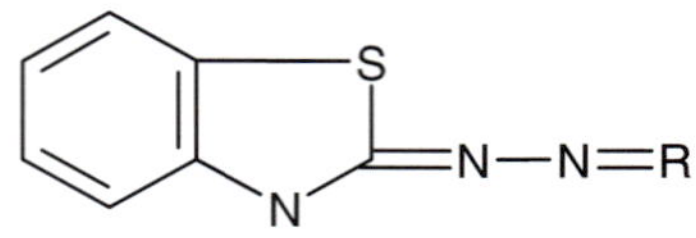

For details, see below

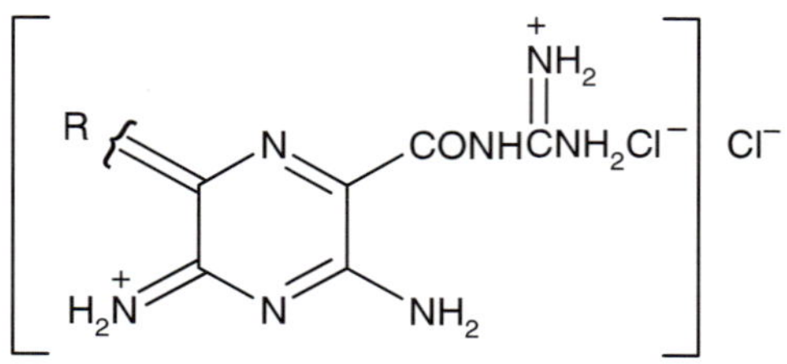

Amiloride

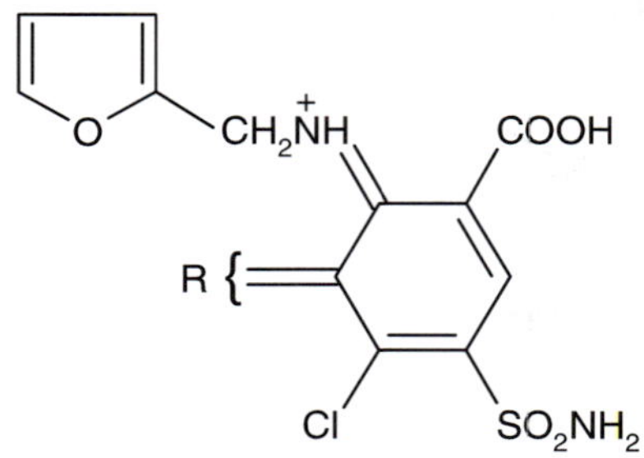

Frusemide

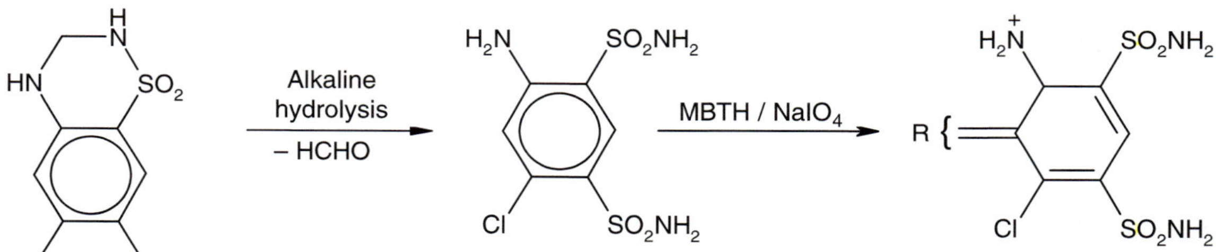

Hydrochlorothiazide Sulphonamide Coloured product

Reference

C.S.P. Sastry, N.V. Prasad, B.S. Sastry & E. Venkata Rao, *Analyst*, **113(2)**, 255-258, 1988.

Belal et al. (1988) have described analytical method based on bromometric titration using N-bromosuccinimide (NBS) and 1,3-dibromo-5,5-dimethylhydantoin (DBH) as analytical reagents.

To sample solution in 0.5 M NaOH, known amount of 0.01 M 'NBS' or 0.005 M DBH reagents are added; then add 20 ml of 10% HCl, shake, after specific time add 10 ml of KI (10%) and titrate the liberated iodine with 0.02 M sodium thiosulphate using starch as indicator.

Probable Reaction Mechanism

In benzothiadiazine derivatives in which thiazide ring is saturated such as hydrochlorothiazide, hydroflumethiazide, methyclothiazide. In this method, hydrogen atom at position-4 and that at position-5 both are replaced by bromine. The hydrogen at position-4 is moderately acidic and we get quite stable N-bromo derivative. The hydrogen at position-5 on the other hand is activated towards electrophilic substitution owing to presence of secondary amino group at position-4, so we get 2 bromo derivatives.

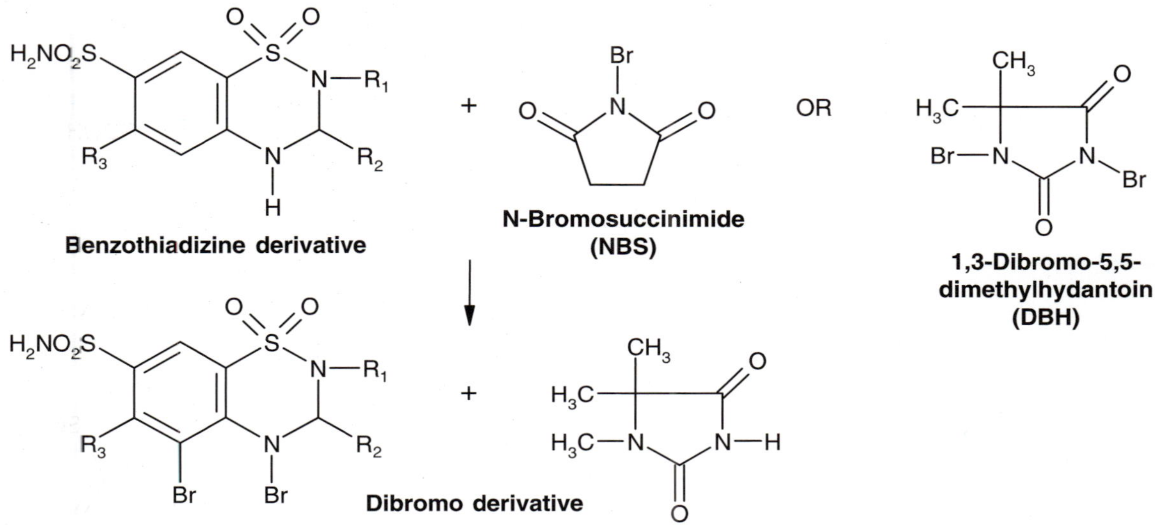

However, benzthiazide shall consume extra volume of the reagent. This is attributed to the reaction of the reagent with thioether group present in the molecule forming corresponding sulphone.

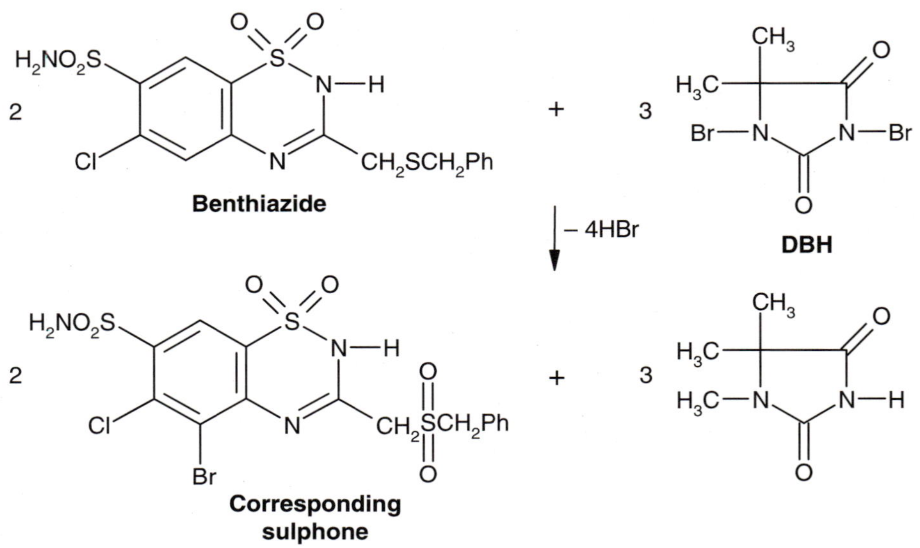

Reference

F. Belal, F. Ibrahim & Amina El-Brashy, *Analyst*, **113(4)**, 637-639, 1988.

Formulation 10

Enalapril maleate, Amlodipine besylate

ESTIMATION

Amlodipine besylate

Reagents

1. 0.1 M sodium hydroxide in methanol.
2. Dimethyl formamide (DMF).

Standard solution

50 mcg/ml of amlodipine besylate in DMF.

Sample solution

Extract appropriate quantity of powdered sample with DMF to get concentration of 50 mcg/ml.

Procedure

To 2 ml each of sample and standard solutions, add 0.2 ml of sodium hydroxide solution and dilute to 10 ml with DMF and measure the absorption of orange chromogen at 450 nm against reagent blank. Calculate the contents of amlodipine by comparison.

Note

For reaction mechanism, see Formulation No. 11.

Enalapril maleate and Amlodipine besylate

Both the compounds were first separated by preparative thin layer chromatography and then subjected to colour development.

Reagents

1. Phthalate buffer, pH 3.1.
2. 1% w/v solution of bromocresol green in buffer, pH 3.1.

Standard solution

1 mg/ml of amlodipine besylate and enalapril maleate prepared separately in methanol.

Sample solution

Accurately weighed quantity of the sample was extracted with methanol to get solution of 1 mg/ml. The solution was centrifuged and clear supernatant used for chromatographic separation.

Stationary phase: TLC pre-coated plates, silica gel $60F_{254}$.
Mobile phase: Chloroform-methanol-acetic acid (8.5 + 1.5 + 0.1, v/v).
Sample volume: 200 μl.
Chamber saturation: 30 min.
Development distance: 70 mm.

Both sample and standard were simultaneously subjected to thin layer chromatography on the same plate. The spots were located under UV and area corresponding to amlodipine was scraped and collected in separate centrifuge tubes each containing 10 ml of methanol, sonicated for 5 min for complete extraction and centrifuged. Blank prepared by scraping silica gel from an equivalent area from upper part of the TLC plate and extracting with 10 ml of methanol.

Amlodipine besylate

Measure the absorption both sample and standard solutions at 237 nm against blank and calculate the results by comparison. Or follow the colour development with methanolic potassium hydroxide as described above.

Enalapril maleate

The spot corresponding to enalapril was scraped and collected in a centrifuge containing 10 ml of buffer, pH 3.1. Shake well and centrifuge. To the entire supernatant, add 1 ml of dye and extract the yellow chromogen with 10 ml of chloroform. Centrifuge the chloroform layer and measure the absorption of both sample and standard at 410 nm against blank prepared by scraping silica gel from equivalent area of the plate and suspending in buffer, followed by addition of dye and extraction.

Note

The method is based on formation of coloured ion-pair complex which is soluble in chloroform.

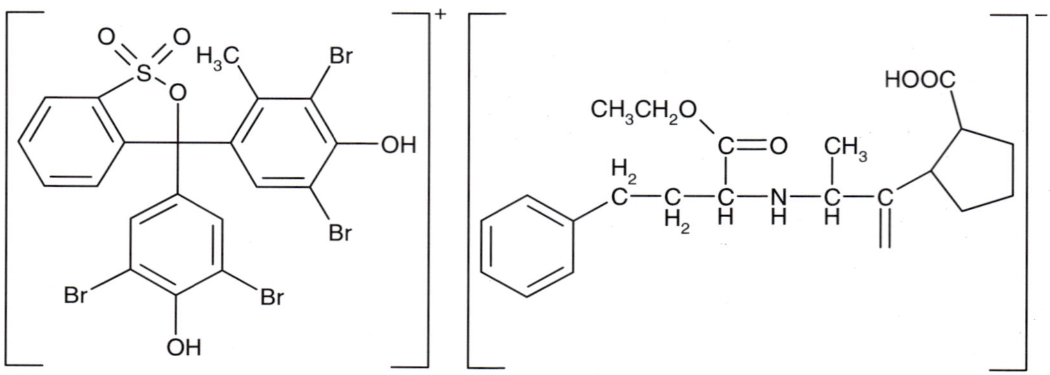

Bromocresol green

Enalapril

Drug-dye ion-pair complex
(λ_{max} 410 nm)

A spectrophotometric method was reported by Razak et al. (2003) based on reaction with Sanger's reagent.

Reagents

1. 0.02 M borate buffer, pH 9.0.
2. 0.2% w/v solution of 2,4-dinitrofluorobenzene (DNFB) in methanol, to be prepared fresh.
3. Silver oxide.

Standard solution

Treat 20 mg of pure substance as under sample.

Sample solution

Powdered sample equivalent to 20 mg of the substance suspended in 50 ml of methanol, add 20 mg of silver oxide, shake for 3 min, dilute to 100 ml with methanol, filter and use the filtrate for assay.

Procedure

To 1 ml each of sample and standard solutions, add 0.2 ml of borate buffer pH 9.0, followed by 2.5 ml of 'DNFB' reagent, place in water-bath for 25 min, cool, dilute to 10 ml with methanol and measure the absorption of the resulting solution at 356 nm against reagent blank.

Probable Reaction Mechanism

To liberate enalapril base, traditional method (alkalinization with sodium hydroxide followed by extraction with organic solvent) was not suitable as the drug contains carboxylic (COOH) group which will form water-soluble alkali salt, hence not extractable with chloroform. Silver oxide (Ag_2O) was used to provide required alkalinity to liberate enalapril base and excess unused Ag_2O removed by filtration.

In borate buffer pH 9.0 nucleophilic aromatic substitution reaction between 'DNFB' and the drug (base) takes place. The secondary amino group present in the molecule provides sufficient basicity to attack 'DNFB'.

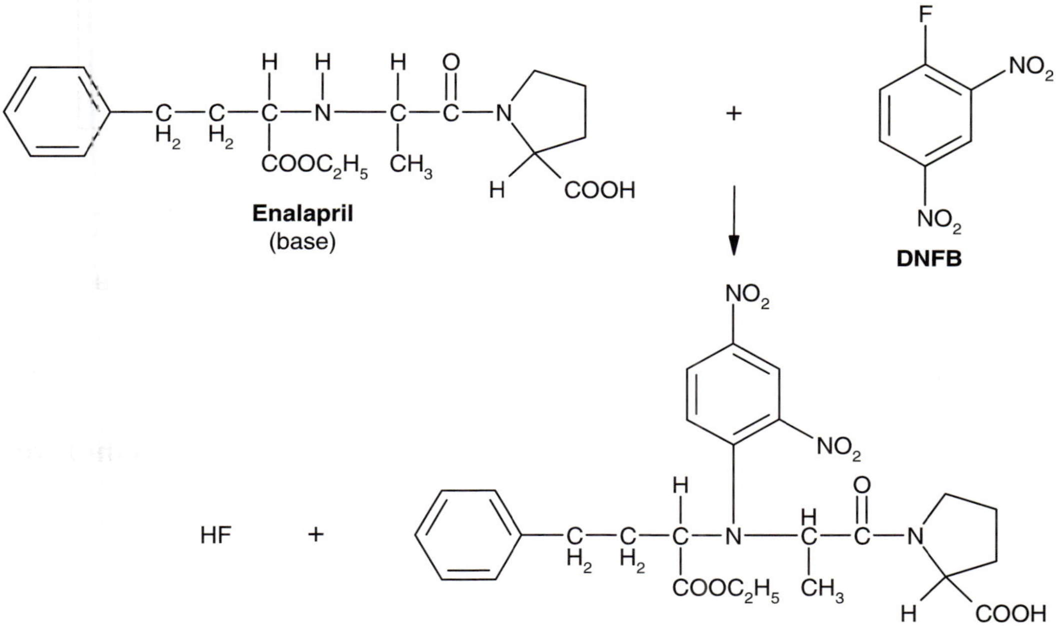

Complex
(λ_{max} 356 nm)

Alternatively, when solution of 'DNFB' in $DMSO_4$ (a dipolar aprotic solvent) is used, reaction occurs simultaneously at room temperature resulting in the formation of Meisenheimer complex, as explained below.

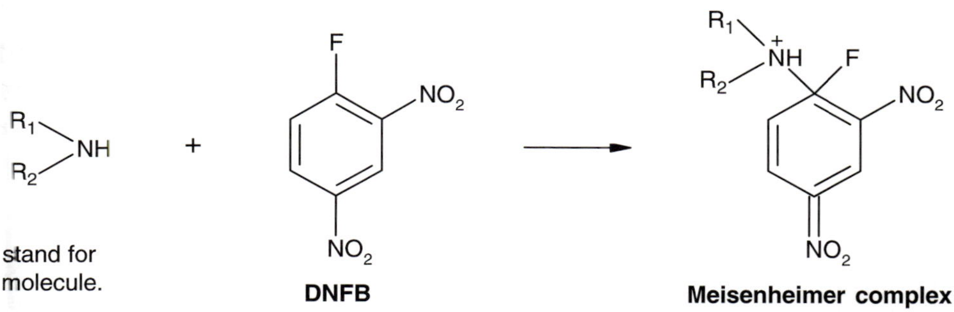

R_1 and R_2 stand for rest of the molecule.

Meisenheimer complex
(λ_{max} 420 nm)

Note

1. Meisenheimer complex stable for 90 min.
2. For details refer to methods described for norfloxacin under chapter on alimentary system.

Amlodipine

Amlodipine, a basic compound, is reported to form ion-pair complex with methyl orange, an acidic dye in acid phthalate buffer pH 4.0. The hydro-alcoholic solutions of the sample/standard were complexed with the dye and the ion-pair complex thus formed extracted into chloroform and absorbance of the yellow-coloured complex measured at 417 nm.

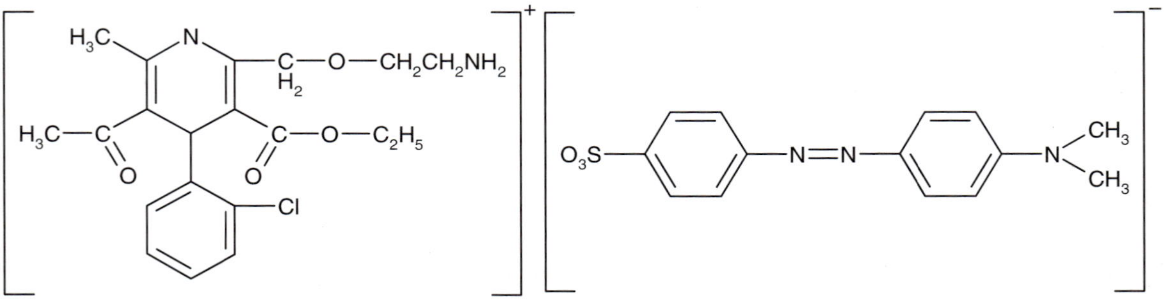

Amlodipine **Methyl orange**

Drug-dye ion-pair complex
(λ_{max} 417 nm)

Reference

Kashmira Gohil, Priti Trivedi and K.I. Molvi. *Ind. J. Pharm. Sci.*, **67(3)**, 376-378, 2005.

A spectrophotometric method has been described by F. Almani et al. (2010) using 2-hydroxy naphthaldehyde as derivatizing reagent.

Reagents

1. 1 M sodium acetate buffer, pH 5.0.
2. 2% w/v solution of 2-OH naphthaldehyde (HN) in alcohol.

Sample and standard solutions

100 µg/ml in alcohol.

Procedure

To 1 ml each of sample and standard solutions, add 1.5 ml of 'HN' reagent and 0.5 ml of acetate buffer, boil in water-bath at 95°C for 15 min, cool, dilute to 5 ml with alcohol and measure the absorbance of both sample and standard solutions at 416 nm against reagent blank and calculate the results.

Probable Reaction Mechanism

The compound forms an imine with the reagent as shown below.

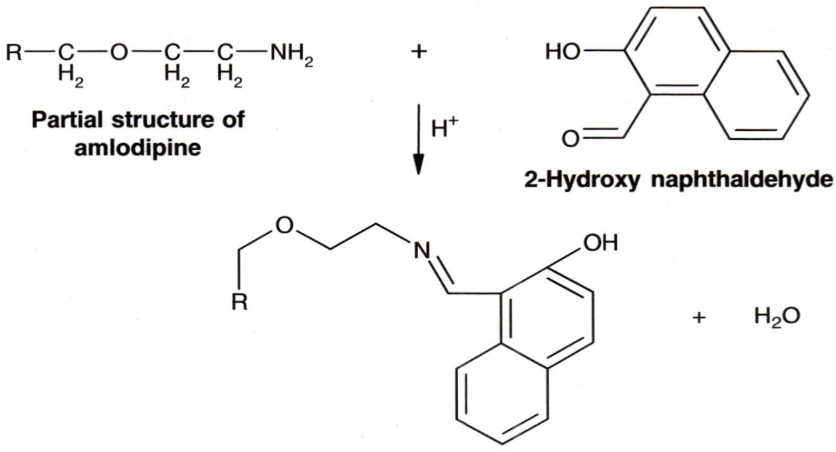

Amlodipine - HN complex, an imine
(λ_{max} 416 nm)

Reference

F. Almani et al. *Asian J. Chem.*, **22(2)**, 1205-1213, 2010.

Formulation 11

Amlodipine besylate, Atenolol

ESTIMATION

Atenolol

Standard solution

100 mcg/ml of atenolol in 0.1 M hydrochloric acid.

Sample solution

Accurately weighed quantity of the sample equivalent to 10 mg of the substance was extracted with 0.1 M hydrochloric acid to get a solution of 100 mcg/ml, centrifuged and supernatant used for estimation.

Measure the absorbance of both sample and standard solutions at maximum at about 276 nm and calculate the results by comparison.

Note

Amlodipine did not interfere.

Amlodipine besylate

Reagent

0.1 M sodium hydroxide in methanol.

Standard solution

50 mcg/ml of amlodipine besylate in DMF.

Sample solution

Accurately weighed quantity of the sample equivalent to 50 mg of the substance extracted with DMF and diluted suitably to produce a solution of 50 mcg/ml.

Procedure

To 2 ml each of sample and standard solutions, add 0.2 ml of sodium hydroxide solution and make up to 10 ml with DMF. Measure the absorption of both sample and standard solutions at 450 nm against reagent blank and calculate the results by comparison. The chromogen is stable for 30 min. The method obeys Beer's law in the range of 25-250 mcg/ml.

In alkaline medium, the compound is hydrolysed to give an orange-coloured product (λ_{max} 450 nm).

Probable Reaction Mechanism

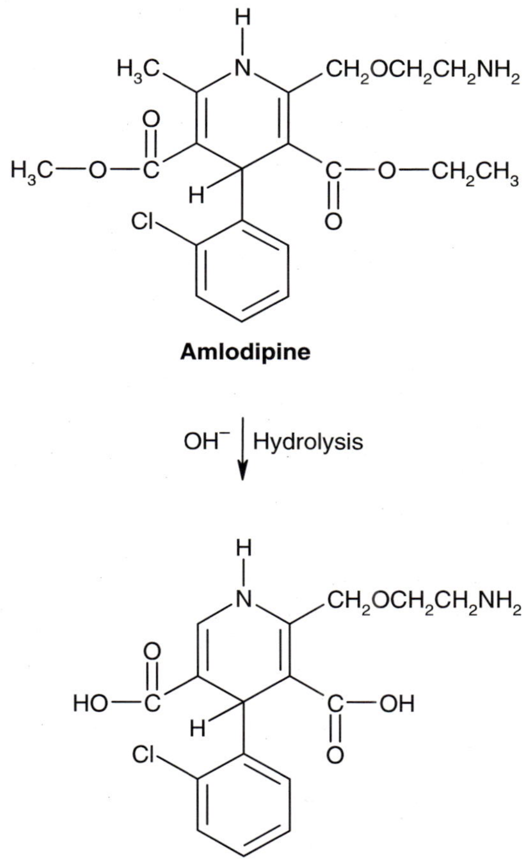

Orange-coloured product
(λ_{max} 450 nm)

METHOD 2

This method is applicable for simultaneous estimation of both the compounds.

Standard solutions

1. Atenolol – 200 μg/ml in methanol.
2. Amlodipine – 20 μg/ml in methanol.

Sample solution

Powdered sample equivalent to 100 mg of atenolol or 10 mg of amlodipine suspended in 70 ml of methanol, sonicate to dissolve, dilute to 100 ml with methanol. Filter and dilute the filtrate appropriately with methanol to get 100 μg/ml (atenolol) and 20 μg/ml (amlodipine).

Procedure

Measure the absorbance of the sample and standard at 276 nm and 361 nm, being λ_{max} of atenolol and amlodipine respectively.

Note

Since there is no mutual interfere at respective maxima, hence no prior separation of individual ingredient required.

Reference

Sukhdev Singh & Ravi Jain. *Indian Drugs*, **34(11)**, 678-679, 1992.

METHOD 3

Reagent

0.2% solution of ascorbic acid (AA): Dissolve 100 mg of AA in 0.5 ml of water and dilute to 50 ml with DMF.

Standard solution

100 μg/ml in DMF.

Sample solution

The sample extracted with DMF, filtered through Whatman filter paper No. 42 and diluted appropriately to get 100 μg/ml.

Procedure

To 1 ml each of sample/standard solutions taken in boiling test tubes add 2.5 ml of AA solution, make up to 5 ml with DMF. Place in water bath (100°C) for 25 min, cool, transfer to 10 ml volumetric flask and dilute to volume with DMF and measure the absorbance at 530 nm. The colour is stable up to 4 hours.

Explanatory Note

On heating, "AA" is converted to dehydroascorbic acid. The carbonyl group then reacts with NH_2 group of amlodipine to form purple-red coloured imino derivative (λ_{max} 530 nm).

Probable Reaction Mechanism

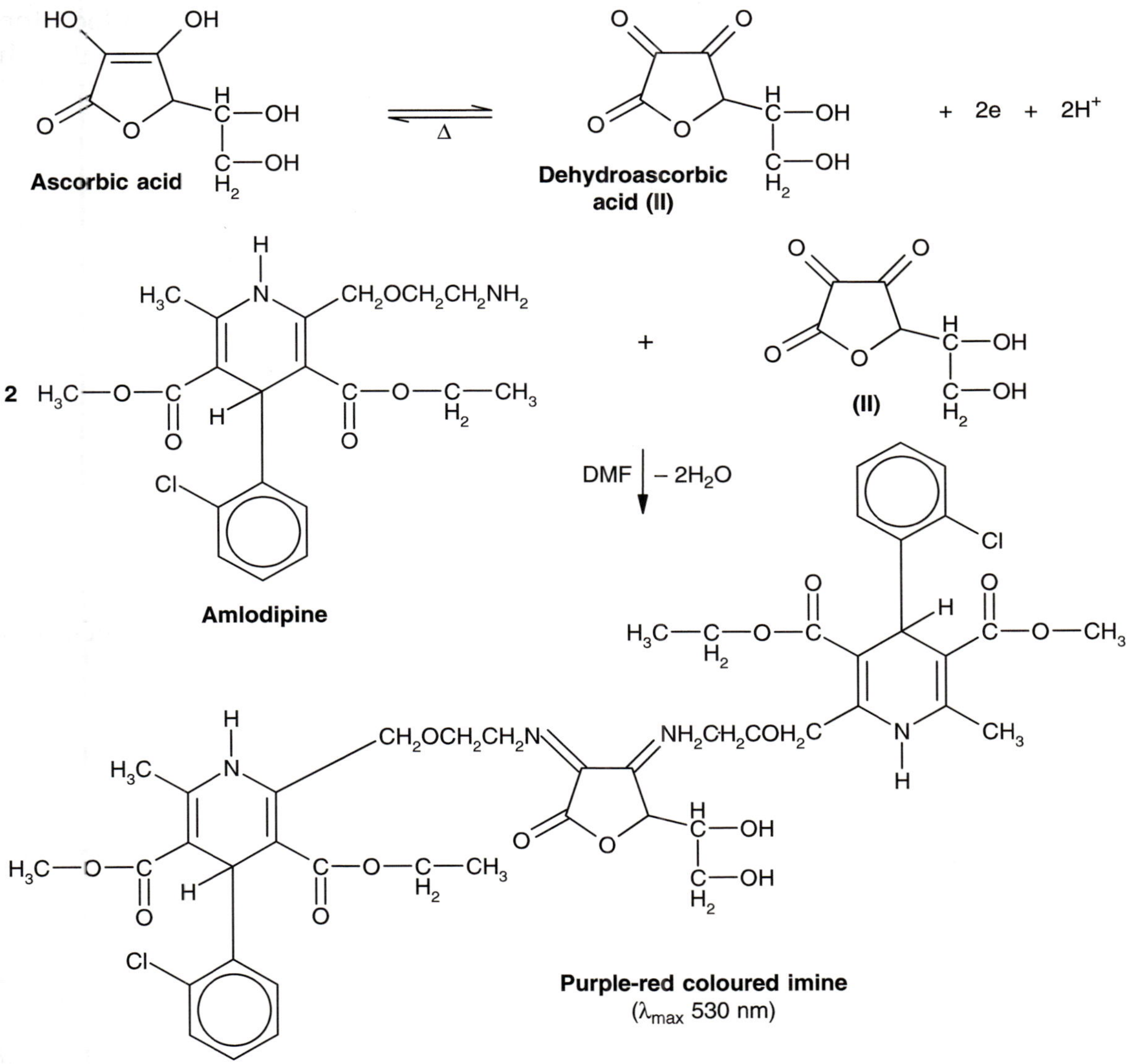

METHOD 4

Reagents

1. 0.5 M sodium carbonate.
2. 0.05% 2,3-dichloro-5,6-dicyano-1,4-benzoquinone in acetonitrile (DDQ) or chloranil.

Standard solution

500 μg/ml (base) in acetonitrile.

Sample solution

The sample was extracted with chloroform and then converted to base as per procedure below.

Conversion of Amlodipine besylate → base (amlodipine)

Take 50 mg of (AB) in chloroform, add sodium carbonate solution, shake, collect organic layer, evaporate, take up the residue in acetonitrile.

Procedure

To 0.5 ml of sample/standard solutions add 1 ml of DDQ reagent to each and dilute to 5 ml with acetonitrile and measure the absorbance at 580 nm. The colour is stable up to 25 min.

Explanatory Note

This is simply interaction between electron donor and acceptor. Amlodipine (base) acts as n donor whereas DDQ is n acceptor, so it readily forms coloured charge transfer complex with absorption maxima at 580 nm.

Probable Reaction Mechanism

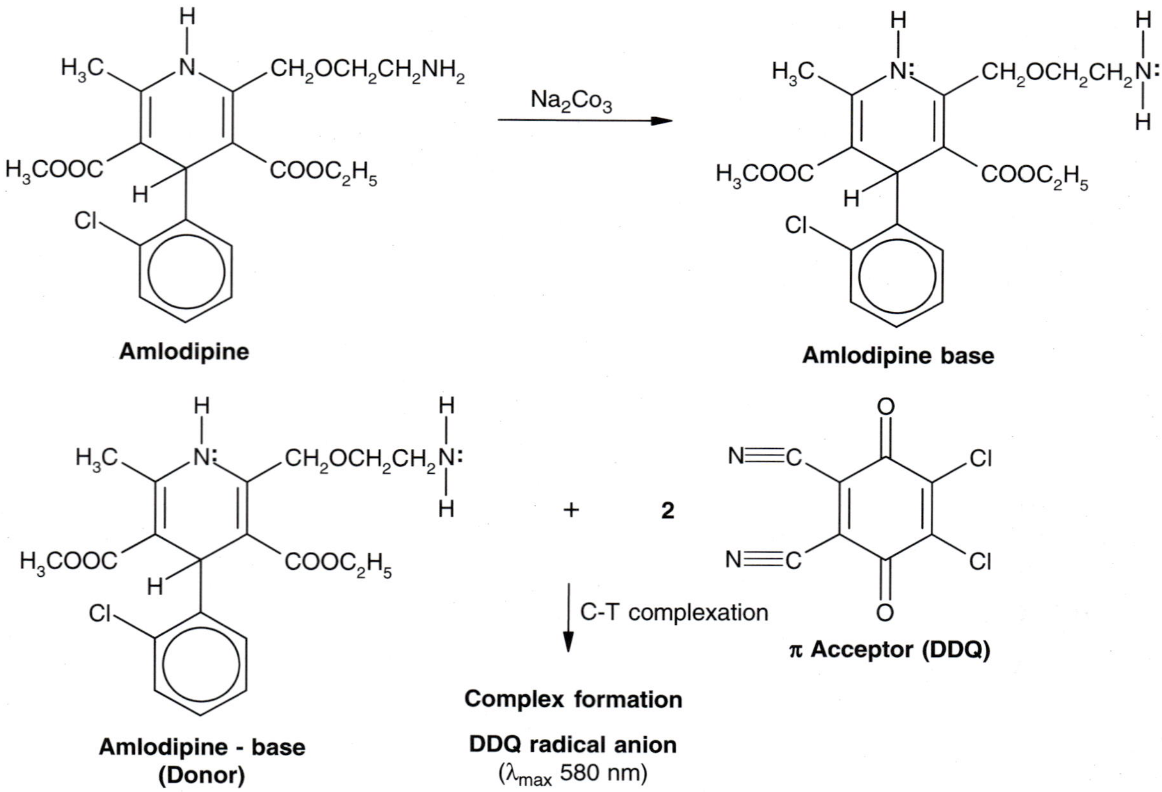

Note

Polar solvent such as acetonitrile promotes complete transfer of charge from donor (D) to π acceptor (A) such as DDQ resulting in the formation of DDQ radical anion as a predominant chromogen.

$$D + A \longrightarrow \underset{\textbf{DA complex}}{[\ddot{D}\text{-}A]} \xrightarrow{\text{Polar solvent}} \underset{\substack{\textbf{Radical}\\ \textbf{anion}\\ \textbf{(coloured)}}}{D^{+} + A^{-}}$$

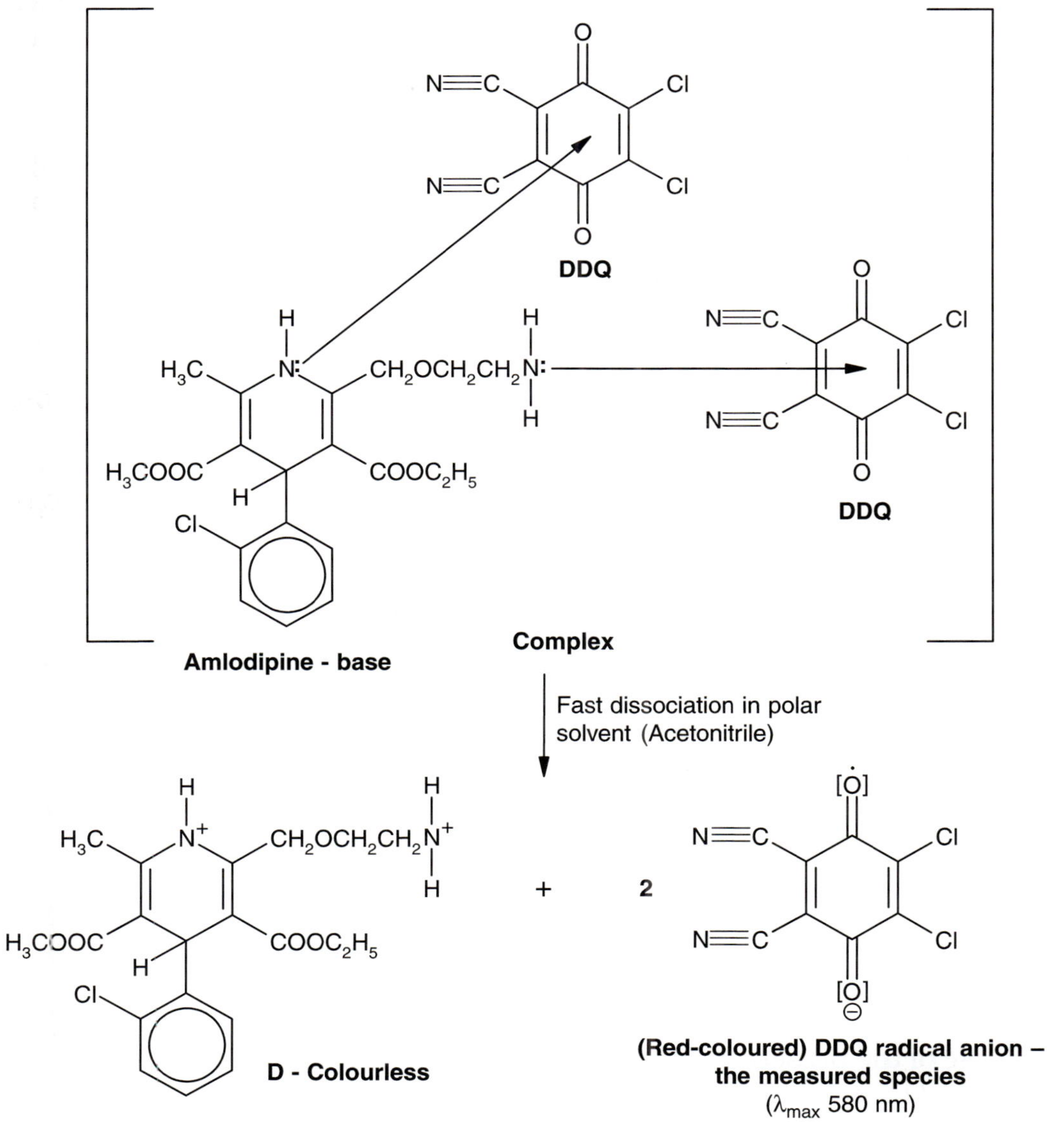

Reference (Methods 3 and 4)

1. Nafisur Rahman and Md. Nasrul Hoda. *J. Pharm. & Biomed. Analysis*, **31**, 381-392, 2003.
2. Lories I. Bebawy, Naglaa El-Kousy, Jihan K. Suddic & Mohamed Shokry. *J. Pharm. & Biomed. Analysis*, **21**, 133-142, 1999.
3. Anu Philips et al. *The Eastern Pharmacist*, p. 111, 2000.

Note

Amlodipine besylate does not react with π acceptors due to non-availability of lone-pair of electrons but the amlodipine base forms the complex.

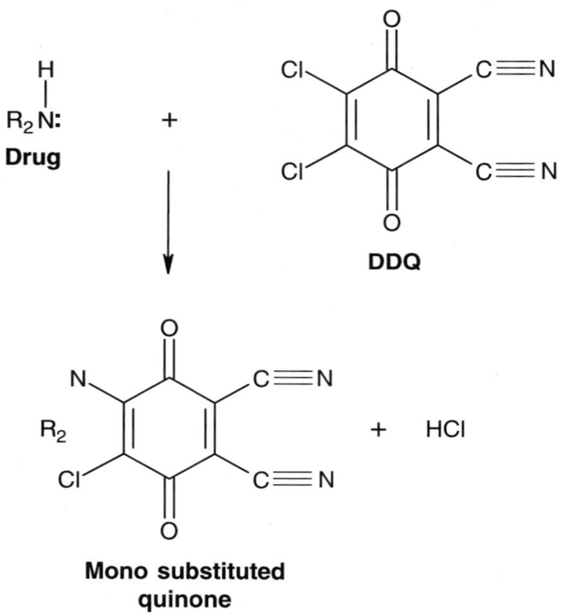

Note

The drug forms complex with chloranil (λ_{max} 362 nm).

The drug forms C-T complex with iodine σ-electron acceptor to form tri-iodide ion-pair. The reaction is as under:

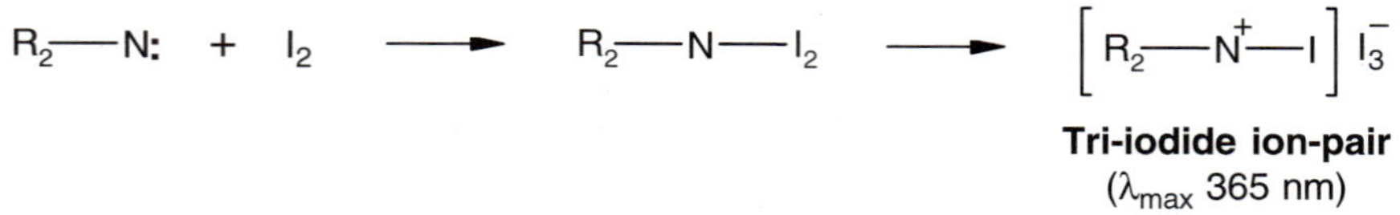

Because of the presence of primary aliphatic amine in the molecule, it answers Folin's test (1,2-naphthoquinone-4-sulphonate sodium) in alkaline medium.

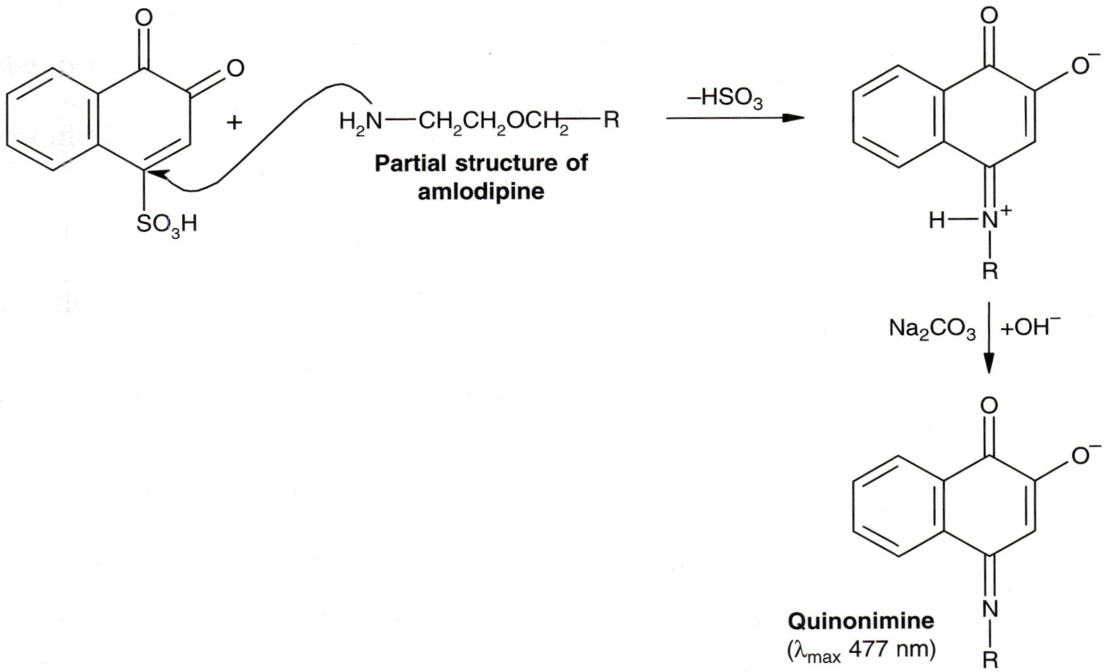

Reference

Anu Philips et al. *Eastern Pharmacist*, p. 111, 2000.

Atenolol

On heating with 0.1 M sodium hydroxide in boiling water-bath (20 min) the compound is converted to a fluorescent species.

Probable Reaction Mechanism

CH_2CONH_2 (acetoamido group) present in the drug on heating with alkali is converted to amine (NH_2) which is highly fluorescent.

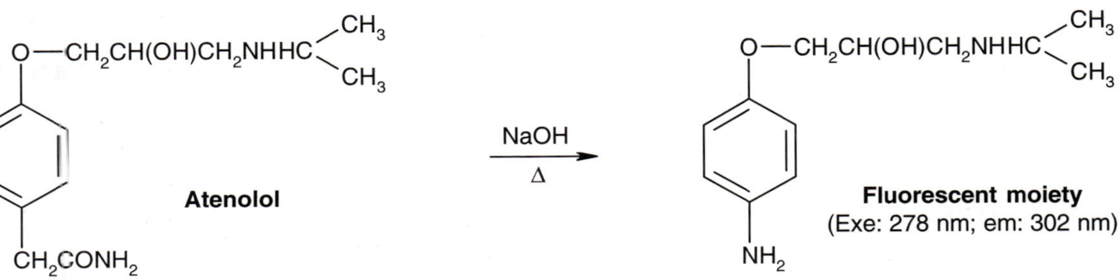

Reference

S.A. Patel, C.N. Patel, I.S. Rathod, B.N. Suhagia & M.M. Patel. *Ind. J. Pharm. Sci.*, **67(2)**, 225-228, 2005.

Formulation 12

Atenolol, Nifedipine

ESTIMATION

Atenolol

Standard solution

20 mcg/ml of atenolol in water.

Sample solution

Accurately weighed quantity of the sample equivalent to 100 mg of the substance is suspended in 100-125 ml water and stirred for 30 min and made up to 250 ml. 5 ml is further diluted to 100 ml with water (20 mcg/ml).

Concomitantly measure the absorbance of both sample and standard solutions at the maxima at about 225 nm using water as blank and calculate the results by comparison.

Nifedipine

METHOD 1

Standard solution

50 mcg/ml of nifedipine in methanol.

Sample solution

Accurately weighed quantity of sample extracted with methanol to get solution of 50 mcg/ml.

Concomitantly measure the absorbance of both sample and standard solutions at 350 nm using methanol as blank and calculate the results by comparison.

METHOD 2

Reagent

1. 2% w/v solution of sodium hydroxide in DMF.

Standard and sample solutions

Prepare the solutions in DMF (200 mcg/ml).

Procedure

To 0.5 ml each of sample and standard solutions, add 0.1 ml of sodium hydroxide solution and dilute to 10 ml with DMF and measure the absorbance of both the solutions at 425 nm against reagent blank and calculate the results by comparison.

Note

Estimation of nifedipine in visible range should be preferred as there are chances of its decomposition in UV range.

Explanatory Note

In alkaline medium, the nifedipine is hydrolysed to give yellow-coloured compound (λ_{max} 425 nm).

Probable Reaction Mechanism

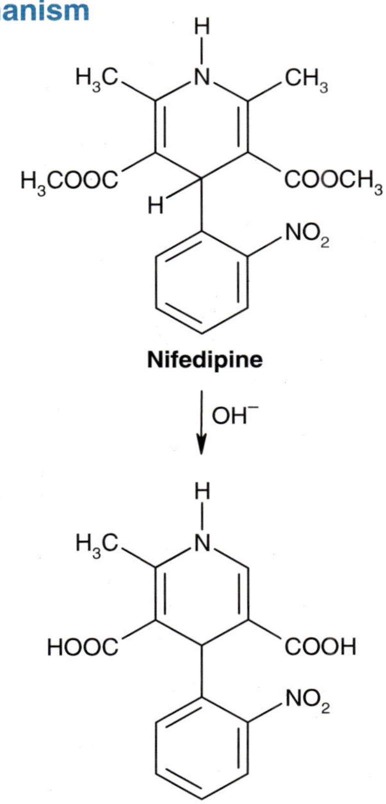

Yellow-coloured compound
(λ_{max} 425 nm)

Alternatively, the nitro group (NO_2) present in the molecule is reduced to amino group by Zn^{++} + HCl and coupled with organic aldehyde (vanillin) to form Schiff's base as under:

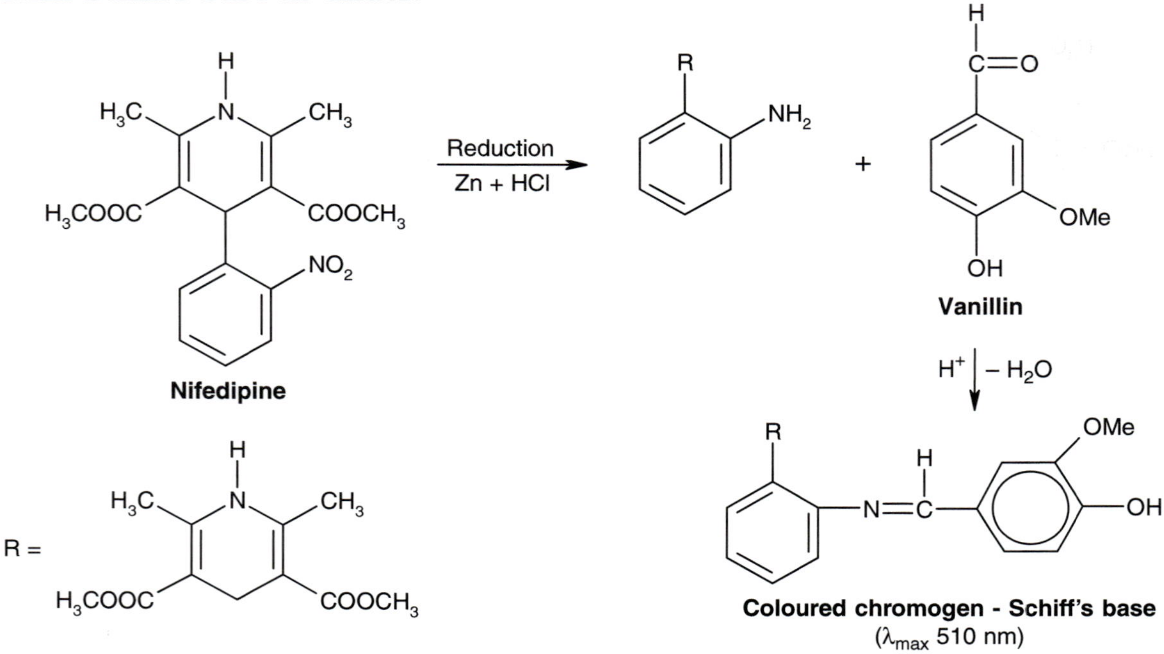

Reference

Indian Drugs, **24(8)**, 415, 1987.

Arvind B. Karadi et al. (2000) have reported coupling of the reduced nifedipine with 3,4,5-trimethoxybenzaldehyde to form Schiff's base.

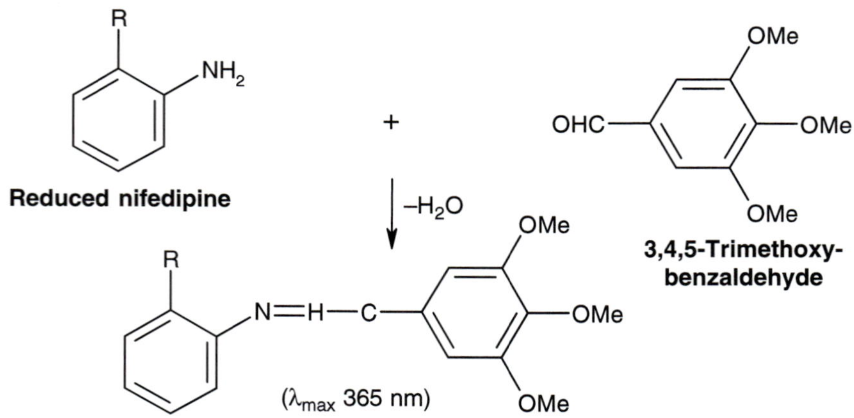

Reference

Arvind B. Karadi et al. *The Eastern Pharmacist*, pp. 117-118, 2000.

Method 3

Nifedipine forms complex with Fe (3) - $K_3Fe(CN)_6$ as shown below.

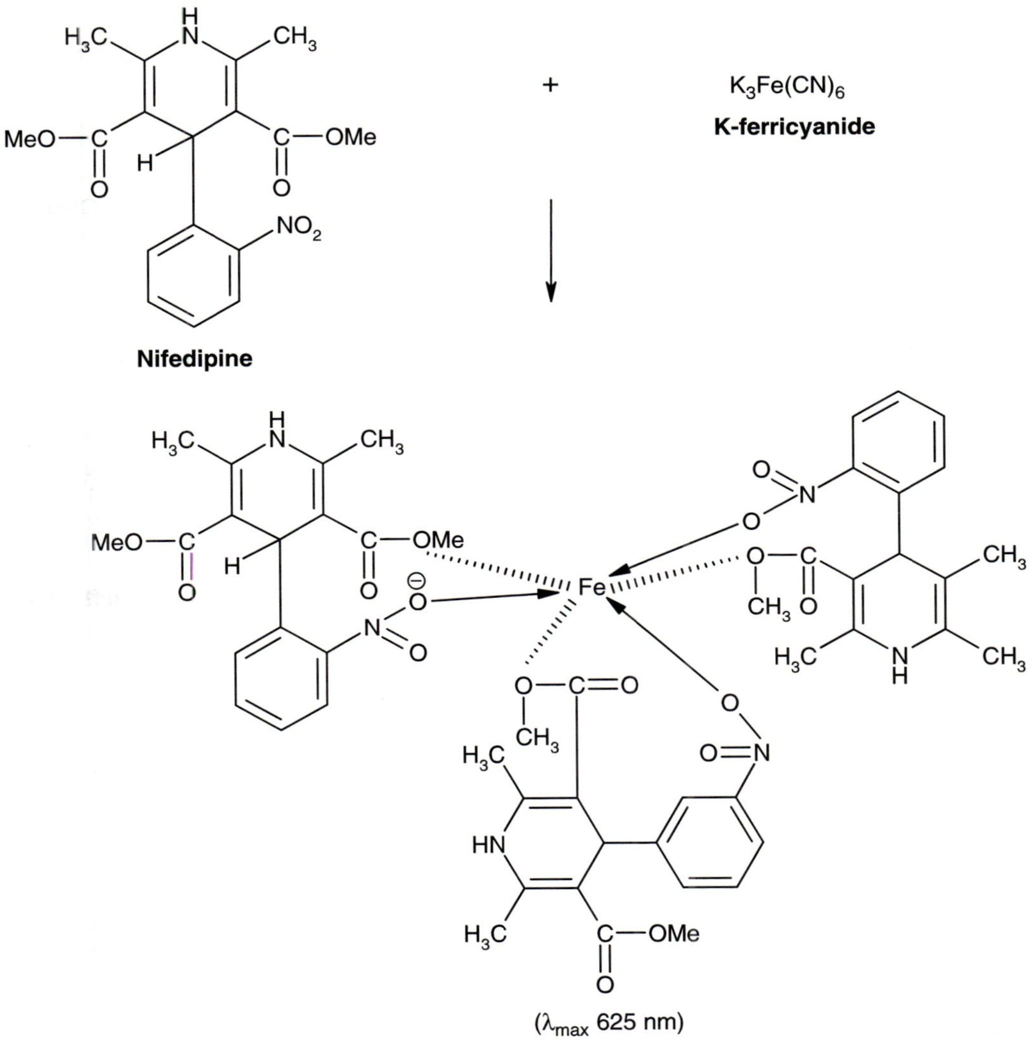

Reference

R.B. Patel, T.P. Gandhi, A.A. Patel, V.C. Patel, S.K. Patel & R.N. Gilbert. *Ind. J. Pharm. Sci.*, May, June, 1984.

Formulation 13

Atenolol, Hydrochlorothiazide, Amiloride hydrochloride

ESTIMATION

Atenolol

METHOD 1

Standard solution

100 mcg/ml of atenolol in methanol.

Sample solution

Weigh accurately powdered sample equivalent 50 mg of the substance and dry extract with 3×30 ml of chloroform. Evaporate the combined chloroform extract and dissolve the residue in 100 ml of methanol by shaking for 5 min. Further dilute 10 ml to 50 ml with methanol.

Determine the absorbance of the sample and standard solutions at 276 nm against blank prepared by evaporating 5 ml of chloroform and 50 ml of methanol. Calculate the results by comparison.

METHOD 2

Atenolol forms ion-pair complex with acidic dyes such as bromophenol blue (BPB), bromothymol blue (BTB), bromocresol purple (BCP), 0.1% w/v solution of each dye in chloroform. The complexes are soluble in chloroform. All other β-blockers with secondary amino group such as timolol and nadolol form ion-pair complexes.

Note

Atenolol, timolol and nadolol make ion-pair complex with acidic sulphophthalein dyes such as bromothymol blue, bromocresol purple and bromophenol blue. All yellow-coloured ion-pair complexes are soluble in chloroform and have λ_{max} at about 415 nm.

Probable Reaction Mechanism

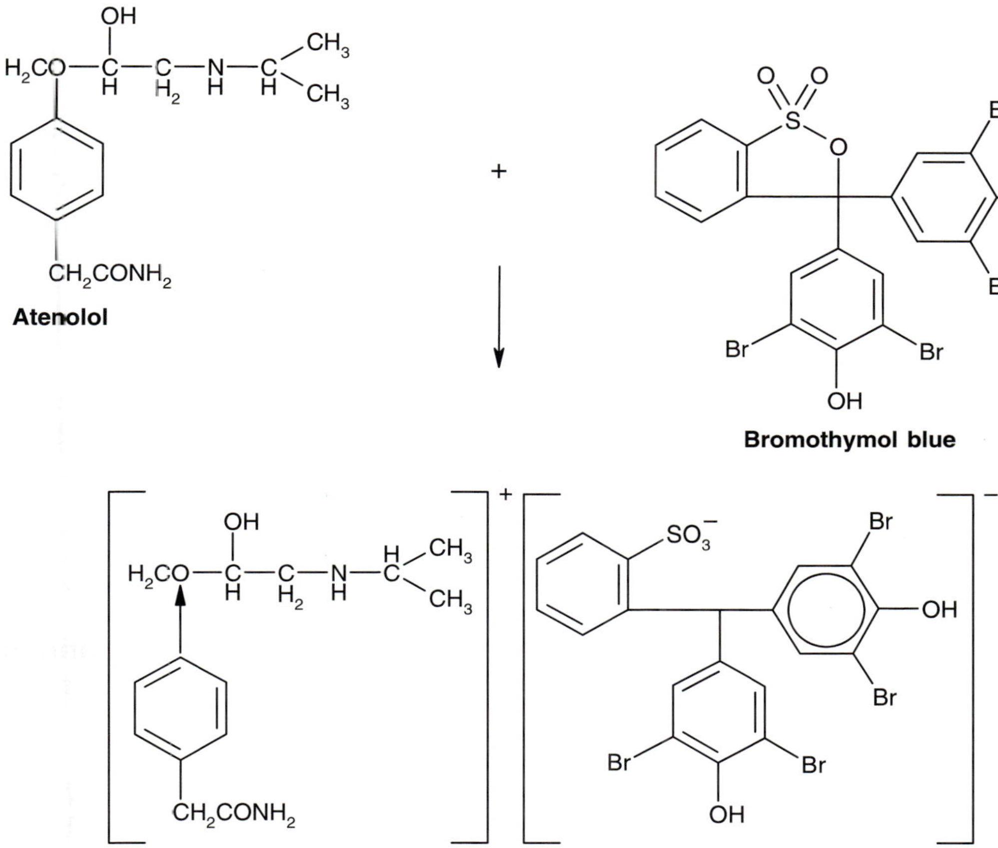

Ion-pair complex
(λ_{max} 415 nm)

Reference

S.M. al-Ghannam. *J. Pharm. Biomed. Analysis*, **40**, 151-156, 2006.

Hydrochlorothiazide

Standard solution

50 mg/ml of hydrochlorothiazide in methanol.

Sample solution

Extract the accurately weighed quantity of the sample equivalent to 25 mg of the substance with 3 × 30 ml acetone by shaking for 5-10 min. Evaporate the combined acetone extract and take up the residue in methanol to produce 100 ml. 10 ml is further diluted to 50 ml with methanol (50 mcg/ml).

Determine the absorbance of both sample and standard solutions at 317 nm against blank (evaporate 5 ml of acetone to dryness and take up in 50 ml of methanol) and calculate the results by comparison.

Amiloride hydrochloride

METHOD 1

Standard solution

5 mcg/ml in 0.1 M hydrochloric acid solution is prepared by heating for 5 min, followed by shaking for 10 min.

Sample solution

Accurately weighed quantity of the sample equivalent to 50 mg of the substance was suspended in 50 ml of 0.1 N hydrochloric acid, heated in water-bath for 5 min, cooled and shaken for 10 min and diluted to 100 ml with 0.1 N hydrochloric acid. 5 ml of the resultant solution is further diluted to 50 ml with 0.1 M hydrochloric acid.

Measure the absorbance of sample and standard at 361 nm using 0.1 N hydrochloric acid as blank. Calculate the results by comparison.

Amiloride in acetic acid has fluorescent properties (Ex. 365, Em 440 nm) which can be used for quantitative extraction.

Reference

Indian Drugs, **23(1)**, 230, Oct. 1985.

METHOD 2

The method is based on the reaction of amiloride with 9,10-phenanthroquinone to give highly fluorescent derivative.

Reagents

1. 1 M sodium hydroxide.
2. Conc. hydrochloric acid.
3. 2 mg/ml solution of 9,10-phenanthroquinone 1 M sodium hydroxide.

Sample and standard solutions

100 μg/ml in water.

Procedure

To 1 ml each of sample and standard solutions, add 2.5 ml of phenanthroquinone reagent and 0.25 ml of 1 M sodium hydroxide solution, allow to stand at room temperature for 45 min and then add 0.25 ml of conc. HCl, dilute to

25 ml with water and measure the fluorescence of the resulting solution (Exc: 360nm; em: 420 nm) and calculate the results by comparison.

Probable Reaction Mechanism

9,10-phenanthroquinone reacts with amiloride, a guanidino derivative, in alkaline medium; an intermediate compound further reacts with one mole of amiloride to give fluorescent compound.

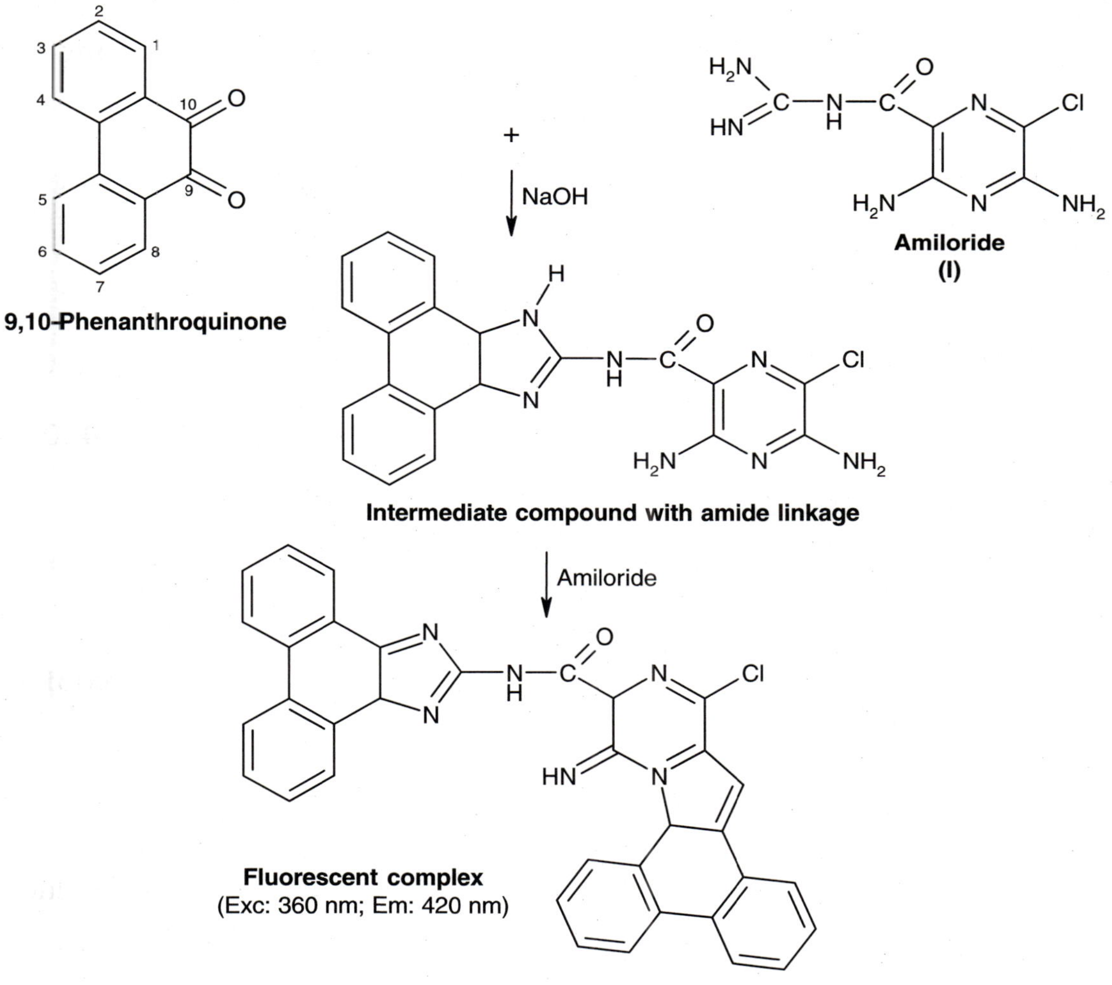

Reference

Mohamed H. Abdel-Hay et al. *Talanta*, **39(10)**, 1369-1375, 1992.

Formulation 14

Captopril, Hydrochlorothiazide

ESTIMATION

Captopril

METHOD 1

Weigh accurately powdered sample equivalent to 200 mg of the substance, add 100 ml of water, warm to 70°C for 5 min with frequent shaking, cool to room temperature, add 10 ml of 1.8 M sulphuric acid and 1 g of potassium iodide and shake to dissolve. Add 2 ml of starch solution and titrate with 0.1 N potassium iodate till dark brown colour persistently for 30 seconds is observed. Each ml of 0.1 N potassium iodate is equivalent to 21.73 mg of captopril.

Probable Reaction Mechanism

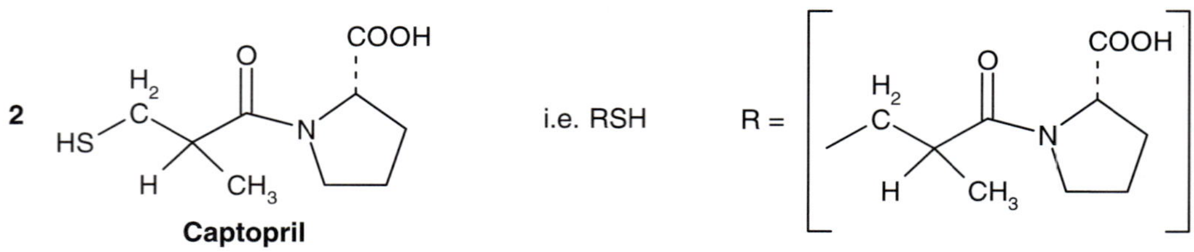

Captopril

$$2\,RSH + I_2 \longrightarrow R{-}S{-}S{-}R + 2\,HI + 2\,e^-$$

This involves iodometric titration.

METHOD 2

Reagents

1. Phosphate buffer, pH 7.2.
2. 4,4-dithiopyridine solution: Dissolve 10 mg of 4,4-dithiopyridine in phosphate buffer, pH 7.2 to produce 100 ml.

Standard solution

10 mcg/ml of the captopril.

Sample solution

An accurately weighed quantity of the sample was extracted with water to get solution of 10 mcg/ml.

Procedure

To 5 ml each of sample and standard solutions, add 3 ml of the reagent and dilute to 10 ml with water. Measure the absorption of both the solutions at 324 nm against reagent blank and calculate the results. The method obeys Beer's law in the range of 0.5-20 mcg/ml.

Probable Reaction Mechanism

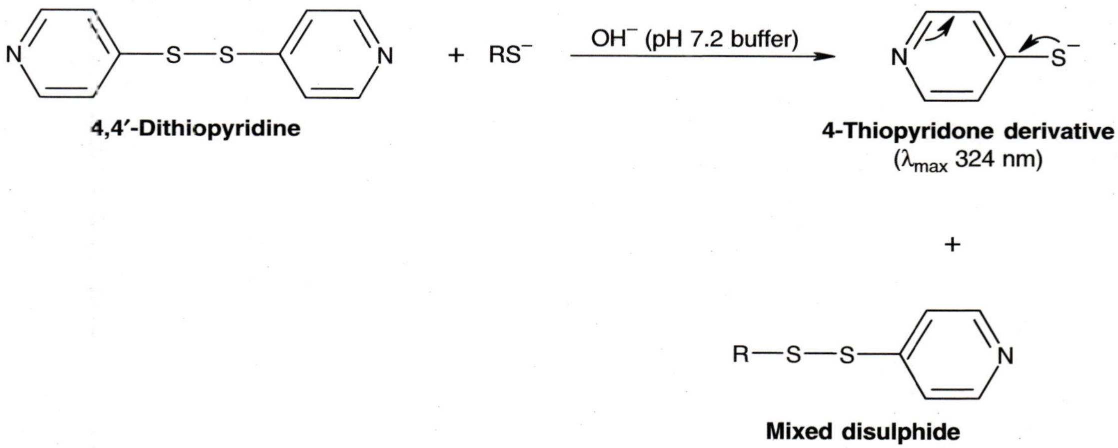

Note

1. Thiol derivative can reduce tetrazolium salt in alkaline medium to give coloured formazone.
2. Thiol can also reduce 2,6-dichlorophenolindophenol to give colourless phenolamines.
3. Thiol reacts with disodiumpentacyanonitrosyl ferrate (II) in alkali; nitrosyl cation gets reduced.

Reference

K.R. Mahadik et al. *Indian Drugs*, **28(11)**, 531, 1991.

METHOD 3

Reagent

1. Dissolve 0.5 g of citric in 4 ml of methanol and dilute to 25 ml with acetic anhydride.

Standard and sample solutions

10 mcg/ml as in method 2, but to be prepared in methanol.

Procedure

To 3 ml each of sample and standard solutions, add 1 ml of the reagent and heat in boiling water-bath for 30 min, cool and dilute to 10 ml with acetic anhydride and measure the absorbance of the chromophore at 570 nm and calculate the results by comparison.

Probable Reaction Mechanism

On heating the substance with citric acid - acetic anhydride, citric acid first reacts with acetic anhydride to give acetyl citric acid anhydride which yields red-violet colour with nitrogen-containing heterocyclic molecule (λ_{max} 570 nm).

METHOD 4

Reagents

1. 0.2% w/v solution of 2,2′-bispyridyl in water.
2. 0.1% w/v solution of ferric chloride in 0.5% HCl.
3. Iodine solution: Dissolve 38 mg of iodine and 80 mg of potassium iodide in 100 ml of water.
4. 0.5% w/v solution of soluble starch in water.
5. 1% w/v solution of sodium fluoride in water.

Standard solution

200 μg/ml in water.

Sample solution

Sample equivalent to 10 mg suspended in 20 ml of water, shake for 10 min, filtered, diluted to get 200 μg/ml.

Procedure

(A) To 1 ml each of sample and standard solutions add 1 ml of ferric chloride solution, mix, add 1 ml of bispyridyl solution, allow to stand for 5 min, add 1 ml of sodium fluoride solution, dilute to 10 ml with water and measure the absorbance at 520 nm against reagent blank. Sodium fluoride is added to quench the interaction after 5 min and get stable absorbance readings.

(B) (i) To 1 ml each of sample and standard solutions add 1 ml of iodine solution, dilute to 10 ml with water and measure the absorbance at 351 nm against reagent blank.

(B) (ii) Repeat the procedure (B-i), add 1 ml of starch solution and measure the absorbance at 620 nm against reagent blank.

Probable Reaction Mechanism

(A) The compound has reducing property due to SH group. Ferric chloride acts as oxidizing agent and itself gets reduced to Fe(II). The Fe(II) is then coupled with 2,2′-bispyridyl to give coloured complex (λ_{max} 520 nm).

Note

This reagent is known as Emmerie Engel reagent and is used for the detection of reducing substances such as vitamin C and vitamin E. Two nitrogen atoms in 2,2′-bispyridyl have one unshared pair of electrons which is shared by Fe(II) as under:

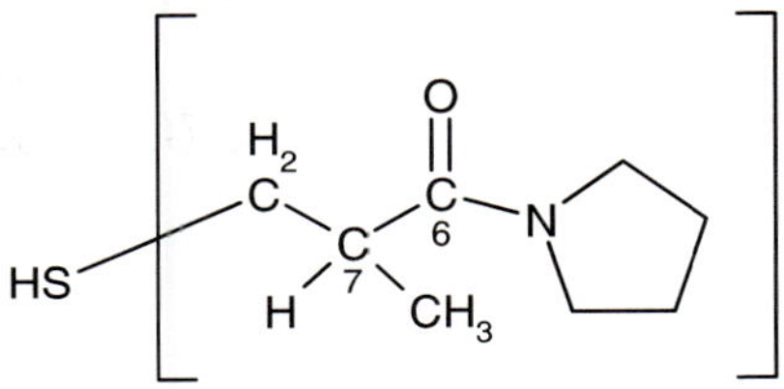

i.e. RSH

$$RSH + FeCl_3 \longrightarrow R{-}S{-}S{-}R + Fe(II)$$

Dimer

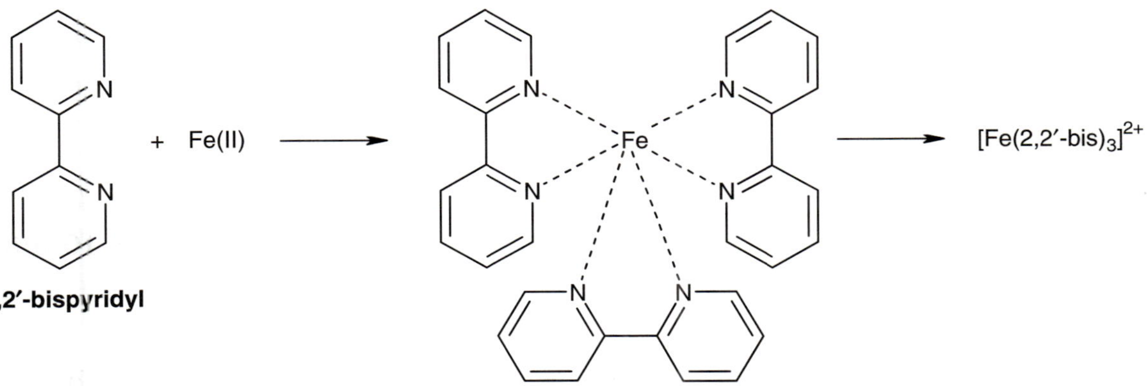

2,2′-bispyridyl

Fe++ - bispyridyl coloured complex
(λ_{max} 520 nm)

Reference

Hassan F. Aksal. *Talanta*, **38(10)**, 1155-1158, 1991.

Note

Fe(II) so produced as a result of oxidation-reduction complex with 1,10-phenanthroline to yield a stable orange red-coloured complex (λ_{max} 510 nm).

Reference

Saad Antakli et al. *Asian J. Chem.*, **22(6)**, 4931-4938, 2010.

Iodine also acts as oxidizing agent. For reaction mechanism see Method 1. Excess iodine is measured at 351 nm as tri-iodide or it is allowed to form complex with starch (λ_{max} 620 nm).

Interestingly, captopril is the only molecule possessing sulphahydryl group among the closely related anti-hypertensive drugs such as ramipril, enalapril and lisinopril, etc.

METHOD 5

A spectrophotometric method reported by Sastry et al. (1985) was based on oxidative coupling of p-aminophenol or metol with thiol (RSH) such as cysteine or captopril.

Probable Reaction Mechanism

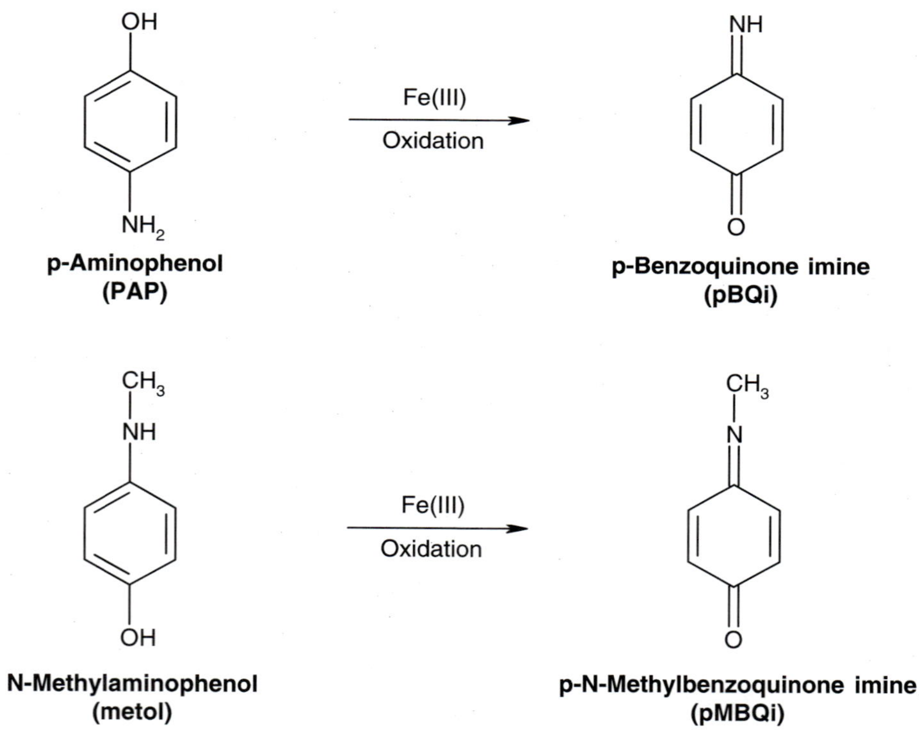

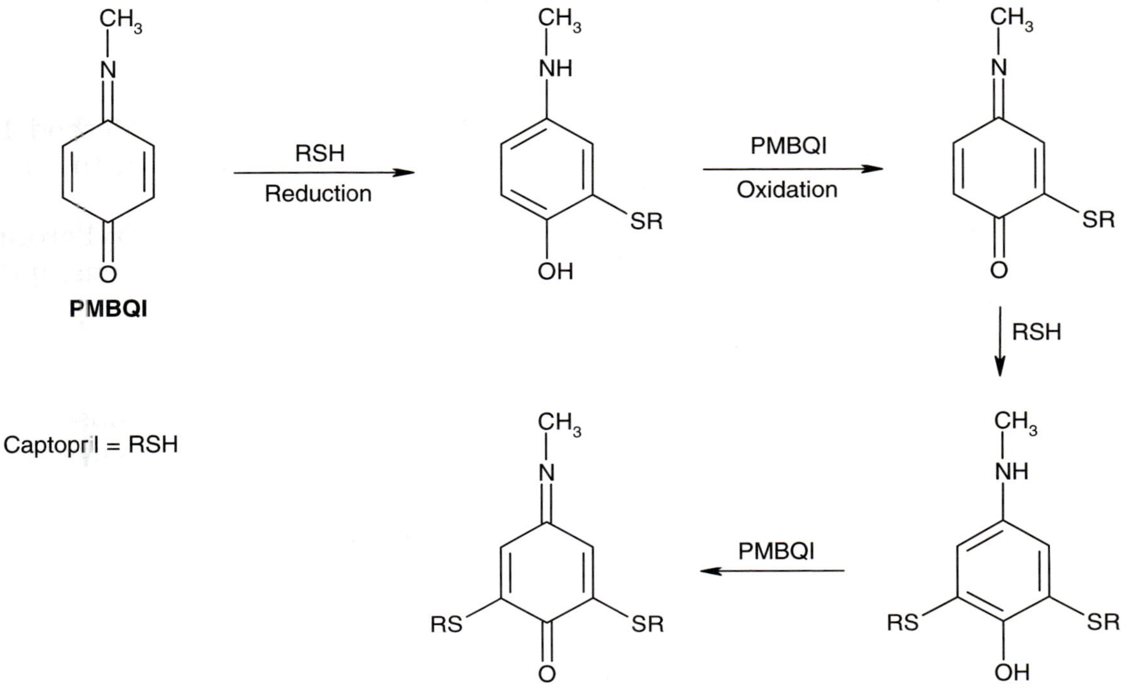

3 : 2 coloured complex
(λ_{max} 580 nm)

Reference

C.S.P. Sastry, P. Satyanarayana & Murli K. Tummuru. *Analyst*, **110(2)**, 189-191, 1985.

A method based on reaction of reducing agent and oxidizing agent for quantitative determination of one of the reactants has been described by N. El-Enany (2009). In this case, captopril acts as reducing agent and potassium permanganate as oxidizing agent.

Either one can measure colour of the manganate radical (λ_{max} 610 nm) or decrease in absorbance of $KMnO_4$ (λ_{max} 525 nm).

Probable Reaction Mechanism

$$\underset{\textbf{Captopril}}{RSH} + KMnO_4 \longrightarrow \underset{\lambda_{max}\ 610\ nm}{Mn^{2+}}$$

Reference

N. El-Enany, F. Belal & M. Rizk. *Analytical Chemistry, An Indian Journal (ACAIJ)*, **8(3)**, 2009.

Hydrochlorothiazide

Standard solution

10 mcg/ml of hydrochlorothiazide in 0.1 M sodium hydroxide.

Sample solution

Suspend accurately weighed quantity of the sample in 50 ml of 0.1 N sodium hydroxide, shake for 5 min and dilute to 100 ml. Filter and dilute further to get solution of 10 mcg/ml.

Measure the absorbance of both sample and standard solutions at 273 nm using 0.1 M sodium hydroxide as blank and calculate the results by comparison.

Formulation 15

Clonidine hydrochloride, Chlorthalidone

ESTIMATION

Clonidine hydrochloride

Reagents

1. 10% w/v acetic acid in water.
2. 0.1% metanil yellow.
3. 1 M hydrochloric acid.

Standard solution

50 mcg/ml of clonidine hydrochloride in water.

Sample solution

Suspend accurately weighed quantity for the sample equivalent to 0.1 mg of the substance in 20 ml of water, add 1 ml of acetic acid and 2 ml of metanil yellow. Shake and allow to stand for 20-25 min. Extract with two 60 ml portions of chloroform. The combined chloroform layer is extracted with three 25 ml portions of 1 M hydrochloric acid (discard chloroform layer) and dilute to 100 ml with 1 M hydrochloric acid.

To 2 ml of the standard solution (100 mcg) add 20 ml of water, 1 ml of acetic acid and 1 ml of metanil yellow solution and proceed as under sample solution.

Measure the absorption of both sample and standard at 530 nm and calculate the results by comparison.

Note

The method is based on ion-pair complex formation, soluble in chloroform, re-extracted with HCl for measurements.

As the hydrogen in the imidazole ring at position 3 is un-substituted it imparts acidic property to the molecule. The same is titratable with 0.1 M ethanolic sodium hydroxide.

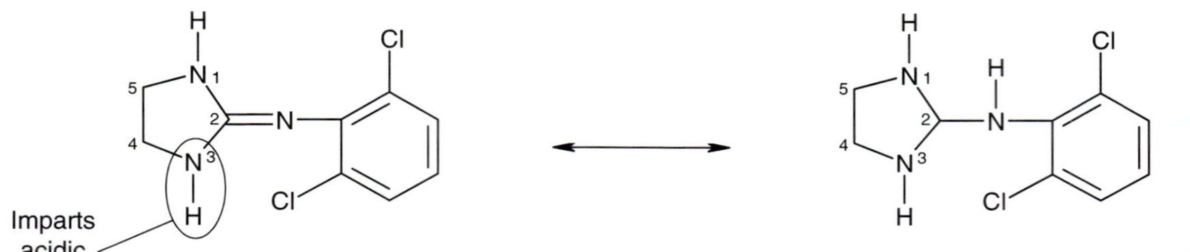

Clonidine (A) **Clonidine (B)**

Clonidine (A) is dominant.

The compound forms ion-pair complex with acidic dyes, i.e. bromophenol blue (phthalate buffer, pH 2.5), bromocresol purple (sodium acetate buffer, pH 6.0) and methyl orange (acetate buffer, pH 4.5). All the ion-pair complexes are extractable into chloroform and have λ_{max} 415 nm for quantitative analysis.

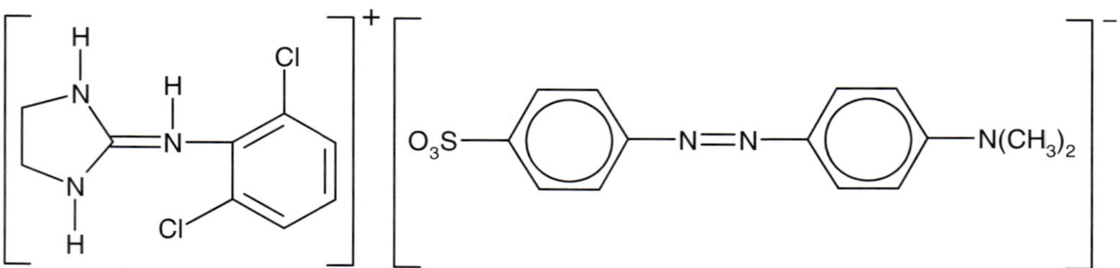

Clonidine **Methyl orange**

Drug-dye ion-pair complex
(λ_{max} 415 nm)

Reference

R.T. Sane & C.H. Thambare. *Indian Drugs*, **18(9)**, 335-337, 1981.

A method based on formation of C-T complex was reported by Fowzya (1986). 2,3-Dichloro-5,6-dicyano-p-benzoquinone (DDQ), an electron acceptor condenses with the drug, an imidazoline derivative and electron donor to give coloured C-T complex (λ_{max} 445 nm).

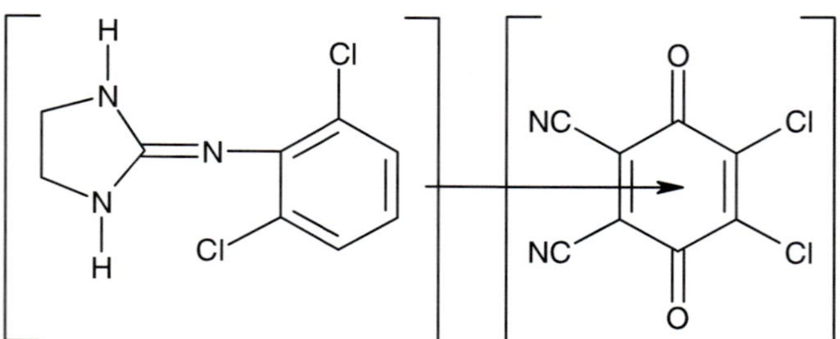

Clonidine **DDQ**

Clonidine - DDQ C-T complex
(λ_{max} 445 nm)

The authors also reported fluorometric method based on reaction of clonidine with dansyl chloride yielding fluorescing dansyl derivative.

Probable Reaction Mechanism

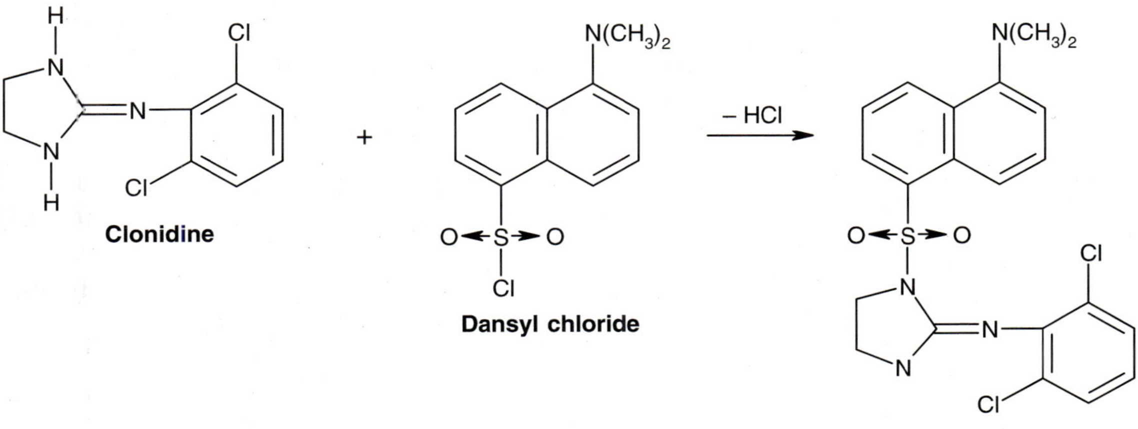

Fluorescing dansyl derivative
(Exc: 345 nm; Em: 445 nm)

Reference

Fowzya El-Yazbi, Mona Bedair & Mohamed A. Korany. *Analyst*, **111**, 477-478, 1986.

Chlorthalidone

Standard solution

1 mg/ml of chlorthalidone in water. To 5 ml add 1 ml of 2 M hydrochloric acid and dilute to 50 ml with methanol (50 mcg/ml).

Sample solution

Accurately weighed quantity of the sample is boiled with 30 ml of methanol for 30 min, and dilute to 100 ml with methanol. To 5 ml of the filtrate, add 1 ml of 2 M hydrochloric acid and dilute to 50 ml with methanol.

Measure the extinction of both the solutions at 275 nm against blank (1 ml of 1 M hydrochloric acid diluted to 50 ml with methanol) and calculate the results by comparison.

On treatment with concentrated sulphuric acid, the compound yields a carbenium ion (λ_{max} 420 nm).

Probable Reaction Mechanism

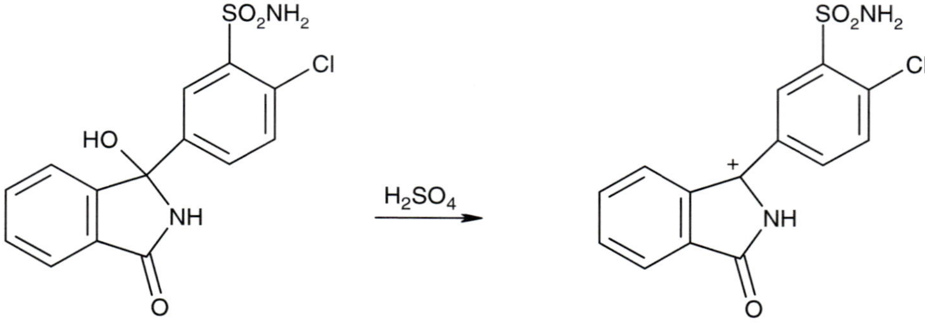

Chlorothalidone **Carbenium ion** (λ_{max} 420 nm)

Reference

Pharmaceutical Chemistry (Vol. 2) by H.J. Roth, p. 449.

NH_2 group of the sulphonamide group present in benzene ring of chlorthalidone forms Schiff's base with PDAB to give yellow complex (λ_{max} 390 nm). This can form the basis for quantitative estimation.

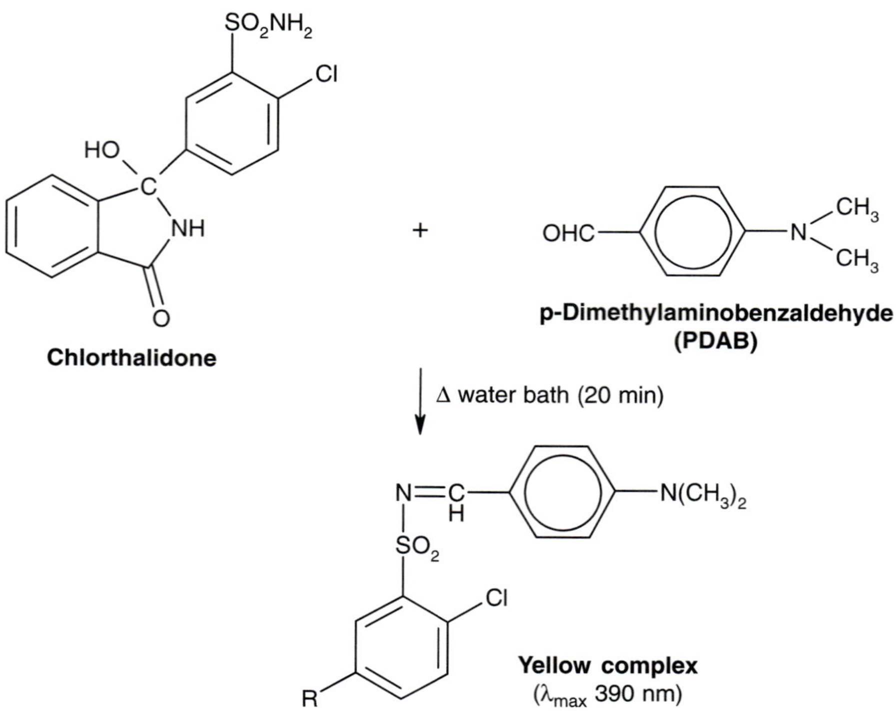

Yellow complex (λ_{max} 390 nm)

Formulation 16

Levodopa, Benserazide hydrochloride

ESTIMATION

Levodopa

Standard solution

30 mcg/ml of levodopa in 0.1 M hydrochloric acid.

Sample solution

Suspend accurately weighed quantity of the sample in 50 ml water. Warm on a boiling water-bath for 5 min, cool and dilute appropriately with 0.1 M hydrochloric acid to get final concentration of 30 mcg/ml.

Measure the absorbance of standard and sample solutions at 280 nm against 0.1 M hydrochloric acid as blank. Calculate the results by comparison.

Levodopa being a o-diphenol reacts with sodium nitrite in acidic medium and gets nitrosated at p-position to OH group by NO^+ ions from HNO_2 formed. By addition of ammonium molybdate, nitrosated compound is oxidized to nitro compound (yellow in colour) which changes to red on addition of NaOH involving deprotonation to red azaxonol.

Probable Reaction Mechanism

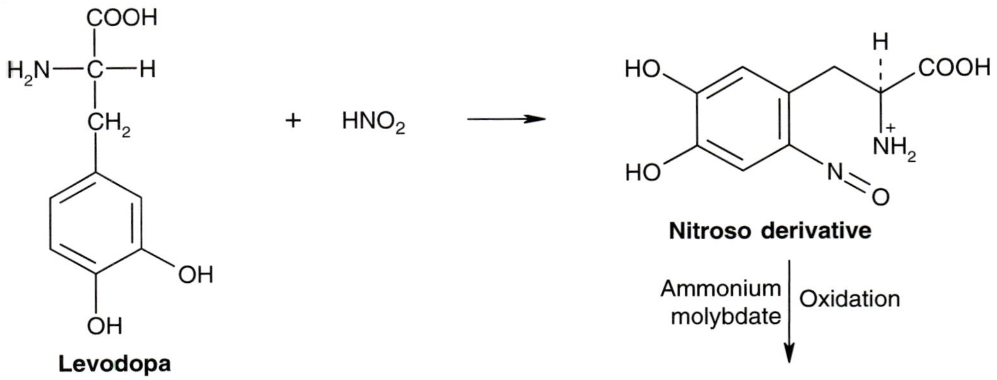

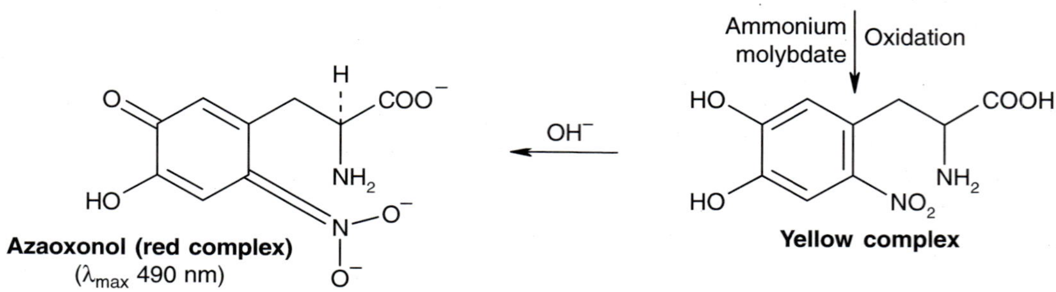

Reaction mechanism of nitrosation reaction

$$Na^+ + NO_2^- + H_3\overset{+}{O} + Cl^- \longrightarrow \underset{\textbf{Nitrous acid}}{HO-N=O} + Na^+ + Cl^-$$

In strongly acidic medium, nitrous acid is protonated, conjugated and then it loses water to give nitrosonium ion and in the presence of halide (Cl^- ions) nitrosyl halide also forms.

$$HO-N=O + H_3\overset{+}{O} \rightleftharpoons H-\underset{+}{\overset{H}{O}}-N=O \longrightarrow H_2O + \underset{\textbf{Nitrosonium ion}}{\overset{+}{N}=O}$$

$$\overset{+}{N}=O + Cl^- \rightleftharpoons \underset{\textbf{Nitrosyl chloride}}{Cl-N=O}$$

$$N\equiv\overset{+}{O} \longleftrightarrow \overset{+}{N}=O$$

Nitrosonium ion is an electrophilic species involved in electrophilic aromatic substitution.

α-Amino group present in the molecule reacts with 4-nitrobenzoyl chloride to give an amide which forms violet-coloured azaoxonol anion on addition of sodium carbonate.

Probable Reaction Mechanism

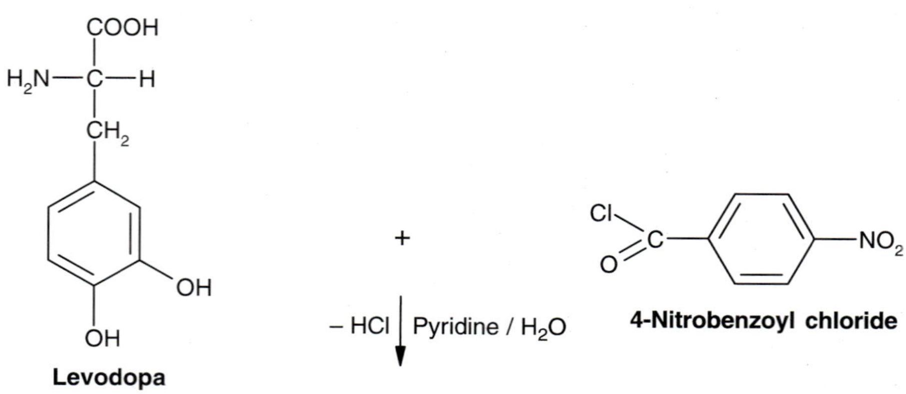

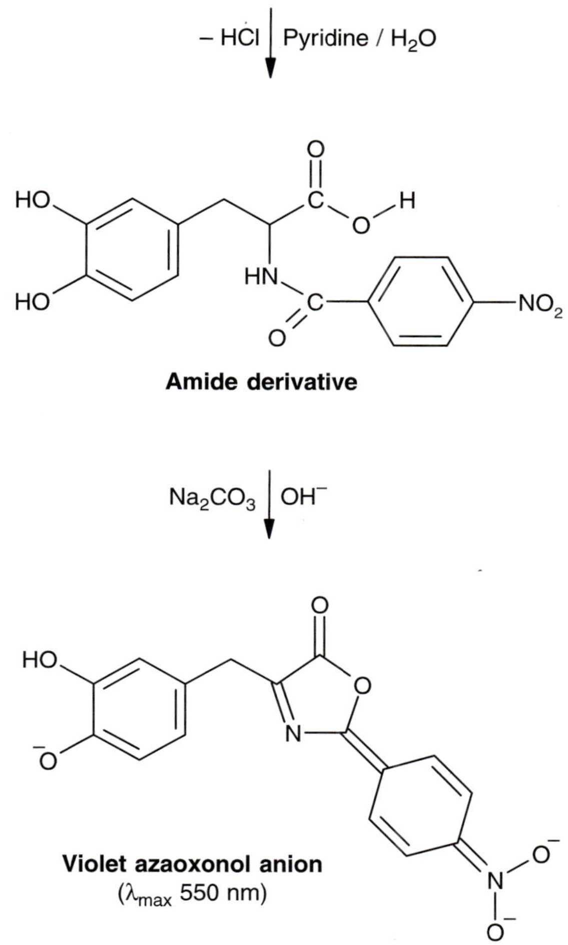

Methyldopa, Levodopa

Reagents

1. 0.4% w/v solution of p-aminophenol (PAP).
2. 10 M ammonium hydroxide.

Sample and standard solutions

100 µg/ml of each compound in 0.1 M hydrochloric acid.

Procedure

To 1 ml each of sample and standard solutions add 1.5 ml of 'PAP' solution and 1.5 ml of ammonium hydroxide, dilute to 10 ml with water and measure the absorbance at 580 nm against reagent blank.

Probable Reaction Mechanism

In alkaline medium, p-aminophenol is first oxidized and then forms indophenol-like complex with methyldopa which is a phenol in itself (λ_{max} 590 nm).

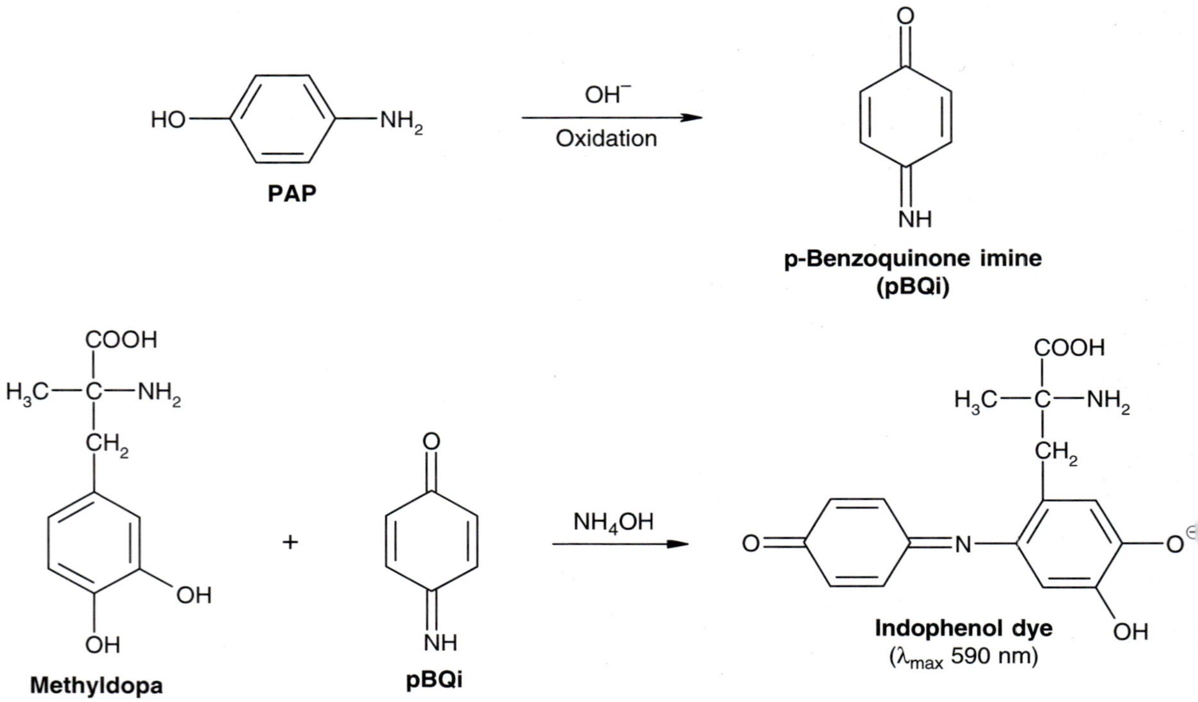

Note

Other reagents used by the authors are resorcinol and p-phenylenediamine dihydrochloride.

Reference

R.T. Sane et al. *Curr. Sci.*, **48(4)**, 158-160, 1979.

The compound undergoes oxidation in acidic conditions with ammonium vanadate to give yellow complex.

Reagents

1. 1% w/v solution of ammonium vanadate in water.
2. Phosphoric acid.

Sample and standard solutions

200 μg/ml solution of each compound in water.

Procedure

To 0.5 ml each of sample and standard solutions add 4 ml of ammonium vanadate solution and 1 ml of phosphric acid, mix, allow to stand for 5 min, dilute to 10 ml with water and measure the absorption of sample and standard solutions at 430 nm against reagent blank.

Probable Reaction Mechanism

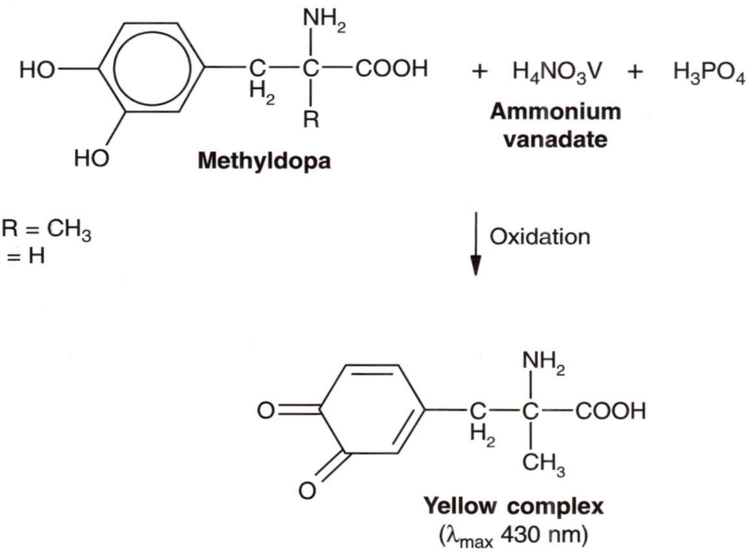

Methyldopa: R = CH_3
Levodopa: R = H

Reference

R.T. Sane, G.J. Bhounsule & S.V. Sawant. *Indian Drugs*, **24(4)**, 207-208, 1987.

A method based on oxidation of the drug with N-bromosuccinimide (NBS) followed by oxidative coupling with INH in alkaline medium was described by Nagaraja et al. (1988). To appropriate quantity of the sample and standard (200 µg) add 0.05% NBS solution, followed by 'INH' solution (0.02%) and then 0.01 M sodium hydroxide solution. Keep aside for 5 min, dilute to 25 ml with water and measure the absorbance of both sample and standard at 480 nm against reagent blank and calculate the results.

Probable Reaction Mechanism

The drug with vicinal dihydroxybenzene derivative is easily oxidized by 'NBS' to ortho-benzoquinone derivative. 'INH' by virtue of its strong electron donating group couples with o-benzoquinone to give oxidized coupled product (λ_{max} 480 nm).

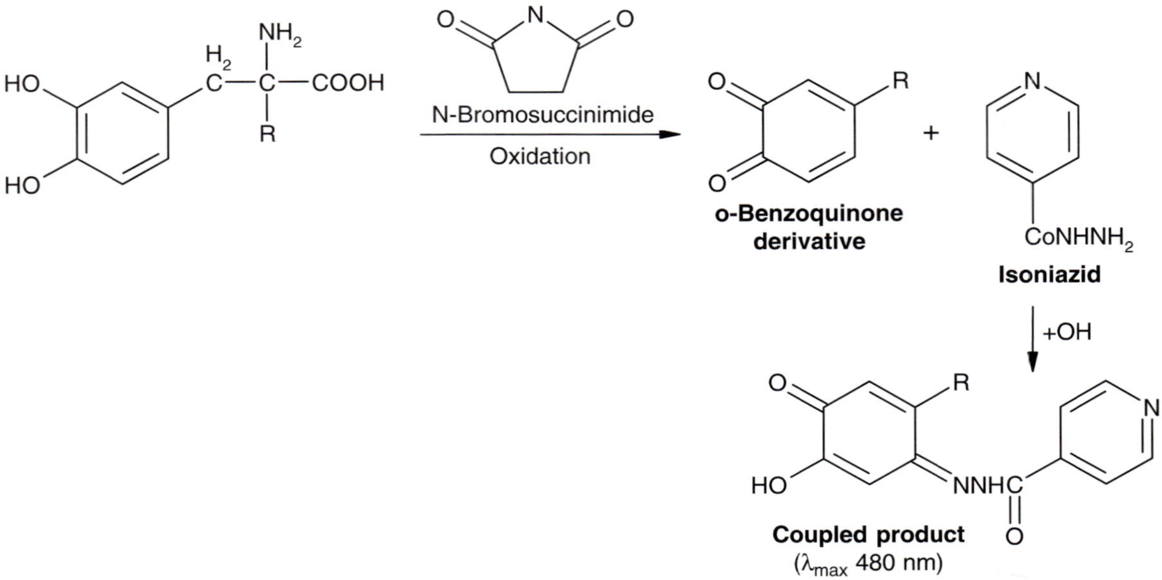

Reference

P. Nagaraja, K.C. Srinivas Murthy, K.S. Rangappa & N.M. Made Gowda. *Talanta*, **46**, 39-44, 1998.

Methyldopa reacts with 'MBTH' in acidic medium in the presence of potassium dichromate ($K_2Cr_2O_7$) or ceric ammonium sulphate [$(NH_4)_4Ce(SO_4)_4$] to give coloured product.

To appropriate quantity of the sample and standard add 1 ml of 'MBTH' reagent (0.4%) and 3 ml of oxidizing reagent, dilute with methanol and measure the absorption at 590 nm ($K_2Cr_2O_7$) and 504 nm [$(NH_4)_4Ce(SO_4)_4$].

Probable Reaction Mechanism

MBTH undergoes oxidative coupling with phenols at the ortho or p-position to the phenolic —OH group. The reaction proceeds in the presence of an oxidizing agent. In the first stages of the reaction MBTH loses two electrons and a proton. The cation so formed will attack the electron-rich centre of the phenol (ortho or para position to the phenolic —OH group) undergoing electrophilic substitution reaction and subsequent oxidation to form the product.

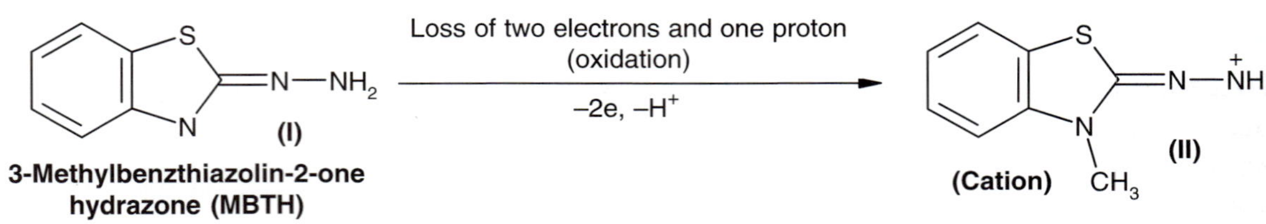

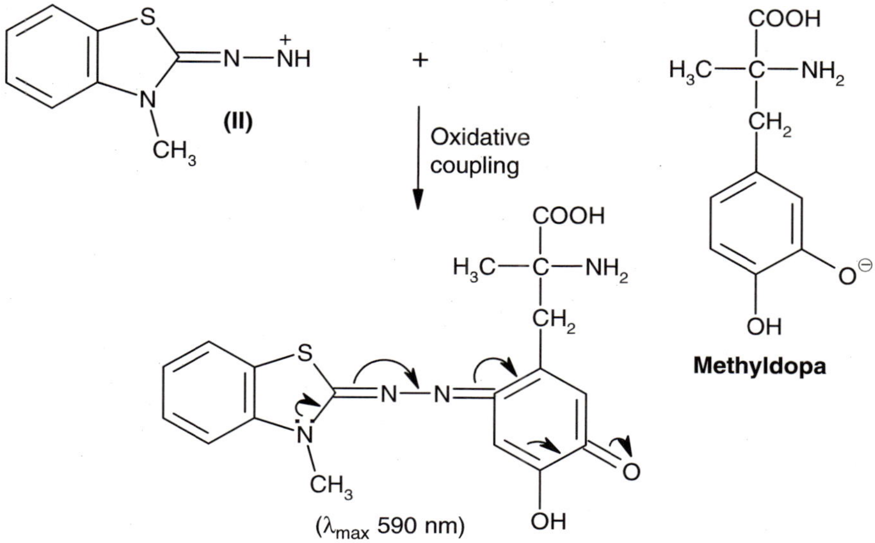

Note

This resonance is possible due to the availability of lone pair of electrons on the 'N' atom.

Reference

1. Pharmaceutical Chemistry (Vol. 2) by H.J. Roth, pp. 74, 75.
2. G. Rama Rao, S. Raghuveer & P. Khadgapathi. *Indian Drugs*, **22(11)**, 597-599, 1981.

A method based on reaction with ninhydrin in acetate buffer pH 5.0 has been described by G. Rama Rao et al. (1982).

Reagents

1. 0.2 M sodium acetate - acetic acid buffer, pH 5.0.
2. 2% w/v solution of ninhydrin, prepared by dissolving 2 g of ninhydrin in 50 ml of methanol, then diluting to 100 ml with pH 5.0 acetate buffer.

Standard and sample solutions

500 μg/ml; dissolve 25 mg of the substance in water, adjust to pH 7.0 with 0.1 M sodium hydroxide, dilute to 50 ml with water.

Procedure

To 2 ml each of sample and standard solutions add 2.5 ml of ninhydrin reagent, heat in boiling water-bath for 40 min, cool to room temperature and dilute to 25 ml with n-propanol and measure the absorbance of both sample and standard solutions at 570 nm against reagent blank.

Probable Reaction Mechanism

Ninhydrin is a stable hydrate of 1,2,3-trioxoindane which has a particularly reactive carbonyl group at the carbon atom 2.

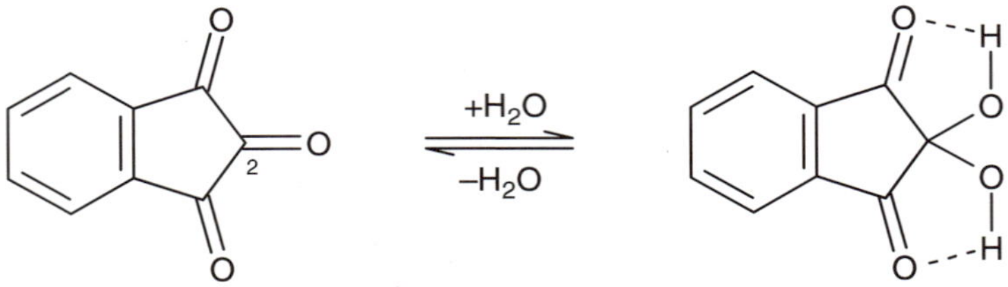

Ninhydrin **Hydrated ninhydrin**

Initially there is formation of semi-aminal which is decomposed to Schiff's base and CO_2 and H_2O.

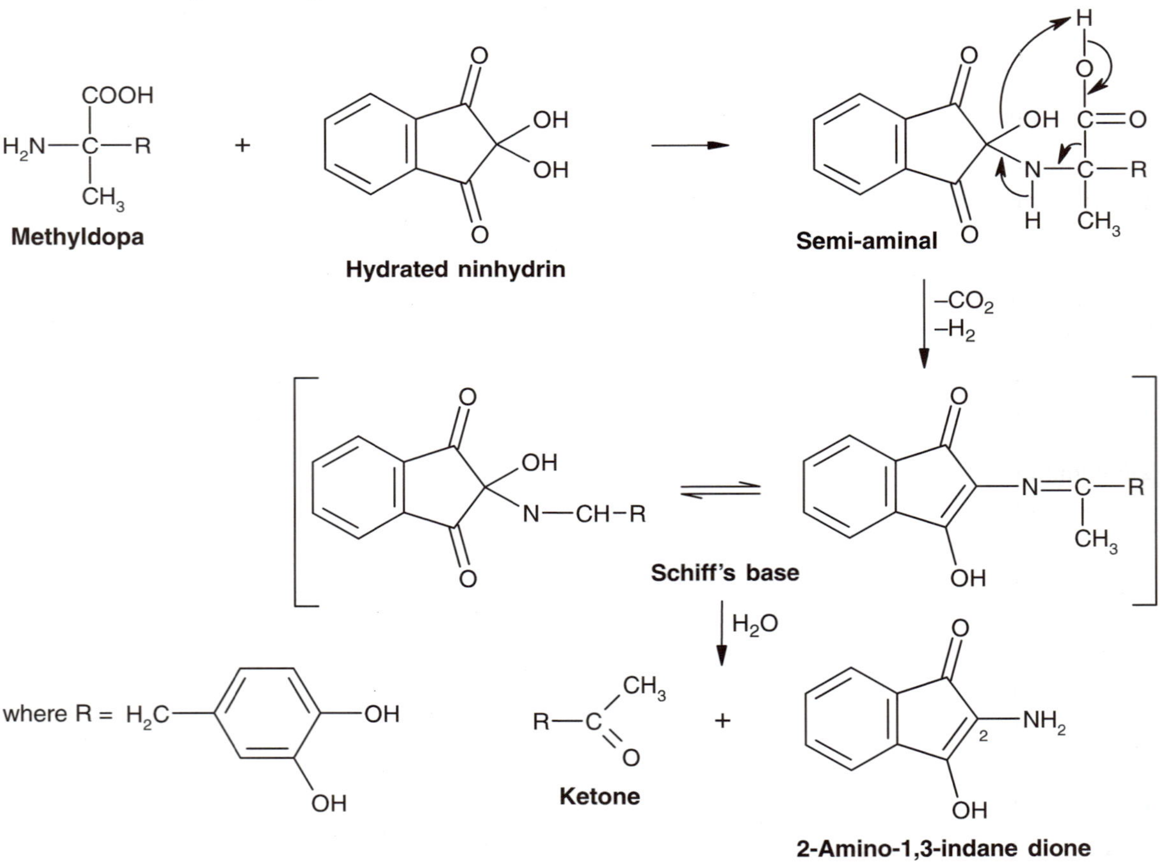

On hydrolysis, the Schiff's base gives 2-amino-1,3-indane dione and ketone as explained above. Further, 2-amino-1,3-indane dione on hydrolysis gives 2-hydroxy indane-1,3-dione.

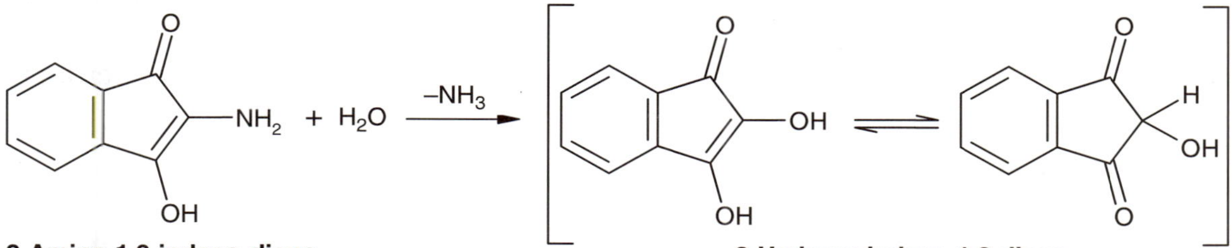

2-Amino-1,3-indane dione **2-Hydroxy indane 1,3-dione**

The 2-amino-1,3-indane dione being a strong reducing agent reduces a part of ninhydrin, then oxidises itself to 2-iminoindane-1,3-dione.

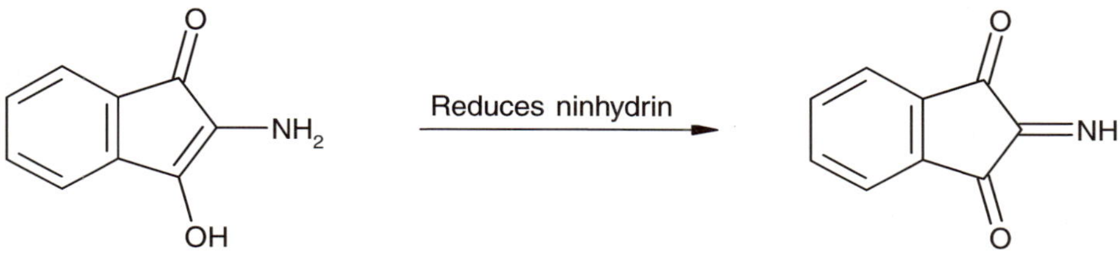

2-Amino-1,3-indane dione **2-Iminoindane-1,3-dione**

Now 2-hydroxy indane-1,3-dione and 2-iminoindane-1,3-dione condense to form azaoxonol which is an anion and responsible for colour.

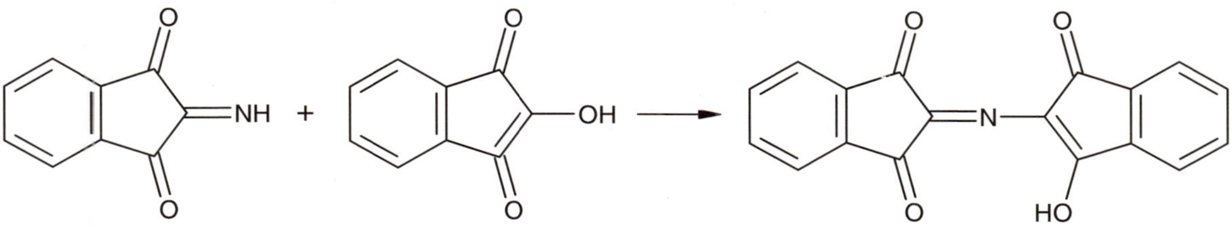

2-Iminoindane-1,3-dione **2-Hydroxyindane-1,3-dione** **Azaoxonol**

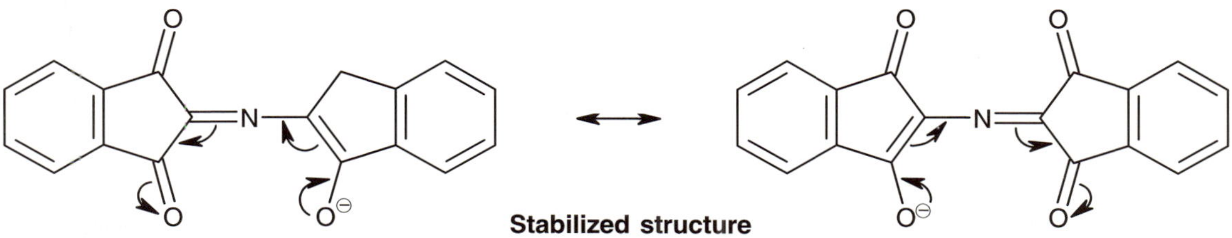

Stabilized structure
(λ_{max} 570 nm)

Reference

1. Pharmaceutical Chemistry (Vol. 2) by H.J. Roth, pp. 212-214.
2. G. Rama Rao & S. Raghuveer. *Eastern Pharmacist*, **25**, 113-114, July 1982.

Methyldopa undergoes Emerson reaction, i.e., reaction with 4-aminophenazone to give coloured product.

Probable Reaction Mechanism

The reaction is based on oxidative coupling in the para position. The presence of an oxidizing agent ($K_3Fe(CN)_6$) is essential for the reaction to proceed. Further, weak alkaline condition (phosphate buffer, pH 8.0) is required for optimal reaction.

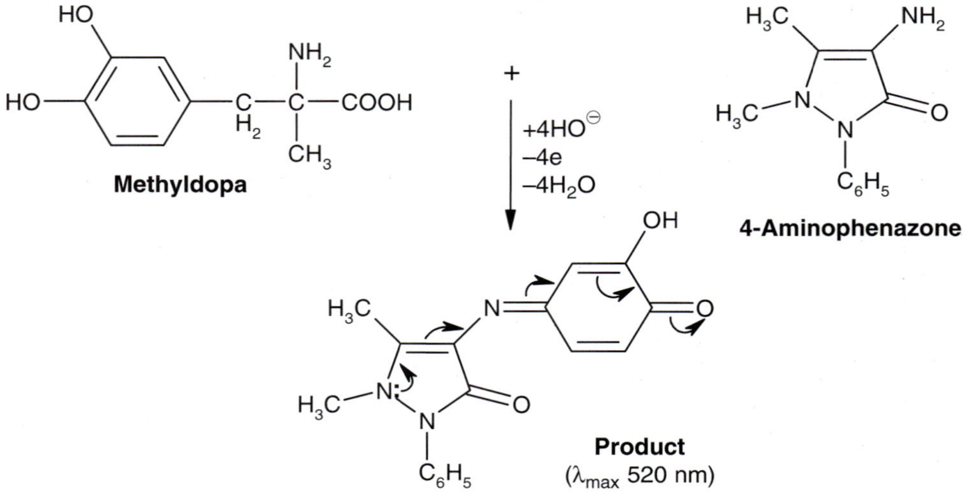

Reference

1. Pharmaceutical Chemistry (Vol. 2) by H.J. Roth, pp. 75-76.
2. *Indian Drugs*, **24(4)**, 199, 1987.

Methyldopa with vicinal phenolic —OH groups couples with Fe(II) in glycine buffer. A chelate is formed as explained below. This chelation has been utilized for quantitative analysis.

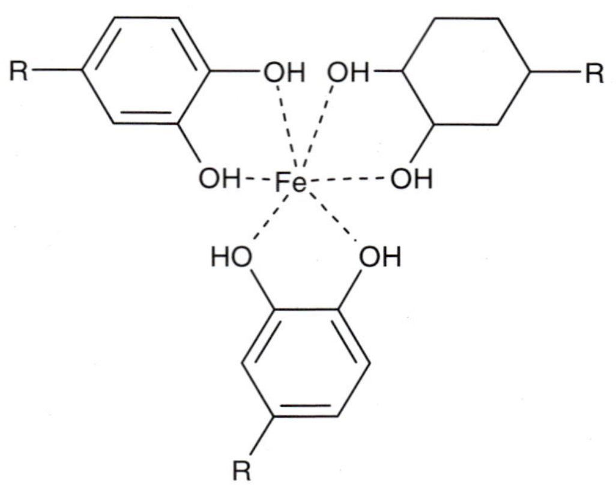

Reference

G. Rama Rao, A. Avadhanulu & R. Giridhar. *Indian Drugs*, **25(9)**, 382, 1988.

Both levodopa and methyldopa react with semicarbazide hydrochloride ($H_2NNHCoNH_2$. HCl) in alkaline medium to give coloured complex (lmax 450 nm). The compound is first oxidized and then couples with the reagent. The reaction is similar to the one described with isoniazid.

Reference

H.D. Devna Siddappa & B. Manju. *Eastern Pharmacist*, p. 117, May 2001.

Benserazide hydrochloride

Suspend accurately weighed quantity of the sample equivalent to 250 mg of the substance in 20 ml of water, add 0.5 ml of nitric acid and titrate with 0.1 N silver nitrate, potentiometrically. Each ml of 0.1 N silver nitrate is equivalent to 29.37 mg of benserazide hydrochloride. 259.21 mg of benserazide ≡ 293.7 mg of benserazide hydrochloride.

The following reactions can be used for the assay of the drug molecule (λ_{max} 272 nm):

1. The primary amine function of hydrazine structure can condense with PDAB to give red Schiff's base.
2. It forms orange-coloured complex with $PdCl_2$.
3. It forms green-coloured complex with $FeCl_3$.

1

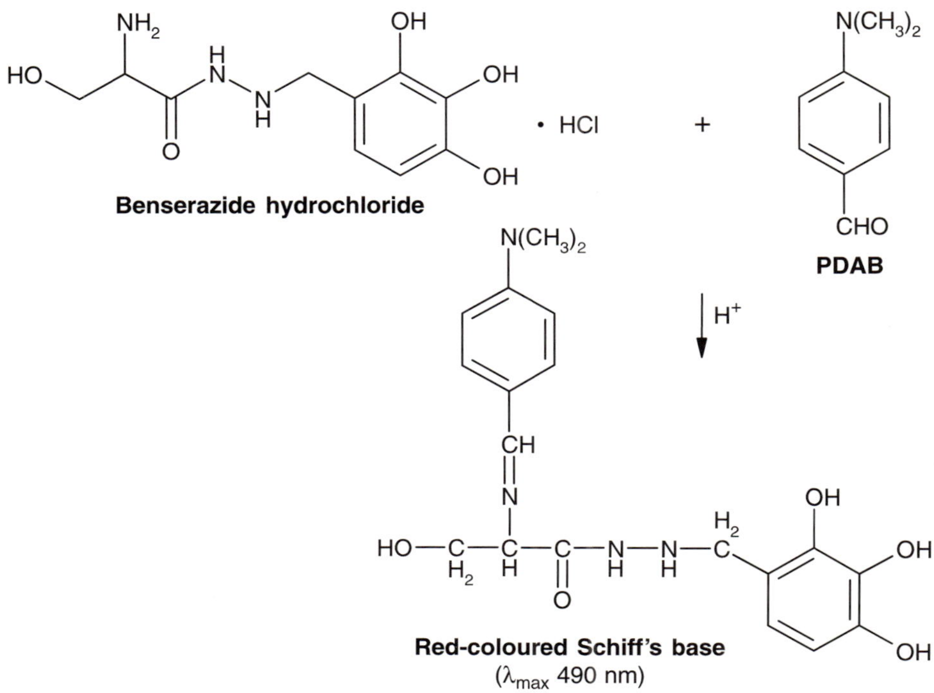

2

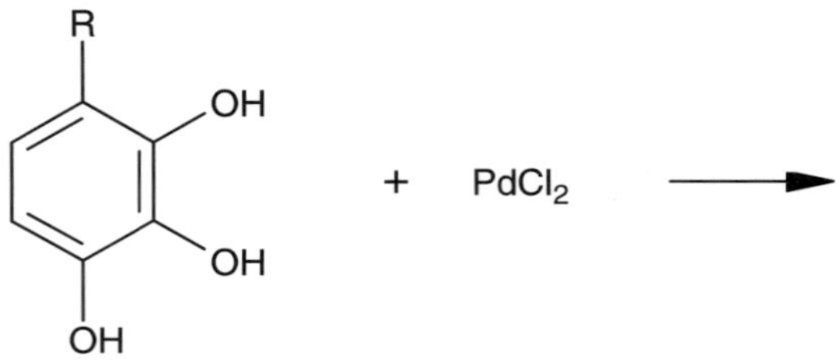

Orange-coloured Pd complex
(λ_{max} 430 nm)

3

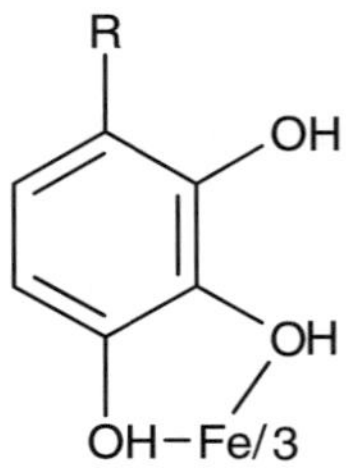

Green iron complex
(λ_{max} 630 nm)

Formulation 17

Isosorbide mono- and di-nitrate, Aspirin

Isosorbide on alkaline hydrolysis (heating in water-bath) yields nitrite salt ($NaNO_2$). Nitrite salt on treating with HCl gives nitrous acid (HNO_2) which causes diazotization of primary amino group of sulphanilic acid. The diazotized product couples with 'NED' to yield coloured product. This indirectly forms the basis of quantitative estimation of isosorbide.

Probable Reaction Mechanism

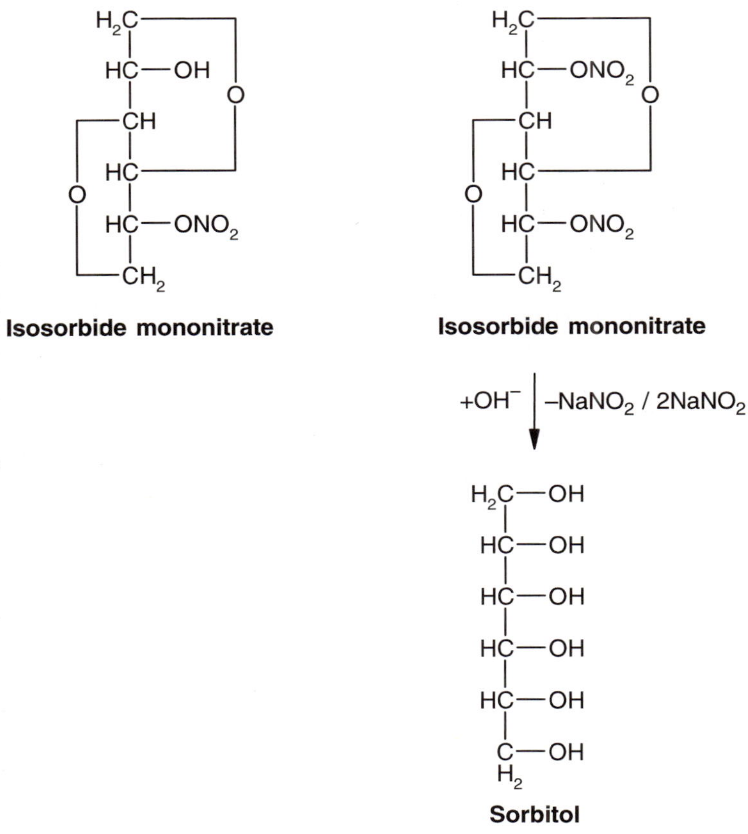

$$NaNO_2 + HCl \longrightarrow HNO_2 + NaCl$$

$$HNO_2 \xrightarrow{H^+} H_2O\overset{+}{N}=O \rightleftharpoons H_2O + \overset{+}{N}=OCl^-$$

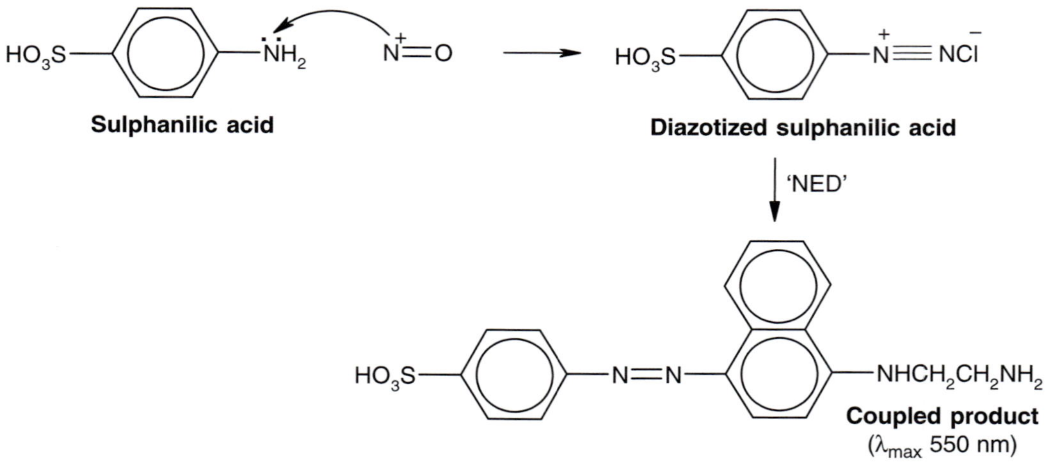

Note

Benzocaine and procaine have also been used for diazotization followed by coupling with 'NED'.

Reference

1. Textbook of Practical Organic Chemistry by Vogel, p. 920.
2. Textbook of Pharmaceutical Analysis by K.A. Connors, p. 225.
3. *Indian Drugs*, **21**, 158, 1984.

Authors have also used benzocaine or procaine as source of primary aromatic amine which can be diazotized as above and coupled with phloroglucinol.

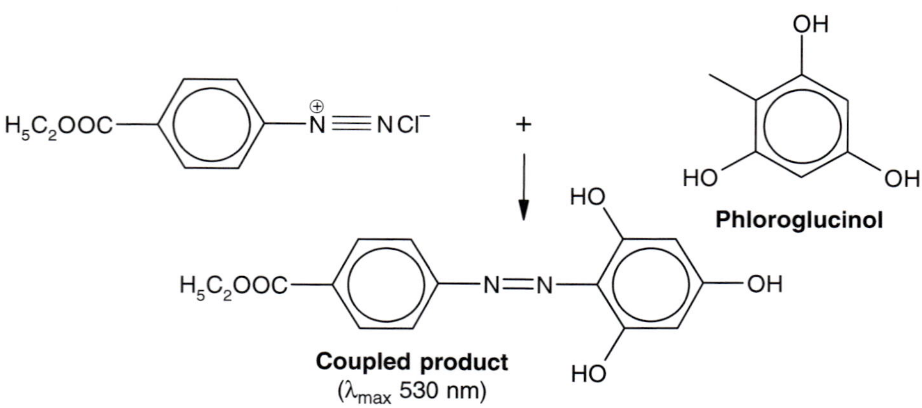

Reference

P.J. Antony & N.M. Sanghavi. Abstract No. C-18, , IPC-1992.

The secondary alcoholic groups of isosorbide are oxidized by the tetrazolium salt in alkaline medium. In this process tetrazolium salt undergoes inductive opening of its heterocyclic ring to give the formazone derivative.

Probable Reaction Mechanism

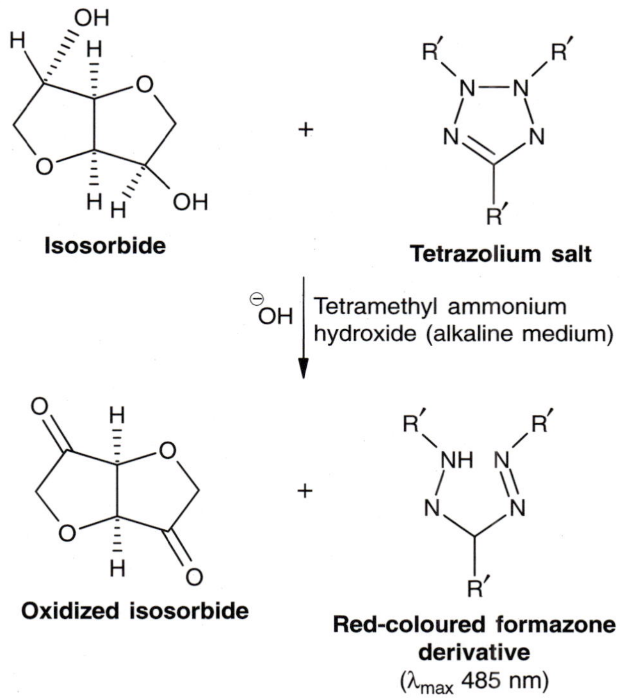

Reference

Indian Drugs, **22(11)**, 237, 1985.

For estimation of aspirin, refer to methods described under chapter on musculoskeletal disorders.

Reaction Mechanism

7

Anti-Inflammatory Drugs

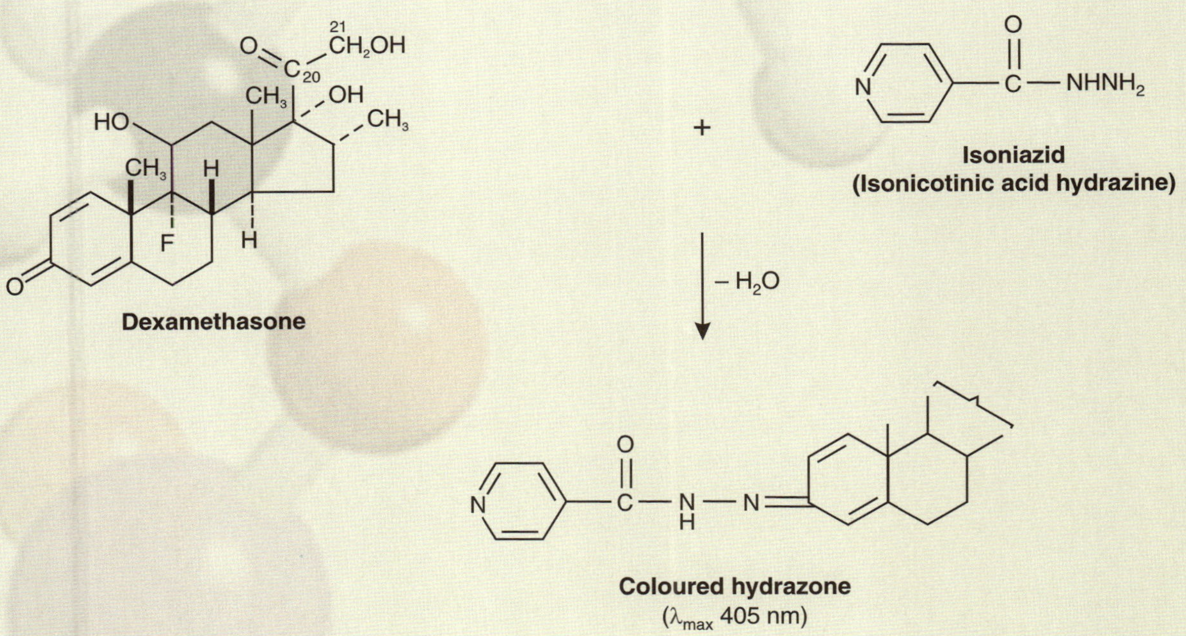

Dexamethasone

Isoniazid (Isonicotinic acid hydrazine)

$- H_2O$

Coloured hydrazone (λ_{max} 405 nm)

Formulation 1

Analgin, Phenylbutazone/Calcium phenylbutazone, Dried aluminium hydroxide gel, Magnesium trisilicate, Diazepam

ESTIMATION

Analgin

METHOD 1

Weigh accurately a quantity of the sample equivalent to 500 mg of analgin and transfer to a 250 ml conical flask. Add 25 ml of alcohol and 5 ml of 0.01 M hydrochloric acid. Shake well to dissolve analgin and titrate immediately with 0.1 N iodine till yellow colour of iodine persists for about 30-60 seconds. Each ml of 0.1 N iodine is equivalent to 0.01757 g of analgin.

The solution is acidified and then slowly titrated with iodine solution. The titration should preferably be carried out below 20°C. Excess of iodine imparts yellow colour to the solution which is end point.

Probable Reaction Mechanism

Another possible reaction mechanism involves oxidation of enolic group present in the molecule.

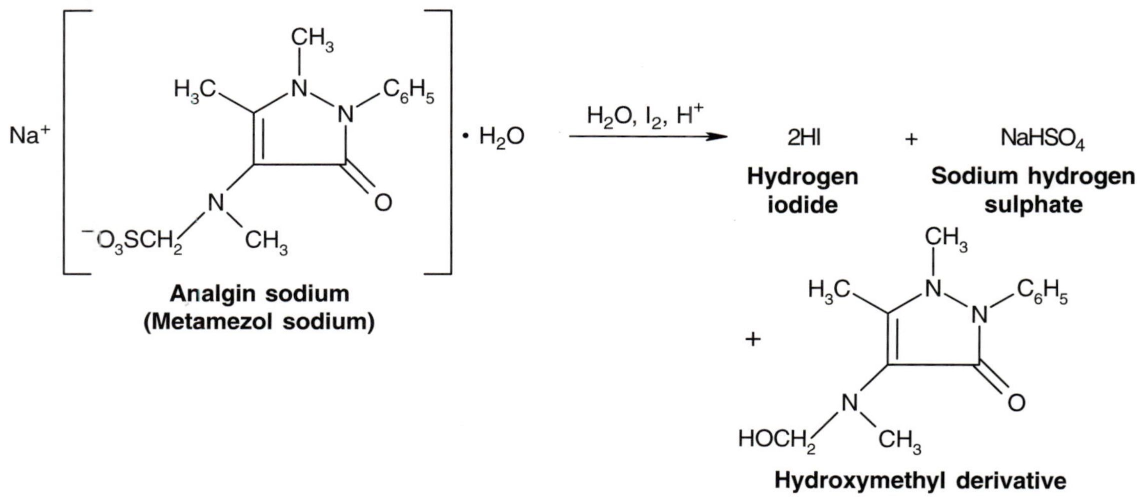

Analgin sodium (Metamezol sodium)

Reference

Pharmaceutical Analysis (Vol. 1), 2nd ed. by A.A. Siddiqui, 2010, pp. 94-95.

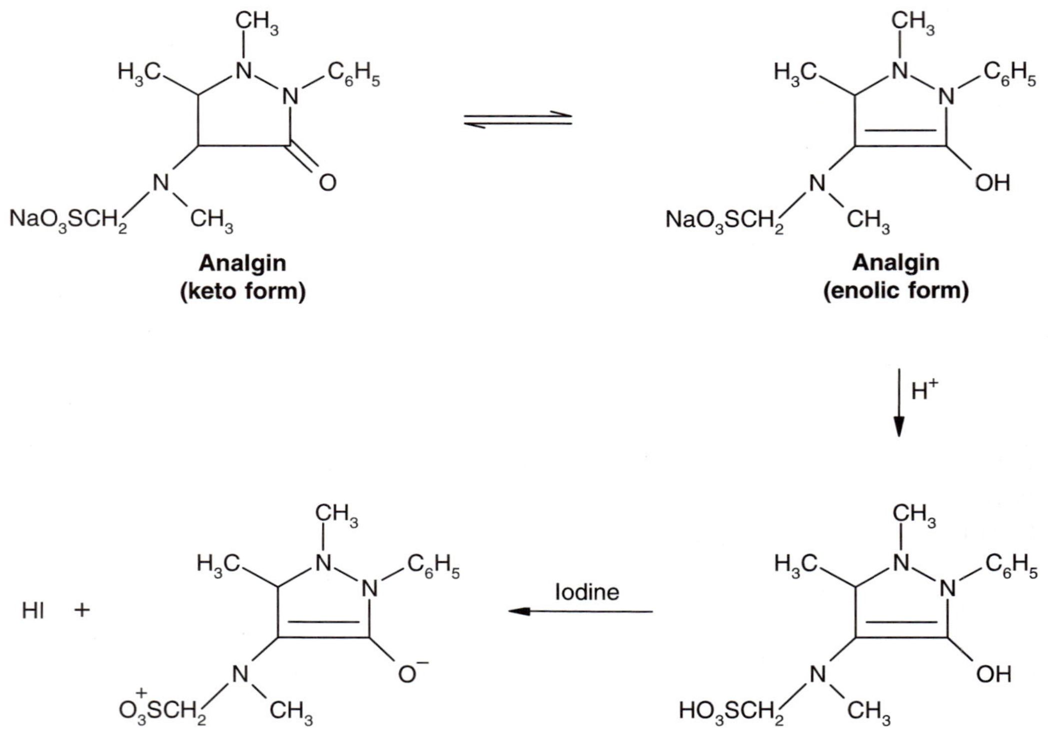

Note

Hydrolysis of aqueous solution yields HCHO, $NaHSO_3$, and methyl amino derivative, hydrolysis being very slow.

METHOD 2

This method involves the formation of formaldehyde which reacts with chromotropic acid to give pink coloured complex with maxima at 550 nm.

Reagents

1. Sulphuric acid (concentrated).
2. 2.5% w/v solution of chromotropic acid (sodium salt) in water.

Standard solution

50 mcg/ml of analgin in water.

Sample solution

Weigh powdered material equivalent to 50 mg of analgin, add about 50 ml of water and allow to stand for 1 hr, shaking occasionally. Make up the volume to 1000 ml with water. Filter, collect the filtrate, rejecting first few millilitres.

Procedure

To 1 ml each of the sample and standard solutions, add drop by drop, 10 ml of sulphuric acid (previously cooled in ice) to each flask, keeping flask in ice-bath. Allow to stand in ice-bath for about 5 minutes. Add 1 ml of chromotropic acid solution and allow to stand in ice-bath for 45 minutes. Bring it to room temperature and measure the extinction of both the solutions at about 550 nm against blank, prepared by using 1 ml of water instead of chromotropic acid solution and calculate the results.

Note

1. Above experiment conducted at room temperature has been found to give reproductive results. The maximum intensity of the colour is obtained within 5 minutes.
2. Paracetamol and caffeine do not interfere.

Probable Reaction Mechanism

On heating the solution to boiling with acid, smell of SO_2 is given off followed by that of formaldehyde. SO_2 can be detected through its reducing action. KIO_3 paper turns blue i.e. SO_2 reduces KIO_3 to iodine which forms blue inclusion complex with starch. Analgin is first hydrolysed to hydroxymethyl derivative and finally to methylamino derivative on loss of HCHO. Formaldehyde so produced as a result of acidic hydrolysis can be estimated by reaction with chromotropic acid or by formation of Schiff's base.

In the first reaction step, formaldehyde condenses with aromatic system of chromotropic acid at ortho position to phenolic-OH in the presence of sulphuric acid acting as dehydrant. In the next step, sulphuric acid acts as oxidizing agent and 3,4,5,6-dibenzoxanthylium cation is formed which is coloured (λ_{max} 530 nm).

The methyl amino derivative, the second hydrolytic product of analgin, reacts with Folin's reagent to give coloured complex which can form the basis of spectrophotometric method of analysis.

Reference

Pharmaceutical Chemistry (Vol. 2) by H.J. Roth, p. 121.

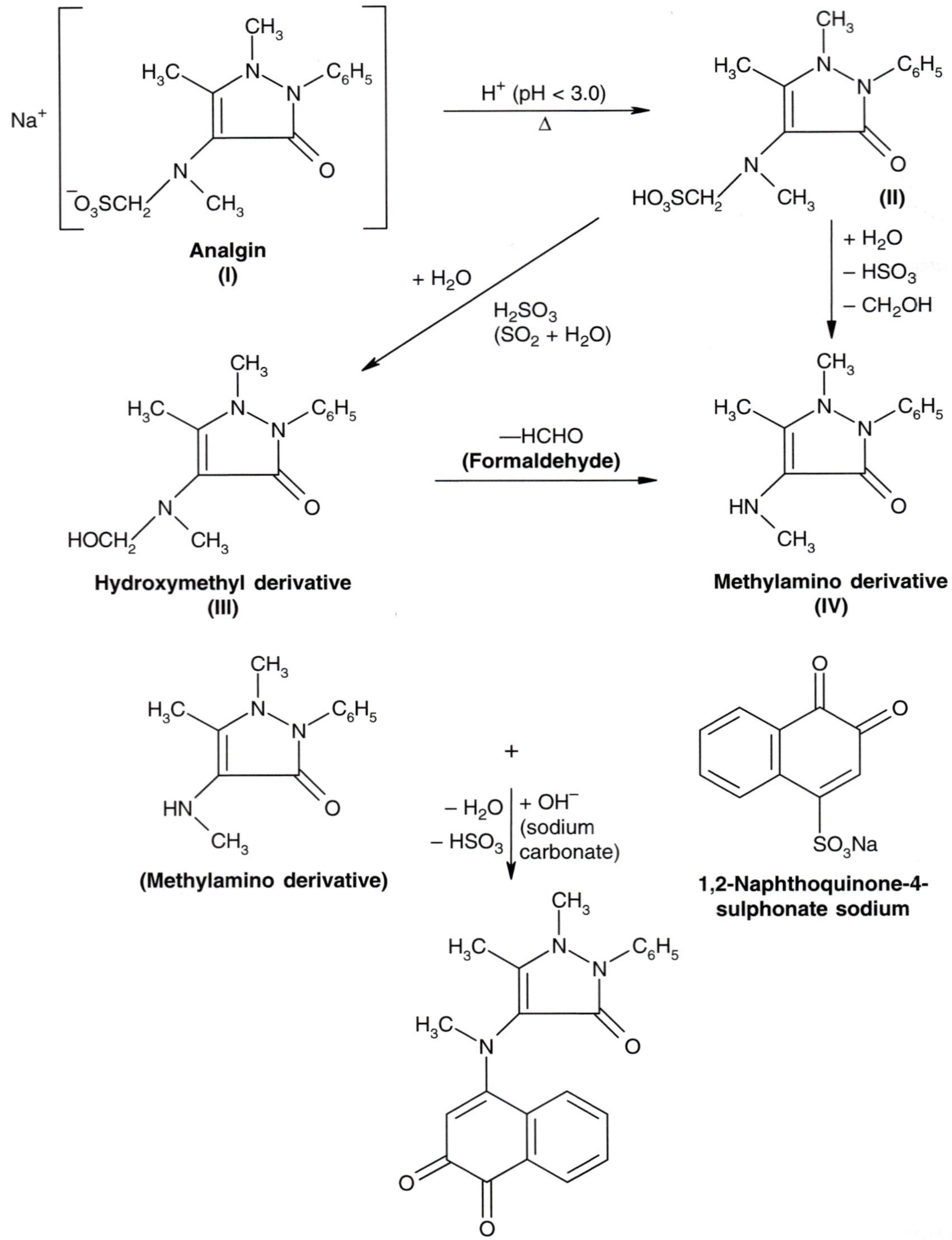

Coloured Michael addition product
(λ_{max} 510 nm)

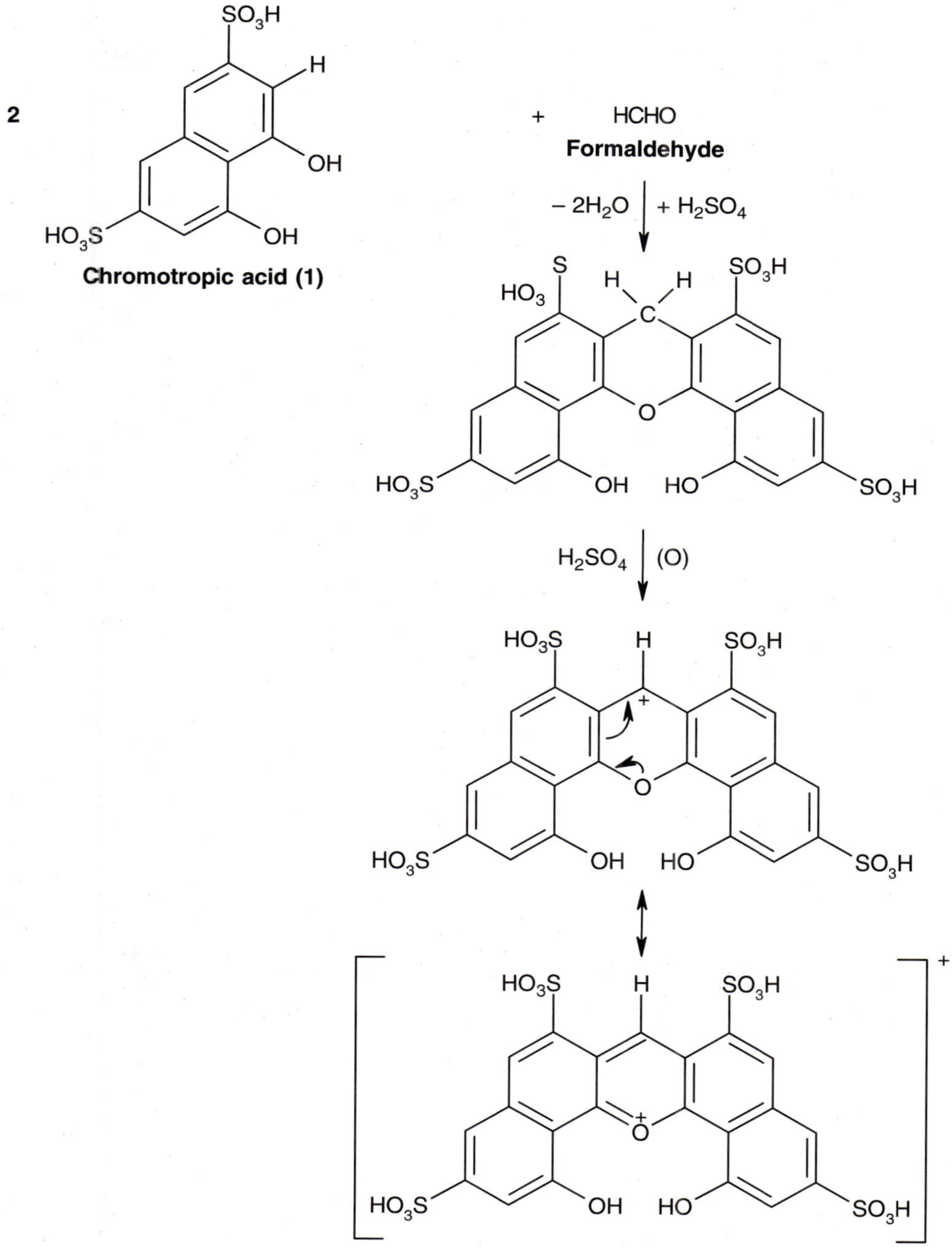

3,4,5,6-Dibenzoxanthylium cation
(λ_{max} 530 nm)

Another possible condensation product, as described by Feigel, is formed by formaldehyde with the para position of phenolic-OH which is also coloured.

Probable Reaction Mechanism

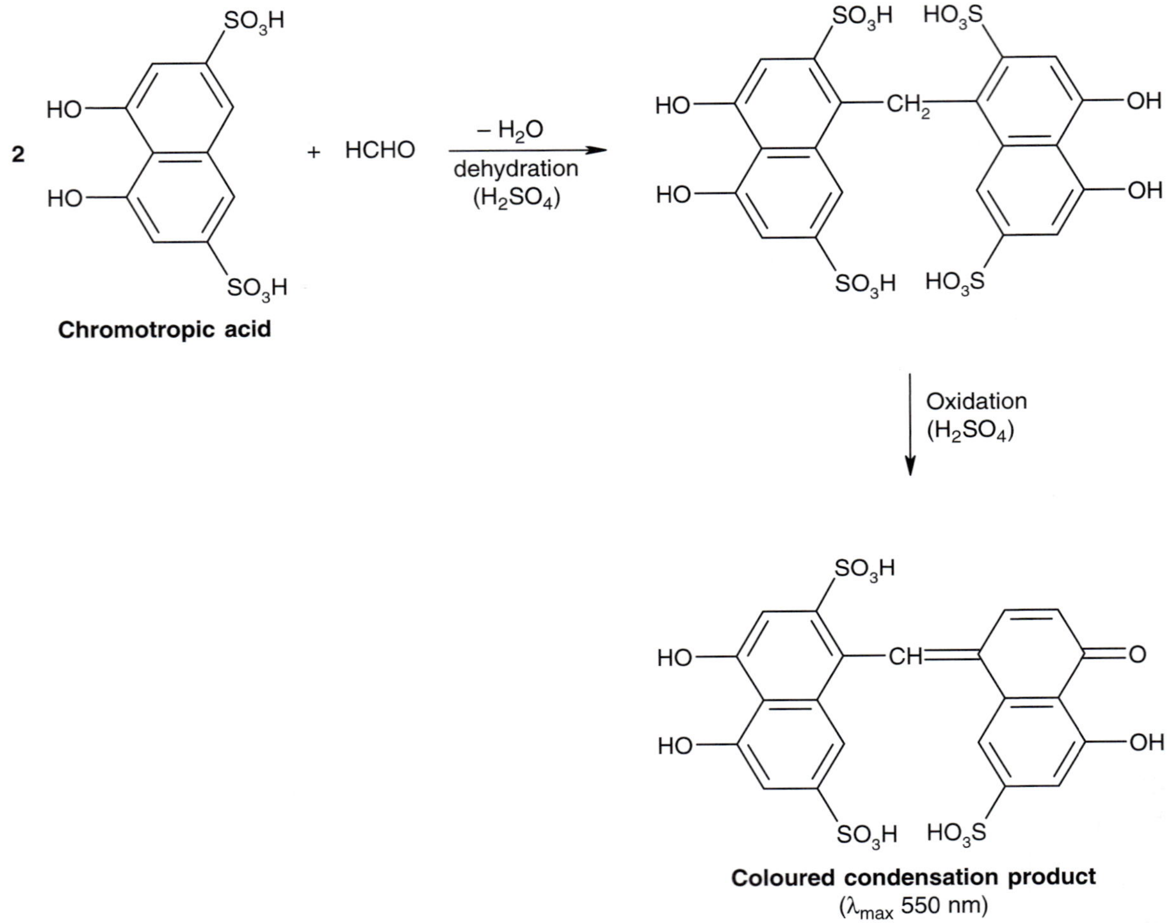

References

1. P.E. Georghiou and C.K. Ho, Canadian J. Chem., 67, 871, 1989.
2. F. Feigel, Spot Tests in Organic Analysis, 7th ed., Elsevier, Amsterdam, pp. 434, 435, 1966.

Analgin undergoes charge-transfer reaction between 7,7,8,8-tetracyano-quinodimethane (TCNQ), π-electron acceptor and the drug (donor) yielding a stable blue colour (λ_{max} 745 nm).

Probable Reaction Mechanism

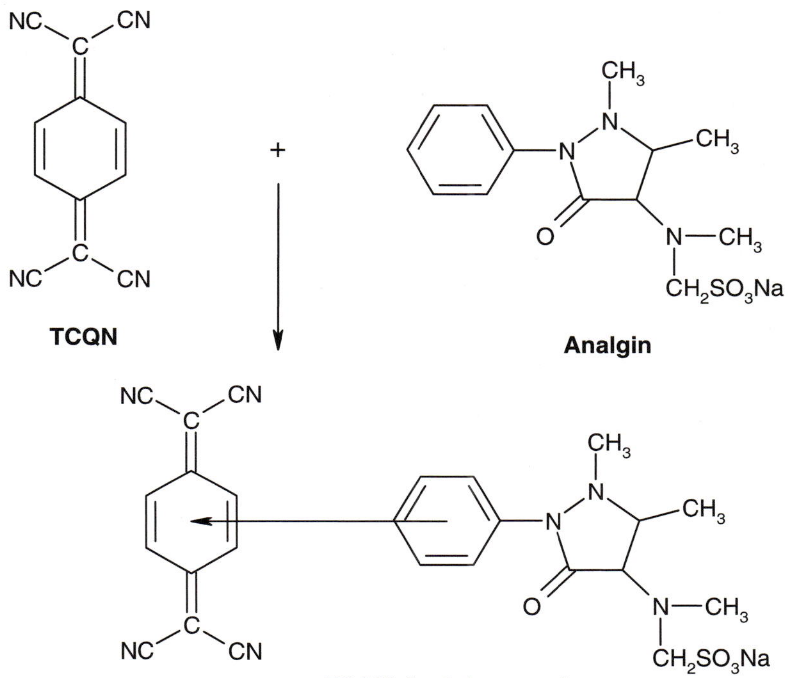

TCQN-Analgin complex
(λ_{max} 745 nm)

Reference

Zhao Feng Lin, Xu Bian-Zhen, Zhang Zhi-Quan & Tong-Shen-Yang. J. Pharm. & Biomed. Analysis, 21, 353-360, 1999.

A spectrophotometric method based on oxidation of analgin by iodate in acidic medium yielding a coloured product has been reported.

Reagents

1. 0.1 M potassium iodate solution.
2. 1 M hydrochloric acid.

Standard solution

500 µg/ml of analgin in water.

Sample solution

Powdered sample equivalent to 2.5 mg of analgin shaken with 30 ml of water for 10 min, filtered through Whatman filter paper No. 42 and the filtrate diluted to 50 ml with water and used for analysis.

Procedure

To 5 ml each of sample and standard solutions, add 0.1 ml of 0.1 M KIO_3, followed by 1 ml of 1 M HCl, allow the reaction mixture to stand at room temperature for 5 min, dilute to 50 ml with water and measure the absorbance of yellow-red colour of both sample and standard solutions at 460 nm against reagent blank.

Note

Aspirin, codeine phosphate, oxyphenbutazone, propyphenazone, phenylbutazone, phenazone, caffeine, diazepam, nicolinemide, dextropropoxyphene, diphenhydramine, dicyclomine and phenobarbitone do not interfere.

Probable Reaction Mechanism

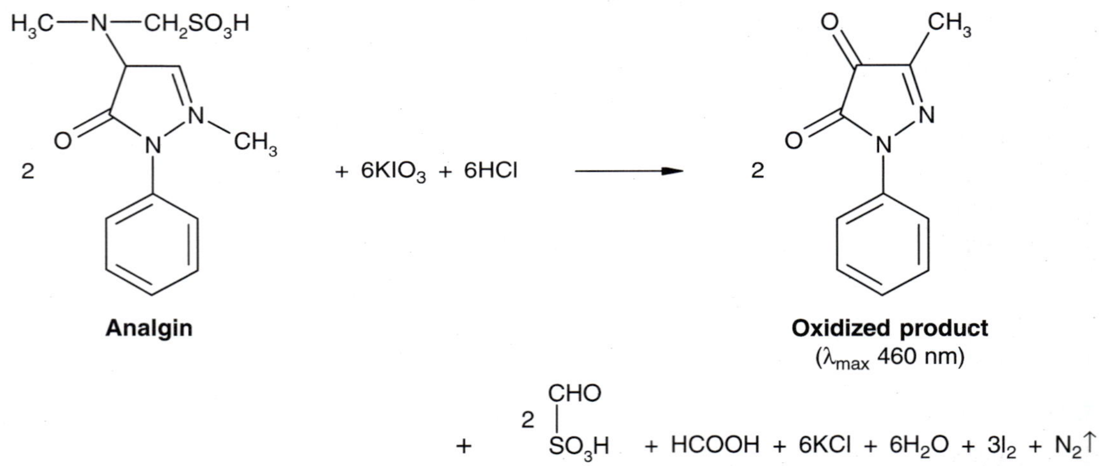

Aluminium hydroxide and Magnesium trisilicate

Preparation of sample solution

Weigh accurately a quantity of the powdered tablets equivalent to 500 mg of aluminium hydroxide in a silica crucible and ash it in a furnace till almost white. Cool and dissolve the ash in 10 ml of concentrated hydrochloric acid. Transfer it into a 100 ml volumetric flask quantitatively, warm if necessary, cool and make up the volume with water.

(a) **Estimation of aluminium** : 25 ml of above sample solution taken in 250 ml conical flask is neutralized with sodium hydroxide solution (Congo red paper). Follow the method 3 for estimation of aluminium described in formulation 1 of the chapter on antacids. Each ml of 0.05 M sodium edetate is equivalent to 0.001349 g of aluminium.

(b) **Estimation of magnesium trisilicate :** To 25 ml of the above sample solution, add 1 g of ammonium chloride and 10 ml or sufficient quantity of triethanolamine to dissolve precipitates. Add 150 ml of water and 5 ml ammonia-ammonium chloride buffer solution. Add few drops of mordant black-II solution as an indicator and titrate immediately with 0.05 M disodium edetate solution till full blue colour is obtained. Each ml of 0.05 M edetate is equivalent to 0.001215 g of magnesium.

Note

Phenylbutazone and oxyphenbutazone tablets are often coated with calcium carbonate which will interfere in the estimation of magnesium as it will consume considerable quantity of edetate solution. The following procedure is recommended in which calcium is first removed as oxalate.

To accurately weighed powder equivalent to 100 mg of magnesium trisilicate, add 2-3 ml of hydrochloric acid and few ml of water. Place on steam-bath for 5-10 minutes to dissolve as much as possible and adjust the volume to 100 ml. Shake well, set aside for 15 minutes and filter. To 15 ml of the filtrate, add 0.5 g of ammonium chloride, 0.5 g of ammonium oxalate and shake to dissolve. Neutralize the solution to litmus paper with dilute ammonia, and then add slight excess. Boil for few minutes and keep at room temperature for 2 h. Filter, wash precipitates 3-4 times with water. The combined filtrate is titrated with 0.02 M edetate for magnesium contents.

Diazepam

METHOD 1

It is hydrolysed to 2-methylamino-5-chlorobenzophenone and yellow colour is measured at 410 nm.

Standard stock solution

Accurately weigh about 100 mg of diazepam standard and transfer to 100 ml volumetric flask, dissolve in alcohol and make volume with alcohol.

Working standard

20 ml of the standard stock solution is diluted to 100 ml with alcohol (200 mcg/ml).

Sample solution

Weigh accurately sample equivalent to 10 mg of diazepam and transfer to 50 ml volumetric flask. Add about 40 ml alcohol, carefully boil for one minute on steam-bath by shaking, cool and dilute to volume with alcohol. Filter solution through Whatman filter paper (No. 1), discard first 10 ml and collect the remaining filtrate.

Procedure

Place 5 ml each of sample and standard solutions in duplicate into separate 100 ml boiling tubes. Add 25 ml of 6 N hydrochloric acid, plug tubes loosely with cotton wool and heat for 1 h in boiling water-bath. Cool to room temperature by dipping in cold water. Extract solution with four 10 ml portions of chloroform. Combine chloroform extracts and make to 50 ml with chloroform in dry volumetric flask. Measure absorbance of both the solutions at about 410 nm against solvent blank. The method obeys Beer's law in the concentration range of 1-30 mcg/ml. Simultaneously take 5 ml aliquot of the sample and standard and treat as above except hydrolysis. Measure their absorbance and subtract the values from the respective hydrolysed values to get net extinction values which are used for calculations.

Note

1. Vitamin B_6, common excipients and colouring agents do not interfere.
2. The method can be applied to other 1,4-benzodiazepines such as chlordiazepoxide.
3. Diazepam usually contains hydrolytic decomposition product. Therefore, to calculate the exact amount of unhydrolysed product before subjecting to acid hydrolysis use unhydrolysed sample as blank.

Explanatory Note

By acidic hydrolysis diazepam decomposes to give 2-methylamino chlorobenzophenone and quinoline derivative. In the analysis of benzodiazepines, the aminobenzophenone which is yellow in colour is important.

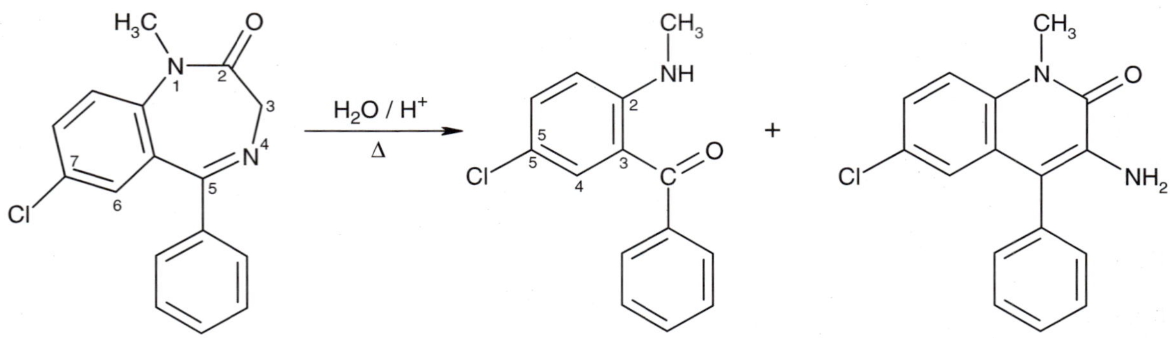

Diazepam **2-Methylamino-5-chlorobenzophenone** (λ_{max} 410 nm) **Quinoline derivative**

Note

2-methylamino-5-chlorobenzophenone so formed can be extracted with chloroform for spectrophotometric analysis.

Reference

T.R. Baggi, S.N. Mahajan & G.R. Rao. J. AoAc, **58**, 875-878, 1979.

METHOD 2

Diazepam hydrolysed to give 2-methylamino-5-chlorobenzophenone and glycine, an amino acid. Method 1 is based on measurement of yellow colour of benzophenone, whereas in this method glycine can be made to react with ninhydrin to give pink colour (λ_{max} 570 nm).

Probable Reaction Mechanism

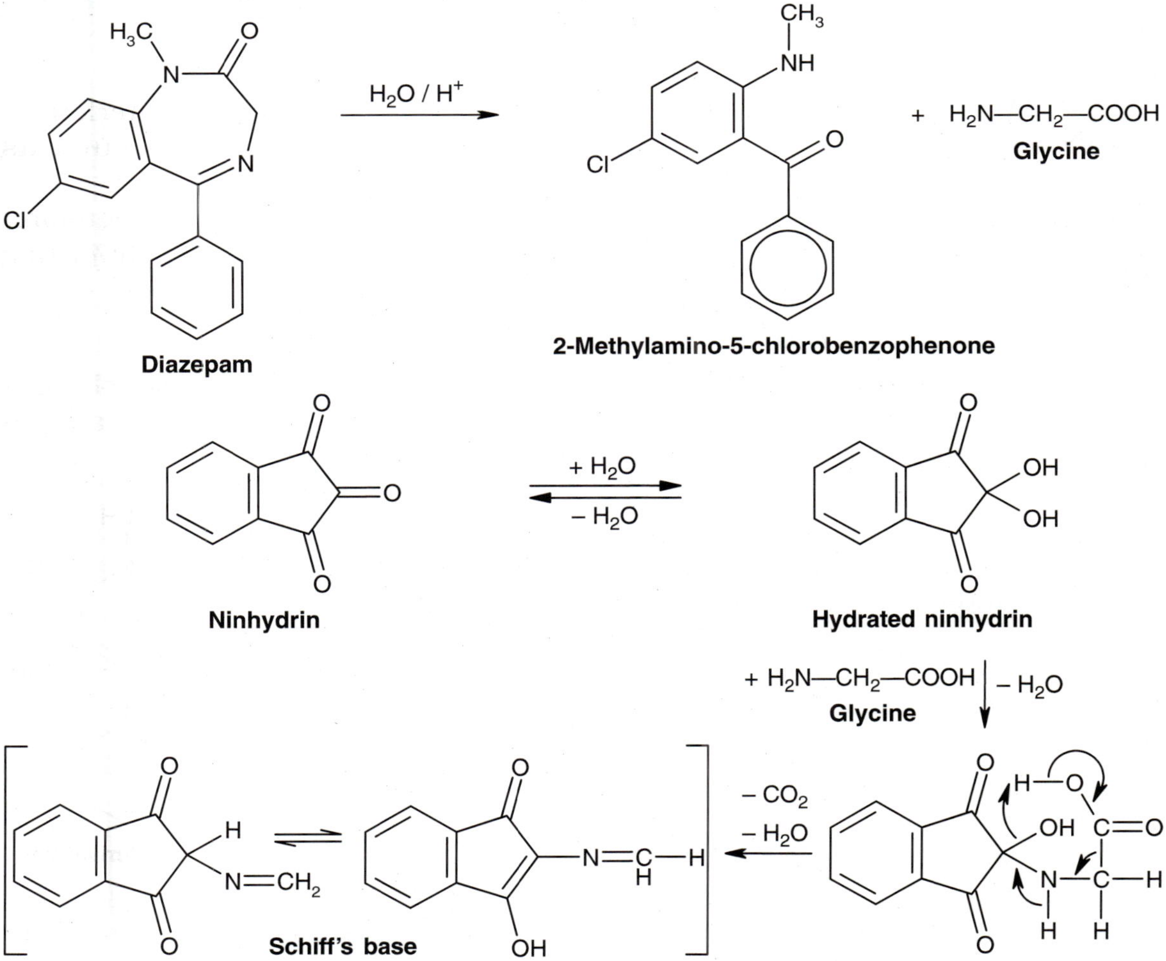

Step 2: The Schiff's base formed gives 2-amino-1,3-indanedione and an aldehyde by hydrolysis.

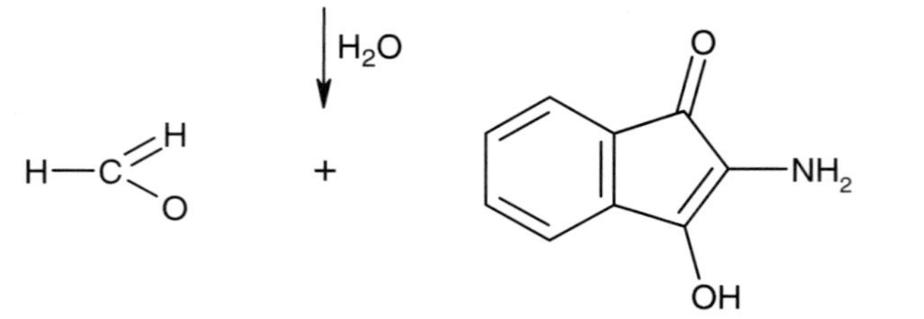

2-Amino-1,3-indanedione (A)

Step 3: Hydrolysis of (A) gives 2-hydroxyindane-1,3-dione (B).

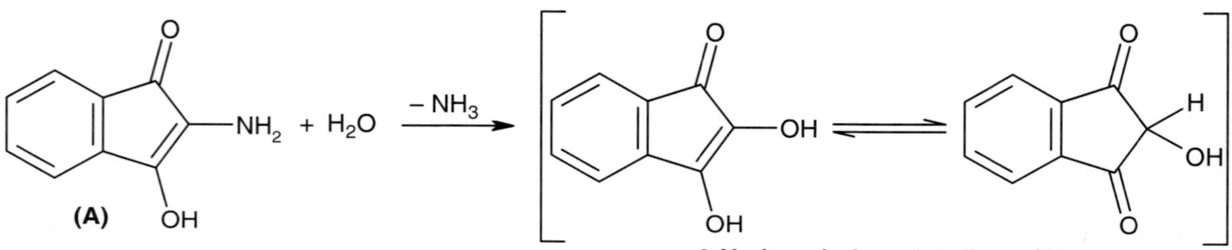

2-Hydroxyindane-1,3-dione (B)

Step 4: (A) i.e. 2-amino-1,3-indanedione behaves as a strong reducing agent and reduces a part of ninhydrin to 2-hydroxyindane-1,3-dione (B).

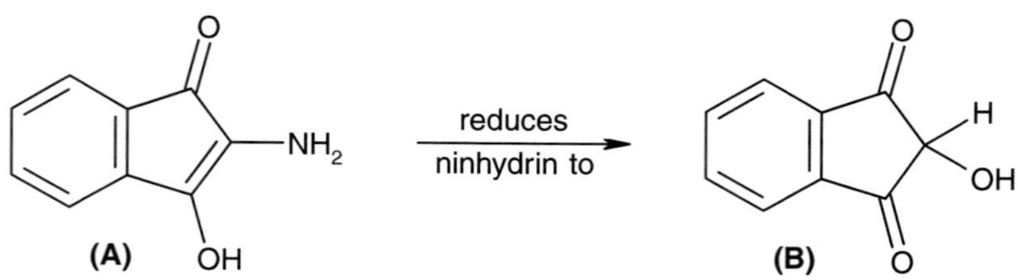

Step 5: 2-hydroxyindane-1,3-dione (A) reduces ninhydrin and oxidizes itself to 2-iminoindane-1,3-dione (C).

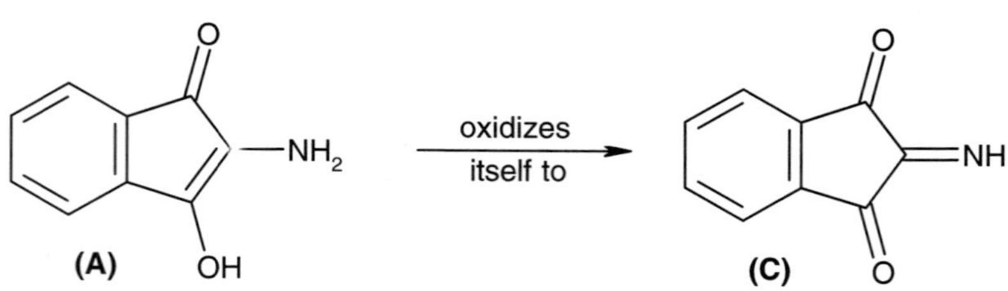

Step 6: (B) and (C) then condense to form azaoxonol which is responsible for the colour. Azaoxonol is an anion and can be represented by mesomeric forms.

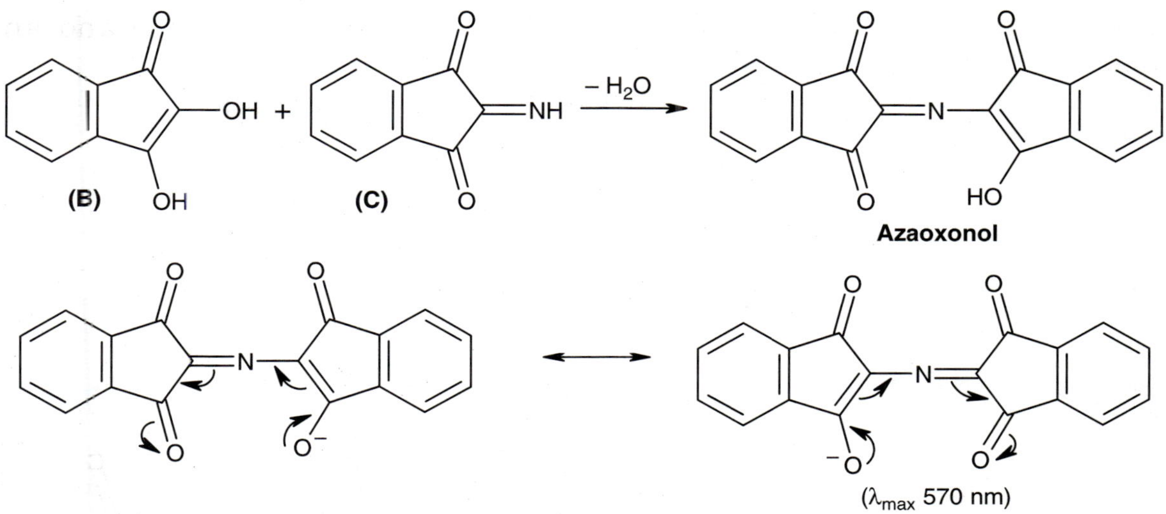

Reference

Pharmaceutical Chemistry (Vol. 2) by H.J. Roth, pp. 212, 213.

On heating with alkali, anion is formed which reacts with m-dinitrobenzene to give coloured derivative.

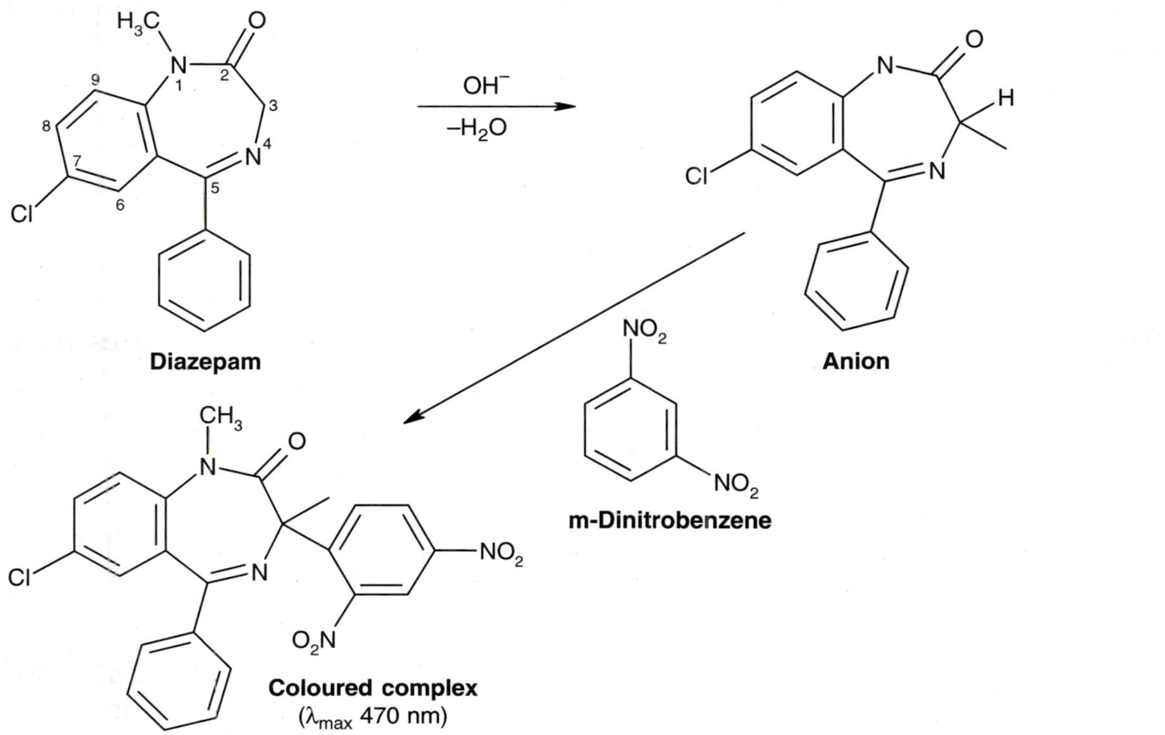

—CH group at position-3 is acidic due to neighbouring oxo-function can also be explored for analytical method. The compounds also react with 2,4-dinitrofluorobenzene in slightly alkaline medium (pH 8.2) to give coloured complex (λ_{max} 368 nm).

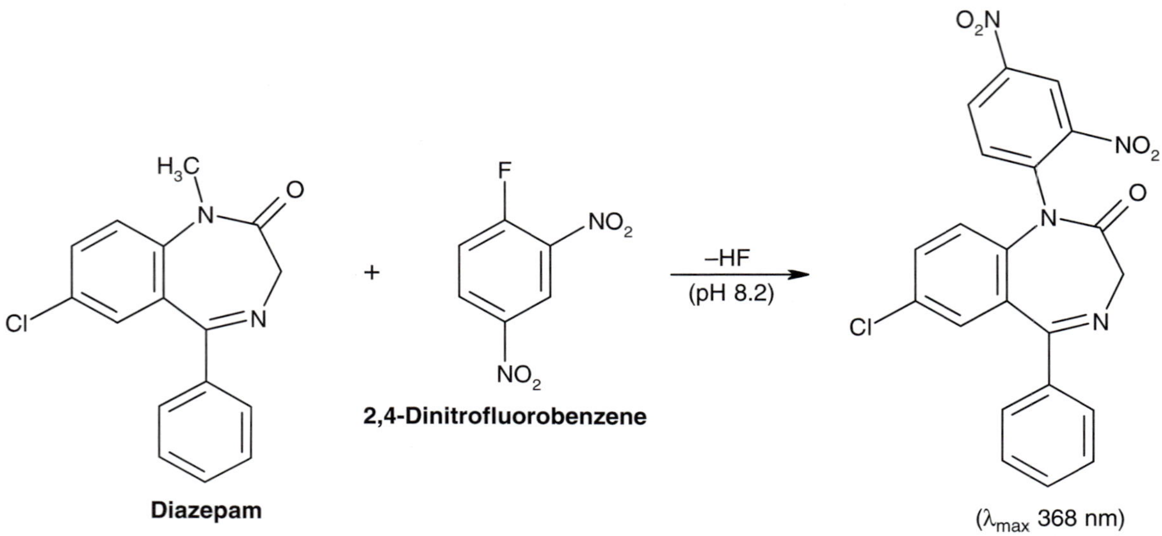

Reference

Indian Drugs, **20(6)**, 232, 1983.

Phenylbutazone/Calcium phenylbutazone

Weigh a quantity of the sample accurately equivalent to 400 mg of phenylbutazone, add 50 ml of neutral acetone (bromothymol blue). Boil on water-bath and filter. Wash the residue with neutral acetone and titrate the combined acetone extract with 0.1 M sodium hydroxide. Each ml of 0.1 M sodium hydroxide is equivalent to 0.03084 g of phenylbutazone or 0.03630 g of calcium phenylbutazone or 0.03302 g of sodium phenylbutazone or 0.03424 g of oxyphenbutazone. Acidimetric titration with sodium hydroxide is based on remarkable 'CH' acidity of phenylbutazone.

Note

1. It has been observed that in formulations containing phenylbutazone and oxyphenbutazone along with magnesium trisilicate, analgin, paracetamol, lower assay values are obtained in respect of phenylbutazone/oxyphenbutazone when determined by the usual method involving acetone extraction, followed by alkaline titration. This problem is more serious

with the older sample. This is probably due to adsorption of phenylbutazone/oxyphenbutazone by magnesium trisilicate. The following method has been found to give satisfactory results:

"Take powder accurately weighed equivalent to 250-300 mg of the substance. Add 25-30 ml of dilute sulphuric acid and heat in boiling water-bath for 30 minutes under reflux condenser. Cool and extract with four 25 ml portions of chloroform or ether. Wash each organic layer with the same 10 ml of water. Evaporate organic layer, the last traces of organic layer should be removed under current of air, otherwise there are chances of decomposition in case of phenylbutazone. Dissolve the residue in neutral acetone and carry out the titration as above. This extraction procedure is also essential for injectible and liquid formulations."

2. Diphenhydramine, salicylamide, thiamine hydrochloride and ascorbic acid do not interfere.
3. Any acidic compound present in the sample shall interfere.

The compound has acid hydrogen at C-4 which can be titrated with NaOH. As an CH-acid compound, it is deprotonated in alkali forming a stabilized anion. Acetone acts as a solvent miscible with water to give homogeneous titration solution.

Probable Reaction Mechanism

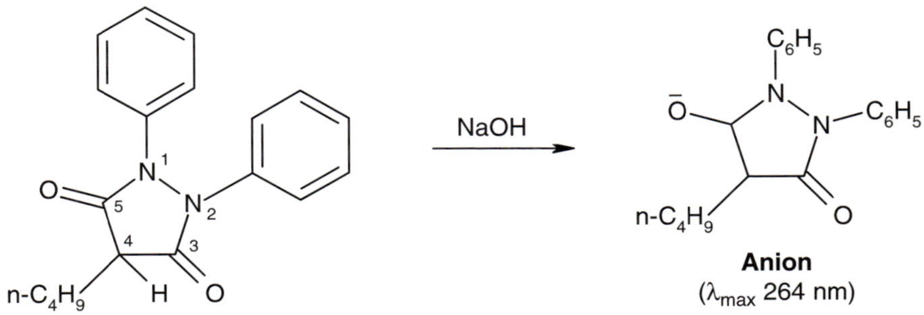

Phenylbutazone

Anion
(λ_{max} 264 nm)

In strong acid solution, the compound undergoes hydrolysis to give butyl malonic acid and hydrazobenzene. Hydrazobenzene so formed undergoes molecular re-arrangement to give benzidine. The benzidine so formed undergoes diazotization followed by coupling with n-(1-naphthyl-ethylene diamine) 2 HCl to give coloured complex (λ_{max} 570 nm), the coupling occurs in position-4.

Probable Reaction Mechanism

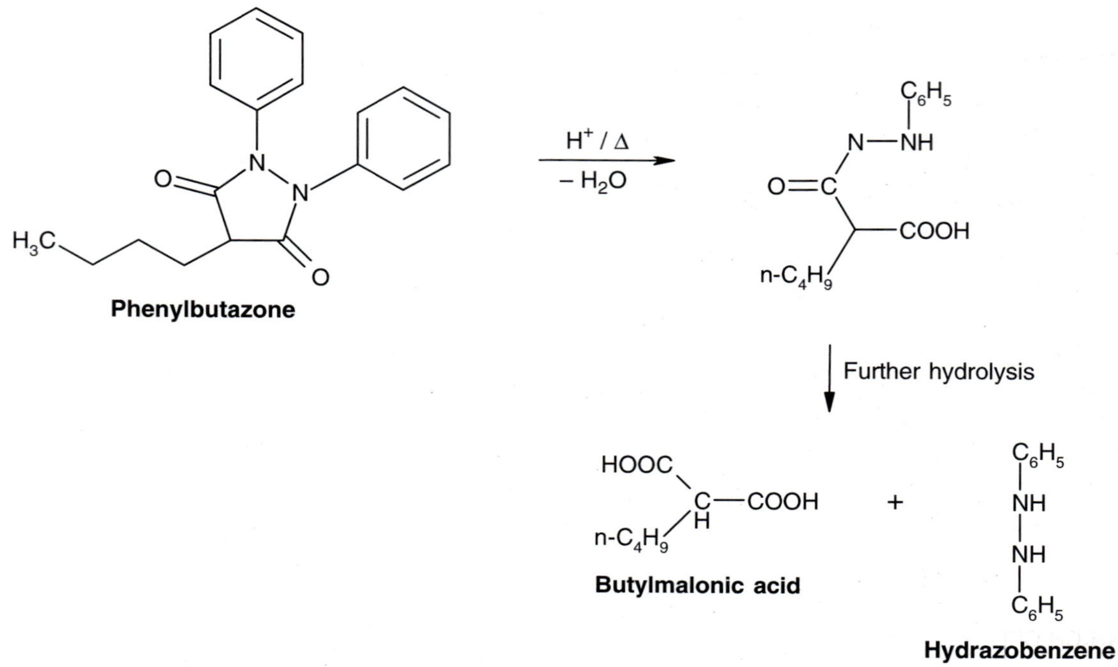

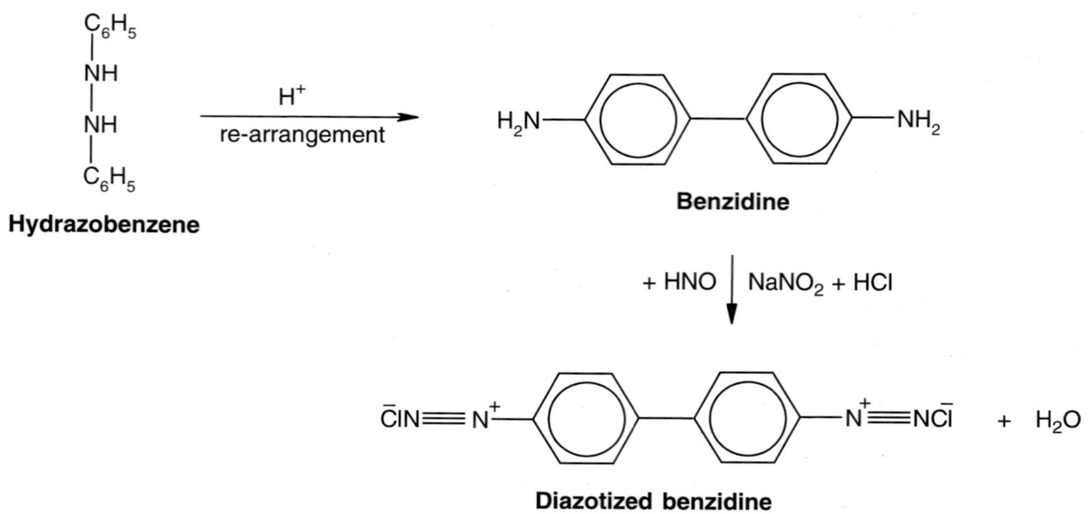

Excess HNO_2 is removed by addition of ammonium sulphamate.

$$HNO2 + H_2NSO_3H \longrightarrow H_2SO_4 + N_2\uparrow + H_2O$$

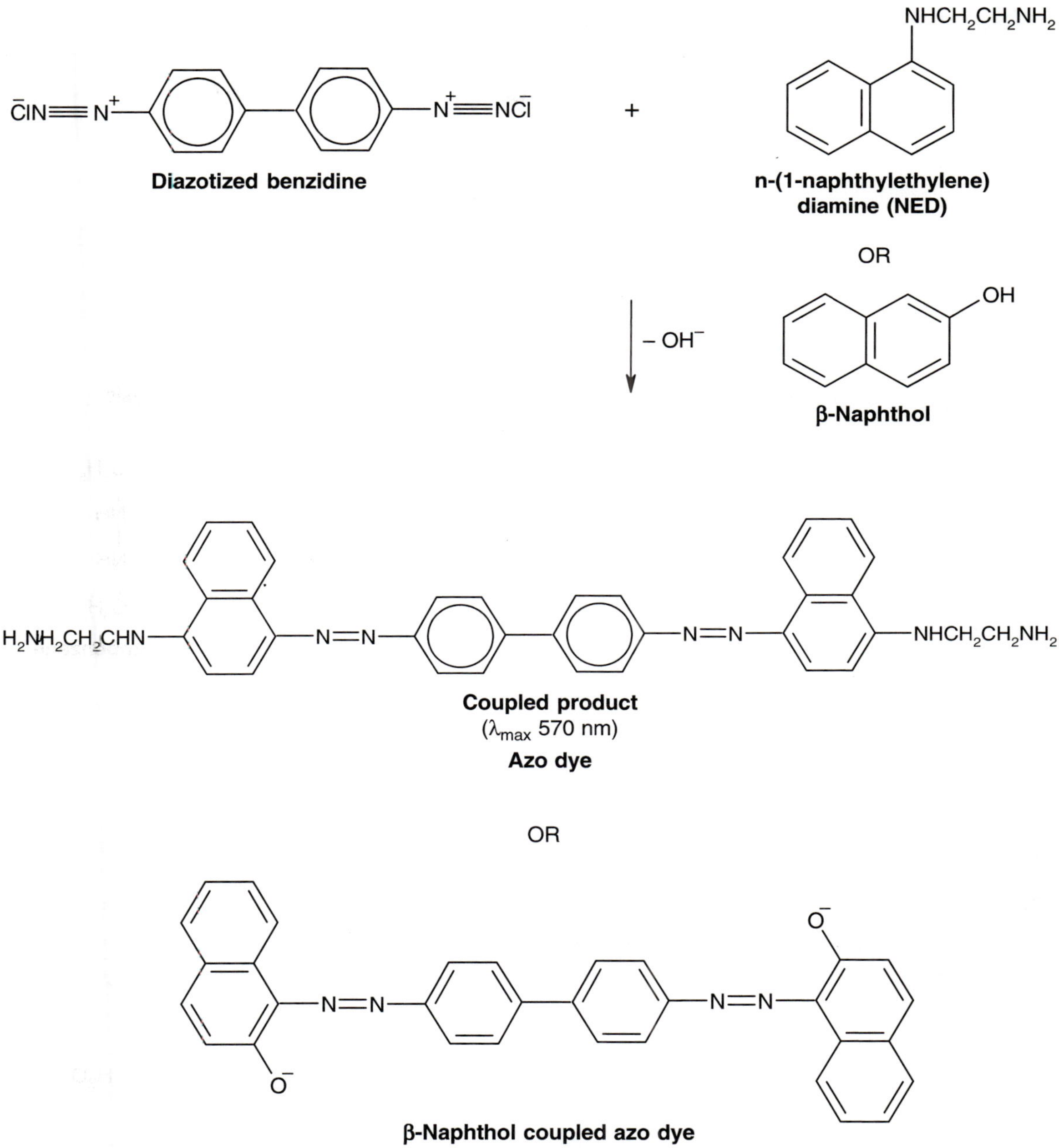

Reference

1. Pharmaceutical Chemistry (Vol. 2) by H.J. Roth, 1991, Ellis Harwood, pp. 510-513, 713.
2. Textbook of Pharmaceutical Analysis by K.A. Connor, 1991, p. 224.

A quantitative colorimetric reaction is possible with diazotized p-nitroaniline in the presence of ethanol and KOH to give an azo dye.

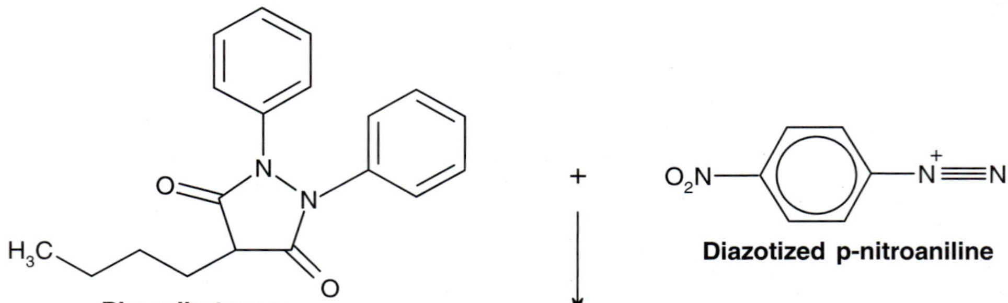

Phenylbutazone

Diazotized p-nitroaniline

As a result of bond cleavage between C_3 and C_4, the following dye with azaoxonol structure is obtained.

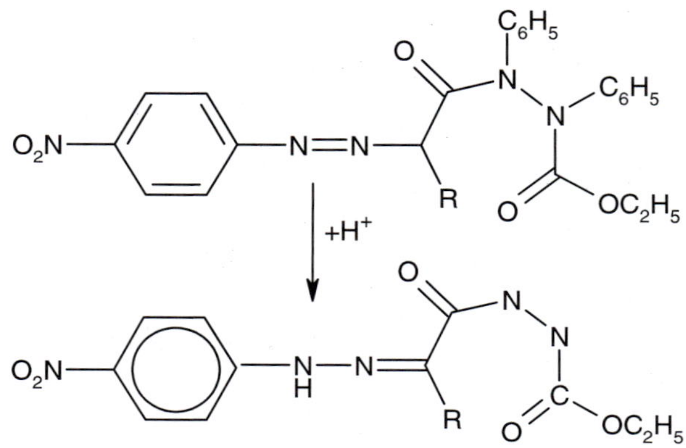

$R = n—C_4H_9$

Reference

Pharmaceutical Chemistry by H.J. Roth, 1991, p. 514.

Note

The compound reacts with electrophilic reagents such as bromine to yield 4-bromophenylbutazone which can form the basis of volumetric analysis.

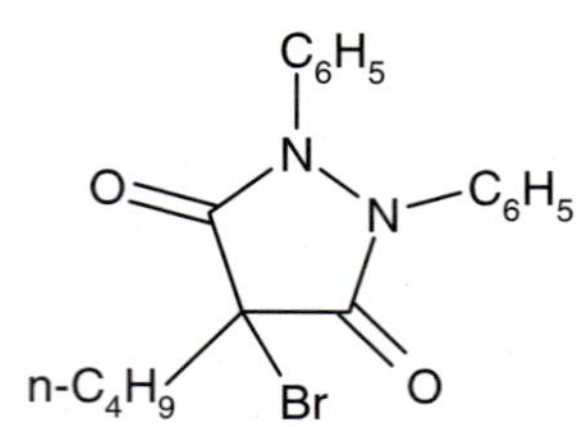

Bromophenylhydrazone

The compound is susceptible to oxidation at C-4 by H_2O, $KMnO_4$, $K_3Fe(CN)_6$ to yield different oxidative products.

Formulation 2

Phenylbutazone, Chloroquine phosphate, Dexamethasone, Meprobamate

ESTIMATION

Phenylbutazone

Accurately weigh and transfer 200 mg of powdered tablets, into a 250 ml separatory funnel. Add 20 ml of water, shake to suspend and acidify. Extract with four 40 ml portions of chloroform and collect all the chloroform extract in one separatory funnel. Wash the chloroform extracts with 40 ml of water. Filter organic layer through anhydrous sodium sulphate into dry 250 ml conical flask. Evaporate the chloroform on water bath (see instructions under 'note' given in estimation of phenylbutazone in formulation-1 of this chapter). Dissolve the residue in 50 ml of hot and previously neutralised acetone. Carry out the titration and calculation as described for this compound in formulation-1 of this chapter.

Chloroquine phosphate

Follow the method described in formulation- of the chapter on anti-diarrhoeals based on the reaction of phosphate moiety of the compound with ammonium molybdate.

Meprobamate

Reagents

1. 1% w/v solution of furfuraldehyde in glacial acetic acid (furfuraldehyde must be distilled before use to get a clear yellow solution).

Standard solution

1 mg/ml of Meprobamate in acetone.

Sample solution

Weigh accurately sample equivalent to 50 mg of meprobamate and extract with acetone to produce 50 ml (1 mg/ml).

Procedure

To 1 ml of sample and standard solutions, add 0.5 ml of furfuraldehyde solution, mix and add 10 ml of hydrochloric acid. Mix and measure the absorbance of both the solutions at maximum at about 585 nm, exactly 45 seconds after addition of concentrated hydrochloric acid.

Probable Reaction Mechanism

The compound forms Schiff's base as explained below:

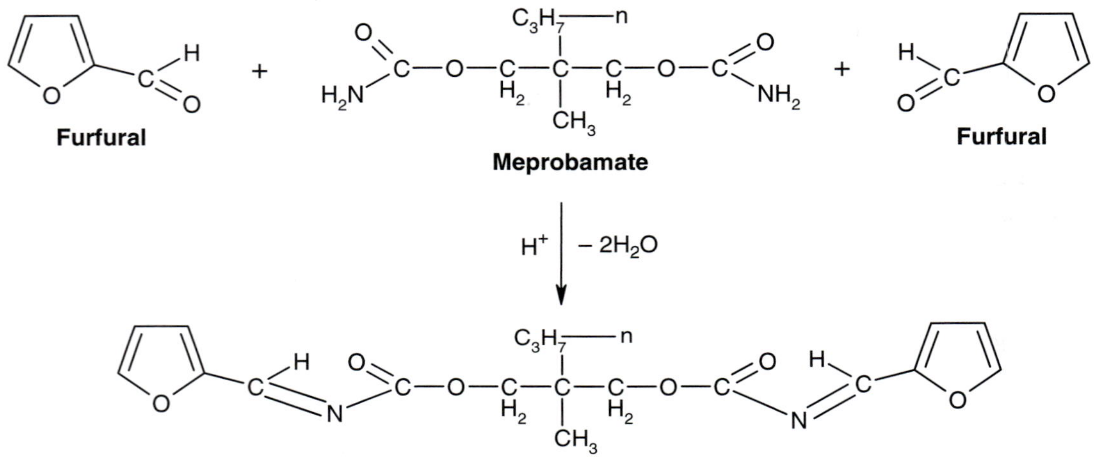

Coloured chromogen
(λ_{max} 585 nm)

On heating with ethanolic potassium hydroxide, cyanate is formed which reacts with Co(2) to give blue tetracyanocobalt (λ_{max} 610 nm).

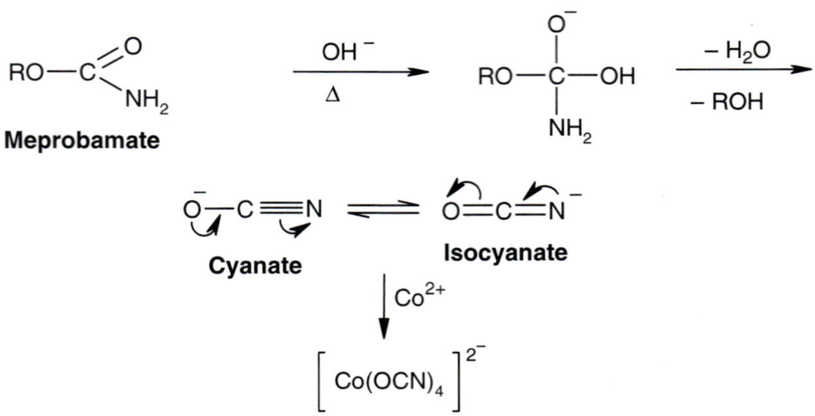

Tetracyanocobalt complex
(λ_{max} 610 nm)

Note

This test can be used for quantitative estimation of meprobamate in formulations.

When treated with conc. acid or alkali, the compound is hydrolysed to give a diol and ammonia which can be estimated (Kjeldahl method).

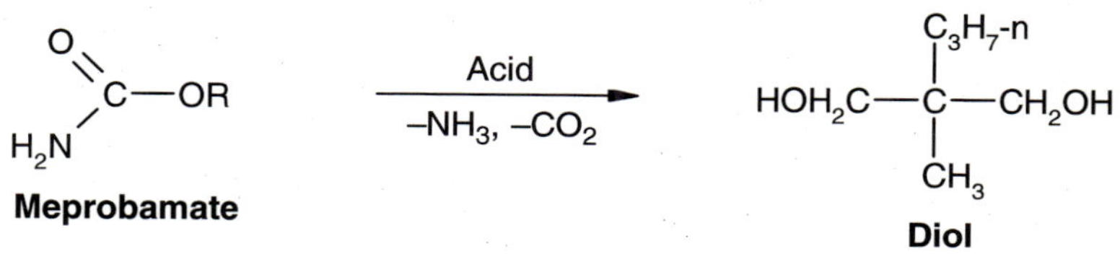

The diol on treating with sulphuric acid is converted to carbonyl compound which condenses with PDAB to give coloured compound (λ_{max} 510 nm).

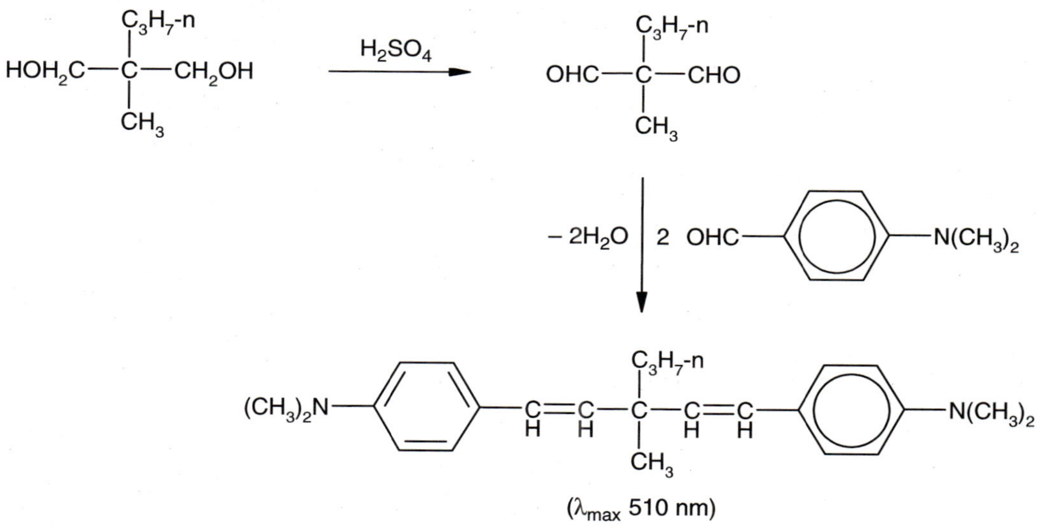

This test is similar to the one for isopropyl alcohol.

Dexamethasone

Reagents

1. Dichloromethane.
2. Isoniazid reagent : Dissolve 500 mg of isoniazid in 250 ml of methanol, add 0.63 ml of hydrochloric acid and adjust the volume to 500 ml with methanol.

Preparation of standard solution

Accurately weigh and transfer 20 mg of dexamethasone, standard to a 200 ml volumetric flask containing 150 ml methanol. Dissolve and make up the volume (100 mcg/ml).

Preparation of sample solution

Accurately weigh and transfer powdered tablets equivalent to 2.5 mg of dexamethasone into 250 ml dry separatory funnel. Add 12 ml of water, shake well to suspend. Extract with 100 ml of dichloromethane for 20 minutes. Allow the organic layer to separate. Filter the dichloromethane layer into another separatory funnel. Repeat extraction with 50 ml of dichloromethane. Filter dichloromethane layer into the same separatory funnel. Extract organic layer with 15 ml 0.1 N sodium hydroxide and reject the alkali layer. Then extract with 15 ml of 0.1 N hydrochloric acid and reject the acid layer. Collect the dichloromethane layer into 250 ml dry conical flask through anhydrous sodium sulphate. Evaporate to dryness on water bath. Dissolve the residue in 10 ml of methanol, shake and transfer into dry 25 ml volumetric flask. Repeat twice each with 5 ml of methanol. Finally make up the volume with methanol. If extract is not clear, filter and use clear filtrate for colour development.

Procedure

To 2 ml each of sample and standard solutions, add 8 ml of methanol and 10 ml of isoniazid reagent, use 10 ml of methanol for blank.

Warm all the flasks in water bath at 50 ± 2°C for 45 minutes. Cool and make up the volume to 25 ml with methanol. Mix and measure extinction of the sample and standard solutions at 410 nm against reagent blank on a suitable spectrophotometer. Calculate the content of dexamethasone by comparison.

Note

1. Prevent incorporation of moisture, as it reduces the intensity of the final colour.
2. Addition of hydrochloric acid to isoniazid reagent should be very accurate as excessive acid reduces the sensitivity of the method.
3. Instead of heating, if after addition of isoniazid reagent, the solutions are kept in the dark at room temperature for 45 minutes and than made up to the volume, the method works equally well. The method obeys Beer's law in the range of 7-17 mcg/ml.
4. Phenylbutazone/oxyphenbutazone, paracetamol, analgin, meprobamate, theophylline, papaverine and chlorzoxazone cause suppression of the colour.

5. Chloramphenicol and diazepam enhance the colour.
6. Chlorpheniramine maleate, atropine sulphate, benzocaine, chlordiazepoxide and antacids do not interfere.
7. If the formulations contain acidic substances like phenylbutazone, the total layer should be shaken twice each with 10 ml 0.1 N sodium hydroxide.
8. If the preparation contain basic substances, the organic layer should be shaken twice each with 10 ml of 0.1 N hydrochloric acid.
9. The aqueous layer will retain neutral substances if present in the formulations.

Probable Reaction Mechanism

The reaction with INH reagent is called Umberger reaction. This reaction is answered by 3-keto steroids and have enone system i.e. α-β-unsaturated ketones and also by steroids with a dienone structure like dexamethasone.

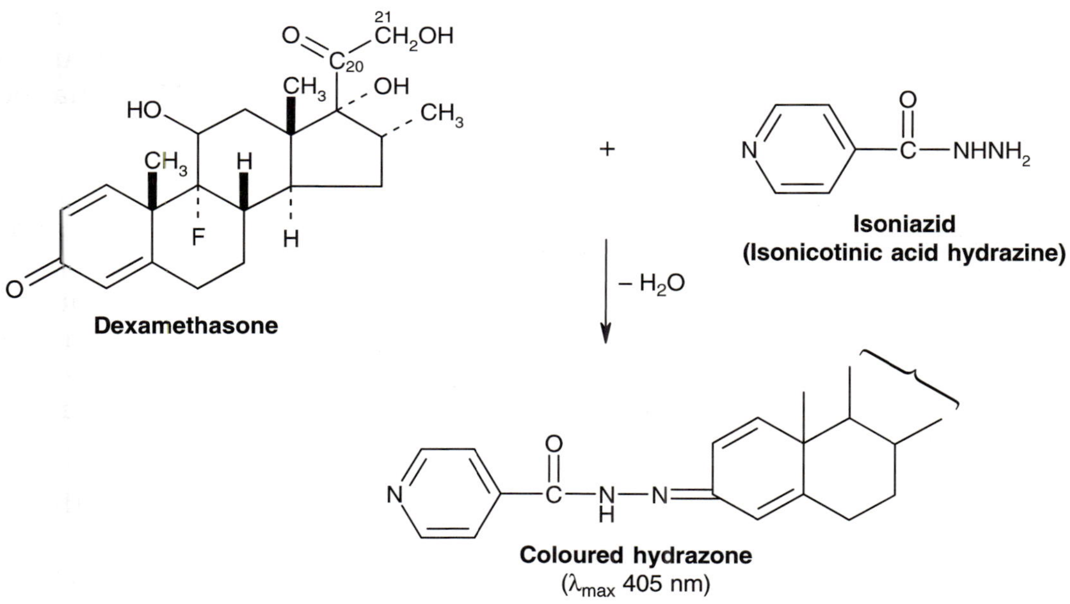

Note

The steroids with dienone structure display a maximum at 238 nm, whereas steroids with enone function i.e. α-β-unsaturated ketone exhibit maximum at 240 nm (239-244 nm). Because of α-ketol structure, all corticosteroids react with triphenyltetrazolium chloride (TTC) in alkaline medium. TTC undergoes reductive opening of heterocyclic ring in alkaline medium to give formazone (λ_{max} 485 nm).

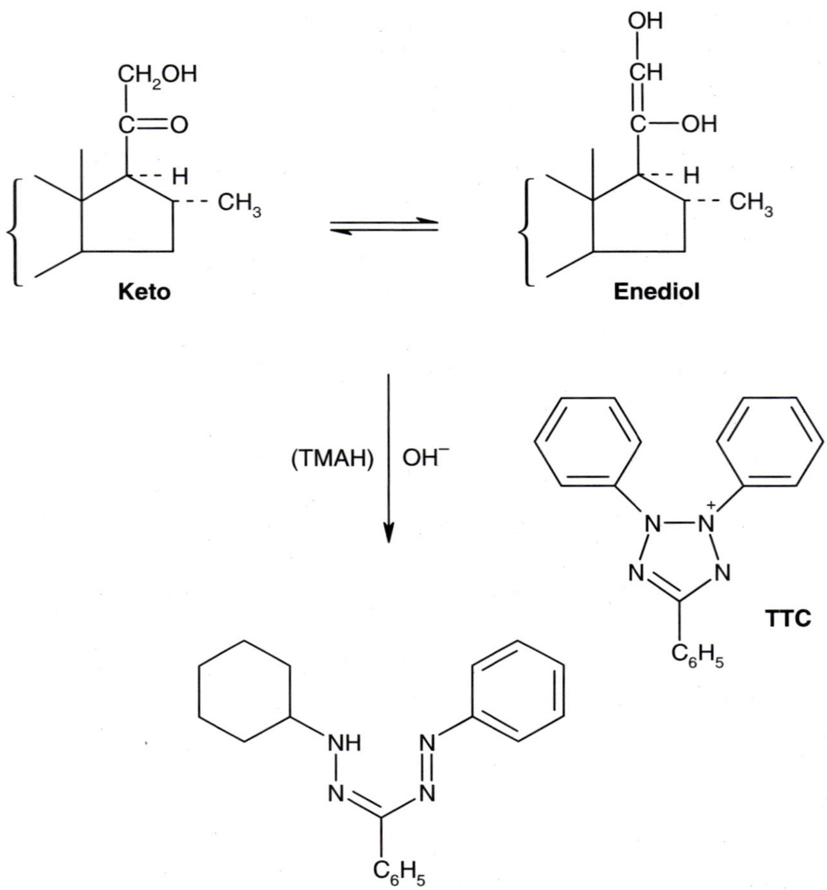

Red triphenylformazone
(λ_{max} 485 nm)

Note

Betamethasone also answers similar reactions.

Reference

Pharmaceutical Chemistry (Vol. 2 - Drug Analysis), H.J. Roth et al., Ellis Harwood, 1991, pp. 465-470.

Both dexamethasone and betamethasone answer Porter-Silber reaction i.e. reaction with phenylhydrazine. On heating with sulphuric acid, CH_2OH group is oxidized to aldehyde (—CHO). This aldehyde couples with phenyl hydrazine to give a stable yellow-coloured cation (λ_{max} 410 nm).

Probable Reaction Mechanism

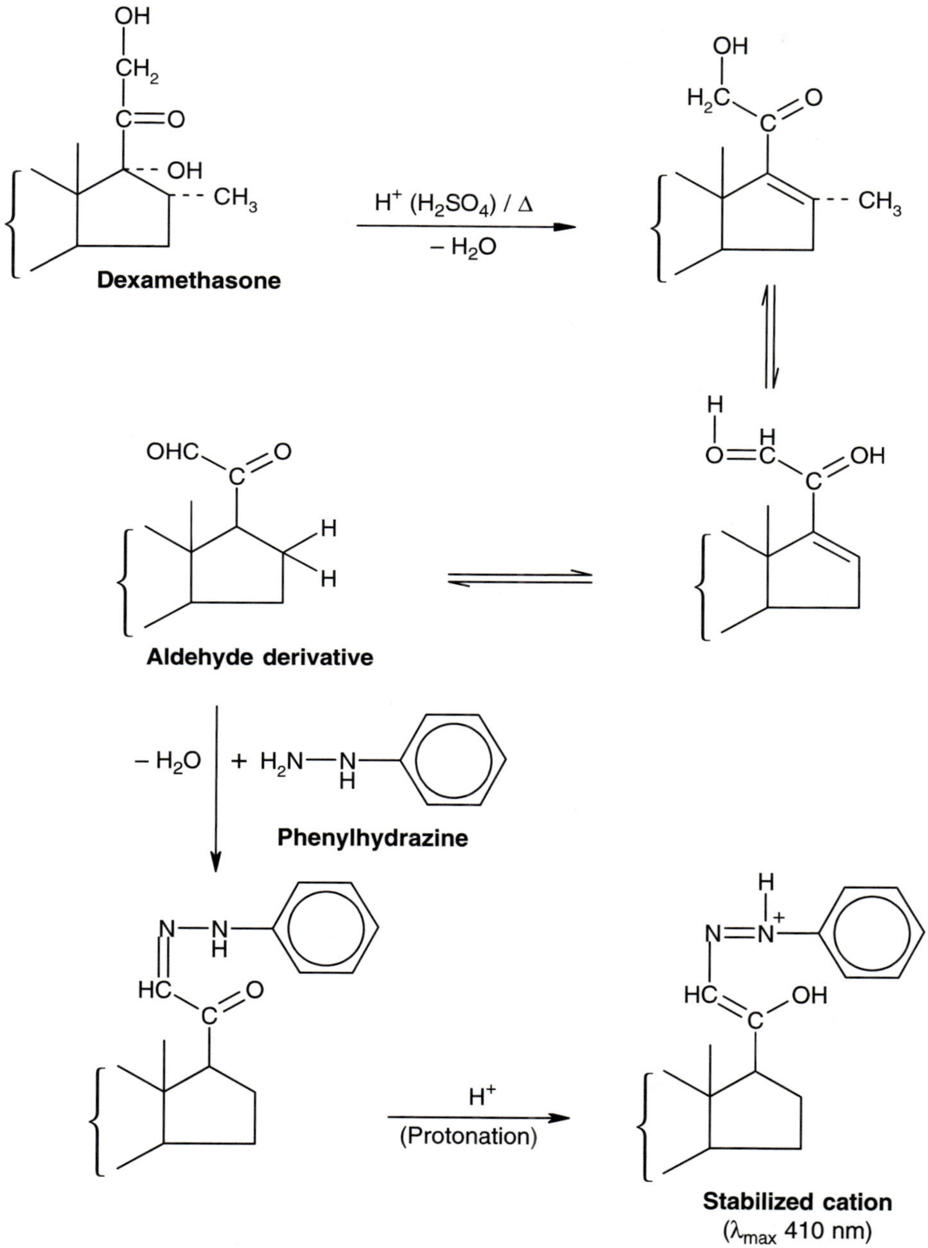

Reference

Pharmaceutical Chemistry (Vol. 2 - Drug Analysis), H.J. Roth et al., Ellis Harwood, 1991, p. 471.

Formulation 3

Aspirin, Oxyphenbutazone, Diazepam, Dried aluminium hydroxide gel

ESTIMATION

Oxyphenbutazone

METHOD 1

This is based on pH induced changes.

Standard solution

20 mg of the pure substance is dissolved in 25 ml of ethyl alcohol and diluted to 200 ml with water, 100 mcg/ml (A).

(a) 5 ml of solution (A) is diluted to 50 ml with 0.01 N sodium hydroxide (10 mcg/ml).

(b) 5 ml of solution (A) is diluted to 50 ml with 0.01 N sulphuric acid (10 mcg/ml).

Sample solution

Accurately weighed quantity of the sample equivalent to 20 mg of oxyphenbutazone is extracted with alcohol and diluted with water to get 100 mcg/ml. Further dilutions are carried out with acid alkali as described under standard solution to get solution (a) and (b).

Procedure

Record the extinction of solution (a) of both standard and sample solutions against solution (b) as blank. Both standard and sample solutions exhibit maximum at about 260 nm. The results are calculated by comparison.

Note

As a CH at position-4 imparts acidic character to the compound, it is depronated in alkali giving λ_{max} at 254 nm. Further, phenolic hydroxy group is also converted to phenolate leading to bathochromic shift in absorption maxima from 254 nm to 264 nm.

METHOD 2

Reagents

1. 1% w/v solution of vanillin in glacial acetic acid.
2. 4% w/v solution of p-dimethylaminobenzaldehyde (PDAB) in glacial acetic acid.

Standard solution

1 mg/ml of oxyphenbutazone in glacial acetic acid.

Sample solution

Weigh accurately sample equivalent to 100 mg of oxyphenbutazone and extract with five 15 ml portions of glacial acetic acid. Filter through G_4 glass sintered funnel, wash the funnel with glacial acetic acid and dilute the filtrate to 100 ml with glacial acetic acid.

Procedure

To 1 ml each of the standard and sample solutions, add 2 ml of hydrochloric acid and keep on water-bath for 30 minutes, cool under running water. To each flask, add 2 ml of either vanillin or 'PDAB' reagent and dilute to 10 ml with glacial acetic acid. Keep for 10 minutes and measure the absorbance of both the solutions as about 424 nm (vanillin reagent) and at 406 nm (dimethylaminobenzaldehyde reagent) using respective reagent blank.

Explanatory Note

Heating the drug with hydrochloric acid in the presence of glacial acetic acid leads to the formation of aniline and p-nitrophenol (first there is cleavage of N-N bond and then hydrolysis of amide structure takes place). Both the products formed can form Schiff's base with vanillin or p-dimethylaminobenzaldehyde.

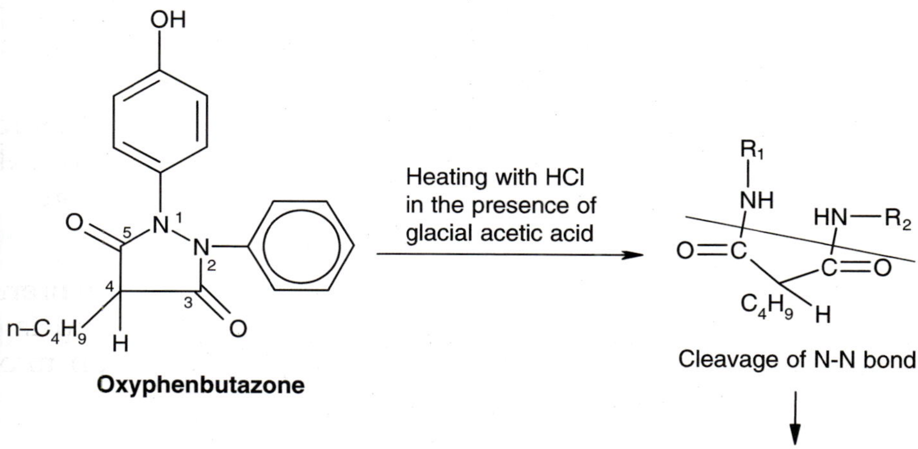

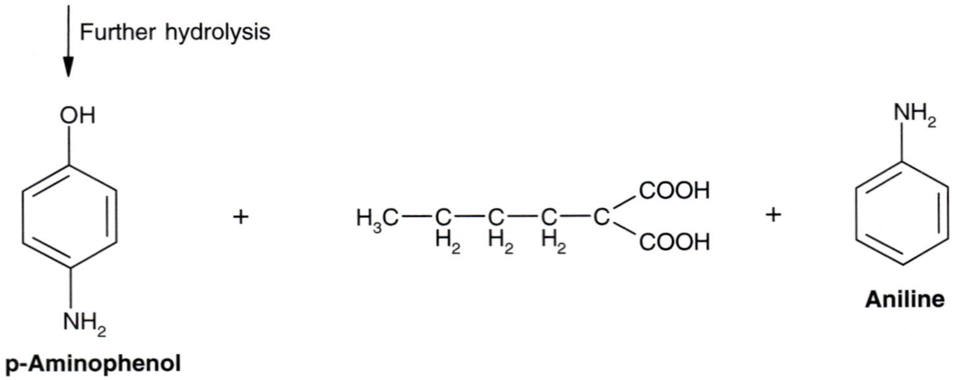

Reference

M. Qureshi, S.Z. Qureshi, H.S. Rathore and A. Mohammed. The J. Physical Chemistry, 79, 116, 1975.

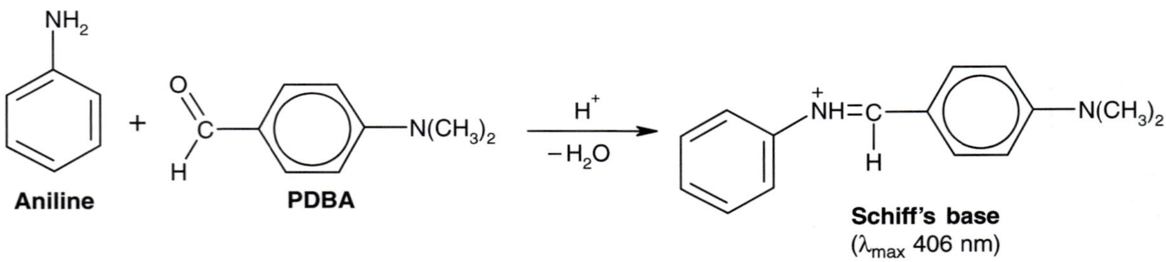

OR

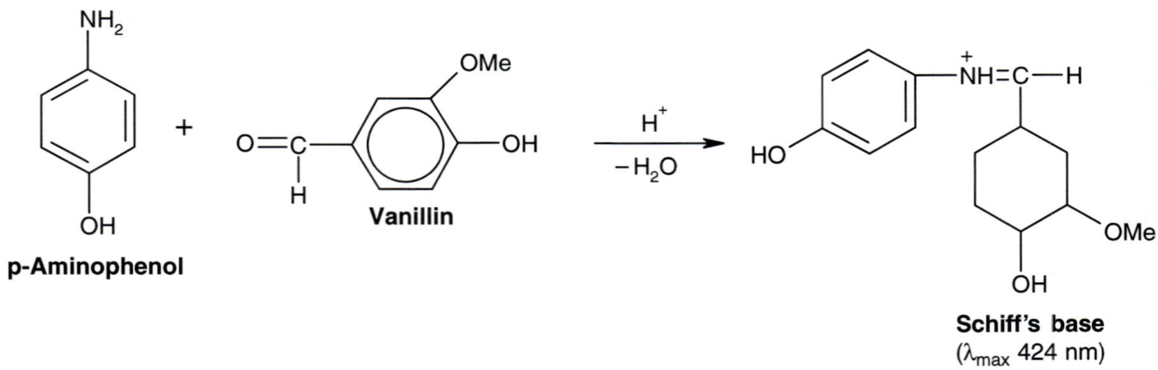

Free phenolic function in the molecule can be made to react in sodium carbonate medium with Gibb's reagent to give phenylogous oxonol (λ_{max} 650 nm). The coupling takes place at free O-position to phenolic-OH.

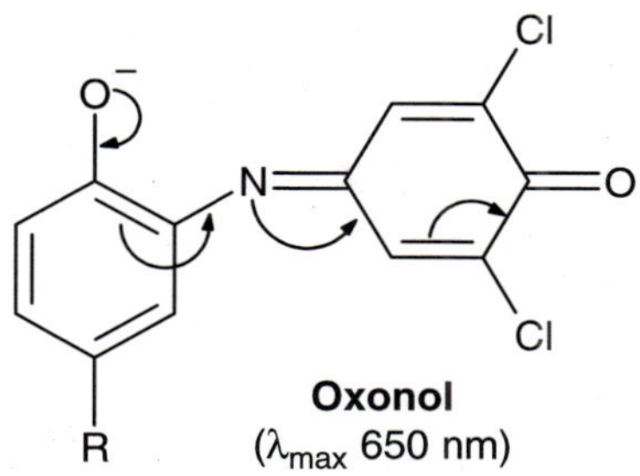

Oxonol
(λ_{max} 650 nm)

Both aniline and p-aminophenol, the hydrolytic products, can be diazotized and coupled with b-naphthol to give orange azo dye.

Reference

Pharmaceutical Chemistry, Vol. 2, H.J. Roth, pp. 515-516, 1991.

METHOD 3

Reagents

1. 0.1 M, 1 M sodium hydroxide.
2. Na_2CO_3 - $NaHCO_3$ buffer, pH 10.2 (1 : 1).
3. 2% v/v of O-cresol in water.

Sample/standard solution

50 μg/ml in water.

Procedure

To 50 ml each of sample/standard solutions add 5 ml of O-cresol solution and 1 drop of 1 N NaOH. When faint blue colour develops, dilute to 50 ml with carbonate buffer pH 10.2. Measure the absorbance of the so developed colour at 600 nm.

Probable Reaction Mechanism

p-aminophenol formed as a result of hydrolysis is spontaneously oxidized in alkaline medium in the presence of O-cresol, which is also a phenol, to form an indophenol dye (λ_{max} 600 nm).

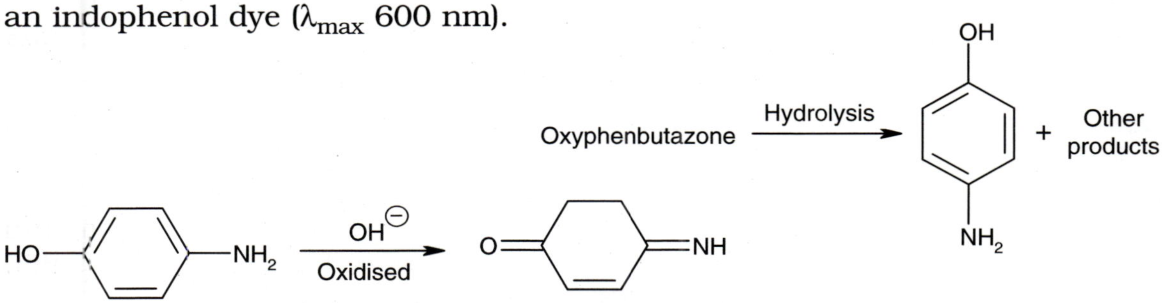

1,4-Benzoquinone monimine

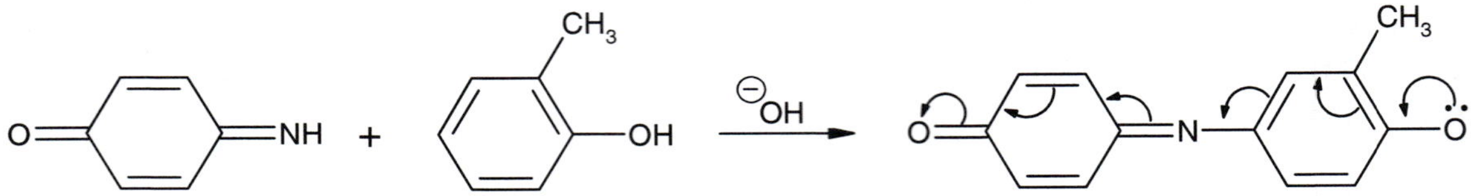

Orthocresol

Indophenol dye (λ_{max} 600 nm)

Some important reactions of oxyphenbutazone of analytical interest

On acid hydrolysis, oxyphenbutazone forms N-4-hydroxyphenyl-N′-phenyl hydrazine which undergoes benzidine re-arrangement to produce 2,4-diamine-5-hydroxybiphenyl, the compound having 4-aminophenol moiety. This couples oxidatively with phenol in alkaline medium to give indophenol (λ_{max} 635 nm).

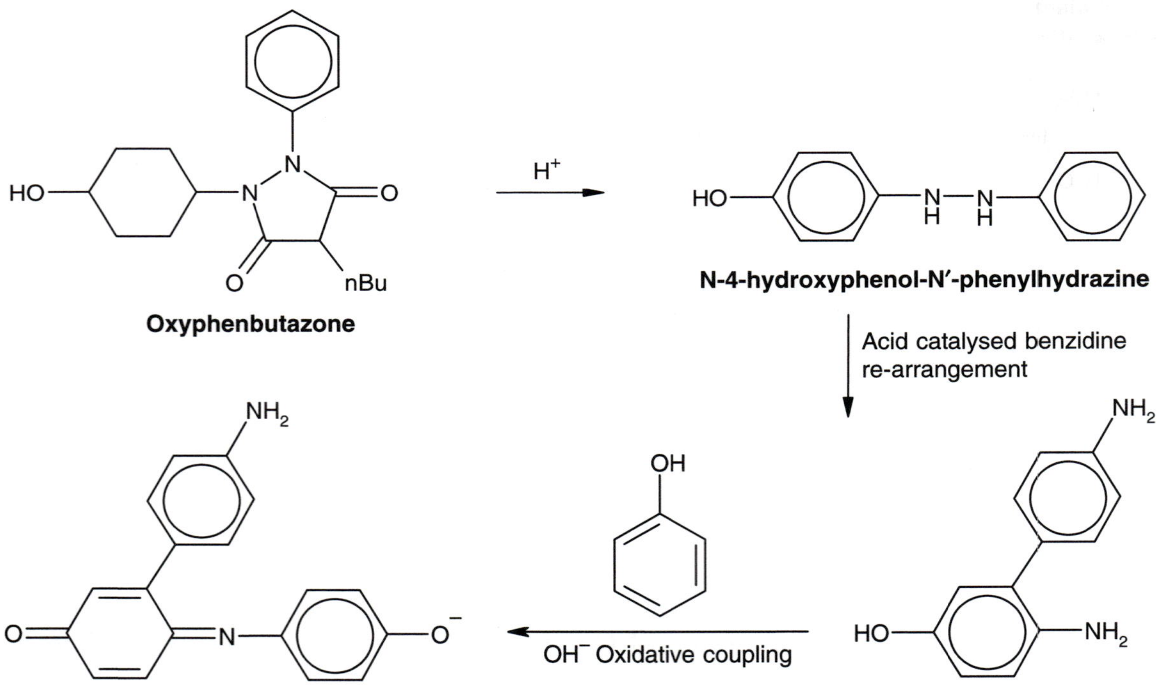

Oxyphenbutazone

N-4-hydroxyphenol-N′-phenylhydrazine

2,4-diamino-5-hydroxyphenyl

Indophenol (λ_{max} 635 nm)

Note

Aspirin and salicylamide do not interfere.

Reference

R.K. Verma and Archana Jain, Analyst, 110, 997-999, 1985; and K.K. Verma and S.K. Sanghi, Farmaco Ed. Pr., 43, 13, 1988.

After acid hydrolysis and as a result of benzidine re-arrangement, the resultant product forms Schiff's base with p-dimethylaminocinnamaldehyde (PDAC) in acidic medium.

Probable Reaction Mechanism

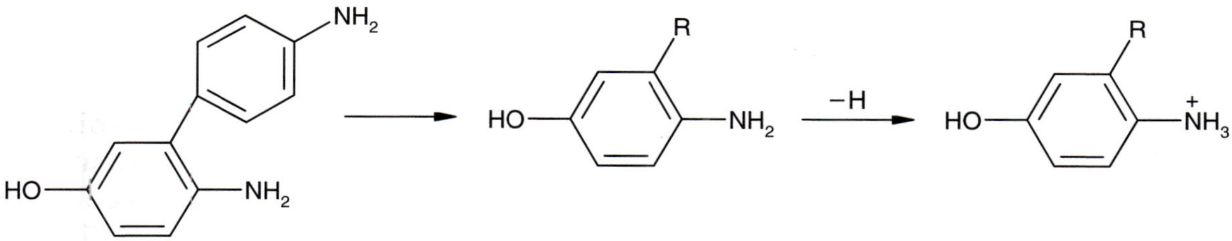

2,4′-diamino-5-hydroxybiphenyl (benzidine re-arrangement product

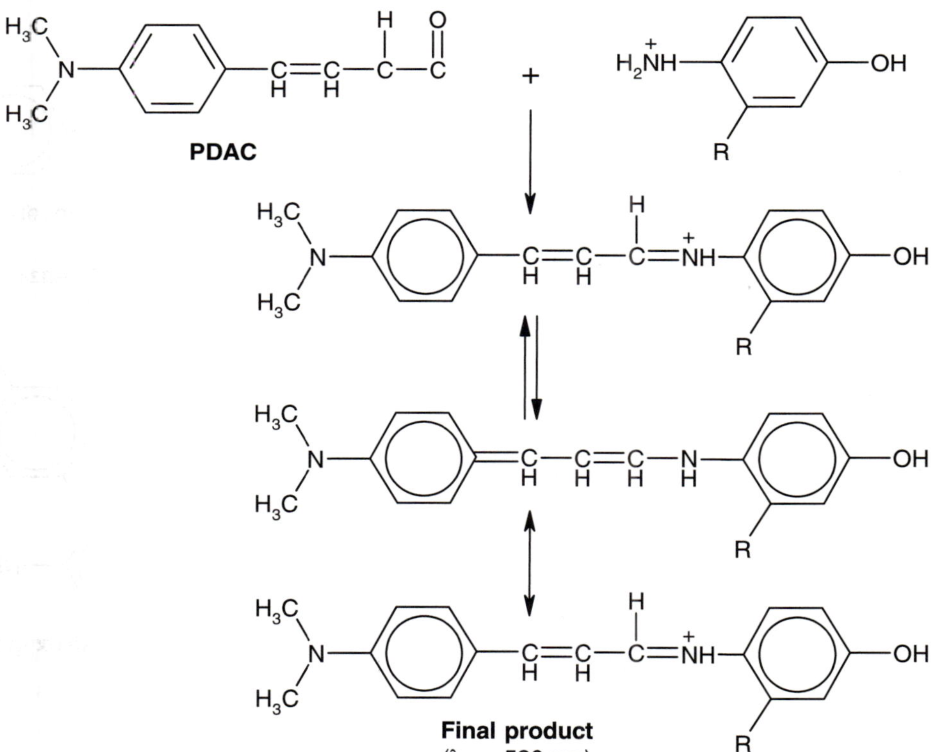

PDAC

Final product
(λ_{max} 520 nm)

Note

Aspirin, salicylamide and propyphenazone do not interfere. If the drug sample contains paracetamol or analgin, then remove these drugs by prior extraction with 2% sulphuric acid.

Reference

Ahsan Saeed, Seema Haque and Saidul Zafar Qureshi. Talanta, 40(12), 1867-1871, 1993.

METHOD 4

Reagents

1. 3% w/v solution of sodium nitrite in water.
2. 0.125 M copper sulphate solution.
3. 1 mg/ml solution of orthoaniline.
4. 0.5% solution of sodium diethyldithiocarbamate solution in methanol.
5. 1 M sodium hydroxide solution.
6. 0.5 M sulphuric acid.

Standard solution

1 mg/ml of oxyphenbutazone in methanol.

Sample solution

The powdered sample extracted with methanol and diluted appropriately with methanol to get

Procedure

(a) To 1 ml of O-aniline solution add 2.5 ml of sodium nitrite solution, mix, allow to stand for 10 min, add 1 ml each of sample/standard solutions to above diazotized reagent, add 3 ml of 1 M sodium hydroxide solution, allow to stand for 5 min, dilute to 25 ml with water and measure the absorbance at 435 nm against reagent blank.

(b) After addition of sample/standard solutions as under procedure (a), add 1 ml of sodium hydroxide solution, allow to stand for 5 min, then add 5 ml of copper sulphate solution and 6 ml of 0.5 M sulphuric acid, extract with chloroform (3×25 ml), filter organic layer through cotton plug, dilute to 100 ml with chloroform and measure the absorbance at 415 nm against blank prepared in the same way but without drug.

(c) To 5 ml of chloroform extract, as obtained under method (b), add 5 ml of dithiocarbamate solution, mix and measure the absorbance of resulting solution at λ_{max} 437 nm.

Probable Reaction Mechanism

(a) Since position of the hydroxyphenyl group in the compound is blocked with nitrogen atom of the phenylpyrazolidine ring, so coupling with diazotized nitroaniline takes place in the position ortho to phenolic-OH group. Since two free positions ortho to phenolic-OH exist, so coupling with diazoaniline to oxyphenbutazone is in the ratio of 2 : 1. The complex is stabilized by addition of sodium hydroxide.

(b) The above coupled compound was chelated with Cu(II) as the coupled compound contains phenolic-OH group with an easily replaceable proton and the diazo group (—N==N—) offers a lone pair of electrons and the two groups are so arranged to include Cu(II) ion in a five-membered ring in the chelate. Since Cu(II) chelate is not easily soluble in water, it can be extracted into chloroform (yellow solution) for measurement. The Cu(II) ion satisfies its 4 coordination valency with two hydroxy group and two diazo group. A slight acidic medium favours quantitative Cu(II) chelate formation, hence addition of sulphuric acid.

(c) Addition of dithiocarbamate to Cu(II) chelate displaces 4-butyl-1-[2,6-di(O-nitrophenylazo)-4-hydroxyphenyl]-phenylpyrazolidine-3,5-dione to give Cu(II)-diethylcarbamate complex with λ_{max} 435 nm.

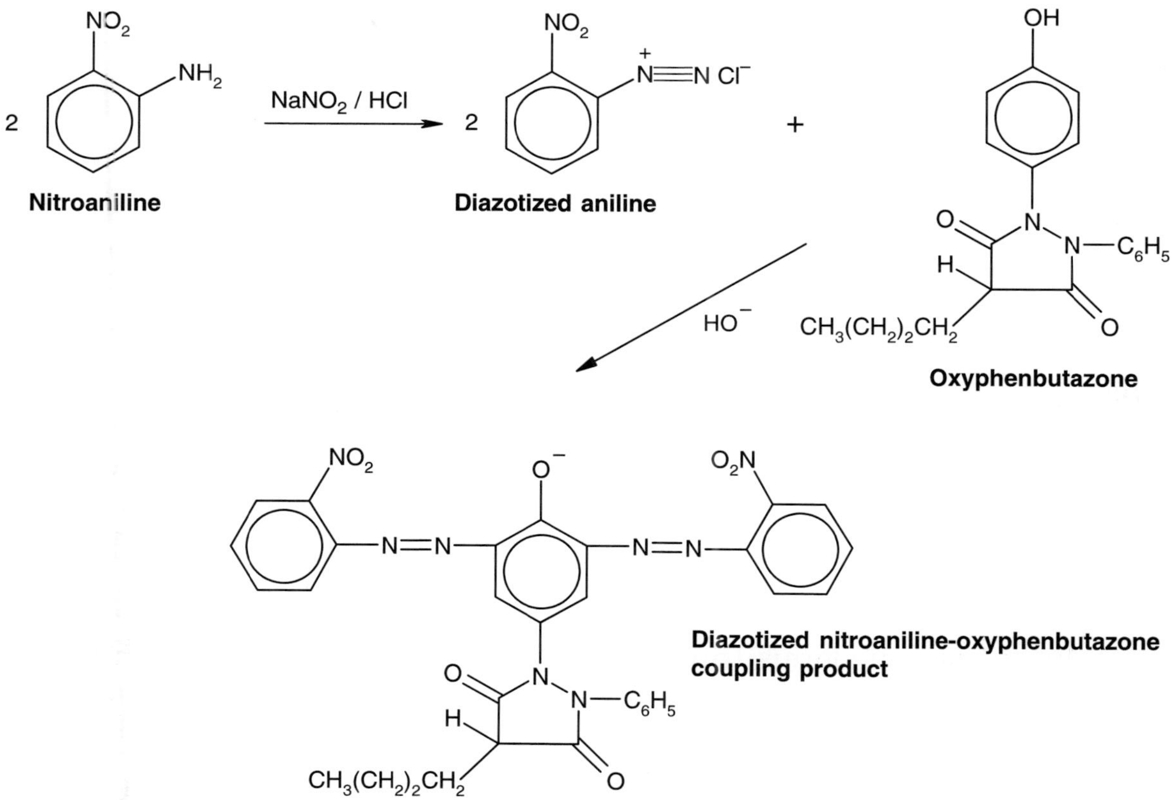

4-Butyl-1[2,6-di(o-nitrophenylazo)4-hydroxyphenyl]phenylpyrazolidine-3,5-dione
(λ_{max} 435 nm)

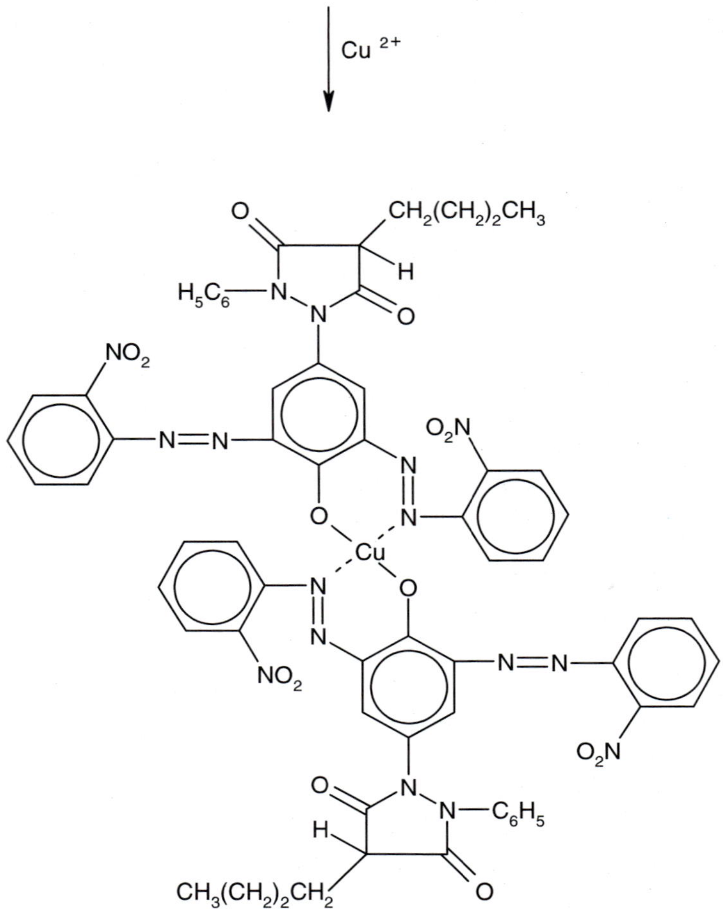

Cu(II) Chelate
(λ_{max} 415 nm)
extractable with chloroform

Reference

S. Belal, A.A. Abou El Kheir and Abdulla El Shanwani. Analyst, 110, 205-210, 1985.

Oxyphenbutazone forms trinitro derivative with HNO_3 and sulphuric acid. The electron deficit polynitro derivative is allowed to react with ketone (acetone), an anion, in alkaline medium to give intense coloured product (λ_{max} 400 nm). These are Meisenheimer type addition products.

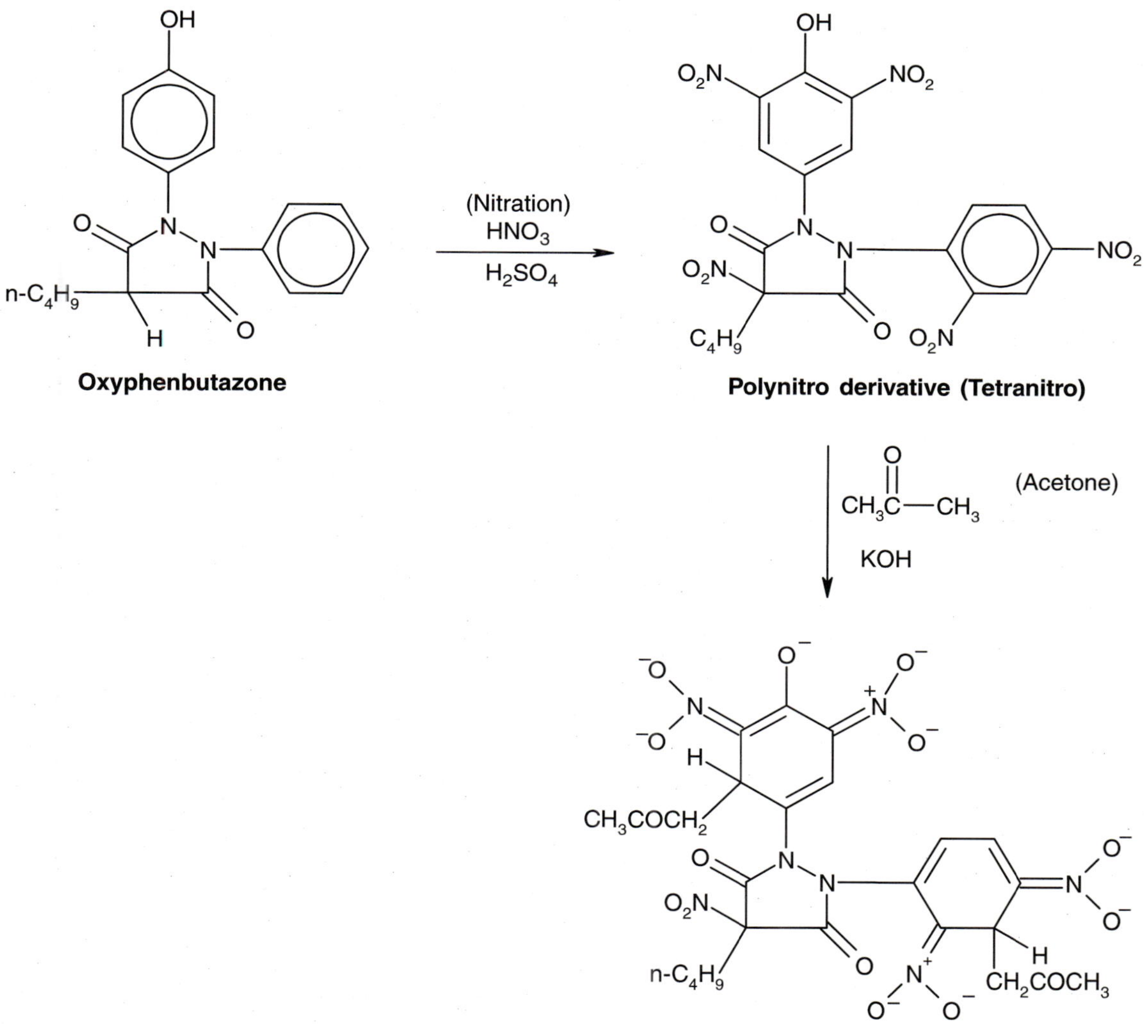

Note

For similar reaction, refer to methods for amoxycillin with phenolic ring.

Reference

Afaf A. El Kheir, S. Belal, Mohammad El Sadek & Abdullah El Shanwani. Analyst, 111, 319-321, 1986.

The compound being phenolic in nature and ortho position being vacant, it can form nitroso derivative. The nitro derivative can form metal (Co^{++}) chelate extractable into isobutylmethyl ketone.

Probable Reaction Mechanism

(a)

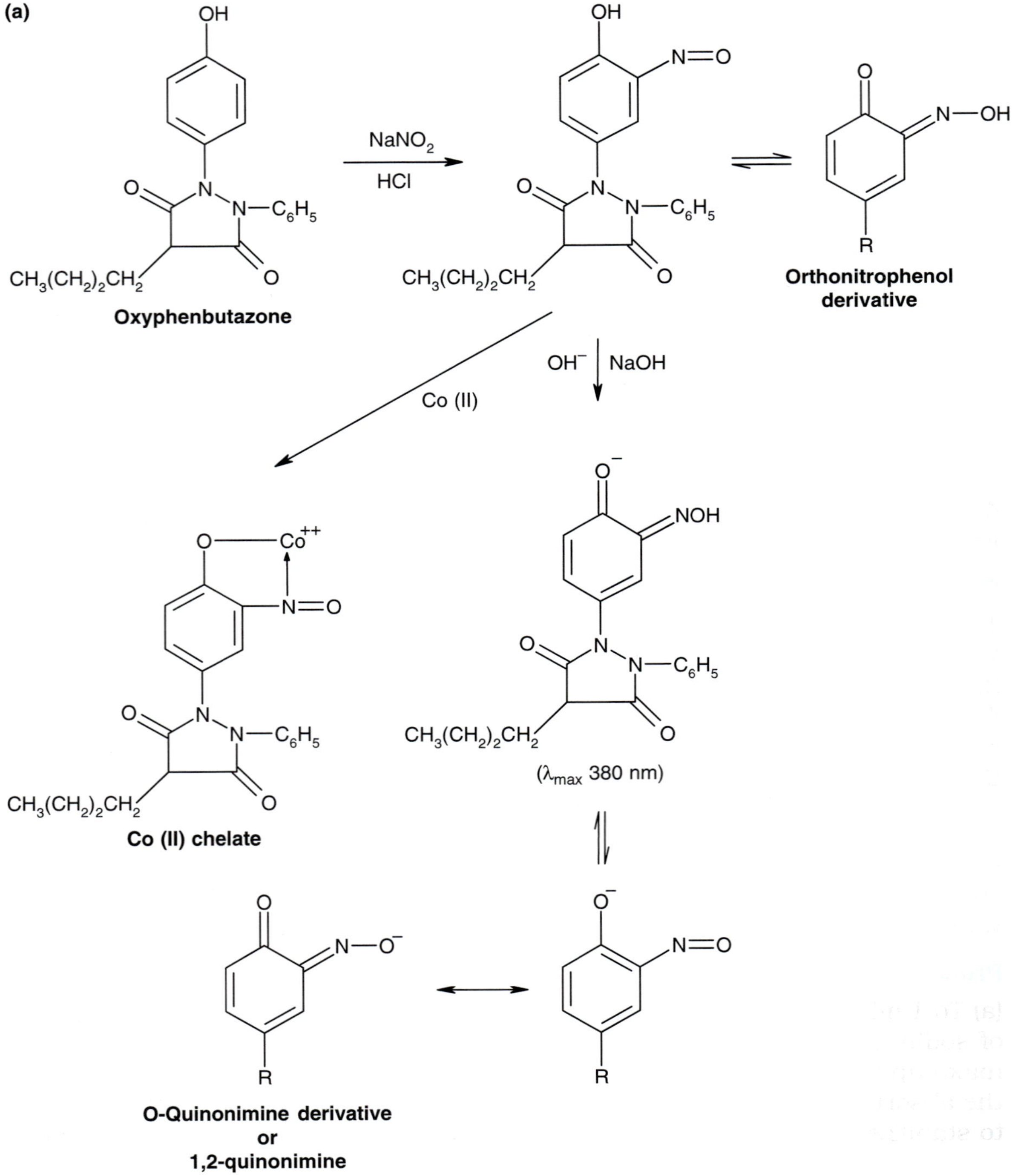

The quinonimine can be stabilized by forming chelate with Hg (II).

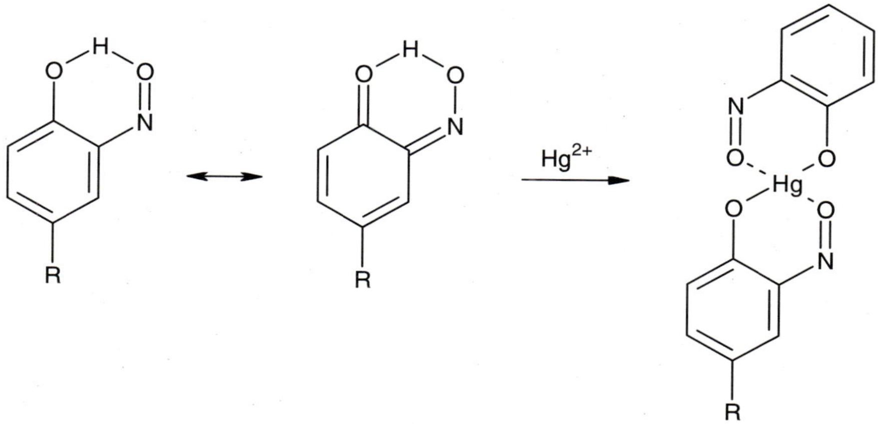

Stabilized mercury chelate

Alternatively, the compound being phenolic in nature, it can condense with 4-aminoantipyrine in the presence of alkaline oxidizing agent. This is based on Emerson's reaction.

Reagents

1. 6 M hydrochloric acid.
2. 10% w/v solution of sodium nitrate.
3. 15% w/v solution of sodium hydroxide.
4. 1% w/v solution of sodium carbonate.
5. 2% w/v solution of 4-aminoantipyrine in methanol.
6. 4% w/v solution of potassium ferricyanide.

Sample/standard solution

Dissolve 100 mg of the substance or sample in 20 ml of 0.1 M sodium hydroxide solution, dilute to 100 ml with water, further dilute 10 ml to 100 ml with water.

Procedure

(a) To 1 ml each of sample/standard solutions add 1 ml of 6 M HCl and 2.5 ml of sodium nitrate solution, keep in boiling water-bath for 35 min, cool and make up the volume to 25 ml with 15% sodium hydroxide solution. Measure the absorbance at 380 nm against reagent blank. Sodium hydroxide is added to stabilize the nitroso derivative.

(b) To 10 ml each of sample and standard solutions, as under method (a), add 1.5 ml of sodium carbonate solution, 0.6 ml of 4-aminoantipyrine solution and 1 ml of $K_3Fe(CN)_6$ solution, dilute to 25 ml with water and measure the absorbance at 500 nm against reagent blank.

Probable Reaction Mechanism

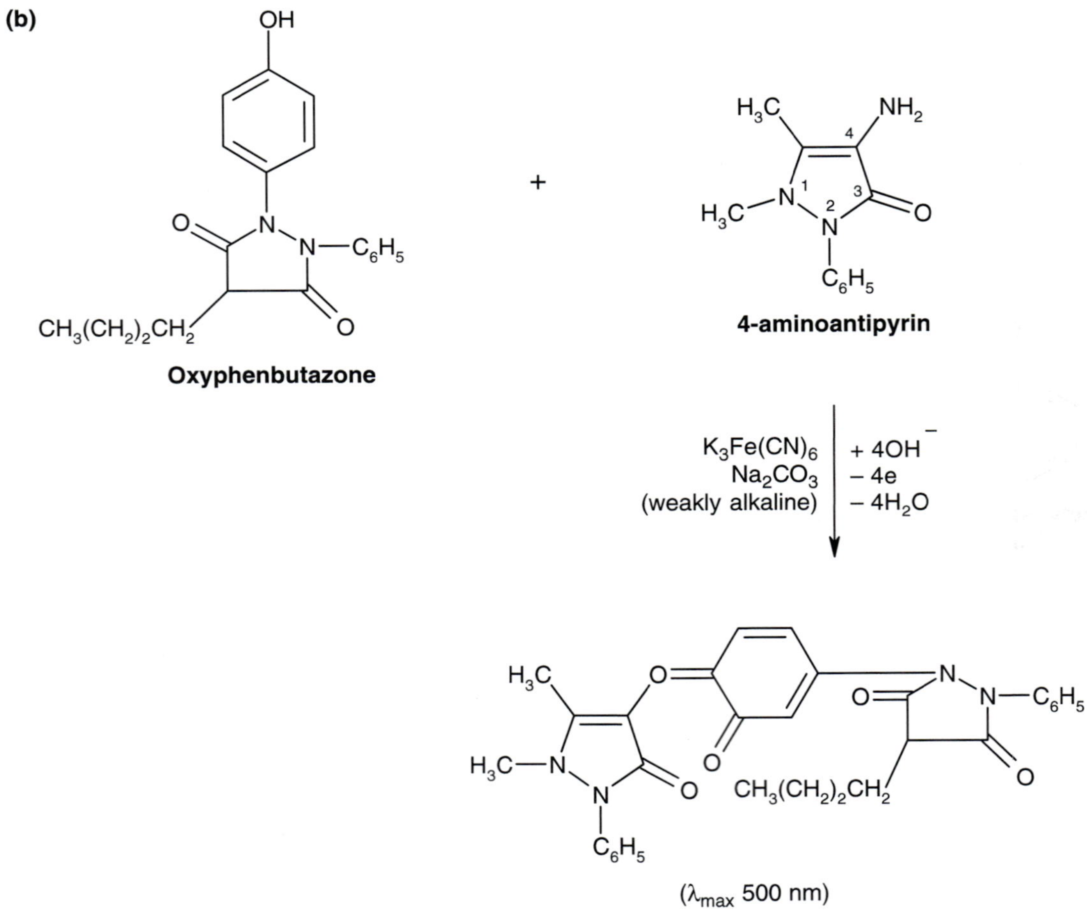

Note

The drug in the presence of oxidizing agent $K_3Fe(CN)_6$ couples with 4-aminoantipyrine in weakly alkaline conditions (Na_2CO_3).

Reference

Ouf, M.I. Walash, S.M. Hassan & S.M. El Sayed. Analyst, 105, 169-173, 1980.

Aspirin

METHOD 1

Extract accurately weighed quantity of the sample equivalent to 10 mg of aspirin with 0.5 M sodium hydroxide by boiling for 10 minutes and dilute to 100 ml with 0.5 M sodium hydroxide. Dilute further with the same solvent to get 20 mcg/ml and measure the extinction at 300 nm. Calculate the results by using a value of 260 as A 1%, 1 cm for salicylic acid at 300 nm.

Explanatory Note

On heating with sodium hydroxide, the aspirin is hydrolysed to salicylic acid (sodium salicylate) and acetic acid (sodium acetate). 300 nm is the λ_{max} of salicylic acid.

Probable Reaction Mechanism

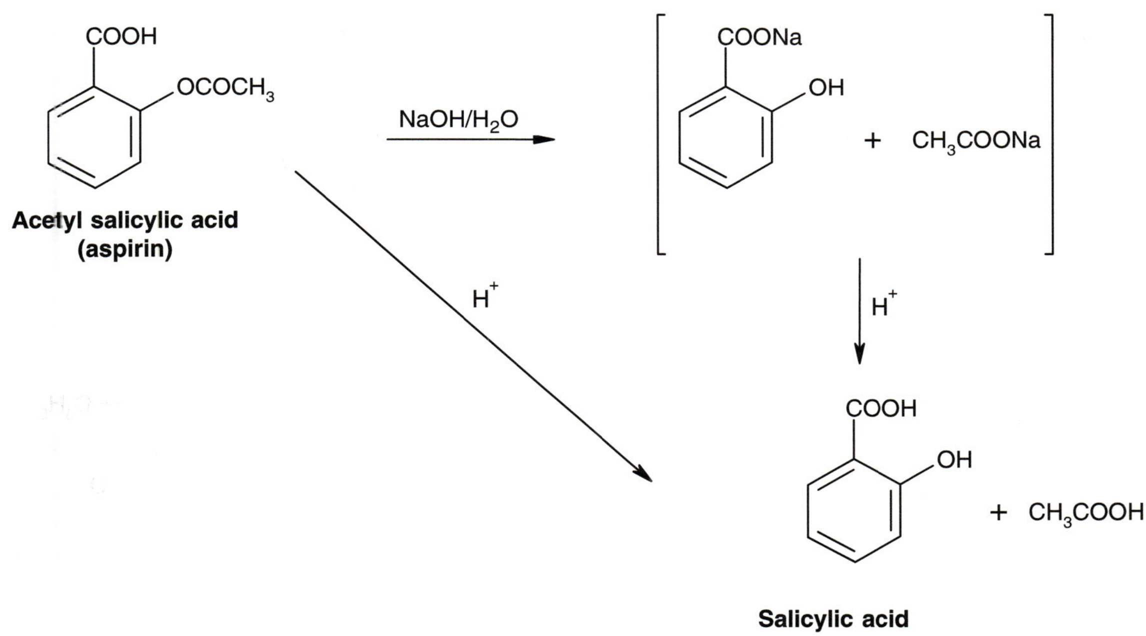

METHOD 2

Standard solution

10 mcg/ml of aspirin in 0.05 M sulphuric acid.

Sample solution

10 mcg/ml of aspirin in 0.05 M sulphuric acid.

Procedure

Measure the extinction of the solutions at maximum at about 230 nm using 0.1 N sulphuric acid as blank. Calculate the results by comparison, 230 nm being the λ_{max} of intact aspirin molecule.

Diazepam

Sample accurately weighed equivalent to 10 mg of diazepam is extracted with ethyl alcohol to get 10 ml. The volume of the sample solution equivalent to 1 mg of the substance is hydrolysed with 6 N hydrochloric acid to give 2-methylamino-5-chlorobenzophenone which is extracted into chloroform and absorbance of yellow colour measured at 410 nm. For reaction details, refer to chapter on analgeics.

Aluminium hydroxide

Follow the sodium edetate titration method described in formulation of the chapter on antacids.

Formulation 4

Phenylbutazone or Oxyphenbutazone, Salicylamide

ESTIMATION

Phenylbutazone and Salicylamide

This method is based on ultraviolet spectrophotometric measurements in 0.1 M sodium hydroxide at their respective maxima i.e. 264 and 328 nm. They do not interfere with each other at their respective maxima and can be estimated without prior separation.

Standard solution of phenylbutazone

10 mcg/ml of phenylbutazone in 0.1 M sodium hydroxide.

Standard solution of salicylamide

10 mcg/ml of salicylamide in 0.1 M sodium hydroxide.

Sample solution

Weigh accurately powdered tablets equivalent to 50 mg of salicylamide and extract with 0.1 M sodium hydroxide to get a concentration of 10 mcg/ml in respect of salicylamide.

Procedure

Measure the extinction of the sample and standard solutions at 264 nm and 328 nm and calculate the results from A 1%, 1 cm values at their respective maxima.

Phenylbutazone exhibits maxima at 264 nm (A 1%, 1 cm = 660) and salicylamide at 328 nm (A 1%, 1 cm = 435).

Oxyphenbutazone in 0.1 M sodium hydroxide exhibits maxima at 254 nm with A 1%, 1 cm value of 750.

Note

Since both oxyphenbutazone and salicylamide shall undergo nitroso reaction, as described earlier under oxyphenbutazone, so this method shall not be applicable, however salicylamide fails to form Co(II) chelate as described under oxyphenbutazone.

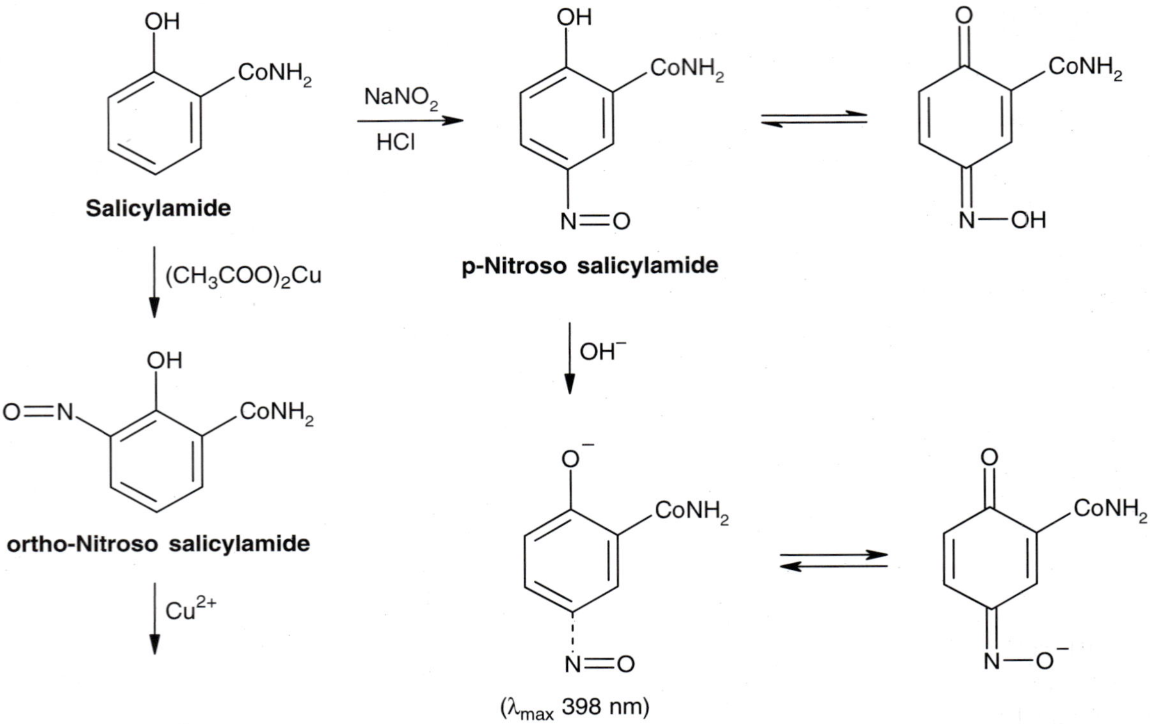

Note

Nitroso derivative is stable in both acidic and alkaline media. p-Nitrosalicylamide will not make Co(II) ion complex like oxyphenbutazone or paracetamol as ortho position is occupied, hence nitrosation occurs at para position to phenolic-OH as shown above. However, in the presence of Cu(II) acetate the nitrosation can occur at ortho position to phenolic-OH leading to formation of coloured copper chelate (λ_{max} 520 nm). For details of reaction mechanism, refer to the above method described under paracetamol.

Reference

S.F. Belal, M. Abdel-Hady El Sayed, A. El Wahly & H. Abdine. Analyst, 104, 919-927, 1979.

The nitration reaction as described for paracetamol and oxyphenbutazone is applicable for salicylamide in the presence of phenylbutazone as it is applicable to compound with phenolic moiety.

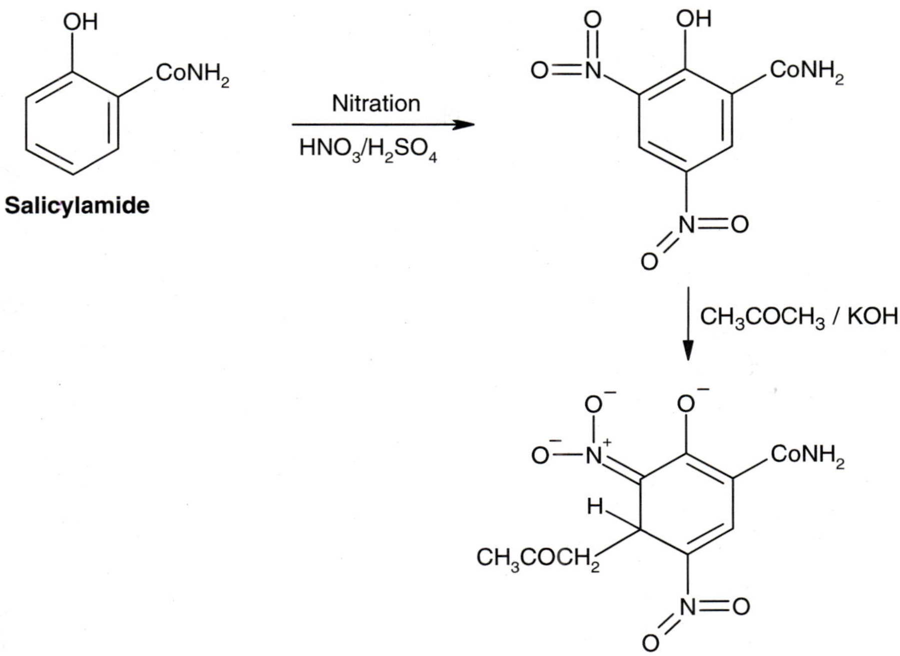

(λ_{max} 390 nm)

Different positions in benzene ring are activated by –OH group and also by carbamoyl ($CoNH_2$) group which facilitate bromination. This can be used for analytical purposes.

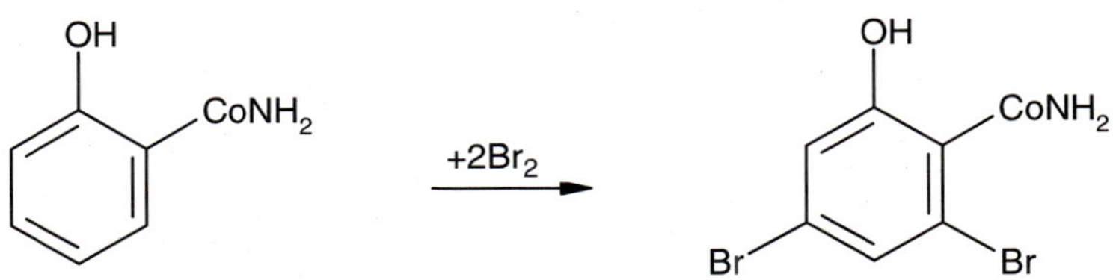

Boron chelate formed with boric acid in the presence of acetic anhydride and sulphuric acid can be used for fluorometric analysis of the compound.

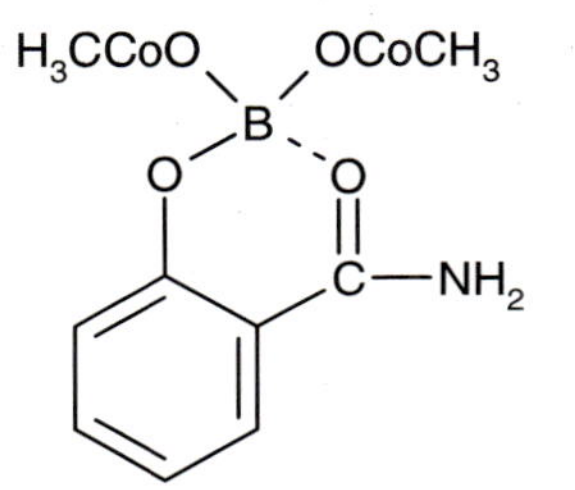

Boron chelate
(Ex. 328 nm; Em. 388 nm)

Reference

Pharmaceutical Chemistry by H.J. Roth, 1991, p. 280.

Since the compound has phenolic function, with p-position free, it reacts with 4-aminophenazone (based on Emerson reagent) to give coloured compound.

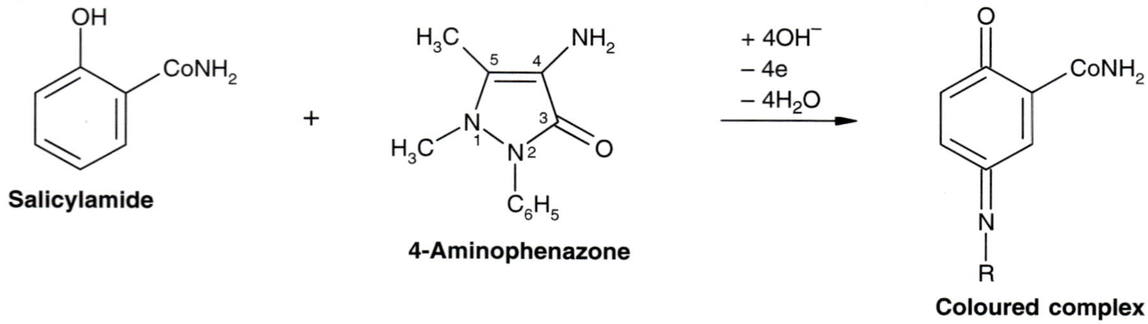

Note

Based on oxidative coupling at p-position.

Reference

Pharmaceutical Chemistry, Vol. 2, H.J. Roth, p. 75.

Formulation 5

Phenylbutazone, Paracetamol

ESTIMATION

Paracetamol

METHOD 1

Weigh accurately a quantity of the sample equivalent to 50 mg of paracetamol, add 50 ml of 0.1 M hydrochloric acid, shake and dilute to 100 ml with acid. Filter and collect the filtrate. To 10 ml of the filtrate, add 10 ml of 0.1 M sodium hydroxide and dilute to 100 ml with water. To 10 ml of the resultant solution, add 10 ml of 0.1 M sodium hydroxide and dilute to 100 ml with water. Mix well and measure absorbance of the above solution at 257 nm against blank prepared by mixing 10 ml of 0.1 M sodium hydroxide with 90 ml of water. Calculate the results taking 715 as value of E 1%, 1 cm of paracetamol at 257 nm.

METHOD 2

This method is based on the formulation of a complex (Schiff's base) with p-dimethylaminobenzaldehyde after hydrolysis, which has absorption maxima at about 440 nm.

Reagents

1. Dilute hydrochloric acid.
2. 3% w/v solution of p-dimethylaminobenzaldehyde (PDAB) in alcohol.

Standard solution

0.5 mg/ml of paracetamol in water, shake to dissolve.

Sample solution

Weigh accurately a quantity of the sample equivalent to 25 mg of paracetamol. Add about 40 ml of water and shake for 10-15 min. Dilute to 50 ml and filter.

Hydrolysis of sample and standard solutions

To 25 ml of the sample and standard solutions as prepared above, add 10 ml of dilute hydrochloric acid. Heat on water-bath for 60 min, cool and dilute to 100 ml with water.

Procedure

To 2 ml of hydrolysed solutions of sample and standard, add 2 ml of dilute hydrochloric acid and 5 ml of (PDAB) reagent. Mix and dilute to 50 ml with alcohol. Measure the extinction of golden yellow complex at about 440 nm against reagent blank, treated similarly.

Note

Analgin, caffeine, phenylbutazone, meprobamate, chloroquine phosphate, oxyphenbutazone, diazepam, dextropropoxyphene and noscapine do not interfere.

Probable Reaction Mechanism

p-Aminophenol as a result of acid hydrolysis reacts with p-dimethylamino-benzaldehyde to give coloured complex (λ_{max} 440 nm).

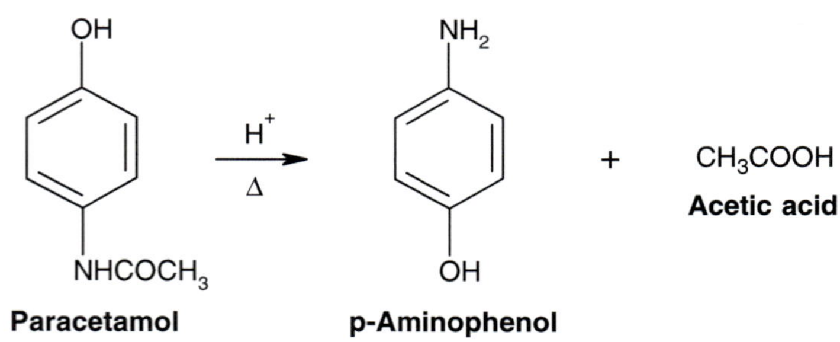

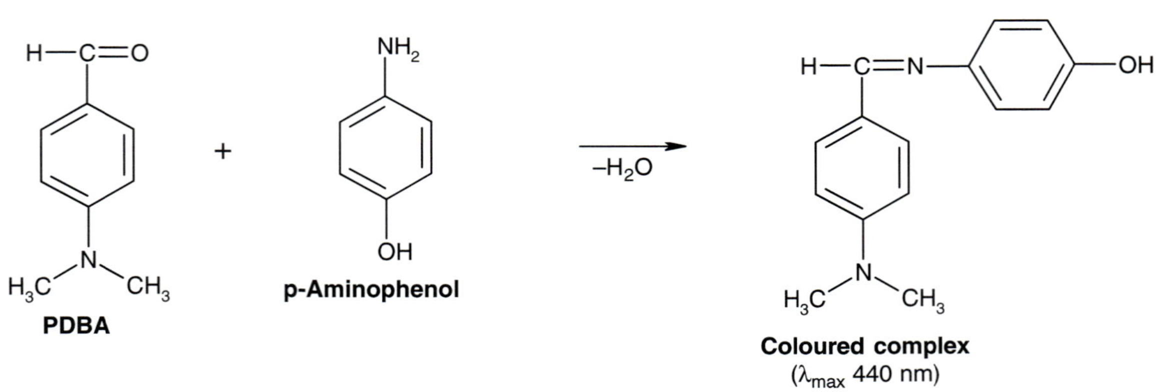

The colorimetric method for paracetamol described in formulation 25 of the chapter on analgesics and antipyretics can be used in such combination. This method involves bathochromic shift from 249 to 463 nm in alkaline medium. The method described in formulation 6 of this chapter can also be used.

Phenylbutazone

Weigh a quantity of the sample, equivalent to 200 mg of phenylbutazone. Extract with four 30 ml portions of chloroform. Combine and evaporate total chloroform extract (see instruction for evaporation under formulation 1 of this chapter). For further details, refer to formulation 1 of this chapter.

Note

For complete extraction from matrix, refer to note under estimation of oxyphenbutazone in formulation 2 of this chapter.

Alternatively, the method based on the fact that paracetamol is soluble in 0.1 M hydrochloric acid, whereas both phenylbutazone and oxyphenbutazone are insoluble in acid. For details of the procedure, refer to formulation 9 of this chapter. Phenylbutazone thus separated can be taken up in 0.1 M sodium hydroxide and contents calculated by using 660 as value of A 1%, 1 cm at 264 nm.

Formulation 6

Paracetamol, Oxyphenbutazone, Magnesium trisilicate

ESTIMATION

Paracetamol

Standard solution

10 mcg/ml of paracetamol in 0.1 M hydrochloric acid.

Sample solution

Extract an accurately weighed quantity of the sample equivalent to about 100 mg of paracetamol with three 25 ml portions of 1 M hydrochloric acid. Filter through G_4 sintered glass funnel. Collect the filtrate and dilute to 100 ml with acid. Dilute appropriately with 0.1 M hydrochloric acid to get a final concentration of 10 mcg/ml. Reserve the residue for estimation of oxyphenbutazone.

Concomitantly measure the extinction of both sample and standard solutions at maxima at about 246 nm using 0.1 M hydrochloric acid as blank. Deduce the results by comparison. In alkaline medium λ_{max} is 257 nm.

Alternatively, the method based on bathochromic shift from 249 to 463 nm in alkaline medium may be used. For details, refer to formulation 25 of the chapter on analgesics and antipyretics.

Oxyphenbutazone

Standard solution

10 mcg/ml of oxyphenbutazone in 0.01 M sodium hydroxide solution.

Sample solution

Use the entire residue left after extraction of paracetamol as described above. Transfer the powder left in the flask and on the top of sintered funnel to 100 ml volumetric flask with the aid of 0.01 M sodium hydroxide. Further dilute appropriately with 0.01 M sodium hydroxide to get a final concentration of 10 mcg/ml.

Simultaneously measure the extinction of both the solutions at maxima at about 254 nm and calculate the results by comparison. Alternatively dissolve the entire residue in neutral (phenolphthalein or bromothymol blue) acetone and titrate with 0.1 M sodium hydroxide. Each ml of 0.1 M sodium hydroxide solution is equivalent to 0.03424 g of oxyphenbutazone.

Note

Acidimetric titration with alkali hydroxide is based on CH acidity of the molecule; acetone is used to dissolve the compound.

Magnesium trisilicate

Follow the method described in formulation 1 of this chapter.

Formulation 7

Oxyphenbutazone, Paracetamol, Diazepam, Dextropropoxyphene hydrochloride

ESTIMATION

Oxyphenbutazone

Transfer powder equivalent to 400 mg of the substance. Extract with acetone and titrate with 0.1 M sodium hydroxide as described under formulation-3 of this chapter.

Paracetamol

METHOD 1

In this method, advantage is taken of the fact that paracetamol is sparingly soluble in water and oxyphenbutazone is insoluble in water.

Standard solution

Dissolve 100 mg of paracetamol in 10 ml of alcohol and dilute with water to 100 ml. 1 ml of this solution is further diluted with water to 100 ml (10 mcg/ml).

Sample solution

Weigh accurately the sample equivalent to 250 mg of paracetamol. Soak the powder with water for 3-4 hours, shaking occasionally. Dilute to 200 ml with water. Filter and dilute 1 ml of the filtrate to 100 ml with water. Oxyphenbutazone being insoluble in water, does not get extracted, hence no inference. The residue can be used for assay of oxyphenbutazone.
Measure the absorbance of both the solutions at 244 nm against blank and calculate the results.

METHOD 2

Suspend accurately weighed amount of the sample equivalent to 50 mg of the compound in 20 ml of water and extract with three 30 ml portions of chloroform, washing each chloroform layer with the same 20 ml of water. Combine aqueous layers, add 50 ml of 0.1 M sodium hydroxide and dilute with water to 200 ml. 2 ml of the resulting solution is further diluted to 200 ml with 0.01 M sodium hydroxide. Measure extinction of the solution at 257 nm and calculate the results by comparing with the standard solution (10 mcg/ml in 0.01 M sodium hydroxide). Alternatively, calculate the amount of paracetamol taking 715 as value of E 1%, 1 cm at 257 nm, see method-1 for paracetamol under formulation-6 of this chapter.

Note

Paracetamol is insoluble in chloroform, hence remains in aqueous layer. The chloroform layer can be used for assay of oxyphenbutazone.

Diazepam

This method is based on the simple fact that at 362 nm; paracetamol does not show any light absorption and oxyphenbutazone is insoluble in 0.1 N hydrochloric acid, the medium used for extraction of diazepam. Hence both the ingredients, oxyphenbutazone and paracetamol, do not interfere in the method described below.

Standard solution

20 mcg/ml of Diazepam in 0.1 M hydrochloric acid.

Sample solution

Weigh accurately powdered material equivalent to 2 mg of diazepam and shake with 0.1 M hydrochloric acid for 10-15 minutes, make up the volume to 100 ml and filter.

Measure the absorbance of both the solutions at 362 nm against 0.1 N hydrochloric acid as blank and calculate the results.

Note

Analgin and diphenhydramine do not interfere in this method.

Dextropropoxyphene hydrochloride

Weigh powdered material accurately equivalent to 350 mg of dextropropoxyphene hydrochloride and suspend in 15-20 ml of water. Add 1 g of sodium chloride and 2 ml of ammonia solution. Extract with four 25 ml portions of chloroform, washing each chloroform layer with the same 20 ml of water. Filter organic layer through anhydrous sodium sulphate and evaporate on a water bath, removing last 5 ml of the extract under current of air. To the residue, add 30 ml of glacial acetic acid and warm on water bath to dissolve. Carry out the non-aqueous titration using crystal violet solution as indicator. From the total volume of 0.1 N perchloric acid consumed in the above titration, subtract the volume equivalent to diazepam contents as estimated above to get net volume of the acid equivalent to dextropropoxyphene contents. Each ml of 0.1 N perchloric acid is equivalent to 37.59 mg of dextropropoxyphene hydrochloride.

Formulation 8

Oxyphenbutazone, Paracetamol, Diazepam, Dextropropoxyphene hydrochloride, Dicyclomine hydrochloride

ESTIMATION

Oxyphenbutazone

Follow the method described in formulation 2 or 3 of this chapter.

Paracetamol

METHOD 1

In this method, advantage is taken of the fact that paracetamol is sparingly soluble in water and oxyphenbutazone is insoluble in water.

Standard solution

Dissolve 100 mg of paracetamol in 10 ml of alcohol and dilute with water to 100 ml. 1 ml of this solution is further diluted with water to 100 ml (10 mcg/ml).

Sample solution

Weigh accurately the sample equivalent to 250 mg of paracetamol. Add 50 ml of water, shake vigorously and dilute to 200 ml with water. Filter and dilute 1 ml of the filtrate to 100 ml with water.
Measure the absorbance of both the solutions at about 244 nm against blank and calculate the results by comparison.

Note

1. By using 0.1 M hydrochloric acid instead of water, better separation is obtained.
2. Dextropropoxyphene hydrochloride being poor UV absorbing compound, does not interfere.

METHOD 2

Suspend accurately weighed amount of the sample equivalent to 50 mg of the compound in 20 ml of water and extract with three 30 ml portions of chloroform, washing each chloroform layer with the same 20 ml of water. Combine aqueous layers, add 50 ml of 0.1 M sodium hydroxide and dilute with water to 200 ml. 2 ml of the resulting solution is further diluted to 200 ml with 0.01 M sodium hydroxide. Measure extinction of the solution at 257 nm and calculate the results by comparing with the standard solution (10 mcg/ml in 0.01 M sodium hydroxide). Alternatively, calculate the amount of paracetamol taking 715 as value of A 1%, 1 cm at 257 nm (see method 1 for paracetamol under formulation 5 of this chapter).

Diazepam

This method is based on the fact that at 362 nm, paracetamol shows no absorption and oxyphenbutazone is insoluble in 0.1 M hydrochloric acid, the medium used for extraction of diazepam. Hence both the ingredients, oxyphenbutazone and paracetamol, do not interfere in the method described below.

Standard solution

20 mcg/ml of diazepam in 0.1 M hydrochloric acid.

Sample solution

Weigh accurately powdered material equivalent to 2 mg of the substance and dilute to 100 ml with acid and filter.

Measure the absorbance of both the solutions at 362 nm against 0.1 M hydrochloric acid as blank and calculate the results by comparison.

Note

Analgin and diphenhydramine do not interfere in this method.

Dextropropoxyphene hydrochloride

Weigh sample accurately equivalent to 350 mg of dextropropoxyphene hydrochloride and suspend in 15-20 ml of water. Add 1 g of sodium chloride and 3.5 ml of 2 M sodium hydroxide. Extract with four 25 ml portions of chloroform, washing each chloroform layer with the same 20 ml of water. Filter organic layer through anhydrous sodium sulphate and evaporate on a water-bath, removing last 5 ml of the extract under current of air. To the residue, add 30 ml of glacial acetic acid and warm on water-bath to dissolve. Carry out the non-aqueous titration using crystal violet solution or α-naphtholbenzein solution as indicator. From the total volume of 0.1 N perchloric acid consumed in the above titration, subtract the volume equivalent to diazepam contents as estimated above to get net volume of the acid equivalent to dextropropoxyphene contents. Each ml of 0.1 N perchloric acid is equivalent to 0.03759 g of dextropropoxyphene hydrochloride.

Note

On basification, both oxyphenbutazone and paracetamol remain in aqueous medium and do not get extracted into chloroform, hence no interference.

Alternatively, the combined chloroform extract after passing through anhydrous sodium sulphate is reduced to 10 ml and subjected to optical measurements for quantitation. For details, refer to formulation 26 of the chapter on analgesics and antipyretics.

Dicyclomine hydrochloride

Reagents

1. 0.04 M sodium lauryl sulphate (SLS). If precipitates appear, discard the solution.
2. Methylene blue 0.25% w/v in water.
3. Colour reagent: To 10 ml of 0.04 M SLS, add 30 ml of chloroform and 1 ml of methylene blue solution. Mix, separate chloroform layer which is blue in colour and is used as colour reagent.
4. Concentrated hydrochloric acid.

Standard solution

Take 20 ml of dicyclomine hydrochloride and transfer to a separatory funnel. Add 10 ml of chloroform.

Sample solution

Transfer finely powdered sample equivalent to 20 mg of dicyclomine hydrochloride to separatory funnel, add 25 ml of water and 1 ml of concentrated hydrochloric acid. Extract 4 × 25 ml portions of chloroform. Pass organic layer through anhydrous sodium sulphate. Evaporate chloroform layer to 10 ml and transfer to a separatory funnel.

Procedure

To each funnel containing sample and standard, add 10 ml of colour reagent and 10 ml of water. Shake and allow the layer to separate. Discard chloroform layer. Measure the absorbance of aqueous layer (blue) of both sample and standard solutions at 590 nm using water as blank and calculate the results.

Note

If the solution is turbid, extract the blue colour into isobutanol and use isobutanol as blank.

Formulation 9

Propyphenazone, Phenylbutazone

ESTIMATION

Propyphenazone (Isopropylphenazone)

METHOD 1

Procedure

Weigh accurately quantity of the sample equivalent to 200 mg of the compound, add 100 ml of glacial acetic acid and 10 ml of acetic anhydride. Warm for few minutes and titrate with 0.1 N perchloric acid using malachite green as indicator, to a yellow end point. Each ml of 0.1 N perchloric acid is equivalent to 0.02303 g of propyphenazone. The oxygen of the vinylogous amide serves as base for non-aqueous titration.

METHOD 2

Reagent

1. Citric acid-acetic anhydride reagent: Dissolve 2 g citric acid monohydrate in 5 ml of methanol and dilute to 100 ml with acetic anhydride, prepare fresh.

Standard solution

100 mcg/ml of propyphenazone in chloroform.

Sample solution

Weigh accurately sample equivalent to 100 mg of the compound and extract with chloroform. Carry out the required dilutions with chloroform to get 100 mcg/ml.

Procedure

Evaporate 1 ml each of the sample and standard solutions to dryness, add 3 ml of citric acid reagent and 7 ml of acetic anhydride. Heat the flasks in boiling water-bath for 30 min, cool to room temperature and dilute to 25 ml with acetic anhydride. Measure the absorbance of both the solutions at about 550 nm against reagent blank. The method obeys Beer's law in the range of 1-12 mcg/ml.

Note

Aspirin, paracetamol, oxyphenbutazone and colouring agents do not interfere. Citric acid reacts with acetic anhydride to give acetyl citric acid - anhydride which gives colour with heterocyclic nitrogen.

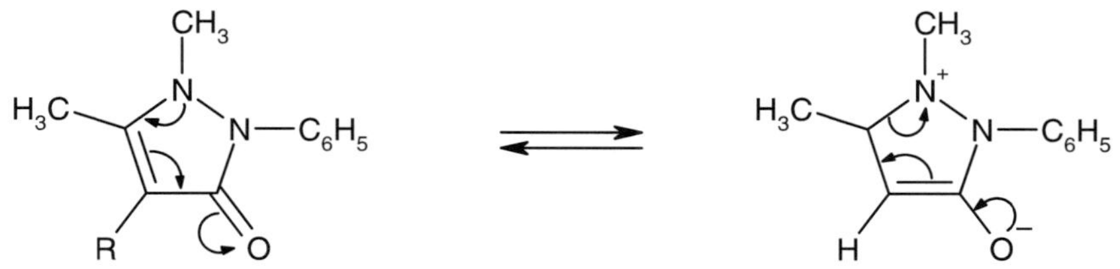

Phenazone: R = H
Propylphenazone: R = i—C_3H_7

Both compounds form complex with iron chloride.

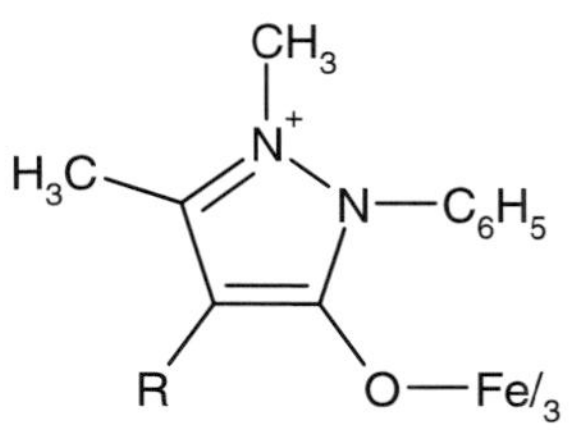

pH-dependent iron (III) complex
(λ_{max} 495 nm)

The compounds can be estimated by iodometric determination in weakly alkaline buffered medium. With excess iodine, 4-iodo derivative is produced. Iodine absorbed can be liberated by treating the compound with HCl and iodine so liberated titrated with sodium thiosulphate.

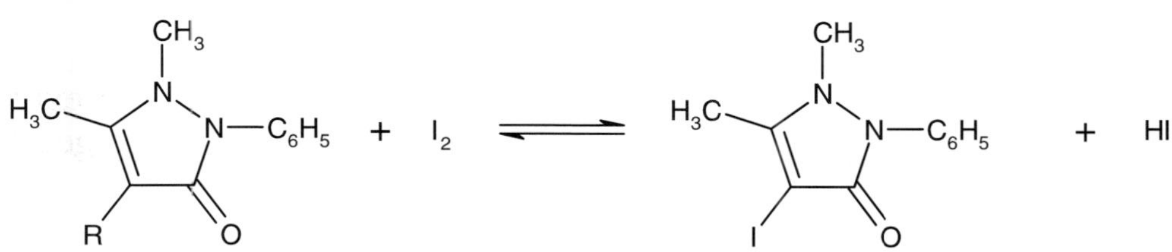

Phenazone **Iodophenazone**

The compounds forms nitroso derivative at position-4 to yield a green-coloured compound as under.

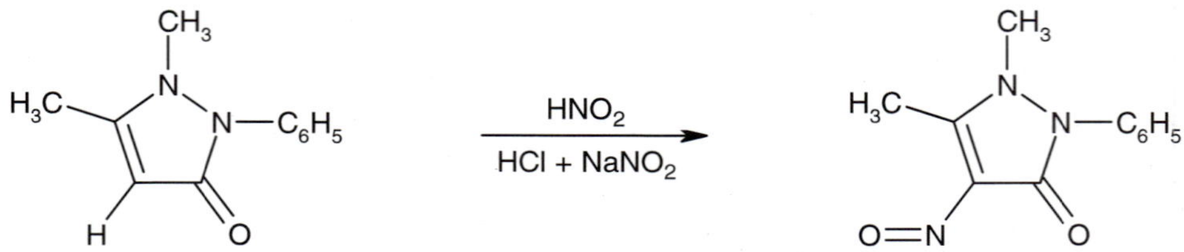

Phenazone **4-Nitrosophenazone**
(λ_{max} 630 nm)

Other electrophilic (E) reagents, which give four substituted derivatives, are No, Cl^-, Br^- and I^-.

Due to presence of enamine group, the compound condenses with PDAB to form coloured compound (λ_{max} 620 nm).

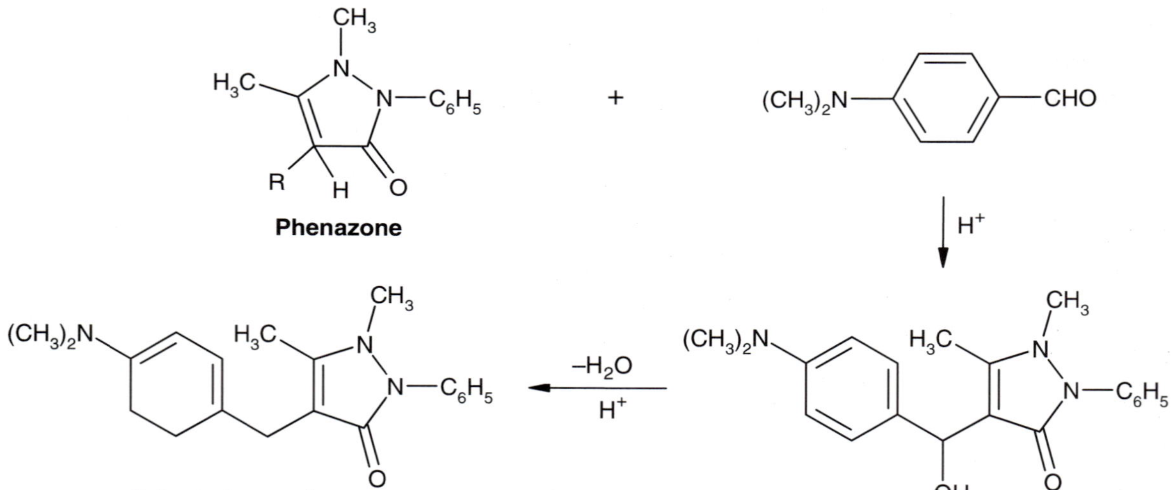

Coloured complex
(λ_{max} 620 nm)

Reference

Pharmaceutical Chemistry by Roth (Vol. 2), 1991, p. 506.

Phenylbutazone

Follow the acetone extraction and alkali titration method. For details refer to the method described in formulation 1 of this chapter.

Formulation 10

Oxyphenbutazone, Isopropyl-phenazone, Paracetamol, Diazepam

ESTIMATION

Oxyphenbutazone

Accurately weighed amount of the sample equivalent to 200 mg of the compound is extracted with acetone and titrated with 0.1 M sodium hydroxide as described in formulation 3 of this chapter.

Isopropylphenazone (Propyphenazone)

Follow the non-aqueous titration method as described in formulation 10 of this chapter. Each ml of 0.1 N perchloric acid is equivalent to 0.02303 g of isopropylphenazone. The method based on reaction with citric acid-acetic anhydride or formation of iron complex as described in formulation 9 of this chapter can be followed.

Paracetamol

Follow the nitroso-derivative method described in formulation 2 of the chapter on analgesics and antipyretics.

Diazepam

Weigh accurately quantity of the sample equivalent to 2 mg of diazepam and carry out the estimation as described in formulation of the chapter on analgesics and antipyretics. Alternatively, follow the method described in formulation 1 of this chapter. The yellow chromophore as a result of acid hydrolysis can be measured directly or extracted into chloroform and then measured at 410 nm.

Formulation 11

Phenylbutazone, Quercetin

ESTIMATION

METHOD 1

Phenylbutazone

Weigh accurately a quantity of the sample equivalent to 100 mg of phenylbutazone and extract dry with three 20 ml portions of toluene. Mix toluene extract with acetone, heat and titrate with 0.1 M sodium hydroxide using phenolphthalein solution as indicator. Each ml of 0.1 M sodium hydroxide is equivalent to 0.03084 g of phenylbutazone. For extraction, chloroform may be used instead of toluene.

Quercetin

The entire toluene insoluble residue obtained above is dissolved in dimethylformamide to get a concentration of 10 mcg/ml in respect of quercetin. Measure the absorbance of the solution at about 377 nm and calculate the results by comparing with standard solution of quercetin dimethylformamide (10 mcg/ml).

METHOD 2

Weigh accurately quantity of the sample equivalent to 25 mg of quercetin and extract with alcohol to get 10 mcg/ml concentration. Measure the extinction of the sample and standard (10 mcg/ml) solutions at about 372 nm using alcohol as blank and calculate the results by comparison.

METHOD 3

Askal et al. (1992) have reported a method based on oxidative reaction of quercetin in neutral aqueous solution with 'NBS' in the presence of phenol to give violet chromogen (λ_{max} 510 nm). The authors have claimed that other flavonoids such as rutin, kaemferol and luteolin do not interfere.

Quercetin	3,5,7,3′,4′-Pentahydroxyflavone
Kaemferol	3,5,7,4′-Tetrahydroxyflavone
Rutin	3-Glucose-rhamnose quercetin
Luteolin	3-Desoxy quercetin

Probable Reaction Mechanism

1. The reaction does not depend on catechol function as rutin has same catechol function as quercetin but sugar moiety at C-3.
2. —OH group at C-5 is essential as quercetin-5-glucose does not give colour with 'NBS'.
3. Kaemferol did not give colour with 'NBS' indicating the necessity of ortho-OH group at C-3′ and C-4′ in ring B.
4. The authors concluded that –OH group at C-3, C-5, C-7, C-3′ and C-4′ are essential for reaction with 'NBS' reagent.

Note

Formed chromogens could not be isolated but the authors have proposed polyquinone structure of quercetin as a result of oxidation.

5-OH flavonoids give coloured adducts with 'NBS'.

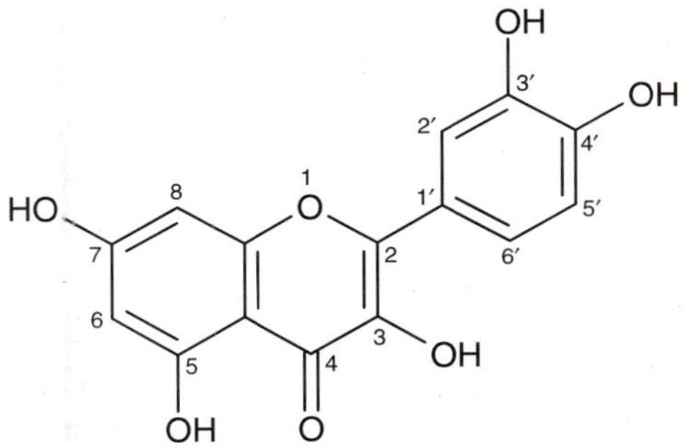

Quercetin
3,5,7,3′,4′-Pentahydroxyflavone

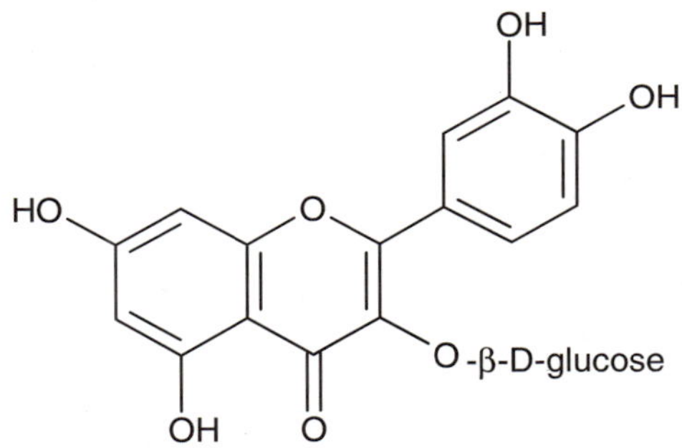

Quercetin-3-glucoside

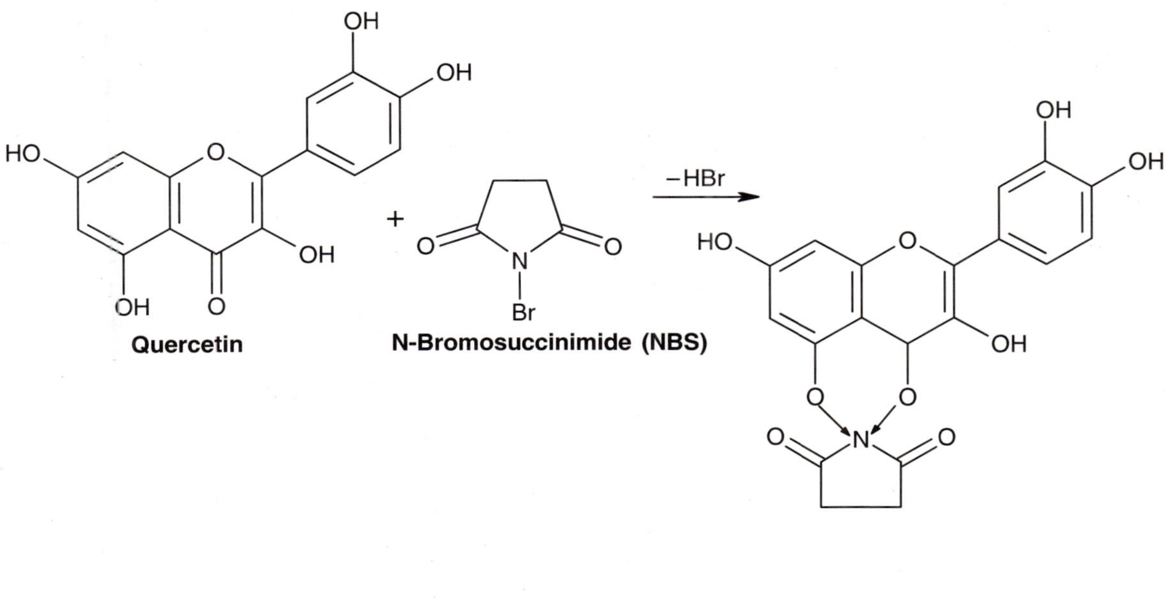

Reference

1. Hassan F. Askal & Gamal A. Saleh. *Talanta*, **39(3)**, 259-263, 1992.
2. K.P. Tiwari, M. Masood. Ind. J. Chem. Soc., 18B, 97-98, 1979.

Like rutin, quercetin also forms fluorescent complex with $AlCl_3$ (P.K. Sengupta & R. Chanda. Easterm Pharmacist, pp. 113-114, June 1980).

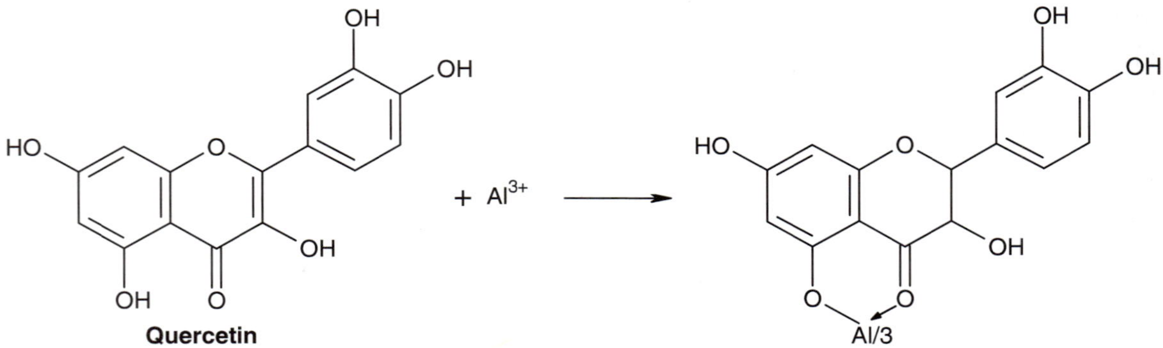

Al - quercetin fluorescent complex

For details, refer to method under rutin. 3-OH flavons also react with flavone reagent (diphenyl boric acid-2-amino ethyl ester) to give a fluorescent complex (λ_{exc} = 365 nm; λ_{em} = 546 nm).

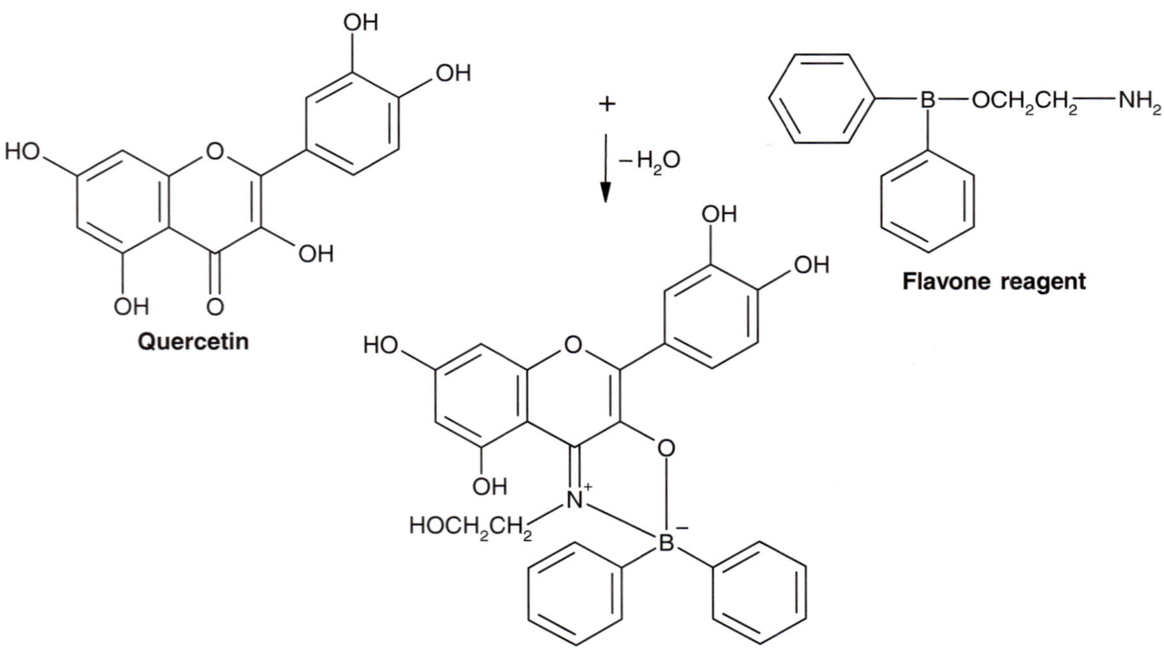

Fluorescent complex
(λ_{exc} = 365 nm; λ_{em} = 546 nm)

Reference

H. Jork et al. Thin Layer Chromatography: Reagents and Identification (Vol. 1a), pp. 277-280, 1990.

Phenylbutazone

Evaporate appropriate volume of the alcoholic extract obtained in method 2 above under quercetin and extract the residue with three 25 ml portions of chloroform. Evaporate combined chloroform extract and take up the residue in 0.1 M sodium hydroxide. Measure the absorbance at 264 nm. Calculate the results taking 660 as value of A 1%, 1 cm at 264 nm.

Formulation 12

Chlorzoxazone, Analgin, Oxyphenbutazone

ESTIMATION

Chlorzoxazone

Standard solution

To accurately weighed 50 mg of the substance, add 20 ml of sodium hydroxide solution (20%). Reflux for 45 minutes directly on a burner, allow it to cool and dilute to 100 ml with water, 20 ml of the resulting solution is further diluted to 100 ml with dilute sulphuric acid.

Sample solution

The sample accurately weighed equivalent to 50 mg of the compound is treated and diluted as under standard solution.

Procedure

To 5 ml each of the sample and standard solutions, add 1 ml of sodium nitrite solution and shake well for one minute. Add 2 ml of ammonium sulphamate solution, shake for two minutes and adjust to 25 ml with water. Measure the extinction of both the solutions at about 405 nm against respective sample blank and calculate the results.

Note

Aspirin, phenylbutazone, paracetamol and indomethacin do not interfere.

Probable Reaction Mechanism

The compound i.e. the drug is hydrolysed to 2-amino-4-chlorophenol by refluxing with NaOH. The amino group of the above obtained product is then diazotized by the addition of $NaNO_2$ and HCl.
Ammonium sulphamate solution is added to destroy the excess of HNO_2 formed during the reaction.

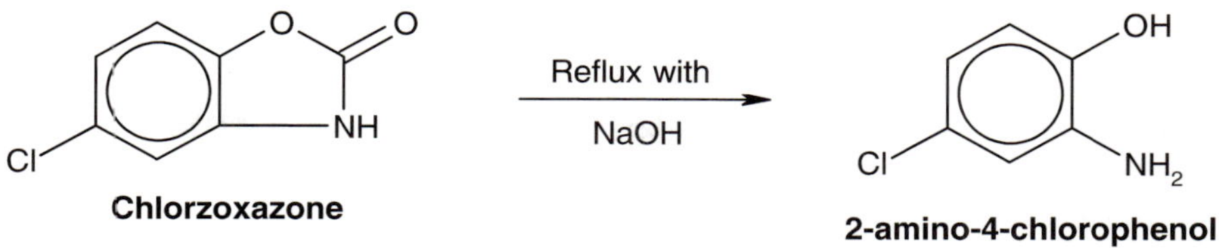

$$NaNO_2 + HCl \longrightarrow NaCl + HNO_2 \xrightarrow{H^+} H_2ONO \quad Cl^- \quad H_2O + Cl^{\ominus}NO^+$$

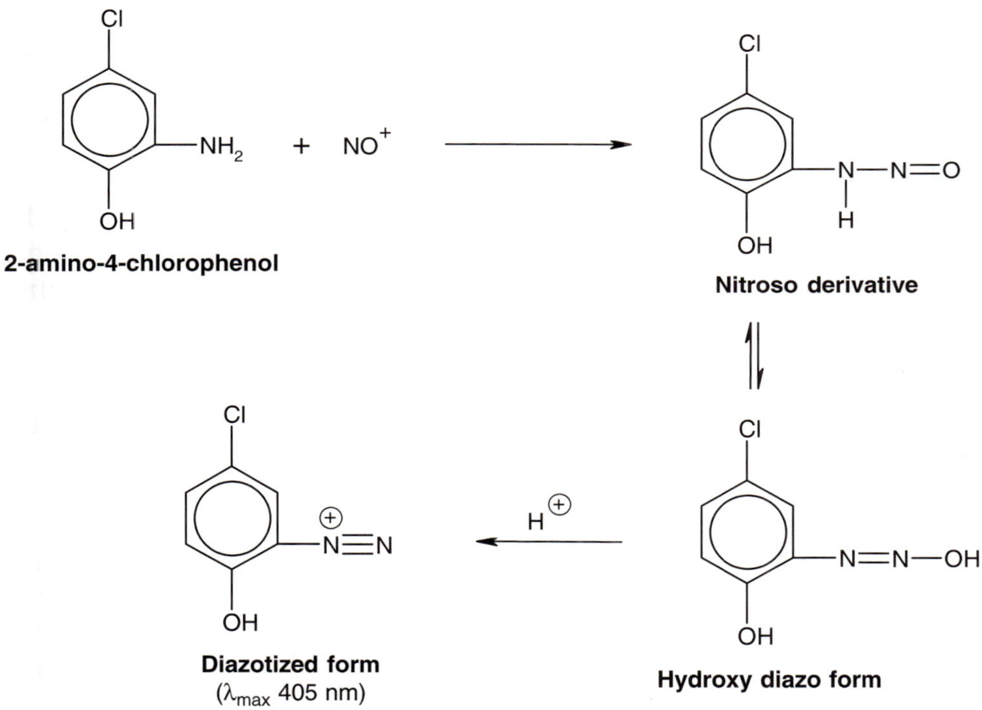

HNO_2	+	H_2NSO_3H	$\longrightarrow$	H_2SO_4	+	$N_2\uparrow$	+	H_2O	(To destroy excess of HNO_2 which shall otherwise interfere.)
Nitrous acid		**Sulphamic acid**							

Note

Hydrolytic product of the molecule having primary aromatic (—NH_2) shall condense with 'PDAB' and Folin's reagent to give coloured product.

Reference

N.M. Sanghvi et al., *Indian Drugs*, **18**, 299-302, 1981.

An indirect analytical method has been suggested by Sastry et al. (2001). The method involves excess of oxidants such as HNO_2, 'NBS' and chloramine T (CAT) and unreacted oxidant estimated spectrophotometrically by reacting with oxidizable dyes such as celestine blue or gallocyanine and measuring the absorbance of the coloured product at 540 nm.

Reference

C.P.S. Sastry et al., *Ind. J. Pharm. Sci.*, **63(3)**, 260-262, 2001.

Analgin

Follow the method involving reaction with p-dimethylaminobenzaldehyde described under formulation 32 of the chapter on analgesics and antipyretics.

Oxyphenbutazone

Follow the extraction with acetone and titration with 0.1 M sodium hydroxide as described for phenylbutazone under formulation 2 of this chapter. Each ml of 0.1 M sodium hydroxide is equivalent to 0.03424 g of oxyphenbutazone.

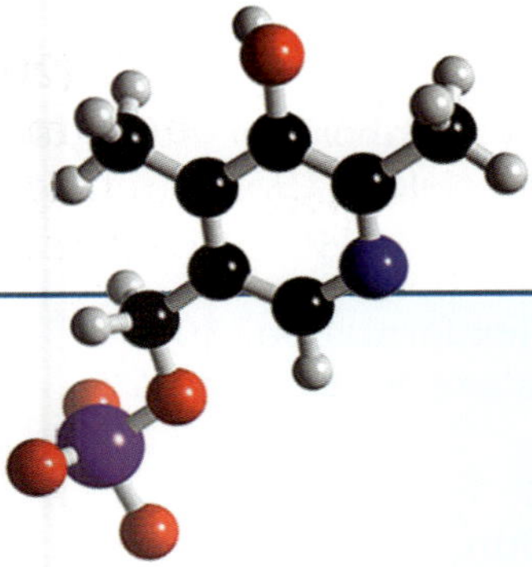

General Index

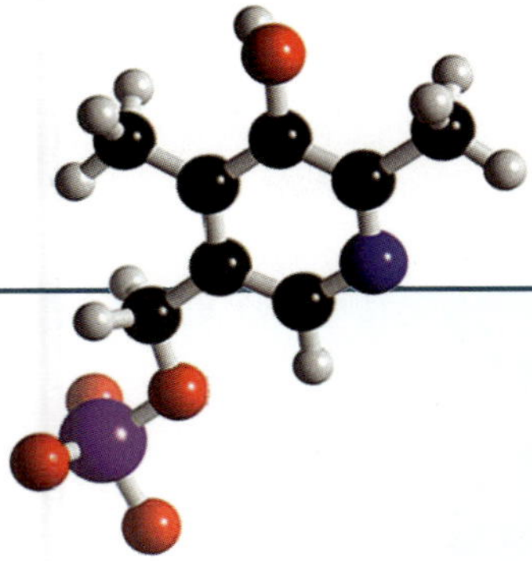

Drug Index

SETHI'S
Quantitative Analysis *of* Pharmaceutical Formulations

SETHI'S

Quantitative Analysis *of* Pharmaceutical Formulations

Methods With Reaction Mechanism

Fourth Edition

Volume 2

Dr. P.D. Sethi
M.Pharm., Ph.D.

CBS

CBS PUBLISHERS & DISTRIBUTORS PVT. LTD.

NEW DELHI • BENGALURU • PUNE • KOCHI • CHENNAI

ISBN : 978-81-239-2187-7

Third Edition : 1997
Reprint : 2003, 2004, 2005, 2008, 2010, 2011
Fourth Edition : 2012

Published by:
Satish K. Jain and produced by Vinod K. Jain for CBS Publishers & Distributors Pvt. Ltd.,
4819/XI Prahlad Street, 24 Ansari Road, Daryaganj, New Delhi - 110002 (India)
E-mail: cbspubs@airtelmail.com, delhi@cbspd.com • www.cbspd.com

Branches:
- ***Bengaluru:*** 2975, 17th Cross, K.R. Road, Bansankari 2nd Stage, Bengaluru - 560070
  Ph.: +91-80-26771678/79
  E-mail: cbsbng@gmail.com, bangalore@cbspd.com
- ***Pune:*** Bhuruk Prestige, Sr. No. 52/12/2+1+3/2, Narhe, Haveli (Near Katraj-Dehu Road By-pass), Pune - 411051
  Ph.: +91-20-64704058/59, 32342277 • E-mail: pune@cbspd.com
- ***Kochi:*** 36/14, Kalluvilakam, Lissie Hospital Road, Kochi - 682018, Kerala
  Ph.: +91-484-4059061-65 • Fax: +91-484-4059065
  E-mail: cochin@cbspd.com
- ***Chennai:*** 20, West Park Road, Shenoy Nagar, Chennai - 600030
  Ph.: +91-44-26260666, 26208620 E-mail: chennai@cbspd.com

Printed at :
Aegean Offset Printers, Greater Noida (UP)

To

Usha, my wife

Although no one is ever born talented nor talent obtained
as a gift or lucky coincidence, it is a resource acquired
through one's own endeavour,
but without her active support and inspiration,
I would never have been an author.

Dedicated to Fellow Analysts, Students, Teachers, Professionals and Mentors

I am quite aware that this compilation may not be flawless, but if I would have waited till it could be done without any error, probably this would never have been possible considering the fact that incompleteness is inevitable feature of any book. I do hope that this compilation will provide adequate stimulus for you to be a sound professional. I would like to appeal the fellow analysts, students, teaching fraternity and professionals to evaluate my efforts in proper perspective. It took me almost 15 years to scan most of the old analytical journals from 1950 onward, the period when analytical methods based on chromogenic reactions were most prevalent. I would like to express my gratitude to fellow analysts, teachers and the mentors in the profession who helped me to shape my ideas for compiling this text. The wide popularity of my books on spectrophotometric analysis, TLC, HPTLC and HPLC among pharmaceutical analysts, students and teachers has been gratifying and encouraging. My aim has never been to use my knowledge as a vehicle but only as a means of sharing my experience with prefessional fraternity.

P.D. Sethi
Pharmaceutical Analyst

"There is no barrier to acquisition of knowledge. Nobody owns it, everybody partakes it and the world becomes richer."

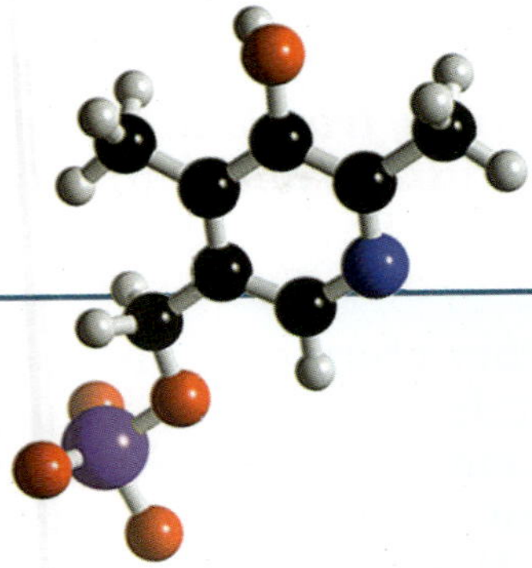

Preface to the Fourth Edition

After the first edition this book appeared in 1985, analytical and teaching fraternity have been of the considered opinion that for professional competency the knowledge of the chemistry involved in the analytical methods i.e. "Reaction Mechanism" needs to be provided, even though not legally mandated, to enable the analysts to perceive the methodology in proper perspective since all aspects of different methods are ultimately founded on chemistry. This is how the idea for contents of this book originated.

Although I had conceptualized the project in 1992 but being busy in compiling books on other subjects of current importance i.e. TLC, HPTLC, HPLC including revision of this title, I could not take up this project due to paucity of time and resources. Further, in view of complexity of the project, I did harbour serious doubts regarding its ultimate completion if and when taken up. If anyone feels that the books can be written by setting an author on his or her way and then waiting for the manuscript to appear, they are delusioned. It needs constant adaptation, definite level of discipline and hunger to keep going. I had been exploring the possibility of associating some teachers with sound knowledge of basic organic chemistry, but met with no success. It has been my ultimate **desire** to complete the project before I close my shop forever.

Knowing fully well that nothing can be achieved without enthusiasm and dedication, being **SCORPIO** decided to accept the challenge with the **SELF BELIEF** and complete the project by myself. I sincerely hope that this series shall find permanent place in every analytical laboratory and teaching institutions with the assurance that such an exhaustive compilation on the subject may never be available.

"Desire is perhaps the starting point of achieving something."

"Belief is the knowledge that we can do something. It is the inner feeling that what we undertake, we can accomplish."

"Scorpio have creative mind with sharp memory, truly explorer of new intelligent horizon, have great stamina and never shy away from challenges, extremely introspective with analytical mind, highly intuitive, determined in pursuit of their goal, passionate about every thing they do, have strong sense of purpose in life with determination to do nothing half-heartedly."

For practical consideration, in addition to introductory chapters, the book has been arranged in 13 principal chapters each containing different multi-component formulations. Analytical methods for each ingredient in a formulation have been described on the pattern similar to 3rd edition using mainly UV-Vis spectroscopy as principal analytical tool. However, as clear from the title, uniqueness of 4th edition is that with each method "probable reaction mechanism" has been described for proper understanding of the methodology as describing methods while ignoring chemistry was considered to be an incomplete endeavour. This should help analysts to integrate fully the analytical methods with the chemistry involved and enable them to transmit the knowledge to others who want to learn. Majority of the reactions included in the text are of the type – addition, elimination, substitution, condensation, rearrangement or oxidation-reduction invariably resulting in the formation of a coloured end product, which could easily be quantified spectrophotometrically in visible region (400-800 nm). This once again established the importance of UV-Vis spectroscopy as an indispensable, reliable and well established analytical tool in spite of steep increase in the use of other physical methods of analysis (HPLC, HPLC/MS, GC, GC/MS, HPTLC, etc.). Analytical methods based on chromogenic reactions have stood the test of time and are still recommended for the fledgling analysts.

Understanding the reaction mechanism allows us to know its specificity and the reaction with the drug being analysed. For drugs having more than one functional group, the methods have been designed depending on the specificity of a particular functional group. With selective chemical reactions, the analyst can manipulate the sample to reveal the desired information and increase the selectivity of the analyte eliminating the possible interference due to other substances present in the formulation while analyzing. It is not

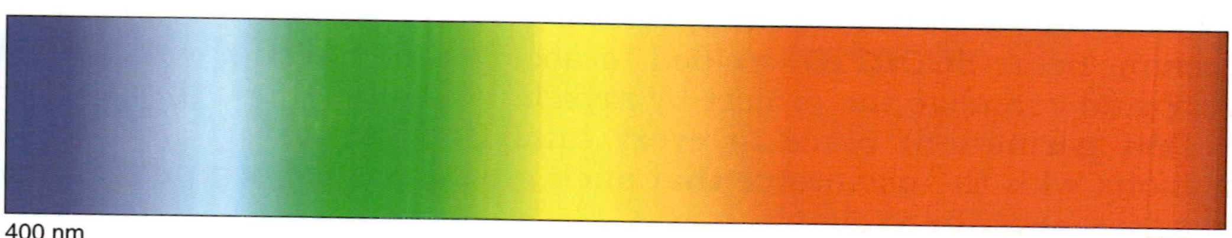

The light that human eye can perceive ranges from deep-violet (short wavelength) through blue, green, yellow and orange to deep red (long wavelength).

"One who never made a mistake never learnt anything."

necessary to learn thousands of individual reactions, instead we can learn few common reactions really well and apply the knowledge to similar cases.

Based on the functional group present in a molecule, the following reagents have been most commonly employed for quantification of the drug molecule: Gibbs' reagent, Bratton-Marshall reagent, Emerson's reagent, Ehrlich's reagent, Pauly's reagent, INH reagent, MBTH reagent, Besthorn's reagent, Folin's reagent, Van Urk's reagent, Wurster's Red reagent, Sanger's reagent, Chromotropic acid reagent, N-Bromosuccinimide reagent and DNPH reagent.

Most of the reaction mechanisms described in the text are as reported by the authors for which relative references have been cited under each reaction. However, the book "Pharmaceutical Chemistry, Vol. 2" by H.J. Roth et al. has been extensively referred to and has been extremely helpful in visualizing the reaction mechanism of several drug substances. Other textbooks of organic chemistry and analytical chemistry invariably consulted have been added under references at the end of introduction.

I am confident that 'Reaction Mechanism' described in this book along with method of analysis shall provide the most stimulating learning experience and will enable you to appreciate the excitement of this fascinating field.

Since newer molecules are invariably chemical modifications of existing drug substances, this compilation should be of help to the analysts in developing suitable method of analysis for newer drug molecules and also understand the chemistry involved and the confidence to tackle newer situations.

Over the years it was observed that at postgraduate level several practical exercises in pharmaceutical analysis were based on the methods described in 1st, 2nd and 3rd editions of this book. The students were invariably keen to know the detailed chemistry involved in methods. I do hope, my attempt in this direction will help students to perform practicals with better understanding. I expect this four-volume book on pharmaceutical analysis with reaction mechanism should make analytical science easier to understand for students, analysts and educators.

The icon representing structure of codeine with "Reaction Mechanism" reflects the underlying concept of this book.

Although I have exerted all my efforts to ensure that the text is free from errors, but it is quite possible that methodology details, certain structures and reaction mechanism may be inaccurate. I hope my efforts shall be evaluated in proper perspective.

It is the analyst who is consistently if not constantly involved with all the aspects of analysis. His/her interest necessarily is not of a curious bystander. This book does not purport to make analysts out of its readers, although it is hoped that some will be "turned on" to such a pursuit.

New Delhi, India

P.D. Sethi, M.Pharm., Ph.D.
Pharmaceutical Analyst

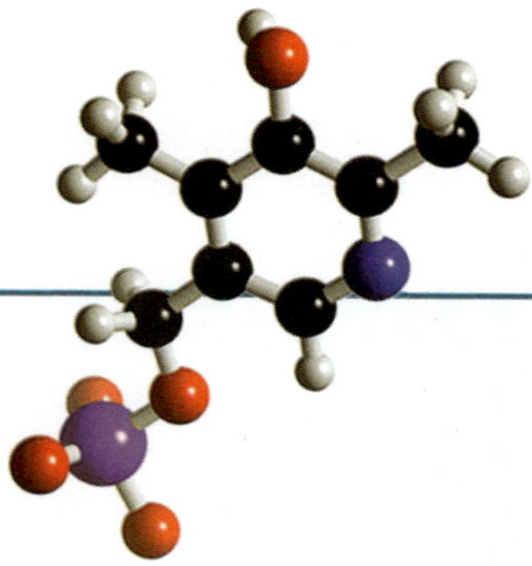

Acknowledgement

I would like to express my most sincere gratitude to analysts, students, teachers and professionals for their continuous support and encouragement and shaping my analytical career and ideas for compiling this book. The support extended by Professor Vijay K. Kapoor, University Institute of Pharmaceutical Sciences, Panjab University, Chandigarh in explaining and correcting several reactions included in the text is sincerely acknowledged. I am deeply indebted to Mr. Dilip Charegaonkar, Managing Director, M/s Anchrom Enterprises (I) Pvt. Ltd., Mumbai for supporting my scientific activities. I would like to convey my appreciation to the management of M/s Anchrom Enterprises (I) Pvt. Ltd., Mumbai and Kongposh Publications Pvt. Ltd., New Delhi for independently establishing life-time annual awards for Best Research Papers in "HPTLC Analysis" and "Pharmaceutical Analysis" respectively in recognition of my contribution in the field of Pharmaceutical Analysis. I am confident, their gesture shall provide impetus to young analysts for their interest in pharmaceutical analysis, currently the most creative and challenging field.

Without the support and untiring efforts of Mr. Dharmvir of 'CBS' my hand-written text particularly the reactions would never have been converted into book, thanks for his dedication and commitment for completing the assignment meticulously. I am thankful to Mr. Satish K. Jain, Managing Director, CBS, for accepting the hand-written manuscript of most challenging project and providing all the required facilities to bring this series to fruition.

New Delhi, India

P.D. Sethi, M.Pharm., Ph.D.
Pharmaceutical Analyst

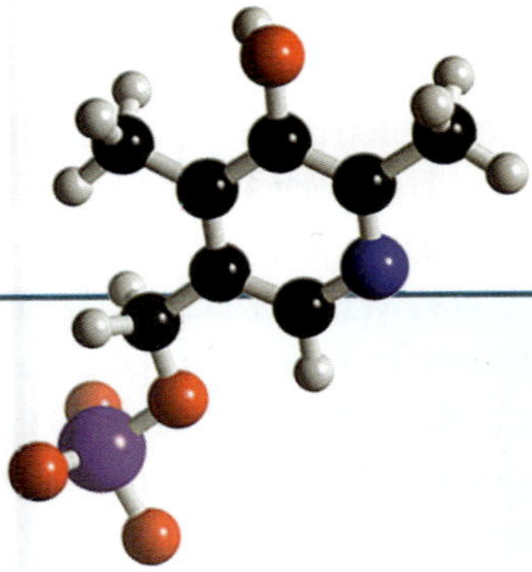

Preface to the First Edition

Devising accurate assay procedures for each ingredient of complex dosage formulations containing several therapeutically and chemically compatible drugs with very similar chemical nature is a monumental undertaking. The very idea of separation, identification and estimation of each ingredient in such complex formulations would make the analyst's hair stand on end. Not only are the multiple active constituents present but they are usually there in widely divergent concentrations depending upon their relative potency and therapeutic need of the patient. The presence of additives, excipients and decomposition products further complicates the development of analytical procedures. Many of the classical tests long regarded as specific for certain substances are now answered by many more compounds. Nevertheless, the therapeutic advantage of such complex drug combinations should take precedence over any potential analytical problem which is ultimately the concern of the analyst. The increasing complexities of pharmaceutical preparations and the marked emphasis on quality control by the ethical manufacturers have placed greater load on the ingenuity of the quality control chemist.

An analyst who is in the need of an analytical method may be obliged to survey tremendous amount of literature in order to select one procedure which may appear to suit his need and facilities available, but when he subjects the selected procedure to actual test, he may find that he cannot reproduce the method. It is, therefore, essential that the practising analyst should have access to analytical procedures which are simple, reliable and workable under routine laboratory conditions.

"No one is ever born talented nor talent obtained as a gift or lucky coincidence. It is a resource acquired through one's own endeavour. In this process, others may provide some help and inspiration, but it is a quality earned by one's own hard endeavour."

Modern analytical techniques rely increasingly on complex techniques of analysis that require expensive equipments and highly specialized personnel. Such methods are not of much help in countries lacking these resources. For the most part, modern analytical techniques merely permit analysis to be carried out more rapidly than the conventional method of analysis, which though not bad are tedious and time-consuming. Even if a manufacturer is ready to procure and install modern instruments/equipments, their maintenance in fittest condition is a herculean task. Non-availability of trained analytical personnel and precise, simple and suitable methods of analysis are major handicaps for pharmaceutical manufacturers in developing countries.

Taking into consideration the technical and economic constraints, it is necessary that the recommended methods should permit their use by drug laboratories located in developing countries. It is significant to stress that even simple instruments like colorimeter and spectrophotometer result in sensitive and accurate measurements with clear advantage of speed, simplicity and easy maintenance. The large volume of literature devoted to their application in almost every field of scientific research constitutes irrefutable evidence of their utility. It is, therefore, reasonable to assume that the analytical procedures involving the use of such simple instruments will find greater application. Selection of analytical method is a very critical point. The method must be accurate, sensitive, selective, reproducible and convenient.

In view of rapid advance during the last several years in the field of pharmaceutical analysis and marketing of ever increasing multi-component formulations, the available texts dealing in pharmaceutical analysis that have been written so far do not in general deal with the analysis of each component in wide range of complex pharmaceutical dosage formulations, particularly in presence of interfering substances. The official compendias are rarely of help in such formulations. To fill the existing gap in literature and keeping in view the economic and technical limitations of drug manufacturers, particularly in medium and small scale sector, it was felt that there exists a need to have a compilation of a simple, suitable and reliable methods for analysis of each ingredient of multi-component drug formulations.

This text, a maiden attempt, is meant to fulfill these needs. Analytical procedures for more than 200 drug formulations of divergent combinations have been compiled to serve as a convenient source of information for analysts and scientists engaged in the field. The focal point for this compilation is the presentation of practical aspect of the methodology using colorimeter and spectrophotometer as the main analytical tools.

For practical considerations, the drug formulations have been classified into 23 different categories based upon their common therapeutic uses as under:

1. Analgesics and antipyretics
2. Antacids and other ulcer healing drugs
3. Antacids, sedatives, antispasmodics
4. Anthelmintics
5. Anti-allergic drugs
6. Antibiotics
7. Anti-diarrhoeals
8. Anti-inflammatory drugs
9. Antimalarials
10. Anti-tuberculous drugs
11. Bronchospasm relaxants (anti-asthma)
12. Enzymes and digestives
13. Expectorants and cough suppressants
14. Eye, ear preparations
15. Keratolytics and cleansers
16. Laxatives, purgatives and lubricants
17. Nasal preparations
18. Oral rehydration salts
19. Rubefacients
20. Sedatives and tranquillisers
21. Topical antifungal, anti-infective preparations
22. Urinary anti-infective preparations
23. Vitamins, minerals and other nutritional additives.

For most of the formulations, several alternative methods have been described for a particular substance so that the analyst can intelligently select and apply the method to suit his need and the laboratory facilities available. Preliminary treatment of the sample for analysis utilizing conventional isolation and extraction procedures have been applied wherever necessary to eliminate the presence of potentially interfering substances. In other cases, the methods are sufficiently specific to permit the analysis of individual ingredients without pre-treatment. The procedures have been described in sufficient details highlighting the important steps in methodology so that these can be reproduced without much difficulty. Merits and demerits of each method and possibility of its application to other formulations have been discussed. To help the analyst and to enhance the book's usefulness, several worked out examples based on actual experimental data have been included. For drug manufacturers, who are interested to set up their independent quality control division, chapter on the profile of a quality control laboratory has been included giving brief outline of different sections.

Its importance for pharmaceutical teachers, students and institutions imparting special course in drug analysis cannot be overestimated. Science graduates interested in pursuing career as analytical chemist will find this compilation invaluable for daily use which will provide ready answers to most of their analytical problems. It is earnest feeling of the author that knowledge of the basic inorganic and organic chemistry tempered by judicious changes and the special skill needed in pharmaceutical analysis and the information included in this text will enable the analyst to overcome most specific problems and he will be able to analyse any viable combination of drug formulations he may encounter in future. It is pertinent to mention that analyst should cautiously choose the method and interpret the results carefully before certifying the product. It is hoped that this text will enable the analyst to take their rightful place in the pharmaceutical industry and in government laboratories concerned with the quality control of medicinal preparations.

The author is indebted to his wife, Usha for her moral support throughout his career.

The author wishes to express his sincere appreciation to Dr. O.P. Ghai, Professor and Head, Department of Pediatrics, All India Institute of Medical Sciences, New Delhi, for his helpful suggestions and guidance.

How far I have succeeded in my attempt, the decision is left to my fellow pharmacists and analysts.

New Delhi, India
1985

P.D. Sethi

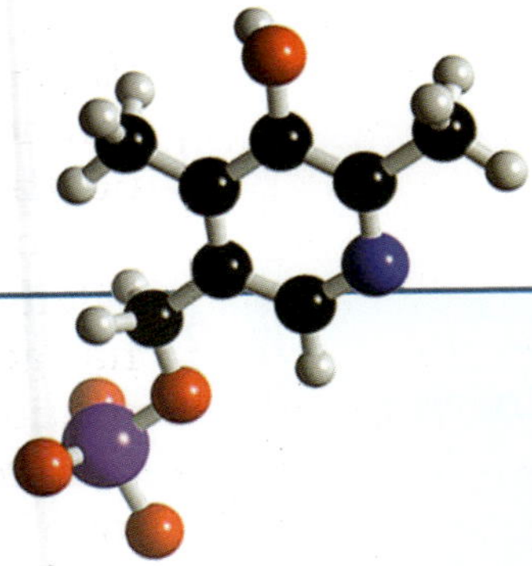

Brief Contents

Volumes I – IV

VOLUME 1

VOLUME 2

VOLUME 3

VOLUME 4

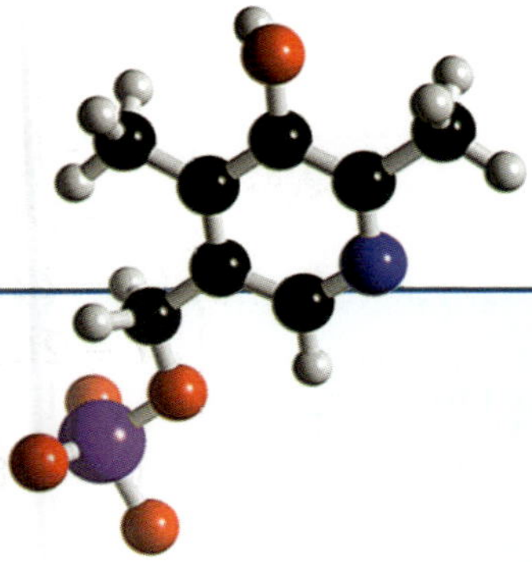

Contents

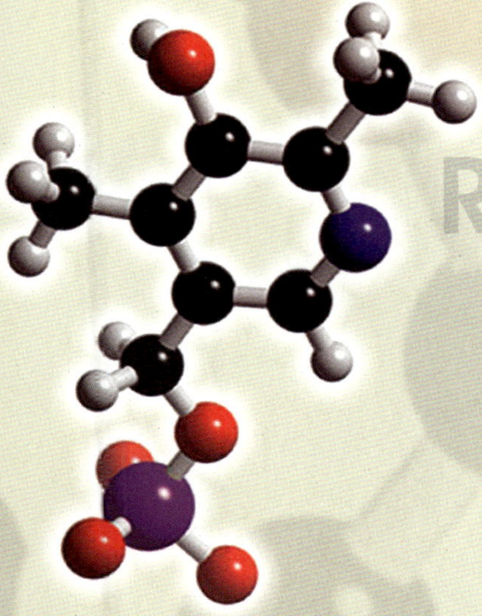

Reaction Mechanism

8

Analgesics and Antipyretics

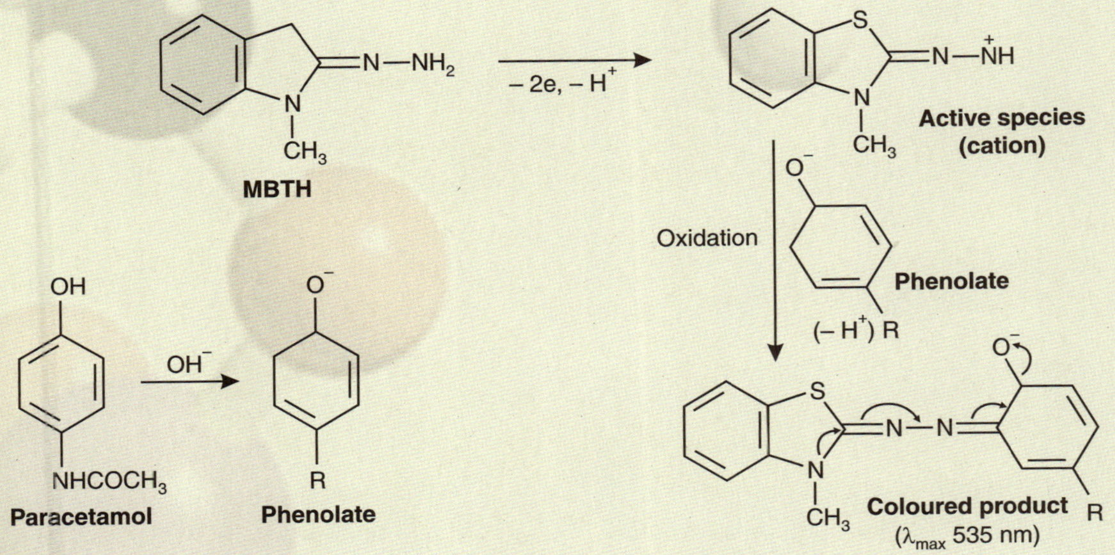

Formulation 1

Aspirin, Caffeine, Phenylephrine hydrochloride, Terpine hydrate, Ascorbic acid

ESTIMATION

Aspirin

Method 1

Standard solution

15 mcg/ml of aspirin in 0.1 M sodium hydroxide.

Sample solution

Transfer accurately weighed portion of the powdered tablets equivalent to 150 mg of aspirin to a 100 ml volumetric flask. Add about 70 ml of 0.1 M sodium hydroxide and heat in a water-bath for 30 min. Cool and adjust the volume with 0.1 M sodium hydroxide. Filter and collect the filtrate after rejecting first 20-25 ml of filtrate. The filtrate is appropriately diluted with 0.1 M sodium hydroxide to get a concentration of 15 mcg/ml in respect of aspirin.

Procedure

Measure the extinction of both the solutions at maximum at about 292 nm using 0.1 M sodium hydroxide as blank and calculate the results by comparison.

Note

The extinction value of standard solution at 292 nm is quite constant on the same instrument and can be used for future estimations. So it is not necessary to run a standard every time.

On boiling with standard NaOH solution, aspirin is hydrolysed to salicylic acid and acetic acid, which in turn reacts with alkali to yield respective sodium salts and excess alkali back titrated with 0.1 M HCl. Each ml of 0.5 M NaOH ≡ 0.04504 g of aspirin.

A novel method has been described by Ahsan Saeed for the estimation of aspirin. The method is based on transacetylation of p-aminophenol by

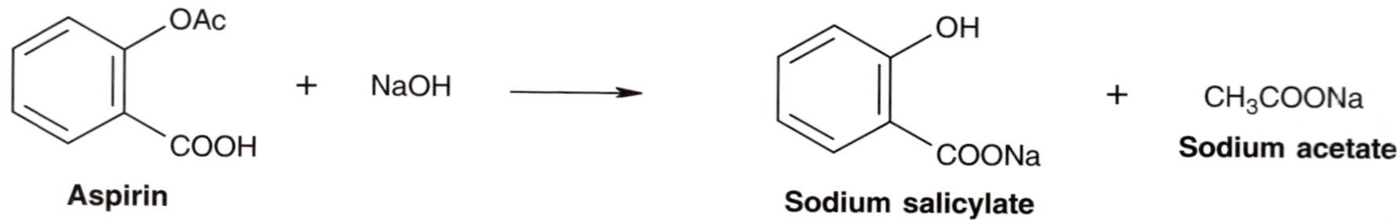

acetylsalicylic acid to give paracetamol which then undergoes alkaline oxidation followed by coupling with m-cresol to produce a blue-coloured product.

Reagents

1. 0.2 M sodium carbonate solution.
2. 0.1% potassium ferricyanide.
3. 0.01 M m-cresol in alcohol.

Procedure

Reflux 100 mg of aspirin with 200 mg of aminophenol in 20 ml of ethanol, dilute to 100 ml with water. Process the sample as above. To 1 ml each of sample/standard solution add 1 ml of sodium carbonate soltion, 2.5 ml of potassium ferricyanide solution, allow to stand for 10 min for complete oxidation, then add 1 ml of m-cresol, keep for another 10 min, dilute to 25 ml with water and measure the absorbance at 640 nm against reagent blank.

Probable Reaction Mechanism

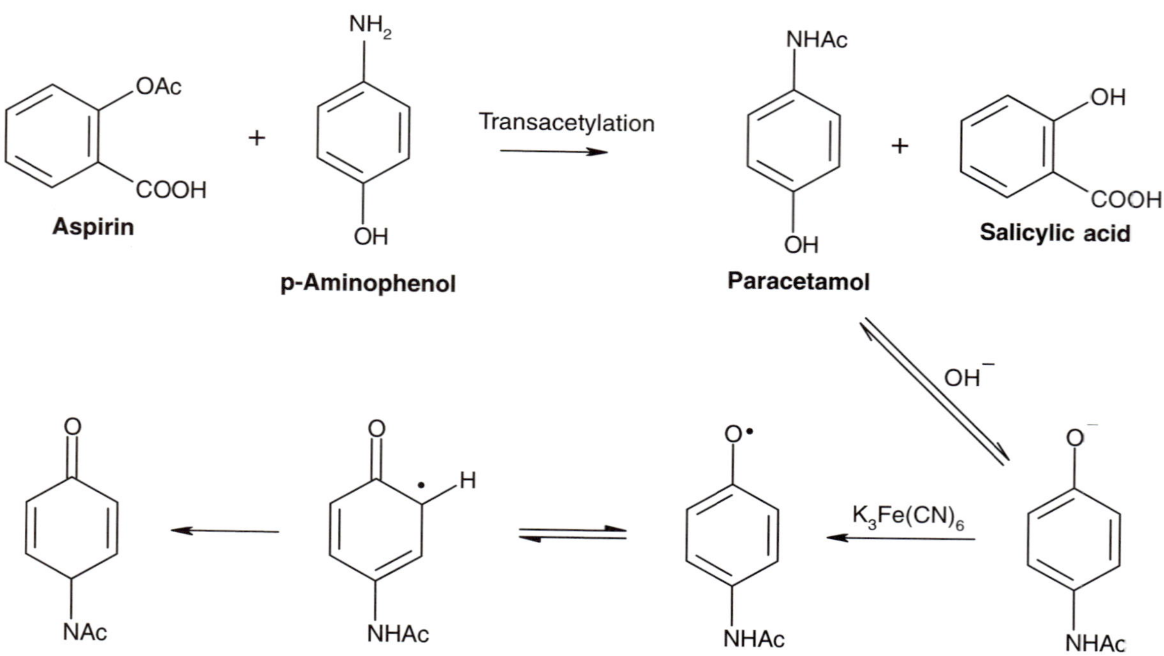

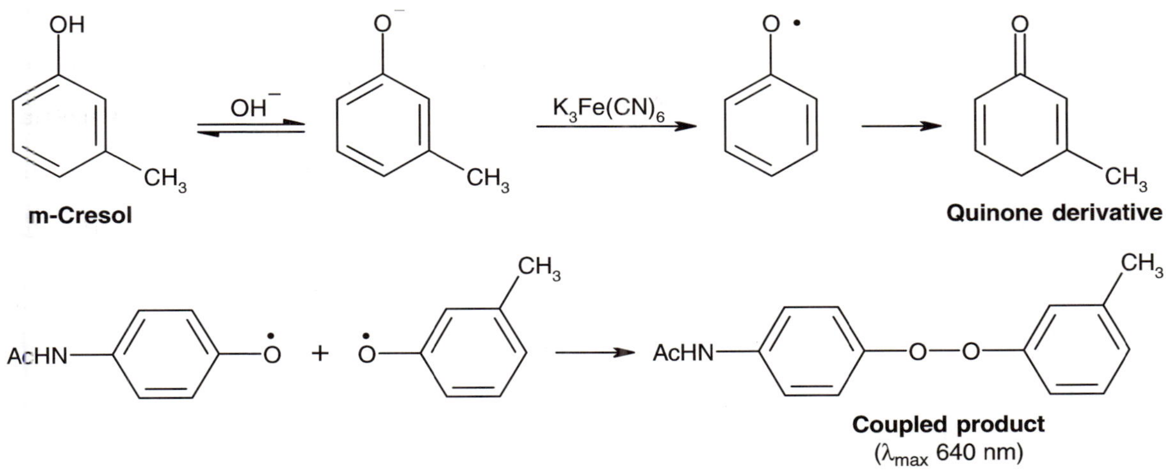

Note

1. This reaction is analogous to oxidation of phenols by $K_3Fe(CN)_6$ in alkaline medium to give aryloxy radical which forms coupled product.
2. Caffeine, phenylephrine, terpine hydrate, chlorpheniramine, ammonium chloride, codeine and barbiturates do not interfere.

Reference

Ahsan Saeed, Indian Drugs, **32(1)**, 15-19, 1995.

Caffeine

METHOD 1

Weigh accurately a quantity of powdered tablets equivalent to 10 mg of caffeine and transfer to a separating funnel. Add 10 ml of water and 10 ml of 1 M sodium hydroxide, shake well and extract with four successive quantities, each of 20 ml of chloroform. Wash each chloroform extract with the same 10 ml of water contained in another separating funnel. Collect in a dry 100 ml volumetric flask after passing through a cotton plug and make up the volume with chloroform. Dilute 10 ml of the aliquot to 100 ml with chloroform. Measure the extinction of this solution at the maximum at about 276 nm using chloroform in the reference cuvette. Calculate the contents of caffeine per tablet from the extinction of a standard caffeine solution (10 mcg/ml) in chloroform run simultaneously with the sample.

METHOD 2

Reagents

1. 0.1 M iodine.
2. 0.1 M sodium thiosulphate.
3. Dilute sulphuric acid.

Procedure

Follow the extraction procedure as described above under method 1 taking sample equivalent to 50 mg of caffeine. Evaporate chloroform layer and dissolve the residue in 30 ml of dilute sulphuric acid. Add 50 ml of 0.1 M iodine and dilute to 100 ml with water. Allow it to stand for 60 min. Filter, discarding the first 20 ml of the filtrate and titrate 25 ml of the filtrate with 0.1 M sodium thiosulphate using starch solution as indicator. Each ml of 0.1 M iodine is equivalent to 4.85 mg of caffeine.

Note

In acidic medium, iodine solution forms brown precipitates with caffeine; probably reaction produces periodite. After precipitation, excess iodine is estimated with sodium thiosulphate. Similarly with bromine solution, it will produce perbromide. Other purine bases react in analogous way.

Method 3

Reagents

1. 5% w/v silicotungstic acid solution in water.
2. A solvent mixture of 1 volume of ethyl alcohol and 5 volumes of anhydrous ether.

Standard solution

0.5 mg/ml of caffeine in alcohol-ether solvent mixture.

Sample solution

Weigh powdered material accurately equivalent to 20 mg of caffeine, add 20 ml of dilute sulphuric acid and 30 ml of water. Reflux for 1 hr, cool and extract with four 25 ml portions of chloroform. Evaporate chloroform layer and dissolve the residue in solvent mixture to produce 50 ml.

Procedure

To 50 ml each of the sample and standard solutions add 10 ml of silicotungstic acid solution, stir and filter through glass sintered funnel G_4. Wash the precipitate with solvent mixture. Dissolve the residue in water and dilute further with water to get 15 mcg/ml solution. Measure the extinction of both the solutions at 265 nm. The method obeys Beer's law over the concentration range of 10-90 mcg/ml.

Note

1. The solvent should be absolutely free from water.
2. Paracetamol, analgin, codeine, salicylamide, atropine, phenobarbitone, vitamin B_1 and niacin do not interfere.

The most specific reaction for caffeine involves alkaline hydrolysis yielding caffeidine by ring opening which forms enamine with acetylacetone. The enamine condenses with PDAB in acidic medium to give polymethine dye (λ_{max} 630 nm).

Probable Reaction Mechanism

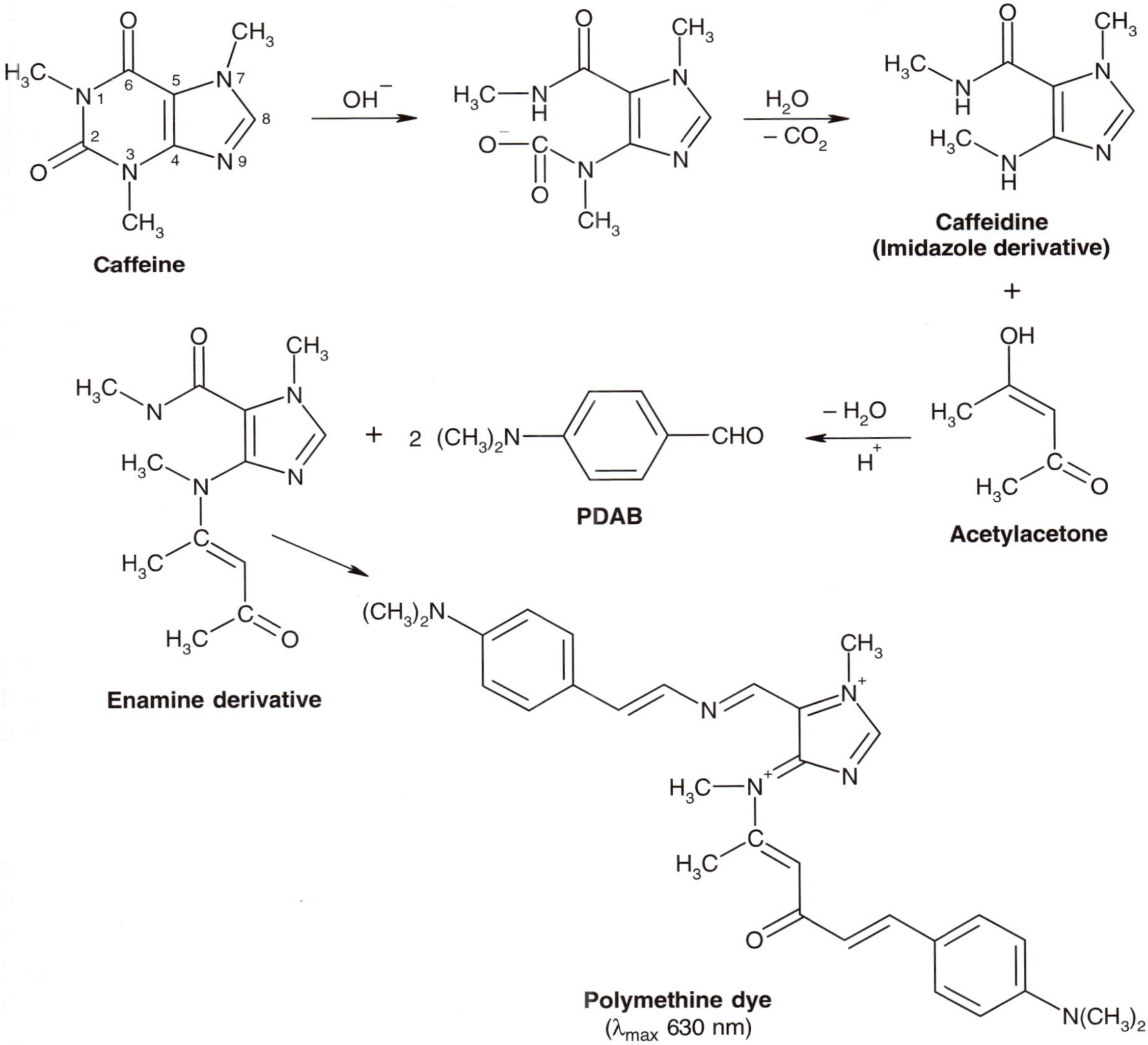

Note

Other xanthine derivatives such as theobromine and theophylline do not interfere.

Reference

Pharmaceutical Chemistry (Vol. 2) by H.J. Roth, 1991, p. 595.

METHOD 4

Reagents

1. 0.01% solution of 4,5-dimethyl-o-phenylene diamine (DMPD) in methanol (solution is stable for 3 days in dark).
2. 0.01% solution of N-bromosuccinimide (NBS) in water.
3. 0.1% solution of sodium thiosulphate in water.
4. 0.6 M acetate buffer, pH 4.3.

Sample and standard solutions of caffeine

10 μg/ml solution in water.

Procedure

To 1 ml each of sample and standard solutions add 1 ml of acetate buffer, 0.2 ml of NBS solution. Keep at 30 C for 20 min, add 0.2 ml of sodium thiosulphate solution and 0.2 ml of DMPD solution. Keep the reaction at 50 C for 30 min and measure the fluorescence against reagent blank. Exc. 390 nm and em 480 nm.

Probable Reaction Mechanism

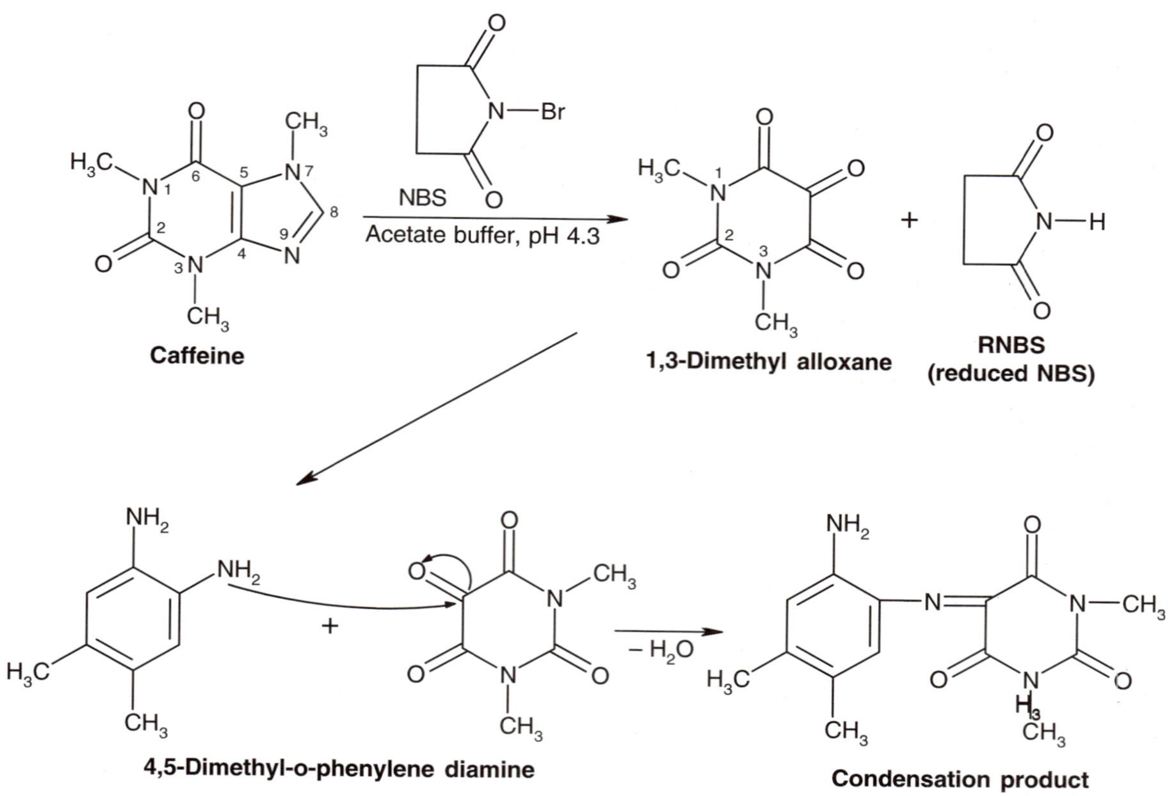

Two of the three adjoining carbonyl groups of 1,3-dimethyl alloxane each form part of a lactam grouping, so only the carbonyl group i.e. at position 1 exhibits ketone properties and therefore can condense with the nucleophilic amine forming a condensation product having fluorescent properties (390/ 480 nm).

Reference

Masatoki Katayama & Hirokazu Taniguchi, Talanta, **36(12)**, 1171-1175, 1989.

Caffeine, a purine derivative, is oxidized by chloramine-T in the presence of hydrochloric acid and forms a purple-red ammonium salt of purpuric acid (murexide) with ammonia.

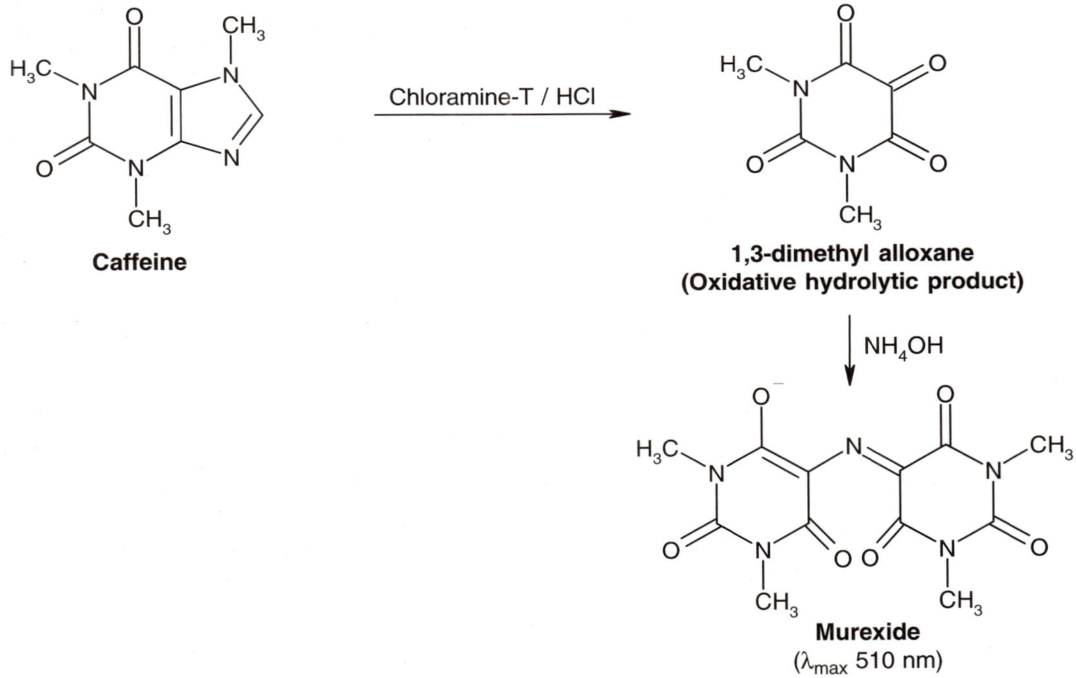

Note

Murexide is a fluorescent compound.

Phenylephrine hydrochloride

METHOD 1

This method is based on alkaline oxidation and coupling with antipyrin.

Reagents

1. 0.5% w/v solution of 4-aminophenazone (4-aminoantipyrin) in water.

2. 8.0% w/v solution of potassium ferricyanide in water.
3. 8.4% w/v solution of sodium bicarbonate in water.

Standard solution

100 mcg/ml of phenylephrine hydrochloride in water.

Sample solution

Weigh accurately a quantity of the powdered tablets equivalent to 10 mg of phenylephrine hydrochloride, dissolve in water to produce 100 ml, filter, reject first 15-20 ml of the filtrate and collect rest of the filtrate.

Procedure

To 10 ml each of sample and standard solutions add 5 ml of the 4-aminophenazone solution, 5 ml of the potassium ferricyanide solution and 1 ml of the sodium bicarbonate solution, allow to stand for half and hour and make up the volume to 100 ml. Read the optical density at 500 nm taking as absorbance of a blank similarly treated but replacing test solution by water. Correct this result by taking a sample blank obtained by diluting 10 ml of the sample filtrate to 100 ml and reading at 500 nm, taking water as blank.

Note

Although the optical density can be measured even after 15 minutes but 30 minutes gives more reproducible results.

Probable Reaction Mechanism

The reaction involves oxidative coupling of 4-aminophenazone in para position to the phenolic function of the molecule. The oxidizing agent used is $K_3Fe(CN)_6$ in weakly alkaline medium (pH 8.0, $NaHCO_3$ buffer)—the optimal reaction conditions. The reaction is known as "Emerson reaction".

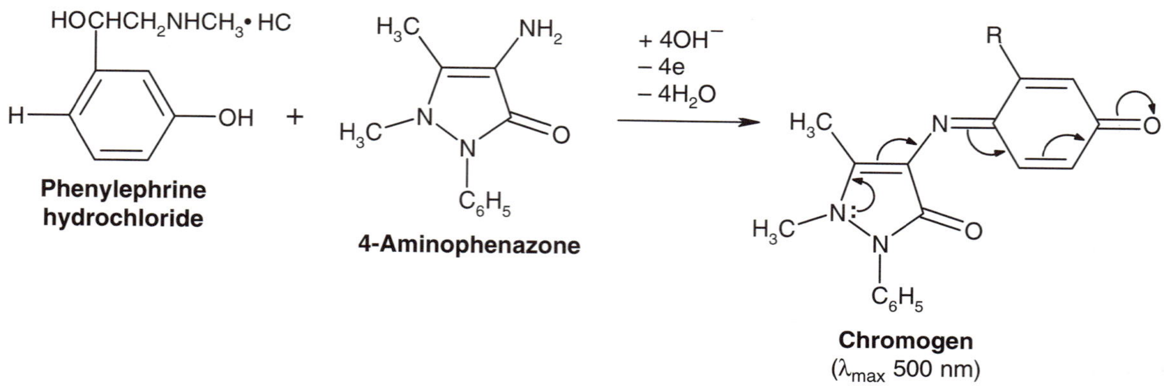

The resonance structure exists because of the lone pair of electrons available with N atom.

Note

The other drugs which answer this reaction are amoxycillin, salbutamol, picroxicam, triamcinolone, guaicolsulphonate, thymol and carvacrol.

Reference

1. C.F. Hiskey & N. Levin, J. Pharm. Sci., **50(5)**, 393-395, 1961.
2. K.T. Koshy & H. Mitchner, J. Pharm. Sci., **52(8)**, 802-803, 1963.
3. Pharmaceutical Chemistry (Vol. 2) by H.J. Roth, 1991, pp. 75-76.

Following conditions must be met for reaction to proceed:

1. Free phenolic —OH groups or a keto enol system in the ring.
2. p-position unsubstituted or with a substituent such as halogen, carboxyl, sulphonic, hydroxy or methoxy groups which are easily oxidatively dissociated.
3. Absence of a nitro group in the o-position which would prevent the reaction.

METHOD 2

Reagents

1. 0.15% w/v solution of nitrosonaphthol in ethyl alcohol.
2. 20% v/v nitric acid.

Standard solution

100 mcg/ml of phenylephrine hydrochloride in water.

Sample solution

Weigh accurately a quantity of powdered tablets equivalent to 10 mg of phenylephrine hydrochloride, extract with 100 ml of water, shake and filter (100 mcg/ml).

Procedure

To 2 ml of sample and standard solutions add 1 ml of nitrosonaphthol reagent and 1 ml of the nitric acid. Heat on a water-bath at 55 C for 30 min, cool and extract with 10 ml of ethylene dichloride. Reject organic layer and read extinction of yellow colour of the aqueous layer at about 420 nm.

Note

Chlorpheniramine maleate which is usually present along with this compound does not interfere.

Probable Reaction Mechanism

Phenylephrine condenses with nitrosonaphthol in acidic medium on heating (55 C) at position para to phenolic function to give yellow-coloured product (λ_{max} 420 nm).

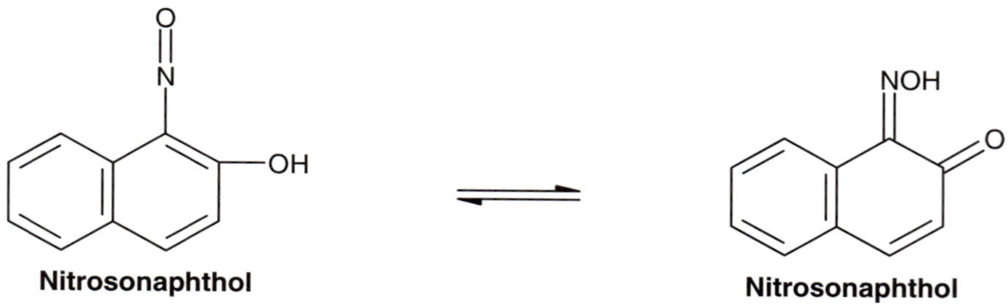

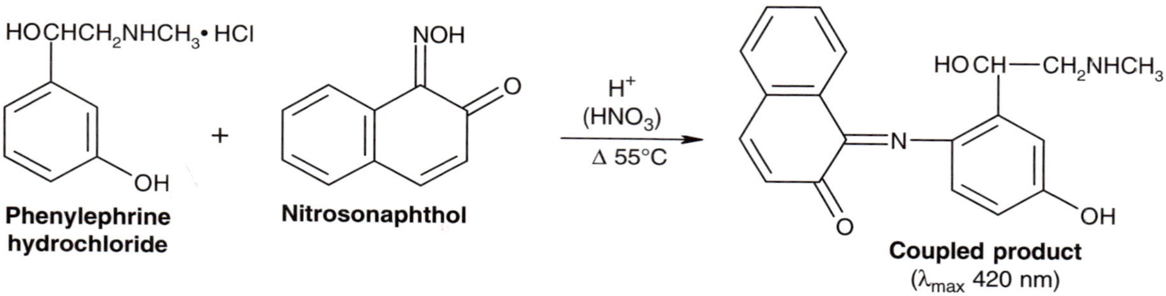

METHOD 3

This method is based on formation of nitroso derivative which is coupled with copper (Cu^{++}) to give pink-coloured complex.

Reagents

1. 5% w/v solution of sodium nitrite in water.
2. 2.5% w/v solution of copper acetate in water.
3. 0.2 M hydrochloric acid.
4. 1% w/v solution of urea in water.

Standard solution

0.5 mg/ml of phenylephrine hydrochloride in water.

Sample solution

Extract the sample with water to get 0.5 mg/ml solution in respect of phenylephrine hydrochloride.

Procedure

To 1 ml each of sample and standard solutions, add 1 ml of sodium nitrite solution, 1 ml of copper acetate solution, 3 ml of 0.2 N hydrochloric acid and

0.5 ml of urea solution, shaking after each addition. Keep in a boiling water bath for 15 minutes. Cool in ice for 1 minute and add 1 ml of 0.2 M hydrochloric acid and dilute to 10 ml with water. Measure the absorbance of both the solutions at about 520 nm. The coloured complex is stable for several hours.

Explanatory Note

Sodium nitrite reacts with hydrochloric acid to give nitrosonium ions. Nitrosonium ion being electron-deficient will attack the ortho position to the phenolic —OH group present in the compound. The complex so formed gives chelate complex with the copper reagent.

Probable Reaction Mechanism

$$NaNO_2 + HCl \longrightarrow NaCl + HNO_2$$

$$H^+ + HNO_2 \longrightarrow H_2ONO^+ \xrightarrow{Cl^{\ominus}} Cl^{\ominus}\ \overset{\oplus}{N}{=}O$$

Nitrosonium ion

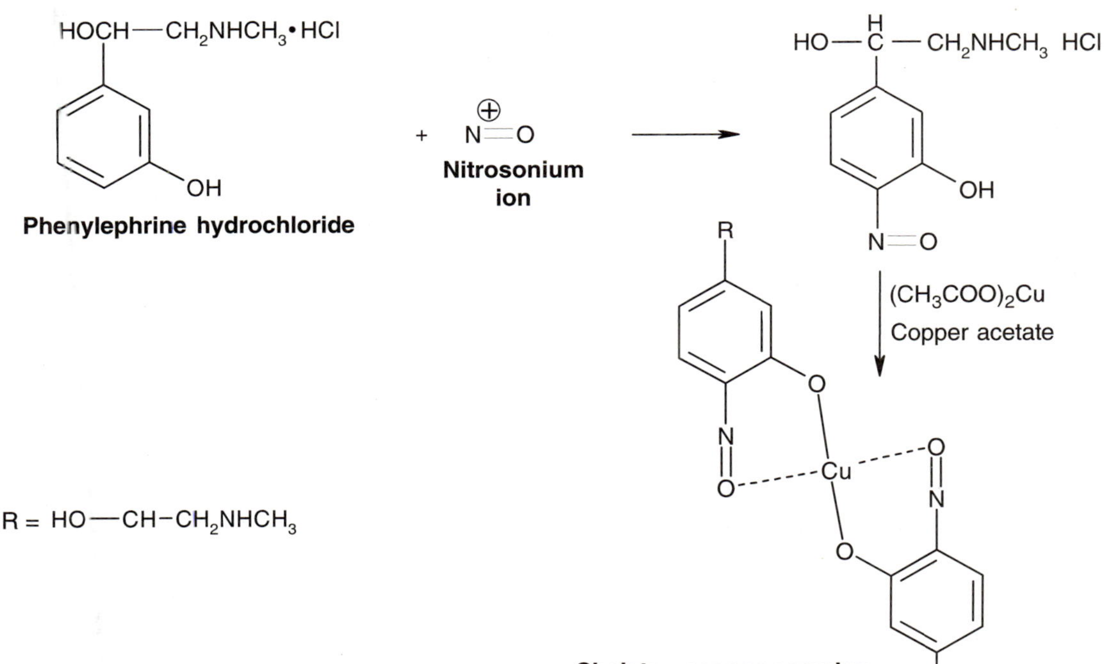

Chelate - copper complex
(λ_{max} 520 nm)

Note

Urea has been added to destroy excess of HNO_2.

Probable Reaction Mechanism

Phenylephrine, being phenylalkylamine derivative, forms Cu^{2+} chelate with with OH and NH_2 group, known as Chen-Kao reaction. The reaction involves formation of chelate between Cu(II) and adjacent placed —OH group and NH_2 group particularly in case of phenylalkylamine. This reaction is known as Chen-Kao reaction. For the reaction to proceed, alkaline conditions are to be maintained.

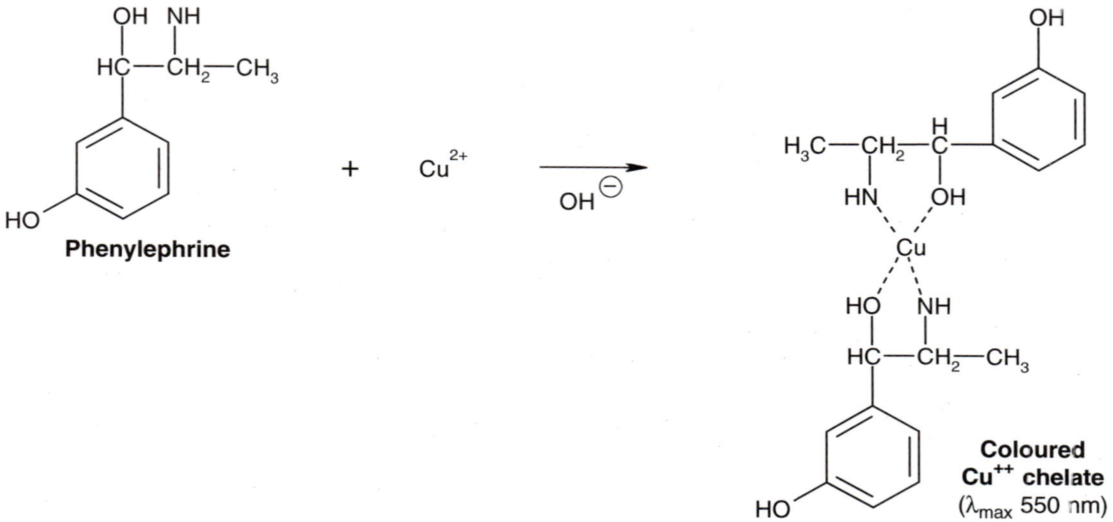

Note

1. This reaction is similar to the one described for ephedrine and other phenylalkylamine derivatives such as adrenaline and salbutamol.
2. Because of its phenolic and amino alcoholic structure it exhibits absorption both in acid and alkaline medium.

Reference

Pharmaceutical Chemistry (Vol. 2) by H.J. Roth, p. 374.

A spectrophotometric method based on ion-pair complex formation was described by Shenoy et al. (1973). The compound formed ion-pair comlex with bromothymol blue in 0.01 M phosphate buffer, pH 6.4. The complex has λ_{max} 420 nm.

Note

Phenylpropanolamine and dextromethorphan did not interfere.

Reference

Bhamy B. Shenoy & V. Das Gupta, J. Pharm. Sci., **62(5)**, 803-804, 1973.

The method described by Sane et al. based on reaction with p-aminophenol in alkaline medium is of analytical interest. The authors have claimed that drugs usually associated (chlorobutol, naphazoline, chlorpheniramine maleate, menthol, caffeine and paracetamol) do not interfere.

Probable Reaction Mechanism

p-Aminophenol reacts at the ortho or para position to the phenolic —OH group in the drug resulting in the formation of indophenol-like product under alkaline condition. The reaction can be represented as under.

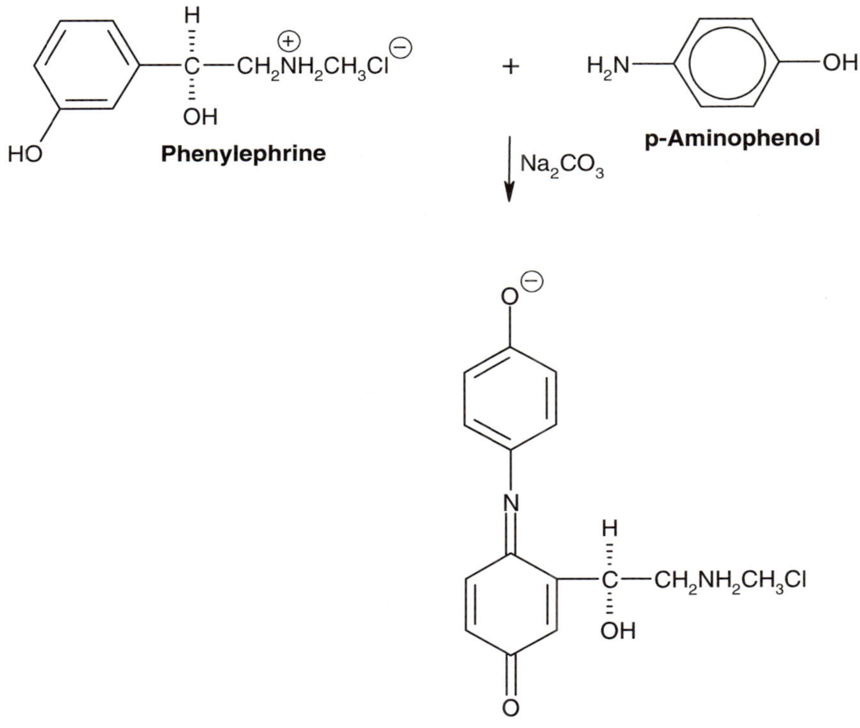

Indophenol-like product
(λ_{max} 640 nm)

Reference

R.T. Sane & V.S. Narkar, Indian Drugs, **18(1)**, 23-24, Oct. 1980.

The coupling reactions involved with following reagents are of analytical interest. All these reagents contain primary aromatic amino group which can be diazotized and then coupled with phenylephrine at para position to the phenolic —OH group present in the drug under basic conditions to give coloured complex.

1. Sulphanilamide 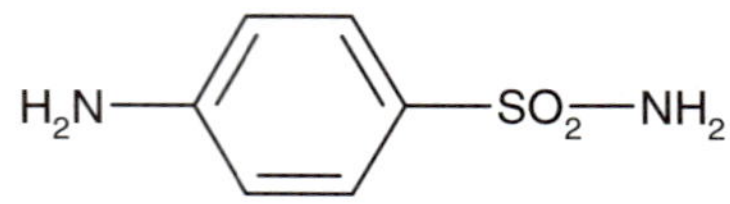 λ_{max} 445 nm

2. Dapsone 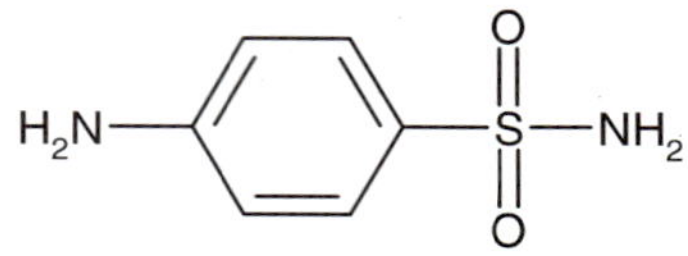 λ_{max} 470 nm

3. p-Aminoacetophenone 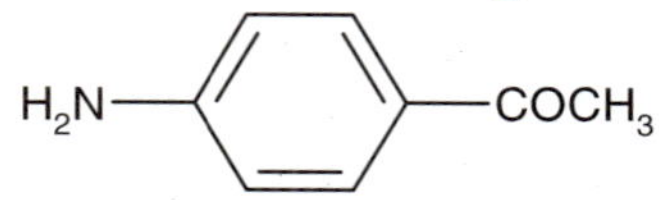 λ_{max} 475 nm

4. Benzocaine 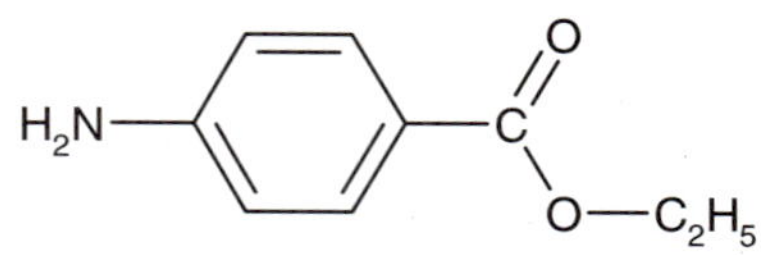 λ_{max} 460 nm

Probable common reaction mechanism for different reagents

Diazotization of the primary amino group of the reagents: To 1 ml of the reagent, add 1 ml of acid mixture; allow to stand for 15 min, then add 2.5 ml of ethyl alcohol to destroy excess of HNO_2 and then proceed with coupling. (Acid mixture: Mix 86 ml of 15% CCl_3 COOH, 20 ml of 2 M H_2SO_4, dilute to 100 ml with water.)

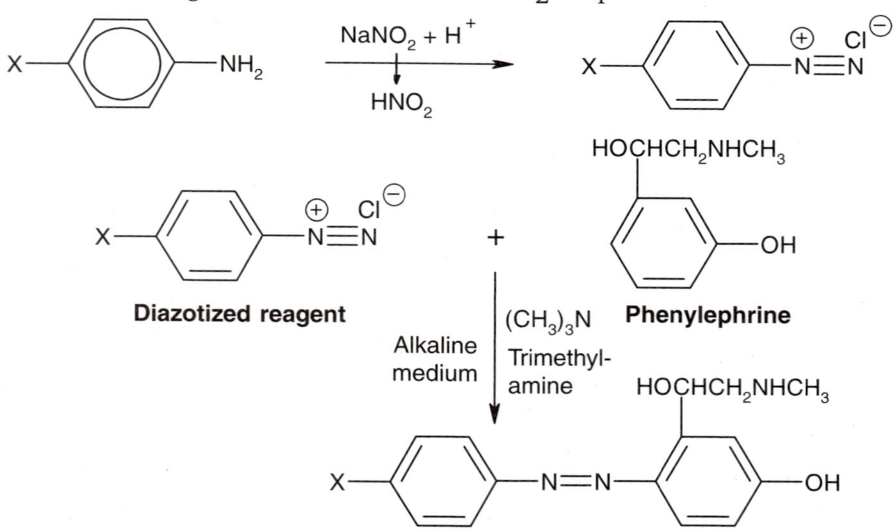

Coupled product

The absorption maxima of the coupled product with different reagents are: Benzocaine - 460 nm, Dapsone - 470 nm, Sulphanilamide - 445 nm, p-Aminoacetophenone - 475 nm.

Reference

1. Textbook of Practical Oraganic Chemistry by Vogel, p. 920.
2. R.T. Sane et al. Indian Drugs, **20(8)**, 337, May 1983.

Terpine hydrate

Reagent

Phosphotungstic - phosphomolybdic acid: To 10 g pure sodium tungstate and 2 g phosphomolybdic acid (free from nitrates and ammonium salts) add 10 g phosphoric acid and 70 ml of water. Boil over free flame for 2 hrs, cool, filter, if necessary, and dilute to 100 ml with water.

Standard solution

Dissolve 50 mg of terpine hydrate in 500 ml of chloroform. Each ml of this solution contains 0.1 mg of terpine hydrate.

Test solution

Transfer a quantity of powdered tablets equivalent to 10 mg of terpine hydrate to a dry 100 ml volumetric flask. Add about 75 ml of chloroform, shake well, make up the volume with chloroform and filter.

Procedure

In a series of 100 ml conical flasks transfer respectively 5 ml each of standard solution, test solution and chloroform (to serve as blank). To each flask add 5 ml water, 2 ml of phosphotungstic - phosphomolybdic acid reagent and shake well for 10 minutes. Evaporate chloroform layer in a water bath at 65-70 C. Cool in the ice-bath, add very slowly 2 ml of ice-cooled sulphuric acid and allow to stand in the ice-bath for half an hour with very light mixing at interval of 10 minutes. Heat the mixture on water-bath (90-95 C) for exactly 10 minutes, with occasional shaking. Cool to room temperature (a turbid solution may be obtained which will subsequently become clear on further dilution). Add about 10 ml of acetone, shake and transfer to a 25 ml volumetric flask with the help of acetone and make up the volume with acetone. Measure the extinction at 630 nm using blank in the reference cuvette. Deduce the results by comparison.

Ascorbic acid

METHOD 1

Reagents

1. 2,6-dichlorophenol - indophenol solution: The dye is dissolved in alcohol to get a concentration of 0.25 mg/ml. The solution is filtered and stored in refrigerator. It is brought to room temperature just before use.
2. Citrate - buffer solution: Dissolve 70 g of citric acid (monohydrate) in 420 ml of 1 N sodium hydroxide and dilute to 1000 ml with water. Adjust the pH to 3.5 and store in refrigerator.

Standardization of the dye solution

Weigh accurately 15 mg of ascorbic acid and transfer to a volumetric flask with the help of sufficient volume of buffer solution to produce 50 ml. To 2 ml of the resulting solution add 10 ml of buffer solution and titrate rapidly with the dye solution with constant shaking till distinct rose-pink colour persists for about 10 seconds. Carry out the blank titration using 12 ml of buffer solution. Express the concentration of the dye solution (per ml) in term of its equivalent (mg) of ascorbic acid.

Sample solution

An accurately weighed/measured quantity of the sample equivalent to about 100 mg of ascorbic acid is shaken with 50 ml of citrate buffer and diluted to 100 ml with the buffer. 2 ml of the resulting solution is titrated with the previously standardized dye solution to a rose-pink end point and the contents of ascorbic acid in the sample are calculated with the help of pre-determined equivalent factor.

Note

1. As ascorbic acid is unstable in citrate buffer, the experiment should be completed within 60 minutes.
2. The dye solution in alcohol is stable for more than 45 days.

This method is based on Tillman's reaction and is still the most important method for assay. Ascorbic acid, being a strong reducing agent, reduces coloured quinonimine system present in the reagent to colourless phenolamine system. However, this reaction is not specific to ascorbic acid but is answered by all reducing agents.

Probable Reaction Mechanism

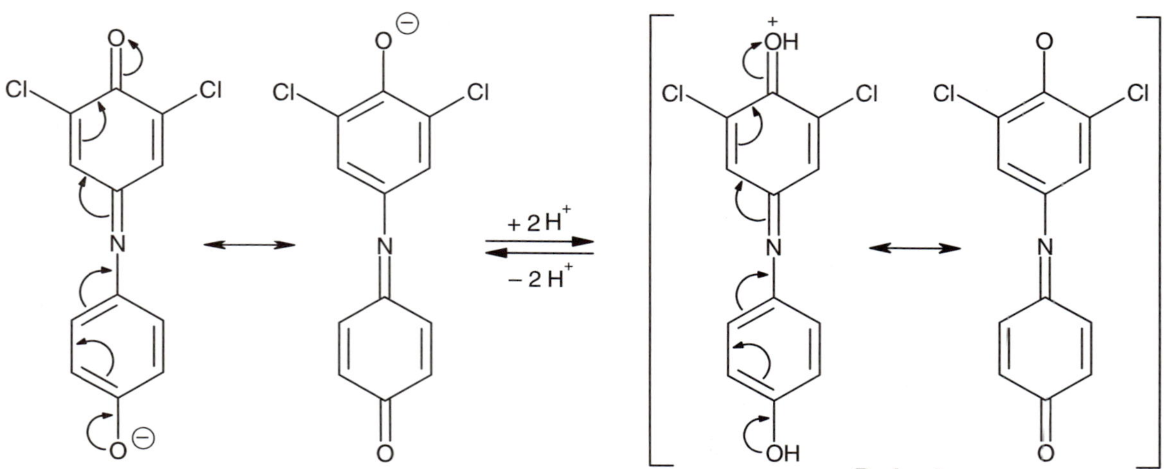

2,6-dichlorophenol - indophenol (deep blue colour)

The above dye can exist in two forms as shown.

Red colour (Protonated form)

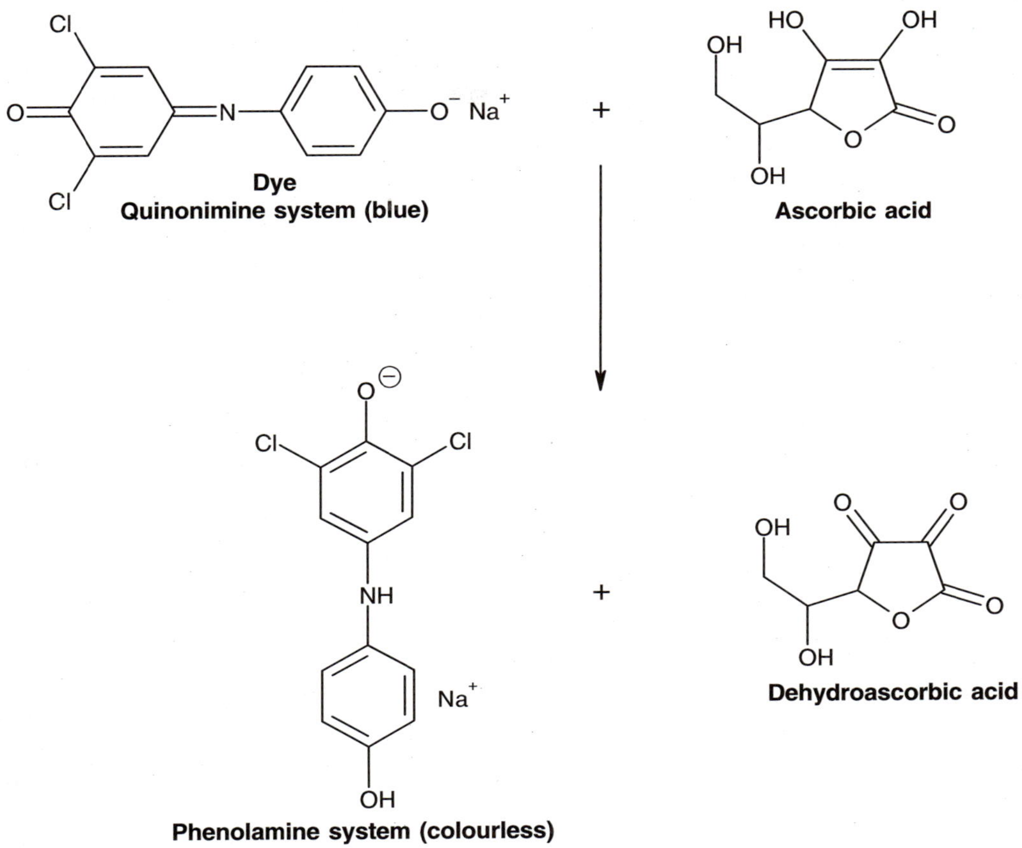

Here the dye 2,6-dichlorophenol - indophenol is reduced by ascorbic acid. In the process of reduction, the red-coloured chromogen (protonated form) is formed (therefore it is stable for 10 seconds). Further reduction by ascorbic acid leads to the formation of a colourless product. Ascorbic acid is at the same time oxidized to dehydroascorbic acid.

METHOD 2

Transfer accurately weighed portion of the powdered tablets equivalent to 250 mg of ascorbic acid, add 25 ml of sulphuric acid (10% v/v) and dilute to 100 ml with water. Filter and titrate 20 ml of the filtrate with N/10 cerric ammonium sulphate using phenanthroline ferrous complex as indicator. Each ml of N/10 cerric ammonium sulphate is equivalent to 0.0088 g of ascorbic acid.

Explanatory Note

Ce - ammonium sulphate, being an oxidizing agent, oxidizes ascorbic acid to dehydroascorbic acid. Once the reaction is complete, excess of Ce - ammonium sulphate will oxidize the indicator phenanthroline ferrous complex (deep red) to phenanthroline ferric complex (pale blue). In this process Ce(IV) gets converted to Ce(III).

$(NH_4)_4\,[Ce(SO_4)_4],\ 2\,H_2O$ +

Ce - ammonium sulphate or ammonium cerium sulphate

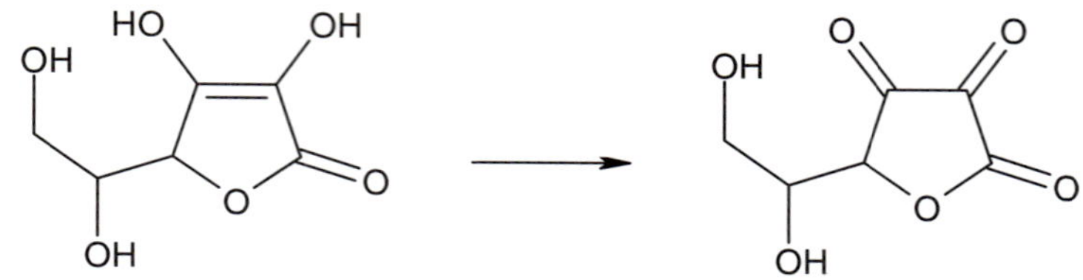

Ascorbic acid → **Dehydroascorbic acid**

$$Ce\ (IV) + e \rightleftharpoons Ce\ (III)$$

$$(C_{12}H_8N_2)_3Fe^{2+} \rightleftharpoons (C_{12}H_8N_2)_3Fe^{3+} + e$$

Phenanthroline ferrous complex ⇌ **Phenanthroline ferric complex**

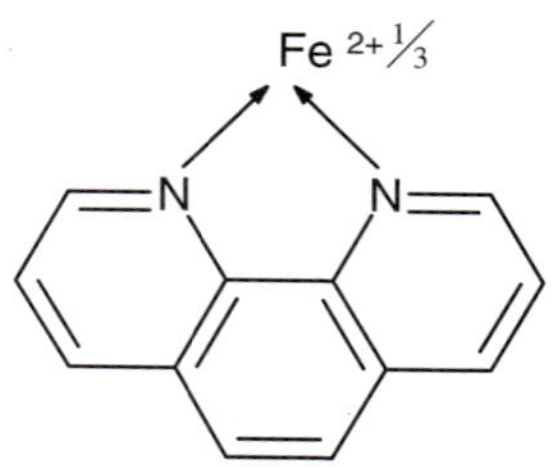

Phenanthroline ferrous complex (ferroin) (used as indicator)

Probable Reaction Mechanism

Amir Besada (1987) has reported that reaction with cerric(IV) is not stoichiometric and varies with time, acidity and temperature and has recommended the use of ferric ammonium sulphate. The Fe(II) produced as a result of oxidizing ascorbic acid to dehydroascorbic acid can react with "Emmerie-Engel reagent" i.e. 2,2′-bispyridine - iron (III) chloride reagent.

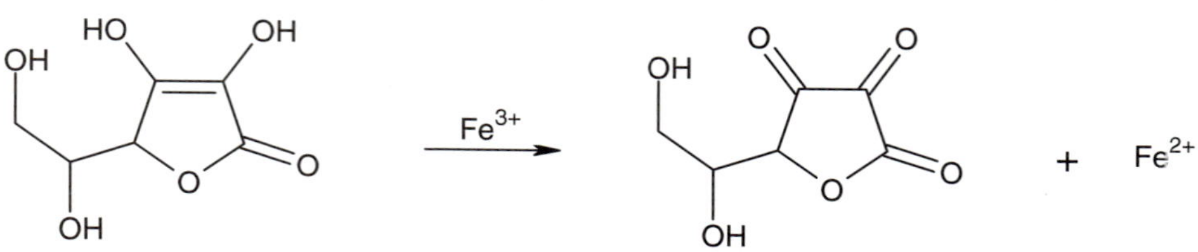

Ascorbic acid → **Dehydroascorbic acid**

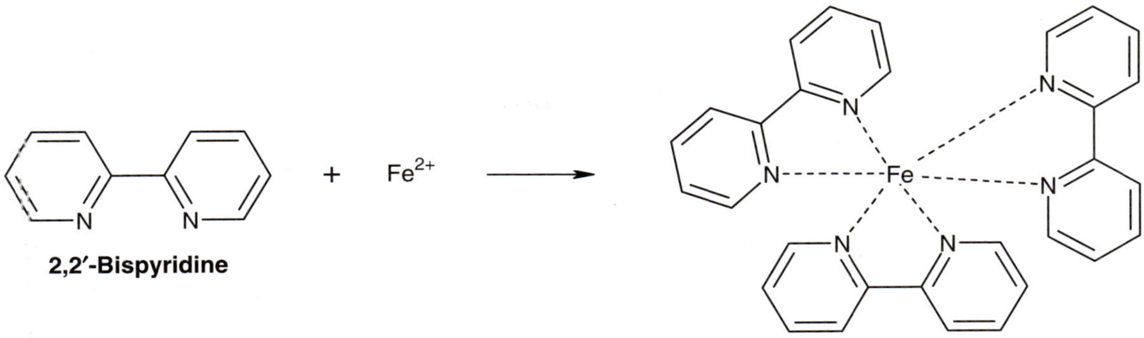

Two nitrogen atoms in bispyridyl have one unshared pair of electrons which can be shared by Fe(II)

Note

Phenols, tocopherols and captopril answer this reaction.

Reference

Amir Besada, Talanta, **34(8)**, 731-732, 1987.

METHOD 3

Reagents

1. 0.1% w/v solution of 4-chloro-7-nitrobenzofuran (NBD-Cl) in acetone, freshly prepared.
2. 0.2 M sodium hydroxide solution.
3. 0.5% citric acid solution.

Standard solution

100 μg/ml in 0.5% citric acid solution.

Sample solution (tablets, capsules, syrup, drops)

The sample was extracted with citric acid by shaking to get final concentration of 100 μg/ml.

Procedure

To 1 ml of the sample/standard solution, add 1 ml of 0.2 M sodium hydroxide solution, 1 ml of NBD–Cl reagent, mix and dilute to 10 ml with citric acid solution. Measure the absorbance of the resulting solution at 582 nm against reagent blank and calculate the results.

Explanatory Note

On addition of sodium hydroxide, ascorbate anion is produced which acts as nucleophile to displace the Cl^- ion from the reagent to give -4-substituted derivative (λ_{max} 582 nm).

Probable Reaction Mechanism

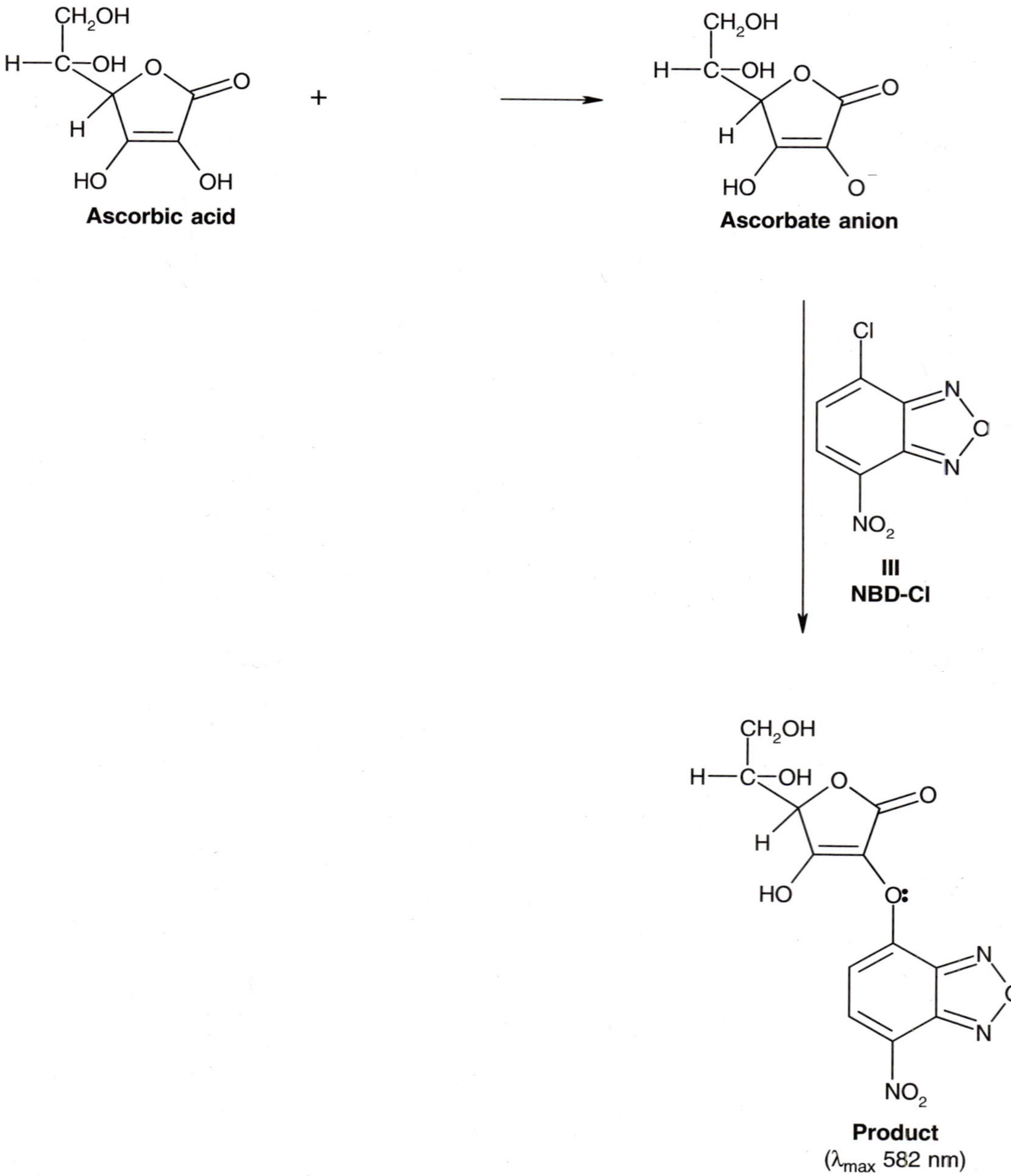

Both ascorbic acid and dehydroascorbic acid react with 1,2-phenylene diamine in acidic medium to yield fluorescent products when heated at 110-120 C for 10-15 min.

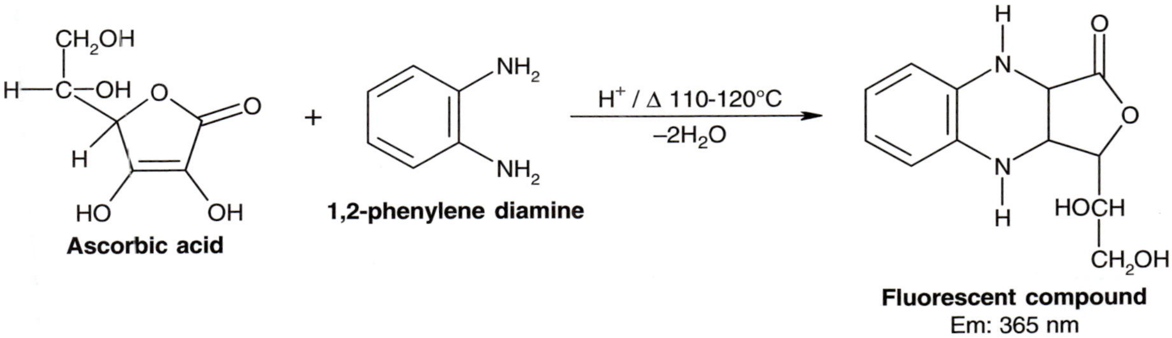

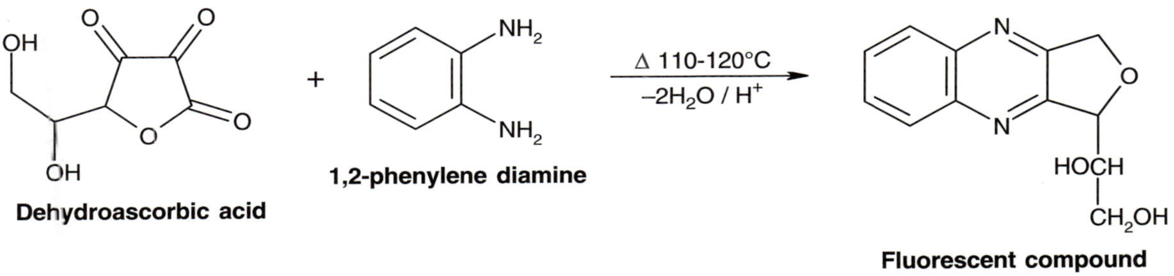

Reference

Thin-Layer Chromatography: Reagents and Detection Methods by H. Jork & others, 1990, Vol. 1a, p. 373.

Formulation 2

Salicylamide, Paracetamol

ESTIMATION

METHOD 1

Standard solution of paracetamol

To 250 mg of paracetamol, accurately weighed, add 10 ml of methyl alcohol and dilute to 250 ml with water.

Standard solution of salicylamide

To 250 mg of salicylamide, accurately weighed, add 10 ml of methyl alcohol and dilute to 250 ml with water.

Solution A: Dilute 3 ml of standard solution of both salicylamide and paracetamol separately to 250 ml with 0.01 N sodium hydroxide (12 mcg/ml).

Solution B: Dilute 3 ml of standard solutions of both salicylamide and paracetamol separately to 250 ml with water (12 mcg/ml).

Sample solution

Weigh accurately a quantity of powdered tablets equivalent to 250 mg of paracetamol, add 10 ml of methyl alcohol, shake and dilute to 250 ml with water. Filter and carry out further dilutions as under standard solution A and B above.

Procedure

Measure the extinction of respective standard solution A at 262.5 nm and 329 nm using respective standard solution B as blank. Use the extinction value at 262.5 nm for calculation of paracetamol and that at 329 nm for calculation of salicylamide.

METHOD 2

Paracetamol

This method involves the formation of nitroso derivative which shows absorption maxima at about 400 nm.

Paracetamol

Reagents

1. 3% w/v solution of sodium nitrite in water.
2. 1 N hydrochloric acid.
3. 1 N sodium hydroxide.
4. 0.12% w/v solution of cobalt (II) bromide or chloride in water.

Standard solution

100 mcg/ml of paracetamol in water.

Sample solution

Weigh accurately powdered tablets equivalent to 50 mg of paracetamol, add 70-80 ml of water. Shake and dissolve paracetamol as completely as possible and dilute to 100 ml with water. Filter and dilute the resulting solution with water to get 100 mcg/ml.

Procedure (a)

To 5 ml of sample and standard solutions add 2 ml of sodium nitrite solution and 1 ml of 1 N hydrochloric acid. Mix and allow to stand for 5 minutes. Add 3 ml of 1 N sodium hydroxide, mix and allow to stand for further 5 minutes. Dilute to 50 ml with water and measure the absorbance of both standard and sample solutions at maximum at about 430 nm. The method obeys Beer's law in the range of 4-36 mcg/ml.

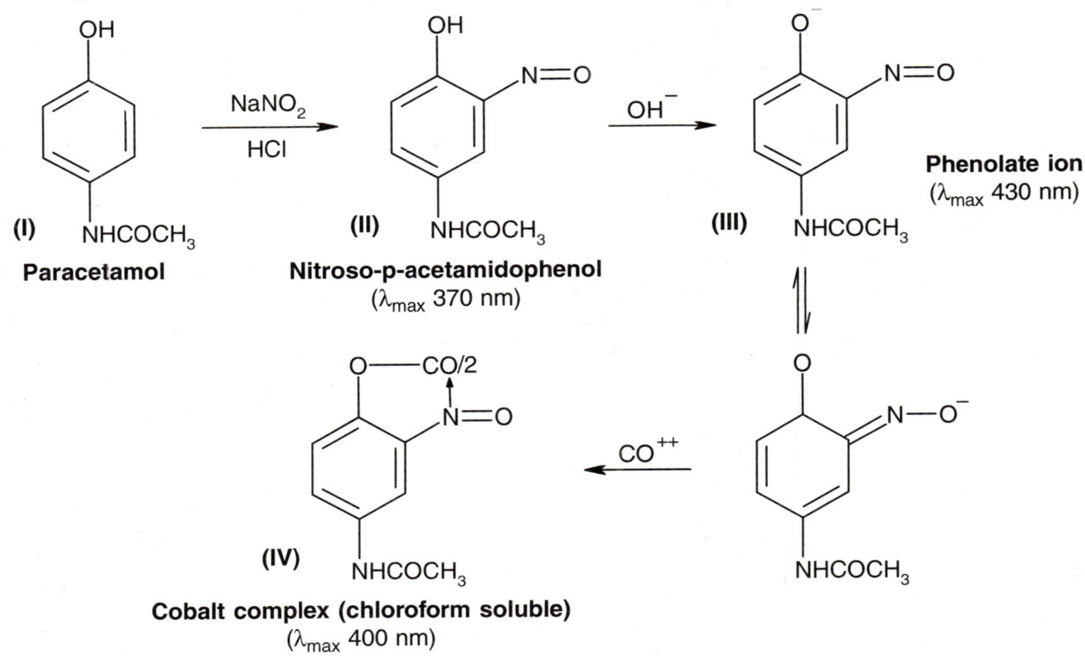

Explanatory Note

Paracetamol, due to the presence of aromatic hydroxyl group, is capable of forming nitroso derivative (yellow chromogen) by reaction with sodium nitrite in acidic medium. Since this yellow-coloured complex is unstable in acidic medium it can be stabilized in methanol. Alkalinisation of medium results in highly stable compound with bathochromic shift along with hyperchromic effect. Nitroso derivative forms complex with Co^{++} which can be extracted into chloroform and absorption measured at 400 nm.

Nitroso-p-acetamidophenol is capable of forming a chelate with Co(II) ion as chelating agent contains a phenolic —OH group (with easily replaceable proton) ortho to the N==O group; the latter offers a lone pair of electrons to the Co(II) ion. This chelate is highly soluble in chloroform, so can be extracted into chloroform and measured at 400 nm.

Reference

S.F. Belal, M. Abdel-Hady El-Sayed, A. El-Walily & H. Abdine, Analyst, **104(10)**, 919-927, 1979.

Formation of yellow-coloured nitroso derivative (λ_{max} 395 nm) was earlier utilized by Inamdar et al. (1969) as a method of analysis for paracetamol. However, nitroso derivative being unstable in acidic medium, its stability was increased by addition of alcohol (M.C. Inamdar & N.N. Kadji, Ind. J. Pharm., **31**, 79-81, 1969).

Lester Chafetz et al. (1971) have claimed that a nitro derivative instead of nitro derivative is produced on treating paracetamol with nitrous acid (HNO_2) and the following reaction was proposed based of spectral analysis.

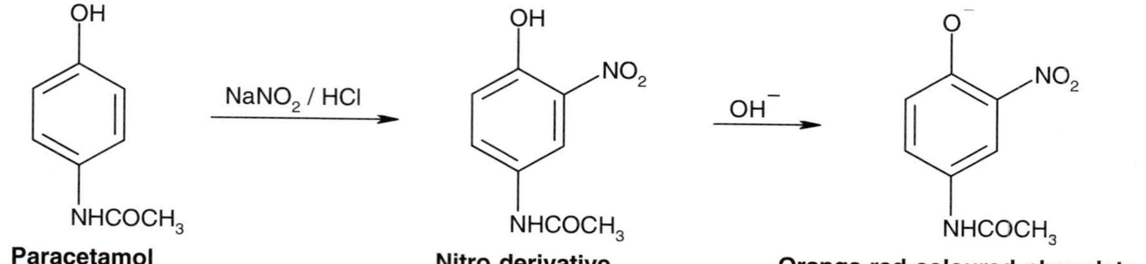

Paracetamol (λ_{max} 246 nm) **Nitro derivative** (λ_{max} 370 nm) **Orange-red coloured phenolate** (λ_{max} 430 nm)

Note

Bathochromic shift 370 nm → 430 nm on addition of alkali.

Reference

Lester Chafetz, Robert E. Daly, Herbert Schriftman & Joseph J. Lomner, J. Pharm. Sci., **60(3)**, 463-466, 1971.

Note

Bathochromic shift on addition of alcohol as observed by Inamdar et al. was 375 nm → 395 nm.

Procedure (b)

Carry out the above procedure till addition of 1 ml of 1 N hydrochloric acid and keeping for 5 minutes. Add 5 ml cobalt bromide/chloride solution and extract with three 5 ml portions of chloroform. Dilute the chloroform layer to 25 ml and measure the absorbance of chloroform extract of both the solutions at about 400 nm against reagent blank. The method obeys Beer's law in the range of 4-36 mcg/ml.

Note

1. Salicylamide does not interfere as it does not yield cobalt derivative. It forms p-nitroso derivative instead of ortho-nitroso derivative.
2. Aspirin, phenobarbitone, glyceryl guaicolate, parabens and phenyl propanolamine did not interfere.

Probable Reaction Mechanism

Paracetamol undergoes hydrolysis in acidic solution to yield p-aminophenol and acetic acid.

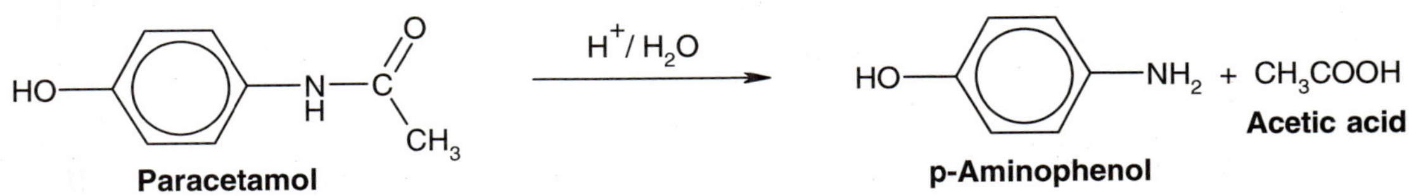

The primary amine group of p-aminophenol is subjected to diazotization reaction by $NaNO_2$ and HCl.

(a) $NaNO_2 + HCl \longrightarrow NaCl + HNO_2 \xrightarrow{H^+} H_2ONO \xrightarrow{Cl^\ominus} H_2O + \overset{\oplus}{NO}\,Cl^\ominus$

(b)

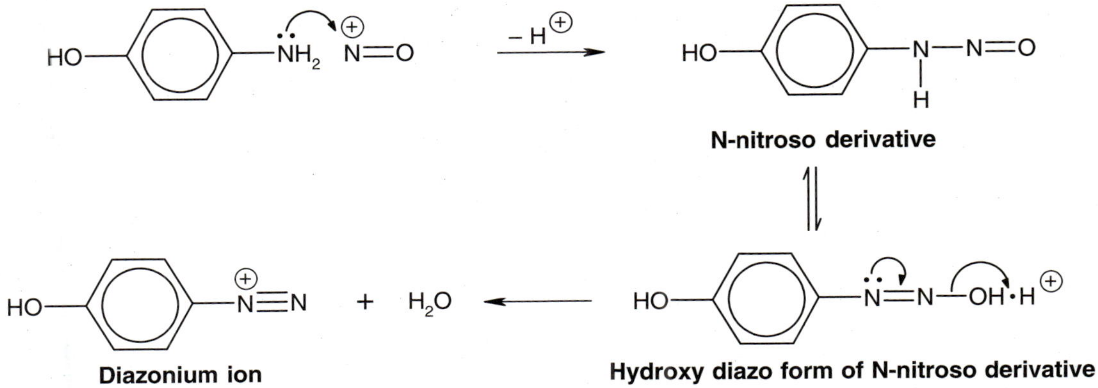

Co(II) chloride forms an octahedral complex as shown below.

(c)

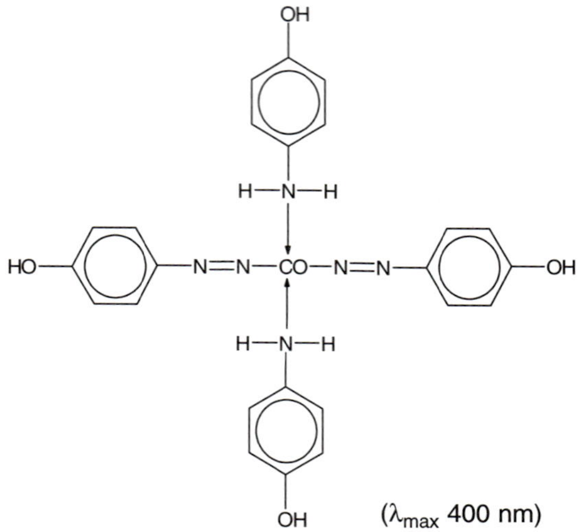

Here the unreacted primary amine group of p-aminophenol i.e. that amino group which has not undergone diazotization acts as a ligand (donates electrons) for the formation of octahedral complex.

Reference

1. Textbook of Practical Organic Chemistry by Vogel, p. 920.
2. Pharmaceutical Chemistry (Vol. 2) by H.J. Roth, pp. 312, 398.

Paracetamol on heating with Millon's reagent produces red colour which is stabilized by forming chelate with Hg^{2+}.

This reaction is specific for phenols in which p-position is occupied.

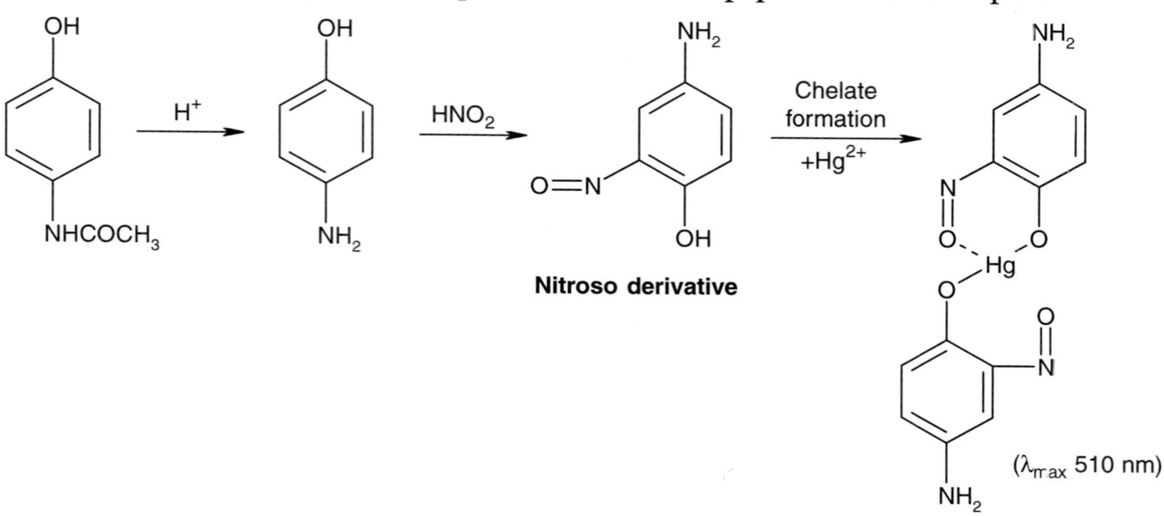

Paracetamol

Reagents

1. 0.135 M potassium dichromate solution in 12 M sulphuric acid.
2. 12 M sulphuric acid.

Sample/standard solution

100 µg/ml of paracetamol in water.

Procedure

Place 10 ml of dichromate solution in 50 ml volumetric flask, add 15 ml of 10 M sulphuric acid, 10 ml of sample/standard solution, mix, dilute to 50 ml with water. Heat in water-bath (80 C) for 15 min, cool and measure the absorbance at 480 nm against reagent blank.

Probable Reaction Mechanism

The authors have proposed that reaction involves deacetylation to p-aminophenol in first step and then to p-benzoquinone.

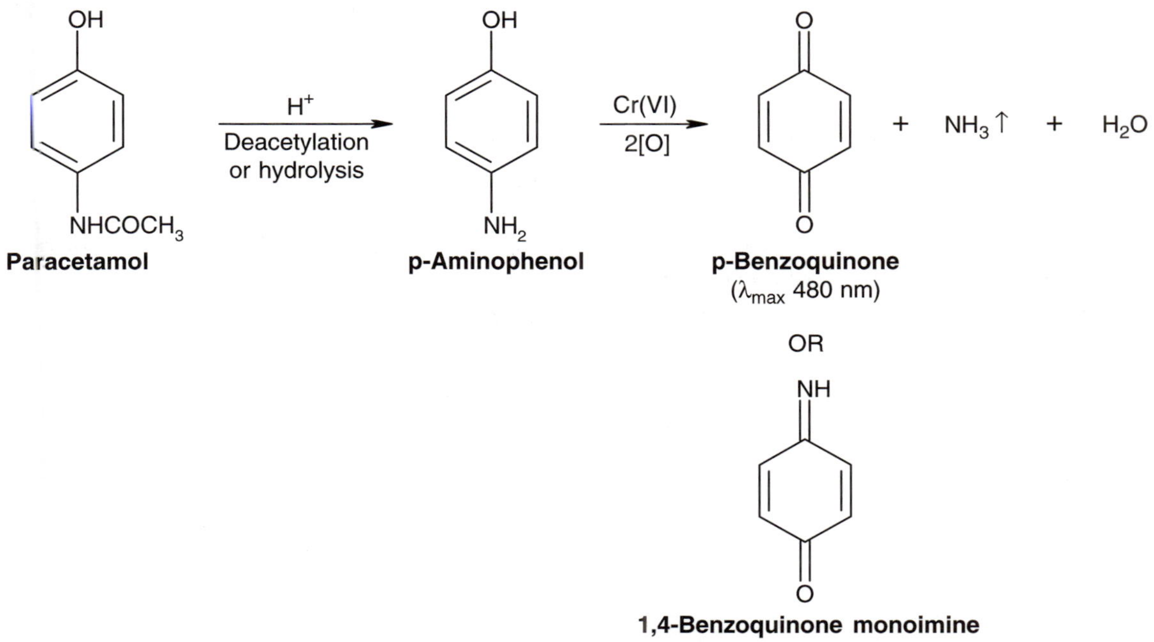

Note

1. Depending on the concentration of sulphuric acid, the colour of the end product varies. While using Ce(IV), the λ_{max} of the end product was 410 nm.
2. $K_3Fe(CN)_6$ has also been proposed as oxidizing agent.

Reference

Salab M. Sultan, Talanta, **34(7)**, 605-608, 1987; Salab M. Sultan, Ibrahim Z. Alzamol Abdullah, M. Aziz Alrahman, Saad A. Allamarals, Yousif Asha, Analyst, **111(8)**, 919-921, 1986; M.K. Srivastava, Saeed Ahmad, Dhirandra Singh & D.C. Shukla, Analyst, **110(6)**, 735-737, 1985.

Another reaction mechanism as described by Roth:

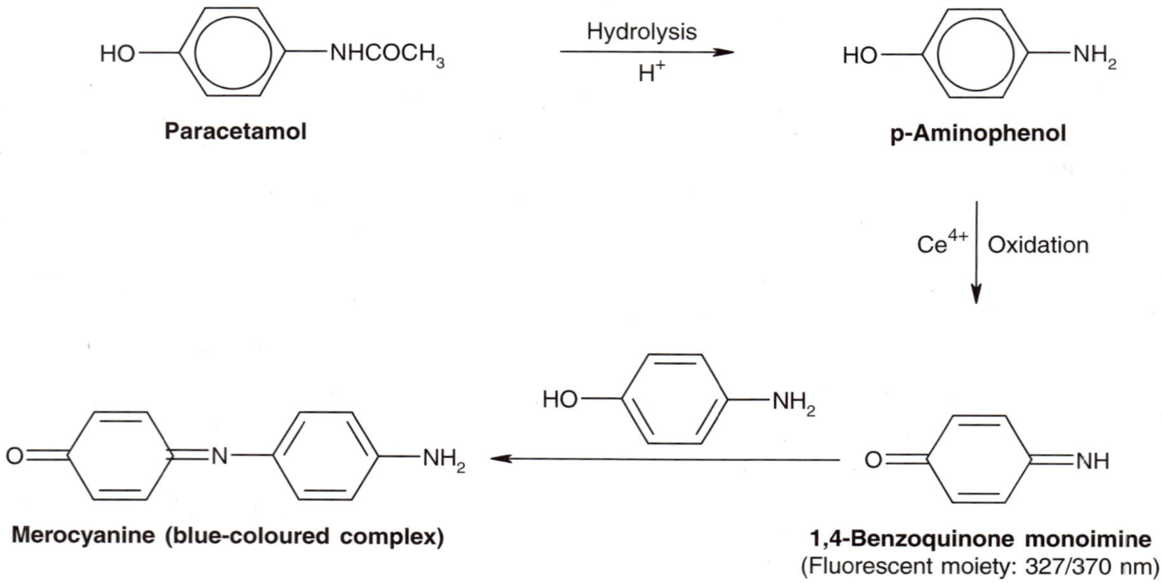

Reference

Pharmaceutical Chemistry (Vol. 2) by H.J. Roth, p. 398-399.

Note

1. Phenylephrine, phenylpropanolamine, pheniramine, nepyramine, caffeine, codeine, noscapine and terpine hydrate do not interfere.
2. Ascorbic acid and aspirin interfere.

Violet-coloured product can be extracted with isobutanol (λ_{max} 500 nm).

Reference

A.K. Basu. Ind. J. Pharmacy, **30(12)**, 280, 1968.

M.A. Korany has proposed a spectrophotometric method for estimation of p-aminophenol, a hydrolytic product of paracetamol in the presence of paracetamol itself.

This is based on reaction of the chromogenic reagent with p-aminophenol in sodium acetate solution to give yellow-coloured product (λ_{max} 410 nm). However, with the addition of chloramine-T (an oxidizing agent), red-coloured (448 nm) product was formed.

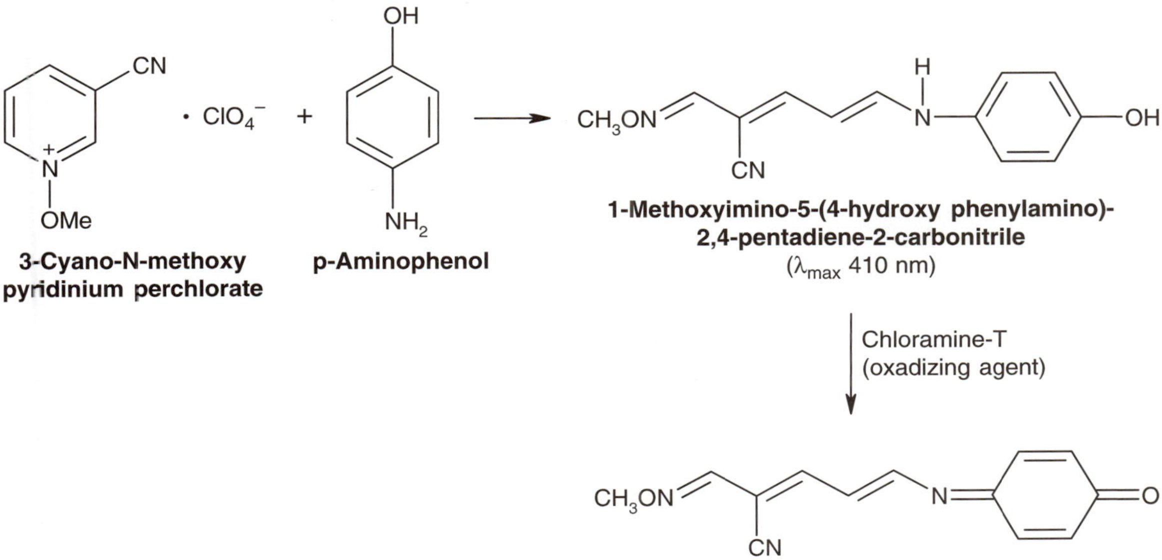

3-Cyano-N-methoxy pyridinium perchlorate

p-Aminophenol

1-Methoxyimino-5-(4-hydroxy phenylamino)-2,4-pentadiene-2-carbonitrile
(λ_{max} 410 nm)

(λ_{max} 448 nm)
Red-coloured p-quinone-imine derivative showing bathochromic shift on addition of chloramine-T from 410 nm to 448 nm

Reference

M.A. Korany, Talanta, **29**, 332-334, 1982.

Note

Nianquin et al. (1995) have stated that p-benzoquinone so formed in 0.12 M sulphuric acid has fluorescent properties which can be used for quantification; exc: 298 nm, emm: 333 nm.

Reference

Nianquin Jie et al., Talanta, **42**, 1575-1579, 1995.

Kalatzis et al. (1976) have described a spectrophotometric method for the estimation of paracetamol. The method is based on acid hydrolysis of paracetamol to p-aminophenol and subsequent Schiff's base formation on condensation with 4-nitrobenzaldehyde or 2,4-dinitrobenzaldehyde. The reaction as proposed by the authors is as under.

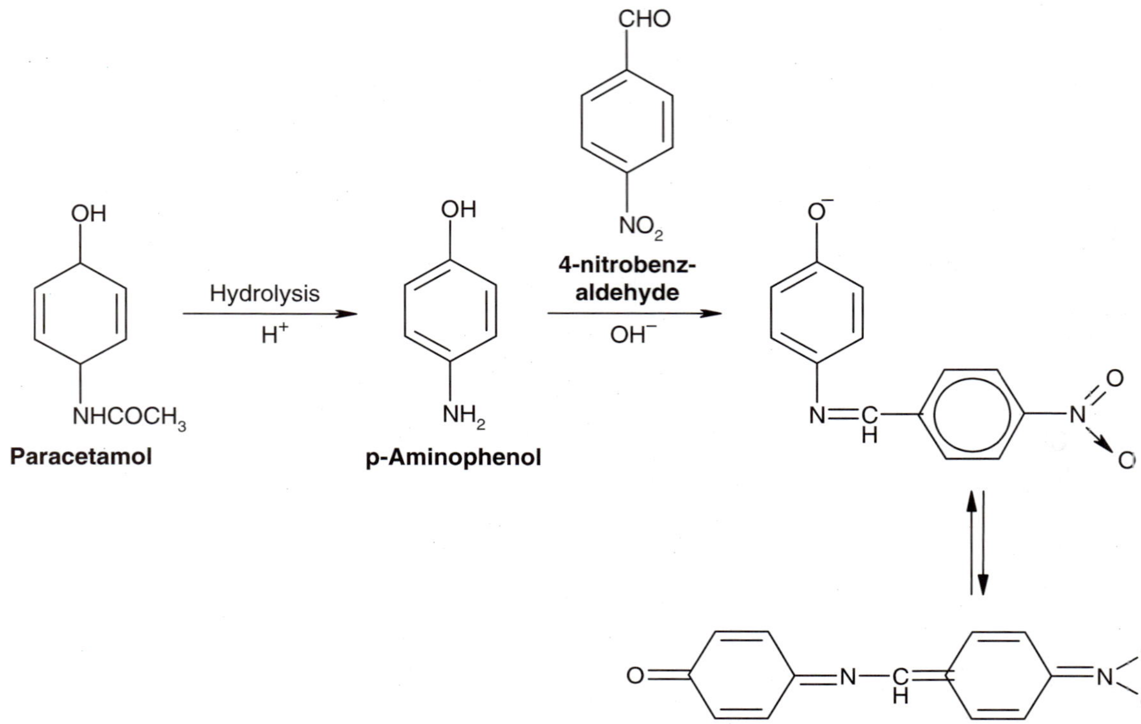

Coloured Schiff's base
(λ_{max} 380 nm)

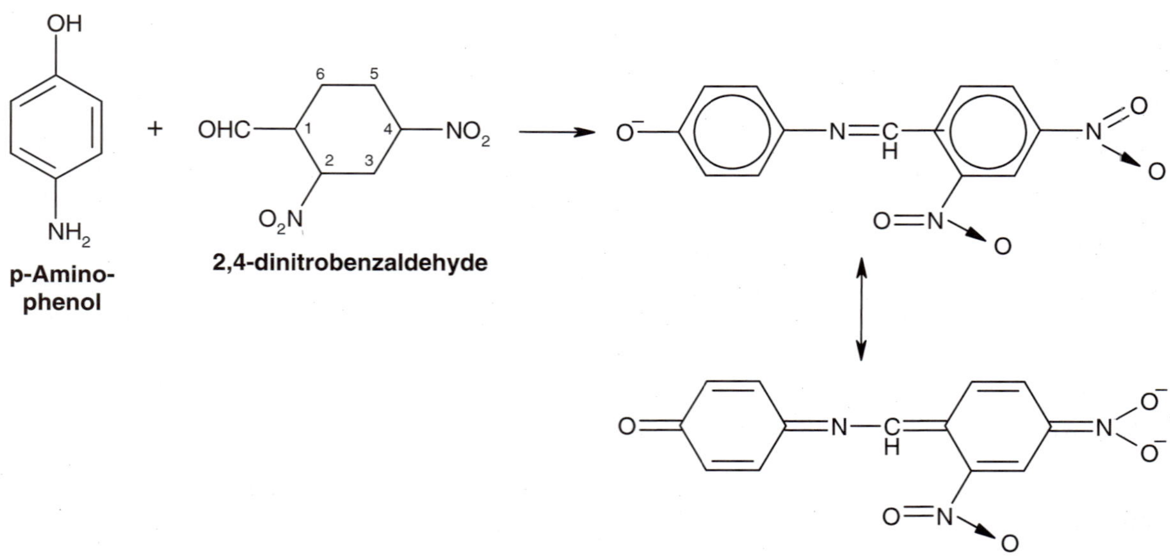

Coloured Schiff's base
(λ_{max} 404 nm)

Reference

Evangelos Kalatzis & Irene Zarbi, J. Pharm. Sci., **65(1)**, 71-75, 1976.

Note

Similarly vanilline in isopropyl alcohol can be used as an aldehyde for formation of Schiff's base (λ_{max} 385 nm) (through Analytical Profiles of Drug Substances by Florey, Vol. 3, p. 49).

A spectrophotometric method based on nitration and subsequent complexation was described by Afaf A. El Kheir et al. (1986).

Reagents

1. 10% w/v solution of potassium hydroxide in water.
2. Concentrated nitric acid.
3. Concentrated sulphuric acid.
4. Acetone.

Sample and standard solutions

To drug equivalent to 25 mg, add 2 ml each of concentrated nitric acid and sulphuric acid, leave for 10 min, cool and dilute to 100 ml with water, further dilute 20 ml to 100 ml with water. To 2 ml each of the diluted solutions add 2.5 ml of acetone and 5 ml of potassium hydroxide solution, dilute to 25 ml with water and measure the absorbance of the resulting solution at 355 nm against reagent blank.

Probable Reaction Mechanism

As proposed by the authors, the nitration of the compound gives dinitro derivative in spite of excess of nitric acid due to steric hindrance. Further heating of electron-deficient polynitro derivative with ketone (acetone) in alkaline medium resulted in coloured complex by interaction with anions such as $CH_3COCH_2^-$. This complex is of "Meisenheimer" type. The low colour intensity and shorter λ_{max} (λ_{max} 355 nm) as observed for complex with paracetamol may be attributed to the auxochrome ($NHCOCH_3$) in para position to the phenolic —OH in contrast to the chromophoric (NO_2) group for the salicylamide (λ_{max} 390 nm).

Note

The colour of the complex is stable for 60 min.

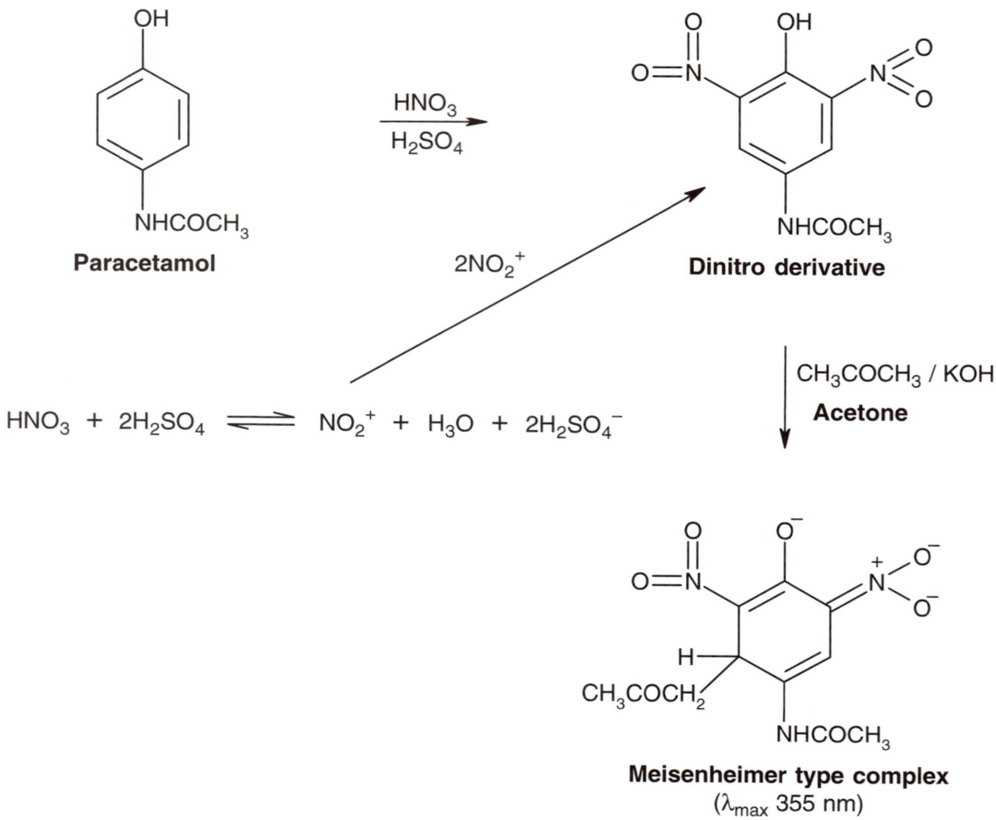

Reference

Afaf A. El Kheir, Saied Belal, Mohammad El Sadek & Abdullah El Shanwani, Analyst, **111(3)**, 319-321, 1986.

Another spectrophotometric method has been reported for estimation of paracetamol by Abdel-Wadod et al. (2005).

Reagents

1. 1.5% w/v solution of N-bromosuccinimide (NBS), freshly prepared.
2. Borate buffer, pH 9.5.

Sample and standard solutions

5 µg/ml solution in methanol.

Procedure

To 1 ml each of sample and standard solutions, add 0.5 ml of borate buffer and 1 ml of 'NBS' reagent, leave at room temperature for 30 min, add 2.5 ml of water and dilute to 25 ml with DMF.

Probable Reaction Mechanism

Since paracetamol is reasonably stable in slightly alkaline medium at room temperature, intact molecule of paracetamol was oxidized by 'NBS' instead of first getting hydrolysed to p-aminophenol as is the case in acidic conditions.

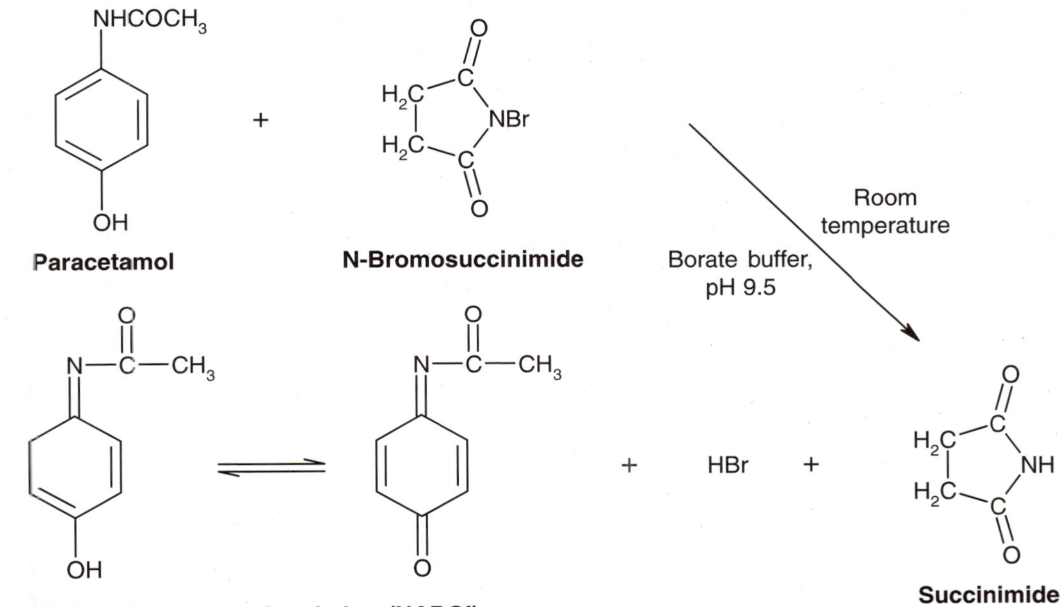

N-Acetyl-p-benzoquinonimine (NABQI)
(Fluorescent moiety: λ_{exc}: 330 nm; λ_{em}: 442 nm)

Note

1. $K_3Fe(CN)_6$ can be used as oxidizing agent in slightly alkaline medium to give similar product (T. Kaito, A. Sagara. J. Pharm. Soc. Japan, **94(5)**, 633, 1974, through Analytical Profile of Drug Substances by K. Florey, Vol. 14, 576-577).
2. Before making up the volume, water was added to avoid precipitation of the drug.
3. Addition of DMF increases intensity of the fluorescence.
4. Co-existing drugs such as CPM, caffeine, aspirin, codeine, ascorbic acid, chloroxazone do not interfere.
5. p-Aminophenol has inherent fluorescence, but has different exc and em spectra (280/370 nm), hence do not interfere.
6. p-Aminophenol is oxidized to fluorescent moiety but with different spectra (327/370 nm), hence no interference. When compared with fluorescent spectra of N-acetyl-p-benzoquinonimine, oxidation produced intact paracetamol molecule.

Reference

Abdel-Wadod, H.M., Mohamed, N.A. & Mohamed, F.A. J. AOAC. Int., **88(6)**, 1626-1636, 2005.

Recently Issa et al. (2008) have described a spectrophotometric method based on reaction with Barton's reagent ($FeCl_3$ - $K_3Fe(CN)_6$ reagent).

Reagents

1. 1 mM ferric sulphate solution in water.
2. 1 mM potassium ferricyanide solution.
3. 1 M HCl.

Standard solution

10 μg/ml of paracetamol in water.

Sample solution

Powdered sample equivalent to 50 mg of paracetamol suspended in water, sonicated, diluted to 50 ml with water, filtered and 1 ml of the filtrate diluted to 100 ml with water.

Procedure

(A) To 2.5 ml each of sample and standard solutions, add 1 ml each of ferric sulphate and $K_3Fe(CN)_6$ solutions, dilute to 5 ml with water and measure the absorbance of both sample and standard solutions at 700 nm against reagent blank after 24 min and calculate the results.

(B) To 2.5 ml each of sample and standard solutions, add 0.5 ml of 1 M HCl and 1 ml of ferric sulphate solutions, heat on water bath at 100 C for 10 min, cool, add 1 ml of $K_3Fe(CN)_6$ solution, dilute to 5 ml with water and measure the absorbance of both sample and standard solutions against reagent blank at 700 nm and calculate the results.

Probable Reaction Mechanism

The reaction with Barton's reagent gives Prussian blue or Turnbull's blue.

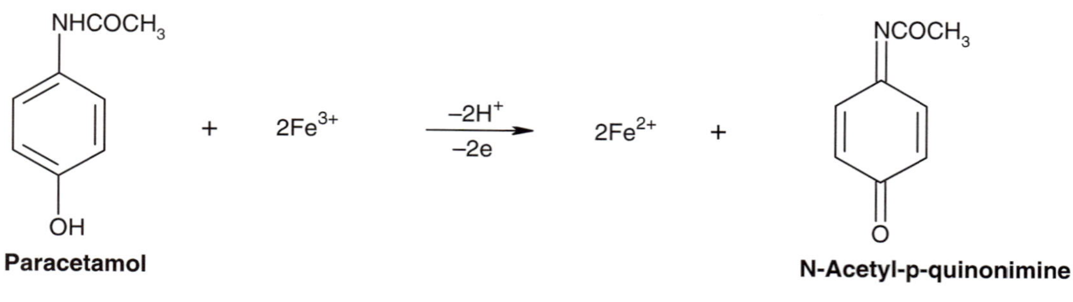

The ferric so produced reacts with $K_3Fe(CN)_6$ to give intense blue colour (λ_{max} 700 nm). The stoichiometry of the reaction was 2 : 1 i.e. 2 mol of Fe(III) and 1 mol of paracetamol.

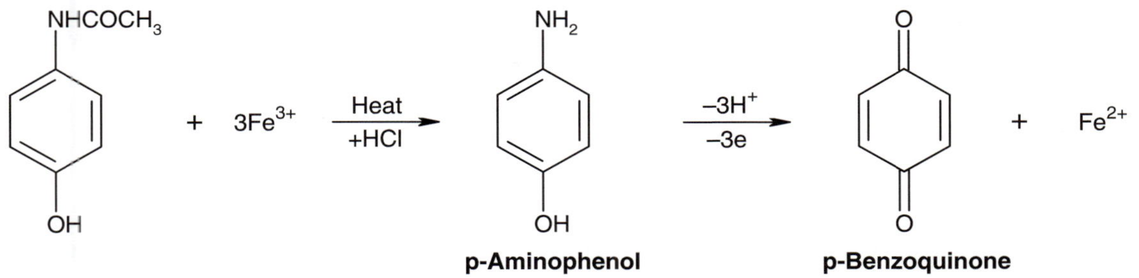

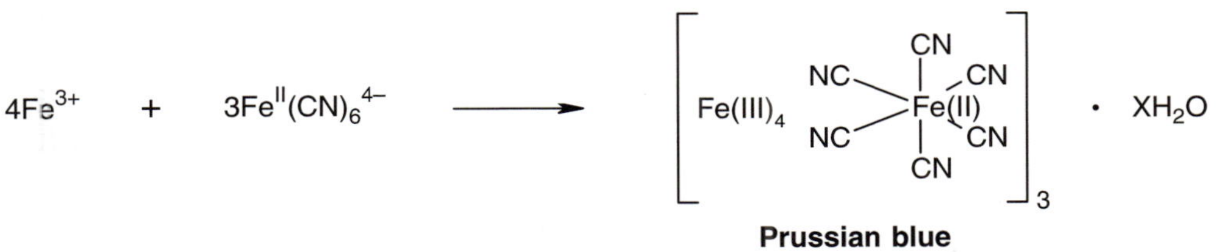

Stoichiometry of this reaction is 3 : 1 as compared to 2 : 1 under method A.

Reference

M.M. Issa, R.M. Nejem, N.S. El-Abadhla, M. Al-Kholy & Akila A. Saleh. Ind. J. Pharm. Sci., **70(3)**, 344-350, 2008.

A rapid spectrophotometric method based on oxidative coupling reaction with p-xylenol (2,3-dimethylphenol) using sodium periodate as catalyst was described by Jalil et al. (2001).

Reagents

1. The solution containing 6.7 mM xylenol and 1.5 mM of $NaIO_4$.
2. 6 M HCl.

Standard solution

1 mg/ml in water.

Sample solution

An appropriate quantity of the powdered sample suspended in water, sonicated, diluted, filtered and the filtrate used for analysis.

Procedure

To 0.2 ml each of sample and standard solutions, add 0.1 ml of 6 M HCl, boil for 10 min, cool under running water, add 3 ml of xylenol-sodium periodate reagent, mix and measure the absorbance of both sample and standard solutions at 635 nm against reagent blank.

Note

The colour is stable for 3 hr.

Probable Reaction Mechanism

It is based on electrophilic aromatic substitution reaction catalyzed by sodium periodate. The presence of OH group para to the amino group in the benzene ring facilitates the oxidative coupling.

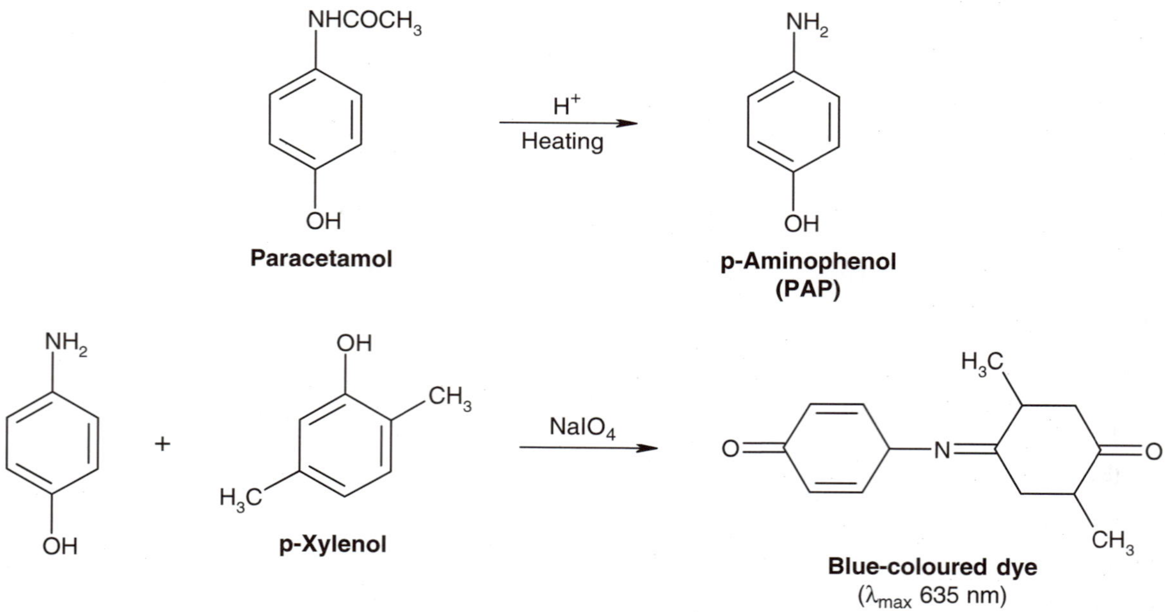

Reference

Jalil Tavakoli Afshari & Tsan-Zon Liu. Analytica Chimica Acta, **443**, 165-169, 2001.

Salicylamide

As salicylamide forms nitroso derivative at position para to phenolic-OH group, hence does not form chelate with Co^{++} as is the case with paracetamol (method 2).

Probable Reaction Mechanism

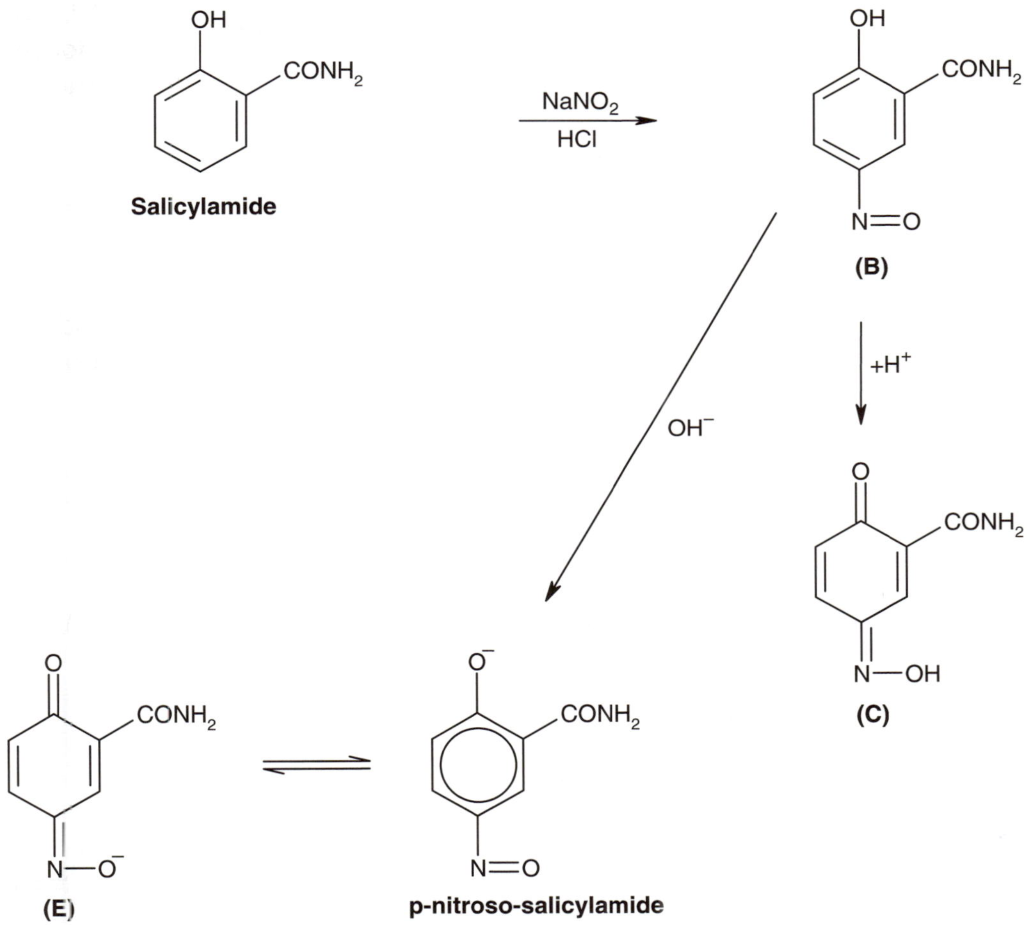

The compound (B) is stable both in acidic and alkaline media, most stable form being p-quinonoidal (C) and (E) structures, have no bathochromic shift is observed in alkaline medium as is the case with paracetamol (method 2).

As explained above, some nitrosation in salicylamide occurs at para position to the phenolic-OH, ortho position being occupied, giving p-nitrosalicylamide, the compound does not form complex with Co^{2+} or Cu^{++}. However, formulation of o-nitroso derivative of both the compounds was achieved by adding copper sulphate solution after sodium nitrite followed by acid. By this procedure, nitrosation by action of nitrous acid at ortho position was possible. Copper salt stabilized the nitrosyl radical and ensuring that ortho and not the para nitroso derivative is formed. Thus, copper chelate of both paracetamol (λ_{max} 535 nm) and salicylamide (λ_{max} 520 nm) was achieved.

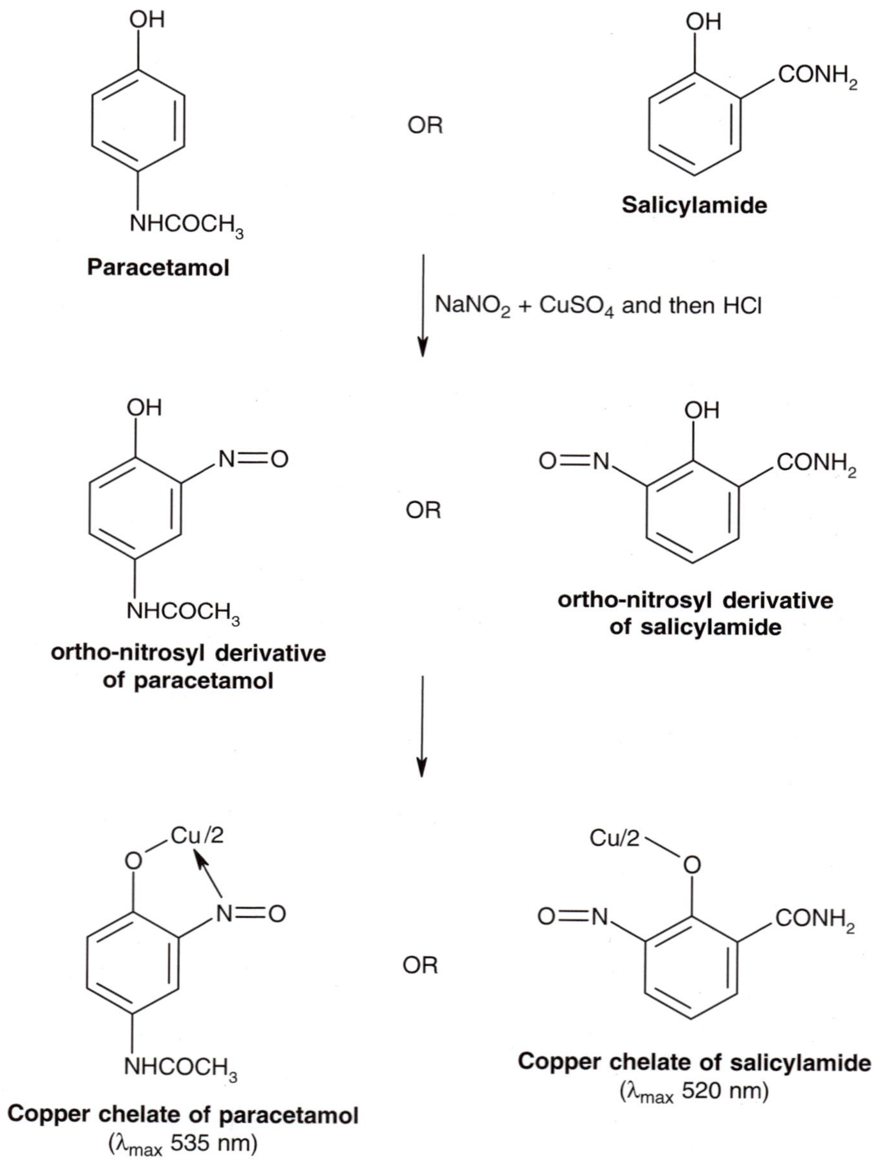

Reference

See method 2 under paracetamol.

Formulation 3

Paracetamol, Salicylamide, Caffeine, Methaqualone hydrochloride, Chlorpheniramine maleate

ESTIMATION

Paracetamol

METHOD

Paracetamol is hydrolysed to p-aminophenol, diazotised and coupled with 'NED' to get pink dye which shows absorption maxima at about 550 nm.

Reagents

1. 0.1% w/v solution of sodium nitrite in water.
2. 0.5% w/v solution of ammonium sulphamate in water.
3. 0.1% w/v solution of N-1-naphthyl-ethylene diamine dihydrochloride (NED) in water.
4. 4 M hydrochloric acid.

Standard solution

Take 250 mg of paracetamol accurately weighed, add 20 ml of hydrochloric acid and 30 ml of water. Reflux on water-bath for 30 minutes, cool and dilute to 100 ml with water. 5 ml of the resultant solution is further diluted to 100 ml with water.

Sample solution

Weigh accurately a quantity of powdered tablets equivalent to 250 mg of paracetamol and proceed with hydrolysis as described above under standard solution.

Procedure

Cool 10 ml of sample and standard solutions in ice-bath, add 0.5 ml of 4 M hydrochloric acid and 1 ml of sodium nitrite solution. Shake vigorously, cool in ice-bath for 3 minutes. Then add 1 ml of ammonium sulphamate solution and keep at room temperature for 2 minutes. (This step ensures complete neutralization of nitrous acid.) Then add 1 ml of 'NED' reagent, shake and keep in water-bath (50°C) for 1 hr. Measure the extinction of both the solutions at 550 nm against reagent blank and calculate the results.

Note

1. Method described in formulation 4 of this chapter involving use of vanillin reagent can also be used.
2. On hydrolysis, free amino group is liberated which can be titrated with sodium nitrite like any free aromatic amino group. Titrate appropriate aliquot of the hydrolysed sample solution as obtained above with 0.1 M sodium nitrite using starch iodide paste as external indicator. Each ml of 0.1 M sodium nitrite is equivalent to 15.12 mg of paracetamol.

Probable Reaction Mechanism

The method is based on reaction of hydrolysed compound with Bratton-Marshall reagent. The compound undergoes hydrolysis under acidic conditions to give p-aminophenol and acetic acid. The primary amino group of p-aminophenol is subjected to diazotization with HNO_2 to give N-nitroso derivative which in turn couples with N-1-naphthylethylene diamine hydrochloride (NED) to give diazo coupled product (λ_{max} 550 nm). Ammonium sulphamate is used to destroy/remove excess of HNO_2 as it interferes in the reaction.

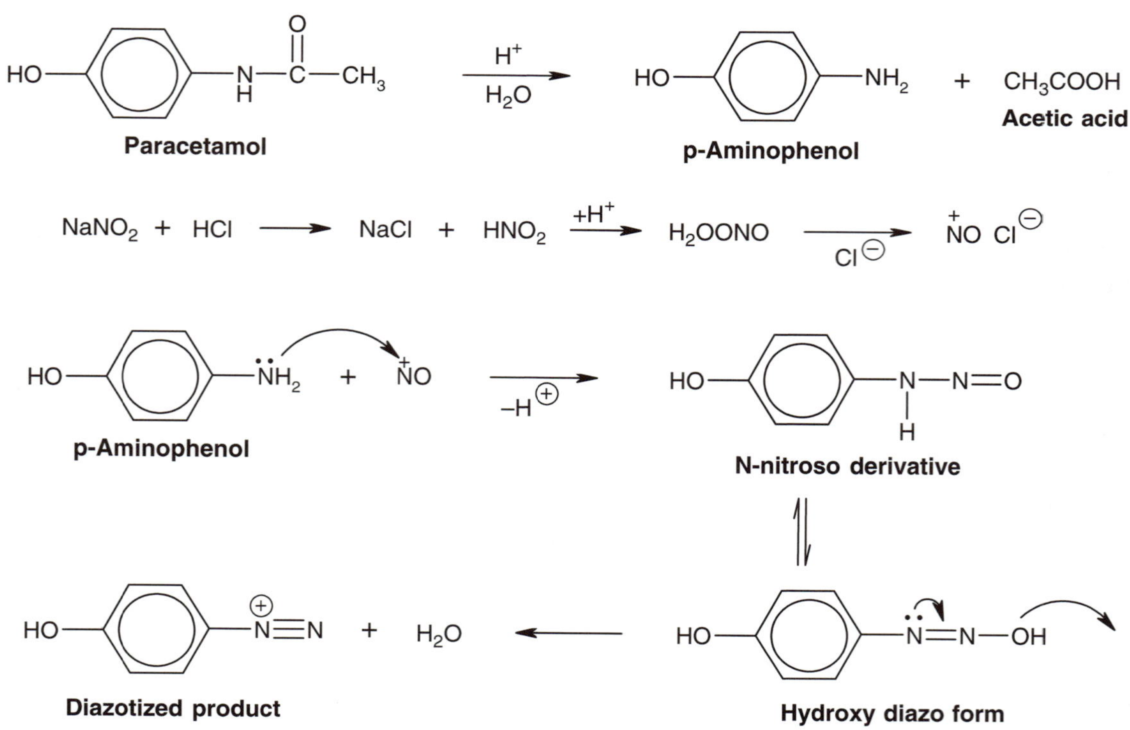

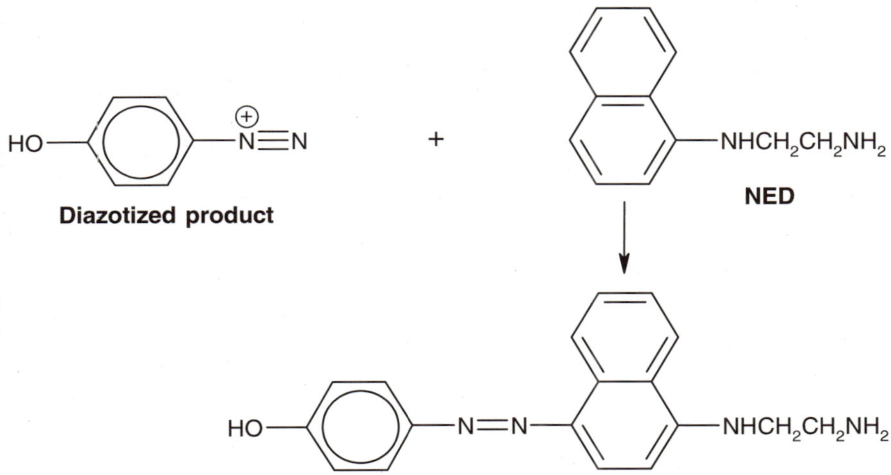

Coupled diazo product
(λ_{max} 550 nm)

$$HNO_2 + \underset{\textbf{Sulphamic acid}}{H_2NSO_3H} \longrightarrow H_2SO_4 + N_2\uparrow + H_2O$$

(Reaction mechanism to destroy excess HNO_2)

Note

Instead of sulphamic acid, ethanol can be used to destroy excess of HNO_2, the end-product being ethyl nitrite.

$$C_2H_5OH + HNO_2 \longrightarrow C_2H_5NO_2\uparrow + H_2O$$

(Textbook of Pharmaceutical Analysis by A.K. Connor, 3rd ed., p. 226.)

S. Belal et al. (1979) described a method based on coupling of diazotized ($NaNO_2$/HCl) o-nitroaniline with paracetamol followed by chelation with Cu(II).

METHOD 2

To diazotized o-nitroaniline, add sample and standard solutions followed by addition of sodium hydroxide solution, keep for 5 min, adjust the volume and measure the absorbance at 430 nm. To get Cu(II) chelate, to the above solution add $CuSO_4$ solution followed by addition of 0.5 M sulphuric acid. Extract the Cu(II) complex with chloroform and measure the absorbance at 400 nm. Chelation with Cu(II) was adopted for increase in selectivity of the method.

Reference

S. Belal, M. Abdel-Hady, El Sayed A. El-Waliely & H. Abdine, J. Pharm. Sci., **68(6)**, 750-752, 1979.

Explanatory Note

Paracetamol as a phenolic compound can couple with diazotized o-nitroaniline. The coloured coupled compound (λ_{max} 430 nm) can be used as chelating agent with Cu^{++} ion (λ_{max} 400 nm). This coupling with diazotized o-nitroaniline occurs ortho to hydroxyl group. Free hydroxyl group has easily replaceable proton and diazo group offers lone electron pair.

Probable Reaction Mechanism

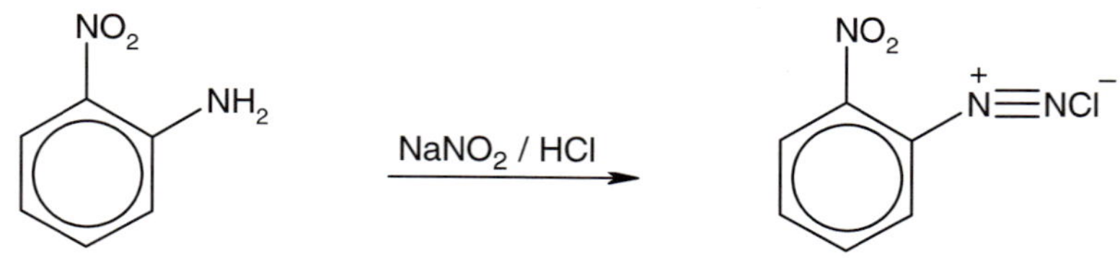

o-Nitroaniline **Diazotized nitroaniline (I)**

Acidic medium favoured formation of Cu^{++} chelate.

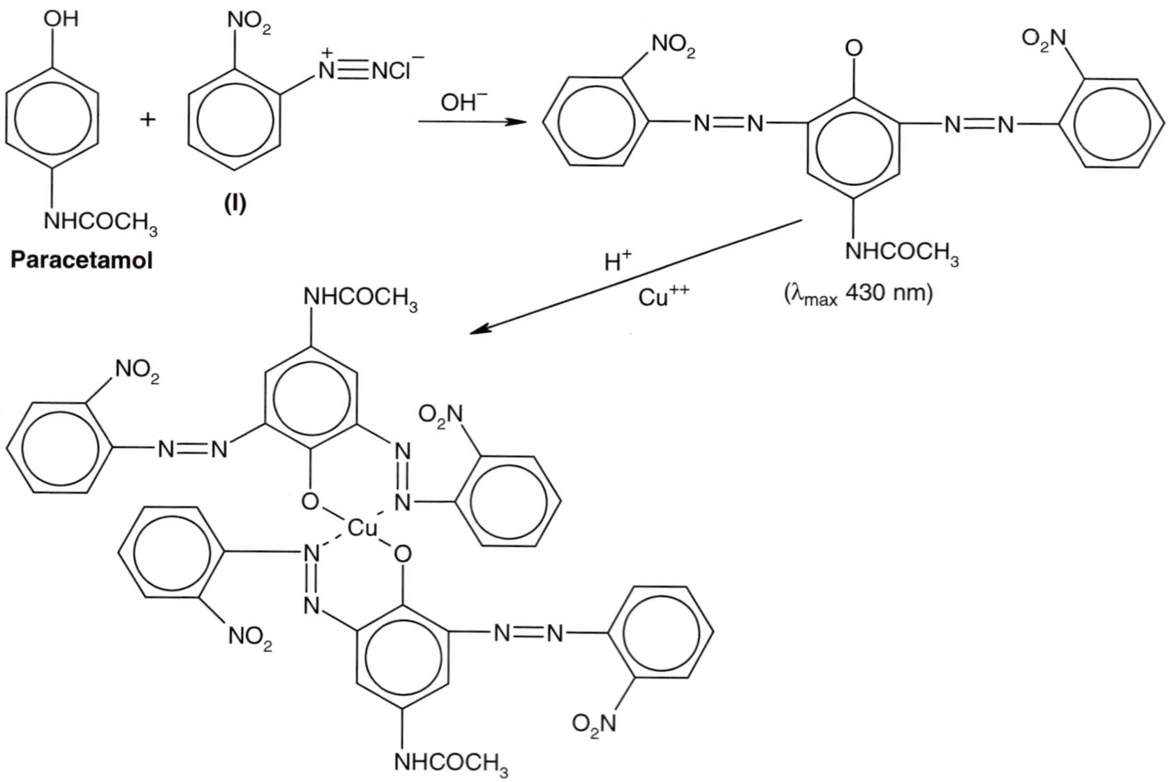

Coloured copper complex extractable into chloroform
(λ_{max} 400 nm)

Similarly, paracetamol shall couple with diazotized sulphanilic acid and p-nitroaniline to give azo dyes with λ_{max} at 480 nm and 425 nm, respectively. (S.M. Hassan et al. JAOAC Int., **64(6)**, 1442, 1981)

Rana et al. have reported that paracetamol couples with diazotized 2-nitroaniline to give red-coloured dye, λ_{max} 520 nm. (N.G. Rana & H.V. Chauhan. Ind. J. Pharmacy, **14(9)**, 184, 1977)

METHOD 3

Reagents

1. 0.1% w/v solution of sodium nitrite in water.
2. 0.5% w/v solution of benzocaine in alcohol.
3. Acid mixture: Mix 86 ml of 15% trichloroacetic acid, 20 ml of 2 M sulphuric acid and 94 ml of water.
4. 60% solution of trimethylamine.

Sample and standard solutions

200 mg/ml in alcohol.

Procedure

To 2 ml of benzocaine solution add 5 ml of acid mixture and 2 ml of sodium nitrite solution, allow to stand for 30 min for diazotization to complete. Then add aliquot of sample and standard solutions containing 200 µg of the drug, allow to stand for 15 min, add 3 ml of trimethylamine solution and dilute to 25 ml with water. Immediately measure the absorbance at 475 nm against reagent blank.

Note

If oxyphenbutazone is present, there is interference. Oxyphenbutazone can be removed by extracting the sample with 1 M hydrochloric acid.

Probable Reaction Mechanism

1. Diazotization of benzocaine

$$NaNO_2 + HCl \longrightarrow NaCl + HNO_2 \xrightarrow{H^+} H_2O\ \overset{\oplus}{N}{=}O \xrightarrow{Cl^{\ominus}} H_2O + \overset{\ominus}{Cl}\ \overset{\oplus}{N}{=}O$$

Nitrosonium ion

2. The nitrosonium ion being electron-deficient, it attacks the primary amine group attached to the aromatic ring as follows:

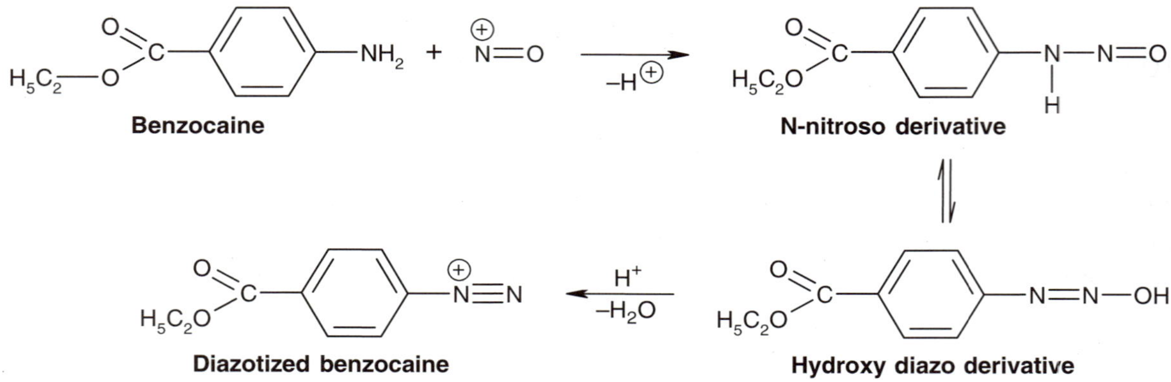

Coupling reaction occurs between the diazotized benzocaine and acetaminophen resulting in the formation of the product.

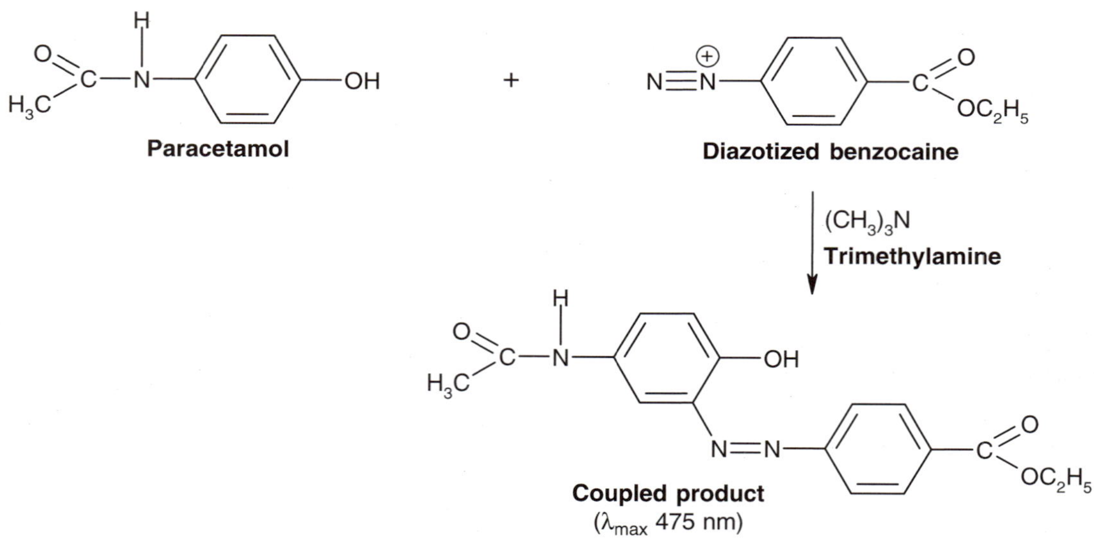

Reference

1. Textbook of Practical Organic Chemistry by Vogel, pp. 920, 946.
2. R.T. Sane & A.B. Ambardekar, Indian Drugs, **19(1)**, 115-117, 1981.

METHOD 4

Reagents

1. 0.002 M solution of 3-methylbenzthiazolin-2-one-hydrazone (MBTH).
2. 0.003 M solution of ceric ammonium sulphate in 0.07 M sulphuric acid.
3. pH 8.0 buffer solution.

Sample and standard solutions

10 µg/ml solution of paracetamol in methanol.

Procedure

To 2 ml of sample and standard solutions, add 10 ml of MBTH reagent, keep aside for 10 min, then add 10 ml of ceric ammonium sulphate solution, allow to stand for 10 min, add 20 ml of buffer solution and extract with chloroform and measure the absorbance of the coloured product at 535 nm against reagent blank.

Probable Reaction Mechanism

The compound undergoes oxidative coupling at ortho position to phenolic —OH group present in the molecule. The presence of oxidizing agents such as potassium ferricyanide or cerric–ammonium sulphate is necessary for this reaction. The reaction proceeds in alkaline conditions.

The coupling reagent:

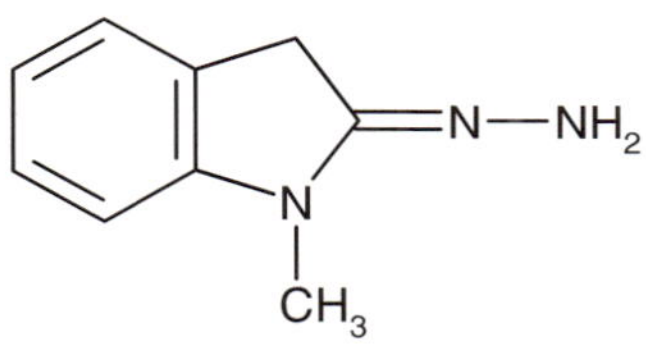

3-Methylbenzthiazolin-2-one-hydrazone (MBTH)

Initially the reagent loses two electrons and a proton and then undergoes oxidative coupling with paracetamol.

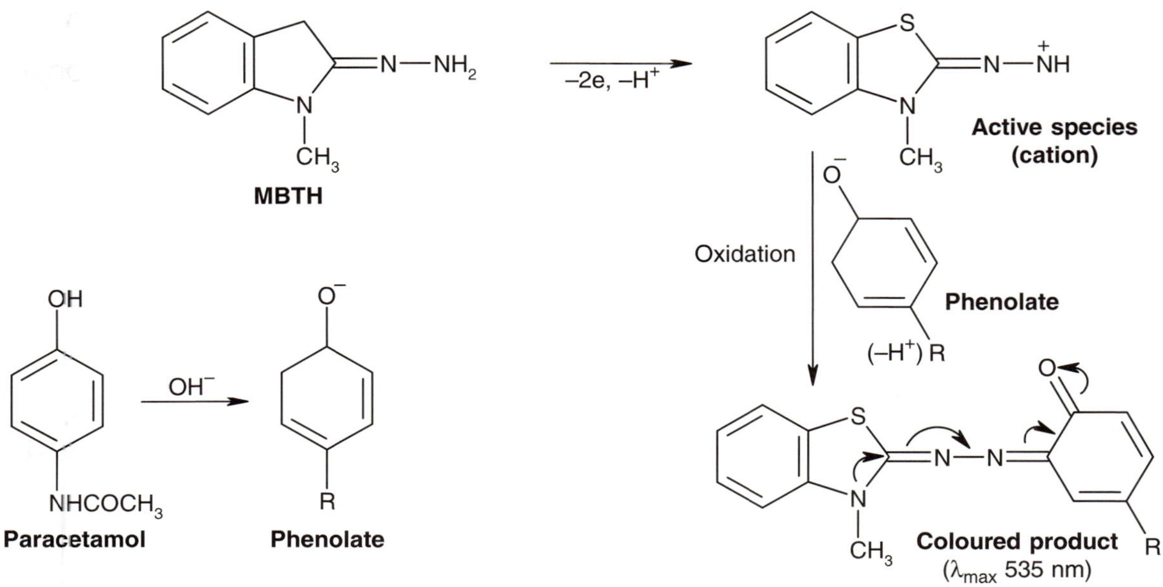

Sanghavi et al. had reported a spectrophotometric method for paracetamol based on the reaction of its hydrolysed product (p-aminophenol) with 1,2-naphthoquinone-4-sulphonate 'NQS' in acid medium to form a Schiff's base (λ_{max} 480 nm) (M.M. Sanghavi & M.G. Pai. Eastern Pharmacist, **17**, 53-54, 1974).

A further improvement of the above method was reported by coupling with 'NQS' in alkaline medium, which yielded a violet-coloured product on addition of 'CTA' (λ_{max} 570 nm).

Reagents

1. 0.02% aqueous solution of 'NQS', freshly prepared.
2. 0.1% aqueous solution of cetyl trimethylammonium bromide (CTA).
3. 2% sodium hydroxide solution in water.

Sample and standard solutions

An appropriate quantity of the sample was hydrolysed with hydrochloric acid to yield p-aminophenol before proceeding with estimation by the proposed method.

Procedure

An appropriate quantity of hydrolysed sample was taken in 25 ml volumetric flask, add 6 ml of 'NQS' reagent, 1 ml of 'CTA' solution and 3 ml of NaOH solution, mix and dilute to volume with water. Measure the absorbance of the sample and the standard solution at 570 nm and calculate the results.

Probable Reaction Mechanism

p-Aminophenol reacts with 'NQS' in alkaline medium to yield a coloured para quinoid imide condensation product (λ_{max} 530 nm). When 'CTA' is added, intense coloured product is formed with bathochromic shift (40 nm) due to substitution of 'CTA' with anionic product.

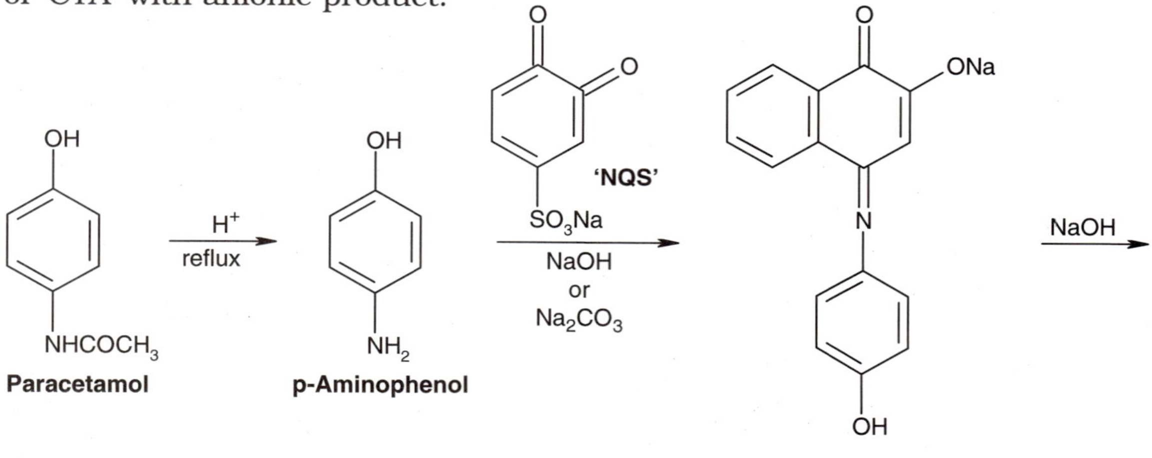

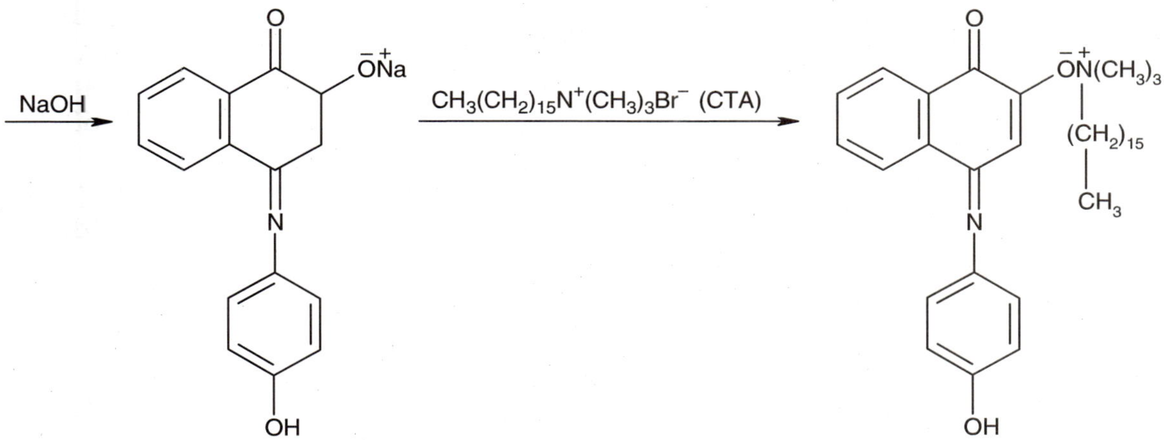

Anionic coloured imide (λ_{max} 530 nm)

Violet-coloured substitution product (λ_{max} 570 nm)

Note

Compounds such as analgin, caffeine, diclofenac and chlorzoxazone do not interfere.

Reference

P. Nagaraja, K.C. Srinivasa Murthy & K.S. Rangappa, J. Pharm. Biomed. Analysis, **17**, 501-506, 1998.

Note

'MBTH', reagent which is also known as 'Besthorn's reagent', was initially introduced as colour reagent for carbonyl compounds. The reaction with carbonyl compounds is as under.

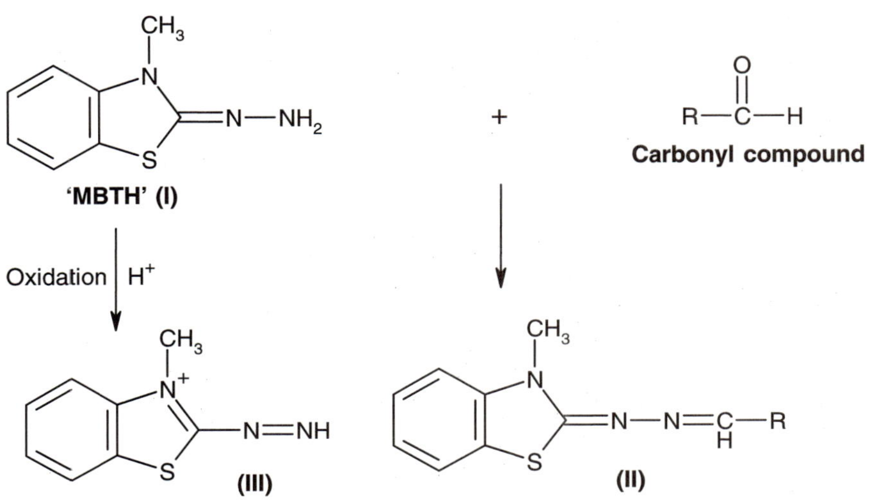

'MBTH' (I)

Carbonyl compound

(III)

(II)

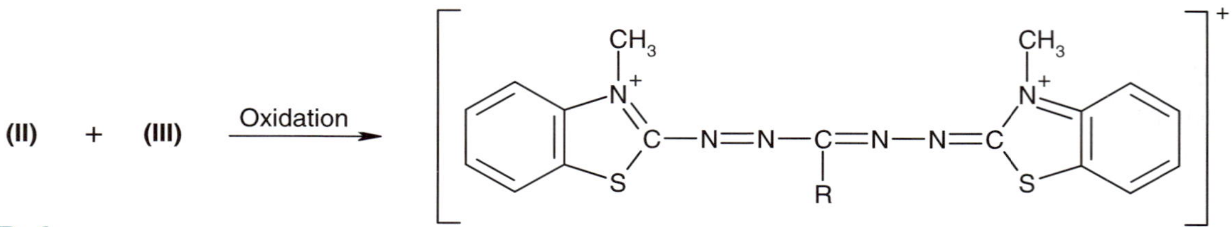

Reference

1. Pharmaceutical Chemistry (Vol. 2) by H.J. Roth, pp. 74, 75.
2. Indian Drugs, **26(8)**, 440, 1989.
3. Analytical Profiles of Drug Substances by K. Florey, Vol. 3, p. 49.

Salicylamide

Reagents

1. 50% w/v solution of sodium hydroxide in water.
2. 4% w/v solution of boric acid in water.
3. 0.1 N sulphuric acid.

Procedure

Weigh accurately a quantity of powdered tablets equivalent to 200 mg of salicylamide and transfer to a distillation flask with the aid of 200 ml of water. Add 50 ml of sodium hydroxide solution and distil. The distillate is absorbed in boric acid solution. Titrate the distillate with 0.1 N sulphuric acid. Each ml of 0.1 N sulphuric acid is equivalent to 0.0137 g of salicylamide.

Explanatory Note

Instead of directly receiving the distillate containing liberated ammonia into standard acid, the distillate is received in solution of boric acid (concentration of boric acid need not be very specific). The ammonia in distillate is fixed as ammonium borate which is then directly titrated as a base with standard acid. This titration is a displacement of the weak acid (boric acid) by strong acid (H_2SO_4). The main advantage of boric acid ammonia fixation method is the use of one instead of two standard solutions.

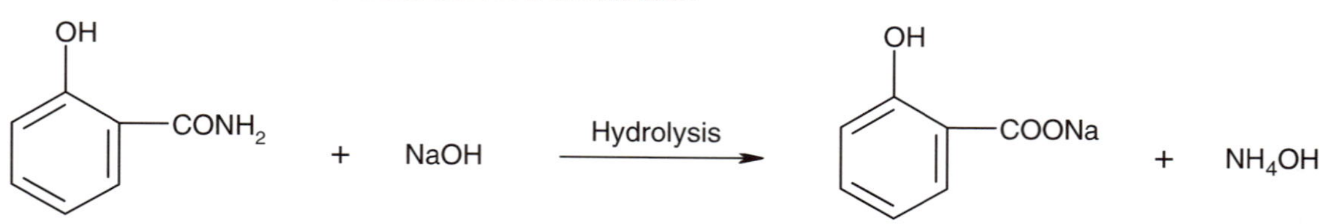

Salicylamide **Sodium salicylate**

$$NH_4OH + H_3BO_3 \longrightarrow (NH_4)_2B_4O_7$$

Ammonium borate (ammonium tetraborate)

Caffeine

Weigh 10 tablets accurately, crush them and take the weight of powder equivalent to 100 mg of caffeine. Extract with successive quantities of dry ether, filter through anhydrous sodium sulphate. Evaporate ether layer to dryness and weigh. Subtract from the total weight, the weight of salicylamide as estimated by above method to find out the contents of caffeine per tablet.

Methaqualone hydrochloride

Dissolve the residue left after extraction of caffeine in methanol and filter. Evaporate the filtrate to dryness and take the weight. Calculate methaqualone hydrochloride per tablet. It is a quinazoline derivative.

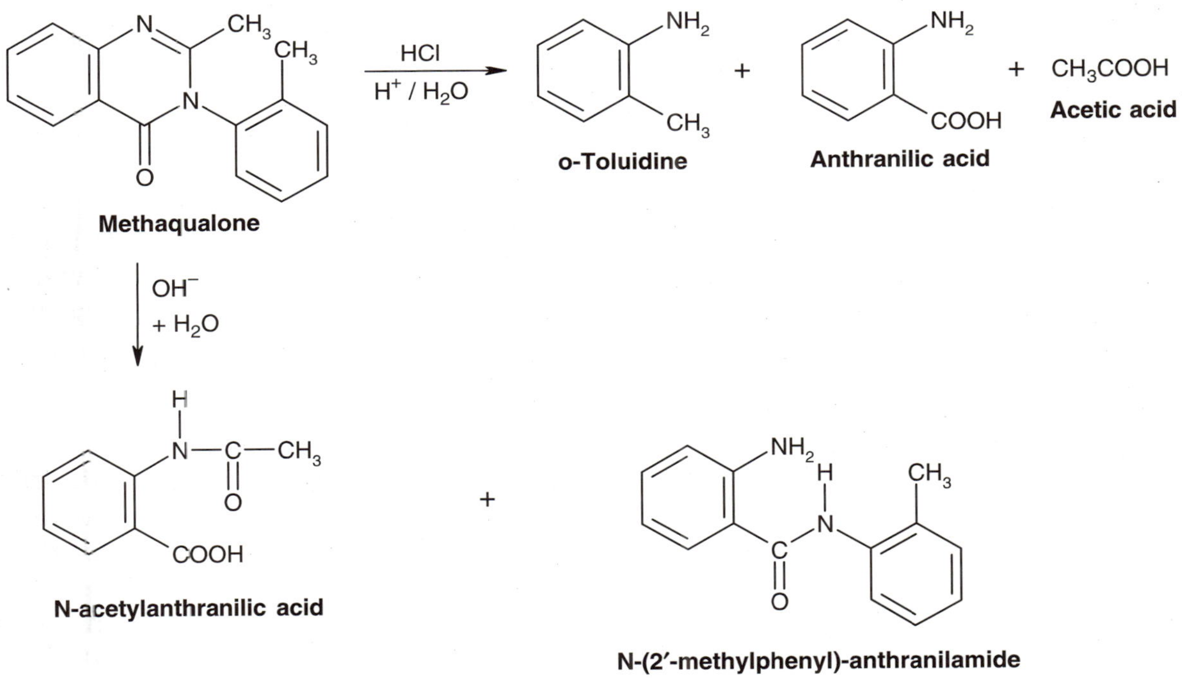

Probable Reaction Mechanism

On heating its ethanolic solution with 'PDAB' in hydrochloric acid (Ehrlich's reagent), an orange-coloured dye is produced. In acidic medium, the compound is protonated which then couples with 'PDAB' to form carbinol followed by dehydration yielding cyanine, an orange dye.

Reference

Pharmaceutical Chemistry (Vol. 2) by H.J. Roth, p. 641.

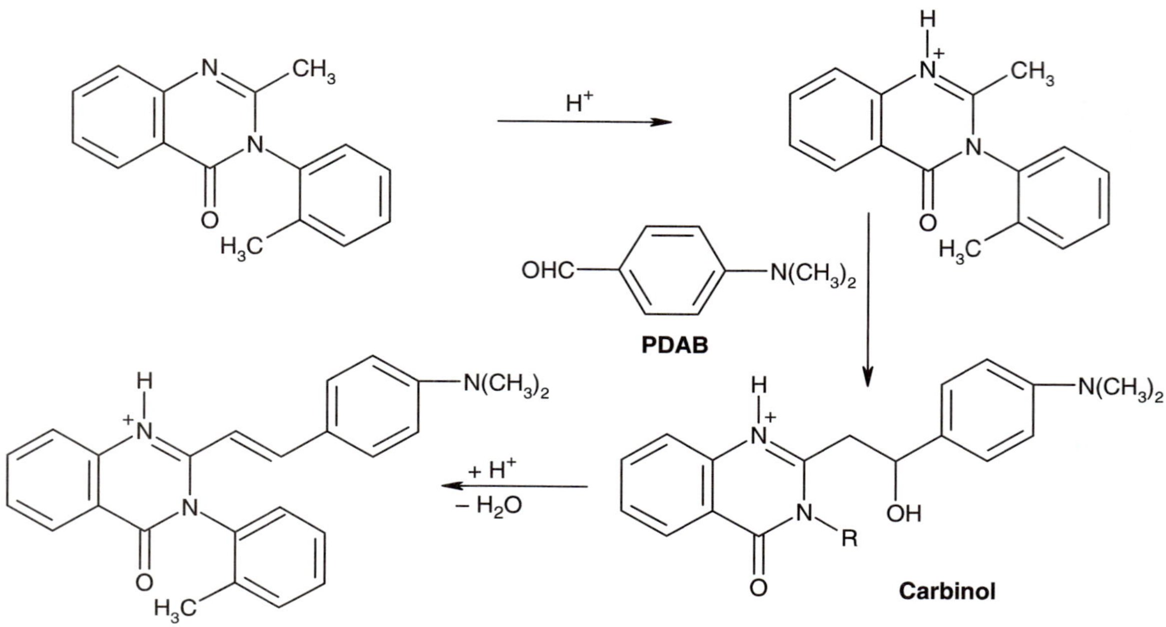

Cyanine (orange dye)
(λ_{max} 503 nm)

Anthranilic acid liberated as a result of acid hydrolysis can be subjected to diazotitration.

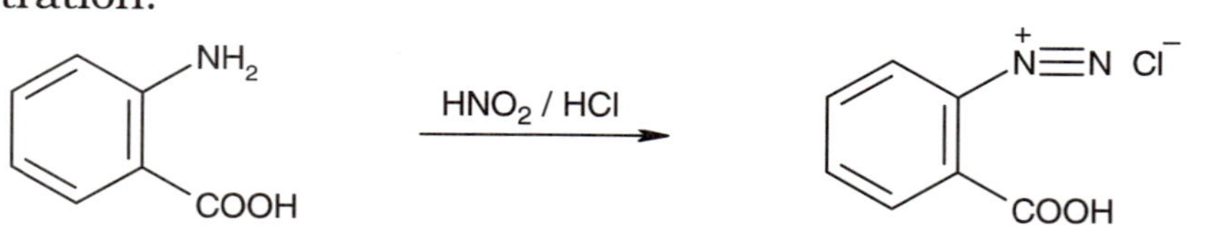

Anthranilic acid **Diazotized anthranilic acid**

Similarly o-toluidine can also be subjected to diazotitration.

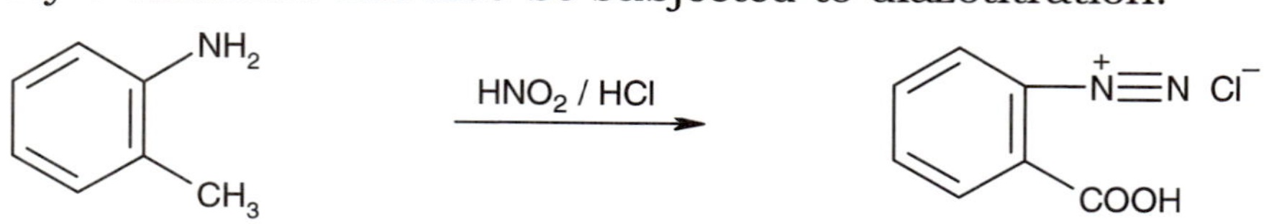

o-toluidine **Diazotized o-toluidine**

Chlorpheniramine maleate

Follow the cyanogen bromide method as described in formulation 1 of the chapter on rubefacients.

Formulation 4

Paracetamol, Caffeine, Chlorpheniramine maleate, Phenylephrine hydrochloride, Ascorbic acid

ESTIMATION

Paracetamol

Method 1

Reagents

1. 1 M hydrochloric acid.
2. 5% w/v solution of vanillin in isopropyl alcohol.

Standard solution

Weigh accurately about 100 mg of pure paracetamol, add 50 ml of 1 M hydrochloric acid. Keep for 20 min and adjust to 100 ml with 1 N hydrochloric acid (1 mg/ml).

Sample solution

Weigh accurately a quantity of powdered tablets equivalent to 100 mg of paracetamol, add 50 ml of 1 M hydrochloric acid and process as per standard to get 1 mg/ml solution.

Procedure

To 2 ml of standard and sample solutions add 5 ml of 1 M hydrochloric acid and heat on boiling water-bath for 5 min. Cool, add 10 ml of vanillin reagent and dilute to 50 ml with water. After 10 min, measure the absorbance of standard and sample solutions at maximum at about 395 nm and calculate the results by comparison.

Probable Reaction Mechanism

Amino group of p-aminophenol generated due to acidic hydrolysis reacts with aldehydic oxygen of vanillin resulting in formation of Schiff's base. On treatment with sodium hydroxide, a fluorescent derivative is formed.

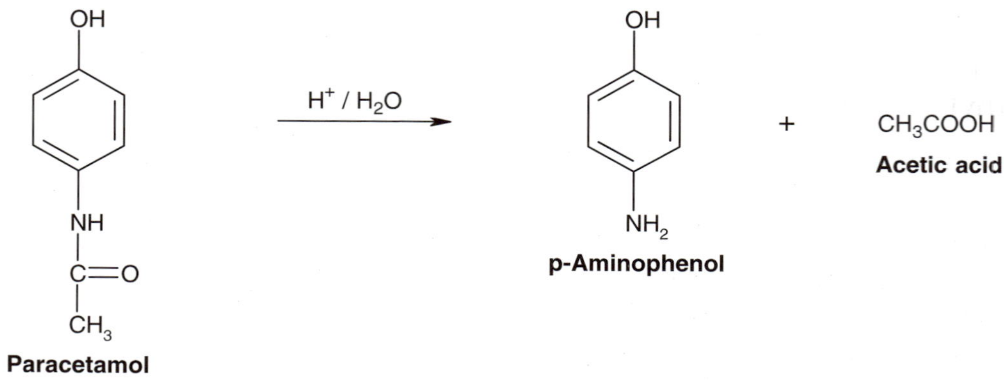

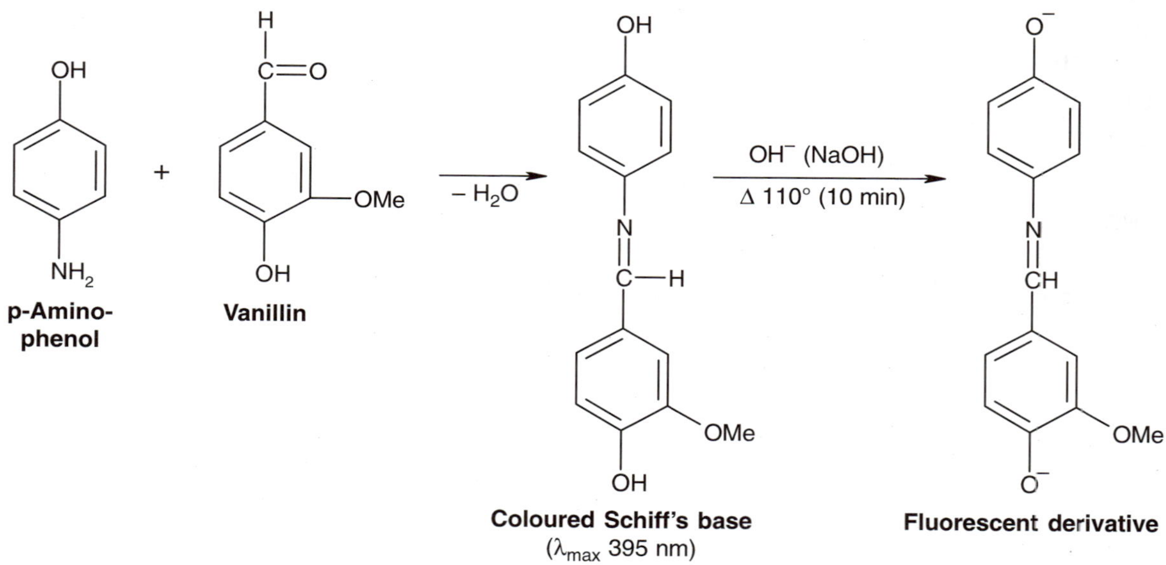

Reference

Analytical Profiles of Drug Substances by K. Florey, Vol. 3, p. 49.

METHOD 2

Reagents

1. 1% w/v solution of 2,4-dinitrobenzeldehyde in 5% v/v sulphuric acid (DNB).
2. 0.1 M and 1 M hydrochloric acid.

Standard solution

Prepare the standard solution of paracetamol according to the method described under sample solution.

Sample solution

Weigh sample accurately equivalent to 150 mg of paracetamol, add 10 ml of methyl alcohol and dilute to 200 ml with 0.1 N hydrochloric acid.

Procedure

To 2 ml each of sample and standard solutions add 5 ml of 1 N hydrochloric acid, heat on water-bath for 30 min, cool, add 10 ml of 'DNB' reagent and after 10 minutes measure the extinction of both the solutions at 430 nm against reagent blank. Calculate the results by comparison.

Probable Reaction Mechanism

Paracetamol undergoes hydrolysis to give p-aminophenol under acidic conditions. The primary amino group of p-aminophenol in turn reacts with aldehydic oxygen of benzaldehyde to form Schiff's base with loss of water. Schiff's base is coloured.

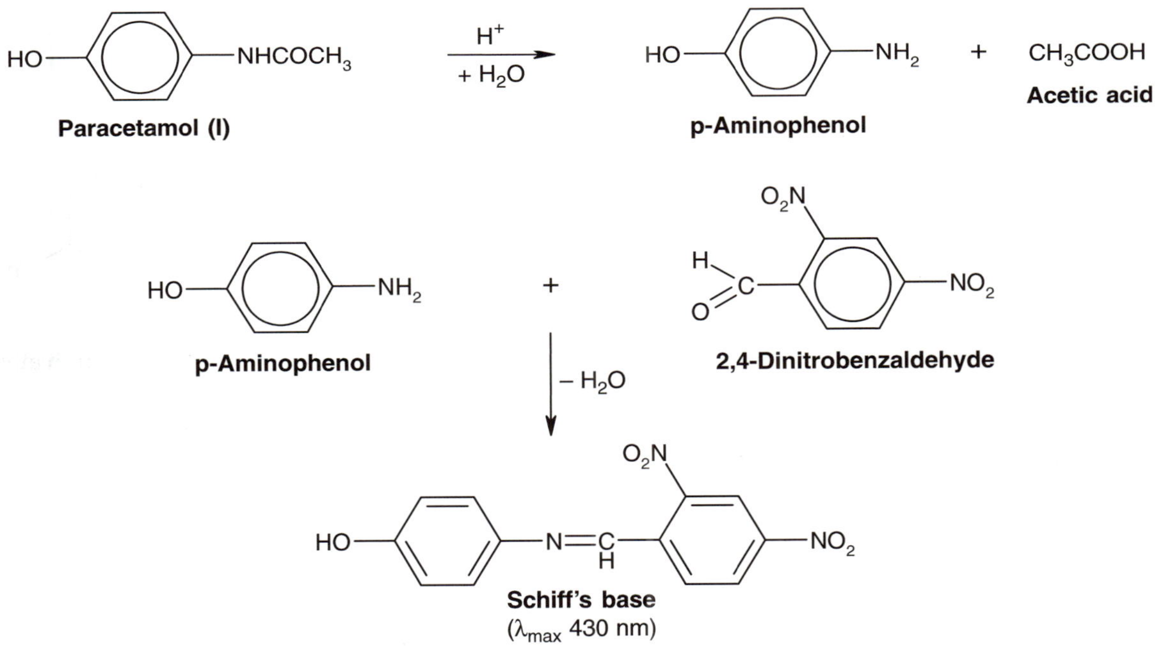

Caffeine

METHOD 1

Weigh accurately a quantity of powdered tablets equivalent to 10 mg and follow the method for estimation of caffeine involving measurement of extinction at 276 nm as described in formulation 1 of this chapter.

METHOD 2

Transfer accurately weighed quantity of the sample and carry out dry extraction with 70 ml of chloroform. Wash the chloroform layer with two 30 ml portions of saturated solution of sodium bicarbonate. Evaporate the organic layer and dissolve the residue in 100 ml of 0.01 N tartaric acid. Carry out further dilution with 0.01 N tartaric acid to get a concentration of 6 mcg/ml. Measure the extinction of the final solution at 271 nm and compare the results with standard solution of caffeine (6 mcg/ml) in 0.01 N tartaric acid.

Chloropheniramine maleate

Follow the cyanogen bromide method as described in formulation 1 of chapter on rubefacients.

Phenylephrine hydrochloride

METHOD 1

Follow the alkaline oxidation with potassium ferricyanide followed by coupling with 4-aminophenazone as described in formulation 1 of this chapter.

METHOD 2

Suspend accurately weighed quantity of the sample in 20 ml of water, basify with ammonia solution and extract with three 20 ml portions of chloroform. Wash the combined chloroform layer with water till free from alkali. Evaporate chloroform layer and dissolve the residue in neutral glacial acetic acid and titrate with 0.01 N perchloric acid. Each ml of 0.01 N perchloric acid is equivalent to 2.037 mg of phenylephrine hydrochloride.

METHOD 3

Reagents

1. 0.1% w/v solution of borax in water, pH 8.2.
2. Dioxane.
3. 1 M hydrochloric acid.
4. Dinitrofluorobenzene (DNFB) reagent: Dilute 2.5 ml to 25 ml with acetone (store in refrigerator). Just before use, dilute 1 ml to 100 ml with borax solution.

Standard solution

100 mcg/ml of the substance in water.

Sample solution

(a) Eye/ear drops/liquid oral (syrups): Directly dilute with water to get 100 mcg/ml.
(b) Ointments: Extract with 10% w/v sodium chloride solution by slight heating for 10 min to get solution of 100 mcg/ml.
(c) Tablets/capsules: Extract with water by heating in boiling water for 5 min, cool and dilute with water to get solution of 100 mcg/ml.

Procedure

To 2 ml each of sample and standard solutions add 2 ml of DNFB reagent. Heat in boiling water-bath for 10 min. Cool, add 1 ml of 1 M hydrochloric acid and 10 ml of dioxane (to dissolve the chromophore) and adjust the volume to 25 ml with water. Measure the absorbance of the sample and standard at about 385 nm against reagent blank. The method obeys Beer's law in the range of 2-10 mcg/ml.

Note

Betamethasone, lignocaine, diphenylpyraline, antipyrine and parabens did not interfere.

Probable Reaction Mechanism

This reagent is known as Sanger's reagent. It reacts with amino group present in alkylamine radical with the loss of one mol of HF to give a coloured complex (λ_{max} 385 nm). The chromophore is soluble in dioxane.

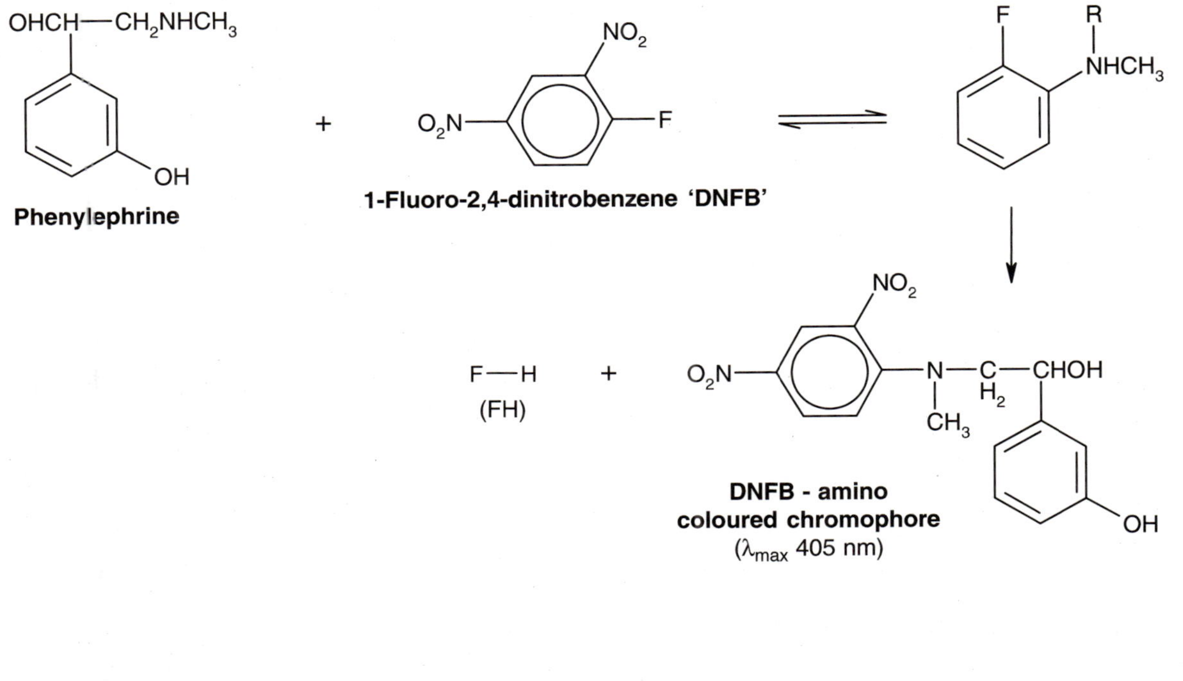

As the reagent is used in excess for reaction to proceed quantitatively, the unreacted 'DNFB' undergoes basic hydrolysis (borax, pH 8.2) to 2,4-dinitrophenolate which is intense yellow in colour. The spectra of both the products is overlapping, hence estimation is not possible as such. However, by acidification after completion of the reaction and the yellow phenolate is turned to colourless phenol, hence no interference and in measuring the colour of the component – 'DNFB' derivative.

Probable Reaction Mechanism

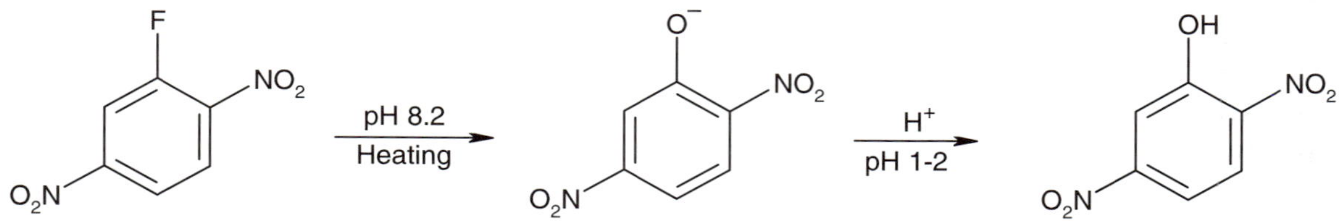

Dinitrophenolate (yellow-coloured)
(λ_{max} 386 nm)

Dinitrophenol
(colourless)

Reference

G. Paraskevas, J. Atta-Politou & M. Kouppavis. J. Pharm. Biomed. Anal., **29**, 865-872, 2002.

A spectrophotometric method has been described based on coupling of diazotized p-nitroaniline with phenylephrine. The coupling takes place at position para to the phenolic —OH group present in the drug.

Probable Reaction Mechanism

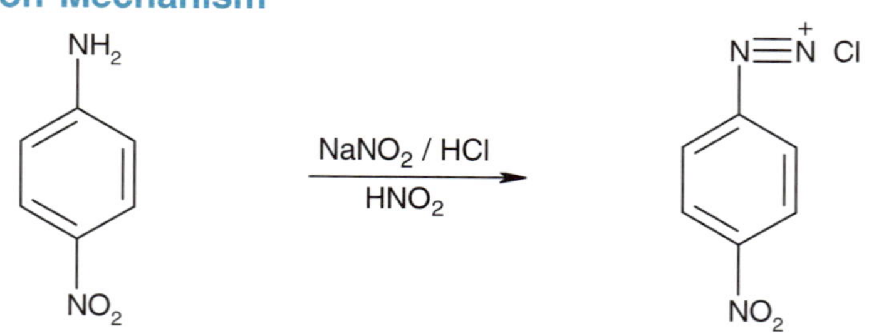

p-Nitroaniline

Diazotized nitroaniline (1)

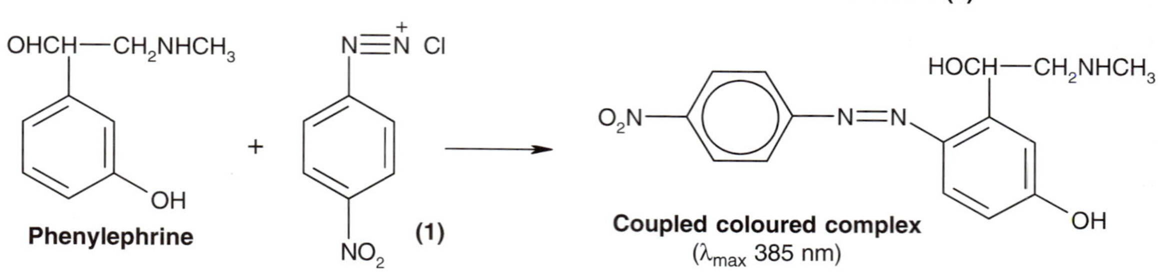

Phenylephrine

Coupled coloured complex
(λ_{max} 385 nm)

Reference

1. M.E. Auerbach, J. Am. Pharm. Assoc., **39**, 50-52, 1950.
2. C.A. Kelly & M.E. Auerbach, J. Pharm. Sci., **50**, 490-493, 1961.

Ascorbic acid

Reagents

1. 85% v/v sulphuric acid in water.
2. 2% w/v solution of 2,4-dinitrophenylhydrazine in 9 N sulphuric acid.
3. 9 N sulphuric acid.
4. 50% w/v solution of oxalic acid in water.
5. Bromine water; saturated aqueous solution.
6. 1% w/v solution of thiourea in oxalic acid solution.

Standard solution

2.5 mg/ml of ascorbic acid in oxalic acid solution. To 1 ml of this solution, add 50 ml of oxalic acid solution and 10-12 drops of bromine water till faint yellow colour. Bubble air till colourless and dilute to 100 ml with oxalic acid solution (25 mcg/ml).

Sample solution

Weigh accurately a quantity of the sample equivalent to 100 mg of ascorbic acid, add 50 ml of water, shake for 15 minutes and dilute to 100 ml with same solvent. Filter, take 2.5 ml (2.5 mg), add 50 ml of oxalic acid solution and treat as per standard solution.

Procedure

To 5 ml each of sample and standard solutions, add 4 ml of thiourea solution and 2 ml of dinitrophenylhydrazine solution. Prepare sample and standard blanks separately, using 5 ml of water instead of sample or standard. Allow all the tubes to stand at 37°C for 3 hrs. Cool in ice-bath and then add 3 ml of 85% sulphuric acid drop by drop in each tube with continuous cooling. Then, add 1 ml of phenylhydrazine reagent to blanks and let all the tubes stand at room temperature for 20-30 minutes. Measure the absorbance at about 550 nm against respective blanks and calculate the results by comparison.

Probable Reaction Mechanism

This method is based on formation of coloured hydrazone as a result of condensation reaction between carbonyl group and the hydrazine.

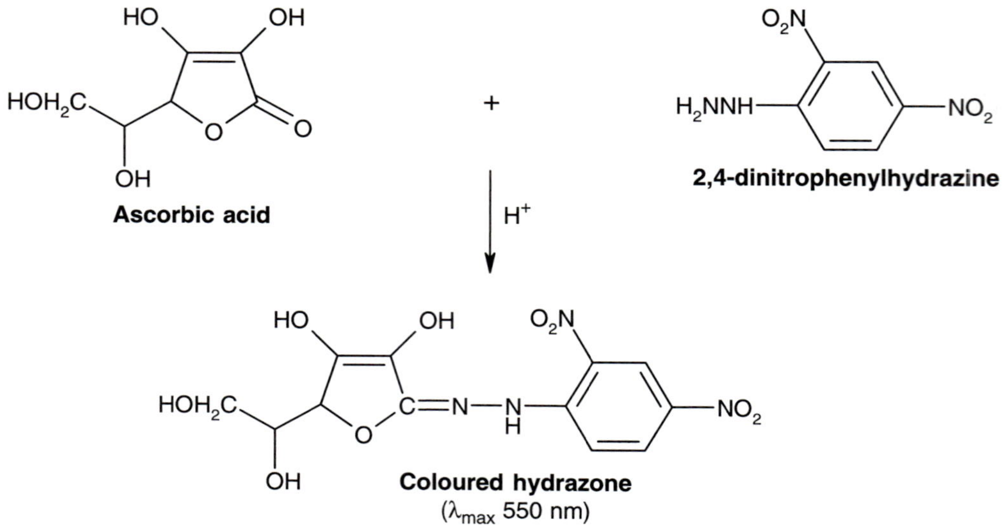

HO
OH
HOH2C
O
O
OH
Ascorbic acid
+
O2N
H2NNH
NO2
2,4-dinitrophenylhydrazine
H+
HO
OH
O2N
HOH2C
C=N—N
H
NO2
O
OH
Coloured hydrazone
(λmax 550 nm)

Formulation 5

Aspirin, Salicylamide, Caffeine, Prednisolone, Codeine phosphate, Paracetamol

ESTIMATION

Codeine phosphate

METHOD 1

Reagents

1. Phosphate buffer, pH 5.0 or phthalate buffer, pH 5.0.
2. 0.1 N sulphuric acid, saturated with ether.
3. 0.1% w/v solution of methyl orange in 20% v/v alcohol.
4. Acidified methanol: 3% v/v sulphuric acid in methanol.

Standard solution

80 mcg/ml of pure codeine phosphate in ether saturated 0.1 N sulphuric acid.

Sample solution

Weigh accurately a quantity of powdered tablets equivalent to 2 mg of codeine phosphate, add 20 ml of 0.1 N sulphuric acid (ether saturated) and extract with four 20 ml portions of chloroform. Collect acid layer and dilute to 25 ml with 0.1 N sulphuric acid.

Procedure

To 5 ml of sample and standard solutions add 5 ml of buffer solution, pH 5.0 and 1 ml of methyl orange solution. Shake and extract with two 10 ml portions of chloroform. Separate chloroform layer and adjust with chloroform to 25 ml. Measure the absorbance of both the solutions at about 410 nm using chloroform as blank.

METHOD 2

Standard solution

80 mcg/ml of codeine phosphate in buffer pH 5.0.

Sample solution

Weigh accurately a quantity of powdered tablets equivalent to 2.0 mg of codeine phosphate, dissolve in ether buffer solution of pH 5.0 to produce 25 ml and filter.

Procedure

Proceed with formation of dye complex and extraction into chloroform as per method 1 above. To 10 ml of the resultant chloroform extract, add 1 ml of acidified methanol and measure the absorbance of both the solutions at 510 nm. This method is more sensitive.

On acidification, the complex decomposes liberating complexed 'MO' which gives red colour (λ_{max} 510 nm) in acidic medium, thus improving the sensitivity of the method.

Probable Reaction Mechanism

The method is based on ion-pair complex formation between the drug and acidic dye, methyl orange at pH 3.5.

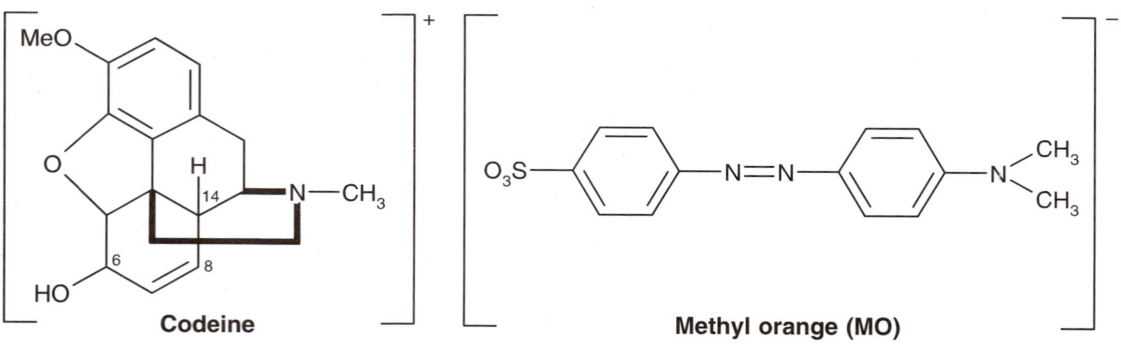

Codeine - methyl orange complex
(λ_{max} 410 nm)

Note

Usually a buffer of pH 3.5 is employed for formation of ion-pair complex but due to presence of aspirin, pH of the extract is slightly lowered, hence the buffer of pH 5.0 is recommended.

Different morphine derivatives with OH group at C-6 and a $\Delta^{7,8}$ double bond such as codeine and ethyl morphine, first undergo an acid catalysed re-arrangement as under.

Here the alcoholic —OH group at C-6 is protonated and then eliminated as water, followed by opening of ether linkage and aromatization of C-ring leading to formation of apomorphine. Apomorphine being an orthodiphenolic structure is a strong reducing agent and in acidic medium forms a blue-coloured orthoquinone with oxidizing agent such as iodine and Fe(III).

The entire reaction sequence is based on oxidation-reduction mechanism.

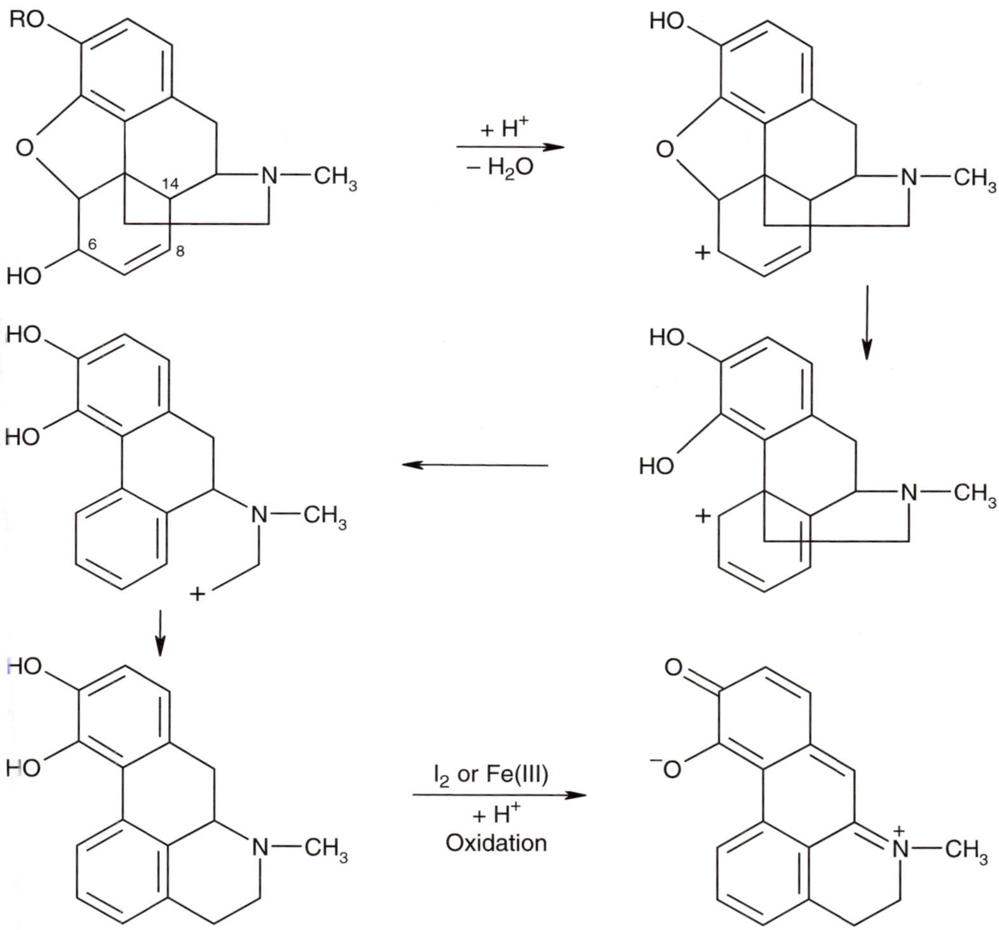

Apomorphine **Blue-coloured orthoquinone structure** (λ_{max} 650 nm)

Formation of red-coloured orthoquinone structure via apomorphine with nitric acid along with nitration of the benzene ring forms the basis of identification test.

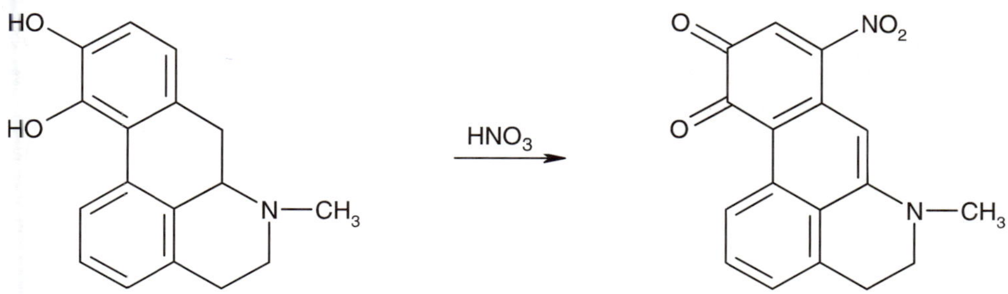

Apomorphine **Orthoquinone** (λ_{max} 510 nm)

In contrast, in alkaline medium apomorphine forms 2 different coloured quinones.

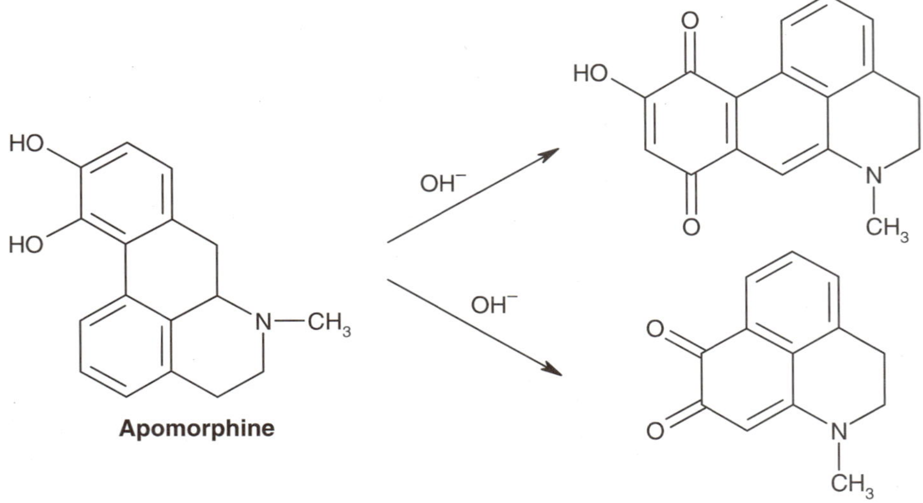

Reference

Thin-Layer Chromatography, Reagents and Detection Methods (Vol. 1b) by H. Jork et al., pp. 63-65.

METHOD 3

Reagents

1. 0.1 M hydrochloric acid.
2. 0.1 M sodium hydroxide.
3. Decalso slurry: Decalso (40-60 mesh) is suspended in water to prepare the slurry for use in column chromatographic separation of codeine phosphate.

Standard solution

0.5 mg/ml of codeine phosphate in water.

Sample solution

Weigh accurately a quantity of the sample equivalent to 50 mg of codeine phosphate, shake with 10 ml of water and filter through sintered funnel. Wash the precipitate with 20-30 ml of water. Adjust the pH of the filtrate to 5.8 ± 0.2 with 0.1 N sodium hydroxide and dilute to 100 ml with water.

Preparation of the column: Fill the glass column with decalso slurry up to 10-12 cm. Wash the column with water. Do not allow the column to dry at any stage. Now the column is ready for use.

Procedure

Transfer 5 ml of the sample solution to the column and allow it to pass slowly. Wash the column with four 5 ml portions of water and discard. Then elute the column with 0.1 N hydrochloric acid and collect 25 ml of the eluate. Treat standard solution similarly and measure the extinction of both the solutions at maximum at about 284 nm and calculate the results.

Salicylamide

Weigh accurately a quantity of powdered tablets equivalent to 15 mg of salicylamide, shake with 25 ml of chloroform and adjust to 100 ml. Carry out further dilution with chloroform to get 10 mcg/ml solution and measure the extinction at maxima at about 308 nm. Calculate the results taking 350 as value of E 1%, 1 cm at 308 nm.

Note

Analgin, phenobarbitone, ascorbic acid, chloroquine, prednisolone and dexamethasone do not interfere.

Alternatively, follow the method described in formulation 3 of this chapter.

Aspirin

Weigh accurately a quantity of the sample equivalent to 150 mg of aspirin. Suspend in 25 ml of ether, shake vigorously for 5 minutes and filter through cotton plug, wash cotton plug with ether. Combine ether extracts and extract with two 25 ml portions of 6% w/v sodium bicarbonate solution. Acidify the alkaline extract with dilute hydrochloric acid, cool and extract with four 20 ml portions of ether. Combine ether layer, wash each layer with the same 10 ml of water. Evaporate ether layer at room temperature under current of air. Dissolve the residue in neutralized methanol and titrate with 0.1 N sodium hydroxide using phenolphthalein as indicator. Each ml of 0.1 N sodium hydroxide is equivalent to 45.05 mg of aspirin.

Paracetamol

Carry out the nitroso derivative method or cobalt derivative method as described in formulation 2 of this chapter.

Note

Salicylamide yields nitroso derivative only on boiling whereas paracetamol gives nitroso derivative in cold, hence is of no analytical problem.

Caffeine

Reagents

1. 15% v/v phosphoric acid in water.
2. Phosphoric acid (1 : 1 v/v) in water.

Standard solution

10 mcg/ml of caffeine in 15% v/v phosphoric acid.

Sample solution

Weigh accurately a quantity of sample equivalent to 5 mg of caffeine and dissolve in water to produce 25 ml. To 5 ml of this solution, add 20 ml of chloroform and extract with 30 ml of phosphoric acid (1 : 1). Collect acid layer, wash it with 20 ml of chloroform. Discard chloroform layer, dilute acid layer to 100 ml with water (10 mcg/ml). Concentration of phosphoric acid in final solution is 15% v/v.

Procedure

Measure the extinction of both standard and sample solutions at maximum at about 269 nm using 15% v/v phosphoric acid as blank and calculate the results by comparison.

Free salicylic acid (FSA)

This special procedure is described as salicylamide if present along with aspirin will interfere in the estimation of free salicylic acid by usual method.

Reagents

1. Petroleum ether (40-60°C).
2. Ferric nitrate solution: Dissolve 2.5 g of ferric nitrate monohydrate in about 200 ml of water. Add 1 ml of concentrated nitric acid and make volume to 250 ml with water. Further dilute 5 ml of the above solution to 100 ml with water.

Standard stock solution of salicylic acid

Weigh accurately 500 mg of salicylic acid and transfer to a dry 50 ml volumetric flask, make up the volume with absolute alcohol.

Working standard

Dilute 5 ml of the standard stock solution of salicylic acid to 100 ml with water. Each ml represents 500 mcg of salicylic acid. Take 1 ml in a 50 ml volumetric flask (A) and proceed for colour development.

Sample preparation

Weigh accurately a suitable quantity of the powdered sample and transfer to a dry 100 ml volumetric flask and make volume to 100 ml with petroleum ether (40-60°C). Shake vigorously for 2 minutes and allow it to stand for 5 minutes. Pipette 25 ml of the filtrate immediately into a 100 ml dry beaker, evaporate off the solvent to dryness at room temperature. Dissolve the residue in 5 ml of absolute alcohol and transfer to a 50 ml volumetric flask (B), rinse the beaker twice with 5 ml of water and proceed further for colour development.

Colour development

Add 5 ml of the diluted ferric nitrate solution to each 50 ml standard and sample flasks (A and B) and make volume with water and mix well. Measure the absorption of the colour on suitable colorimeter at 540 nm against water as blank and calculate the results.

Prednisolone

Reagents

1. 0.1% w/v solution of 2,4-dinitrophenylhydrazine (DNPH) in hydrochloric acid : methanol (1 : 3) mixture. Keep in cool place and change after every 7 days.
2. 0.1 M sodium bicarbonate solution.
3. Acidic ferric chloride solution.
4. 4 M sodium hydroxide.

Standard solution

10 mcg/ml prednisolone in methyl alcohol.

Sample solution

Weigh accurately a quantity of powdered tablets equivalent to 1 mg of prednisolone. Add 30 ml of methyl alcohol, keep it in water-bath maintained at nearly boiling point for 30 minutes with occasional stirring. Allow to cool, filter and adjust to 100 ml with methanol.

Extraction procedure

This procedure is specially designed to remove interfering substances. Evaporate 50 ml of sample and standard solutions to dryness on a steam-bath with the help of air current. Subject the residue from sample solution to following extraction procedure: To each of three 100 ml separating funnels add 5 ml of acidic ferric chloride solution. Add 15 ml of water to separators 2 and 3. Transfer the residue from the sample to separator 1. Wash the residue with 20 ml of chloroform and add to separator 1. Shake for 1 minute and allow to separate. Take chloroform layer and transfer to separator 2. Shake, separate and then transfer chloroform layer to separator 3. If the aqueous layer is still purple, extract chloroform layer with more water and acidic ferric chloride solution. Repeat the extraction of first separator with two more 20 ml portions of chloroform and pass through each separator. Shake chloroform layer with two 20 ml portions of 0.1 N sodium bicarbonate solution. Wash chloroform layer with water and evaporate to 50 ml (A).

Procedure

Evaporate chloroform extract (A) equivalent to 100 mcg of prednisolone (avoid excessive heating). Dissolve the residue in 5 ml methanol, add 2 ml of 'DNPH' reagent and heat on constant temperature water-bath maintained at 60°C for 2 hours, add 2 ml of 4 N sodium hydroxide and dilute to 10 ml with methanol. Mix and allow to stand for 30 minutes and measure the absorbance at maximum at about 480 nm. The residue from standard solution equivalent to 100 mcg is dissolved in methanol and processed for colour development as per procedure described for the sample. The results are calculated by comparison.

Probable Reaction Mechanism

Prednisolone is a keto steroid with α-β unsaturated ketone at C-3. This method is based on reaction of the keto group with Porter–Silber reagent in acidic conditions. This is similar to the reaction with 'INH' i.e. Umberger's reagent.

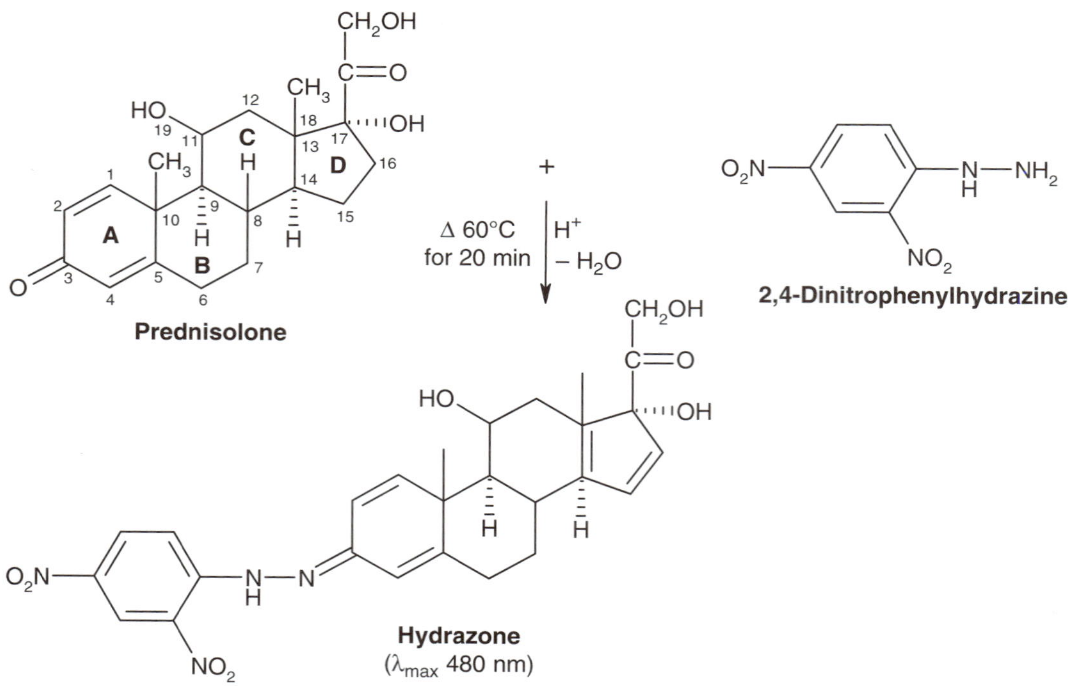

Reference

1. Pharmaceutical Chemistry (Vol. 2) by H.J. Roth, p. 463.
2. Thin-Layer Chromatography: Reagents and Detection Methods by H. York, p. 274.

Other compounds which react with this reagent to give hydrazones: allantoin, nitrofurantoin, dexamethasone, ofloxacin, menadione, ofloxam and rifampin.

Note

Prednisolone having methyl keto group at C-17 answers Janovsky reaction forming coloured Meisenheimer complex in basic condition with m-dinitrobenzene.

General Reaction Mechanism

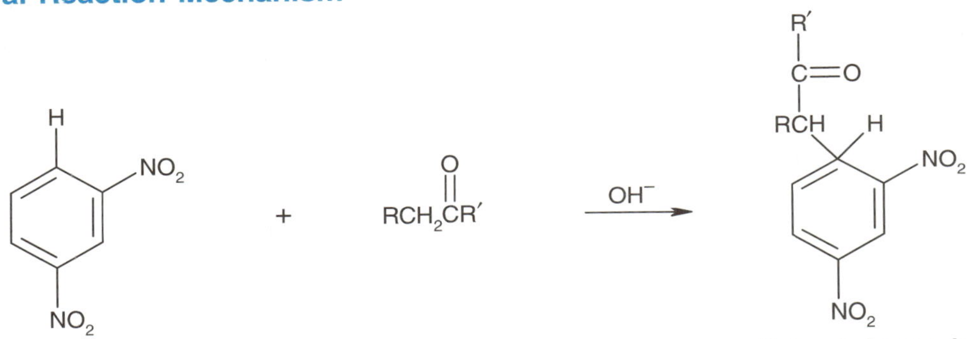

Meisenheimer salt

Compounds such as atropine, ephedrine undergo this reaction after nitration.

Prednisolone can be oxidized to give ketone and formaldehyde. Formaldehyde can be analysed by reaction with chromotropic acid and ketone by formation of Meisenheimer salt with m-dinitrophenol.

Probable Reaction Mechanism

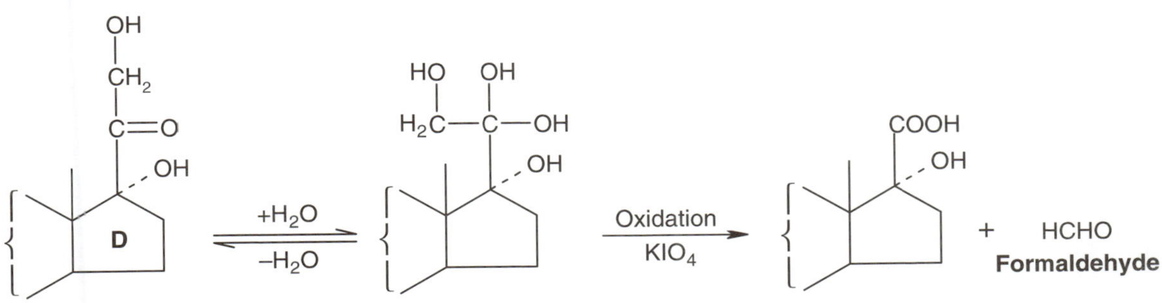

Partial structure of Prednisolone **Hydrated derivative** **Hydroxycarboxylic acid derivative**

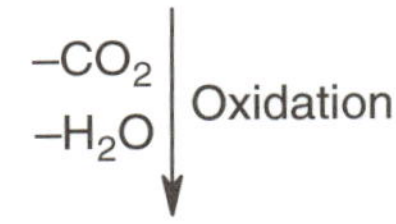

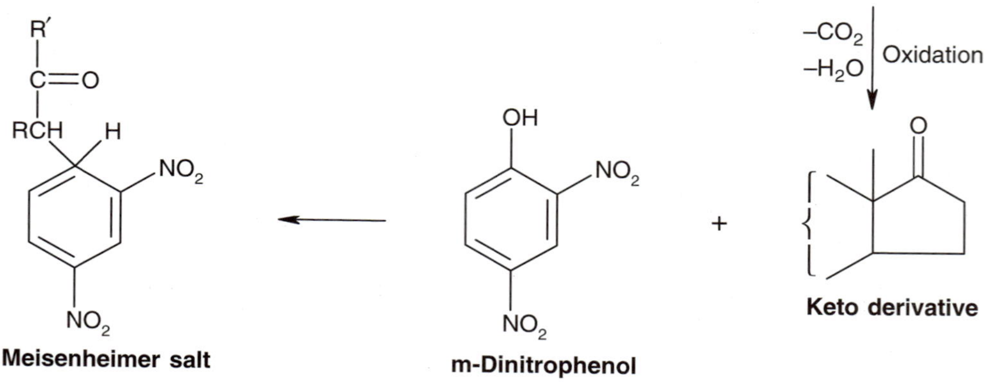

Reference

Pharmaceutical Chemistry (Vol. 2) by H.J. Roth, p. 469.

Formulation 6

Aspirin, Chlorpheniramine maleate, Salicylamide

ESTIMATION

Aspirin

Extract accurately weighed quantity of the powdered sample equivalent to 500 mg of aspirin with neutral acetone and titrate with 0.1 N sodium hydroxide using phenolphthalein solution as indicator.

Each ml of 0.1 N sodium hydroxide is equivalent to 45.05 mg of aspirin. For estimation of free salicylic acid in the formulation, follow the method given in formulation 5 of this chapter.

Chlorpheniramine maleate

Follow the cyanogen bromide method as described in formulation 1 of the chapter on rubefacients.

Salicylamide

METHOD 1

Reagents

1. 0.1% 2,6-dichloroquinone chlorimide in isopropyl alcohol (Gibbs' reagent).
2. Buffer solution, pH 9.2 (borate or phosphate).
3. Isopropyl alcohol : water (1 : 1) mixture.

Standard solution

50 mcg/ml of salicylamide in alcohol-water solvent mixture.

Sample solution

Weigh accurately powdered tablets equivalent to 50 mg of salicylamide and extract with isopropyl alcohol–water mixture to make 100 ml. Dilute appropriately with the same solvent to get 50 mcg/ml solution.

Procedure

To 2 ml of standard and sample solutions add 2 ml of buffer solution, pH 9.2, 5 ml of isopropyl alcohol and 1 ml of chlorimide reagent. Shake for 1 minute and allow to stand for 30 minutes. Measure the absorbance of both the solutions at maximum at about 650 nm and calculate the results.

Probable Reaction Mechanism

Buffer solution of pH 9.2 causes hydrolysis of the reagent. This hydrolysed reagent acts as oxidizing agent and attacks the para position to the phenolic —OH present in the molecule. This reaction is answered by all phenols with free para position. This is called Gibbs' reaction.

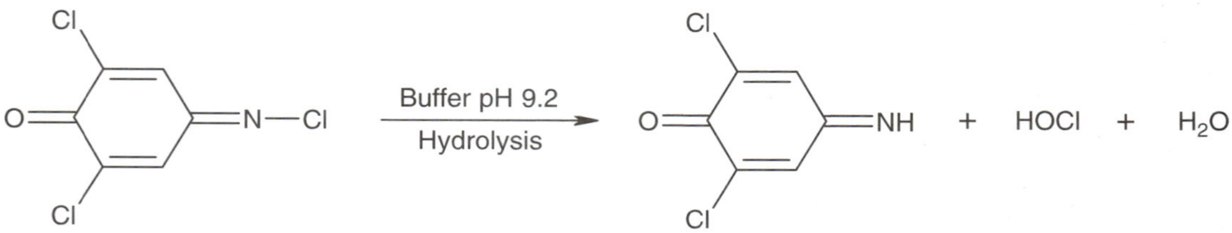

2,6-dichloroquinone chlorimide (1) **2,6-dichloroquinonimine (2)**

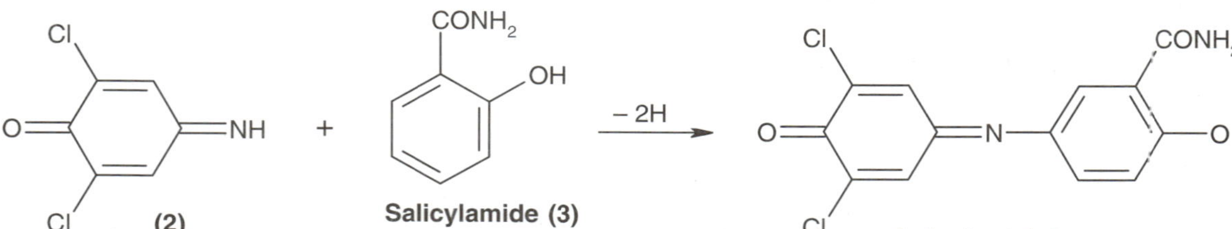

(2) **Salicylamide (3)** **Indophenol dye** (λ_{max} 650 nm)

Note

1. Other drugs which react with this reagent are vitamin B_6, primary and secondary amines and barbiturates.
2. Chlorimide is not the reacting reagent, it is dichloroquinonimine which is rapidly produced from chlorimide in aqueous solution. The reagent is of low stability and has to be prepared fresh. Its recrystallization from n-heptane and storage in dark improves its quality. The hydrolysis of the reagent to quinonimine is quick at pH 8.5, slow at pH 7.5 and at pH 10.0 chlorimide reacts with itself producing indophenol dye; so pH 10.0 is not suitable. Hence, buffer of around 9 has been selected. Ammonia buffers and glycine buffers are not suitable as they react with the reagent.

Reference

Pharmaceutical Chemistry (Vol. 2) by H.J. Roth, 1991, p. 73.

El-Kheir et al. (1986) described a method for estimation of salicylamide based on nitration followed by complexation.

METHOD 2

Reagents

1. Concentrated nitric acid.
2. Concentrated sulphuric acid.
3. 10% w/v solution of potassium hydroxide.
4. Acetone.

Sample and standard solutions

1 mg/ml in methanol.

Procedure

To 5 ml each of sample and standard solutions add 2 ml each of nitric acid and sulphuric acid, leave to stand for 10 min, cool, dilute to 100 ml with water.

Note

Care must be taken during handling of nitration mixture. To 2 ml of the aliquot add 2.5 ml of acetone and 5 ml of potassium hydroxide solution, dilute to 25 ml with water. Measure the absorbance of resulting solution at 390 nm against reagent blank.

Probable Reaction Mechanism

The nitration of the compound gave dinitro derivative. Further treatment of electron-deficient dinitro derivative with ketone (acetone) in alkaline medium gives coloured complex by interaction with anions such as $CH_3COCH_2^-$. These complexes are of Meisenheimer type. The coloured complex is stable for 60 min.

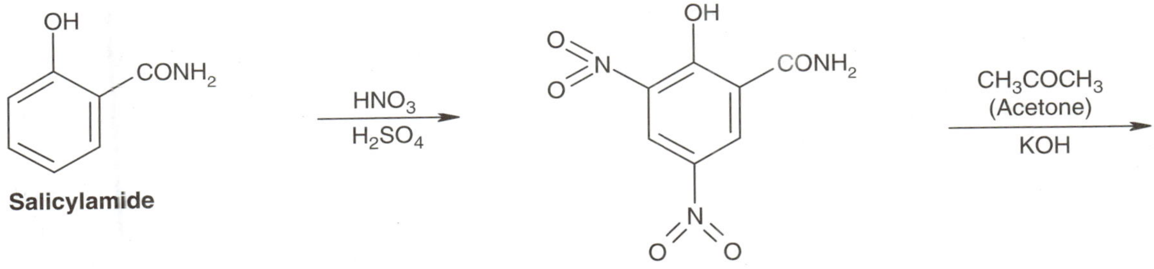

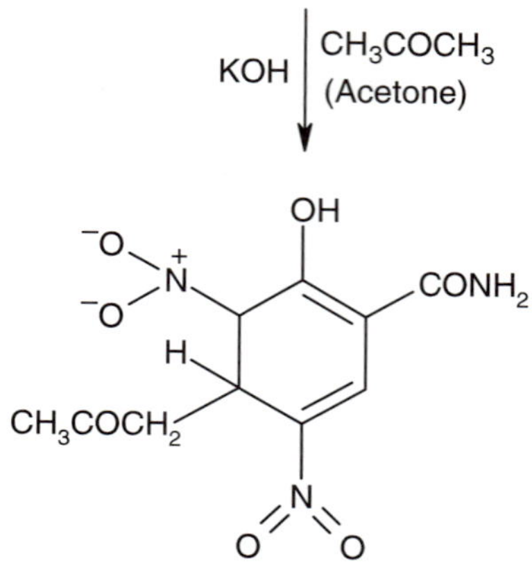

Meisenheimer complex
(λ_{max} 390 nm)

Reference

Afaf A. El Kheir, Saied Belal, Mohammad El Sadek & Abdullah El Shanwani, Analyst, **111(3)**, 319-321, 1986.

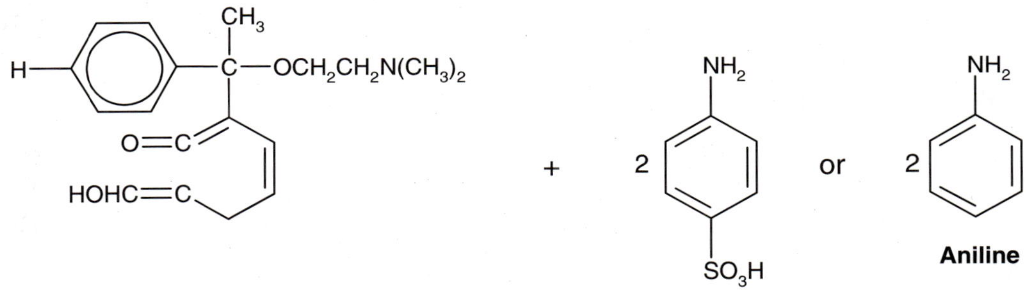

Sulphanilic acid

Aniline

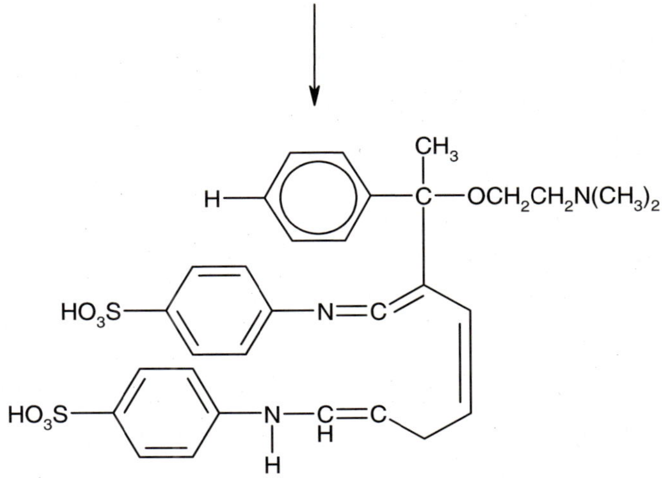

Polymethine dye
(λ_{max} 490 nm)

Note

1. It is reported that addition of micellar anion like sodium dodecyl sulphate in the reaction medium enhances sensitivity, stabilizes the complex and shortens the coupling time.
2. The above method is applicable to carbinoxamine as well.

Formulation 11

Paracetamol, Dicyclomine hydrochloride, Clidinium bromide

ESTIMATION

Clidinium bromide

Follow the method 1 or 2 described under formulation 1 of the chapter on sedatives and tranquilizers.

Paracetamol

Follow the method 1 or 2 described under formulation 2 of this chapter.

Dicyclomine hydrochloride

Follow the method described under formulation 20 of this chapter.

Alternatively, its complexation with cobalt thiocyanate in acid medium can be used for quantitative estimation.

Probable Reaction Mechanism

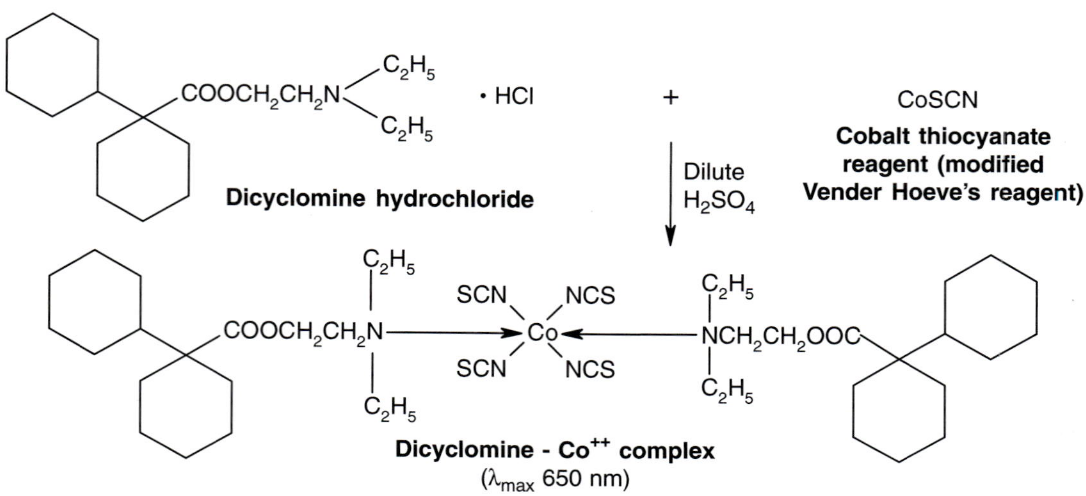

The complex is extractable into benzene.

Kale et al. (1998) have proposed another method of analysis based on coupling with potassium dichromate in acidic buffer.

Reagents

1. 1% w/v solution of potassium dichromate.
2. Buffer solution, pH 1.2, containing 0.2 M HCl and 0.2 M KCl.

Sample and standard solutions

200 µg/ml in pH 1.2 buffer.

Procedure

To 2 ml each of sample and standard solutions add 5 ml of dichromate solution and 10 ml of toluene. Shake for 10 min and separate toluene layer and measure the absorbance at 357 nm against reagent blank.

Note

Tinidazole and diloxamide did not interfere.

Probable Reaction Mechanism

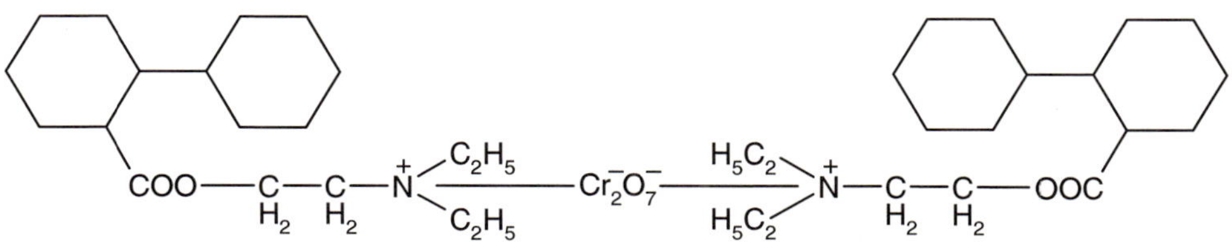

Dicyclomine - dichromate complex
(λ_{max} 357 nm)

Reference

A.D. Kale, S.J. Kachhwaha, G.P. Jadhav & Piyush Trivedi, *Indian Drugs*, **35(11)**, 718-720, 1998.

Raggi et al. have described a spectrophotometric method based on ion-pair complex formation in pH 3.0 sodium citrate - HCl buffer with bromocresol green. The complex was extractable into chloroform and has λ_{max} 415 nm.

Reference

M.A. Raggi, V. Cavrini & A.M. DiPietra, J. Pharm. & Biomed. Analysis, **3(3)**, 287-291, 1985.

Formulation 12

Ibuprofen, Colchicine

ESTIMATION

Ibuprofen

Accurately weighed quantity of the powdered sample equivalent to 400 mg of the substance was suspended in 25 ml of 1 M hydrochloric acid and extracted with three 20 ml portions of chloroform (reserve the acid layer for estimation of colchicine). Evaporate combined chloroform layer, take up the residue in neutral (phenol red) methanol and titrate with 0.1 N sodium hydroxide. Each ml of 0.1 M sodium hydroxide is equivalent to 20.63 mg of ibuprofen.

The method is based on acid-base titration; carboxyl (COOH) group present in the side chain reacts with alkali.

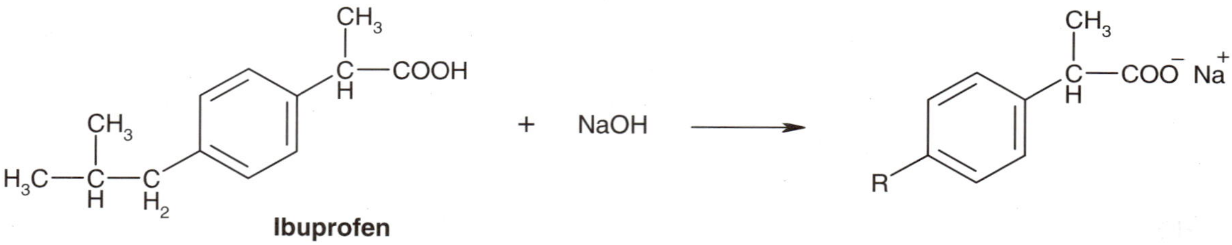

Note

On acidification, the ibuprofen gets extracted into chloroform, whereas colchicine, an alkaloid with basic properties, remains in acidic layer which can be subjected to spectrophotometric analysis.

Colchicine

The acidic extract retained during estimation of ibuprofen was diluted to 50 ml with methanol and extinction measured at absorption maxima at about 243 nm. Calculate the results by comparing with the standard (5 mcg/ml) or by taking 730 as value of A 1%, 1 cm at 243 nm.

A spectrophotofluorometric method has been reported by Arai et al. (1975) exc. 350 nm, em. 425 nm (Arai T. & Okuyania, T., Anal. Biochem., **69**, 443, 1975).

After acid hydrolysis, the compound gives orange-red colour with $FeCl_3$ (470 nm). This can form the basis of quantitative estimation.

Probable Reaction Mechanism

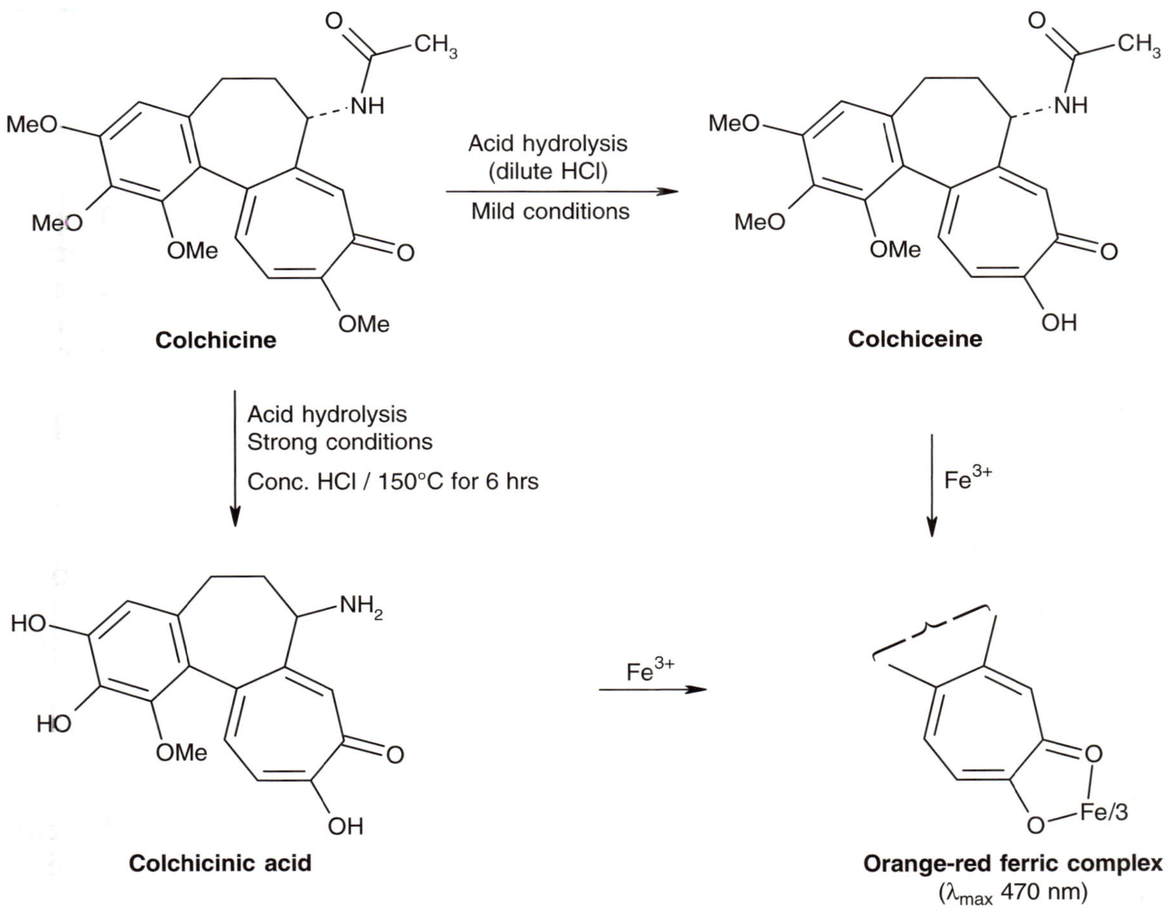

Reference

J.S. King, *J. Amm. Pharm. Assoc.*, **40**, 424, 1951.

Formulation 13

Paracetamol, Promethazine hydrochloride

ESTIMATION

METHOD 1

Standard solution

1. Paracetamol: 10 mcg/ml in 0.1 M hydrochloric acid.
2. Promethazine hydrochloride: 40 mcg/ml in 1% v/v sulphuric acid.

Promethazine hydrochloride

Take a measured volume of suspension equivalent to 100 mg (10 ml) of promethazine hydrochloride in a 250 ml separator. Add 5 ml of 1 M sodium hydroxide, mix thoroughly. Immediately extract the promethazine base with four 25 ml portions of chloroform. Collect the total chloroform in a second separator. The aqueous layer is acidified with 1 M hydrochloric acid and preserved for paracetamol estimation. The chloroform extract is washed with 2 × 10 ml of 1 in 9 hydrochloric acid and collect the chloroform extract in a 250 ml conical flask. Wash the acid portion with 25 ml chloroform and add this 25 ml chloroform to total chloroform layer. Evaporate the chloroform on a boiling water bath to dryness. Add 5-10 ml of methanol and evaporate. Dissolve the residue in 1 in 100 sulphuric acid and dilute to get a final concentration of 40 mcg/ml. Measure the absorbance at 298 nm and calculate the result by comparing with standard. Carry out the entire procedure under low actinic light.

Paracetamol

The above preserved solution is taken and warmed slightly on water bath till it is free from smell of chloroform. Dilute with 0.1 M hydrochloric acid to get a final concentration of 40 mcg/ml. Measure the extinction at 244 nm and calculate the results by comparing with standard solution (10 mcg/ml) (final concentration of 7.5 mcg/ml is preferable).

Typical laboratory analysis

1. Promethazine hydrochloride

Weight of standard promethazine hydrochloride = 0.0630 g

0.063 g of standard promethazine hydrochloride $\xrightarrow{\text{1 in 100 } H_2SO_4}$ 50 ml

1.6 ml $\xrightarrow{\text{1 in 100 } H_2SO_4}$ 50 ml (40 mcg/ml)

Sample:

10 ml of suspension equivalent to 0.010 g of promethazine → Extraction, evaporation and residue $\xrightarrow{\text{1 in 100 } H_2SO_4}$ 250 ml (40 mcg/ml)

Absorbance at 298 nm:

Standard reading – 0.398 Sample reading – 0.391

$$\text{Promethazine hydrochloride mg/5 ml} = \frac{0.391}{0.398} \times \frac{0.063}{50} \times \frac{1.6}{50} \times \frac{250 \times 5}{10}$$

$$= 4.95 \text{ mg}$$

Claim = 5 mg

2. Paracetamol

0.0249 g of standard paracetamol $\xrightarrow{\text{0.1 N HCl}}$ 50 ml

1 ml $\xrightarrow{\text{0.1 N HCl}}$ 50 ml (10 mcg/ml)

10 ml of suspension equivalent to 0.5 g of paracetamol $\xrightarrow{\text{1 N NaOH}}$ basified, extracted, acidic extract $\xrightarrow{\text{0.1 N HCl}}$ 100 ml

1 ml $\xrightarrow{\text{0.1 N HCl}}$ 50 ml

5 ml $\xrightarrow{\text{0.1 N HCl}}$ 50 ml (10 mcg/ml)

Absorbance at 245 nm:

Standard reading – 0.760 Sample reading – 0.780

$$\text{Paracetamol mg/5 ml} = \frac{0.780}{0.760} \times \frac{0.0249}{50} \times \frac{1}{50} \times \frac{100}{0.50} \times \frac{50}{1} \times \frac{50}{5} \times \frac{5}{10} = 255 \text{ mg}$$

$$\text{Claim} = 250 \text{ mg}$$

METHOD 2

Paracetamol

Reagents

1. 1 M hydrochloric acid
2. 1 M sodium hydroxide
3. 10% w/v solution of sodium nitrite in water.
4. 10% w/v solution of sulphamic acid in water.

Standard solution

Dissolve 100 mg of the substance in 50 ml of 1 M hydrochloric acid and dilute to 500 ml with water.

Sample solution

Accurately measured quantity of the sample equivalent to 100 mg of the substance is suspended in 50 ml of 1 M hydrochloric acid and diluted to 500 ml with water.

Procedure

To 5 ml each of sample and standard solutions add 5 ml of sodium nitrite solution, shake and allow to stand for 5 min. Add 5 ml of sulphamic acid solution drop by drop with constant shaking till the effervescence clears. Allow to stand for 5 min and dilute to 50 ml with 1 M sodium hydroxide. Measure the absorbance of both sample and standard solutions at about 430 nm against reagent blank and calculate the results by comparison.

Probable Reaction Mechanism

Two alternate reactions are proposed:

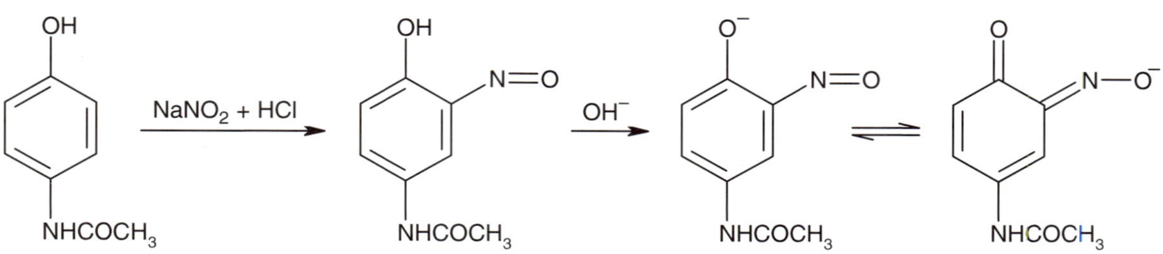

Paracetamol (λ_{max} 370 nm) (λ_{max} 430 nm)

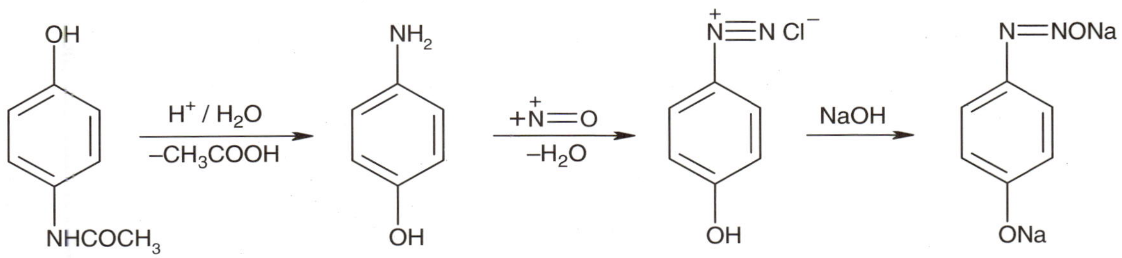

Paracetamol p-Aminophenol Dizonium salt (λ_{max} 430 nm)

Reference

1. Textbook of Practical Organic Chemistry by Vogel, p. 920.
2. Pharmaceutical Chemistry (Vol. 2) by H.J. Roth, p. 398.

Promethazine hydrochloride

METHOD 1

Reagents

1. Buffer solution pH 2.7: 6 g of citric acid and 3.9 g of disodium dihydrogen phosphate dissolved in about 900 ml of water, pH adjusted to 2.7-2.8 with citric acid and diluted to 1000 ml.
2. Bromocresol green solution: 69.8 mg of dye was dissolved in 2 ml of 0.1 N sodium hydroxide and made to 1000 ml with buffer solution.

Standard solution

1 mg/ml of promethazine hydrochloride in water.

Sample solution

The sample (suspension) containing 5 mg/5 ml of the substance was used as such.

Procedure

To 2 ml each of sample and standard solutions, add 50 ml of water, 25 ml dye solution. Mix and extract with three 30 ml portions of chloroform. Pass the chloroform layer through anhydrous sodium sulphate (already moistened with chloroform), make up to 100 ml. Measure the absorbance of both sample and standard solutions at about 415 nm using chloroform as blank and calculate the results.

Note

Complex ratio of the drug and the dye was 1 : 1 but for complete complexation and quantitative extraction it was 1 : 3.

Probable Reaction Mechanism

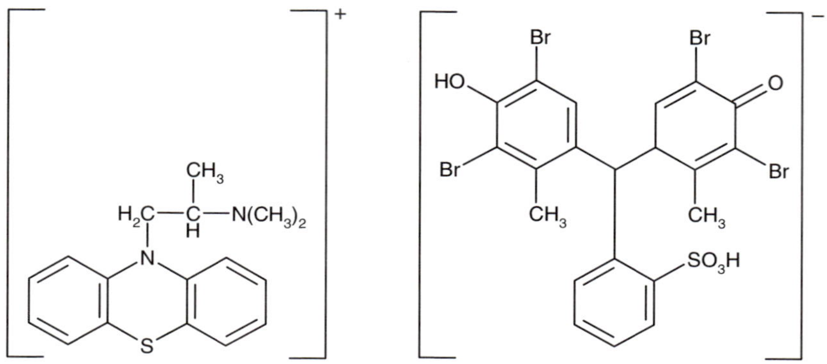

Promethazine **Bromocresol green**

1 : 1 Drug-dye ion-pair complex
(λ_{max} 415 nm)

Reference

Abdol-Ali M. & Emami K., *J. Pharm. Sci.*, **72(6)**, 704, 1983.

METHOD 2

The method is based on reaction with 'PDAB' in acidic medium. Position C-2 of phenothiazine is readily attacked by electrophilic (electron-loving species) i.e. PDAB resulting in the formation of a complex (λ_{max} 520 nm). $FeCl_3$ acts as a catalyst to facilitate the reaction.

Probable Reaction Mechanism

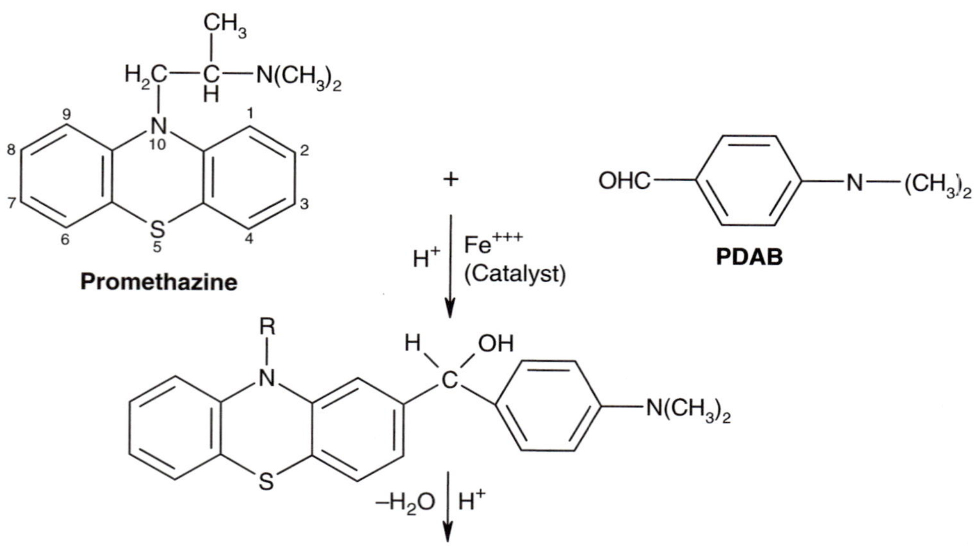

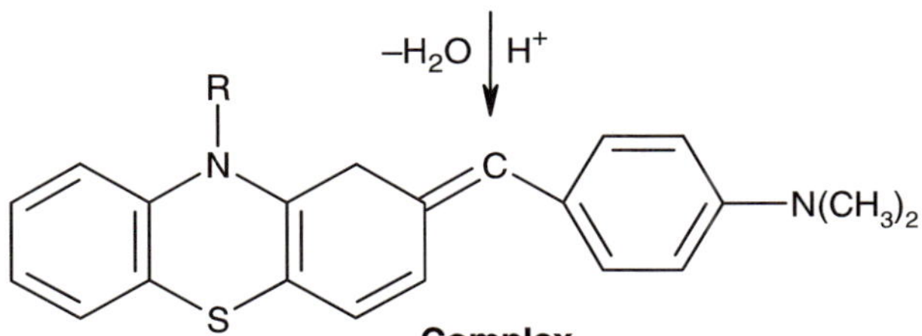

Complex
(λ_{max} 520 nm)

References

1. T.P. Gandhi, M.R. Patel, A.A. Patel, V.C. Patel & R.N. Gilbert, *Ind. J. Pharm.*, July 1979, p. 1.
2. G.N. Singh, V.P. Singh & R.P. Gupta, *Ind. J. Pharm. Sci.*, May-June 1984, pp. 124-126.
3. Pharmaceutical Chemistry (Vol. 2) by H.J. Roth, pp. 694-698.

Note

Different electrophilic groups as substituents at C-2 are H, Cl^-, CF_3, OCH_3, SCH_3 and CN.

A spectrofluorometric method has been reported by Fardous et al. This involves oxidation of the molecule by cerric (IV) ammonium sulphate (CAS) in acidic medium. The oxidized molecule exhibits strong fluorescence (Exc. 254 nm; Em. 355 nm) which can be utilized for quantitative analysis.

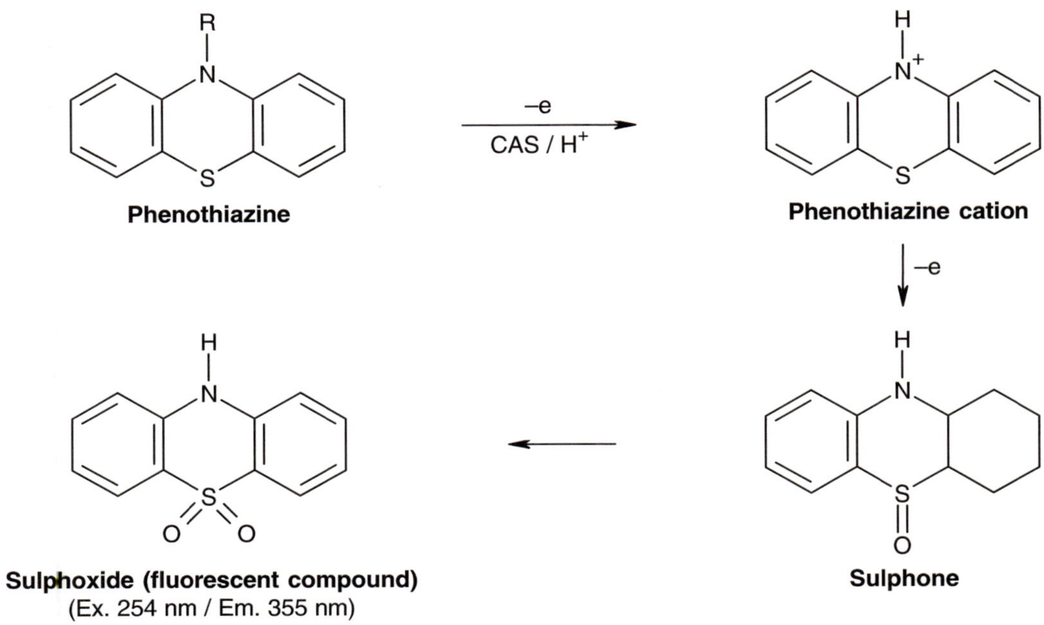

Reference

Fardous A. Mohamed, H.A. Mohamed, Samila A. Hussein, Smeh A. Ahmed, *J. Pharm. Biomed. Anal.*, **39**, 139-146, 2005.

METHOD 3

Reagents

1. 0.01% N-bromosuccinimide (NBS) in water.
2. 0.1% ortho-toluidine (OTD) in methanol.
3. 6 M ammonia solution.
4. 0.1 M hydrochloric acid.

Standard solution

1 mg/ml of promethazine hydrochloride in water. Further dilutions made to get 100 μg/ml.

Sample solution

Powdered sample equivalent to 70 mg of the drug suspended in water, shake for 10 min, filter and dilute to 100 ml with water. The samples of elixirs (10 ml) are made alkaline (litmus) with 6 M ammonia, extract with 3 × 15 ml chloroform, evaporate organic layer and take up the residue in 0.1 M HCl to get 200 μg/ml.

Procedure

To 1 ml each of sample and standard solutions, add 4 ml of NBS solution, 3 ml of OTD solution, dilute to 20 ml with water. Add 10 ml of chloroform, shake well, collect chloroform layer, pass through anhydrous sodium sulphate and measure the absorbance of red colour at 516 nm.

Probable Reaction Mechanism

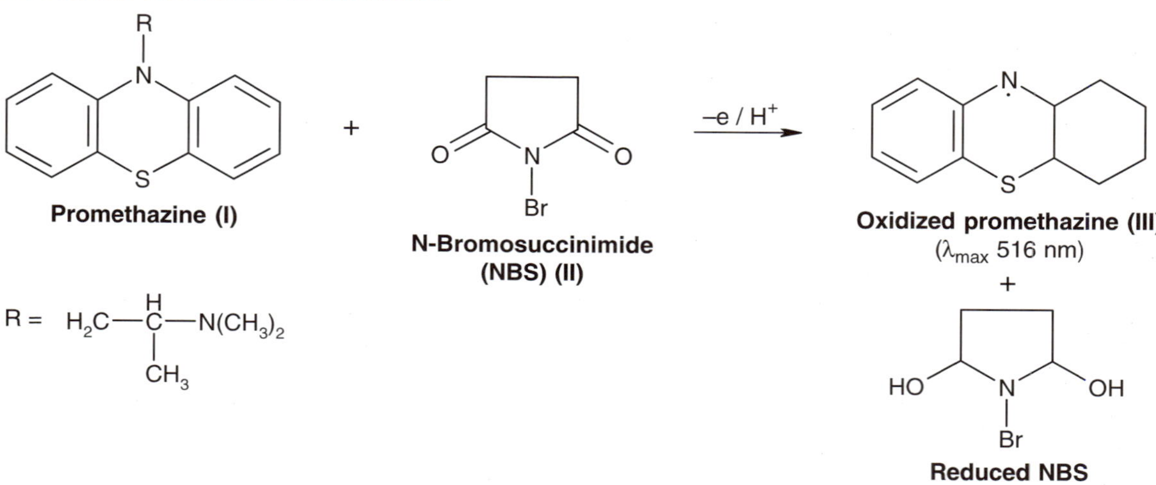

NBS oxidizes promethazine eliminating the side chain giving an unstable red-coloured complex (III) and itself gets reduced. On addition of 'OTD' a stable intense green colour is produced (λ_{max} 580 nm). However, the colour intensity decreases when the coloured complex is extracted into chloroform and a stable red-coloured product (λ_{max} 516 nm) is obtained.

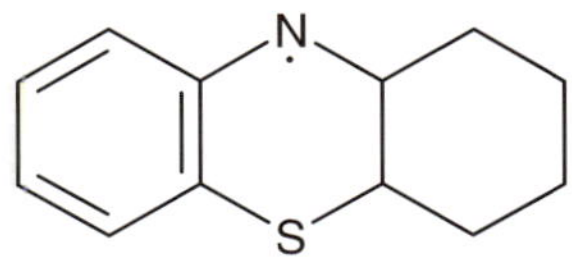

Oxidized promethazine

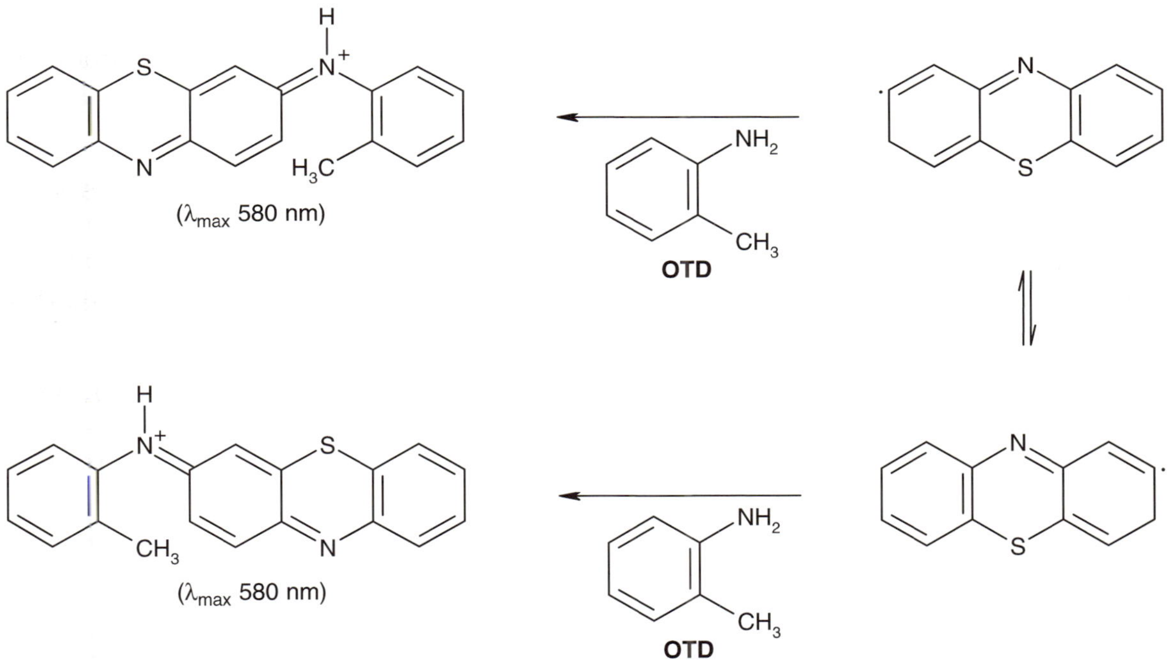

Reference

K.C. Ramesh, B.G. Gowda & J. Keshavayya, *Ind. J. Pharm. Sci.*, **65(4)**, 432-435, 2003.

Taha et al. (1983) had earlier reported spectrophotometric method for promethazine and some other phenothiazine using N-bromosuccinimide (NBS) in strong sulphuric acid. It was reported that NBS oxidizes the phenothiazine to yield stable pink or violet-coloured semiquinonoid radical by oxidizing the phenothiazine. The following reaction mechanism was proposed by the author:

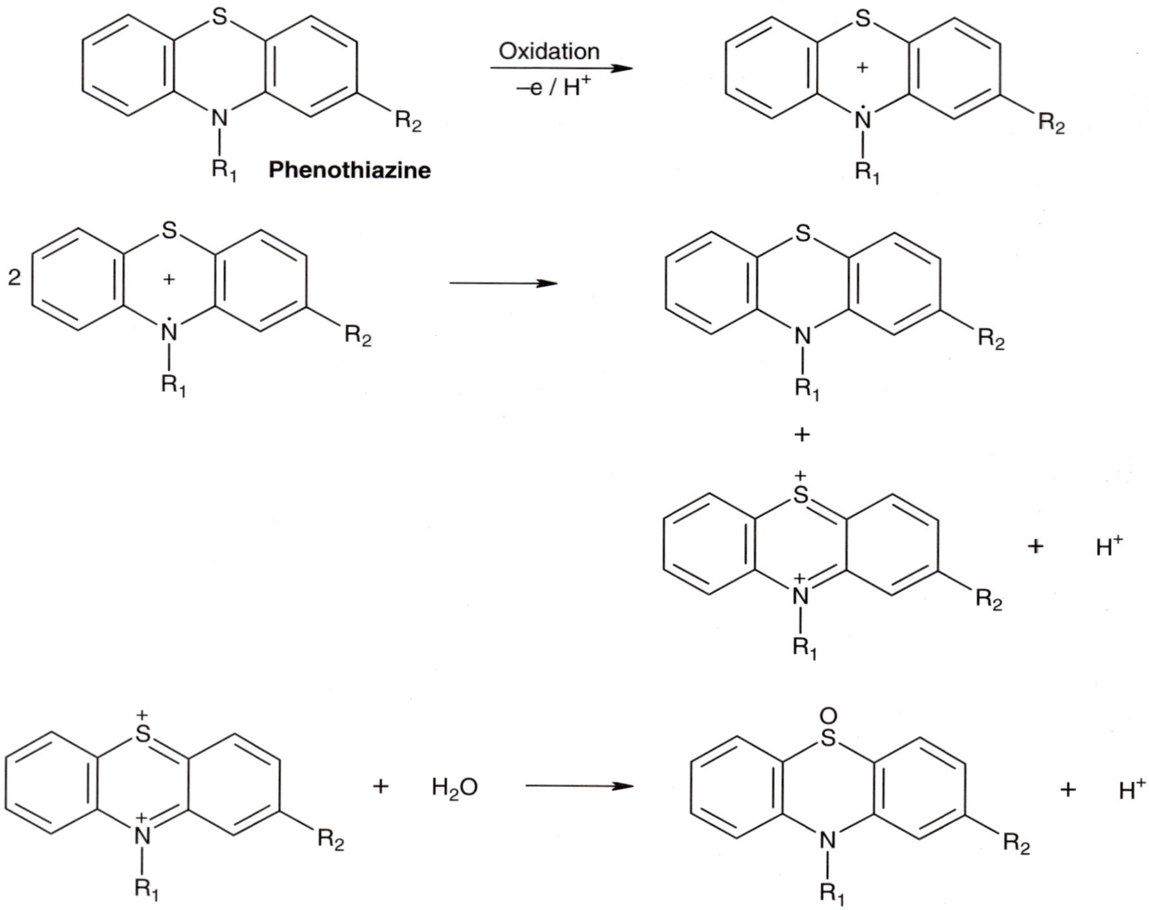

Reference

Aly M. Taha, Nawal A. El-Rabbat & Michael E. El-Kommos, *Analyst*, **108**, 1500-1505, 1983.

METHOD 4 (Promethazine hydrochloride and Promethazine theoclate)

Reagents

Formaldehyde - sulphuric acid reagent (Marquis reagent).

Standard solution

100 μg/ml of promethazine in 0.1 M hydrochloric acid.

Sample solution

Powdered sample equivalent to 10 mg of the drug suspended in water, shake and finally dilute with 0.1 M HCl.

Procedure

To 2 ml each of sample and standard solutions, add 0.2 ml of formaldehyde solution (40%), followed by 4 ml of conc. H_2SO_4, cool in ice-cold water, dilute to 10 ml with water and measure the absorbance at 550 nm and calculate the results.

Note

λ_{max} for hydrochloride salt is 520 nm.

Probable Reaction Mechanism

The method is based on Marquis reaction. The molar ratio of promethazine and HCHO is 2 : 1. Aromatic ring present in the molecule is attacked by HCHO resulting in condensation reaction between the two compounds.

Now sulphuric acid acts as an oxidizing agent resulting in the formation of quinoid phenothiazin-3-one which is the coloured product.

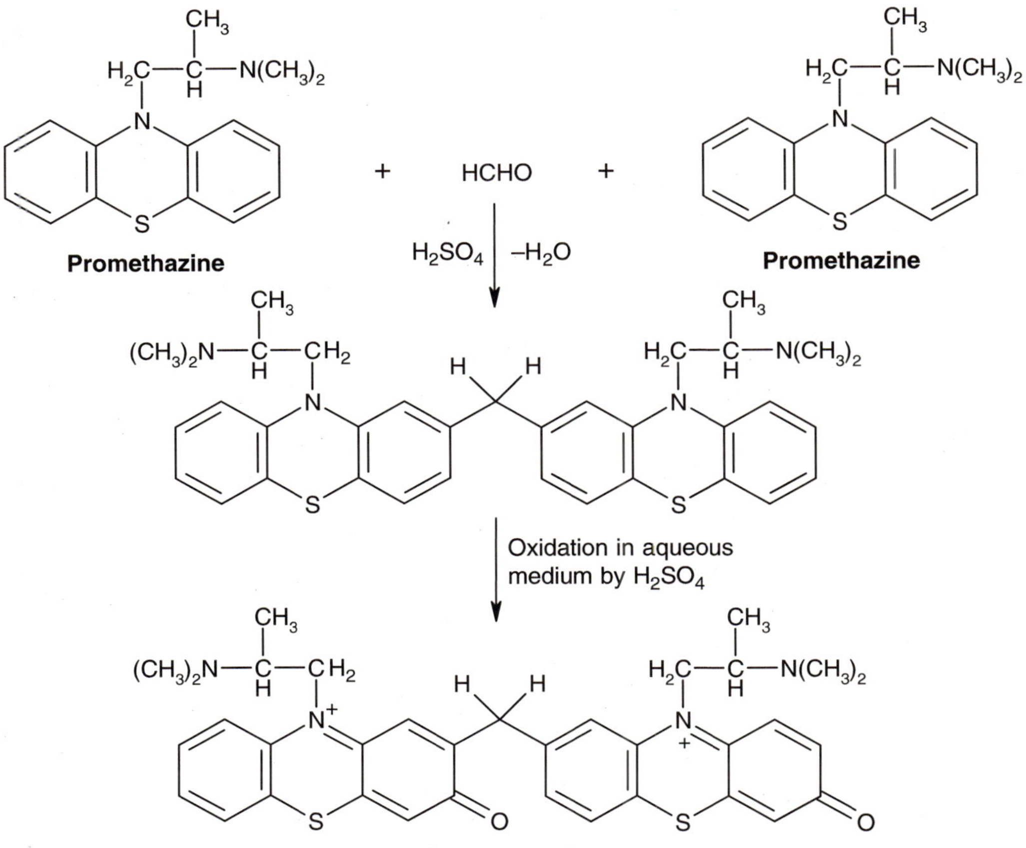

(λ_{max} 520 nm)

Reference

S.S. Zarapakar, Kishor R. Athalye, *Indian Drugs*, **26(1)**, 32-36, 1989.

METHOD 5

Reagents

1. 10% w/v solution of sodium nitrite in water.
2. Conc. hydrochloric acid.
3. Conc. sulphuric acid.
4. Sulphuric acid (1 :1) in water.

Sample and standard solutions

100 μg/ml in water.

Procedure

To 0.75 ml each of sample and standard solutions, add to each 1 ml of methanol, 0.5 ml of sodium nitrite solution and 1.5 ml of conc. HCl. Shake and then add slowly and with shaking 1.5 ml of conc. sulphuric acid, allow to stand at room temperature for 5 min and measure the absorbance at 565 nm against reagent blank.

Probable Reaction Mechanism

$$NaNO_2 + HCl \longrightarrow HCl + NaNO_2$$

Nitrous acid

$$NaNO_2 + HCl \longrightarrow \overset{+}{N}{=}O + HCl + NaNO_2$$

Nitrosonium ion

Nitrosonium ion being electron deficit will attack C-2 being electrophilic (other electrophilic groups are Cl^-, CF_3, OCH_3, CN, etc.) and will result in the formation of nitroso derivative. In the presence of conc. H_2SO_4, being an oxidizing agent, promethazine is oxidized to nitrosoquinoid structure which has violet colour (λ_{max} 565 nm).

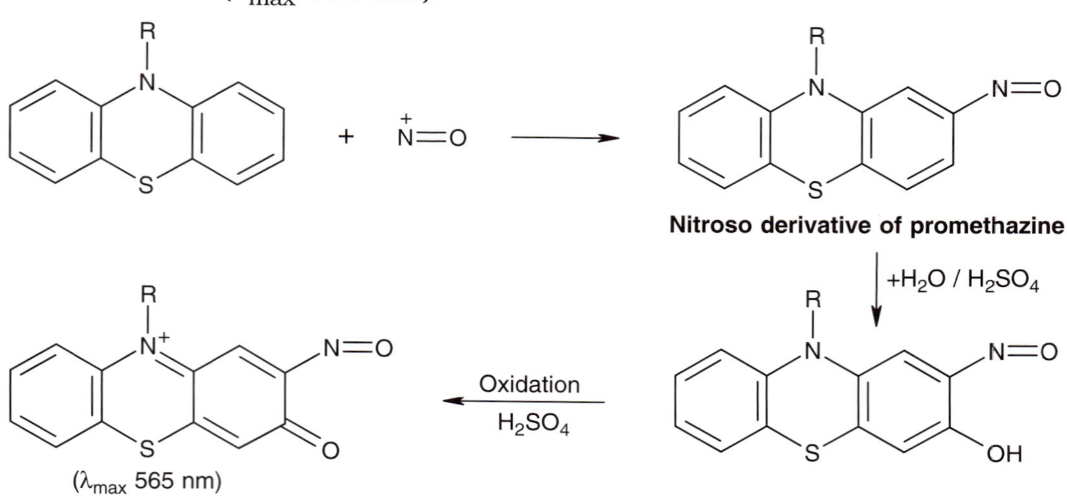

METHOD 6

This method is based on formation of ion-pair complex (salt).

Reagents

1. 0.5% solution of brilliant blue and orange-II in water.
2. 0.1 M hydrochloric acid.

Sample and standard solutions

100 μg/ml in water.

Procedure

(a) To 1 ml each of sample and standard solutions, add 1 ml of dye solution (brilliant blue), dilute to 10 ml with water. To each, add 15 ml of chloroform, shake for 2 min, separate chloroform layer, pass through anhydrous sodium sulphate and measure the absorbance at 620 nm against reagent blank.

(b) To 5 ml each of sample and standard solutions, add 2 ml each of 0.1 M HCl and orange-II, dilute to 10 ml with water and proceed further as under procedure (a). Measure the absorbance at 495 nm against reagent blank.

Probable Reaction Mechanism

Method (a)

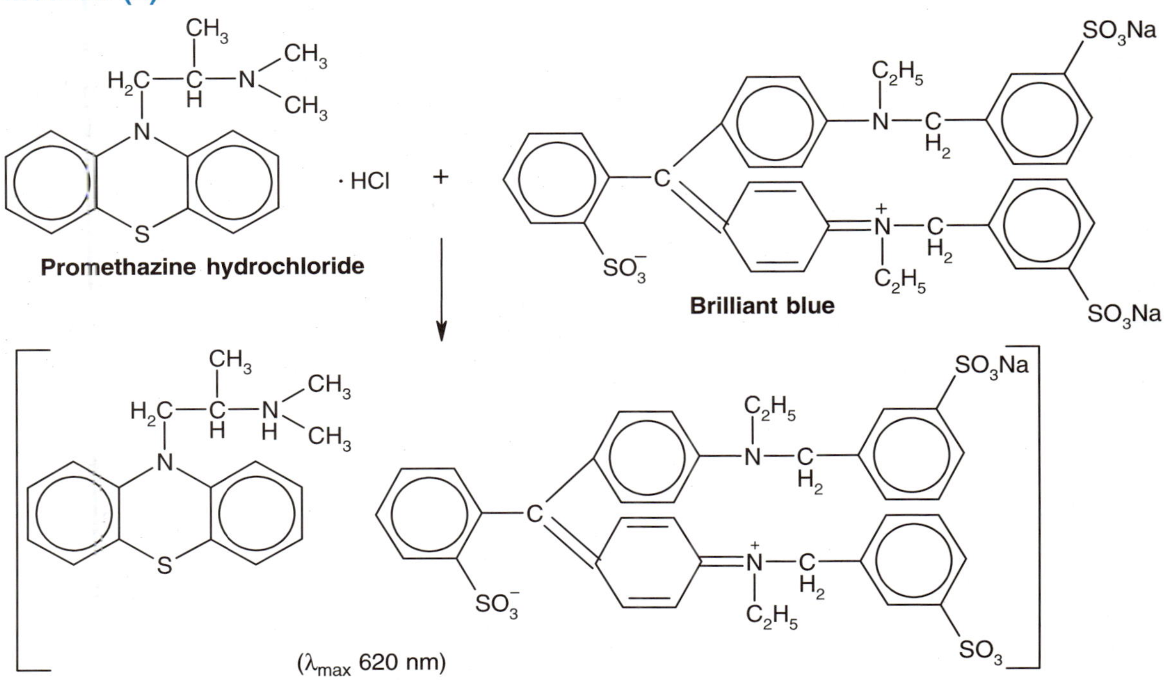

Drug-dye complex + NaCl

Method (b)

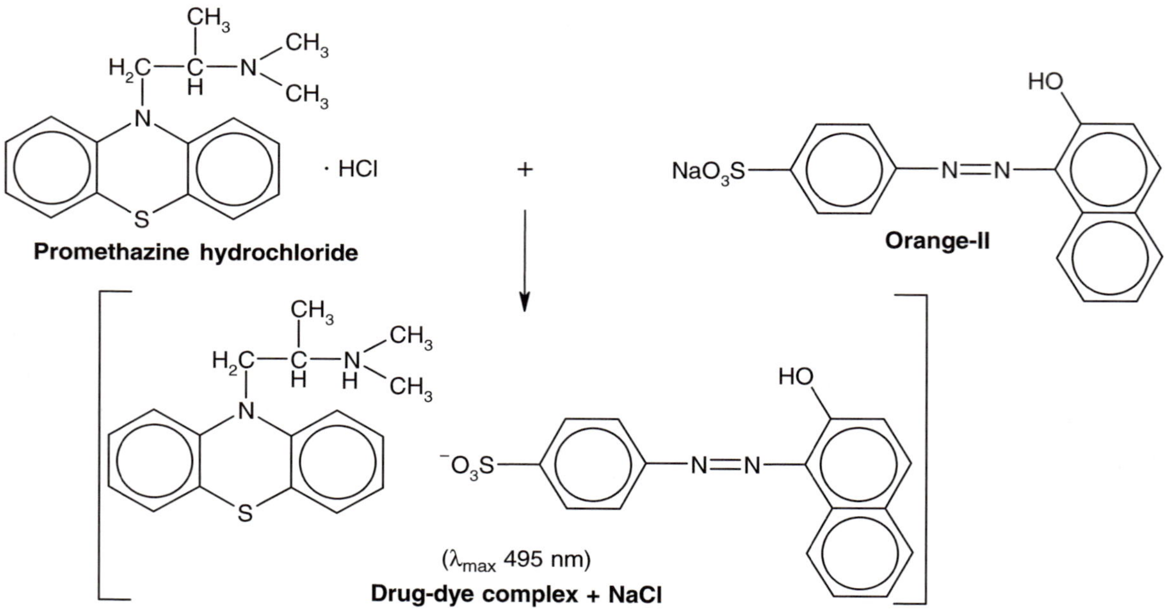

Structure of brilliant blue and orange-II and their respective complexes with promethazine hydrochloride

Note

Chlorpromazine, prochlorperazine, thioridazine, trifluoperazine, trimeperazine, fluophenazine and phenothiazine derivatives form ion-pair complexes.

Reference

S.L. Bhongade & A.V. Kasture, *Talanta*, **40(10)**, 1525-1528, 1993.

Probable Reaction Mechanism

The tertiary 'N' atom present in the side chain of the drug forms a complex with $Co(SCN)_6$ resulting in the formation of the product.

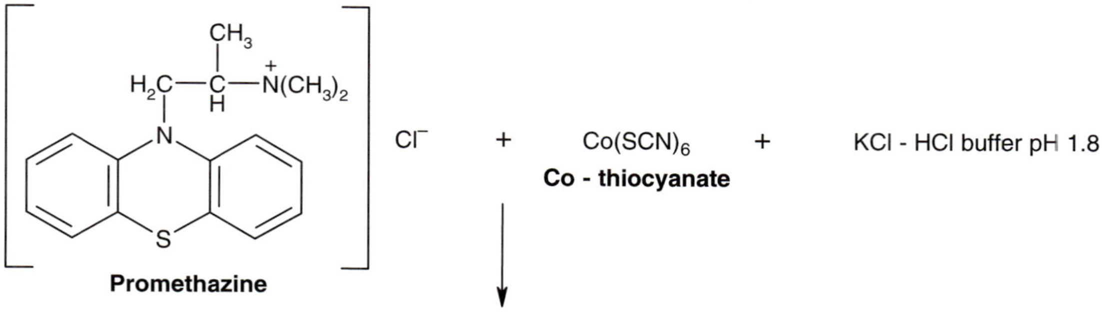

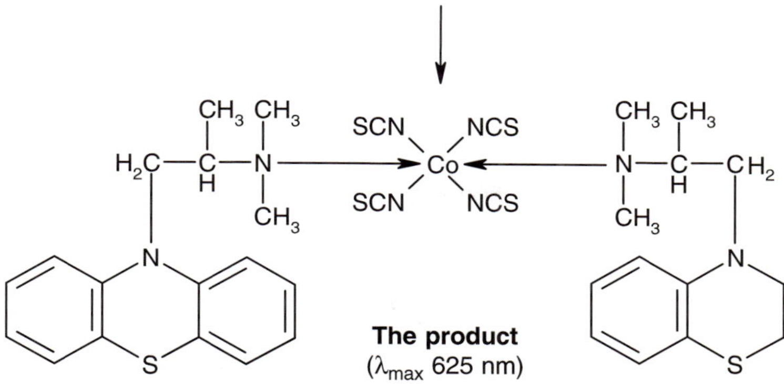

The product
(λ_{max} 625 nm)

Since there is high electron density at 'S', it is oxidized easily. Thus, on treatment with oxidizing agent such as $FeCl_3$ in the presence of HCl, intense red-coloured product is formed. This reaction can be used for analysis of the drug in formulation.

Probable Reaction Mechanism

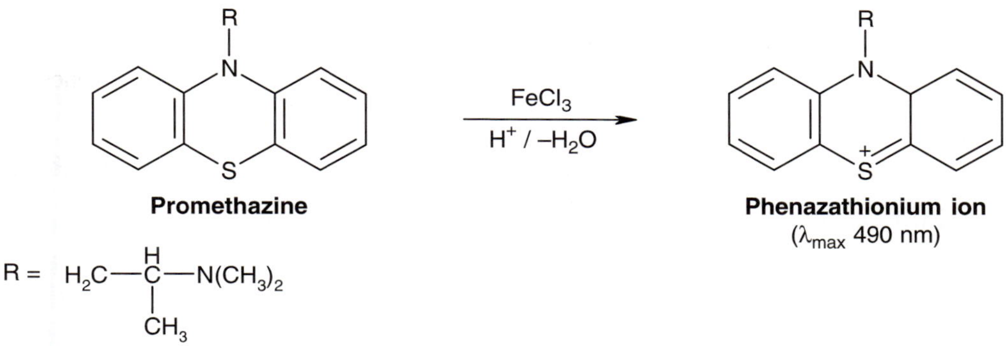

Reference

M.K. Youseff & I.A. Attia, *Ind. J. Pharm.*, **37**, 121, 1975.

Formulation 14

Aspirin, Dipyridamole

ESTIMATION

Aspirin

METHOD 1

Follow the method described in formulation 5 of this chapter.

METHOD 2

Standard solution

20 mcg/ml of aspirin in 0.1 N sulphuric acid. Solution is prepared by heating in boiling water-bath.

Sample solution

Weigh accurately powdered sample equivalent to 100 mg of aspirin, suspend in 60-70 ml of 0.1 N sulphuric acid. Heat in a boiling water-bath, cool and make the volume to 100 ml with 0.1 N sulphuric acid. Dilute further to get solution of 20 mcg/ml. Measure the absorbance of both sample and standard solutions at about 229 nm using 0.1 N sulphuric acid as blank and calculate the results by comparison.

Dipyridamole

Standard solution

15 mcg/ml of dipyridamole in 0.1 N sulphuric acid.

Sample solution

Weigh accurately equivalent to 75 mg of dipyridamole, suspend in about 150 ml of 0.1 N sulphuric acid. Shake for 10 min and make up the volume to 250 ml with 0.1 N sulphuric acid. Further dilutions are appropriately done with 0.1 N sulphuric acid to get final dilution of 15 mcg/ml. Measure the absorbance of both sample and standard solutions at about 285 nm using 0.1 N sulphuric acid as blank and calculate the results by comparison.

Formulation 15

Ibuprofen, Paracetamol, Chlorzoxazone

ESTIMATION

Paracetamol

Follow the method described in formulation 2 of this chapter.

Ibuprofen

Follow the method described in formulation 12 of this chapter.

A.K. Sanyal et al. have described spectrophotometric method based on measurement of iodine released by ibuprofen from iodide - iodate mixture. The measurement was done at 352 nm.

Probable Reaction Mechanism

The drug being propionic acid derivative liberates iodine from KI - KIO_3 mixture through hydrogen ion mediated reaction by virtue of free carboxyl group.

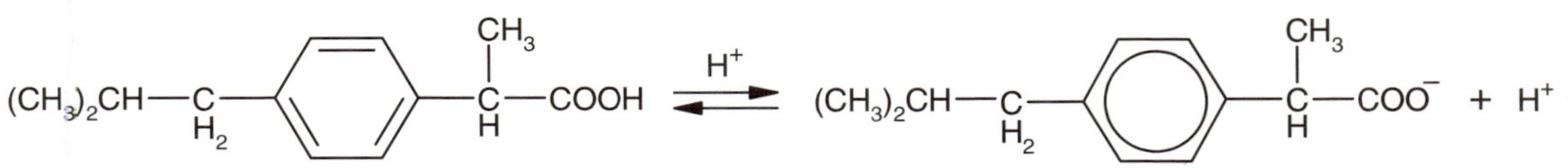

Ibuprofen

$$IO_3 + 5I^- + 6H^+ \longrightarrow 3I_2 + H_2O$$

Reference

A.K. Sanyal & Dinabandhu Laha, *JAOAC*, **77(5)**, 1108, 1994.

Chlorzoxazone

Standard solution

20 mcg/ml of chlorzoxazone in methanol.

Sample solution

Suspend accurately weighed quantity of powdered sample equivalent to 50 mg of the substance in slightly warm water. Cool and extract with diethyl ether (4 × 20 ml). Combined ethereal layer is washed twice with water (2 × 20 ml) and passed through a bed of anhydrous sodium sulphate. Organic layer is evaporated to dryness and residue taken up in methanol to produce a working solution of 20 mcg/ml for analysis. Measure the absorbance of both the solutions at about 282 nm and calculate the results by comparison.

Note

The compound shows λ_{max} 282 nm (methanol) and λ_{max} 289 nm (NaOH).

Reference

Analytical Profile of Drug Substances (Vol. 16) by Klaus Florey, p. 140, 1987.

The compound has intrinsic (native) fluorescence, its chloroform solution. exc: 286 nm; em: 310 nm; no interference from paracetamol. This property has been used for analysis of formulations.

Reference

J.T. Stewart & C.W. Chan, J. Pharm. Sci., **68**, 910-912, 1979.

The compound reacts with dansyl chloride, fluorescamine, 2,4-dihydroxy-benzaldehyde and salicylaldehyde to form fluorophores (exc: 370 nm; em: 505 nm).

Alternatively, chlorzoxazone on alkaline hydrolysis yields o-amino derivative which gives fluorophore moiety with fluorogenic reagent.

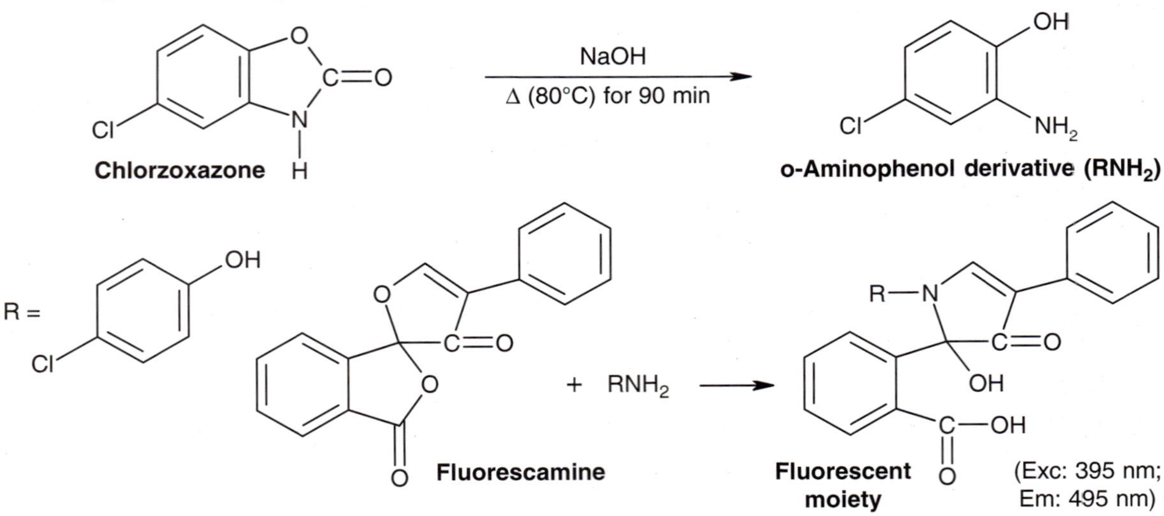

OR

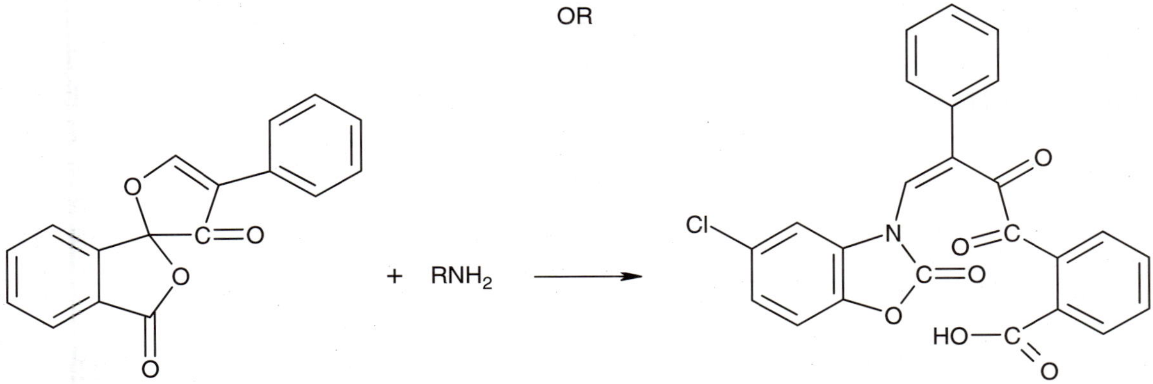

Fluorescamine

Fluorescent moiety
(Exc: 370 nm; Em: 505 nm)

Primary amines, secondary amines and phenolic hydroxyls are dansylated to yield fluorescent moiety. However, tertiary amines and alkyl hydroxyls are not dansylated.

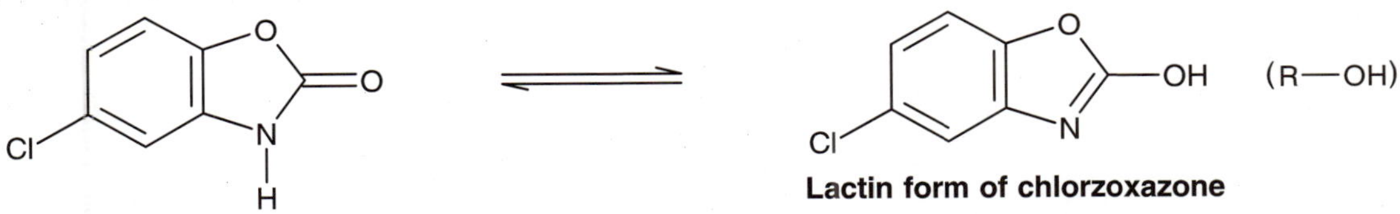

Chlorzoxazone

Lactin form of chlorzoxazone

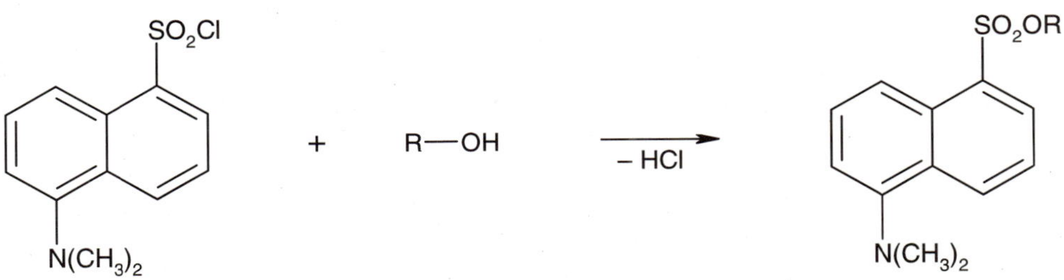

Dansyl chloride
(1-dimethylaminonaphthalene-5-sulphonic acid chloride)

Fluorescent moiety
(Extractable into benzene)
(Exc: 350 nm; Em: 500 nm)

Reference

J.T. Stewart & Che.W. Chan, Analytical Letters, **B-11(9)**, 667-680, 1978.

After hydrolysis, yielding primary (—NH_2) aromatic compound, shall condense with 'PDAB', Folin's reagent and shall undergo diazotization as well.

Formulation 16

Paracetamol, Serratiopeptidase

Since paracetamol gives positive test with Folin's reagent and being the larger component of the formulation, it interferes in the assay of the enzyme. The method involves extraction of the sample with acetone whereby the enzyme being composed of polypeptide is precipitated whereas paracetamol is extracted into acetone.

Extraction procedure

Weigh finely powdered sample equivalent to 25 mg of the enzyme, place on G_4 sintered funnel, add 15 ml of acetone, stir with glass rod, filter under slight vacuum, repeat the procedure further with 2 × 15 ml acetone, collect acetone layer, make it up to 100 ml with acetone and use for assay of paracetamol; follow any one of the methods reported in the book. To dissolve the residue left on the funnel, add 10 ml of warm (40°C) water, stir, filter under vacuum, repeat with further 2 × 5 ml water, collect water layer, make up to 25 ml with water to get 1 mg/ml. Further dilute with water to get 200 μg/ml and read at 230 nm and compare with the standard. Or, to 1 ml each of sample and standard solutions (1 mg/ml) add 5 ml of Fehling's solution. After 10 min measure the absorbance at 620 nm.

Fehling's solution: Prepared by mixing 1 ml each of solution (A) and (B) and diluting to 25 ml with water.

or

Reagents

All reagents to be freshly prepared.

1. Borate buffer, pH 9.0: Dissolve 9.5 g of borax in 450 ml of water, adjust the pH to 9.0 with 1 M HCl, dilute to 500 ml with water.
2. Trichloric acid solution: Dissolve 1.8 g in 3 g of sodium acetate and 2 ml of glacial acetic acid, dilute to 100 ml with water.
3. Folin's reagent: Prepared by diluting the reagent with water (1 : 2).
4. 5% ammonium sulphate solution in water.
5. 6% sodium carbonate solution in water.

Preparation of substrate

Dissolve 1.2 g of casein (Hammerstein grade) in 100 ml of borate buffer, pH 9.0, keep in boiling water-bath for 1-2 min to get clear solution, filter through cotton plug and dilute to 200 ml with borate buffer, pH 9.0.

Standard solution

15 μg/ml of tyrosine in water.

Standard enzyme solution

100 mg —(5% ammonium sulphate solution)→ 100 ml

100 ml ↓ 1 ml

1 ml —(Borate buffer, pH 9.0)→ 200 ml

Enzyme sample solution

Suspend powdered sample in 75 ml of ammonium sulphate solution, shake and keep for 5 min, dilute to 100 ml with borate buffer. Further dilute 1 ml to 200 ml with borate buffer and use for assay.

Procedure

	Standard	Test	Standard blank	Sample blank
Standard/sample	1 ml	1 ml	1 ml	1 ml
Casein solution	5 ml	5 ml	×	×
TCA reagent	×	×	5 ml	5 ml

Shake and keep for 20 min at 37°C and then proceed.

	Standard	Test	Standard blank	Sample blank
TCA reagent	5 ml	5 ml	×	×
Casein solution	×	×	5 ml	5 ml

Shake and keep for 30 min at 37°C, cool and filter through Whatman filter paper No. 42 and proceed for estimation as under.

	Standard	Test	Standard blank	Sample blank
Standard/test	2 ml	2 ml	2 ml	2 ml
Sodium carbonate solution	5 ml	5 ml	5 ml	5 ml
Folin's reagent	1 ml	1 ml	1 ml	1 ml

Shake and keep for 30 min at 37°C and measure the absorbance at 660 nm.

Note

TCA solution is added to remove the substrate to avoid further action of the enzyme on the substrate.

Formulation 17

Paracetamol, Dicyclomine hydrochloride, Activated Dimethicone

ESTIMATION

Paracetamol

Follow the method described in formulation 2 of this chapter.

Dicyclomine hydrochloride

Reagent

Picric acid solution: 20 mg of picric acid and 2.90 g of sodium acetate anhydrous are dissolved in 70-80 ml of water, add 4 ml of glacial acetic acid and dilute to 100 ml with water.

Standard solution

20 mcg/ml of dicyclomine hydrochloride in 0.1 M hydrochloric acid.

Sample solution

Accurately weighed quantity of powdered sample is extracted with 0.1 M hydrochloric acid to get a final concentration of 20 mcg/ml in respect of dicyclomine hydrochloride.

Procedure

To 20 ml each of sample and standard solutions add 5 ml of picric acid solution, shake and extract with chloroform (2 × 10 ml) passing each extract through bed of anhydrous sodium sulphate. Make up the volume to 25 ml and measure the absorbance of both the solutions at 405 nm against reagent blank and calculate the results by comparison.

Alternatively, follow the method described in formulation 21 of this chapter. Being tertiary nitrogen compound, it forms complex with Co(II).

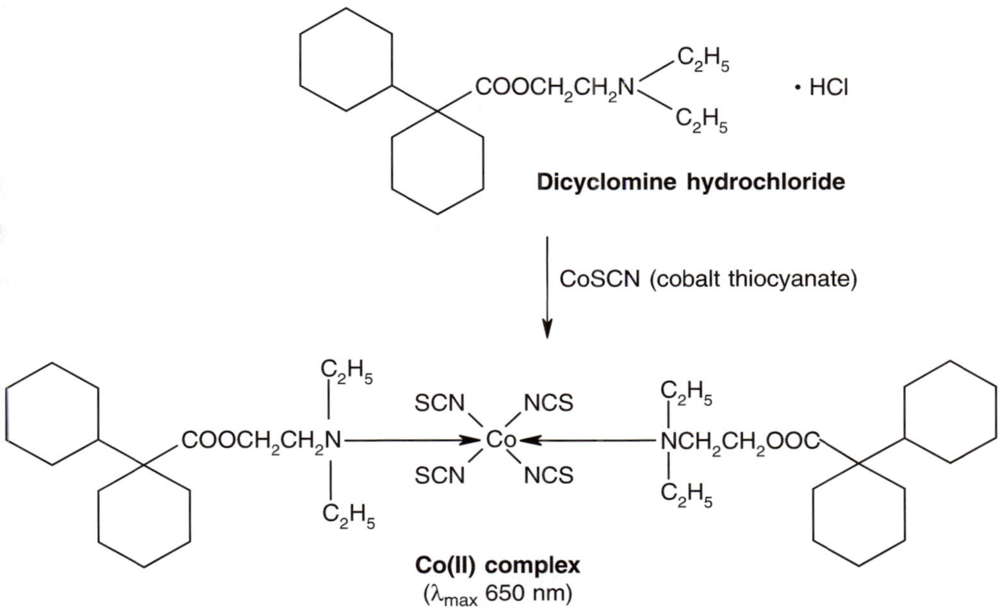

Reference

D.M. Shingbal & Uday G. Barad, Indian Drugs, **22(11)**, 609-610, 1985.

Activated Dimethicone (Dimethylpolysiloxane) (DMP)

Weigh sample equivalent to 40 mg of the DMP, add 15 ml of concentrated hydrochloric acid. Digest on water-bath for 15 min till all the foam has disintegrated and emulsifying action has been destroyed. Extract the contents with four 40 ml portions of chloroform–ether (2 : 6) mixture. Wash the pooled organic layer with three 15 ml portions of 1 N sodium hydroxide followed by 3 × 15 ml of water. Pass the organic layer through cotton plug and evaporate to dryness at 150°C for 45 min. Cool and weigh. The weight of the residue obtained represents the amount of DMP present in the sample initially taken for analysis.

Note

Washing with sodium hydroxide removes parabens; this step can be omitted if parabens are absent.

Formulation 18

Mefenamic acid, Dicyclomine hydrochloride

ESTIMATION

Mefenamic acid

Weigh accurately powdered sample equivalent to 250 mg of mefenamic acid, suspend in 50-60 ml water and shake for 5 min and filter through G_3 glass sintered funnel, discard the filtrate. Wash the residue with water, rejecting the filtrate. Dissolve the residue in 100 ml of methanol (phenol red) and titrate with 0.1 M sodium hydroxide. Each ml of 0.1 M sodium hydroxide is equivalent to 0.02413 g of mefenamic acid.

Sodium lauryl sulphate (SLS) acts as titrant for quaternary and tertiary amines. These amines form slightly dissociated salt with 'SLS' on acid side.

Reference

K. Marcali, Analytical Chem., **27**, 1586, 1955.

Explanatory Note

Mefenamic acid, being insoluble in water, remains as residue which is dissolved in warm methanol and the carboxylic group present in the molecule is titrated with sodium hydroxide.

Mefenamic acid also forms nitroso derivative. Nitrosonium ion attacks at secondary amine group of the compound resulting in the formation of nitroso derivative.

$$2NaNO_2 + H_2SO_4 \longrightarrow Na_2SO_4 + 2HNO_2$$

$$HNO_2 \xrightarrow{H^+} \overset{+}{N}{=}O \xrightarrow{Cl^-} H_2O + Cl^- \; N{=}O$$

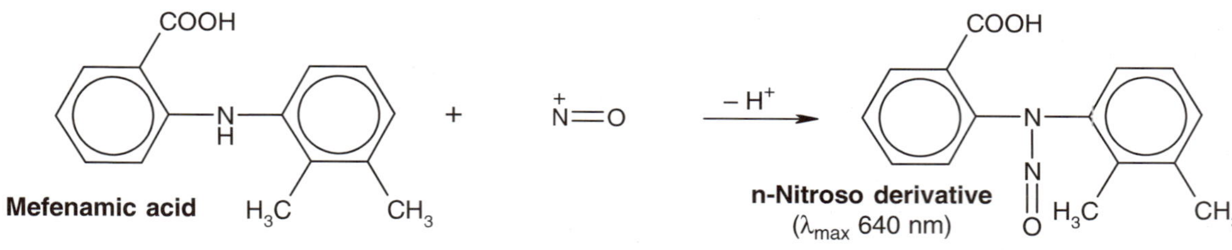

Reference

Textbook of Practical Organic Chemistry by Vogel, p. 920; Indian Drugs, **22(12)**, 653, 1986.

Alternatively, as the ring containing 2 methyl is richer in electrons due to the presence of 2 methyl group, it can be attacked by nitro to give nitro derivative.

$$KNO_3 + HCl \longrightarrow NO_2^{\oplus}$$

Nitronium ion

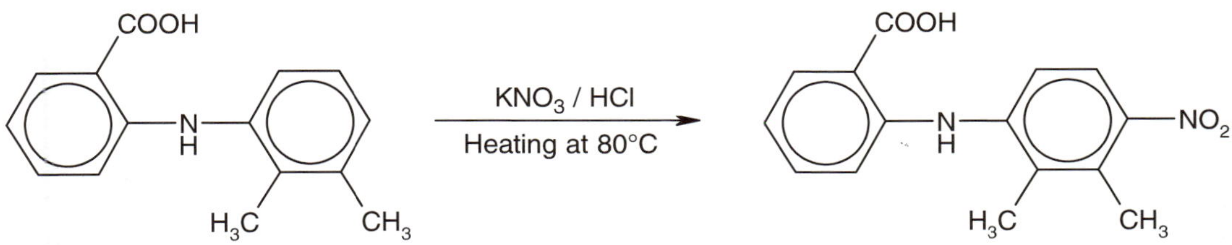

Nitro derivative
(λ_{max} 360 nm)

Mefenamic acid has strong absorption at 350 nm with high molar absorptivity but has poor solubility in most of the organic solvents. 1,4-dioxane, being good solvent for the drug, was used for spectrophotometric assay by Mathai et al. (G. Mathai, J.T. Moolayil, K.B. Jose & V.S. Sebastian. *Ind. J. Pharm. Sci.*, **72(4)**, 525-526, 2010).

Mefenamic acid, an N-phenylanthranilic acid derivative, has native fluorescence in organic solvents. This property has been utilized for quantitative estimation of the compound. The compound showed fluorescence only in organic solvent with low dielectric constant such as dioxan.

Note

1. Other anthranilic acid derivatives such as flufenamic acid and meclofenamic acid also have similar native fluorescence. The excitation/ emission wavelengths (nm) are:

Mefenamic acid	Dioxan	350/440 nm
	Chloroform	365/460 nm
Flufenamic acid	Dioxan	334/410 nm
	Chloroform	340/410 nm
Meclofenamic acid	Dioxan	334/390 nm
	Chloroform	340/406 nm

2. Their solution in water, 0.1 M NaOH, 0.1 M H_2SO_4 and 95% ethanol did not show fluorescence.

Reference

1. Anil C. Mehta & Stephen G. Schulman, Talanta, **30**, 702-703, 1973.
2. Advance Organic Chemistry by Jerry March, pp. 468, 469.

A spectrophotometric method has been described by several authors. Secondary aromatic amine $\left(R-\underset{H}{\underset{|}{N}}-R \right)$ present in the molecule condenses with 'PDAB' in acidic medium to yield coloured complex.

Reagents

1. 3% w/v solution of p-dimethylaminobenzaldehyde (PDAB) in methanol.
2. Conc. H_2SO_4.

Standard and sample solutions

1 mg/ml in methanol.

Procedure

To 2 ml each of sample and standard solutions, add 2 ml of 'PDAB' reagent and 0.6 ml of conc. H_2SO_4, heat at 90°C for 90 sec in water-bath, cool, dilute to 10 ml with methanol and measure the absorbance of both the sample and standard solutions at 590 nm against reagent blank and calculate the results.

Probable Reaction Mechanism

The compound reacts with 'PDAB' to give imminium salt.

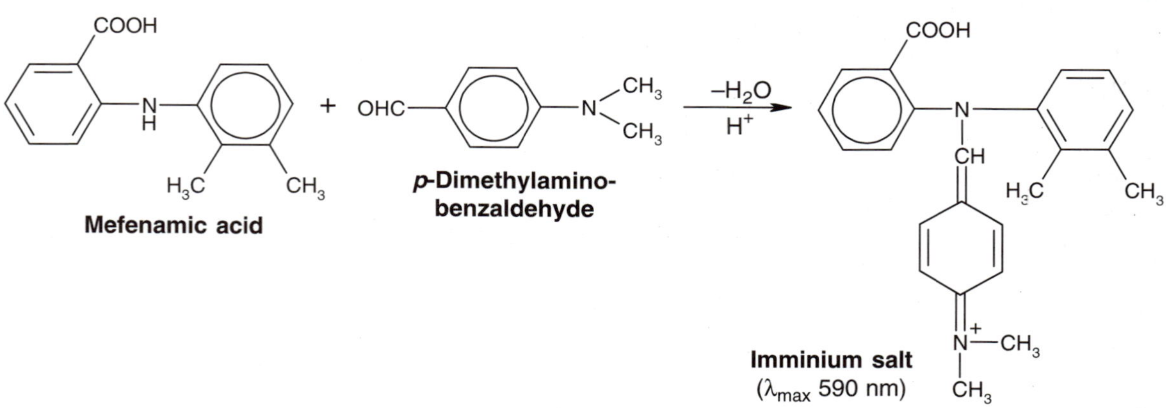

Reference

1. Tehseen A., Kazi A.A. & B. Maken, *Analytical Letters*, **38**, 1899-1912, 2005.
2. Z.A. El-Sherif et al., *Analytical Letters*, **30(10)**, 1881-1886, 1997.
3. N.H. Zawilla et al., *J. Pharm. Biomed. Analysis*, **27**, 243-251, 2002.

It has been reported that mefenamic acid reacts with 4-aminophenazone in the presence of oxidizing agent in weakly alkaline medium to give coloured chromogen (λ_{max} 590 nm).

Probable Reaction Mechanism

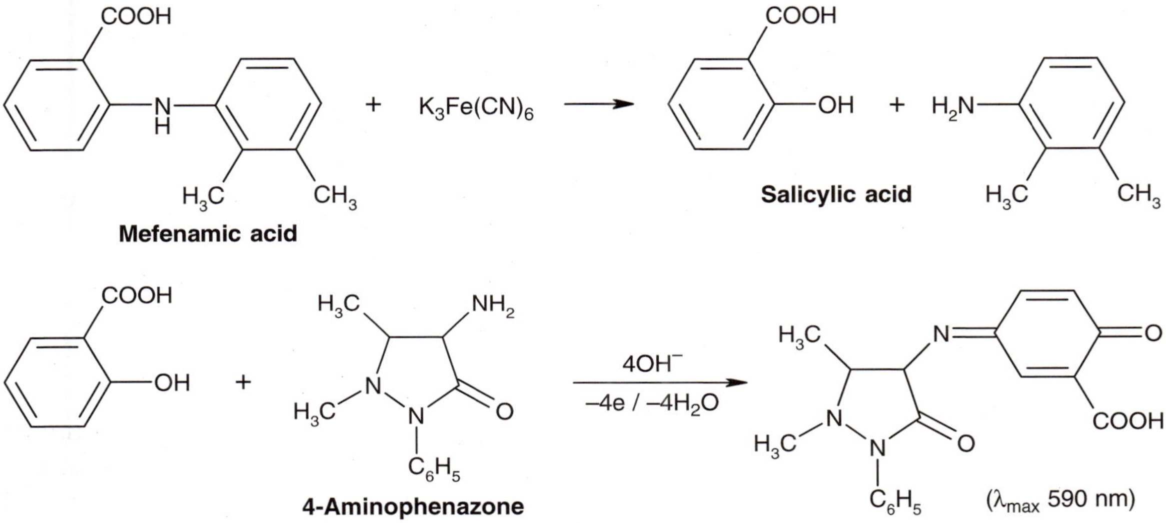

Idowu, S.O. et al. (2002) had reported use of 4-amino-3,5-dinitrobenzoic acid as coupling reagent with mefenamic acid after oxidation with $K_3Fe(CN)_6$ (for reaction mechanism, see above).

Reference

1. S. Khanna Babu et al., *Eastern Pharmacist*, p. 129, 1995.
2. S.O. Idowu, S.C. Tambo & A.O. Adegoke, *Trop. J. Pharm. Res.*, 1, 15-22, 2002.

Mefenamic acid is oxidized by ferric chloride to give salicylic acid. Fe(II) ion so formed complexes with potassium ferricyanide to give prussian blue colour (λ_{max} 730 nm) → Barton's reaction.

Probable Reaction Mechanism

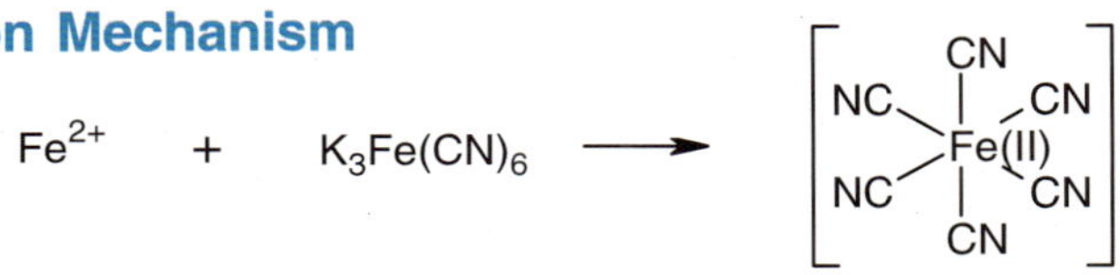

Blue colour
(λ_{max} 730 nm)

Reference

M.M. Langade, Analytical Chemistry, An Indian Journal (ACAIJ), **8(4)**, 2009.

The compound undergoes oxidative coupling with MBTH reagent in the presence of oxidizing reagent.

Probable Reaction Mechanism

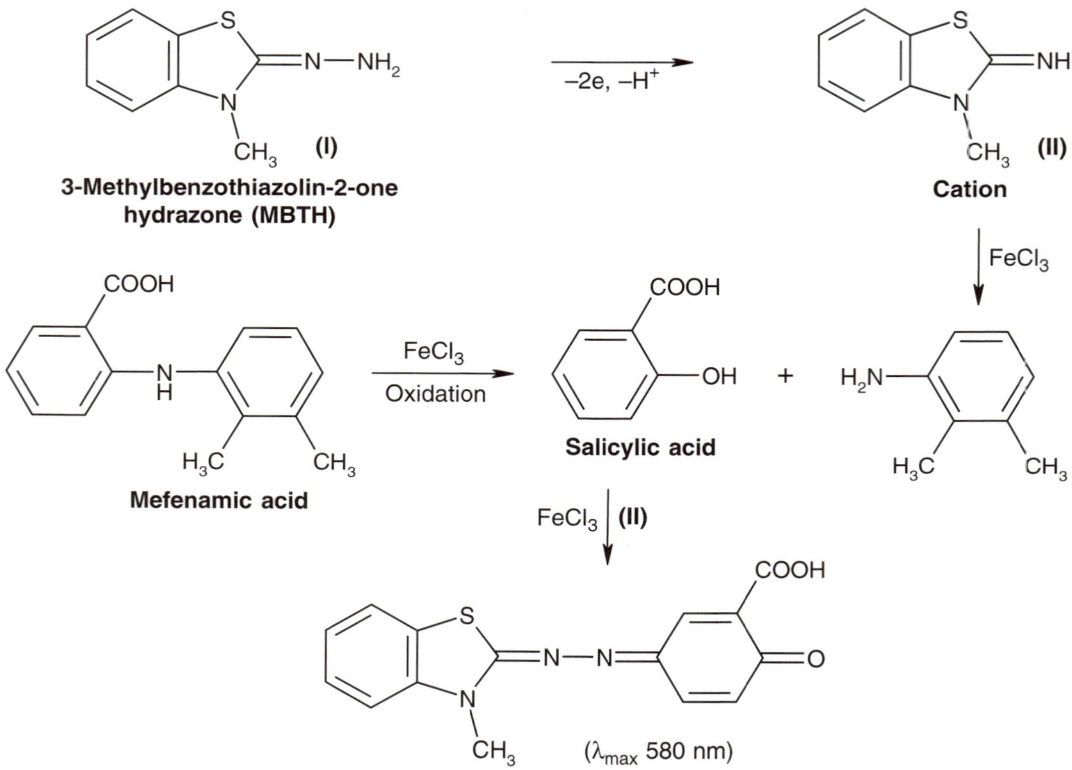

Reference

Indian Drugs, **24(6)**, 30, 1987.

Dicyclomine hydrochloride

Suspend accurately weighed quantity of finely powdered sample equivalent to about 10 mg of dicyclomine hydrochloride in 40-50 ml of water. Shake for 5-10 min, add 10 ml of 1 N sulphuric acid and 1 ml of potassium permanganate solution (0.1%). Allow the mixture to stand for 2 min, add 0.1 ml of dimethyl yellow solution (indicator) and 25 ml of chloroform. Shake and titrate with 0.004 M sodium lauryl sulphate to permanent pink colour in chloroform layer. Each ml of 0.004 M sodium lauryl sulphate is equivalent to 0.001384 g of dicyclomine hydrochloride.

Formulation 19

Aspirin, Chlorpheniramine maleate, Salicylamide

ESTIMATION

Aspirin

Extract accurately weighed quantity of the powdered sample equivalent to 500 mg of aspirin with neutral acetone and titrate with 0.1 N sodium hydroxide using phenolphthalein solution as indicator. Each ml of 0.1 N sodium hydroxide is equivalent to 0.018016 g of aspirin. For estimation of free salicylic acid in the formulation, follow the method given in formulation 1 of this chapter.

Chlorpheniramine maleate

Follow the cyanogen bromide method as described in formulation 1 of the chapter on rubefacients.

Salicylamide

Reagents

1. 0.1% w/v solution of 2,6-dichloroquinone chlorimide in isopropyl alcohol (DCQ) (Gibbs' reagent).
2. Buffer solution, pH 9.2.
3. Isopropyl alcohol : water (1 : 1) v/v mixture.

Standard solution

50 mcg/ml of salicylamide in alcohol–water solvent mixture.

Sample solution

Weigh accurately powdered tablets equivalent to 50 mg of salicylamide and extract with isopropyl alcohol–water mixture to make 100 ml. Dilute appropriately with the same solvent to get 50 mcg/ml solution.

Procedure

To 2 ml each of standard and sample solutions add 2 ml of buffer solution, pH 9.2, 5 ml of isopropyl alcohol and 1 ml of chlorimide reagent. Shake for 1 minute and allow to stand for 30 minutes. Measure the absorbance of both the solutions at about 650 nm and calculate the results by comparison.

Probable Reaction Mechanism

This is based on oxidative coupling; DCQ acts as oxidizing agent in alkaline medium.

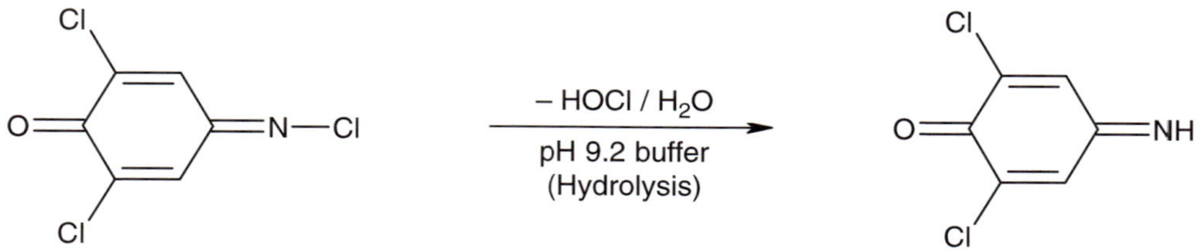

2,6-dichloroquinone chlorimide (I) **Active species (II)**

Buffer solution of pH 9.2 causes hydrolysis of the reagent. The hydrolysed reagent acts as an oxidizing agent and attacks at the free para position to the phenolic —OH to give indophenol dye. This reaction is answered by phenolic compounds with free para position.

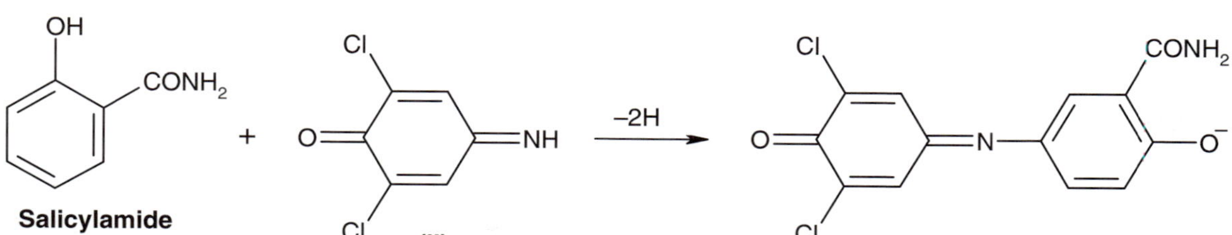

Salicylamide

(II)
Hydrolysed reagent
2,6-Dichloroquinonimine

Indophenol dye
(λ_{max} 650 nm)

It is a typical reaction of phenols. Since p-position is free in salicylamide, the coupling takes place at position para to the phenolic function. 2,6-dibromo derivative can be substituted for dichloro derivative. In this reaction, hydrolysis of I → II is essential for reaction to proceed and this is quickest at pH around 9.0.

Salicylamide also couples with 'MBTH' at free para position giving a red dye.

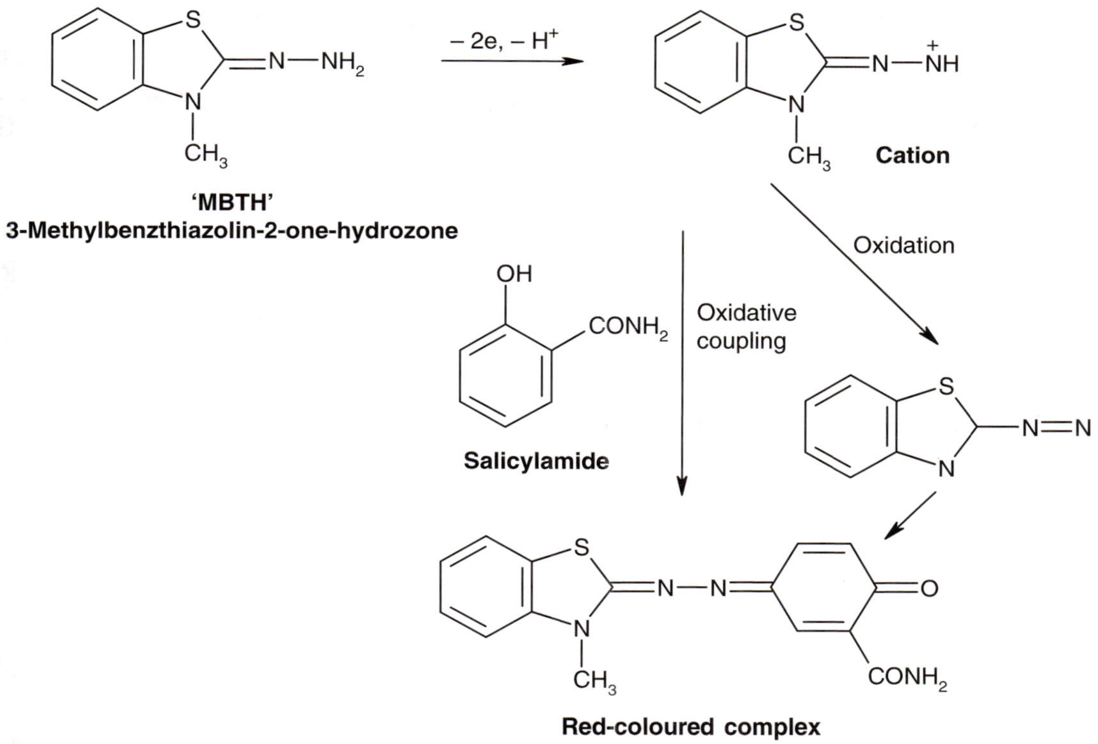

Salicylamide also undergoes Emerson reaction i.e. oxidative coupling with 4-aminoantipyrin.

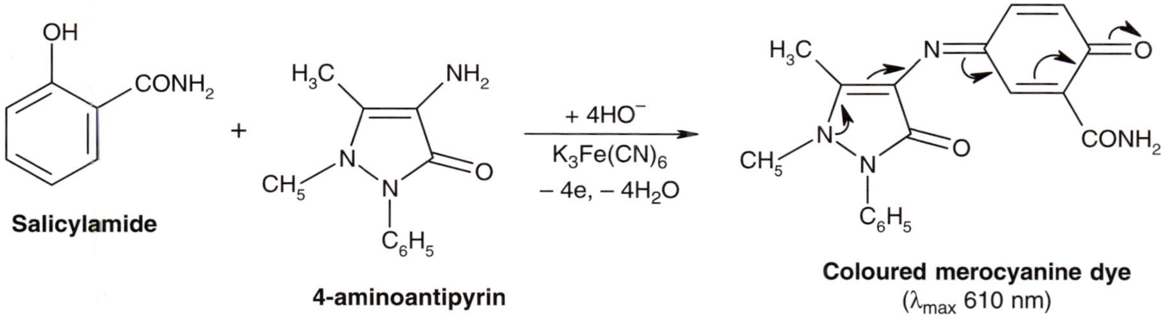

Note

Salicylic acid does not interfere since phenolate formation is masked by a strong hydrogen bridge bonding.

Reference

Pharmaceutical Chemistry (Vol. 2) by H.J. Roth, p. 267.

Like salicylic acid, salicylamide forms complex with Fe(III).

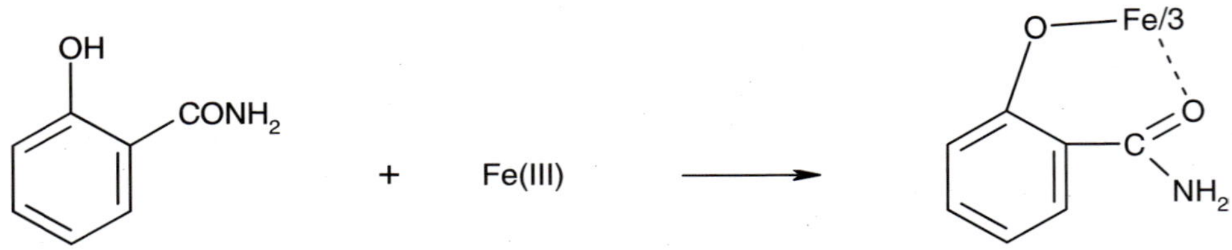

Salicylamide **Violet-red coloured complex**
(λ_{max} 505 nm)

Salicylamide forms chelate with boric acid in the presence of acetic anhydride and sulphuric acid. Boron chelate has fluorescent properties (exc: 328 nm; exe: 388 nm).

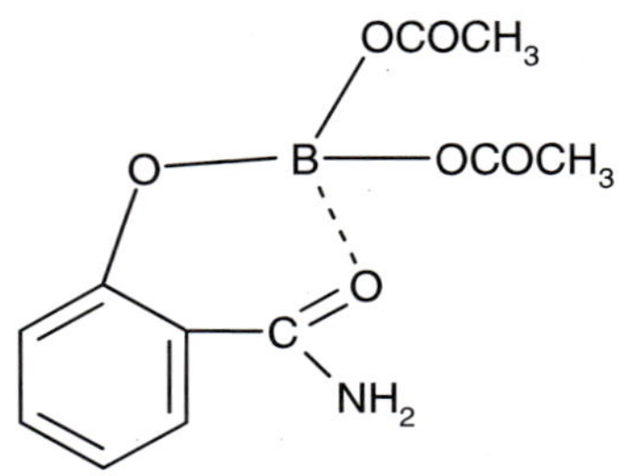

Salicylamide - boron fluorescent chelate

Formulation 20

Dextropropoxyphene napsylate, Paracetamol, Diazepam

ESTIMATION

Dextropropoxyphene napsylate

METHOD 1

Weigh accurately a quantity of powdered tablets equivalent to about 500 mg of dextropropoxyphene napsylate, add 10 ml of water and 3 ml of 10% w/v solution of sodium hydroxide. Extract with four 30 ml portions of chloroform. Wash combined chloroform extract with water till washings are free from alkali. Pass organic layer through anhydrous sodium sulphate and titrate with N/10 perchloric acid using crystal violet solution as indicator (change of colour from violet to blue). Each ml of N/10 perchloric acid is equivalent to 56.58 mg of dextropropoxyphene napsylate.

METHOD 2

Reagents

1. Buffer solution, pH 4: To 50 ml of 0.2 M potassium hydrogen phthalate add 0.1 ml of 0.2 N hydrochloric acid and dilute to 200 ml with water. Check and adjust the pH to 4.0.
2. Bromocresol green solution: 0.01% w/v solution of the dye in water. Glasswares should be thoroughly washed with water before preparing the dye solution.

Standard solution

20 mcg/ml of dextropropoxyphene napsylate.

Sample solution

Extract accurately weighed quantity of the sample equivalent to 20 mg of dextropropoxyphene with water to make 100 ml. Dilute further with water to get 20 mcg/ml solution.

Procedure

To 10 ml of sample and standard solutions add 5 ml of pH 4.0 buffer solution and 2.5 ml of the dye solution. Mix and extract with two 10 ml portions of chloroform and dilute organic layer to 25 ml with chloroform. Measure the absorbance of both the solutions at about 420 nm using chloroform as blank.

METHOD 3

In acidic medium, the compound forms chelate with cobalt thiocyanate (CoSCN) which can be extracted into benzene (λ_{max} 620 nm).

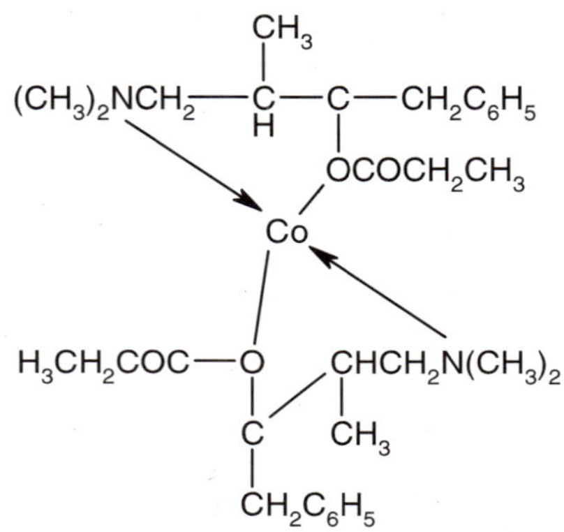

OR

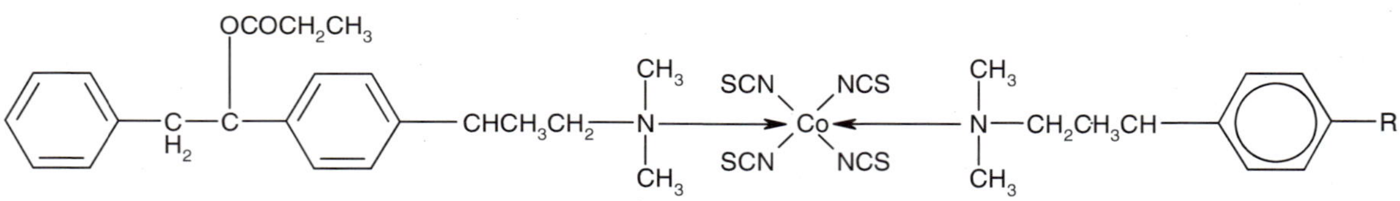

(λ_{max} 620 nm)

Paracetamol

METHOD 1

Add an accurately weighed quantity of the powdered sample equivalent to about 0.15 g of paracetamol to 50 ml of 0.1 M sodium hydroxide taken in a 200 ml volumetric flask. Add 100 ml of water, shake for 15 minutes and add sufficient water to produce 200 ml. Mix, filter and dilute 10 ml of the filtrate to 100 ml with water. Add 10 ml of the resulting solution to 10 ml of 0.1 M sodium hydroxide and dilute to 100 ml with water. Measure the extinction of the resulting solution at 257 nm and calculate the results taking 715 as value of E 1%, 1 cm.

METHOD 2

This method is based on bathochromic shift from 249 nm to 460 nm as a result of alkaline hydrolysis.

Reagent

10% w/v solution of sodium hydroxide in water.

Standard solution

100 mg of paracetamol is dissolved in methanol to get 100 ml (1 mg/ml).

Sample solution

1 mg/ml of the compound in methyl alcohol.

Procedure

To 1 ml of sample and standard solutions add 1 ml of sodium hydroxide solution and keep in boiling water-bath for 15 minutes. Remove and add immediately 1.5 ml of water and mix. Allow to stand for 60 minutes and dilute to 5 ml with water. Measure the absorbance at maximum about 460 nm using reagent blank.

Note

Aspirin, caffeine, oxyphenbutazone and phenobarbitone do not interfere.

Explanatory Note

On treatment with NaOH, due to the excitation of the proton attached to oxygen, a quinoid-like structure is formed which is responsible for the bathochromic shift in absorption λ_{max} (460 nm).

Probable Reaction Mechanism

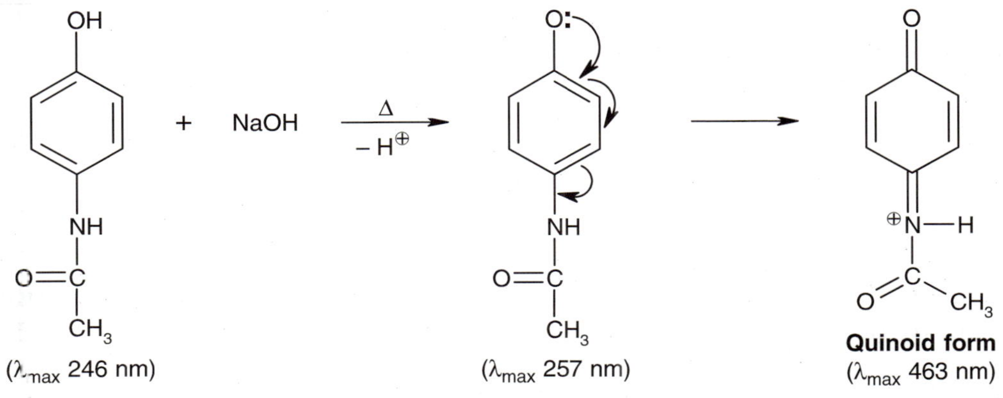

Reference

R.T. Sane & S.S. Kamal, J. Ass. Off. Anal. Chem., **63(6)**, 1189-1190, 1980.

Note

Other oxidizing agents can be used to give similar products.

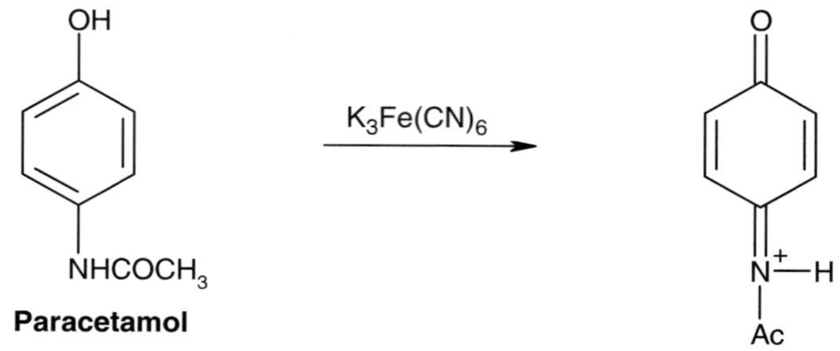

Reference

K.K. Verma, A.K. Gulati, S. Palod & P. Tyagi, Analyst, **109(6)**, 735-737, 1984.

Diazepam

Reagents

1. Acidified methanol: 3% sulphuric acid in methanol.
2. Phosphate buffer, pH 7.0.
3. Anaesthetic ether.
4. 10% w/v solution of sodium hydroxide in water.

Standard solution

50 mg of diazepam is dissolved in acidified methanol to get 40 mcg/ml solution.

Sample solution

Weigh accurately a quantity of powdered tablets equivalent to 2 mg of diazepam, add 20 ml of buffer solution, pH 7.0 and extract with four 30 ml portions of ether. The combined ether layer is washed with 10 ml of sodium hydroxide solution and then with water to get free of alkali. Pass through sodium sulphate, anhydrous. Evaporate ether layer and dry at 105°C. Cool and take up the residue in acidified methanol to get 50 ml (40 mcg/ml).

Procedure

Measure the absorbance of yellow colour of standard and sample solutions at maximum at about 368 nm and compare the results.

Probable Reaction Mechanism

In strong alkali, the anion is formed which is extracted into ether (λ_{max} 368 nm).

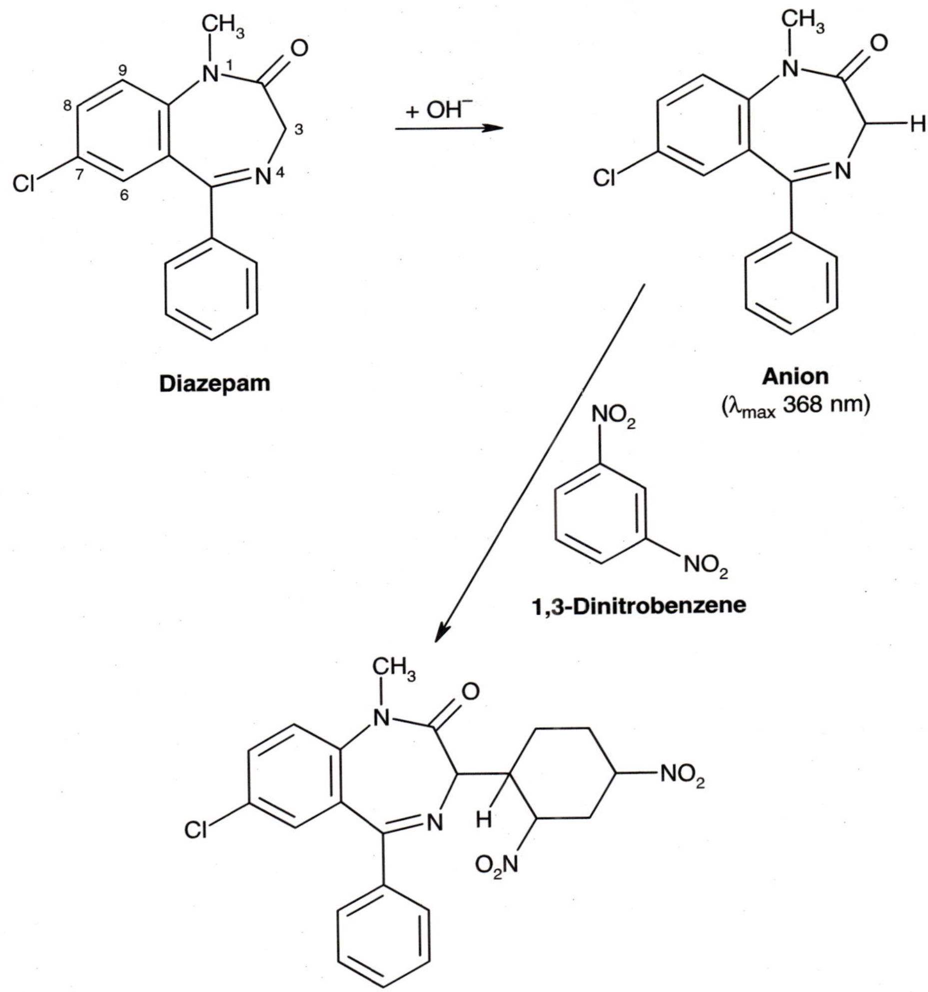

Reference

1. Vinay Nevrekar, *Indian Drugs*, **21(5)**, 219, 1984.
2. Pharmaceutical Chemistry (Vol. 2) by H.J. Roth, 1991, p. 667.

Formulation 21

Paracetamol, Dicyclomine hydrochloride, Phenylisopropyl pyrazolone, Ethylmorphine hydrochloride

ESTIMATION

Paracetamol

Carry out the nitroso-derivative method described in formulation 2 of this chapter or the method described in formulation 2 of this chapter.

Dicyclomine hydrochloride

Follow the method described in formulation 11 of this chapter.

Phenylisopropyl pyrazolone / Isopropyl antipyrine / Isopropyl phenazone

Follow the method described in formulation 10 of the chapter on anti-inflammatory drugs.

Ethylmorphine hydrochloride

Reagents

1. Dilute sulphuric acid (75% v/v).
2. 1 N sodium hydroxide.
3. 1.0% w/v solution of p-dimethylaminobenzaldehyde (PDAB) in 75% v/v sulphuric acid.

Standard solution

80 mcg/ml of ethylmorphine hydrochloride in dilute sulphuric acid.

Sample solution

Measure appropriate quantity of the sample equivalent to 5 mg of the compound. Saturate the solution with sodium chloride and make alkaline with 1 N sodium hydroxide. Extract the alkaline solution with five 40 ml portions of chloroform. Wash the combined chloroform layers with 10 ml of sodium chloride solution.

Dry chloroform extract over anhydrous sodium sulphate and evaporate to 25 ml. To 10 ml of the above solution, add 5 ml of dilute sulphuric acid and evaporate on water-bath till the smell of chloroform is not perceptible. Dilute to 25 ml with dilute sulphuric acid.

Procedure

To 0.5 ml each of sample and standard solutions add 8 ml of the 'PDAB' reagent, mix and allow the flasks to stand at room temperature for one hour in the dark. Measure the absorption of both solutions at about 450 nm against reagent blank. Results are calculated by comparison.

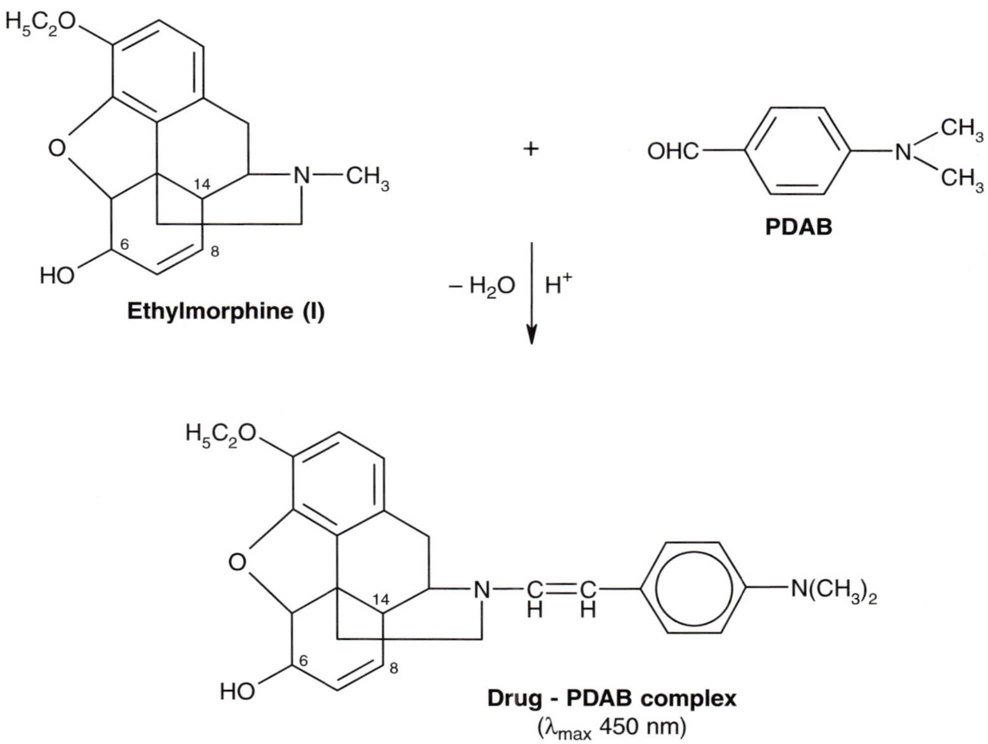

Note

This is similar to the reaction of analgin with 'PDAB'.

Ethylmorphine and codeine form coloured 'C-T' complex with 7,7,8,8-tetracyanoquinone dimethane, a π electron acceptor, using acetonitrile as solvent.

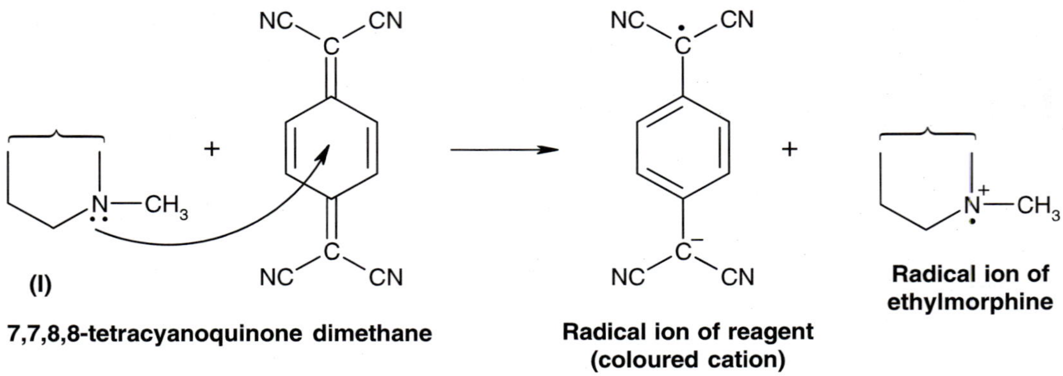

For reaction mechanism, see also under codeine.

Note

Most of the reactions are similar to codeine.

Reference

Pharmaceutical Chemistry (Vol. 2) by H.J. Roth, p. 629.

Formulation 22

Ascorbic acid, Analgin

ESTIMATION

Analgin

METHOD 1

Reagent

1% w/v solution of p-dimethylaminobenzaldehyde in 5% v/v sulphuric acid.

Standard solution

1 mg/ml of analgin in water.

Sample solution

Appropriate weight of the powdered sample is extracted with water to get 1 mg/ml of analgin.

Procedure

To 5 ml each of sample and standard solutions add 5 ml of p-dimethylaminobenzaldehyde reagent. Keep for 5 minutes and make up the volume to 25 ml with water. Measure the absorbance of both the standard and sample solutions at maximum at about 420 nm and calculate the results by comparison.

Analgin undergoes hydrolysis in the presence of sulphuric acid through two different routes. The ease with which the compound undergoes hydrolysis is attributed to the aminomethane sulphonic acid side chain present in the molecule. One of the hydrolytic products reacts with 'PDAB' to give coloured product (λ_{max} 430 nm).

Probable Reaction Mechanism

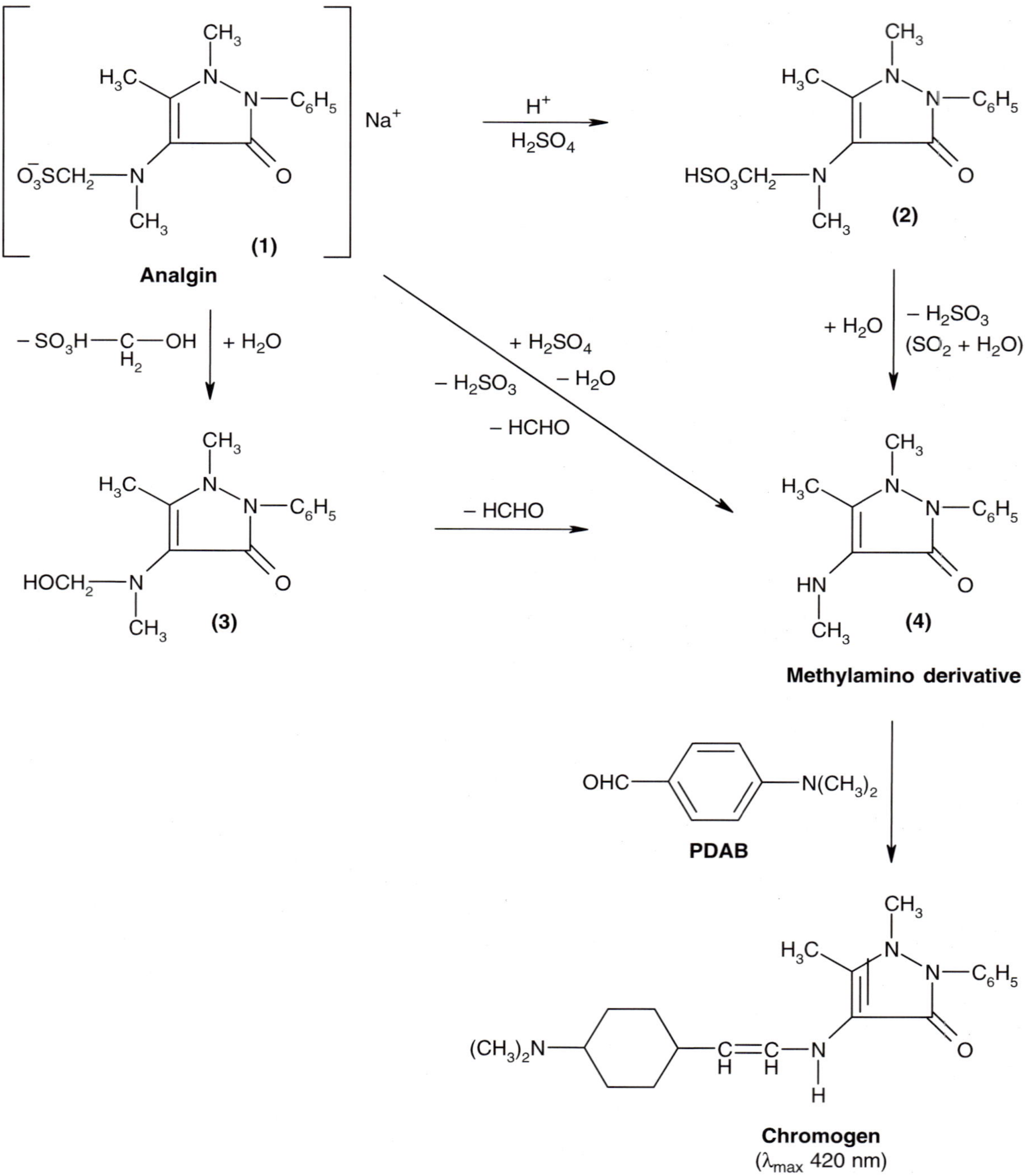

OR

$$(1) \xrightarrow[H^+]{+ H_2O} (4) + HCHO + NaHSO_3$$

METHOD 2

This method is based on charge transfer between the reagent, the electron acceptor and the benzene ring of the drug which is most rich in electrons, so a π-π CT complex is formed.

Reagent

0.2% w/v solution of 7,7,8,8-tetracyanoquinodimethane (TCNQ) in acetone.

Sample and standard solutions

1 mg/ml of the drug in acetone.

Procedure

To 1 ml each of sample and standard solutions add 2 ml of 'TCNQ' reagent, keep at 35°C for 30 min, dilute to 10 ml with acetone and measure the absorbance at 740 nm against reagent blank.

Probable Reaction Mechanism

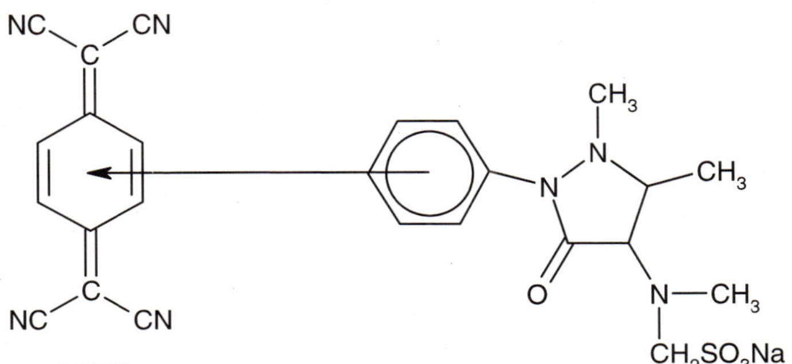

TCNQ

Analgin

TCNQ - Analgin C-T complex
(λ_{max} 740 nm)

Reference

Zhao Feng-Lin, X. U. Bian-Zhen, Zhang Zhi-quan & Tong Shen-Yang, J. Pharm. & Biomed. Analysis, **21**, 355-360, 1999.

While describing the titrimetric determination of analgin, Srivastava et al. (1983) used potassium ferricyanide as titrant and excess titrant estimated indirectly by titrating the liberated iodine from potassium iodide with sodium thiosulphate. The authors suggested the use of zinc sulphate in titration which acts as a catalyst by shortening the reaction time by forming complex with $K_3Fe(CN)_6$ - $K_2Zn_3[Fe(CN)_6]_2$. The method is based on Redox titration. The reaction took about 25 min for completion, i.e. oxidation of methyl (CH_3) group to carboxylic (—COOH) group. One mole of the drug reacted with 6 mols of the reactant $Fe(CN)_6^{-3}$. The following reaction mechanism was proposed by the authors.

Probable Reaction Mechanism

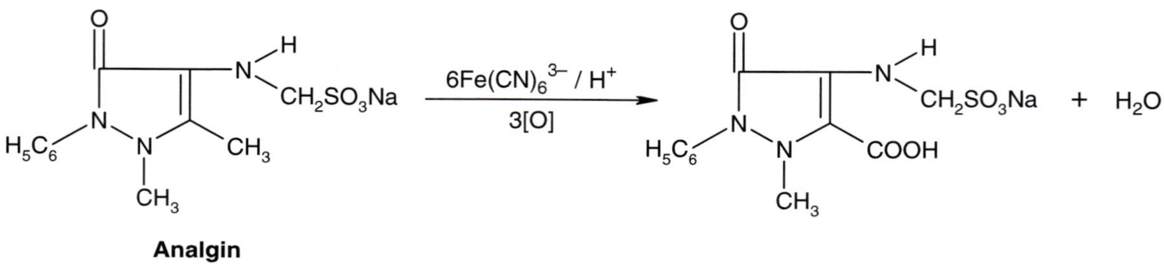

Reference

M.K. Srivastava, Saeed Ahmad, Dhirendra Singh & Ishwar C. Shukla, Analyst, **110(6)**, 735-737, 1985.

Ascorbic acid

Carry out the method involving titration with standard 2,6-dichlorophenol-indophenol solution. For preparation of indophenol solution, refer to formulation 1 of this chapter.

Note

Iodine titration method is not applicable in this formulation as both analgin and ascorbic acid react with iodine.

Formulation 23

Dicyclomine hydrochloride, Paracetamol, Isopropylantipyrin, Chlordiazepoxide

ESTIMATION

Chlordiazepoxide

Reagents

1. Dilute hydrochloric acid.
2. 0.5% hydrochloric acid.
3. 2% w/v solution of p-dimethylaminobenzaldehyde (PDAB) in alcohol.

Standard solution

Weigh accurately 50 mg of chlordiazepoxide, add 25 ml of dilute hydrochloric acid and heat on water bath for 30 minutes; cool, dilute to 50 ml with water. 5 ml of the resulting solution is further diluted to 100 ml with water (50 mcg/ml).

Sample solution

Weigh accurately a quantity of the sample equivalent to 50 mg of the substance and proceed as for standard solution.

Procedure

To 1 ml each of sample and standard solutions add 1.5 ml each of dilute hydrochloric acid and 'PDAB' reagent. Shake and dilute to 10 ml with water. Measure the absorbance of both the solutions at about 450 nm against reagent blank.

Probable Reaction Mechanism

By acid hydrolysis, first amidine group is converted to an amide group yielding demoxepam and methylamine. Further hydrolysis gives 2-amino-5-chlorobenzophenone and glycine-N-oxide. In the analysis of benzodiazepine, 2-aminobenzophenone plays the key role for analytical colour reaction. It undergoes following reactions:

(a) The amino group present can be diazotized and coupled with n-(1-naphthylethylene diamine) to give violet azo dye (Bratton–Marshall reaction) (λ_{max} 550 nm).

(b) The amino group can undergo condensation reaction with 'PDAB' to form coloured product (λ_{max} 450 nm).

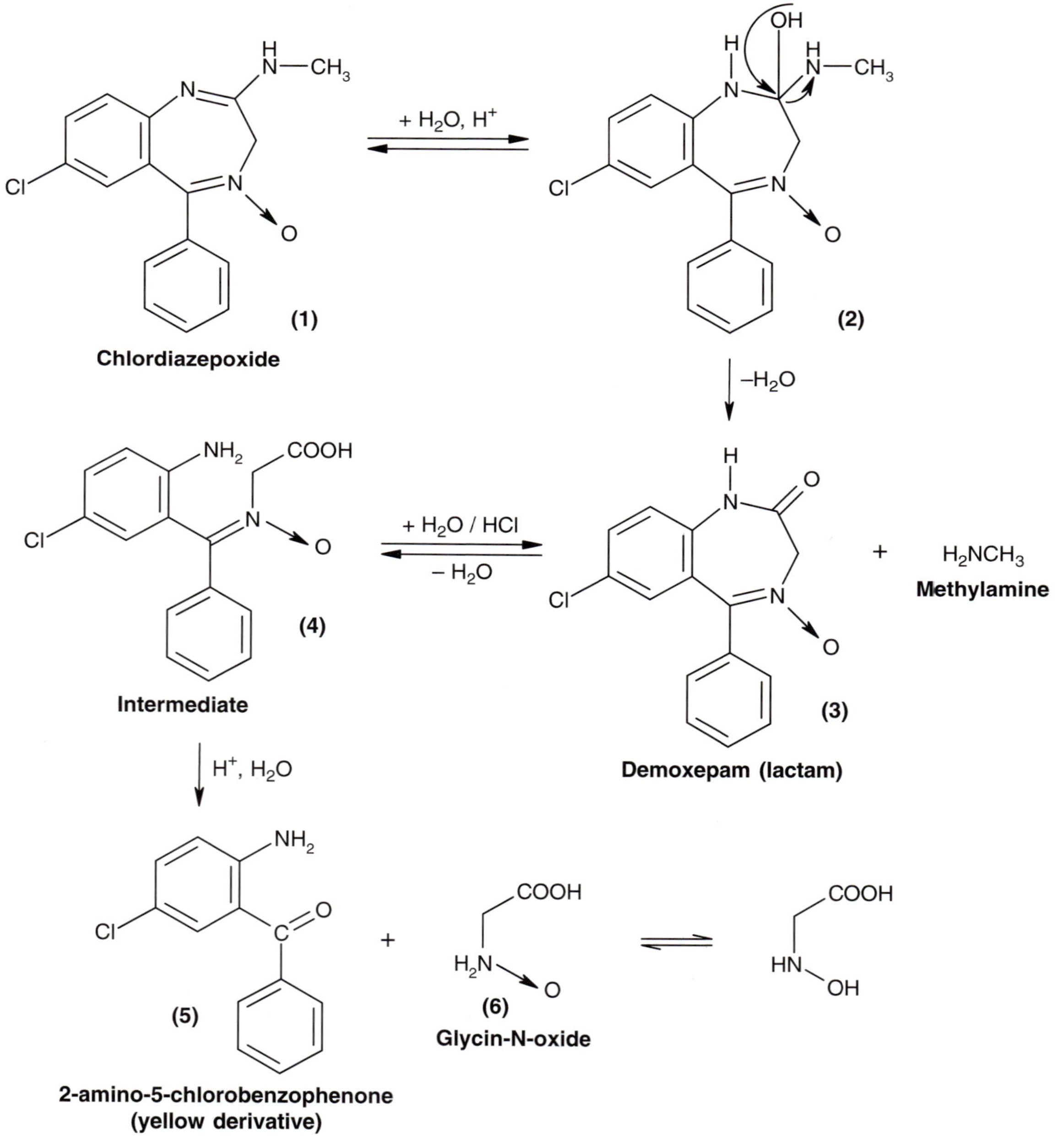

Diazotization and coupling with 1-naphthylamine, thiocol, 1-naphthol, 8-hydroxyquinoline and thymol are some of the other analytical reactions. Reaction with 1,2-naphthoquinone-4-sulfonate is of analytical interest as well.

Note

Methylamine, one of the hydrolytic products, can serve as sensitive method for estimation of chlordiazepoxide as it reacts with fluorescamine to give intense fluorescent pyrrolidone derivative like amino acids.

1.

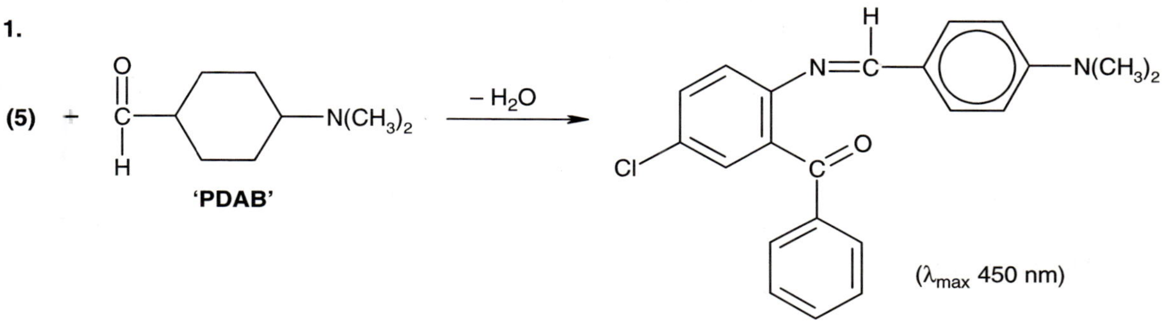

2.

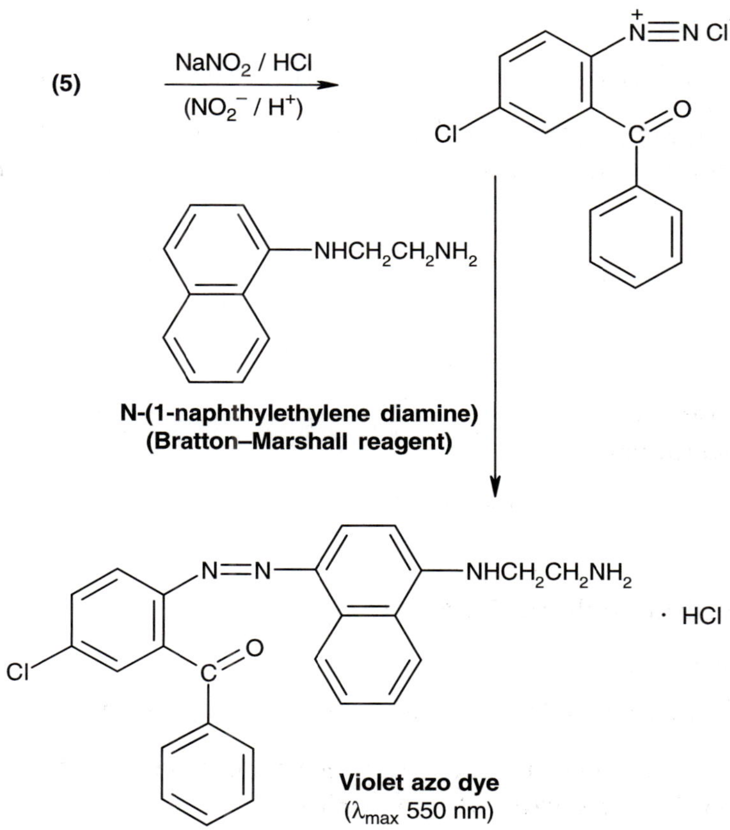

Reference

1. Jiri Gasparic & Jiri Zimak, J. Pharm. & Biomed. Analysis, **1(3)**, 259-279, 1983.
2. Pharmaceutical Chemistry (Vol. 2) by H.J. Roth, pp. 663, 664.

Mild hydrolysis of chlordiazepoxide yields lactam which on photolytic rearrangement in alkaline medium gives a compound with 4,5-epoxide group which exhibits intense fluorescence. This reaction is specific for 1,4-benzodiazepine containing N→O group such as chlordiazepoxide.

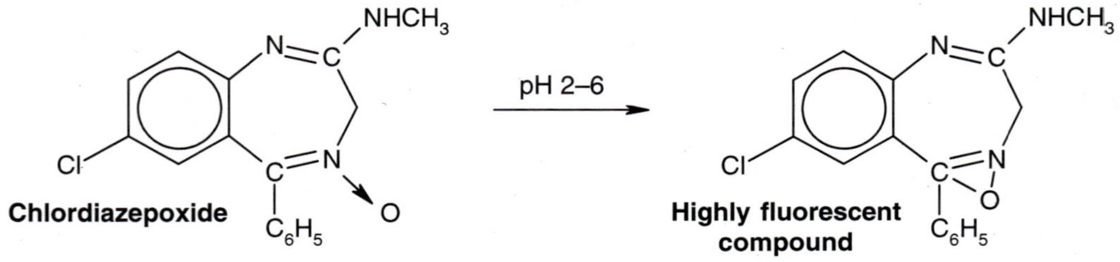

Reference

M.A. Schwartz & E. Postma, J. Pharm. Sci., **55**, 1358-1362, 1966.

Methylamine liberated by acid hydrolysis can be determined fluorometrically by reacting with fluoroscamine. The hydrolysis step has been discussed above.

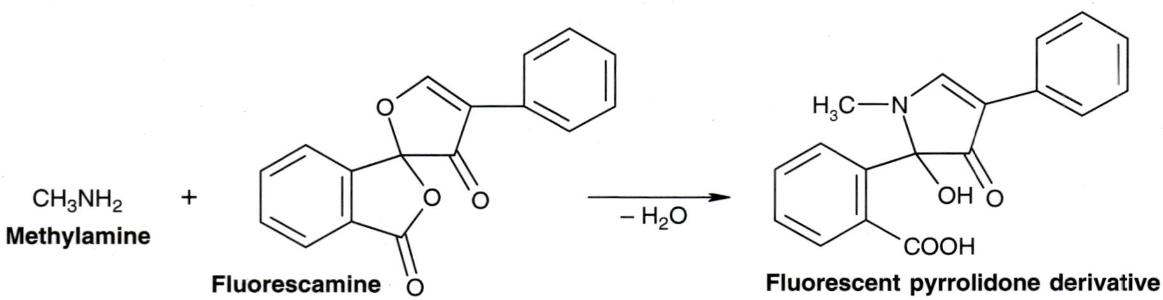

Note

Amino acids undergo similar reaction.

Reference

J.T. Stewart & J.L. Williamson, Anal. Chem., **48**, 1182-1185, 1976.

Chlordiazepoxide undergoes Polonvski rearrangement when heated with acetic anhydride at 100-105°C.

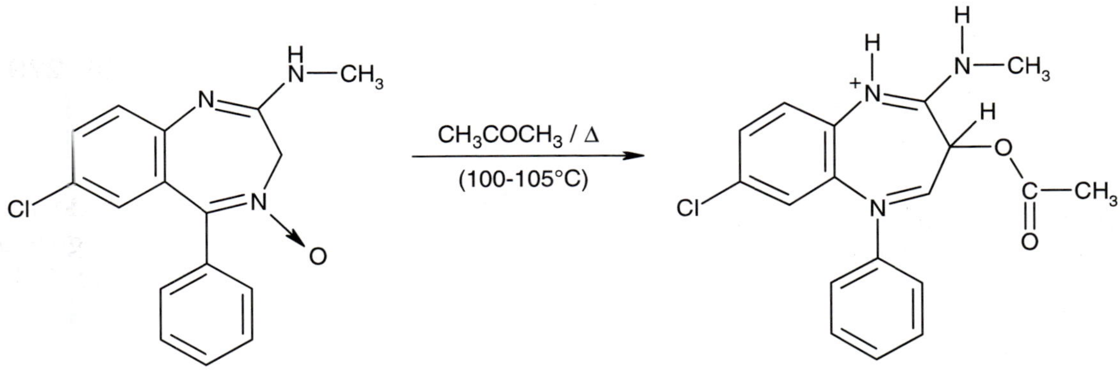

Chlordiazepoxide

The compound forms ion-pair complex with fast green (dye) and orange-II in pH 5 phosphate buffer. Both these ion-pair complexes can be extracted into chloroform for spectrophotometric measurements.

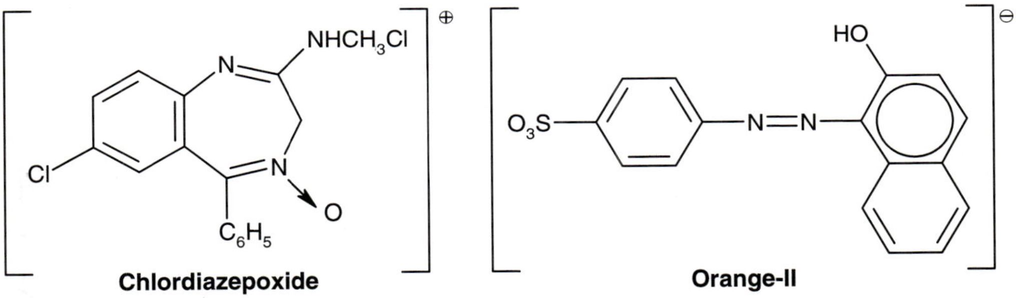

Chlordiazepoxide **Orange-II**

Drug - dye ion-pair complex
(λ_{max} 495 nm)

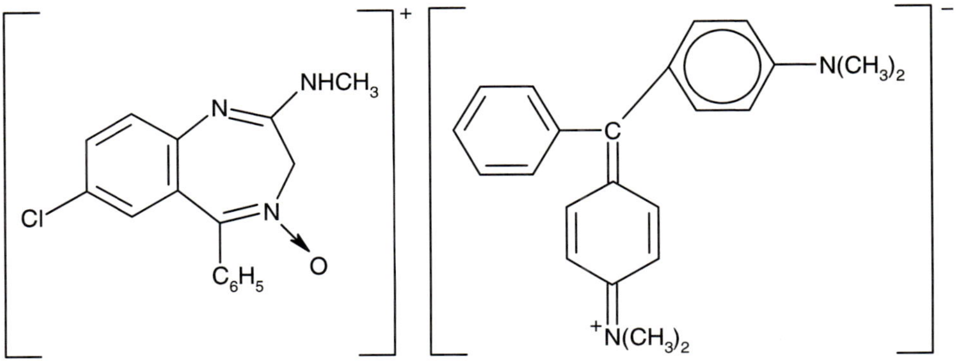

Chlordiazepoxide **Fast-green**

Drug - dye ion-pair complex
(λ_{max} 630 nm)

Reference

Indian Drugs, **27(12)**, 617, 1990.

Isopropylantipyrin (Propyphenazone)

Follow the method described under formulation 11 of the chapter on anti-inflammatory drugs.

Note

4-aminoantipyrin, an important pyrazolane derivative, has often been used as analgesic and antipyretic in certain situations where salicylates may not work such as Hodgkin's disease in place of 4-isopropylantipyrin. In addition to general reaction of amino group, a spectrophotometric method of estimation has been described by Al-Abachi et al. (1988) involving coupling with diazotized p-nitroaniline in acidic medium. It was established by the authors that it is 1 : 1 complex formation between the drug and the reagent as under.

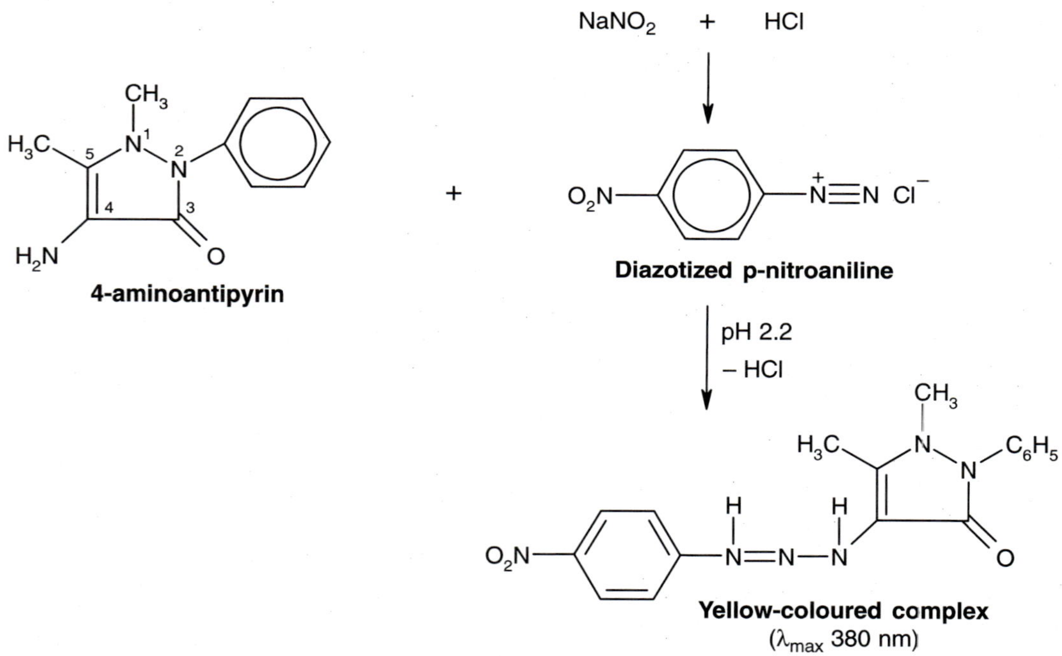

Note

1. The colour is stable for 24 hrs.
2. Antipyrin did not interfere.

Reference

Mouayed Q. Al-Abachi, A.M.S. Al-Delami & S. Al-Najafi, Analyst, **113(11)**, 1661-1663, 1988.

Paracetamol

Follow the method described in formulation 2 of this chapter. The method is based on conversion of paracetamol to p-aminophenol, followed by alkaline oxidation with sodium nitroprusside.

Dicyclomine hydrochloride

Follow the method described in formulation 21 of this chapter. Each ml of 0.004 M sodium lauryl sulphate is equivalent to 0.001384 g of dicyclomine hydrochloride.

Formulation 24

Paracetamol, Caffeine citrate, Phenyldimethylisopropylpyrazolone, Diethyldioxotetrahydropyridine

ESTIMATION

Paracetamol

Follow the nitroso derivative method described under formulation 2 of this chapter.

Caffeine citrate

Reagents

1. Saturated solution of sodium bicarbonate in water.
2. 0.01 N tartaric acid.
3. Chloroform.

Standard solution

7.5 mcg/ml caffeine citrate in 0.01 N tartaric acid.

Sample solution

Weigh powdered sample accurately equivalent to about 20 mg of caffeine citrate, carry out dry extraction of the sample with four 25 ml portions of chloroform. Wash the combined chloroform layer with 25 ml of sodium bicarbonate solution. Discard the aqueous layer, the chloroform layer is evaporated and the residue is taken up in 0.01 N tartaric acid and further diluted with the acid to get final concentration of 7.5 mcg/ml.

Measure the extinction of both the sample and standard solutions at maxima at about 271 nm against solvent blank. Calculate the results by comparison.

Note

Although paracetamol is practically insoluble in chloroform, to remove traces the chloroform extract is shaken with sodium bicarbonate solution.

Phenyldimethylisopropylpyrazolone (Propyphenazone / Isopropylantipyrin / Isopropylphenazone)

Propyphenazone exists as Zwitter-ion and reacts with ferric chloride to give reddish-violet colour. The colour being pH-dependent disappears on addition of sulphuric acid.

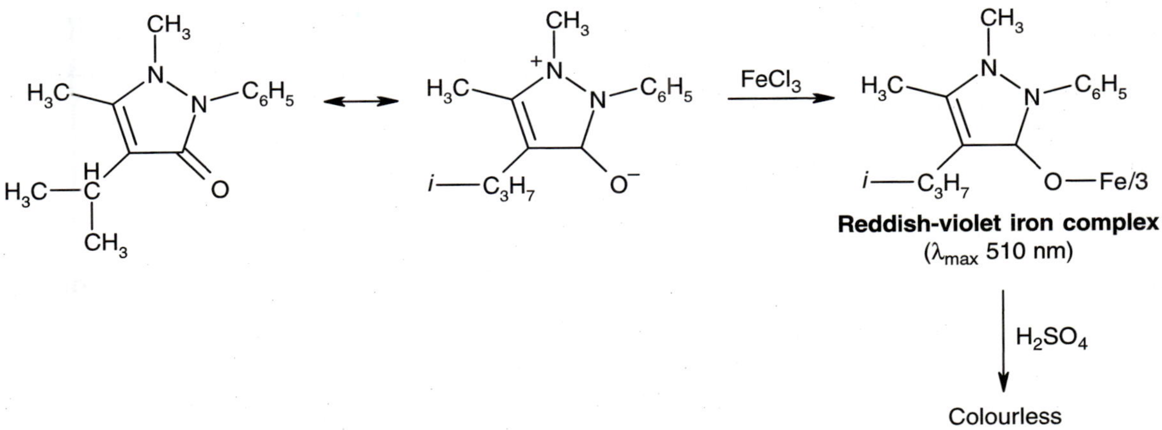

The compound undergoes oxidation with sodium metaperiodate with cleavage between C_4/C_5 to produce oxalic acid derivative.

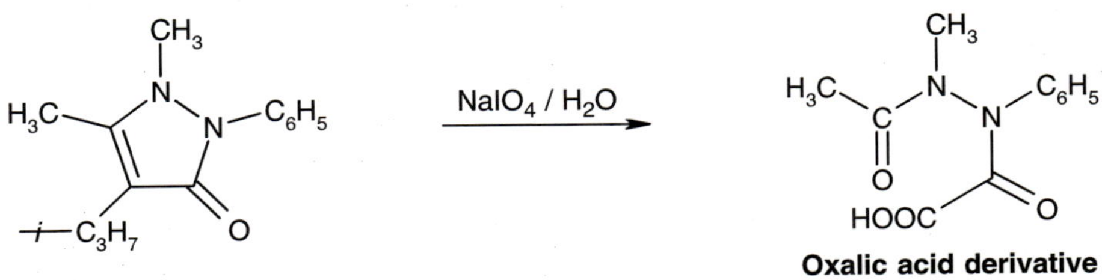

Diethyldioxotetrahydropyridine

METHOD 1

Standard solution

10 mcg/ml of substance in methanol.

Standard solution

Accurately weighed quantity of the sample equivalent to 20 mg of the substance is extracted with methanol and made up to 100 ml. The resultant solution is further diluted appropriately to get final concentration of 10 mcg/ml.

The extinction of both the solutions is measured at 310 nm using methanol as blank. The results are calculated by comparison.

Note

Although maxima of the compound in methanol is observed at 305 nm, but at this wavelength, there is slight interference from paracetamol and propyphenazone. However, at 310 nm, the interference due to above ingredients is almost nil, hence, the latter wavelength is preferred for estimation.

METHOD 2

Follow the above method using 0.1 M sodium hydroxide instead of methanol. Measure the extinction of both the sample and standard solutions at about 366 nm and calculate the results by comparison.

Formulation 25

Ergotamine tartrate, Caffeine, Paracetamol, Prochlorperazine maleate

ESTIMATION

Ergotamine tartrate

METHOD 1

Reagents

1. 0.125% w/v solution of tetrazolium blue in alcohol.
2. Tetramethyl ammonium hydroxide, 0.25% v/v: Mix 0.5 ml of tetramethyl ammonium hydroxide (10%) with ethyl alcohol to produce 20 ml.
3. 20% w/v sodium hydroxide solution in water.

Standard solution

Accurately weigh and transfer 20 mg of ergotamine tartrate to 50 ml dry volumetric flask containing 40 ml ethyl alcohol. Dissolve and make up the volume with ethyl alcohol. Dilute 5 ml of the resulting solution to 50 ml with ethyl alcohol (40 mcg/ml).

Sample solution

Accurately weigh and transfer a quantity of tablet powder equivalent to 2 mg of ergotamine tartrate to 40 ml of water, shake for 5 minutes and dilute to 50 ml with water. Transfer 25 ml of the clear filtrate to 250 ml separatory funnel. Add 1 ml of sodium hydroxide solution and extract with four 30 ml portions of chloroform. Wash the combined chloroform extracts with 10 ml of water. Pass chloroform extracts through anhydrous sodium sulphate. Wash the sodium sulphate layer with 20 ml of chloroform. Evaporate the chloroform on water-bath. Dissolve the residue in sufficient ethyl alcohol to produce 25 ml. Use clear solution for colour development.

Procedure

Transfer 3 ml each of ethyl alcohol (blank), standard solution and sample solution to separate 10 ml dry volumetric flasks. Add 2 ml of tetrazolium blue reagent and mix. Add 2 ml of tetramethyl ammonium hydroxide, mix and wait for 60 minutes. Make up the volumes with ethyl alcohol, mix and measure absorption of sample and standard solutions against reagent blank at about 525 nm. Calculate the content by comparison.

Probable Reaction Mechanism

In alkaline medium, tetrazolium blue oxidizes ergotamine and itself gets reduced to coloured or fluorescent formazan (λ_{max} 525 nm).

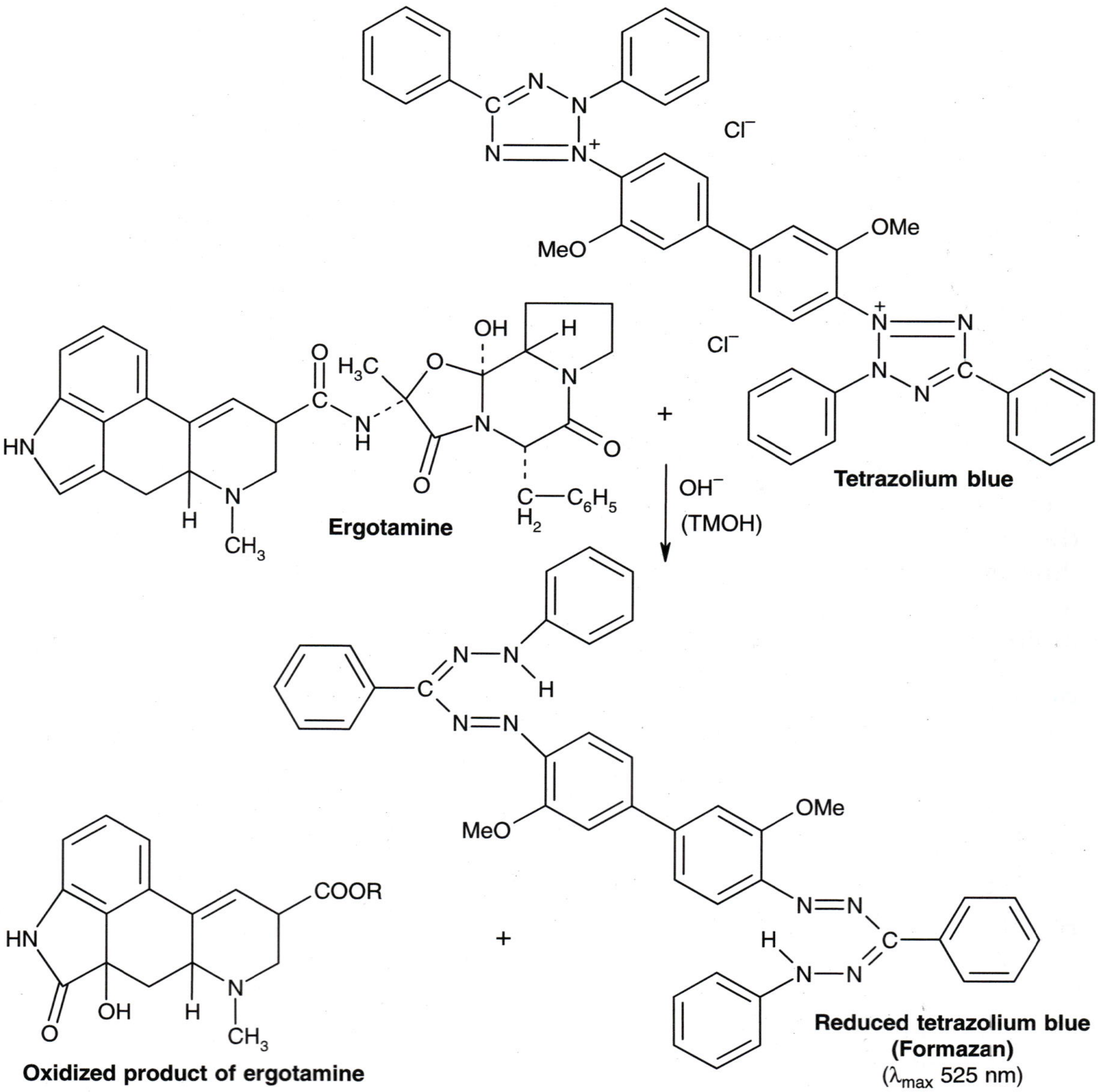

METHOD 2

Reagents

1. 0.125% w/v solution of p-dimethylaminobenzaldehyde (PDAB) in water.
2. 2% w/v tartaric acid in water.

Standard solution

60 mcg/ml of ergotamine tartrate in 2% tartaric acid.

Sample solution

Weigh accurately a quantity of powdered tablets equivalent to 3 mg of ergotamine tartrate, add 25 ml of dilute ammonia solution and extract with three 25 ml portions of solvent ether. Wash the combined ether layer with 10 ml of dilute ammonia solution. Pass ether layer through anhydrous sodium sulphate. Evaporate the ether layer on water-bath. Cool and dissolve the residue in 2% tartaric acid to make 50 ml (60 mcg/ml).

Procedure

To 2 ml each of standard and sample solutions add 4 ml of 'PDAB' solution and keep at room temperature for 30 minutes. Measure the absorbance of both the solutions at 650 nm against reagent blank. Calculate the results by comparison.

The ergot alkaloids in general give blue colour with 'PDAB' reagent in acidic medium (Van–Urk reagent). This is nucleophilic substitution at position 2 of the indole nucleus (rings A and B). Other drugs which react with 'PDAB' under different conditions are terbutaline, paracetamol, chlordiazepoxide, analgin, amoxycillin, oxyphenbutazone, isoniazid, benzocaine, phenothiazine, aminophylline, urea, sulphonamide and tropane alkaloids.

Probable Reaction Mechanism

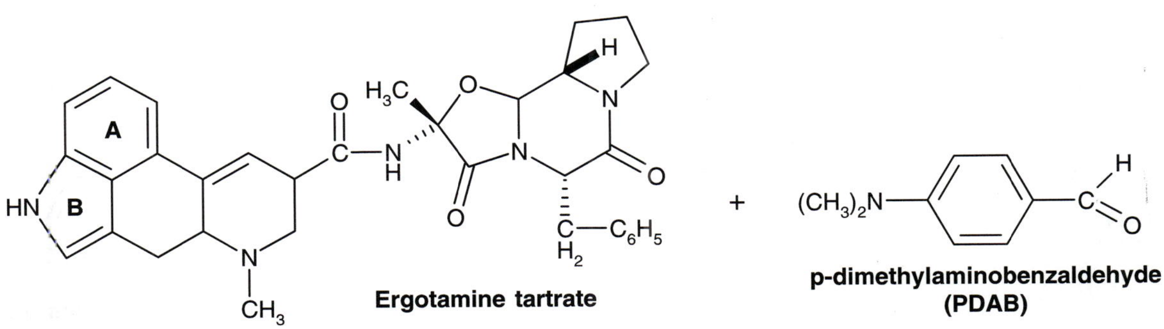

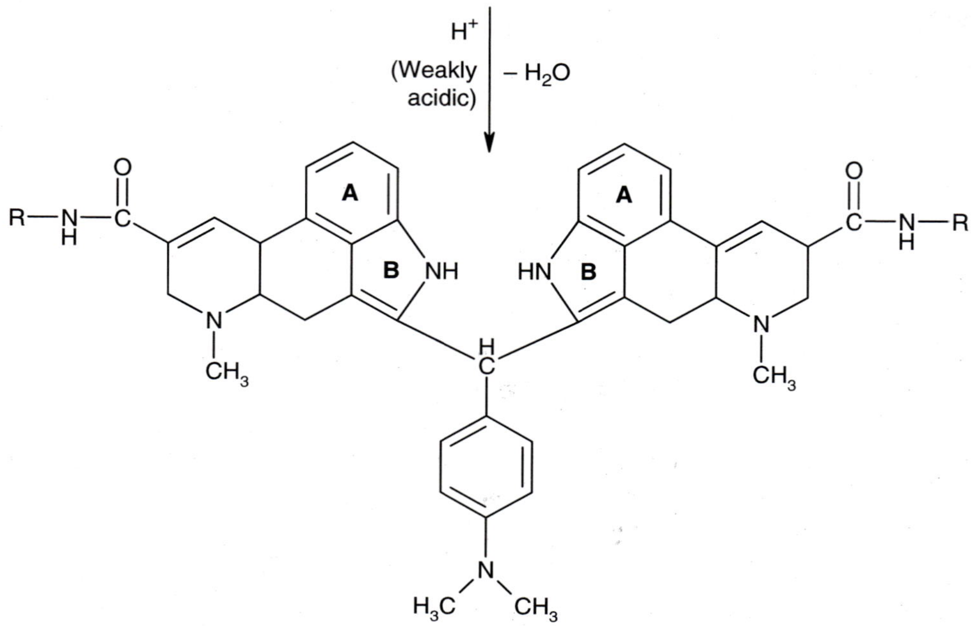

Colourless

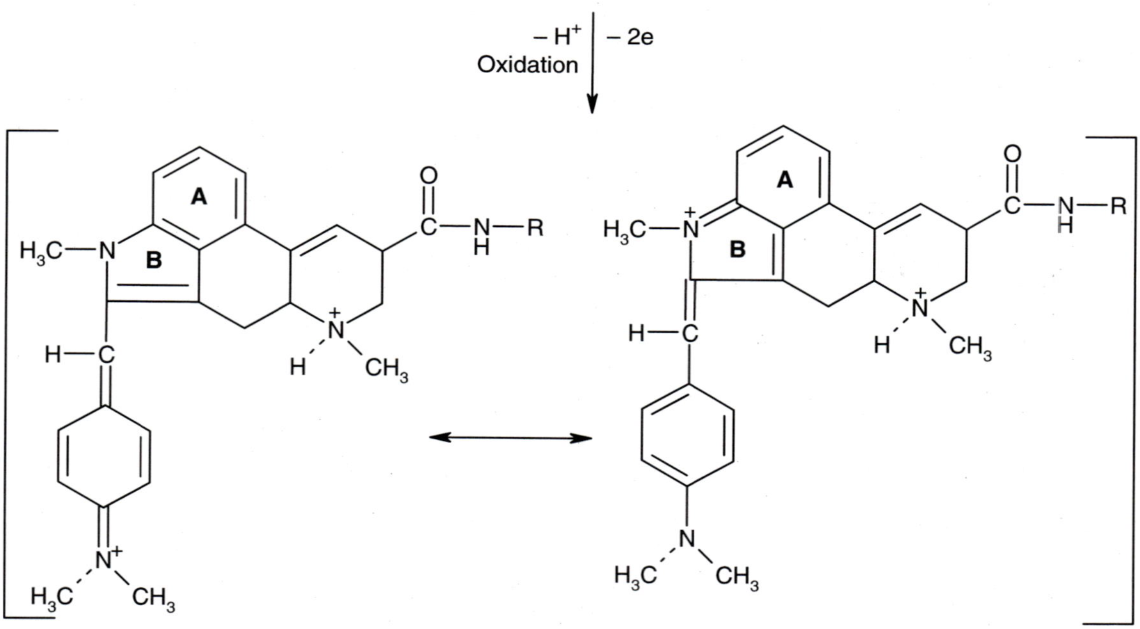

Cyanin dye
(λ_{max} 650 nm)

In strong acid, the reagent forms yellow complex with the alkaloid.

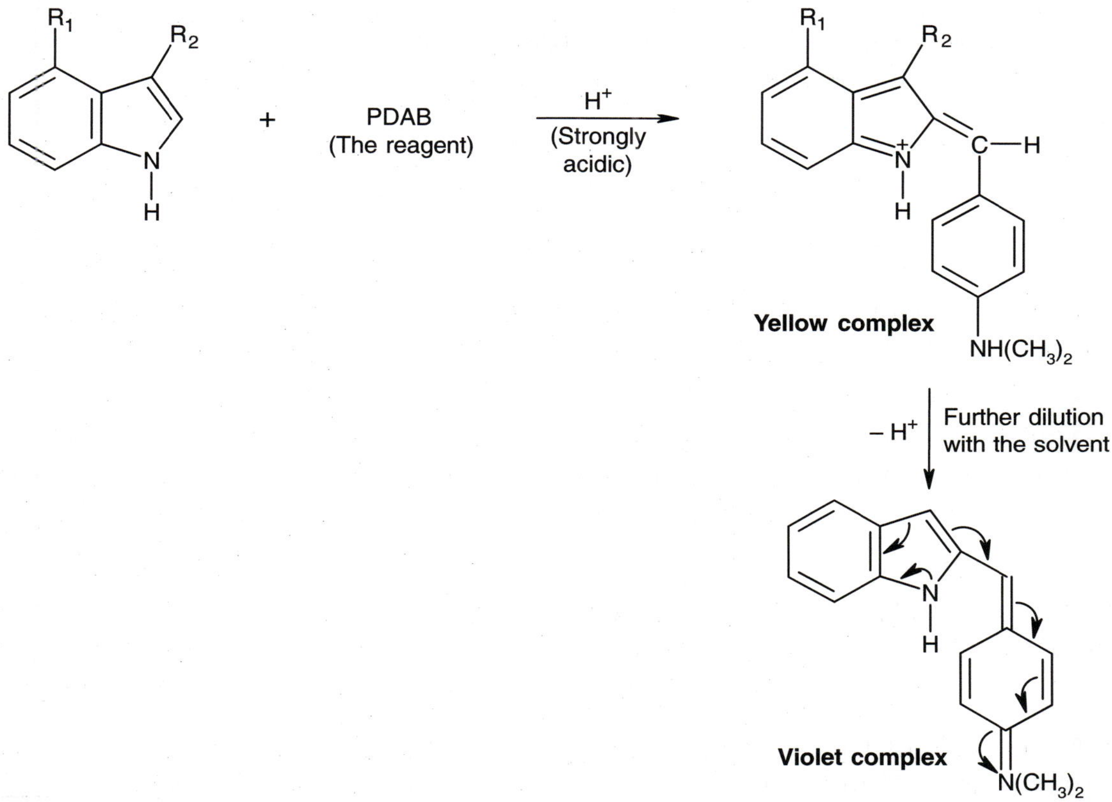

Note

The reaction of indole alkaloid with 'PDAB' is influenced by reaction conditions.

Reference

Pharmaceutical Chemistry (Vol. 2) by H.J. Roth, p. 568.

Caffeine citrate

Accurately weigh and transfer tablet powder equivalent to 100 mg of caffeine to 100 ml round bottom flask. Add 10 ml dilute sulphuric acid and reflux on low flame for one hour. Cool and transfer the contents to a 250 ml separatory funnel with the aid of 10 ml water. Extract with three 50 ml portions of chloroform. Wash the combined chloroform extracts with two 10 ml portions of water. Pass chloroform extracts through anhydrous sodium sulphate layer into 250 ml dry weighed conical flask. Wash the sodium sulphate layer and separatory funnel with 25 ml of chloroform and mix along with main chloroform extracts. Evaporate the chloroform extracts and dry the conical flask along with residue at 105°C for one hour or till constant weight. Cool the flask in dessicator and re-weigh. Weight of the residue represents amount of caffeine present in the weight of the sample taken for analysis or dissolve the residue in 0.01 N tartaric acid (7.5 mcg/ml) for spectrophotometric analysis. For further details refer to formulation of this chapter.

Paracetamol

METHOD 1

Reagents

1. 4% w/v solution of sodium nitroprusside in water.
2. 4% w/v solution of sodium hydroxide in water.

Standard solution

To 100 mg of paracetamol add 50 ml of concentrated hydrochloric acid and boil for 60 minutes in water-bath. Cool, filter and adjust to 100 ml with water. Dilute 1 ml of the resultant solution to 100 ml with water (10 mcg/ml).

Sample solution

Weigh accurately sample equivalent to 100 mg of paracetamol and treat as under standard solution (conversion to p-aminophenol).

Procedure

To 5 ml each of the sample and standard solutions add 0.5 ml of sodium nitroprusside solution and adjust to 10 ml with sodium hydroxide solution. Keep at room temperature for 10 minutes and measure the absorbance of both the solutions at about 725 nm. Calculate the results by comparison.

Note

1. Aspirin, phenobarbitone, phenylbutazone, chlorpheniramine maleate and ephedrine hydrochloride do not interfere.
2. Phenols with substitution as para-position except p-aminophenol do not interfere.

Probable Reaction Mechanism

Step 1: Hydrolysis of paracetamol to p-aminophenol and acetic acid under acidic conditions.

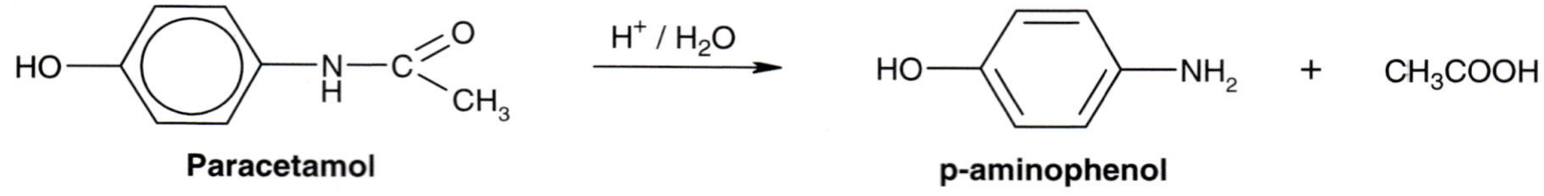

Step 2: The p-aminophenol formed now reacts with Na–nitroprusside solution, known as disodium pentacyanonitrosyl ferrate (II), in alkali medium to form the complex and sodium nitroprusside gets reduced.

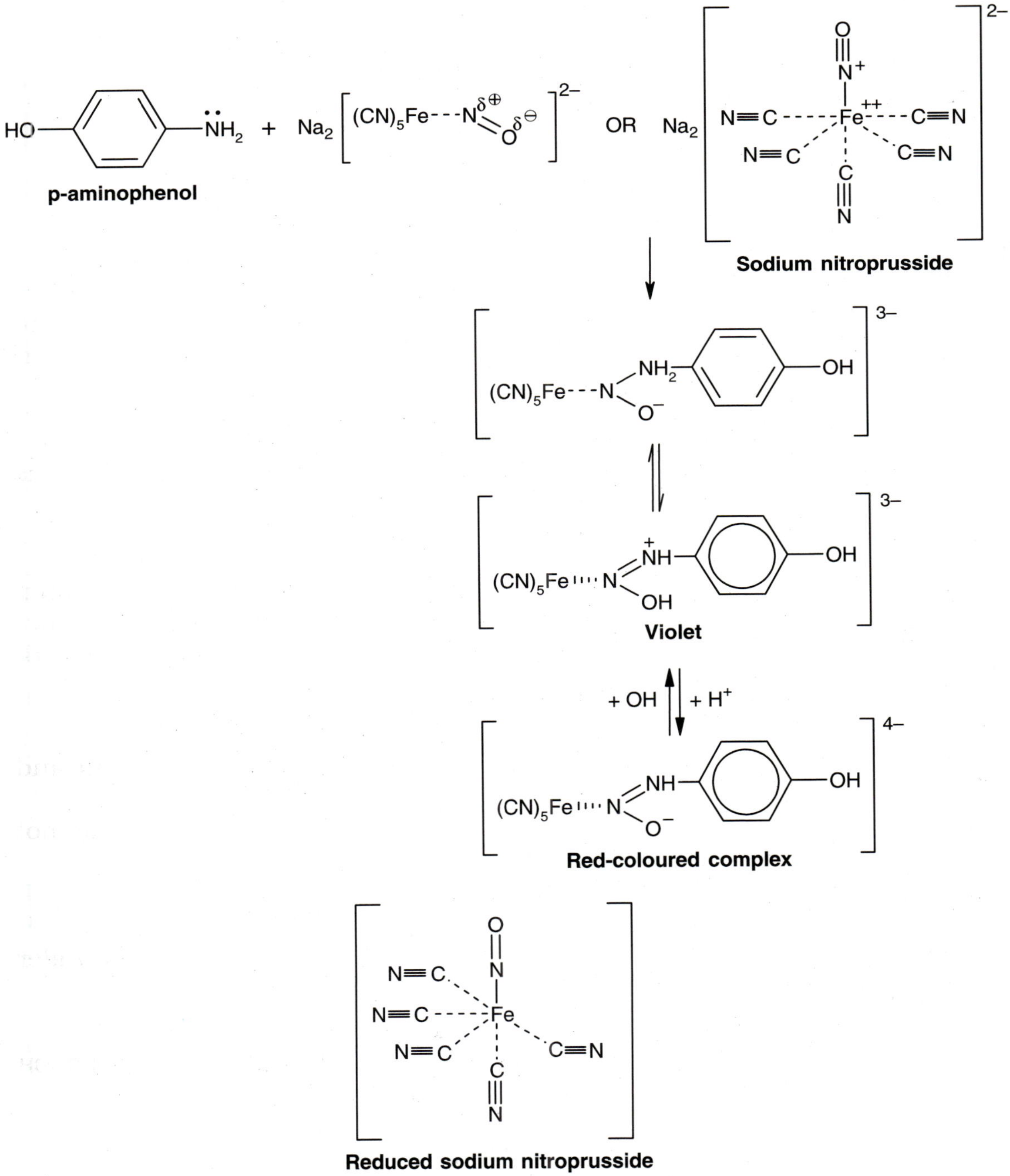

Reference

Pharmaceutical Chemistry (Vol. 2) by H.J. Roth, p. 133.

METHOD 2

Follow the method described in formulation of this chapter. This method is based on acid hydrolysis to p-aminophenol, diazotization and coupling with 'NED'.

Prochlorperazine maleate

METHOD 1

Reagent

0.05% w/v solution of 1,2-naphthoquinone-4-sulphonate (Na^+) (NQS) in 62.5% v/v sulphuric acid. The reagent should be freshly prepared (Folin's reagent).

Standard solution

Weigh accurately 50 mg of prochlorperazine maleate and dissolve in water by heating to produce 100 ml. 10 ml of the resultant solution may be further diluted with water to produce 50 mcg/ml.

Sample solution

Weigh accurately powdered tablets equivalent to 10 mg of prochlorperazine maleate and dissolve in boiling water to produce 200 ml (50 mcg/ml).

Procedure

To 4 ml each of standard and sample solutions add 8 ml of the 'NQS' reagent. Mix and allow to stand at room temperature for 30 minutes. Measure the absorbance of both the solutions at about 520 nm and calculate the results by comparison.

Probable Reaction Mechanism

1,2-naphthoquinone-4-sulphonate (Na^+) is a strong oxidizing agent. It oxidizes prochlorperazine and itself gets reduced to 1,2-naphthoquinol-4-sulphonic acid. Phenothiazine with three carbon atoms separating two nitrogen atoms such as chlorpromazine or prochlorperazine are preferentially oxidized to sulphoxide without elimination of side chain, whereas phenothiazine with two carbon atoms separating N—N side chain is eliminated as a result of oxidative reaction giving phenothiazone derivative.

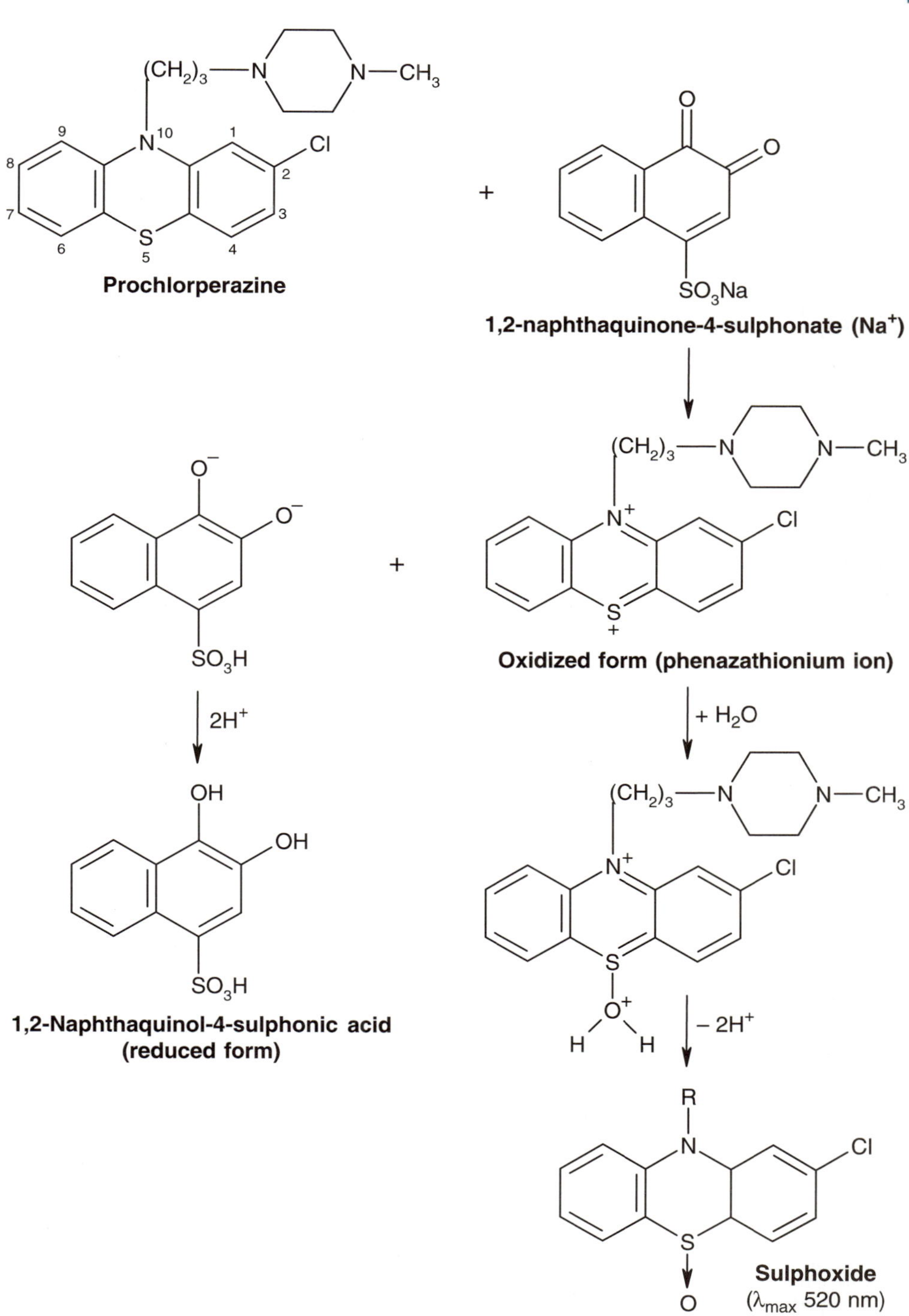

Reference

1. Pharmaceutical Chemistry (Vol. 2) by H.J. Roth, p. 697.
2. H.T. Fawzy, I.A. Saad & L.N. Gadel-Rub, Pharmazie, **28**, 322, 1973.

METHOD 2

Reagents

1. 0.1 M hydrochloric acid.
2. 2% w/v solution of ferric chloride in 0.1 M HCl.
3. 0.05% w/v solution of p-benzoquinone in 50% sulphuric acid.
4. 50% v/v solution of sulphuric acid in water.

Sample/standard solution

To 1 ml each of sample and standard solutions add 4 ml of water, 1 ml of benzoquinone reagent and 5 ml of sulphuric acid, dilute to 10 ml with water and measure the absorbance at λ_{max} 528 nm.

Probable Reaction Mechanism

In the presence of p-benzoquinone, an oxidizing agent prochlorperazine is oxidized to 3,7-dihydroxyphenathiazonium benzohydroxyquinone. The phenothiazine ring present in the drug prochlorperazine is easily susceptible to oxidation and hence oxidation is carried out at room temperature. The reaction can be represented as follows:

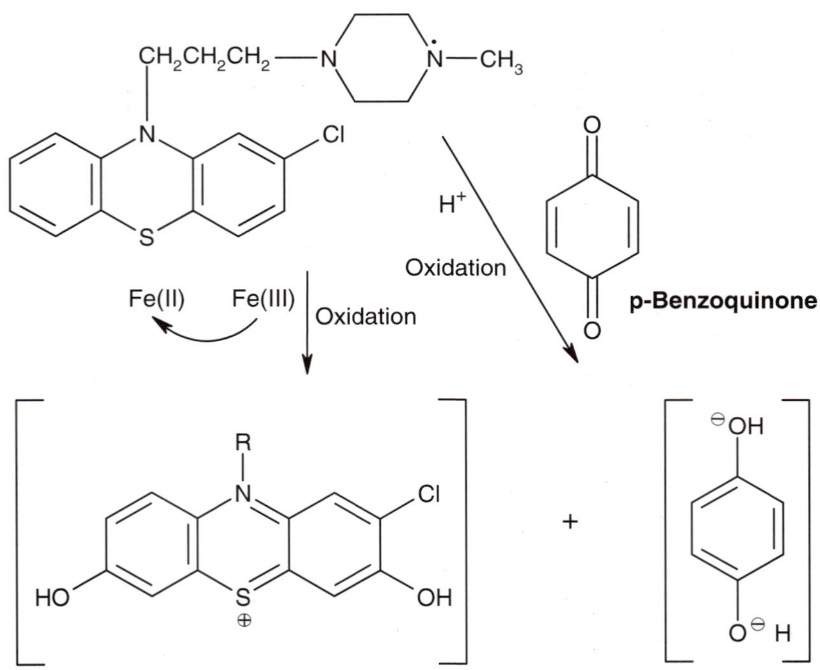

3,7-dihydroxyphenathiazonium benzohydroxyquinone (λ_{max} 528 nm)

Hydroxyquinone

Similarly with $FeCl_3$ in acidic medium oxidation of the phenathiazine ring takes place resulting in the formation of similar product as above.

Reference

1. Pharmaceutical Chemistry (Vol. 2) by H.J. Roth, p. 701.
2. J. Emmanuel & E. Silva Dias, Indian Drugs, **25(8)**, 343-345, 1988 and *Indian Drugs*, **25(6)**, 252, 1988.

METHOD 3

Reagents

1. 1% w/v solution of p-aminobenzoic acid (PABA) in methanol.
2. 1% w/v solution of potassium persulphate in water.

Sample and standard solutions

Sample and standard solutions in water.

Procedure

To 1 ml each of sample and standard solutions add 4 ml of 'PABA' solution, 2 ml of potassium persulphate, dilute to 25 ml with water, allow to stand at room temperature for 5 min and measure the absorbance at 560 nm against reagent blank.

Reference

Indian Drugs, **21(3)**, 119, 1983.

Probable Reaction Mechanism

Quantitative oxidation of phenothiazine skeleton of the drug occurs with potassium persulphate which is stabilized by p-aminobenzoic acid to give a violet-coloured chromophore. The reaction can be represented as follows:

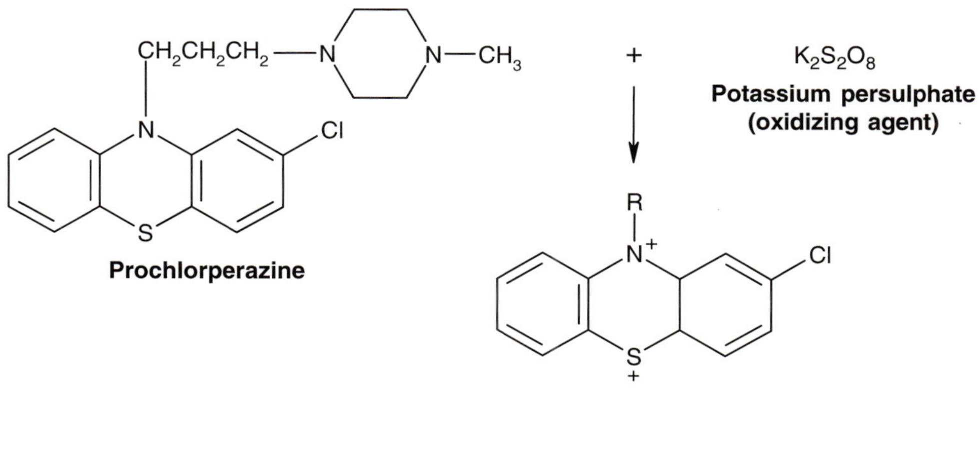

Since water is present in the medium

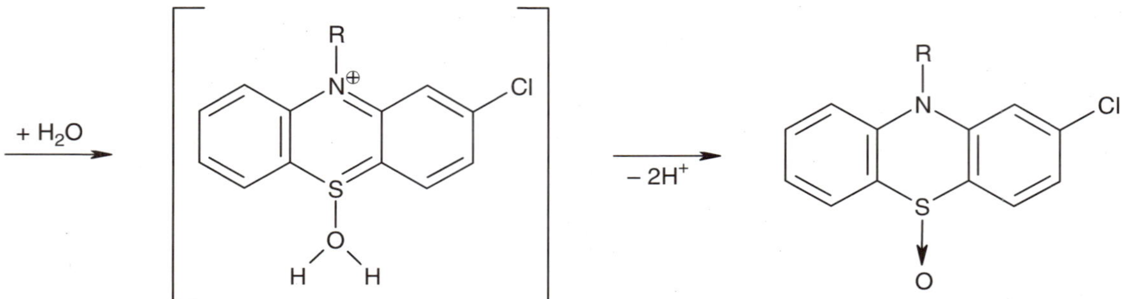

Sulphoxide (the product)
(λ_{max} 560 nm)

Reference

Pharmaceutical Chemistry (Vol. 2) by H.J. Roth, pp. 694, 695, 696.

The drug forms Schiff's base with 'PABA' (λ_{max} 520 nm). Paracetamol, caffeine and CPM do not interfere.

METHOD 4

Reagents

1. 5% w/v solution of ferric chloride in water.
2. PDAB reagent: Dissolve 125 mg of PDAB in 65% v/v mixture of sulphuric acid - water, cool, add 0.1 ml of ferric chloride solution, further cool.

Sample and standard solutions

100 μg/ml in dilute hydrochloric acid.

Procedure

To 1 ml each of sample/standard solutions add 8 ml of 0.1 M HCl and 2 ml of the PDAB reagent, allow to stand for 15 min and measure the absorbance at 520 nm against reagent blank.

Probable Reaction Mechanism

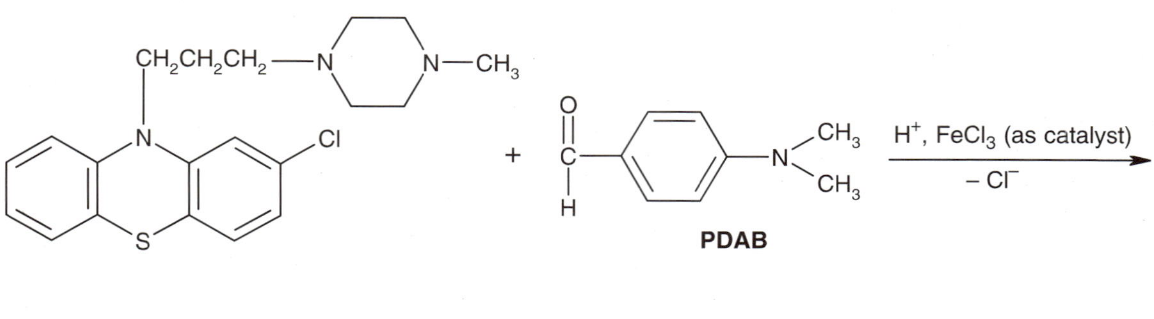

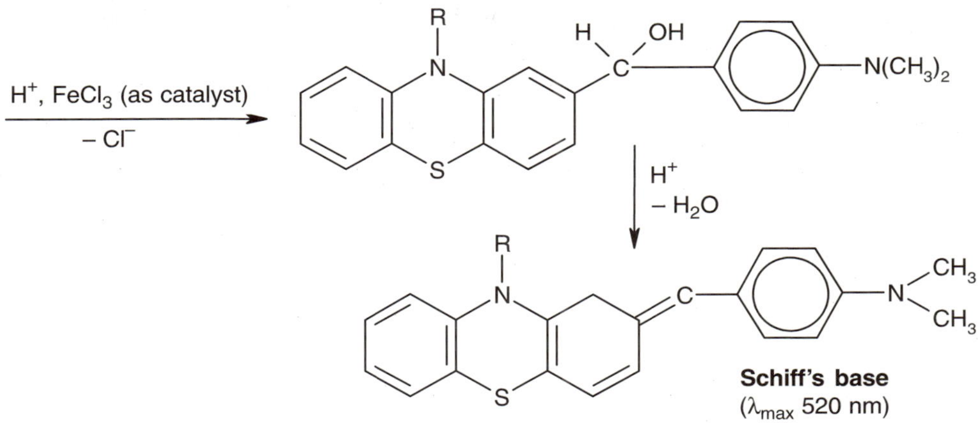

Schiff's base
(λ_{max} 520 nm)

Reference

T.P. Gandhi, M.R. Patel, A.A. Patel, V.C. Patel & R.N. Gilbert, Indian Drugs, **16(10)**, 242-244, 1979.

The drug will form ion-pair complexes with acidic dyes such as brilliant green and orange-II in acidic medium. Both complexes are soluble in chloroform and exhibit maxima at 620 nm and 595 nm.

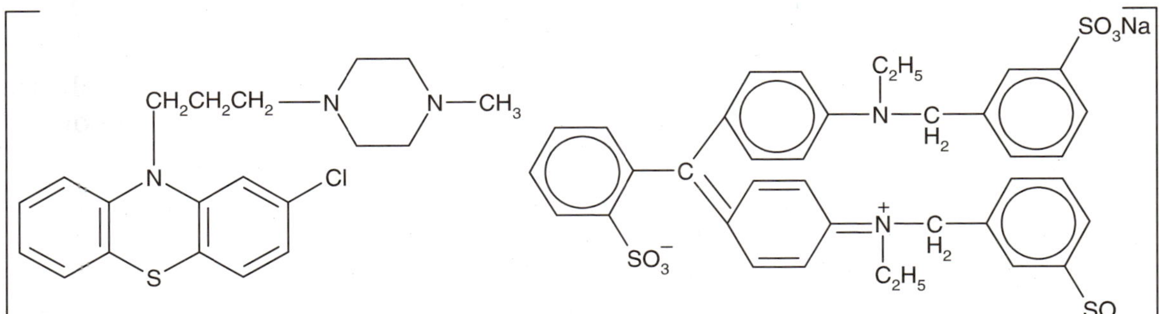

Brilliant green

Prochlorperazine - dye complex + NaCl
(λ_{max} 620 nm)

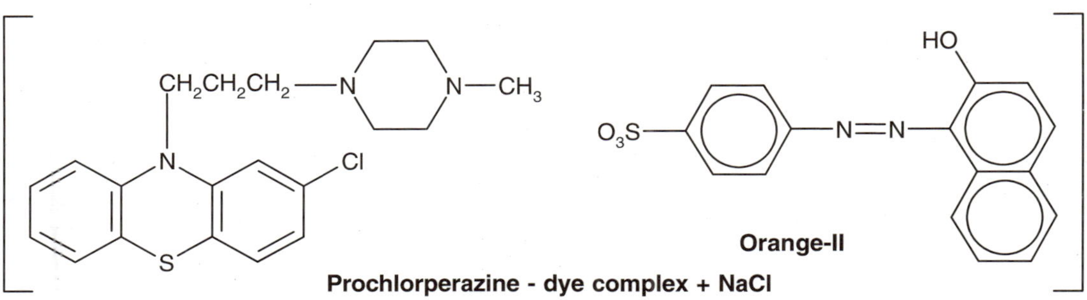

Orange-II

Prochlorperazine - dye complex + NaCl
(λ_{max} 595 nm)

Having electrophilic group (Cl^-) at C-2, the compound forms nitroso derivative which in the presence of sulphuric acid, an oxidizing agent, is converted to nitrosoquinoid derivative which is coloured and forms the basis of analytical method. For details, refer to trifluoperazine under chapter on tranquillizers and sedatives.

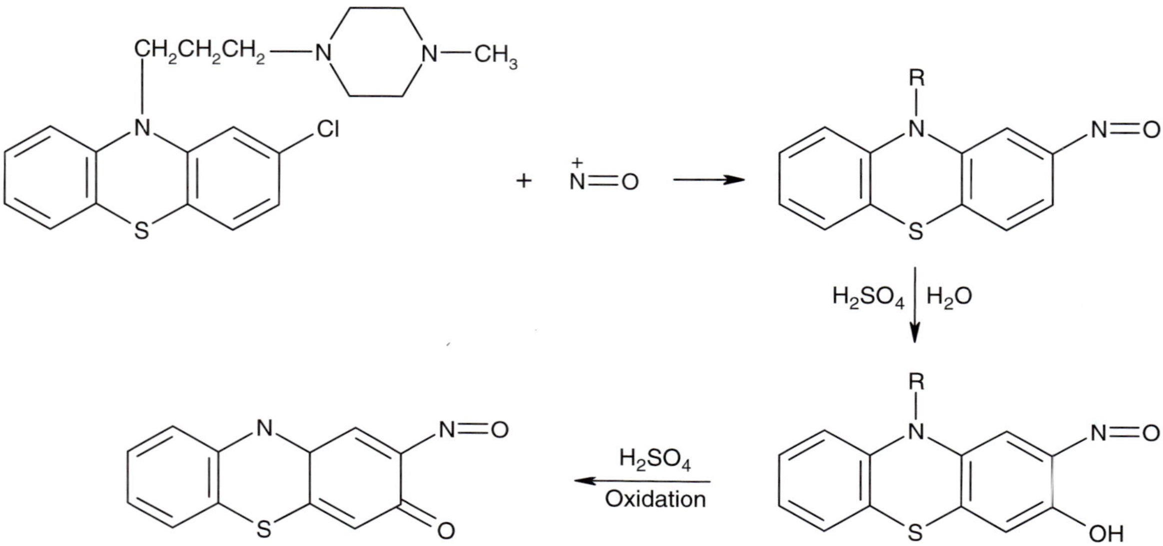

Nitrosoquinoid phenothiazine derivative

Formulation 26

Ergotamine tartrate, Cyclizine hydrochloride, Caffeine citrate

Preparation of test solution

Transfer finely powdered quantity of sample equivalent to about 20 mg of ergotamine tartrate into a volumetric flask. Add 2.5 g of tartaric acid and 100 ml of water. Shake for 30 minutes and dilute to 250 ml with water. Filter, collect the filtrate rejecting first few ml of the filtrate.

ESTIMATION

Cyclizine hydrochloride

Transfer 10 ml of test solution into separating funnel, make alkaline with 5 N sodium hydroxide and extract with three 25 ml portions of cyclohexane. Wash the combined organic layer with two 10 ml portions of 0.1 N sodium hydroxide. Extract the organic layer with four 25 quantities of 0.05 N sulphuric acid. Dilute the combined acidic layer to 100 ml. Further dilution may be done with 0.05 N sulphuric acid to get a concentration of 10 mcg/ml. Measure the extinction at maximum at 225 nm using acid as blank. Calculate the results taking 390 as value of A 1%, 1 cm at 225 nm.

Alternatively, ion-pair complex formation method can be used.

Hom & Ebert (1977) have described a spectrophotometric method for estimation of meclizine and cyclizine. The method is based on formation of ion-pair complex with acidic dye methyl orange in pH 2.8 MacIlvaine buffer. The ion-pair complex extracted with chloroform was found to be 1 : 1 complex and has λ_{max} 422 nm.

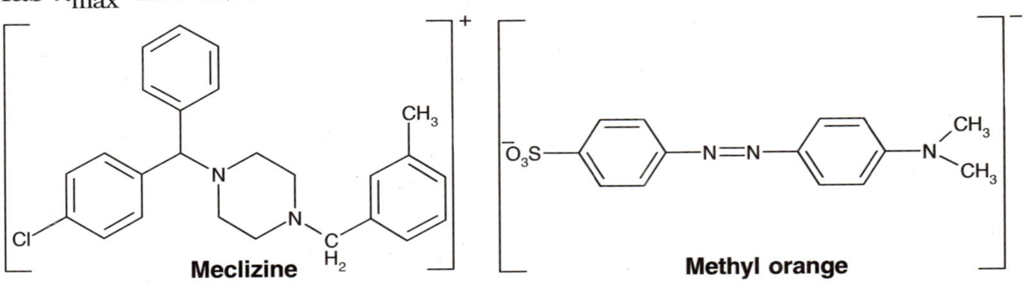

Drug - methyl orange ion-pair complex
(λ_{max} 422 nm)

OR

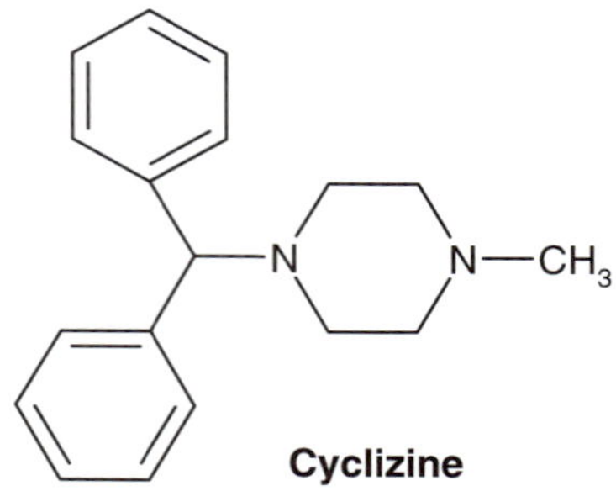

Cyclizine

Reference

F.S. Hom & W.R. Ebert, J. Pharm. Sci., **66(5)**, 710-712, 1977.

Caffeine citrate

Dilute the test solution with water to get concentration of 10 mcg/ml. Measure the absorbance of final solution at maximum at about 272 nm and calculate the results using 500 as value of A 1%, 1 cm. Each g of caffeine anhydrous is equivalent to 1.092 g of caffeine monohydrate.

Ergotamine tartrate

Standard solution

40 mcg/ml of ergotamine tartrate in 1% v/v acetic acid in methanol.

Sample solution

To accurately weighed quantity of the sample equivalent to about 4 mg of the substance add 1 ml of glacial acetic acid and about 80 ml of methanol, place in ultrasonic bath for 10 min and dilute to 100 ml with methanol.

Concomitantly, measure the extinction of both the solutions at maximum at about 320 nm using 1% v/v solution of glacial acetic acid in methanol as blank and calculate the results by comparison. Use amber-coloured glass apparatus. The absorption maximum is explainable in relation to the indole component of the molecule and the conjugated double bond associated with it.

Formulation 27

Paracetamol, Pentazocine

ESTIMATION

Pentazocine

METHOD 1

Weigh powdered tablets accurately equivalent to 60 mg of pentazocine, add 20 ml of 1 N sodium hydroxide and extract with four 25 ml portions of chloroform. Pass chloroform layer through anhydrous sodium sulphate. Evaporate chloroform layer and take the residue (A) in 25 ml glacial acetic acid and titrate with 0.02 N perchloric acid using crystal violet as indicator.

Each ml of 0.02 N perchloric acid is equivalent to 5.708 mg of pentazocine.

METHOD 2

Dissolve the residue (A) obtained in above method in 0.1 N hydrochloric acid or 0.1 N sodium hydroxide to get 50 mcg/ml solution. Measure the extinction at 278 nm (acidic solution) or at 298 nm (alkaline solution). Calculate the contents of pentazocine using value of 69 as E 1%, 1 cm for acidic solution and 108 for alkaline solution. The method obeys Beer's law in the concentration range of 10-200 mcg/ml.

Probable Reaction Mechanism

Under acidic conditions, pentazocine undergoes no structural change, however under basic condition, quinoid-like structure formation takes place resulting in an increase in absorption.

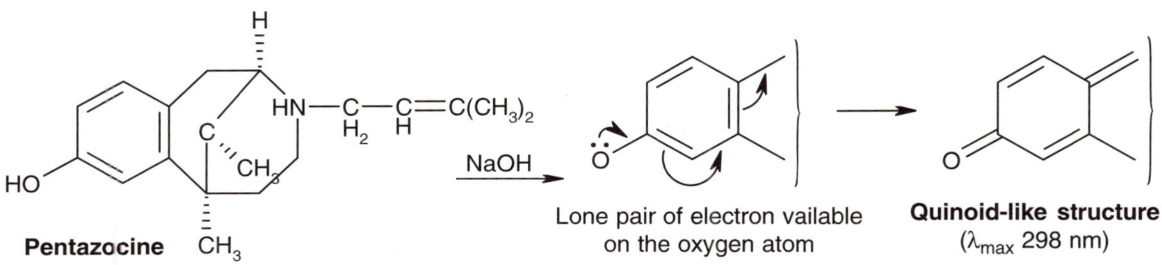

Reference

P.K. Chatterjee, P.D. Sethi & Y. Kumar, Indian Drugs, **22(5)**, 277-278, 1985.

METHOD 3

Reagents

1. 0.1 M and 1 M hydrochloric acid.
2. 1 M sodium hydroxide.
3. 3% w/v freshly prepared solution of sodium nitrite in water.

Standard solution

0.2 mg/ml of pentazocine in 0.1 N hydrochloric acid.

Sample solution

(a) **Tablets and injections:** An accurately weighed or measured aliquot of the preparation is extracted and suitably diluted with 0.1 N hydrochloric acid to give a concentration of about 200 mcg/ml of pentazocine. Filter, if necessary.

(b) **Pentazocine in presence of paracetamol:** An accurately weighed amount of the sample equivalent to 20 mg of pentazocine is extracted with chloroform as described under method 1. The chloroform layer is evaporated and the residue is taken in 0.1 N hydrochloric acid to produce 100 ml.

Procedure

To 5 ml of sample and standard solutions add 2 ml of sodium nitrite solution and 1 ml of 1 N hydrochloric acid. Heat the mixture on water-bath for 30 minutes, cool and add 3 ml of 1 M sodium hydroxide. Allow the mixture to stand at room temperature for five minutes and dilute to 25 ml with water. Measure the extinction of both the solutions at about 434 nm against reagent blank. Pentazocine may be converted into its hydrochloride salt by multiplying with a factor of 1.1278. The method follows Beer's law in the concentration range of 50-500 mcg/ml.

Probable Reaction Mechanism

Step 1:

(a) $$NaNO_2 + 2HCl \longrightarrow HNO_2 + NaCl$$

(b) $$H^+ + HNO_2 \rightleftharpoons H_2ONO^+ \xrightarrow{Cl^\ominus} Cl^\ominus \overset{\oplus}{N}{=}O + H_2O$$

Nitrosonium ion $\longrightarrow \overset{\oplus}{N}{=}O$

Step 2: The nitrosonium ion formed will attack electrophilically at the ortho position to the phenolic —OH present in pentazocine to yield the nitroso derivative as shown below:

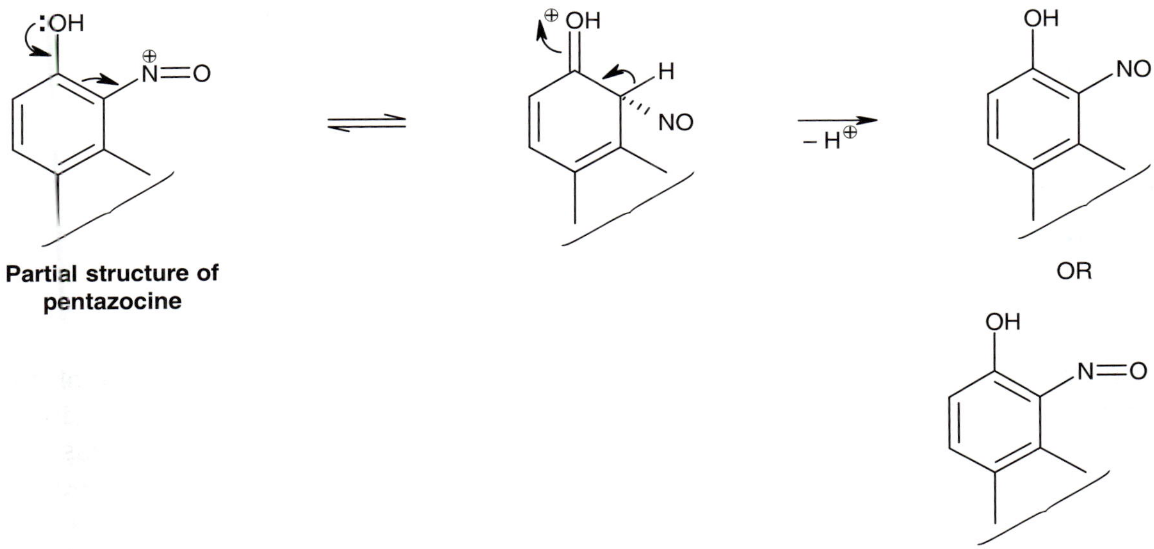

Partial structure of pentazocine

Nitroso derivative

Step 3: When the nitroso derivative is treated with alkali, it loses a molecule of H_2O and the reaction proceeds as shown below:

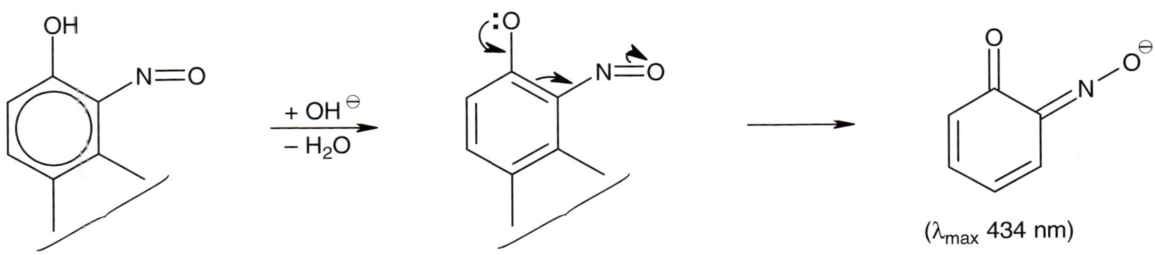

(λ_{max} 353 nm)

(λ_{max} 434 nm)

Alkalisation of the medium after nitrosation resulted in the formation of a highly stable compound with bathochromic shift together with hyperchromic effect. This is probably due to the contribution of an extra pair of unshared electron in the interaction with aromatic nucleus i.e. because of extended conjugation.

Reference

P.K. Chatterjee & P.D. Sethi, Indian Drugs, **22(7)**, 391-392, 1985.

METHOD 4

Reagents

1. 1% w/v solution of p-nitroaniline in 1 : 9 hydrochloric acid.
2. 2% w/v solution of sodium nitrite in water.
3. 5% w/v solution of sodium hydroxide.

Sample and standard solutions

To 2 ml of sample and standard solutions add 5 ml of diazotized p-nitroaniline and 4 ml of sodium hydroxide solution, dilute to 25 ml with water and measure the absorbance at 475 nm against reagent blank.

Sodium nitrite in acidic conditions generates nitrous acid which in acidic conditions generates nitrosonium ions which are electron-deficient. These nitrosonium ions then attack the primary aromatic amino group of p-nitroaniline generating the diazotized product. Reactions are represented as under:

$$NaNO_2 + HCl \longrightarrow NaCl + HNO_2 \xrightarrow{H^+} H_2O\ \overset{\oplus}{N}{=}O \xrightarrow{Cl^-} H_2O + Cl^{\ominus}\ \underset{\oplus}{N}{=}O$$

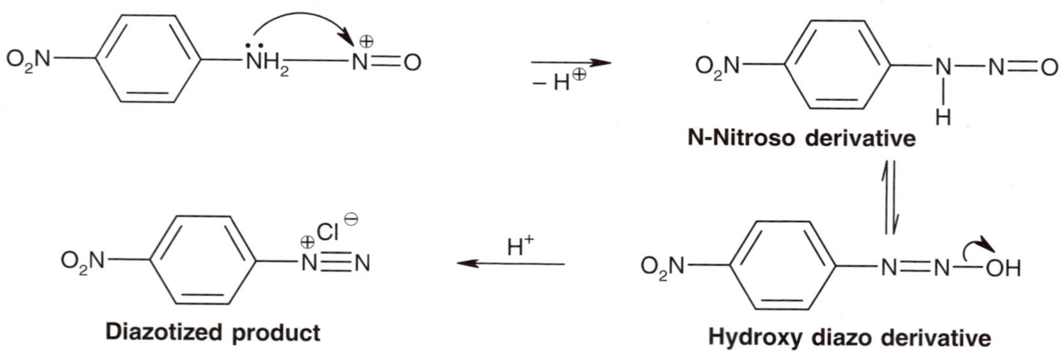

The diazotized product so formed couples with the drug under basic conditions resulting in the formation of the product.

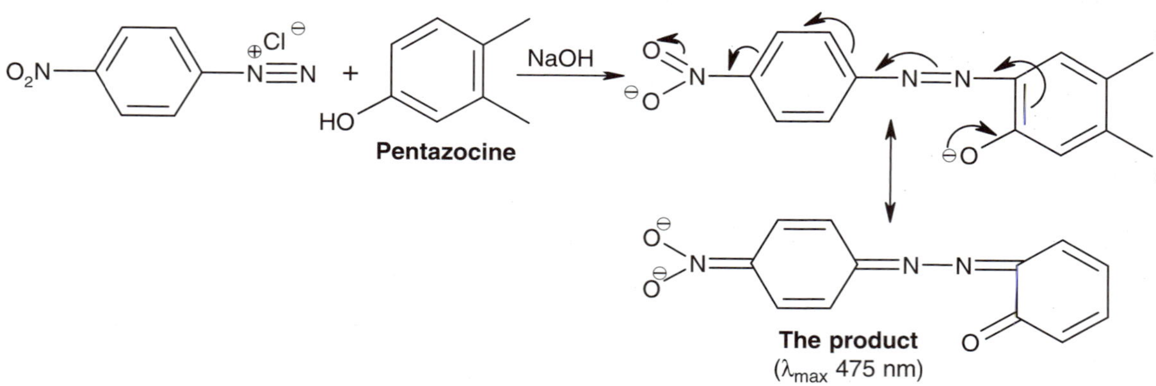

Reference

1. Textbook of Practical Organic Chemistry by Vogel, p. 920.
2. D.M. Shingbal & Girish D. Sardesai, Indian Drugs, **24(7)**, 359-360, 1987.

Paracetamol

Standard solution

10 mcg/ml of paracetamol in 0.1 N hydrochloric acid.

Sample solution

Extract powdered tablets equivalent to 10 mg of paracetamol with 0.1 N hydrochloric acid to produce 100 ml. Filter and dilute 10 ml of the filtrate to 100 ml with same solvent.

Procedure

Measure the extinction of both sample and standard solutions at absorption maximum at about 244 nm using 0.1 N hydrochloric acid as blank. Pentazocine does not interfere at this wavelength.

Formulation 28

Aspirin, Caffeine citrate

ESTIMATION

Caffeine citrate

Standard solution

10 mcg/ml of caffeine citrate in water.

Sample solution

Dissolve powder equivalent to 30 mg of caffeine in 2 ml of water by gentle shaking and filter through a sintered glass funnel G_4 (retain the residue for estimation of aspirin). Dilute 0.5 ml of the filtrate with water suitably to produce a final concentration of about 10 mcg/ml of caffeine citrate.

Measure the extinction at maximum at about 272 nm taking water as blank. Calculate the results by comparison.

Note

The total filtrate so obtained should be presumed to be 2 ml and contains 30 mg of caffeine and further dilutions are done accordingly.

Aspirin

Standard solution

10 mcg/ml of aspirin in 7% v/v ammonia.

Sample solution

Dissolve entire insoluble residue obtained above under caffeine in 6 ml of 7% ammonia solution and filter. Dilute the filtrate suitably with 7% ammonia solution to produce concentration of about 10 mcg/ml.

Measure the extinction of sample and standard solutions at maximum at about 240 nm taking 7% ammonia solution as blank. Calculate the results by comparison.

Note

1. The above method has been extensively used with excellent results. In the opinion of the author, the method can be adopted for regular use by manufacturers of above combination.
2. The methods based on differential solubilities have been extensively used under different methods described in this book for separation and quantitative estimation of individual component in several formulations. These methods are suitable for routine quality control.

Formulation 29

Aspirin, Paracetamol, Caffeine

ESTIMATION

Aspirin

Follow the method as described in formulation 5 of this chapter.

Caffeine

Carry out chloroform extraction, followed by spectrophotometric measurement at 276 nm as described in formulation 1 of this chapter.

Paracetamol

Follow the nitroso-derivative method as described in formulation 2 of this chapter.

Working Example

Each tablet contains:

Paracetamol	250 mg
Aspirin	250 mg
Caffeine	30 mg

Average weight = 0.599 g

Estimation of Aspirin:

(Method followed: See formulation 5 of this chapter.)

Weight of sample taken for analysis = 0.486 g
Volume of 0.1 N sodium hydroxide consumed = 11.2 ml

$$\text{Aspirin, mg/tablet} = \frac{11.2 \times 0.180 \times 0.599}{0.486}$$

$$= 249 \text{ mg}$$

Claim = 250 mg

Estimation of Caffeine citrate:
(Method followed: Basification, followed by chloroform extraction, see formulation 1 of this chapter.)

Dilutions, to be done with chloroform

Standard	0.0133 g	→	100 ml;	10 ml	→	100 ml
Sample	0.602 g	→	250 ml;	10 ml	→	100 ml

	Sample	Standard
Extinction values at 276 nm	0.56	0.66

$$\text{Caffeine, mg/tablet} = \frac{0.56}{0.66} \times \left(\frac{0.0133}{100} \times \frac{10}{100} \times \frac{250}{0.602} \times \frac{100}{10} \right) \times 0.599$$

$$= 28 \text{ mg}$$

$$\text{Claim} = 30 \text{ mg}$$

Estimation of Paracetamol:
(Method followed: Nitroso-derivative, followed by coupling with cobalt—see formulation 2 of this chapter.)

Dilutions, to be done with water

Standard	0.293 g	→	50 ml;	1 ml	→	100 ml
Sample	0.059 g	→	25 ml;	1 ml	→	100 ml

	Sample	Standard
Extinction values at 395 nm	0.420	0.400

$$\text{Paracetamol, mg/tablet} = \frac{0.420}{0.400} \times \left(\frac{0.059}{25} \times \frac{1}{100} \times \frac{50}{0.293} \times \frac{100}{1} \right) \times 0.599$$

$$= 253.2 \text{ mg}$$

$$\text{Claim} = 250 \text{ mg}$$

Formulation 30

Analgin, Salicylamide

ESTIMATION

Method 1

Analgin

Weigh a quantity of powdered tablets equivalent to 200 mg of analgin and dissolve in water to produce 200 ml (1 mg/ml). Prepare standard solution of analgin of same concentration (1 mg/ml) and follow the colorimetric method involving the use of p-dimethylaminobenzaldehyde. The coloured complex exhibited absorption maxima at 420 nm. For details, refer to formulations 8 and 31 of this chapter.

Method 2

Reagents

1. 0.2% ferric chloride solution in 0.1 M HCl.
2. 0.1 N HCl.
3. 0.2% solution of 3-methyl-2-benzothiazolidone hydrochloride in 0.1 M HCl (MBTH).

Sample/standard solution

150 μg/ml in water.

Procedure

To 1 ml each of sample and standard solutions add 1 ml of MBTH reagent followed by 1 ml of ferric chloride solution, set aside for 15 min and measure the absorbance at 630 nm and calculate the results by comparison.

MBTH on oxidation with $FeCl_3$ loses two electrons and one proton. Analgin on hydrolysis gives methylamino derivative and HCHO. Formaldehyde reacts with oxidized MBTH to give Schiff's base.

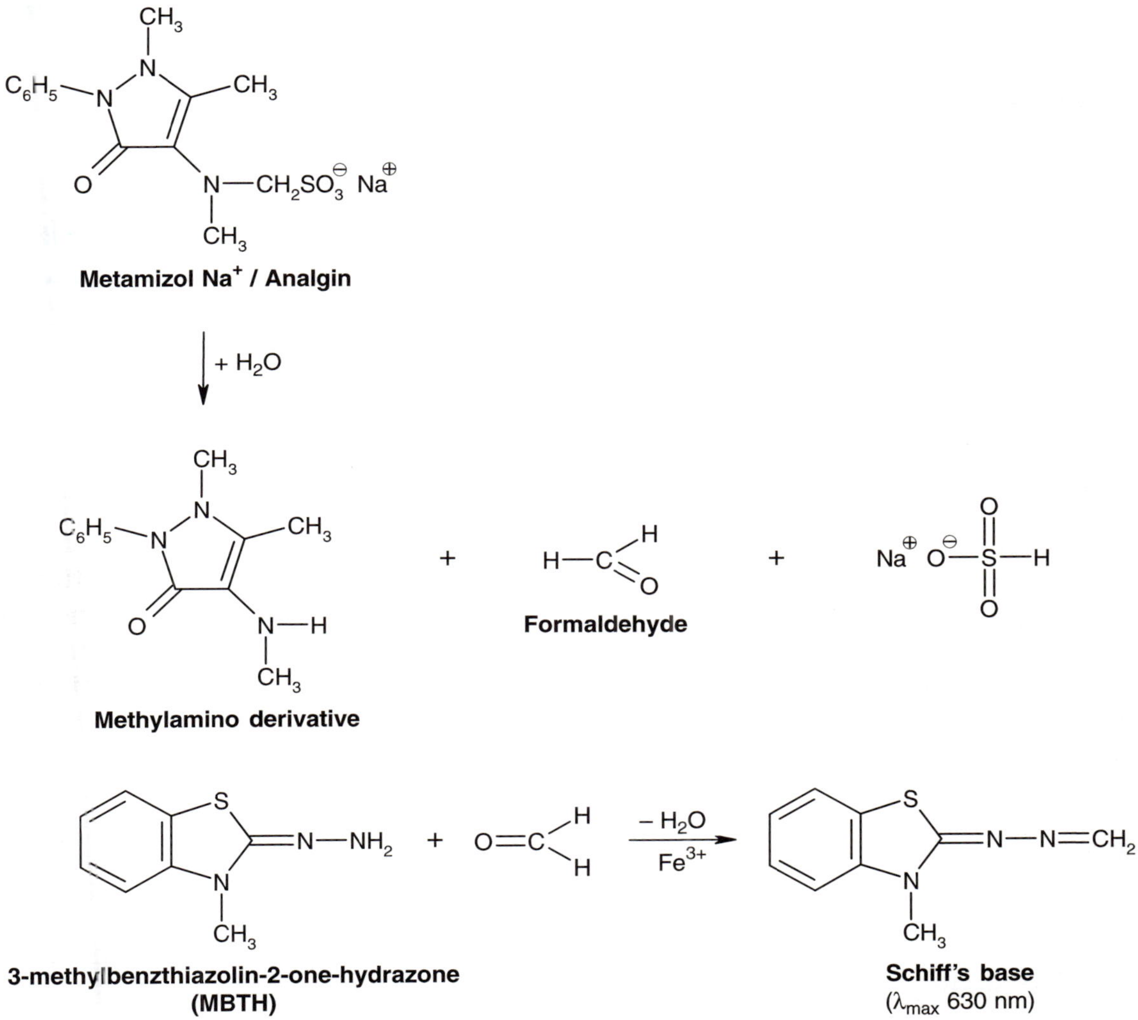

Salicylamide

Standard solution

10 mcg/ml of pure salicylamide in 1 N sodium hydroxide.

Sample solution

Weigh a quantity of powdered tablets equivalent to 100 mg of salicylamide, extract with 1 N sodium hydroxide and dilute appropriately with the same solvent to get a concentration of 10 mcg/ml.

Standard and sample solutions exhibit maximum at 328 nm. The results are calculated by comparing with the standard.

Formulation 31

Analgin, Paracetamol, Caffeine citrate, Codeine phosphate

ESTIMATION

Analgin

Reagents

1. 0.2 M phthalate buffer, pH 4.0.
2. 0.5% w/v solution of 1,2-naphthoquinone-4-sulphonic acid (sodium salt) in water.

Standard solution

1 mg/ml of analgin in water.

Sample solution

Weigh accurately a quantity of powdered tablets equivalent to 250 mg of analgin and extract with water to produce 250 ml (1 mg/ml).

Procedure

To 2 ml each of sample and standard solutions add 10 ml of buffer solution and 1 ml of naphthoquinone reagent. Heat in water bath at 50°C for 60 minutes. Cool and extract with three 20 ml portions of chloroform. Combine chloroform layer, pass through anhydrous sodium sulphate and adjust to 100 ml with chloroform. Measure the absorbance of both standard and sample solutions at about 475 nm. Deduce the results by comparison.

Probable Reaction Mechanism

In the presence of sulphuric acid, analgin undergoes hydrolysis. Since pH of the solution is less than 3.0, methylamino derivative is expected to be directly formed with the release of HCHO.

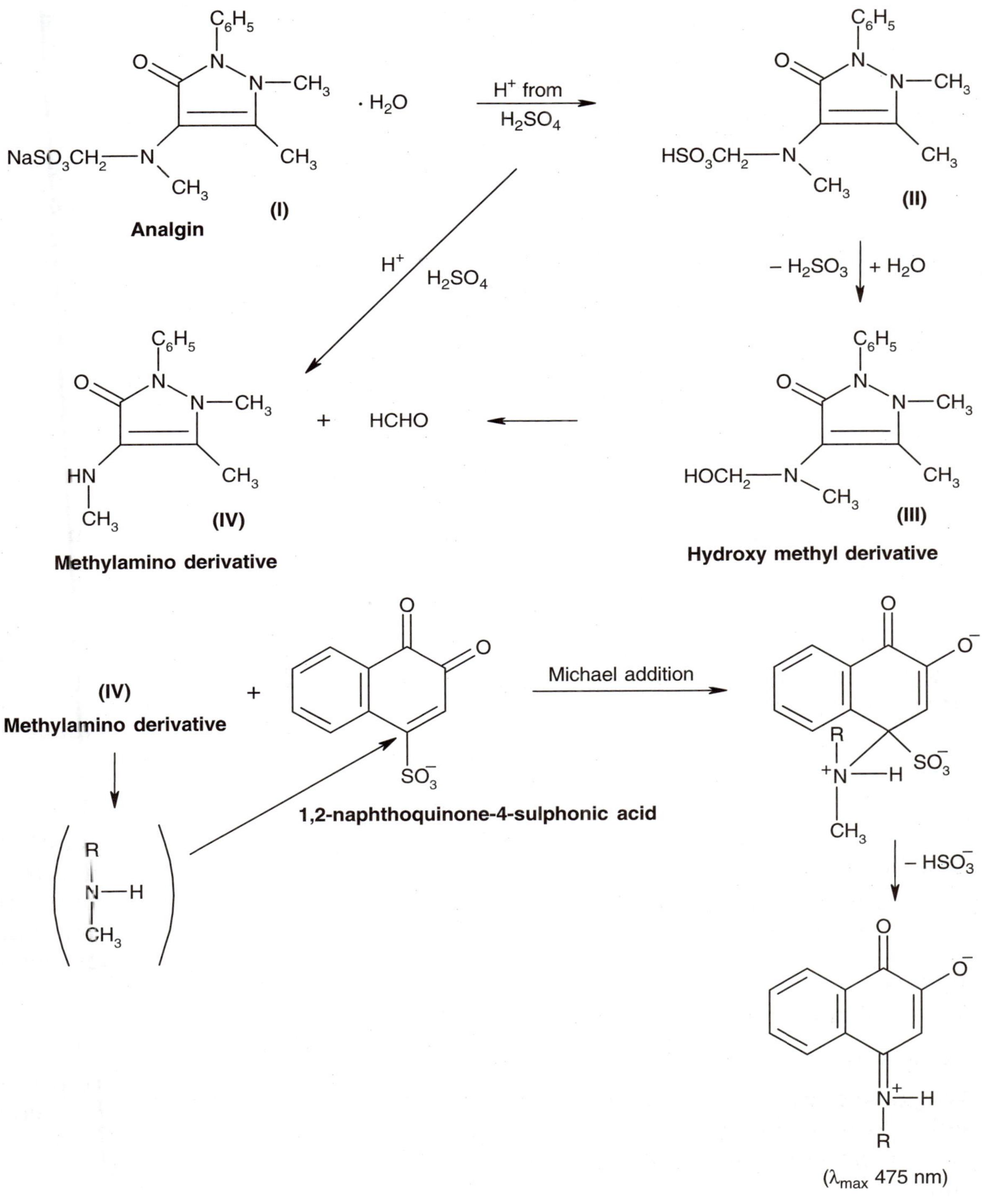

Analgin
(I)
· H2O
H+ from
H2SO4
(II)
– H2SO3
+ H2O
H+
H2SO4
(IV)
Methylamino derivative
+ HCHO
(III)
Hydroxy methyl derivative
(IV)
Methylamino derivative
+
1,2-naphthoquinone-4-sulphonic acid
Michael addition
– HSO3−
(λmax 475 nm)

Michael addition takes place with the elimination of monohydrogen sulphite radical giving quinoimine derivative.

A method has been reported based on the reaction of formaldehyde with 2,4-pentadione forming a yellow product (λ_{max} 415 nm).

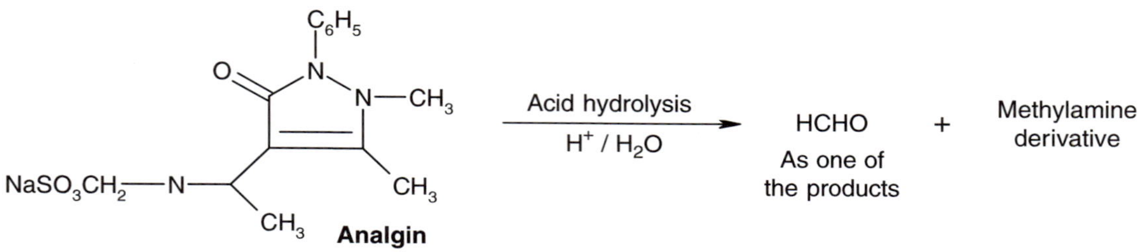

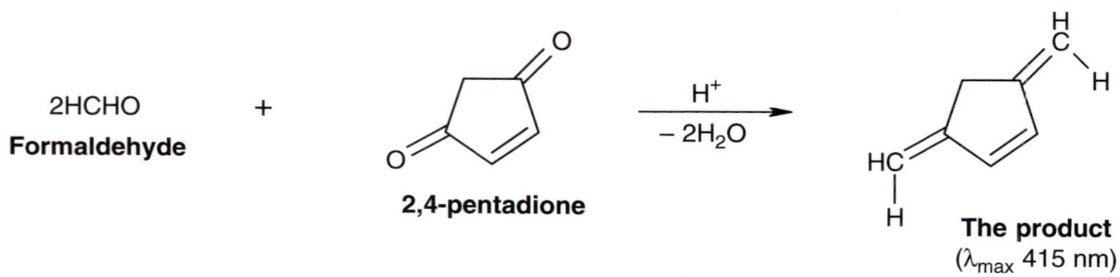

Reference

K.K. Vishwanath, A. Sivaprasada Rao & M.V. Sivaramakrishnan, Indian Drugs, **25(1)**, 25-27, 1987.

Caffeine citrate

METHOD 1

Reagents

1. 10% w/v solution of phosphomolybdic acid in water.
2. 1 M hydrochloric acid.

Standard solution

1 mg/ml of caffeine in water.

Sample solution

Weigh accurately sample equivalent to 100 mg of caffeine, add 50 ml of chloroform or dichloromethane and boil on water-bath for few minutes. Filter hot, evaporate organic layer and dissolve the residue in water to produce 100 ml.

Procedure

To 25 ml each of sample and standard solutions add 15 ml of 1 N hydrochloric acid and 3 ml of phosphomolybdic acid solution. Boil for 3 minutes, chill for 30 minutes. Filter the precipitates through dry glass sintered funnel G_4. Wash the residue with dilute hydrochloric acid till filtrate is colourless. Allow the acid layer to drain off completely. Dissolve the residue in acetone to produce 25 ml. Measure the absorbance of both standard and sample solutions at 440 nm, and calculate the results. The method obeys Beer's law in the range of 1-5 mg/ml.

METHOD 2

Reagents

1. 5% w/v solution of silicotungstic acid in alcohol–ether solvent mixture.
2. A solvent mixture of ethyl alcohol and anhydrous ether (1 : 5) v/v.

Procedure

Weigh accurately a quantity of powdered tablets equivalent to 30 mg of caffeine, extract with 100 ml of alcohol–ether solvent mixture. Filter and add 10 ml of silicotungstic acid reagent. Allow to stand for 10 minutes, filter through G_4 sintered glass funnel, wash the precipitates with the solvent mixture and dry at 105°C to a constant weight.

$$\text{Weight of caffeine (g)} = \text{Weight of the precipitates (g)} \times 0.1701$$

The precipitates obtained above can be dissolved in water to get a concentration of 10 mcg/ml in respect of caffeine which exhibits maxima at above 265 nm. For details, refer to the method for estimation of caffeine described under formulation 1 of this chapter.

Codeine phosphate

METHOD 1

This is based on estimation of phosphate moiety of the compound.

Reagents

1. 10 N sulphuric acid.
2. Stannous chloride solution: To 1 g stannous chloride add 5 ml of concentrated hydrochloric acid. Heat on boiling water-bath till clear solution is obtained. Just before use, dilute 1 ml of this solution to 100 ml with water.
3. Ammonium molybdate solution: To 6.4 g of ammonium molybdate add 40 ml of water and 50 ml of 10 N sulphuric acid. Make up to 100 ml with water.

Standard solution

100 mcg/ml of codeine phosphate in water.

Sample solution

Weigh accurately powdered material equivalent to 10 mg of codeine phosphate and extract with water to produce 100 ml.

Procedure

To 10 ml each of sample and standard solutions add 50 ml of water, 10 ml of 10 N sulphuric acid and 10 ml of ammonium molybdate solution. Then, add 5 ml of stannous chloride solution with care and shake. Keep at room temperature for 60 minutes and dilute with water to 100 ml. Measure the absorbance of both the solutions at 675 nm and calculate the results by comparison.

Formulation 32

Paracetamol, Oxyphencyclimine hydrochloride

ESTIMATION

Paracetamol

Reagents

1. 1 N sodium hydroxide.
2. 0.2% w/v solution of sodium nitroprusside in water.

Standard solution

Weigh 100 mg of standard paracetamol, add 50 ml of dilute hydrochloric acid.

Sample solution

Powdered sample equivalent to 100 mg of paracetamol is transferred to 100 ml volumetric flask, add 50 ml of dilute hydrochloric acid.

Procedure

Keep both sample and standard solutions in boiling water-bath for one hour. Cool and dilute to 100 ml with water. Filter and dilute 1 ml of the filtrate to 100 ml with water.

To 5 ml each of sample and standard solutions add 0.5 ml of sodium nitroprusside solution and 4.5 ml of sodium hydroxide solution. Measure the absorbance of both the solutions at 730 nm after 10 minutes and calculate the results by comparison.

Explanatory Note

p-aminophenol formed reacts with sodium nitroprusside (disodium pentacyano-nitrosylferrate) in alkaline medium to form the complex.

Probable Reaction Mechanism

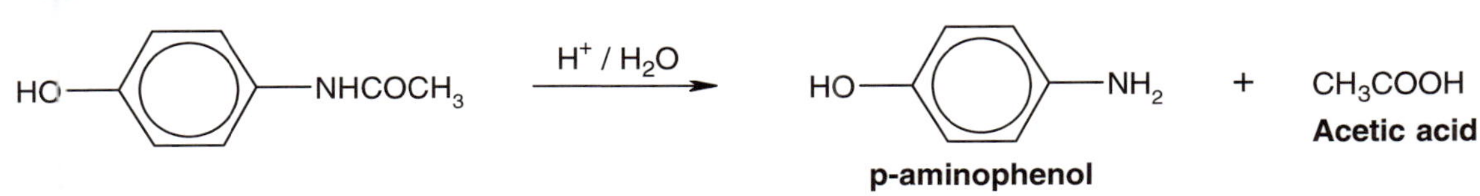

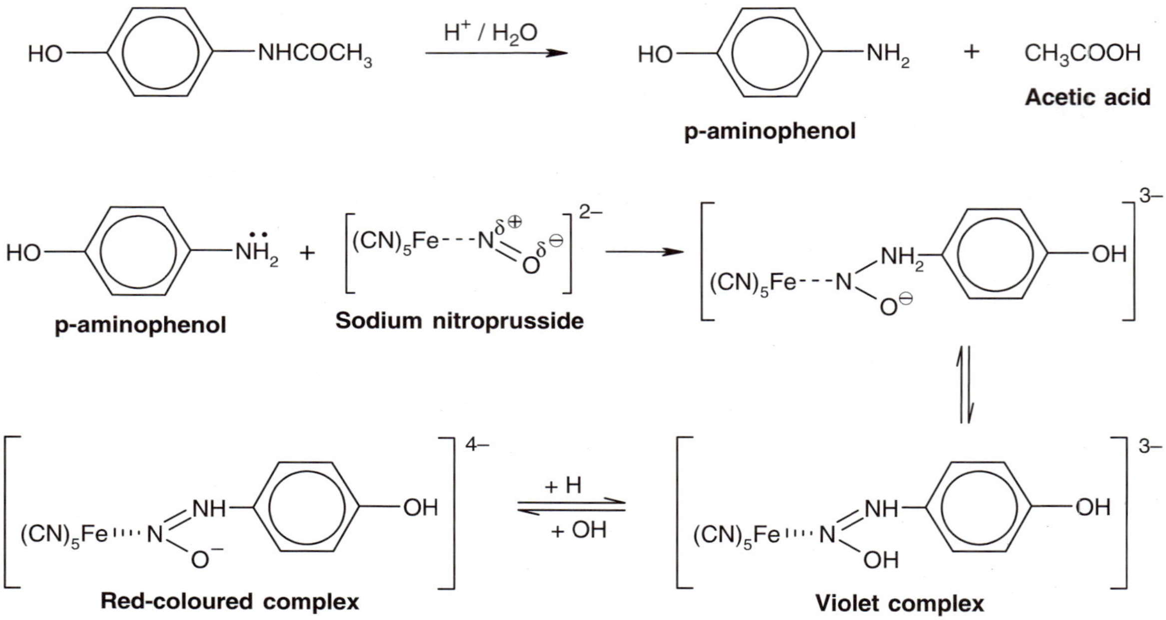

Oxyphencyclimine hydrochloride

Procedure

Transfer accurately weighed quantity of the powdered tablets equivalent to about 25 mg of oxyphencyclimine hydrochloride to a separator. Basify with sodium hydroxide solution (5% w/v). Extract with five 25 ml portions of chloroform. Pass chloroform extract through anhydrous sodium sulphate and evaporate the combined chloroform extract on water-bath till the volume is reduced to about 2 ml. Cool, add 5 ml of acetic anhydride and 10 ml of glacial acetic acid. Carry out non-aqueous titration with 0.02 N perchloric acid using crystal violet solution as indicator. Each ml of 0.02 N perchloric acid is equivalent to 0.0076189 g of oxyphencyclimine hydrochloride.

Formulation 33

Paracetamol, Diclofenac sodium

ESTIMATION

Paracetamol

Standard solution

10 mcg/ml of paracetamol in 0.1 M hydrochloric acid.

Sample solution

Weigh accurately powdered sample equivalent to about 100 mg of paracetamol. Carry out the dry extraction with three 25 ml portions of 0.1 M hydrochloric acid, filtering through G_4 sintered glass funnel. Dilute the combined filtrate to 100 ml with acid. Dilute further appropriately with the acid to get final concentration of 10 mcg/ml.

Measure the extinction of both sample and standard solutions at maxima at about 244 nm and deduce the results by comparison. Alternatively, follow the method described in formulation 3 of this chapter.

Diclofenac sodium

METHOD 1

Standard solution

The entire residue left after the extraction of paracetamol as described above is used for estimation of diclofenac sodium. Transfer the residue left in the conical flask and on the top of sintered funnel quantitatively to 100 ml volumetric flask with the help of 0.1 M sodium hydroxide. Make up the volume and carry out the further dilutions appropriately with sodium hydroxide to get final concentration of 10 mcg/ml.

Measure the extinction of standard and sample solutions at maxima at about 276 nm using 0.1 M sodium hydroxide solution as blank. Deduce the results by comparison.

Note

Diclofenac sodium can be neutralized to obtain its free COOH group which will dissolve in solution of Na_2CO_3 with evolution of CO_2 and formation of non-metallic salt by displacement of 'H' of the carboxyl group. Paracetamol containing phenolic-OH does not react with Na_2CO_3. Since hydrogen atoms of both acidic-OH and phenolic-OH groups are displaced by the metal, we can employ Na_2CO_3 to selectively estimate diclofenac sodium without any interference from paracetamol whereas paracetamol is hydrolysed in dilute HCl by refluxing to liberate p-aminophenol which behaves like primary amine and estimation by diazotization without any interference from diclofenac.

Reference

P. Parimoo et al., *The Eastern Pharmacist*, pp. 111-112, April 1997.

METHOD 2 (a & b)

Reagents

1. 0.2% w/v solution of ferric chloride in methanol.
2. 2,2′-bipyridine solution: 0.5% w/v solution in methanol.
3. Ammonia - ammonium chloride buffer, pH 9.4: Prepared by mixing equal volumes of 1 M ammonia and ammonium chloride and adjusting the pH with sodium hydroxide or hydrochloric acid.
4. Methylene blue solution: 0.032% w/v solution in pH 9.4 buffer (extract with chloroform and discard organic layer).

Standard solution

(a) 25 mcg/ml of diclofenac sodium in water.
(b) 50 mcg/ml of diclofenac sodium in buffer.

Sample solution

Accurately weighed quantity of the powdered sample equivalent to 500 mg of diclofenac sodium was shaken for 5 min with 30 ml of water, made up to 50 ml and filtered.

(a) Dilute 5 mg of the filtrate to 200 ml with water.
(b) Dilute 5 ml of the filtrate to 100 ml with buffer.

Procedure

(a) To 5 ml each of sample and standard solutions, marked "a" above, add 1 ml each of ferric chloride and 2,2′-bipyridine solution, keep in water-bath for 5 min, cool to room temperature and dilute to 10 ml with water. Measure absorbance of both sample and standard solutions at 520 nm against reagent blank and calculate the results by comparison.

(b) To 10 ml each of sample and standard solutions, marked "b" above, add 5 ml of methylene blue solution and 1 ml of pH 9.4 buffer. The complex extracted with chloroform (10 + 10 + 5 ml) passing each extract through anhydrous sodium sulphate, diluted to 25 ml with chloroform. Absorbance of the resulting solution was measured at 650 nm against reagent blank and results calculated by comparison. The compound forms ion-pair complex extractable into chloroform.

Note

Both these methods were found to be suitable for gels also.

Alternatively, diclofenac sodium can be estimated by non-aqueous titration by dissolving the powdered sample equivalent to 250 mg of the substance in 50 ml of glacial acetic acid and titrating with 0.05 N perchloric acid (crystal violet).

Each ml of 0.05 N perchloric acid is equivalent to 15.905 mg of diclofenac sodium.

Paracetamol in the above combination can be directly estimated by UV method described in formulation 25 or 32 of this chapter.

Diclofenac sodium has insignificant absorption at 257 nm, the absorption maxima of paracetamol. However, if contents of diclofenac sodium are more than 10% of the paracetamol contents, it will interfere in the assay of paracetamol.

Probable Reaction Mechanism (2a)

The compound is oxidized with Fe(III). Fe(II) so produced complexes with bispyridine to give coloured complex (λ_{max} 520 nm). Several ligands with

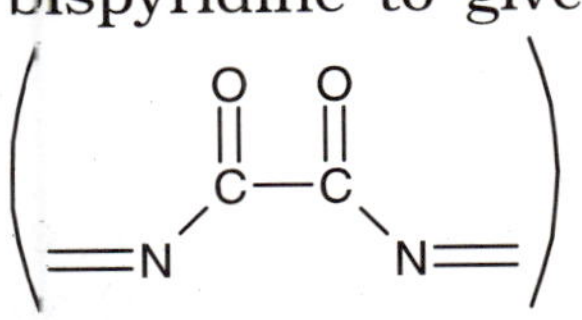

grouping is the most effective reagent for spectrophotometric estimation of Fe^{++} ion. The most widely used ligands are 1,10-phenanthroline and 2,2′-bispyridine.

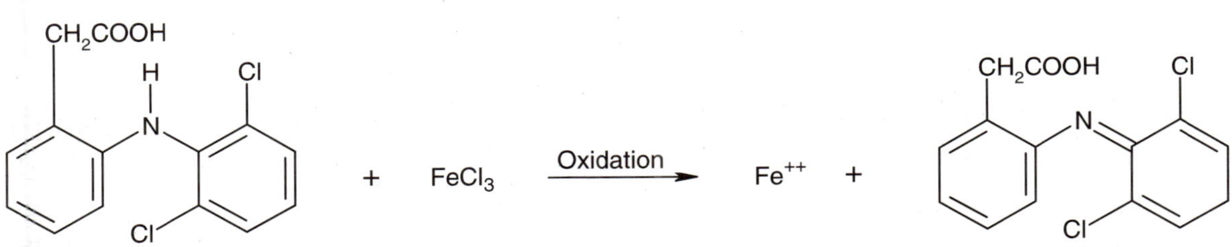

Diclofenac **Oxidized diclofenac**

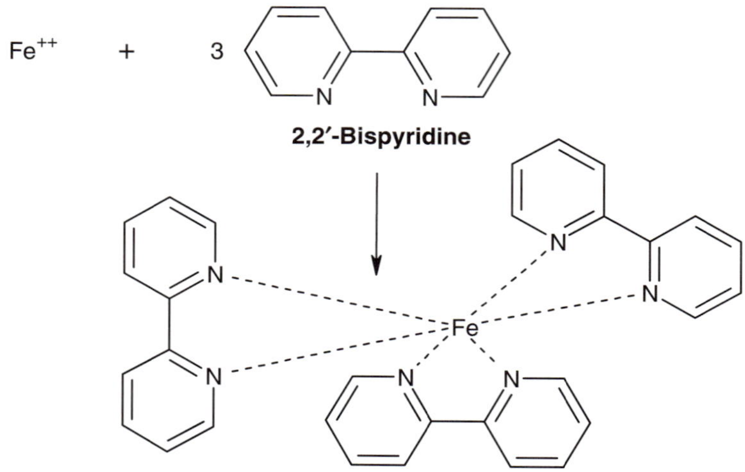

(λ_{max} 520 nm)

Two nitrogen atoms in 2,2′-bispyridyl have one unshared pair of electrons which can be shared by Fe(II) to give coloured complex.

Note

2,2′-bipyridine – $FeCl_3$ reagent is called "Emmerie–Engel reagent". Other compounds reacting with reagent giving coloured complexes are phenolic substances, vitamin E (tocopherol), ascorbic acid, captopril, methionine and cysteine.

Probable Reaction Mechanism (2b)

The compound forms ion-pair complex with 2 dyes. The complexes are extractable into chloroform.

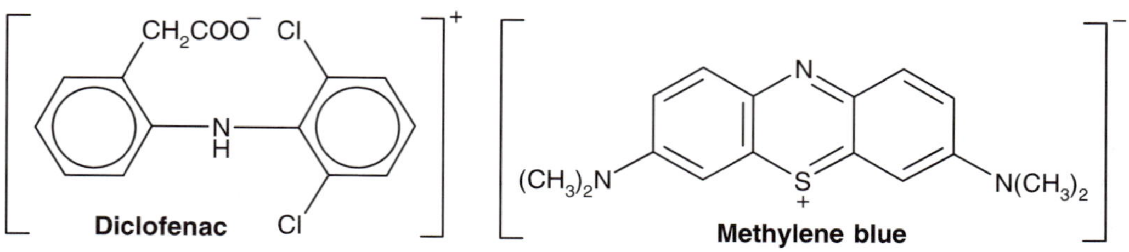

Diclofenac - methylene blue ion-pair complex
(λ_{max} 450 nm)

Reference

Julio C. Botello & Guadalupe Perez–Caballero, *Talanta*, **42(1)**, 105-108, 1995.

Note

Ion-pair complex with methylene violet in 0.067 M phosphate buffer, pH 7.6, is reported. The ion-pair complex is extractable into chloroform and has λ_{max} 540 nm.

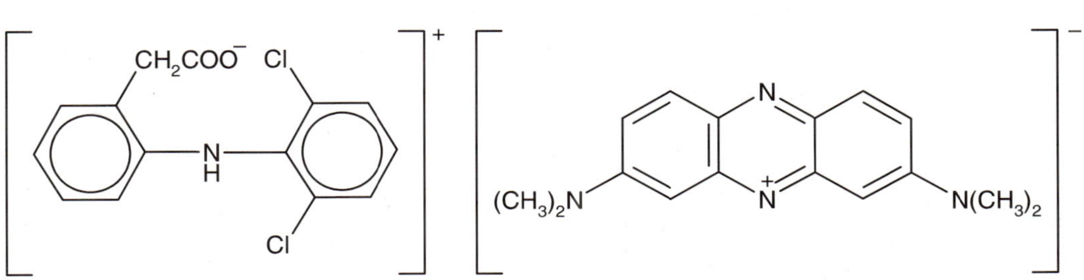

Diclofenac **Methylene violet**

Diclofenac - methylene violet ion-pair complex
(λ_{max} 540 nm)

Reference

C.S.P. Sastry, A.S.R. Prasad Tipirneni & M.V. Saryanarayana, *Analyst*, **114**, 513-515, 1989.

Note

The method has been applied for estimation of ketoprofen, ibuprofen, piroxicam, mefenamic acid and enfenamic acid.

METHOD 3

To 1 ml each of sample and standard solutions (1 mg/ml in water) add 5 ml of methanol, 1 ml of orthophosphoric acid and 1 ml of 0.25% solution of sodium cobaltinitrite. Heat in a water-bath at 45-50°C for 30 min, cool and dilute to 10 ml with methanol. Measure the absorbance of both sample and standard solutions at 368 nm against reagent blank and calculate the results by comparison.

Probable Reaction Mechanism

The drug forms cobalt complex to give yellow-coloured product (λ_{max} 368 nm).

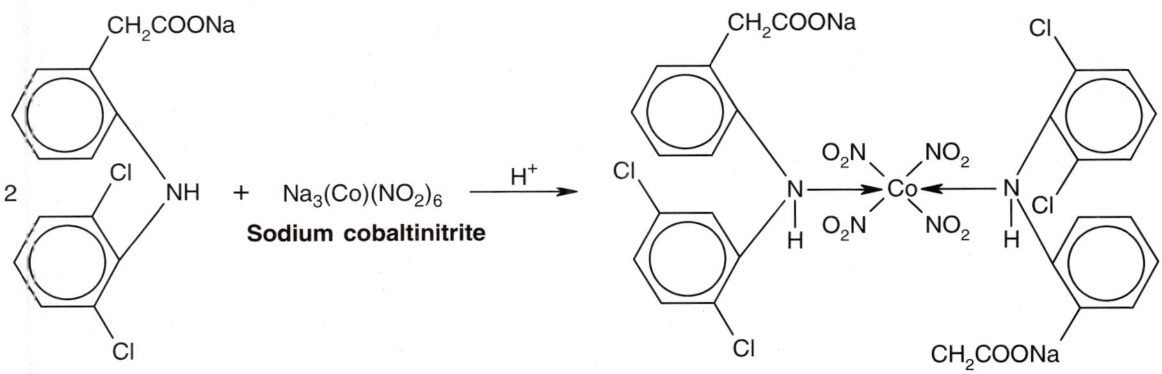

Diclofenac sodium

Yellow-coloured complex
(λ_{max} 368 nm)

Reference

Ashok K.S., K. Gopal & P. Mishra, *Ind. J. Pharm. Sci.*, **54(1)**, 44-46, 1991.

METHOD 4

Reagents

1. 2% w/v solution of ferric chloride in 0.1 N hydrochloric acid, filter if necessary.
2. 0.1 N solution of 3-methyl-2-benzothiazolinone hydrazone hydrochloride (MBTH).

Standard solution

25 mcg/ml solution of diclofenac sodium in 0.01 N sodium hydroxide.

Sample solution

Sample is extracted with 0.01 M sodium hydroxide, filtered and used for analysis.

Procedure

To 3 ml each of sample and standard solutions add 1 ml of 1 N hydrochloric acid, 1 ml of ferric chloride solution, shake and add 1 ml of the hydrazone reagent. Heat in a water-bath at 40°C for 15 min, cool and dilute to 250 ml with acetone. Measure the absorbance of sample and standard solutions at 590 nm against blank and calculate the results by comparison.

Probable Reaction Mechanism

Oxidative coupling occurs at the para position to the secondary amino group in the drug in the presence of an oxidizing agent. The oxidizing agent used here is $FeCl_3$. In the initial stages of the reaction, MBTH loses 2 electrons and a proton to give electrophilic intermediate (II) which is postulated to be active coupling species. It reacts with diclofenac by electrophilic attack on the most nucleophilic site in the aromatic ring of the compound i.e. para position of the secondary amino group resulting in coloured species. The reaction can be represented as under:

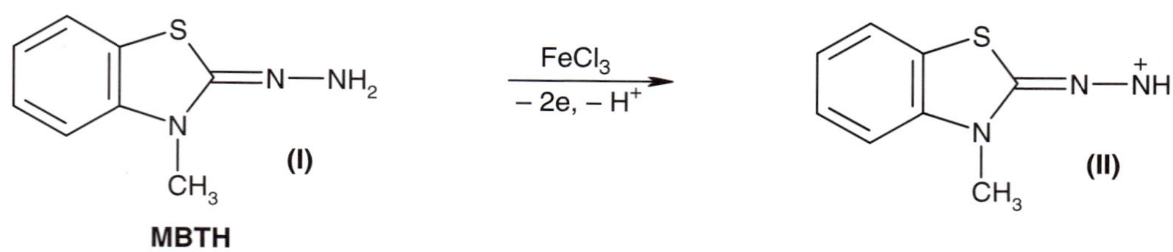

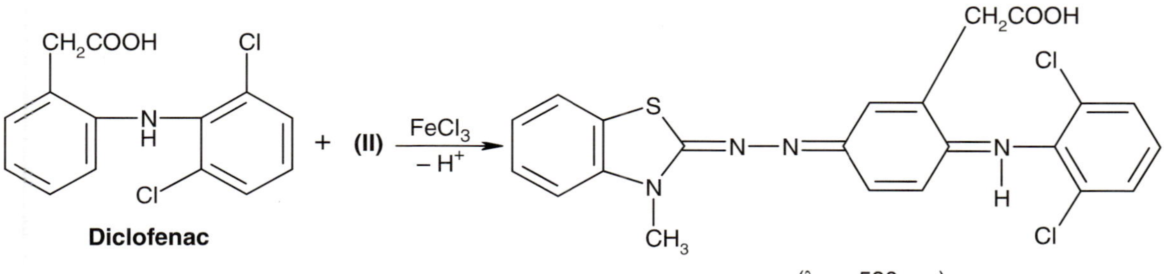

Garcia et al. (1998) have described spectrophotometric method based on formation of coloured compound with MBTH using ceric (IV) as oxidizing agent.

Reagents

1. 9 M sulphuric acid.
2. Ceric ammonium nitrate solution in 9 M H_2SO_4.
3. MBTH solution – 200 μg/ml in water.

Standard solution

100 μg/ml solution of diclofenac sodium in water.

Sample solution (Tablets, suppositories, gel and injection)

Extracted with water by sonication.

Probable Reaction Mechanism

Diclofenac sodium containing a diphenylamine group reacts with MBTH in presence of an oxidizing agent to form a coloured oxidative coupling product. Preliminaries studies showed that in diluted sulphuric acid medium (1.5×10^{-2} M) and employing Ce(IV) as oxidant, the product formed presented an absorption maximum at 580 nm. Mixtures of MBTH and oxidant (reagent blank) or DCF and oxidant show low or no absorbance at this wavelength. The absorbance was measured at 580 nm in all subsequent studies.

Under the reaction conditions MBTH (**I**) loses two electrons and one proton on oxidation forming an electrophilic intermediate (**II**) which has been postulated to be the active coupling species. The intermediate reacts with diclofenac (**III**) by electrophilic attack on the most nucleophilic site on the aromatic ring of the diclofenac, p-position to secondary amino group, and the resulting intermediate is spontaneously oxidized with Ce(IV) to form the coloured species.

Reference

M. Soledad Garcia et al., *J. Pharm. Biomed. Analysis*, **17**, 267-273, 1998.

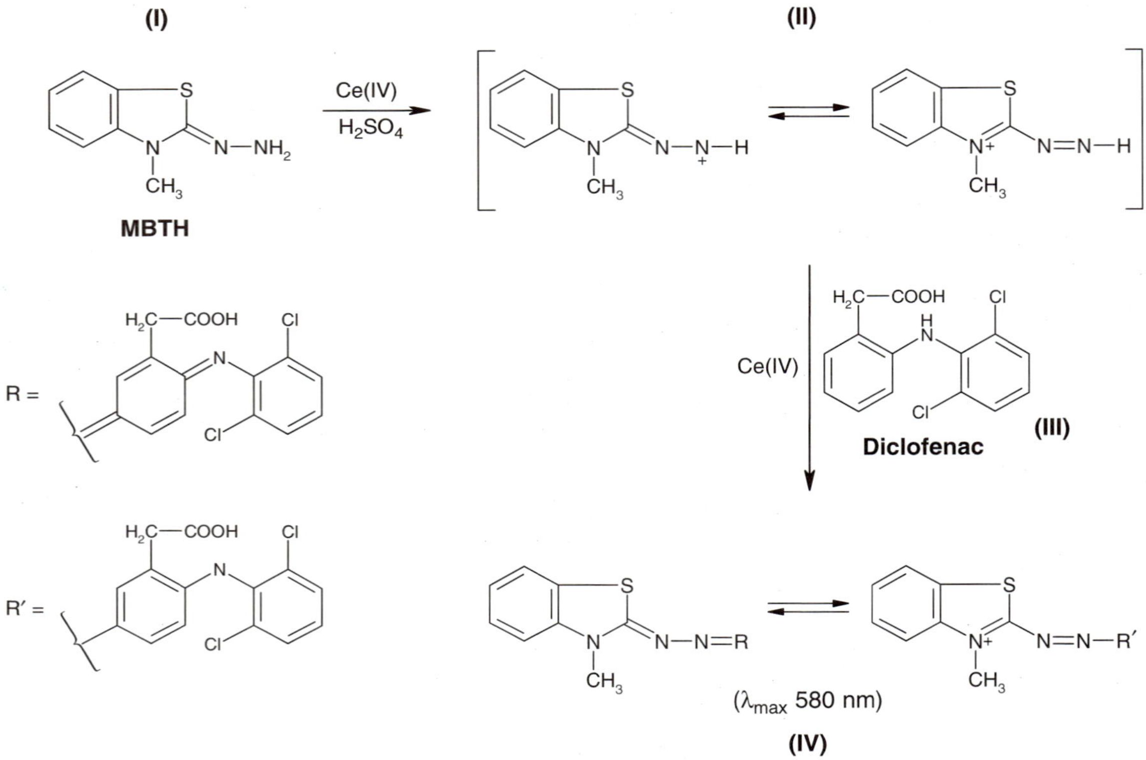

Reaction between diclofenac – MBTH – Ce(IV)

METHOD 5

Reagent

Copper chloride solution: Dissolve 3 g of copper (II) chloride in 25 ml of pyridine and dilute to 100 ml with water.

Standard solution

1 mg/ml of diclofenac sodium in water.

Sample solution

Extract accurately weighed quantity of the sample with warm water to get final concentration of 1 mg/ml.

Procedure

To 4 ml each of sample and standard solutions add 6 ml of copper chloride solution, shake and extract the complex with 10 ml of chloroform shaking intermittently for 10 min. Separate chloroform layer and measure its absorbance at about 730 nm against blank prepared by following above procedure except the sample. The method obeys Beer's law in the concentration range of 1-10 μg/ml of diclofenac sodium.

Probable Reaction Mechanism

The drug forms chelate with Cu^{++} in alkaline medium (pyridine). Pyridine also stabilizes the copper complex.

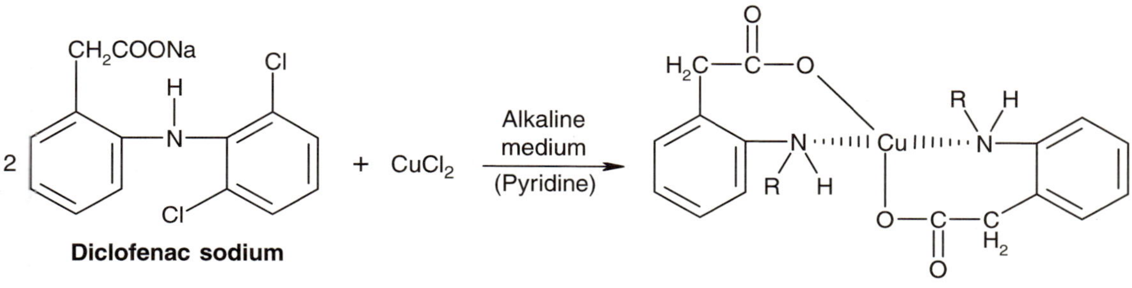

Copper complex
(λ_{max} 730 nm)

R =

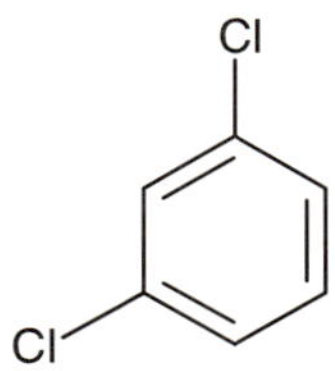

Reference

M.S. Bhatia & S.R. Dhaneshwar, *Eastern Pharmacist*, p. 133, Feb. 1995.

Turbino et al. have described gravimetric method for estimation of diclofenac from formulations based on reaction with Cu^{2+} (copper acetate) in pH 5.3 acetate buffer. Light green complex with copper (1 : 2) is soluble in organic solvents but insoluble in water. The precipitates are filtered through G_3 sintered glass funnel, heat at 130°C for 60 min to ensure complete loss of water and weighed. Excess copper acetate should be added to ensure complete precipitation.

Reference

Mathieu Turbino & Rafael L. De Souza, *JAOAC Int.*, **88(6)**, 1684-1687, 2005.

Z.A. El-Sherif reported that secondary aromatic amine of the drug condenses with 'PDAC' in acidic medium (CCl_3COOH) and forms the basis for quantitative estimation. The following reaction was proposed.

Probable Reaction Mechanism

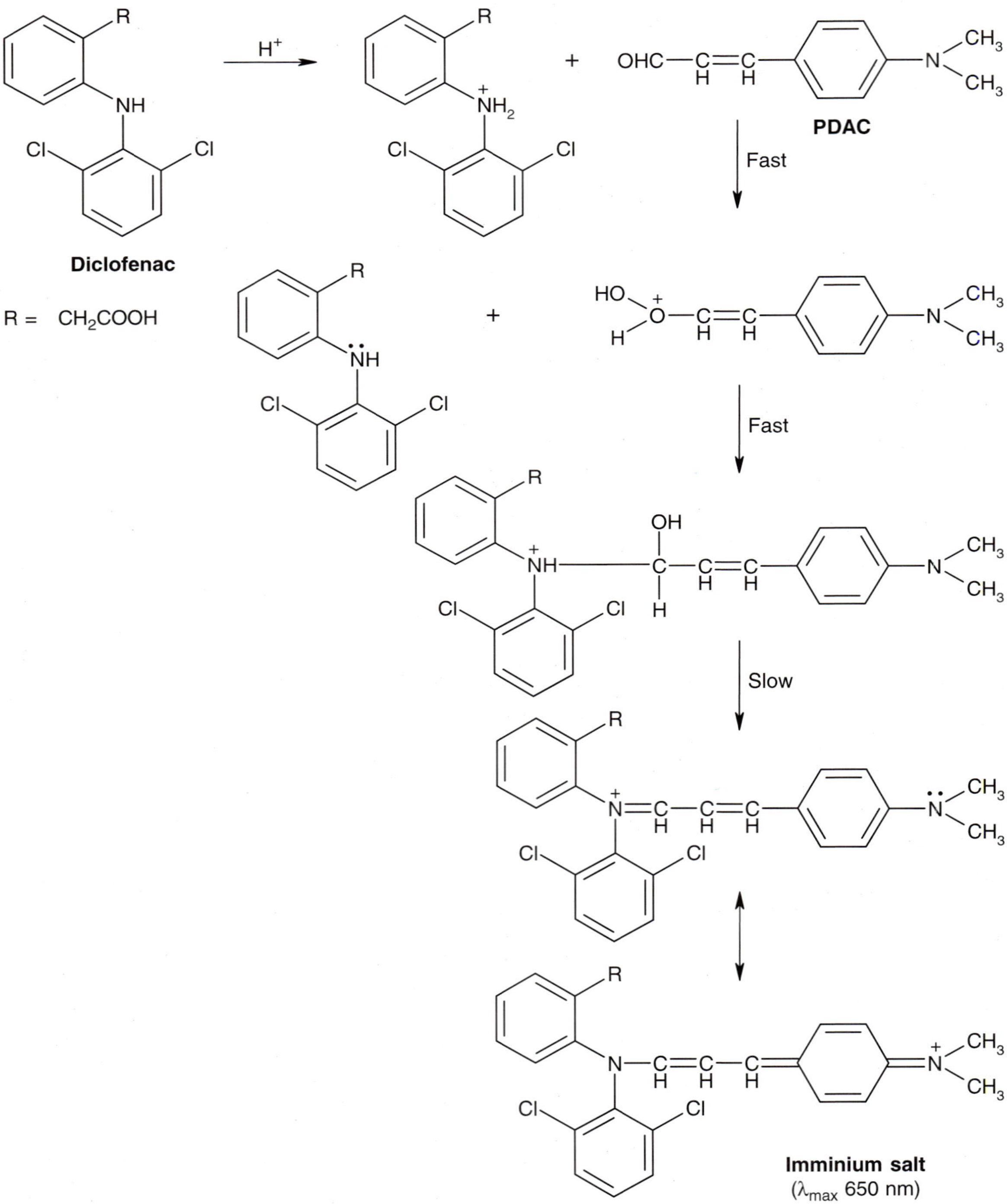

Reference

Z.A. El Sherif, M.I. Walash, M.F. El Tarras & A.O. Oman, *Analytical Letters*, **30(10)**, 1881-1896, 1997.

Similar method is reported for aceclofenac in formulations (N.H. Zawilla, M. Abul Azim Mohamaad, N.M. El Kousy & S.M. El-Moghazy, *J. Pharm. & Biomed. Analysis*, **27**, 243-251, 2002).

Diclofenac is reported to form complex with $K_3Fe(CN)_6$ in alkaline medium to give orange-coloured complex (λ_{max} 450 nm).

Probable Reaction Mechanism

The drug solution (100 μg/ml) is mixed with $K_3Fe(CN)_6$ (1%) and sodium hydroxide (5%), diluted with water. The orange colour is measured at 450 nm.

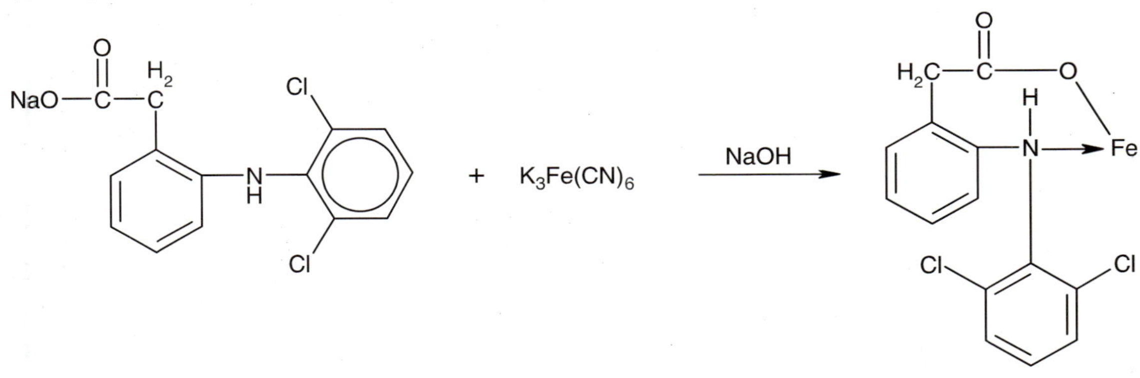

(λ_{max} 450 nm)

Reference

R.T. Sane, R.S. Sawant & V.G. Nayak, *Indian Drugs*, **24(3)**, 161-162, 1986.

The drug undergoes nitrosation reaction at secondary amine. The nitrosonium ion being electron-deficient attacks the secondary amine resulting in the formation of nitroso derivative (λ_{max} 378 nm).

Probable Reaction Mechanism

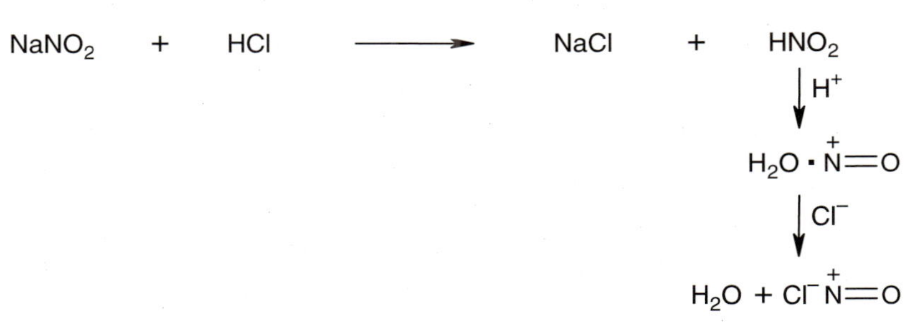

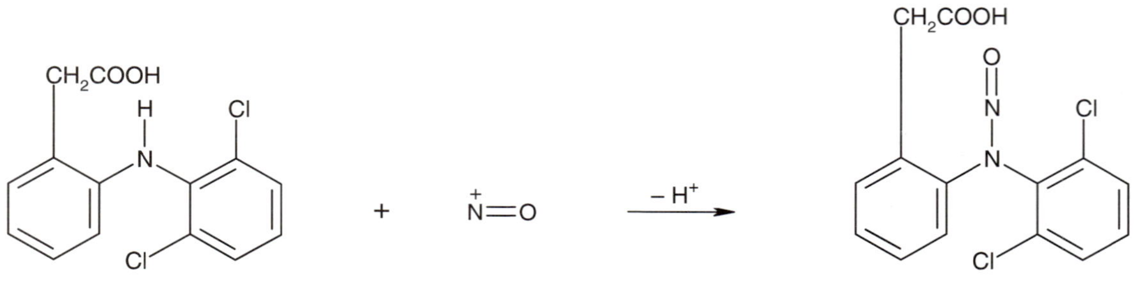

N-Nitroso derivative
(N-nitrosamine)
(λ_{max} 378 nm)

Note

The drug reacts with sodium cobaltinitrite to give similar product (λ_{max} 368 nm)—see method 3.

Reference

1. K.S. Ashok, K. Gopal & Pardeep Mishra, Ind. J. Pharm. Sci., **54(1)**, 44-46, 1991.
2. S.C. Mathur, Y. Kumar, P.B.N. Prasad, A.C.S. Rao, Y.K.S. Rathor & S.C. Gupta, Indian Drugs, **31(9)**, 447-448, 1994.
3. Textbook of Practical Organic Chemistry by Vogel, p. 920.

N-nitrosamine formed above can undergo Fischer–Hepp re-arrangement to give n-nitrosation product i.e. we may get mixture of N-nitroso derivative and C-nitroso derivative as explained below.

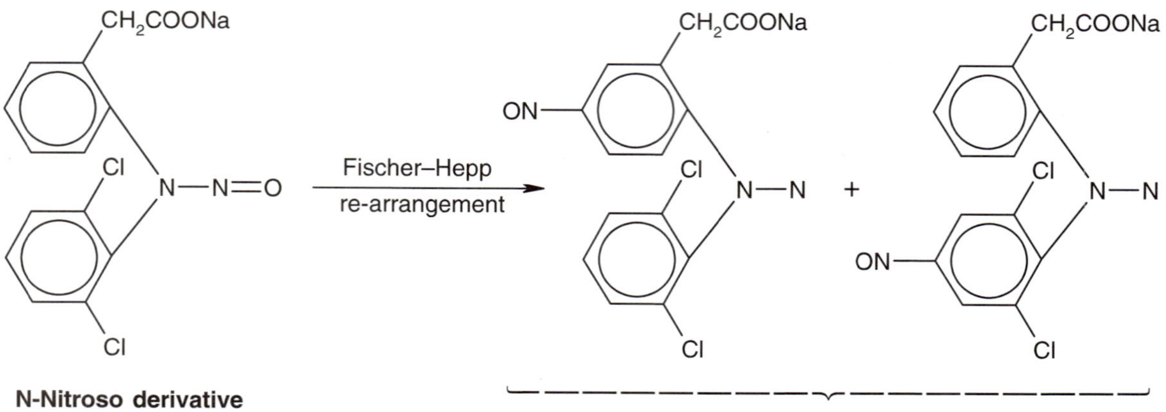

N-Nitroso derivative

C-nitrosation product

Reference

Advanced Organic Chemistry by Jerry March, pp. 470, 502.

Note

A similar method for compounds with secondary amine group (mefenamic acid) has been described using 'PDAB' as chromogenic reagent.

Reference

Tehseen Aman et al., *Analytical Letters*, **38**, 1899-1912, 2005.

Diclofenac gets oxidized with ferric chloride and itself gets converted to Fe^{2+} which in turn reacts with potassium ferricyanide to give prussian blue colour (λ_{max} 700 nm).

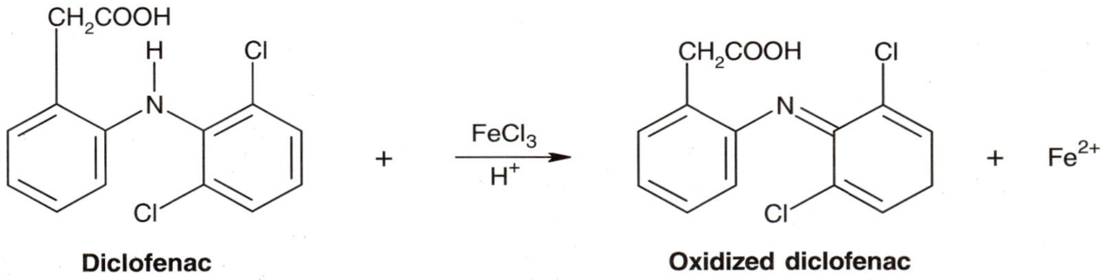

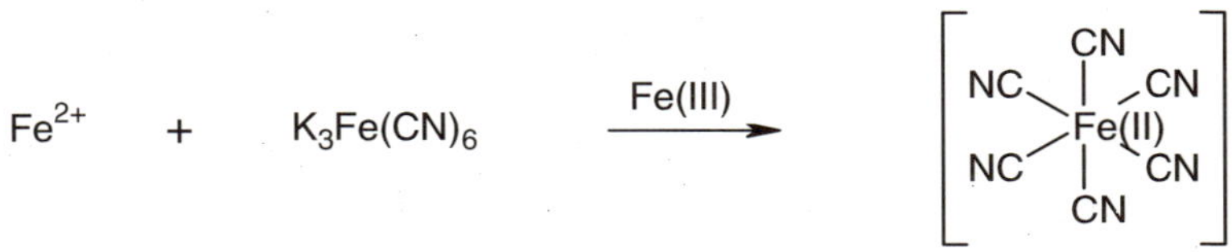

Prussian blue colour
(λ_{max} 700 nm)

Note

A similar reaction is described for aceclofenac, a related compound giving blue colour (λ_{max} 760 nm).

Reference

M.M. Langade, *Analytical Chemistry, An Indian Journal (ACAIJ)*, **8(2)**, 2009.

Formulation 34

Paracetamol, Metoclopramide hydrochloride

ESTIMATION

Paracetamol

Standard solution

10 mcg/ml of paracetamol in 0.01 M sodium hydroxide.

Sample solution

Weigh accurately sample equivalent to about 50 mg of paracetamol. Add 25 ml of 0.1 M sodium hydroxide and shake for 10-15 min, dilute to 100 ml with water, mix and filter. Dilute further appropriately with 0.01 M sodium hydroxide solution to get final concentration of 10 mcg/ml.

Measure the extinction of both sample and standard solutions at 257 nm. Calculate the results by comparison or by using 715 as value of A 1%, 1 cm at 257 nm.

Metoclopramide hydrochloride

METHOD 1

Reagents

1. Bromothymol blue solution: Dissolve 150 mg of bromothymol blue and 150 mg of anhydrous sodium carbonate in water to make 100 ml.
2. Citric acid – phosphate buffer, pH 5.7: Buffer is prepared by mixing appropriately 10% w/v solutions of citric acid and disodium phosphate or phosphate buffer, pH 6.2.
3. 2% w/v solution of boric acid in methanol.

Standard solution

100 mcg/ml of metoclopramide hydrochloride in water.

Sample solution

Weigh accurately a quantity of the sample equivalent to about 10 mg of the substance. Add about 50 ml of water and warm in a warm-bath for 20-25 min to effect complete solution. Cool to room temperature and adjust the volume to 100 ml with water.

Procedure

To 5 ml each of sample and standard solutions add 1 ml of dye solution and 20 ml of phosphate buffer solution. Mix and extract with three 25 ml portions of chloroform. Pass each chloroform layer through anhydrous sodium sulphate. Add 25 ml of boric acid solution and dilute to 100 ml with chloroform. Measure the absorbance of both the solutions at about 425 nm using chloroform as blank. Calculate the results by comparison.

Note

1. Allow complete separation of layers after each extraction.
2. Extract the dye solution with chloroform till chloroform layer is colourless before using the dye for colour development; this will reduce the blank value.
3. Centrifuge the chloroform layer for consistent results.

Explanatory Note

It is based on the formation of ion-pair complex between the drug and the dye in pH 5.7 buffer solution with λ_{max} 425 nm.

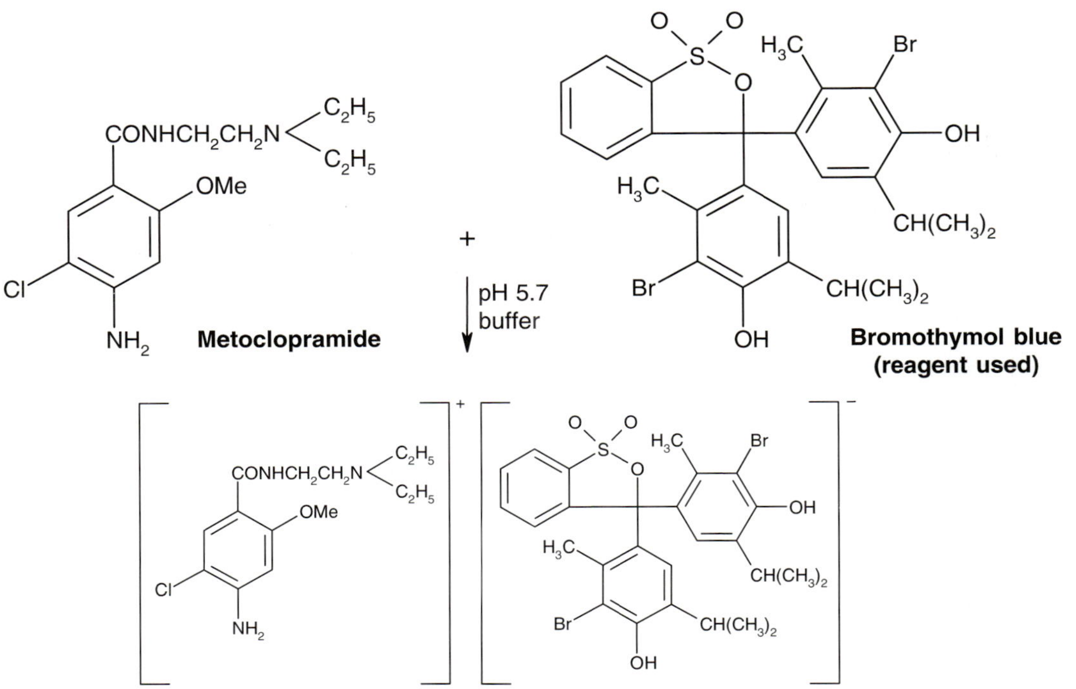

Yellow-coloured ion-pair complex extractable into chloroform
(λ_{max} 425 nm)

Reference

D.M. Shingbal & V.S. Velingkar, *Indian Drugs*, **25(12)**, 529-531, 1988.

But at higher pH, the colour of the dye changes to blue. This is because of the following change occurring in the structure of the dye in alkaline medium (pH 7.6). This can be utilized for quantitative analysis by diluting the $CHCl_3$ layer (containing the complex) with alkaline methanol (pH > 7.6) and λ_{max} at about 620 nm.

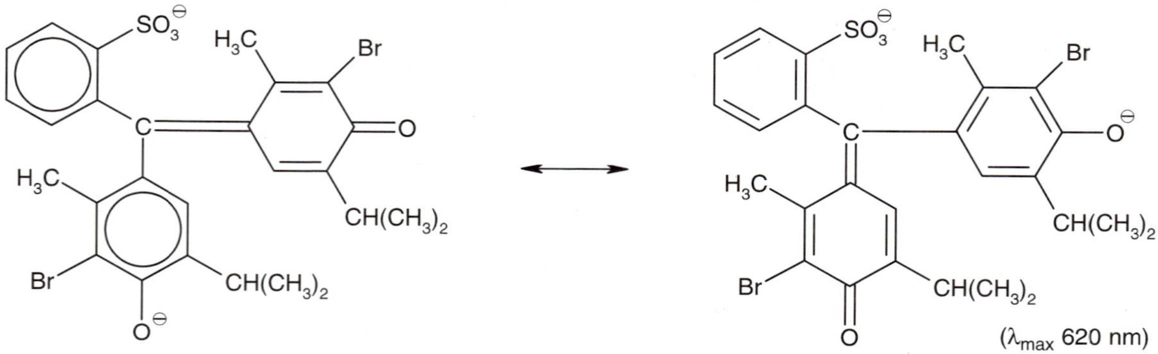

Reference

Indian Drugs, **20**, 490, Sept. 1983.

METHOD 2

Reagents

1. 1% solution of p-dimethylaminobenzaldehyde in 0.05 M sulphonic acid (Ehrlich's reagent).
2. 0.1% alkaline solution of β-naphthol in 1 M sodium hydroxide.
3. 0.05 M sulphuric acid in methanol.

Standard solution

(a) 500 μg/ml in methanol; and (b) 100 μg/ml in water.

Sample solution

Powdered sample dissolved in methanol (a) or water (b) to get respective concentration.

Procedure

(a) To 1 ml each of sample or standard solution add 1 ml of Ehrlich's reagent and 0.5 ml of methanolic sulphuric acid, keep aside for 2 min and dilute to 10 ml with methanol and measure the absorbance of resulting solution at 438 nm against reagent blank.

(b) To 1 ml of diazotized metoclopramide solution add 0.5 ml of β-naphthol solution, dilute to 10 ml with water and measure the absorbance at 550 nm against reagent blank.

Probable Reaction Mechanism

In method (a) the compound forms Schiff's base with PDAB whereas in method (b) the diazotized compound couples with β-naphthol.

Method (a)

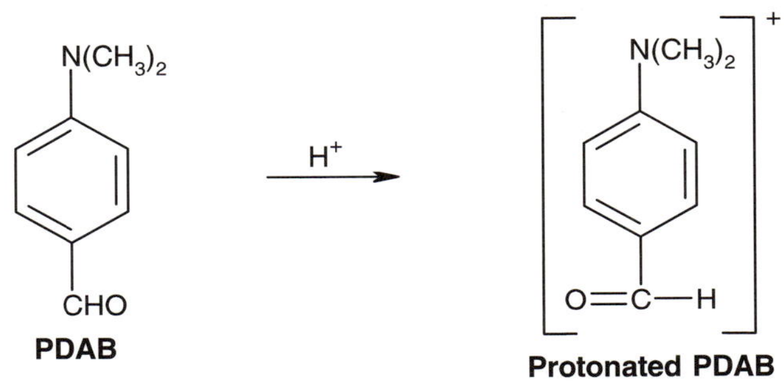

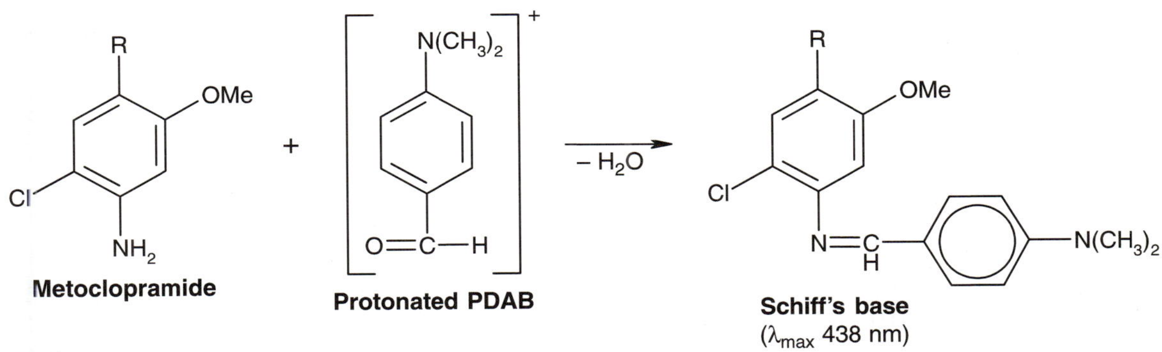

Reference

W. Baeyens, *Analyst*, **103**, 359, 1978.

Method (b)

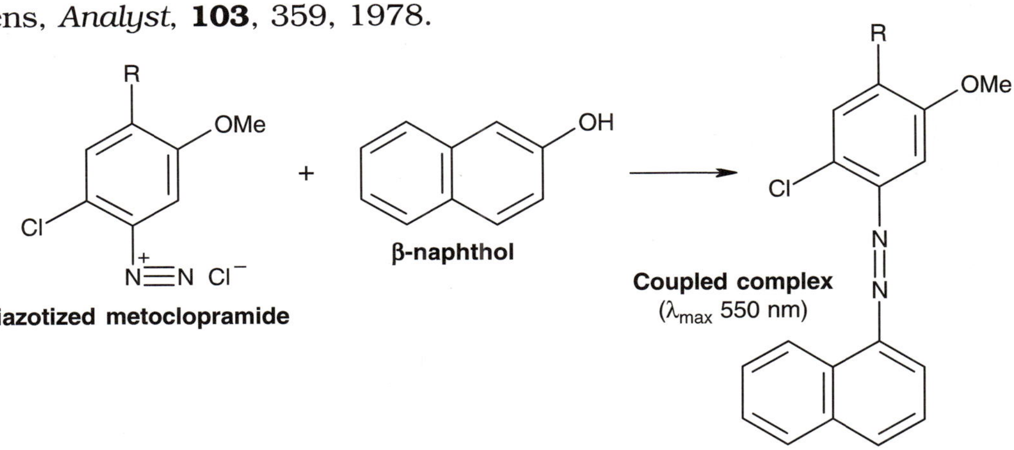

Reference

1. S.A. Patel, C.N. Patel & M.M. Patel, *Ind. J. Pharm. Sci.*, **68(3)**, 397-399, 2006.
2. D.M. Shingal & K.V. Sawat, *Indian Drugs*, **19**, 239, 1982.
3. R.T. Sane, A.Y. Dhamankar, U.R. Pandit & A.B. Ambardekar, *Indian Drugs*, **20(2)**, 73, Nov. 1982.

METHOD 3

Reagents

1. 3% w/v solution of sulphamic acid in water.
2. 0.1% sodium nitrite solution in water.
3. 4 M NaOH.
4. 1 M HCl.
5. Acetylacetone (AA).

Standard solution

Initial solution was made in methanol. Further dilutions done with water to get 25 μg/ml.

Sample solution

The sample extracted with methanol and then further dilutions made with water.

Procedure

To 2 ml of the sample/standard solutions add 2 ml of sodium nitrite solution and 1 ml of 1 M HCl. After 3 min add 1 ml of sulphamic acid, then add 4 ml each of AA and 4 M NaOH, dilute to 25 ml with methanol, mix and after 10 min measure at 430 nm.

Probable Reaction Mechanism

Diazotized metoclopramide couples with active methylene group of acetylacetone in alkaline medium to produce azo dye (λ_{max} 430 nm). Compounds containing active methylene (CH_2) group such as acetylacetone (AA) can be used as a reagent for determination of primary amines after diazotization by means of electrophilic substitution in alkaline medium as shown below.

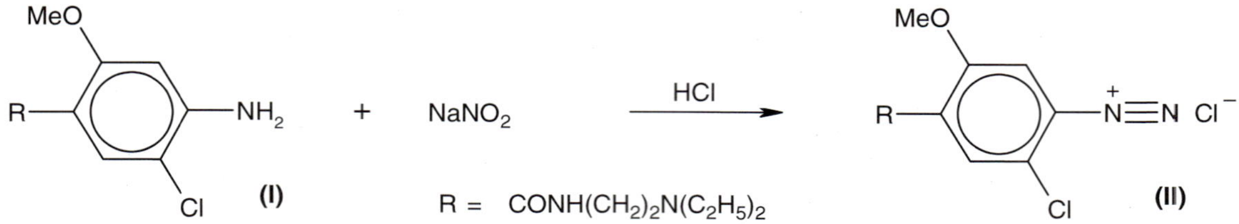

Metoclopramide **Diazotized metoclopramide**

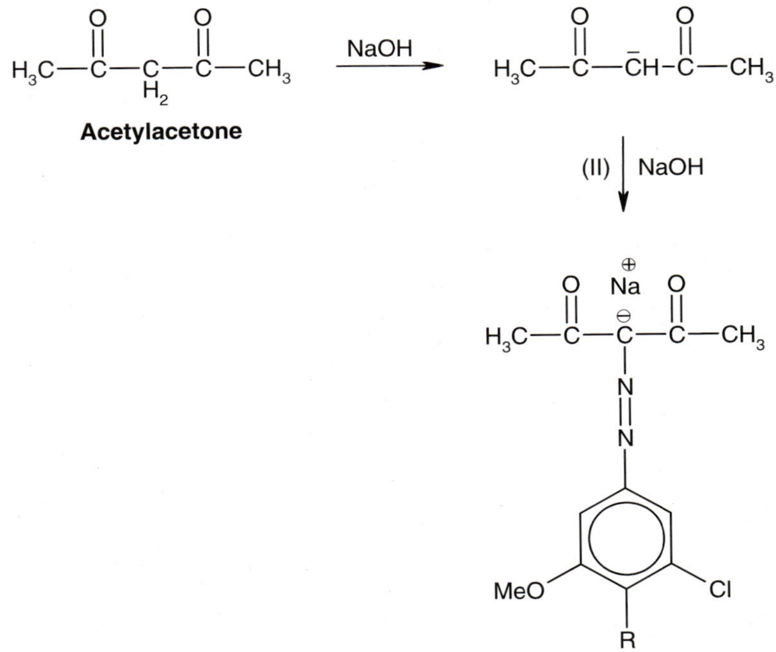

Coloured product
(λ_{max} 430 nm)

Note

Instead of acetylacetone, ethylacetoacetate can also be used as coupling reagent.

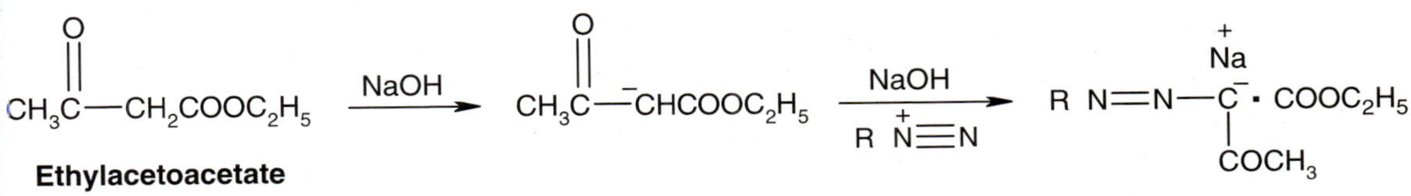

Coloured product
(λ_{max} 400 nm)

Reference

1. K. Ramakrishnam Raju, S.R.K.M. Akella, J.V.S. Murthy & U.T. Bhalerao, *Talanta*, **43**, 577-581, 1996.
2. H.D. Revanasiddapa & B. Manju, *Drugs Development & Ind. Pharmacy*, **28(5)**, 515-521, 2002.

In addition to coupling with acetylacetone or ethylacetoacetate, the compound after diazotization is made to couple with active methylene (CH_2) group in dibenzoyl methane in alkaline medium to give azo dye (λ_{max} 440 nm).

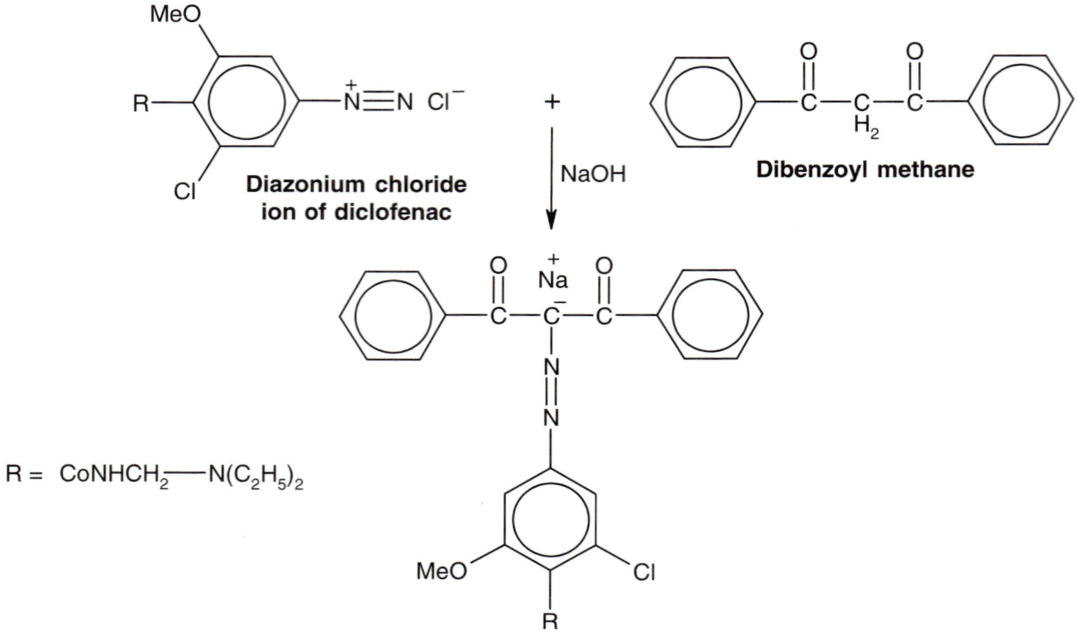

Azo dye
(λ_{max} 440 nm)

Reference

H.D. Revanasiddapa & B. Manju, *J. Pharm. Biomed. Analysis*, **25**, 631-637, 2001.

Another important reaction of the compound with p-dimethylaminocinnamaldehyde (PDAC) to give red-coloured Schiff's base is suitable for analysis.

Probable Reaction Mechanism

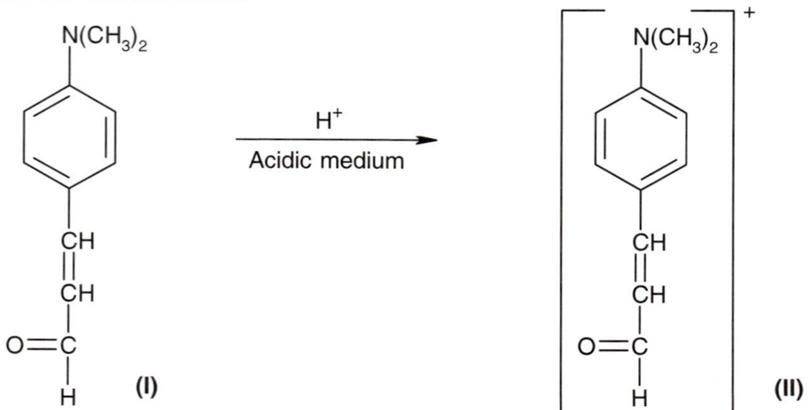

p-dimethylaminocinnamaldehyde (PDAC)

Protonated PDAC

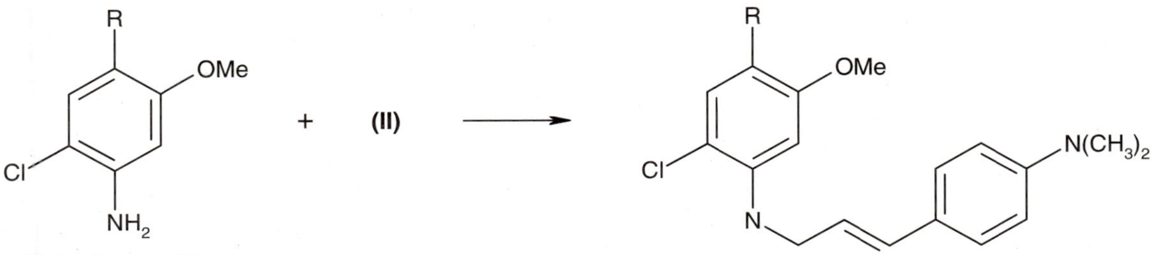

Metoclopramide

R = $CONHCH_2CH_2N(C_2H_5)_2$

Schiff's base
(λ_{max} 548 nm)

Reference

Bahia A. Moussa, *J. Pharm. & Biochem. Analysis*, **23**, 1045-1055, 2000.

Note

In buffer pH 2.0, the substance exhibits fluorescence properties (λ_{exc}: 310 nm; λ_{em}: 360 nm).

METHOD 4

Reagents

1. 1% w/v solution of sodium nitrite in water.
2. 5% w/v solution of ammonium sulphamate.
3. Dilute hydrochloric acid.

Sample and standard solutions

50 μg/ml in 0.1 M HCl.

Procedure

To 1 ml each of sample and standard solutions add 1 ml of dilute HCl and 1 ml of sodium nitrite solution. Mix and allow to stand for 5 min at room temperature, then add 1 ml of ammonium sulphamate solution and measure the absorption at 375 nm.

Probable Reaction Mechanism

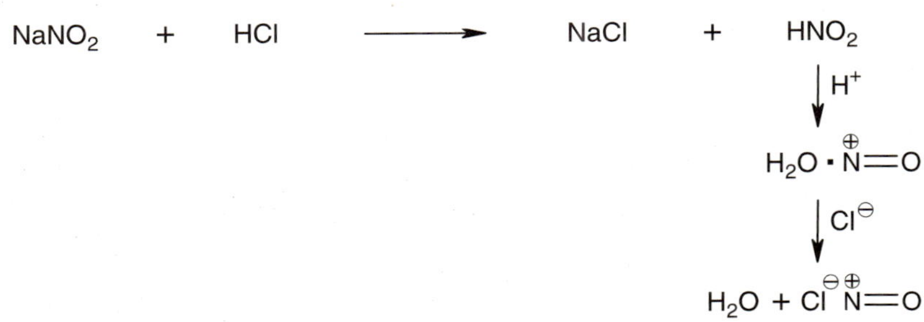

The nitrosonium ion so formed being electron-deficient will attack the aromatic amino group of the drug resulting in the formation of diazotized product.

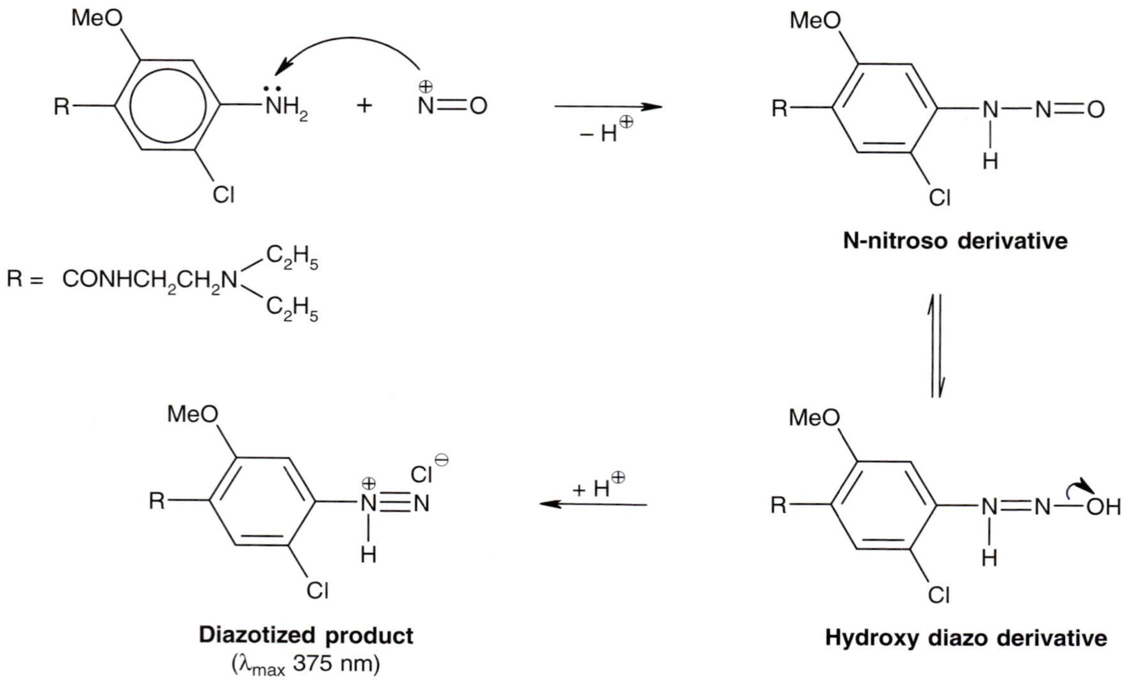

Reference

1. D.M. Shingbal & S.D. Naik, *Indian Drugs*, **18**, 441, 1981.
2. Practical Organic Chemistry by Vogel, p. 920.
3. Pharmaceutical Analysis by K.A. Connors, p. 225.

Ammonium sulphamate is added to destroy the excess of HNO_2 formed to H_2O, H_2SO_4 and N_2.

$$H_2NSO_3H + HNO_2 \longrightarrow H_2O + H_2SO_4 + N_2\uparrow$$

METHOD 5

Reagents

1. 1% w/v solution of borax in water.
2. 0.2% w/v solution of Na–1,2-naphthoquinone-4-sulphonate (Folin's reagent).
3. 10% aq. solution of HCl.

Sample and standard solutions

50 μg/ml of the drug.

Procedure

To 1 ml each of sample and standard solutions add 1 ml of borax solution and 3 ml of naphthoquinone reagent, then add 0.5 ml of dilute HCl, measure absorption at 470 nm after 10 min.

Reference

1. *Indian Drugs*, **25(2)**, 75, 1987; **28(2)**, 108, 1990..
2. Pharmaceutical Chemistry (Vol. 2) by H.J. Roth, p. 378.

Probable Reaction Mechanism

Primary aromatic amino group of the drug undergoes Michael addition, eliminating the monohydrogen sulphite radical and forming the product.

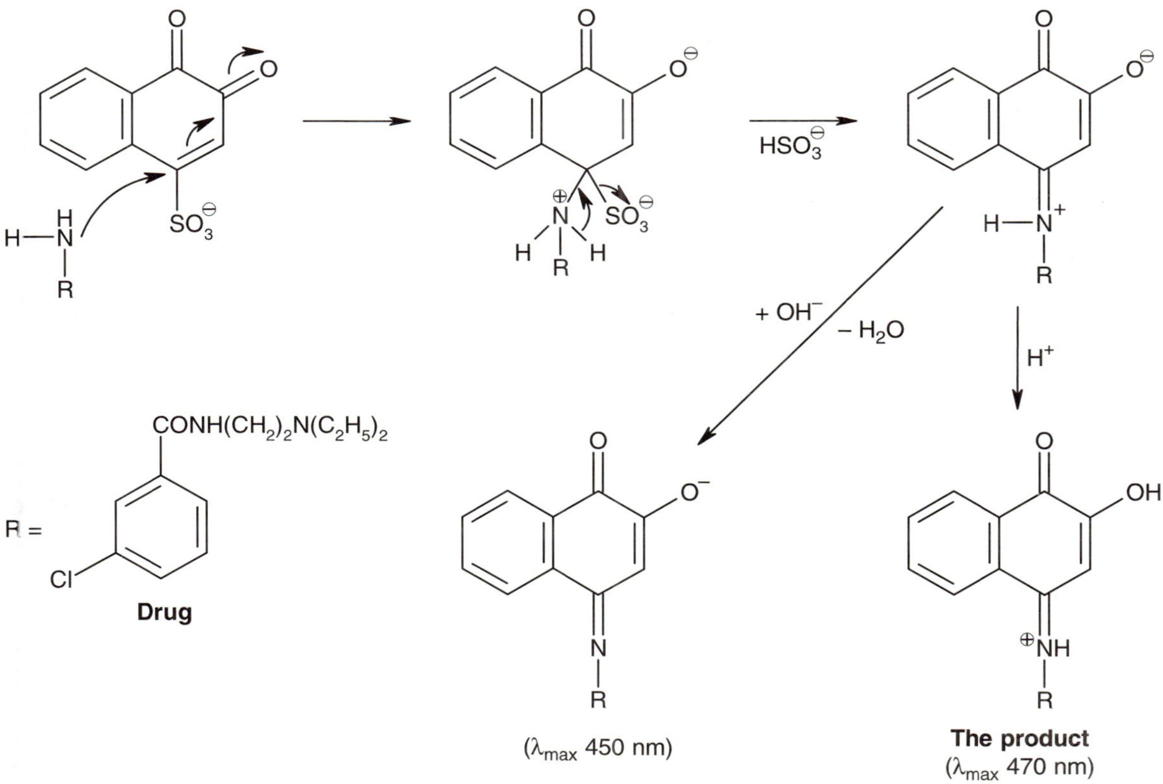

Reference

S.S. Zarapkar, *Indian Drugs*, **25(2)**, 75, 1987.

Note

Diazotized product can couple with thymol in alkaline medium at para position to the phenolic —OH group present in thymol (λ_{max} 495 nm) (Ref. Indian Drugs, **20(7)**, 298, 1983) undergoes Bratton–Marshall reaction (λ_{max} 525 nm) (D.M. Shingbal & K.V. Sawant, Indian Drugs, **19(6)**, 239, 1982), couples with p-aminosalicylic acid at ortho position to phenolic —OH (λ_{max} 440 nm) (Ref. Indian Drugs, **20(9)**, 387, June 1983).

The diazotized drug couples with α-naphthylamine and thiobarbituric acid resulting in the formation of coupled product.

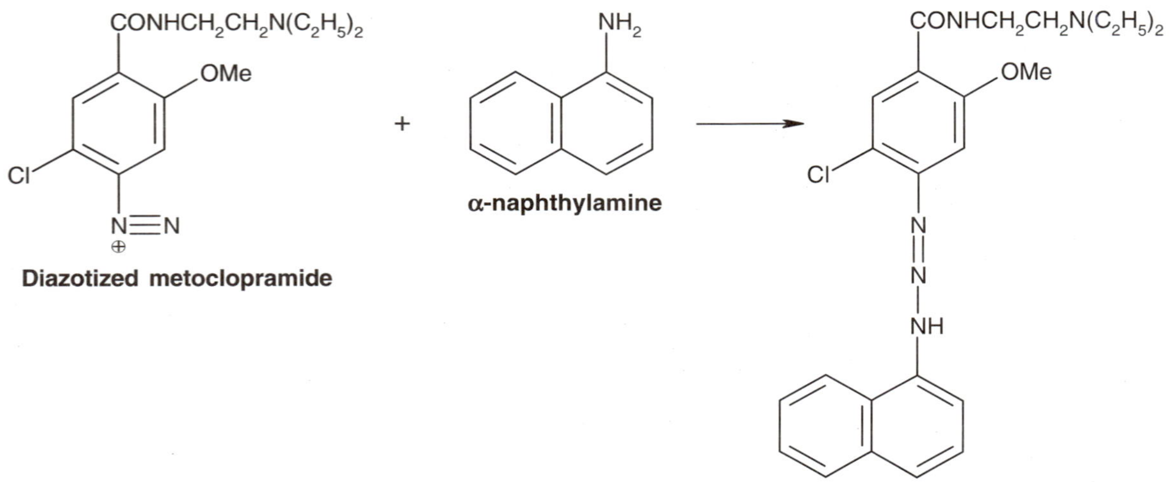

Diazotized metoclopramide

α-naphthylamine

Coupled product
(λ_{max} 510 nm)

Reference

O.S. Kamalapurkar & Sanjay R.S. Priolkar, *Indian Drugs*, **20(3)**, 108-110, 1982.

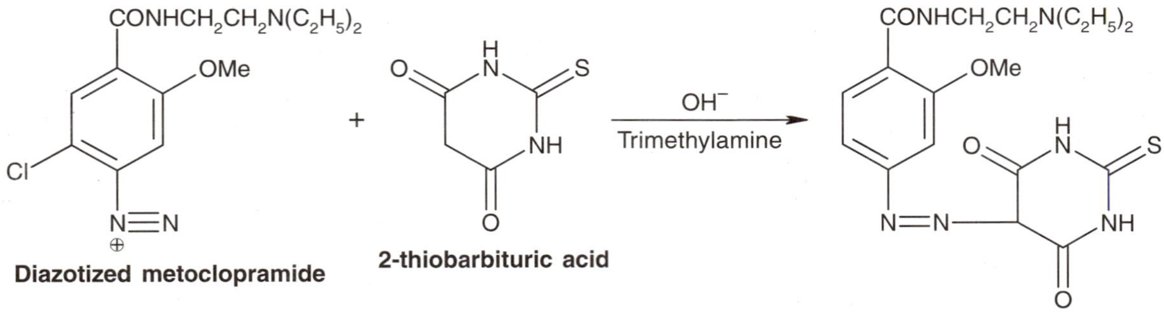

Diazotized metoclopramide

2-thiobarbituric acid

Coupled product
(λ_{max} 430 nm)

Reference

R.T. Sane, A.Y. Dhamankar, U.A. Pandit & A.B. Ambardekar, *Indian Drugs*, **20(2)**, 73, 1982.

Due to the presence of tertiary amine, the compound forms Co(II) complex (λ_{max} 620 nm).

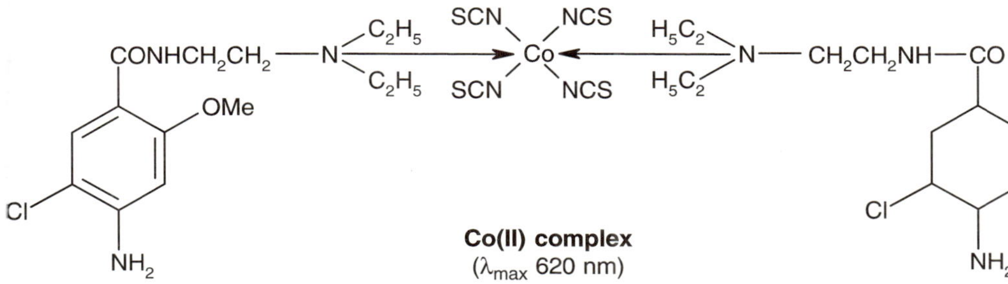

Co(II) complex
(λ_{max} 620 nm)

Diazotized metoclopramide couples with various reagents such as 'NED' reagent, m-aminophenol, resorcinol, iodochlorhydroxyquinoline, orcinol, R-salt of β-naphthol, thymol, p-aminosalicylic acid in alkaline medium to give coloured products.

Probable Reaction Mechanism

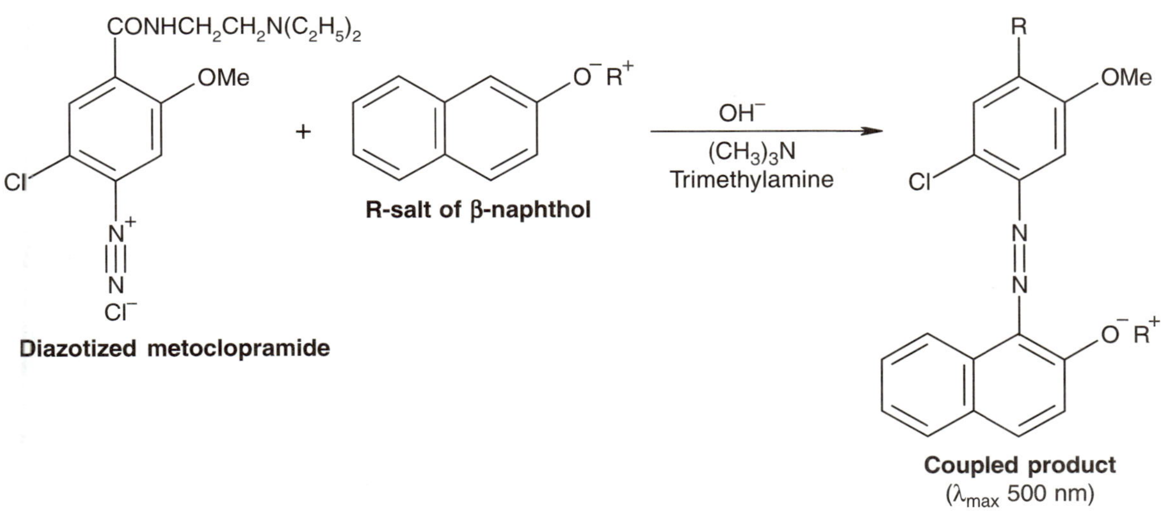

Reference

R.T. Sane, A.B. Ambardekar, P.G. Anaokar & S.S. Zarapkar, *J. of University of Bombay*, Science, Vol. L_1 - L_{11}, No. 78-79, 1982-83.

H.L. Rao et al. (1991) have described a fluorometric method based on inherent property of the compound. The sample in water shows fluorescence (λ_{exc} : 310 nm; λ_{em} : 360 nm).

Reference

H.L. Rao, A.R. Aron & P. Gundu Rao, *Indian Drugs*, **28(4)**, 195-196, 1991.

METHOD 6

Ramappa et al. (1999) have described two analytical methods based on reaction of diazotized drug with chromotropic acid in alkaline medium and oxidation coupling with MBTH in the presence of ceric ammonium sulphate (Ce^{4+}).

Reagents

1. 1 M sulphuric acid.
2. 1 M hydrochloric acid.
3. 3% sodium nitrite.
4. 5% sulphamic acid.
5. 0.2% chromotropic acid (CTA) solution.
6. 0.003 M ceric (IV) ammonium sulphate in 1 M sulphuric acid.
7. 4 M sodium hydroxide solution.
8. 'MBTH' reagent.

Sample and standard solutions

100 µg/ml.

Procedure

(a) To 2 ml each of sample and standard solutions add 2 ml of MBTH solution and 4 ml of Ce (IV) solution, leave at room temperature for 15 min, dilute to 25 ml with water and measure the absorption at 560 nm against reagent blank.

(b) To 2 ml each of sample and standard solutions add 1 ml of sodium nitrite solution followed by 1 ml of 1 M HCl. Keep for 3 min and then add 4 ml of sulphamic acid, 2.5 ml of CTA solution and 1.5 ml of 4 M NaOH solution, dilute to 25 ml with water and measure the absorption at 540 nm against reagent blank after 10 min.

Probable Reaction Mechanism

(a)

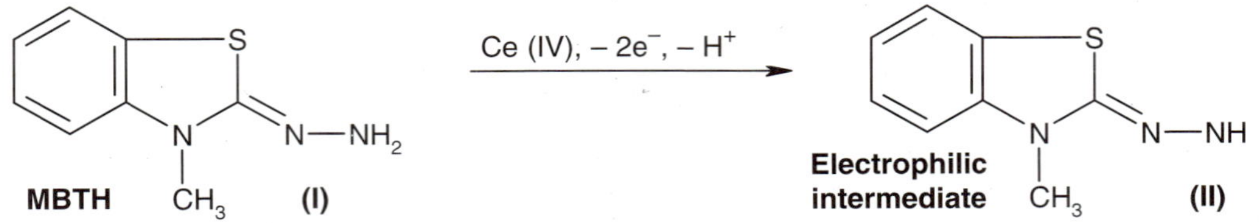

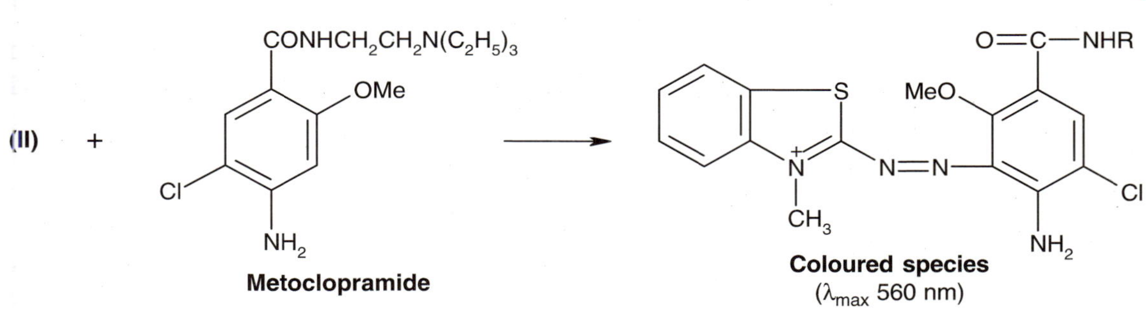

(b)

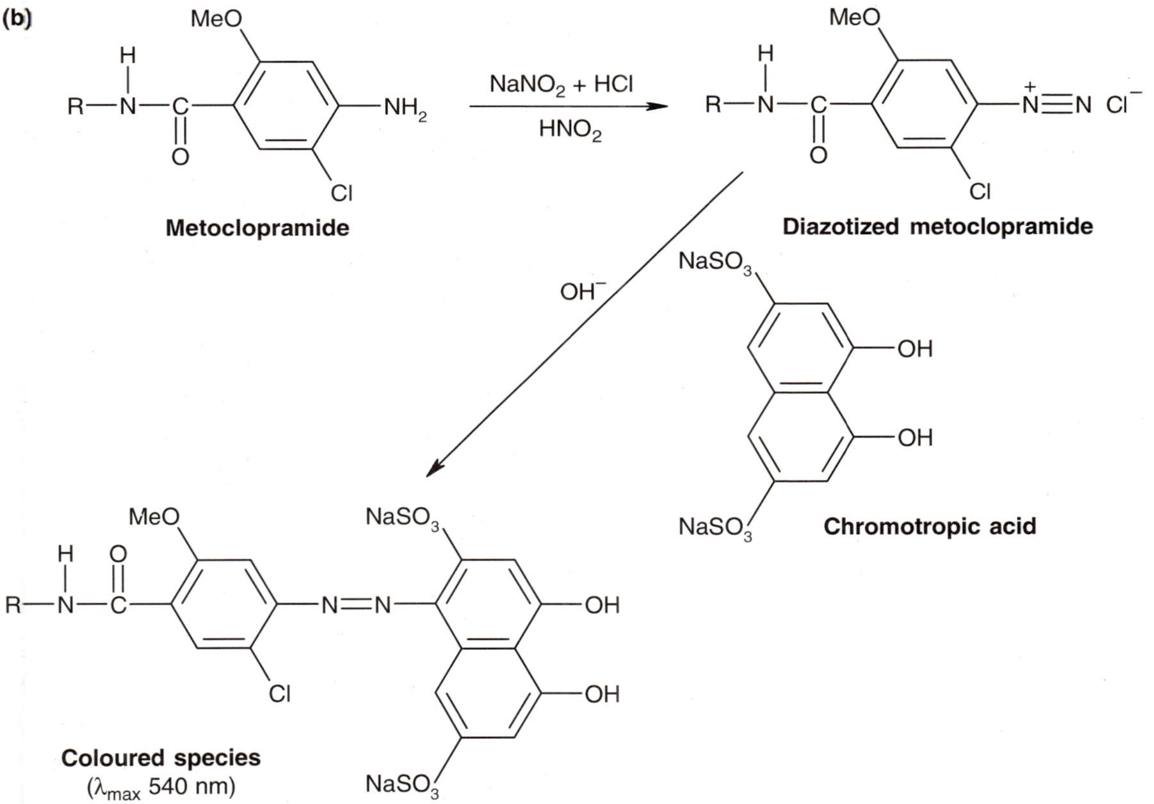

Reference

P.G. Ramappa, Somashekara & H.D. Revanasiddappa, Indian Drugs, **36(6)**, 381-384, 1999.

Formulation 35

Paracetamol, Mefenamic acid

ESTIMATION

Paracetamol

METHOD 1

Standard solution

10 mcg/ml of paracetamol in 0.1 M hydrochloric acid.

Sample solution

Weigh accurately powdered sample equivalent to about 100 mg of paracetamol. Dry extract with three 25 ml portions of 1 N hydrochloric acid filtering through G_4 sintered glass funnel (reserve the residue left on the funnel for estimation of mefenamic acid). Collect the filtrate and dilute to 100 ml with the acid. Further dilutions are done appropriately with the acid to get a concentration of 10 mcg/ml.

Measure the extinction of sample and standard solutions at 244 nm and deduce the results by comparison.

Note

As the mefenamic acid is insoluble in acid, it does not interfere in estimation of paracetamol.

METHOD 2

Follow the nitroso derivative method as described in formulation 2 of this chapter.

Mefenamic acid

METHOD 1

Standard solution

10 mcg/ml of mefenamic acid in 0.1 M sodium hydroxide.

Sample solution

Dissolve the entire residue obtained on the sintered funnel during the estimation of paracetamol in 1 N sodium hydroxide by slowly adding the alkali on the top of funnel and filtering by slow suction, dilute to 100 ml. Dilute 10 ml of the resultant solution to 100 ml with water. Further dilutions are done with 0.1 M sodium hydroxide to get 10 mcg/ml concentration.

Measure the extinction of both sample and standard solutions at 284 nm using 0.1 M sodium hydroxide as blank. The results may be deduced by comparison.

METHOD 2

Standard solution

10 mcg/ml of mefenamic acid in 0.1 M methanolic hydrochloric acid.

Sample solution

Dissolve accurately weighed quantity of the sample equivalent to about 100 mg of mefenamic acid in 100 ml of 0.1 M methanolic hydrochloric acid. Filter, rejecting first few ml of the filtrate. Dilute the filtrate suitably with 0.1 M methanolic hydrochloric acid to get concentration of 10 mcg/ml.

Measure the extinction of both sample and standard solutions at maxima at about 350 nm using methanolic hydrochloric acid as blank. Deduce the results by comparison.

Note

Paracetamol has no absorption at 350 nm, hence no interference.

METHOD 3

Weigh accurately powdered sample equivalent to about 500 mg of mefenamic acid, dissolve in neutralized (phenol red) methanol by slight warming. Titrate with 0.1 M sodium hydroxide using phenol red as indicator. Each ml of 0.1 M sodium hydroxide is equivalent to 0.02413 g of mefenamic acid. Paracetamol does not interfere.

METHOD 4

Reagents

1. 1% w/v solution of potassium ferricyanide in water.
2. 0.1% solution of aminophenazone in water (freshly prepared).

Standard solution

50 mcg/ml of mefenamic acid in methanol.

Sample solution

Accurately weighed quantity of the powdered tablets equivalent to 100 mg of mefenamic acid was extracted with methanol and finally diluted to get a solution of 50 mcg/ml.

Procedure

To 1 ml each of sample and standard solutions add 2 ml of phenazone reagent and 5 ml of potassium ferricyanide. The contents were mixed and allowed to stand for 15 min and diluted to 25 ml with water. The absorbance was measured at 590 nm against reagent blank and results calculated by comparison. The chromogen was stable for 45 min. The method obeyed Beer's law in concentration range of 0.5-4 mcg/ml.

Probable Reaction Mechanism

The method is based on oxidative coupling with the reagent.

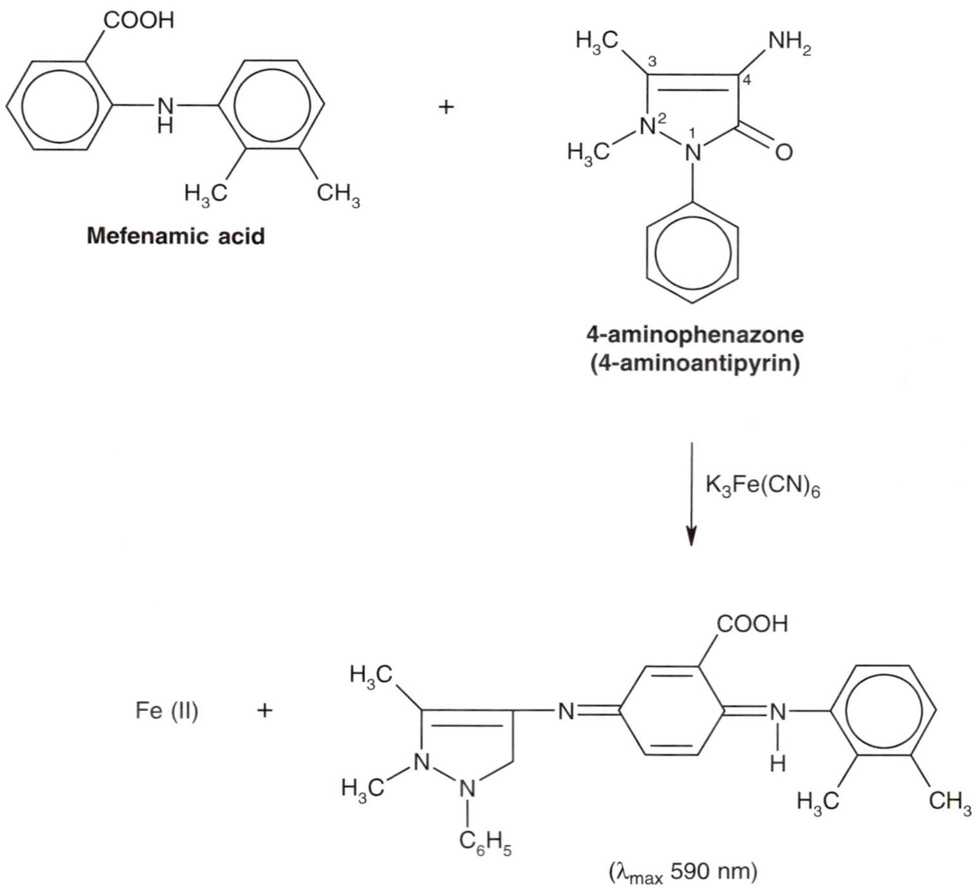

The compound undergoes oxidative coupling with 'MBTH' to give coloured product.

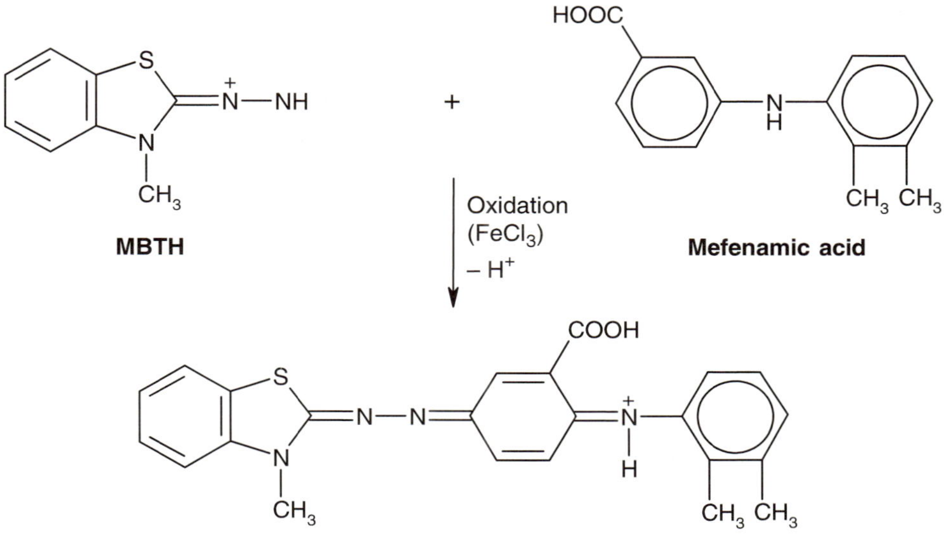

Reference

Indian Drugs, **24(6)**, 303, 1986.

Note

Orhan et al. have described non-aqueous titrimetric method for certain acidic anti-inflammatory drugs such as ibuprofen, diclofenac using tetrabutylammonium hydroxide as titrant in acetonitrile medium.

Reference

Orhan Cakirer et al., *J. Pharm. Biomed. Anal.*, **20**, 19-26, 1999.

Formulation 36

Nimesulide, Tinazidine hydrochloride

ESTIMATION

Nimesulide and Tizanidine

Procedure

Suspend powdered sample in 0.1 M hydrochloride, shake with 3 × 25 chloroform (reserve aqueous acidic layer for estimation of tizanidine hydrochloride). Combine chloroform extract, dilute to 100 ml (10 μg/ml) and measure the absorbance at 300 nm. Calculate the results by comparing with the standard.

Tizanidine hydrochloride

Dilute the acidic layer appropriately and subject to spectrophotometric mesurements at 320 nm. Calculate the results by comparing with the standard.

Note

Since nimesulide is totally insoluble in acidic medium, it gets extracted into chloroform layer whereas tizanidine remains in aqueous acidic medium.

Note

This method is based on differential solubility of the two compounds.

Reduced nimesulide reacts with 'MBTH' reagent to give blue green azo dye. This is based on oxidative coupling of 'MBTH' reagent with aromatic amine (Huning et al., *Ann. Chim.*, **143**, 609, 1957).

Probable Reaction Mechanism

MBTH on oxidation loses 2 electrons and one proton forming electrophilic intermediate – active species. This allows the reduced nimesulide at ortho position (p position is occupied).

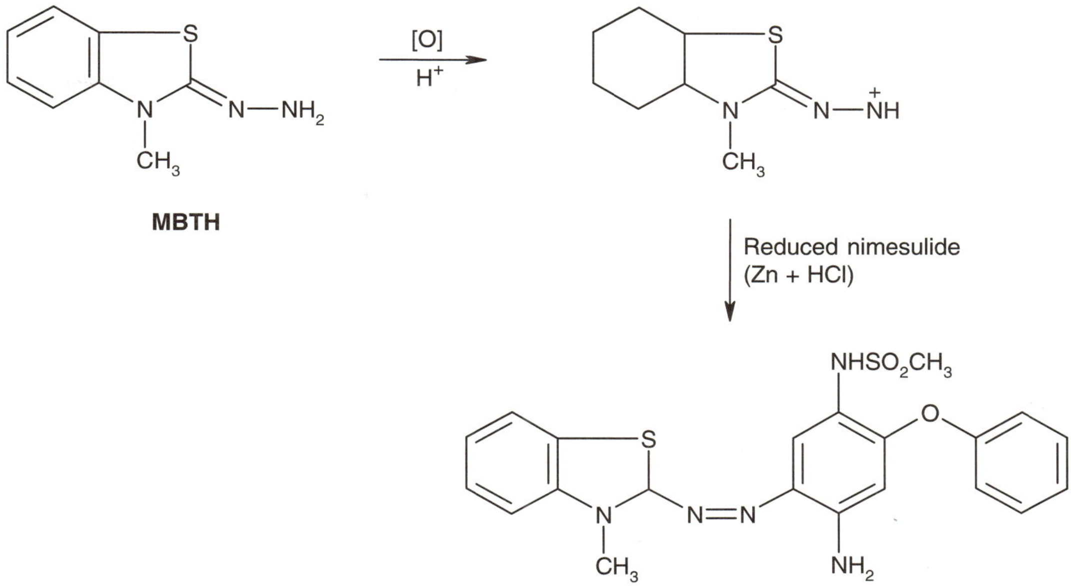

Blue-green azo dye
(λ_{max} 600 nm)

P. Nagaraja et al. (2002) have described two very sensitive spectrophotometric methods based on coupling of reduced nimesulide (NIME) with iminodibenzyl and o-aminophenol (AP) in acidic medium.

Reagents

1. 1% w/v solution of iminodibenzyl (IDB) in methanol.
2. 1% w/v freshly prepared solution of 3-aminophenol in water.
3. 1% w/v aqueous solution of sodium nitrite.
4. 2% v/v solution of sulphuric acid.

Procedure

(a) To the reduced and diazotized solutions of sample/standard, add 3 ml of IDB solution, heat on water-bath for 5 min, cool, add 3 ml of methanol and dilute to 10 ml with sulphuric acid (1 : 1), mix and measure the coloured complex at 600 nm within 60 min.

(b) For (AP) method, add 2 ml of (AP) solution to the diazotized sample/standard solution, heat on boiling water-bath for 5 min, cool, add 2 ml of 0.1 M HCl, dilute to 10 ml with water and measure the absorbance at 470 nm.

Reference

P. Nagaraja, H.S. Yathirajan, H.R. Arunkumar & R.A. Vasantha, *J. Pharm. & Biomed. Analysis*, **24**, 277-282, 2002.

Probable Reaction Mechanism

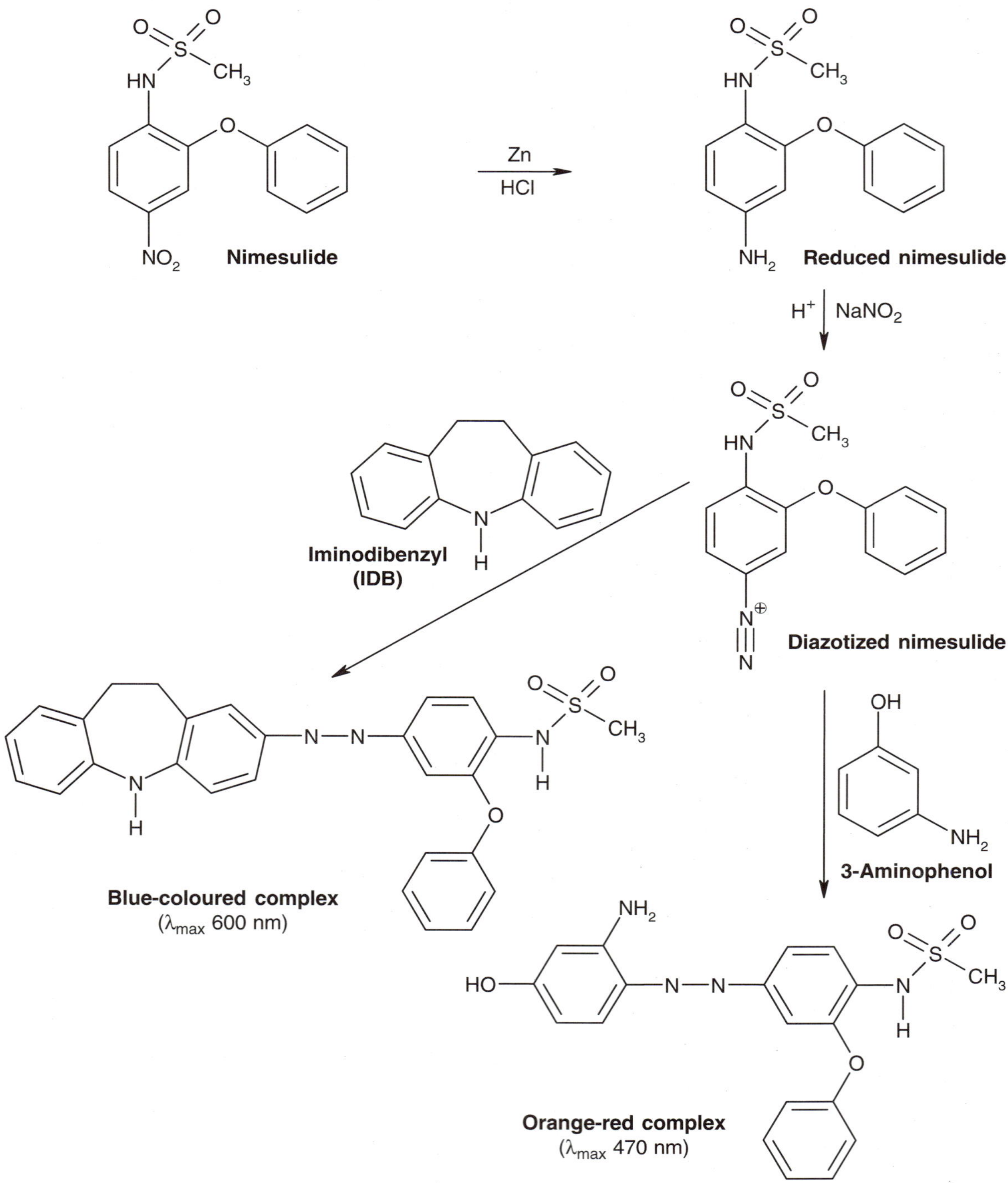

Note

Reduced and diazotized drug coupled with 'NED' to form a stable purple-coloured chromogen (λ_{max} 560 nm) formed the basis of spectrophotometric method.

Reference

1. K.P.R. Chowdary, G. Devala Rao & I. Sudheer Babu, *Indian Drugs*, **37(7)**, 396, 1997.
2. Sadhana J. Rajput & Gitanjali R., *Eastern Pharmacist*, p. 113, July 1997.

Note

C.S.R. Lakshmi et al. have described spectrofluorometric method for the estimation of nimesulide based on quenching of native fluorescence of 'NED' by reaction with reduced and diazotized nimesulide (Exc : 309 nm; em : 427 nm).

Methanolic solution of the compound was subjected to reduction (Zn + HCl) followed by diazotization ($NaNO_2$ + HCl), after adding ammonium sulphamate to remove excess of HNO_2, reacted with 'NED' to yield fluorescent moiety which formed the basis of quantitative estimation of the compound in formulation.

Reference

C.S.R. Lakshmi, M.N. Reddy & Pelia Y. Naidu, *Indian Drugs*, **35(8)**, 519-520, 1998.

Reduced nimesulide can condense with organic aldehyde i.e. p-dimethyl-aminocinnamaldehyde to form Schiff's base (λ_{max} 525 nm).

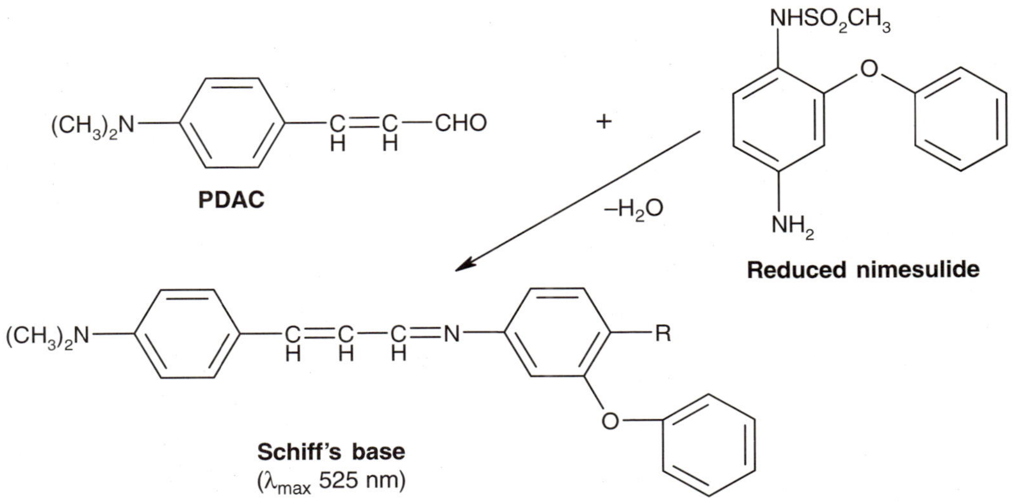

Reference

M. Narayana Reddy et al., *Eastern Pharmacist*, p. 119, March 1998.

Formulation 37

Paracetamol, Methocarbamol

ESTIMATION

Methocarbamol

METHOD 1

Transfer accurately weighed quantity of the powdered sample equivalent to 400 mg of methocarbamol to a separating funnel with the aid of 5-10 ml of water. Basify with 2-3 ml of 1 M sodium hydroxide solution. Extract with 4 × 25 ml of chloroform. Shake the combined chloroform layer with 20 ml of water, add washing to the alkaline layer (reserve for estimation of paracetamol). Pass the combined chloroform layer through anhydrous sodium sulphate placed over cotton plug and pre-moistened. Evaporate the chloroform on a steam-bath, finally drying in an oven at 50°C to a constant weight. From the weight initially taken for analysis, calculate the contents of methocarbamol (mg) in each tablet.

METHOD 2

Standard solution

100 mg of the substance accurately weighed and dissolved in chloroform to make 100 ml. 5 ml of the resultant solution is diluted to 50 ml with methanol (100 mcg/ml).

Sample solution

Extract the powdered sample equipment to 100 mg of the substance with chloroform after basifyin with 1 N sodium hydroxide. The chloroform layer is made up to 100 ml. 5 ml of the solution is further diluted to 50 ml with methanol (100 mcg/ml).

Measure the extinction of both the sample and standard solutions at 274 nm against solvent blank and calculate the results by comparison.

Methocarbamol, a carbamate derivative has free aliphatic amino group. It can undergo condensation reaction with PDAB in acidic medium to give coloured product. The reaction is similar to the one described for meprobamate as described under formulation of the chapter on bronchospasm relaxants.

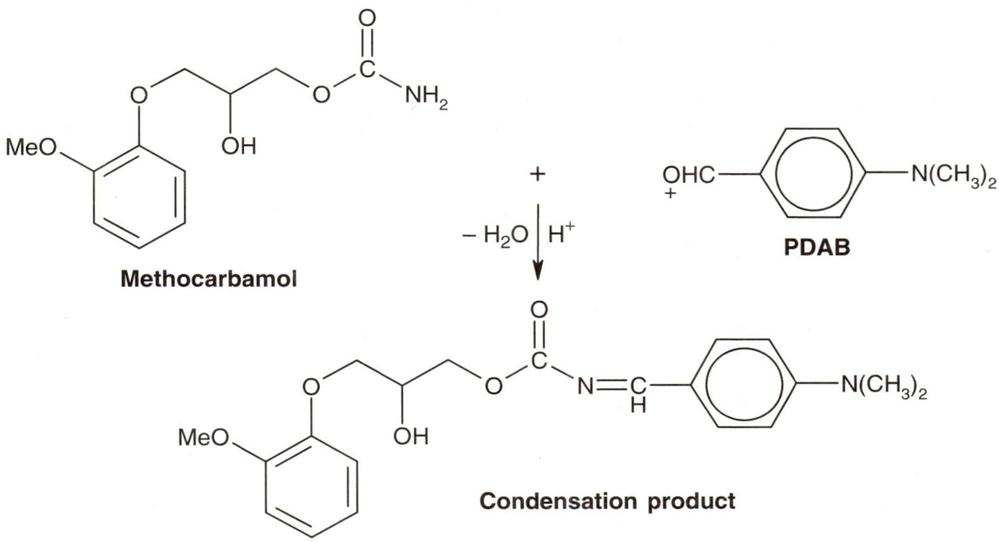

Morgan et al. (1957) have described a method based on alkaline hydrolysis of amide, extraction into chloroform to remove carbamate ester, followed by oxidation with KIO_4 resulting in the formation of formaldehyde. The aldehyde so formed is estimated by reaction with chromotropic acid or by coupling with acetylacetone in the presence of ammonia; see under mephenesin.

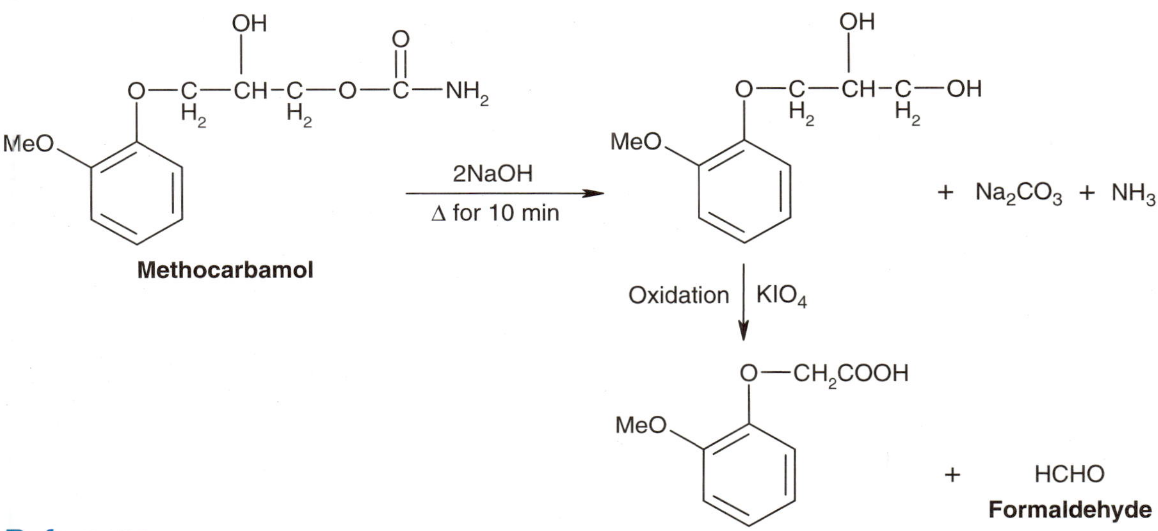

Reference

A.M. Morgan, E.B. Truitt & J.M. Little, J. Amm. Pharm. Assoc., **46**, 374-377, 1957.

Note

The method is suitable for mephenesin and guaiacol glyceryl ether.

The method described by Titus et al. (1948) involves extraction into chloroform after basification and then reacting with diazotized dinitroaniline resulting in the formation of orange-red complex (λ_{max} 490 nm).

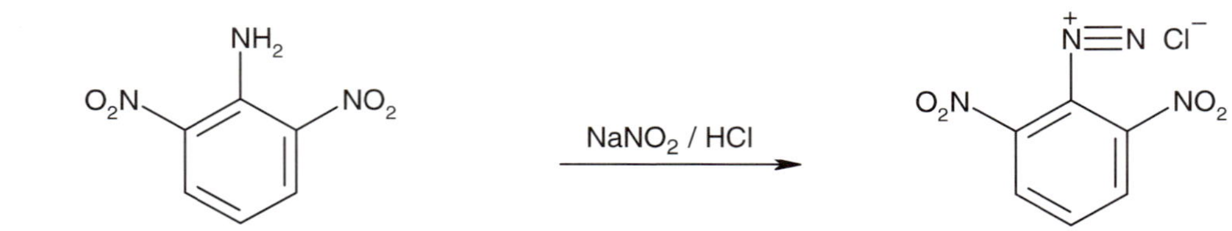

Dinitroaniline   Diazotized dinitroaniline

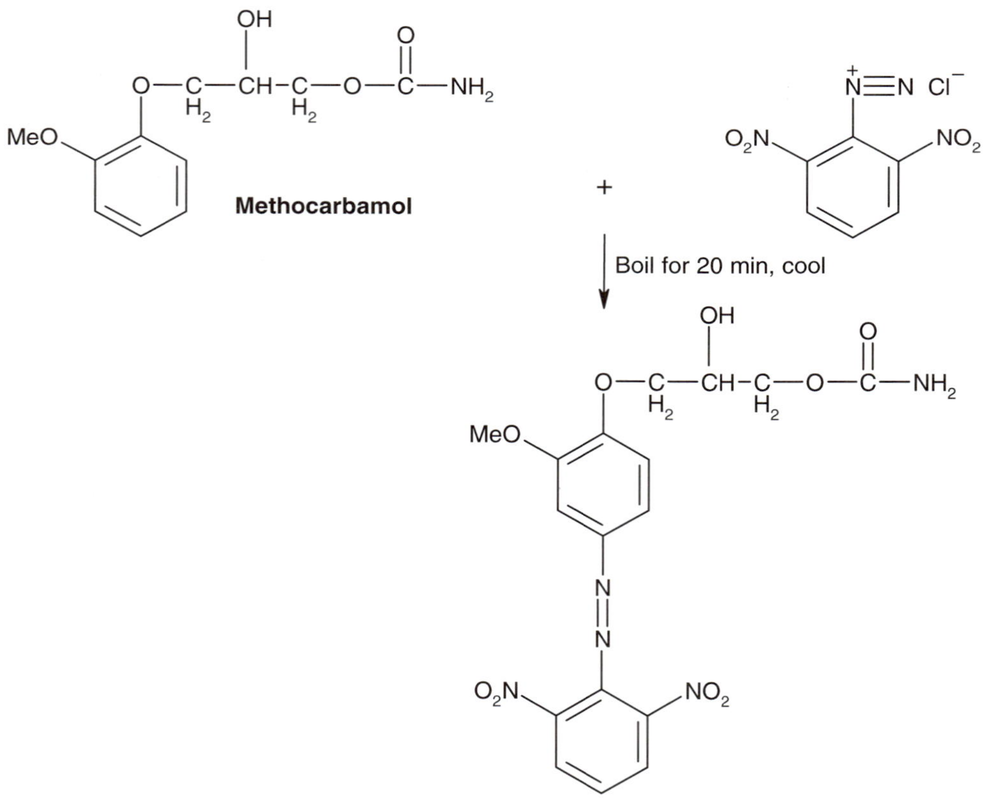

Methocarbamol

Orange-red complex (λ_{max} 490 nm)

Note

The sample is basified (2 M NaOH), extracted into chloroform and back extracted into phosphoric acid (85%) and acidic layer used for analysis.

Reference

E. Titus, S. Ulik & A.P. Richardson, J. Pharmacol. Expt. Therapeutics, **93**, 129-134, 1948.

Paracetamol

To the combined alkaline aqueous layer obtained during estimation of methocarbamol (method 1) add 2.5 ml of 1 M sodium hydroxide solution and dilute to 250 ml with water. Further dilutions are made appropriately with 0.1 M sodium hydroxide to obtain a solution of 10 mcg/ml. Measure extinction of the resulting solution at 257 nm against reagent blank. Calculate the results by using 715 as value of A 1%, 1 cm at 257 nm.

Formulation 38

Paracetamol, Methionine

ESTIMATION

Paracetamol

Follow the nitroso derivative method as described in formulation 2 of this chapter.

Methionine

METHOD 1

Weigh accurately powdered sample equivalent to 150 mg of methionine and transfer to iodine flask containing 50 ml of water. Add 2.5 g of potassium dihydrogen phosphate and 1 g of potassium iodide. Shake to dissolve the contents. Add 25 ml of 0.1 N iodine, seal the flask tightly with glass stopper and allow to stand for 30 min. Immerse in ice water and titrate excess of iodine with 0.1 N sodium thiosulphate using starch as indicator. Run the blank. Each ml of 0.1 N iodine consumed is equivalent to 7.461 mg of methionine.

Methionine could also be assayed by formol titration using phenolphthalein or thymol blue as indicator.

Note

The method involving oxidation with sodium nitroprusside as described in the chapter on vitamins is not applicable as paracetamol will interfere.

Probable Reaction Mechanism

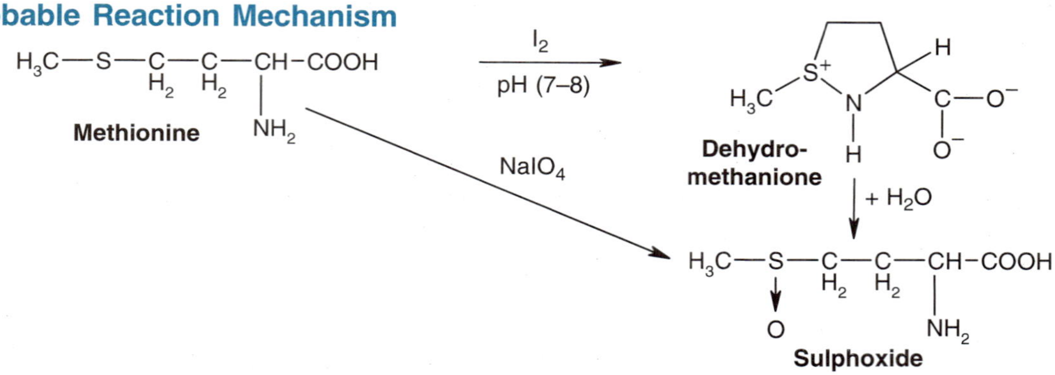

Note

Reaction with Br_2/H_2O forms sulphoxide or sulphone depending on the reaction conditions.

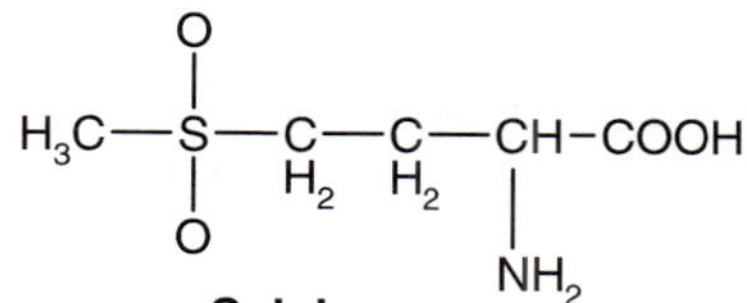

Sulphone

Due to the presence of both amino functions and a carbonyl group, both basic and acidic properties of α-amino acids is expected. In aqueous solution, α-amino acids occur as Zwitterion.

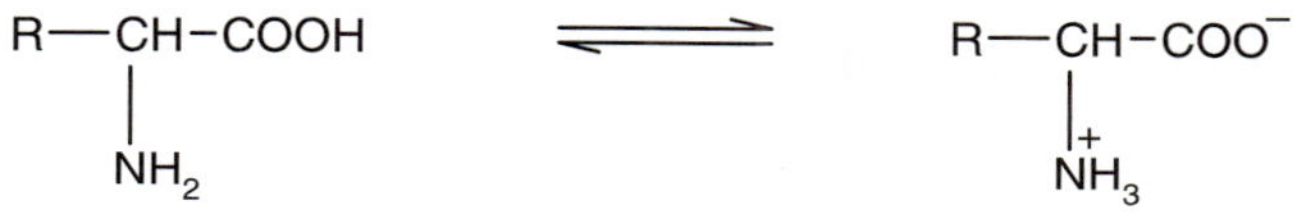

However, in the presence of formaldehyde (HCHO) Schiff's base is formed with amino group, allowing titration of the amino acid as an acid. The reactions proposed by different authors are as under. This is called formol titration.

(a)

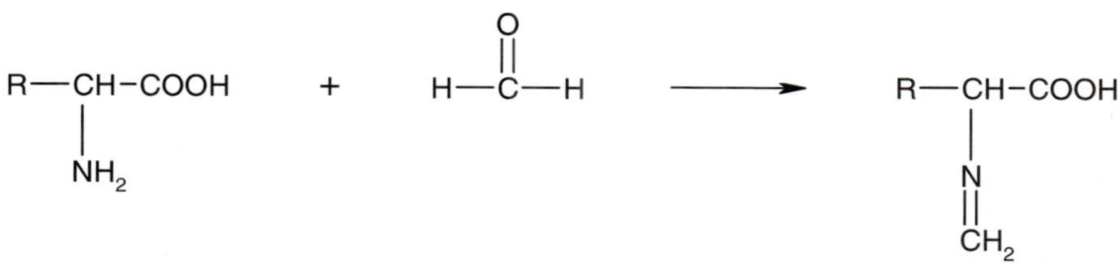

(Sørensen, S.P.L., 1907)

(b)

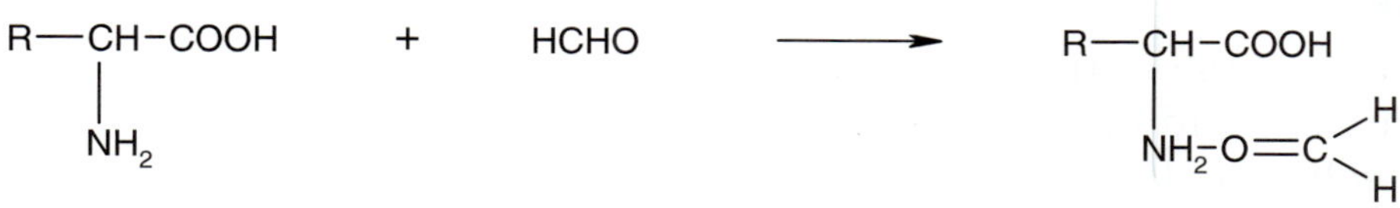

(Harris, L.J., J. Biochem., 24, 1080, 1930)

(c)

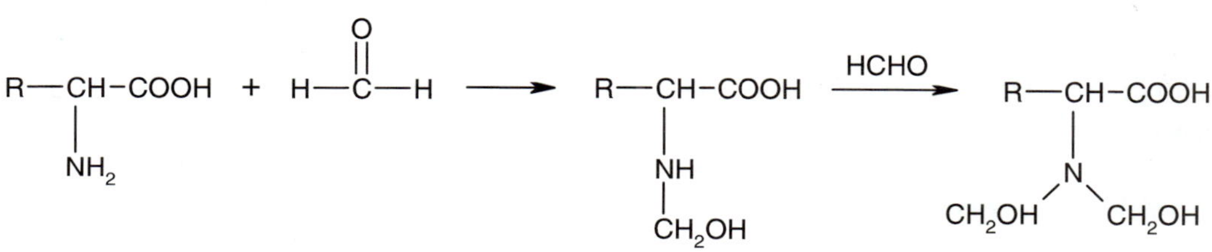

(Levy, M.J., Biol. Chem., 99, 767, 1933)

Reference

Pharmaceutical Analysis by T. Higuchi et al., p. 269-270, 1961.

A titrimetric method was described by Verma (1980) using iodine trichloride ICl_3) as titrant. To the solution of amino acid in water 5 ml of carbon tetrachloride was added and then titrated with ICl_3 until the colour of the organic layer has maximum intensity. Shake and add 20 ml of 6 M hydrochloric acid and continue titration till the organic layer is colourless.

Probable Reaction Mechanism

ICl_3 oxidizes methione to sulphoxide.

$$RSR + ICl_3 + H_2O \longrightarrow R{-}\underset{\underset{O}{\|}}{S}{-}R + ICl + 2HCl$$

Note

This method is suitable for estimation of biotin as well.

Reference

K.K. Verma, Talanta, **27**, 541-544, 1980.

METHOD 2

Another analytical method involving oxidation of the amino acid with charamine-T has been described by Gowda et al. (1977).

Reagents

1. 0.02 M chloramine-T (CAT) solution.
2. 0.1% aqueous solution of indigo carmine.
3. Glacial acetic acid.

Procedure

To the sample equivalent to 2 mg of the sample in water add 1 ml of glacial acetic acid and 0.2 ml of the indicator solution. Titrate with 0.02 M CAT to the pale-yellow colour.

Alternatively, to the sample solution add excess of 'CAT' solution in iodine flask containing enough NaOH to give overall alkalinity of 0.1 M NaOH, shake the reaction mixture and allow to stand for 60 min, then add 20 ml of 1 M H_2SO_4 and 20 ml of 20% KI solution and titrate the liberated iodine with sodium thiosulphate.

Probable Reaction Mechanism

(a) Direct titration

$$CH_3SRH + RNClNa + H_2O \longrightarrow \underset{\text{Methionine sulphoxide}}{H_3C{-}\underset{\underset{O}{\|}}{S}{-}RH} + \underset{\text{Sulphonamide}}{RNH_2} + NaCl$$

$R = p\text{-}CH_3C_6H_4SO_2$

(b) Back titration

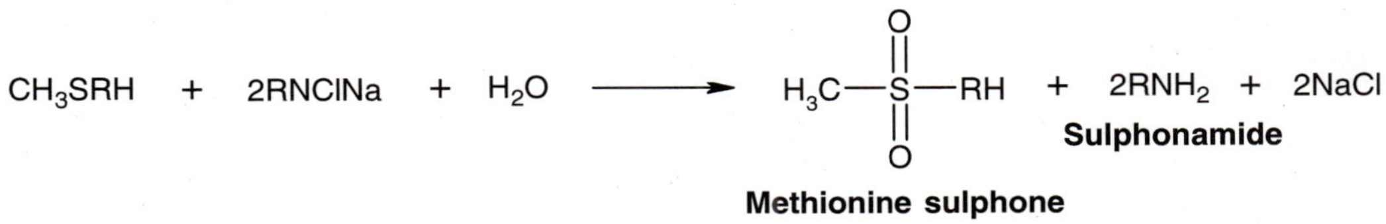

Reference

N.M.M. Gowda & D.S. Mahadevappa, Talanta, **24**, 470-472, 1977.

Krishna & Gupta (1981) have described titrimetric method by using iodine monochloride as titrant. The titration procedure was almost similar to the one described above.

Probable Reaction Mechanism

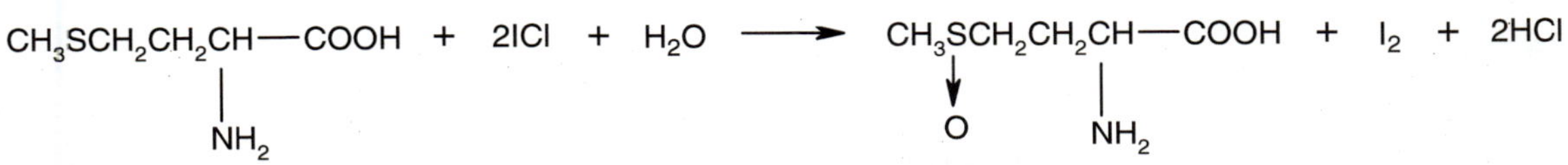

Sulphide group present in methionine is oxidized to sulphoxide in the above titration procedure.

Reference

K.K. Verma & A.K. Gupta, Talanta, **28**, 849-852, 1981.

Formulation 39

Paracetamol, Phenylpropanolamine hydrochloride, Caffeine citrate, Chlorpheniramine maleate

ESTIMATION

Paracetamol

Follow the nitroso derivative method described under formulation 2 of this chapter.

Caffeine citrate

Transfer accurately weighed quantity of powdered tablets equivalent to 20 mg of caffeine citrate to a separating funnel. Add 20 ml of saturated solution of sodium chloride, shake to disperse. Extract with three 25 ml portions of chloroform, washing each extract with same 10 ml of saturated solution of sodium bicarbonate (reserve aqueous layer for estimation of phenylpropanolamine hydrochloride). Filter the combined chloroform layer through moistened cotton plug and make up to 100 ml with chloroform. Take 5 ml of chloroform extract into volumetric flask, evaporate, take up the residue in 0.01 N tartaric acid and follow the method described in formulation 60 of this chapter.

Phenylpropanolamine hydrochloride

METHOD 1

Reagents

1. 2% w/v solution of sodium carbonate in water.
2. 2% w/v solution of sodium metaperiodate in water.
3. 6 M hydrochloric acid.

Standard solution

1.5 mg/ml of the substance in water. To 10 ml of this solution add 40 ml of saturated solution of sodium bicarbonate, 30 ml of 6 M hydrochloric acid, stir to remove carbon dioxide and dilute to 200 ml with water.

Sample solution

To the aqueous extract reserved during estimation of caffeine add 30 ml of 6 M hydrochloric acid and dilute to 200 ml with water.

Procedure

To 10 ml each of sample and standard solutions add 10 ml each of sodium carbonate and sodium metaperiodate solutions, mix, allow to stand. Make slightly acidic with hydrochloric acid. Extract with three 30 ml portions of dichloromethane, passing each extract through same layer of anhydrous sodium sulphate. Dilute to 100 ml with dichloromethane. Concomitantly measure the absorbance of both standard and sample solutions at about 242 nm against solvent blank and calculate the results by comparison.

Explanatory Note

Sodium carbonate is added to remove hydrochloride associated with the drug and then excess Na_2CO_3 removed by addition of hydrochloric acid. Na–metaperiodate is an oxidizing agent which brings about the cleavage of C—C bond in compounds having one or two hydroxyl groups and an amino group attached to adjacent carbon atoms. This reaction is called "Malaprade reaction". In phenylpropanolamine, a hydroxyl group and an amino group are attached to adjacent carbon atoms, hence cleavage of this C—C bond which results in the formation of benzaldehyde in addition to ammonia. After the reaction is complete, ammonia so liberated is neutralized with hydrochloric acid. Benzaldehyde being highly soluble in dichloromethane is extracted into this organic solvent and its absorption measured at 242 nm for quantitative analysis.

Probable Reaction Mechanism

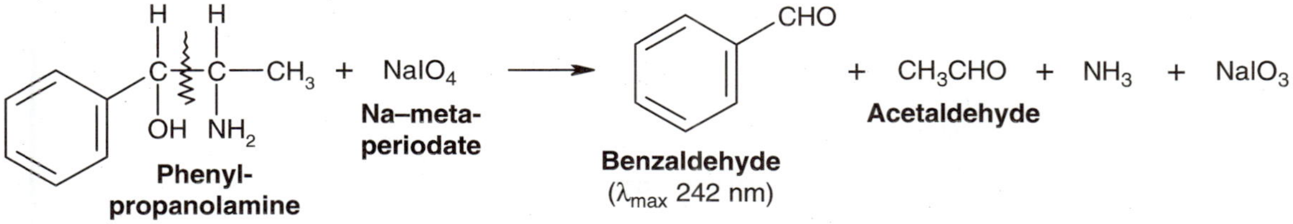

METHOD 2

Reagents

1. 1.5% w/v solution of ninhydrin in pyridine : methanol mixture (1 : 1).
2. 0.05% w/v solution of ascorbic acid in water.

Standard solution

50 mcg/ml of phenylpropanolamine hydrochloride in water.

Sample solution

Weigh the powdered sample equivalent to 25 mg of the substance, dissolve in 200-300 ml of water by mechanical stirring, dilute to 500 ml with water.

Procedure

To 2 ml each of sample and standard solutions add 1 ml of ascorbic acid solution and 2 ml of ninhydrin solution. Place the test tubes in boiling water-bath for 25 minutes, cool in ice-bath and dilute to 25 ml with water. After 10 minute measure at about 570 nm against reagent blank and deduce the results by comparison.

Probable Reaction Mechanism

Step 1

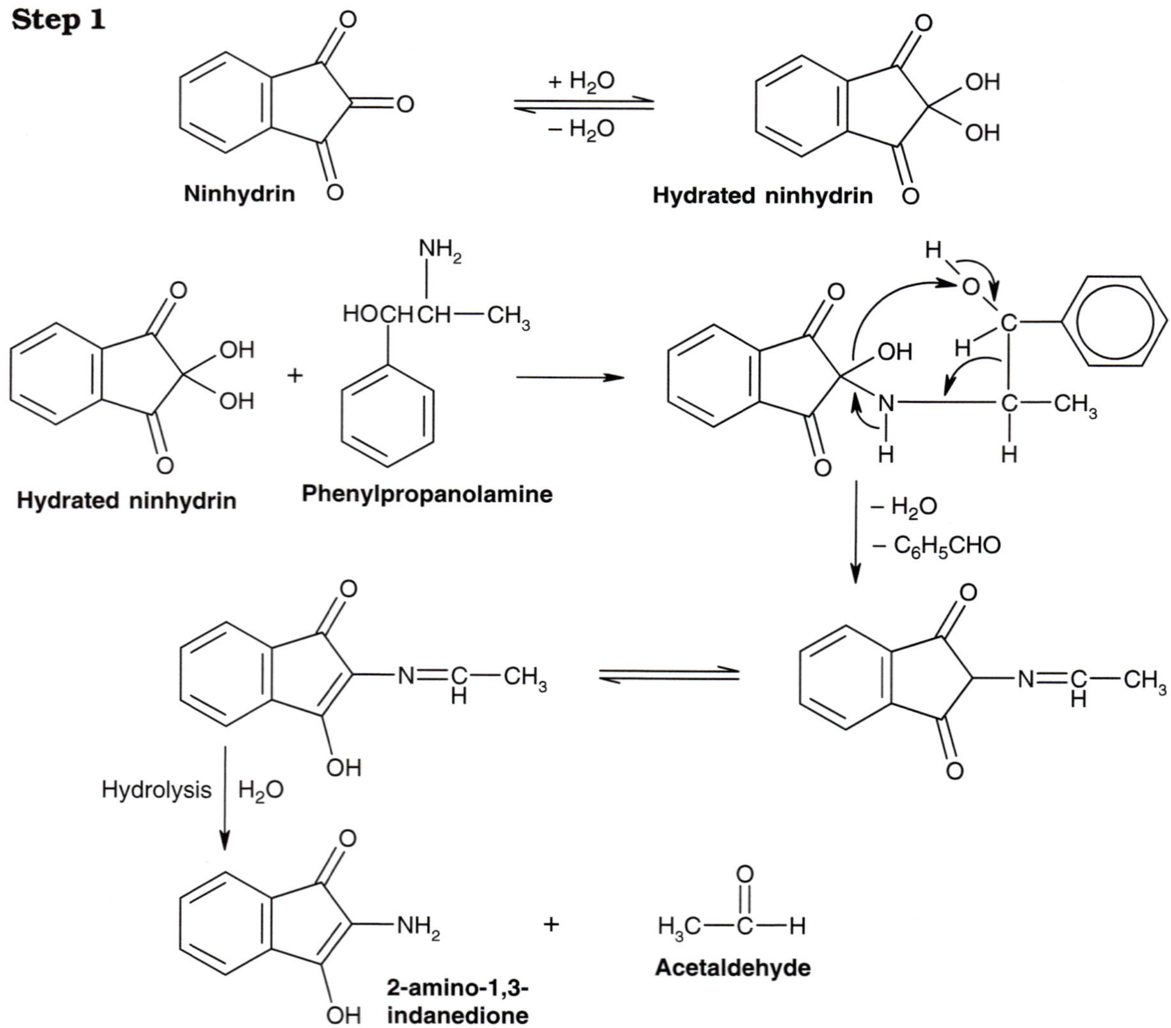

Step 2: 2-amino-1,3-indanedione further undergoes hydrolysis.

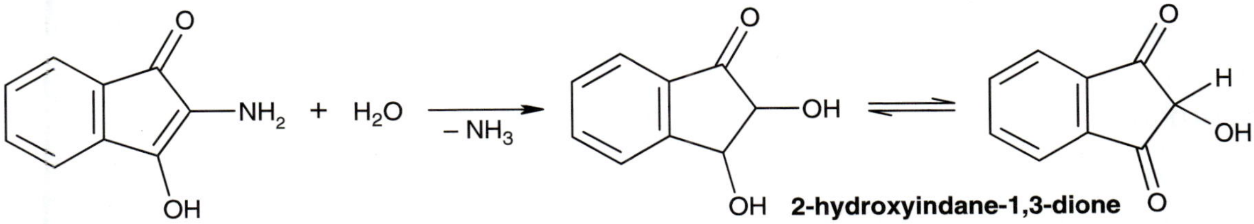

Step 3: 2-amino-1,3-indanedione reduces part of ninhydrin to 2-hydroxy-indane-1,3-dione and itself is oxidized to 2-iminoindane-1,3-dione.

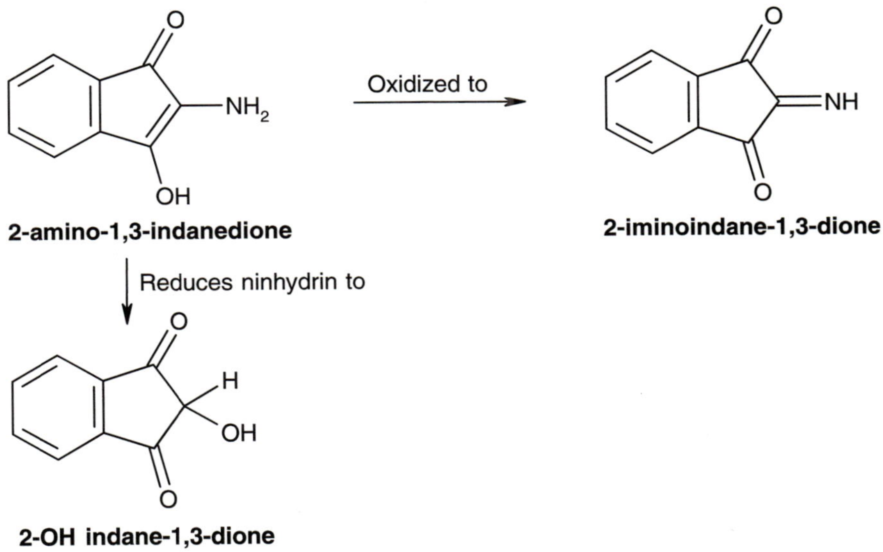

Step 4: Now 2-OH indane-1,3-dione and 2-iminoindane-1,3-dione condenses to form azaoxanol which is responsible for the final colour.

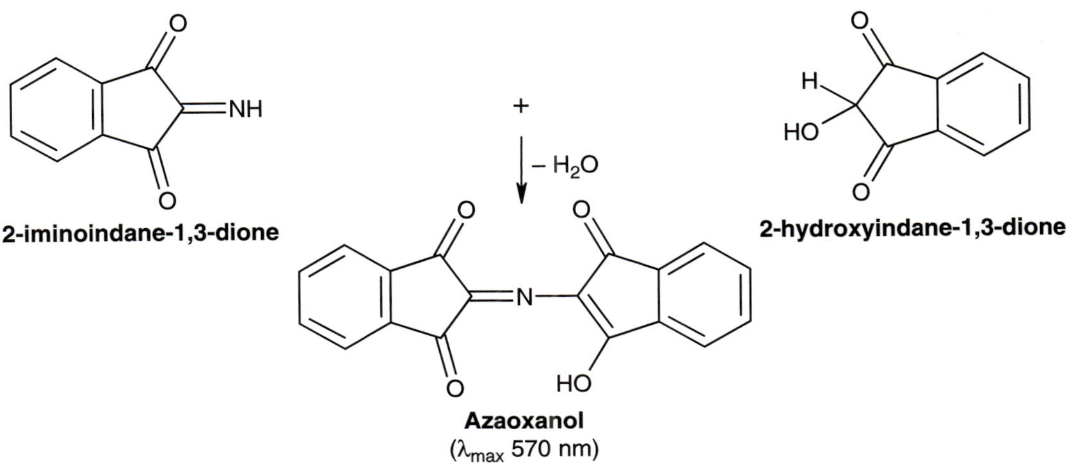

Chlorpheniramine maleate

Standard solution

Weigh accurately 20 mg of the substance, add 10 ml of water, 2.5 ml of 1 M hydrochloric acid and dilute to 50 ml with water.

Sample solution

Transfer accurately weighed quantity of the powdered sample equivalent to 20 mg of chlorpheniramine maleate to 100 ml volumetric flask. Add 10 ml of water, 2.5 ml of 1 M hydrochloric acid and dilute to 50 ml with water.

Follow the cyanogen bromide method described under formulation 1 of the chapter of rubefacients.

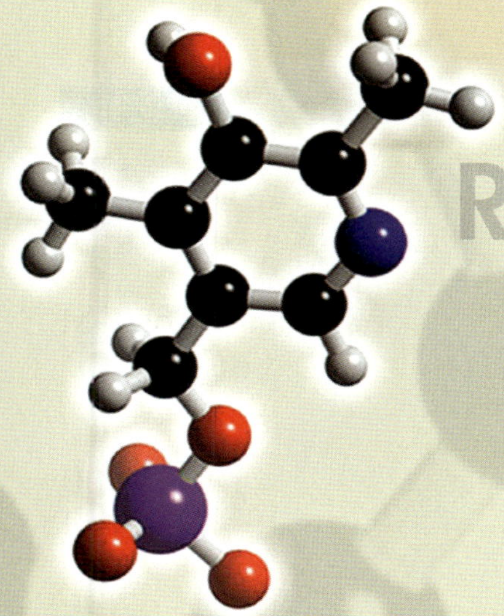

Reaction Mechanism

9

Antibiotics

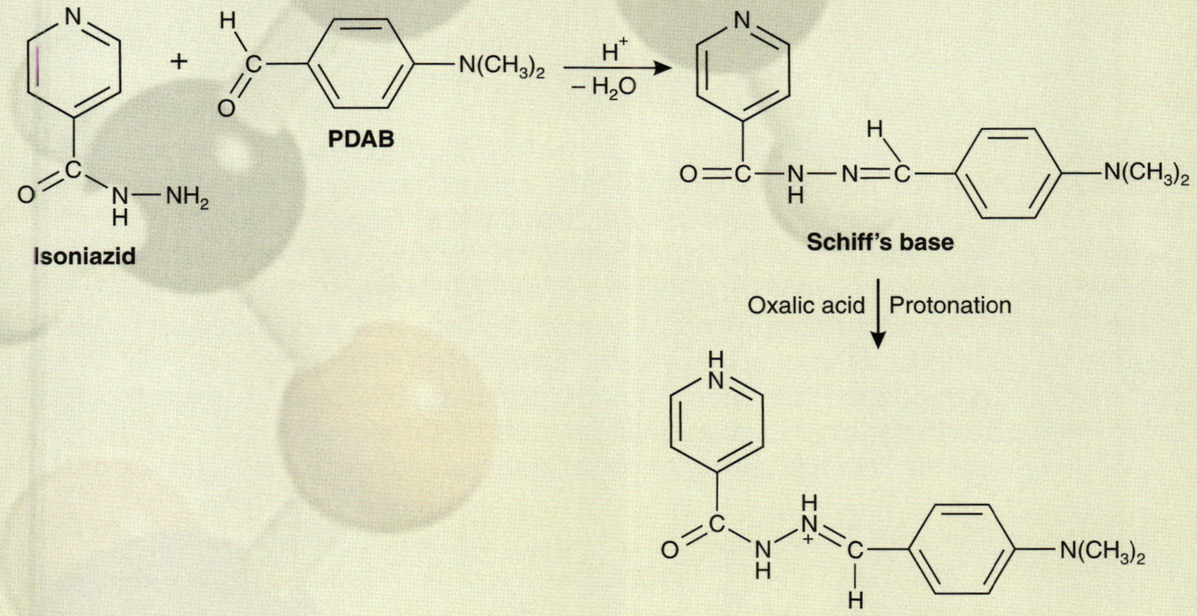

Yellow-coloured Schiff's base
(Pronated hydrazone)
(λ_{max} 395 nm)

Formulation 1

Isoniazid, Calcium gluconate, Pyridoxine hydrochloride

ESTIMATION

Isoniazid

METHOD 1

To sample accurately measured or weighed equivalent to 50 mg of isoniazid, add 50 ml of distilled water and 1.5 of sodium bicarbonate. Add 50 ml of 0.1 N iodine solution, stopper and allow to stand for 90 minutes. Cautiously add 20 ml of dilute hydrochloric acid and titrate excess iodine with 0.1 N sodium thiosulphate. Each ml of 0.1 N iodine is equivalent to 0.003429 g of isoniazid.

Probable Reaction Mechanism

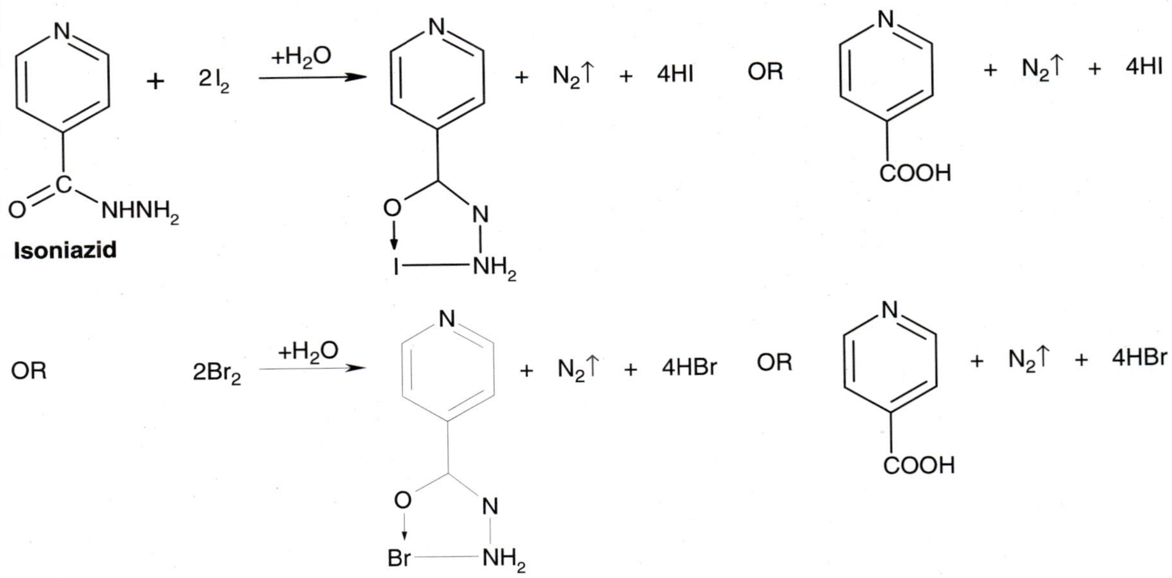

Reference

Practical Pharmaceutical Chemistry, 4th ed., by A.H. Beckett & J.B. Stenlake, p. 194, 2005.

METHOD 2

Reagents

1. Ammonia-ammonium chloride buffer, pH 10.8.
2. 0.33% w/v solution of 2,3-dichloro-1,4-naphthoquinone in absolute alcohol.

Standard solution

100 mcg/ml of isoniazid in water.

Sample solution

Sample equivalent to 100 mg of the substance is extracted and diluted with water to produce 100 mcg/ml.

Procedure

To 2 ml each of sample and standard solutions, add 1 ml of buffer solution, 6 ml of naphthoquinone reagent and dilute to 25 ml with water. Cool the mixture in ice-bath for 40 min. Measure the absorbance of purple blue complex of both sample and standard solutions at 610 nm against reagent blank. The method obeys Beer's law in the concentration range of 2-14 mcg/ml. The colour is stable for more than 2 hours. Thiacetazone and PAS do not interfere.

Note

If isoniazid is present as calcium methane sulphonate, estimate on the basis of calcium contents by the method: Extract the powdered sample with warm water to produce 2 mg/ml. Take aliquot equivalent to 200 mg (100 ml) and titrate with 0.1 M sodium edetate using erochrome-T as indicator.

Each ml of 0.1 M sodium edetate is equivalent to 0.025 g of calcium methane sulphonate of isoniazid.

In isoniazid there are two nucleophilic nitrogen atoms of which the sp^3 hybridized hydrazide nitrogen is more nucleophilic under alkaline conditions i.e. pH 10.8. It attacks nucleophilically at the chlorine-bearing C atom resulting in the formation of coloured product as shown.

Probable Reaction Mechanism

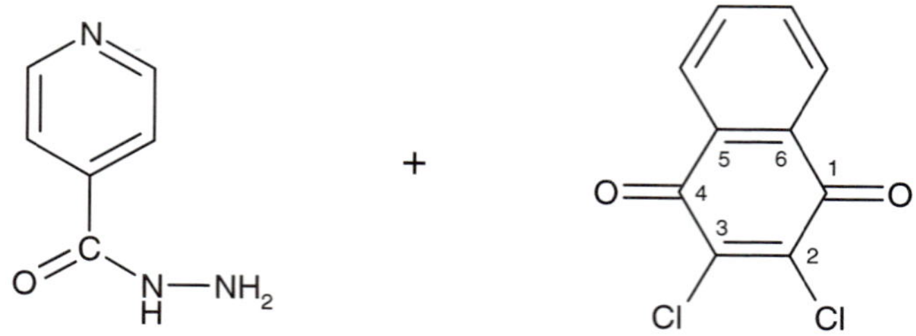

Isoniazid

2,3-dichloro-1,4-naphthaquinone (Dichlone)

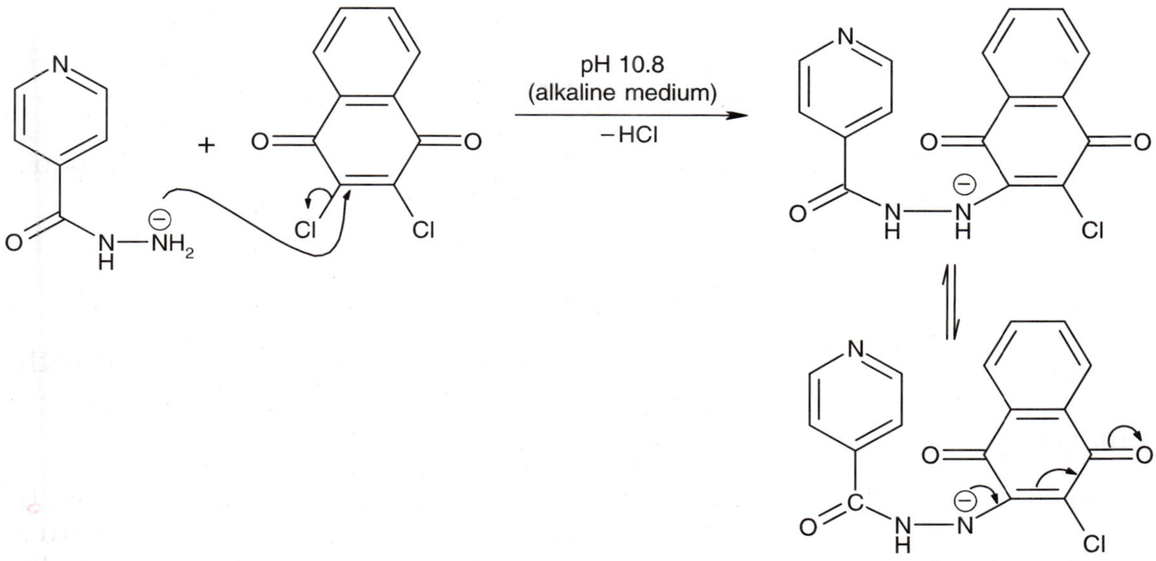

Note

Thiacetazone and PAS did not interfere.

Reference

M.B. Devani, C.J. Shishoo, M.A. Patel & D.D. Bhalara. *J. Pharm. Sci.*, 67(5), 661-663, 1978; A.A. Abou-Ouf, A.M. Taha & Sidhom. *J. Pharm. Sci.*, 62, 1700, 1973; and M.B. Devan et al. *Ind. J. Pharm. Sci.*, 42(6), 179-181, 1980.

Note

This method is suitable for estimation of isoniazid in the presence of hydrazine formed as a result of interaction between isoniazid and lactone in tablet formulation.

METHOD 3

Reagents

1. 2% w/v solution of p-dimethylaminobenzaldehyde (PDAB) (Ehrlich's reagent).
2. 1% oxalic acid in methanol.

Standard solution

100 mcg/ml of isoniazid in alcohol.

Sample solution

Extract the accurately weighed quantity of the sample equivalent to 50 mg of isoniazid with alcohol to get 1 mg/ml. Dilute further with alcohol to get 100 mcg/ml.

Procedure

To 1 ml each of sample and standard solutions, add 2 ml of 'PDAB' solution. Allow to stand at room temperature for 10 min, add 15 ml of methanol, 10 ml of oxalic acid and dilute to 50 ml with methanol. After 10 min, measure absorbance of yellow complex at about 395 nm against reagent blank. The method obeys Beer's law in the concentration range of 2-8 mcg/ml.

Note

Thiacetazone does not interfere.

Condensation takes place between the drug and aldehyde part of the reagent to form Schiff's base. Addition of oxalic acid results in protonation of structure (III) leading to the formation of yellow-coloured product.

Probable Reaction Mechanism

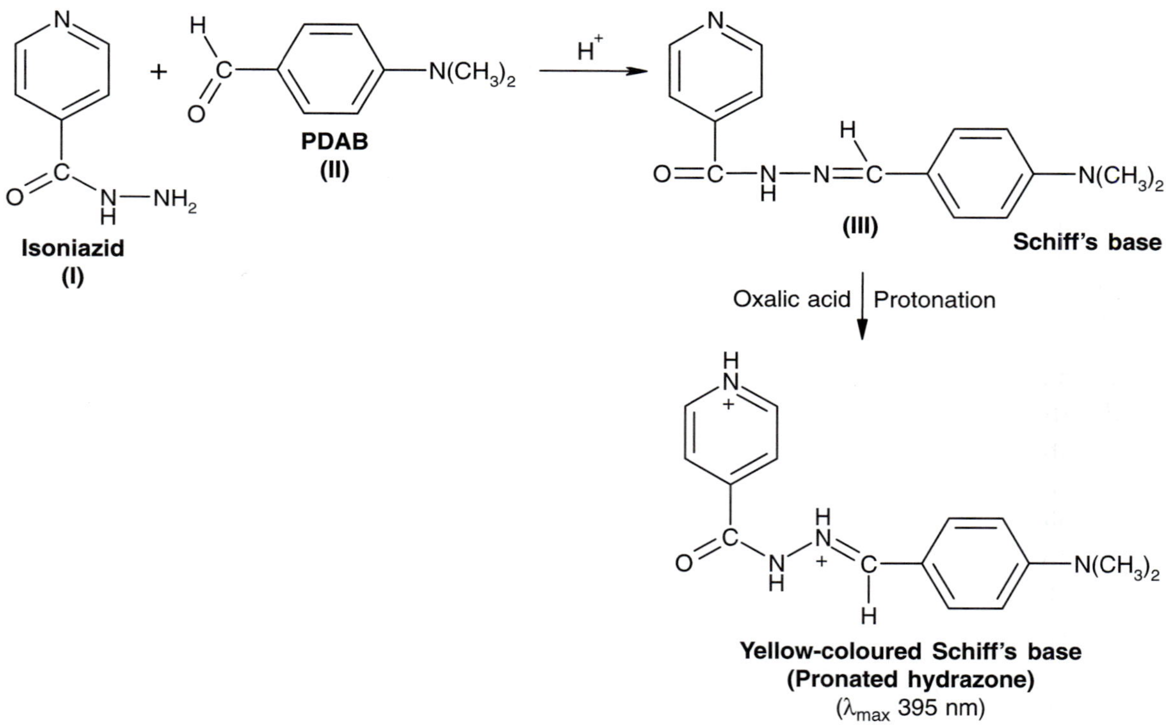

Note

Vanillin can also be used as aldehyde.

Reference

H.G. Boxenbaum & S. Riegelman, *J. Pharm. Sci.*, **63**, 1191, 1974.

On alkaline hydrolysis, isonicotinate and hydrazine are produced. Hydrazine reacts with 2 moles of PDAB to give orange-red coloured complex.

Probable Reaction Mechanism

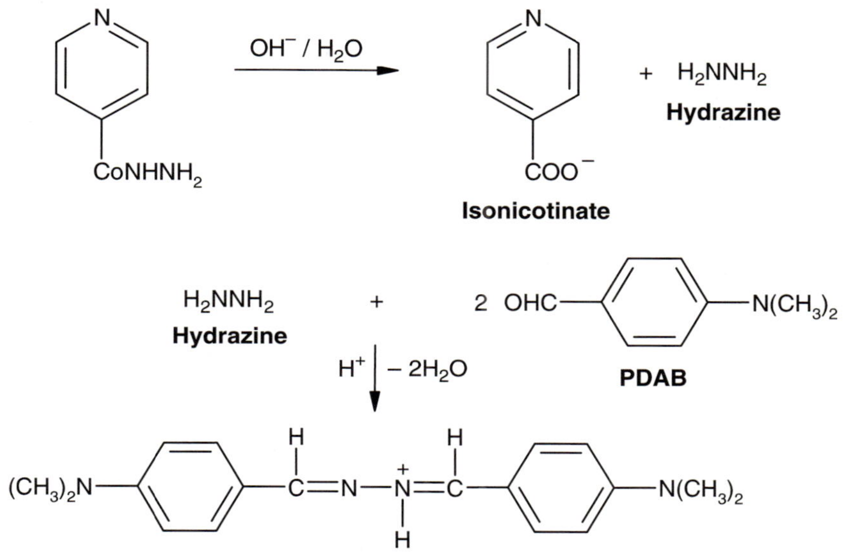

Orange-red coloured complex
(λ_{max} 450 nm)

METHOD 4

Reagents

1. Buffer solution, pH 6.0.
2. Modified Grote's reagent: 10 ml of solution of sodium nitroprusside and 5 ml of hydroxylamine hydrochloride solution are taken in 50 ml beaker, mixed and allowed to stand for 2 min. Then, add 10 ml of the sodium bicarbonate solution, 1 ml of bromine is slowly added and after 10 min, 5 ml of the phenol solution is added. The reagent is allowed to stand at room temperature for 5-12 h. Filter and store at 5°C. This stock solution is stable for 75 days. Dilute one part of the reagent with 19 parts of buffer solution, pH 6 just before use.
3. 5% w/v solution of sodium nitroprusside in water.
4. 10% w/v solution of sodium bicarbonate in water.
5. 2% w/v solution of phenol in water.
6. 10% w/v solution of hydroxylamine hydrochloride in water.

Standard solution

500 mcg/ml of isoniazid in pH 6.0 buffer.

Sample solution

Extract accurately weighed amount of the powdered tablets with pH 6.0 buffer to get concentration of 500 mcg/ml.

Procedure

To 0.5 ml each of sample and standard solutions, add 5 ml of diluted Grote's reagent and dilute to 10 ml with pH 6.0 buffer. Shake and after 5 min, measure the absorbance of both the solutions at about 440 nm against reagent blank.

Probable Reaction Mechanism

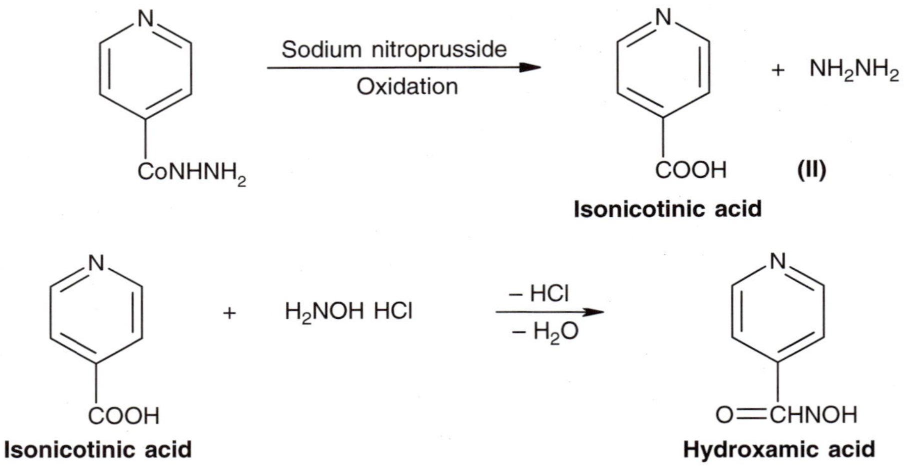

Note

In addition to calcium gluconate and vitamin B_6, vitamin D_2, proteolysed liver, lysine and common colouring agents do not interfere.

METHOD 5

Reagents

1. 0.1% w/v solution of 6,7-dichloroquinoline-5,8-dione (DCQD) in methanol.
2. 0.1 M sodium bicarbonate solution.

Standard solution

200 μg/ml of isoniazid in water.

Sample solution

Powdered sample equivalent to 50 mg of isoniazid suspended in water, dissolved in sufficient water to produce 50 ml, filtered and filterate diluted to get 200 μg/ml.

Procedure

To 1 ml each of sample and standard solutions, add 0.5 ml of DCDQ reagent and 1 ml of sodium bicarbonate solution, allow to stand for 5 min at room temperature with occasional shaking, dilute to 10 ml with methanol and measure the absorbance at 545 nm against reagent blank.

Probable Reaction Mechanism

Nucleophilic attack of amino group of the hydrazide moiety of isoniazid on 'DCQD' gives 6-hydrazoquinoline derivative. This reaction is analogous to the reaction under method 2 of isoniazid. The 6-hydrazoquinoline derivative tautomerizes in alkaline medium to form enolate ion which is responsible for green colour (λ_{max} 645 nm).

Probable Reaction Mechanism

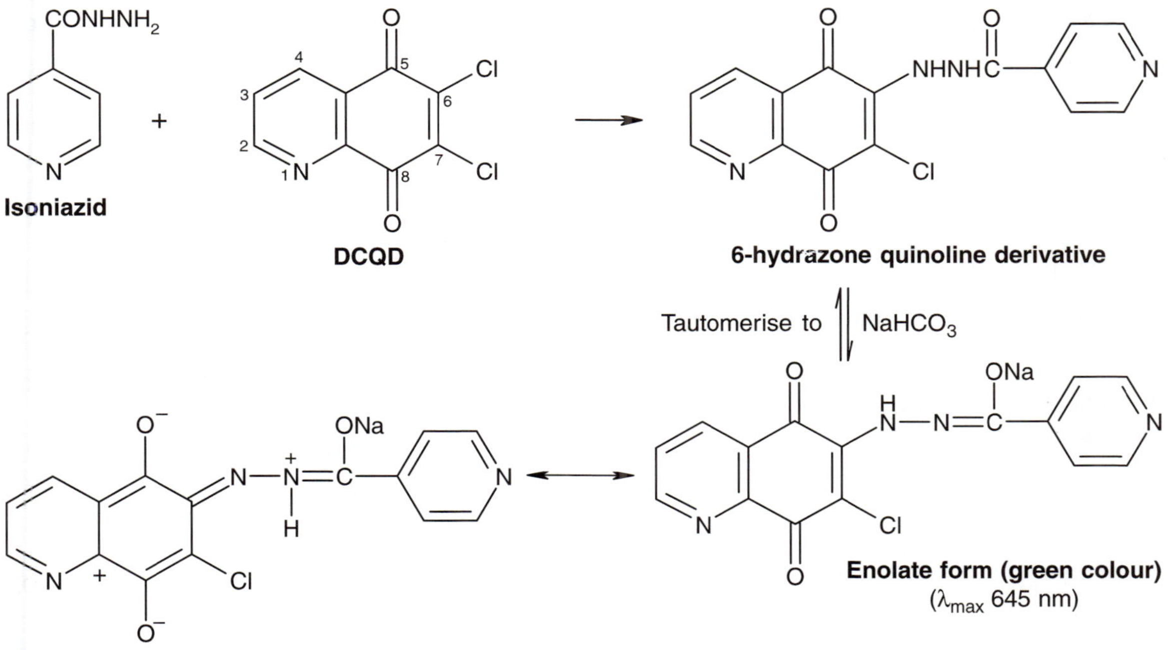

Note

As compared to 2,3-dichloronaphthoquinone as in method 2, the electron withdrawing effect of ring nitrogen in 6,7-dichloroquinoline-5,8-dione renders the α-carbonyl group in the latter more electron-dependent than the β-carbonyl group, thus increasing the probability of coupling.

Reference

Michael E. El Kommos & Amal S. Yanni. Analyst, 113, pp. 1091-95, 1988.

METHOD 6

Reagents

1. 0.05% w/v solution of potassium periodate (PPI).
2. 0.5% tiron solution (4,5-dihydroxy-1,3-benzene disulphonic acid sodium).
3. 0.1 M sodium hydroxide.

Standard solution

200 μg/ml in water.

Sample solution

Powdered sample equivalent to 50 mg of 'INH' suspended in water, shake for 5 min and dilute to volume. Filter and further dilute to get 200 μg/ml.

Procedure

To 1 ml each of sample and standard solutions, add 1 ml of 'PPI' solution, 0.5 ml of tiron solution and 1 ml of sodium hydroxide solution, dilute to 10 ml with water and measure the absorbance at 505 nm against reagent blank.

Probable Reaction Mechanism

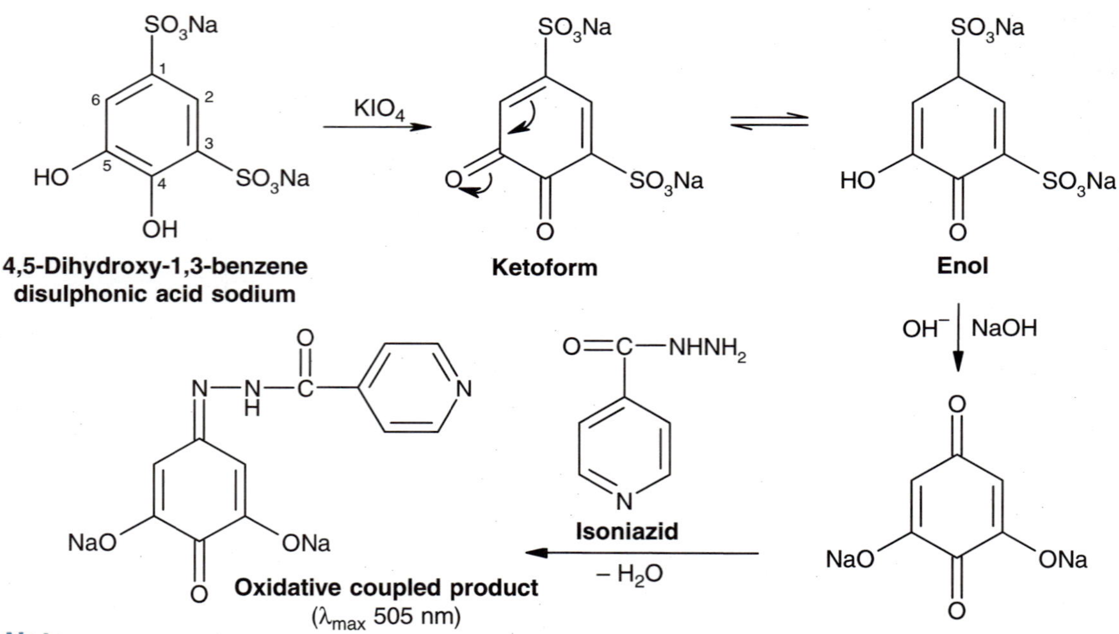

Note

1. Other oxidizing agents such as chloramine-T and potassium iodate do not give red colour.
2. N-bromosuccinimide, $K_3Fe(CN)_6$, ceric ammonium sulphate gave less intense coloured products.

Reference

1. B.G. Gowda, M.B. Melwanki, K.C. Ramesh & J. Keshavayya, *Ind. J. Pharm. Sci.*, **65(1)**, 86-90, 2003.
2. P. Nagaraja, Srinivasa Murthy & H.S. Yathirajan, *Talanta*, **43**, 1075, 1996.

METHOD 7

Reagents

1. 0.04% w/v solution of p-aminophenol (PAP) in methanol.
2. 1 M sodium hydroxide solution.

Sample and standard solutions

100 μg/ml of isoniazid in water.

Procedure

To 3 ml each of sample and standard solutions, add 1 ml of sodium hydroxide solution and then add 0.2 ml of PAP reagent, adjust the volume to 10 ml and measure the absorbance after 15 min at 420 nm against reagent blank.

Note

1. PAP solution should be freshly prepared.
2. Catechol also reacts similarly.

Probable Reaction Mechanism

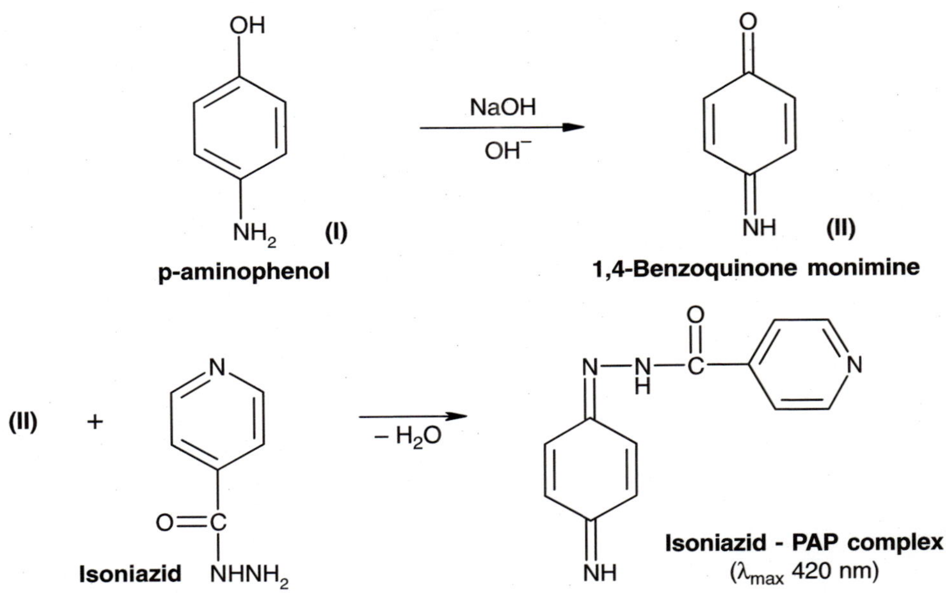

Reference

R.T. Sane & C.H. Thombare, *Curr. Sci.*, **48(23)**, 1030-1031, 1979.

Isoniazid can be estimated titrimetrically. Iodine liberated from iodine monochloride (ICl) is titrated with iodine trichloride (ICl_3). This reaction is based on the reducing property of acid hydrazide group present in the molecule which reacts with iodine monochloride to produce iodine.

Probable Reaction Mechanism

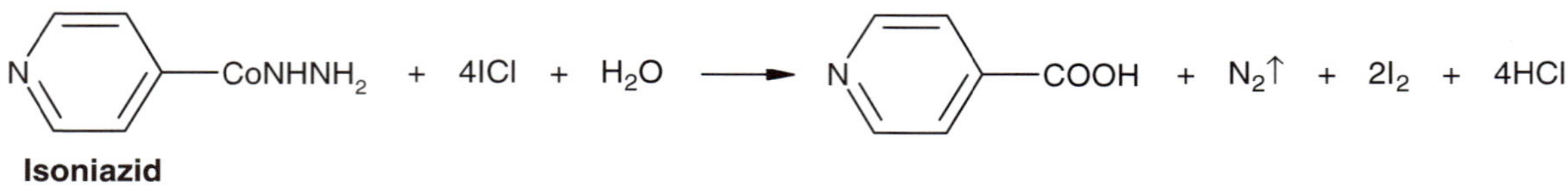

$$2I_2 + 2ICl_3 \longrightarrow 6ICl$$

Reference

K.K. Verma & A.K. Gupta, *Talanta*, **28**, 849-852, 1981.

A spectrophotometric method based on interaction of the drug in alkaline medium with 1-chloro or 1-fluoro-2,4-dinitrobenzene has been described by Scott et al. (1952). The end product is dinitrophenyl hydrazide. INH has two nucleophilic nitrogen atoms of which hydrazide nitrogen is more nucleophilic; so it attacks at chlorine-bearing carbon to produce hydrazide.

Probable Reaction Mechanism

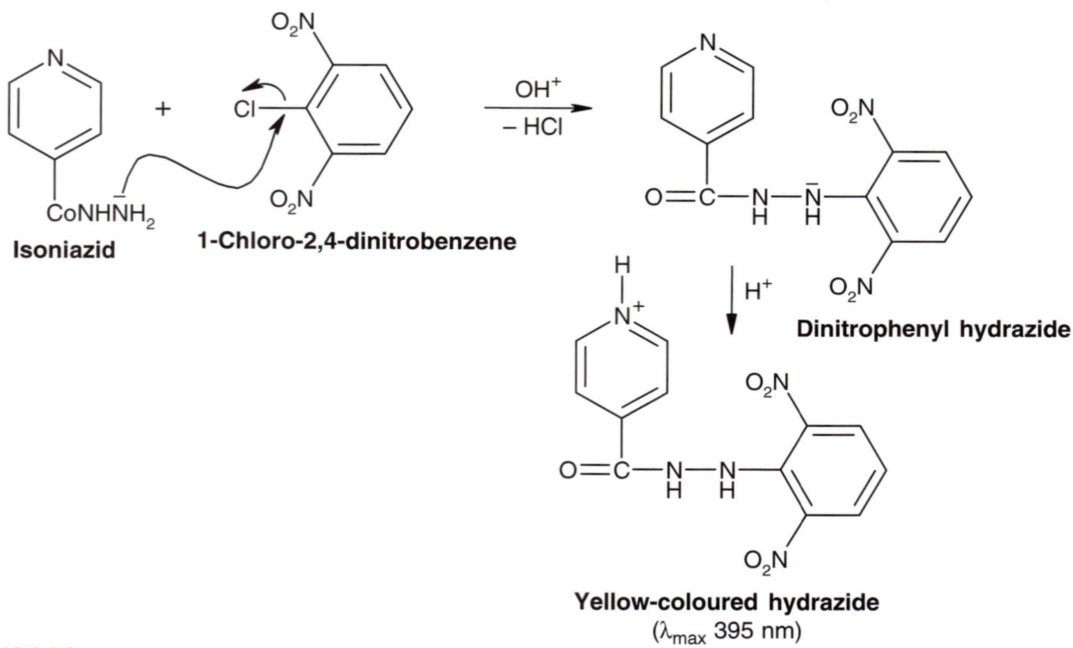

Reference

P.G.W. Scott, *J. Pharm. & Pharmacol.*, **4**, 681, 1952.

Reaction with 4-chloro-7-nitrobenzofuran in alkaline medium has also been used for spectrophotometric estimation of isoniazid.

Probable Reaction Mechanism

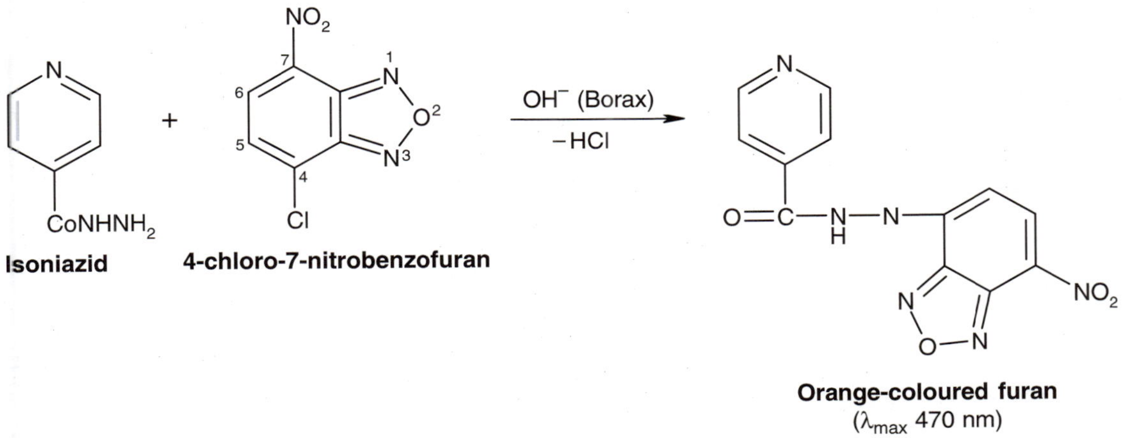

Reference

Pharmaceutical Chemistry (Vol. 2) by H.J. Roth, p. 545.

Nagaraja et al. (1996) have proposed a spectrophotometric method for the estimation of drug. The method is based on reaction of the component with 1,2-naphthoquinine-4-sulphonate (NQS) and cetyltrimethyl ammonium bromide (CTA) in alkaline medium.

To appropriate quantity of the sample and standard, add 4 ml of 0.006% 'NQS' solution, 3 ml of 1% CTA soluton and 2 ml of 1 M sodium hydroxide solution. The solution is diluted to 25 ml and absorbance measured at 500 nm against reagent blank.

Probable Reaction Mechanism

Orthoquinoidal 'NQS' in alkaline medium reacts with 'INH', a compound with two removable hydrogen atoms attached to one nitrogen atom, giving an orange-coloured paraquinoid imide (λ_{max} 485 nm). However, when 'CTA' was added, an intense red-coloured product was obtained with bathochromic shift of 15 nm (λ_{max} 500 nm).

Note

1. 'CTA' stabilizes the colour and also increases sensitivity.
2. Streptomycin, vitamin B_6 and nicotinamide did not interfere.

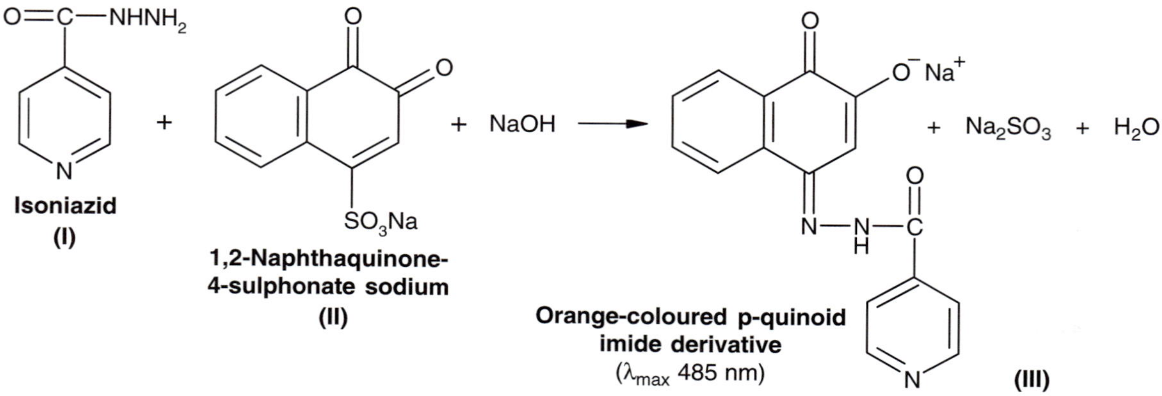

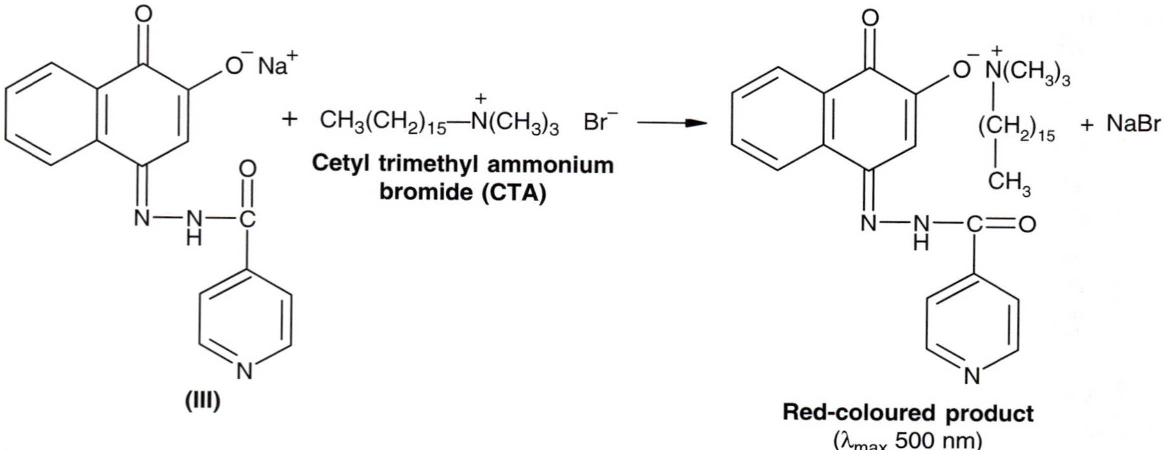

Reference

P. Nagaraja, K.C. Srinivasa Murthy & H.S. Yathirajan, *Talanta*, **43**, 1075-1080, 1996.

C.S.P. Sastry et al. (1992) have proposed the following reaction mechanism between oxidized metol and isoniazid. Metol is first oxidized by N-bromo-succinimide in acidic medium to give monoimine which reacts with isoniazid to give a coloured complex (λ_{max} 620 nm).

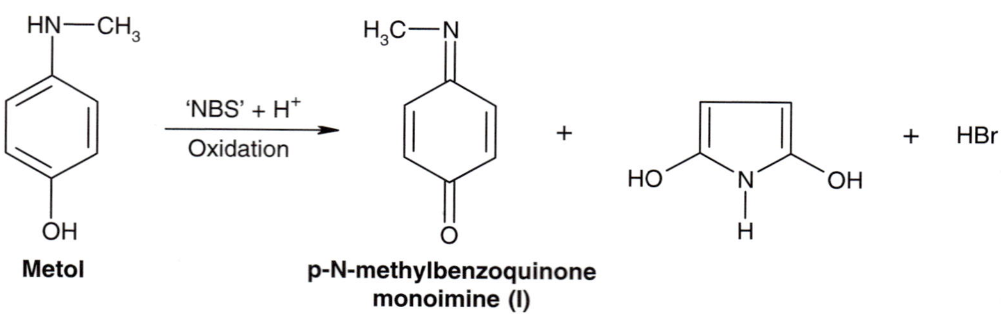

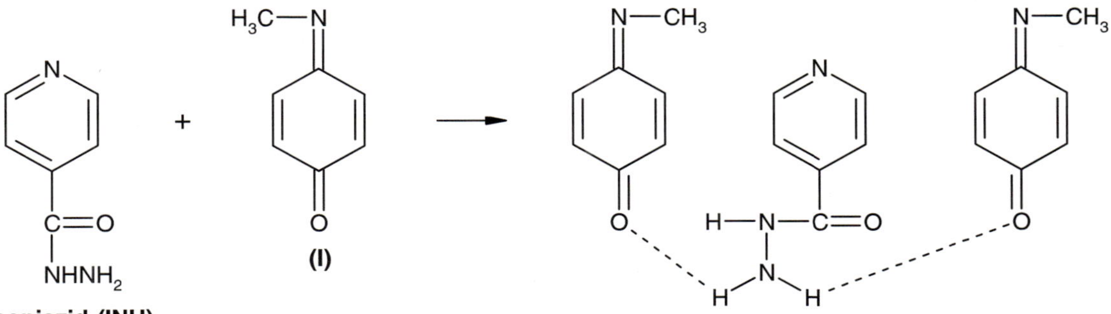

Isoniazid (INH)

(I)

(λ_{max} 620 nm)

Note

Ammonium vanadate (λ_{max} 605 nm) or $K_3Fe(CN)_6$ (λ_{max} 610 nm) could be used as oxidizing agents.

Reference

1. C.S.P. Sastry, B.S. Reddy & B.G. Rao, *Indian. J. Pharm. Sci.*, **43**, 118, 1981.
2. C.S.P. Sastry, A. Sailaja, T.T. Rao & D. Murali Krishna, *Talanta*, **39(6)**, 709-713, 1992.
3. P. Siraj, R. Rama Krishna, S.S.N. Murthy, B.S. Reddy & C.S.P. Sastry, *Talanta*, **28**, 477-481, 1981.

Stewart et al. (1975) have described an analytical method based on reaction of the drug with 9-chloroacridine. This chromogenic reagent was earlier reported to have been used for spectrophotometric estimation of aromatic amines. The reaction of the drug with the reagent suggests that a free amino (NH_2) function being present in the molecule.

Probable Reaction Mechanism

As suggested by the authors, the following reaction mechanism is possible.

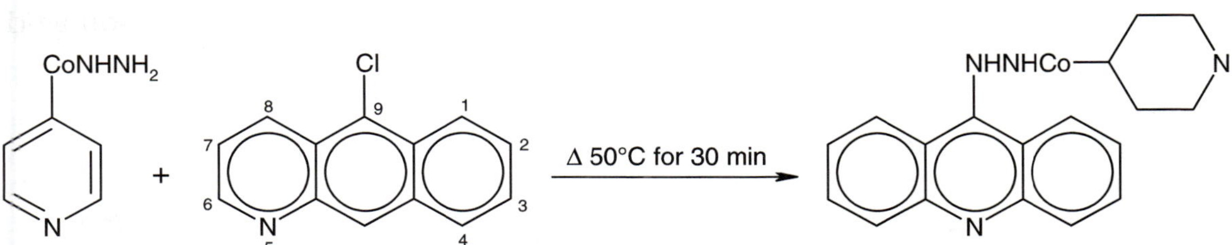

Isoniazid

9-chloroacridine

Isoniazid - acridine complex
(λ_{max} 500 nm)

Reference

James T. Stewart & David A. Settle, *J. Pharm. Sci.*, **64(8)**, 1403-1405, 1975.

Isoniazid reacts with $CuCl_2$ in hydrochloric acid to give green-coloured complex. Excess Cu (II) can be estimated with EDTA.

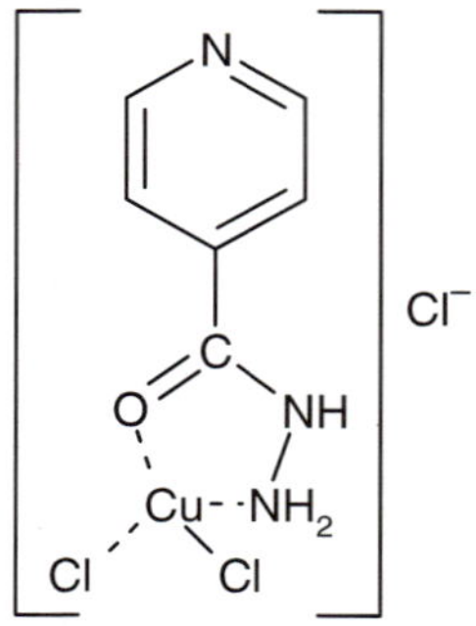

For quantitative estimation, volumetric method involving titration with nitrite (HNO_2) has also been used.

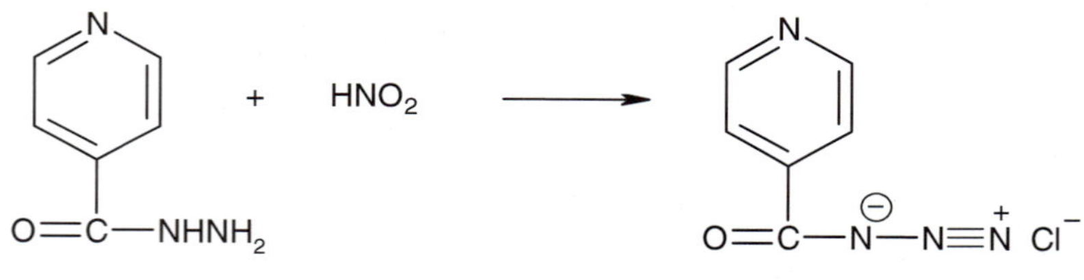

Isonicotinic acid azide

For oxidimetry, several oxidizing reagents such as Br_2, $KMnO_4$, $K_2Cr_2O_7$, cerric (IV) sulphate, KIO_3, KIO_4, chloramine-T, N-bromosuccinimide have been used.

Reference

Pharmaceutical Chemistry (Vol. 2) by H.J. Roth, p. 544.

METHOD 8

Two colorimetric methods for the estimation of isoniazid are developed. The first method depends on coupling of isoniazid with diazotized 1-amino anthraquinone zinc chloride salt (fast red AL salt) to form a red colour (λ_{max} 510 nm). The second one is based on the formation of a green complex (λ_{max} 655 nm) between the acid hydrazide and 2,6-dimethoxy-1,4-benzoquinone (DMBQ). All measurements of the two procedures were carried out in the presence of sodium hydroxide at room temperature (20 ± 3°C). The two methods are applied for the determination of isoniazid in the presence of congenial drugs, vitamins and additives normally encountered with it in pharmaceutical dosage forms.

Method 8A

Reagents

1. 0.2% w/v solution of diazotized 1-amino anthraquinone in water, prepared freshly and protected from light.
2. 0.4% and 10% w/v solutions of sodium hydroxide in water.

Standard solution

50 µg/ml solution of isoniazid in ethanol.

Sample solution

Extract the powdered sample with water to get 100 µg/ml solution.

Procedure

To 1 ml each of sample and standard solutions, add 1 ml of anthraquinone solution, mix and allow to stand for 10 min, add 1 ml of 10% sodium hydroxide solution and dilute to 10 ml with ethanol and measure the absorbance of both the solutions at 510 nm against reagent blank.

Probable Reaction Mechanism

Diazotized anthraquinone reacts with isoniazid in molar ratio of 1 : 1 to form red colour with maximum absorption at 510 nm. After adding the reagent, the solution must be allowed to stand for 10 min before adding sodium hydroxide solution. The colour is stable for 20 min.

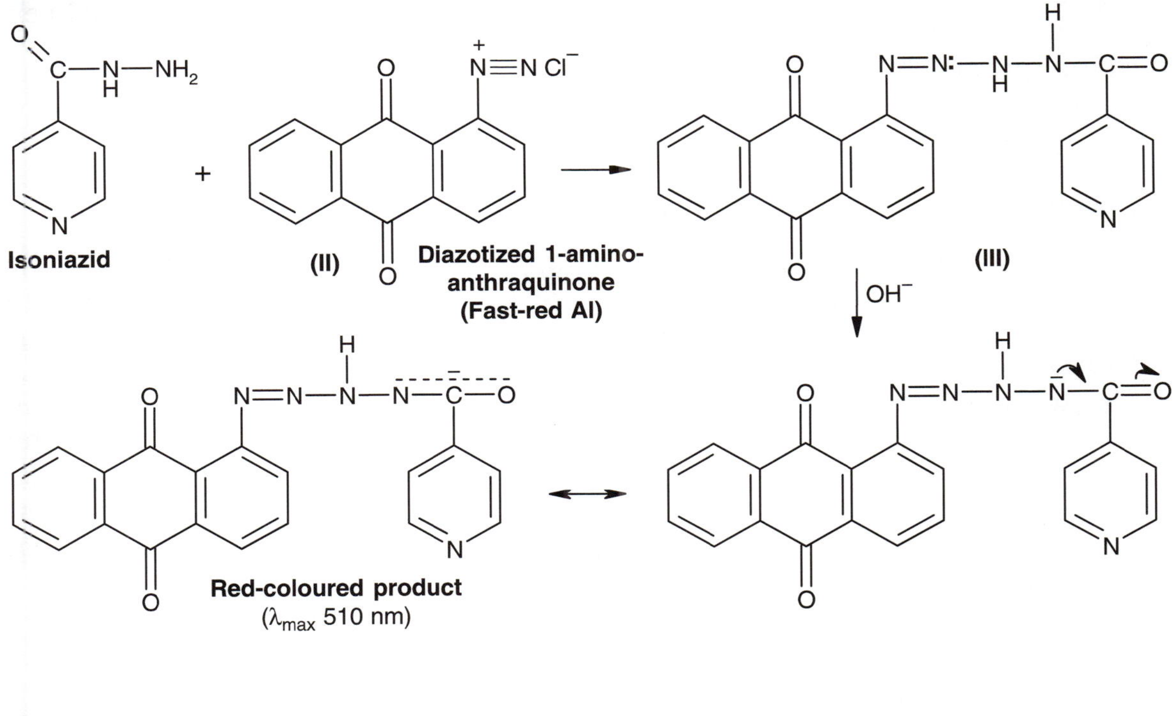

Method 8B

Reagents

1. 0.1% solution of 2,6-dimethoxy-1,4-benzoquinone in ethanol (DMBQ).
2. 0.4% sodium hydroxide solution in water.

Standard solution

As under method 8A.

Sample solution

50 µg/ml solution of sample in water.

Procedure

To 1 ml of the sample and standard solutions, add 1 ml of benzoquinone reagent and 0.1 ml of sodium hydroxide solution, mix and allow to stand the contents for 10 min at room temperature and then dilute to 10 ml with ethanol. Measure the absorbance of both the solutions at 655 nm against reagent blank.

Note

For complete formation of colour in method A, allow the solution to stand for 10 min before addition of alkali, whereas in method B, solution is allowed to stand for 10 min after the addition of alkali.

Probable Reaction Mechanism

Isoniazid, being a hydrazine derivative, is a strong reducing agent in alkaline medium. It reacts with DMBQ and reduces the latter to hydroquinone derivative forming quinone-hydroquinone (charge-transfer or donor-acceptor complex – λ_{max} 655 nm).

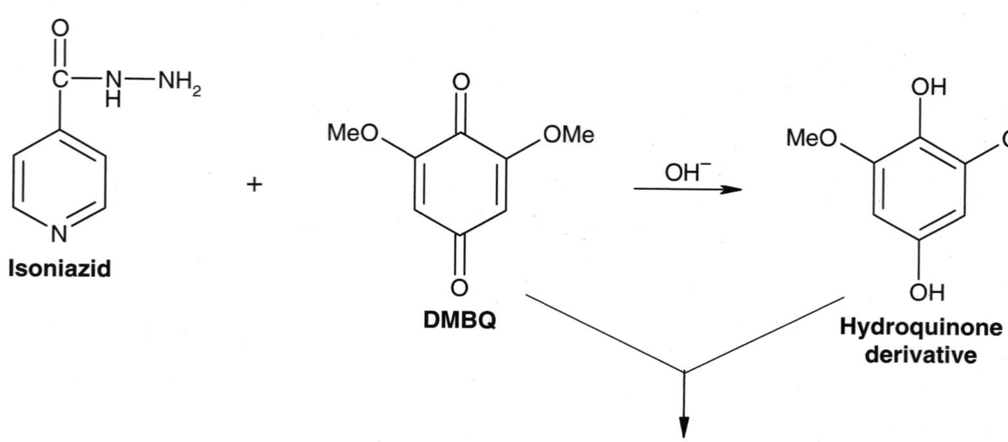

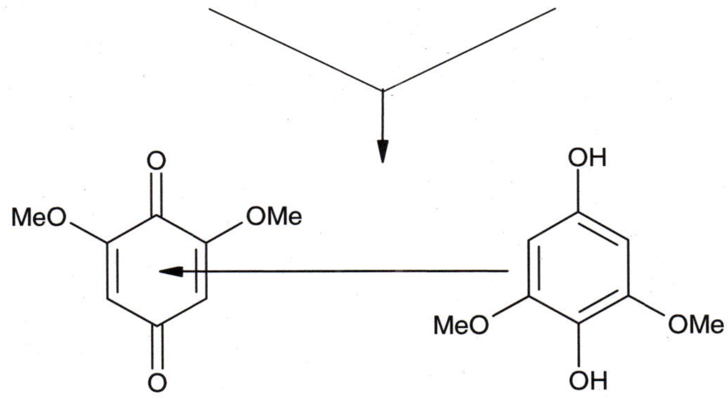

Green-coloured quinone-hydroquinone charge-transfer complex
(λ_{max} 655 nm)

Reference

Nadia M.A. Mahfouz & Kamla M. Emara, *Talanta*, **40(7)**, 1023-1029, 1993.

Calcium gluconate

To sample equivalent to 200 mg of calcium gluconate, add 3 ml of hydrochloric acid. Bring to boiling and add hot ammonium oxalate solution, followed by dilute ammonia solutions. Heat on water-bath for 1 hr and cool. Transfer precipitates to G_4 sintered funnel with the aid of 0.1% w/v ammonium oxalate solution. Wash precipitates with water till free of chloride. Dissolve the precipitates in dilute sulphuric acid, heat to 70°C and titrate with 0.1 N potassium permanganate maintaining solution at 70°C throughout titration. Each ml of 0.1 N potassium permanganate is equivalent to 0.02242 g of calcium gluconate, pentahydrate.

Pyridoxine hydrochloride

Follow method 1 or 3 as described in general methods for estimation of pyridoxine hydrochloride.

Formulation 2

Thiacetazone, Isoniazid

ESTIMATION

METHOD 1

This involves spectrophotometric method for estimation of both the components without prior separation.

Standard solution

25 mg each of thiacetazone and isoniazid were accurately weighed, separately dissolved in methanol and diluted to 250 ml with the solvent. 5 ml of each solution was further diluted to 100 ml with 0.1 N methanolic hydrochloric acid.

Sample solution

A quantity of sample equivalent to 50 mg of isoniazid was accurately weighed, dissolved in methanol and diluted to 100 ml with the solvent. 2 ml of the solution was further diluted to 100 ml with 0.1 N methanolic hydrochloric acid.

Procedure

The extinction of the sample and standard solutions was immediately measured at 268 nm and 328 nm, the absorption maxima of isoniazid and thiacetazone respectively. The concentration of thiacetazone in the sample was directly calculated by using predetermined absorptivity value with standard thiacetazone solution in methanolic hydrochloric acid at 328 nm. Isoniazid does not interfere at this wavelength. The concentration of isoniazid was calculated by applying the following equation:

$$C_1 = \frac{E_1 \times A_2 - E_2 \times A_1}{A_2 \times B_1}$$

where C_1 = concentration (g/L) of isoniazid in the final sample solution;
E_1 and E_2 = extinction values of the sample solution at 268 nm and 328 nm respectively;
A_1 and A_2 = absorptivity values of thiacetazone at 268 and 328 nm respectively;
B_1 = absorptivity value of isoniazid at 268 nm.

The values of A_1, A_2 and B_2 were found to be 18, 188 and 37 respectively.

Note

1. The extinction value of thiacetazone in acidic methanol tends to decrease if the solution is stored at room temperature beyond 30 minutes. It is, therefore, desirable that the extinction should be measured immediately after the preparation of the solutions.
2. Vitamins commonly present in such formulations interfere in the estimation of isoniazid but no such interference is observed in the estimation of thiacetazone.

METHOD 2

This method is based on the fact that isoniazid is highly soluble in water, whereas thiacetazone is practically insoluble.

Isoniazid

Weigh accurately quantity of the sample equivalent to 100 mg of isoniazid. Extract with three 25 ml portions of 0.01 N hydrochloric acid filtering each portion through the same sintered glass funnel (G_4), the filtrate is diluted to 100 ml with 0.01 N hydrochloric acid. Further dilutions are done appropriately with 0.01 N hydrochloric acid to final concentration of 10 mcg/ml. Measure the extinction of resultant solution at maxima at about 266 nm and calculate the results taking 378 as value of A 1%, 1 cm at 266 nm.

Thiacetazone

METHOD 1

The entire residue left after the extraction of isoniazid as described above is used for estimation. The residue is transferred to a volumetric flask with the aid of ethanol, used in small portions and diluted to 100 ml and filtered. The filtrate is appropriately diluted with ethanol to get final concentration of 10 mcg/ml. Measure the extinction of resulting solution at maxima at about 328 nm using ethanol as blank. Calculate the results taking 580 as value of A 1%, 1 cm at 328.

METHOD 2

Acid hydrolysis of thiacetazone is carried out by heating the drug solution in H_2O bath. The drug being a thiosemicarbazone, it undergoes hydrolysis resulting in the formation of an aldehyde. The aldehyde so formed undergoes condensation reaction with p-toluidine resulting in the formation of Schiff's base.

Probable Reaction Mechanism

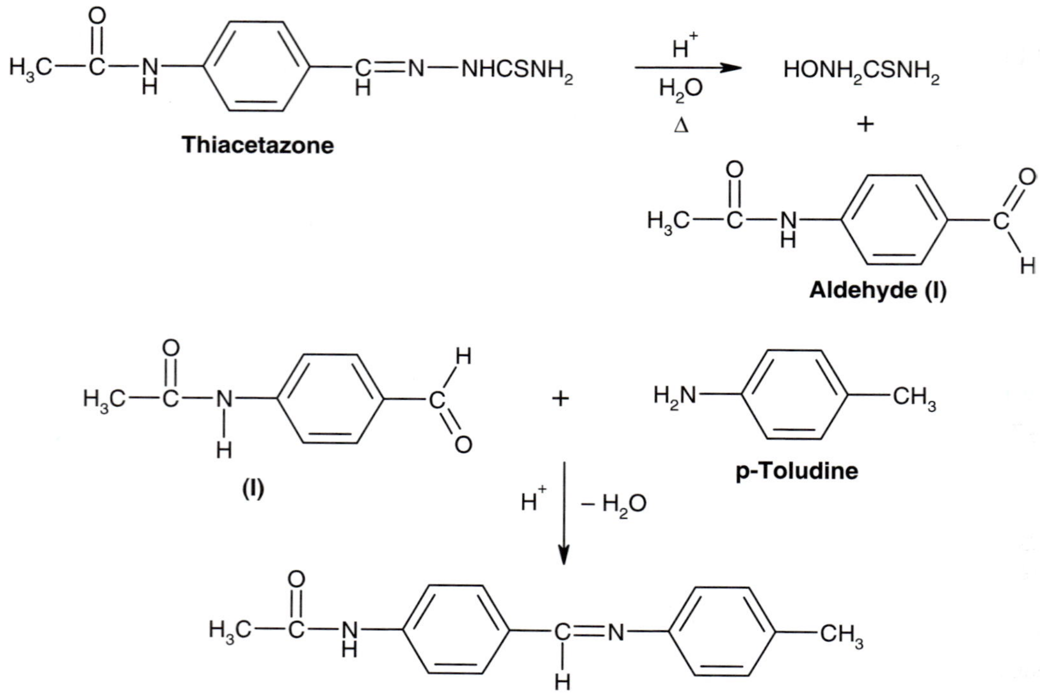

Schiff's base

Formulation 3

Ethambutol hydrochloride

METHOD 1

Reagents

1. 1.67×10^{-4} M Iodine in anhydrous chloroform.

Standard solution

50 mg of pure ethambutol hydrochloride is processed as per sample to get standard solution (50 mcg/ml).

Sample solution

Transfer powdered tablets equivalent to 50 mg of ethambutol accurately weighed to a separating funnel. Add 3 ml of 3 N sodium hydroxide to dissolve and extract with five 15 ml portions of dry chloroform (shake for 5 minutes for each extraction). Dry total chloroform layer over anhydrous sodium sulphate previously washed with chloroform and dilute to 100 ml with the same solvent. 5 ml of the resultant solution is further diluted to 50 ml with chloroform (50 mcg/ml).

Procedure

To 1 ml of the sample and standard solutions, add 5 ml of the iodine reagent and dilute to 10 ml with anhydrous chloroform. Allow to stand in dark for 1 h and measure the extinction of both sample and standard solutions at 293 nm. The method follows Beer's law in the final concentration range of 1.6-5.8 mcg/ml.

Note

Although, we observe peak at 293 and 360 nm but the one at 293 nm is quite linear.

Probable Reaction Mechanism

Ethambutol is non-UV/poor UV absorbing compound. Iodine is a mild oxidizing agent, it probably oxidizes the primary alcoholic groups in ethambutol to the aldehydic group thus increasing the UV absorption. In this process I_2 is reduced to iodide.

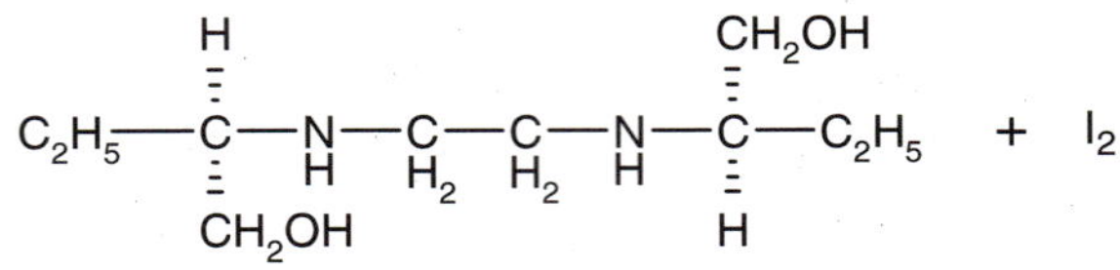

Ethambutol

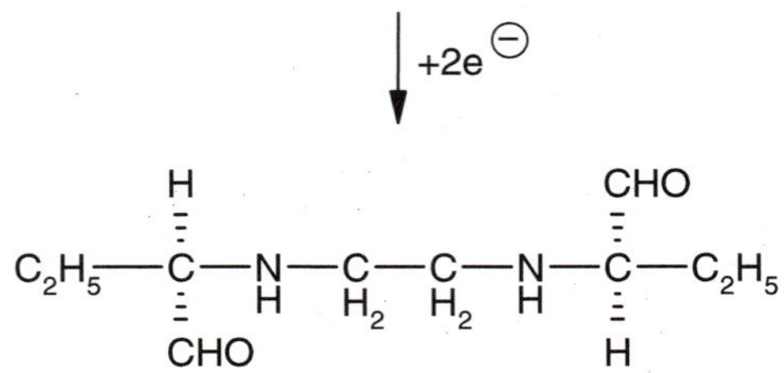

(λ_{max} 295 nm)

$$I_2 + 2e \rightleftharpoons 2I^{\ominus}$$

Reduced iodine form

Tan et al. (1977) have suggested that amines being lone-pair (n) electron donors can interreact with sacrificial electron acceptors such as iodine form charge-transfer (C-T) complexes. Estimation of ethambutol is based on above explanation. The sample is first basified and liberated base extracted with chloroform before proceeding with (C-T) complex formation. The complex formation is different for slow oxidation reaction of iodine with amines by being instantaneous. After complex formation, ethambutol exhibited blue shifted iodine bands at 293 nm and 360 nm, the peak at 293 nm being more intense. The (C-T) complex formed showed 1 : 2 molar ratio of ethambutol : iodine.

Note

For (C-T) complex formation, chloroform should contain ≥ 0.02% water for use as medium; no complex is formed when water content is more than 0.02%. Since the binding energy of charge-transfer (C-T) complex is usually small, addition of solvent with higher water content causes decomposition of the complex.

Reference

Henry S.I. Tan, Eric D. Gerlach & Anthony S. Diamattio, *J. Pharm. Sci.*, **66(6)**, 766-769, 1977.

METHOD 2

Ethambutol forms coloured complex with copper, nickel and cobalt in alkaline medium, pH 11.0. This forms the basis for quantitative estimation of ethambutol in dosage formulations.

Reagents

1. 1% w/v solution of copper sulphate, nickel sulphate and cobalt chloride in water.

Standard solution

10 mg/ml of pure ethambutol hydrochloride in water.

Sample solution

Weigh a quantity of powdered tablets equivalent to 500 mg of ethambutol hydrochloride. Extract with water to produce 50 ml (10 mg/ml).

Procedure

To 50 ml of sample and standard solutions, add 6 ml of any one of the three reagents and 25 ml of water. The pH is adjusted to 11.0 with 0.2 N sodium hydroxide. Filter the solution to remove precipitate of metal hydroxide. Adjust the filtrate to 50 ml and measure the absorbance of both sample and standard solutions at 625 nm (blue) for copper sulphate; 480 nm (orange) for nickel sulphate and 560 nm (violet) for cobalt chloride. The method obeys Beer's law in the concentration range of 0.2 to 2 mg/ml.

Note

Excess metal solution should not be used owing to heavy amount of metal hydroxide being precipitated.

On treating aqueous solution of ethambutol with Cu(II) and adding NaOH solution a blue colour is obtained due to the formation of Cu complex. This reaction is typical of compounds with a 1,2-amino alcohol or 1,2-diamine structure and is known as 'Chen Kao reaction'. The reaction can be represented as:

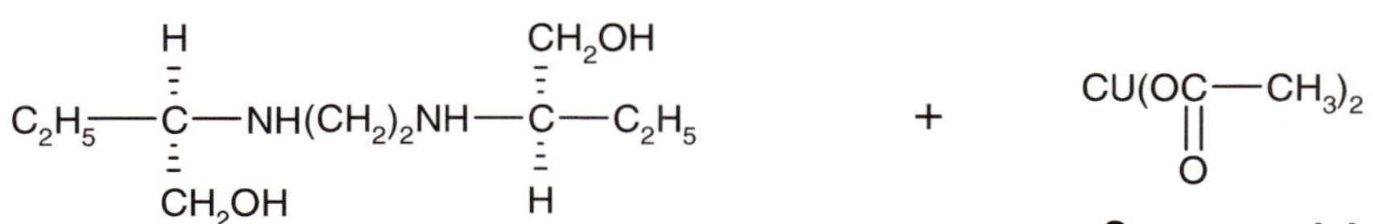

Ethambutol **Copper acetate or $CuSO_4$**

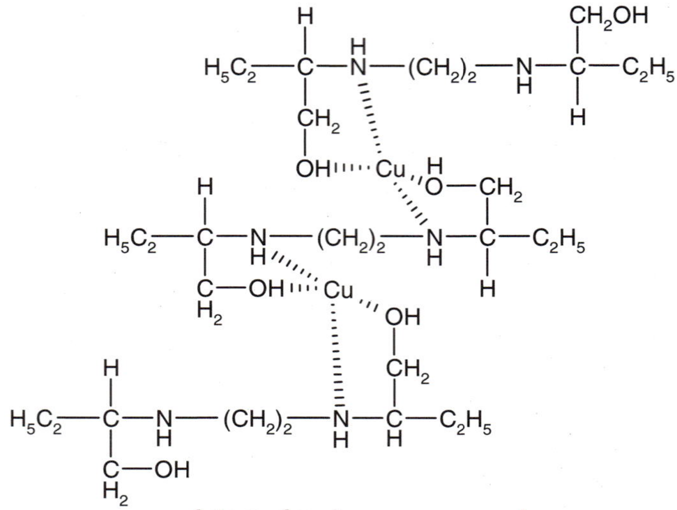

Intermolecular copper complex
(λ_{max} 680 nm and λ_{max} 260 nm)

Note

Similar reaction with other transition metals like $Ni(2)^+$ (orange colour - λ_{max} 480 nm) and $Co(2)^+$ (violet colour - λ_{max} 560 nm).

Reference

1. R.G. Bhattacharya & V.K. Paul, *Ind. J. Pharm. Sci.*, **43(6)**, 219-221, 1981.
2. R.B. Patel, A.A. Patel, T.P. Gandhi, V.C. Patel & R.N. Gilbert, *Indian Drugs*, **15(10)**, 191-194, 1978.

Alternative chelation of ethambutol and $Cu(II)^+$ is reported. This forms the basis for UV spectrophotometric method (λ_{max} 260 nm).

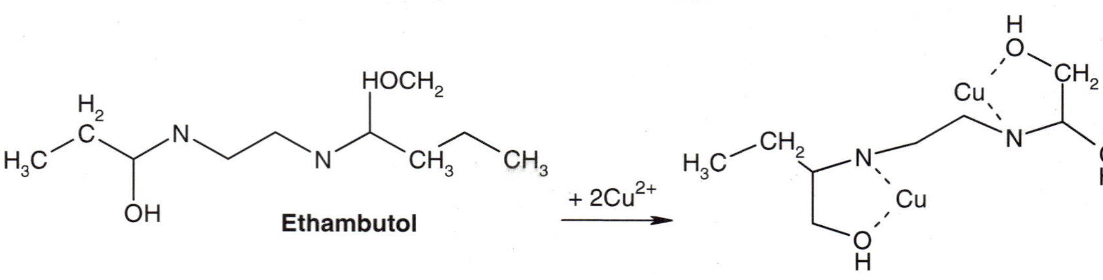

Intramolecular ethambutol - $Cu(2)^+$ complex
(λ_{max} 260 nm)

Reference

Z. Jiang, H. Wang & D.C. Locke. *Analytica Chemica Acta*, 456, 189-192, 2002.

Gupta et al. have also reported chelation of ethambutol with $Cu(II)^+$ in alkaline medium giving chelate complex with molecular formula ($C_{10}H_{22}N_2O_2Cu$).

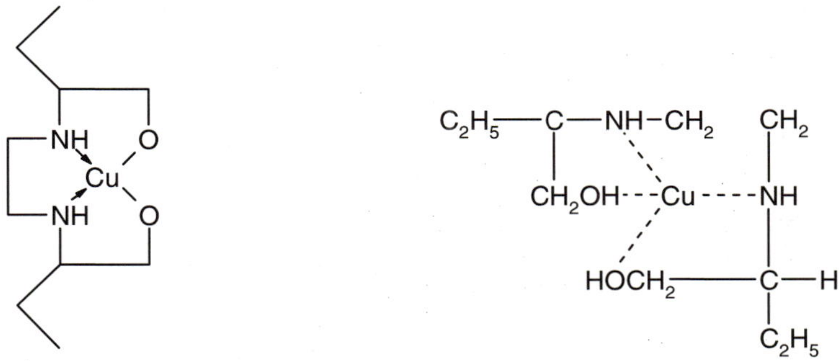

Intramolecular ethambutol - copper blue chelate
(λ_{max} 620 nm)

Reference

V.K. Gupta, R. Prasad & Azad Kumar, *Talanta*, **60**, 149-160, 2003.

The compound forms ion-pair complex with acidic dye (bromothymol blue) in pH 7.0 buffer. The complex is extractable into chloroform and has λ_{max} 410 nm. The method is suitable for solid dosage form.

Reference

E.H. Girgies, Z. Gad & M. Maran, *J. Pharm. Sci.*, **63(11)**, 1764-1766, 1974.

METHOD 3

This is based on iodometric estimation of the substance.

Reagents

1. 0.5 N periodic acid solution; Dissolve 5.5 g of pure periodic acid solution in water to produce 500 ml. Store in dark glass bottle and standardize before use.
2. 0.2 N sodium thiosulphate.
3. 20% w/v solution of potassium iodide in water.

Procedure

Weigh accurately, a quantity of powdered tablets equivalent to 200 mg of ethambutol. Dissolve in water, followed by 5 ml of 1 N sodium hydroxide. Add 24 ml of periodic acid solution and keep for 1 hr. Then, add 15 ml of potassium iodide solution and 20 ml of dilute sulphuric acid and titrate against 0.2 N sodium thiosulphate solution using starch as indicator. Each ml of 0.1 N sodium thiosulphate is equivalent to 0.00698 g of ethambutol hydrochloride.

Note

PAS, thiacetazone and rifampicin do not interfere in this procedure.

Excess HIO_4 liberates iodine (I_2 from KI) which is titrated with sodium thiosulphate.

Comments on method official in BP, 1980

1. Filtration of chloroform extract through filter paper as given in BP gives lower assay values because of absorption by filter paper.
2. Basification with 2 N sodium hydroxide requires more chloroform for complete extraction. (71% is extracted with single extraction of 25 ml of chloroform). It is recommended that :
   (a) Filter chloroform extract through 20 g layer of anhydrous sodium sulphate instead of filter paper.
   (b) Use 3 N sodium hydroxide for basification for better extraction (89.5% is extracted with single extraction of 25 ml of chloroform).

METHOD 4

$NaIO_4$ has a selective oxidising action on compounds having an hydroxyl and an amino group attached to adjacent carbon atom. This C—C bond is cleaved and the reaction is known as **Malaprade reaction**. The cleavage results in the formation of aldehydes with which MBTH can react resulting in the colour formation.

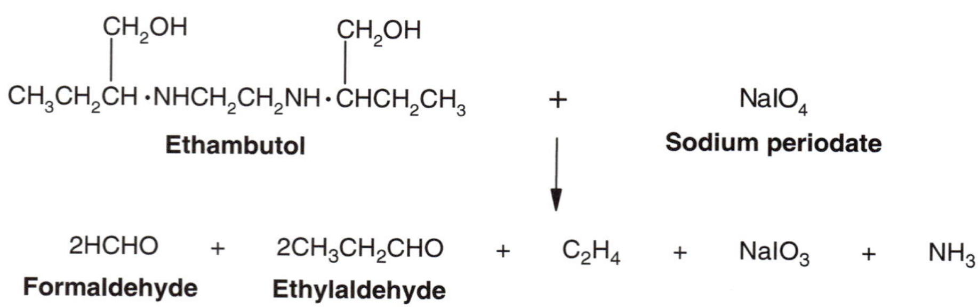

Both aldehydes react with MBTH to give corresponding products.

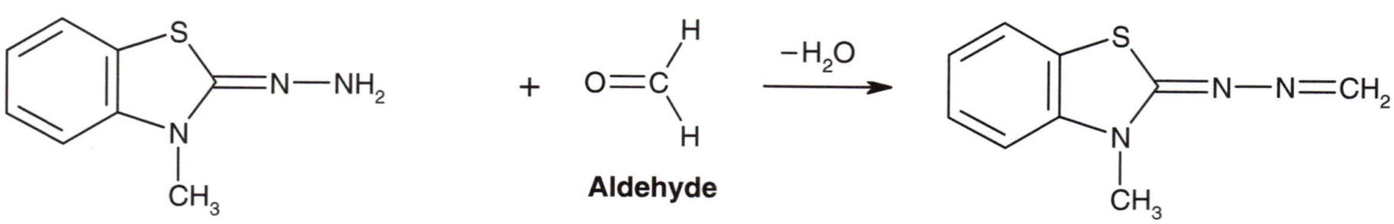

3-methyl-2-benzothiazolinone hydrazone (MBTH)

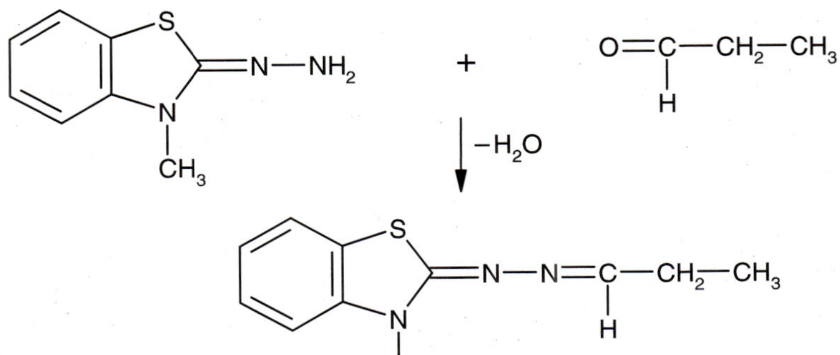

Coloured complex
(λ_{max} 630 nm)

Reference

G. Rama Rao, S.S.N. Murthy & P. Khadgapathi, *Eastern Pharmacist*, **141**, March 1981.

Formulation 4

Ethambutol hydrochloride, Isoniazid

METHOD 1

Reagent

1.67×10^{-4} M iodine in anhydrous chloroform.

Standard solution

50 mcg/ml of ethambutol hydrochloride in chloroform is processed as per sample to get standard solution (50 mcg/ml).

Sample solution

Transfer sample equivalent to 50 mg of ethambutol accurately weighed to a separating funnel. Add 3 ml of 3 N sodium hydroxide and extract with five 15 ml portions of dry chloroform (shake for 5 minutes for each extraction). Dry total chloroform layer over anhydrous sodium sulphate previously washed with chloroform and dilute to 100 ml with the same solvent. 5 ml of the resultant solution is further diluted to 50 ml with chloroform (50 mcg/ml).

Procedure

To 1 ml each of the sample and standard solutions, add 5 ml of the iodine reagent and dilute to 10 ml with anhydrous chloroform. Allow to stand in dark for 1 h and measure the extinction of both sample and standard solutions at 293 nm. The method follows Beer's law in the final concentration range of 1.5-7.5 mcg/ml.

Note

Although the peaks are observed at 293 and 360 nm but the one at 293 nm is quite linear.

For reaction mechanism see Formulation 3 of this chapter.

METHOD 2

This is based on iodometric estimation of the substance.

Reagents

1. 0.5 N periodic acid solution: Dissolve 5.5 g of pure periodic acid in water to produce 500 ml. Store in dark glass bottle and standardize before use.
2. 0.2 N sodium thiosulphate.
3. 20% w/v solution of potassium iodine in water.

Procedure

Weigh accurately, a quantity of powdered tablets equivalent to 200 mg of ethambutol. Dissolve in water, followed by 5 ml of 1 N sodium hydroxide. Add 25 ml of periodic acid solution and keep for 1 hr. Then, add 15 ml of potassium iodide solution and 20 ml of dilute sulphuric acid and titrate against 0.2 N sodium thiosulphate solution using starch as indicator. Each ml of 0.1 N sodium thiosulphate is equivalent to 0.00698 g of ethambutol hydrochloride. Excess periodic acid oxidizes KI to iodine which is finally titrated with thiosulphate.

Note

PAS, thiacetazone and rifampicin do not interfere in this procedure.

Comments on assay method official in IP, 1996

1. Filtration of chloroform extract through filter paper will give lower assay values because of absorption by filter paper; filtration through layer of anhydrous sodium sulphate is recommended.
2. Basification with 2 N sodium hydroxide requires more chloroform for complete extraction (71% is extracted with single extraction of 25 ml of chloroform); use 3 N sodium hydroxide for basification for better extraction (89.5% is extracted with single extraction of 25 ml of chloroform).

METHOD 3

The method is based on non-aqueous titration of the molecule with perchloric acid.

Reagents

1. 3 N sodium hydroxide.
2. 0.1 N perchloric acid.

Sample solution

Weigh accurately a quantity of the sample equivalent to 200 mg of ethambutol hydrochloride. Add 10 ml of 3 N sodium hydroxide solution and extract with five 25 ml portions of chloroform. Pass the combined chloroform layer through anhydrous sodium sulphate and evaporate to dryness and take up the residue in 100 ml of glacial acetic acid and titrate with 0.1 N perchloric acid using α-naphtholbenzein or crystal violet as indicator. Each ml of 0.1 N perchloric acid is equivalent to 0.01386 g of ethambutol hydrochloride.

Note

For extraction and filtration, follow instructions described in formulation 3 of this chapter.

Isoniazid

Follow the methods described in formulation 1 of this chapter.

Formulation 5

Pyrazinamide, Rifampicin, Isoniazid

ESTIMATION

Pyrazinamide

METHOD 1

Weigh accurately quantity of the sample equivalent to about 300 mg of pyrazinamide, suspend in 25 ml of chloroform and extract with five 30 ml portions of 0.1 N hydrochloric acid. Discard the chloroform layer. Transfer the combined acidic layer to ammonia distillation flask, add 100 ml of water and 100 ml of sodium hydroxide solution (50% w/v). Carry out ammonia distillation, collecting the distillate in 0.1 N sulphuric acid. Titrate excess acid with 0.1 N sodium hydroxide using methyl red as indicator. Each ml of 0.1 N sulphuric acid is equivalent to 0.01231 g of pyrazinamide.

METHOD 2

Pyrazinamide is converted to piperazine by heating with zinc + hydrochloric acid. Piperazine so formed interacts with 2 mol of ninhydrin to give coloured complex (λ_{max} 560 nm).

Probable Reaction Mechanism

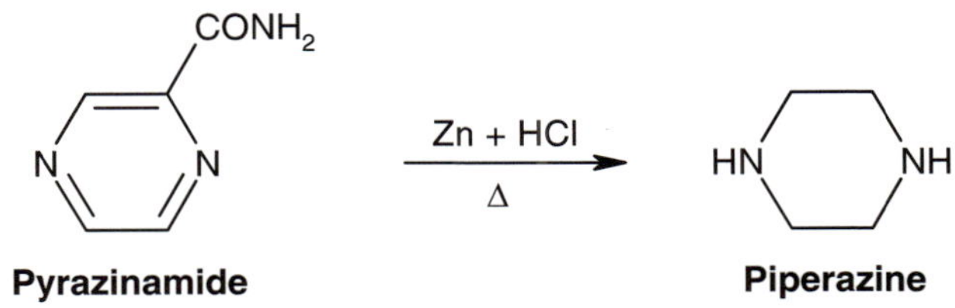

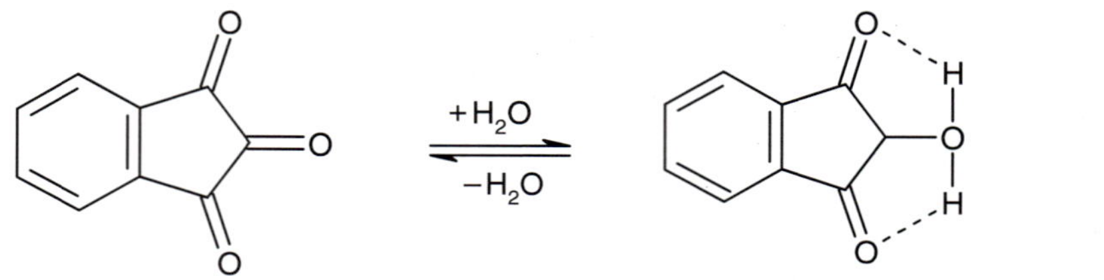

Ninhydrin (1,2,3-trioxoindane)

Hydrated form (intramolecular hydrogen bond)

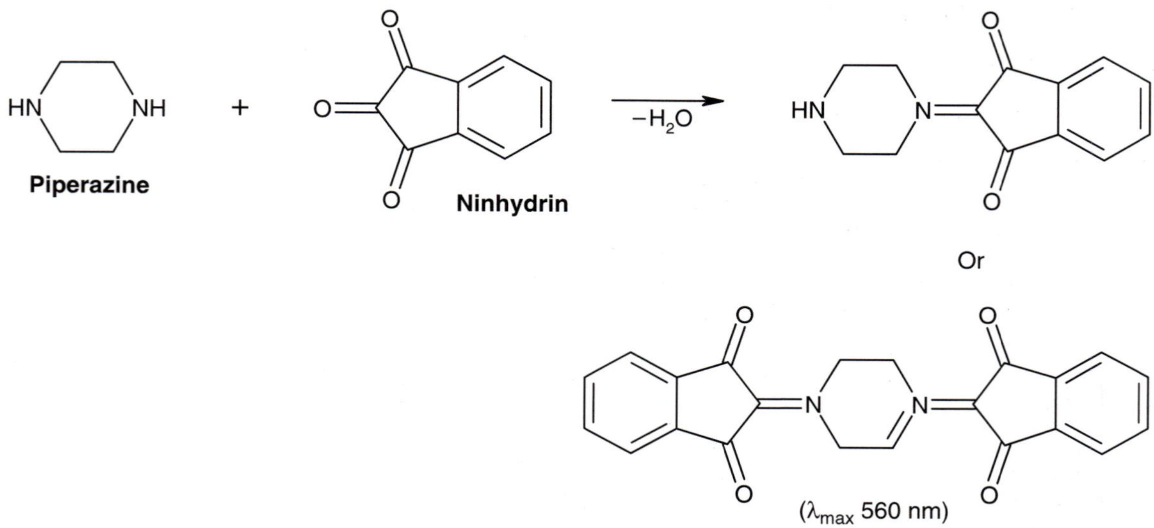

Since both the forms of ninhydrin are in equilibrium in the presence of water and co-exist, other possible reaction products are also likely.

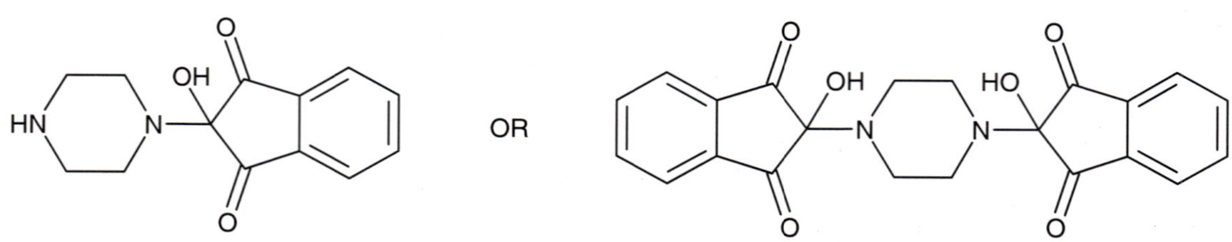

Reference

E. Venkata Rao, S.S.N. Murthy & G. Rama Rao, *Indian Drugs*, **22(5)**, 269-270, 1985.

METHOD 3

Pyrazinamide can couple with MBTH in the presence of ferric chloride (oxidizing agent) to give a complex (λ_{max} 635 nm).

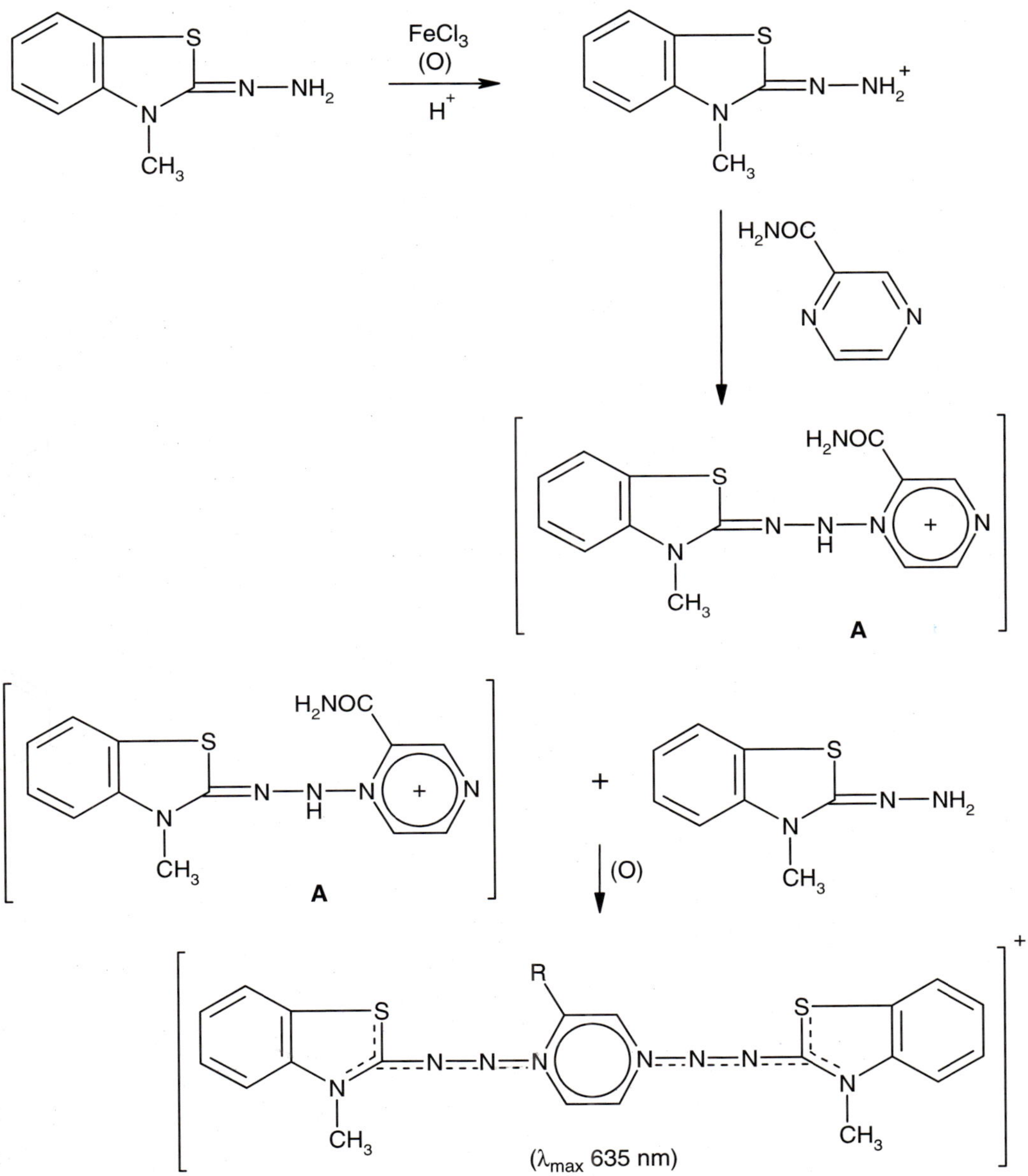

Note

Nicotinamide, nicotinic acid and piperazine do not answer this reaction; hence no interference.

Reference

G. Rama Rao, S.S.N. Murthy, P. Khadgapathi & E. Venkata Rao. Indian Drugs, 26(7), 362-365, 1989.

Rifampicin

METHOD 1

Reagents

1. 5.0% w/v solution of potassium dichromate in water.
2. Phosphate buffer, pH 7.4.
3. Methyl isobutyl ketone (solvent).

Standard solution

1 mg/ml of rifampicin in methanol.

Sample solution

Weigh accurately the sample equivalent to about 100 mg of the rifampicin, add 50 ml of methyl alcohol, shake and make up to 100 ml with methyl alcohol.

Procedure

Take 5 ml each of potassium dichromate solution and buffer solution in two separators. Add 2 ml each of sample and standard solutions. Stir well and after 1 minute, extract with two 10 ml portions of methyl isobutyl ketone. Make up the volume to 25 ml with the solvent. Measure the absorbance of resulting solutions at about 540 nm against reagent blank. Deduce the results by comparison.

$K_2Cr_2O_7$ is an oxidizing agent. It probably oxidizes the naphthohydroquinone to quinone resulting in the increased absorption.

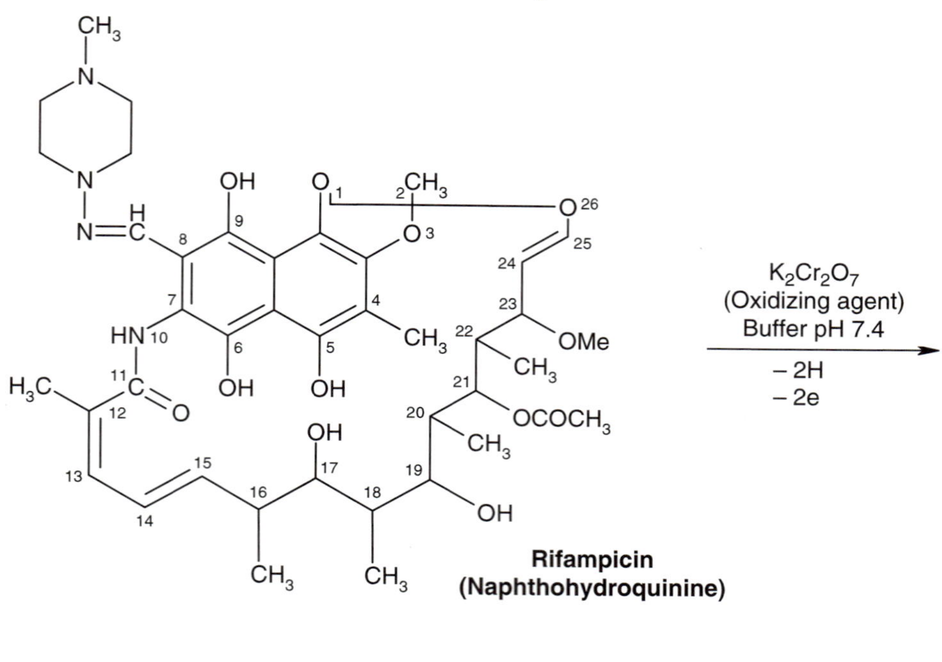

Rifampicin (Naphthohydroquinine)

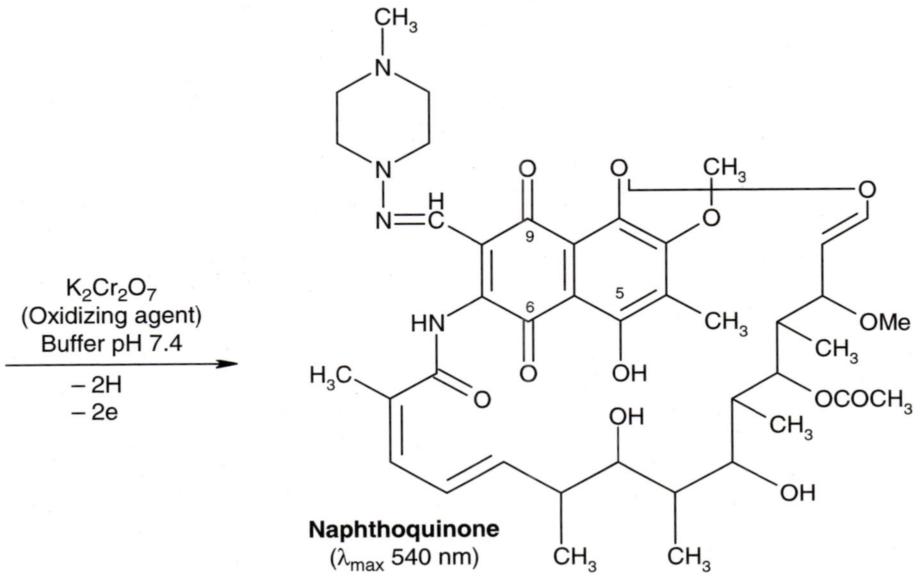

Oxidation of rifampicin with $K_2Cr_2O_7$ of OH group at C-6 and C-9.

Reference

R.B. Patel et al. Ind. J. Pharmacy, 41(1), 40-42, 1979.

Rifampicin also reacts with phenylhydrazine to give coloured product (λ_{max} 410 nm). Carbonyl function at C-1 condenses with amino group of the reagent.

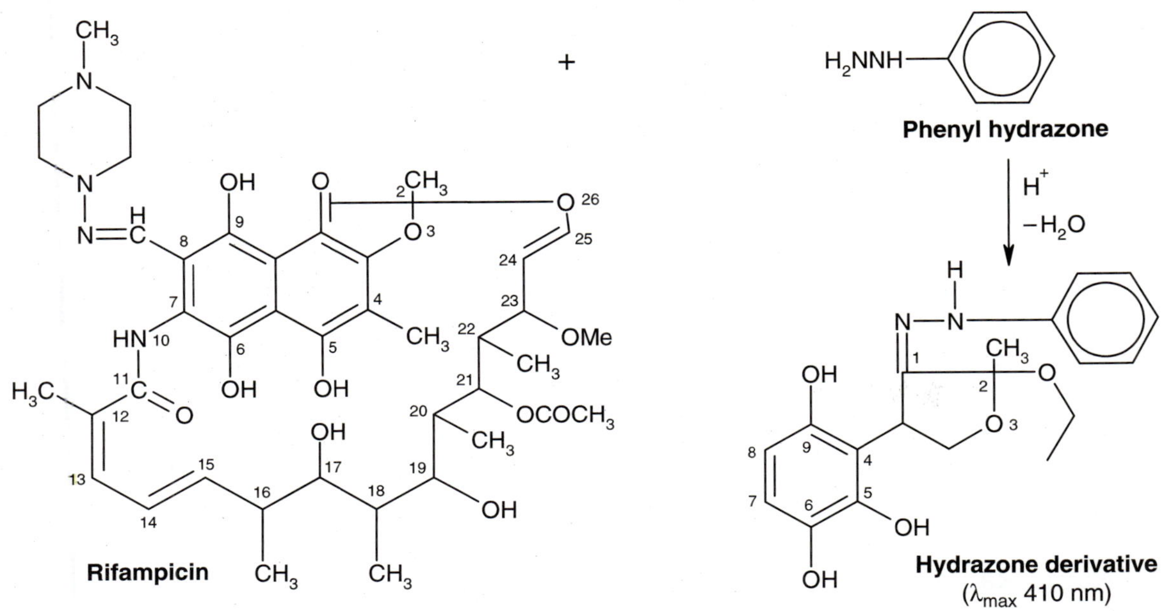

Note

Isoniazid, pyrizinamide, PAS and ethambutol do not interfere.

Reference

B.B. Patel, T.P. Gandhi, A.A. Patel, V.C. Patel & R.N. Gilbert, *Ind. J. Pharm. Sci.*, **41(1)**, 40-42, 1979.

Rifampicin also reacts with chlorimide reagent to form indophenol dye. The coupling takes place with 'N' at position 10.

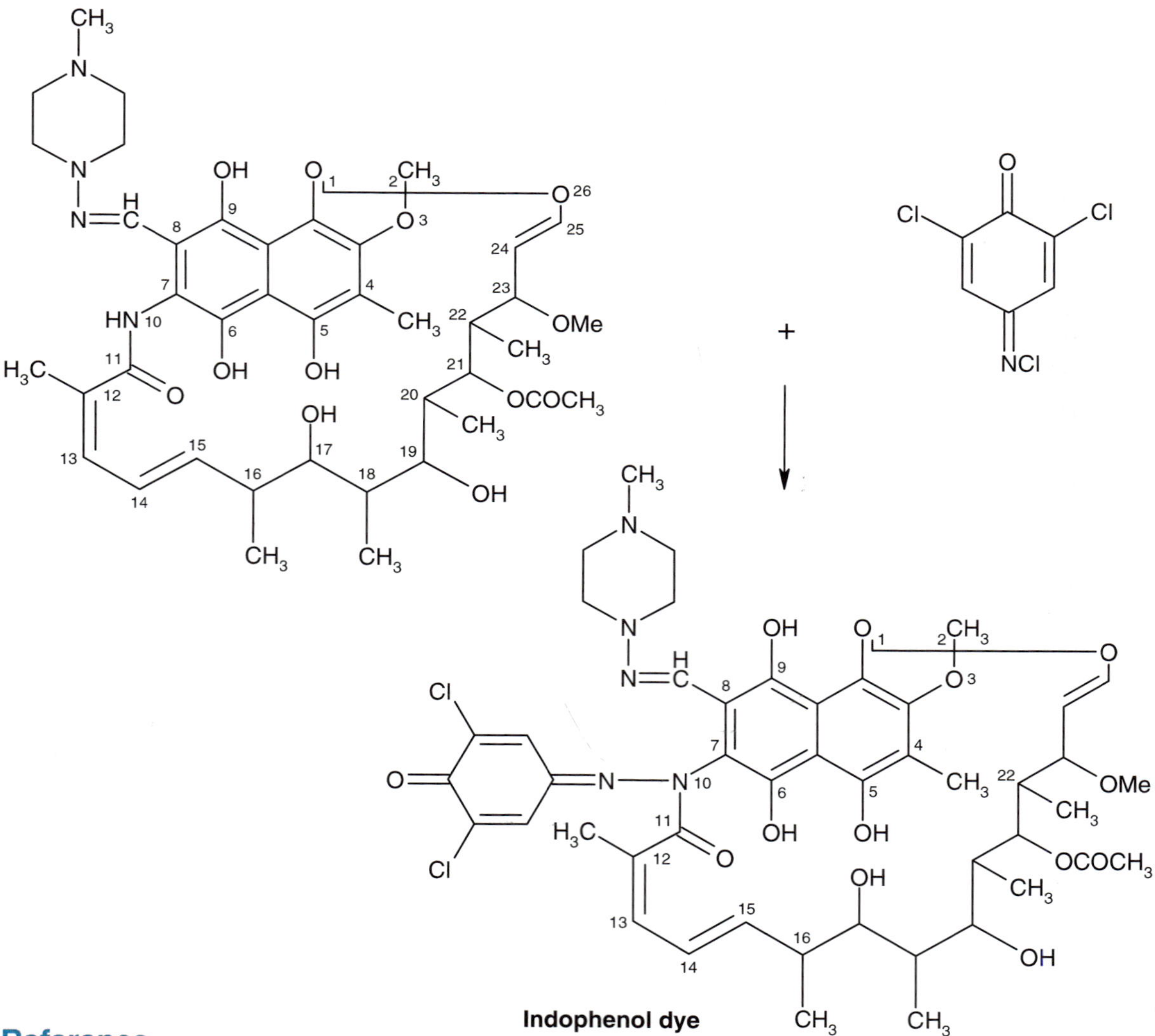

Indophenol dye

Reference

G. Rama Rao, S.S.N. Murty & E. Venkata Rao, *Indian Drugs*, **22(9)**, 483–488, 1985.

The compound forms chelate with vanadium (NH_3-metavandate), Ni($NiCl_2$) which forms the basis of analytical method. Keto pyrazinamide, ethambutol and PAS do not interfere.

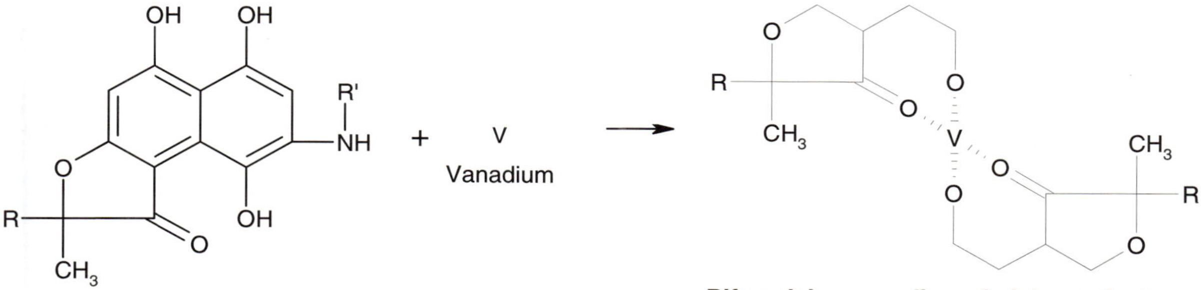

Rifampicin - vanadium chelate product
(λ_{max} 540 nm)

Note

Chelate with Ni^{2+} (580 nm), Zn^{2+} (525 nm) and Ce^{3+} (520 nm).

METHOD 2

Prepare solution of sample in methanol (1 mg/ml). Further dilution is done with pH 7.4 buffer (prepared as per IP 1996) to get final concentration of 20 mcg/ml. Measure the extinction at about 475 nm and calculate the results taking 187 as the value of A 1%, 1 cm at 475 nm.

Isoniazid

Reagents

1. 10% w/v solution of potassium iodide in water.
2. 0.1 N sodium thiosulphate.
3. 0.1 N bromine solution.
4. 0.1 M hydrochloric acid.
5. Starch solution (indicator).

Procedure

Weigh accurately quantity of the sample equivalent to about 25 mg of isoniazid. Suspend in 20 ml of 0.1 N hydrochloric acid and extract with five 50 ml portions of dichloromethane, allowing the layers to separate completely after each extraction. Transfer the combined acidic layer to iodine flask, cool, add 10 ml of concentrated hydrochloric acid and 25 ml of bromine solution, allow to stand for 30 min. Add 20 ml of potassium iodide solution, allow it to stand for 10 min and titrate with sodium thiosulphate solution using starch solution as indicator. Each ml of 0.1 N bromine is equivalent to 0.003429 g of isoniazid. Run a blank to calculate volume of bromine consumed by the drug.

Note

Acidic solution can be directly titrated with 0.1 N bromine solution using methyl red as indicator or potentiometrically.

The following reactions are of analytical interest:

(a) The compound condenses with aromatic aldehydes such as vanillin or PDAB, PDAC.

(b) It undergoes König reaction i.e. reaction with BrCN and then coupling with arylamine.

(c) The compound reacts with copper citrate or $CuCl_2$ to give coloured precipitate or complex.

(d) It reacts with nitrite to give INH-azide.

(a)

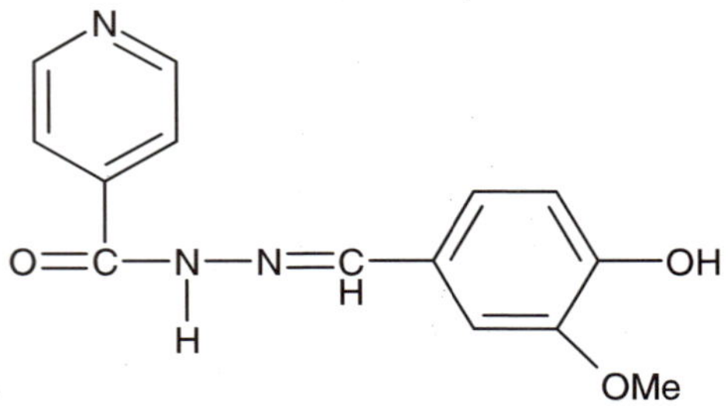

INH - vanillin condensation product

(b) See detailed reaction mechanism under nicotinamide.

(c)

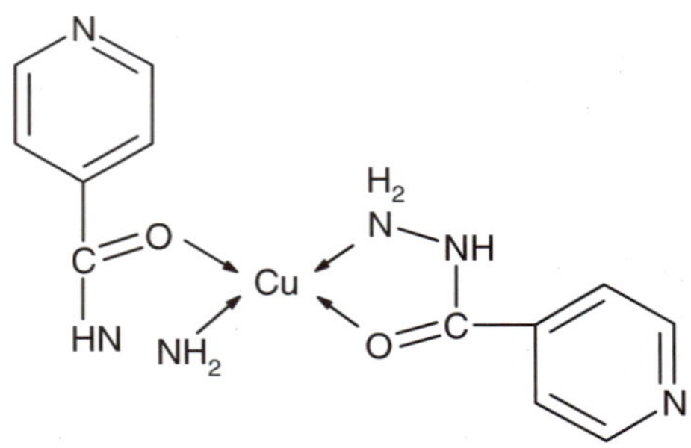

INH - copper complex (2 : 1)

Or

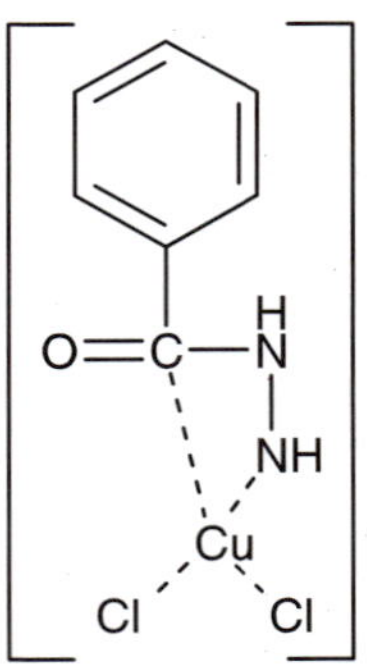

INH - $CuCl_2$ complex (1 : 1)

Note

The compound forms complexes with Co^{2+}, Zn^{2+}, Cd^{2+} and Ni^{2+}.

Reference

Pharmaceutical Chemistry (Vol. 2) by H.J. Roth, p. 542.

Formulation 6

Isoniazid, Rifampicin, Pyridoxine hydrochloride

ESTIMATION

Isoniazid

Follow the method 3 described in formulation 1 of this chapter based on reaction with aldehyde reagent. Alternatively, suspend the sample in 0.01 N hydrochloric acid and extract with 2 × 40 ml portions of chloroform. Chloroform layer may be washed with 25 ml of 0.1 N hydrochloric acid. The acidic layers are combined and diluted appropriately to get solution of 10 mcg/ml. See method 2 under formulation 2 of this chapter.

Rifampicin

Follow the method 2 described in formulation 5 of this chapter. The extinction of the substance is measured at 475 nm in phosphate buffer.

Pyridoxine hydrochloride

Follow the method based on the reaction with chlorimide reagent as described for estimation of pyridoxine hydrochloride.

Formulation 7

Ampicillin

Penicillins

METHOD 1

Reagents

1. 0.1 M hydrochloric acid.
2. 0.1% w/v solution of ninhydrin in 0.1 N hydrochloric acid.
3. Ethyl alcohol.

Standard solution

1 mg/ml of ampicillin in 0.1 M hydrochloric acid.

Sample solution

(a) Capsule and tablets: Contents are accurately weighed and dissolved in 0.1 N hydrochloric acid to produce 1 mg/ml of ampicillin, and filter.

(b) Dry syrup: The granules are just diluted with water to the desired volume. Aliquot equivalent to 100 mg of the compound is taken and diluted to 100 ml with 0.1 N hydrochloric acid.

Procedure

To 0.3 ml each of sample and standard solutions (300 mcg), add 5 ml of 0.1 M hydrochloric acid and 5 ml of ninhydrin solution. Keep the flask in water-bath for 30 minutes ensuring uniform heating of all the flasks. Take out and immediately add 10 ml of ethyl alcohol, shake and rapidly cool to room temperature and dilute to 50 ml with 0.1 M hydrochloric acid. After 10 minutes, measure the absorption at about 490 nm. The method obeys Beer's law in the concentration range of 2-10 mcg/ml. The colour is stable for more than 1 h.

Note

1. Addition of ethyl alcohol, immediately after the reaction is over, is necessary to prevent formation of precipitates.

2. Other semisynthetic penicillins such as benzyl penicillin, oxacillin, cloxacillin do not give measurable colour with this reagent.
3. Ensure that all the flasks are uniformly heated, failing which unsatisfactory results are obtained. This is the major drawback with this method.

Explanatory Note

Ninhydrin is the stable hydrate of 1,2,3-trioxoindane which has reactive carbonyl group at C-2 atom. Both forms of ninhydrin can react with amines and existence of these two forms of ninhydrin are dependent on the solvent used.

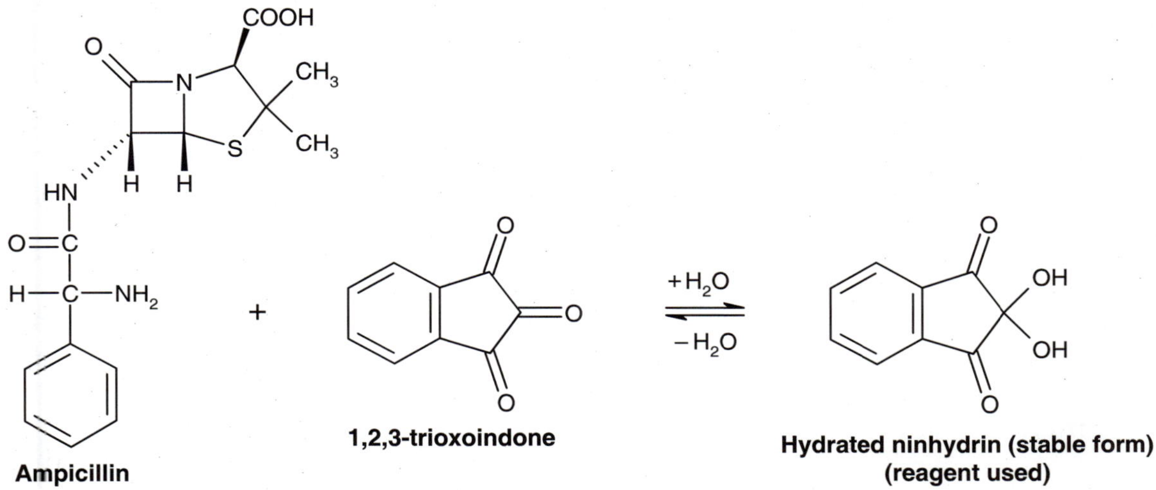

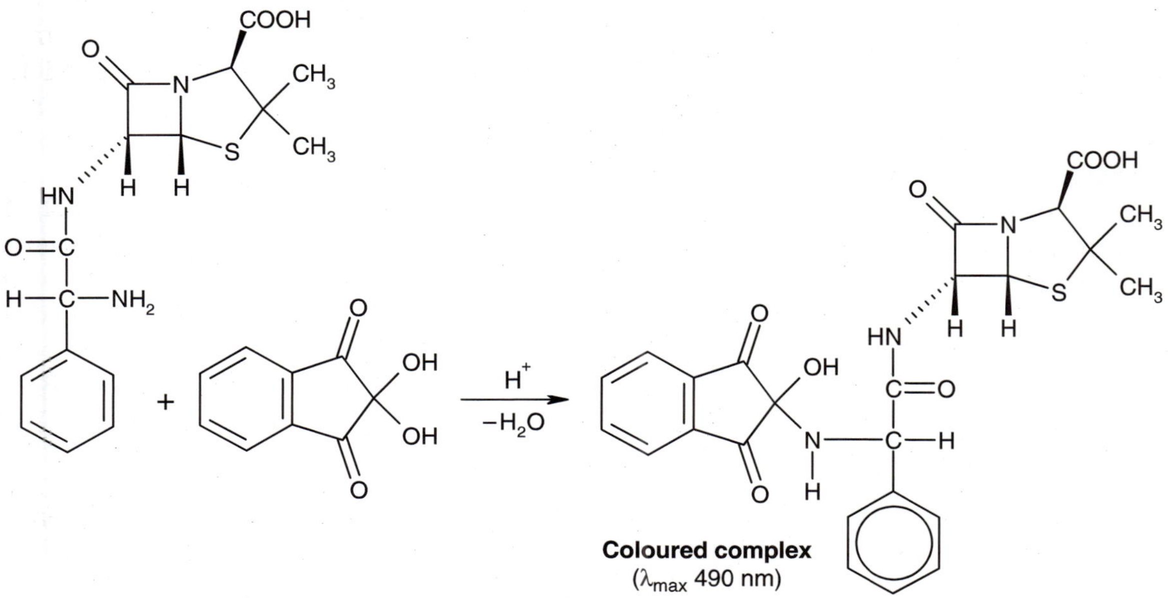

Reference

1. C. Chowdhary et al. *Ind. J. Pharm.*, **38(5)**, 124-126, 1976.
2. Przyborowski, *Farm* Poland, **39(9)**, 527-530, 1983.
3. S.K. Mukerji & M.K. Majumdar, *Indian Drugs*, **26**, 370, 1989.

METHOD 2

Reagent

Fehling reagent: Prepared by mixing 2 ml of Fehling solution A and 2 ml of Fehling solution B and diluting to 50 ml with water.

Standard solution

Dissolve accurately weighed quantity of ampicillin (anhydrous) in water to produce 1 mg/ml.

Sample solution

(a) Raw material: 1 mg/ml in water.
(b) Accurately weigh powder from capsule equivalent to 100 mg of ampicillin, add 80 ml of water, shake and dilute to 100 ml.
(c) Dry syrup: Add sufficient water so as to represent the labelled volume. Shake and keep for 45 minutes. Transfer aliquot of the syrup equivalent to 100 mg of anhydrous ampicillin, adjust the pH to 6.8-7.0, dilute to 100 ml and shake to mix.

Procedure

To 2 ml each of sample and standard solutions, add 3.5 ml of water. To all the tubes, add 0.5 ml of Fehling reagent. After 2 minutes, measure the absorbance of all the solutions at about 558 nm using 5.5 ml of water instead of drug solution as blank. The method obeys Beer's law over the concentration range of 50-350 mcg/ml.

This method is highly specific as 6-aminopenicillinic acid, penicillin G sodium, phenoxymethyl penicillin and degradation products of ampicillin do not react with this reagent.

Note

Nucleophilic species which will produce hydrobromic acid are likely to interfere in this method.

Explanatory Note

Fehling's solution is alkaline in nature. Since the reaction is carried out in alkaline medium, heteroatom i.e. 'N' may lose acidic proton resulting in a structure which can easily form a complex with Cu(2).

Probable Reaction Mechanism

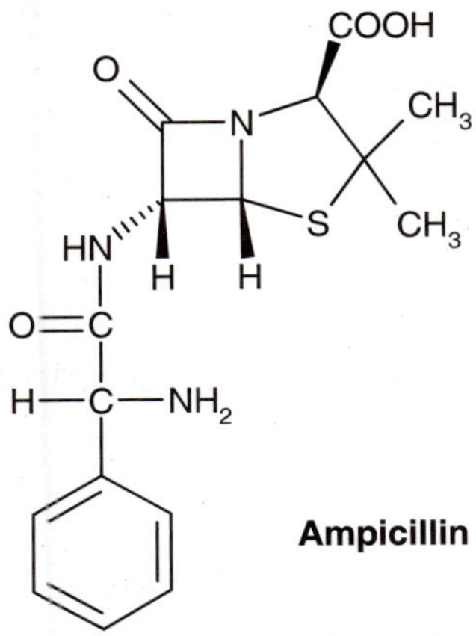

Ampicillin

+

$K_2CuC_4H_4O_6$

Potassium cupritartarate
(component of Fehling's solution which is alkaline in nature)

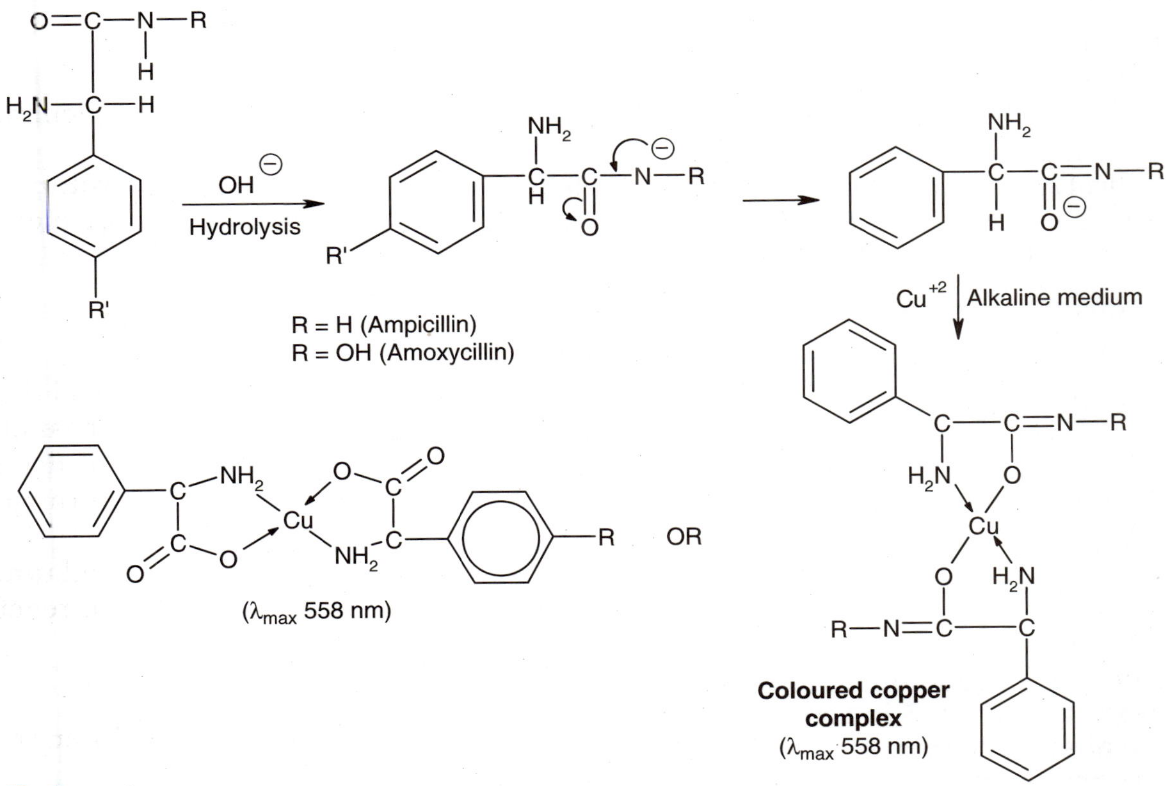

Reference

1. A.A. Patel, T.P. Gandhi, P.R. Patel, M.R. Patel & V.C. Patel. *Ind. J. Pharm. Sci.*, pp. 64-66, March-April 1978.
2. U. Saha, *Analyst*, **111**, 1179-1181, 1986.
3. Textbook of Practical Organic Chemistry by Vogel, pp. 1230, 31.

P.B. Issopoulos (1988) while reporting the analysis of β-lactam antibiotics (cephalexin, ampicillin, amoxycillin) has suggested the existence of the following Cu^{2+} chelates.

(a)

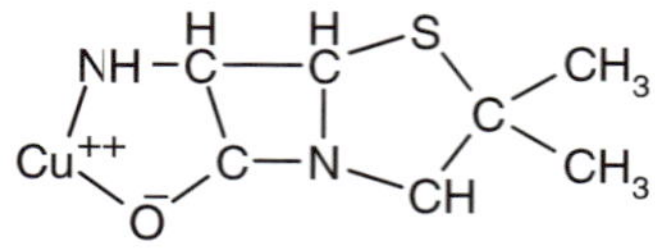

(b)

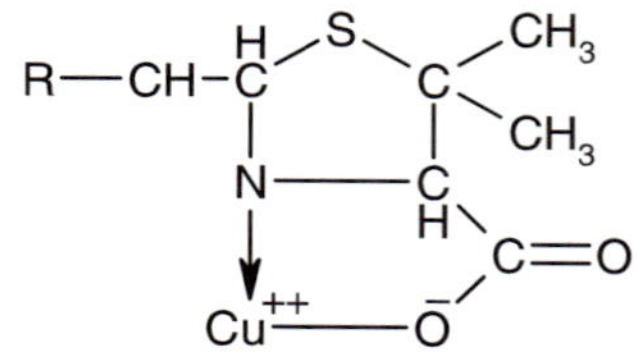

Note

The method involves reaction of antibiotics with Cu^{++} in 0.2 M sodium acetate at ambient temperature. The absorbance is measured after 10 min. Cephalexin - Cu (II) complex — 670 nm; Cephradine - Cu (II) complex — 650 nm; Ampicillin - Cu (II) complex — 640 nm; Amoxycillin - Cu (II) complex — 650 nm.

Reference

P.B. Issopoulos, *J. Pharm. Biomed. Anal.*, **6(3)**, 321-327, 1988.

METHOD 3

This method has been found to give good results for capsules. The acidic hydrolysis of ampicillin with 1% formaldehyde in 0.3 N hydrochloric acid yields a degradation product identified as 2-hydroxy-3-phenyl-6-methyl pyrazine, which has a well-defined UV absorption at 352 nm.

Reagent

1% v/v formaldehyde in 0.3 N hydrochloric acid.

Standard solution

1 mg/ml of ampicillin in the solvent.

Sample solution

Accurately weigh about 100 mg of the material from the capsules and dilute with the solvent to 100 ml.

Procedure

Dilute 1 ml each of sample and standard solutions to 50 ml with the solvent, heat at 90°C ± 0.5 in constant temperature bath for 60 min, cool and measure the absorbance of both the solutions at 380 nm using solvent as blank. Calculate the result in comparison with standard. The Beer's law is obeyed in the concentration range between 10^{-4} and 10^{-6} M.

Note

It is absolutely essential that the temperature is maintained within specified limits.

Probable Reaction Mechanism

The function of HCHO can be understood by the following:

$$RNH_2 + H^+ \rightleftharpoons \underset{\text{Cationic form}}{RNH_3^+}$$

This cationic form has low nucleophilic ability due to unavailability of electrons on nitrogen. HCHO forms Schiff's base.

$$RNH_2 + O{=}C\begin{smallmatrix}H\\H\end{smallmatrix} \xrightarrow{-H_2O} R{-}N{=}C\begin{smallmatrix}H\\H\end{smallmatrix}$$

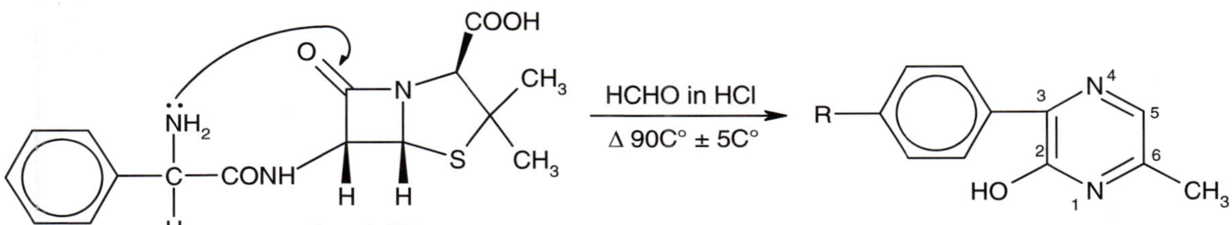

Ampicillin **2-OH-3-phenyl-6-methyl pyrazine** (λ_{max} 380 nm)

Reference

1. Juan A. Squella, Luis J. Nunez-Vergara & Maxima Aros, *JAoAC*, **63(5)**, 1049, 1980.
2. P.P. Shirke, P.C. Balasubramanya, A.R. Samant, V.B. Tirodkar & P.D. Sethi, *Indian Drugs*, **31(8)**, 370, 1994.

Explanatory Note

This involves intramolecular aminolysis; in acidic medium α-amino benzoyl group present in the side chain (β-lactam ring) nucleophilically attacks carbonyl group present in the β-lactam ring, thus ring closure and formation of pyrazine derivative. Under acidic conditions, primary amino group is in cationic form (RNH_3^+), thus significant decrease in its nucleophilic activity, hence decrease in pyrazine formation. HCHO forms Schiff's base with free NH_2 which being unstable in acidic medium releases unionized form of NH_2 which in turn reacts with carbonyl (C==O) group of β-lactam ring resulting in enhanced formation of pyrazine derivative.

METHOD 4

Reagents

1. Acetic acid, glacial.
2. Copper acetate reagent: 1 g of copper (II) acetate, 50 ml water and 0.9 ml of glacial acetic acid are diluted to 100 ml with water.

Standard solution

1 mg/ml of ampicillin in water. (80.84 mg of ampicillin trihydrate = 70 mg of ampicillin anhydrous)

Sample solution

In case of syrups, first add water as specified on the label and then dilute appropriate volume of syrup with water to produce 1 mg/ml. Filter and use for estimation.

Procedure

To 10 ml each of sample and standard solutions, add 1 ml of copper acetate reagent and dilute with water to 20 ml. Heat at 75°C for 30 min, cool immediately and make up to 100 ml with water. Measure the absorbance at 428 nm against reagent blank. The complex is stable for 2 h and Beer's law is obeyed in the range of 50-75 mcg/ml.

Probable Reaction Mechanism

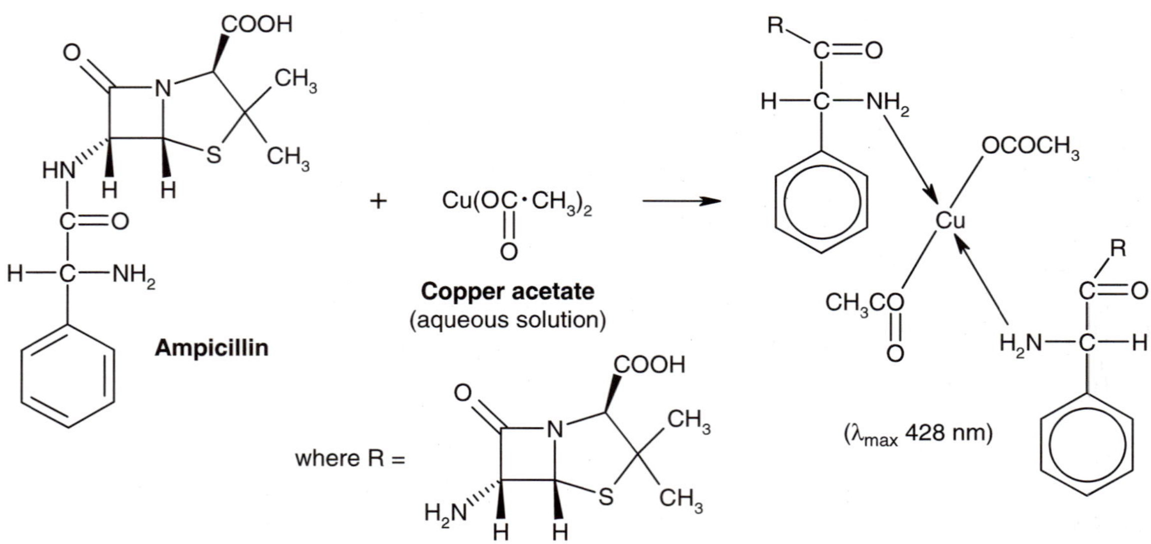

Explanatory Note

Cu(2) being divalent, it can form complex with side chain of the molecule which is coloured (λ_{max} 428 nm).

METHOD 5

Ampicillin couples with 1,2-naphthoquinone-4-sulphonic acid sodium. The drug solution is heated with the reagent. The coloured complex has λ_{max} 475 nm.

Explanatory Note

The aliphatic amino group present in the side chain of ampicillin forms a Michael addition like product, eliminating the monohydrogen sulphite radical and resulting in the formation of the product. The reaction can be represented as follows:

Probable Reaction Mechanism

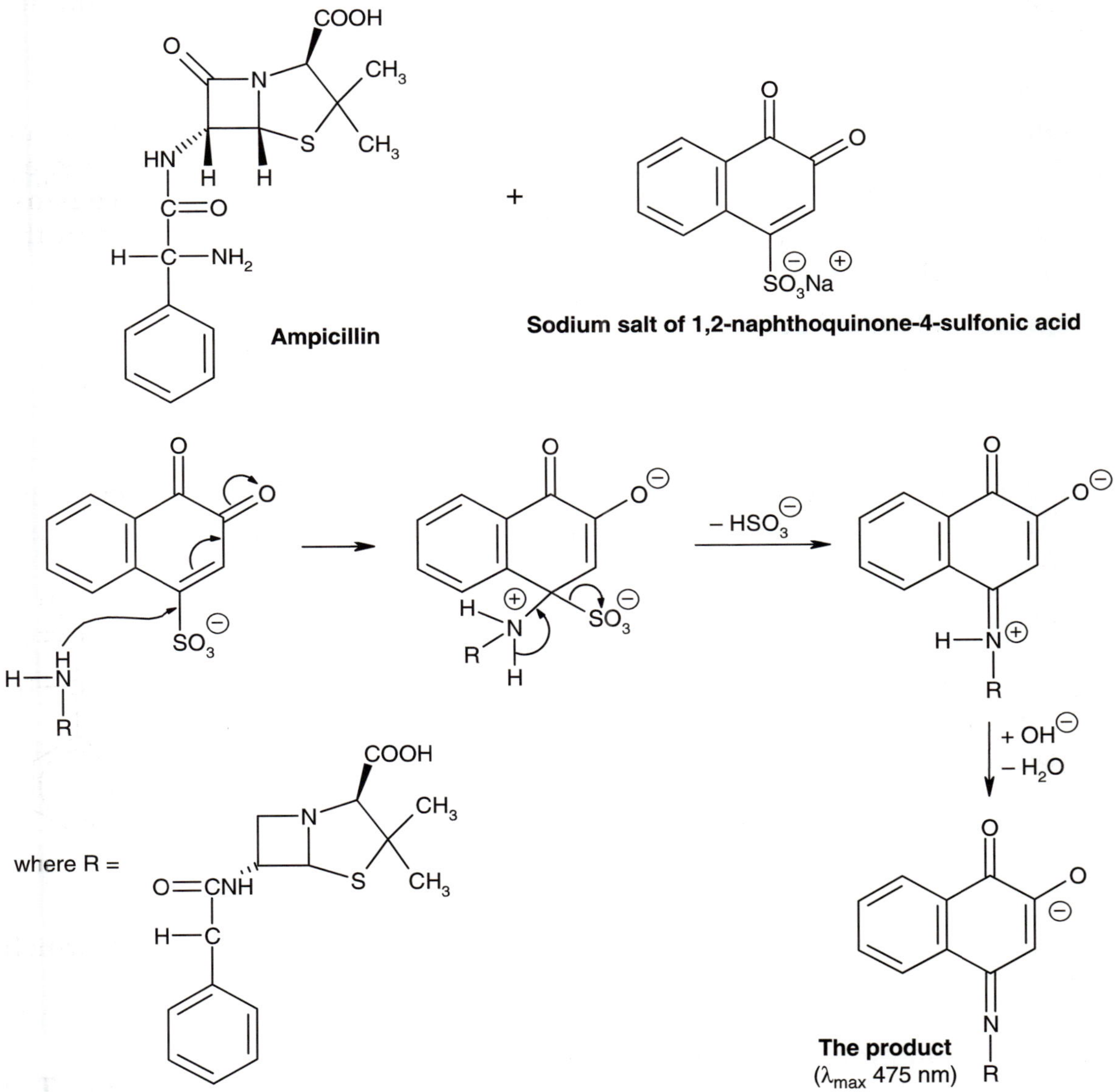

Reference

Indian Drugs, **25(6)**, 249, 1988.

A titrimetric method is reported which involves reaction of phenacyl bromide with ampicillin resulting in the formation of phenacyl ampicillinate hydrobromide, which is finally titrated with sodium carbonate (Na_2CO_3) using thymol blue as indicator. To increase the stability of the end-point, use of sodium thiosulphate is recommended. It reacts with excess of phenacyl bromide.

Reference

Indian Drugs, **18(3)**, 111, 1980.

METHOD 6

Reagent

Acetylacetone formaldehyde reagent: Mix 7.8 ml of freshly distilled acetylacetone with 15 ml of formaldehyde (36%), 16 ml 0.2 M sodium acetate and 34 ml 0.2 M acetic acid. Keep in boiling water-bath for 5 min, cool to room temperature, adjust the pH to 4.3, dilute to 100 ml with water.

Sample and standard solutions

100 µg/ml in water.

Procedure

To 1 ml each of sample/standard solutions add 4 ml of the acetylacetone formaldehyde reagent, keep the reaction mixture in water-bath at 37°C for 30 min, dilute to 25 ml with water and measure the absorbance at 400 nm against reagent blank.

Probable Reaction Mechanism

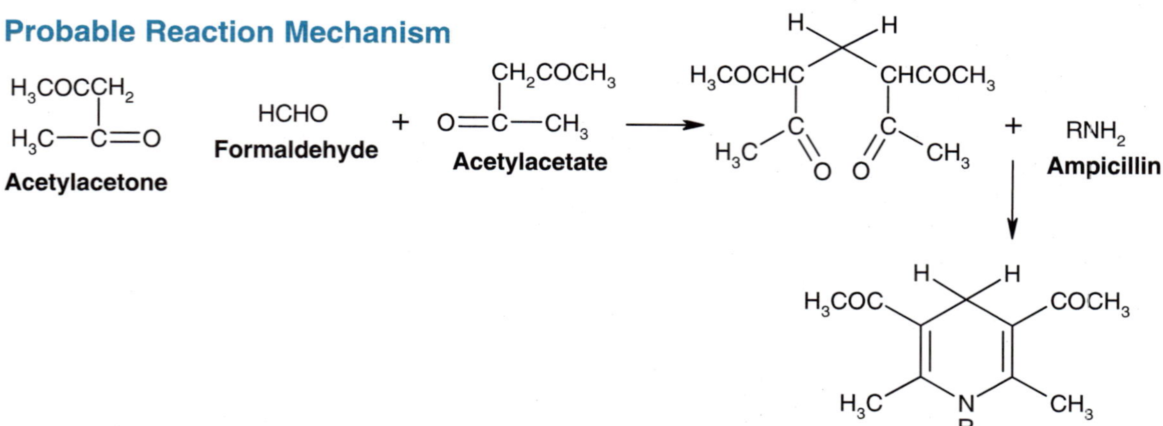

(λ_{max} 400 nm)

Note

Cloxacillin and probenecid do not interfere.

Reference

M.B. Devani, Ila T. Patel & T.M. Patel. *Talanta*, **39(10)**, 1391-1394, 1992.

Bundgaard et al. (1972 & 1973) have described a UV-spectrophotometric method for the estimation of ampicillin. The compound is first acetylated with acetic anhydride and then coupled with mercuric mercaptide having λ_{max} 325 nm.

Probable Reaction Mechanism

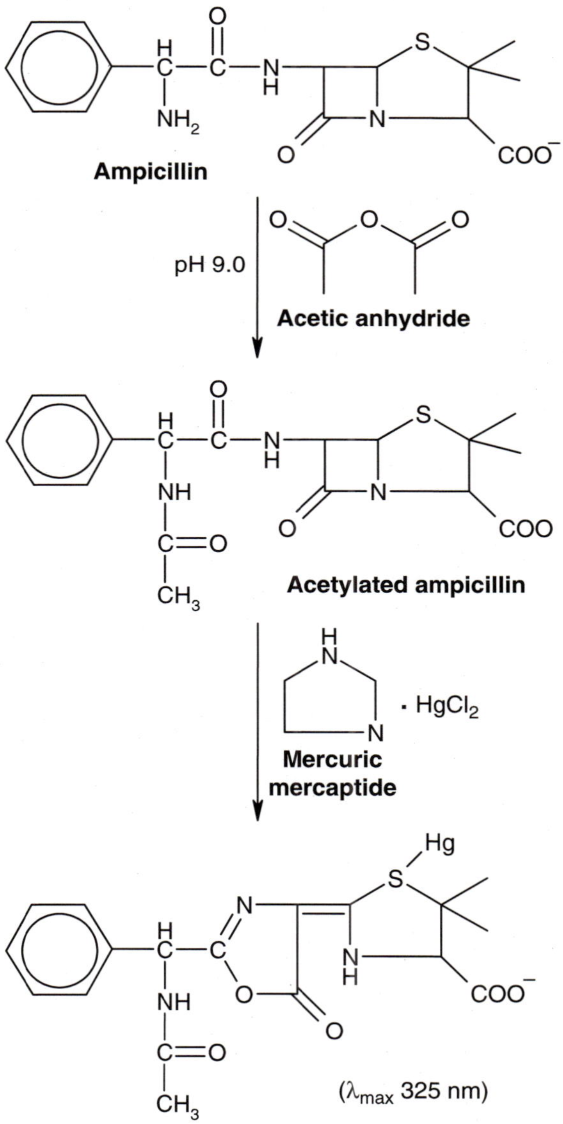

Reference

Bundgaard et al., *J. Pharm. Pharmacol.*, **24**, 790, 1972; **26**, 385, 1973.

Formulation 8

Amoxycillin

ESTIMATION

All the methods described below are based on phenolic function of the molecule, hence ampicillin does not interfere.

METHOD 1

Reagent

p-Dimethylaminobenzaldehyde (PDAB) reagent: Weigh 400 mg of p-dimethylamino-benzaldehyde, add 10 ml of ethyl alcohol, 2 ml of concentrated sulphuric acid and dilute to 50 ml with water.

Standard solution

1 mg/ml of amoxycillin in water.

Sample solution

Weigh material accurately equivalent to 25 mg of amoxycillin, add 15 ml of water and heat on water-bath to dissolve, adjust to 25 ml with water.

Procedure

To 2 ml of the standard and sample solutions, add 4 ml of 'PDAB' reagent and heat on water-bath at 65°C for 1 hr. Cool to room temperature and adjust to 10 ml with water. Measure the absorbance of both the solutions at about 410 nm. The method obeys Beer's law in the concentration range of 10-600 mcg/ml.

Note

1. Penicillin G sodium and ampicillin do not give similar colour reaction.
2. 6-aminopenicillinic acid (6-APA), an impurity gives colour reaction at very high concentration, above 600 mcg/ml. For aged samples, it would be necessary to ascertain that 6-APA is not present in such samples in quantities greater than 600 mcg/ml.

Explanatory Note

Condensation reaction occurs between p-dimethylaminobenzaldehyde and side chain of amoxycillin. Here reaction occurs between the aldehydic group (—CHO group) of PDAB and the amino group of the side chain of amoxycillin as shown:

Probable Reaction Mechanism

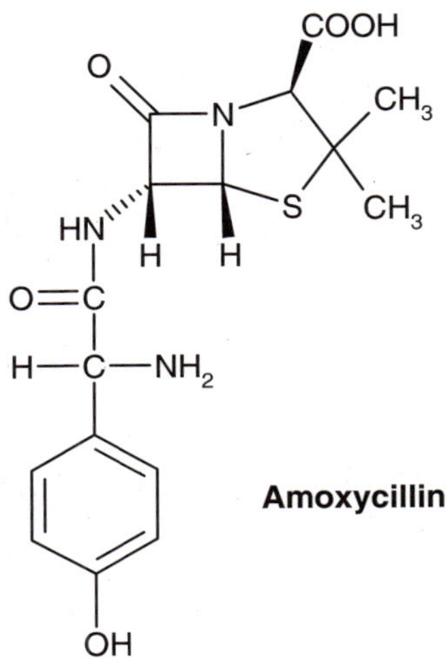

Amoxycillin

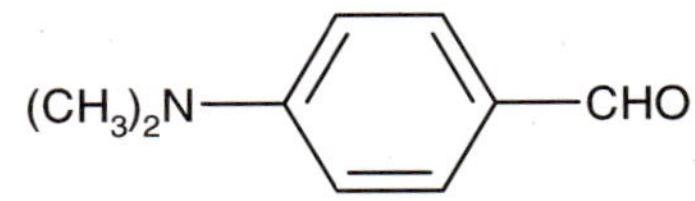

p-dimethylaminobenzaldehyde (PDAB)
(reagent used)

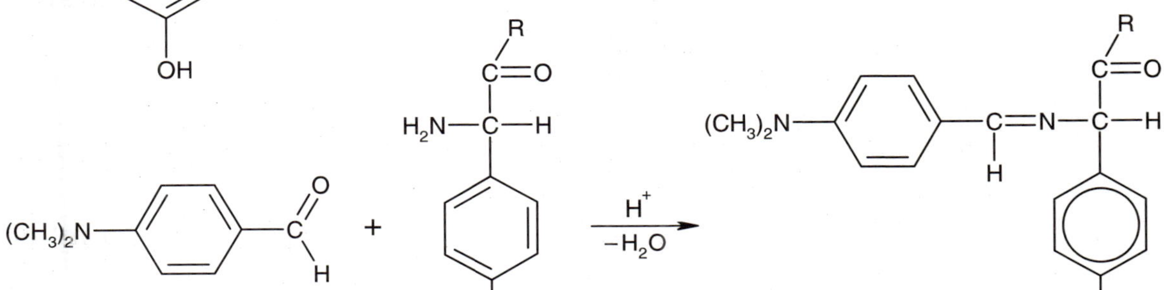

PDAB + **Amoxycillin** $\xrightarrow[-H_2O]{H^+}$ **Coloured chromogen** (λ_{max} 410 nm)

where R =

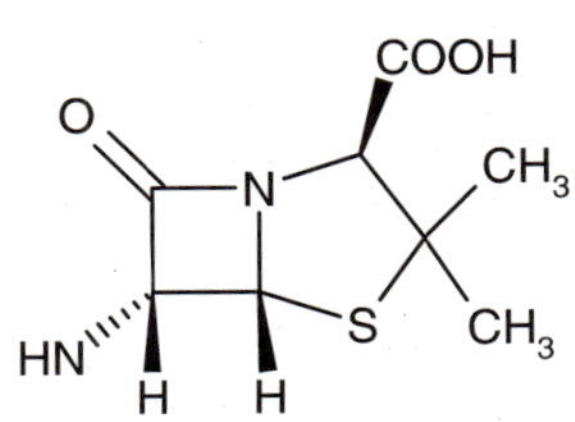

Reference

A.A. Patel, T.P. Gandhi, P.R. Patel, M.R. Patel & V.C. Patel, *Ind. J. Pharm. Sci.*, **41(6)**, 229-230, 1979.

METHOD 2

Reagents

1. 0.1% w/v solution of p-dimethylaminocinnamaldehyde (PDAC) in isopropyl alcohol.
2. Acetic acid-isopropanol mixture (2 : 3 v/v).

Standard solution

1 mg/ml of amoxycillin in acetic acid-isopropanol mixture.

Sample solution

Dissolve accurately measured or weighed quantity of the sample in acetic acid-isopropanol mixture to produce 1 mg/ml.

Procedure

Dilute 1 ml aliquot each of the standard and sample solutions as obtained above to 25 ml with isopropanol. To 1 ml of these solutions, add 1 ml of 'PDAC' reagent, followed by 1 ml of acetic acid. Immerse all the flasks in water-bath for 2 min, cool and dilute to 10 ml with isopropanol. Measure the absorbance at about 480 nm against a reagent blank. The colour is stable for 15 min.

Note

1. This method has advantage over method 1 as more stable colour is obtained.
2. This method requires only two minutes of heating while the method 1 requires longer heating period.

Here also condensation occurs between aldehydic group of the reagent (PDAC) and amino group present in the side chain of the drug.

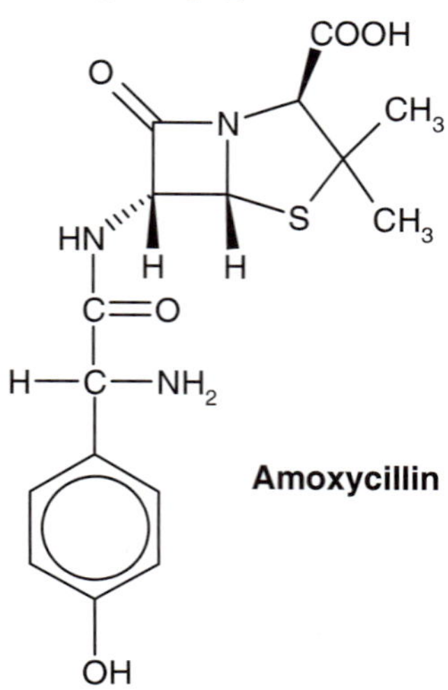

Amoxycillin

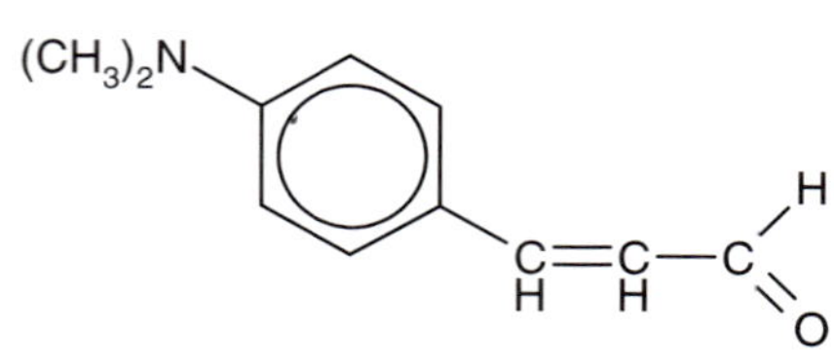

p-dimethylaminocinnamaldehyde (PDAC)

Probable Reaction Mechanism

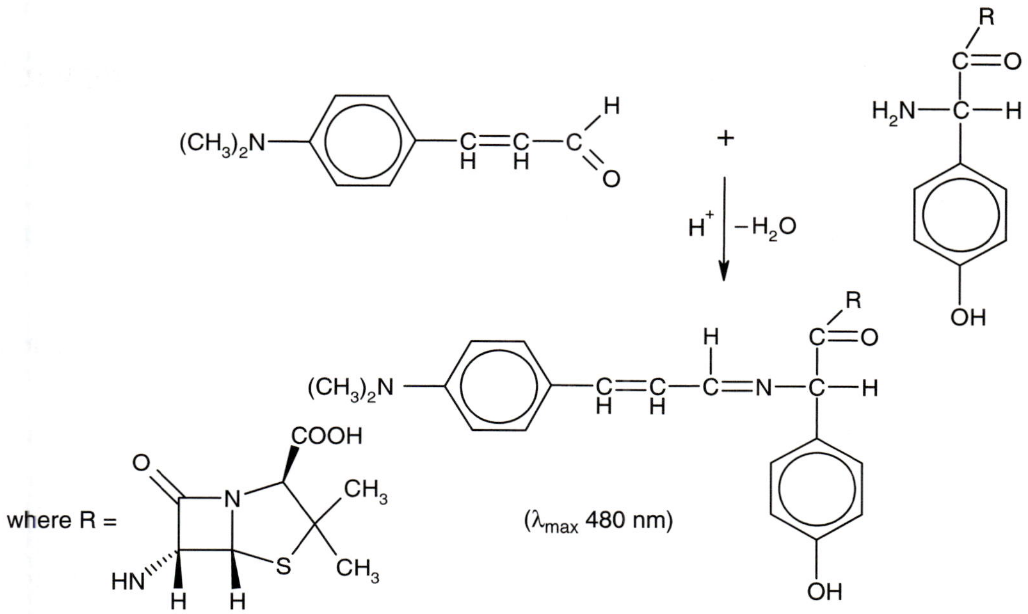

Reference

1. G. Rama Rao, Geeta Kanjhal & K. Rama Mohan, *Indian Drugs*, **19(8)**, 326-327, 1982.
2. A.P. Patel et al., *Ind. J. Pharm. Sci.*, **41(6)**, 229-230, 1979.

Advantage of the use of p-dimethylaminocinnamaldehyde over p-dimethylaminobenzaldehyde is that the resultant product formed in the later case i.e. by the use of PDAC has extended conjugation. Hence, it will not only absorb at a greater wavelength but is also more stable.

METHOD 3

Reagents

1. 5% w/v solution of sodium cobaltinitrite in water.
2. 20% w/v solution of sodium hydroxide in water.

Standard solution

0.5 mg/ml of anhydrous amoxycillin in water.

Sample solution

Weigh accurately a quantity of sample equivalent to 250 mg of anhydrous compound and dissolve in water to produce 500 ml. Shake well and filter. Use the filtrate for estimation.

Procedure

(a) To 2 ml each of the sample and standard solutions, add 5 ml of water, 2 ml of glacial acetic acid and 2 ml of sodium cobaltinitrite solution. Heat the solution in water-bath for 15 min, cool and dilute to 50 ml with water. Measure the absorbance of both the solutions at about 370 nm against reagent blank.

(b) Proceed as under method (a) above. After heating for 15 minutes, cool and add 20 ml of sodium hydroxide solution. Filter, wash the precipitates with three 5 ml portions of water, collect the filtrate and dilute to 50 ml with water. Measure the absorption at about 430 nm against reagent blank.

Note

1. 6-APA does not interfere.
2. Procedure (b) is more sensitive.
3. Procedure (b) is not applicable to dry syrups due to interference of excipients present.

Explanatory Note

Na-cobaltinitrite forms a complex with amoxycillin as shown below. There are 2 types of complex possible depending on the atoms which take part in the formation of the complex.

Probable Reaction Mechanism

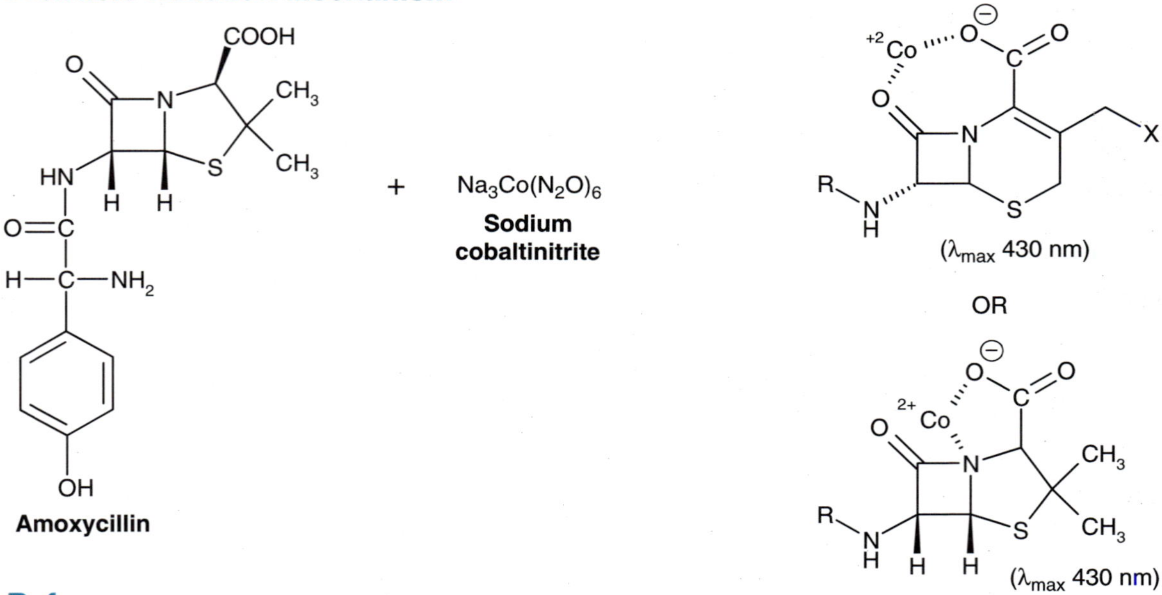

Reference

N.G. Rama, H.K. Dhyoni, M.R. Patel & B.J. Shah, *Indian Drugs*, **17(5)**, 142-144, 1980.

METHOD 4

Reagents

1. 0.04% w/v solution of 2,6-dichloroquinone chlorimide in isopropyl alcohol. The solution is stable for 7 days if stored in refrigerator (Gibbs' reagent).
2. Borate buffer, pH 9.4.

Standard solution

100 mcg/ml of amoxycillin in water.

Sample solution

Accurately weighed quantity of the powdered material is extracted with water to produce 100 mcg/ml.

Procedure

To 2 ml each of standard and sample solutions, add 1.5 ml of buffer and 1.5 ml of the chlorimide reagent. Allow to stand for 5 minutes at room temperature and then dilute to 10 ml with water. Measure the absorption of blue indophenol derivative at about 620 nm against reagent blank. Calculate the results by comparison. Blue chromophore is stable for 24 h and the method obeys Beer's law in the range of 0.5-6 mcg/ml.

Explanatory Note

2,6-dichloroquinone chlorimide is converted into 2,6-dichloroquinonimine in the presence of aqueous solution. Next step involves oxidative coupling reaction between 2,6-dichloroquinonimine and the side chain of the drug. The reaction site offered by the drug is ortho position to the phenolic-OH group present in the side chain.

Probable Reaction Mechanism

Step 1

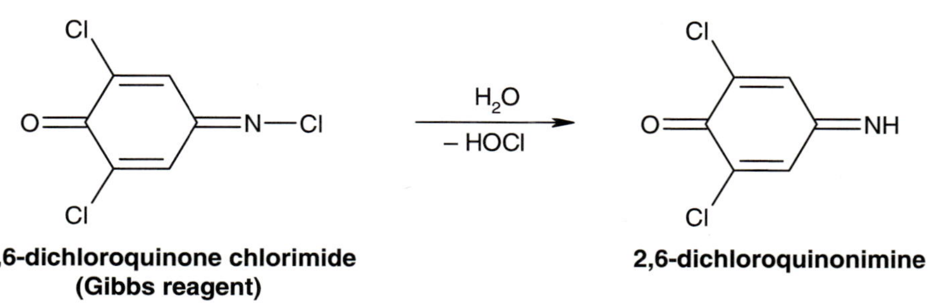

Step 2

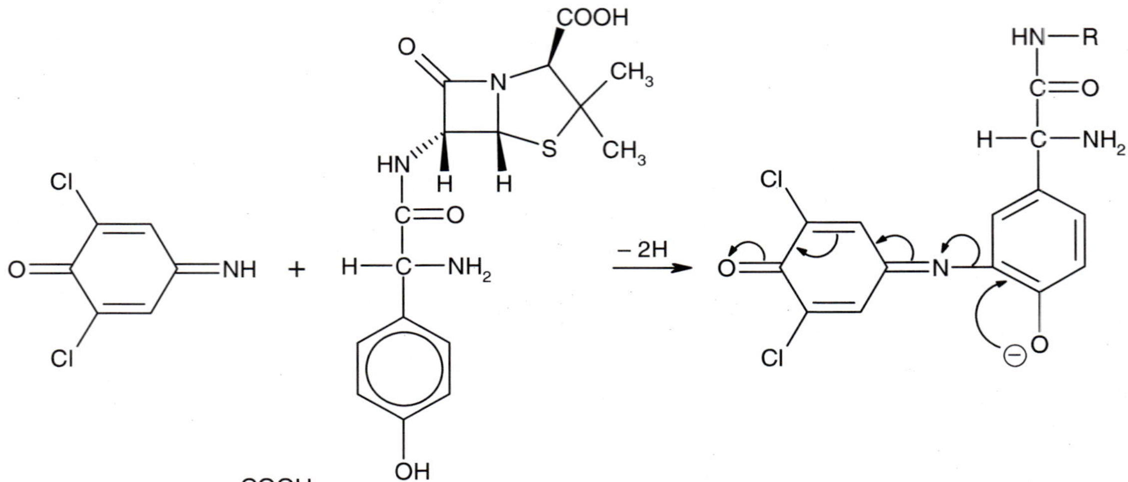

where R = 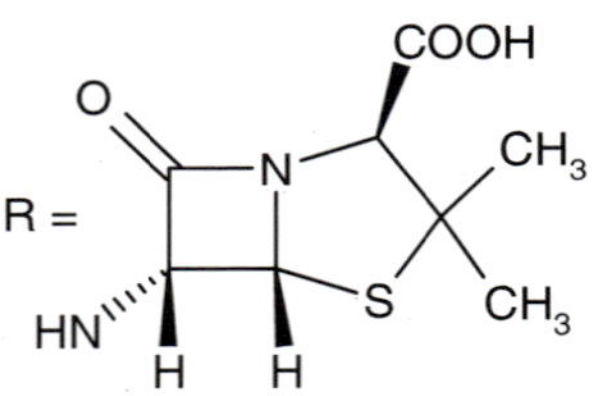

Reference

R.T. Sane, V.B. Malkar & V.G. Nayak, *Indian Drugs*, **20(11)**, 462-463, 1983.

METHOD 5

This method is based on alkaline oxidation, followed by condensation with 4-aminophenazone. The complex has absorption maximum at about 505 nm. This is called "Emerson's reaction".

Reagents

1. 1% w/v solution of sodium carbonate in water.
2. Methanol: water mixture (1 : 3 v/v)—solvent.
3. 0.5% w/v solution of 4-aminophenazone in the solvent.
4. 2% w/v solution of potassium ferricyanide in water.

Standard solution

200 mcg/ml of amoxycillin in water.

Sample solution

Accurately weighed or measured aliquot of the sample equivalent to 10 mg of amoxycillin is dissolved in water to get 50 ml (200 mcg/ml).

Procedure

To 1 ml each of sample and standard solutions, add 1 ml each of aminophenazone solution, potassium ferricyanide solution and sodium carbonate solution, dilute to 25 ml with water. The absorbance of the resulting solutions is measured at 505 nm against reagent blank. The colour reaches maximum intensity within 5 min and is stable for more than 2 h. Beer's law is obeyed in the concentration range of 4-24 mcg/ml. Other penicillins do not interfere in this method.

Explanatory Note

The drug condenses with 4-amino antipyrine in the presence of alkaline oxidizing agent.

Probable Reaction Mechanism

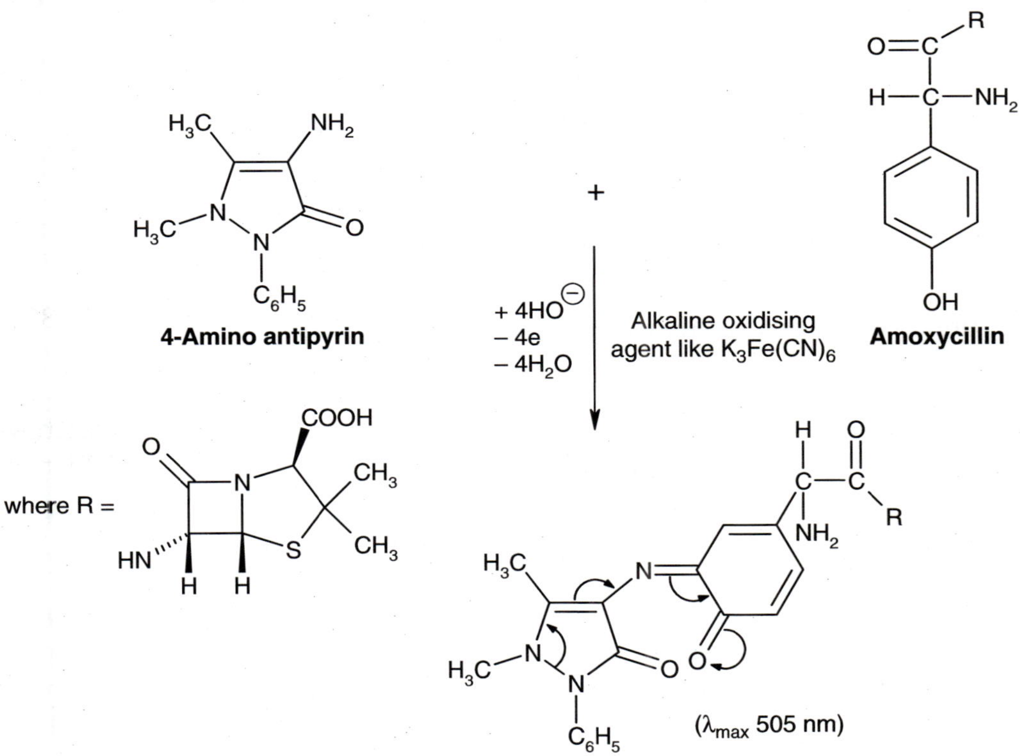

Reference

1. Pharmaceutical Chemistry (Vol. 2) by H.J. Roth, p. 76.
2. R.T. Sane, V.G. Nayak, V.B. Malkar, D.S. Sapre, A.D. Nadkarni, U.R. Pandit & V.J. Doshi, *Indian Drugs*, **21(2)**, 76-78, 1983.
3. R.G. Bhatkar et al., *Indian Drugs*, **21(2)**, 70-71, 1983.

METHOD 6

Reagents

1. 0.05% w/v solution of N-chlorosuccinimide (NCS) or N-bromosuccinimide (NBS) in water (prepare fresh).
2. 0.1 N sodium hydroxide.

Standard solution

Dissolve 50 mg of the substance in 1 ml of methanol and dilute to 50 ml in water. Further dilutions are done with water to get solution of 50 mcg/ml.

Sample solution

Accurately weighed or measured amount of the sample equivalent to 100 mg of the substance is dissolved in 2 ml of methanol and final volume made up to 100 ml with water. Further dilutions are carried out with water to get solution of 50 mcg/ml.

Procedure

To 1 ml each of sample and standard solutions, add 1 ml of sodium hydroxide solution immediately followed by 1 ml of NCS or NBS reagent. Mix well and dilute to 10 ml with methanol. Measure the absorbance of both the solutions at 395 nm against reagent blank.

Note

1. The intense yellow colour is stable for at least 30 min.
2. The method obeys Beer's law in the range of 1-20 mcg.
3. Amoxycillin and cefadroxil, the only phenolic compounds among the β-lactam antibiotics behave differently from the penicillins and cephalosporins on oxidation with NCS or NBS in alkaline medium.
4. The method is applicable to the estimation of cefadroxil, a phenolic compound.
5. Potassium clavulanate, cloxacillin, dicloxacillin, flucloxacillin and other related penicillins or structurally related degradation products such as penicillic acid, 6-aminopenicillinic acid and D-penicillamine do not interfere.
6. Amoxipenicilloic and amoxipenicillenic acid, alkaline and acid hydrolysis products interfere. Their interference can be eliminated by adding 0.4 ml of 0.025% methanolic solution of iodine and allowing the mixture to stand for 5 min before proceeding with the method involving oxidation with NCS or NBS.

Explanatory Note

N-bromosuccinimide/N-chlorosuccinimide, both being oxidizing agents, cause selective oxidation of the secondary OH group to keto (C==O) group in alkaline medium.

Probable Reaction Mechanism

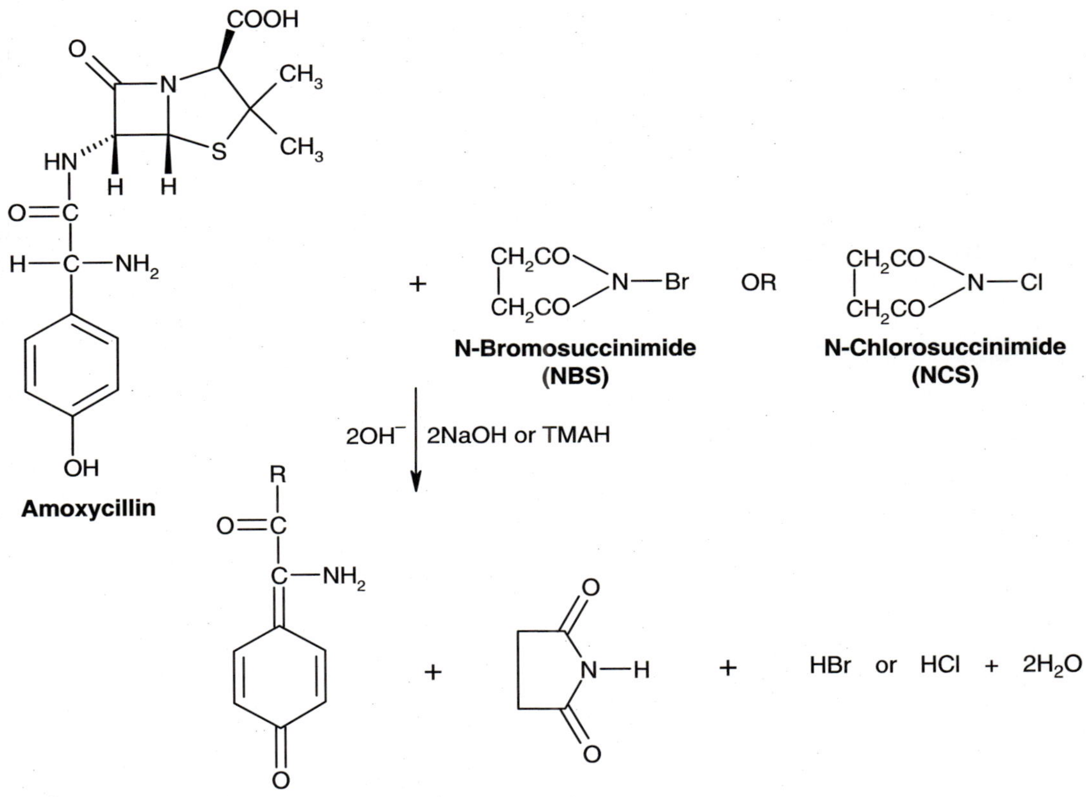

(λ_{max} 395 nm)

Note

Cefadroxil also reacts with 'NBS' or 'NCS' in a similar way. This reaction is positive for penicillins having phenolic-OH group such as cefperazone, cefprozil intense yellow colour.

Reference

Gamal A. Saleh. Analyst, 121, 641-645, 1996.

METHOD 7

Reagents

1. Borate buffer pH 10.
2. 5% sodium nitrite solution.
3. 1 M hydrochloric acid.
4. Diazotized phenylhydrazine-4-sulphonic acid (DPHS).
5. Ethyl alcohol.

Sample and standard solutions

100 µg/ml in water. Diazotized phenylhydrazine-4-sulphonic acid. To 50 mg of phenylhydrazine-4-sulphonic acid (Na) add 5 ml of water, 5 ml of 1 N HCl, cool to 10°C, add 1 ml of $NaNO_2$ solution, cool, allow to stand for 5 min, dilute to 25 ml with water.

Procedure

To 2 ml of DPHS solution add 5 ml of ethyl alcohol, allow to stand for 5 min. Add 5 ml each of sample and standard solutions and 50 ml of borate buffer. Allow to stand for 15 min and measure the absorbance at 440 nm.

Probable Reaction Mechanism

Coupling takes place between the DPHS and side chain of amoxycillin i.e. ortho to phenolic-OH group as explained.

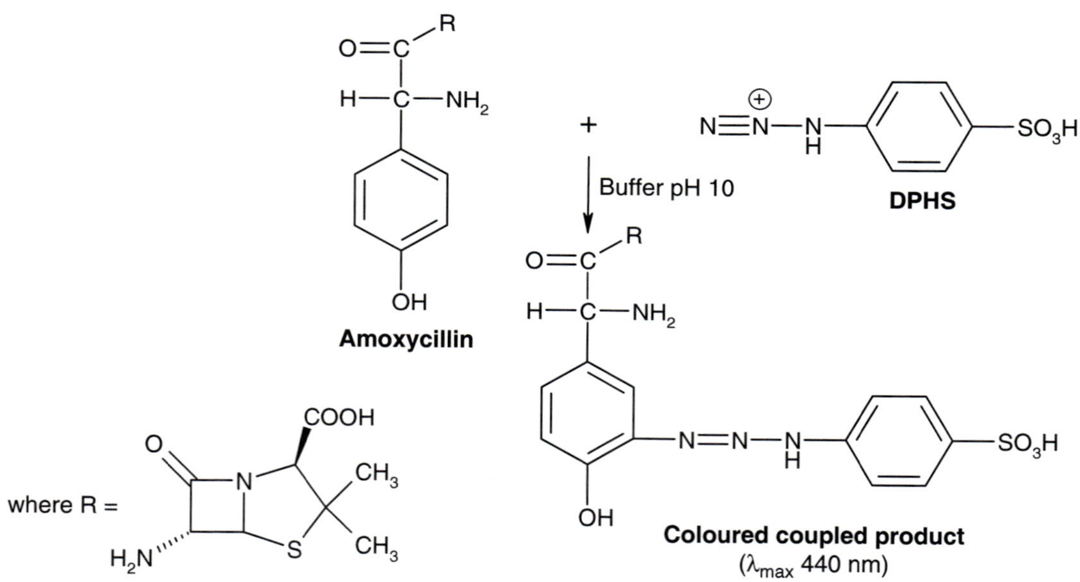

Reference

A. Sivaprasada Rao & M.V. Sivaramakrishnan, *Indian Drugs*, **23(8)**, 475-476, 1986.

METHOD 8

Reagents

1. 0.001% w/v solution of 4-nitrophenol (I), 2,4-dinitrophenol (II) or 3,5-dinitrobenzoic acid (III) in acetone.
2. Borate buffer pH 9.0.

Sample and standard solutions

Dissolve 50 mg of the sample/standard in 5 ml of methanol and then dilute to 250 ml with water (200 μg/ml).

Procedure

To 2 ml of any of the reagents, add 5 ml of borate buffer pH 9.0, 1 ml of acetone and 1 ml of sample/standard solution, dilute to 10 ml with water, keep at room temperature for 5 min and measure the absorbance at 336 nm. In case of reagents (I) and (II), the solution should be heated at 50°C for 30 min and then allow to stand for 10 min.

Probable Reaction Mechanism

In this case, the drug acts as donor whereas nitro derivatives act as acceptor to form charge transfer complex.

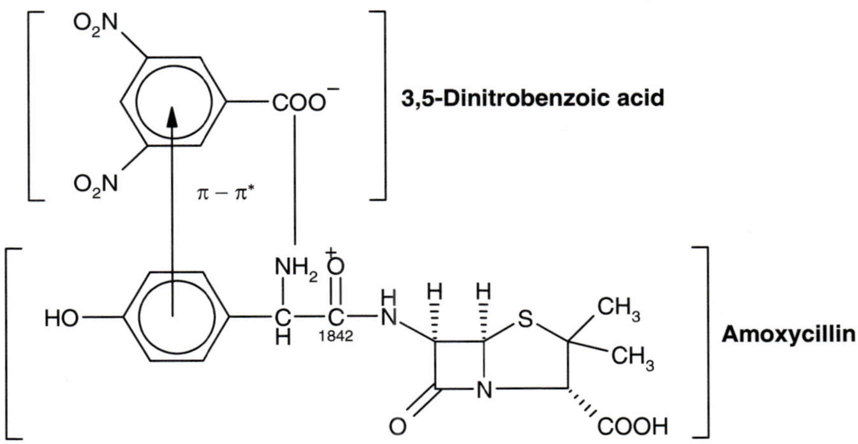

Note

Ampicillin, cloxacillin and the degradation products of amoxycillin (penillo-aldehyde) do not interfere.

Reference

A.S. Amin, A.L. El-Ansary & Y.M. Issa, *Talanta*, **41(5)**, 691-699, 1994.

METHOD 9

Reagents

1. 0.2% w/v solution of 1,2-naphthoquinone-4-sulphonate sodium in water.
2. pH 9.0 phosphate buffer.

Standard solution

1 mg/ml solution of amoxycillin in water.

Sample solution

Suspend accurately weighed quantity of the sample in water and dilute to get 1 mg/ml solution, filter and use for analysis.

Procedure

To 2 ml each of sample and standard solutions add 4 ml of naphthoquinone reagent, followed by 4 ml of buffer pH 9.0, dilute to 25 ml with water. Keep at room temperature for 25 min and measure the absorption of both the solutions at 468 nm against reagent blank.

Probable Reaction Mechanism

Amino group present in the drug having lone pair of electrons on nitrogen nucleophilically attack electron-dependent centre in 1,2-naphthoquinone because of C==C bond attached to the sulphonate molecule. Therefore, amoxycillin reacts with naphthoquinone to form coloured n-alkyl-amino naphthoquinone (λ_{max} 468 nm). At pH <4.0, the protonated amino salt $-NH_3^+$ loses nucleophilic activity, hence chromogenic reaction cannot take place at lower pH, whereas at pH >9.0 the amount of –OH ions increases and –OH being more basic than amino group, the nucleophilic activity of –OH is far more stronger than amino group and thus OH^- ion shall compete heavily with amino group to attack sulphonate and holds back the reaction between amoxycillin and chromogenic reagent. Hence pH 9.0 was found most suitable medium for reaction.

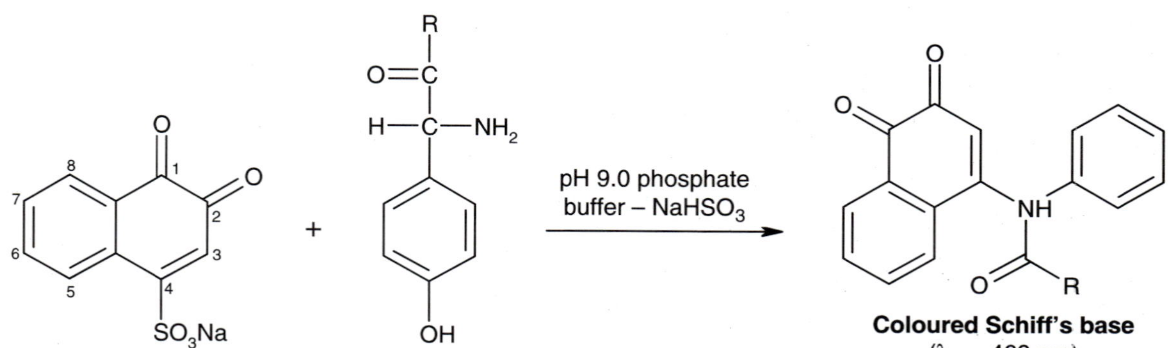

1,2-Naphthoquinone-4-sulphonate sodium

Amoxycillin

Coloured Schiff's base (λ_{max} 468 nm)

Reference

Q. Li & Z. Yang, *Analytical Letters*, **39**, 763-775, 2006.

METHOD 10

This is a common method for different phenolic β-lactam antibiotics* such as cefoperazone sodium, cefadroxil and cefprozil in different pharmaceutical dosage forms. Potassium clavulanate does not interfere if present. Different methods involved are:

(a) Nitration and subsequent chelation with a nucleophilic reagent.
(b) Nitrosation and metal chelation.
(c) Coupling with diazo reagent.
(d) Reaction with copper (II).

Probable Reaction Mechanism

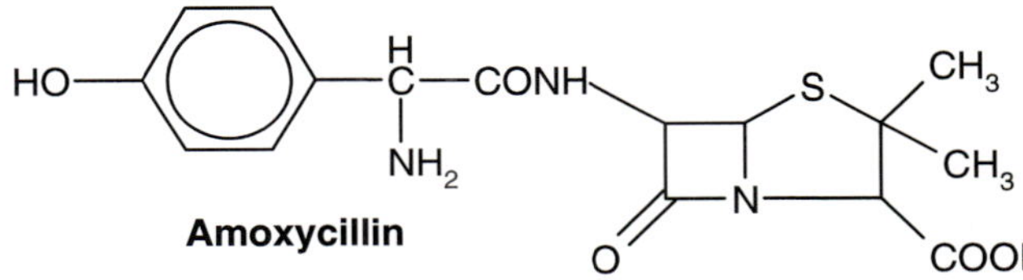

Amoxycillin

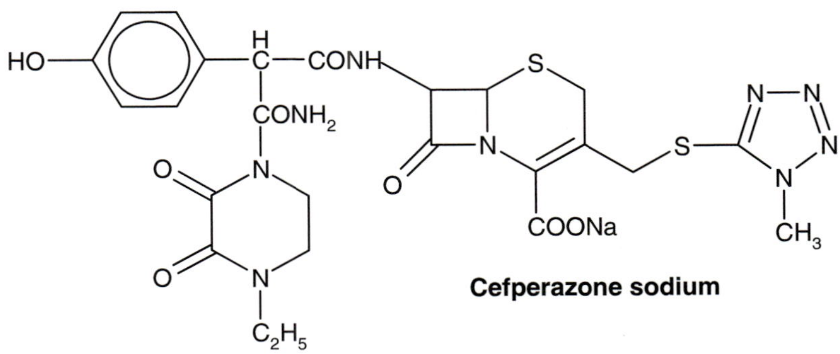

Cefperazone sodium

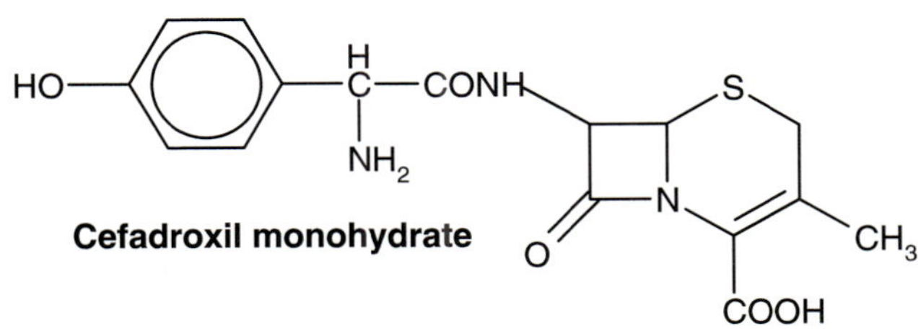

Cefadroxil monohydrate

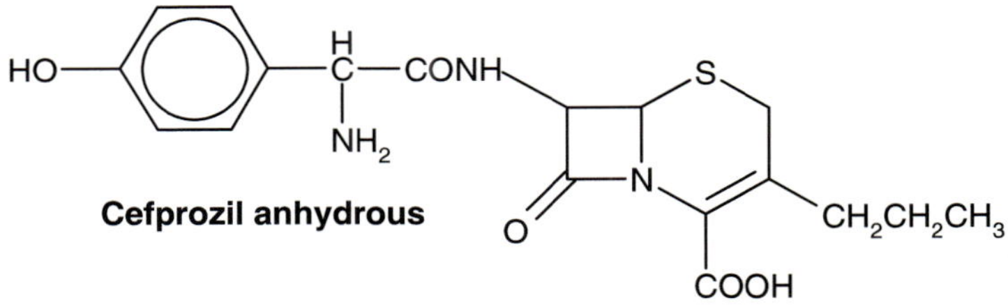

Cefprozil anhydrous

General formula

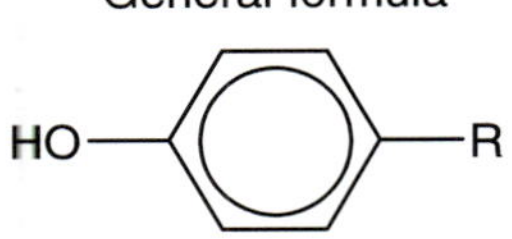

(a) Nitration results in dinitro derivative in two ortho positions to phenolic-OH. The so formed complex being electron deficit, it reacts with acetone-carbanion to give intense coloured complex (λ_{max} 390 nm). This complex is of Meisenheimer type. (M.J. Strauss. Chem. Rev., 70, 667, 1970)

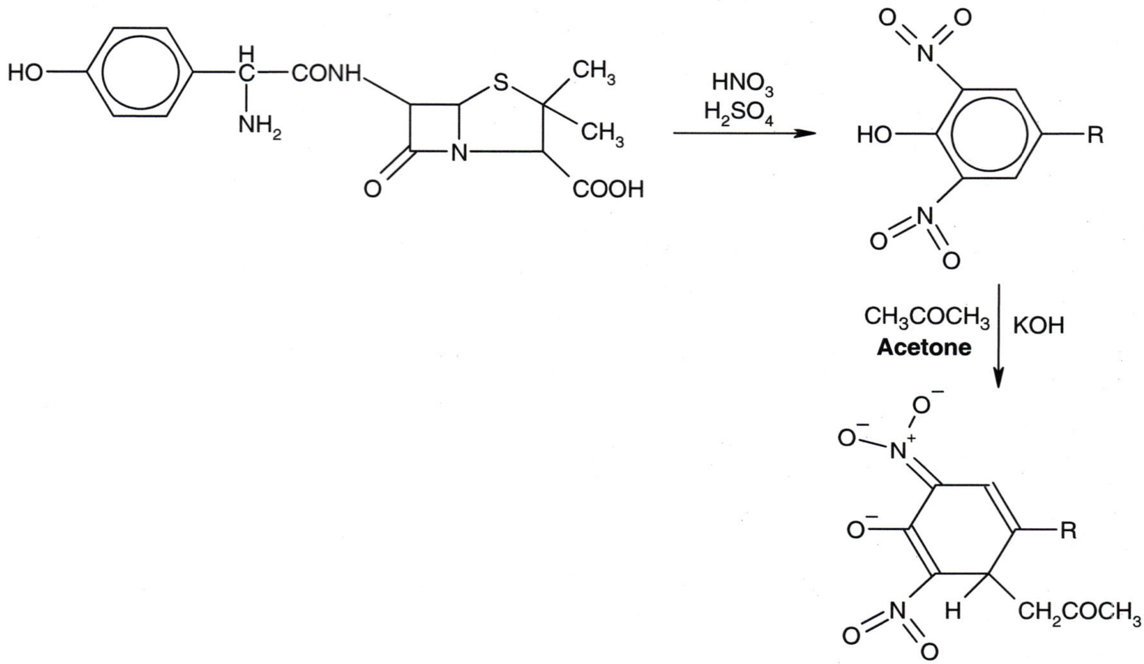

Meisenheimer type complex with acetone (λ_{max} 390 nm)

Reference

M.J. Strauss, *Chem. Rev.*, **70**, 667, 1970.

(b) Nitrosation and metal chelation.

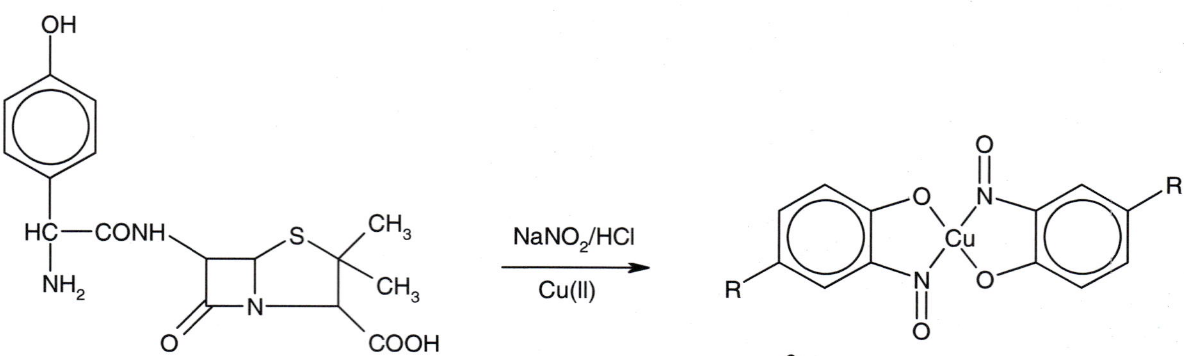

Cu^{2+} chelate of nitroso derivative (λ_{max} 520 nm)

(c) Diazo coupling with nitroaniline. Diazotized nitroaniline is used as chromogenic reagent.

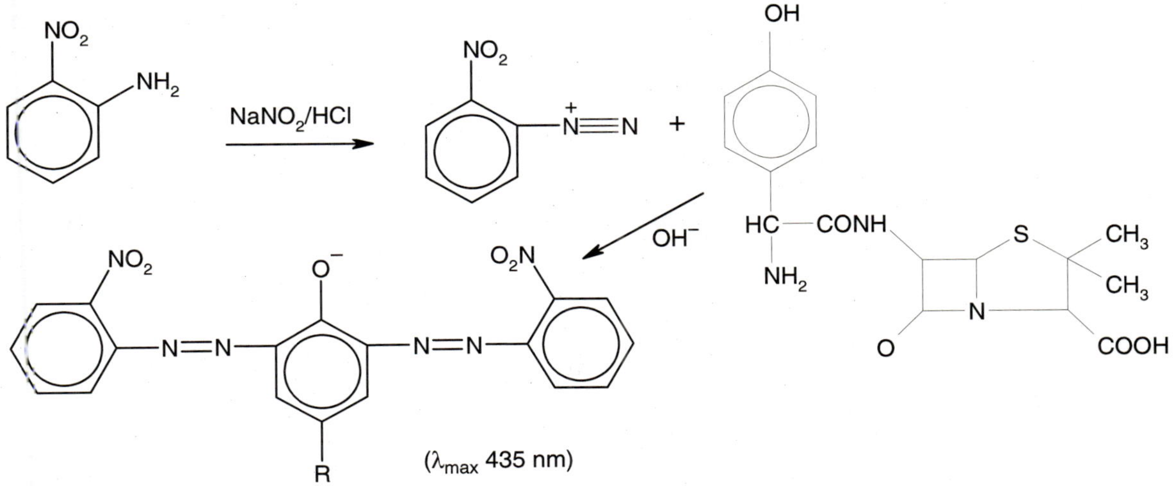

(d) Diazo coupling with subsequent chelation. The diazotized nitroaniline derivative (c) was complexed with Cu(II) to give chloroform extractable yellow-coloured complex (λ_{max} 415 nm).

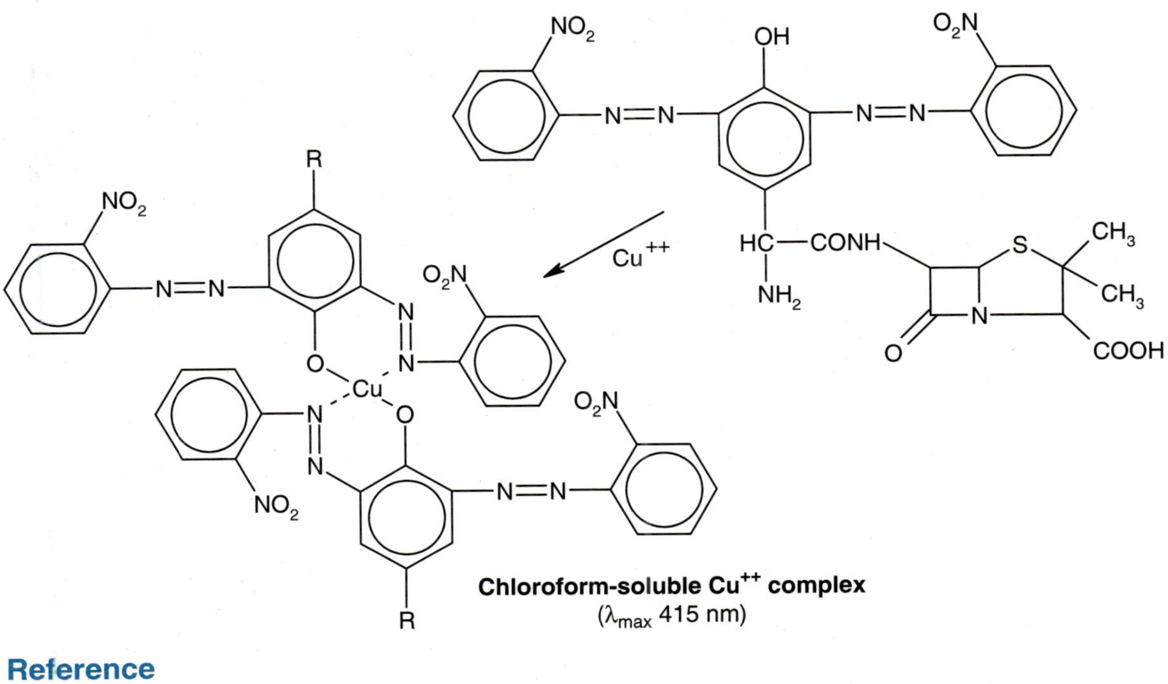

Reference

Hesham Salem, *Analytica Chimica Acta*, **515**, 331-341, 2002.

Amoxycillin and ampicillin an anion forms ion-pair association complex with 1,10-phenanthroline-Fe(III) – λ_{max} 515 nm. This is extractable into organic solvent.

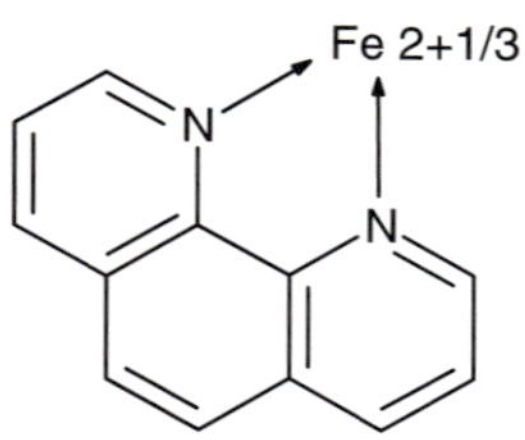

Ferroin

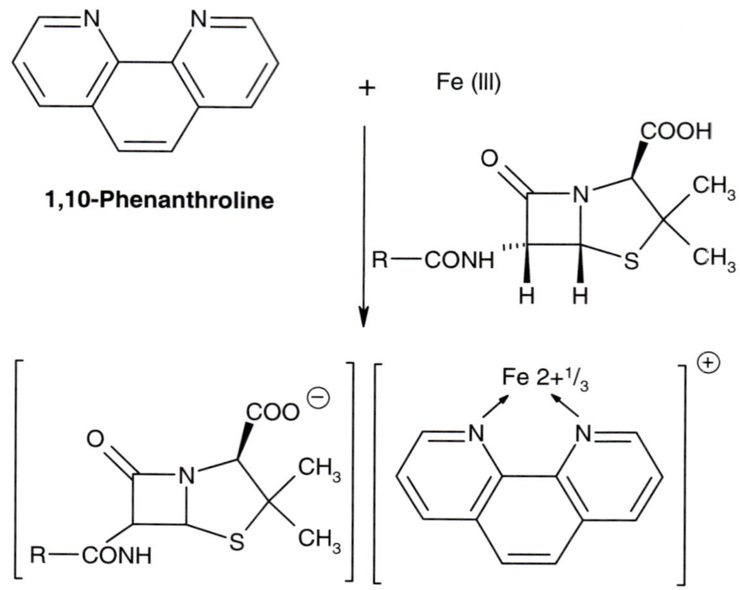

Ion-pair complex
(λ_{max} 515 nm)

The drug reacts with Emmerie-Engel reagent which involves oxidation of the drug with Fe^{3+} and in turn Fe^{3+} gets reduced to Fe^{2+}. Fe^{2+} so formed reacts with 2,2′-bispyridine to give red-coloured complex $[Fe(bipy)_3]^{2+}$ (λ_{max} 522 nm).

Probable Reaction Mechanism

Two nitrogens present in the reagent have one unshared pair of electrons which can be shared by Fe^{2+} to give complex.

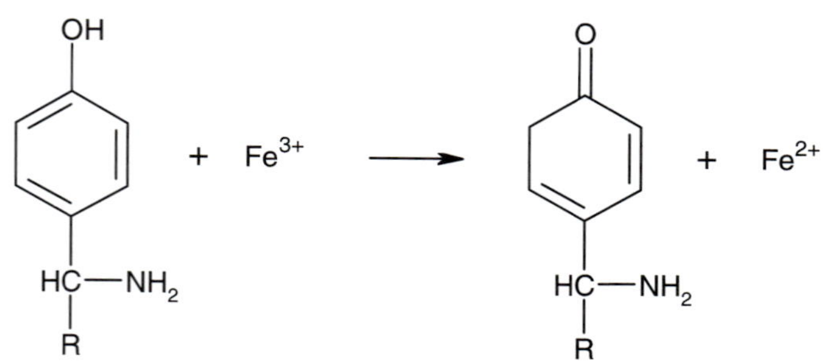

Amoxycillin

Reference

B.S. Nagaralli, J. Seetharamappa & M.B. Melwanki, *J. Pharm. Biomed. Anal.*, **29**, 859-864, 2002.

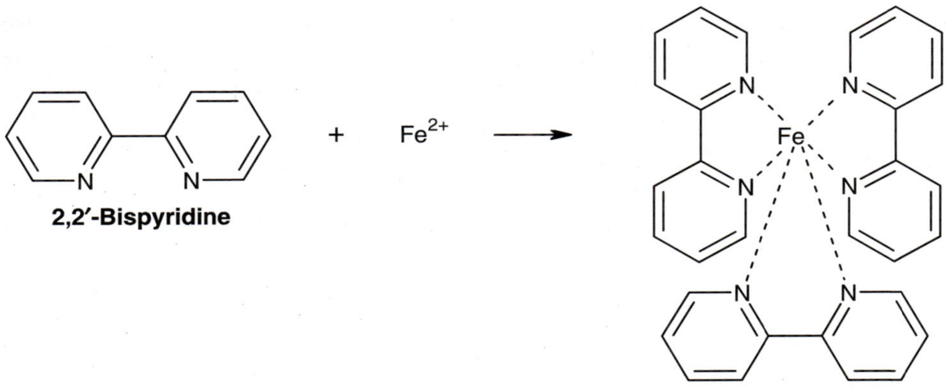

[Fe(bipy)$_3$]$^{2+}$ complex
(λ_{max} 522 nm)

Amoxycillin undergoes oxidative coupling with p-N,N-dimethyl phenylenediamine (DMPD) at ortho to the phenolic OH group present in the molecule. This has been used for quantitative analysis of the compound.

Probable Reaction Mechanism

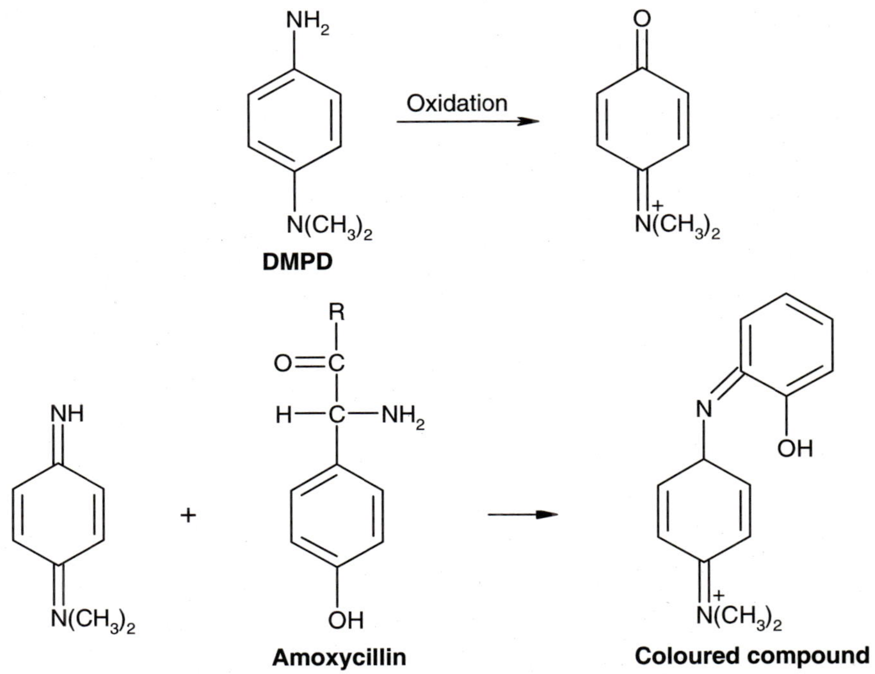

Reference

R.T. Sane, R.S. Samant, S.V. Desai, M.L. Kubal, V.G. Nayak & A.D. Nadkarni, *Indian Drugs*, **22**, 592, 1988.

A spectrophotometric method for the estimation of ampicillin and amoxycillin reported by Korany et al. (1989) is based on reaction with carboxylic (–COOH) group present in the penicillin moiety. It involves reaction with 2-nitrophenyl-hydrazine (2-NPH) in the presence of dicyclohexylcarbodiimide (DCC) and pyridine. The resultant acid hydrazide has λ_{max} 546 nm. The reaction was carried out in non-aqueous mixed solvent.

Probable Reaction Mechanism

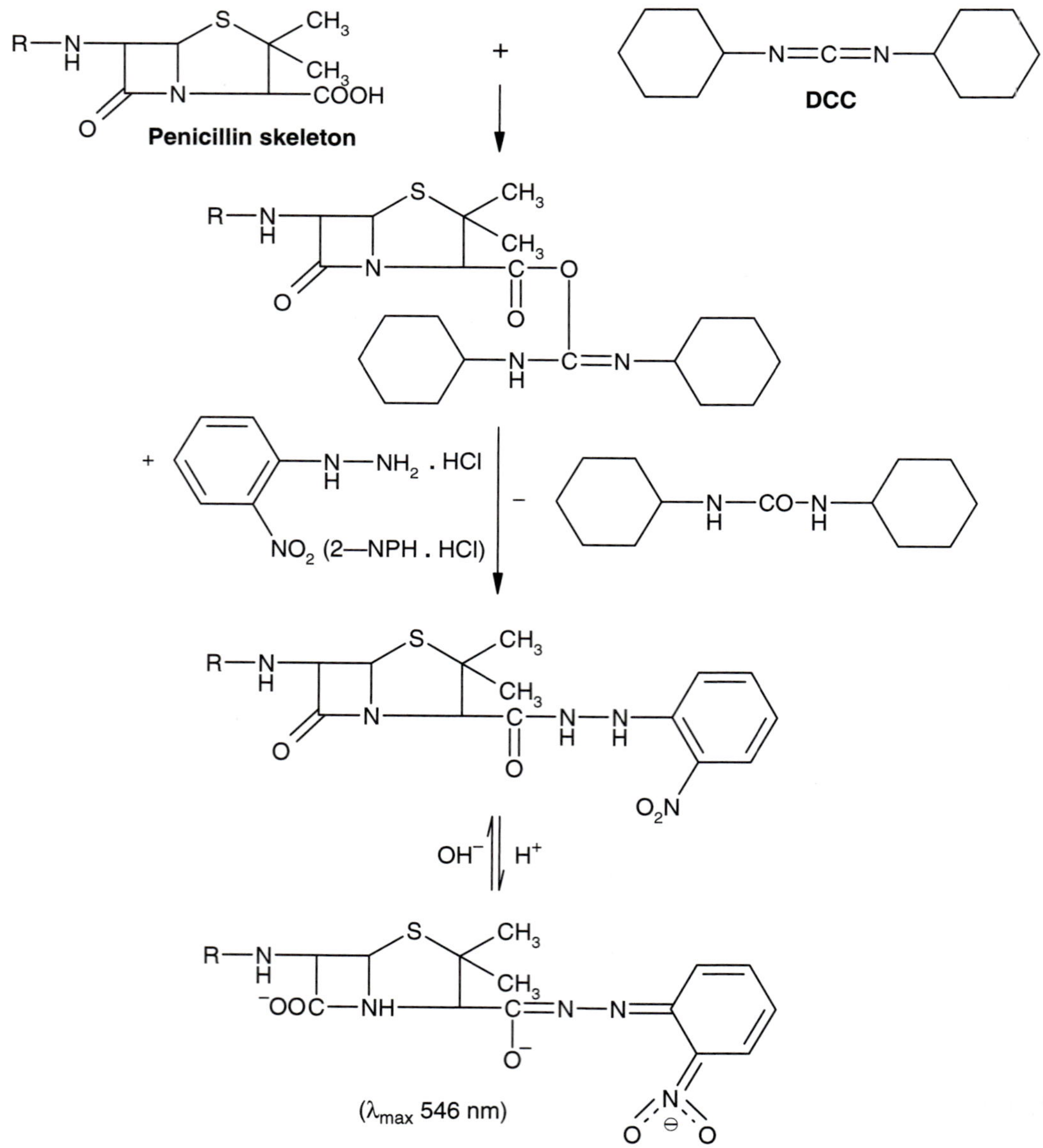

Reference

Mohamed A. Korany, Mohamed H. Abdel-Hay, Mona M. Bedair & Azza A. Gazy, *Talanta*, **36(12)**, 1253-1257, 1989.

An analytical method based on formation of charge-transfer (C-T) complex with 2,3-dichloro-5,6-dicyano-p-benzoquinone (DDQ) was reported by Askal et al. (1991). 'DDQ' is electron acceptor whereas the drug is electron donor.

Probable Reaction Mechanism

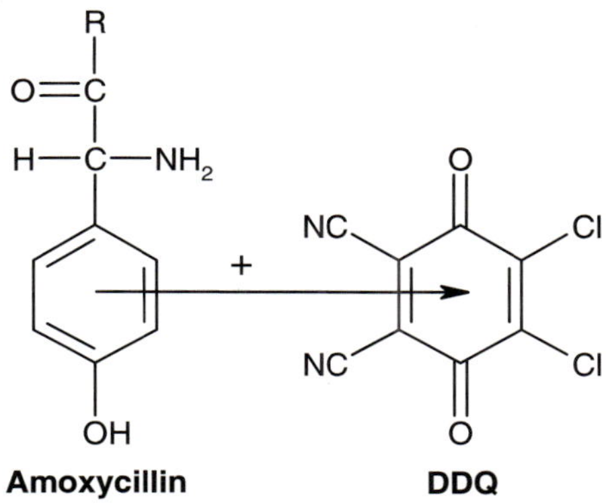

Amoxycillin - DDQ C-T complex
(λ_{max} 460 nm)

Reference

H.F. Askal, G.A. Saleh & N.M. Omar, *Analyst*, **116**, 387-390, 1991.

Note

1. Other electron-accepting reagents for analysis through C-T complexes are p-chloranil and p-bromanil.
2. Authors have reported the analysis of several penicillins (ampicillin, methicillin, oxacillin) with this reagent.

Both ampicillin and amoxycillin containing primary amino group shall react with Sanger's reagent. The reagent having electron withdrawing group (NO_2) ortho and para to halogen (F) activates the halogen for nucleophilic substitution.

Reference

1. D.M. Shingbal & R.R. Naik, *Indian Drugs*, **22(5)**, 271-272, and **22(7)**, 383-384, 1985.
2. Organic Chemistry by Seyhar Edge (2nd ed.) pp. 957, 1128.

Probable Reaction Mechanism

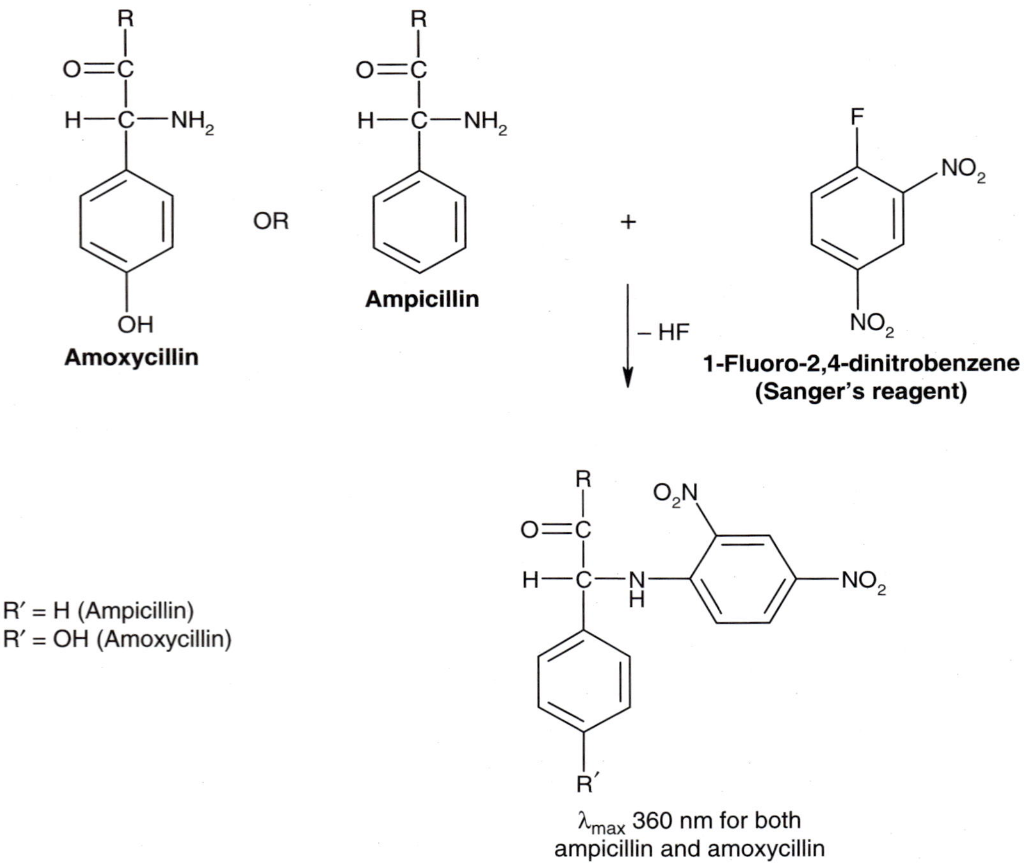

An alternate reaction based on Michael addition giving coloured quinonimine is as under.

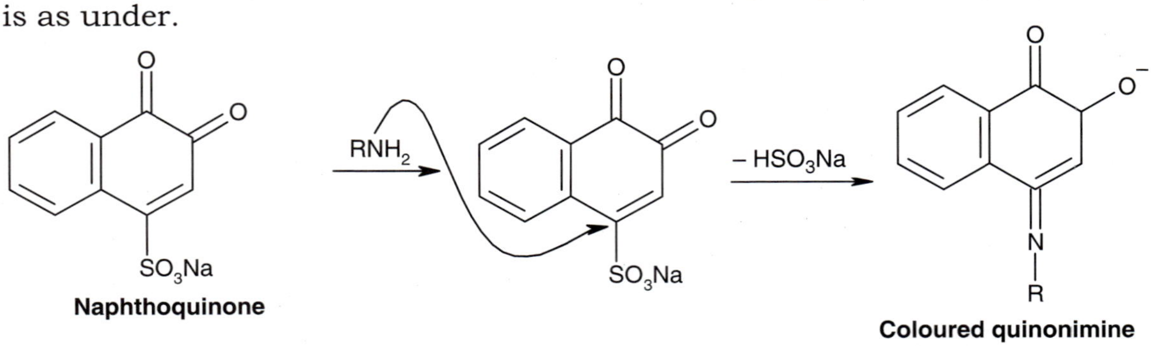

Reference

Pharmaceutical Chemistry (Vol. 2) by H.J. Roth, p. 377.

Hydroxylamine as nucleophile opens the penicillin ring and forms hydroxamic acid derivative which gives characteristic colour with Fe(III) chloride in acid solution. The method has been official in several compendia.

Probable Reaction Mechanism

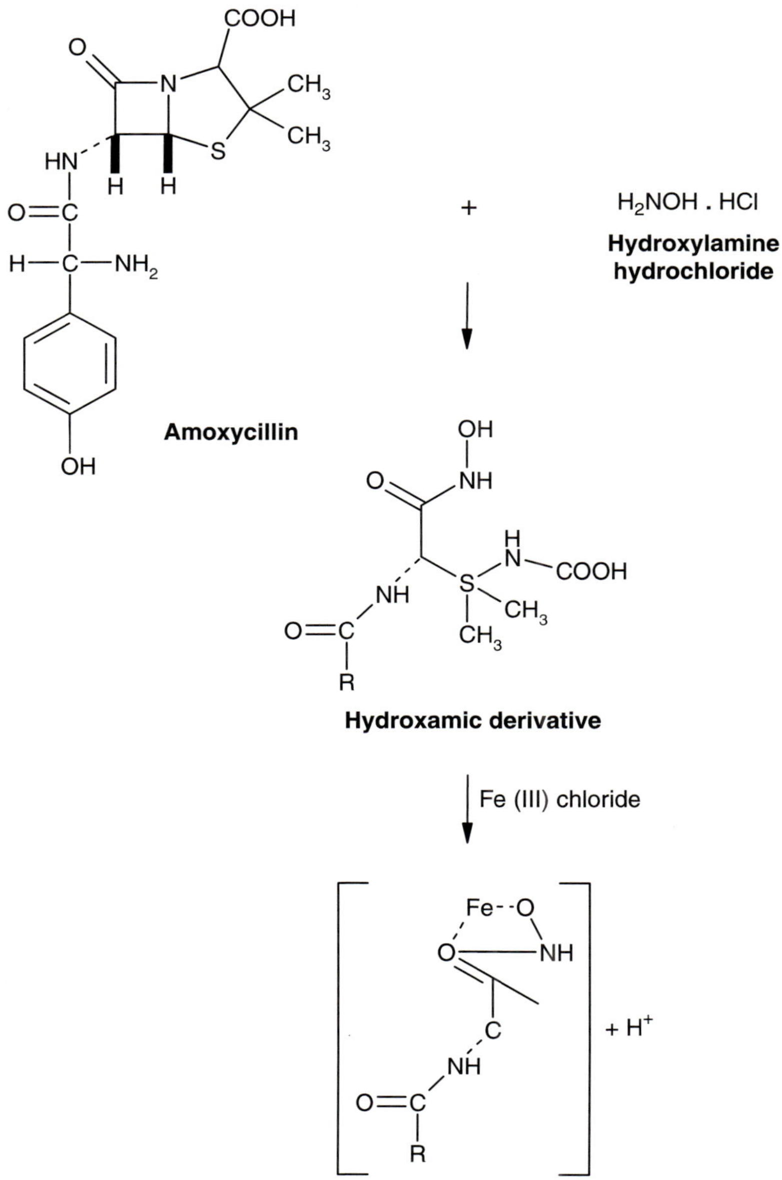

1 : 1 Fe (III) - hydroxamic acid complex

(λ_{max} 490 nm)

Amoxycillin gives positive test with Millon's reagent (test for phenols with free ortho position). This test is not answered by ampicillin.

Probable Reaction Mechanism

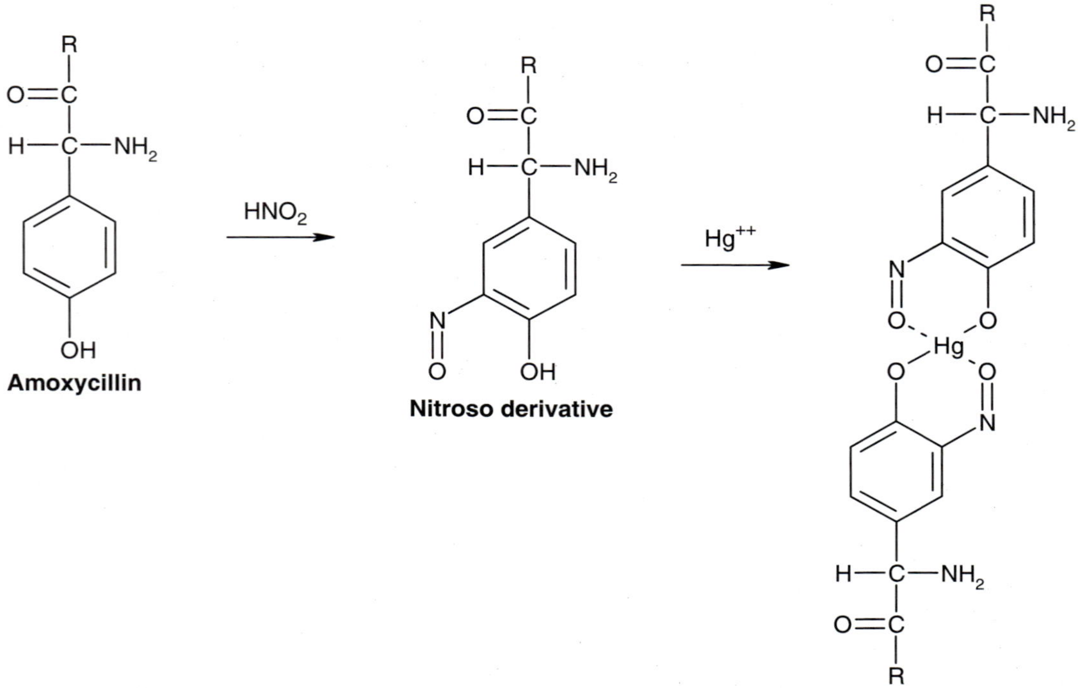

Amoxycillin

Nitroso derivative

Stabilized coloured chelate with Hg^{2+}

Formulation 9

Ampicillin/Amoxycillin, Cloxacillin sodium

ESTIMATION

Ampicillin/Amoxycillin

METHOD 1

Reagents

1. 0.1 M sodium hydroxide.
2. 0.1 M hydrochloric acid.
3. Phenolphthalein solution (indicator).

Procedure

Weigh accurately quantity of the sample equivalent to about 0.25 g of ampicillin and transfer to a conical flask. Add about 25 ml of freshly boiled, cooled and neutralized (phenolphthalein) water. Slightly warm in boiling water-bath and titrate immediately with 0.1 N sodium hydroxide using phenolphthalein solution as indicator till faint pink colour appears. Warm slightly and continue titration till distinct pink colour persists. The volume of 0.1 N sodium hydroxide used in the titration represents the amount of ampicillin present in the sample. Each ml of 0.1 N sodium hydroxide is equivalent to 0.03495 g of ampicillin (anhydrous) or 0.03654 g of amoxycillin.

Reference

Y. Kumar, S.C. Mathur, N. Murgesan, A.C.S. Rao, Y.K. Rathor & P.D. Sethi. *Indian Drugs*, **29(11)**, 478-480.

METHOD 2

The method is based on formation of Schiff's base.

Reagents

1. 0.1% w/v solution of p-dimethyl aminocinnamaldehyde (PDAC) in methanol.
2. 50% w/v solution of trichloroacetic acid (TCA) in methanol.

Standard solution

50 mcg/ml of ampicillin in water.

Sample solution

Accurately weighed quantity of the sample was extracted with water to get a concentration of 50 mcg/ml.

Procedure

To 2 ml each of sample and standard solutions in 100 ml volumetric flasks, add 2 ml of PDAC reagent, followed by 10 ml of TCA, shake and allow to stand for 10 min and dilute to 100 ml with methanol. Keep the final diluted solution to stand at room temperature for 60 min and measure the absorbance of both sample and standard solutions at absorption maxima at about 500 nm and calculate the results by comparison. For reaction mechanism, see method 2 under amoxycillin in this chapter.

Cloxacillin

METHOD 1

To the solution obtained after completing the titration for ampicillin/amoxycillin (method 1), add exactly 50 ml of 0.1 N sodium hydroxide solution and heat in a boiling water-bath for not less than 30 min. Cool and titrate excess of alkali with 0.1 N hydrochloric acid till the pink colour disappears.

From the volume of sodium hydroxide consumed in the second titration, subtract the volume of alkali used in the first titration i.e. for ampicillin. The difference represents the volume of alkali consumed by cloxacillin present in the sample. Each ml of 0.1 N sodium hydroxide is equivalent to 0.04350 g of cloxacillin.

Note

1. The method gives excellent results with solid dosage forms (capsules). However in case of dry syrups, colour present tends to interfere. Charcoal treatment can remove interference to great extent.
2. The method is not suitable if ampicillin is present as sodium salt.

METHOD 2

Reagents

1. 0.3 M hydrochloric acid.
2. 1% v/v solution of formaldehyde in 0.3 N hydrochloric acid.

Standard solution

500 mcg/ml of ampicillin, amoxycillin or cloxacillin in water.

Sample solution

Accurately weighed quantity of the sample (capsule, syrup) equivalent to 50 mg of the substance is suspended in 70-80 ml of water and sonicated for 5 min or slightly warm in boiling water-bath to ensure complete dissolution. Dilute with water to 100 ml, filter and use the filtrate for analysis.

Procedure

Dilute 2 ml each of the standard and sample solutions to 50 ml with formaldehyde reagent and proceed as under:

(a) Maintain part of both the solutions at room temperature and after 20 min measure the absorbance of sample and standard solutions at 346 nm against reagent blank and calculate the contents of cloxacillin in the sample by comparison.

(b) Heat other portion of both the sample and standard solutions at 90°C (± 0.5°C) in constant temperature water-bath for 60 min, cool to room temperature and measure the absorbance at 380 nm (ampicillin) and 397 nm (amoxycillin) against reagent blank and calculate the contents by comparison.

Note

1. On treatment with acidic formaldehyde, β-lactam ring of penicillin present in cloxacillin opens up resulting in the formation of penicillinic acid, an intermediate compound having absorption maximum at 346 nm. Penicillinic acid being unstable undergoes further degradation to form D-penicillamine and penaldic acid, both of which have negligible absorbance. This explains the reason for decrease in absorbance after 20 min.
2. In case of ampicillin/amoxycillin, intra-molecular aminolysis occurs; as a result, a-aminobenzoyl group present in the side chain of both the drugs attack nucleophilically carbonyl group present in the b-lactam ring resulting in formation of pyrazine derivative.
3. Formaldehyde plays no role in the acid hydrolysis of cloxacillin.
4. Under acidic conditions, the free amino group is in its cationic form $R–NH_3^+$ resulting in decrease in its nucleophilic ability and hence formation of pyrazine derivative. On addition of formaldehyde, the free amino group forms Schiff's base which being unstable in acidic medium releases unionised form of amino group which reacts with carbonyl group present in the b-lactam ring, resulting in enhanced formation of pyrazine derivative.

Probable Reaction Mechanism

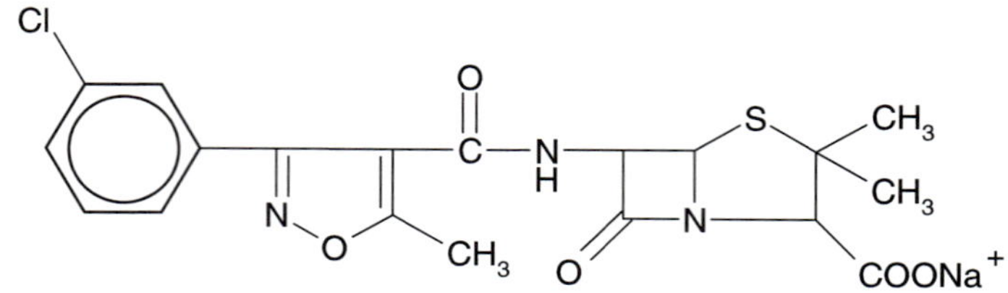

Cloxacillin sodium

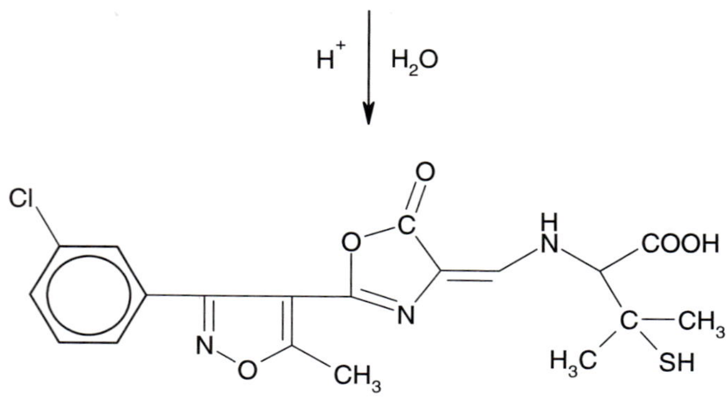

Penicillinic acid
(λ_{max} 346 nm)

This being unstable, it further degrades to

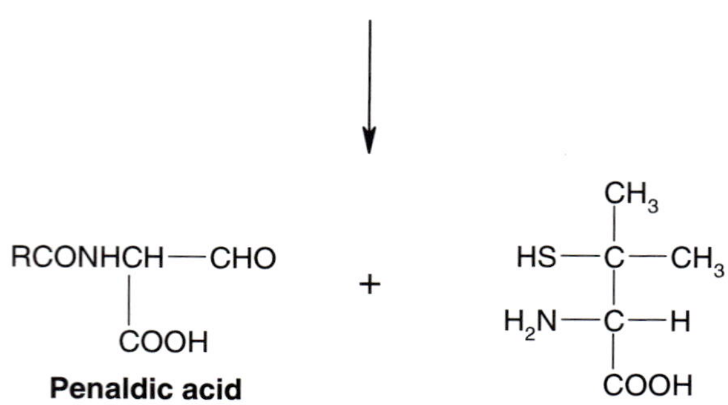

Penaldic acid + **D-Penicillamine**

Note

The absorption decreases after 12 min. This is explained by degradation of penicillinic acid and both the degradation products have negligible absorption.

METHOD 3

Cloxacillin can also be estimated by reaction with hydroxylamine under alkaline conditions. The carboxylic group present in the penicillin ring structure of cloxacillin will react with hydroxyammonium chloride under alkaline condition resulting in the formation of hydroxamic acid. The hydroxamic acid yields a red chelate with Fe(III) ions.

Probable Reaction Mechanism

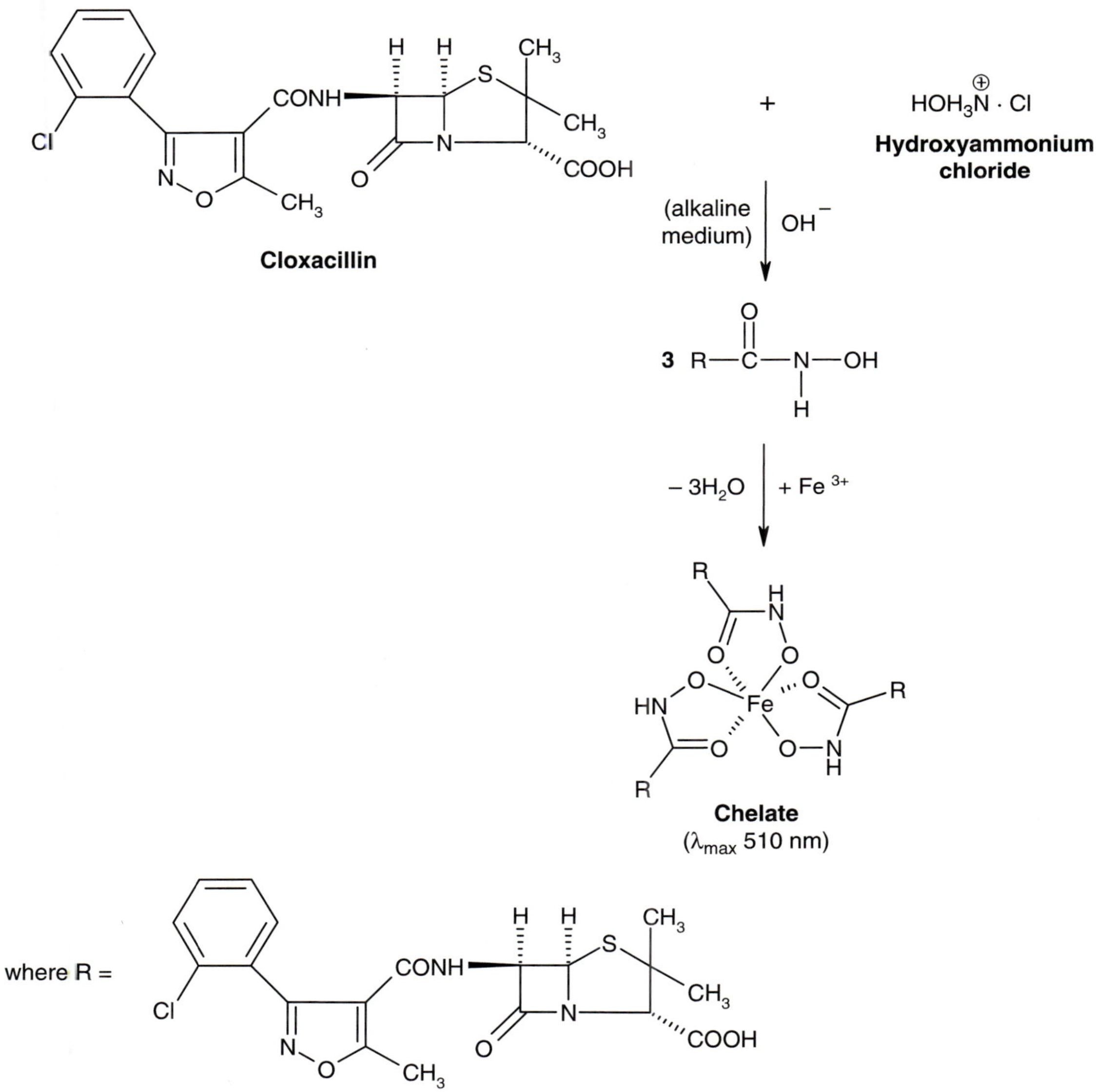

Formulation 10

Ampicillin, Probenecid

ESTIMATION

Probenecid

Reagents

1. Chloroform.
2. 0.1 N methanolic hydrochloric acid.

Standard solution

Prepare 100 mcg per ml solution of probenecid in chloroform. Evaporate 5 ml of it and dissolve the residue in 50 ml of 0.1 N methanolic hydrochloric acid (10 mcg/ml).

Sample solution

Weigh accurately the powdered sample equivalent to 100 mg of probenecid, extract the dry powder with three 25 ml portions of chloroform, filtering each through the same G_4 sintered glass funnel. Dilute the combined filtrate to 100 ml with chloroform. Evaporate 5 ml of the filtrate on a water-bath and take up the residue in 0.1 N methanolic hydrochloric acid to get a final concentration of 10 mcg per ml.

Measure the extinction of the sample and standard solutions at the maximum at about 248 nm using 0.1 N methanolic hydrochloric acid as blank and deduce the results by comparison.

Ampicillin

Reagents

1. 0.3 N hydrochloric acid.
2. 1% v/v formaldehyde in 0.3 N hydrochloric acid.

Standard solution

1 mg/ml of ampicillin in 0.3 N hydrochloric acid.

Sample solution

Use the entire residue left after the extraction of probenecid as described above. Dissolve the residue left in the G_4 sintered funnel in 100 ml of 0.3 N hydrochloric acid.

Procedure

Dilute 2 ml each of standard and sample solutions to 50 ml with 1% v/v formaldehyde in 0.3 N hydrochloric acid. Heat on a water-bath at 90 ± 0.5°C for 60 minutes. Cool to room temperature and measure the absorbance of both standard and sample solutions at the maximum at about 380 nm using 1% v/v formaldehyde in 0.3 N hydrochloric acid treated in the same manner as the blank and deduce the results by comparison. For further details, refer to method 2 in formulation 2 of this chapter.

For reaction mechanism, see under ampicillin in this chapter.

Formulation 11

Amoxycillin, Probenecid

ESTIMATION

Probenecid

Follow the method described under formulation 10 of this chapter. The method makes use of the fact that probenecid is soluble in chloroform whereas amoxycillin is totally insoluble in chloroform. The solution of the compound in 0.1 N methanolic hydrochloric acid exhibits maxima at about 248 nm. Sample equivalent to about 100 mg of probenecid is initially taken for analysis.

Amoxycillin

The residue obtained after extraction of probenecid is subjected to quantitative analysis for amoxycillin contents. For estimation, follow the method 8 described under formulation 8 of this chapter.

Formulation 12

Cephalexin, Probenecid

ESTIMATION

Probenecid

Follow the method described under formulation 9 of this chapter. Probenecid is soluble in chloroform. Cephalexin, ampicillin and amoxycillin are insoluble in chloroform.

Cephalexin

METHOD 1

Standard solution

10 mcg/ml of cephalexin in 0.1 N methanolic hydrochloric acid.

Sample solution

The entire residue left after extraction of probenecid with chloroform is used for analysis of cephalexin. The residue left on sintered funnel is taken in 0.1 N methanolic hydrochloric acid and further diluted appropriately to get a concentration of 10 mcg/ml.

Measure the extinction of both sample and standard solutions at maxima at about 258 nm using 0.1 N methanolic hydrochloric acid as blank and calculate the results by comparison.

METHOD 2

Reagents

1. 50% v/v sulphuric acid.
2. 0.1% w/v solution of ninhydrin in 50% sulphuric acid.

Standard solution

200 mcg/ml of cephalexin in water.

Sample solution

The residue left after extraction of probenecid was taken up in water.

Procedure

To 1 ml each of sample and standard solutions, add 2 ml of water, 1 ml of 50% sulphuric acid. Heat in steam-bath for 5 min, then add 2 ml of ninhydrin solution. Heat for another 10 min, cool and extract with chloroform (2 × 10 ml). Dilute the combined chloroform layer to 25 ml and measure the absorbance of both the sample and standard solutions at 520 nm within 10 min and calculate the results by comparison.

Probable Reaction Mechanism

On heating with sulphuric acid, the compound is hydrolysed to give 7-amino derivative. The amino group so liberated reacts with ninhydrin to give violet colour (λ_{max} 520 nm). For general reaction of amino group with ninhydrin, see under neomycin or under ampicillin.

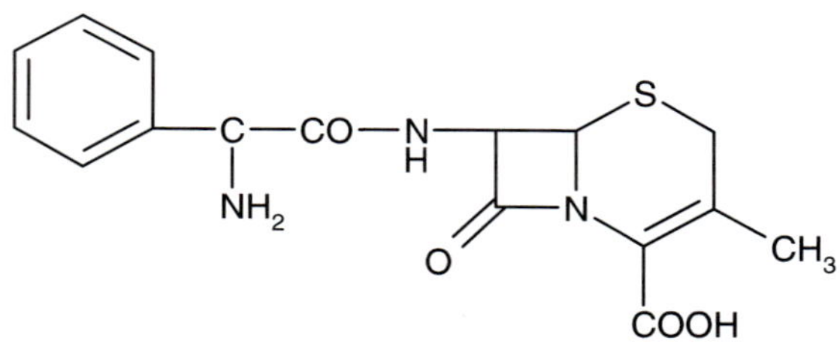

Cephalexin

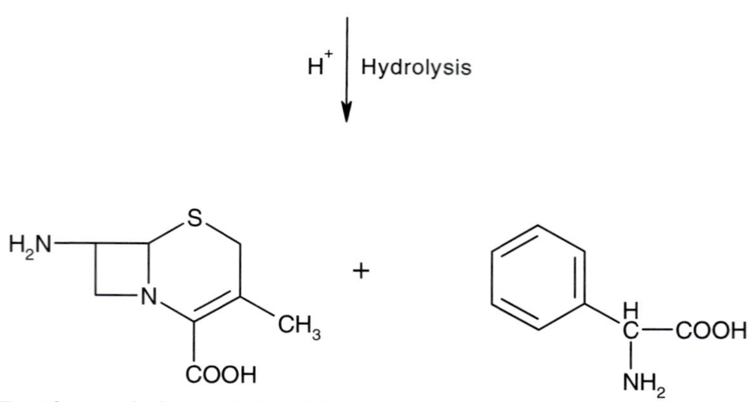

7-aminocephalosporinic acid
(I)

Amino group at position 7 can also form Schiff's base with PDAB or PDAC.

Probable Reaction Mechanism

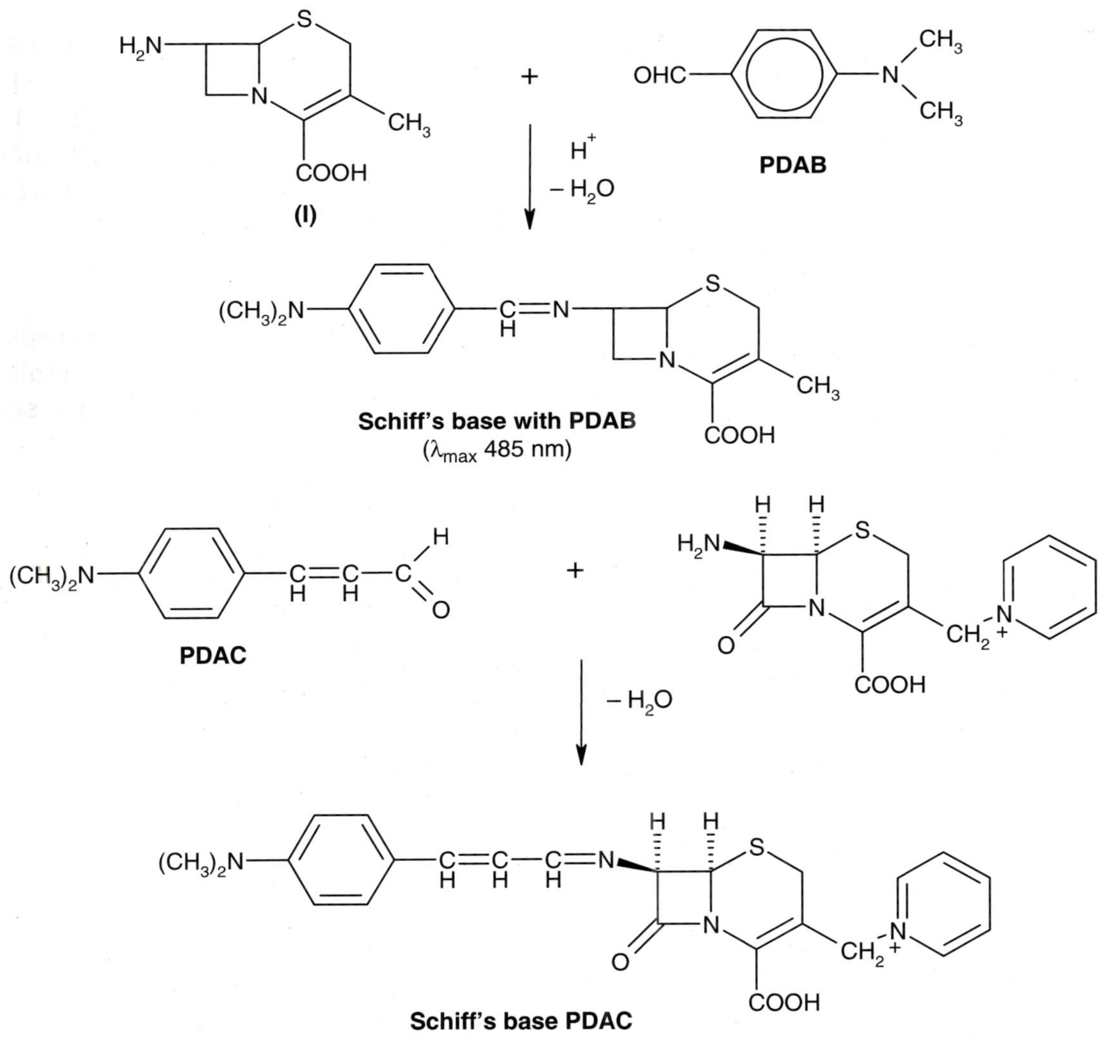

Reference

G. Rama Rao & S. Raghuveer. *J. Inst. Chem.*, **55**, 61-62, 1983.

METHOD 3

Reagents

1. 1.5% solution of 2,4-dinitrofluorobenzene in acetone (DNFB).
2. 2.5% solution of borax in water.

3. Combine 1 and 2 in ratio of 1 : 10 to get reagent solution.
4. Acidic dioxane [hydrochloric acid dioxane (5 : 95, v/v)].

Sample and drug sample

200 µg/ml.

Procedure

To 1 ml of sample/standard solution, add 1 ml of reagent solution (3), heat at 75°C for 40 min, cool, add 35 ml of acidic dioxane and dilute to 100 ml with water. Measure at 385 nm for quantitative analysis.

Probable Reaction Mechanism

This reagent 1-fluoro-2,4-dinitrobenzene is known as Sanger's reagent. The amino group of caphalexin bahaves as a nucleophilic and attacks the position at which fluoride is present in the reagent resulting in the formation of the product as shown in the reaction below.

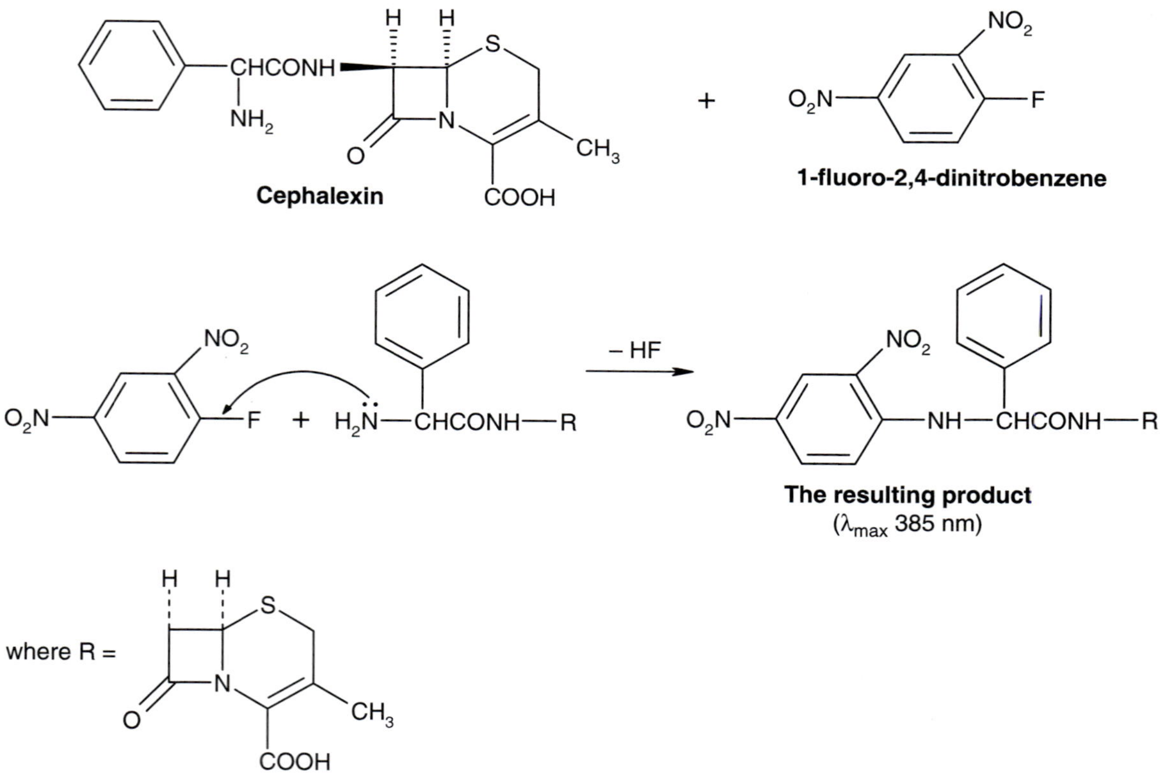

Reference

J. Emmanuel & E. Silva Dias, *Indian Drugs*, **24(7)**, 357-358, 1987.

Note

A method using p-nitrobenzene as reagent has been reported to give coloured compound (λ_{max} 390 nm).

Reference

Indian Drugs, **24(7)**, 367, 1987.

METHOD 4

Cephalexin reacts with p-dinitrobenzene on heating with NaOH for 10 min.

Probable Reaction Mechanism

The NaOH added i.e. the base extracts a proton from the position next to sulphur resulting in the formation of carbanion (i.e. carbon with negative charge). Then attack of the reagent occurs at that position resulting in the formation of the product.

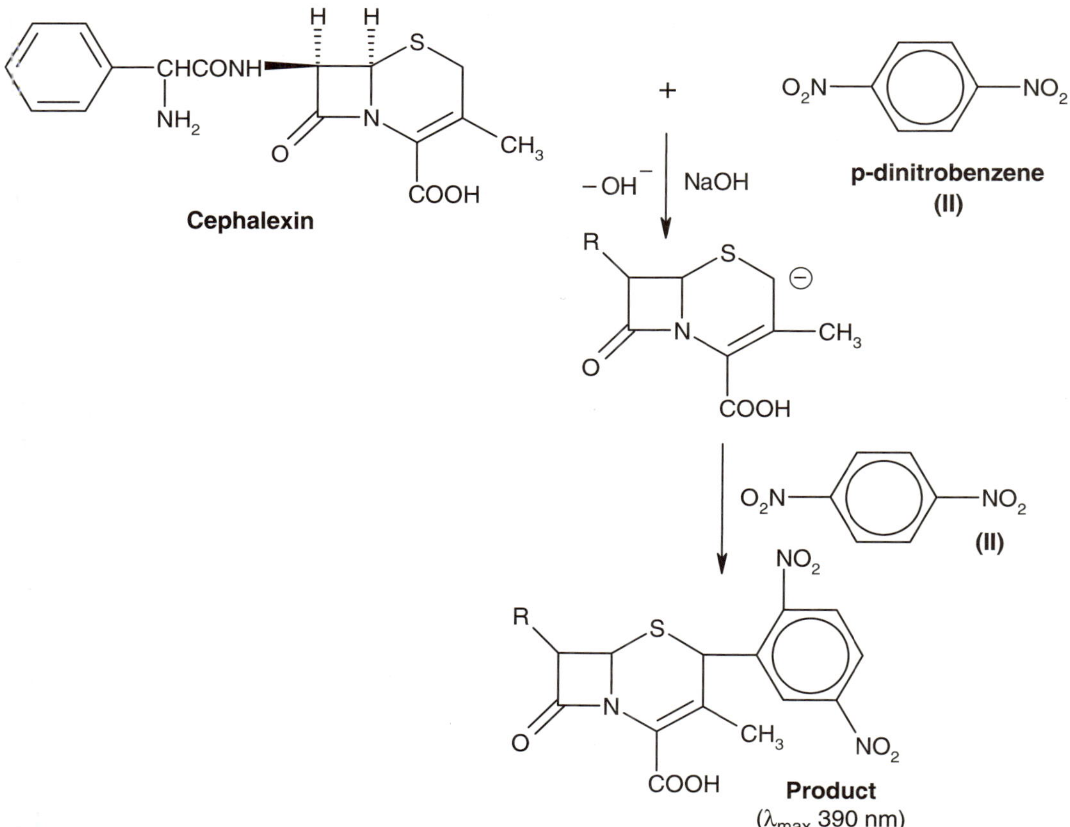

Reference

D.M. Shingbal & S.B. Bangle, *Indian Drugs*, **24(7)**, 367-368, 1987.

A spectrophotometric method based on reaction of cephalosporins with 2-nitrophenyl hydrazine in the presence of dicyclohexylcarbodiimide (DCC) and pyridine has been reported by Korany et al. (1989). The reaction mechanism as proposed by the authors is as follows: The method involves determination of carboxylic (–COOH) moiety of the molecule based on DDC coupled reaction of 2-nitrophenylhydrazine HCl (2-NPH HCl) and carboxylic (–COOH) group in non-aqueous mixed solvent.

Probable Reaction Mechanism

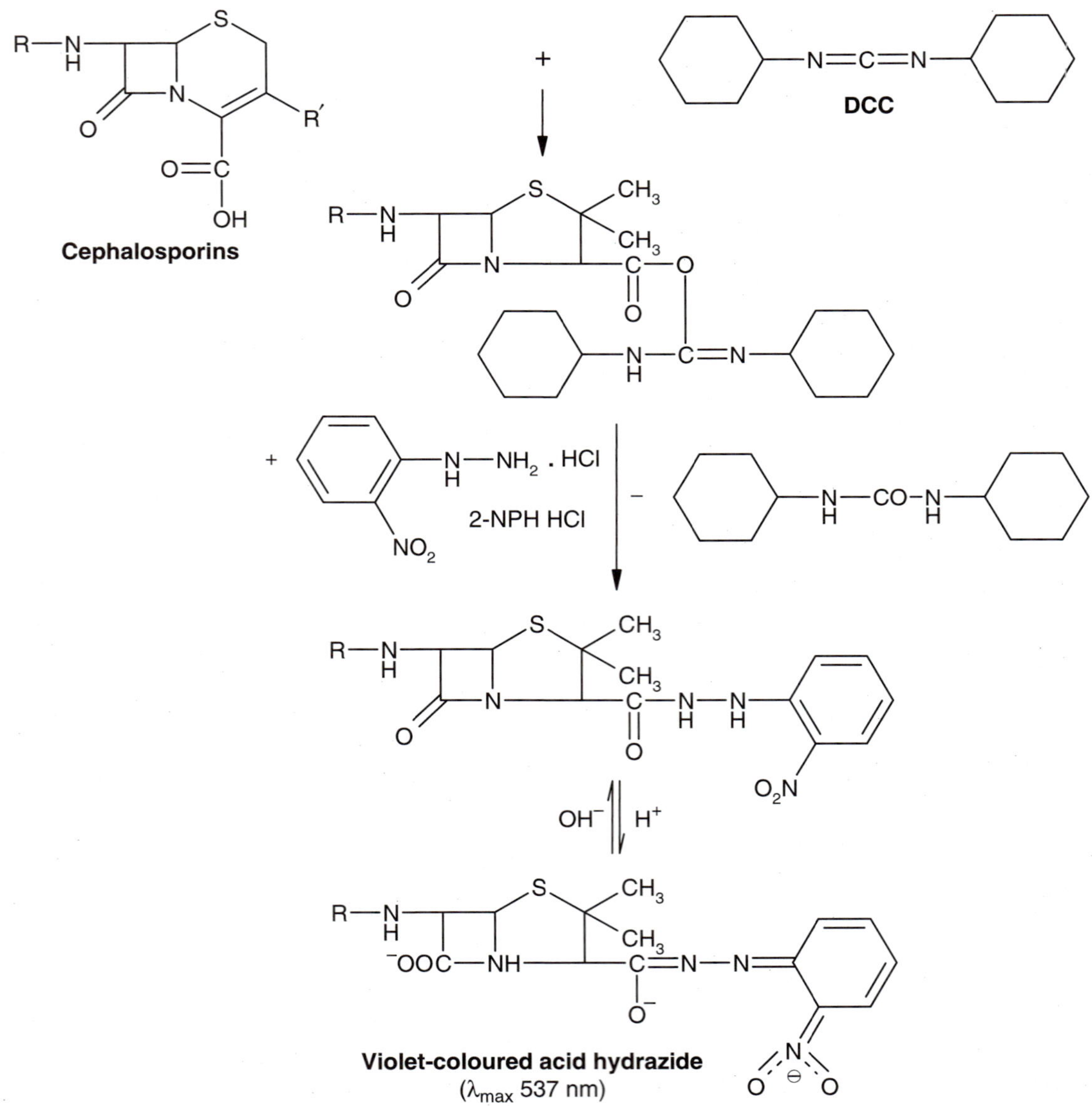

Reference

Mohamed A. Korany, Mohamed H. Abdel-Hay, Mona M. Bedair & Azza A. Gazy, *Talanta*, **36(12)**, 1253-1257, 1989.

Note

Different cephalosporins analysed were cephalexin, cefotaxine, cefazolin and cefoperazone.

Another spectrophotometric method was reported by Sengün and Fedai (1986) for the determination of cephalosporins. After heating the drug with sodium hydroxide, it was reacted with Ellman's reagent in pH 7.2 phosphate buffer to give yellow-coloured product (λ_{max} 410 nm). Various cephalosporins analysed were cephalexin, cephacetrile, ceftizoxime and cephalothin. Ellman's reagent reacts with free thiol group liberated as a result of alkaline hydrolysis. The reaction proposed by the authors is as follows: Based on the work of Fogg et al. that sulphide is the alkaline degradation product of cephalosporins, determination with Ellman's reagent is based on cleavage of the S-S band of the reagent by another thiol component producing the yellow anion of 5-thio-2-nitrobenzoic acid.

Probable Reaction Mechanism

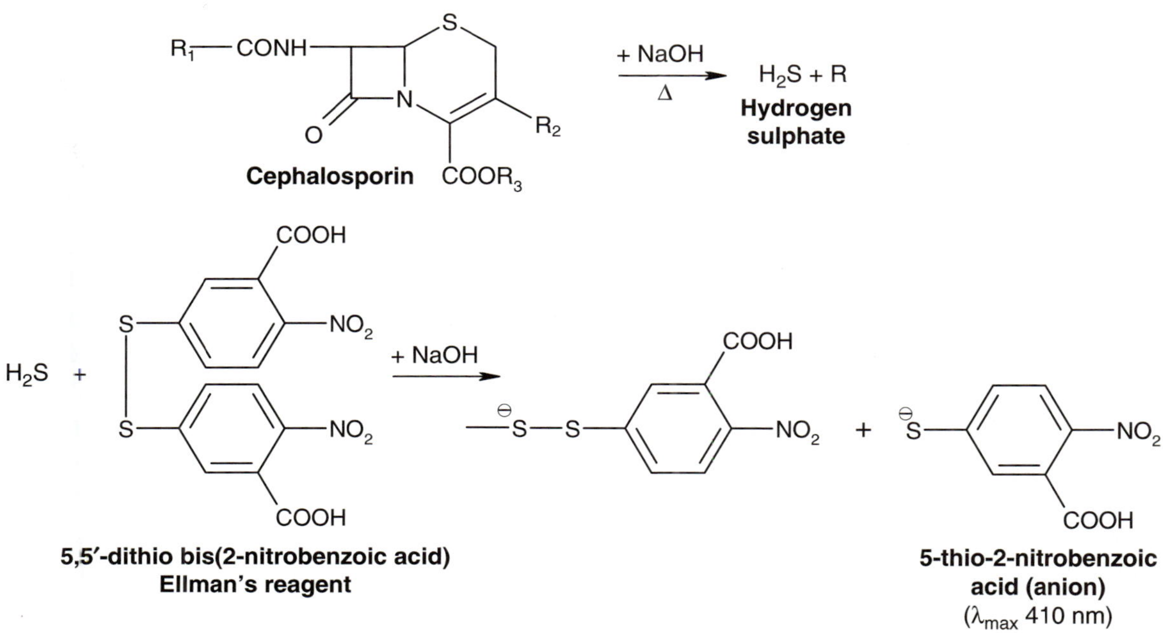

Reference

1. F. Inci Sengün & Inci Fedai, *Talanta*, **33(4)**, 366-369, 1986.
2. A.G. Fogg, N.M. Fayad & R.N. Goyal, *J. Pharm. Pharmacol.*, **32**, 302, 1980.

Formulation 13

Piperazine and its salts (Hexahydrate, Adipate and Citrate)

METHOD 1

Reagents

1. Phosphate buffer, pH 5.7.
2. Bromothymol blue solution: 10^4 M solution in phosphate buffer of pH 5.7. The dye solution is shaken with chloroform and chloroform layer, which may be coloured, is rejected.
3. Chloroform.

Standard solution

0.4 mg/ml of piperazine in water.

Sample solution

The sample is appropriately diluted with water to get a concentration of 0.4 mg/ml of piperazine hexahydrate.

Procedure

To 10 ml of the sample and standard solutions, add 10 ml of the dye solution, mix and add 15 ml of chloroform and shake vigorously for one min. Separate chloroform layer and measure the extinction of both the solutions at 420 nm against reagent blank prepared by substituting water for piperazine solution. The method obeys Beer's law in the concentration range of 100 to 400 mcg/ml of piperazine hexahydrate.

Piperazine being basic in nature may cause the ring opening in bromothymol blue resulting in coloured complex.

Probable Reaction Mechanism

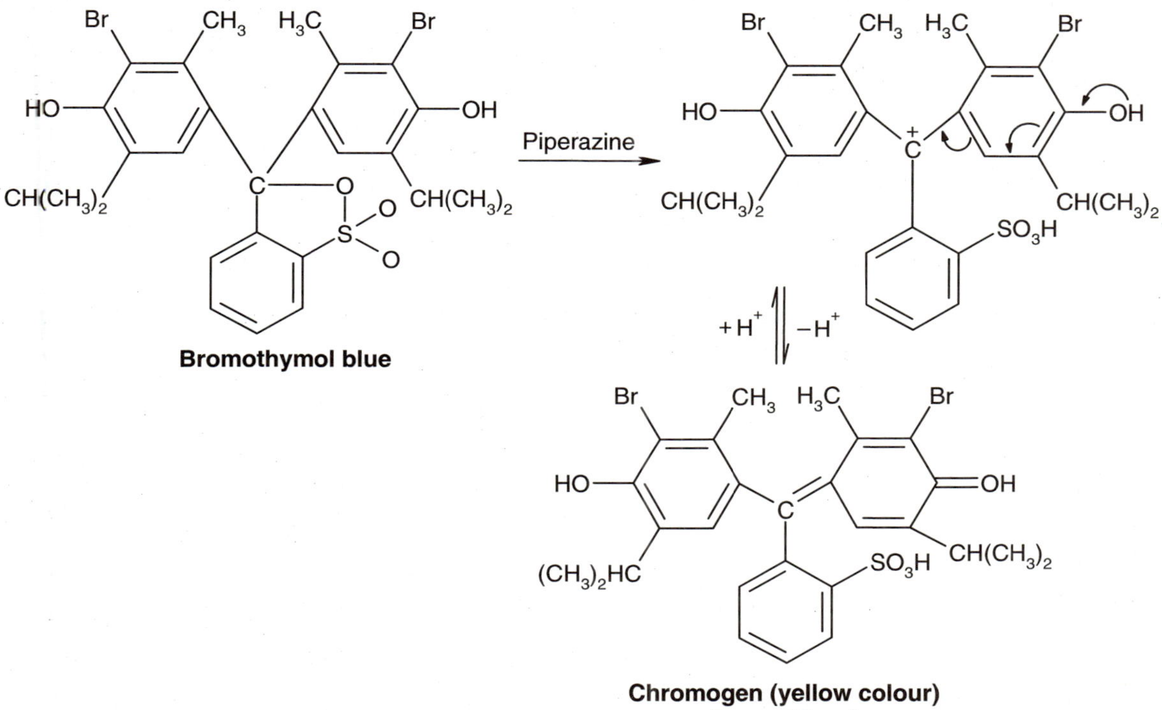

(λ_{max} 410 nm)

METHOD 2

The method is based on spectrophotometric measurement of N-nitroso derivative formed by interaction of piperazine with nitrous acid.

Reagents

1. 1% w/v solution of sodium nitrite in water.
2. 5% w/v solution of ammonium sulphamate in water.
3. Ethyl alcohol.
4. Britton-Robinson buffer, pH 2.3.
5. 4 N hydrochloric acid.

Standard solution

100 mcg/ml of piperazine or its equivalent of citrate, adipate or phosphate salts.

Sample solution

Accurately weigh or measure composite sample (syrup, tablets, granules) equivalent to about 50 mg of piperazine (base), add 30 ml of water, shake thoroughly (in case of effervescent granules, wait until effervescence ceases; stir for 1 h in case of tablets) and dilute to 500 ml with water.

Procedure

To 5 ml of the standard and sample solutions, add 1 ml of buffer solution and 0.5 ml of sodium nitrite solution. Heat at 80°C for 15 minutes on water-bath and cool. Add 1 ml of 4 N hydrochloric acid, 1 ml of ammonium sulphamate solution and 5 ml of ethyl alcohol. Shake and dilute to 100 ml with water and measure the extinction at 239 nm against blank prepared by substituting water for the sample. The method obeys Beer's law in the concentration range of 1-15 mcg/ml of piperazine.

Explanatory Note

Piperazine has two secondary amino groups. Nitrous acid formed can generate nitrosonium ion i.e. $N^+{=}{=}O$ which is deficient in electron. This nitrosonium ion will attack the secondary amino group of piperazine forming N-nitroso derivative. Ammonium sulphamate is used to destroy excess nitrous acid.

Probable Reaction Mechanism

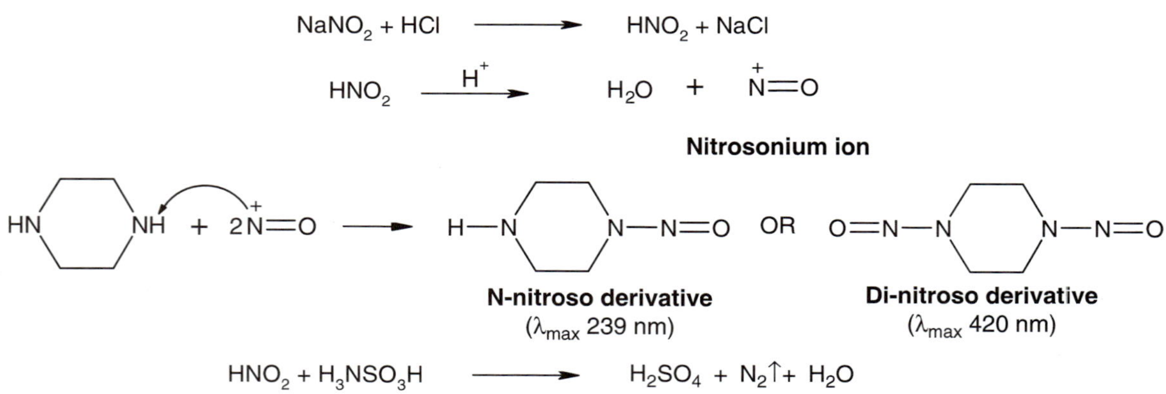

Reference

Abdel M. Abou-Ouf, Mohamed I. Walash, Mohamd S. Rizk. *J. AOAC*, **62(5)**, 1138-39, 1979.

METHOD 3

Reagents

1. Saturated solution of ammonium reineckate in water, prepare fresh on the day of use.
2. Wash solution - dilute 2 ml of saturated solution of ammonium reineckate to 1000 ml with water.
3. Hydrochloric acid.
4. Acetone.

Standard solution

1 mg/ml of piperazine hexahydrate or its equivalent of citrate, phosphate or adipate in water.

Sample solution

Accurately weigh or measure quantity of the sample equivalent to about 100 mg of the compound, add 50-60 ml water, shake and filter. Make up the volume to 1000 ml with water (1 mg/ml).

Procedure

To 20 ml of the standard and sample solutions, add 3 ml of hydrochloric acid and 25 ml of saturated solution of ammonium reineckate. Mix and allow to stand for 15 min. Filter the precipitates through G_4 sintered glass funnel. Wash the precipitates with 4 ml of wash solution. Transfer the precipitates into 50 ml volumetric flask with the help of acetone and adjust the volume with acetone. Measure the absorbance at 525 nm using acetone as blank.

Note

Piperazine is precipitated as reineckate. The precipitates are freely soluble in acetone and the resulting coloured solution is measured spectrophotometrically.

METHOD 4

Reagents

1. 4% w/v solution of 2,6-dichloroquinone chlorimide in isopropyl alcohol (Gibbs' reagent).
2. Isopropyl alcohol.
3. Hydrochloric acid.

Standard solution

3 mg/ml of piperazine or its corresponding salt in water. Dilute 5 ml of this solution to 100 ml with water. Dilute further 5 ml of the solution to 100 ml with water (7.5 mcg/ml).

Sample solution

(a) Tablets or granules: Accurately weigh a quantity of crushed tablets equivalent to about 0.3 g of the piperazine. Add 20 ml of water and shake for 1 h. Filter, wash the residue with five 15 ml portions of water and dilute the combined filtrate to 100 ml. Further dilute the solution with water to get a concentration of 7.5 mcg/ml.

(b) Syrups: Dilute with water as described under standard solution (7.5 mcg/ml).

Procedure

To 5 ml of the sample and standard solutions, add 1 ml of chlorimide reagent. Heat gently on water-bath for 30 minutes, cool to room temperature and add 1 ml of hydrochloric acid. Adjust the volume to 25 ml with water and measure the extinction at 525 nm against reagent blank. The method obeys Beer's law in the concentration range of 5-50 mcg/ml.

Explanatory Note

Piperazine reacts with Gibbs' reagent to give a complex (λ_{max} 525 nm).

Probable Reaction Mechanism

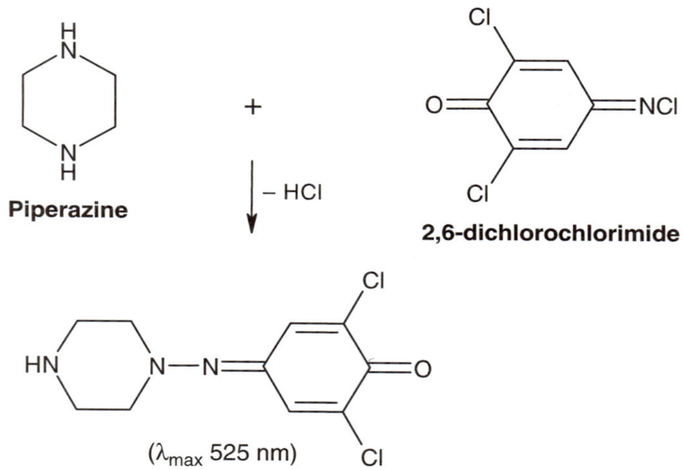

Reference

Tulsidas R. Baggi & Surinder N. Mahajan, *J. AOAC*, **57(5)**, 1144-1146, 1974.

METHOD 5

Reagents

1. 1% w/v solution of trinitrophenol (picric acid) in water.
2. 10% sulphuric acid: 5 ml of concentrated sulphuric acid is diluted to 100 ml with water.
3. Piperazine dipicrate wash solution: To 200 mg of piperazine in a beaker add 10 ml 1 N sulphuric acid, 20 ml of water, mix and add 100 ml of trinitrophenol solution. Allow to stand for two hours and filter through a medium porosity (G_2) sintered glass crucible. Wash the precipitates with water until the filtrate is free of sulphate. Transfer the residue to a 2 litre bottle, add 2 litres of water and shake for two hours. Filter this solution and use as wash liquid as described in the procedure.

Procedure

Transfer 5 ml of homogeneous suspension of the sample to a 50 ml volumetric flask rinsing the pipette with water into the flask, add water to volume, mix and filter.

To 5 ml of the sample filtrate in a beaker, add 10 ml of 10% sulphuric acid, 15 ml water, mix and add 100 ml of trinitrophenol solution. Allow to stand for two hours and filter through a pre-tared medium porosity (G_2) sintered glass crucible, washing the beaker and crucible with five 20 ml portions of piperazine dipicrate wash solution. Dry the residue at 105°C for 2 hours, cool and weigh.

Anhydrous piperazine (mg) = mg of the residue × 0.1582 × dilution factor.

Working example

Each 5 ml of the sample is labelled to contain 750 mg of piperazine citrate.
Quantity of the sample taken for analysis = 2 ml.
Weight of the precipitates obtained (as dipicrate) = 0.659 g
Each g of the precipitate (dipicrate) is equal to 0.357 g of piperazine hexahydrate.
Contents of piperazine hexahydrate/5 ml of the sample

$$= \frac{0.659 \times 0.357 \times 5}{2} = 0.5878 \text{ g}$$

0.5874 g of piperazine hexahydrate = 0.734 g of piperazine citrate. OR 100 mg of piperazine hexahydrate = 125 mg of piperazine citrate.

$$\text{Contents of piperazine citrate} = \frac{0.659}{2} \times \frac{0.357}{1} \times \frac{5}{1} \times \frac{125}{100} = 734 \text{ mg}$$

Claim = 750 mg.

METHOD 6

Reagents

1. 2 mg/ml solution of tetrachloro-o-benzoquinone in chloroform.
2. 10% w/v solution of sodium hydroxide in water.

Standard solution

0.25 mg/ml of piperazine in chloroform.

Sample solution

Piperazine salts such as hexahydrate, phosphate, adipate or citrate, equivalent to 25 mg of piperazine (base) are quantitatively brought into solution with the aid of 20-30 ml of water. To each sample, add 10 ml of sodium hydroxide solution and extract with three 30 ml portions of chloroform. The combined organic extract is made up to 100 ml with chloroform.

Procedure

To 2 ml of sample and standard solutions, add 1 ml of benzoquinone reagent, mix and dilute to 10 ml with chloroform. After 3 minutes, measure the absorbance of both the solutions at maximum at about 590 nm using reagent blank. The method obeys Beer's law in the concentration range of 5-30 mcg/ml and the coloured complex is stable for 24 hrs.

Explanatory Note

It is a charge transfer complex between piperazine and tetrachloro-o-benzoquinone.

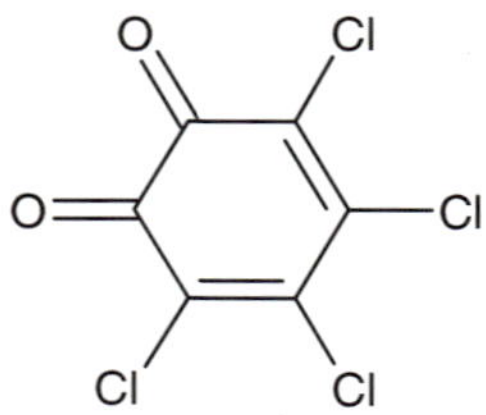

Tetrachloro-o-benzoquinone
(2)

or

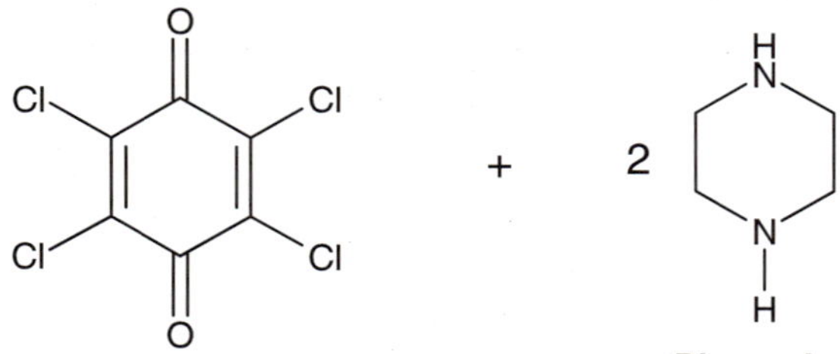

Tetrachloro-p-benzoquinone
(3)

Piperazine
(1)

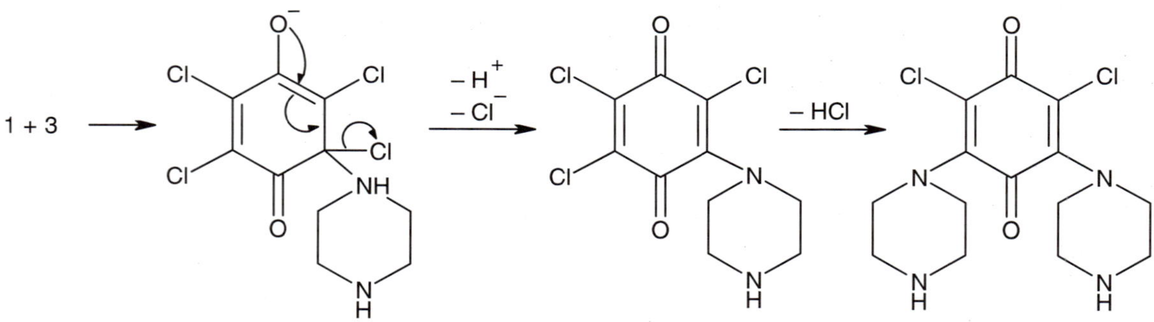

(λ_{max} 380 nm)

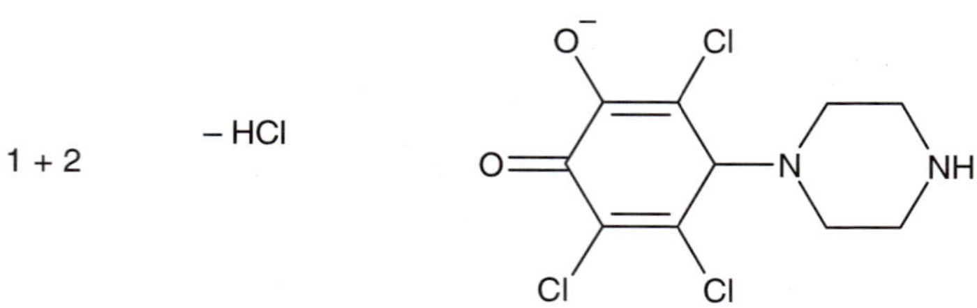

(λ_{max} 590 nm)

Reference

U. Muralikrishna, N. Someswara Rao & M. Krishnamurthy, *Ind. J. Pharm. Sci.*, **45(1)**, 28-29, 1983; *Analyst*, **109**, 1278-1279, 1984; and Abdel-Aziz M. Wahbi, Mohammad Abdu Nassif & El-Rasheed A. Gad Karim, *Analyst*, **109**, 1513-1514, 1984.

Note

The drug can form charge complex with 2,3-dichloro-5,6-dicyanobenzoquinone (DDQ), the reaction being similar to tetrachlorobenzoquinone.

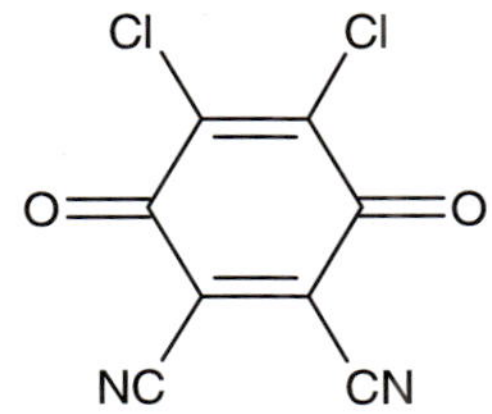

DDQ reagent

Reference

E.M. Abdel Gawad et al., *J. Pharm. & Biomed. Analysis*, **15(11)**, 1679, 1997.

It was earlier reported that condensation takes place between amine and benzoquinone at position 2 or 2 & 5 but the work of above authors have confirmed that the ratio of the reagent to piperazine to be 4 : 1 which can be explained to oxidation-reduction reaction as shown below. This reaction was possible at room temperature.

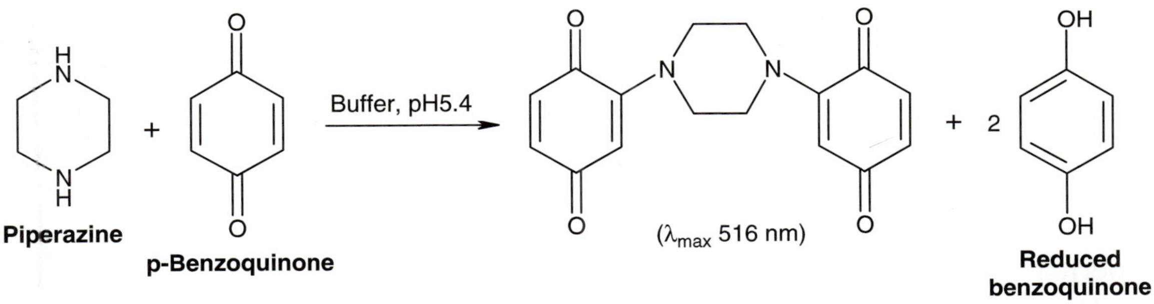

Reference

1. Abdel-Aziz et al., *Talanta*, **33(2)**, 179-181, 1986.
2. M. Senthilraja, *Ind. J. Pharm. Sci.*, **68(6)**, 643-644, 2006.

METHOD 7

Two secondary amino groups of piperazine condense with acetaldehyde to form N,N-divinylpiperazine which interacts with 'DDQ' to give coloured substituted quinone.

Reagents

1. 10% w/v solution of acetaldehyde in dioxane.
2. 0.5% w/v solution of dichlorodicyanobenzoquinone (DDQ) in dioxane.

Standard solution

100 mcg/ml of piperazine in dioxane or dichloromethane.

Sample solution

Dilute or extract appropriate aliquot of the sample with dioxane or dichloromethane to get 100 mcg/ml concentration.

Procedure

To 1 ml of sample and standard solutions, add 0.1 ml of acetaldehyde solution and 0.1 ml of benzoquinone reagent. Heat for 3 minutes in water-bath maintained at 70°C, cool to room temperature and dilute to 100 ml with dioxane or dichloromethane. Measure the absorbance of both the solutions at about 570 nm (dioxane) or 600 nm (dichloromethane) using reagent blank prepared with 1 ml of the solvent. The method obeys Beer's law in the concentration range of 1-12 mcg/ml.

Note

1. The method is insensitive for primary and ternary amines.
2. The coloured product exhibits two maxima; at 330 and 570 nm in dioxane and at 330 and 600 nm in dichloromethane.
3. The developed chromogen is stable at least for 1 hr.
4. Methanol, ethanol, acetone, n-butanol, benzene, dioxane, dichloromethane, isopropanol have been examined as solvents for dilution, but dioxane and dichloromethane have been found to be best as they yield highest absorption values and most stable coloured complex.

Explanatory Note

Piperazine, a secondary amine, reacts with acetaldehyde to form vinylamine, which being strong nucleophilic moiety displaces chloro group from the reagent to give coloured complex (λ_{max} 570 nm).

Probable Reaction Mechanism

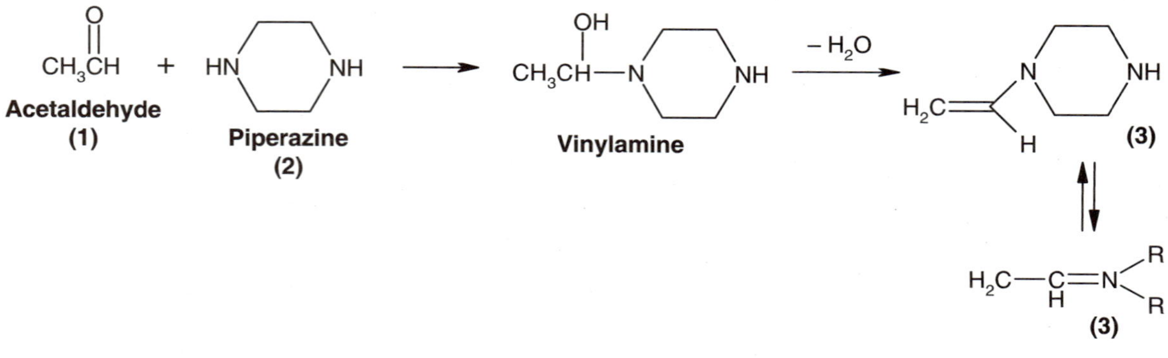

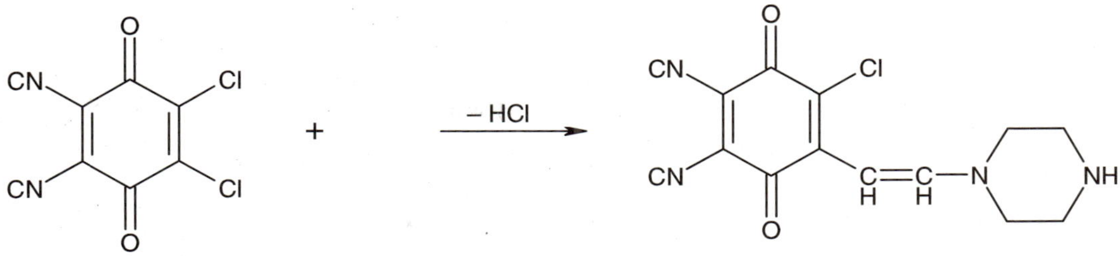

Dichloro-dicyanobenzoquinone (DDQ)

(λ_{max} 570 nm)

2,3-dichloro-1,4-naphthoquinone (dichlone) also gives similar reaction carried out in DMSO, the final product being.

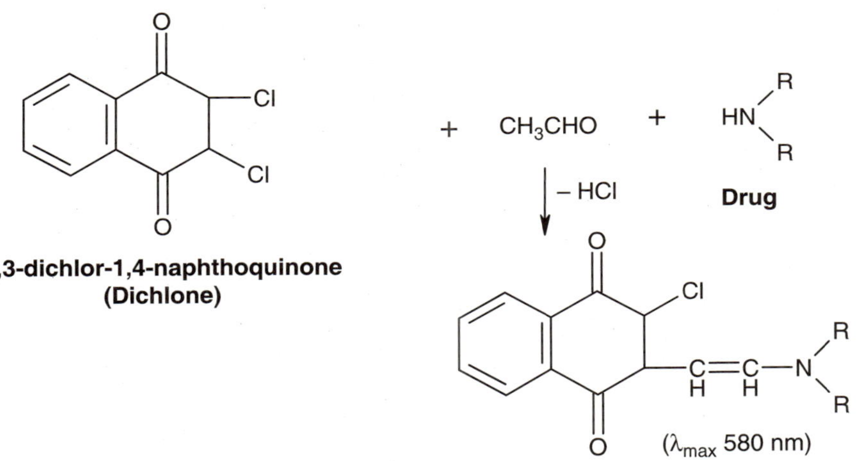

2,3-dichlor-1,4-naphthoquinone (Dichlone)

(λ_{max} 580 nm)

Reference

Y.M. Dessouky & S.A. Ismail, *Analyst*, **99**, 482, 1979.

METHOD 8

Reagents

1. Ninhydrin reagent in 2-methoxyethanol.
2. Isopropanol.

Sample and standard solutions

20 μg/ml of piperazine in water.

Procedure

To 5 ml each of sample and standard solutions, add 5 ml of 2-methoxyethanol and 4 ml of ninhydrin reagent. Heat in boiling water-bath for 45 min, cool, dilute to 25 ml with methoxyethanol and measure the absorbance of sample and standard solutions at 570 nm against reagent blank.

Probable Reaction Mechanism

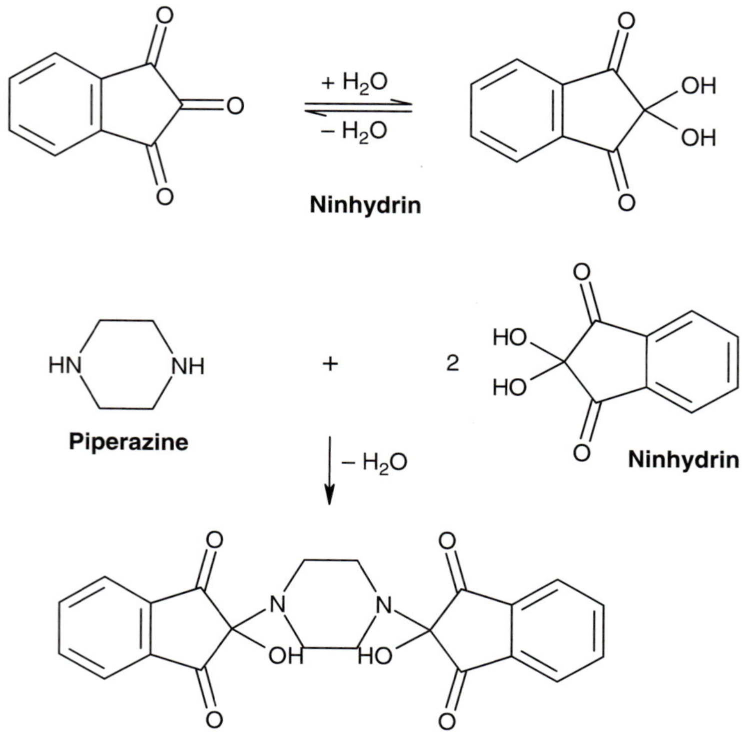

The product
(λ_{max} 570 nm)

Reference

1. Pharmaceutical Chemistry (Vol. 2) by H.J. Roth, p. 124.
2. G. Rama Rao, S.S.N. Murthy & R.K. Raju, *Indian Drugs*, **24(12)**, 558-560, 1987.

Formulation 14

Piperazine, Pyrvinium pamoate

ESTIMATION

Pyrvinium pamoate

Standard solution

Weigh accurately about 57 mg of pyrvinium pamoate and transfer quantitatively into 50 ml volumetric flask. Dissolve in and dilute to volume with dimethylformamide. Pipette 1 ml of this solution into 100 ml volumetric flask and dilute to volume with the same solvent. Use low actinic glassware in preparing solutions of pyrvinium pamoate.

Sample solution

Transfer a volume of homogeneous sample suspension equivalent to 57 mg of pyrvinium pamoate into a 100 ml volumetric flask. Wash the pipette with two 3 ml portions of water, followed by three 20 ml portions of dimethylformamide into the flask to ensure complete transfer of the contents. Mix the contents and heat on a water-bath until all of the pyrvinium pamoate is dissolved (it takes about 30 minutes). Cool to about 25°C, add dimethylformamide to volume and mix. Centrifuge a portion of this mixture and dilute 3 ml of the clear supernatant liquid to 100 ml with dimethylformamide, mix.

Concomitantly measure the absorbance of the sample and standard solutions against dimethylformamide as blank at about 508 nm.

Note

1. Complete the procedure without prolonged interruption.
2. Since the compound is orange-red in colour, spectrophotometric method is based on measurement of absorption of the solution of the compound in DMF.

Calculations

$$\text{Pyrvinium base (mg) per ml} = \frac{A_u}{A_s} \times \frac{0.6644}{1} \times \frac{S}{V} \times d_f$$

where A_u = absorbance of the sample solution;
A_s = absorbance of the standard solution;
V = volume of the sample taken for analysis;
S = weight of the standard taken for analysis;
d_f = dilution factor.

0.6644 is the factor for the conversion of anhydrous pyrvinium pamoate (575.71) to the formula weight of pyrvinium base (382.53) ratio.

$$\frac{382.53}{575.71} = 0.6644$$

Piperazine

Follow method 5 as described under formulation 13 of this chapter.

Formulation 15

Mebendazole

ESTIMATION

Mebendazole

METHOD 1

Reagents

1. 1% w/v solution of hydroxylamine hydrochloride in water.
2. 2% dicyclohexylcarbodiimide (DCC).
3. 5% w/v solution of ferric chloride hexahydrate in water.
4. Formic acid (90%).
5. Isopropanol.
6. Absolute alcohol.

Standard solution

To 100 mg of mebendazole, accurately weighed, add 3 ml of formic acid and dilute to 100 ml with isopropyl alcohol. 1 ml of this solution is further diluted to 100 ml with isopropanol (10 mcg/ml).

Sample solution

Weigh a quantity of powdered tablets equivalent to 100 mg of the compound and process as under standard solution.

Procedure

Take 2 ml of standard and sample solutions in two separate 25 ml volumetric flasks, add 2 ml of isopropanol, 1 ml of hydroxylamine hydrochloride solution and 2 ml of dicyclohexylcarbodiimide reagent. Heat at 70°C for 20 minutes, cool, add 2 ml of ferric chloride solution and make up the volume with alcohol. Measure the absorbance of both the solutions at about 495 nm against reagent blank.

Explanatory Note

The drug and DCC form activated acid derivative which reacts with hydroxylamine to form hydroxamic acid. Hydroxamic acid forms red chelate with Fe(3) ions.

Probable Reaction Mechanism

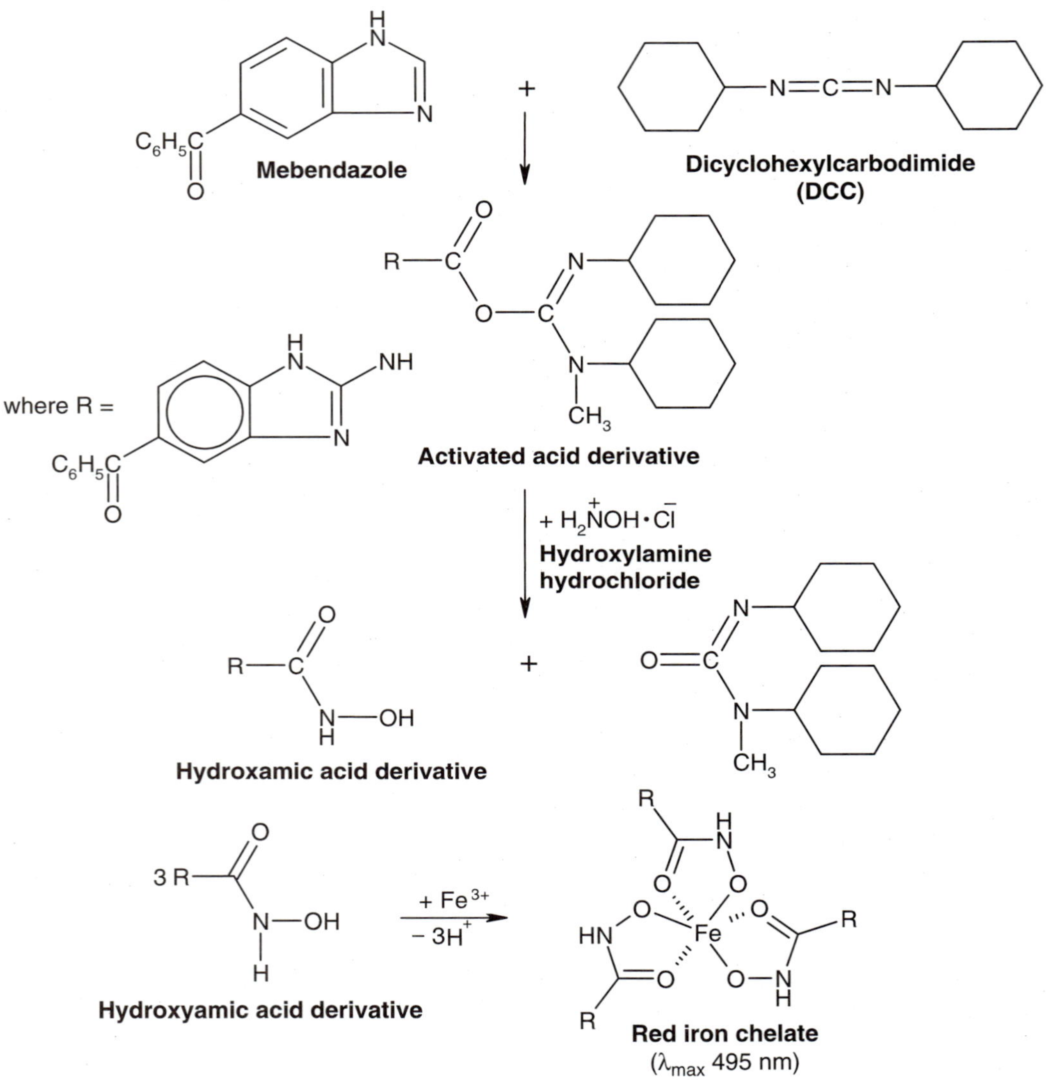

METHOD 2

This involves alkaline hydrolysis of the compound to 2-amino-5-benzyol benzimidazole and measurement of the resultant yellow colour at 420 nm.

Reagents

1. Formic acid (90%).
2. Formic acid-isopropyl alcohol mixture (1 : 9 v/v).
3. Methanol.
4. 30% w/v solution of potassium hydroxide in water.

Standard solution

To 25 mg of mebendazole, accurately weighed, add 2.5 ml of formic acid, shake to dissolve and make up the volume to 25 ml with isopropyl alcohol (1 mg/ml).

Sample solution

Weigh accurately a quantity of powdered tablets equivalent to 50 mg of the compound. Add 40 ml of formic acid-isopropanol mixture, shake for 5 minutes and filter. Wash the residue with two 5 ml portions of the mixture and adjust the volume to 50 ml with above mixture (1 mg/ml).

Procedure

Take 2 ml of standard and sample solutions. To each, add 3 ml of methanol and 3 ml of potassium hydroxide solutions. Allow to stand for 30 minutes for maximum colour to develop. The absorbance of both the solutions is measured at 420 nm against reagent blank on suitable spectrophotometer. The method obeys Beer's law in the concentration range of 25-250 mcg/ml.

Probable Reaction Mechanism

(a) In the presence of alkali, the acidic hydrogen present on the 'N' atom are removed resulting in the formation of a product as shown below.

(b) The anilide side chain is broken during alkaline hydrolysis resulting in an increase in λ_{max} (288 nm → 420 nm).

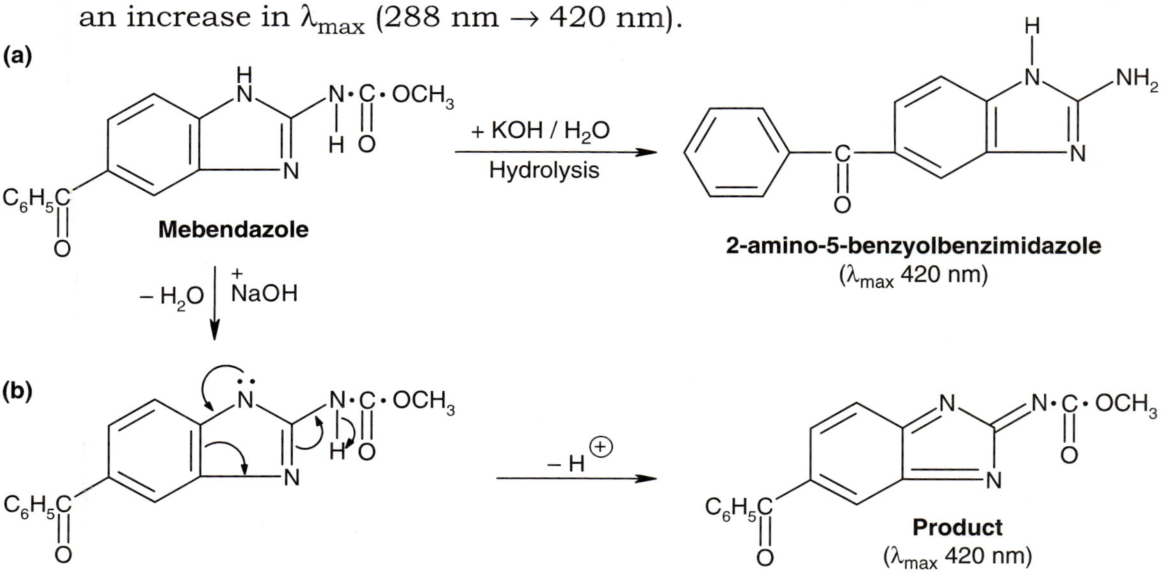

Reference

A.A. Patel, T.P. Gandhi, P.R. Patel & V.C. Patel, *Ind. J. Pharm.*, p. 76, March 1978.

METHOD 3

Standard solution

To 50 mg of pure compound, accurately weighed, add 10 ml of perchloric acid, shake and dilute to 50 ml with water (1 mg/ml). 1 ml of this solution is further diluted to 100 ml with water (10 mcg/ml).

Sample solution

Powdered tablets equivalent to 50 mg of the compound are accurately weighed and to this 10 ml of perchloric acid (70%) is added. Shake for 10 minutes and dilute to 50 ml with water. 1 ml of this solution is further diluted with water to get 10 mcg/ml of mebendazole.

Blank solution : 0.2 ml of perchloric acid and 89.8 ml of water are mixed.

Measure the extinction of sample and standard solutions at 288 nm against blank. The method obeys Beer's law in the range of 5-15 mcg/ml.

METHOD 4

When dissolved in appropriate solvent, mebendazole exhibits either basic or acidic properties.

(a) **Basic equivalent:** Accurately weigh a quantity of sample equivalent to about 250 mg of mebendazole and dissolve in 125 ml of glacial acetic acid. Warm, cool, filter, wash the residue in the flask and filter with two 10 ml portions of glacial acetic acid. Titrate the combined filtrate with N/10 perchloric acid using crystal violet solution as indicator. Each ml of N/10 perchloric acid is equivalent to 29.52 mg of mebendazole.

(b) **Acid equivalent**

Reagents

1. 0.1% w/v solution of thymol blue in ethyl alcohol.
2. Neutral dimethylformamide: Add 10 drops of thymol blue solution to 50 ml of dimethylformamide and neutralize to blue end point with 0.02 N sodium methoxide.

Procedure

Accurately weigh powdered tablets equivalent to 50 mg of mebendazole, dissolve in neutralized dimethylformamide and titrate with 0.02 N sodium methoxide to a green end point. Each ml of 0.02 N sodium methoxide corresponds to 5.906 mg of mebendazole.

A method based on nitration of benzene ring has been described by Sanghavi et al. (1980) giving coloured nitroso derivative.

$$H_2SO_4 + KNO_3 \longrightarrow KSO_4^- + H_2NO_3$$

$$H_2NO_3 \xrightarrow{-H_2O} O{-}\overset{+}{N}{-}O$$

Nitronium ion

Sulphuric acid protonates nitrate to give H_2NO_3 which loses water (H_2O) to give nitronium ion ($\overset{+}{N}O_2$). Further H_2SO_4 helps in the reaction by taking up water molecule. Nitronium ion so formed attacks the benzene ring to form coloured derivative which forms the basis of spectrophotometric method of analysis.

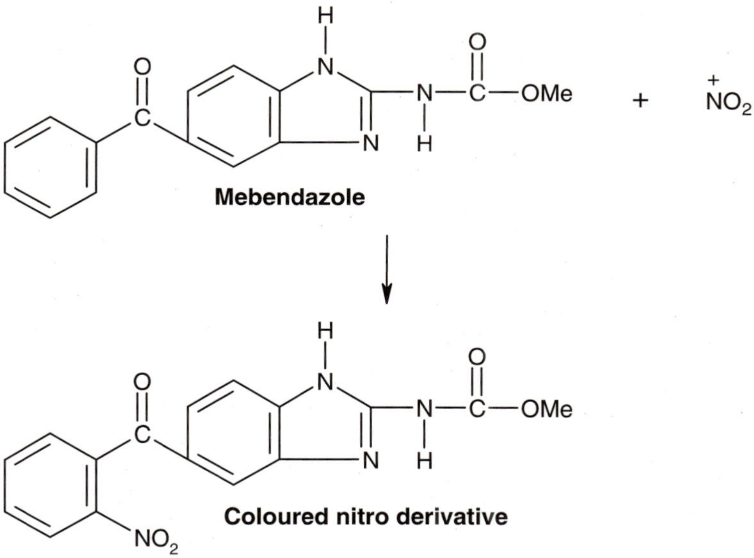

Reference

N.M. Sanghavi & Varsha Tane, *Indian Drugs*, **30(3)**, 136-137, 1980.

Formulation 16

Mebendazole, Levamisole hydrochloride

ESTIMATION

Mebendazole

METHOD 1

Standard solution

To an accurately weighed about 50 mg of the substance, add 10 ml of formic acid, keep in boiling water-bath for few minutes. Add 70 ml of isopropyl alcohol, cool to room temperature and make up the volume (100 ml). Dilute further appropriately with isopropyl alcohol to get 10 mcg/ml.

Sample solution

Weigh powdered sample accurately equivalent to 50 mg of the substance. Add 10 ml of formic acid and keep in boiling water-bath and make up to 100 ml with isopropyl alcohol. Shake well and centrifuge at moderate speed to get clear solution. The resultant clear solution is further diluted appropriately with isopropyl alcohol to get 10 mcg/ml. Measure the extinction of both sample and standard solutions at maximum at about 310 nm using isopropyl alcohol as blank. Calculate the results by comparison.

METHOD 2

The residue obtained during dry extraction of levamisole under method 2, is taken up in glacial acetic acid for non-aqueous titration using crystal violet as indicator. Each ml of 0.1 N perchloric acid is equivalent to 0.02953 g of mebendazole.

Levamisole hydrochloride

METHOD 1

Reagents

1. 6% w/v solution of sodium hydroxide in water.

2. 5% w/v solution of sodium nitroprusside in water.
3. 2% w/v boric acid in water.

Standard solution

250 mcg/ml of levamisole hydrochloride in water.

Sample solution

Transfer accurately weighed powdered sample equivalent to 50 mg of levamisole to a 200 ml volumetric flask. Add about 150 ml of water, shake well and make up the volume. Centrifuge and use the clear supernatant solution for estimation (250 mcg/ml).

Procedure

To 1 ml each of sample and standard solutions, add 0.5 ml of sodium hydroxide solution and 1 ml of nitroprusside solution, followed by 5 ml of boric acid solution. Shake well and allow to stand for 2 minutes, dilute to 10 ml with water. The absorption of resultant purple coloured solution is measured at about 540 nm against reagent blank. Calculate the results by comparison. Each g of levamisole hydrochloride is equivalent to 0.8486 g of levamisole (base).

Probable Reaction Mechanism

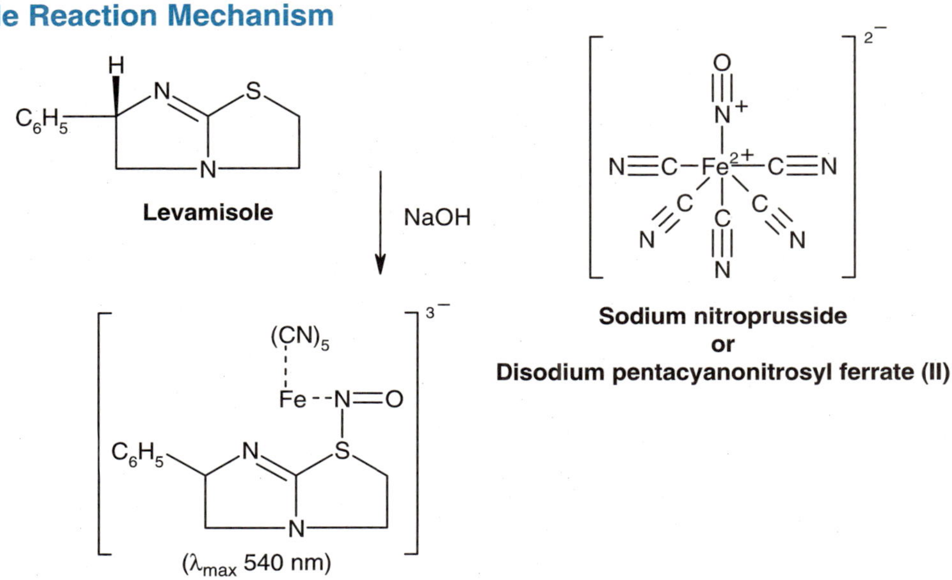

DL-form is called tetramisole.

In alkaline medium, nitrosyl cation of the reagent (sodium nitropruside) is reduced giving a complex with λ_{max} 540 nm.

Its reactivity is based on the positive nitrosyl group ($N^{+}\equiv O$) reacting with nucleophilic species mostly in alkaline medium. Nucleophilic agents are primary and secondary aliphatic amines, amino acids, anilins, indols, ketones, phenols, quinones, sulphite and thiols (in case of thiols, it interacts with 'S' group of the drug.

Reference

1. R.T. Sane, S.V. Sawant, V.J. Joshi & J.G. Mhalal, *Indian Drugs*, **20(11)**, 460-461, 1983.
2. D.M. Shingbal & S.V. Joshi, *Indian Drugs*, **21(9)**, 396-397, 1984.

Note

(a) The drug is reported to form ion-pair complex with several dyes (bromothymol blue, bromophenol blue, bromocresol purple, bromocresol green – all λ_{max} 420 nm, all complexes extractable into chloroform.
(b) Solochrome Dark blue, Solochrome Black-T – λ_{max} 520 nm.

Reference

R.T. Sane, D.S. Sapre & V.G. Nayak, *Talanta*, **32(2)**, 148-149, 1985.

METHOD 2

Weigh accurately powdered sample equivalent to 100 mg of levamisole. Extract the dry powder with four 25 ml portions of chloroform (retain the residue for estimation of mebendazole). Pass the organic layer through anhydrous sodium sulphate. Evaporate to about 50 ml, add glacial acetic acid. Carry out non-aqueous titration using brilliant green solution as indicator. Each ml of 0.1 N perchloric acid is equivalent to 0.02408 g of levamisole.

Formulation 17

Diethylcarbamazine citrate, Chlorpheniramine maleate

ESTIMATION

Diethylcarbamazine citrate

Reagent

20% w/v sodium hydroxide solution in water.

Procedure

Take the powdered sample equivalent to about 30 mg of diethylcarbamazine citrate in a 250 ml separating funnel. Add 75 ml of water and 5 ml of sodium hydroxide solution and extract with three 25 ml portions of chloroform. Dry combined chloroform layer by passing through anhydrous sodium sulphate and titrate with 0.1 N perchloric acid using thymol blue as indicator. Each ml of 0.1 N perchloric acid is equivalent to 0.03914 g of diethylcarbamazine citrate.

Explanatory Note

On addition of sodium hydroxide, free base is librated which is extracted into chloroform which can be subjected to non-aqueous titration.

Alternatively, the chloroform layer is evaporated, residue taken up in methanol and then heated with MAA reagent (10% malonic acid in acetic anhydride) for 30 min and diluted with ethanol.

Probable Reaction Mechanism

It is based on catalysed condensation of mixed anhydride of organic acid and ternary amine which acts as basic catalyst.

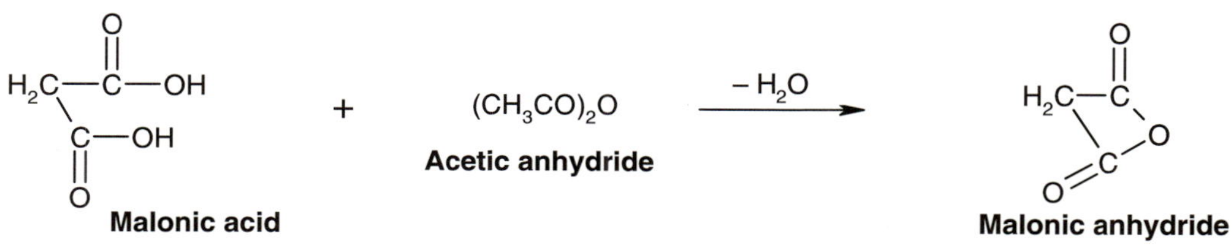

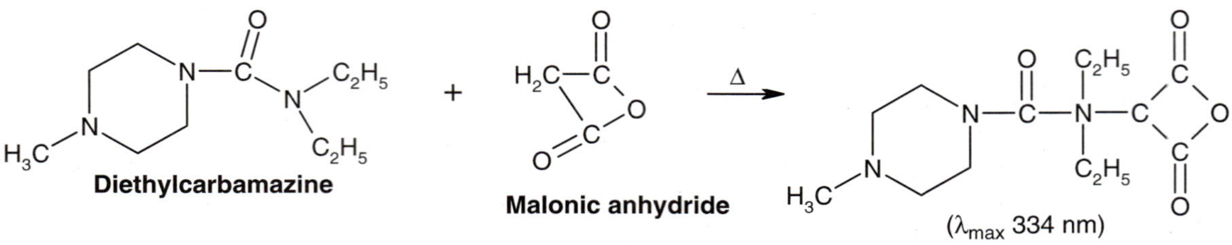

Note

1. For colour development, the amine must be soluble in 'MAA' reagent; insoluble amines do not catalyse the condensation reaction.
2. The final condensation product has fluorescent property which can be exploited for analytical purpose.

Reference

M.V. Bulbule, A.V. Kasture & S.G. Wadodkar, *Indian Drugs*, **19(1)**, 27-28, 1981.

Chlorpheniramine maleate

Procedure

Take the sample equivalent to about 10 mg of chlorpheniramine maleate, add solution of sodium hydroxide (50% w/v) to produce pH of about 11.0. Transfer the mixture to a 500 ml separator with the aid of three 10 ml portions of saturated solution of sodium chloride and extract with two 50 ml portions of n-hexane. Shake gently to avoid formation of emulsion. Wash the combined organic extract with 2×10 ml of water. Wash the aqueous layer with 2×20 ml of n-hexane and discard the aqueous layer. Pass the combined hexane layer through cotton and evaporate to dryness. To the residue, add 5 ml of acetic anhydride and 25 ml of glacial acetic acid and allow to stand for 15 minutes. Add 2 drops of indicator and titrate with 0.01 N perchloric acid. Each ml of 0.01 N perchloric acid is equivalent to 0.001945 g of chlorpheniramine maleate.

Alternatively, follow the cyanogen bromide method. For method and reaction mechanism refer to Formulation 1 under chapter on rubefacients. This is based on König's reaction (W.J. König. *J. Prakt. Chem.*, 70, 19, 1904).

Formulation 18

Sulphadoxine, Pyrimethamine

ESTIMATION

Sulphadoxine

METHOD 1

Reagents

1. 0.5 N hydrochloric acid.
2. 0.1% w/v solution of sodium nitrite in water.
3. 0.5% w/v solution of ammonium sulphamate in water.
4. 0.1% w/v solution of N-1-naphthyl-ethylenediamine dihydrochloride in water.
5. Dilute ammonia solution.

Standard solution

Weigh accurately 80 mg of standard Sulphadoxine, add 10 ml of dilute ammonia, shake and dilute to 100 ml with water. Dilute further appropriately with water to produce a concentration of 40 mcg/ml.

Sample solution

Weigh accurately a quantity of powdered tablets equivalent to 80 mg of sulphadoxine, add 10 ml of dilute ammonia solution, shake and make upto 100 ml with water. Filter, reject first few ml of the filtrate and dilute the filtrate appropriately with water to get 40 mcg/ml.

Procedure

To 5 ml of the sample and standard solutions taken in 2 separate volumetric flasks, add 5 ml of 0.5 N hydrochloric acid and 5 ml of sodium nitrite solution. Allow to stand for 3 minutes, then, add 5 ml of ammonium sulphamate solution, wait for 1 minute, add 5 ml of n-naphthyl ethylenediamine solution and dilute with water to 100 ml. Measure the absorbance of both the solutions at 545 nm against reagent blank. Deduce the results by comparison. For detailed reaction mechanism, see under general reactions for sulphonamides.

METHOD 2

Weigh accurately a quantity of powdered tablets equivalent to 500 mg of sulphadoxine, add 50 ml of hydrochloric acid (1 : 1 v/v), cool to 0°C and titrate with 0.1 N sodium nitrite solution, previously cooled to 0°C, using starch-iodine paste as external indicator. Each ml of 0.1 N sodium nitrite is equivalent to 28.02 mg of sulphadoxine.

Pyrimethamine

METHOD 1

The method is based on direct UV spectrophotometric measurement of chloroform solution of the compound at about 272 nm.

Standard solution

10 mcg/ml of pure pyrimethamine in chloroform.

Sample solution

Weigh accurately 25 mg of pure pyrimethamine, add 50-60 ml 0.1 N hydrochloric acid, warm to dissolve, cool and dilute to 100 ml with the same solvent. 5 ml of the resulting solution is further diluted to 100 ml with 0.1 N hydrochloric acid (12.5 mcg/ml).

Measure the extinction of both the solutions at maximum at 272 nm using chloroform as blank. Calculate the results by comparison.

METHOD 2

Standard solution

Weigh accurately 25 mg of pure Pyrimethamine, add 50-60 ml 0.1 N hydrochloric acid, warm to dissolve, cool and dilute to 100 ml with the same solvent. 5 ml of the resulting solution is further diluted to 100 ml with 0.1 N hydrochloric acid (12.5 mcg/ml).

Sample solution

Weigh accurately powdered tablets equivalent to 25 mg of pyrimethamine, add 20 ml of dilute ammonia solution and shake. Extract with five 30 ml portions of chloroform, wash total chloroform layer with 20 ml of dilute ammonia solution. Filter organic layer through anhydrous sodium sulphate supported on cotton plug. Dry organic layer to dryness on water bath and take up the residue in 0.1 N hydrochloric acid. Dilute further with 0.1 N hydrochloric acid to get a concentration of 12.5 mcg/ml.

Both the solutions show absorption maximum at about 272 nm in 0.1 N hydrochloric acid. Calculate the results by comparison.

METHOD 3

This method is based on the complex formation with the dyes.

Reagents

1. 0.04% w/v solution, each of bromophenol blue (BPB), picric acid (PA), bromocresol purple (BCP), bromothymol blue (BTB), methyl orange (MO) in distilled water.
2. Buffer solution : Phthalate buffer of pH 2 to 4.5
3. Potassium chloride-hydrochloric buffer of pH-1 in water.

Standard solution

200 mcg/ml of pure pyrimethamine in ethyl alcohol.

Sample solution

Accurately weighed powdered tablets equivalent to 20 mg of pyrimethamine is extracted with ethyl alcohol to produce 100 ml (200 mcg/ml).

Procedure

To 0.5 ml of sample and standard solutions, add 5 ml of buffer solution, 5 ml of dye solution, shake to mix. Extract the coloured complex with 10 ml of chloroform by vigorous shaking. Absorbance values of both the chloroform solutions are measured at respective maxima as shown below :

Reagent (Dye)	Maximum (nm)	pH	Beer's law range (mcg/ml)
BPB	420	2.5	1-9
BCP	420	3.5	1-9
BTB	415	3.8	1-12
MO	420	4.5	1-12
PA	415	1.0	4-24

It has been observed that reagents 'BPB', 'BCP' are more sensitive in the determination of pyrimethamine.

Reference

R.T. Sane & A.Y. Dhamankar, *Indian Drugs*, **19(2)**, 80-82, 1981.

The compound can be diazotized and coupled with orcinal at ortho position to phenolic-OH in alkaline medium to give coloured complex.

Probable Reaction Mechanism

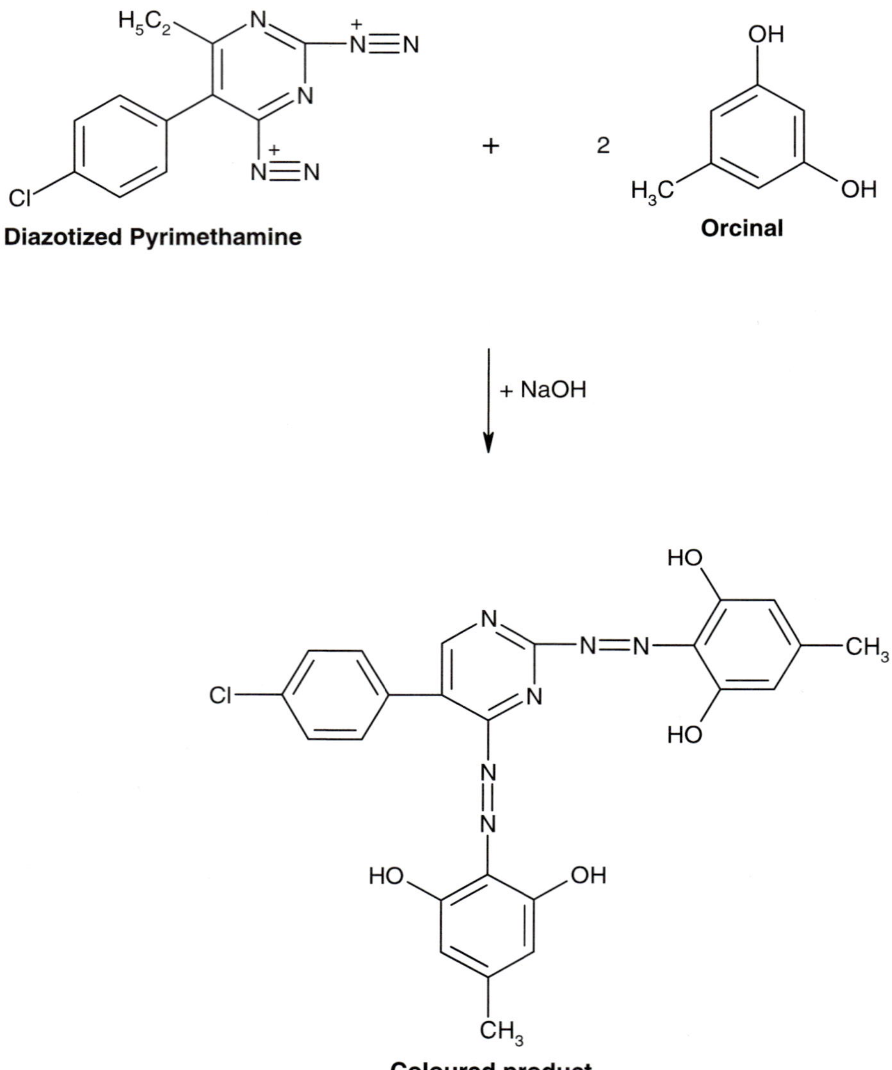

Coloured product
(λ_{max} 455 nm)

Reference

S.S. Zarapkar, *Indian Drugs*, **26(12)**, 721, 1989.

Primary aromatic amine group of the compound undergoes Michael addition with 1,2-naphthoquinone-4-sulphonic acid with elimination of HSO_3 and giving a yellow-coloured quinoimine.

Probable Reaction Mechanism

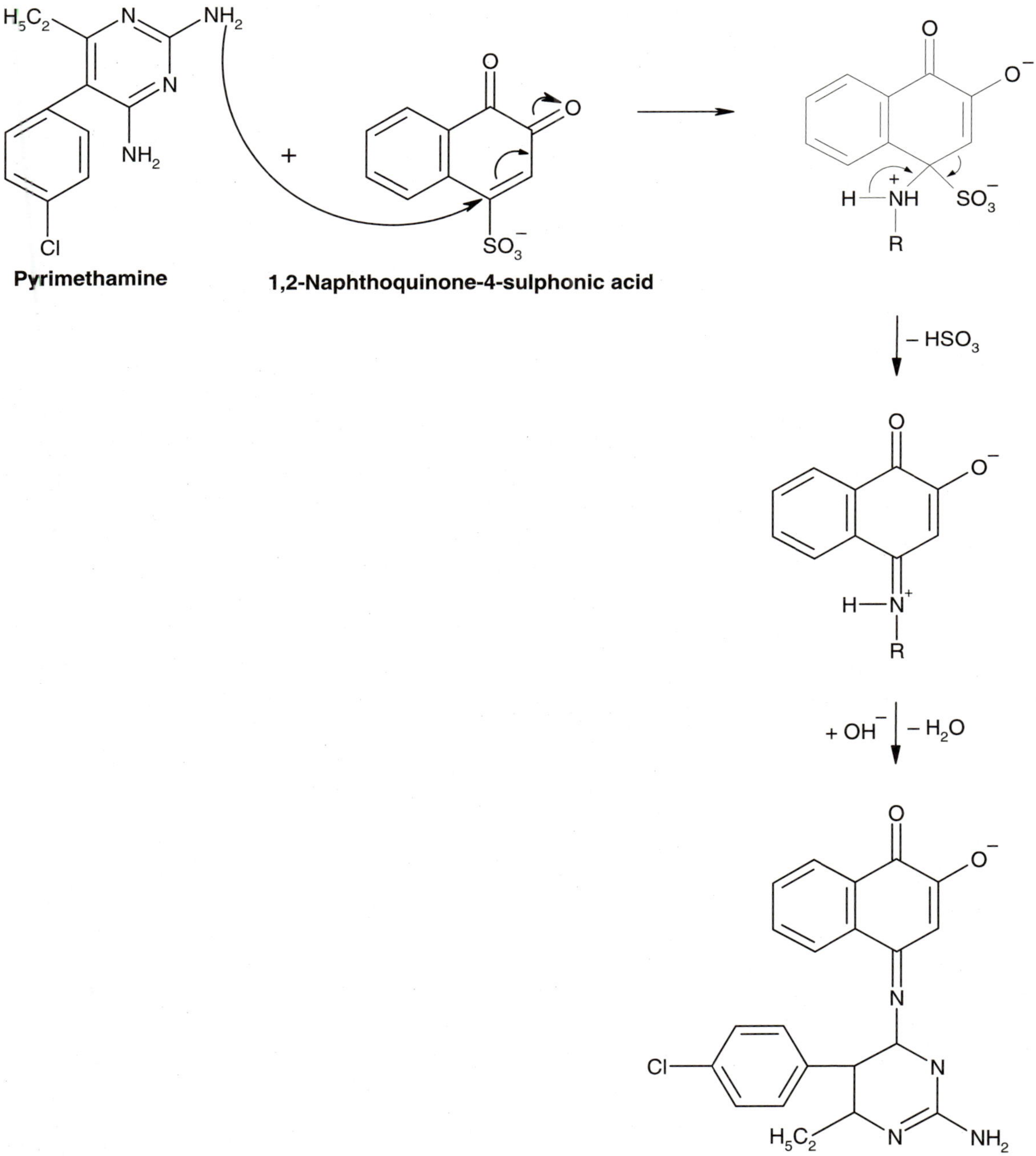

Coloured addition product
(λ_{max} 415 nm)

The primary amine group of the molecule can add to p-chloranil resulting in the formation of Michael addition with loss of HCl.

Probable Reaction Mechanism

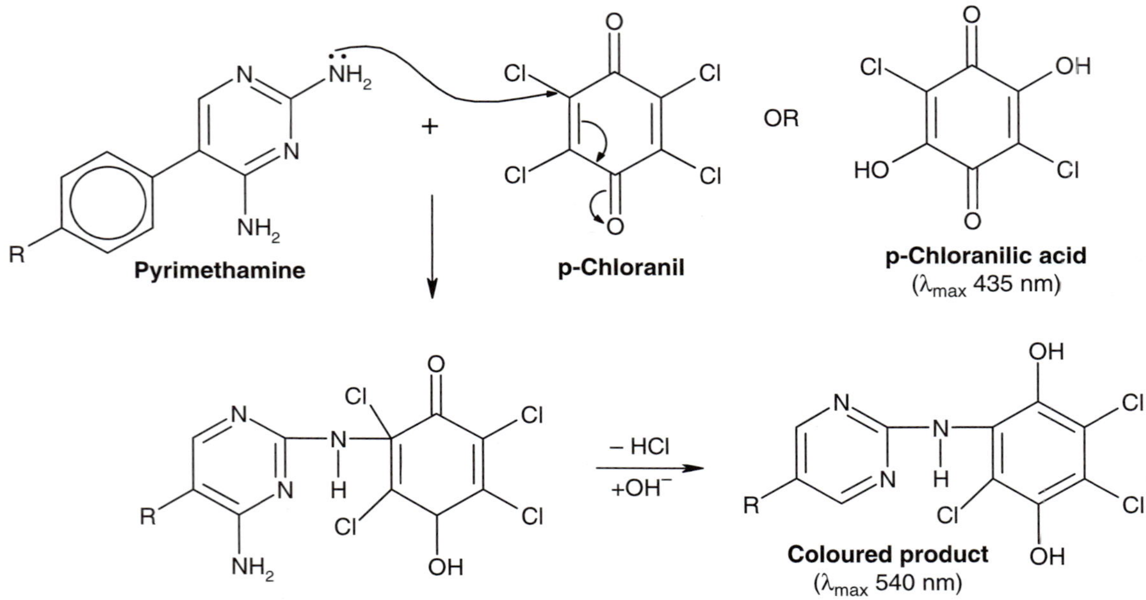

p-Chloranilic acid in undissociated form (H_2A^-) has λ_{max} 435 nm, but in alkaline medium it has violet colour (HA^-) i.e. ion-pair salt obtained dissociates to give purple HA anion (λ_{max} 540 nm).

$$H_2A \rightleftharpoons H^+ + HA^- \text{ (Violet)}$$

$$B + H^+ \rightleftharpoons BH^+ \text{ (Colourless)}$$

Reference

J. Emmanuel & E. Silva Dias, *Indian Drugs*, **24(7)**, 371-372, 1987.

Note

p-Chloranilic acid has been reported as chromogenic reagent for the estimation of several antimalarial drugs such as quinine sulphate, primaquine, amodiaquine, pyrimethamine and trimethoprim based on above reaction mechanism.

Reference

M.S. Mahrous, M. Abdel Salem, A.S. Issa & M. Abdel-Hamid, *Talanta*, **33(2)**, 185-186, 1986.

Formulation 19

Primaquine phosphate

METHOD 1

Reagents

1. 0.2% w/v solution of 2,6-dichloroquinone chlorimide in isopropyl alcohol (Gibbs reagent).
2. 0.4% w/v solution of 1,2-Naphthoquinone-4-sulphonic acid (sodium salt).
3. 0.5 M sodium acetate.

Method-1 (a)

Primaquine phosphate reacts with chlorimide reagent to give an emerald-green coloured complex with maxima at 7000 nm. The above complex formation is affected by pH of the medium. In acidic medium, red colour is formed which fades rapidly, whereas in alkaline medium, a blue colour is produced which also fades rapidly. However, if the medium is buffered to pH between 3.5 and 10.5, the intensity of the colour does not vary. Maximum intensity obtained after 5 minutes, is stable for more than 3 h. Heating does not affect the colour intensity. The coloured complex is soluble in chloroform with no change in maxima, but absorbance is slightly decreased.

Standard solution

100 mcg/ml primaquine phosphate in water.

Sample solution

Accurately weighed quantity of the sample equivalent to 10 mg of primaquine phosphate is shaken with water to effect dissolution, then dilute to make 100 ml (100 mcg/ml).

Procedure

To 2 ml of the sample and standard solutions, add 1 ml of chlorimide reagent and dilute to 25 ml with isopropyl alcohol. Allow to stand at room temperature for 10 min., and measure the absorbance of both the solutions at 700 nm against reagent blank, prepared by using 2 ml of water instead of sample.

Calculate the results by comparison. The method obeys Beer's law in the range of 2-20 mcg/ml of primaquine phosphate.

Explanatory Note

The reagent 2,6-dichloroquinone chlorimide attacks at C-4 of the quinoline ring resulting in the formation of complex (λ_{max} 700 nm).

Probable Reaction Mechanism

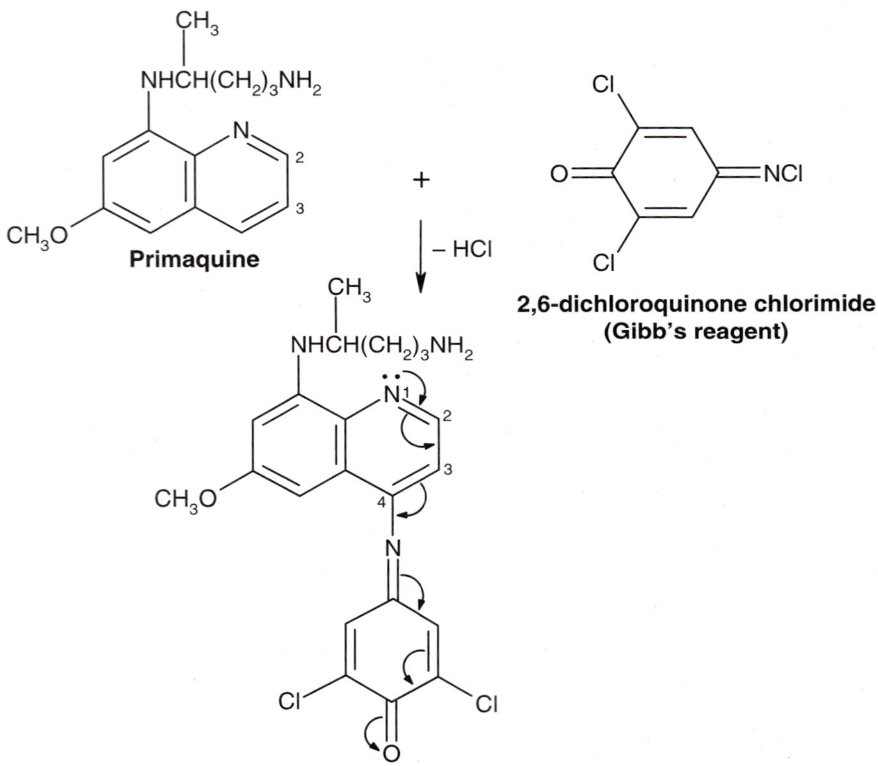

Coloured complex
(λ_{max} 700 nm)

Method-1 (b)

Naphthoquinone reagent reacts with primary amines to give coloured complex.

Standard solution

250 mcg/ml of primaquine phosphate in water.

Sample solution

250 mcg/ml of primaquine phosphate in water, to be prepared as under method-1 (a).

Procedure

To 4 ml of the sample and standard solutions, add 3 ml of naphthoquinone reagent and 5 ml of sodium acetate solution. Heat on water-bath for 15 min, cool to room temperature, add 7 ml of glacial acetic acid and dilute to 25 ml with water. Measure the extinction of both the solutions at 478 nm against blank, prepared by adding reagents to 4 ml of water instead of sample. The colour is stable for more than 1 h and can not be extracted into common organic solvents. The method obeys Beer's law in the range of 10-100 mcg/ml of primaquine phosphate.

Note

1. The mean values of E 1%, 1 cm with two reagents are 590 and 110 respectively. Therefore the method with chlorimide reagent is about five times more sensitive than the method using naphthoquinone reagent.
2. Amodiaquine, chloroquine, quinine and trimethoprim cause no analytical problem in these two methods.

Explanatory Note

Primary aliphatic amine undergoes Michael addition eliminating monohydrogen sulphite radical resulting in an orange-red quinonimine.

Probable Reaction Mechanism

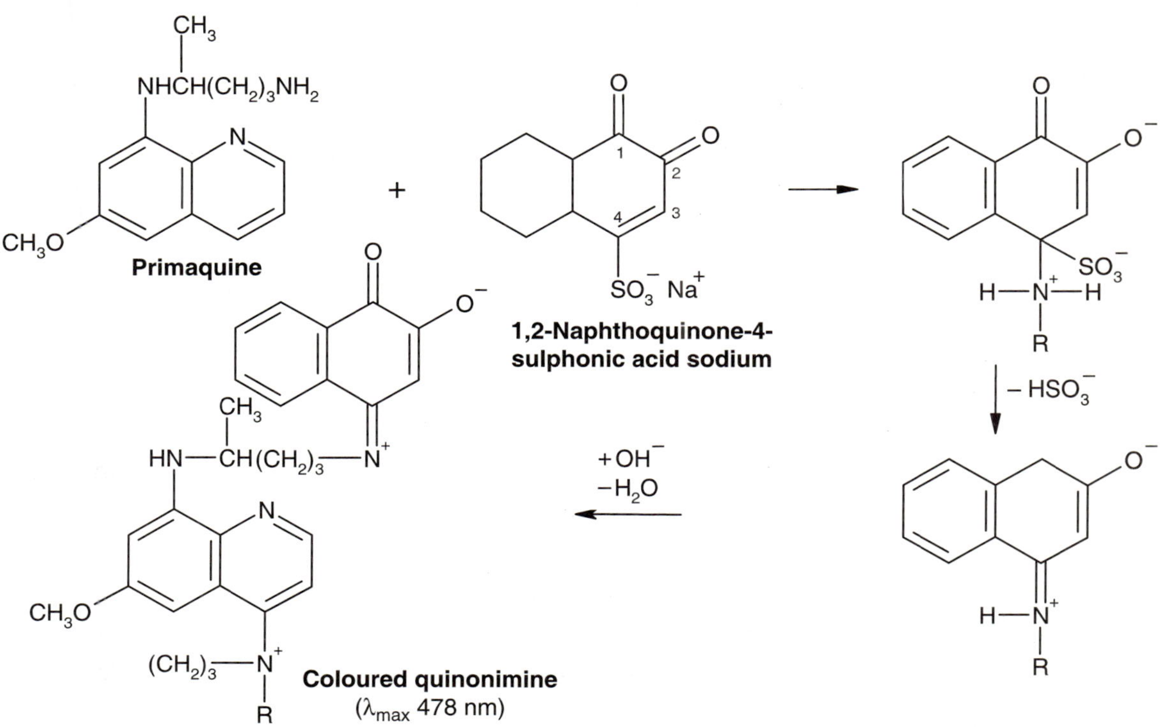

Reference

1. 1(a) & 1(b): A.A. Abou Ouf, S.M. Hassan & M.E.S. Metwally, *Analyst*, **105**, 1113-1118, 1980.
2. Pharmaceutical Chemistry (Vol. 2) by H.J. Roth, pp. 378 & 600.

METHOD 2

Reagents

1. Buffer solution, pH 3.0: Mix 6 ml of 2 M sodium hydroxide with 10 ml of 2 M citric acid and dilute to 100 ml with water.
2. Cobalt thiocyanate reagent: Dissolve 6.8 g of cobalt-(II) chloride, hexahydrate and 4.3 g of ammonium thiocyanate in 100 ml of water.

Standard solution

1 mg/ml of pure primaquine phosphate in water.

Sample solution

Weigh/measure accurately sample equivalent to 100 mg of the compound, add about 50 ml of water, shake to dissolve and dilute to 100 ml with water.

Procedure

Transfer 2 ml of aliquot of sample and standard solutions, add 3 ml of cobalt reagent and 10 ml of pH 3 buffer solution. Add 10 ml of nitrobenzene and shake for 1 min. Separate nitrobenzene layer and measure the absorbance of both the solutions at 625 nm against blank prepared by using 2 ml of water instead of sample and following above procedure. The colour is stable even for several weeks. The method obeys Beer's law in the range of 0.1-0.8 mg/ml.

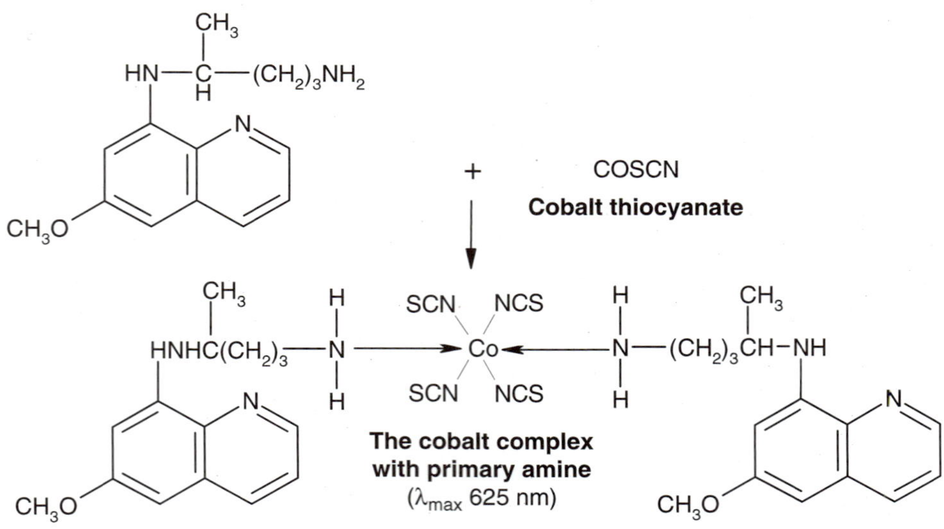

Note

1. The above procedure is also applicable for estimation of Chloroquine phosphate and Amodiaquine hydrochloride. Beer's law is obeyed in the range of 0.05 to 0.4 mg/ml.
2. Trimethoprim gives positive reaction.
3. Lactose, starch, stearate, preservatives and bacteriostatics (used in parenteral preparations) do not interfere.

The complex is extractable into nitrobenzene. The cobalt complexes with primary amine (λ_{max} 625 nm).

OR

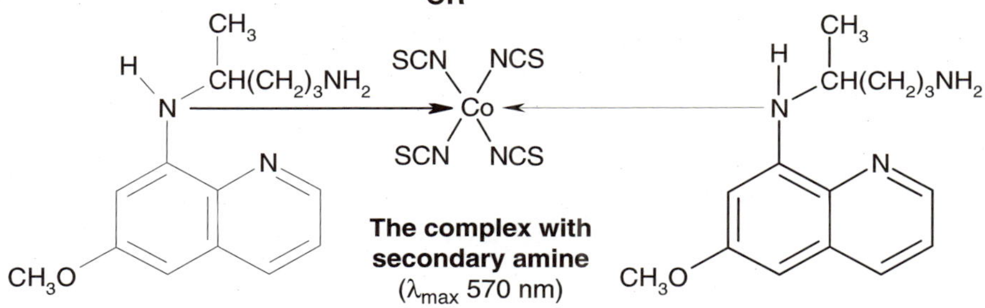

The complex with secondary amine (λ_{max} 570 nm)

METHOD 3

Reagents

1. 0.1 N sodium vanadate reagent: Weigh 12.0 g of ammonium metavanadate and 11.5 g of sodium carbonate and transfer to a 500 ml beaker containing 200 ml of water. Boil till the vapours do not give reaction of ammonia, making up the lost water by addition of water. Cool to room temperature.
2. 5 N perchloric acid

Sample and standard solution

100 mcg/ml of the compound, to be prepared as described under method-1(a).

Procedure

Pipette 2 ml of the sample and standard solutions to 10 ml volumetric flasks containing 0.3 ml of 5 N perchloric acid and 0.5 ml of sodium vanadate. Shake and dilute to 10 ml with water. Measure the extinction of both the solutions at 550 nm against reagent blank within 10 minutes. The method obeys Beer's law in the range of 2-30 mcg/ml. The colour is stable only for 10 minutes.

Probable Reaction Mechanism

This reaction is analogous to reaction based on Mandelin's test i.e. redox reaction in acidic medium using ceric ammonium sulphate as oxidizing agent. In this case, ammonium metavanadate is used as oxidizing agent. The compound is oxidized to quinolinic acid derivative and vanadyl (V) ion is transformed to vanadyl (IV) ion.

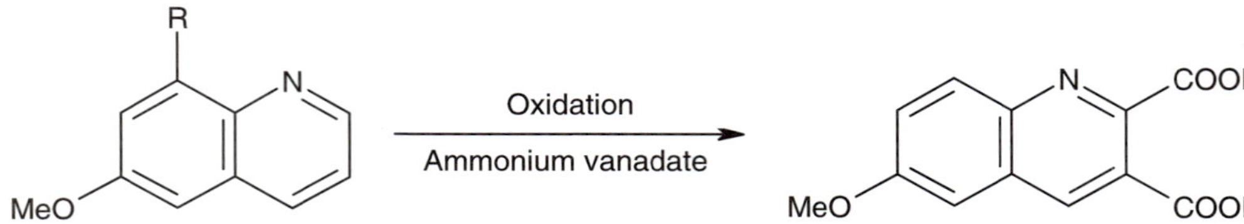

Primaquine

Quinolinic acid derivative
(λ_{max} 550 nm)

Reference

1. John Thomas, Shobha Rani & D.R. Hirematt, *Indian Drugs*, **33(6)**, 393, 1996.
2. Organic Chemistry by I.L. Finar, 6th ed., p. 859.

B.S. Sastry (1990) had suggested a method based on reaction of oxidized brucine with aliphatic amine through nucleophilic substitution.

Probable Reaction Mechanism

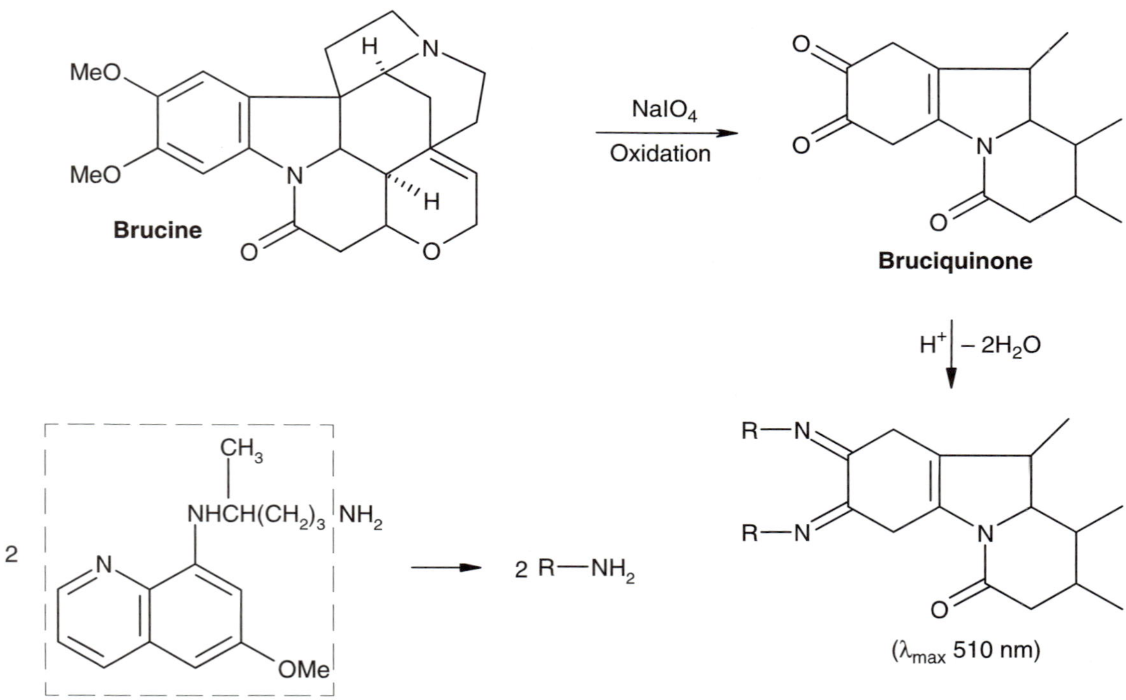

Brucine

Bruciquinone

(λ_{max} 510 nm)

Primaquine

Note

The colour was developed by heating in boiling water-bath after adding all the reagents.

Reference

B.S. Sastry et al., *Indian Drugs*, **27(4)**, 260, 1990.

G. Rama Rao (1988) had suggested a method based on reaction of amine group present in the compound with ninhydrin.

Probable Reaction Mechanism

Ninhydrin, a stable hydrate of 1,2,3-trioxidane, has a particularly reactive carbonyl group at position 2. The 2 forms shown above are found depending on the solvent and both the forms can react with the primary amine group of the drug resulting in the formation of the product. The reaction is represented as:

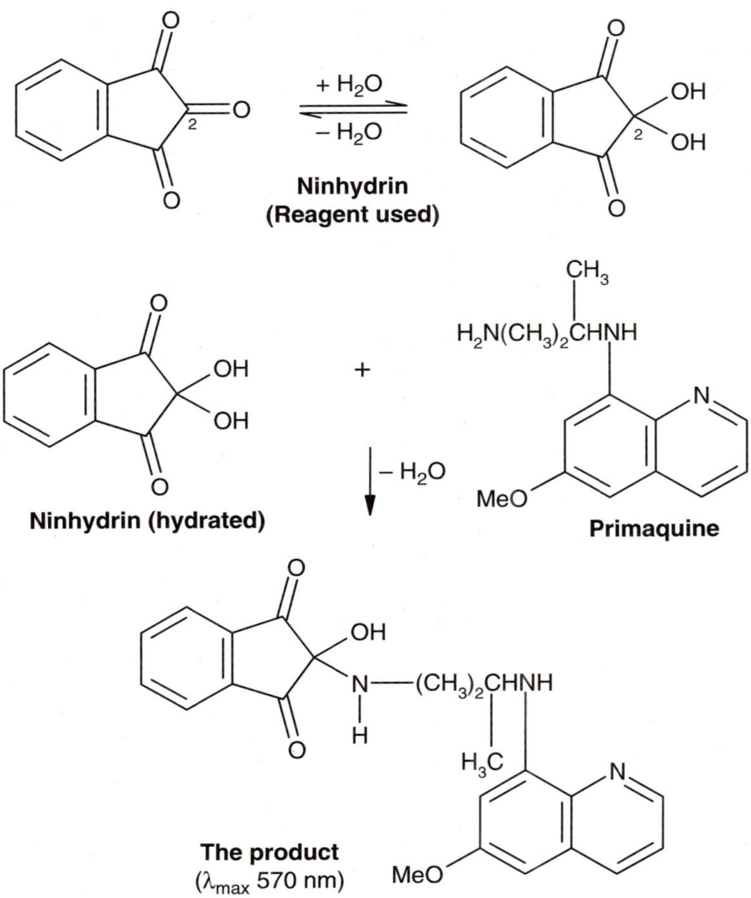

The reaction can also occur with the other form of ninhydrin as shown below.

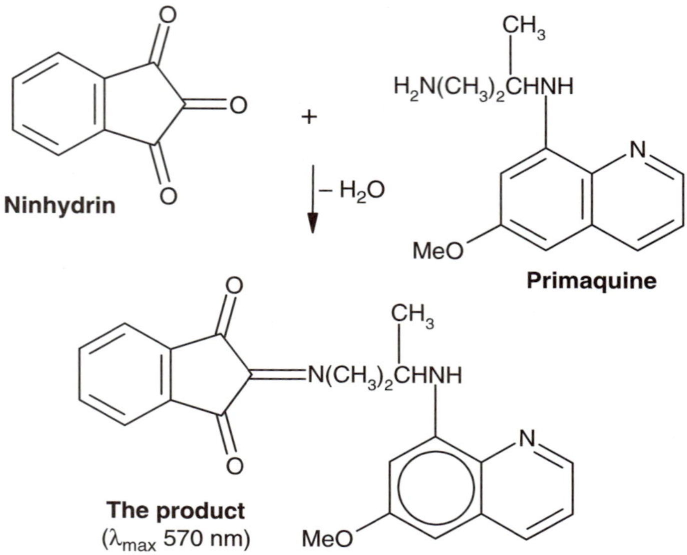

Reference

G. Rama Rao, S.S.N. Murthy & I.R.K. Raju, *Indian Drugs*, **26(2)**, 86, 1988.

Formulation 20

Amodiaquine hydrochloride, Primaquine phosphate

METHOD A

(a) Estimation of Amodiaquine hydrochloride

Reagents

1. Buffer solution (Britton-Robinson buffer) pH 7.6: Prepared by adding 0.2 M sodium hydroxide solution to a mixed acid solutions, 0.04 M in respect of phosphoric acid, boric acid and acetic acid to get a pH of 7.6 (use pH meter).
2. 0.05 M chloramine-T solution in water.

Standard solution

1 mg/ml of pure amodiaquine hydrochloride in water.

Sample solution

Weigh a quantity of powdered material equivalent to 10 mg of the compound, add about 50 ml of water, shake to effect dissolution and dilute to get 1 mg/ml concentration.

Procedure

To 4 ml of sample and standard solutions, add 5 ml of pH. 7.6 buffer solution, 5 ml of chloramine-T reagent and dilute with water to 50 ml. Extract with four 10 ml portions of chloroform. Dry the organic extract over anhydrous sodium sulphate, make up to 50 ml with same solvent and measure the absorbance at 442 nm against reagent blank. The method obeys Beer's law in the range of 1-200 mcg/ml of amodiaquine hydrochloride.

Note

1. The absorption maxima and absorbance values are influenced by the solvent used for extraction of coloured complex.
2. Chloroform and carbon tetrachloride are the suitable solvents.
3. Chloroquine phosphate and primaquine phosphate do not interfere in this method.

Explanatory Note

Chloramine-T oxidises the phenolic hydroxyl group of amodiaquine resulting in the formation of the product as shown in the reaction.

Based on IR and NMR spectroscopy, the authors have suggsted that the final reaction product contains sulphonamide group i.e. SO_2N of the reagent and quinoid form being absent in the drug after treatment with the reagent, it was inferred that sulphonamide group of the reagent (chloramine-T) must be attached either to oxygen of the phenolic-hydroxyl group in the drug or to the 'N' atom present in the drug. If the sulphonamide is linked with oxygen atom of the phenolic-OH group of the drug, then the structure of the final product shall be:

Probable Reaction Mechanism

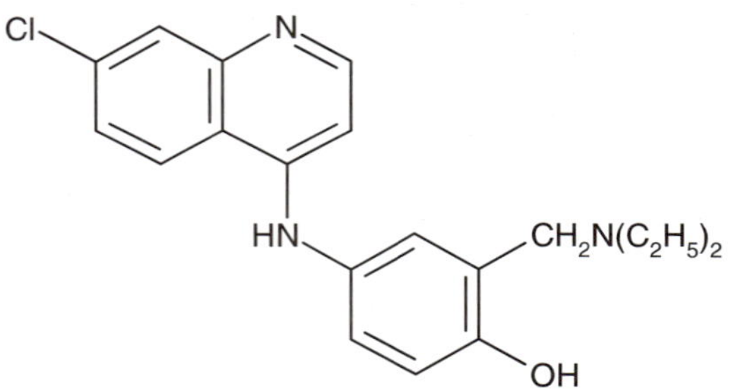

Amodiaquine

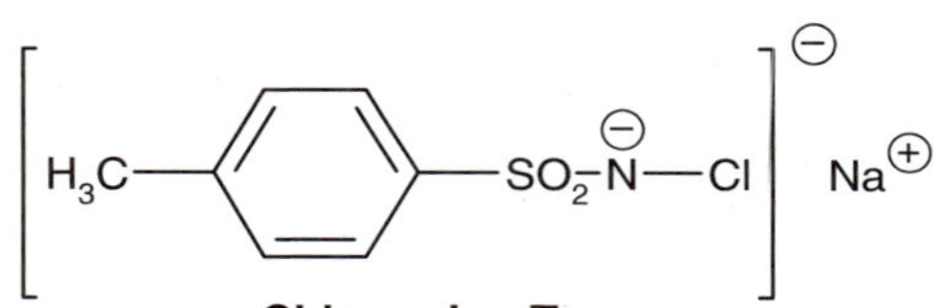

Chloramine-T (reagent used)

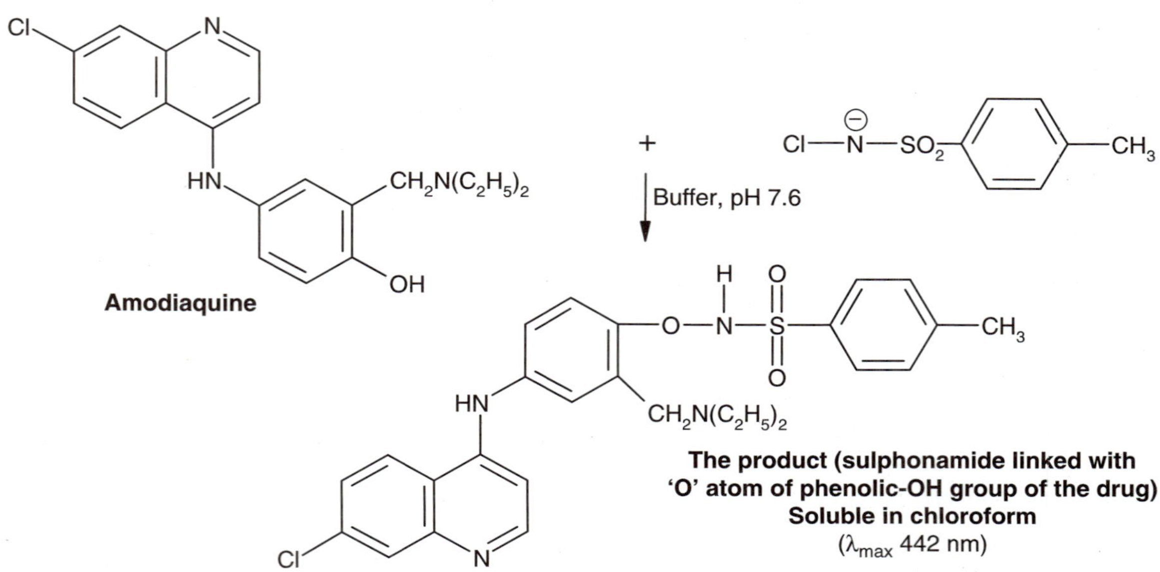

The product (sulphonamide linked with 'O' atom of phenolic-OH group of the drug) Soluble in chloroform

(λ_{max} 442 nm)

OR

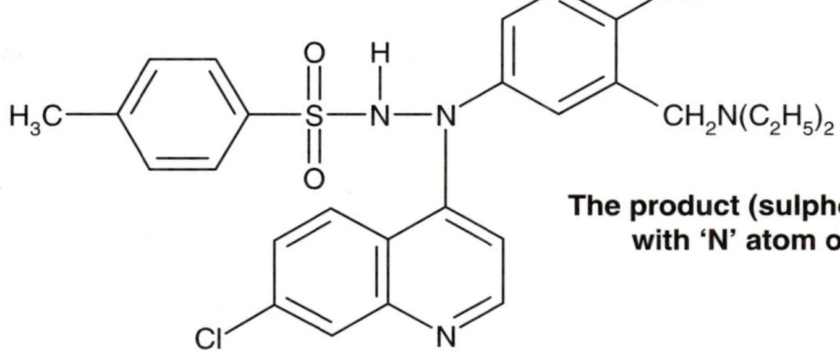

The product (sulphonamide linked with 'N' atom of the drug)

Reference

G. Rama Rao, Y. Pulla Rao & I.R.K. Raju, *Analyst*, **107**, 776-780, 1982.

Methods 2, 3 and 4, where reaction mechanisms are explained, are of analytical interest.

METHOD 2

Nitrosonium ion, being electron deficient, can attack secondary amine (NH) group present in the molecule (amodiaquine) thus giving N-nitroso derivative (λ_{max} 430 nm).

Reagent

10% sodium nitrate solution in water.

Probable Reaction Mechanism

$$NaNO_2 + HCl \longrightarrow NaCl + HNO_2$$

$$HNO_2 \xrightarrow{+H^+} H_2\overset{+}{O}NO \xrightarrow{Cl^-} H_2O + \overset{+}{N}{=}O$$

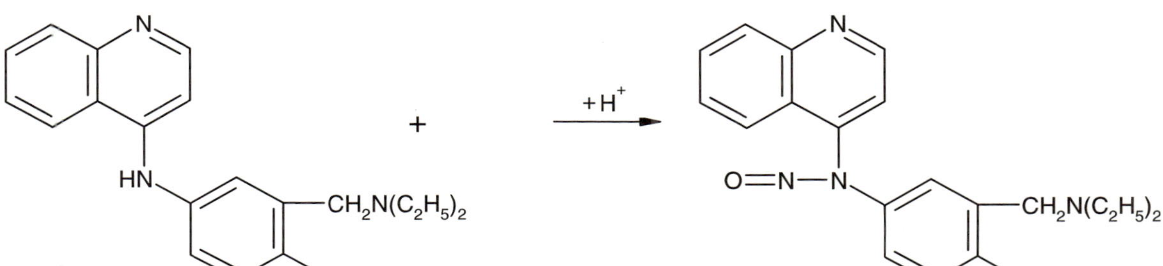

Amodiaquine (λ_{max} 430 nm)

Sulphamic acid is required to remove excess of HNO_2 so formed.

$$HNO_2 + H_2NSO_3H \longrightarrow H_2SO_4 + N_2\uparrow + H_2O$$

Sulphamic acid

Reference

1. Gopal Krishan, S.K. Talwar, S.C. Sharma & R.G. Sharma, *Indian Drugs*, **28(5)**, 236-237, 1991.
2. Practical Organic Chemistry by Vogel, p. 920.

METHOD 3

This method is based on coupling of diazotized sulphanilic acid with the drug at ortho position to the phenolic-OH present in the drug in alkaline medium.

Probable Reaction Mechanism

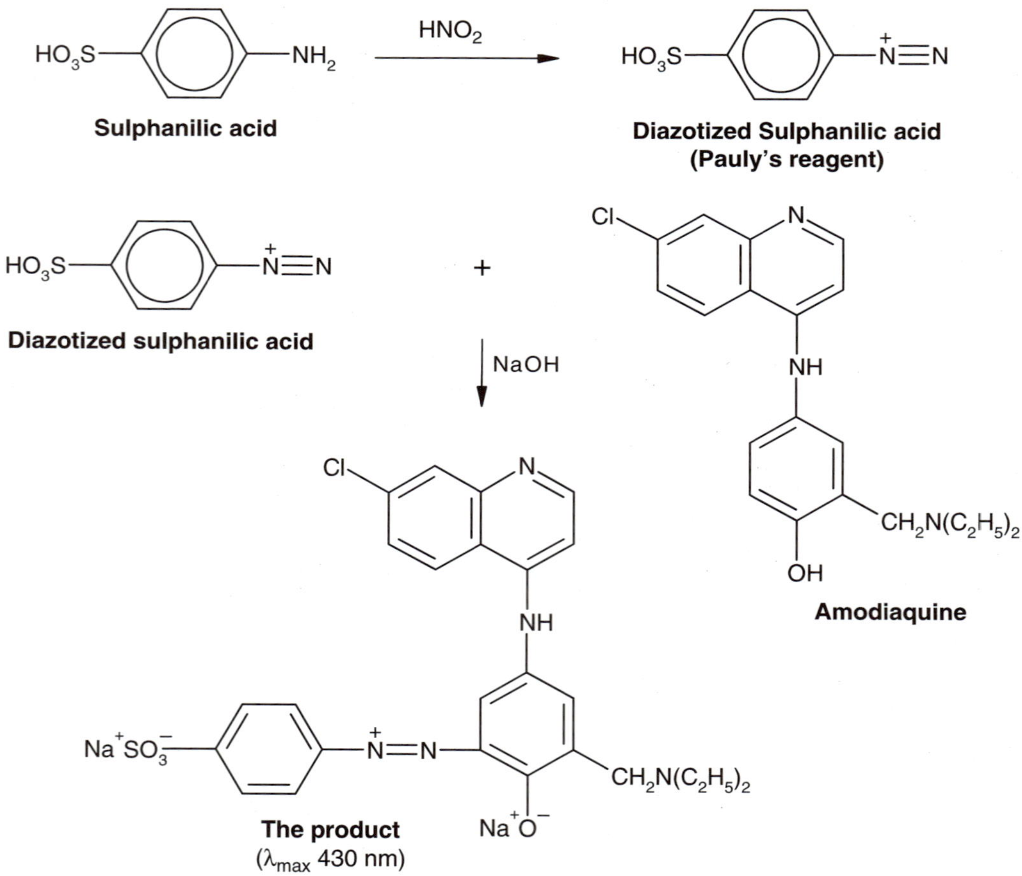

Note

Diazotized p-nitroanaline can also be used.

Reference

Pharmaceutical Chemistry (Vol. 2) by H.J. Roth, p. 519.

METHOD 4

N-bromosuccinimide causes oxidation of the hydroxyl group to ketone resulting in the formation of the coloured product (λ_{max} 450 nm).

Reagent

0.01 M potassium acid phthalate - sodium hydroxide buffer pH 5.2.

Probable Reaction Mechanism

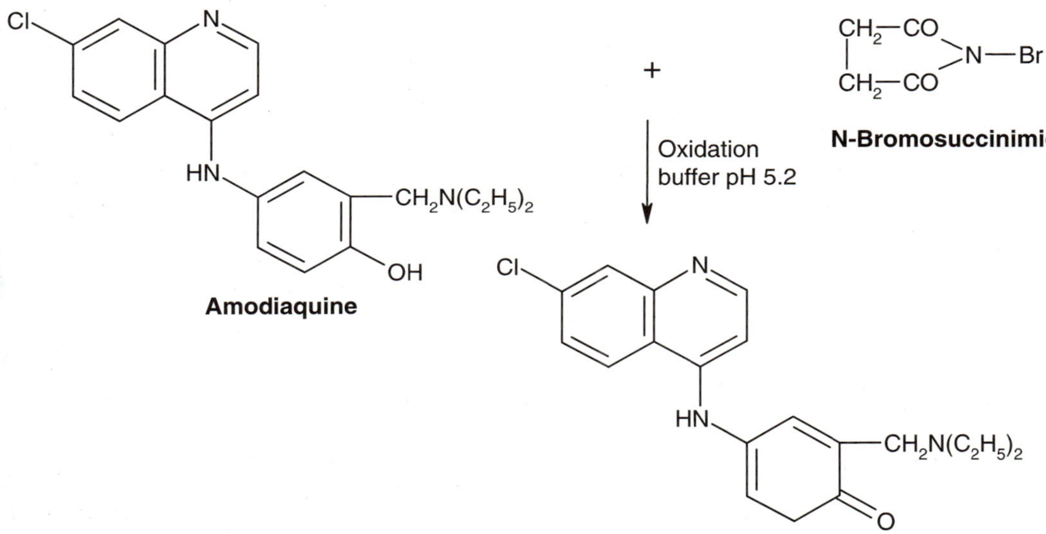

Amodiaquine

N-Bromosuccinimide

Orange-red coloured product
(λ_{max} 450 nm)

Reference

1. B.S. Sastry, E. Venkata Rao & C.S.P. Sastry, *Indian Drugs*, **22(10)**, 550, 1985.
2. Advance Organic Chemistry by Jerry Marsh, p. 1059.

The drug undergoes oxidative coupling with 'MBTH' reagent. The coupling takes place at ortho position to phenolic-OH to give red-coloured complex (λ_{max} 507 nm).

Probable Reaction Mechanism

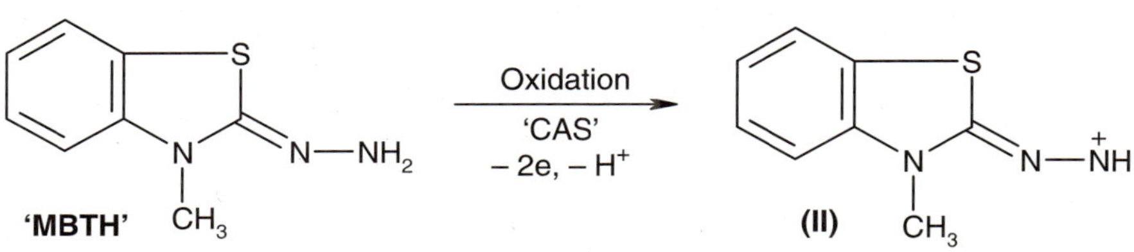

'MBTH' **(II)**

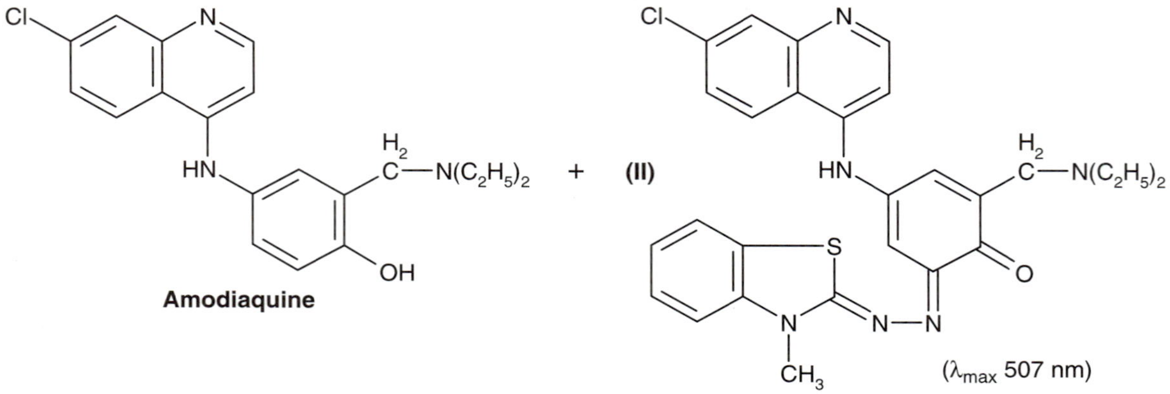

Reference

G. Rama Rao et al., *Indian Drugs*, **27(1)**, 75, 1989.

(b) Estimation of Primaquine phosphate

Follow the method-1 (a or b) as described under formulation-2- of this chapter.

METHOD B

(a) Estimation of Amodiaquine hydrochloride

Sample solution

Weigh a quantity of powdered tablets equivalent to 20 mg of amodiaquine hydrochloride and extract with 0.1 N hydrochloric acid to produce 100 ml. Filter, dilute 10 ml of the filtrate to 100 ml with 0.1 N hydrochloric acid (10 mcg/ml).

Measure the absorbance at the maxima at 342 nm using 0.1 N hydrochloric acid as blank. Calculate the results using 436 as value of E, 1% 1 cm at 342 nm.

Note

Primaquine phosphate has negligible absorption at 342 nm. A solution containing 10 mcg/ml of primaquine shows an absorbance of about 0.006 at 342 nm. It hardly interferes at the concentration (1 : 20) usually present along with amodiaquine.

Estimation of Primaquine phosphate

Weigh powdered tablets equivalent to 60 mg of primaquine, add 50-60 ml water and 5 ml of hydrochloric acid. When on water bath till tablets have completely disintegrated. Cool in ice bath to below 15°C and titrate with 0.01 M sodium nitrite solution. Each ml of 0.02 M sodium nitrite is equivalent to

5.187 mg of primaquine (base). Perform blank and carry out the necessary correction to calculate nett volume of 0.02 M sodium nitrite consumed by the sample.

METHOD C

Simultaneous spectrophotometric determination of amodiaquine and primaquine in mixture

Both the components can be determined without prior separation by measuring the extinction at 282 and 342 nm in 0.1 N hydrochloric acid and by solving 2 simultaneous equations based on Vierordt's method. Primaquine shows another peak at 266 nm but this peak is unsuitable for analysis of the mixture as it coincides with sharply sloping part of amodiaquine spectrum. The following 2 equations are applied for calculation of concentration of each ingredient.

$$\text{Concentration of Primaquine phosphate (PP)} = \frac{(A_1\beta_2 - A_2\beta_1)}{(\alpha_1\beta_2 - \alpha_2\beta_1)}$$

$$\text{Concentration of Amodiaquine hydrochloride (AH)} = \frac{(A_2\alpha_1 - A_1\alpha_2)}{(\alpha_1\beta_2 - \alpha_2\beta_1)}$$

A_1 and A_2 are the absorbance values of the sample mixture at 282 and 342 nm respectively; a and b represent the absorptivity values of Primaquine phosphate and Amodiaquine hydrochloride respectively at the relevant wavelength. These constant values may be determined with pure compounds and substituted in the equations. This method is applicable only to the ratios within 1 : 7.5 (PP : AH) because at the ratios 1 : 10 and 1 : 15, the method shows large error.

Procedure

Accurately weighed amount of crushed tablets equivalent to 150 mg of amodiaquine hydrochloride is shaken with 50 ml of 0.1 N hydrochloric acid to dissolve the drug. Dilute to 100 ml with the same solvent, filter and subsequently dilute to get 15 mcg/ml. The absorbance of the mixture is measured at 282 and 340 nm against 0.1 N hydrochloric acid as blank. Contents of each ingredient are calculated from the two equations described above by substituting the values thus obtained.

METHOD D

This method based on the work of the author involves quantitative separation of primaquine and amodiaquine by selective precipitation. Amodiaquine is quantitatively precipitated from alkaline medium whereas primaquine is soluble in excess of ammonia.

Procedure

Accurately weighed quantity of powdered material equivalent to 2.5-5 mg of primaquine but not containing more than 100 mg of amodiaquine is suspended in about 175 ml of 0.01 N hydrochloric acid and shaken vigorously to ensure proper dispersion. 10 ml of 4 N ammonia is slowly added with continuous stirring. The precipitate is filtered through glass sintered funnel, the filtrate and washing adjusted to 250 ml with water. The filtrate is further diluted appropriately with 0.1 N hydrochloric acid and the extinction measured at 282 nm. The results are compiled by using 572.2 as a value of E, 1 per cent, 1 cm of the base. The residue obtained above is dissolved in 0.1 N hydrochloric acid and contents of amodiaquine determined by the procedure described in method-B above.

Note

1. The above method is applicable even when the ratio of primaquine : amodiaquine is up to 1 : 40.
2. The higher amount of amodiaquine yields low results in respect of primaquine as on precipitation with ammonia, the primaquine gets trapped in the precipitated amodiaquine. Hence the amount of sample taken for analysis should not contain more than 100 mg of amodiaquine.

Methods 2, 3 and 4 where reaction mechanisms are explained are of analytical interest.

Reference

P.K. Chatterjee, C.L. Jain & P.D. Sethi, *Indian Drugs*, **23(10)**, 563-565, 1986.

Formulation 21

Pyrvinium pamoate, Piperazine citrate

ESTIMATION

Pyrvinium pamoate

Standard solution

Weigh accurately about 57 mg of Pyrvinium pamoate and transfer quantitatively into 50 ml volumetric flask. Dissolve in and dilute to volume with dimethylformamide. Pipet 1 ml of this solution into 100 ml volumetric flask and dilute to volume with the same solvent. Use low actinic glassware in preparing solutions of Pyrvinium pamoate.

Sample solution

Transfer a volume of homogeneous sample suspension equivalent to 57 mg of pyrvinium pamoate into a 100 ml volumetric flask. Wash the pipet with two 3 ml portions of water, followed by three 20 ml portions of dimethylformamide into the flask to ensure complete transfer of the contents. Mix the contents and heat on a water bath until all of the pyrvinium pamoate is dissolved (it takes about 1 h). Cool to about 25°C, add dimethylformamide to volume and mix. Centrifuge a portion of this mixture and dilute 3 ml of the clear supernatant liquid to 100 ml with dimethylformamide, mix.

Concomitantly determine the absorbance of the sample and standard solutions against dimethylformamide as blank in a spectrophotometer at wavelength of maximum absorbance at about 508 nm. The compound is orange-red in colour, hence method based on measuring colour intensity of the solution.

Note

Complete the procedure without prolonged interruption.

Calculations

$$\text{Pyrvinium base (mg) per ml} = \frac{A_u}{A_s} \times \frac{0.6644}{1} \times \frac{S}{v} \times \text{df. of sample}$$

where A_u = Absorbance of the sample solution
A_s = Absorbance of the standard solution
V = Volume of the sample taken for assay
df = Dilution factor

0.6644 is the factor for the conversion of one half of the molecular weight of anhydrous pyrvinium pamoate (575.71) to the formula weight of pyrvinium base (382.53) ratio $\frac{382.53}{575.71} = 0.6644$

Piperazine

Follow method-5 as described under formulation 13 of this chapter.

Formulation 22

Sulphamethoxazole, Trimethoprim

METHOD A

(a) Estimation of Trimethoprim

Method 1

Reagents

1. Chloranil reagent, 0.5% w/v solution of chloranil in dioxan.
2. 0.1 M Sodium hydroxide.

Standard solution

0.4 mg/100 ml of trimethoprim in chloroform.

Sample solution

Weigh accurately, a quantity of powdered tablets or measure sample volume equivalent to 40 mg of trimethoprim. Add 30 ml of 0.1 N sodium hydroxide, shake and extract with four 50 ml portions of chloroform. Wash combined chloroform extract twice with 10 ml of 0.1 N sodium hydroxide. Concentrate chloroform extract to 80 ml and make up the volume to 100 ml with chloroform.

Procedure

Evaporate 5 ml of the sample and standard solutions on boiling water bath. Treat the residue with 2 ml of chloranil reagent. Heat the mixture on a boiling water bath for 10 minutes, cool and adjust to 10 ml with chloroform. Read extinction of red coloured complex at about 480 nm against reagent blank. The method obeys Beer's law in the concentration of 50-350 mcg/ml.

Note

1. The red coloured chromophore is stable for more than 1 h.
2. As moisture affects the stability of the colour, the experiment should be carried out in non-aqueous conditions.

Probable Reaction Mechanism

Primary amine group of the molecule can add to chloranil resulting in the formation of Michael addition with loss of HCl.

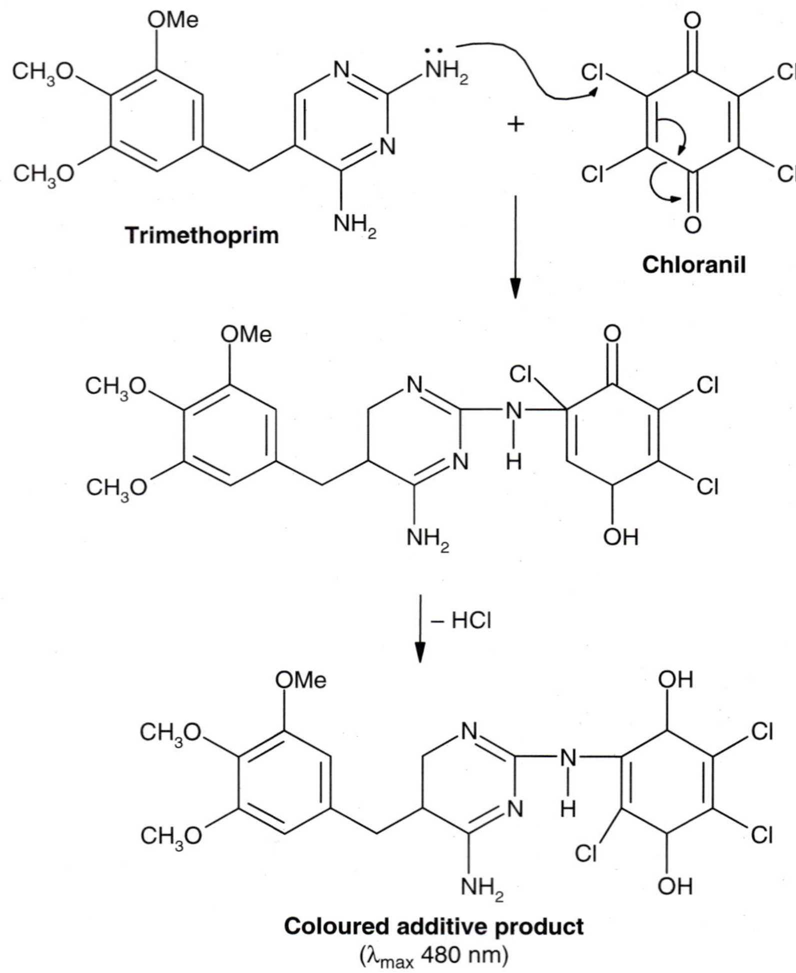

Reference

J. Emmanuel & T.V. Yegyanarayanan, *Indian Drugs*, Sept. 1982, p. 503.

METHOD 2

The above method is applicable for estimation of trimethoprim by using citric acid-acetic anhydride reagent instead of chloranil reagent.

Citric acid-acetic anhydride reagent : To 1.2 g of citric acid, add 5 ml of methanol and make up the volume to 100 ml with acetic anhydride.

Procedure

Carry out the procedure as given under method-1 above. After evaporation of the chloroform layer, treat the residue obtained both with the sample and standard solutions with 10 ml of the reagent and heat in a boiling water bath for 30 minutes. Cool to room temperature and adjust the volume to 100 ml with acetic anhydride. Read the absorbance of both the solutions at maxima at about 560 nm against reagent blank. The method obeys Beer's law in the range of 1-40 mcg/ml. The intensity of the colour is affected by moisture, hence dry conditions should be adhered to throughout the experiments.

METHOD 3

Reagents

1. 0.1 M Dipotassium hydrogen phosphate.
2. 0.025% w/v aqueous solution of dyes: bromocresol red, bromocresol green or bromothymol blue.

Standard solution

Weigh accurately about 5 mg of the pure Trimethoprim, add 10 ml of 0.1 M phosphate solution and dilute to 100 ml with water.

Sample solution

Weigh or measure accurately a quantity of the sample equivalent to 5 mg of trimethoprim, add 10 ml of 0.1 M phosphate solution and make up to 100 ml with distilled water. Stir to mix and keep on water bath (50°C) for 30 minutes for complete dissolution and filter.

Procedure

To 0.5 ml of the sample and standard solutions, add 1 ml of the dye solution and 5 ml of chloroform. Shake the mixture for 2 minutes and allow the chloroform layer to separate. Measure the absorbance of organic layer at about 420 nm. The method obeys Beer's law in the concentration range of 1-5 mcg/ml.

METHOD 4

Standard solution

20 mcg/ml of Trimethoprim in chloroform.

Sample solution

Transfer accurately weighed portion of the sample equivalent to 40 mg of trimethoprim to a separating funnel. In case of suspensions, shake the sample well for 10 minutes before withdrawing the sample for analysis. Add 10 ml of 1 N sodium hydroxide and shake for 1 min. Extract the aqueous phase with three 20 ml portions of chloroform. Retain aqueous layer for estimation of sulphamethoxazole. Pass the combined chloroform layer through anhydrous sodium sulphate into a 100 ml volumetric flask. Rinse the sodium sulphate layer with chloroform and make up the volume. 5 ml of the resulting solution is diluted to 100 ml with chloroform (20 mcg/ml).

Measure the extinction of sample and standard solutions at 289 nm using chloroform as blank. The solution also exhibits a sharp maxima at 242 nm which can be used for quantitative estimation.

(b) Estimation of Sulphamethoxazole

METHOD 1

Standard solution

1 mg/ml of sulphamethoxazole in 1 N sodium hydroxide. Further dilutions are done with water to get 10 mcg/ml.

Sample solution

Collect quantitatively alkaline layer retained during assay of trimethoprim under method-4 above and dilute to 100 ml with 1 N sodium hydroxide. Further dilutions are done with water to get a concentration of 10 mcg/ml.

Measure the extinction of both the sample and standard solutions at maxima at about 260 nm and calculate the results by comparison.

METHOD 2

This involves colour reaction of sulphamethoxazole with p-dimethylaminobenz-aldehyde in acidic medium to give a yellow colour which shows maximum absorbance at about 450 nm.

Reagents

1. p-Dimethylaminobenzaldehyde solution: 200 mg of p-dimethylaminobenz-aldehyde is dissolved in 25 ml of acetone or methanol, 5 ml of 1 N hydro-chloric acid is added and then diluted to 100 ml with distilled water.
2. 25% v/v solution of acetone or methanol in water.

Standard solution

Weigh accurately about 200 mg of Sulphamethoxazole dissolve in 25 ml of acetone or methanol and adjust the volume to 100 ml with distilled water. 5 ml of the resultant solution is further diluted to 100 ml with aqueous acetone or methanol (100 mcg/ml).

Sample solution

Accurately weigh, a quantity of crushed tablets or measure volume (injections or suspensions) equivalent to 200 mg of sulphamethoxazole. In case of syrups or suspensions, wash the pipette with two 5 ml portions of water and mix with the main solution. Add 25 ml of acetone, shake and dilute to 100 ml with water. 5 ml of the resultant solution is further diluted with aqueous acetone or methanol to 100 ml (100 mcg/ml).

Procedure

To 5 ml of sample and standard solutions, add 10 ml of the reagent and make up the volume to 25 ml with acetone. Allow to stand for 40 minutes at room temperature and measure the absorbance of both the solutions at 450 nm against reagent blank. Calculate the results by comparison. The method obeys Beer's law in the range of 4-32 mcg/ml.

Note

Sulphamoxole can also be estimated by this method.

The compound forms Schiff's base with PDAB in acidic medium.

Probable Reaction Mechanism

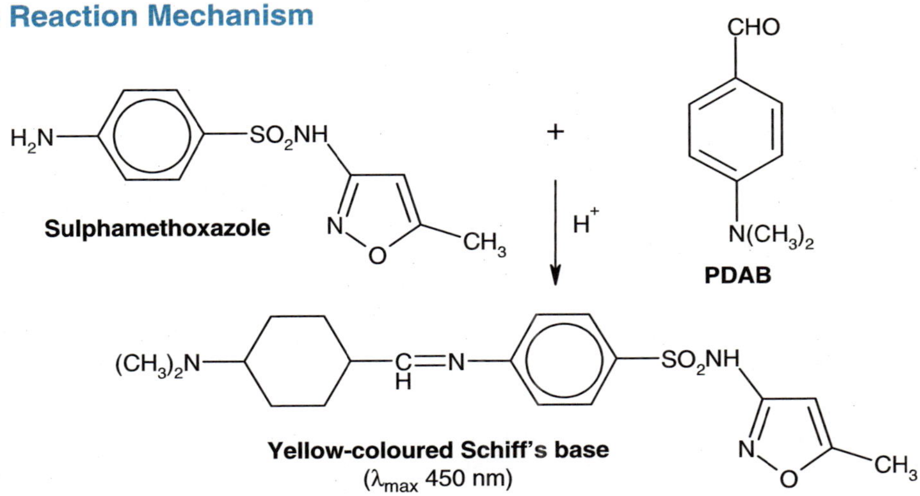

Other general reactions of sulphonamide can be used for assay of this compound.

METHOD B

This method is based on simultaneous estimation of trimethoprim (TMP) and sulphamethoxazole (SMX) by isoabsorption point method. This is a rapid spectrophotometric assay method for each ingredient without the need for prior separation. The absorption spectra of solutions of 'TMP' and 'SMX' in 0.1 N hydrochloric acid when recorded separately are not markedly different. However, they exhibit an isoabsorption point at 240.5 nm in solution of pH 7.2 (Isoabsorption point is the wavelength at which spectra of the two compounds at same concentration exhibit same absorbancy).

Preparation of standard solution of Trimethoprim and Sulphamethoxazole

Weigh accurately 50 mg each of 'TMP' and 'SMX' and dissolve in 0.1 N hydrochloric acid to make 500 ml. These acidic solutions are suitably diluted and adjusted to pH 7.2 with 0.1 N sodium hydroxide to give a concentration of 10 mcg/ml of each compound. The spectra of standard solutions is recorded from 220 to 360 nm. The isoabsorption point occurs at 240.5 nm and 'SMX' has absorption maxima at 255 nm. Both 'TMP' and 'SMX' obeys Beer's law separately in the concentration range of 6-14 mcg/ml at 240.5 and 255 nm. The absorbance ratio method is applied to the mixture of these compounds by solving two equations (i) and (ii) as given below :

$$C_I = \frac{Q_0 - Q_{II}}{Q_I - Q_{II}} \times \frac{A_I}{a_I} \qquad \text{...(i)}$$

$$C_{II} = \frac{Q_0 - Q_I}{Q_{II} - Q_I} \times \frac{A_I}{a_I} \qquad \text{...(ii)}$$

C_I, C_{II} = concentration (g/1) of component I and II present in the sample;

Q_o = ratio of absorbance values of binary mixture (sample) at two different wavelengths, one of which is isoabsorption point (240.5 nm) and the other is a wavelength at which one of the drug absorbs more strongly (255 nm for SMX);

Q_i, Q_{II} = absorbance ratio values of components I and II at two wavelengths (225 : 240.5);

A = absorption value of the sample at isoabsorption wavelengths (240.5 nm);

a = absorptivity of the components at isoabsorption wavelengths - 240.5 nm (it is the absorbance of a solution containing 1 g/litre of the substance, it is 1/10th the value of E 1%, 1 cm.

Preparation of sample solution

The crushed tablets accurately weighed equivalent to 25 mg of 'TMP' are dissolved in 0.1 N hydrochloric acid and made up to 500 ml. Acidic solution is suitably diluted and adjusted to pH 7.2 with 0.1 N sodium hydroxide to get solution of 2 mcg/ml of 'TMP'. Absorbance values of the resultant solution is measured at 240.5 and 255 nm to calculate Q_0.

The average values for 3 estimations of each 'TMP' (Q_I) and 'SMX' (Q_{II}) and A are calculated.

Working example

Each tablet contains 80 mg of 'TMP' and 400 mg of 'SMX';

Q_I (255 : 240.5 nm) = 0.212
Q_{II} (255 : 240.5 nm) = 1.378
a (240.5 nm) = 47.00
A (240.5 nm) = 0.548
Q_0 (255 : 240.5 nm) = 1.177

$$\text{Concentration (g/L) of 'TMP'} (C_1) = \frac{Q_0 - Q_{II}}{Q_I - Q_{II}} \times \frac{A}{a_I} = \frac{1.177 - 1.378}{0.212 - 1.378} \times \frac{0.548}{47.0} = 0.00207 \text{ g/L}$$

Claim = 0.002 g/L

$$\text{Concentration (g/L) of 'SMX'} (C_2) = \frac{Q_0 - Q_I}{Q_{II} - Q_I} \times \frac{A}{a_I} = \frac{1.177 - 0.212}{1.166} \times \frac{0.548}{47.0} = 0.0098 \text{ g/L}$$

Claim = 0.010 g/L

METHOD C

This method is direct colorimetric estimation of both the components without prior separation. The estimation of trimethoprim (TMP) is based on its ion-pair formation with bromophenol blue and subsequent measurement of absorbance of yellow complex at 418 nm. Sulphamethoxazole (SMX) is estimated by Bratton-Marshall reaction.

Reagents

1. Citrate-phosphate buffer, pH 3.2.
2. 0.1% w/v solution of sodium nitrite in water.
3. 0.5% w/v solution of ammonium sulphamate in water.
4. 0.1% w/v solution of N-1-(naphthyl)-ethylenediamine dihydrochloride (NED).
5. 0.4% w/v solution of bromophenol blue in buffer, pH 3.2.
6. 0.1 N, 4 N Hydrochloric acid.

Preparation of standard solution

Accurately weighed amount of each of 'TMP' and 'SMX' are dissolved in 2 ml methanol and diluted to 100 ml with water (200 mcg/ml). The above stock solutions are diluted with water separately to get concentration of 40 and 3 mcg/ml of 'TMP' and 'SMX' respectively.

Preparation of sample solution

Accurately weighed/measured portion of the sample equivalent to 8 mg of 'TMP' and 40 mg of 'SMX' are mixed with 150 ml of water and warmed on water bath for 15 min. with intermittent shaking. The solution is cooled, 0.8 ml methanol is added and diluted with water to 200 ml. This serves as the final sample solution for 'TMP'. However, for 'SMX', 1.5 ml of above solution is diluted to 200 ml with water.

Estimation of Trimethoprim

To 2.5 ml of the sample and standard solutions, add 1.5 ml water, 2 ml bromophenol blue solution and 20 ml of chloroform. Instantaneously formed ion-pair complex is extracted into organic layer by shaking for 1 min. The layers are allowed to separate and the absorbance of the organic layer is measured at 418 nm against reagent blank.

Estimation of sulphamethoxazole

5 ml of the sample and standard solutions are acidified with 1.5 ml 4 N hydrochloric acid, 0.5 ml of sodium nitrite solution is added and the mixture is allowed to stand for 3 min. 0.5 ml of ammonium sulphamate solution is added to neutralise excess of nitrous acid and after 2 min, 0.5 ml of Bratton Marshall reagent is added and allowed to stand for 10 mins for complete colour development. The absorbance of both the solutions is measured at 545 nm against reagent blank.

Note

The yellow chromophore of the ion-pair complex is stable for 24 h and the method follows Beer's law up to 80 mcg/ml of chloroform layer. Common preservatives such as hydroxybenzoates usually presents in oral preparations do not interfere in the analysis of both the components.

Probable Reaction Mechanism

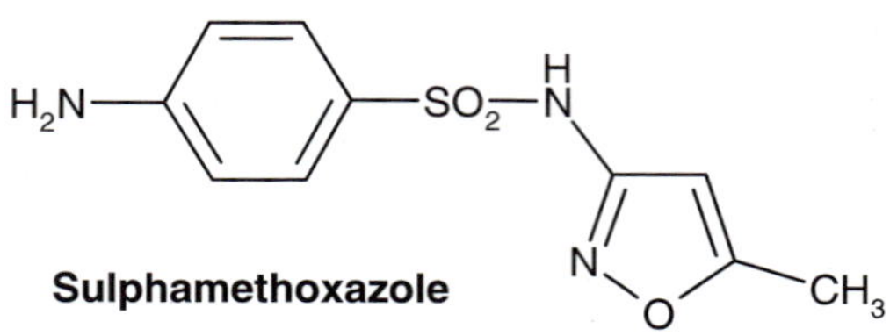

Sulphamethoxazole

$$NaNO_2 + HCl \longrightarrow NaCl + HNO_2 \xrightarrow{H^+} H_2\overset{+}{O}N{=}O \xrightarrow{Cl^-} \bar{Cl}\ \overset{+}{N}{=}O^- + H_2O$$

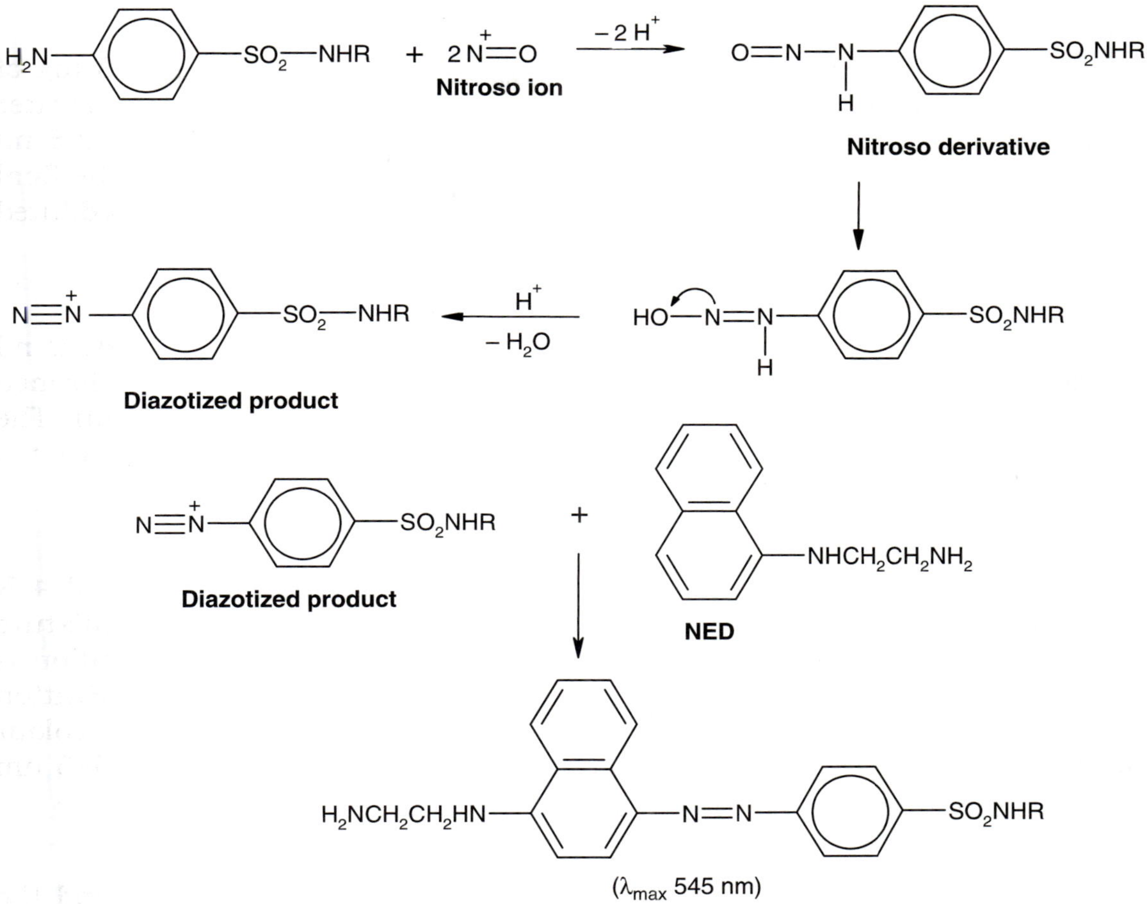

Excess HNO_2 is removed by ammonium sulphomate.

$$HNO_2 + H_2NSO_3H \longrightarrow H_2SO_4 + N_2\uparrow + H_2O$$

Formulation 23

Nitrofurantoin, Deglycyrrhizinised liquorice, Trimethoprim

ESTIMATION

Nitrofurantoin

METHOD 1

Reagents

1. Dimethylformamide (DMF)
2. Solvent: It contains 1.8% w/v sodium acetate and 0.14% v/v glacial acetic acid in water.

Procedure

Weigh and powder 20 tablets. To a quantity of the powdered sample equivalent to 30 mg of nitrofurantoin, add 50 ml of dimethylformamide, shake for 5 minutes and add sufficient water to produce 500 ml, mix thoroughly. Dilute 10 ml from the above solution to 100 ml with the solvent and filter through G-4 sintered glass funnel. Collect 20 ml portion after discarding first 15 to 20 ml of the filtrate. Measure the optical density in a suitable spectrophotometer at 367 nm using 1% v/v solution of dimethylformamide as blank. Calculate the contents of nitrofurantoin per tablet by taking 765 as the value of E (1% 1 cm) at 367 nm.

Note

Since the compound is poorly soluble in water and in most organic solvents, 'DMF' is the solvent of choice.

METHOD 2

Reagents

1. 0.1% w/v solution of resorcinol in water.
2. 1.5 M Sodium hydroxide.

Standard solution

100 mcg/ml of nitrofurantoin in water.

Sample solution

Accurately weighed or measured quantity of the sample (tablets, capsule or suspension) equivalent to 10 mg of nitrofurantoin is shaken with 50-60 ml of water, filtered and volume adjusted to 100 ml with water.

Procedure

To 1 ml of the standard and sample solutions, add 1.4 ml of resorcinol reagent and 1 ml of 1.5 N sodium hydroxide. Immerse the flask in boiling water bath for 15 minutes, cool and adjust to 10 ml with water. The absorption of pink colour is measured at 535 nm against reagent blank. The method obeys Beer's law in the range of 2-14 mcg/ml.

Explanatory Note

5-Nitrofurfural derivatives give red colour with the addition of aqueous alkaline solution resulting in shift of absorption maximum from UV region to visible region. Since the red colour so formed is unstable, addition of phenol (resorcinol) renders the colour stable for several hours. The red colour in alkaline solution is because of electron attacking character of nitro group at position 5. Further, the hydrogen attached to the nitrogen placed between two carbonyl (C==O) groups is very acidic and on addition of alkali it loses its acidic character resulting in the formation of resonically stabilized anion. The acidic property of the compound can be used for quantitative analysis by titrating with alkali using 'DMF' as solvent.

Probable Reaction Mechanism

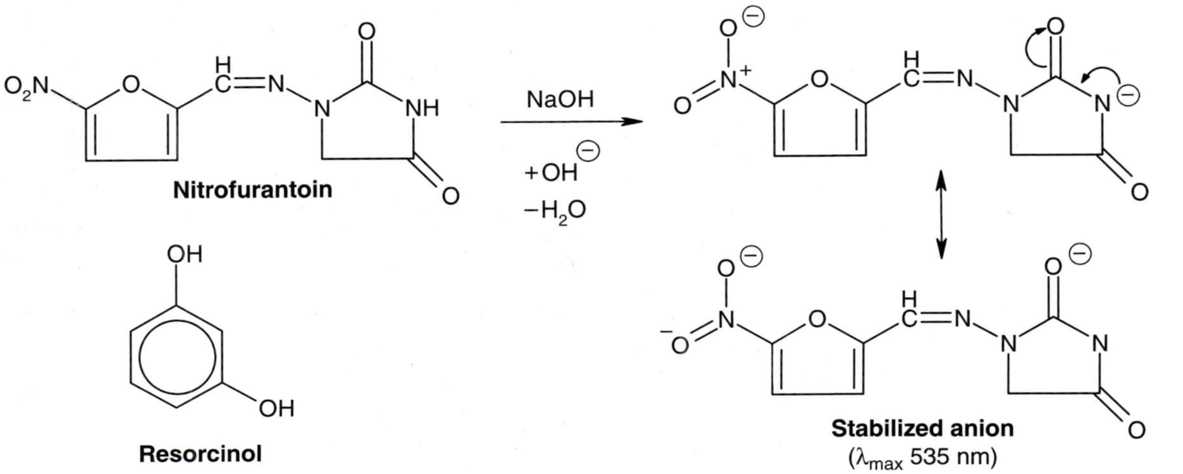

Reference

R.G. Bhatkar & S.K. Chodankar, *Ind. J. Pharm. Sci.*, **42(1)**, 23, 1980.

METHOD 3

Reagents

1. 0.05 w/v solution of isoniazid in water.
2. 0.1 N Sodium hydroxide.

Standard solution

100 mcg/ml of nitrofurantoin in distilled water.

Sample solution

Weigh accurately sample equivalent to 10 mg of nitrofurantoin, add 50 ml of water, shake for 5 minutes and filter. Wash the residue twice with 25 ml of water, mix the filtrate and dilute to 100 ml with water.

Procedure

To 0.5 ml of the sample or standard solution, add 0.5 ml of isoniazid reagent and 2.0 ml of 0.1 N sodium hydroxide and dilute to 10 ml with water. Read the absorbance of the colour after 5 minutes at 390 nm against reagent blank. The method obeys Beer's law in the concentration range of 1-10 mcg/ml of final solution. Yellow colour is stable for 30 minutes.

Condensation reaction occurs between nitrofurantoin and isoniazid resulting in the formation of the product.

Probable Reaction Mechanism

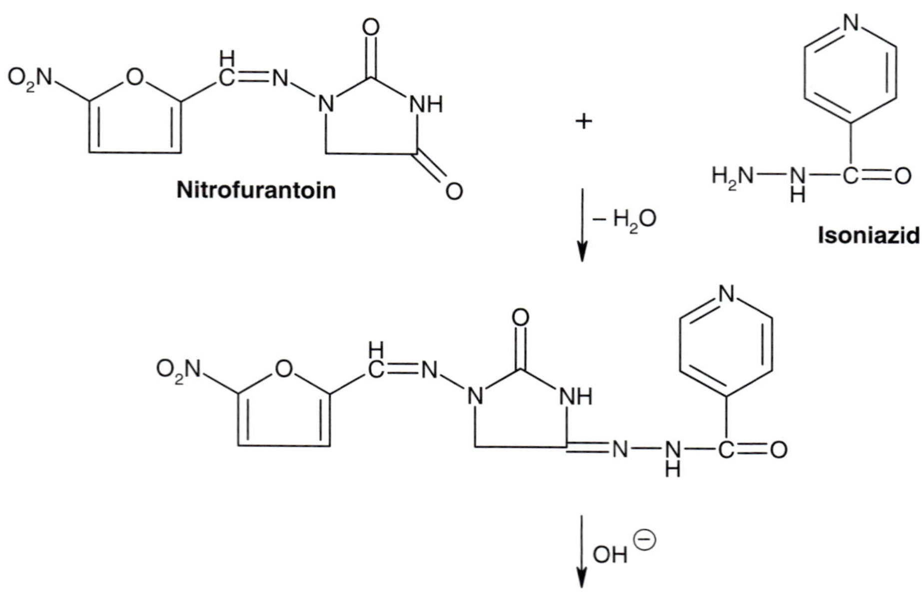

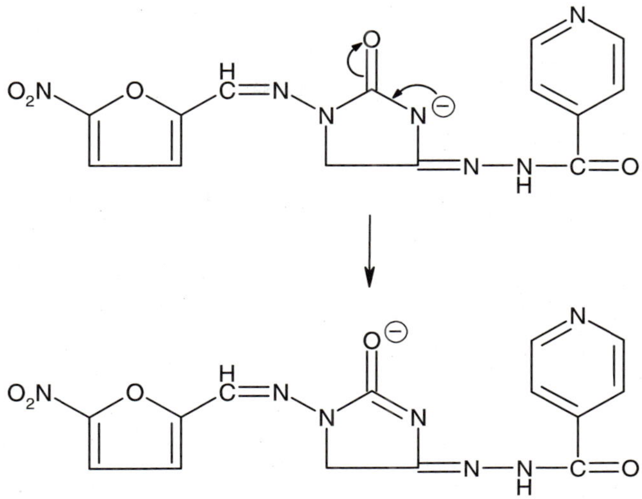

Condensation product
(λ_{max} 390 nm)

Reference

D.M. Shingbal et al. *Eastern Pharmacist*, **XXIII(265)**, 117-118, 1980.

METHOD 4

Reagents

1. Dimethylformamide (DMF): Before use treat with activated charcoal (2 g/100 ml) for 5 min and filter).
2. 0.1 M Tetraethyl ammonium hydroxide in methyl alcohol (TEAH).
3. 0.1% v/v acetone in DMF.

Standard solution

20 mcg/ml of Nitrofurantoin in DMF.

Sample solution

Sample equivalent to 50 mg of nitrofurantoin is extracted with 'DMF' and suitably diluted with DMF to get a concentration of 25 mcg/ml.

Procedure

To 1 ml of sample and standard solutions, add 8 ml of DMF, 0.2 ml of acetone solution, 0.5 ml of 'TEAH' reagent and dilute to 10 ml with DMF. Read the absorbance of both the solutions after 8 minutes at about 520 nm against reagent blank. The method obeys Beer's law in the concentration range of 1-60 mcg/ml.

Note

1. The colour was stable for 30 min.
2. By using aqueous TEAH, colour faded quickly, hence methanolic TEAH.
3. The entire method should be carried out in low actinic light.
4. The method can also be applied to creams, ointments and dusting powders containing nitrofurantoin.

The reaction is carried out in alkaline medium. The acidic proton attached to 'N' can easily be removed. Since the 'N' atom is placed between two carbonyl groups which are electron withdrawing, the resultant product is resonically stabilized anion.

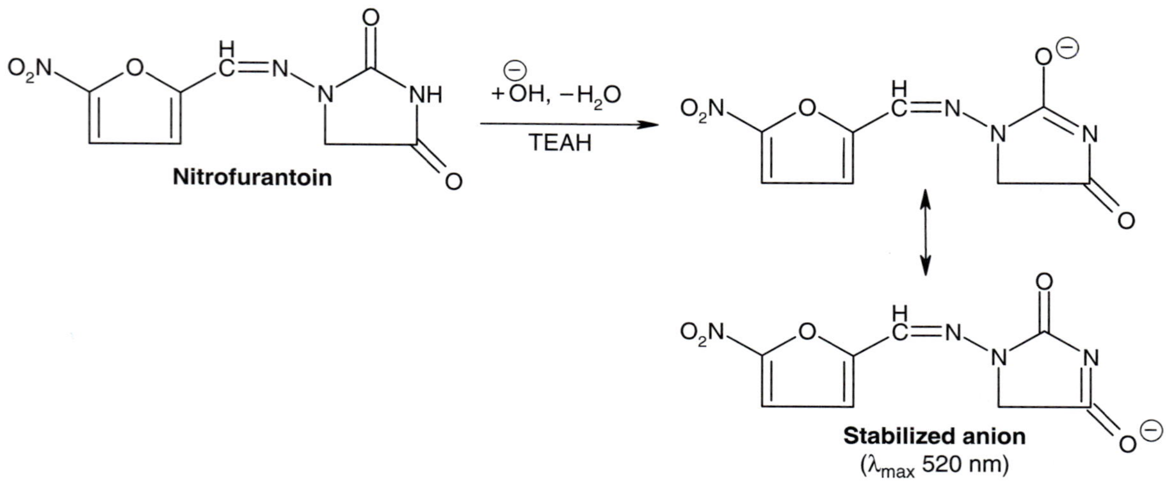

Reference

1. G. Rama Rao et al. *Ind. J. Pharm.*, **29(4)**, 83-85, 1977.
2. G. Rama Rao, S. Raghuveer, S.S.N. Murthy & B. Rajrangrao. *Indian Drugs*, **17(2)**, 50-51, 1979.

Furan part of the molecule undergoes coupling with diazonium salt to yield azo dye. The coupling preferably occurs at C-2 or C-5 positions but since both these positions are occupied, the coupling takes place at positions C-3 or C-4 as explained below.

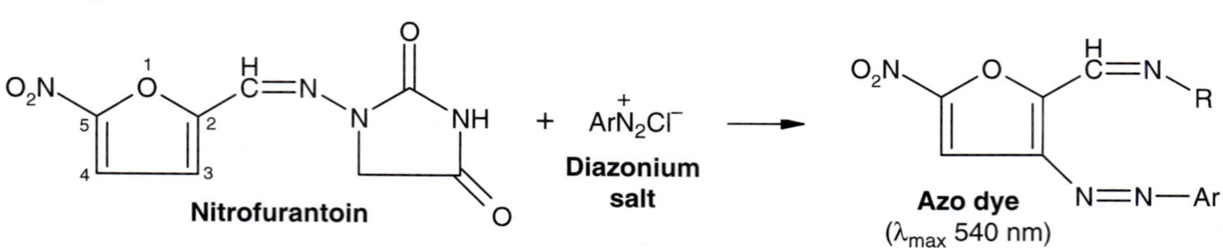

METHOD 5

Reagents

1. 5 M hydrochloric acid.
2. 0.25% 2,4-dinitrophenylhydrazine (DNPH).

Procedure

To 1 ml of sample and standard solutions add 1 ml of DNPH reagent and 5 ml of 5 M HCl. Heat in a water-bath (80°C) for 10 min, cool, dilute to 100 ml with water and measure at 475 nm.

Probable Reaction Mechanism

Condensation reaction occurs between the carbonyl group of the drug and the amino group of the reagent resulting in the formation of Schiff's base in acidic condition.

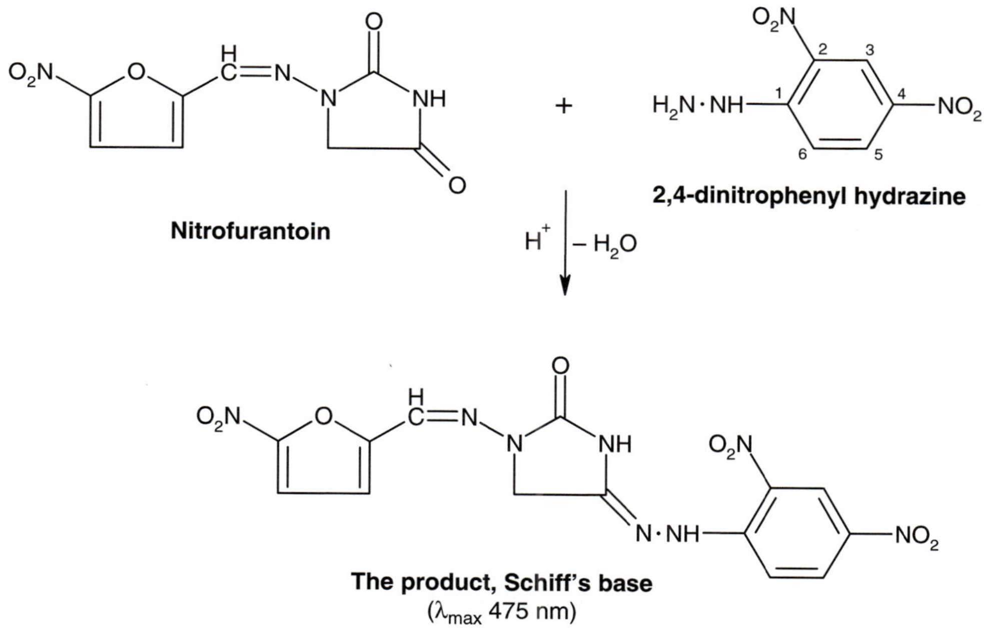

Reference

Indian Drugs, **22(9)**, 482, 1985.

Walari et al. (1980) have described a spectrophotofluorometric method for assay of nitrofurantoin. The method is based on reaction of 2-furfural obtained by acidic hydrolysis of nitrofurantoin with O-amino thiophenol giving a fluorescent moiety i.e. 2-(5-chloro-2-furyl)benzothiazole.

Probable reaction as proposed by the authors

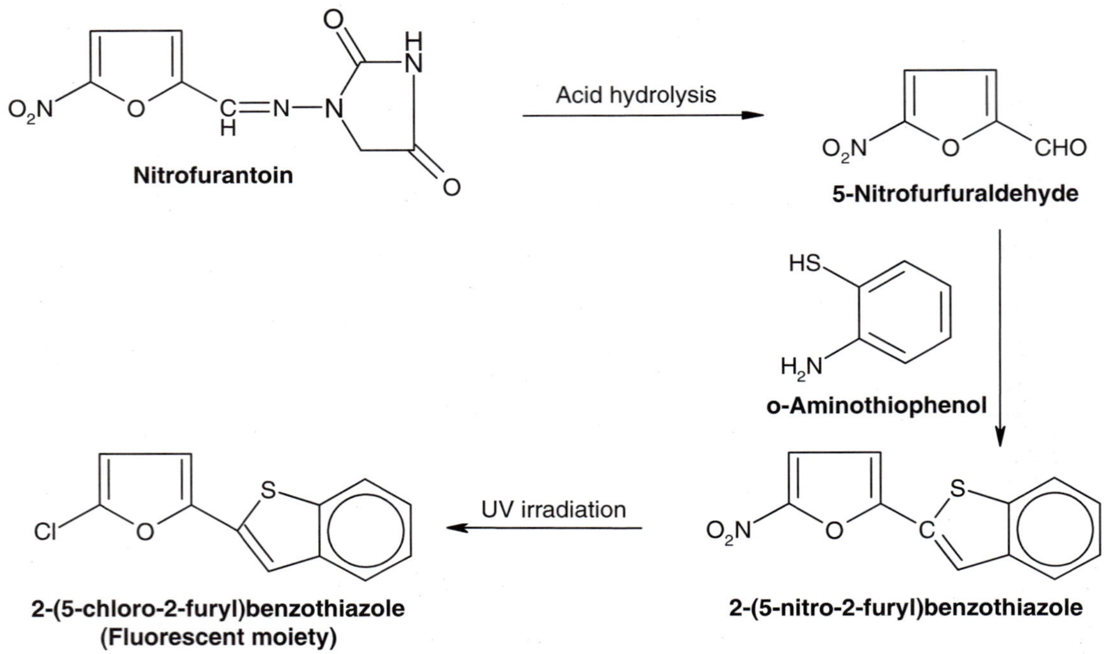

Reference

Nobutoshi Walari, Tomoo Funaki & Nobuyoshi Kaneniwa. *J. Pharm. Sci.*, **69(1)**, 106-108, 1980.

Estimation of Liquorice Deglycyrrhizinated (estimated as Glycyrrhizic acid)

METHOD 1

Reagent

3% w/v solution of trichloroacetic acid in acetone.

Procedure

Weigh and powder 20 tablets. Weigh a portion equivalent to 1 g of liquorice and transfer to a 250 ml beaker. Add 50 ml hot trichloroacetic acid solution and keep it for 20 minutes, stir with glass rod. Allow the mixture to stand for 3 minutes and decant the liquid into filter paper No. 41. Repeat the extraction two more times by adding 25 ml of hot trichloracetic acid solution and steeping for 15 minutes each time. With the third extraction, transfer the solids and liquid to the filter paper. Wash the beaker and filter paper containing residue with 25 ml of acetone. Collect the extracts in 250 ml beaker, add drop by drop strong ammonia solution and stir until an abundant cheesy precipitates are formed. Adjust pH to 8.3 to 8.6, transfer the precipitates together with the mother liquor to a sintered glass funnel. Wash the residue with 50 ml of acetone in 3-4 stages. Pass water through sintered funnel to the flask in which precipitation is made and transfer the resultant solution quantitatively to 250 ml volumetric flask. Dilute 20 ml of the resulting solution to 100 ml with water and determine the optical density on a spectrophotometer at 258 nm against water as blank.

$$\text{Content of Glycyrrhizic acid (X)} = \frac{D \times 822 \times 100 \times 100 \times 250}{a \times b \times 11000 \times 1000}$$

X = Glycyrrhizic acid content.
D = Optical density of the final solution.
a = Weight of the sample taken for analysis.
b = Volume (ml) of final solution taken for analysis.
822 = Molecular weight of glycyrrhizic acid.
11000 = Molar index of absorption.

Note

Do not use ordinary filter paper, as it is difficult to wash the residue free of nitrofurantoin which will otherwise contribute to absorption at 258 nm.

METHOD 2

The method is based on coupling of acidic genin, β-glycyrrhetinic acid with a basic dye, methylene blue.

Reagents

1. 0.1% w/v solution of methylene blue in water.
2. Citrate-phosphate-borate buffer, pH 9.2.
3. 6 N Sulphuric acid.
4. Ethyl alcohol.

Standard solution

5 mg/100 ml of pure glycyrrhetinic acid in chloroform.

Sample solution

Weigh sample accurately equivalent to 1 g of liquorice, add 20 ml of boiling water. Transfer the contents to a separating funnel and wash the residue with further two 10 ml portions of boiling water, cool, add 5 ml of ethyl alcohol and 1 ml of 6 N sulphuric acid. Shake gently with three 20 ml portions of chloroform. Discard chloroform layer, transfer aqueous phase and the residue to boiling flask with the help of 5 ml of water and 10 ml of 6 N sulphuric acid. Heat in boiling water bath for 20 minutes. While hot, transfer to a separator and extract with four 20 ml portions of chloroform. Pass chloroform through 2 g of anhydrous sodium sulphate and dilute to 100 ml with chloroform.

Procedure

To 20 ml of chloroform layer of sample solution, add 20 ml of buffer pH 9.2 and 2 ml of dye solution. Shake for 1 minute and allow to separate (after separation, the aqueous layer must be blue in colour, if it has greenish or yellow colour, add 1 ml more of dye solution and re-shake). Separate chloroform layer and shake with 5 ml of pH 9.2 buffer and separate chloroform layer. Continue the extraction of the dye complex with further 10, 5, 5 ml portions of chloroform, shaking each layer in turn with the same 5 ml of pH 9.2 buffer solution. All chloroform layers are combined (do not pass chloroform extract through sodium sulphate at this stage) and diluted to 100 ml with ethanol. To 5 ml of standard solution (50 mcg/ml of glycyrrhetinic acid), add 15 ml of chloroform and couple with the dye as above. The absorbance of the extracted ion-pair complex of both standard and sample solution is measured at maximum at about 640 nm against a blank prepared at the same time and by same coupling procedure but with 20 ml of chloroform. The method obeys Beer's law in the range of 5-10 mcg/ml.

Calculation

$$\%\ \text{glycyrrhizin} = \frac{a_u \times 1.75 \times \text{average weight of the tablet}}{a_s \times \text{weight of sample taken}}$$

1.75 = transformation factor of glycyrrhetinic acid to glycyrrhizin.

Note

The first chloroform extraction in the procedure for sample preparation ensures elimination of free acidic constituent such as simple organic acid, sugar acid and free glycyrrhetinic acid. The procedure ensures complete glycyrrhizic acid hydrolysis and extraction of liberated glycyrrhetinic acid.

Estimation of Trimethoprim

Weigh accurate quantity of the sample equivalent to 200 mg of trimethoprim. Extract with three 50 ml portions of boiling chloroform, filtering through sintered glass funnel (G_4). Evaporate the combined chloroform extract to 20 ml and titrate with 0.05 N perchloric acid using α-naphtholbenzein as indicator. Each ml of 0.05 N perchloric acid is equivalent to 0.01451 g of trimethoprim.

Formulation 24

Nalidixic acid, Metronidazole/ Metronidazole benzoate

In oral suspension, metronidazole benzoate is used because of its being tasteless, whereas in solid oral dosage form, metronidazole is used.

METHOD 1

Estimation of Nalidixic acid

Standard solution

12 mcg/ml of nalidixic acid in 0.1 N sodium hydroxide.

Sample solution

Shake the sample gently and then transfer accurately measured volume of the sample equivalent to 300 mg of nalidixic acid to separating funnel. Add 10 ml of 1 N sodium hydroxide and extract with four 25 ml portions of chloroform. Wash the combined chloroform layer with 15 ml of water containing 0.1 ml of 0.1 N sodium hydroxide (reserve the chloroform layer for estimation of metronidazole). Transfer the alkaline layer and washings to a 250 ml volumetric flask and dilute to volume with water. Further dilutions are done appropriately with 0.1 N sodium hydroxide to get a concentration of 12 mcg/ml in respect of nalidixic acid.

Measure the extinction of both sample and standard solutions at maxima at about 334 nm and calculate the results by comparing.

Estimation of Metronidazole benzoate

Standard solution

Dissolve accurately weighed quantity of metronidazole benzoate in 0.1 N methanolic sulphuric acid to get a solution of 15 mcg/ml in respect of metronidazole.

Sample solution

Transfer the combined chloroform extract reserved in the estimation of nalidixic acid to a dry 100 ml volumetric flask by passing through anhydrous sodium sulphate. Dilute to volume. Further dilutions are done with 0.1 N methanolic sulphuric acid to get a concentration of 15 mcg/ml in respect of metronidazole. Measure the extinction of both samples and standard solutions at maxima at about 277 nm using 0.1 N methanolic sulphuric acid as blank. Calculate the results by comparison.

Metronidazole benzoate may be converted to metronidazole by applying the factor $\frac{171.2}{275.3}$

METHOD 2

This method is used when metronidazole is present as base (not as benzoate) as in solid dosage forms.

Estimation of Metronidazole

Standard solution

1 mg/ml of metronidazole in 0.1 N hydrochloric acid. Further dilution is done quantitatively with 0.1 N hydrochloric acid to get a solution of 15 mcg/ml of metronidazole.

Sample solution

Transfer accurately weighed quantity of the sample equivalent to 45 mg of metronidazole to a separator. Add 25 ml of 0.1 N hydrochloric acid and extract with four 25 ml portions of chloroform. Wash the combined chloroform layer with three 30 ml portions of 0.1 N hydrochloric acid (reserve the chloroform layer for estimation of nalidixic acid). Dilute the combined acid layer and washings to 250 ml with 0.1 N hydrochloric acid. Filter and dilute further appropriately with 0.1 N hydrochloric acid to get a concentration of 15 mcg/ml in respect of metronidazole.

Measure the extinction of both sample and standard solutions at maximum at about 277 nm using 0.1 N hydrochloric acid as blank and calculate the results by comparison.

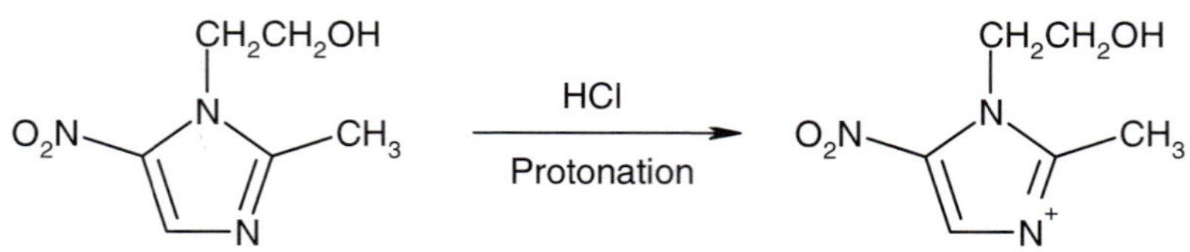

Metronidazole **Protonated metronidazole (cationic species)** (λ_{max} 277 nm)

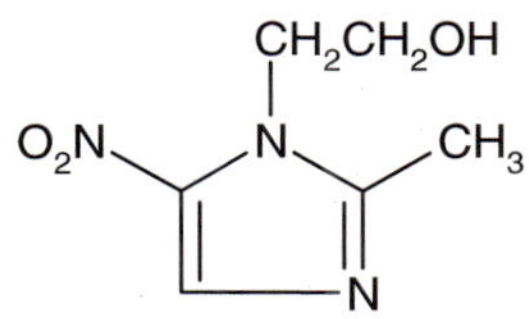

Metronidazole alcoholic solution
(λ_{max} 310 nm)

METHOD 3

In case of solid dosage forms (capsules and tablets), the following simple and inexpensive method can be used with reasonable accuracy and precision.

Standard solution

15 mcg/ml of metronidazole in water.

Sample solution

Weigh accurately a quantity of the sample equivalent to 150 mg of metronidazole. Extract the dry powder with three 25 ml portions of water, filtering each through the same G_2 sintered glass funnel. Dilute the combined filtrate to 100 ml with water.

Measure the extinction of both the solutions at about 310 nm using water as blank. Deduce the results by comparison.

Note

In hydrochloric acid, metronidazole exists as cationic acid. UV absorption maximum of this cationic species is 277 nm whereas in neutral medium (water, ethanol) the longest wavelength maximum i.e. 310 nm is observed.

Estimation of Nalidixic acid

METHOD 1

Standard solution

About 9.5 mcg/ml of nalidixic acid in chloroform.

Sample solution

Pass the combined chloroform layer reserved in the estimation of metronidazole through anhydrous sodium sulphate (pre-moistened with chloroform) and make upto 100 ml with chloroform. Dilute further appropriately with chloroform to get a concentration of about 10 mcg/ml.

Measure the extinction of both sample and standard solutions at maxima at about 334 nm using chloroform as blank and calculate the results by comparison.

Note

Nalidixic acid exhibits the same maxima i.e. 334 nm both in alkaline medium as well in chloroform.

METHOD 2

Use the entire residue left after the extraction of metronidazole as above. Dissolve the residue left in sintered funnel in 2 N sodium hydroxide and follow the procedure described under method-1 of this formulation.

Alternatively, the residue is taken up in neutral (phenolphthalein) methanol and titrated with 0.1 N sodium hydroxide. Each ml of 0.1 N sodium hydroxide is equivalent to 0.02322 g of nalidixic acid. This involves titration of carboxylic group present in the molecule.

METHOD 3

Nalidixic acid forms chelate with ferric nitrate with λ_{max} at 430 nm.

Probable Reaction Mechanism

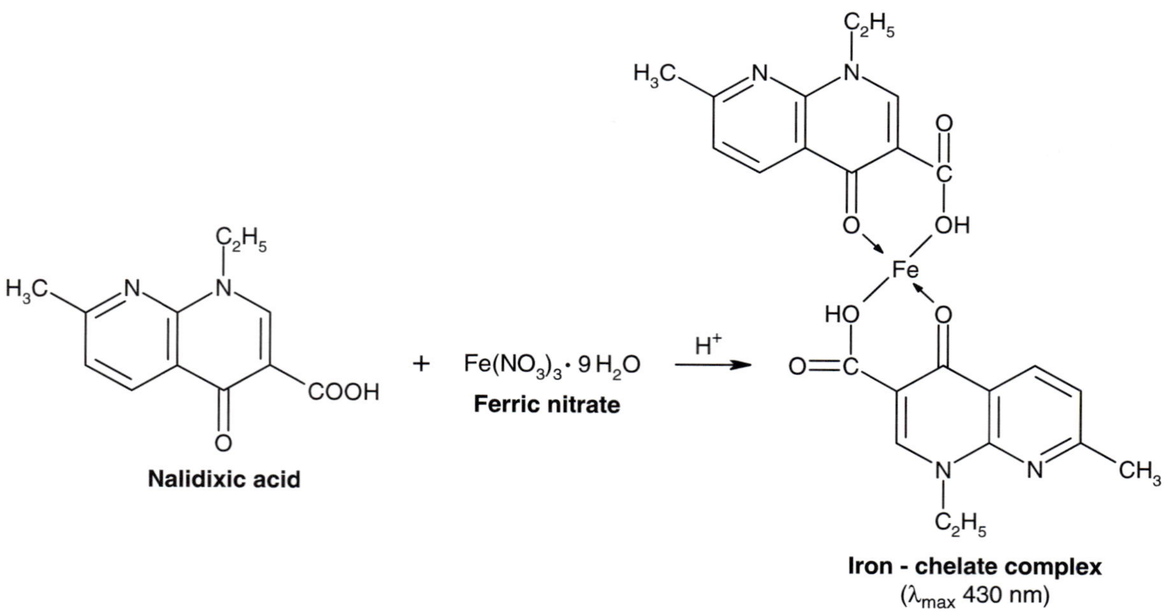

Reference

K.P.R. Chowdary & P. Venkateshwara Rao. *Indian Drugs*, **28(12)**, 569-570, 1991.

Nalidixic acid chelate with Fe(III) in DMF/methanol medium as reported by the authors has following formulae.

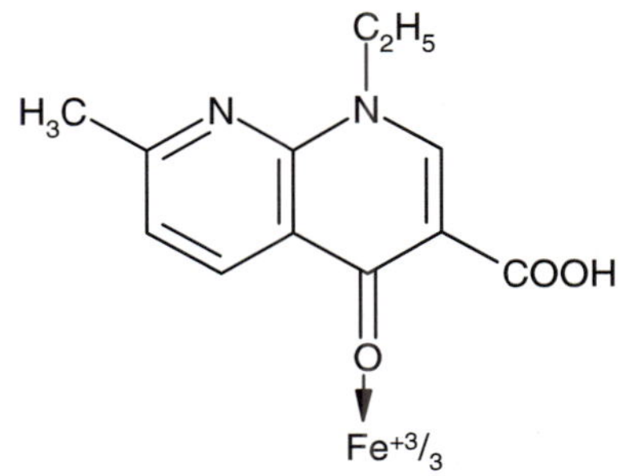

G. Rama Rao et al. have also reported analytical method based on oxidative coupling with MBTH. The method is similar to the one reported for norfloxacin and ciprofloxacin under chapter on alimentary system.

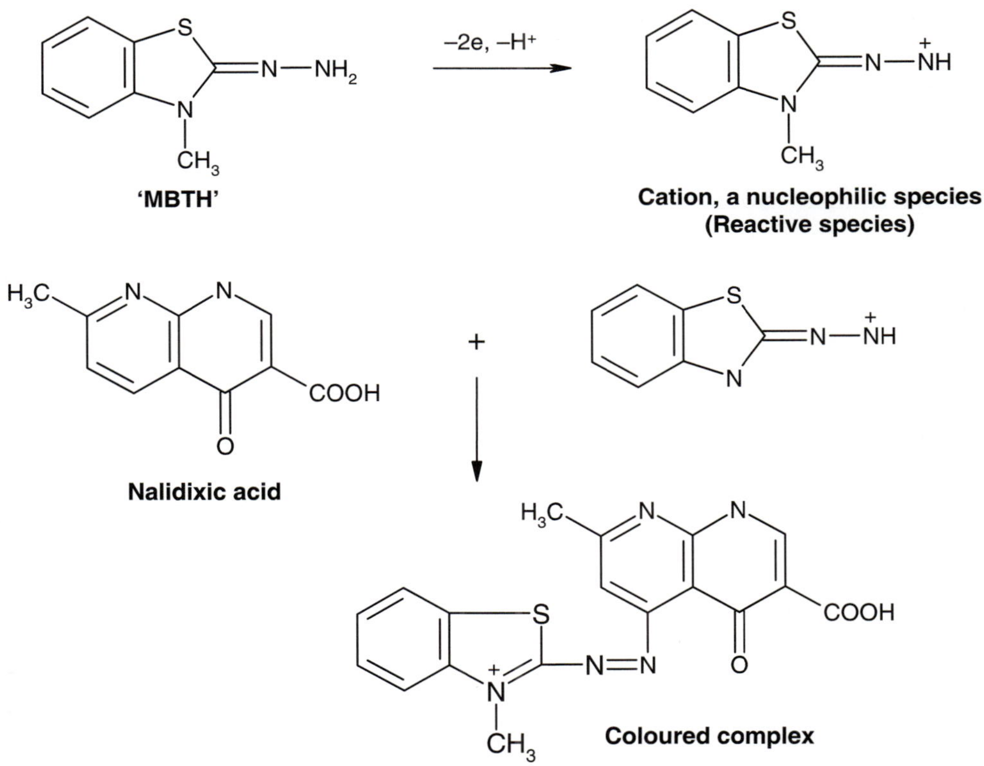

The cation will attack at p-position as ortho being occupied.

Reference

G. Rama Rao, A.B. Avadhanulu & D.K. Valsa. *Indian Drugs*, **27**, 532, 1990.

Formulation 25

Phenazopyridine hydrochloride, Nalidixic acid

ESTIMATION

Phenazopyridine hydrochloride

Standard solution

6 mcg/ml of phenazopyridine hydrochloride in chloroform.

Sample solution

Transfer accurately weighed sample equivalent to 100 mg of phenazopyridine hydrochloride to a separator, add 50 ml of 1 M sodium hydroxide solution. Extract with four 50 ml portions of chloroform. (Reserve alkaline layer for estimation of Nalidixic acid). Pass organic layer through anhydrous sodium sulphate and make up the volume to 250 ml with chloroform. Transfer 3 ml of the solution and dilute to 200 ml with chloroform (6 mcg/ml).

Measure the extinction of both the solutions at maxima at about 390 nm using chloroform as blank. Calculate the results by comparison.

Nalidixic acid

Standard solution 8 mcg/ml of nalidixic acid in 1 M sodium hydroxide.

Sample solution

Dilute sodium hydroxide layer obtained during the estimation of phenazopyridine above appropriately with 1 M sodium hydroxide to get 8 mcg/ml.

Measure the extinction of both sample and standard solutions at maxima at about 258 nm and calculate the results by comparison.

Note

These two compounds PPZ and NLA are usually formulated in the ratio 1 : 10 and there is no mutual interference at their respective maxima.

The following simple method can also be applied to such formulations without prior separation or extraction of each ingredient.

Nalidixic acid and phenazopyridine hydrochloride are usually present in the ratio of 10 : 1.

Common sample solution

Weigh accurately the powdered sample equivalent to 25 mg of nalidixic acid and transfer to 100 ml volumetric flask. Add 70-80 ml of chloroform : methanol (80 : 20) mixture, warm gently to ensure complete solution of both the ingredients, cool and dilute to 100 ml with above solution.

Estimation of Nalidixic acid

Standard solution

7.5 mcg/ml of nalidixic acid in chloroform-methanol (80 : 20) v/v mixture.

Sample solution

Dilute the common sample solution prepared above appropriately with the solvent to get final concentration of 7.5 mcg/ml of the substance.

Measure the extinction of both the sample and standard solutions at maxima at about 258 nm against solvent blank and calculate the results by comparison.

Estimation of Phenazopyridine hydrochloride

Standard solution

7.5 mcg/ml of substance in chloroform : methanol (80 : 20) mixture.

Sample solution

Dilute the common sample solution prepared above appropriately with the solvent to get final concentration of 7.5 mcg/ml of the substance.

Measure the extinction of both the sample and standard solutions at maxima at about 390 nm and calculate the results by comparison.

Note

At their respective maxima, there is no significant interference by the other component, so estimation can be done without prior separation or extraction.

Alternatively, the following method is recommended.

Estimation of Nalidixic acid

Standard solution

Weigh accurately about 85 mg of nalidixic acid and transfer to a separating funnel containing about 25 ml 1 M hydrochloric acid.

Sample solution

Weigh accurately quantity of the sample equivalent to 85 mg of nalidixic acid and transfer to separating funnel. Add 25 ml of 1 M hydrochloric acid and shake to disperse the powder.

Extract both sample and standard solutions with three 25 ml portions of chloroform. Wash combined chloroform layer with 25 ml of 1 M hydrochloric acid and use the combined acidic layer for estimation of phenazopyridine hydrochloride by spectrophotometric analysis.

Extract the washed chloroform layer with five 20 ml portions of 1 M sodium hydroxide. Combine the alkaline aqueous layer and dilute to 100 ml with 1 M sodium hydroxide.

Solutions of both sample and standard in 1 M sodium hydroxide are further diluted appropriately to get a concentration of 5 mcg/ml.

Measure the extinction of resulting solutions at maxima at about 258 nm using water as blank. Calculate the contents of nalidixic acid by comparison.

Nalidixic acid forms complex with Fe^{3+} to give yellow-coloured iron chelate (λ_{max} 430 nm). For detailed reaction mechanism, see formulation of this chapter.

Estimation of Phenazopyridine hydrochloride

Method 1

Standard solution

Accurately weigh and transfer about 50 mg of phenazopyridine hydrochloride to a 250 ml separating funnel containing 25 ml of 1 M sodium hydroxide.

Sample solution

Transfer accurately weighed quantity of the sample equivalent to 50 mg of the substance to a separating funnel containing 25 ml of 1 M sodium hydroxide. Shake to disperse. Saturate both sample and standard solutions placed in separating funnel with sodium chloride. Extract with three 25 ml portions of chloroform. Combine the chloroform layer and wash with 25 ml 0.1 M sodium hydroxide. Extract the combined chloroform layer with five 20 ml portions of 0.1 M hydrochloric acid and filter the acid layer through filter paper and make up to 100 ml with the acid. Solutions of both sample and standard are further diluted appropriately with the acid to get final concentration of 7.5 mcg/ml.

Measure the extinction of resulting solutions at maxima at about 390 nm using acid as blank, calculate the results by comparison.

Alternatively accurately weighed quantity of the sample is extracted dry with three 25 ml portions of 0.1 M hydrochloric acid, filtering each through the same G_2 sintered glass funnel. Dilute the combined filtrate to 100 ml with 0.1 N hydrochloric acid and use for estimation of phenazopyridine by methods discussed above. Dissolve the insoluble residue in 0.1 N sodium hydroxide and use for estimation of nalidixic acid by methods discussed above.

METHOD 2

Reagents

1. 2% w/v solution of sodium nitrite in water.
2. 5% w/v solution of ammonium sulphamate in water.
3. 0.1% w/v solution of N-(1-naphthylethylenediamine dihydrochloride (NED).
4. 1 M Hydrochloric acid.

Standard solution

50 mcg/ml of phenazopyridine hydrochloride in water.

Sample solution

An accurately weighed quantity of powdered sample equivalent to 5 mg of the substance was extracted with water and diluted to 100 ml, filtered.

Procedure

To 5 ml each of sample and standard solutions, add 1 ml of 1 M hydrochloric acid and 2 ml of sodium nitrite solution. Keep aside for 10 min then add 2 ml of ammonium sulphamate solution. Keep aside for 5 min and add 1 ml of 'NED' reagent. Dilute to 25 ml with water. Measure the absorbance of both the solutions at about 550 nm after 15 min against reagent blank prepared by taking 5 ml of water instead of sample. Deduce the results by comparison.

Explanatory Note

Diazotization of the drug is carried out with HNO_2. The nitrosonium ion formed attacks the amino group present in the drug resulting in the formation of diazotized product. As usual, the diazotized product answers Bratton-Marshall reaction resulting in the formation violet azo dye.

Probable Reaction Mechanism

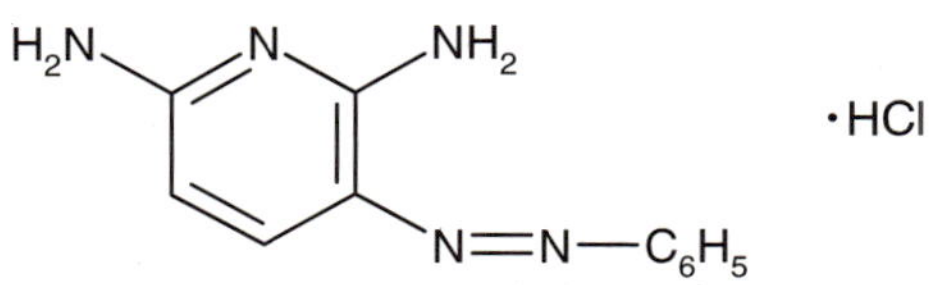

Phenazopyridine hydrochloride

$$NaNO_2 + HCl \longrightarrow NaCl + HNO_2 \xrightarrow{H^+} H_2\overset{+}{O}N{=}O \xrightarrow{Cl^-} Cl^- \overset{+}{N}{\equiv}O^- + H_2O$$

Nitroso ion

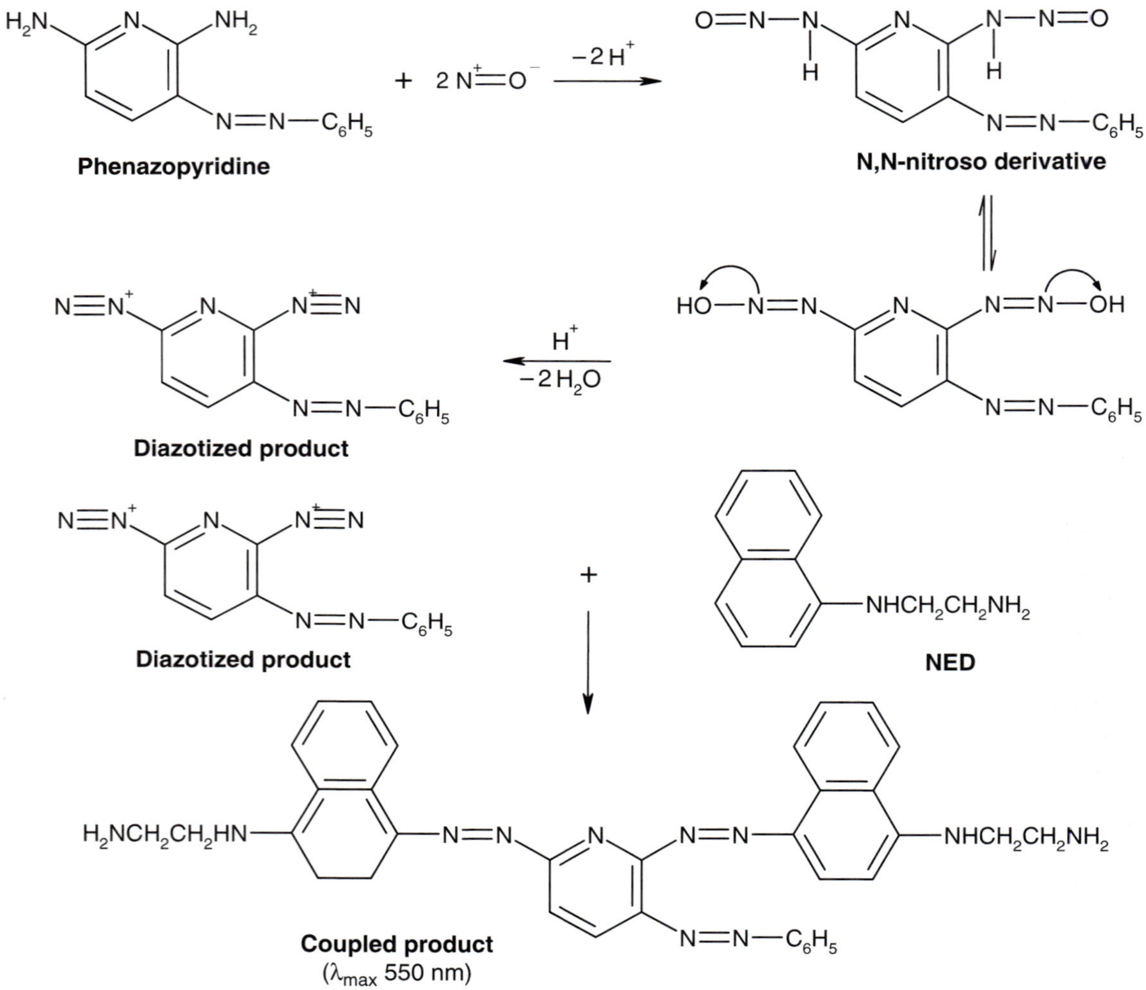

The excess HNO_2 is destroyed by ammonium sulphamate.

$$HNO_2 + H_2NSO_3H \longrightarrow H_2SO_4 + N_2\uparrow + H_2O$$

Note

If the quantity of the diazotization reagent is restricted, diazotization and coupling shall take place at only one amino group.

Reference

S.C. Mathur, Y. Kumar, N. Murugesan, Y.K.S. Rathor & P.D. Sethi. *Eastern Pharmacist*, pp. 189-190, August 1992; *Indian Drugs*, **29(5)**, 375-376, 1992.

Formulation 26

Trimethoprim, Sulphadiazine

ESTIMATION

Trimethoprim

Weigh accurately a quantity of the sample equivalent to 50 mg of trimethoprim. Add about 30 ml of 0.1 N sodium hydroxide, mix to suspend. Extract with four 50 ml portions of chloroform, washing each extract with the same two 10 ml portions of 0.1 N sodium hydroxide, wash the combined chloroform layer with water till washings are neutral. (Combine the alkaline layer and washings and reserve for estimation of sulphadiazine). Evaporate chloroform layer to dryness, take up the residue in glacial acetic acid with the aid of gentle heat. Titrate with 0.1 N perchloric acid using crystal violet as indicator. Each ml of 0.1 N perchloric acid is equivalent to 0.02903 g of trimethoprim. Alternatively, take up the residue in dilute acetic acid and dilute appropriately and stepwise to get concentration of 15 mcg/ml. Measure the extinction of the solution at 271 nm and calculate the contents of trimethoprim taking 204 as value of E 1%, 1 cm at 271 nm.

Sulphadiazine

Standard solution

5 mcg/ml of sulphadiazine in 0.1 N sodium hydroxide.

Sample solution

Combine the alkaline aqueous layer and the washings reserved during estimation of trimethoprim and dilute with 0.1 N sodium hydroxide to produce 100 ml. Dilute further appropriately with 0.1 N sodium hydroxide to get concentration of 5 mcg/ml. Measure the extinction of both the solutions at about 240 nm and calculate the results by comparison. Alternatively, the sample can be taken up in water and hydrochloric acid and titrated with 0.1 M sodium nitrite. Each ml of 0.1 M sodium nitrite is equivalent to 0.02503 g of sulphadiazine.

Note

Owing to inductive effect of SO_2 group, N—H group has acidic property; so the compound dissolves in sodium hydroxide.

Probable Reaction Mechanism

$$NaNO_2 + HCl \longrightarrow NaCl + HNO_2$$

$$HNO_2 + H_2O \xrightarrow{H^+} \overset{+}{N}{=}O$$

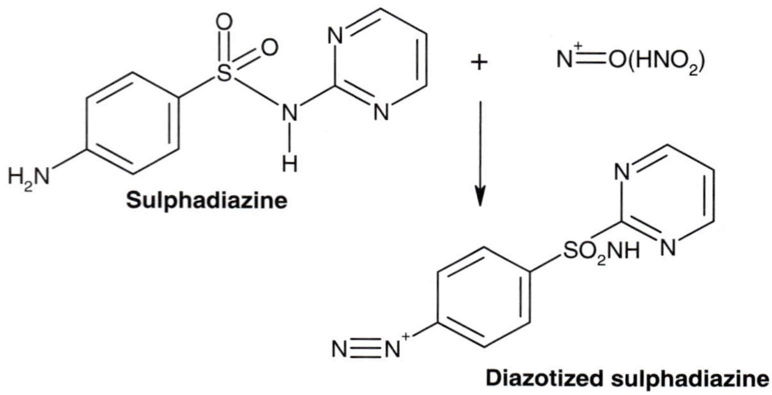

Excess HNO_2 librates iodine from starch-iodide paper giving blue colour, the end point.

Note

Sulphonamides are amphoteric compounds. They have weakly basic property due to aniline structure and thus can form salt with strong acids. Due to inductive effect of 'SO_2' group they have an available —N—H acidity and thus dissolve in alkali hydroxide solutions, extent of solubility being dependent on degree of substitution on the sulphonamide group.

Reported reactions of sulphonamides for analytical interest

Detailed analytical methods have been reported by different authors, the reference for the same has been cited. Probable reaction mechanism for each method has been explained.

METHOD 1

Primary aromatic amino group present in the drugs undergoes Michael addition with the reagent eliminating the monohydrogen sulphite radical giving the final product.

Probable Reaction Mechanism

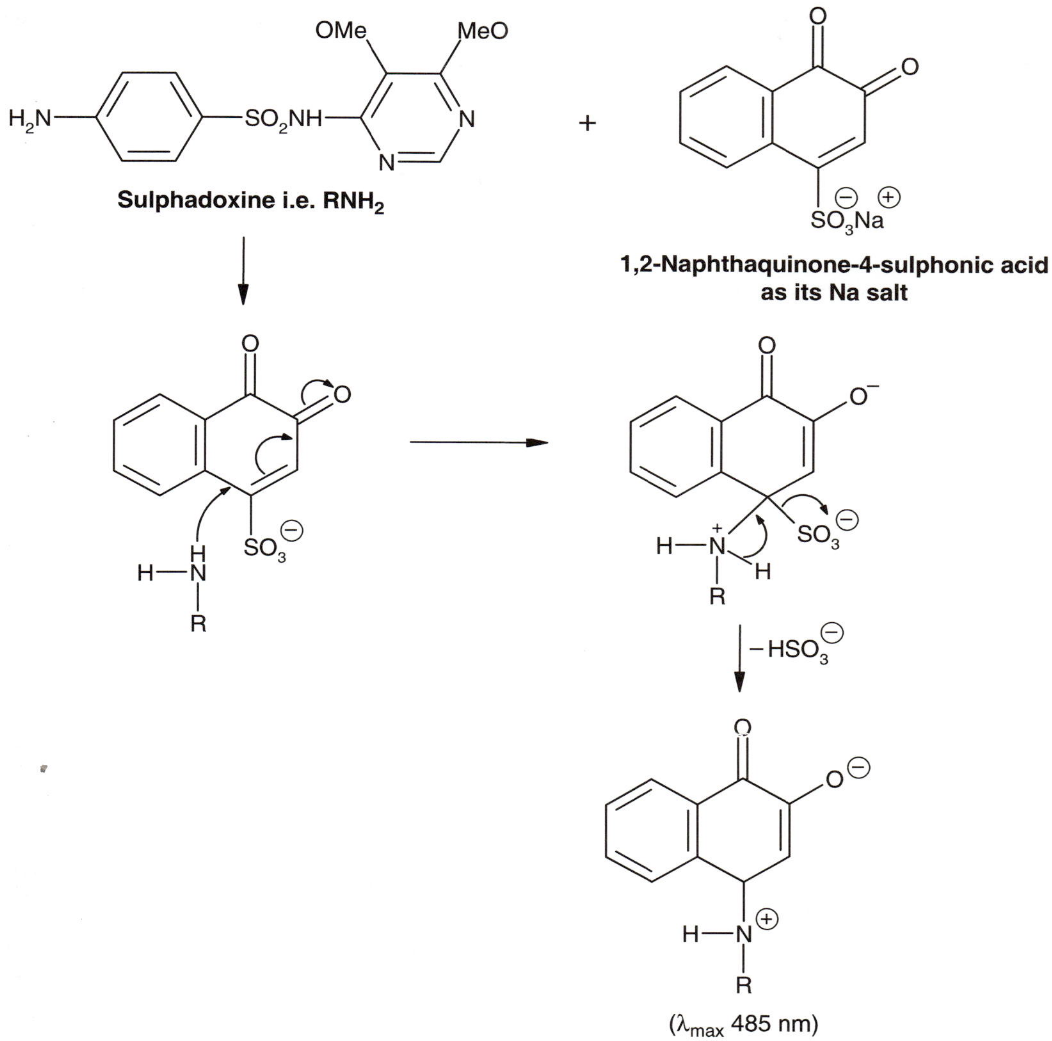

Reference

G. Rama Rao, S.S.N. Murthy & I.R.K. Raju. *Eastern Pharmacist*, pp. 185-186, Aug. 1989.

METHOD 2

In the presence of an oxidising agent like ammonium cerium (IV) sulphate or Fe(III), MBTH can result in the formation of a diazonium salt which can attack the electron-rich i.e. nucleophilic amino group of the drug resulting in the formation of the corresponding product.

The NH_2 group of sulphadoxine may be responsible for the reaction with MBTH. Phthalylsulphathiazole in which the NH_2 group is blocked by phthalyl group will not yield any colour under the experimental conditions.

Probable Reaction Mechanism

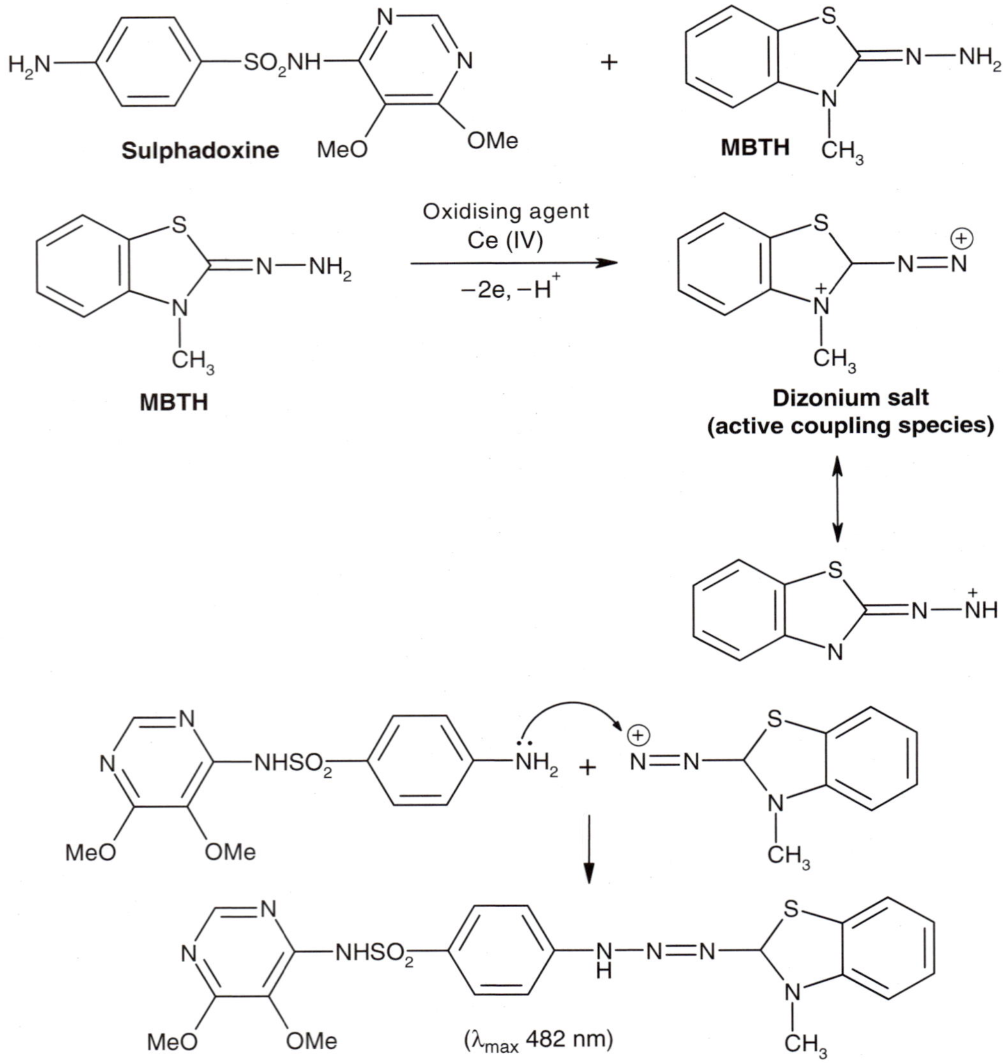

Reference

1. Pharmaceutical Chemistry (Vol. 2), 1991 by H.J. Roth, pp. 74, 75.
2. Textbook of Practical Organic Chemistry by Vogel, p. 948.
3. G. Rama Rao, S.S.N. Murthy & I.R.K. Raju. *Eastern Pharmacist*, pp. 137-138, Sept. 1987.

METHOD 3

The amine group of the drug being a nucleophile adds to chloranil resulting in the loss of a HCl molecule and formation of Michael type addition product.

Probable Reaction Mechanism

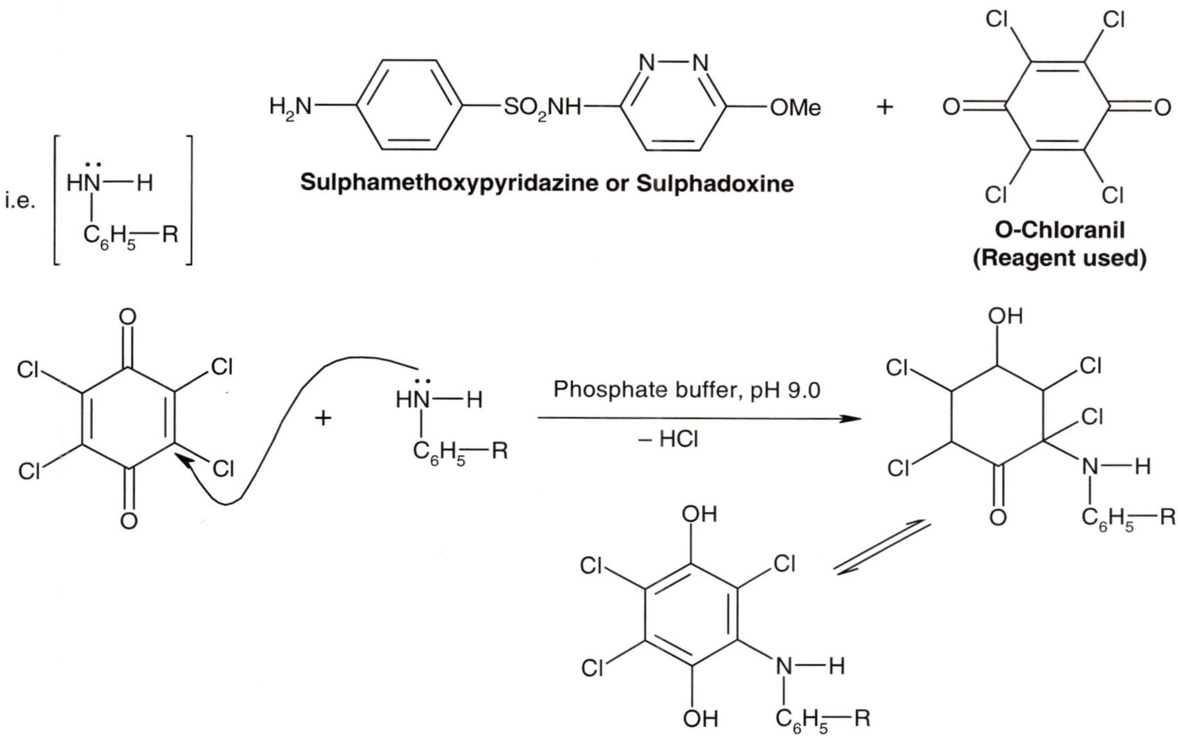

The product
(λ_{max} 525 nm)

The product may undergo oxidation if there is presence of excess of hydroxyquinone in the medium.

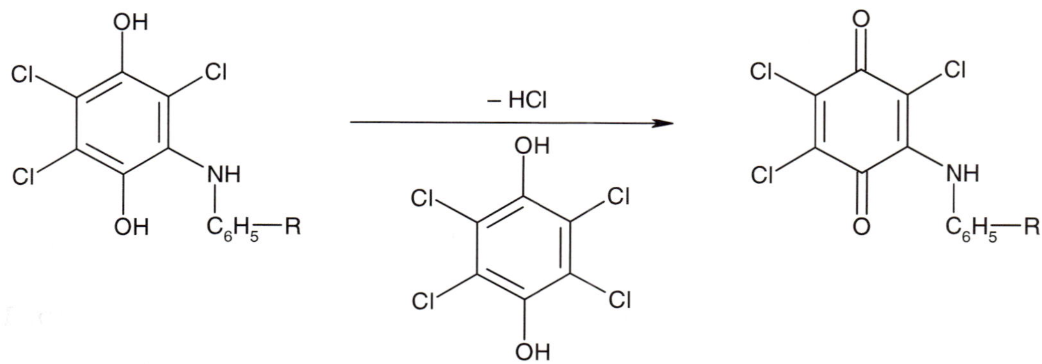

Reference

1. G. Rama Rao, S.S.N. Murthy, I.R.K. Raju & P. Jagannadha. *Indian Drugs*, **26(5)**, 237, 1989; 26(8), 414, 1989.
2. Pharmaceutical Chemistry (Vol. 2) by H.J. Roth, pp. 106, 107.

METHOD 4

Amino group present in the molecule forms Schiff's base in acidic medium with PDAB and PDAC.

Probable Reaction Mechanism

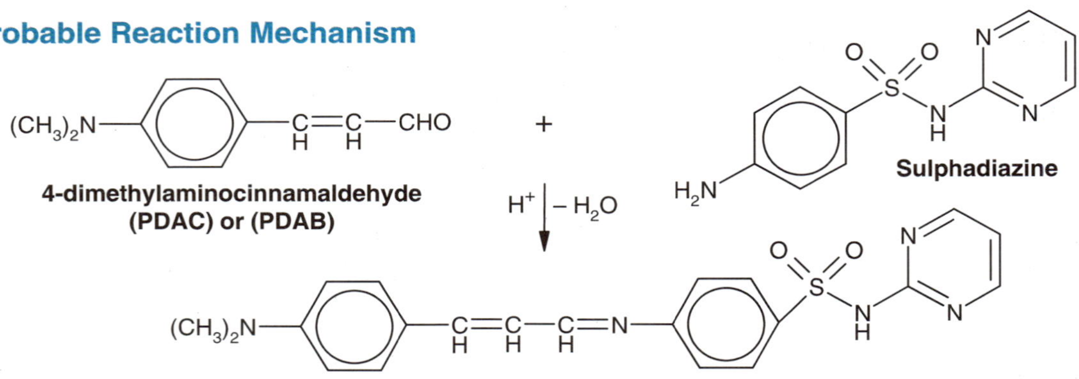

PDAC complex (Red chromogen)
(λ_{max} 545 nm)

Similar to the reaction with 'PDAC' and 'PDAB', the sulphonamides react with furfural to give Schiff's base. In the presence of acetic acid, hydrolytic dissociation occurs to give dicarbonyl compound whose end-point —CHO group reacts with one more mole of sulphonamide to give red dye.

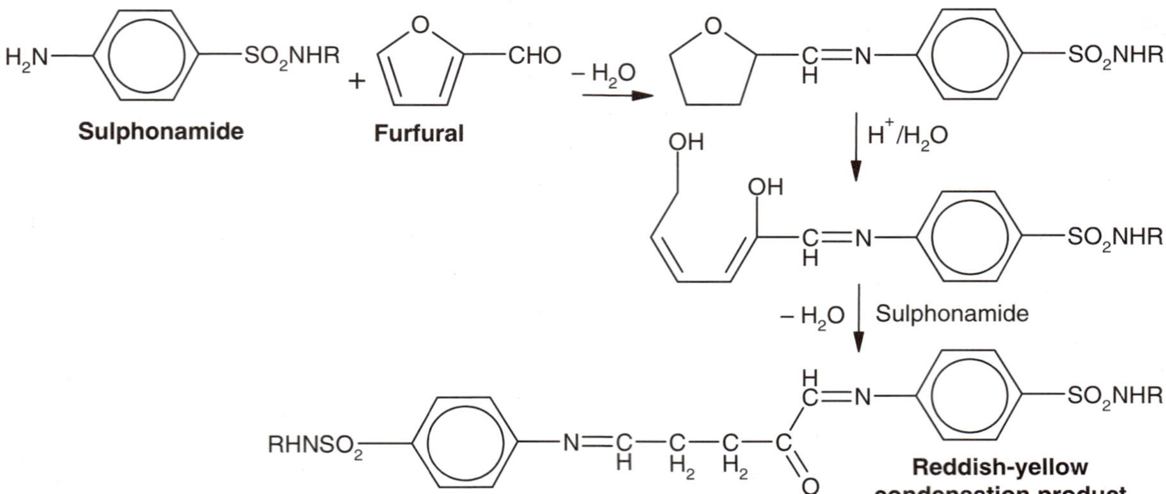

Reddish-yellow condensation product
(λ_{max} 485 nm)

Reference

1. Pharmaceutical Chemistry (Vol. 2) by H.J. Roth, p. 432.
2. N.M. Sanghavi & Varsha Tandel, *Indian Drugs*, **30(3)**, 132-137, 1993; and S. Raghuveer, I.R.K. Raju, D.K. Vatsa & C.M.R. Srivastava, *Indian Drugs*, **30(4)**, 191-193, 1992.

Note

Trimethoprim present in the same formulation with sulphadiazine does not interfere in spite of free amino group being available. As in this compound the amino group is attached to the pyrimidine ring as shown in the structure. Pyrimidine ring is electron deficient and hence the amino group will not react to form Schiff's base.

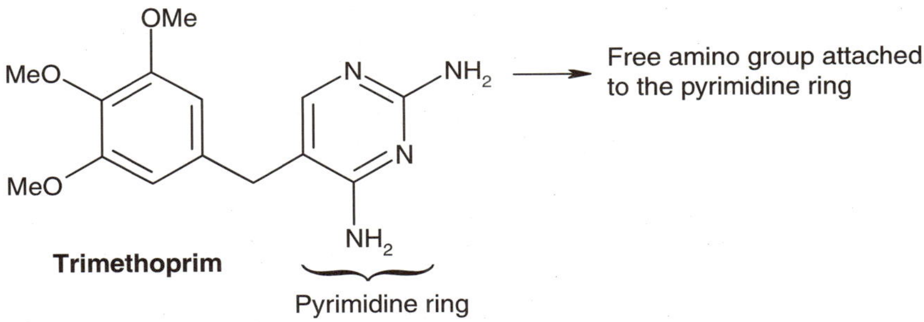

Trimethoprim

METHOD 5

In the presence of oxidising agent i.e. Na-metaperiodate, oxidative coupling occurs between the reagent and the ortho position to the amino group in the drug resulting in the formation of the product.

Probable Reaction Mechanism

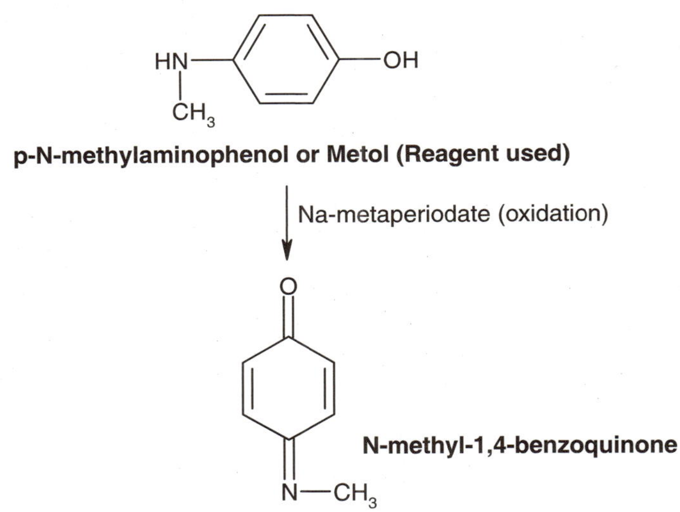

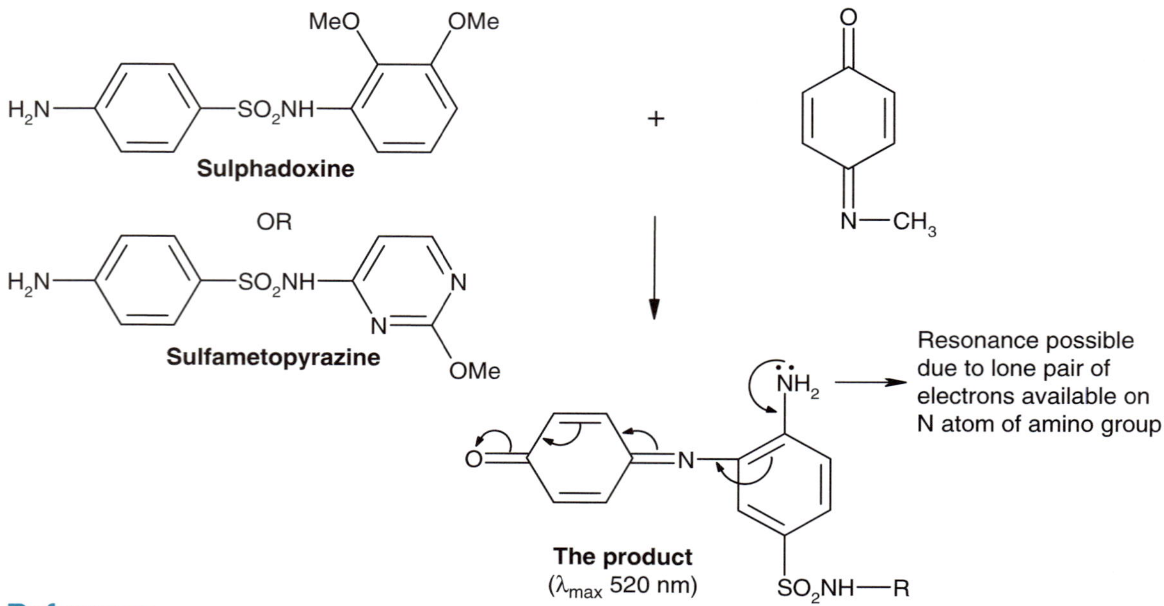

Reference

1. G. Rama Rao, S.S.N. Murthy & I.R.K. Raju, *Indian Drugs*, **26(8)**, pp. 417-420, 1989.
2. Pharmaceutical Chemistry (Vol. 2) by H.J. Roth, pp. 398, 433.

Note

Both the drugs, pyrimethamine and trimethoprim, do not interfere as they do not contain a free ortho position next to the amino group.

R. Ramakrishna & Sastry (1979) have reported the use of potassium dichromate as oxidising agent for estimation of several drugs with primary aromatic amine such as sulphonamide, benzocaine, chloramphenicol (after reduction with Zn + HCl).

Reference

1. R. Ramakrishna & C.S. Sastry, *Talanta*, **26**, 861-865, 1979.
2. C.S.P. Sastry, T.M.K. Reddy & B.G. Rao, *Indian Drugs*, 145-152, 1984.

METHOD 6

The undermentioned reaction has been studied in respect of sulphadiazine, sulphacetamide, sulphanilamide, sulphasomidine and sulphadimidine. These drugs can be represented as

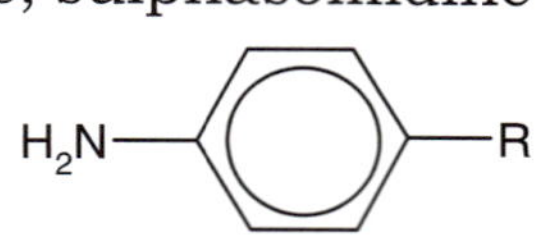

Probable Reaction Mechanism

All these drugs contain a primary aromatic group which is initially diazotized by using $NaNO_2$ and HCl. The diazotized product then couples with orcinol, resulting in the formation of the product.

Diazotization of the primary aromatic amino group of the drug

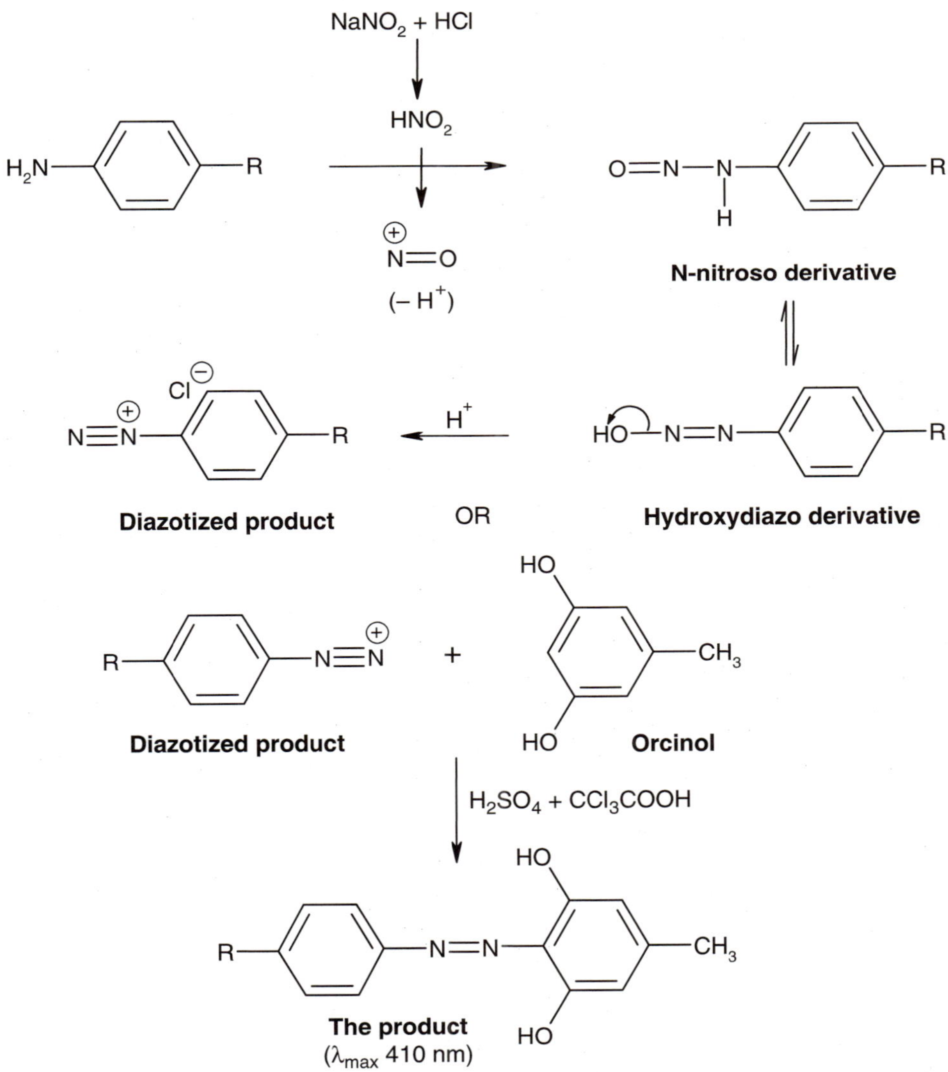

A general method based on reaction of primary aromatic amines with 9-chloroacridine can also be applied for estimation of sulphonamides with free amino groups or amino group released as a result of hydrolysis. The reaction yields a coloured product with λ_{max} at about 435 nm.

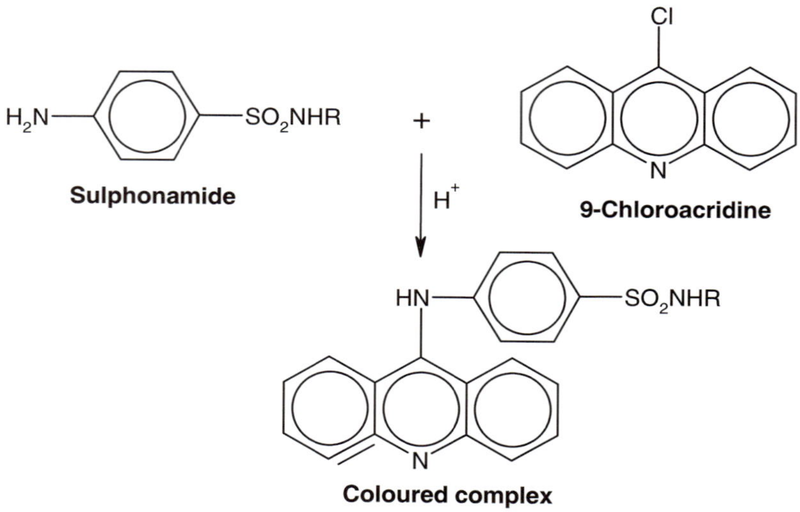

Reference

1. James T. Stewart & D.M. Lotti, *J. Pharm. Sci.*, 59(6), 838-840, 1970.
2. James T. Stewart & David A. Settle, *J. Pharm. Sci.*, 64(8), 1403-1405, 1975.

Sulphonamide undergoes oxidation reaction with cerric (IV) in acidic medium to yield a chromogen (λ_{max} 460 nm).

Probable Reaction Mechanism

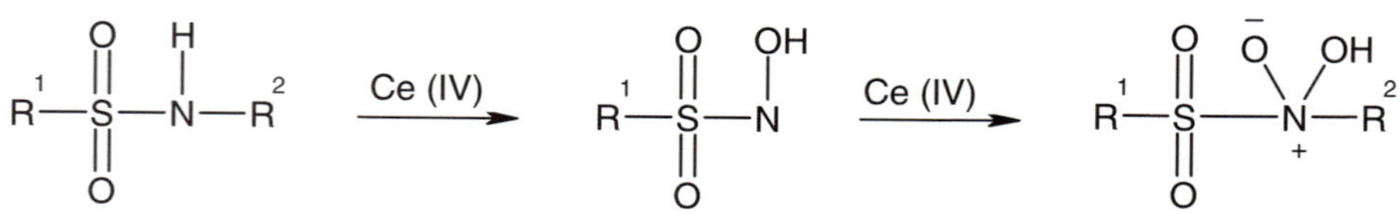

Note

Trimethoprim did not interfere.

Reference

Sajid Hussain, A.S.R. Krishnamurthy, P. Ravi Prasad & R. Sekar, *Indian Drugs*, **32(7)**, 336-339, 1999.

Sane et al. have described spectrophotometric method for several sulphonamides (sulphadiazine, sulphaphenazole, sulphasomidine, sulphanilamide, sulphacetamide sodium, sulphathoazole, sulphaguainidine, sulphadimidine, sulphamethoxazole) based on reaction of diazotized sulphonate with Bratton-Marshall reagent and some other coupling reagents.

Reagents

1. 0.1% solution of sodium nitrite in water.
2. Acid mixture: Mix 86 ml of trichloroacetic acid and 20 ml of 2 M sulphuric acid and dilute to 20 ml with water.
3. Alcohol.

Coupling reagents

(a) α-naphthylamine (0.1% in alcohol).
(b) m-aminophenol (0.4% in water).
(c) N-1-naphthyl ethylene diamine dihydrochloride (NED) (0.1% in water).

Sample and standard solutions

250 μg/ml of respective sulphonamide in water.

Procedure

To 1 ml each of sample and standard solutions, add 5 ml of acid mixture and 0.5 ml of sodium nitrite solution, allow to stand for 5 min till diazotization is complete. Then add 5 ml of alcohol (to remove excess of HNO_2) and stabilize the diazotized product and remove turbidity, if any. Then add 0.5 ml of NED reagent, dilute the solution to 50 ml with water and measure the absorbance at 545 nm against reagent blank.

Probable Reaction Mechanism

Diazotization of the primary aromatic amino group of the drug is carried using nitrous acid obtained by the reaction of sodium nitrite in acid mixture.

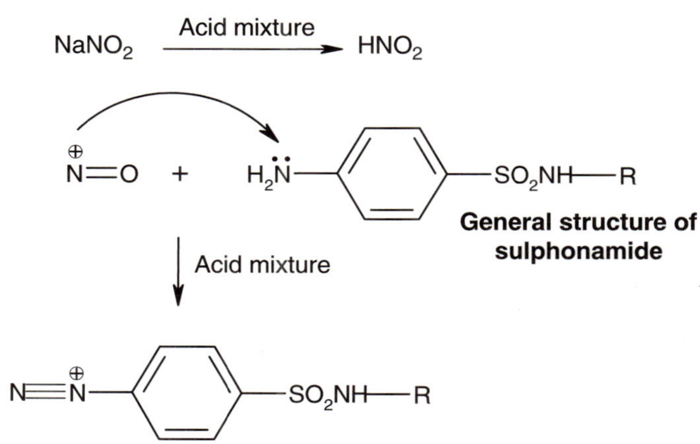

Diazotized product

Diazotized sulphonamide couples with α-naphthylamine and N-(naphthyl-ethylenediamine) (NED) at para position to give coloured product as shown.

Probable Reaction Mechanism

(a)

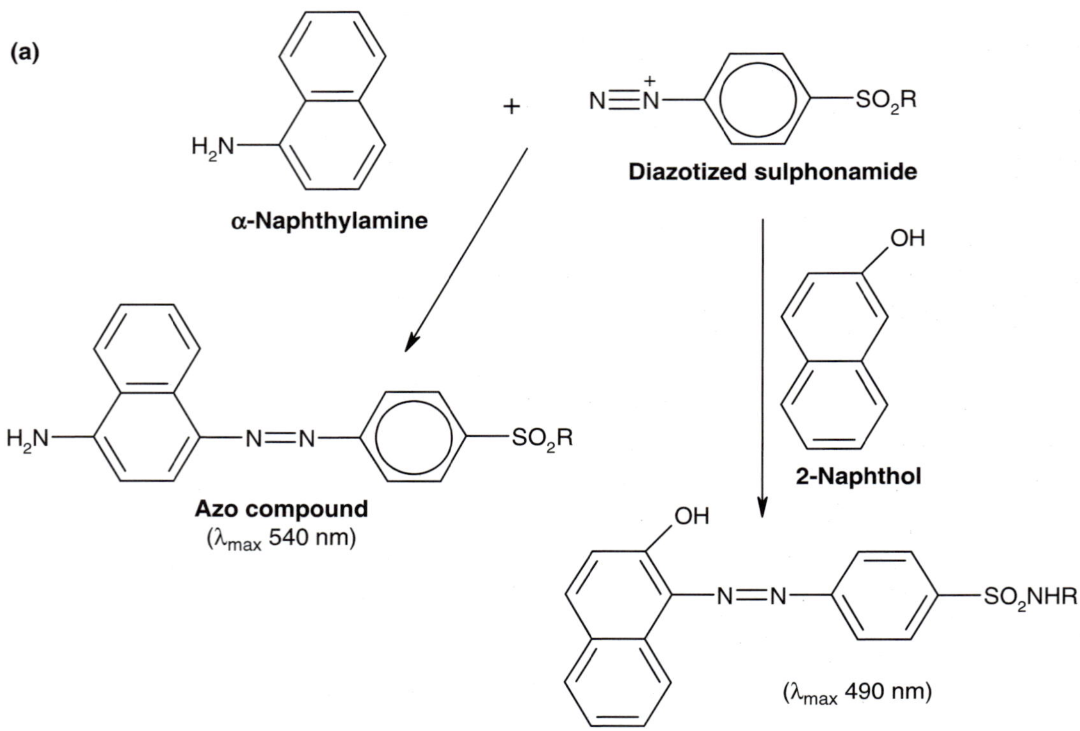

(b)

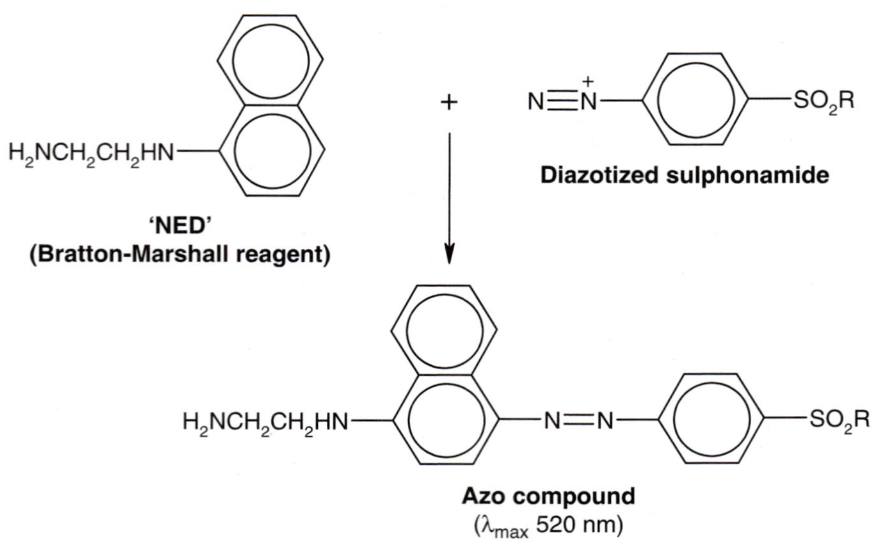

Reference

R.T. Sane & V.G. Nayak, *Indian Drugs*, **19(5)**, 206-210, 1982.

Note

1. Hydroxyl (OH) or amino groups (NH_2) if they are ortho or para to azo bond such as 2-naphthol, they intensify the colour of azo compounds.
2. The compounds in which azo linkage is between 2 aromatic rings are highly coloured since these compounds have extended conjugation system.
3. The method is similar for eye and ear drops, tablets, ointments, creams and lotions, etc.

Note

The amino group couples oxidatively with 4-aminophenol to give coloured product (λ_{max} 465 nm).

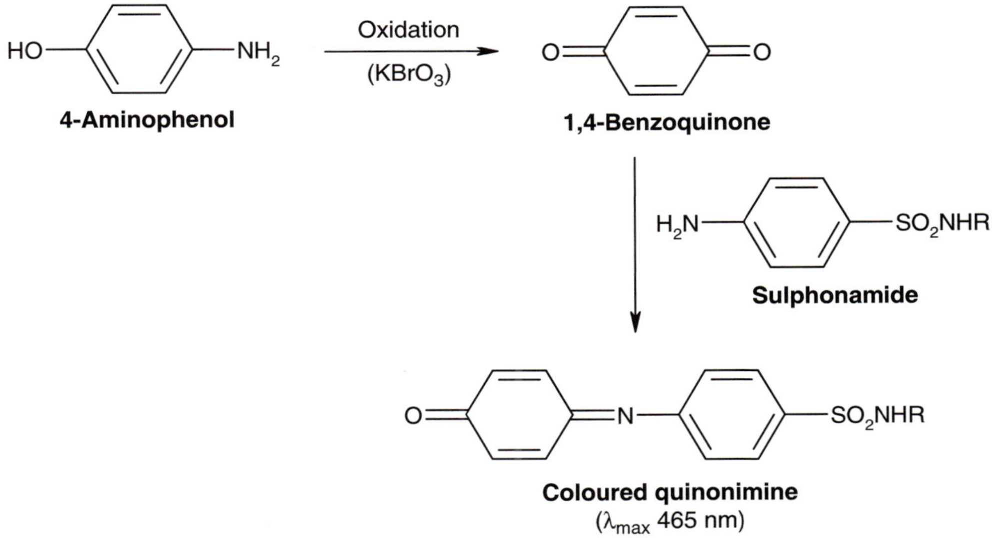

Reference

Pharmaceutical Chemistry (Vol. 2) by H.J. Roth, p. 433.

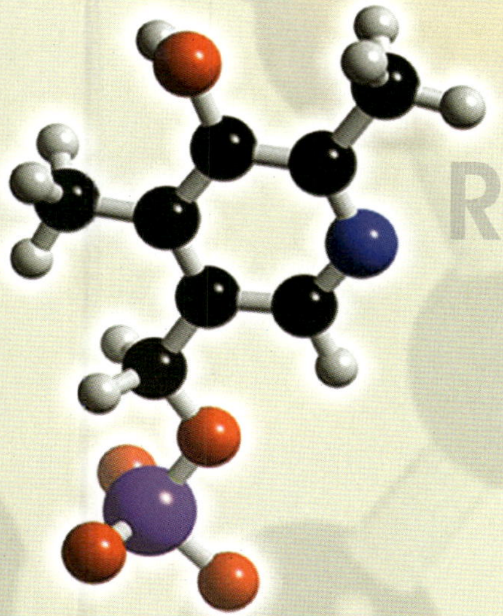

Reaction Mechanism

10

Sedatives and Tranquillisers

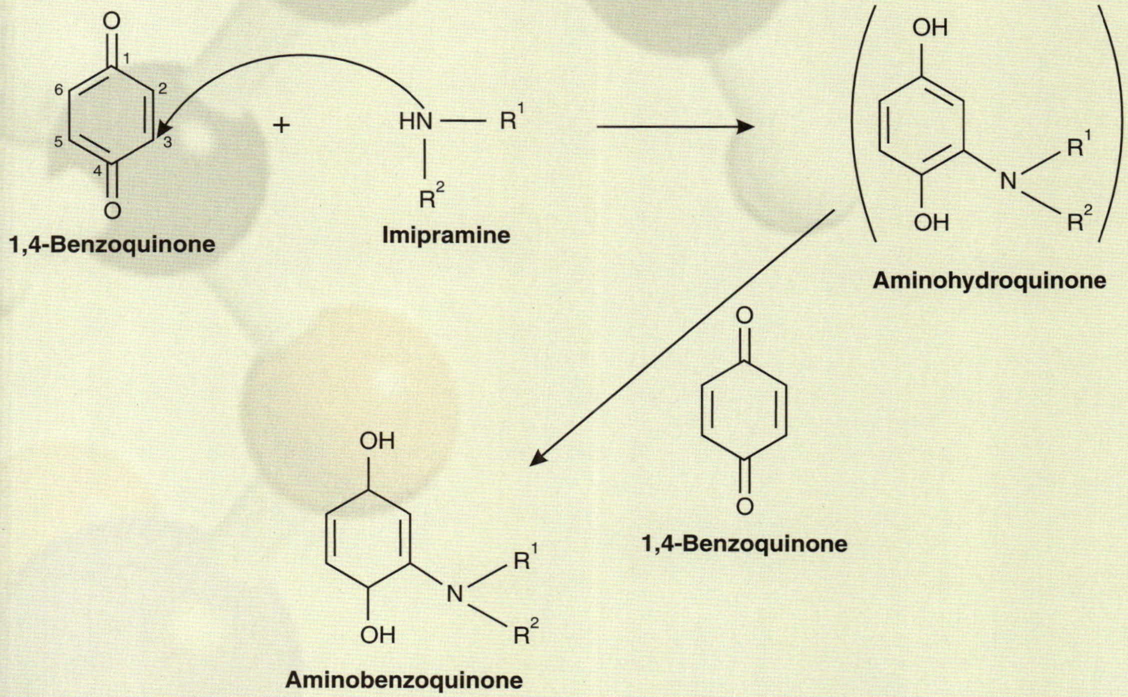

Formulation 1

Chlordiazepoxide hydrochloride, Clidinium bromide

ESTIMATION

Chlordiazepoxide hydrochloride

METHOD 1

Standard solution

20 mcg/ml of chlordiazepoxide hydrochloride in 0.1 N hydrochloric acid.

Sample solution

Shake a quantity of the sample powder equivalent to 20 mg of chlordiazepoxide hydrochloride with 150 ml of 0.1 N hydrochloric acid, make volume to 200 ml and filter. Dilute 10 ml of the filtrate to 50 ml with 0.1 M hydrochloric acid (20 mcg/ml). Measure the extinction of standard and test solutions at the maximum at about 308 nm. Calculate the content of chlordiazepoxide hydrochloride by comparison.

METHOD 2

Reagents

1. 1% w/v solution of vanillin in acetone.
2. Hydrochloric acid.

Standard solution

100 mcg/ml of the compound in glacial acetic acid.

Sample solution

Extract accurately weighed quantity of the sample with glacial acetic acid and dilute to get 100 mcg/ml.

Procedure

To 2 ml of the sample and standard solutions, add 2 ml of vanillin reagent and 2 ml of hydrochloric acid. Heat on water bath for 10 minutes, cool to room temperature and dilute to 10 ml with water. Measure the absorbance of both the solutions at about 530 nm. The method obeys Beer's law in the range of 40-200 mcg/ml.

On heating with hydrochloric acid the product gets hydrolysed to 2-amino-5-benzophenone and glycine-N-oxide. The amino derivative couples with vanillin to give coloured Schiff's base (λ_{max} 530 nm). For detailed reaction mechanism see method 3 of this formulation.

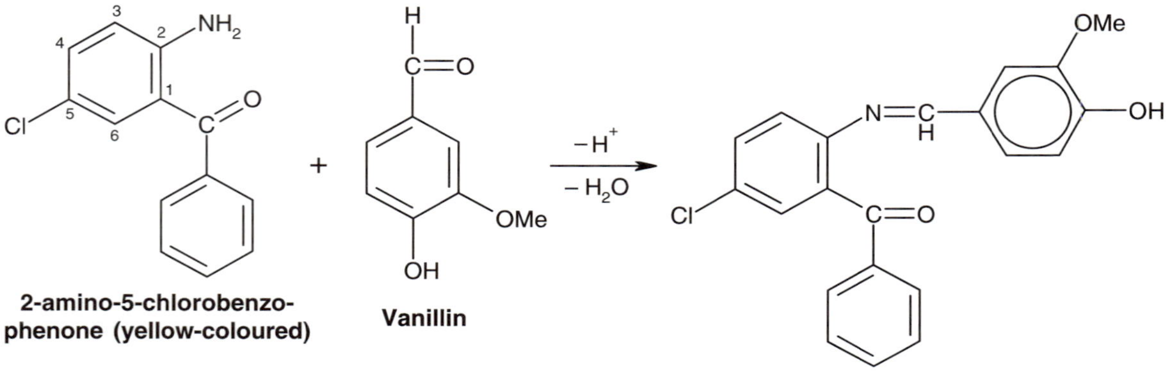

2-amino-5-chlorobenzophenone (yellow-coloured)

Vanillin

Coloured Schiff's base
(λ_{max} 530 nm)

Interestingly 2-amino-5-chlorobenzophenone is itself yellow in colour (λ_{max} 410 nm) and can form the basis for quantitative estimation of the compound.

METHOD 3

Reagents

1. Dilute hydrochloric acid.
2. 0.5% w/v hydrochloric acid.
3. 2% w/v solution of p-dimethylaminobenzaldehyde in alcohol.

Standard solution

Weigh accurately 100 mg of the compound, add 50 ml of dilute hydrochloric acid and heat on water bath for 40 minutes. Cool and dilute to 100 ml with water. 5 ml of the resultant solution is further diluted with water to 100 ml.

Sample solution

Weigh accurately aliquot of the sample equivalent to 100 mg of the compound and proceed as per standard solution.

Procedure

To 1 ml of sample and standard solutions, add 1.5 ml of dilute hydrochloric acid and 1.5 ml of aldehyde reagent. Shake and dilute to 10 ml with water. The absorbance of both the solutions is measured at about 452 nm against blank (0.5% hydrochloric acid). The method obeys Beer's law in the range of 2.5 to 7 mcg/ml.

Heating the drug with 0.5% HCl for 30 minutes causes the complete hydrolysis of the drug. Here, initially, by the acid hydrolysis amidine group is converted to an amide group. The amide group then gives demoxepam and methylamine. Further hydrolysis causes demoxepam to be broken down into an intermediate which then converts itself into 2-amino-5-chlorobenzophenone and glycin-N-oxide. The 2-amino-5-chlorobenzophenone formed undergoes condensation reaction with p-dimethylaminobenzaldehyde to form the coloured product.

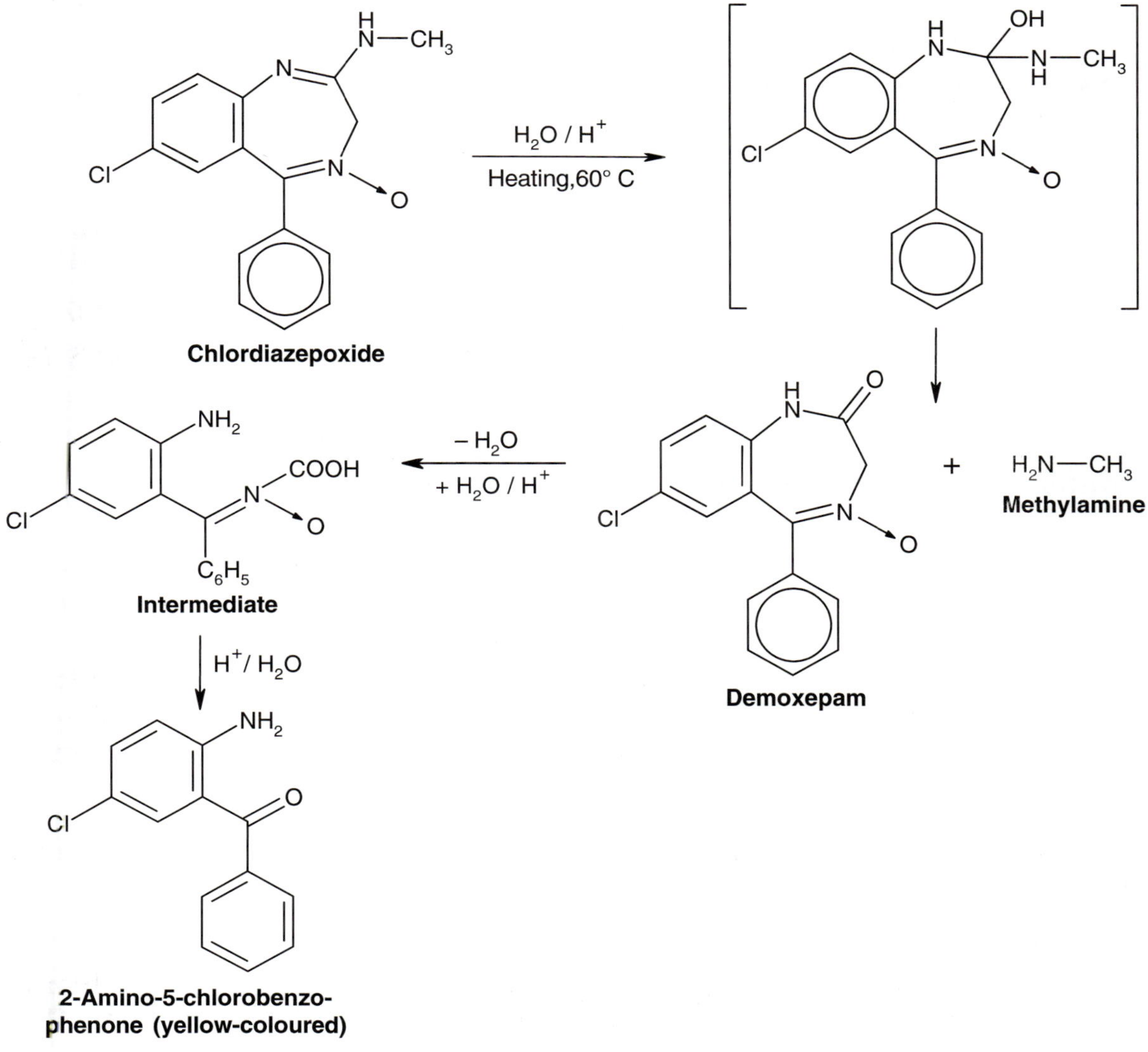

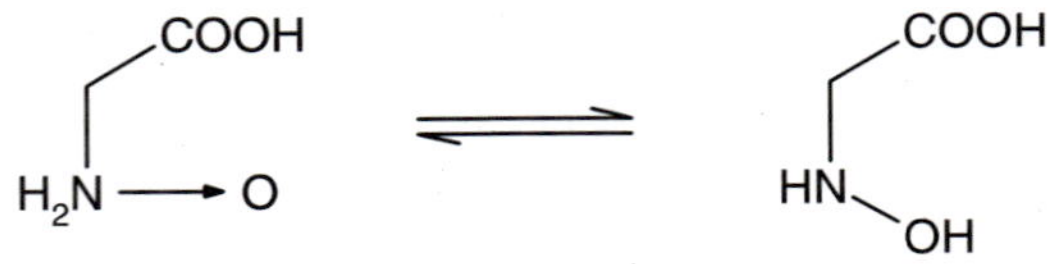

Glycine-N-oxide

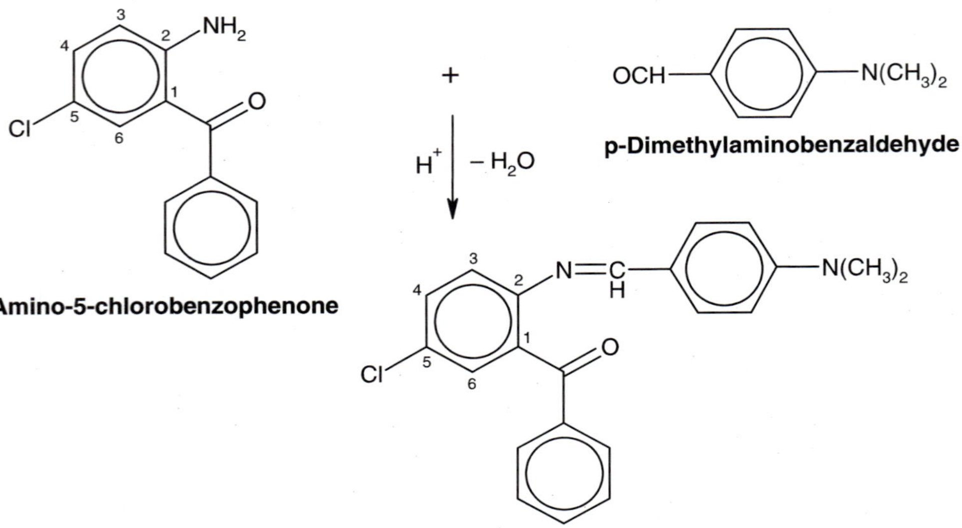

Coloured Schiff's base
(λ_{max} 452 nm)

Note 1

2-aminobenzophenone so produced can be diazotized and then answers Bratton-Marshall reaction to produce violet azo dye.

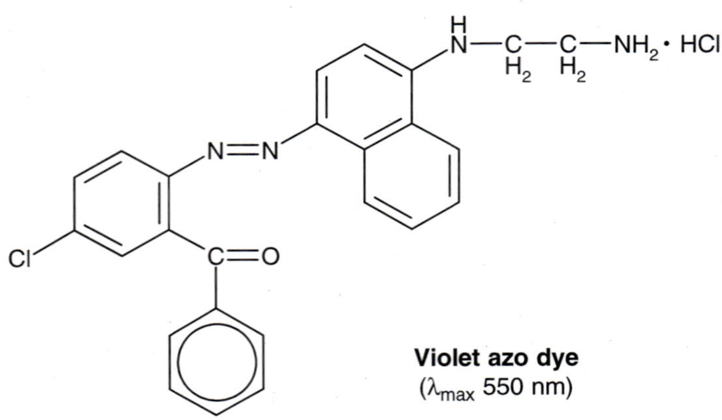

Violet azo dye
(λ_{max} 550 nm)

Reference

Pharmaceutical Chemistry (Vol. 2) by H.J. Roth, p. 663.

Note 2

Methylamine liberated as a result of hydrolytic decomposition of chlordiazepoxide reacts with fluorescamine to give highly fluorescent compound which can form the basis for quantitative determination of the compound.

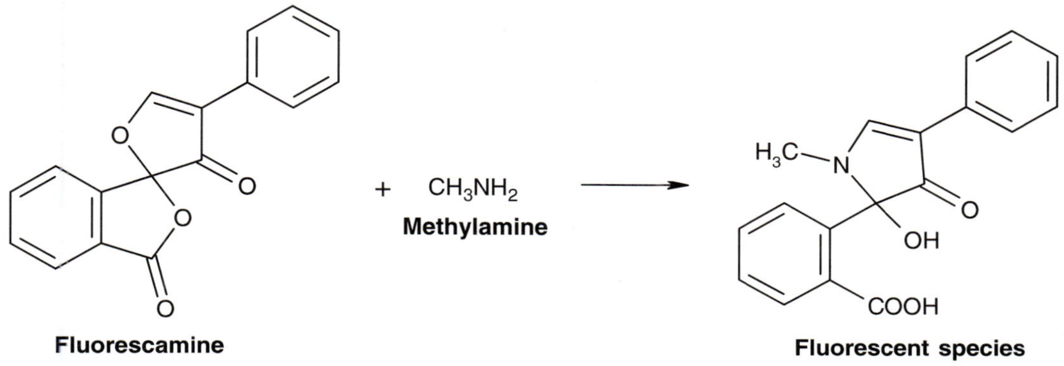

Clidinium bromide

Reagents

1. Buffer solution, pH 7.0 : To 104.5 ml of 0.2 M sodium phosphate dibasic, add 85.5 ml of 0.2 M potassium phosphate monobasic and water to make 1000 ml.
2. Bromocresol purple solution (buffered) : Weigh about 80 mg of the dye and dissolve in few drops of methyl alcohol. Add 50 ml of buffer solution, pH 7.0 and make up the volume to 100 ml with water. Wash the dye solution with chloroform till chloroform washings are colourless. This treatment reduces the blank values.

Standard solution

100 mcg/ml of clidinium bromide in water.

Sample solution

Transfer the powdered sample accurately weighed equivalent to 10 mg of the compound to a 100 ml volumetric flask. Shake with 50 ml of water for five minutes, add sufficient water to produce 100 ml and filter.

Procedure

Transfer 5 ml aliquot of the sample and standard solutions to separating funnel and add 10 ml of buffered dye solution. Extract it with three 15 ml portions of chloroform. Pass the chloroform into a 50 ml dry volumetric flask through a cotton plug previously moistened with chloroform. Add sufficient chloroform to make the volume. Measure the absorbance of the standard and test solutions at 420 nm. Calculate the content of clidinium bromide by comparison.

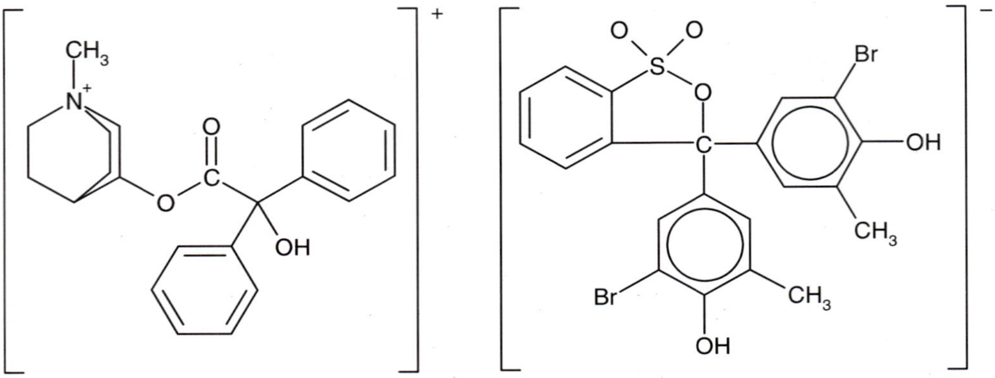

Clidinium - bromocresol purple complex
(λ_{max} 420 nm)

Note

1. The method is based on ion-pair complex formation which is extractable into chloroform.
2. Centrifugation of chloroform layer gives consistent results.
3. The substance can be estimated by non-aqueous titration; each ml of 0.1 M $HClO_4$ is equivalent to 43.24 mg of the substance.

Formulation 2

Dicyclomine hydrochloride, Chlordiazepoxide, Clidinium bromide

ESTIMATION

Dicyclomine hydrochloride

Reagents

1. 0.004 M SLS.
2. 10% w/v of sodium hydroxide sodium.
3. 1.0% w/v of dimethyl yellow solution.
4. Dilute sulphuric acid solution.

Procedure

Weigh accurately a quantity of tablet powder equivalent to 20 mg of dicyclomine hydrochloride in a separator, add 25 ml of water and 10 ml of sodium hydroxide solution and extract it with 3 × 25 ml of chloroform. Wash the chloroform layer with water to get it free from alkali. Pass the chloroform layer through anhydrous sodium sulphate into a dry stoppered iodine flask. Evaporate the chloroform on water-bath. To the residue, add 10 ml methanol, 10 ml dilute sulphuric acid, 10 ml of water, 1 ml of dimethyl yellow solution and 50 ml of chloroform. Shake and titrate it against 0.04 M SLS, shaking vigorously after each addition and allowing the layer to separate until the colour of the chloroform layer changes to red. Each ml of 0.004 M SLS is equivalent to 1.384 mg of dicyclomine hydrochloride.

Chlordiazepoxide

Standard solution

Weigh accurately about 100 mg of chlordiazepoxide working standard in a 100 ml volumetric flask. Dissolve it in 0.1 M HCl and make up the volume with the same. Mix well and filter it. Pipette 2 ml of the filtrate into another 100 ml volumetric flask and make up the volume to the mark with 0.1 M HCl. Designate this as standard solution.

Test solution

Weigh and powder 20 tablets. Weigh accurately a quantity of the tablet powder equivalent to about 5 mg of chlordiazepoxide into a 250 ml volumetric flask. Add about 100 ml of 0.1 M HCl, shake for about 5 minutes to dissolve and make up the volume to the mark with the same. Mix well and filter it. Designate this as Test solution.

Procedure

Measure the absorbance of both the standard and test solution at the maxima at about 308 nm using 0.1 M HCl as blank.

Clidinium bromide

Reagents

1. Phosphate buffer pH 8.8 : Weigh about 26.8 g of dibasic sodium phosphate and dissolve it in water to produce 200 ml. Adjust the pH to 8.8 with phosphoric acid or sodium hydroxide.
2. Thymol blue solution : Weigh 100 mg of thymol blue, add 2.5 ml of 1.0 N NaOH and dissolve it in water to produce 100 ml. Adjust the pH to 8.8 with HCl or NaOH solution.

Standard solution

Weigh accurately about 100 mg of clidinium bromide working standard in a 100 ml volumetric flask. Dissolve it in water and make up the volume with the same. Mix well and filter it. Pipette 10 ml of the filtrate into another 100 ml volumetric flask and make up the volume with water. Designate this as standard solution.

Sample solution

Weigh and powder 20 tablets. Weigh accurately a quantity of tablet powder equivalent to about 10 mg of clidinium bromide a 100 ml volumetric flask. Add about 50 ml of water, shake for about 5 minutes to dissolve and make up the volume to the mark with water. Mix well and filter it. Designate this as test solution.

Procedure

Pipette 10 ml each of standard and test solution into two different 250 ml separator, add 10 ml of pH 8.8 buffer and 5 ml of thymol blue solution and extract it with 3 × 30 ml of chloroform. Combine the extract into a dry 100 ml volumetric flask and make up the volume with chloroform. Measure the absorbance at about 410 nm using chloroform as the blank. The method is based on formation of ion-pair complex extractable into chloroform.

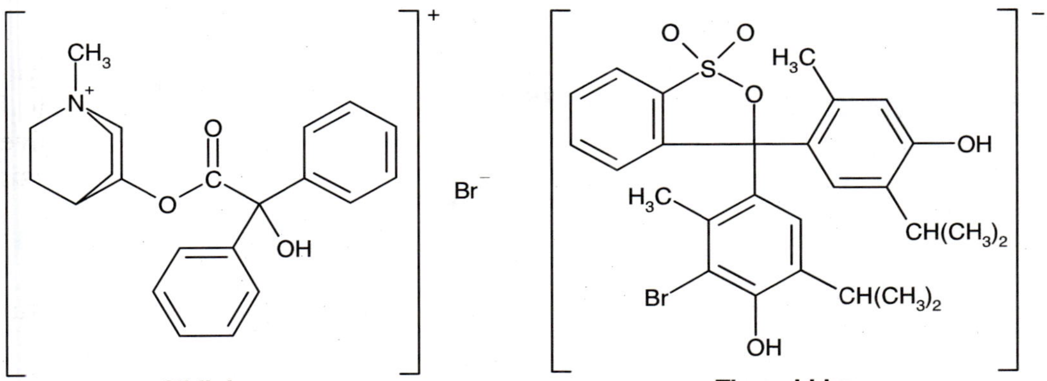

Clidinium **Thymol blue**

Drug - dye ion-pair complex in pH 8.8 buffer
(λ_{max} 410 nm)

Formulation 3

Imipramine hydrochloride, Diazepam

METHOD A

(a) Determination of Imipramine hydrochloride

METHOD 1

Weigh accurately powdered tablets equivalent to about 25 mg of imipramine hydrochloride and extract and adjust the volume to 50 ml with ether saturated water. Shake total aqueous extract with 10 ml of ether. Allow the layers to separate. Retain ether layer for estimation of diazepam. Dilute aqueous layer with 0.1 N sulphuric acid to get 20 mcg/ml and measure the extinction at 251 nm. Calculate the contents of imipramine hydrochloride taking 264 as value of E 1%, 1 cm.

METHOD 2

Reagents

1. Cobalt thiocyanate reagent : Dissolve 4.3 g of ammonium thiocyanate and 6.8 g of cobalt chloride in 100 ml of water.
2. Britton and Robinson buffer, pH 1.98.

Standard solution

1 mg/ml of imipramine hydrochloride in water.

Sample solution

Transfer powdered sample accurately weighed equivalent to 100 mg of the compound into a 100 ml volumetric flask. Shake with water, filter and adjust to volume.

Procedure

Transfer 10 ml of the sample and standard solutions to separatory funnels. Add 1 ml of buffer, followed by 5 ml of cobalt thiocyanate reagent. Extract the aqueous layer with 10, 5 and 5 ml of toluene. The combined organic layer is centrifuged and diluted to 25 ml with chloroform. Measure the absorbance of blue coloured chromogen at 625 nm against reagent blank. The method obeys Beer's law in the concentration range of 20-560 mcg/ml.

Explanatory Note

The compound forms complex with cobalt thiocyanate. The complex can be extracted into organic layer (benzene) and blue colour measured at 625 nm.

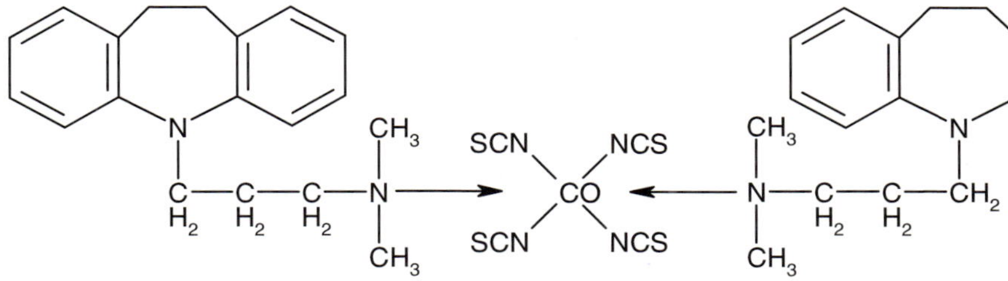

Cobalt thiocyanate complex of imipramine
(λ_{max} 625 nm)

Several other drugs are reported to form cobalt thiocyanate complex: naphazoline nitrate, oxymetazoline hydrochloride, antazoline hydrochloride, xylometazoline hydrochloride, tetramisole hydrochloride, chlorpheniramine maleate and amitriptyline hydrochloride. In case of all these drugs, cobalt complex is formed in pH 4.0 buffer and most of them are extractable either in chloroform or toluene.

Reference

R.T. Sane, B.R. Shinde, A.K. Parikh & S.P. Tikekar, Indian Drugs, **21(6)**, 257-260, 1984.

METHOD 3

Reagents

Brilliant blue solution: 0.1% w/v solution of the dye in water.

Standard solution

50 μg/ml of the substance in water.

Sample solution

Accordingly weighed quantity of the powdered sample was extracted with water to get final concentration of 50 μg/ml of the substance.

Procedure

To 2 ml each of sample and standard solutions, add 3 ml of dye solution and make up to 10 ml with water. Add 10 ml of chloroform to each and shake for not less than 2 min. Allow the layers to separate and centrifuge. Measure the absorbance of chloroform layer at 620 nm chloroform using chloroform as blank. The method following linearity with range of 2-20 μg.

Note

1. Common excipients present in tablets, capsules did not interfere.
2. Diazepam, chlordiazepoxide and amitriptyline do not interfere.

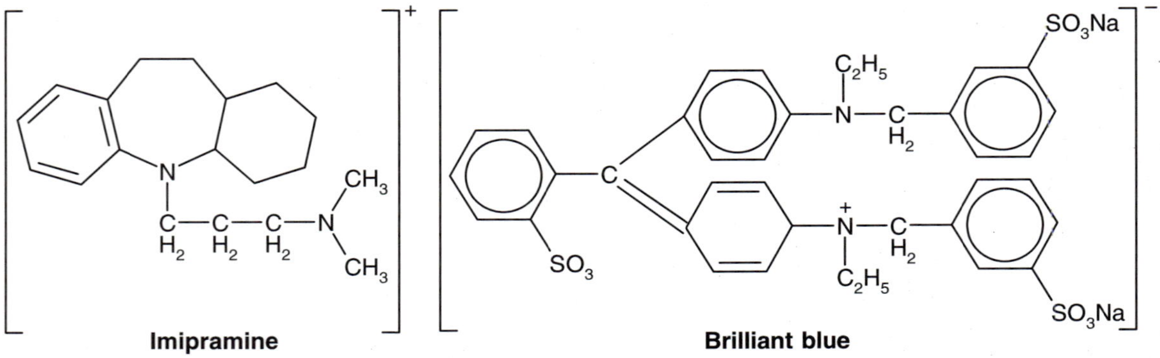

Brilliant blue dye complex
(λ_{max} 620 nm)

Reference

S.L. Bhongade, P.A. Thakurdesai & A.V. Kasture, Indian Drugs, **31(5)**, 219-221, 1994.

Recently, Fardous et al. have reported spectrophotometric method for some psychoactive drugs including imipramine. The drugs are oxidized by Ce(IV) in sulphuric acid medium and relative fluorescence intensity measured at λ_{ex} 254 nm and λ_{em} 355 nm.

Reagents

1. 0.001 M cerric (IV) ammonium sulphate in 0.25 M sulphuric acid.

Sample and standard solutions

100 μg/ml in water.

Procedure

To 1 ml each of sample and standard solutions add 1 ml of Ce(IV) solution, heat in boiling water-bath at 100°C for 20 min, cool, dilute to 10 ml with water and measure the fluorescence (254/355 nm).

Imipramine and dibenzazepine derivative: The compound is first oxidized to form a radical cation and finally gives a dimeric species which is fluorescent.

Probable Reaction Mechanism

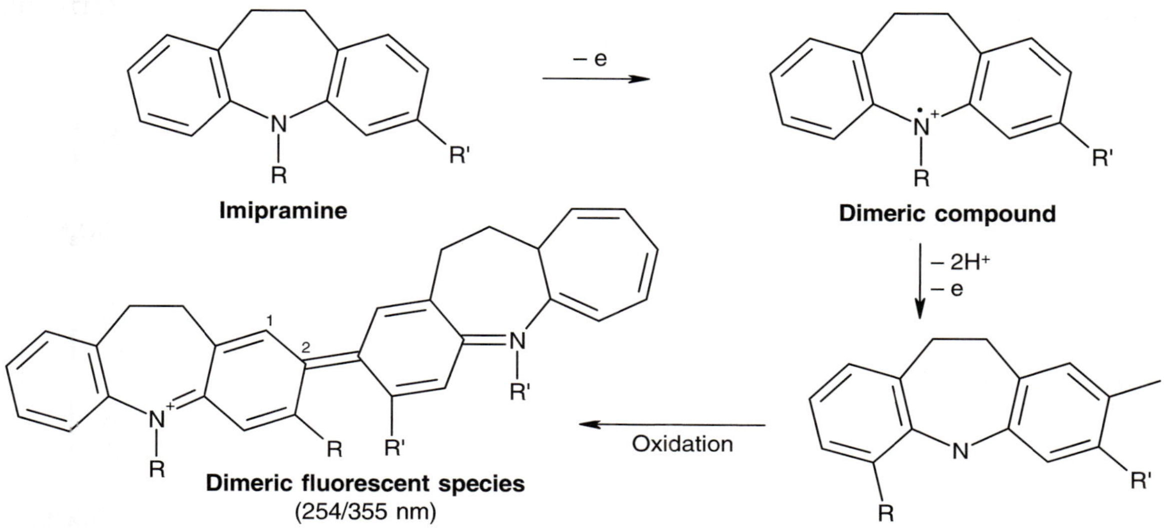

Reference

Fardous A. Mohamed, Horria A. Mohamed, Samiha A. Hussain & Sameh A. Ahmed, J. Pharm. & Biomed. Analysis, **39**, 139-146, 2005.

In a manner similar to Michael addition imipramine adds at the enone system (1,4-benzoquinone) which ultimetely changes to hydroquinone. Excess of benzoquinone oxidizes hydroquinone to quinone.

Probable Reaction Mechanism

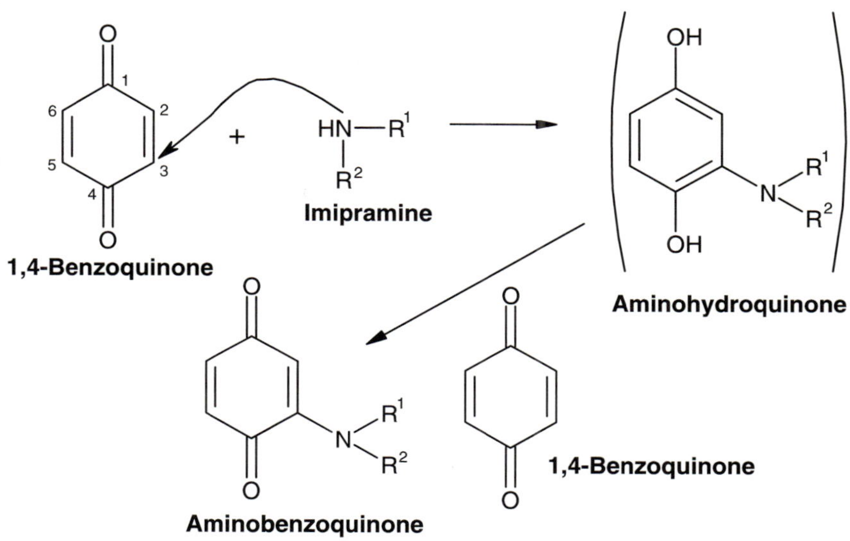

Reference

Pharmaceutical Chemistry (Vol. 2) by H.J. Roth, p. 663.

Hussain et al. (1989) have described two spectrophotometric methods for the estimation of imipramine hydrochloride, a dibenzazepine derivative. In these methods, diazotized p-nitroaniline and MBTH have been employed as chromogenic agents.

Reagents

1. 0.16% solution of diazotized p-nitroaniline (DPNA).
2. 0.4% solution of 'MBTH' in water.
3. 1% solution of ammonium iron (III) sulphate in 0.1 M hydrochloric acid.
4. Conc. hydrochloric acid.
5. 5 M hydrochloric acid.

Standard solution

50 μg/ml solution of imipramine hydrochloride in water.

Sample solution

Powdered sample equivalent to 50 mg of the substance suspended in 75 ml of water, shake for 10 min, dilute to 100 ml with water. Filter and dilute the filtrate suitably with water to get 50 μg/ml solution of imipramine.

Procedure

(a) DPNA method: To 1 ml each of sample and standard solutions, add 2 ml of 'DPNA' reagent, followed by 1 ml of conc. hydrochloric acid, mix well, keep in water-bath (70-75°C) for 20 min, cool, dilute to 10 ml with 5 M hydrochloric acid and measure the absorbance of both the solutions at 575 nm against reagent blank and calculate the results by comparison.

(b) MBTH method: To 1 ml each of sample and standard solutions, add 2 ml of 'MBTH' reagent and 2 ml of ammonium iron (III) sulphate. Mix well, keep at room temperature for 15 min, dilute to 10 ml with water and measure the absorbance of both the solutions at 630 nm against reagent blank and calculate the results by comparison.

Probable Reaction Mechanism

Electron density in the dibanzazepine derivative (imipramine hydrochloride) is highest at positions C-2 and C-8, which permits electrophilic attack by the two proposed reagents.

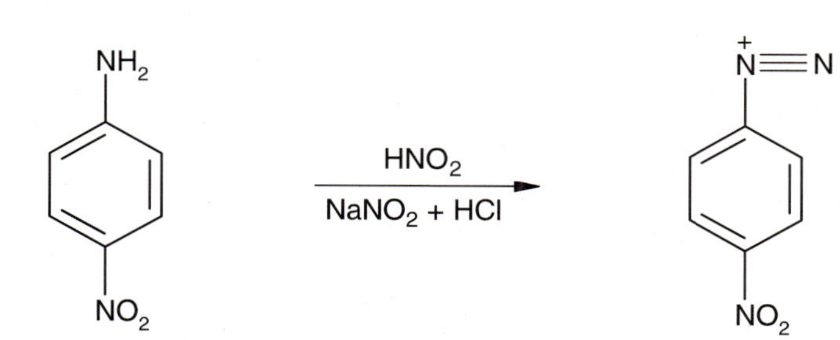

p-Nitroaniline **Diazotized p-nitroaniline (DPNA)**
Reagent A

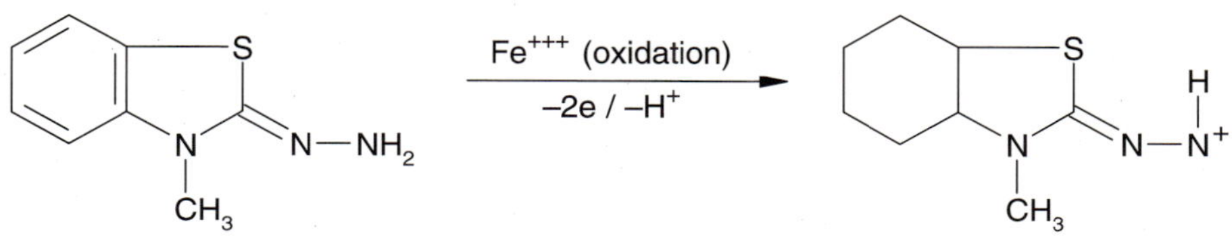

MBTH **Oxidized MBTH (active species)**
Reagent B

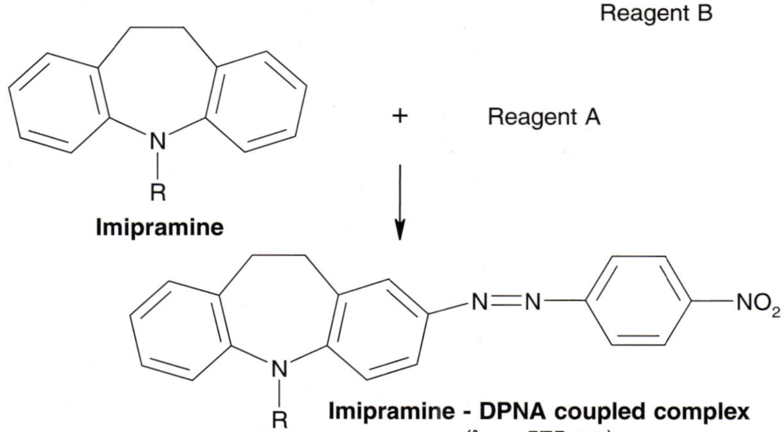

Imipramine - DPNA coupled complex
(λ_{max} 575 nm)

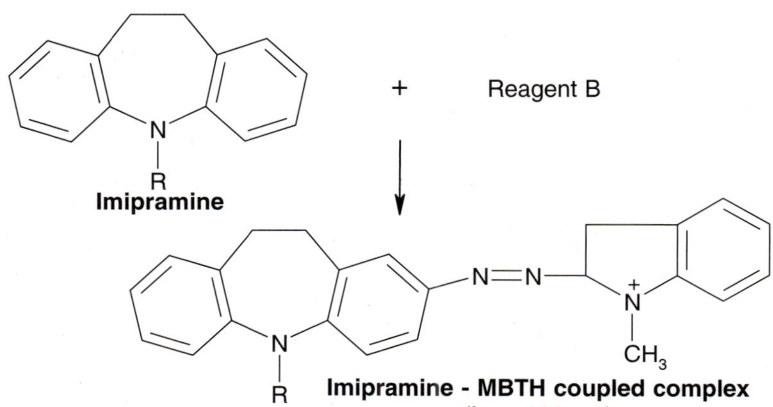

Imipramine - MBTH coupled complex
(λ_{max} 630 nm)

Reference

S.A. Hussain, Michael E. El-Kommos, Hoday Hassan & Abdel-Maboud I. Mohamed, Talanta, **36(9)**, 941-944, 1989.

Another spectrophotometric method was proposed by Hussain et al. (1989) for the determination of dibenzazepine including imipramine hydrochloride based on charge transfer (C-T) method. Other dibenzazepine derivatives studied were trimipramine maleate, desipramine hydrochloride and clomipramine hydrochloride.

Reagents

1. 0.5% solution of picryl chloride in acetonitrile.

Standard solution

Dissolve 100 mg of imipramine hydrochloride in water, basify with ammonia, extract free base with 3 × 25 chloroform. Pass combined chloroform layer through anhydrous sodium sulphate, dilute to 250 ml with chloroform. Further dilute 5 ml to 50 ml with chloroform to get 4 μg/ml solution of the compound.

Sample solution

Powdered sample equivalent to 25 mg of the compound suspended in 40 ml of water, shake for 10 min, dilute to 50 ml with water, filter and proceed with basification and extraction with chloroform as described under standard solution to get final concentration of 4 μg/ml in respect of the substance.

Procedure

To 1 ml each of sample and standard solutions, add 1 ml of picryl reagent, dilute to 10 ml with chloroform and measure the absorbance of both the solutions at 395 nm against reagent blank and calculate the results.

Probable Reaction Mechanism

The drug being "donor" and the reagent being electron acceptor, it forms C-T complex.

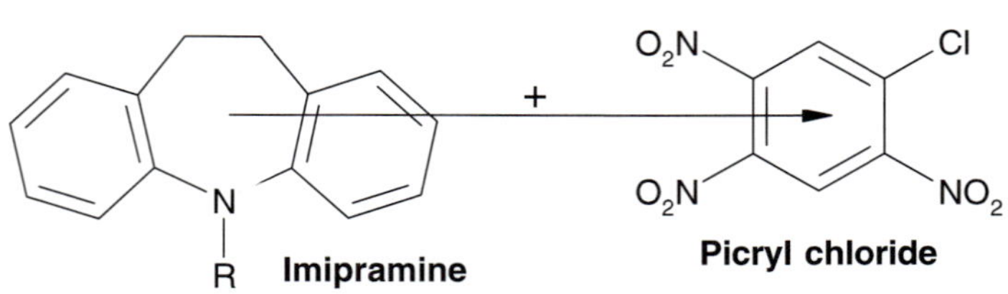

Imipramine - picryl chloride C-T complex
(λ_{max} 395 nm)

Reference

S.A. Hussain, et al., Talanta, **36(11)**, 1147-1149, 1989.

Determination by simultaneous spectrophotometric method does not involve prior separation of two drugs. The absorbance of a mixture of drugs at any wavelength is the sum of the absorbance of the individual drug at that wavelength.

Standard solution of Imipramine hydrochloride

15 mcg/ml of authentic sample of imipramine hydrochloride in 0.1 N sulphuric acid.

Standard solution of Diazepam

15 mcg/ml of authentic sample of diazepam in 0.1 N sulphuric acid. Record the spectra of both the components in UV range (200-360 nm).

It is observed that imipramine hydrochloride (x) exhibits absorption maxima at 251 nm, whereas diazepam (y) has two maximas i.e. 241 and 285 nm. The absorptivity indices of both the compounds at 251 and 285 nm calculated on the basis of average of five observations with 15 mcg/ml solutions are given below :

	Absorptivity indices	
Compound	251 nm	285 nm
Imipramine hydrochloride (X)	26	15
Diazepam (Y)	68	44

Preparation of sample solution

Weigh accurately powdered tablets equivalent to about 25 mg of imipramine hydrochloride. Extract and adjust the volume to 200 ml with 0.1 N sulphuric acid. 8 ml of the resultant solution is further diluted to 100 ml with 0.1 N sulphuric acid. The extinction of the sample solution is measured at 251 and 285 nm. The amount of each component is calculated from the following two analogous equations :

$$C_x \text{ (Concentration of Imipramine, mg)} = \frac{a_3A_2 - a_1A_1}{a_3a_4 - a_1a_2}$$

$$C_x \text{ (Concentration of Imipramine, mg)} = \frac{a_4A_1 - a_2A_2}{a_3a_4 - a_1a_2}$$

a_1 = Absorptivity of y at 285 nm
a_2 = Absorptivity of x at 251 nm
a_3 = Absorptivity of y at 251 nm

a_4 = Absorptivity of x at 285 nm
A_1 = Absorptivity of the final sample solution at 251 nm
A_2 = Absorptivity of the final sample solution at 285 nm

Note

For differential spectroscopy, following conditions are required to be fulfilled:

1. Only bicomponent mixtures can be subjected to this differential treatment.
2. Two components of the mixture should be unreactive with each other.
3. Each component should follow Beer's law separately in the concentration range employed for analysis.
4. The spectral graph of each component should be available to determine the exact maxima.
5. Absorptivity values for each component should be sufficiently different at chosen wavelengths and should be easily and accurately determined.
6. The absorption value of the mixture should be accurately determined.

Determination of Diazepam

Evaporate ether layer as obtained in method 1 for the estimation of imipramine hydrochloride, dissolve the residue in 0.1 N sulphuric acid to get a solution of about 3 mcg/ml. Measure the extinction at 241 nm and calculate the contents of diazepam taking 1402 as E 1%, 1 cm.

Diazepam hydrolysis with alkali gives anion which reacts with m-dinitrobenzene giving a coloured complex.

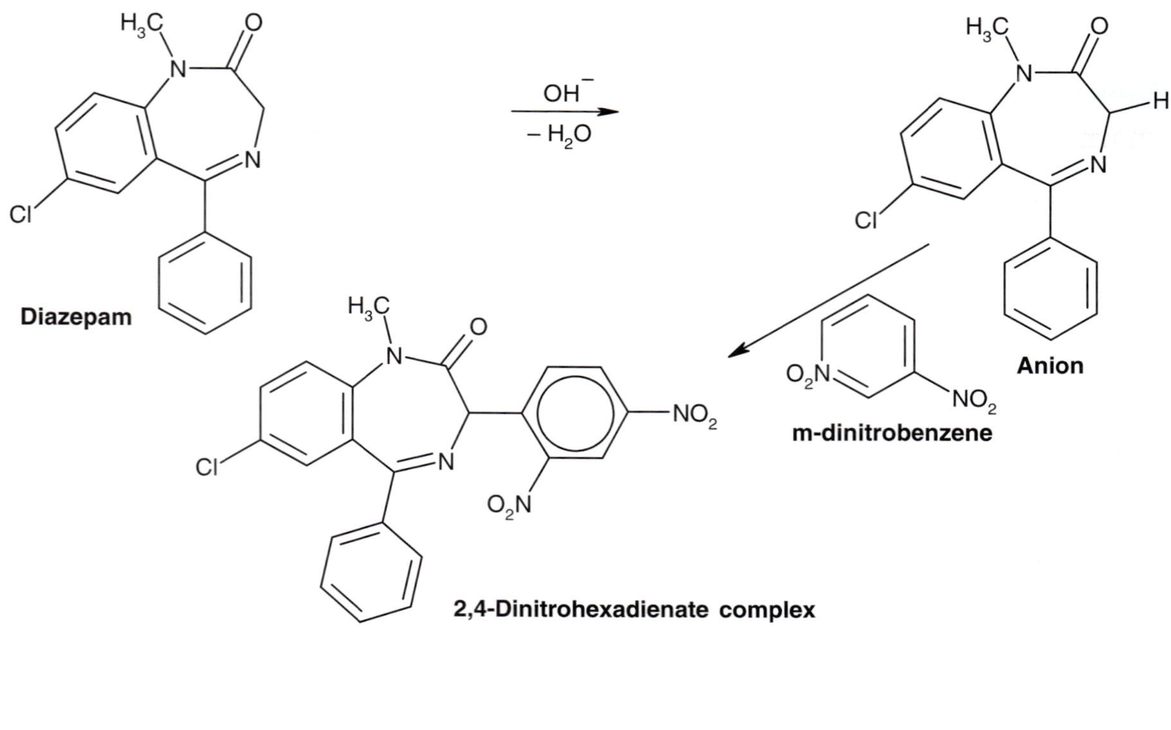

2,4-Dinitrohexadienate complex

On acid hydrolysis, as under chlordiazepoxide, aminobenzophenone is formed which undergoes intramolecular rearrangement in the presence of sodium carbonate and DMF to give fluorescent acridone derivative.

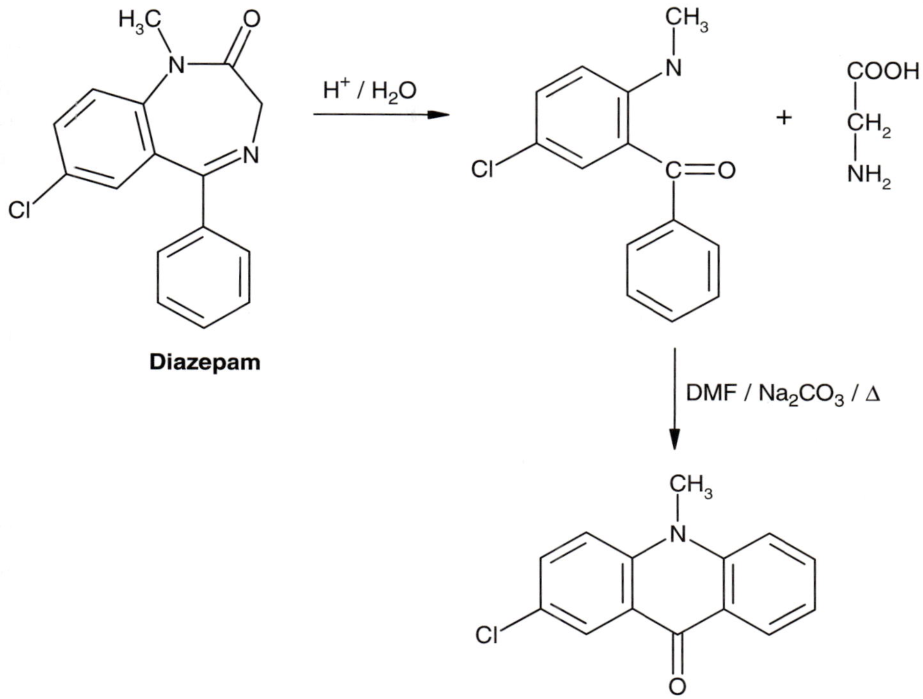

Diazepam

Fluorescent acridone derivative

Reference

Pharmaceutical Chemistry (Vol. 2—Drug Analysis) by H.J. Roth, p. 667-668.

Formulation 4

Trifluoperazine hydrochloride, Trihexyphenidyl

ESTIMATION

Trifluoperazine hydrochloride

Reagents

1. 0.1% w/v ammonium vanadate or ammonium metavanadate solution (slight warming is necessary to get quick solution).
2. Dilute hydrochloric acid (1 : 1 and 1 : 4 v/v).

Standard solution

200 mcg/ml of authentic trifluoperazine hydrochloride in 0.1 N hydrochloric acid.

Sample solution

Accurately weigh powdered tablets equivalent to about 10 mg of trifluoperazine hydrochloride, add 25 ml of 0.1 N hydrochloric acid. Shake and adjust the volume to 50 ml with 0.1 N hydrochloric acid (200 mcg/ml).

Procedure

To each 25 ml volumetric flask, add 0.5 ml of ammonium vanadate solution and 1 ml of dilute hydrochloric acid (1 : 1). Mix and allow to stand for 1 minute. Add 5 ml of standard and sample solutions to each flask and make up the volume with dilute hydrochloric acid (1 : 5). Concomitantly measure the absorbance of both the solutions at absorption maximum at about 525 nm against reagent blank. Calculate the results by comparison.

Probable Reaction Mechanism

Phenothiazine with three carbon atoms separating 2 nitrogen are preferably oxidized to sulphoxide without elimination of side chain. The sulphoxide so produced reacts in a form of Smiles rearrangement to give hydroxylated ring which is further oxidized to quinoid phenothiazine-3-one.

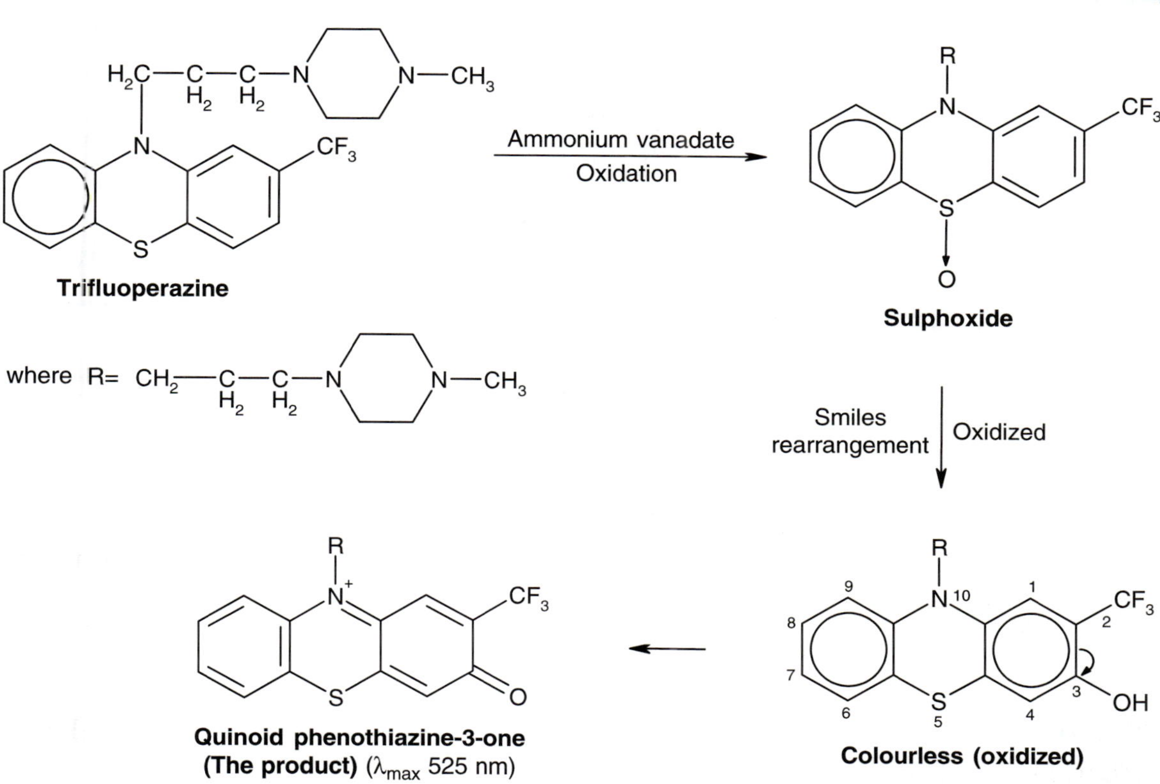

Reference

Pharmacuetical Chemistry (Vol. 2) by H.J. Roth, p. 698.

Typical calculations

$$\text{Trifluoperazine (mg/tab)} = \frac{A_u}{A_s} \times \frac{W_s}{W_u} \times d_f \times \text{Av. wt.} \times 1000 \times 0.85$$

$$= \frac{0.294}{0.288} \times \frac{0.1001}{0.076} \times 0.256 \times \frac{1}{20} \times 1000$$

$$= 1.03$$

Claim = 1.0 mg as base
Multiply with 0.85 to convert salt and base.

Another reaction mechanism reported is that electron density at sulphur is very high and as a result can be easily oxidized resulting in the formation of a highly coloured cationic species. The oxidizing agent used in this case is sodium vanadate ($NaVO_3$) in acidic medium (H_2SO_4/HCl or H_3PO_4).

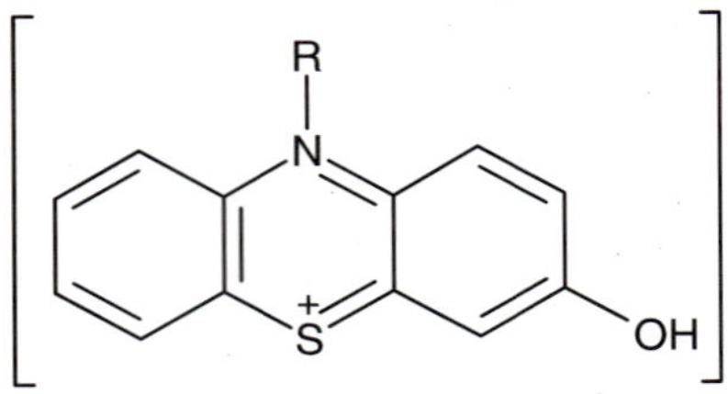

Reference

Indian Drugs, **24(9)**, 441, 1987.

In acidic medium p-benzoquinone also acts as oxidizing agent converting the drug into quinoid phenothiazine-3-one with the formation of cation radical.

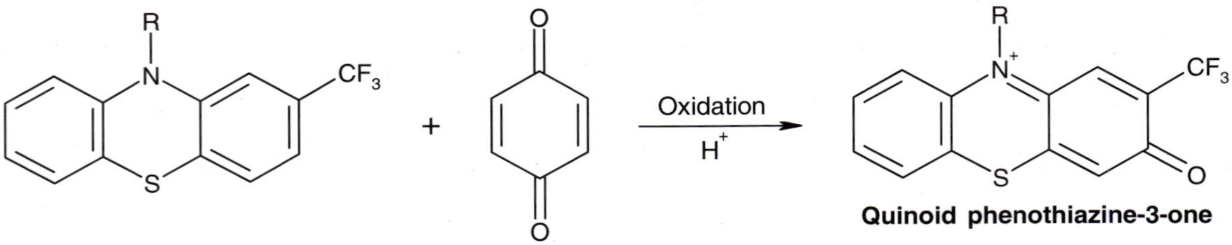

Quinoid phenothiazine-3-one

Reference

Indian Drugs, **25(12)**, 528, Sept. 1988.

Murthy et al. (2000) have suggested the following reaction mechanism for oxidation of phenothiazines by p-benzoquinone. The compound undergoes one electron reversible oxidation by p-benzoquinone in acidic medium to give radical cation. The formation of cation radical was also confirmed by ion-exchange studies.

Suggested Reaction Mechanism

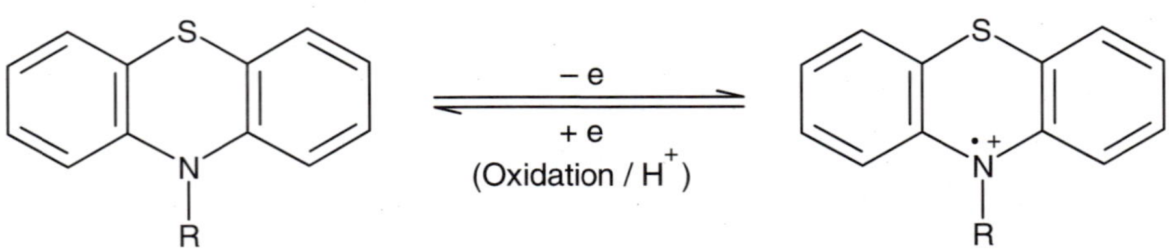

Red-coloured cation radical
(λ_{max} 480 nm)

Reference

K.C. Srinivasa Murthy & J. Seetharamappa, Ind. J. Pharm. Sci., **62(4)**, 273-276, 2000.

Zarapakar et al. have described an analytical method based on reaction with Marquis reagent.

Reagent

Formaldehyde - sulphuric acid reagent.

Sample and standard solutions

To 2 ml each of sample and standard solutions add 2 ml of formaldehyde solution (< 37%) followed by 4 ml of conc. sulphuric acid, cool in ice-bath and then dilute to volume with water. Measure the absorption of resulting solution at 560 nm against reagent blank.

Probable Reaction Mechanism

Aromatic ring of the molecule is attacked by formaldehyde in acidic solution to yield a condensation product. Now sulphuric acid acts as oxidizing agent resulting in the formation of quinoid i.e. phenothiazine-3-one which is coloured.

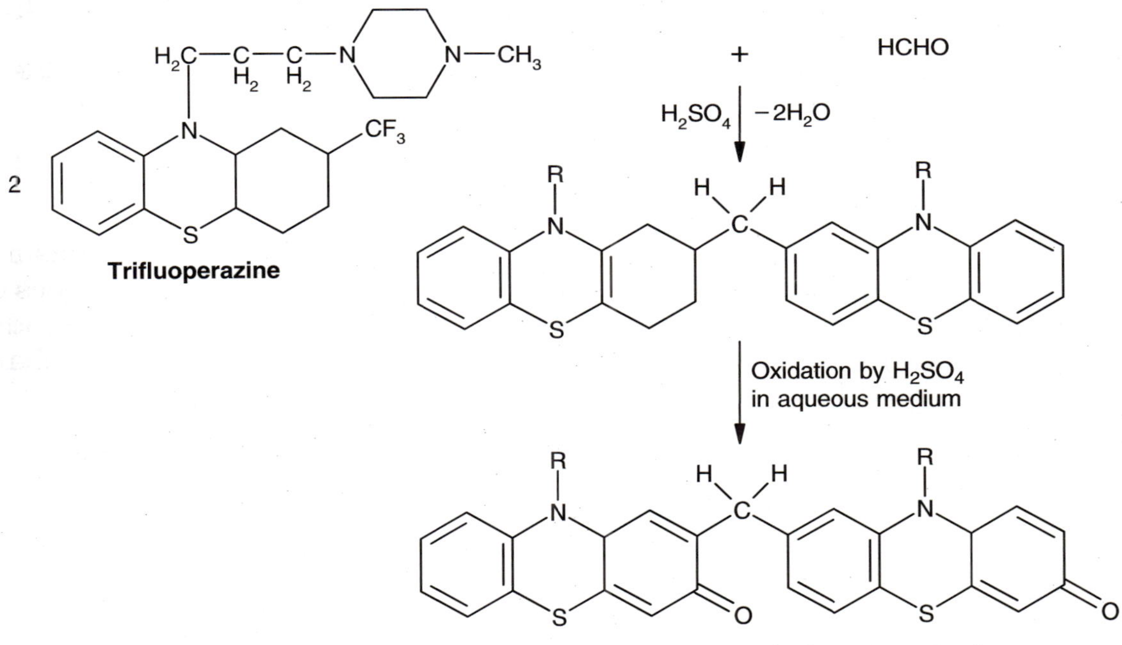

Phenothiazine-3-one (coloured product)
(λ_{max} 560 nm)

Note

Mole ratio of phenothiazine : HCHO is 2 : 1 i.e. 2 moles of phenothiazine condense with 1 mole of formaldehyde as shown above.

Reference

S.S. Zarapakar et al., *Indian Drugs*, **26(1)**, 32-36, 1989.

R.T. Sane et al. (1980) have described a method based on formation of nitroso derivative.

Reagents

1. 10% w/v solution of sodium nitrite.
2. Conc. HCl.
3. Conc. H_2SO_4.

Sample and standard solutions

100 μg/ml in water.

Procedure

To 0.5 ml each of sample/standard solution add 1.5 ml of methanol, 0.5 ml of sodium nitrate solution, 1.5 ml of conc. HCl, then add 2 ml of H_2SO_4 slowly with gentle heating, cool and dilute to 10 ml with sulphuric acid (1 : 1) and keep at room temperature for 5 min and then measure the absorbance at 538 nm against reagent blank.

Probable Reaction Mechanism

$$NaNO_2 + HCl \longrightarrow NaCl + HNO_2 \text{ (Nitrous acid)}$$

$$HNO_2 + H_2SO_4 \quad \overset{+}{N}{=}O + H_2O + HSO_4^-$$

Nitrosonium ion

The nitrosonium ion so formed being electron deficient will attack the aromatic ring of phenothiazine at position 2 and result in the formation of nitroso derivative as shown below.

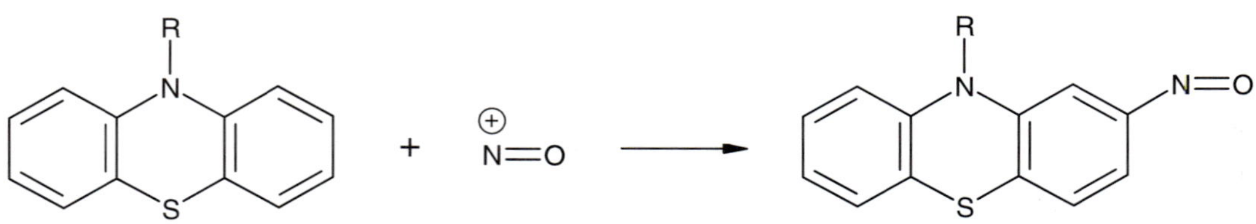

Nitroso derivative

Since conc. H_2SO_4 is added, it being a strong oxidizing agent and H_2O also present in the reaction medium, phenothiazine ring is oxodized to give the following nitroso-quinoid product which is responsible for the colour.

Note

Different electrophilic groups as substituents at C-2 are I^-, H, Cl^-, CF_3, OCH_3, CN, SCH_3.

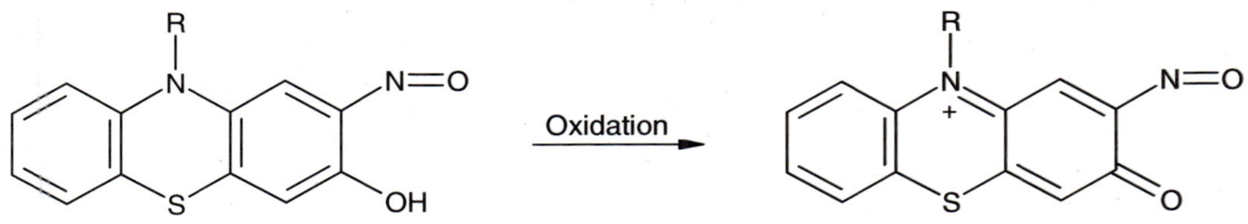

Nitroso quinoid product
(λ_{max} 538 nm)

Reference

R.T. Sane, S.S. Kamat, V.S. Narkar, A.Y. Sathe & J.G. Mhalas, Indian Drugs, **18(1)**, 19-22, 1980.

The drug forms ion-pair complexes with dyes such as brilliant green and orange-II.

Both these dye complexes can be extracted into chloroform and subjected to spectrophotometric measurements at their respective minimum wavelengths. For detailed experimental conditions, see under promethazine hydrochloride.

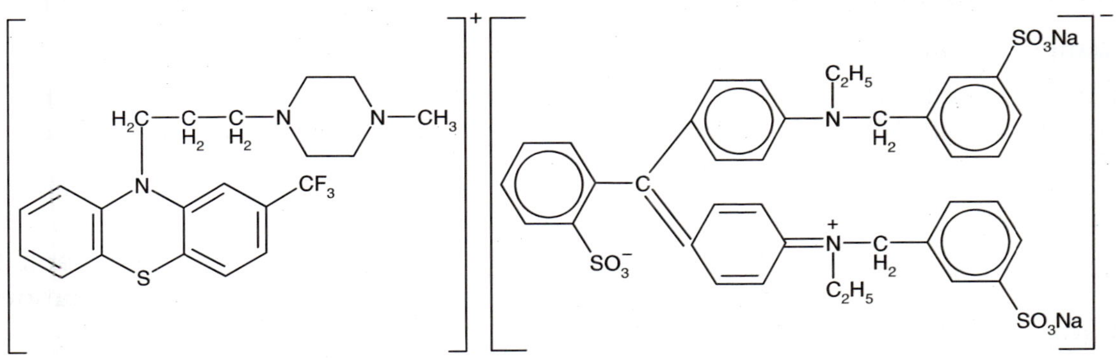

Drug - brilliant blue dye complex
(λ_{max} 620 nm)

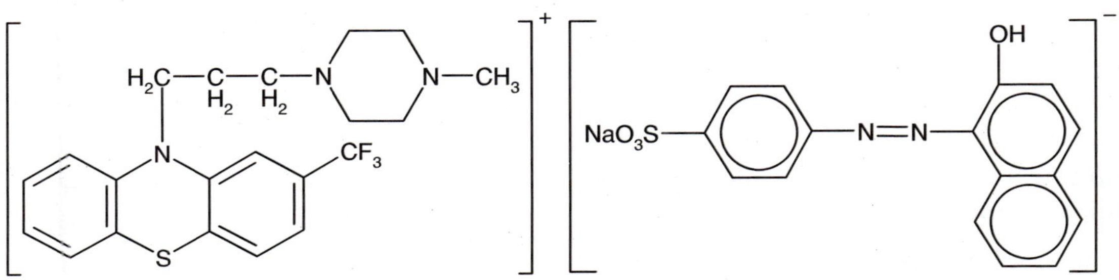

Drug - orange-II dye complex
(λ_{max} 495 nm)

Reference

S.L. Bhongade & A.V. Kasture, Talanta, **40(10)**, 1525-1528, 1993.

Trihexyphenidyl

Its determination requires thin layer chromatographic separation, followed by colour complex with bromocresol purple.

Reagents

1. Phosphate buffer solution, pH 5.3.
2. 0.4% w/v solution of bromocresol purple in water.
3. Chloroform.
4. TLC glass plates (20 × 20 cm), coated (0.25 mm) with silica gel G and activated at 105°C for 20 minutes.
5. Developing solvent.
   (i) Benzene : Acetone : Strong ammonia (8 : 4 : 1 v/v).
   (ii) Chloroform : Methyl alcohol (9 : 1 v/v).
   (iii) Acetone-water (85 + 15 v/v).

Standard solution

100 mcg/ml of pure trihexyphenidyl in chloroform.

Sample solution

Weigh accurately powdered tablets equivalent to about 10 mg of the compound, add 25 ml of chloroform, shake and filter. Wash the residue with chloroform and adjust the filtrate to 100 ml.

Procedure

Apply with the help of a microsyringe 4 ml each of standard and sample solutions, 1.5 cm from the lower edge of the plate and 1.5 cm apart. Apply also 1 ml of the standard solution to serve as a guide. The plate is developed in either of the solvents to a distance of 10 cm. The plates are dried and spot obtained with 1 ml of standard solution is located with the help of Dragendorff's reagent. Using this as a guide, the corresponding areas of standard as well as sample are marked and extruded on a butter paper. To each extruded portion, add 5 ml of phosphate buffer solution, pH 5.3 and 5 ml of bromocresol purple solution and shake. It is then shaken with 10 ml of chloroform. Chloroform layer is allowed to separate and absorbance of the yellow complex in organic layer is measured at absorption maximum at about 410 nm. The results are calculated by comparison. For ion-pair complex, see formulation 5 of this chapter.

It has been reported that aromatic nucleus of the drug is first nitrated, then (NO_2) group reduced with Zn + HCl and then amino group coupled with Bratton-Marshall reagent to yield purple-coloured chromophore (λ_{max} 537 nm). The method obeys Beer's law in the range of 1-40 mcg/ml and colour being stable for more than 2 h.

Probable Reaction Mechanism

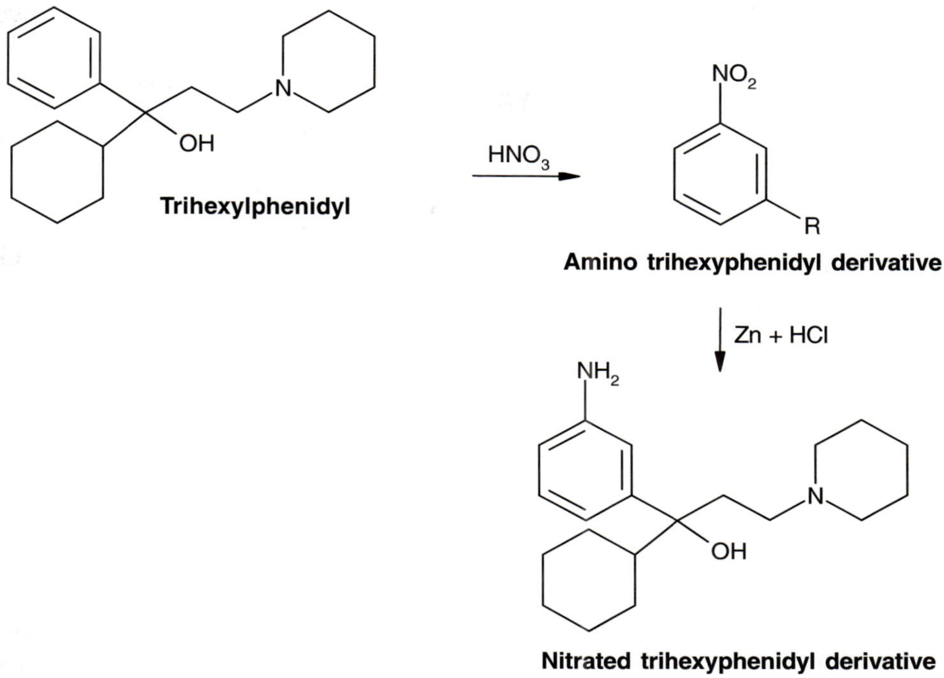

Note

The amino group can be diazotized and coupled with different reagents such as β-naphthol or 'NED' to give coloured chromophore.

Reference

Hemant Kumar, M.D. Karvekar, Sanjay Pai P.N. & Gopal Krishan Rao, 52nd IPC, Abstract No. GP-26.

Formulation 5

Methaqualone hydrochloride, Diphenhydramine hydrochloride

METHOD A

(a) Determination of Methaqualone hydrochloride

Preparation of standard solution

5 mcg/ml of methaqualone reference standard in 0.1 N hydrochloric acid.

Preparation of sample solution

Weigh accurately a portion of the powdered sample, equivalent to about 80 mg of methaqualone. Transfer to a 100 ml volumetric flask, and add 50 ml of 0.1 N hydrochloric acid. Shake the flask for 15 minutes, dilute to volume with 0.1 N hydrochloric acid, mix and filter. Further dilute the solution with 0.1 N hydrochloric acid, to get 5 mcg/ml.

Measure the absorbance of the sample and the standard preparations in a suitable spectrophotometer at the maximum at about 234 nm against 0.1 N hydrochloric acid as a blank. Calculate the quantity (mg) of methaqualone per tablet by comparison.

Determination of Diphenhydramine hydrochloride

Reagents

1. Phosphate-citrate buffer solution, pH 5.0: 48.5 ml of 0.1 M citric acid and 51.5 ml of 0.1 M disodium acid phosphate are mixed.
2. 0.05% w/v methyl orange solution in phosphate-citrate buffer, pH 5.0.
3. Acidified methanol : 1% w/v sulphuric acid in methanol.

Preparation of standard solution

Weigh accurately 50 mg of diphenhydramine hydrochloride and dissolve in chloroform to produce 100 ml. Dilute further with chloroform to get 5 mcg/ml concentration.

Preparation of sample solution

Weigh accurately powdered tablets equivalent to about 5 mg of diphenhydramine hydrochloride and add 70 ml of chloroform. Shake for 2 minutes and adjust with chloroform to 100 ml. Dilute 5 ml of the resultant solution to 50 ml with chloroform (5 mcg/ml).

Procedure

To 20 ml of standard and sample solutions, add 10 ml of methyl orange solution and shake for 30 seconds. Allow chloroform layer to separate. Take 10 ml of chloroform layer and add 3 ml of acidified methanol. Concomitantly measure the absorbance of both the solutions at absorption maxima at about 525 nm against reagent blank and compare the results.

METHOD B

(a) Determination of Methaqualone hydrochloride

Reagents

1. Saturated solution of ammonium vanadate in water : Dissolve sufficient quantity of ammonium vanadate in water and allow to stand for 24 hrs before use.
2. Dragendorff's reagent, modified: Boil a mixture of 25 ml of acetic acid, 2.5 g of basic bismuth carbonate and 7 g of sodium iodide for a few minutes. Keep for 12 hrs and filter through G_4 sintered glass funnel. Mix 20 ml of above filtrate with 80 ml of ethyl acetate and 0.5 ml of distilled water.

Preparation of standard solution

Weigh accurately 40 mg of pure methaqualone, add 1 ml of hydrochloric acid and few ml of water. Dissolve and dilute to 100 ml with water (0.4 mg/ml).

Preparation of sample solution

Weigh accurately powdered tablets equivalent to about 200 mg of methaqualone and suspend in 20 ml of water. Extract with four 20 ml portions of toluene. Dry the toluene layer under reduced pressure and dry the residue in desiccator. Methaqualone is quantitatively extracted into toluene layer. Retain the aqueous layer for estimation of diphenhydramine hydrochloride. Weigh accurately 40 mg of the residue obtained above, add 1 ml of hydrochloric acid to dissolve and dilute to 100 ml with water.

Procedure

Transfer 10 ml of standard and sample solutions to 25 ml volumetric flask, add 0.5 ml of saturated solution of ammonium vanadate and 1 ml of dragendorff's reagent. Shake for 1 minute and allow to stand for 1 h. Filter through G_4 glass sintered funnel. Transfer the precipitate quantitatively to the funnel. Wash thoroughly with distilled water till filtrate is colourless. Dissolve the precipitate (red complex) by passing acetone through the funnel to produce 100 ml. Dilute appropriately with acetone and measure the absorbance of the sample and standard solutions at absorption maximum at about 470 nm against reagent blank (10 ml of water treated as per sample or standard solutions). The colour is stable for 24 hours at room temperature. The method obeys Beer's law in the concentration range of 2-45 mcg/ml.

Note

Aspirin, phenacetin, meprobamate and salicylamide do not interfere in this method.

(b) Determination of Diphenhydramine hydrochloride

Filter the aqueous extract obtained during the extraction of methaqualone with toluene. Wash the residue with water to produce 100 ml. Dilute further appropriately with water to produce 100 mcg/ml solution.

Procedure

To 1 ml of sample solution, add 20 ml of chloroform and follow the method described for determination of diphenhydramine hydrochloride under method-A of this formulation.

METHOD C

(a) Determination of Methaqualone hydrochloride

Reagents

1. Saturated solution of ammonium reineckate in water.
2. 0.02% w/v ammonium reineckate solution in water, wash solution.

Preparation of standard and sample solutions

Prepare the standard and sample solutions as described under method-B of this formulation for determination of methaqualone. Retain aqueous extract obtained during extraction of sample with toluene for determination of diphenhydramine hydrochloride.

Procedure

Transfer 10 ml of standard and sample solutions to a stoppered flask, add 5 ml of saturated solution of ammonium reineckate. Shake for 5 minutes and filter through G_4 sintered funnel. Wash the precipitate with ammonium reineckate-wash solution and dry the precipitate under reduced pressure.

Dissolve the residue by passing acetone through funnel to produce 100 ml. Dilute further appropriately with acetone and measure its absorbance at absorption maximum at about 525 nm. The colour of complex is stable for 3 hr. The method obeys Beer's law in the concentration range of 2-20 mcg/ml.

Note

Aspirin, paracetamol, analgin, meprobamate and salicylamide do not interfere in this method.

(b) Determination of Diphenhydramine hydrochloride

Filter the aqueous extract obtained during extraction of methaqualone with toluene and follow the method-A for determination of diphenhydramine hydrochloride.

METHOD D

(a) Determination of Methaqualone hydrochloride

Reagents

1. 5% w/v solution of phosphomolybdic acid in absolute alcohol-ether mixture.
2. 1% w/v solution of hydrazine hydrate.
3. Absolute alcohol-ether (1 : 5 v/v) mixture.

Preparation of standard solution

25 mg/100 of pure methaqualone in absolute alcohol-ether mixture.

Preparation of sample solution

Extract the sample with toluene to get methaqualone. For details, see preparation of the sample solution under method-B in this formulation. The residue of methaqualone thus obtained is dissolved in absolute alcohol-ether mixture to get 25 mg/100 ml.

Retain the aqueous layer for determination of diphenhydramine hydrochloride.

Procedure

To 10 ml of sample and standard solutions, add 5 ml of phosphomolybdic acid reagent. Filter the precipitate through G_4 sintered funnel and wash the residue with alcohol-ether mixture till free from the reagent. Add to the crucible, 3 ml of hydrazine hydrate solution and 10 ml of water. Filter and wash the crucible with water. Add 10 ml of dilute sulphuric acid to the filtrate and adjust with water to 250 ml. Dilute this solution further appropriately and read at 725 nm. The molybdenium-complex shows no sharp maxima but a broad band of absorption in the range of 715-740 nm is observed. The method obeys Beer's law in a concentration range of 5-30 mcg/ml.

On heating alcoholic solution of the drug with PDAB in (hydrochloric acid - 'Ehrlich' reagent), an orange red dye is produced.

Probable Reaction Mechanism

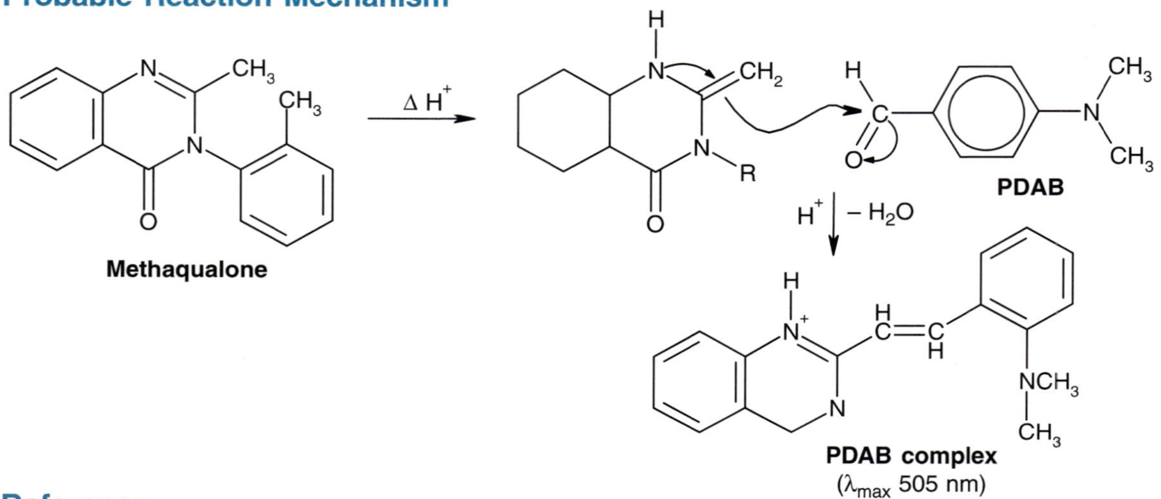

Reference

Pharmaceutical Chemistry (Vol. 2) by H.J. Roth, p. 641.

Another analytical method suggested is based on nitrite titration i.e. after hydrolysis the compound yields o-toluidine, anthranilic acid and acetic acid. o-toluidine being lipophilic is extractable into chloroform and anthranilic acid is quantitatively estimated nitrometrically using potassium iodide—starch paper as indicator.

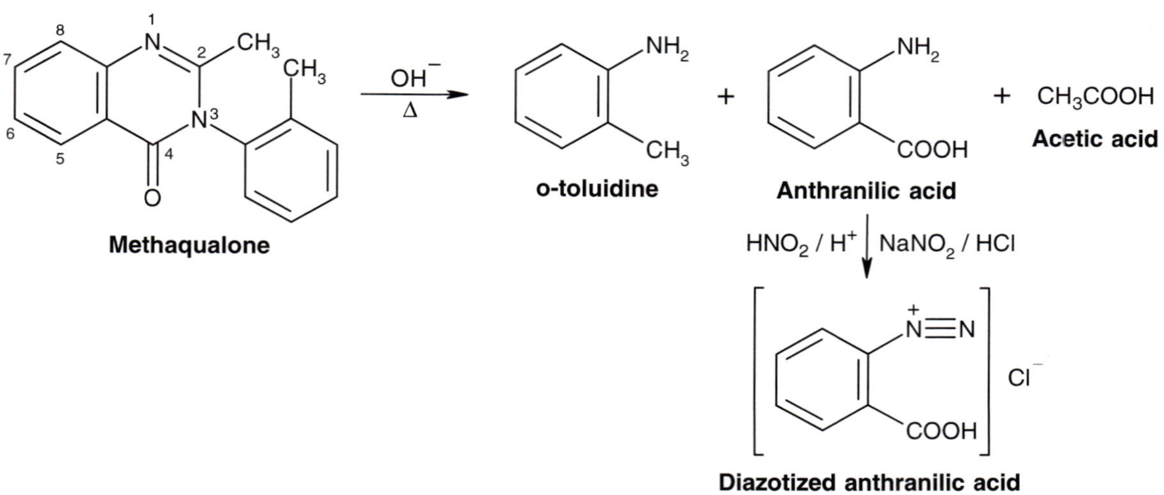

Excess HNO_2 reacts with KI oxidizing it to I_2 which reacts with starch giving blue inclusion complex.

(b) Determination of diphenhydramine hydrochloride

Filter the aqueous layer obtained above during extraction of methaqualone and follow the method described for determination of diphenhydramine hydrochloride under method-A of this formulation.

Formulation 6

Diazepam, Diphenhydramine hydrochloride

ESTIMATION

Diazepam

Standard solution

5 mcg/ml of diazepam in methanol.

Sample solution

Accurately weighed quantity of the powdered sample equivalent to 5 mg of diazepam extracted with 20 ml of dry ether by shaking for 5 min. The ether layer evaporated to dryness and residue taken up in methanol to get a solution of 5 mcg/ml.

The absorbance of both sample and standard solutions measured at 245 nm and results calculated by comparison.

Diphenhydramine hydroxide

Standard solution

200 mcg/ml of diphenhydramine hydroxide in methanol.

Sample solution

The residue left after extraction of the powdered sample with dry ether as under estimation of diazepam was taken up in methanol and diluted to get final concentration of 200 mcg/ml in respect of the substance.

The absorbance of both sample and standard was measured at 255 nm using methanol as blank and results calculated by comparison.

Formulation 7

Haloperidol, Trihexyphenidyl

ESTIMATION

Haloperidol

Accurately weighed quantity of powdered sample is suspended in 30 ml of ether (saturated with water). Extract with 4 × 15 ml portion of 0.25 M sulphuric acid. Combine the acid extracts and heat in a water-bath till there is no perceptible odour of ether. Dilute to 100 ml with 0.25 M sulphuric acid. To 25 ml of the sample, add 5 ml of methanol and sufficient 0.25 M sulphuric acid to get 50 ml.

Measure the absorbance of the resulting solution at 245 nm and calculate the results using 340 as value of A 1%, 1 cm.

Note

1. In methanol, λ_{max} 245 nm.
2. By extraction procedure, any interference due to parabens gets removed.

The compound reacts with 2,4-dinitrophenyl hydrozone yielding hydrazone derivative.

Probable Reaction Mechanism

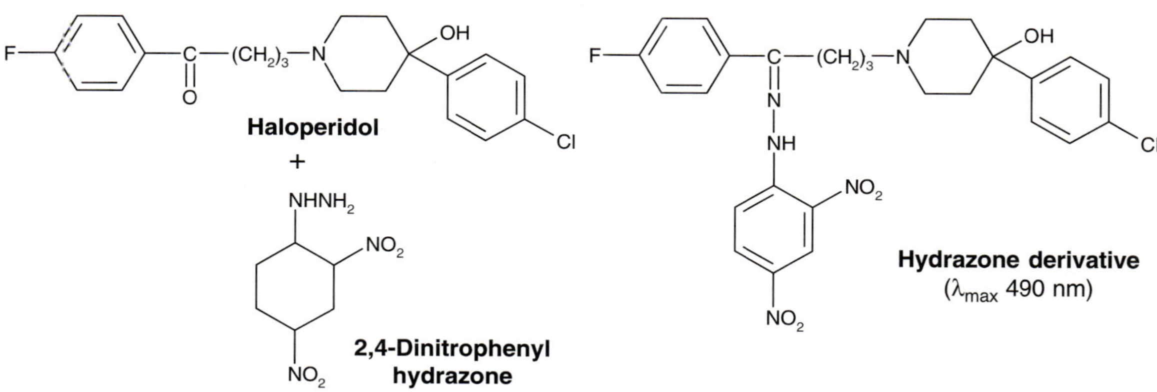

A method had been proposed by Haemers et al. (1969) based on formation of Meisenheimer salt as discussed under diazepam. In strong alkali anion is formed which reacts with 2,4-dinitrobenzoic acid to yield coloured salt (λ_{max} 525 nm).

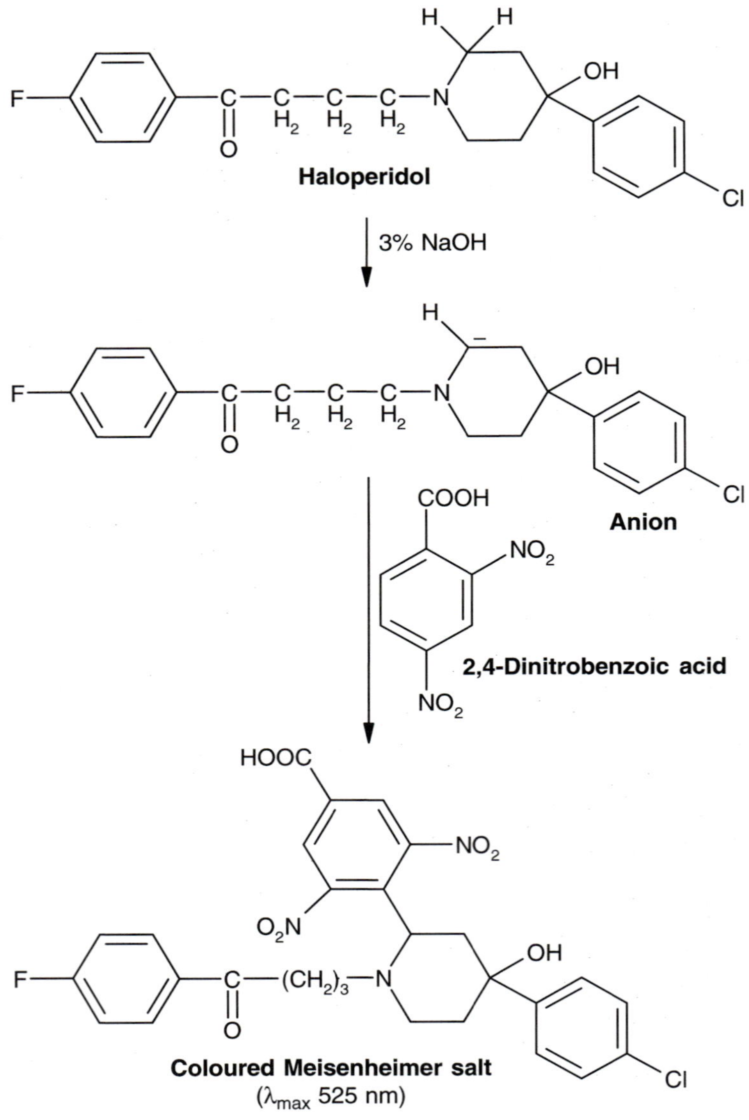

Note

Substitution of hydrogen in haloperidol by a nucleophile does not occur in benzene, but in the presence of nitro group it is sufficient to activate ortho or para positions. Nitrobenzene is itself a mild oxidizing agent, so the reaction proceeds without adding any oxidizing agent.

Reference

1. A. Haemers & W. van Bosschie, J. Pharm. Pharmacol., **21**, 531-532, 1969.
2. Pharmaceutical Chemistry (Vol. 2) by H.J. Roth, 1991, p. 132.
3. Organic Chemistry by I.L. Finar, 9th ed., p. 628.

An ion-pair complex formation with the drug and the dye (methyl orange) at pH 5.0 had been proposed by Janicki et al. (1974). The complex was extractable into chloroform, which in turn was acidified with methanolic hydrochloric acid to give coloured complex (λ_{max} 525).

Alcoholic solution of the compound on treatment with $KMnO_4$ in acidic medium was oxidized to give a compound which has fluorescent properties.

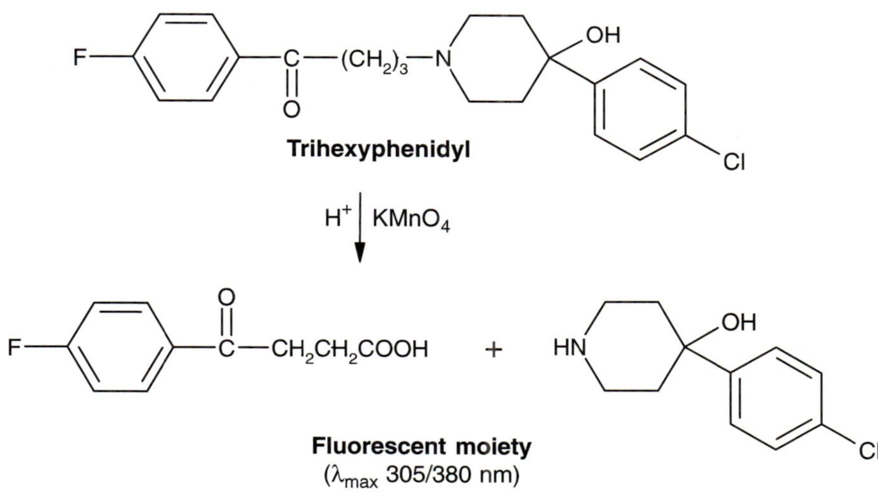

Reference

W. Baeyens & P. De Moerloox, Pharmazie, **32**, 764, 1977 through Analytical Profile of Drug Substances, Vol. 9, p. 364.

Trihexyphenidyl

Reagents

1. Phosphate buffer solution, pH 5.3 ± 0.1 : To 55 ml of solution of dipotassium hydroxide phosphate (8.7%), add 20 ml of citric acid solution (9.6%).
2. Bromocresol purple solution : Dissolve 400 mg of the dye in 30 ml of water, add 6.3 ml of 0.1 N sodium hydroxide and dilute to 500 ml with water.

Standard solution

10 mcg/ml of the substance in water (solution is usually affected by heating).

Sample solution

Accurately weighed quantity of the powdered sample equivalent to 2 mg of the substance is suspended in 40 ml of hot water. Heat slightly with swirling and make up the volume to 100 ml.

Procedure

To 2 ml each of sample and standard, add 5 ml of buffer and 5 ml of dye solution, shake to mix and to each add 10 ml of chloroform. Shake and allow the layers to separate. Measure the absorbance of chloroform layer at 420 nm using chloroform as blank.

The method is based on ion-pair complex in pH 5.3 buffer. The complex is extractable into chloroform.

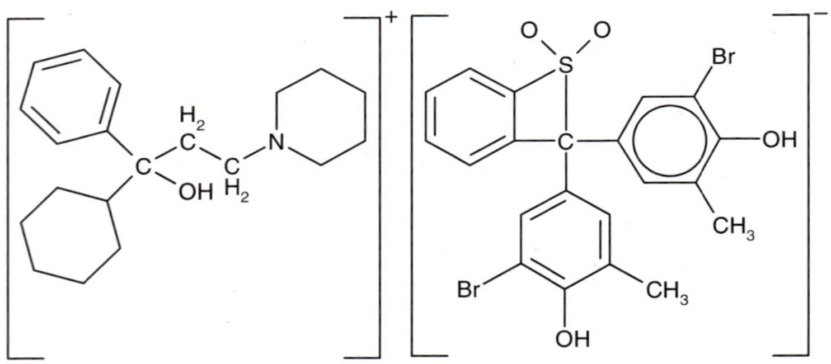

Trihexyphenidyl - Bromocresol purple ion-pair complex
(λ_{max} 420 nm)

Formulation 8

Haloperidol, Propantheline bromide

ESTIMATION

Haloperidol

Standard solution

200 mcg/ml of haloperidol in methanol. 5 ml of this solution is diluted to 100 ml with 1 N sulphuric acid (10 mcg/ml).

Sample solution

Weigh accurately powdered sample equivalent to 1 mg of the substance and suspend in 20 ml of 1 N sulphuric acid. Make it distinctly alkaline with 1 N sodium hydroxide and extract with 5 × 40 ml of chloroform, washing each chloroform layer with same 2 × 25 ml of water. Discard the aqueous layer and extract the organic layer with 4 × 20 ml of 1 N sulphuric acid, collecting the acid extract in 100 ml volumetric flask. Add 5 ml of methanol and dilute to volume with 1 N sulphuric acid.

Measure the absorbance of both sample and standard solutions at about 245 nm using 5% v/v methanol or 1 N sulphuric acid as blank. Calculate the results in term of mg/tablet. λ_{max} is 245 nm in methanol.

The carbonyl group present in the compound reacts with 2,4-dinitrophenyl hydrazine to give yellow-coloured hydrazone.

Probable Reaction Mechanism

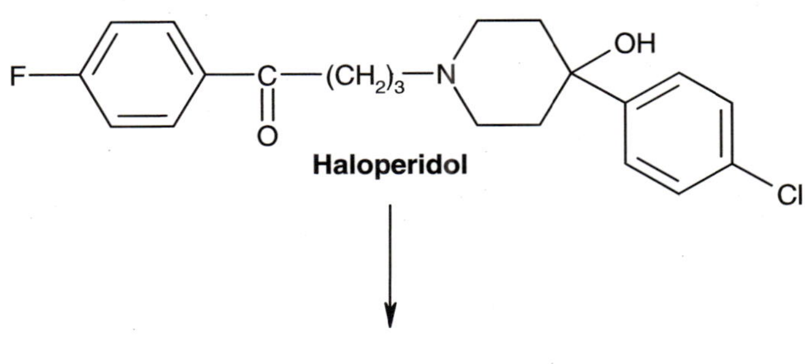

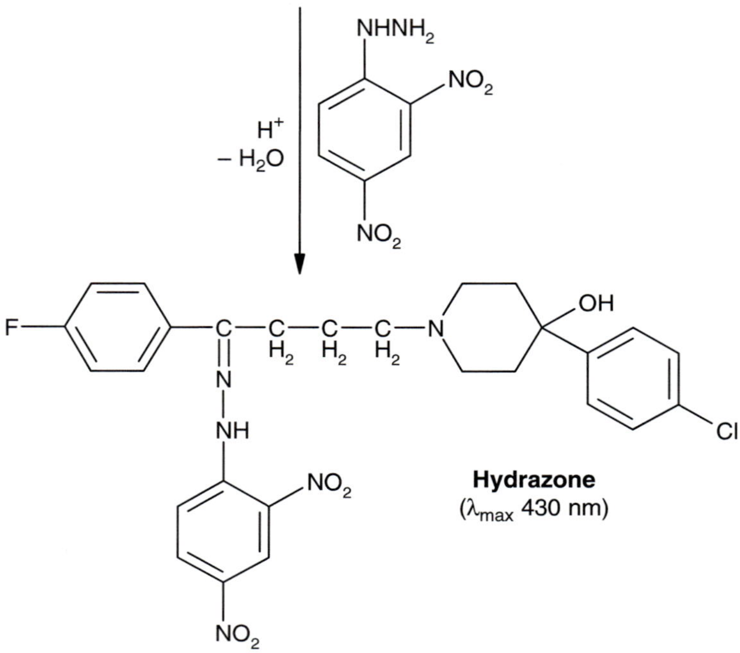

Its reaction with 3,5-dinitrobenzoic acid in alkaline medium can form the basis for colorimetric method.

Probable Reaction Mechanism

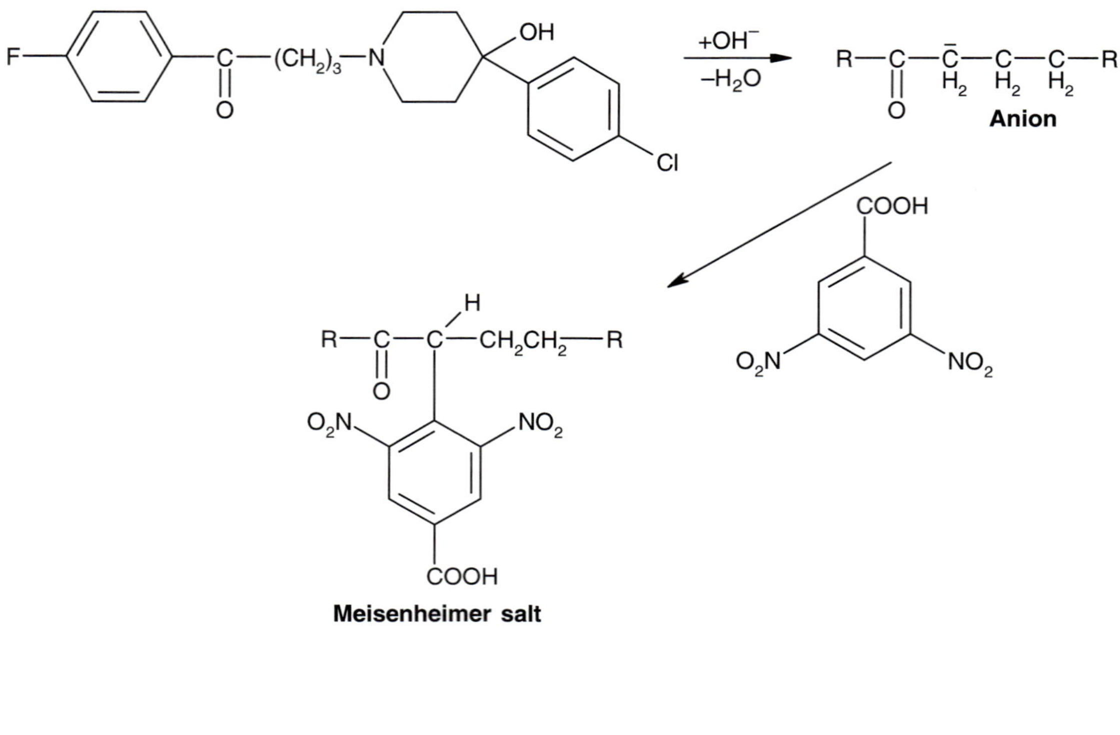

Reference

Pharmaceutical Chemistry (Vol. 2) by H.J. Roth, 1991, pp. 134 & 667.

Propantheline bromide

Transform accurately weighed quantity of the powdered sample equivalent to 250 mg of propantheline bromide to a G_3 sintered glass funnel. Water the powdered material with 4 × 20 ml portions of anaesthetic ether, removing ether each time by mild suction. Extract the powder on sintered funnel with 6 × 25 ml chloroform. Evaporate the combined chloroform layer and take up the residue in 50 ml of glacial acetic acid. Warm gently to affect the solution. Add 6 ml of mercuric acetate (6%) and dilute with 0.05 N perchloric acid using crystal violet as indicator. Carry out the blank titration. Each ml of 0.05 N perchloric acid is equivalent to 14.948 of propantheline bromide.

Formulation 9

Trifluoperazine, Isopropamide iodide

ESTIMATION

Isopropamide

Reagent

Methyl orange buffer solution: Dissolve 200 mg of methyl orange in phosphate-sodium carbonate buffer (pH 10.2) by heating in steam-bath and constant stirring and finally diluting to 200 ml with buffer.

Standard solution

100 mcg/ml of isopropamide iodide in 0.1 N sulphuric acid.

Sample solution

Weigh accurately powdered sample equivalent to 10 mg of isopropamide iodide, suspend in 60-70 ml of 0.1 N sulphuric acid, shake for 20 min and dilute to 100 ml with 0.1 N sulphuric acid (100 mcg/ml).

Procedure

To 5 ml each of sample and standard solutions, add 60 ml of chloroform and 30 ml of methyl orange buffer solution. Shake well for 3-4 min and allow to stand to ensure complete separation of two phases. Separate chloroform layer and repeat the extraction with 2×50 ml of chloroform. Combine the chloroform layer and extract with 3×25 ml of 10% hydrochloric acid. The acid layers are separated and diluted to 10 ml.

Measure the absorbance of both sample and standard at 510 nm using 10% hydrochloric acid as blank.

Note

Although the ion-pair complex in chloroform layer is yellow in colour it is extracted with acid to increase its sensitivity i.e. red colour (510 nm).

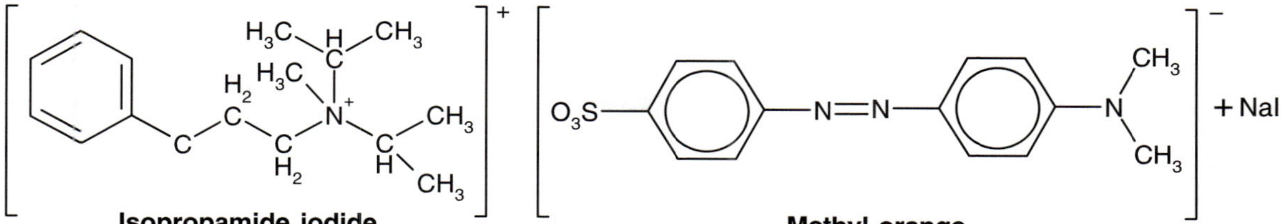

Isopropamide - methyl orange ion-pair complex in acid
(λ_{max} 510 nm)

Note

Before extracting the organic layer with hydrochloric acid, λ_{max} 415 nm, extraction with acid increases the sensitivity.

Reference

L.G. Chatten & K.O. Okamura, J. Pharm. Sci., **62**, 1328, 1973.

Trifluoperazine

METHOD 1

Accurately weighed quantity of the sample is suspended in 0.1 M hydrochloric acid to get final solution of 10 mcg/ml in respect of trifluoperazine. Measure the absorption of the solution at about 256 nm and calculate the results.

Note

Isopropamide has negligible absorbance at 256 nm (A 1%, 1 cm = 9.1) and interferes to the extent of about 5%.

Alternatively, 25 ml of the solution is made alkaline with 2 N sodium hydroxide (about 1.5 ml) and extracted with 3 × 25 ml of ether. The combined ether layer is in turn extracted with 0.1 M hydrochloric acid (3 × 25 ml) and diluted to 100 ml.

The absorption of both sample and standard (100 mcg/ml in 0.1 N hydrochloric acid) may be measured at 256 nm for final calculation.

METHOD 2

Reagents

1. 0.04% solution of bromophenol blue in water.
2. Buffer, pH 3.5, potassium hydrogen phthalate.

Standard solution

100 mg of trifluoperazine (base) and 40 mg of trihexyphenidyl is diluted in 50 ml of methanol. 10 ml of the resultant solution is diluted to 50 ml with methanol.

Sample solution

Accurately weighed quantity of the powdered sample equivalent to 20 mg of trifluoperazine is suspended in 30-35 ml of methanol. Shake vigorously for 15-20 min and make up to 50 ml with methanol, centrifuge.

Chromatographic parameters

TLC plates (aluminium) pre-coated with silica gel 60F_{254}.
Mobile phase : Acetone-water (85 + 15 v/v)
Development distance : 100 mm
Amount spotted : 80 ml of both sample and standard
Detection : Iodine chamber

After developing, the plate was dried and evaporated to iodine vapours. The spots were marked and plate was slightly heated to remove iodine. The separated marked spots to trifluoperazine and trihexyphenidyl were separately extracted with 5 ml of phosphate buffer (pH 3.5). To this add 5 ml of dye solution and 10 ml of chloroform. Shake and then allow the layers to separate. Measure the absorption of chloroform layer at 410 nm using chloroform as blank. The method is based on formation of ion-pair complex extracted into chloroform.

Formulation 10

Trifluoperazine, Chlordiazepoxide hydrochloride

ESTIMATION

Trifluoperazine

Follow the method for determination of trifluoperazine described under formulation 3 of this chapter. It has been experimentally observed that chlordiazepoxide hydrochloride does not interfere in the assay of trifluoperazine even when present 10 times its concentration.

Chlordiazepoxide hydrochloride

METHOD 1

Weigh powdered tablets accurately, equivalent to 100 mg of chlordiazepoxide. Extract and adjust the volume to 100 ml with 0.1 M hydrochloric acid. Dilute the resultant solution appropriately with 0.1 M hydrochloric acid to get a concentration of 5 mcg/ml. Measure the extinction at about 246 nm and calculate the results taking 1020 as value of A 1%, 1 cm.

Note

Trifluoperazine is normally present 1/10th of chlordiazepoxide in formulations and in such concentration, it has been observed that interference by trifluoperazine is even less than 3%.

METHOD 2

Being 1,4-benzodiazepines derivative, the compound can be subjected to acid hydrolysis (6 N hydrochloric acid) and the resulting yellow colour can be measured at about 410 nm. For details, refer to the method as described for diazepam in formulation 1 of the chapter on anti-inflammatory drugs.

Formulation 11

Diazepam, Propranolol hydrochloride

ESTIMATION

Diazepam

This method is based on acid hydrolysis of diazepam to 2-methylamino-5-chlorobenzophenone and the resultant yellow colour is measured at 410 nm. Methanolic solution of sample and standard (200 mcg/ml) is used for the acidic hydrolysis. For details refer to formulation 1 of the chapter on anti-inflammatory drugs.

Propranolol hydrochloride

Standard solution

10 mcg/ml of propranolol hydrochloride in methanol.

Sample solution

Accurately weighed quantity of the powdered sample is extracted with methanol to get a concentration of 10 mcg/ml. Measure the extinction of both sample and standard at 290 nm using methanol as blank.

Note

Interference due to diazepam in this method is less than 4%.

Typical laboratory analysis

Diazepam

Average weight of the tablet = 0.276 g

$$\text{Diazepam (mg/tab)} = \frac{A_v}{A_s} \times \frac{W_s}{W_u} \times d_f \times \text{Av. wt.} \times 1000$$

$$= \frac{0.230}{0.235} \times \frac{0.1018}{0.545} \times \frac{1}{20} \times 0.276 \times 1000$$

$$= 2.52 \text{ mg}$$

Claim = 2.5 mg

Propranolol hydrochloride

$$\text{Propranolol hydrochloride (mg/tab)} = \frac{0.490}{0.460} \times \frac{0.1044}{0.1432} \times \frac{1}{20} \times 0.276 \times 1000$$

$$= 20.74 \text{ mg} \qquad \text{Claim} = 20 \text{ mg}$$

A spectrophotometric method has been reported for estimation of propanolol in tablets. The method is based on using diazotized 4-amino-3,5-dinitrobenzene and 'ADBA' as the chromogenic reagent resulting in the formation of azo dye (λ_{max} 470 nm). The solution of 'ADBA' in conc. sulphuric acid was diazotized and reacted with propanolol (100 µg/ml in glacial acetic acid). The reaction was terminated after 5 min by placing the reaction mixture in ice-bath. The aqueous solution was extracted with ethyl acetate and the absorption of the organic layer was measured at 470 nm against reagent blank. The diazo coupling gave blue colour instantly which changed to purple and later to reddish pink within 5 min. This bathochromic shift is due to blank reagent in the underivitized drug.

Probable Reaction Mechanism

Diazonium ion is reported to couple with phenolic ether such as anisole. The p-position to the naphthoxy oxygen is favoured as it is typical of α-naphthol.

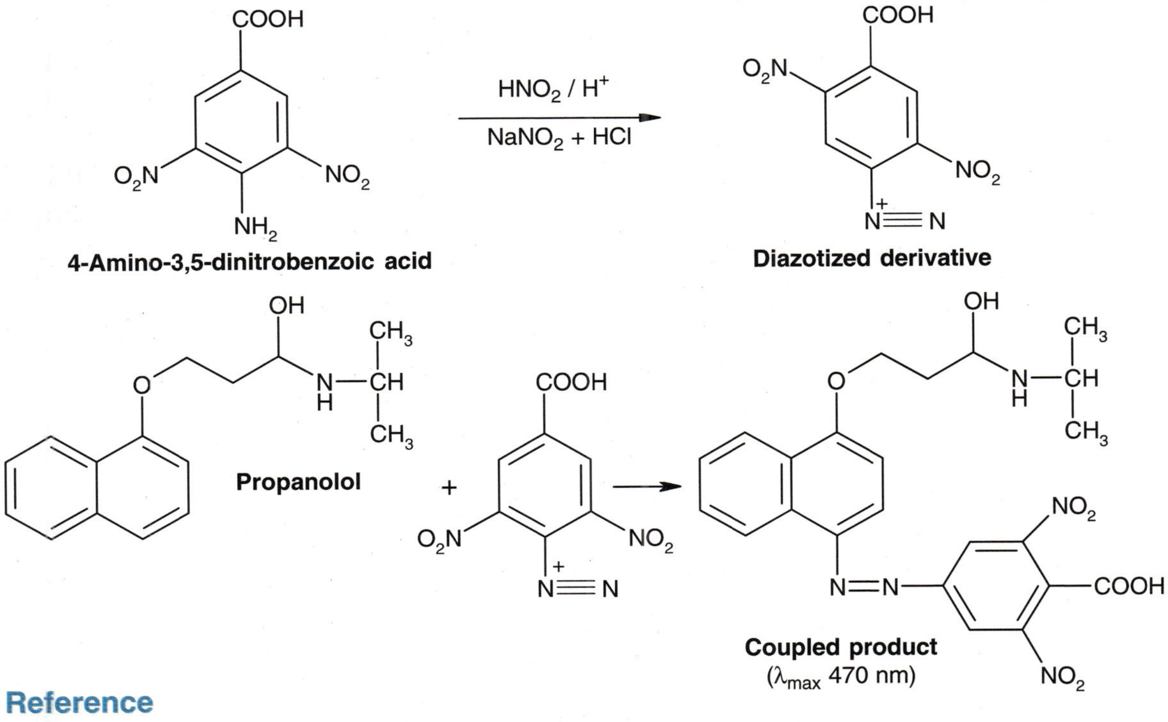

Reference

O.S. Idowu, O.A. Adegoke & A.A. Olaniyi, JAoAc. Int., **87(3)**, 573-578, 2004.

Formulation 12

Oxyphenbutazone, Diazepam, Pyridoxine hydrochloride

ESTIMATION

Oxyphenbutazone

Weigh accurately a quantity of the sample equivalent to 400 mg of oxyphenbutazone, add 4 ml of hydrochloric acid, 1 g of sodium chloride and extract with ether or chloroform. Evaporate organic layer and take up the residue in neutral acetone (bromothymol blue) and titrate with 0.1 M sodium hydroxide. Each ml of 0.1 M sodium hydroxide is equivalent to 0.03424 g of oxyphenbutazone.

Note

If the sample is first suspended in appropriate quantity of 0.1 M sodium hydroxide, filtered and then acidified for extraction, it will ensure complete extraction of the substance from matrix (see formulation 2 of this chapter).

Diazepam

Weigh accurately quantity of the sample equivalent to 2 mg of diazepam and carry out the estimation as described in formulation 9 of the chapter on analgesics and antipyretics, involving extraction from buffer solution, pH 7.0 or 9.0, followed by extinction at 368 nm in acidified methanol.

Note

Diazepam solution in acidified methanol exhibits maxima at 284 and 368 nm. Pyridoxine hydrochloride having maxima at 291 nm will interfere at 284 nm, hence extinction should be taken at 368 nm.

Alternatively the compound can be subjected to acid hydrolysis and the coloured product measured at 410 nm. For details refer to formulation 1 of this chapter.

Pyridoxine hydrochloride

Follow the method 3 for estimation of pyridoxine hydrochloride as described under general analytical methods for vitamins.

Formulation 13

Some Important General Reactions of Phenothiazine Derivatives

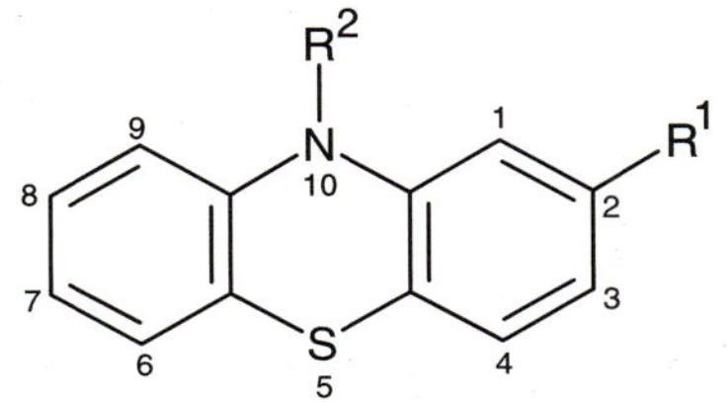

Phenothiazine derivatives

R^1 and R^2 are the substituents.
Reagents: $NaNO_2$, HCl.
$R^1 = Cl^-$, CF_3, OCH_3, CN, H
$R^2 = -(CH_2)_2, -N(CH_3)_2, -(CH_2)_3, -N(CH_3)_2$

Probable Reaction Mechanism

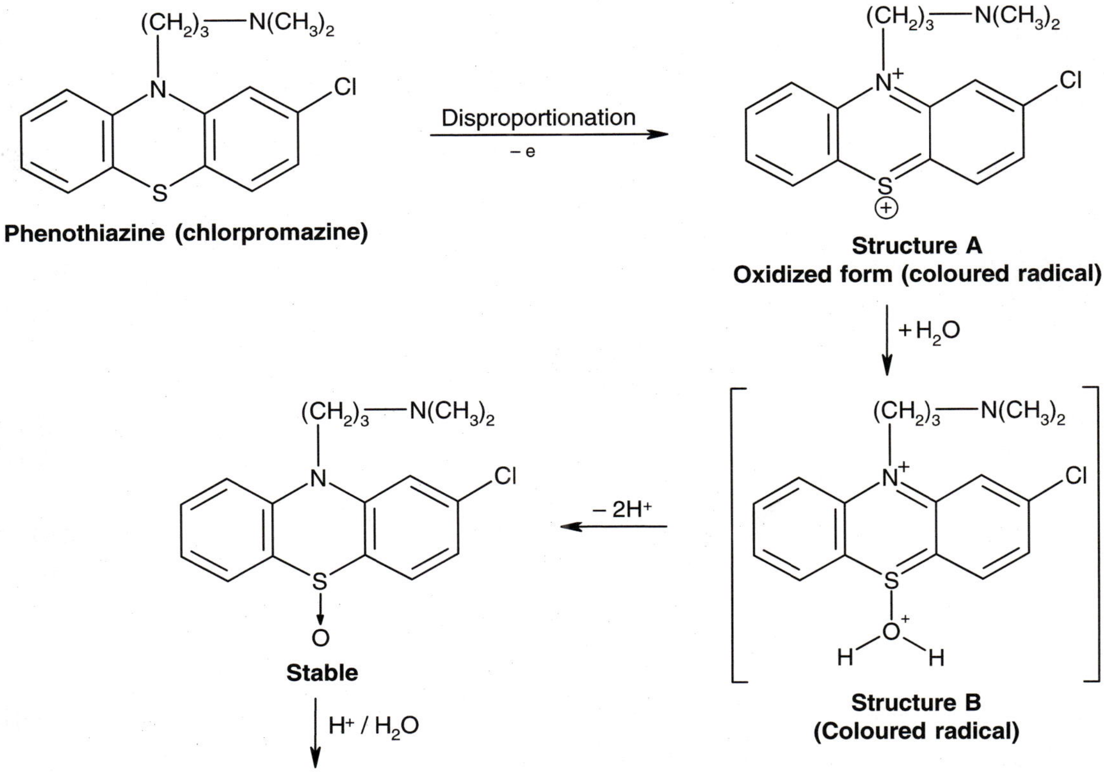

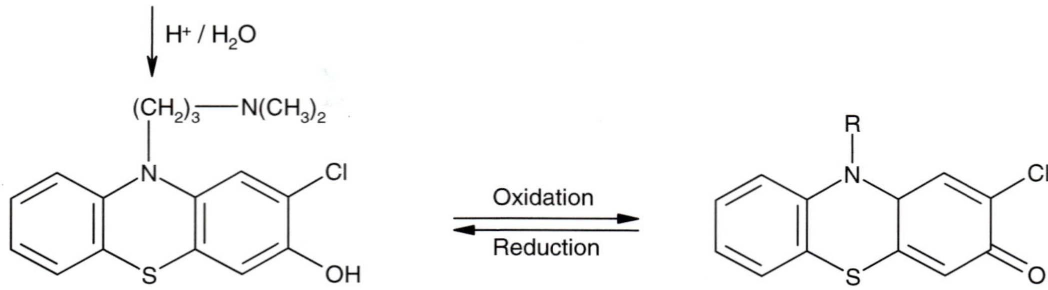

Structure C
(Colourless)

Phenothiazine-3-one (Quinoid)
(λ_{max} 490 nm)

Structure C so obtained contains a phenolic-OH group. Thus the nitrosonium ion generated from nitrous acid in acidic medium will attack the ortho position to the phenolic-OH group resulting in the formation of the product.

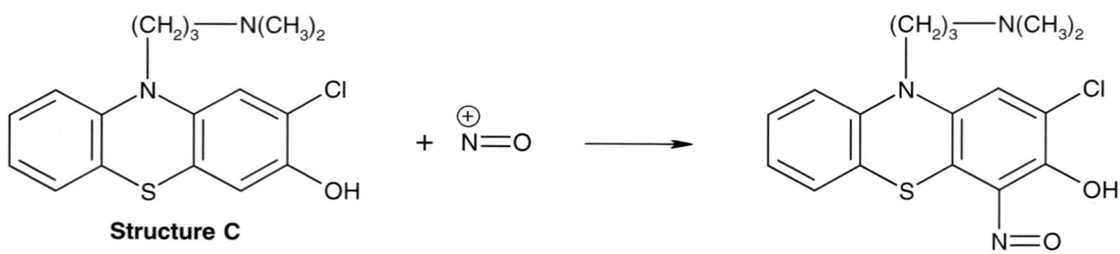

Structure C

But 'C' being unstable is rapidly oxidized to the quinoid form which is the final coloured product.

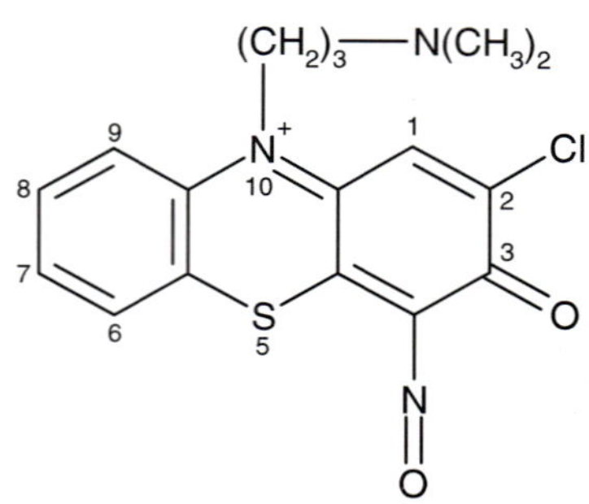

Phenothiazines are oxidized by Ce(IV) in acidic medium to yield fluorescent compound.

Probable Reaction Mechanism

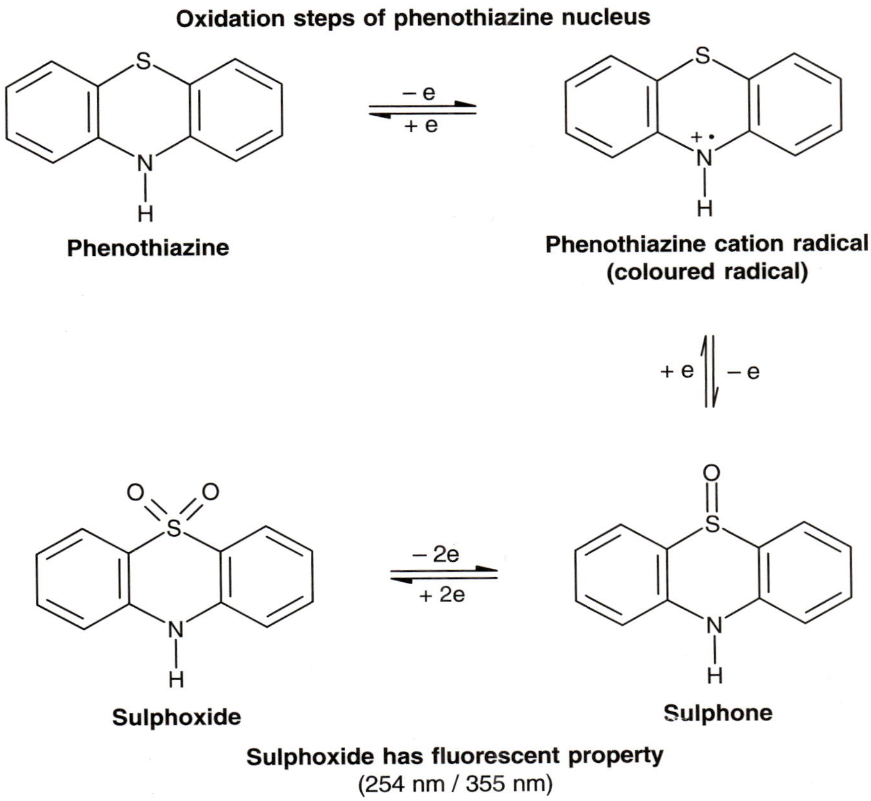

Reference

Fardous A. Mohamed et al., J. Pharm. & Biomed. Analysis, **39**, 139-146, 2005.

Chatten et al. (1971) while proposing a titrimetric method of analysis for phenothiazine derivatives using ceric sulphate and cupric perchlorate have suggested the following reaction mechanism. The oxidation proceeds through two successive distinct one-electron steps. A highly coloured free radical or semiquinone (II) results from first oxidation step. The loss of another electron gives phenazathionium ion (III) which reacts with water to give sulphonium base (IV). The base loses a proton to yield phenothiazine sulphoxide (V). Oxidation upto first step i.e. formation of semiquinone or free radical formed the basis of photometric method of assay and colourless end point was for titrimetric method of analysis. The authors have proposed the following reaction scheme.

Oxidation pathway of N-substituted phenothiazine derivative

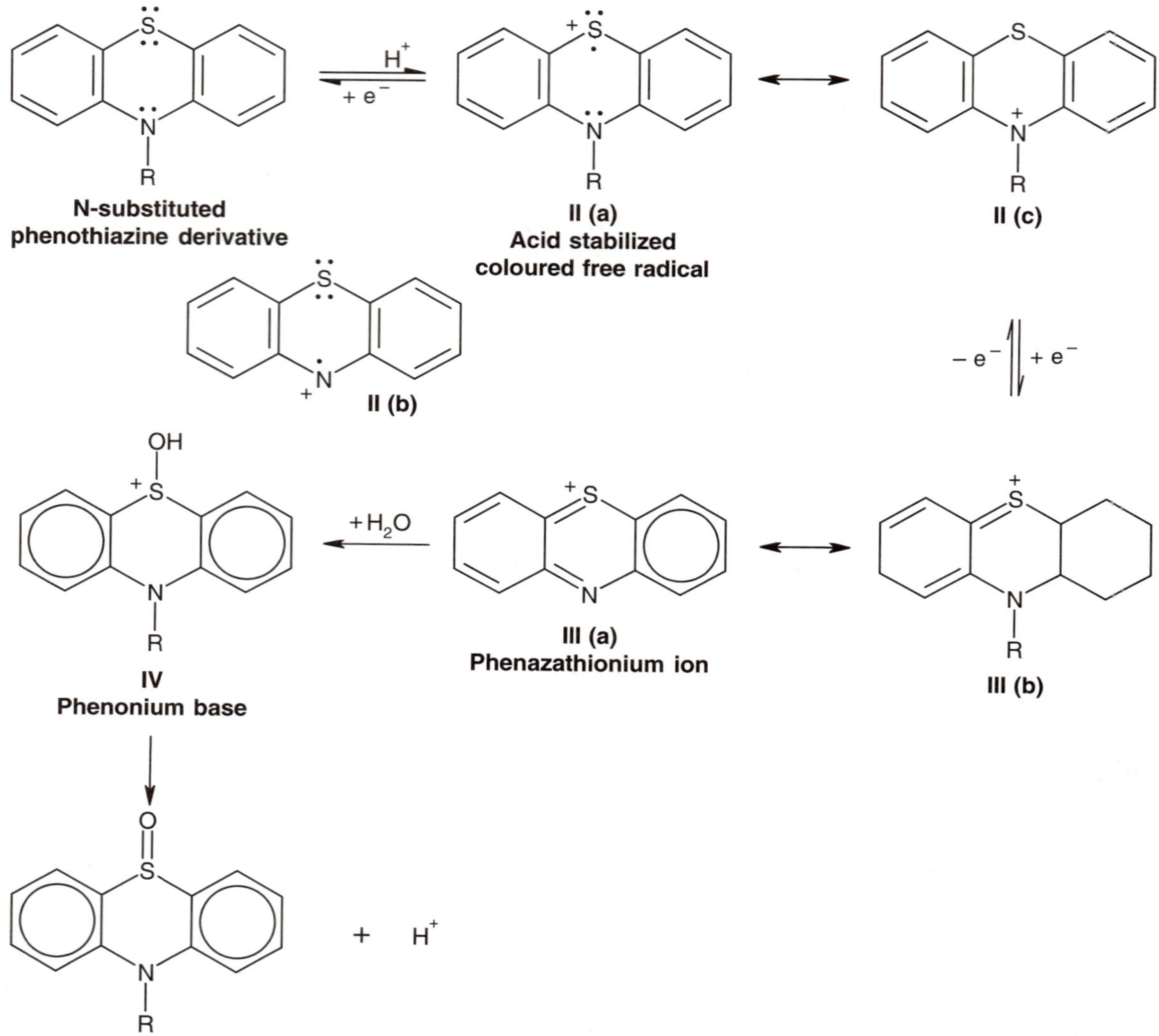

Phenothiazine sulphoxide

Reference

L.G. Chatten, R.A. Locock & R.D. Krause, J. Pharm. Sci., **60(4)**, 589-592, 1971.

Reagents

1. Van Urk's reagent: Dissolve 0.125 g of PDAB in cooled mixture of 65 ml of conc. sulphuric acid, 35 ml of water and 0.1 ml of 5% ferric chloride (should be allowed to stand for 24 h before use).

Sample and standard solutions

200 μg/ml in water.

Procedure

To 1 ml each of sample and standard solutions add 4 ml of the reagent, dilute to 10 ml with water and measure the absorbance of sample and standard solutions at 515 nm against reagent blank.

Probable Reaction Mechanism

In this case, Van Urk's reagent attacks at C-2 of the phenothiazine. Due to greater electron availability on the S atom the reaction proceeds as under.

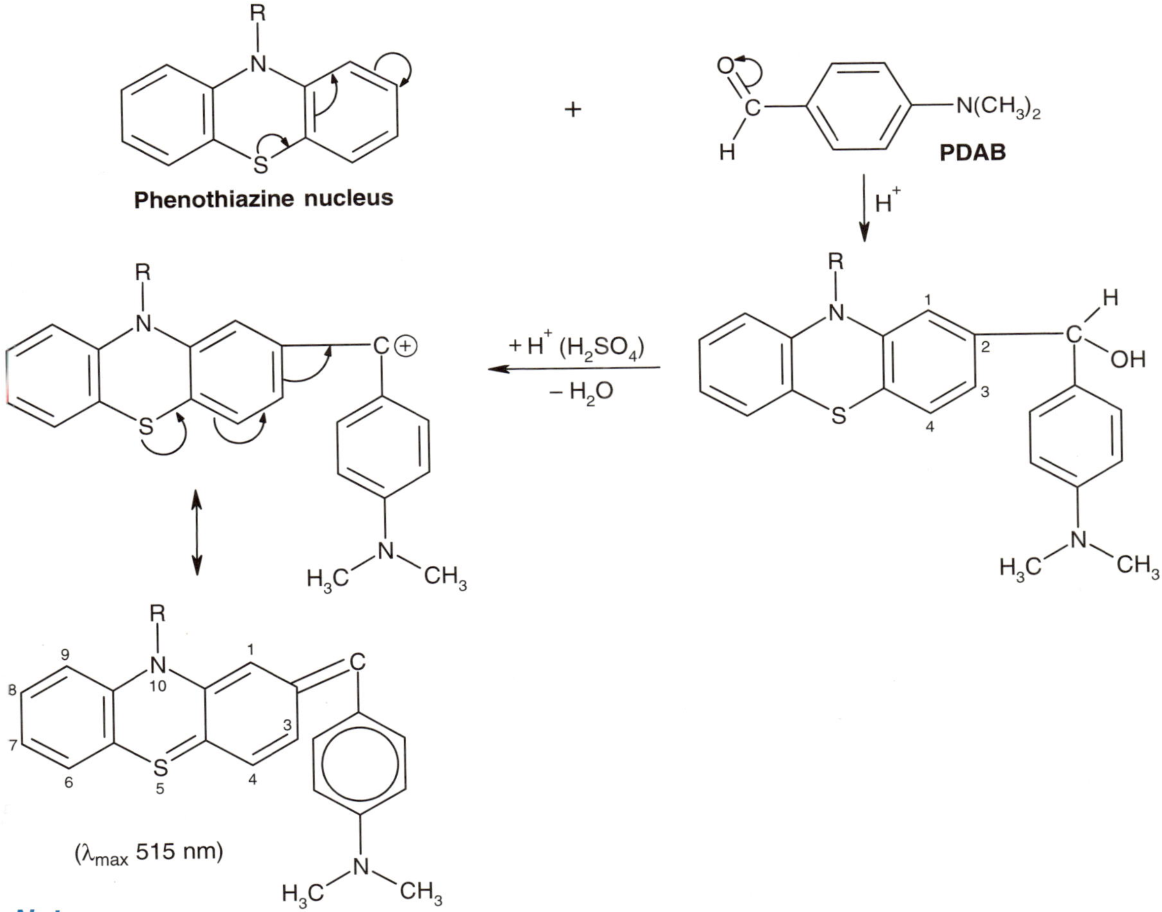

Note

This reaction is similar to the one proposed for methdialzine, a phenothiazine derivative (S. Emmuel & Roy Mathew, Indian Drugs, **22(11)**, 601-603). See also Pharmaceutical Chemistry (Vol. 2) by H.J. Roth, pp. 365, 694, 695.

Phenothiazines: Promethazine, Promazine, Mepazine and Trifluopromazine

Reagents

1. 0.02 M solution of picric acid (PA).
2. Methanol.

Sample and standard solutions

100 μg/ml in water.

Procedure

To 10 ml of 'PA' solution add solution of the sample and standard till there is no precipitate. Yellow-gold C-T complex of phenothiazine with PA filtered, washed with water till the filtrate is colourless. Dry in vacuum.

Prepare 50 μg/ml solution of phenothiazine - PA C-T complex in methanol and measure the absorbance at 360 nm. This absorption originates from picryl component of C-T complex.

Probable Reaction Mechanism

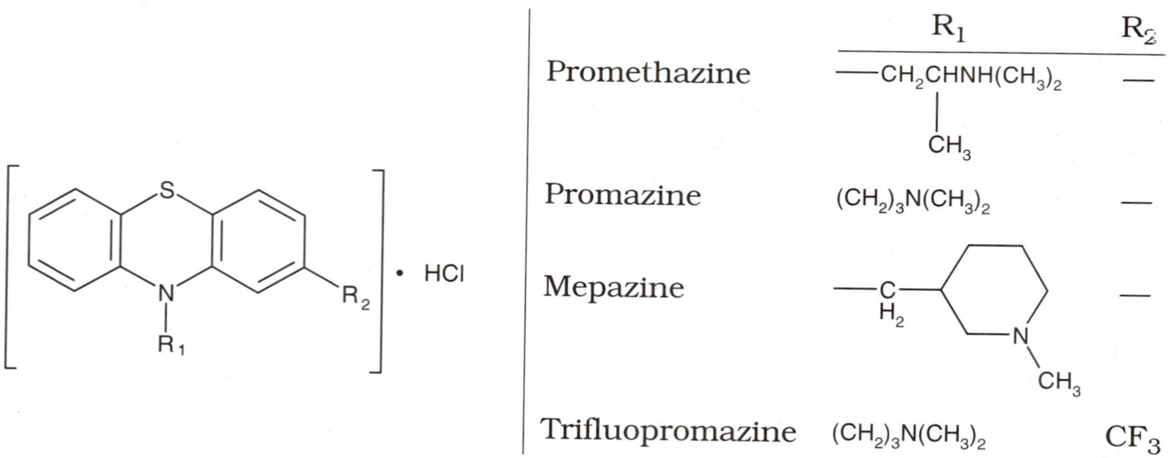

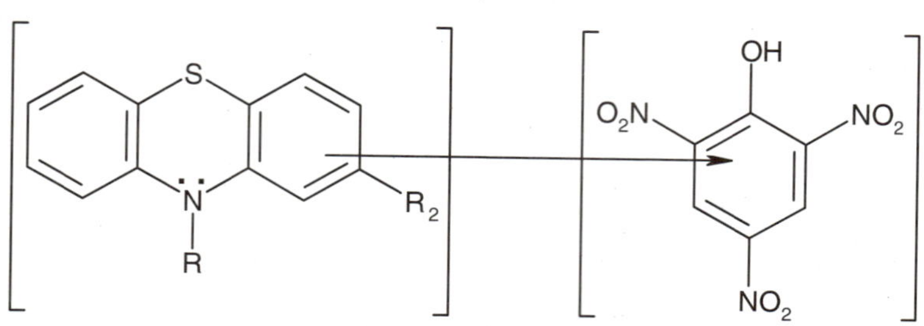

2,4,6-trinitrophenol picric acid (PA)

Phenothiazine - PA C-T complex

(λ_{max} 360 nm)

Reagent

5% w/v solution of phosphomolybdic acid prepared by dissolving in hot water by stirring and filtering if necessary.

Sample and standard solutions

200 μg/ml solution of each compound in 0.1 M HCl.

Procedure

To 1 ml each of sample/standard solutions add 1 ml of phosphomolybdic acid solution, shake, allow to stand for 10 min and dilute to 10 ml with water and measure the absorbance at respective wavelength against reagent blank. Promethazine (525 nm); Chlorpromazine (540 nm); Prochlorperazine (540 nm); Trifluoperazine (510 nm).

Probable Reaction Mechanism

By I.R. studies the authors have postulated that the reaction between phenothiazine and phosphomolybdic acid is accompanied by anion exchange at the main 'N' atom in the side chain as is the case with organic bases in general. Due to oxidative action of phosphomolybdic acid, phenothiazine is converted to free radical and a phosphomolybdate of cationic radical is formed by this oxidation. This is supported by the colour obtained corresponding to that reported in literature for free radicals formed by oxidation.

Note

The authors have established that derivatives with hydrogen at C-2 have λ_{max} 525 nm; chlorine at C-2 (perchlorperazine) causes bathochromic effect shifting λ_{max} to 540 nm; CF_3 group (trifluoperazine) causes hypsochromic shift (λ_{max} 510 nm).

Reference

Maria Stan, V. Dorneanu & G.H. Ghimicescu, Talanta, **24**, 140-142, 1977.

Sane et al. have reported spectrophotometric method for several compounds using phosphomolybdic acid (10%) reagent in alkaline medium (10% NaOH). All the compounds studied gave blue colour with λ_{max} between 660 to 690 nm. The compounds studied were terbutaline sulphate, vitamin B_1, levadopa, methyldopa, orciprenaline sulphate and ninhydrin hydrochloride.

Reference

R.T. Sane et al., Indian Drugs, **21(6)**, 254-256, 1984.

A spectrophotometric method based on interaction of nitroso-R salt to form 1 : 1 complex which can be extracted into chloroform has been described by Jayarama et al. (1986). Phenothiazines studied were promethazine, trifluoperazine, chlorpromazine hydrochloride, promazine hydrochloride in different dosage forms (tablets, injections, syrup, elixir, etc.).

Reagent

0.2% solution of nitroso-R salt (disodium 1-nitroso-2-naphthol-3,6-disulphonate) 'NRS' in water.

General Procedure

Transfer appropriate quantity of the sample/standard solution to a separating funnel. Add 3 ml of 'NRS' solution, mix, extract with 3 × 5 ml chloroform. Combine the entire layer, dilute to 25 ml with chloroform and measure the absorbance between 380 and 385 nm depending on the type of phenothiazine.

Probable Reaction Mechanism

Phenothiazines play a dual role in their action with 'NRS' acting both as electron donor in the charge-transfer interaction and as a hydrogen bonding through tertiary amino nitrogen atom in the side chain. A possible structure is as under.

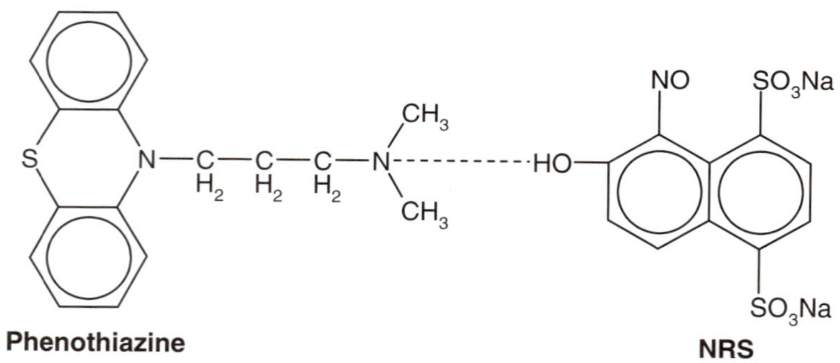

Possible structure of phenothiazine - NRS complex
(λ_{max} 385 nm)

Reference

Jayarama M., Violet D'Souza, H.S. Yathirajan & Rangaswamy, Talanta, **33(4)**, 352-354, 1986.

A method based on 'C.T.' using chloranilic acid as electron acceptor and phenothiazine (base) as donor in pharmaceutical formulations has been suggested by Zakhari et al. (1986). Chloranilic acid in organic solvent (acetonitrile) exists in un-ionized form and phenothiazine derivative has a lone pair of electrons which acts as a donor resulting in the formation of charge-transfer complex of π-π type which finally leads to the formation of radical ion.

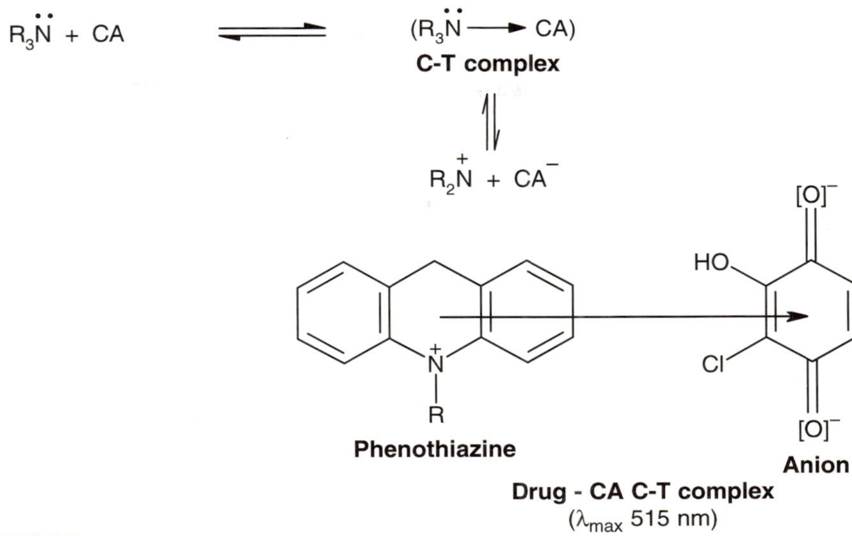

Reference

N.A. Zakhari, M. Rizk, F. Ibrahim & M.I. Walash, Talanta, **33(2)**, 111-114, 1986.

A spectrophotometric method for estimation of phenothiazines (promethazine, chlorpromazine, promazine) was proposed by Mahrous et al. (1984). The method involves use of sodium coballinitrite as oxidizing agent in acidic medium resulting in the formation of cation radical. The reaction mechanism is similar to the one proposed by Srinivasa et al. (2000) described earlier.

Reference

M.S. Mahrous & M.M. Abdel-Khalek, Talanta, **31(4)**, 289-291, 1984.

Promethazines are strong electron donors and are reported to form highly coloured charge-transfer (C-T) complexes with electron-acceptor reagents. The following reagents being electron-acceptors can be used for spectrophotometric analysis of different promethazines (promethazine, prochlorperazine, trifluperazine, chlorpromazine, etc.).

1. p-Benzaquinone
2. Chloranil
3. 7,7,8,8-Tetracyanoquinodimethane (TCNQ)
4. 2,4,7-Trinitro-9-fluorenone (TNF)
5. Tetracyanoethylene (TCNE)
6. 1,3,5-Trinitrobenzene (TNB)

Reference

Janet E. Forrest & R.A. Heacock, J. Chromatogr., **75**, 156-160, 1973.

A spectrophotometric method has been reported by Nagaraja et al. (1999) for the estimation of phenothiazines with specific refernce to promethazine. The method is based on oxidation with N-bromosuccinimide (NBS) followed by coupling with 4-aminobenzoic acid (ABA) giving coloured complex extractable into chloroform.

Probable Reaction Mechanism

Promethazine (I) is first oxidized by 'NBS' to give phenothiazinyl-free radical (II) and then to PMH cation having resonating forms (III, IV and V). The lowest electron density found at positions C-3, C-7 and S-5 which permits nucleophilic attack at position 3 or 7 by ABA. 'NBS' attacks at position 2 to form coloured compounds VI and VII (λ_{max} 510 nm).

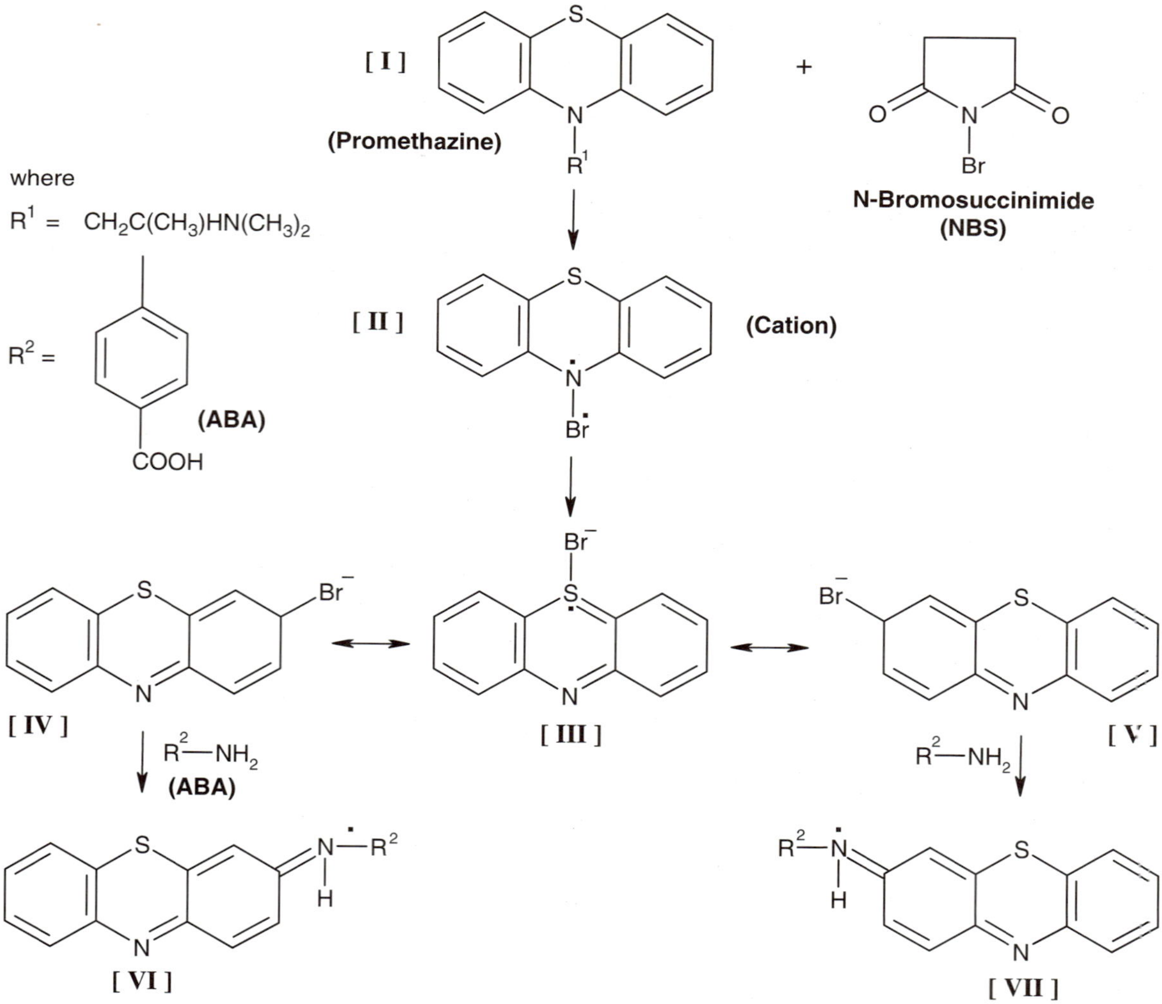

Reference

P. Nagaraja, K.C. Srinivasa Murthy & K.S. Rangappa, Eastern Pharmacist, pp. 103-105, June 1999.

Michael et al. (1988) have reported a spectrophotometric method for the estimation of N-substituted phenothiazines. The method is based on oxidative coupling of 3-methylbenzoline-2-one hydrazone (MBTH) with phenothiazines in the presence of oxidizing agent (Fe^{3+}) salt.

Under the reaction concluding, MBTH loses two electrons and one proton forming the electrophilic intermediate active coupling species which acts as chromogenic reagent. At the same time phenothiazine derivative is oxidized to a phenothiazinyl-free radical. This free radical has maximum electron density at C-2 and C-8 atoms. Finally electrophilic substitution takes place by the attack of 'MBTH' active species at position 2 or 8 of free radical giving conjugated methylene blue like dye stuff (λ_{max} 700-740 nm) depending on the drug under analysis. Phenothiazines react with MBTH in the ration of 1 : 1.

Reagents

1. 0.4% MBTH solution in water.
2. 0.5% Ferric (III) ammonium sulphate solution prepared in 0.5 M HCl.

Standard solution

500 μg/ml in 0.5 M HCl.

Sample solution (powders, tablets, drops and injections)

Extracted or diluted with 0.5 M HCl to get desired concentration.

Reaction mechanism as proposed by the authors

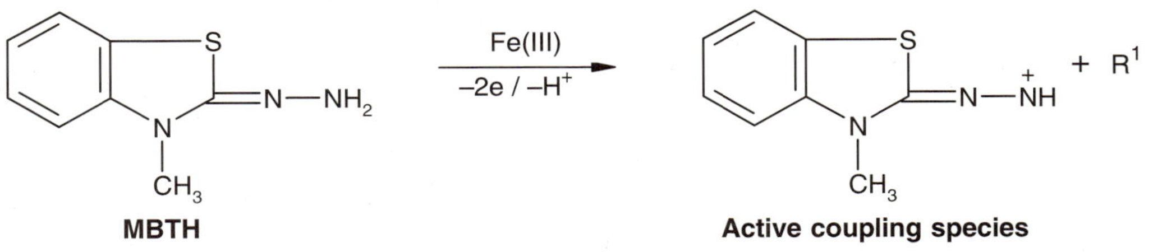

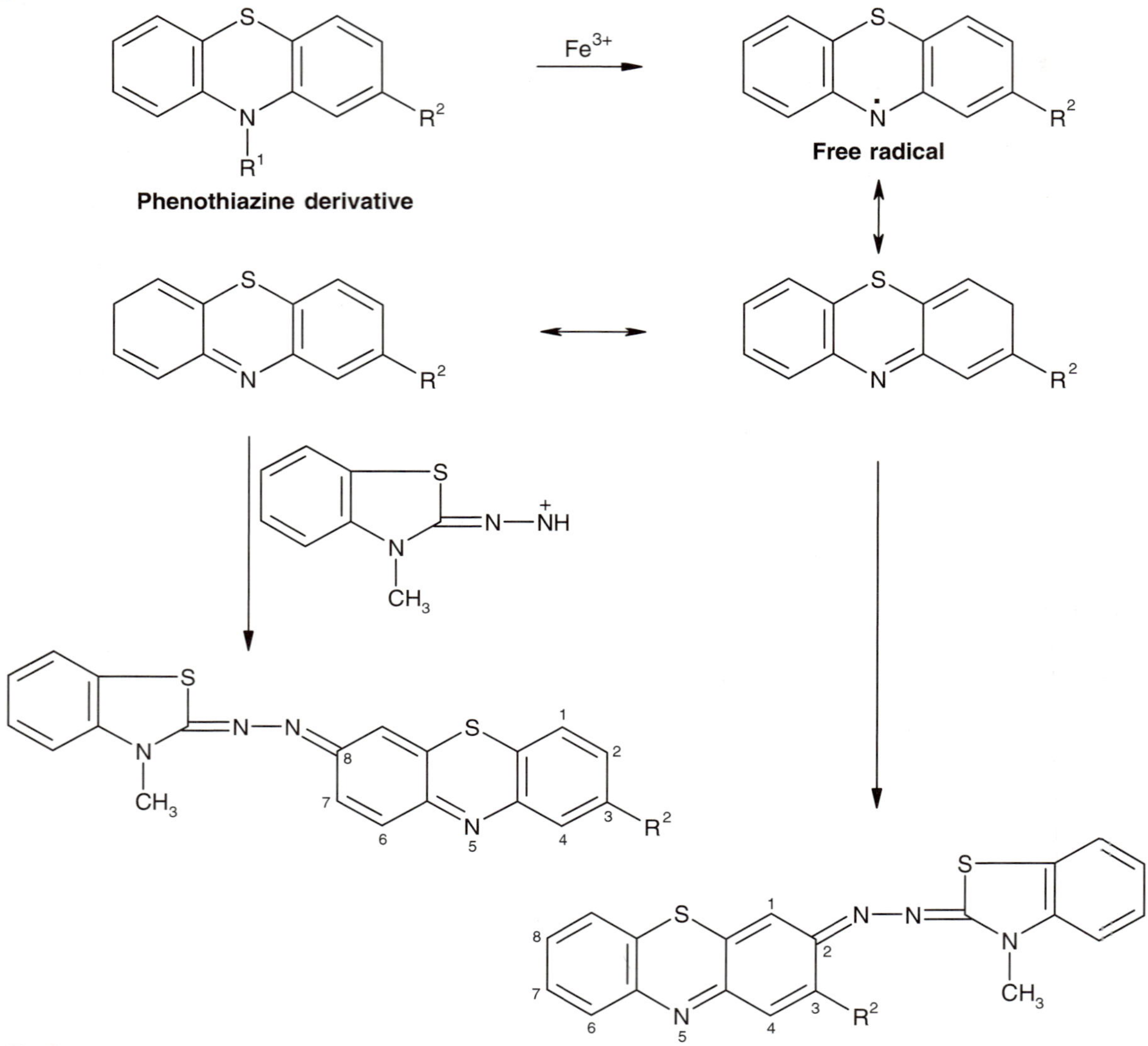

Reference

Michael E. El-Kommos & Kamla M. Emara, Analyst, **113**, 1267-1271, 1988.

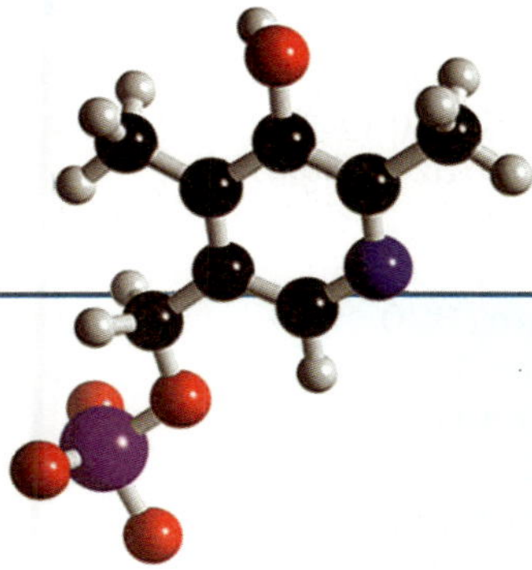

Drug Index

L

M

N

O

P

R

S

T

SETHI'S

Quantitative Analysis *of* Pharmaceutical Formulations

SETHI'S
Quantitative Analysis *of* Pharmaceutical Formulations

Methods With Reaction Mechanism

Fourth Edition

Volume 3

Dr. P.D. Sethi
M.Pharm., Ph.D.

CBS

CBS PUBLISHERS & DISTRIBUTORS PVT. LTD.
NEW DELHI • BENGALURU • PUNE • KOCHI • CHENNAI

ISBN : 978-81-239-2187-7

Third Edition : 1997
Reprint : 2003, 2004, 2005, 2008, 2010, 2011
Fourth Edition : 2012

Published by:
Satish K. Jain and produced by Vinod K. Jain for CBS Publishers & Distributors Pvt. Ltd.,
4819/XI Prahlad Street, 24 Ansari Road, Daryaganj, New Delhi - 110002 (India)
E-mail: cbspubs@airtelmail.com, delhi@cbspd.com • www.cbspd.com

Branches:
- ***Bengaluru:*** 2975, 17th Cross, K.R. Road,
  Bansankari 2nd Stage, Bengaluru - 560070
  Ph.: +91-80-26771678/79
  E-mail: cbsbng@gmail.com, bangalore@cbspd.com
- ***Pune:*** Bhuruk Prestige, Sr. No. 52/12/2+1+3/2,
  Narhe, Haveli (Near Katraj-Dehu Road By-pass), Pune - 411051
  Ph.: +91-20-64704058/59, 32342277 • E-mail: pune@cbspd.com
- ***Kochi:*** 36/14, Kalluvilakam, Lissie Hospital Road, Kochi - 682018, Kerala
  Ph.: +91-484-4059061-65 • Fax: +91-484-4059065
  E-mail: cochin@cbspd.com
- ***Chennai:*** 20, West Park Road, Shenoy Nagar, Chennai - 600030
  Ph.: +91-44-26260666, 26208620 E-mail: chennai@cbspd.com

Printed at :
Aegean Offset Printers, Greater Noida (UP)

To

Usha, my wife

Although no one is ever born talented nor talent obtained
as a gift or lucky coincidence, it is a resource acquired
through one's own endeavour,
but without her active support and inspiration,
I would never have been an author.

Dedicated to Fellow Analysts, Students, Teachers, Professionals and Mentors

I am quite aware that this compilation may not be flawless, but if I would have waited till it could be done without any error, probably this would never have been possible considering the fact that incompleteness is inevitable feature of any book. I do hope that this compilation will provide adequate stimulus for you to be a sound professional. I would like to appeal the fellow analysts, students, teaching fraternity and professionals to evaluate my efforts in proper perspective. It took me almost 15 years to scan most of the old analytical journals from 1950 onward, the period when analytical methods based on chromogenic reactions were most prevalent. I would like to express my gratitude to fellow analysts, teachers and the mentors in the profession who helped me to shape my ideas for compiling this text. The wide popularity of my books on spectrophotometric analysis, TLC, HPTLC and HPLC among pharmaceutical analysts, students and teachers has been gratifying and encouraging. My aim has never been to use my knowledge as a vehicle but only as a means of sharing my experience with prefessional fraternity.

P.D. Sethi
Pharmaceutical Analyst

"There is no barrier to acquisition of knowledge. Nobody owns it, everybody partakes it and the world becomes richer."

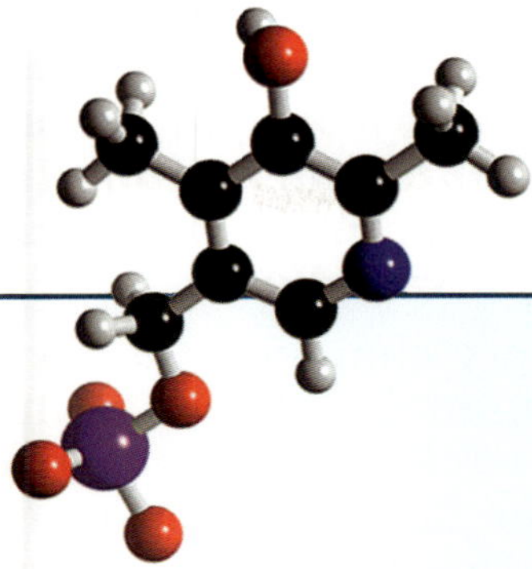

Preface to the Fourth Edition

After the first edition this book appeared in 1985, analytical and teaching fraternity have been of the considered opinion that for professional competency the knowledge of the chemistry involved in the analytical methods i.e. "Reaction Mechanism" needs to be provided, even though not legally mandated, to enable the analysts to perceive the methodology in proper perspective since all aspects of different methods are ultimately founded on chemistry. This is how the idea for contents of this book originated.

Although I had conceptualized the project in 1992 but being busy in compiling books on other subjects of current importance i.e. TLC, HPTLC, HPLC including revision of this title, I could not take up this project due to paucity of time and resources. Further, in view of complexity of the project, I did harbour serious doubts regarding its ultimate completion if and when taken up. If anyone feels that the books can be written by setting an author on his or her way and then waiting for the manuscript to appear, they are delusioned. It needs constant adaptation, definite level of discipline and hunger to keep going. I had been exploring the possibility of associating some teachers with sound knowledge of basic organic chemistry, but met with no success. It has been my ultimate **desire** to complete the project before I close my shop forever.

Knowing fully well that nothing can be achieved without enthusiasm and dedication, being **SCORPIO** decided to accept the challenge with the **SELF BELIEF** and complete the project by myself. I sincerely hope that this series shall find permanent place in every analytical laboratory and teaching institutions with the assurance that such an exhaustive compilation on the subject may never be available.

"Desire is perhaps the starting point of achieving something."

"Belief is the knowledge that we can do something. It is the inner feeling that what we undertake, we can accomplish."

"Scorpio have creative mind with sharp memory, truly explorer of new intelligent horizon, have great stamina and never shy away from challenges, extremely introspective with analytical mind, highly intuitive, determined in pursuit of their goal, passionate about every thing they do, have strong sense of purpose in life with determination to do nothing half-heartedly."

For practical consideration, in addition to introductory chapters, the book has been arranged in 13 principal chapters each containing different multi-component formulations. Analytical methods for each ingredient in a formulation have been described on the pattern similar to 3rd edition using mainly UV-Vis spectroscopy as principal analytical tool. However, as clear from the title, uniqueness of 4th edition is that with each method "probable reaction mechanism" has been described for proper understanding of the methodology as describing methods while ignoring chemistry was considered to be an incomplete endeavour. This should help analysts to integrate fully the analytical methods with the chemistry involved and enable them to transmit the knowledge to others who want to learn. Majority of the reactions included in the text are of the type – addition, elimination, substitution, condensation, rearrangement or oxidation-reduction invariably resulting in the formation of a coloured end product, which could easily be quantified spectrophotometrically in visible region (400-800 nm). This once again established the importance of UV-Vis spectroscopy as an indispensable, reliable and well established analytical tool in spite of steep increase in the use of other physical methods of analysis (HPLC, HPLC/MS, GC, GC/MS, HPTLC, etc.). Analytical methods based on chromogenic reactions have stood the test of time and are still recommended for the fledgling analysts.

Understanding the reaction mechanism allows us to know its specificity and the reaction with the drug being analysed. For drugs having more than one functional group, the methods have been designed depending on the specificity of a particular functional group. With selective chemical reactions, the analyst can manipulate the sample to reveal the desired information and increase the selectivity of the analyte eliminating the possible interference due to other substances present in the formulation while analyzing. It is not

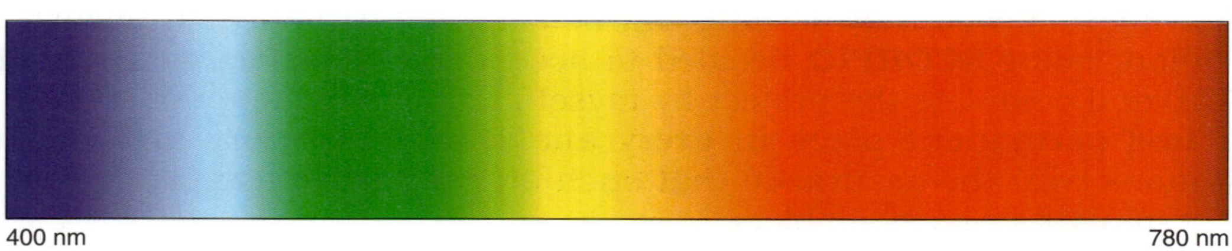

The light that human eye can perceive ranges from deep-violet (short wavelength) through blue, green, yellow and orange to deep red (long wavelength).

"One who never made a mistake never learnt anything."

necessary to learn thousands of individual reactions, instead we can learn few common reactions really well and apply the knowledge to similar cases.

Based on the functional group present in a molecule, the following reagents have been most commonly employed for quantification of the drug molecule: Gibbs' reagent, Bratton-Marshall reagent, Emerson's reagent, Ehrlich's reagent, Pauly's reagent, INH reagent, MBTH reagent, Besthorn's reagent, Folin's reagent, Van Urk's reagent, Wurster's Red reagent, Sanger's reagent, Chromotropic acid reagent, N-Bromosuccinimide reagent and DNPH reagent.

Most of the reaction mechanisms described in the text are as reported by the authors for which relative references have been cited under each reaction. However, the book "Pharmaceutical Chemistry, Vol. 2" by H.J. Roth et al. has been extensively referred to and has been extremely helpful in visualizing the reaction mechanism of several drug substances. Other textbooks of organic chemistry and analytical chemistry invariably consulted have been added under references at the end of introduction.

I am confident that 'Reaction Mechanism' described in this book along with method of analysis shall provide the most stimulating learning experience and will enable you to appreciate the excitement of this fascinating field.

Since newer molecules are invariably chemical modifications of existing drug substances, this compilation should be of help to the analysts in developing suitable method of analysis for newer drug molecules and also understand the chemistry involved and the confidence to tackle newer situations.

Over the years it was observed that at postgraduate level several practical exercises in pharmaceutical analysis were based on the methods described in 1st, 2nd and 3rd editions of this book. The students were invariably keen to know the detailed chemistry involved in methods. I do hope, my attempt in this direction will help students to perform practicals with better understanding. I expect this four-volume book on pharmaceutical analysis with reaction mechanism should make analytical science easier to understand for students, analysts and educators.

The icon representing structure of codeine with "Reaction Mechanism" reflects the underlying concept of this book.

Although I have exerted all my efforts to ensure that the text is free from errors, but it is quite possible that methodology details, certain structures and reaction mechanism may be inaccurate. I hope my efforts shall be evaluated in proper perspective.

It is the analyst who is consistently if not constantly involved with all the aspects of analysis. His/her interest necessarily is not of a curious bystander. This book does not purport to make analysts out of its readers, although it is hoped that some will be "turned on" to such a pursuit.

New Delhi, India

P.D. Sethi, M.Pharm., Ph.D.
Pharmaceutical Analyst

Acknowledgement

I would like to express my most sincere gratitude to analysts, students, teachers and professionals for their continuous support and encouragement and shaping my analytical career and ideas for compiling this book. The support extended by Professor Vijay K. Kapoor, University Institute of Pharmaceutical Sciences, Panjab University, Chandigarh in explaining and correcting several reactions included in the text is sincerely acknowledged. I am deeply indebted to Mr. Dilip Charegaonkar, Managing Director, M/s Anchrom Enterprises (I) Pvt. Ltd., Mumbai for supporting my scientific activities. I would like to convey my appreciation to the management of M/s Anchrom Enterprises (I) Pvt. Ltd., Mumbai and Kongposh Publications Pvt. Ltd., New Delhi for independently establishing life-time annual awards for Best Research Papers in "HPTLC Analysis" and "Pharmaceutical Analysis" respectively in recognition of my contribution in the field of Pharmaceutical Analysis. I am confident, their gesture shall provide impetus to young analysts for their interest in pharmaceutical analysis, currently the most creative and challenging field.

Without the support and untiring efforts of Mr. Dharmvir of 'CBS' my hand-written text particularly the reactions would never have been converted into book, thanks for his dedication and commitment for completing the assignment meticulously. I am thankful to Mr. Satish K. Jain, Managing Director, CBS, for accepting the hand-written manuscript of most challenging project and providing all the required facilities to bring this series to fruition.

New Delhi, India

P.D. Sethi, M.Pharm., Ph.D.
Pharmaceutical Analyst

Preface to the First Edition

Devising accurate assay procedures for each ingredient of complex dosage formulations containing several therapeutically and chemically compatible drugs with very similar chemical nature is a monumental undertaking. The very idea of separation, identification and estimation of each ingredient in such complex formulations would make the analyst's hair stand on end. Not only are the multiple active constituents present but they are usually there in widely divergent concentrations depending upon their relative potency and therapeutic need of the patient. The presence of additives, excipients and decomposition products further complicates the development of analytical procedures. Many of the classical tests long regarded as specific for certain substances are now answered by many more compounds. Nevertheless, the therapeutic advantage of such complex drug combinations should take precedence over any potential analytical problem which is ultimately the concern of the analyst. The increasing complexities of pharmaceutical preparations and the marked emphasis on quality control by the ethical manufacturers have placed greater load on the ingenuity of the quality control chemist.

An analyst who is in the need of an analytical method may be obliged to survey tremendous amount of literature in order to select one procedure which may appear to suit his need and facilities available, but when he subjects the selected procedure to actual test, he may find that he cannot reproduce the method. It is, therefore, essential that the practising analyst should have access to analytical procedures which are simple, reliable and workable under routine laboratory conditions.

"No one is ever born talented nor talent obtained as a gift or lucky coincidence. It is a resource acquired through one's own endeavour. In this process, others may provide some help and inspiration, but it is a quality earned by one's own hard endeavour."

Modern analytical techniques rely increasingly on complex techniques of analysis that require expensive equipments and highly specialized personnel. Such methods are not of much help in countries lacking these resources. For the most part, modern analytical techniques merely permit analysis to be carried out more rapidly than the conventional method of analysis, which though not bad are tedious and time-consuming. Even if a manufacturer is ready to procure and install modern instruments/equipments, their maintenance in fittest condition is a herculean task. Non-availability of trained analytical personnel and precise, simple and suitable methods of analysis are major handicaps for pharmaceutical manufacturers in developing countries.

Taking into consideration the technical and economic constraints, it is necessary that the recommended methods should permit their use by drug laboratories located in developing countries. It is significant to stress that even simple instruments like colorimeter and spectrophotometer result in sensitive and accurate measurements with clear advantage of speed, simplicity and easy maintenance. The large volume of literature devoted to their application in almost every field of scientific research constitutes irrefutable evidence of their utility. It is, therefore, reasonable to assume that the analytical procedures involving the use of such simple instruments will find greater application. Selection of analytical method is a very critical point. The method must be accurate, sensitive, selective, reproducible and convenient.

In view of rapid advance during the last several years in the field of pharmaceutical analysis and marketing of ever increasing multi-component formulations, the available texts dealing in pharmaceutical analysis that have been written so far do not in general deal with the analysis of each component in wide range of complex pharmaceutical dosage formulations, particularly in presence of interfering substances. The official compendias are rarely of help in such formulations. To fill the existing gap in literature and keeping in view the economic and technical limitations of drug manufacturers, particularly in medium and small scale sector, it was felt that there exists a need to have a compilation of a simple, suitable and reliable methods for analysis of each ingredient of multi-component drug formulations.

This text, a maiden attempt, is meant to fulfill these needs. Analytical procedures for more than 200 drug formulations of divergent combinations have been compiled to serve as a convenient source of information for analysts and scientists engaged in the field. The focal point for this compilation is the presentation of practical aspect of the methodology using colorimeter and spectrophotometer as the main analytical tools.

For practical considerations, the drug formulations have been classified into 23 different categories based upon their common therapeutic uses as under:

1. Analgesics and antipyretics
2. Antacids and other ulcer healing drugs
3. Antacids, sedatives, antispasmodics
4. Anthelmintics
5. Anti-allergic drugs
6. Antibiotics
7. Anti-diarrhoeals
8. Anti-inflammatory drugs
9. Antimalarials
10. Anti-tuberculous drugs
11. Bronchospasm relaxants (anti-asthma)
12. Enzymes and digestives
13. Expectorants and cough suppressants
14. Eye, ear preparations
15. Keratolytics and cleansers
16. Laxatives, purgatives and lubricants
17. Nasal preparations
18. Oral rehydration salts
19. Rubefacients
20. Sedatives and tranquillisers
21. Topical antifungal, anti-infective preparations
22. Urinary anti-infective preparations
23. Vitamins, minerals and other nutritional additives.

For most of the formulations, several alternative methods have been described for a particular substance so that the analyst can intelligently select and apply the method to suit his need and the laboratory facilities available. Preliminary treatment of the sample for analysis utilizing conventional isolation and extraction procedures have been applied wherever necessary to eliminate the presence of potentially interfering substances. In other cases, the methods are sufficiently specific to permit the analysis of individual ingredients without pre-treatment. The procedures have been described in sufficient details highlighting the important steps in methodology so that these can be reproduced without much difficulty. Merits and demerits of each method and possibility of its application to other formulations have been discussed. To help the analyst and to enhance the book's usefulness, several worked out examples based on actual experimental data have been included. For drug manufacturers, who are interested to set up their independent quality control division, chapter on the profile of a quality control laboratory has been included giving brief outline of different sections.

Its importance for pharmaceutical teachers, students and institutions imparting special course in drug analysis cannot be overestimated. Science graduates interested in pursuing career as analytical chemist will find this compilation invaluable for daily use which will provide ready answers to most of their analytical problems. It is earnest feeling of the author that knowledge of the basic inorganic and organic chemistry tempered by judicious changes and the special skill needed in pharmaceutical analysis and the information included in this text will enable the analyst to overcome most specific problems and he will be able to analyse any viable combination of drug formulations he may encounter in future. It is pertinent to mention that analyst should cautiously choose the method and interpret the results carefully before certifying the product. It is hoped that this text will enable the analyst to take their rightful place in the pharmaceutical industry and in government laboratories concerned with the quality control of medicinal preparations.

The author is indebted to his wife, Usha for her moral support throughout his career.

The author wishes to express his sincere appreciation to Dr. O.P. Ghai, Professor and Head, Department of Pediatrics, All India Institute of Medical Sciences, New Delhi, for his helpful suggestions and guidance.

How far I have succeeded in my attempt, the decision is left to my fellow pharmacists and analysts.

New Delhi, India **P.D. Sethi**
1985

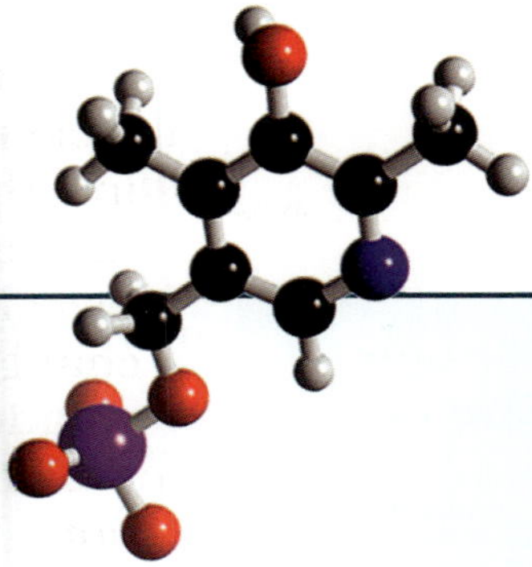

Brief Contents
Volumes I – IV

VOLUME 1

VOLUME 2

VOLUME 3

VOLUME 4

Contents

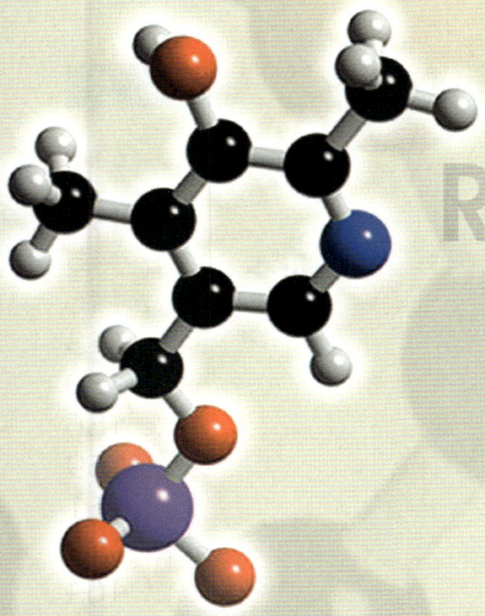

Reaction Mechanism

11

Expectorants, Cough Suppressants and Anti-Allergics

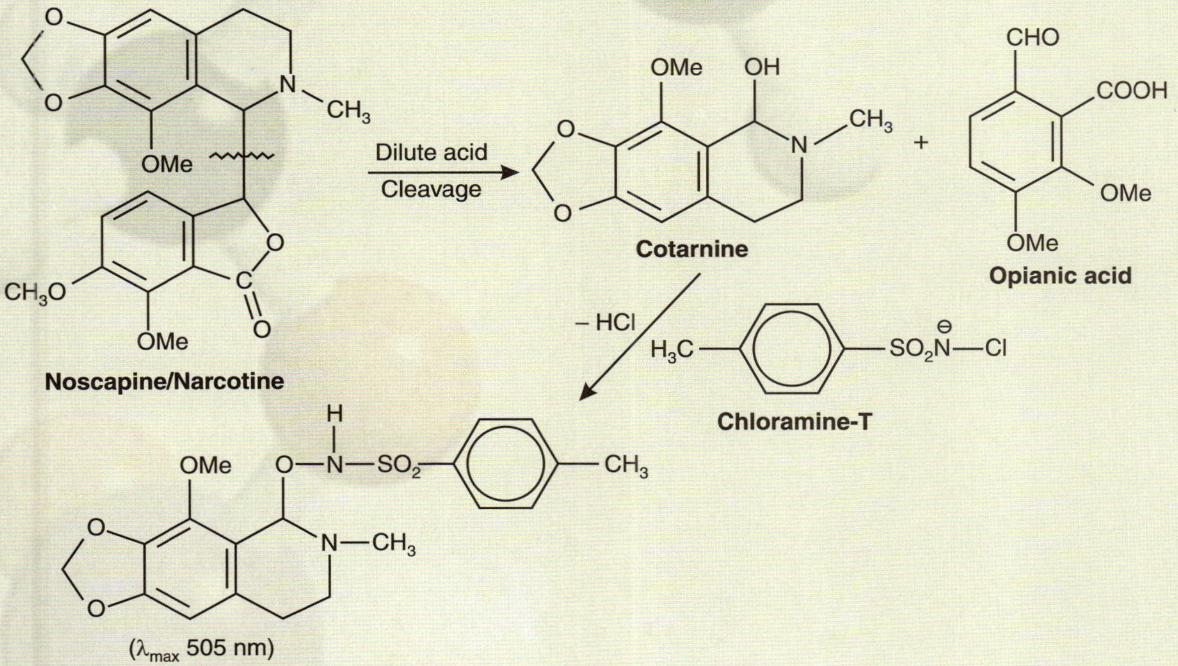

Formulation 1

Codeine phosphate, Ephedrine hydrochloride, Sodium citrate, Alcohol

ESTIMATION

Codeine phosphate

METHOD 1

Reagents

1. 2% and 4% v/v sulphuric acid.
2. 25% w/v sodium hydroxide solution in water.
3. Hexane-chloroform (3 : 1 v/v), solvent mixture.

Standard solution

150 mcg/ml of codeine phosphate in 2% sulphuric acid.

Sample solution

Dilute accurately measured volume of the sample equivalent to 7.5 mg of codeine phosphate to 50 ml with 4% sulphuric acid (150 mcg/ml).

Procedure

Transfer 5 ml of sample solution into a 250 ml separating funnel, add 15 ml of 2% sulphuric acid and swirl to mix. Extract the acid solution with three 30 ml portions of chloroform. Combine the chloroform extracts and extract with 5 ml of 2% sulphuric acid. Discard the chloroform layer and make the total acidic solution strongly alkaline with sodium hydroxide solution. Extract the solution using gentle shaking with 50 ml of solvent mixture. Transfer the organic layer into another 250 ml separating funnel containing 50 ml 2% sulphuric acid. Continue the extraction with an additional four 25 ml portions of the solvent mixture, gently shaking each time for 10-15 seconds. Allow for a clean separation each time and transfer organic solvent through cotton plug into separating funnel containing sulphuric acid. Shake the separating funnel containing acid and solvent layers vigorously for one minute to extract codeine back into the acid layer. Allow the phases to separate and centrifuge the aqueous phase to clarify the solution. Determine the absorbance of the standard codeine phosphate solution and of the sample solution obtained above by extraction procedure at 285 and 360 nm using 285 nm to obtain the net absorbance due to codeine and calculate the results by comparing with the standard solution.

METHOD 2

The acidic extract obtained in the method 1 above can be subjected to the following method.

Reagents

1. Buffer solution: The solution is prepared by dissolving 300 g of monosodium hydrogen phosphate and 9 g of sodium hydroxide in water and the volume is made to 750 ml with water.
2. 1% w/v solution of picric acid in water.

Standard solution

10 mcg/ml of codeine phosphate in water.

Sample solution

The sample solution (acidic extract as obtained in method 1 above) is diluted appropriately with water to get a concentration of 10 mcg/ml.

Procedure

To 5 ml each of the sample and standard solutions, add 5 ml of buffer solution, 5 ml of picric acid solution and 10 ml chloroform. Shake for 5-10 seconds and allow the chloroform layer to separate. Filter organic layer through cotton plug and measure the absorbance of both the solutions at about 430 nm against reagent blank and calculate the results by comparison.

Probable Reaction Mechanism

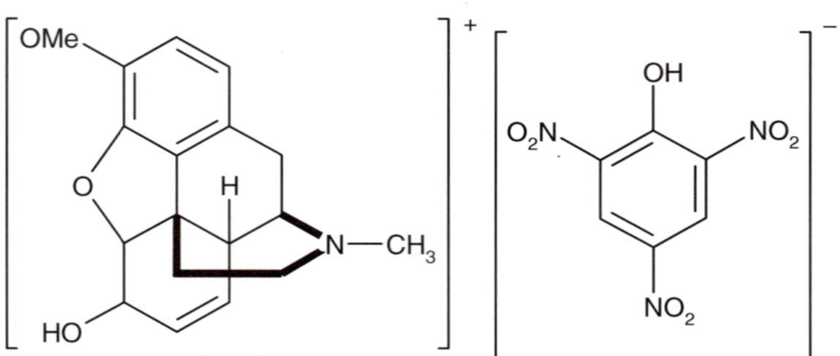

Codeine **Picric acid**

Drug - Picric acid complex

(λ_{max} 430 nm)

Ephedrine hydrochloride

Reagents

1. Sodium metaperiodate, 0.75 M: Dissolve 1.6 g of sodium metaperiodate in 100 ml of water, prepare each day.
2. 50% w/v solution of sodium hydroxide in water.

Standard solution

30 mcg/ml of ephedrine hydrochloride in 0.1 N hydrochloric acid.

Sample solution

Transfer aliquot of the cough syrup (sample) equivalent to 60 mg of ephedrine hydrochloride into a 500 ml separating funnel and add 10 g of sodium chloride. Shake well to dissolve sodium chloride. Make the solution alkaline with sodium hydroxide solution. Extract alkaline aqueous solution with three 50 ml portions of ether. Collect ether extracts and wash with 20 ml of saturated solution of sodium chloride. Extract the ether solution with three 50 ml portions of 0.1 N hydrochloric acid. Collect all the acid extracts in a 250 ml beaker and warm on steam-bath to expel the dissolved ether from the acid. Dilute the acid solution to 200 ml in a volumetric flask. Further dilute 10 ml of the solution to 100 ml with 0.1 N hydrochloric acid. Designate this as sample solution (30 mcg/ml).

Procedure

Transfer 5 ml each of the sample and standard solutions to 25 ml volumetric flasks. Add 2 ml of water and three drops of phenolphthalein indicator solution to the flask containing standard solution. Add 2 ml of sodium metaperiodate solution and 3 drops of phenolphthalein solution to the flask containing sample solution. Add 1 N sodium hydroxide solution dropwise to each of the flasks until a permanent pink colour appears. The alkali should be added so as not to wet the neck. Add 2 drops of excess alkali and then swirl to mix the solution. Immediately, add 10 ml of n-hexane to each flask and stopper. After 5 minutes, shake both the flasks vigorously for 15 seconds and allow the phases to separate. Carefully open the flasks and dilute to volume with hexane, stopper and mix thoroughly by shaking. Allow the phases to separate before decanting the hexane solution into a 1 cm absorption cell. Determine the differential ultraviolet absorbance of the sample solution at 240 and 260 nm using hexane layer from the standard solution in the reference cell. Absorbance due to benzaldehyde is determined by subtracting the values at 260 nm (minimum) from that observed at 240 nm (maximum). Repeat the above analytical procedure using the standard solution (30 mcg/ml) for comparative purposes. It is preferable if the standard is processed simultaneously with the sample.

Note

This method involves alkaline periodate oxidation of ephedrine to benzaldehyde, acetaldehyde and methylamine. Absorbance due to benzaldehyde is responsible for analysis.

Probable Reaction Mechanism

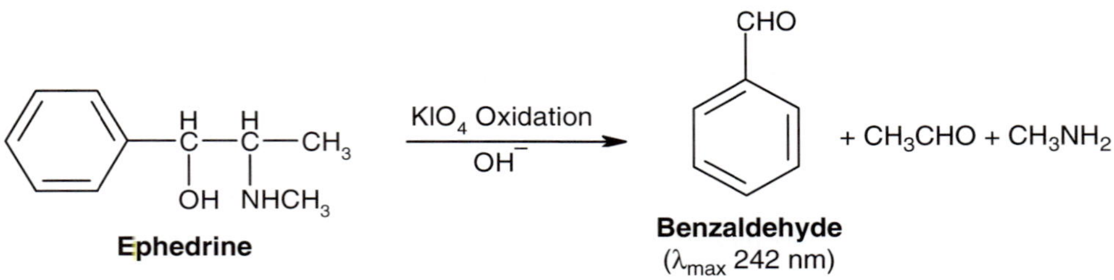

For detailed reaction mechanism, refer to chapter on anti-asthma drugs.

Sodium citrate as total citrate

Follow methods described in formulation 7 of this chapter.

Formulation 2

Codeine phosphate, Ephedrine hydrochloride, Potassium guaiacolsulphonate

ESTIMATION

Ephedrine hydrochloride

Weigh or measure accurately a quantity of the sample equivalent to 20 mg of ephedrine hydrochloride. Basify with dilutes solution of ammonia and extract with four 30 ml portions of ether. Reserve aqueous layer for the estimation of codeine phosphate. Evaporate the ether layer at low temperature, dissolve the residue in 40 ml of glacial acetic acid and follow the method 2 involving nonaqueous titration described for estimation of ephedrine in formulation 8 of this chapter. Each ml of 0.1 N perchloric acid is equivalent to 0.02017 g of ephedrine hydrochloride.

Codeine phosphate

This method is based on phosphate-moiety of the molecule.

Reagents

1. Molybdate reagent: To 5 g of ammonium molybdate, add 80 ml of water and 25 ml of sulphuric acid. Warm to dissolve, cool and dilute to 100 ml with water.
2. Metol-bisulphite reagent: To 50 ml of water, add 0.1 g of sodium metabisulphite and 0.35 g of metol. Shake to mix, add 20 g of sodium metabisulphite and dilute with water to 100 ml.

Standard solution

20 mcg/ml of codeine phosphate in water.

Sample solution

Take the entire aqueous layer reserved during estimation of ephedrine, warm to expel dissolved ether and adjust the volume with water to get 20 mcg/ml in respect of codeine phosphate.

Procedure

To 5 ml each of the sample and standard solutions, add 4 ml of dilute sulphuric acid, 1 ml of molybdate reagent and 1 ml of metol-bisulphite reagent. Keep at room temperature for 30 minutes and measure the extinction of both the solutions at about 725 nm against reagent blank and calculate the results by comparison.

Note

Metol reduces the molybdate complex to molybdinium blue (λ_{max} 725 nm).

Potassium guaiacolsulphonate

Reagents

1. Borate buffer, pH 9.4.
2. 0.04% w/v solution of 2,6-dichloroquinone chlorimide in isopropyl alcohol.

Standard solution

100 mcg/ml of potassium guaiacolsulphonate in water.

Sample solution

Dilute appropriate quantity of the sample with water to get 100 mcg/ml of the substance.

Procedure

To 1 ml each of the sample and standard solutions, add 1 ml of borate buffer solution, pH 9.4, 2 ml of isopropyl alcohol and 1 ml of water. Add 1 ml of chlorimide reagent to each tube and keep aside for 15 minutes at room temperature. Measure the absorbance of both the solutions at about 650 nm against reagent blank and calculate the results by comparison. The method obeys Beer's law in the concentration range of 10-20 mcg/ml.

Note

1. Phenolic compounds, if present, will interfere.
2. If ascorbic acid is present, reflux the sample with 0.1 N hydrochloric acid to destroy it.
3. The colour attains its maximum intensity within 10 minutes and is stable for 20 minutes.

Probable Reaction Mechanism

Potassium guaiasulphonate is a mixture of 3-hydroxy-4-methoxy benzene sulfonic acid monopotassium salt and 4-hydroxy-3-methoxy benzene sulfonic acid monopotassium salt.

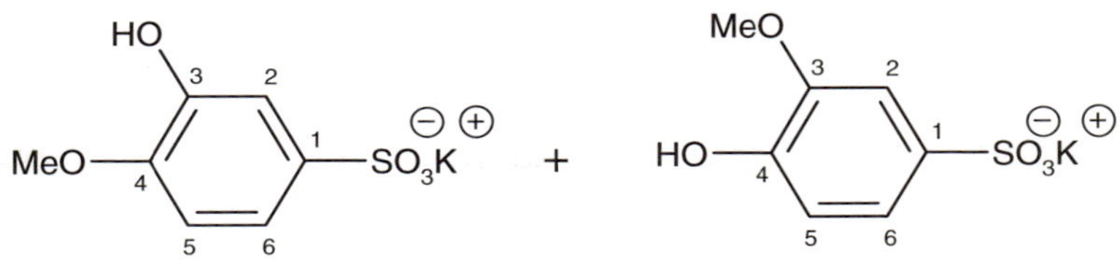

Potassium guaiacol sulphonate (1)

Explanatory Note

Oxidative coupling occurs at the ortho position to the phenolic-OH group of any of the salts in the above mixture. Buffer solution is required for the reaction to proceed.

In the presence of H_2O, dichloroquinone chlorinide is converted into 2,6-dichloroquinonimine.

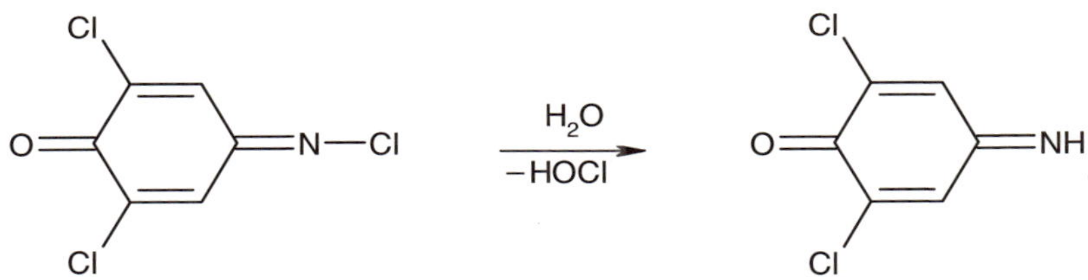

Dichloroquinone chlorinide **2,6-Dichloroquinonimine (reactive species)**

The 2,6-dichloroquinonimine so formed will further react as shown below.

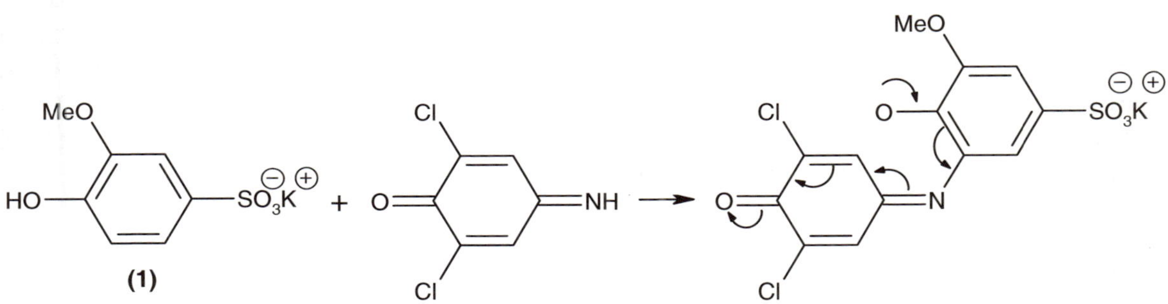

(1) **2,6-Dichloroquinonimine** (λ_{max} 650 nm)

Codeine and Ephedrine (total alkaloids as ephedrine hydrochloride)

Weigh or measure sample accurately equivalent to 20 mg of ephedrine hydrochloride, basify with 1 N sodium hydroxide and proceed for extraction and estimation of total alkaloids as described under formulation 18 of this chapter.

Working example

Each 5 ml of the preparation contains 10 mg of ephedrine hydrochloride and 1.5 mg of codeine phosphate. Total alkaloids in term of ephedrine hydrochloride can be estimated as under. Convert the claimed contents of codeine phosphate to ephedrine and express the total alkaloids in term of ephedrine hydrochloride.

- 1 ml of 0.1 N sulphuric acid is equivalent to 20.17 mg of ephedrine hydrochloride.
- 1 ml of 0.1 N sulphuric acid is equivalent to 39.74 mg of codeine phosphate.
- 39.74 mg of codeine phosphate = 20.17 mg of ephedrine hydrochloride.
- 1.5 mg of codeine phosphate = 0.76 mg of ephedrine hydrochloride.
- Total alkaloids as ephedrine hydrochloride = 10 + 0.76 = 10.76 mg

After the titration with sodium hydroxide is complete, as described in formulation 18 of this chapter, add further 5 ml of 0.1 N sodium hydroxide and subject the contents to steam distillation. Estimate ephedrine in the distillate by acid, base titration. This procedure will give the contents of ephedrine present in the sample.

Note

Addition of sodium hydroxide after completion of titration generates ephedrine (base) which being volatile is steam distilled, distilate being received in acid and finally subjected to acid-base titration.

Formulation 3

Codeine phosphate, Glyceryl guaiacolate, Phenylephrine hydrochloride, Chlorpheniramine maleate

ESTIMATION

Codeine phosphate

Follow the method 1 as described under formulation 1 of this chapter.

A spectrophotometric method based on chrge-transfer was reported. 7,7,8,8-Tetracyanoquinodimethane (TCQN) acts as electron acceptor whereas codeine being electron donor. Stable charge-transfer complex in acetone (λ_{max} 643 nm), i.e. as a result of complex formation, there is bathochromic shift i.e., 216 nm to 643 nm.

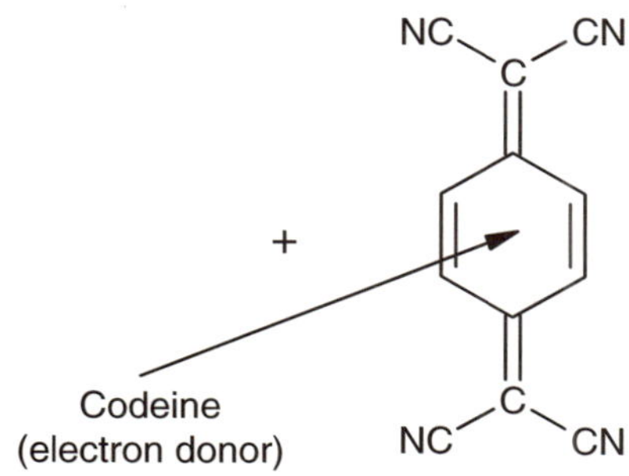

7,7,8,8-Tetracyanoquinone dimethane
(electron acceptor)

Glyceryl guaiacolate

Reagent

1. 20% w/v solution of sodium hydroxide in water.

Standard solution

Prepare a standard solution by dissolving 300 mg of glyceryl guaiacolate in 100 ml chloroform. Pipette 2 ml aliquot into 100 ml volumetric flask and dilute to volume with anhydrous methyl alcohol (60 mcg/ml).

Sample solution

Transfer accurate volume of the sample equivalent to 300 mg of glyceryl guaiacolate into 250 ml, separating funnel. Add 10 ml of sodium hydroxide solution and extract with four 40 ml portions of petroleum ether, reject ether layer. Collect the aqueous layer and extract with four 20 ml portions of chloroform. Filter the chloroform through a small cotton pledget into a 100 ml volumetric flask. Rinse the funnel and cotton with chloroform. Dilute to volume with chloroform. Transfer 2 ml aliquot into a 100 ml volumetric flask and dilute to volume with anhydrous methanol (60 mcg/ml).

Procedure

Determine the absorbance of the sample and standard solutions at 275 nm using anhydrous methanol as blank and calculate the results by comparison.

Phenylephrine hydrochloride

METHOD 1

Follow the method based on alkaline oxidation and coupling with antipyrine. For details, refer to formulation 1 of the chapter on analgesics and antipyretics.

METHOD 2

Follow the method 2 for estimation of phenylephrine as described in formulation 11 of this chapter.

Chlorpheniramine maleate

Reagents

1. Buffered solution of sulphanilic acid: Dissolve 2.5 g of sulphanilic acid and 10 g of anhydrous sodium acetate in 40 ml methanol and make volume to 200 ml with methanol.
2. 25% w/v sodium hydroxide solution in water.
3. Saturated solution of cyanogen bromide in water.

Stock standard solution

Accurately weigh 100 mg of chlorpheniramine maleate into 100 ml volumetric flask, dissolve and dilute to volume with 0.1 N hydrochloric acid.

Working standard

Dilute 10 ml of the stock solution to 250 ml with 0.1 N hydrochloric acid (40 mcg/ml).

Sample solution

Transfer sample equivalent to 10 mg of the substance into a 250 ml separatory funnel, rinse the pipette. Add 15 ml of sodium hydroxide solution and extract with four 50 ml portions of petroleum ether. Collect and combine the ether extracts. Wash the combined ether extract twice with 25 ml water. Reject the aqueous extract and washings. Extract the combined ether extract with five 20 ml portions of 0.1 N hydrochloric acid. Collect the combined acidic extract and dilute to 250 ml with 0.1 N hydrochloric acid (40 mcg/ml).

Procedure

To 5 ml each of sample and standard solutions, add 5 ml of buffered sulphanilic acid solution, 2 ml of cyanogen bromide solution and 1 ml of 0.25 N sulphuric acid. Prepare separate sample and standard blank. Allow all the tubes to stand for 10 min, and measure the absorbance of the sample and standard solutions against respective reagent blanks at about 480 nm and calculate the amount of chlorpheniramine maleate in the sample by comparison.

Note

Ephedrine, diphenhydramine, aminophylline, pyrilamine maleate and naphazoline hydrochloride do not interfere.

For complete reaction mechanism see formulation 1 of the chapter on rubefacients.

Formulation 4

Codeine phosphate, Chlorpheniramine maleate, Terpine hydrate, Potassium guaiacolsulphonate, Glycerin, Menthol, Tincture ipecac

ESTIMATION

Terpine hydrate

METHOD 1

Follow the method described in formulation 1 of the chapter on analgesics and antipyretics.

METHOD 2

1. 1% w/v solution of phosphomolybdic acid in water.
2. Concentrated sulphuric acid, ice cooled.

Standard solution

100 mcg/ml of terpine hydrate in chloroform.

Sample solution

Take sample equivalent to about 10 mg of terpine hydrate, add 10 ml of water and shake with 30 ml of petroleum ether (40-60°). Separate aqueous layer and then extract with four 20 ml portions of chloroform. Combine chloroform layer and dilute to 100 ml with chloroform.

Procedure

To 10 ml each of the sample and standard solutions, add 10 ml of chloroform, 5 ml of water and 2 ml of phosphomolybdic acid. Shake for 10 minutes, allow the layers to separate and discard chloroform layer. Keep aqueous layer on water-bath to remove traces of chloroform, cool and add slowly 2 ml of ice cooled sulphuric acid. Allow to remain in ice-bath for 30 minutes with occasional shaking. Now keep on water-bath for 10 minutes, cool and dilute to 25 ml with acetone. Measure the absorbance of both the standard and sample solutions at about 610 nm and calculate the results by comparison.

Chlorpheniramine maleate

Standard solution

25 mcg/ml of substance in 0.5 N sulphuric acid.

Sample solution

Take a quantity of the sample equivalent to 20 mg of the compound, acidify with hydrochloric acid and extract with three 50 ml portions of ether. Discard ether layer, make acidic layer alkaline with 5 N sodium hydroxide solution and extract with three 50 ml portions of ether. Wash combined ether extract with water till free of alkali. Extract combined ether layer with three 50 ml portions of 0.5 N sulphuric acid. Dilute the acidic extract to 200 ml (100 mcg/ml). Dilute further appropriately with 0.5 N sulphuric acid to get 20 mcg/ml.

Measure the absorbance of standard and sample solutions at maximum at about 264 nm using 0.5 N sulphuric acid as blank and calculate the contents of chlorpheniramine maleate by comparison.

Potassium guaiacolsulphonate

METHOD 1

Follow the chlorimide reagent method for estimation of the compound as described in formulation 2 of this chapter.

METHOD 2

To a quantity of the sample equivalent to 500 mg of the compound, add 50 ml of water, and 20 ml of concentrated nitric acid with caution. Heat the mixture for 1 h on very low flame. Cool to room temperature and cautiously add 500 mg of potassium carbonate. Evaporate the solution to dryness with low flame to remove nitric acid, if any. Dissolve the residue in water and acidify with dilute hydrochloric acid, boil and cool. Add 10% w/v barium chloride solution till the precipitation is complex. Digest the mixture on water bath for 1 h and filter through filter paper. Wash precipitates with water till free from barium. It is ignited to constant weight and contents of potassium guaiacolsulphonate calculated. Each 1 g of the residue is equivalent to 1.038 g of potassium guaiacolsulphonate.

Note

Sulphur (S) from sulphonic acid moiety of the compound is precipitates as $BaSO_4$ and estimated gravimetrically.

Codeine phosphate

Reagents

1. Hydrochloric acid.
2. 0.1 N sulphuric acid.
3. 0.1 N sodium hydroxide.
4. 0.5 N sodium hydroxide.
5. Anhydrous sodium sulphate, granular.

Procedure

Transfer sample equivalent to 100 mg of codeine phosphate into a separatory funnel. Add 10 to 15 ml of water, 2 ml hydrochloric acid and mix well. Extract thrice each with 50 ml portions of ether and discard the ether extracts. Add 0.5 N sodium hydroxide till the aqueous layer is distinctly alkaline. Extract again with three 50 ml portions of chloroform. Wash the combined chloroform extract thoroughly with water till it is free from alkali. Filter the chloroform extract into a dry 250 ml conical flask through anhydrous sodium sulphate placed over cotton plug. Evaporate the chloroform extract to complete dryness and dissolve the residue in exactly 10 ml of 0.1 N sulphuric acid. Titrate the excess acid with 0.1 N sodium hydroxide using methyl red as indicator. Each ml of 0.1 N sulphuric acid is equivalent to 0.03974 of codeine phosphate.

Total alkaloids as emetine

Tincture ipecac contains about 0.2% of total alkaloids calculated as emetine. It has been observed that about 2 ml of tincture ipecac is usually present in 100 ml of different liquid formulations of cough mixtures.

Reagents

1. McLivaine buffer, pH 5.0: 48.5 ml of 0.1 M citric acid monohydrate and 51.5 ml of 0.02 M disodium phosphate are mixed. Check and adjust the pH to 5.0.
2. Buffered methyl orange solution: 10 mg/100 ml of methyl orange in buffer solution, pH 5.0.
3. Acidified alcohol: To 70 ml of ethyl alcohol, add 1 ml of 1 N hydrochloric acid and dilute to 100 ml with water.

Standard solution

400 mcg/ml of emetine in buffer solution, pH 5.0.

Sample solution

Take sample equivalent to 1 ml of the tincture ipecac, basify with ammonia and extract with ether. Evaporate the ether layer and take up the residue in 5 ml of McLivaine buffer, pH 5.0.

Procedure

To 2 ml each of the standard and sample solutions, add 10 ml of the dye solution and shake with 10 ml chloroform. Allow the layers to separate. Extract aqueous layer further with three 10 ml portions of chloroform. Shake combined chloroform layer with 10 ml of 0.1 N sodium hydroxide for 15 seconds. Wash the chloroform layer with another 10 ml of 0.1 N sodium hydroxide. Combine the alkaline layers and dilute to 25 ml with 0.1 N sodium hydroxide (C). Shake chloroform layer with 10 ml of 0.1 N sulphuric acid and dilute the acid layer to 25 ml with 0.1 N sulphuric acid (D). Measure the absorbance of the sample and standard solutions (C) at about 460 nm and calculate the percentage of total alkaloids as emetine. The measurement of extinction of solutions (D) of both standard and sample at maxima at about 283 nm gives non-phenolic alkaloids calculated as emetine.

Note

Belladonna alkaloids, if present, do not interfere in this determination as at 283 nm, belladonna alkaloids have insignificant absorbance.

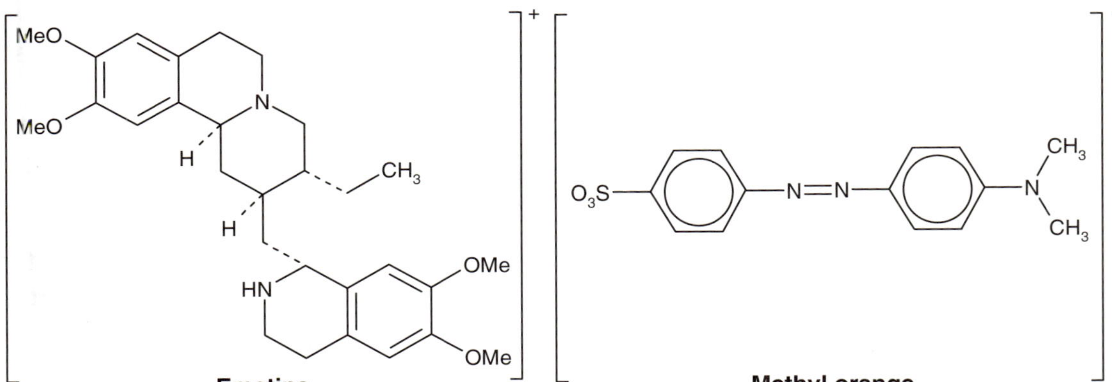

Emetine **Methyl orange**

Drug - Dye ion-pair complex
(λ_{max} 460 nm)

Since both phenolic and non-phenolic alkaloids form ion-pair complex, dye complexation of phenolic alkaloids can be extracted into alkali whereas non-phenolic alkaloid breaks down and remains in chloroform and can be extracted into acid which corresponds to emetine (λ_{max} 283 nm).

Menthol

Follow the method involving reaction with p-dimethylaminobenzaldehyde for estimation of menthol in formulation 5 of this chapter.

Glycerin

The assay involves Malaprade cleavage, followed by determination of formic acid produced by titration with sodium hydroxide.

Probable Reaction Mechanism

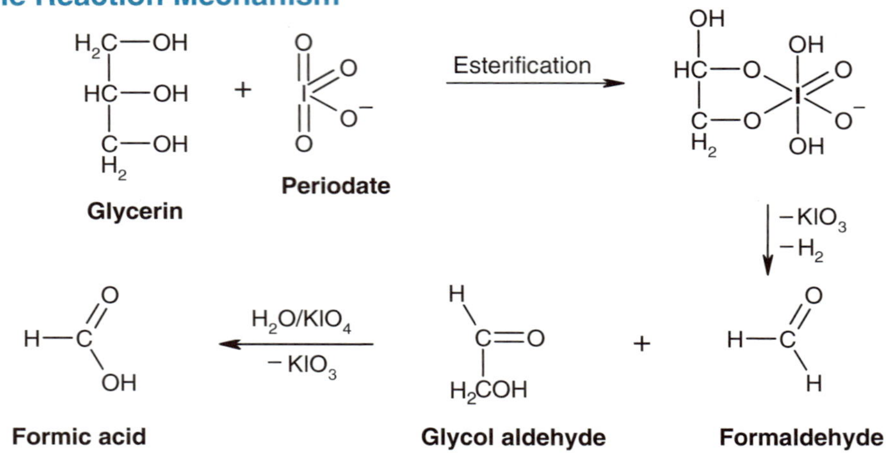

Note

The assay method involves the use of ethylene glycol before titration of formic acid. This is required to remove excess of periodate by reducing it to iodate as periodate at pH above 7.0 uses hydroxy ion; hence, we may get higher assay values.

Reference

Pharmaceutical Chemistry (Vol. 2) by H.J. Roth, p. 63.

Formaldehyde produced during reaction can be estimated by its reaction with chromotropic acid in the presence of sulphuric acid to form coloured product.

Probable Reaction Mechanism

Here HCHO condenses with the aromatic system of chromotropic acid in the O-position to the phenolic hydroxy group in the presence of H_2SO_4 to form the following product.

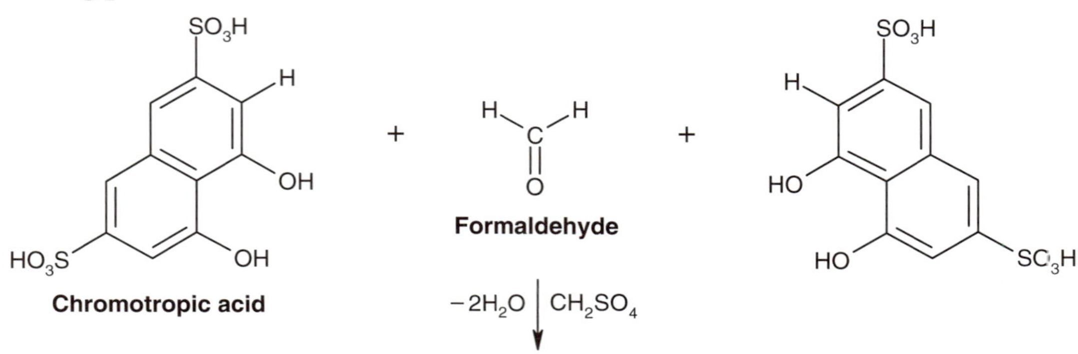

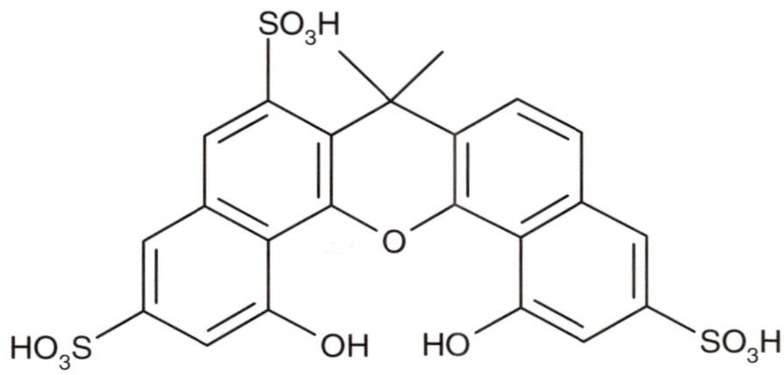

H_2SO_4 acts as an oxidising agent in the next step resulting in a stabilized 3,4,5,6-dibenzoxanthylium cation.

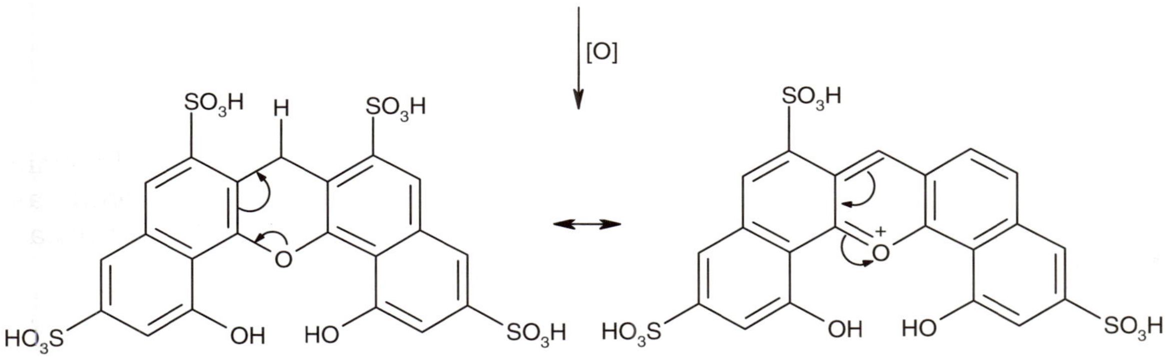

3,4,5,6-dibenzoxanthylium cation

Reference

1. Pharmaceutical Chemistry (Vol. 2), H.J. Roth, p. 121.
2. J. Pharm. Sci., 68, 1064-1068, 1979.

Formulation 5

Codeine phosphate, Terpine hydrate, Ammonium bromide, Potassium antimony tartrate

ESTIMATION

Potassium antimony tartrate

Reagents

1. Concentrated sulphuric acid.
2. Hydrochloric acid.
3. Hydrogen peroxide (100 volumes).
4. 6 N Hydrochloric acid—sulphuric acid (1 : 1 v/v) mixture.
5. 5% w/v solution of sodium nitrite in water.
6. 10% w/v solution of urea in water.
7. 0.05% w/v solution of brilliant green.
8. Toluene.

Standard solution

To 0.110 g of antimony trioxide, add 550 ml hydrochloric acid and dilute with water to 1000 ml (100 mcg/ml of antimony). Dilute further 10 ml with 6 N hydrochloric acid (10 mcg/ml of antimony).

Sample solution

Accurately take sample equivalent to 1 mg of antimony in a Kjeldahl's flask. Add carefully 10 ml of concentrated sulphuric acid, cool and further add 30 ml of concentrated sulphuric acid. Heat slowly at low temperature till all organic matter is dissolved. Then, add hydrogen peroxide drop by drop into hot solution till the solution is totally decolorised. Dilute to 100 ml with 6 N hydrochloric acid.

Procedure

To 2 ml of the sample and standard solutions, add 13 ml of hydrochloric acid-sulphuric acid mixture and 1 ml of sodium nitrite solution. Mix and add 2 ml of urea solution. Allow the gas to escape and then add 5 ml of brilliant green solution. Add exactly 15 ml of toluene and extract the coloured complex. Allow the toluene layer to separate. Discard the aqueous layer. Measure the absorbance of organic layer of both the solutions at maxima at about 640 nm and calculate the results.

Terpine hydrate

Follow the method 2 for estimation of terpine hydrate described in formulation 4 of this chapter.

Ammonium bromide

Follow the silver nitrate titration method as described in formulation-9 of this chapter for ammonium chloride. Each ml of 0.1 N silver nitrate is equivalent to 9.795 mg of ammonium bromide.

Codeine phosphate

Follow the method 1 as described under formulation 1 of this chapter.

Formulation 6

Codeine phosphate, Papaverine hydrochloride, Diphenhydramine hydrochloride, Ammonium chloride, Menthol

ESTIMATION

Diphenhydramine hydrochloride

Standard solution

200 mcg/ml of diphenhydramine hydrochloride in water.

Sample solution

Weigh accurately a quantity of the sample equivalent to 20 mg of diphenhydramine hydrochloride, add 15 ml of water and make alkaline with 1 N sodium hydroxide. Extract with three 50 ml portions of petroleum ether (40-60°). Filter organic layer through sodium sulphate, anhydrous, supported on a cotton plug. Reduce the volume to 10 ml, add 10 ml of 0.1 N hydrochloric acid and evaporate ether completely. Cool and make alkaline the acidic layer with 1 N sodium hydroxide. Add 20 ml of saturated aqueous solution of ammonium reineckate. Filter through G_4 sintered funnel, wash the precipitates with water till the filtrate is colourless. Dissolve the precipitates in acetone to produce 25 ml. Take 10 ml of standard solution and process as per sample.

Measure the absorption of samples and standard solutions at about 525 nm and calculate the results. Chlorpheniramine does not interfere.

Note

The compound precipitated as reineckate is soluble in acetone.

Papaverine hydrochloride

Take volume of the sample syrup, equivalent to 5 mg of papaverine hydrochloride, add 5 ml of 1 N hydrochloric acid and extract with three 25 ml portions of chloroform. Extract combined chloroform extract with 10 ml of 1 N sodium hydroxide. Reject aqueous layer, evaporate chloroform layer and dry the residue at about 75°C till free from the smell of menthol. Dissolve the residue in 1 N hydrochloric acid with the aid of slight warming to produce 250 ml. Filter and measure the extinction of the solution at 310 nm using 1 N hydrochloric acid as blank. Calculate the results using 228 as value of A 1%, 1 cm at 310 nm.

Codeine phosphate

Reagents

1. 3% w/v solution of potassium permanganate in water.
2. 5% w/v solution of sodium nitrite in water.
3. 10% w/v solution of ferrous ammonium sulphate in water, prepare fresh.
4. 15% w/v solution of sodium hydroxide in water.
5. 1% w/v solution of sodium bicarbonate in water.
6. Diazotised sulphanilic acid. To 1 g of sulphanilic acid, add 20 ml of hydrochloric acid, digest on burner for 5 minutes, cool and filter. Take 1.5 ml of the filtrate, cool in ice-bath and add 1.5 ml of sodium nitrite solution. Wait for 5 minutes, again add 5 ml of sodium nitrite solution and make up the volume to 50 ml with water.

Standard solution

2 mg/ml of codeine phosphate in water. From this solution, take 10 ml, make it alkaline with sodium hydroxide solution and proceed as under sample solution below.

Sample solution

Measure syrup (sample) equivalent to 2 mg of codeine phosphate, make it alkaline with sodium hydroxide solution. Extract with three 30 ml portions of chloroform. Filter combined chloroform extract through anhydrous sodium sulphate. Wash sodium sulphate layer with 10 ml of chloroform. Evaporate combined chloroform layer completely and take up the residue in 10 ml solution of sodium bicarbonate with slight warming for 5-10 minutes. Cool and adjust to 250 ml with water. Filter and use this solution for colour development.

Procedure

To 10 ml each of sample and standard solutions, add 1 ml of potassium permanganate solution. Keep exactly for 15 seconds, add 5 ml of ferrous ammonium sulphate solution. Keep for 3 minutes, add 5 ml of sodium hydroxide solution and 10 ml of water. After 60 minutes, filter the solution. To 10 ml of the filtrate from standard and sample solutions, add 2 ml of diazotised sulphanilic acid, shake and measure the absorbance of both the solutions at about 490 nm within 3 minutes of addition of diazotised reagent against reagent blank and deduce the results by comparison.

Probable Reaction Mechanism

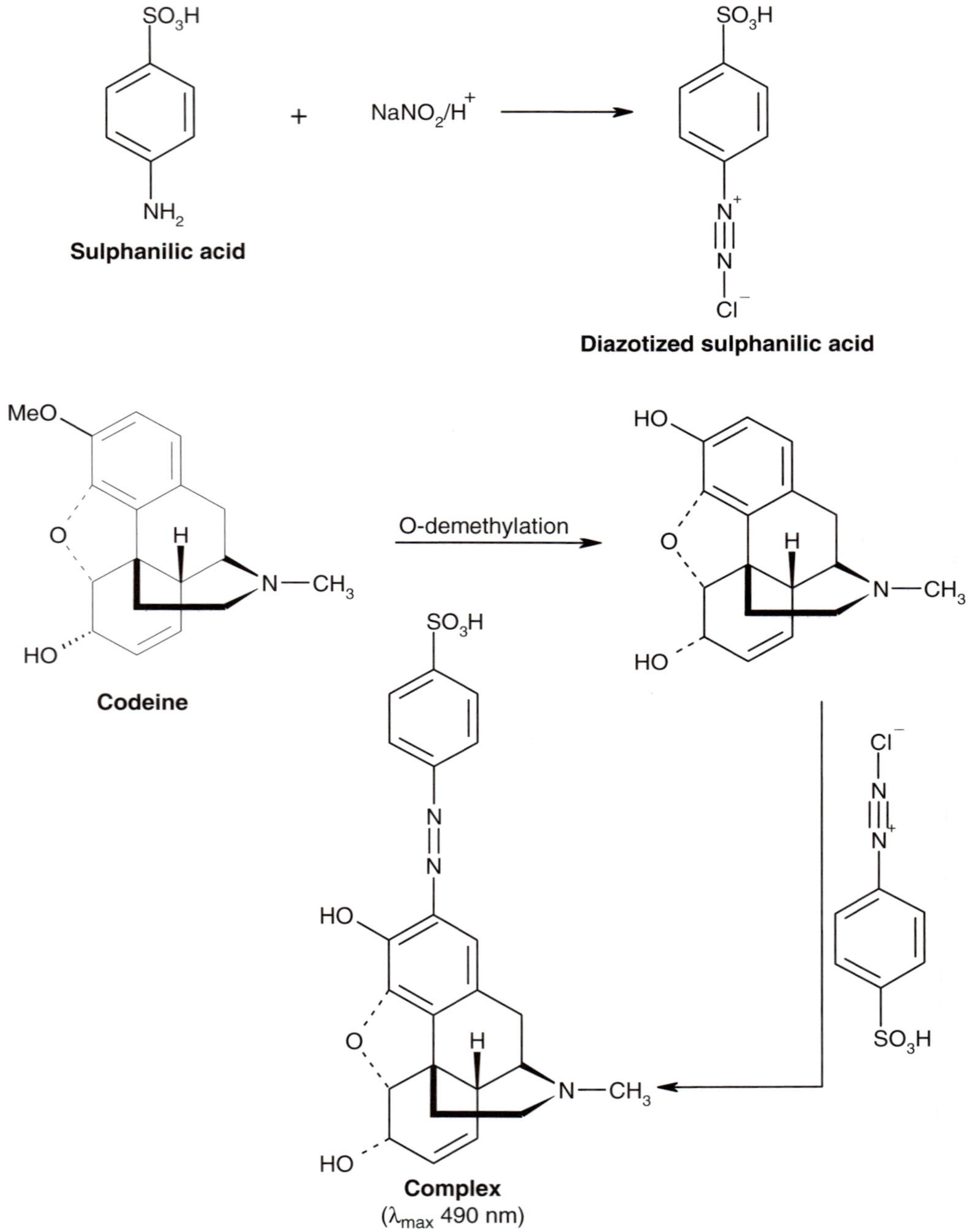

Note

Ferrous ammonium sulphate is added to remove excess of $KMnO_4$.

Menthol

Reagents

1. Dilute sulphuric acid (prepared by mixing 68 parts of sulphuric acid with water to produce 100 ml.
2. 0.5% w/v solution of p-dimethylaminobenzaldehyde in ice-cold dilute sulphuric acid. Always store in refrigerator.

Standard stock solution

1 mg/ml of menthol in methyl alcohol.

Standard working solution

5 ml of the stock solution is diluted to 100 ml with 50% v/v methanol.

Sample solution

Take syrup equivalent to about 4.5 mg of menthol, add 100 ml of water, 25 ml of methanol and glass bead to avoid bumping. Dip the tip of receiver in 25 ml of methanol contained in 100 ml volumetric flask. Distil slowly till 70 ml of the distillate is collected. Rinse condenser and adapter with 25 ml of methanol, add to distillate and make up the final volume to 100 ml with water.

Note

Keep the receiving flask in ice water throughout distillation.

Procedure

To 2 ml each of standard and sample solutions, add 5 ml of ice cold p-dimethylamino-benzaldehyde reagent. Heat in a boiling water-bath for exactly 2 minutes, cool and measure the absorbance of both the solutions at about 550 nm after 15 min using reagent blank and calculate the results.

Note

1. Use phosphoric acid instead of grease for glass joints.
2. Glass joints should be air tight to avoid loss of menthol during distillation.

Probable Reaction Mechanism

This method is based on isopropyl moiety of the molecule. This reaction is analogous to isopropanol. Isopropyl moiety on reaction with sulphuric acid gets oxidized and then condenses with aldehyde (PDAB) to give coloured condensation product (λ_{max} 550 nm).

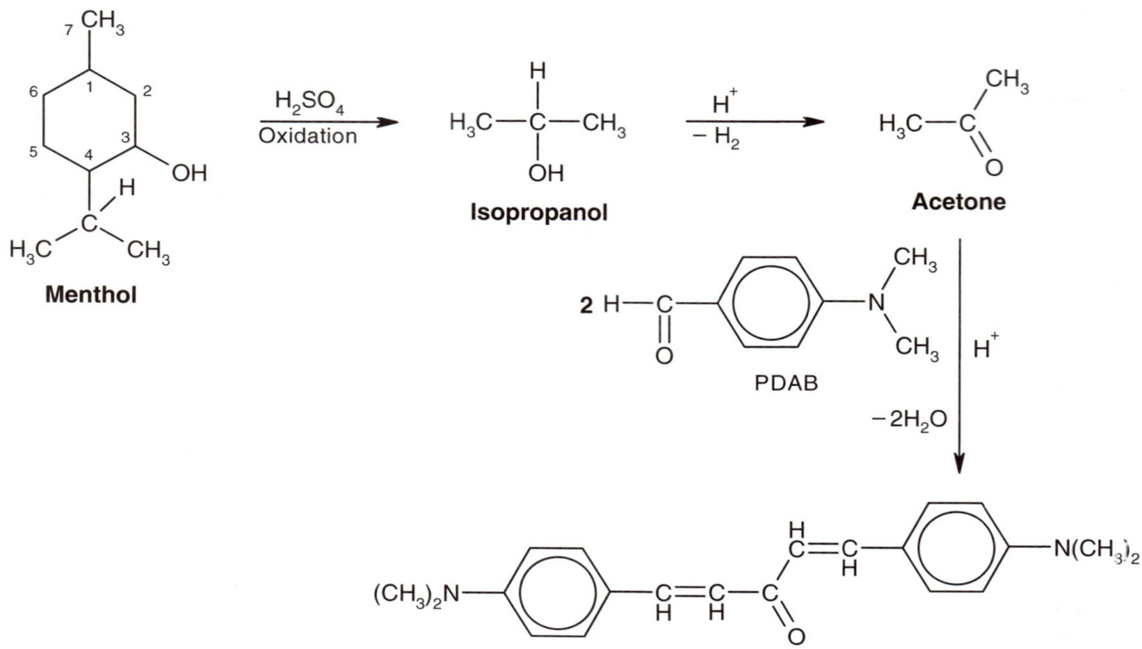

Disubstituted aldehyde product
Drug - PDAB condensation product
(λ_{max} 550 nm)

Note

This reaction is similar to the one for isopropyl alcohol.

Reference

Pharmaceutical Chemistry (Vol. 2) by H.J. Roth, p. 53.

Ammonium chloride

Follow the ammonia distillation method or silver nitrate titration method as described in formulation 9 of this chapter.

Formulation 7

Diphenhydramine hydrochloride, Chlorpheniramine maleate, Ephedrine hydrochloride, Ammonium chloride, Sodium citrate, Menthol

ESTIMATION

Diphenhydramine hydrochloride

METHOD 1

Reagents

1. Cobalt thiocyanate solution: Dissolve 6.8 g cobalt chloride and 4.3 g ammonium thiocyanate in sufficient water to make 100 ml. This solution should be freshly prepared.

Sample and standard solutions

750 mcg/ml of diphenhydramine hydrochloride in water.

Procedure

Transfer 10 ml each of the sample and standard solutions into a 250 ml separating funnel, add 10 ml cobalt thiocyanate solution and mix. Extract with three 25 ml portions of chloroform, filtering each chloroform extract through anhydrous sodium sulphate into 100 ml dry volumetric flask. Make up the volume to 100 ml and mix. Transfer 2 ml to a 50 ml dry volumetric flask and evaporate the chloroform to dryness. To the residue, add 10 ml concentrated sulphuric acid, mix and make up the volume to 50 ml with concentrated sulphuric acid. Measure the extinction at 430 nm using concentrated sulphuric acid as blank. Calculate the results by comparison.

Probable Reaction Mechanism

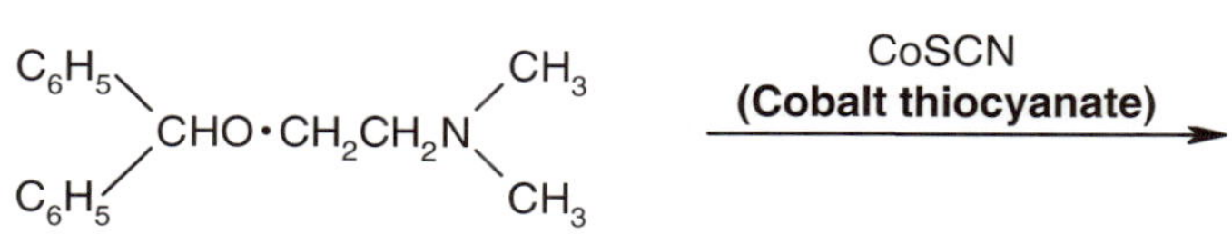

Diphenhydramine

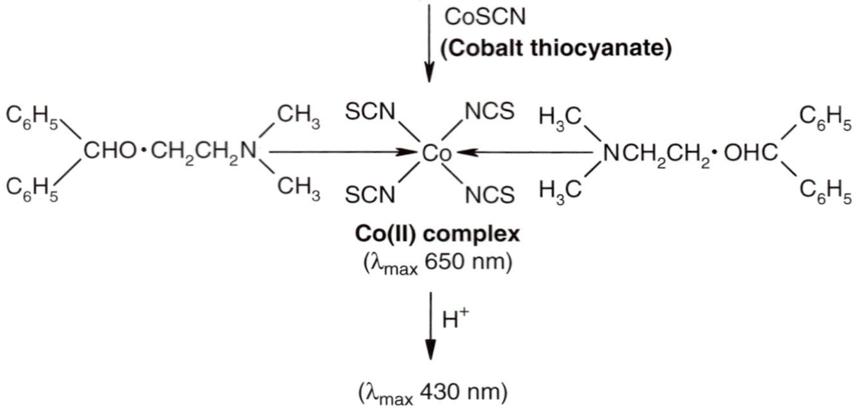

Reference

D.M. Shinghal & Uday G. Barad, *Indian Drugs*, **22(11)**, 609, 19.

METHOD 2

Follow ammonium reineckate method as described in formulation 6 of this chapter. Chlorpheniramine maleate does not interfere in this method.

METHOD 3

Reagents

1. Buffer solution, pH 3.0: 100 ml of 0.1 N potassium hydrogen phthalate and 40.6 ml of 0.1 N hydrochloric acid are mixed and diluted to 200 ml with water, check pH with pH meter.
2. Bromocresol green solution: Dissolve 69.8 mg of the dye in 2 ml of 0.1 N sodium hydroxide and dilute to 1000 ml with water.

Standard solution

25 mcg/ml of diphenhydramine hydrochloride in water.

Sample solution

Weigh accurately a quantity of the sample equivalent to 20 mg of the compound and dissolve in water (20 mcg/ml).

Procedure

Take aliquots from sample and standard solutions equivalent to 100 mcg of the compound in separating funnel, add 20 ml of dye solution and 2-3 drops of 1 N sodium hydroxide or 1 N hydrochloric acid to obtain yellow colour. Then, add 10 ml of buffer solution and extract the yellow complex with 5, 3 and 2 ml of chloroform. Combine chloroform layers and dilute to 10 ml with chloroform (do not pass through sodium sulphate). Measure the absorption of sample and standard solutions at 415 nm against reagent blank. The complex is stable as long as 10 days.

Note

1. Ammonium chloride, menthol, sodium citrate, paracetamol, saccharine, vitamin C, phenylephrine do not interfere.
2. Under acidic conditions, most substances with ternary amino group or quaternary ammonium salts make yellow complex with the dye, extractable with chloroform.

It has been suggested by Rahman et al. that dyes like bromocresol green and bromophenol blue having sulphonic acid group undergo dissociation in acidic medium, thus opening of lactoid ring and formation of quinoid group and it is the quinoid molecules which form ion-pair complex with the drugs having tertiary amino group.

Probable Reaction Mechanism

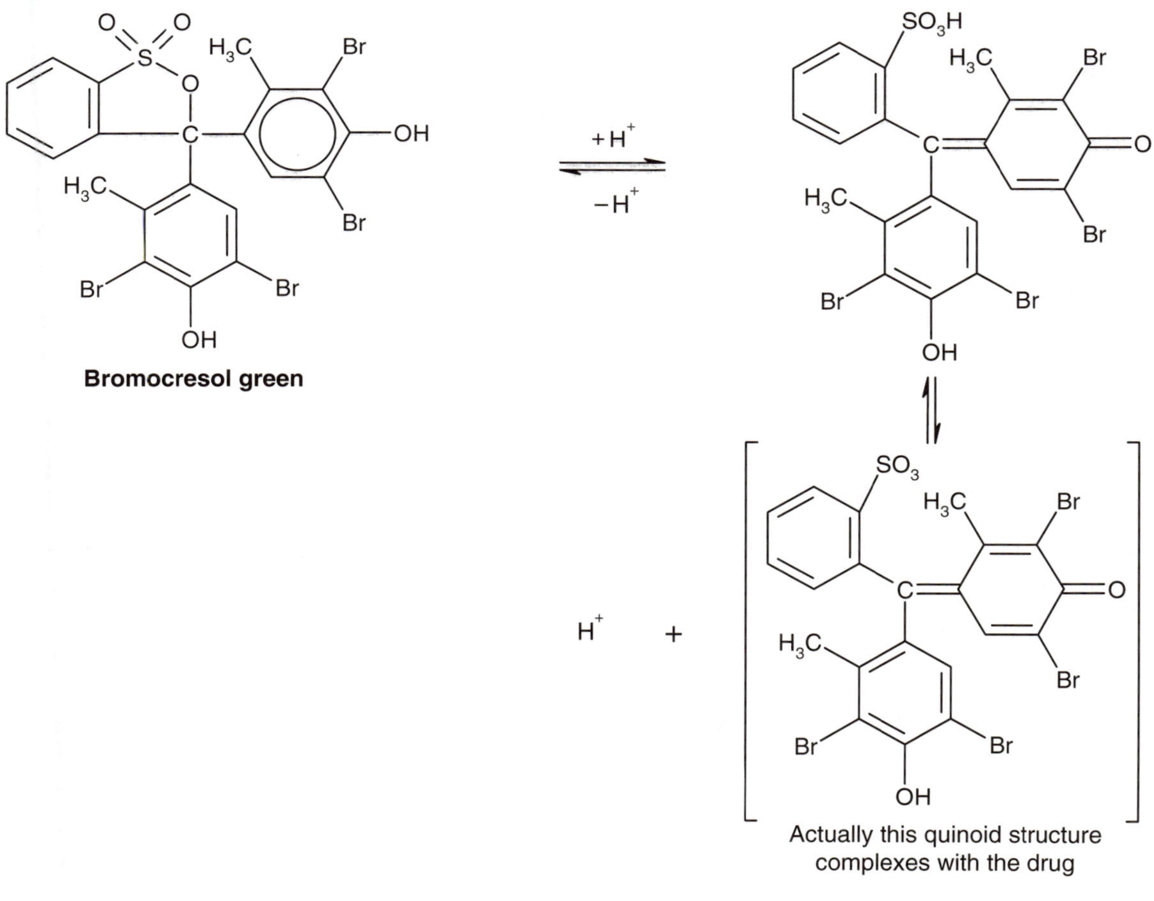

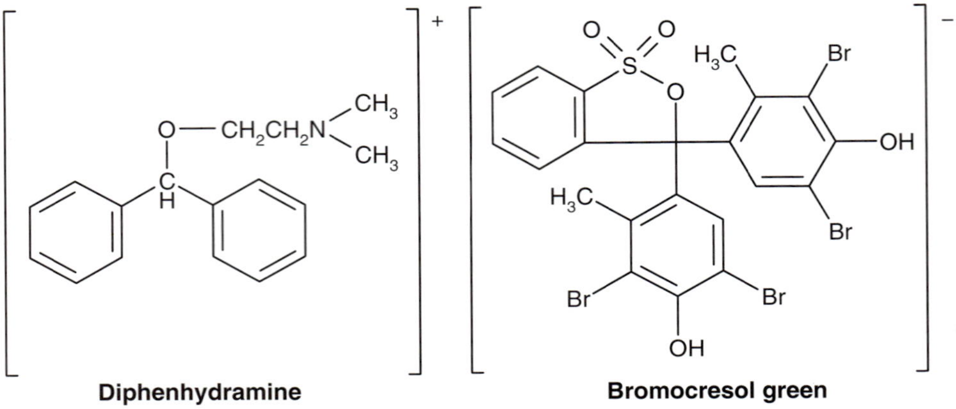

Drug - dye ion-pair complex at pH 3.0 extractable into chloroform
(λ_{max} 415 nm)

Note

Other sulphonaphthalein type of dyes behave like that.

Reference

Nafisur Rahman & Syed Najmul Hejar-Azmi, *J. Pharm. & Biomed. Analysis*, **24**, 33-41, 2000.

METHOD 4

Reagent

10% malonic acid in acetic anhydride (MAA reagent).

Sample/standard solution

5 µg/ml of the substance in water.

Procedure

To 5 ml each of the sample/standard solution, add 5 g of sodium chloride, basify with NaOH, extract the base with 5 × 25 ml ether. Combine organic layer, evaporate to dryness, add 3 ml of 'MAA' reagent, heat in water-bath at 80°C for 20 min, cool, dilute to 25 ml with methanol and measure the absorbance at 334 nm against reagent blank.

Probable Reaction Mechanism

Step 1: Acetic anhydride is used as a dehydrating agent. Here it may dehydrate malonic acid resulting in the formation of malonic anhydride with active methylene group (CH_2).

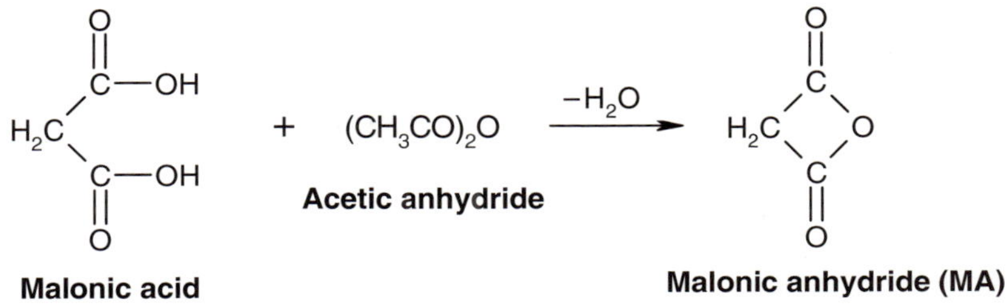

According to suggested mechanism malonic acid in acetic anhydride yields a highly coloured alcohol-soluble complex with tertiary amine which shows a maximum absorption at 334 nm. The principle is a base catalysed condensation of mixed anhydrides of organic acids where a tertiary amine functions as the basic catalyst and coloured complex is formed.

The structure of the complex is as follows:

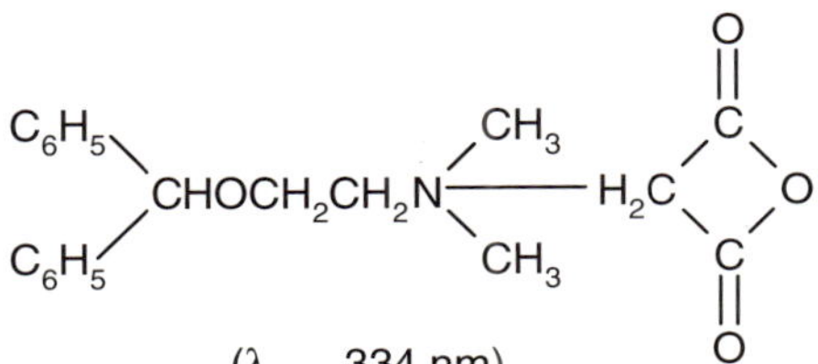

(λ_{max} 334 nm)

Reference

A.V. Kasture, M.V. Balbule & M.R. Tajne. Indian Drugs, **22(1)**, 42, 1984.

A spectrophotometric method has been described by Adikwu Mu & Ezengwu Ac (2006) based on charge transfer (C-T) complex formation. Diphenhydrone, a tertiary amine, acts as electron donor whereas chloranilic acid is electron acceptor. The C-T complex has λ_{max} 484 nm.

On basification with sodium hydrochloride the base was extracted with chloroform and chloroform extract was used for C-T complex formation. Solution of chloranilic acid was prepared in 1,4-dioxan.

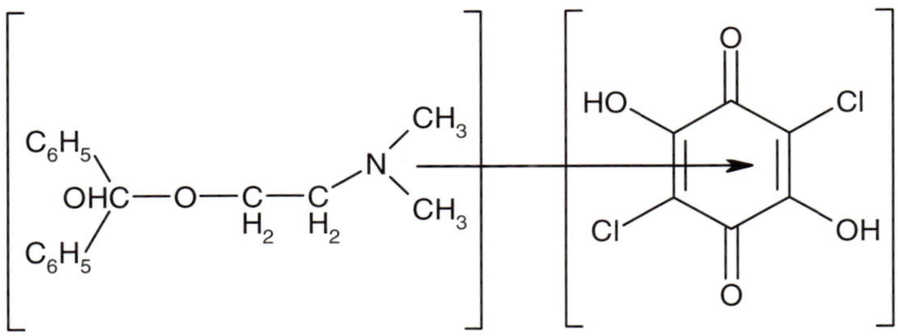

Diphenhydrone - chloranilic acid (C-T) complex
(λ_{max} 484 nm)

Note

The authors have also suggested a titrimetric method i.e. the base after extraction with alkaline medium with chloroform is taken up in known volume of 0.05 M H_2SO_4 and excess acid back titrated with 0.1 M NaOH (melly-red).

Reference

Adikwu Mu & Ezengwu Ac. *J. Pharm. Research*, **5(3)**, 74-78, 2006.

In acid medium, the compound is hydrolysed to benzhydrol which on further oxidation yields benzophenone. This can be used for spectrophotometric analysis of the compound.

Probable Reaction Mechanism

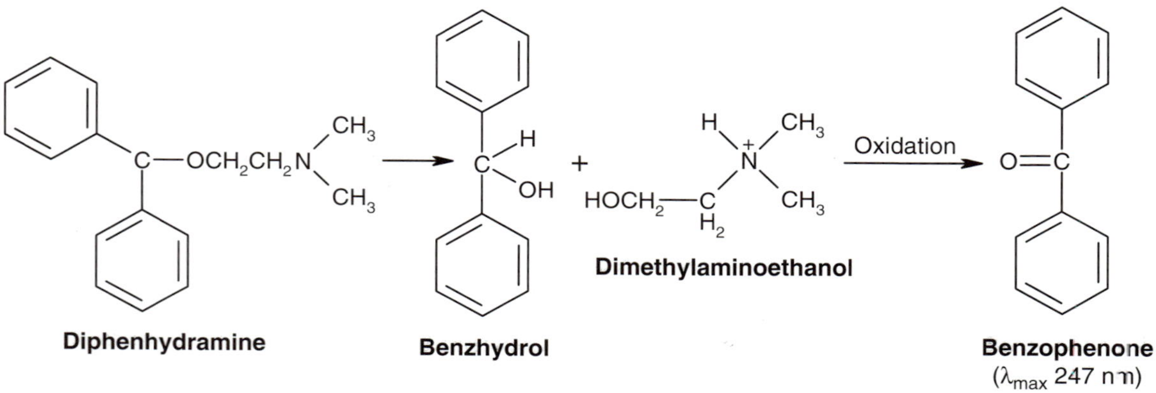

Chlorpheniramine maleate

Follow the cyanogen bromide method as described in formulation 3 of this chapter.

Ephedrine hydrochloride

Follow the ammoniacal copper sulphate method as described in formulation 1 of the chapter on anti-asthma drugs.

Ammonium chloride

Follow ammonia distillation method as described in formulation 6 of this chapter. Each ml of 0.1 N hydrochloric acid is equivalent to 0.005349 g of ammonium chloride. For calculation, subtract the volume of 0.1 N hydrochloric acid equivalent to ephedrine hydrochloride present in the quantity of the sample taken for analysis. Each ml of 0.1 N hydrochloric acid is equivalent to 0.02017 g of ephedrine hydrochloride.

$$NH_4Cl + NaOH \longrightarrow NaCl + NH_3 + H_2O$$

Ammonia is distilled, received into flask containing boric acid to form ammonium borate and then titrated with hydrochloric acid.

Sodium citrate

METHOD 1

Reagent

0.05 M calcium chloride solution.

Procedure

Take sample equivalent to 120 mg of sodium citrate in a beaker and dissolve in 20 ml water. Add 25 ml of calcium chloride solution and adjust the pH of the mixture between 7.0 to 7.5 by pH meter. Add a volume of alcohol approximately equal to that of the solution in the beaker and digest the precipitates on boiling water-bath for 30 minutes covering the beaker with a watch glass. Cool and filter the precipitates through a Whatman filter paper No. 1 or 4, wash with four 10 ml portions of 50% v/v alcohol and dry carefully. Carbonise the residue in silica dish first on low flame and then strongly. Cool, add 50 ml of 0.1 N hydrochloric acid, boil and filter through a plug of cotton wool. Wash the dish 2 to 3 times each with 20 ml water and filter the washings through the same cotton wool. Add 3-4 drops of methyl red, indicator and titrate the excess acid against 0.1 N sodium hydroxide. Perform blank with 50 ml of acid. Each ml of 0.1 N hydrochloric acid is equivalent to 0.0098 g of sodium citrate.

If ammonium chloride is present in the formulation along with sodium citrate, above method with slight modification may be used.

Explanatory Note

The citrate ion is first precipitated as calcium citrate, ignited to CaO and then dissolved in hydrochloric acid and excess acid back titrated with sodium hydroxide.

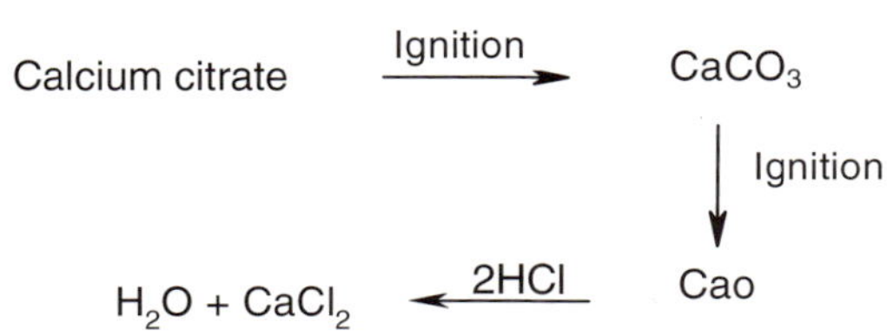

METHOD 2

Add calculated amount of 0.1 N silver nitrate equivalent to chloride of ammonium chloride to precipitate chloride as silver chloride. Filter and wash the precipitates. Evaporate the filtrate to dryness and carbonise. Take the residue in known volume of 0.1 N hydrochloric acid (50 ml), boil and cool.

Titrate the excess acid with 0.1 N sodium hydroxide using methyl red as indicator. Each ml of 0.1 N hydrochloric acid consumed is equivalent to 0.0108 g of potassium citrate, 0.0098 g of sodium citrate, or 0.0064 g of total citrates.

METHOD 2 (a)

Take accurately 2 ml of the sample preparation in a platinum crucible and heat gently with care, then heat to a temperature not exceeding 450°C until free from carbon. Cool and boil the residue with about 50 ml of water. Cool and filter the solution into a 100 ml volumetric flask. Wash the platinum crucible and the filter paper with water until the last washing is neutral to litmus. Combine the washings with main filtrate. Make up the volume to 100 ml with water, mix and mark the solution as sample solution.

Solution 1: Take 50 ml of the sample solution and titrate with 0.1 N sulphuric acid using methyl red-methylene blue solution (Teshiro's indicator). Each ml of 0.1 N sulphuric acid is equivalent to 0.0098 g of sodium citrate.

Solution 2: Take 25 ml of the sample solution, add 3 ml of nitric acid, 5 ml of nitrobenzene and 25 ml of 0.1 N silver nitrate solution. Shake vigorously for one minute and titrate with 0.1 N ammonium thiocyanate, using solution of ferric ammonium sulphate as indicator. Each ml of 0.1 N silver nitrate is equivalent to 0.0098 g of sodium citrate.

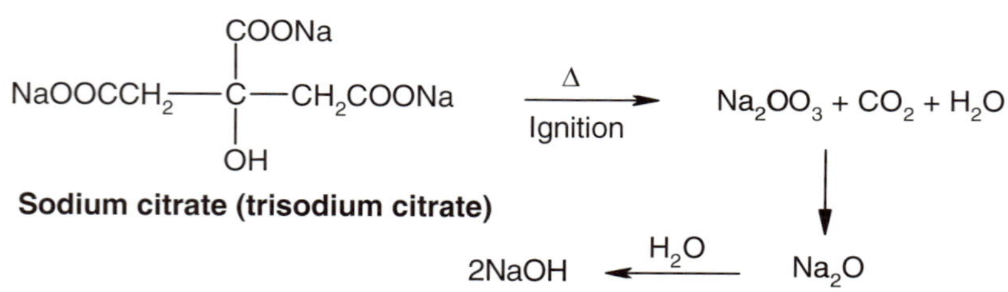

Sodium citrate (trisodium citrate)

In method 2(a), it is sodium hydroxide which is titrated with sulphuric acid.

Note

During ignition, NH_4Cl present in the formulation decomposes to give NH_3 + HCl. HCl so generated reacts with Na_2CO_3 as shown above to give NaCl + CO_2 + H_2O.

Therefore, at the end of complete ignition, we get NaOH and HCl. For estimation of total citrate, we need to estimate both NaOH and NaCl and then add up both.

The calculations shown in the formulation are based on above explanation.

Calculations

Amount of sodium citrate (g/5 ml) = X × 0.0098 × 5(a)—from solution 1

X = Volume (ml) of 0.1 N sulphuric acid consumed in the titration.

Amount of sodium citrate (g/ml) = $Y \times 0.0098 \times \dfrac{5}{0.5}$ (b)—from solution 2

Y = Volume (ml) of 0.1 N silver nitrate used in the titration.
Total sodium citrate = (a) + (b)

Note

1. Other sodium salts of the substances usually present in the formulation such as sodium benzoate, methyl paraben, propyl paraben (sodium salt) will interfere as they will finally get converted into sodium hydroxide on ignition as described in method 1 (a) and will get titrated with sulphuric acid.
2. However, citric acid usually added to adjust the pH of the preparation will not interfere in this method.

METHOD 3

Reagent

1. Pyridine-acetic anhydride (3 : 1) mixture.

Standard solution

1 mg/ml of sodium citrate in water.

Sample solution

Measure accurately the volume of the sample and dilute with water to get a concentration of 1 mg/ml of sodium citrate.

Procedure

Take 3 test tubes and mark them as standard, sample and sample blank. Pipette out 1 ml each of standard and sample solutions in respective tubes, add 2 ml water in each tube. Cool the tubes and the pyridine-acetic anhydride mixture to 5 to 10°C. Add 10 ml of pyridine-acetic anhydride mixture each to standard and sample tubes and 10 ml water to sample blank tube. Mix gently and measure absorbance of both the solutions at 450 nm against reagent blank between 3 to 4 minutes after the addition of reagent and calculate the results.

Note

1. Higher results are obtained due to presence of citric acid in the formulation.
2. Temperature should not exceed 10°C during the entire experiment.

Explanatory Note

The method involves acetylation of hydroxyl group present in citric acid by acetic anhydride, pyridine being catalyst. However, it has been suggested by

Bonner et al. that acetic anhydride first reacts with pyridine through hydrogen bonding and then final acetylation takes place.

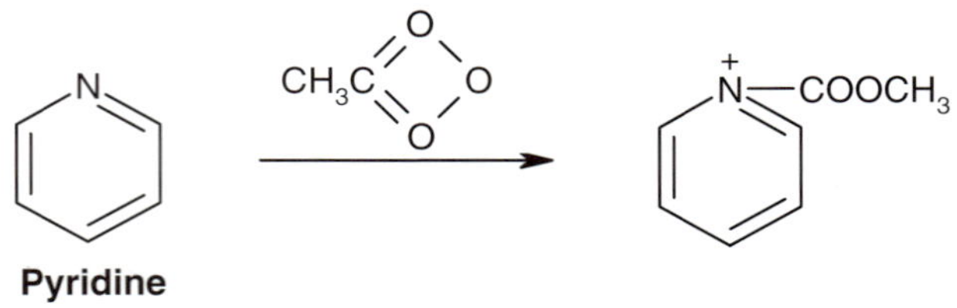

The above step is pre-requisite for acetylation of OH group present in citric acid.

Reference

Organic Chemistry (Vol. 1), 6th ed. by I.L. Finar, pp. 183, 851.

METHOD 4

Reagent

0.05% w/v solution of ferric chloride in 0.1 N hydrochloric acid (freshly prepared).

Standard solution

1 mg/ml of sodium citrate in water, prepare fresh.

Sample solution

Dilute the sample appropriately with water to get 1 mg/ml concentration.

Procedure

To 2 ml each of the sample and standard solutions, add 10 ml of 0.01 N hydrochloric acid and 5 ml of ferric chloride solution and dilute to 25 ml with 0.01 N hydrochloric acid. Mix and measure absorbance of standard and sample solutions at about 380 nm against blank prepared with 2 ml of sample solution but without ferric chloride solution.

Note

This method measures total citrate including citric acid present in the sample.

Probable Reaction Mechanism

Ferric (III) chloride may react with citric acid to give a complex of indefinite composition freely soluble in water, the solution being yellow in colour (λ_{max} 380 nm). The iron (III) may form a chelate complex between COOH and OH which is represented below. This needs confirmation.

Note

Ferric chloride reacts with lactic acid to give a coloured complex (λ_{max} 380 nm).

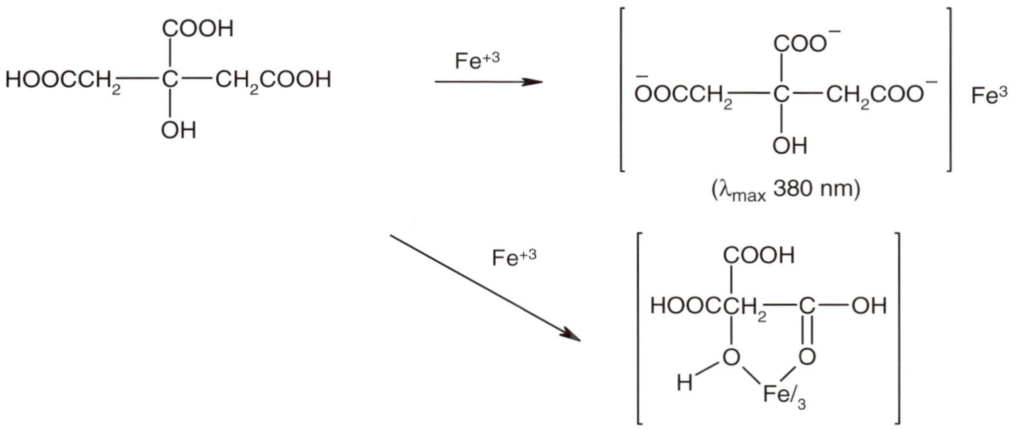

Iron (III) complex

METHOD 5

Most of the methods described for estimation of sodium citrate are based on reaction of citrate ions, hence obviously will estimate total citrate. Amount of citric acid to be added to adjust the pH will vary from batch to batch depending on pH of the initial formulation, hence amount of citric acid to be added cannot be pre-determined. The following method gives satisfactory results and can be employed.

Procedure

The appropriate quantity of the sample equivalent to 100 mg of sodium citrate is evaporated on water-bath to remove completely the water. Allow it to cool and add 20-25 ml of anhydrous methanol. Triturate to dissolve citric acid. Keep in refrigerator overnight and decant as completely as possible. Methanolic extract contains citric acid and can be used for estimation of citric acid by titration with 0.1 N hydroxide using phenolphthalein as indicator.

The residue insoluble in methanol is taken up in water to produce 100 ml (1 mg/ml). Amount of sodium citrate present in the sample is estimated by reaction with ferric chloride. For details, follow the method 5 described below.

Alternatively, one may titrate the sample to pH 1.55 with hydrochloric acid to determine the contents of sodium citrate and with 0.1 N sodium hydroxide (phenolphthalein) for citric acid. However, the suitability of this method has to be verified on individual formulation.

Menthol

Follow the method for estimation and reaction mechanism of menthol involving reaction with p-dimethylaminobenzaldehyde (PDAB) as described in formulation 6 of this chapter.

Formulation 8

Sodium iodide, Sodium salicylate, Caffeine, Ephedrine hydrochloride, Total belladonna alkaloids

ESTIMATION

Sodium iodide

Reagents

1. M/20 Potassium iodate.
2. Hydrochloric acid.
3. Chloroform.

METHOD

Pipet into an iodine flask 5 ml of the sample, add 20 ml of water, 30 ml of hydrochloric acid and 5 ml of chloroform. Titrate with M/20 potassium iodate solution until the purple colour of iodine disappears from the chloroform layer. Add the last portion of the iodate solution dropwise, shaking the mixture vigorously. After the chloroform has been decolorised, allow the mixture to stand for 5 minutes. If the chloroform layer again develops a purple colour, titrate further with the iodate solution. Each ml of M/20 potassium iodate solution is equivalent to 14.99 mg of sodium iodide.

Explanatory Note

Potassium iodate oxidizes iodide to free iodine.

Caffeine

Reagents

1. 30% w/v sodium hydroxide solution in water.
2. 0.1 N Sodium hydroxide.

Procedure

Take 25 ml of the sample in a separator and add 20 ml of water. Extract it with two 30 ml portions of chloroform. To the pooled chloroform extract, add 5 ml of sodium hydroxide solution, 20 ml water and shake well. Caffeine will remain in the chloroform layer and sodium salicylate will pass into the aqueous layer. Combine the aqueous layer and reserve for assay of sodium salicylate.

Take the chloroform extract in a beaker and evaporate it on a water-bath and dry to constant weight at 105°C. Cool in a desiccator and weigh, which represents caffeine.

Sodium salicylate

Acidify the aqueous layer reserved during assay of caffeine with hydrochloric acid and extract it with five 30 ml portions of chloroform. Wash the combined chloroform extract with two 10 ml portions of water. Transfer the chloroform extract to a conical flask. Carefully evaporate on a water-bath. When the chloroform is completely removed, dissolve the residue (salicylic acid) in 20 ml of ethanol. Titrate the ethanolic solution with 0.1 N sodium hydroxide solution using phenol-red as indicator. Each ml of 0.1 N sodium hydroxide is equivalent to 16 mg of sodium salicylate.

Explanatory note

On acidification, salicylic acid is liberated, extracted into chloroform. Since salicylic acid tends to sublime, extreme care should be observed while evaporating the chloroform layer.

Ephedrine hydrochloride

Reagents

1. 30% w/v solution of sodium hydroxide in water.
2. 0.1 N Sodium hydroxide.
3. 0.1 N Sulphuric acid.
4. Sodium chloride solution, saturated.

METHOD

Take appropriate volume of the sample equivalent to 100 mg of ephedrine in a 250 ml separator and add 5 ml of sodium hydroxide solution. Extract the ephedrine with four 30 ml portions of ether. Combine the ethereal extracts, wash it with saturated sodium chloride solution until free from alkali (test with litmus paper). Take the combined ethereal extract in a 250 ml conical flask, add 10 ml of 0.1 N sulphuric acid. Evaporate the ether on a water-bath and titrate the excess of sulphuric acid with 0.1 N sodium hydroxide solution using methyl-red as indicator. Each ml of 0.1 N sulphuric acid consumed is equivalent to 20.17 mg of ephedrine hydrochloride.

Total Belladonna Alkaloids

Follow the method for estimation of total belladonna alkaloids as described in the chapter on alimentary drugs.

Formulation 9

Noscapine, Chlorpheniramine maleate, Ephedrine hydrochloride, Ammonium chloride, Caramel

ESTIMATION

Noscapine and Chlorpheniramine maleate

Procedure

Weigh sample accurately, equivalent to 10 mg of noscapine, add 20 ml of water and adjust the pH to 9.0 with dilute solution of ammonium hydroxide. Extract the alkaline solution with four 25 ml portions of chloroform. Combine chloroform layers and evaporate on water-bath. Dissolve the alkaloidal residue in 0.1 N hydrochloric acid to make 250 ml (A). Shake the total acidic extract with 50 ml of ether. Methyl and propyl parabens present as preservatives which absorb at 265 nm and 310 nm get removed by this step. Measure the extinction of acidic extract at 265 nm and 310 nm and calculate the content of noscapine and chlorpheniramine maleate (CPM) by the following method.
Noscapine (mg)/ 15 ml of the sample

$$= \frac{A\ 310}{89.4} \times \frac{\text{Weight per ml}}{\text{Weight of sample taken}} \times 15$$

Extinction of "CPM" at 310 nm is negligible i.e. 0.03. Correction, if necessary, can be applied.
CPM (mg)/ 15 ml of the sample

$$= \frac{(A_{265} - A_{310}) \times 0.413}{212} \times \frac{\text{Weight per ml}}{\text{Weight of sample taken}} \times 15$$

89.4 = E 1%, 1 cm of Noscapine at 310 nm, reported value is 90.7.
212 = E 1%, 1 cm of 'CPM' at 265 nm.
0.413 = It is the ratio between A_{310} and A_{265} of Noscapine and 'CPM'.

Chlorpheniramine maleate (CPM)

Use appropriate volume of the solution (A) obtained above for estimation of 'CPM' by cyanogen bromide method as described in formulation 3 of this chapter.

Ephedrine hydrochloride

Follow the periodate oxidation method as described in formulation 1 of this chapter.

Ammonium chloride

METHOD 1

Transfer volume of the sample equivalent to 100 mg of ammonium chloride in a conical flask. Add 100 ml of 0.1 N silver nitrate solution, 30 ml of water and 3 ml of nitric acid. Boil for ten minutes or until the solution turns yellow. Cool, add 10 ml of nitrobenzene and titrate with 0.1 N ammonium thiocyanate, using ferric alum as indicator. Each ml of 0.1 N silver nitrate is equivalent to 0.005349 g of ammonium chloride.

METHOD 2

Reagents

1. 40% w/v solution of sodium hydroxide in water.
2. 5% w/v solution of boric acid in water.
3. 0.1 N hydrochloric acid.
4. Indicator solution : 80 mg of methylene blue and 125 mg of methyl red are dissolved in alcohol to produce 100 ml. (This is called Teshiro's indicator solution.)

Procedure

Transfer volume of the sample equivalent to 100 mg of ammonium chloride into a Kjeldahl distillation flask. Add through the funnel about 70 ml of sodium hydroxide solution, rinse the funnel with a small portion of water. Tightly close the flask and start distillation. Collect the distillate in about 50 ml of boric acid solution containing few drops of indicator solution. Add sufficient water to cover the end of the condensing tube. Continue the distillation until the distillate measures about 200 ml. Remove the absorption flask, rinsing the end of the condensing tube with a small quantity of water. Titrate the distillate (ammonia-boric acid complex) with 0.1 N hydrochloric acid. The end point is the first persistent purple colour that follows a grey colour.

Each ml of 0.1 N hydrochloric acid is equivalent to 0.005349 g of ammonium chloride.

Note

Necessary correction for ephedrine solution be made both in methods 1 and 2.

Each ml of 0.1 N hydrochloric acid is equivalent to 0.02017 g of ephedrine hydrochloride.

Boric acid is added to stabilize ammonia as ammonium borate before titrating with hydrochloric acid. Usually ammonia is received directly into standard acid and excess acid back titrated with standard alkali but the main advantage of adding boric acid to fix ammonia is that we need only one standard solution i.e. 0.1 M HCl.

METHOD 3

Reagents

1. Dilute sulphuric acid.
2. 0.1 N, 1 N sodium hydroxide.
3. 0.1 N potassium permanganate.
4. Formaldehyde solution, previously neutralized.

Procedure

Pipet out the sample equivalent to 150 mg of ammonium chloride into 250 ml conical flask. To it, add 50 ml water and 10 ml dilute sulphuric acid. To this mixture, add 0.1 N potassium permanganate solution dropwise till solution becomes colourless or pale yellow. Neutralize the resultant solution with 1 N sodium hydroxide using phenolphthalein as indicator. To the neutralized solution, add 20 ml of previously neutralised formaldehyde solution and then titrate it with 0.1 N sodium hydroxide.

Each ml of 0.1 N sodium hydroxide is equivalent to 5.349 mg of ammonium chloride.

Explanatory note and reaction mechanism

Alkalimetric titration of amino acids, so called formol titration, is applicable to alkalimetric titration of ammonium salts such as ammonium chloride in the presence of formaldehyde, however, the products of ammonia formaldehyde reaction is hexamethylenetetramine (methamine) rather than an imine as is the case in case of amino acids. Methamine is much weaker base than ammonia itself, so reaction of the acid with alkali proceeds favourably.

$$NH_4Cl \longrightarrow NH_3 + HCl$$

$$3NH_3 + 6HCHO \longrightarrow$$

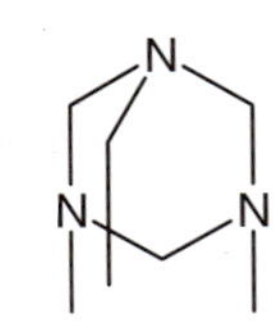

Methamine

$$HCl + NaOH \longrightarrow NaCl + H_2O$$

Identification test for Caramel

To 5 ml of the sample, add 1 ml of 1% pectin solution, 5 drops of hydrochloric acid and 40 ml of alcohol. Mix and centrifuge. Decant and dissolve the precipitates in 10 ml water. Add acid and alcohol as above, shake well, centrifuge and decant. Repeat the operation until supernatant liquid is colourless. Finally dissolve gelatinous residue in 10 ml hot water. If the solution is brown, caramel is present. Add 1 ml of 2,4-dinitrophenylhydrazine solution, mix and heat for 30 minutes in boiling water. If precipitate is formed, caramel is confirmed. The precipitates so formed are of hydrazone, confirming the presence of sugars.

Formulation 10

Noscapine, Ephedrine hydrochloride, Potassium guaiacolsulphonate

ESTIMATION

Ephedrine hydrochloride

METHOD 1

Follow the method as described in formulation 1 of chapter on anti-asthma drugs or in formulation 1 of this chapter.

METHOD 2

Weigh sample accurately equivalent to 20 mg of ephedrine hydrochloride, basify with dilute solution of ammonia and extract with four 25 ml portions of ether. Evaporate ether layer, take up the residue in 40 ml of glacial acetic acid and add 10 ml of 10% w/v solution of mercuric acetate. Titrate with 0.1 N perchloric acid using crystal violet as indicator. Each ml of 0.1 N perchloric acid is equivalent to 0.02017 g of ephedrine hydrochloride.

Noscapine

Reagents

1. Hydrochloric acid-sodium chloride buffer solution, pH 1.0 : Mix 50 ml of 0.2 M solution of sodium chloride with 97 ml of 0.2 N solution of hydrochloric acid and dilute to 200 ml with water.
2. Citrate-phosphate buffer solution : Mix 39.8 ml of 0.1 M solution of citric acid and 10.2 ml of 0.2 M solution of disodium phosphate and dilute to 100 ml with water.
3. Dye solution : Dissolve 54 mg of bromocresol purple (acid form) in citrate-phosphate buffer solution and dilute to 100 ml.
4. 1% v/v solution of hydrochloric acid in water.

Standard solution

Dissolve 30.0 mg of noscapine in hydrochloric acid-sodium chloride buffer solution to produce 250 ml (120 mcg/ml).

Sample solution

Accurately weigh the sample equivalent to 30 mg of noscapine and dilute to 250 ml with hydrochloric acid-sodium chloride buffer solution.

Procedure

Take 1 ml each of sample and standard solutions in a 50 ml stoppered cylinder. Add 50 ml of hydrochloric acid-sodium chloride buffer solution, 5 ml of dye solution and 10 ml of chloroform. Shake for 1 minute and centrifuge about 7.5 ml portion of chloroform layer rapidly to effect complete clarification. Measure the absorbance of the supernatant layer at 410 nm against reagent blank prepared following the same procedure but without sample preparation. The result may be obtained by comparing.

Note

The method is based on the formation of ion-pair complex extractable into chloroform.

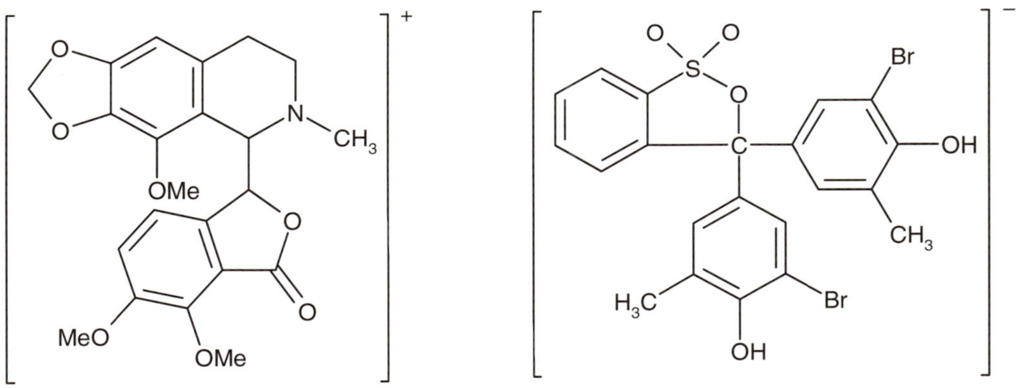

Noscapine / Narcotine **Bromocresol purple**

Drug - dye ion-pair complex extractable in chloroform
(λ_{max} 410 nm)

Potassium guaiacolsulphonate

Reagents

1. 1% v/v trihexylamine in chloroform.
2. Citrate buffer, pH 4.2 : Prepare by mixing equal volumes of 0.5 M citric acid and 0.5 M sodium citrate, adjust the pH to 4.2 with citrate.
3. Adsorbent, celite-545, acid washed.
4. 0.1 M phosphoric acid.
5. Chloroform, saturate with water before use.

Standard solution

20 mcg/ml of substance in 0.1 N sodium hydroxide.

Sample solution

Dilute the sample with citrate buffer, pH 4.2, to get 2.5 mg/ml of the compound.

Preparation of column: Mix 2 g of celite-545 with 1 ml of phosphoric acid, transfer to the column with tempering using gentle pressure. Take 2 ml of the sample solution (5 mg), add 5 mg of sodium hydrosulphite and 3 g of celite. Mix and transfer to the column by tapping with light pressure. Scrap beaker with 1 g of celite and 2-3 drop of buffer and transfer to the column. Cover the top of the column with a pad of cotton wool.

Procedure

Pass 100 ml chloroform, water saturated and discard the eluate. Elute the column with 100 ml of trihexylamine solution. Collect the eluate in separating funnel containing 25 ml of 0.1 N sodium hydroxide, previously saturated with chloroform. Shake the total eluate and allow to stand for 10 minutes for complete separation. Dilute 10 ml of the aqueous phase to 100 ml with 0.1 sodium hydroxide (20 mcg/ml).

Record the extinction of both sample and standard solutions at maximum at about 290 nm using 0.1 N sodium hydroxide as blank and compare the results.

Note

Dextromethorphan, codeine, morphine, noscapine, antihistamines, diphenhydramine, phenylephrine, alcohol and glycerin do not interfere.

Formulation 11

Noscapine, Chlorpheniramine maleate, Phenylephrine hydrochloride, Ephedrine hydrochloride, Ascorbic acid

ESTIMATION

Noscapine

To volume of the syrup equivalent to 40 mg of noscapine, add 25 ml of water, 2.0 g of sodium chloride and make the solution alkaline with sodium hydroxide solution. Extract with anaesthetic ether thrice each with 50 ml. Combine the ether extract and wash with water till free from alkali (test with litmus paper). Evaporate the ether and to the residue, add 50 ml of 0.1 N hydrochloric acid, warm to dissolve. Transfer to a 100 ml volumetric flask and make up the volume with water. Further dilute 5 ml to 50 ml with water and measure the extinction at 310 nm against the blank. Calculate the results taking 90.7 as valve of E 1%, 1 cm at 310 nm.

Note

1. λ_{max} observed at 291 nm and 310 nm in alcohol; ratio of 310 : 291 being 1.2.
2. Noscapine can be estimated by non-aqueous titration with 0.1 M HCl; equivalent factor being 0.04134 g of $C_{22}H_{23}NO_7$.

Ascorbic acid

Weigh accurately, syrup equivalent to 150 mg of ascorbic acid. Add to this, 10 ml acetic acid and 20 ml water. Titrate with 0.1 N iodine using starch as indicator. Each ml of 0.1 N iodine is equivalent to 0.008806 g of ascorbic acid.

Explanatory Note

Iodine is a mild oxidizing agent. It oxidizes ascorbic acid to dehydroascorbic acid and end point being determined by formation of blue-coloured iodine-starch inclusion complex.

Chlorpheniramine maleate

Follow cyanogen bromide method as described in this chapter.

Phenylephrine hydrochloride

METHOD 1

The method is based on alkaline oxidation of phenolic group and then coupling with 4-aminoantipyrine as described in formulation 1 of the chapter on analgesics and antipyretics. Ascorbic acid present in this formulation will interfere as it is a strong reducing agent. However, the use of 10% w/v solution of potassium ferricyanide will overcome this problem.

METHOD 2

Reagents

1. 1% w/v solution of sodium carbonate in water.
2. 0.1% w/v solution of p-aminophenol in ethyl alcohol, prepare fresh.

Standard solution

250 mcg/ml of phenylephrine hydrochloride in water.

Sample solution

Dilute accurately measured volume of the sample with water to get 250 mcg/ml concentration of phenylephrine hydrochloride.

Procedure

To 2 ml each of sample and standard solutions, add 5 ml of sodium carbonate solution, 0.5 ml of p-aminophenol solution and dilute to 10 ml with water. Mix and allow to stand for 25 minutes. Read the absorbance of both the standard and sample solution at about 640 nm. The colour is stable up to 50 min and obeys Beer's law in the concentration range of 10-80 mcg/ml.

Note

Caffeine, paracetamol, pheniramine maleate, chlorpheniramine maleate, menthol, chlorobutol and naphazoline do not interfere in this method.

Probable Reaction Mechanism

p-Aminophenol reacts at ortho or para position to the phenolic-OH present in the drug resulting in the formation of indophenol-like product under alkaline conditions. Phenolic-OH being ortho or para directing with preference for para position.

Reference

R.T. Sane & V.S. Narkar, *Indian Drugs*, **18(1)**, 23-24, 1980.

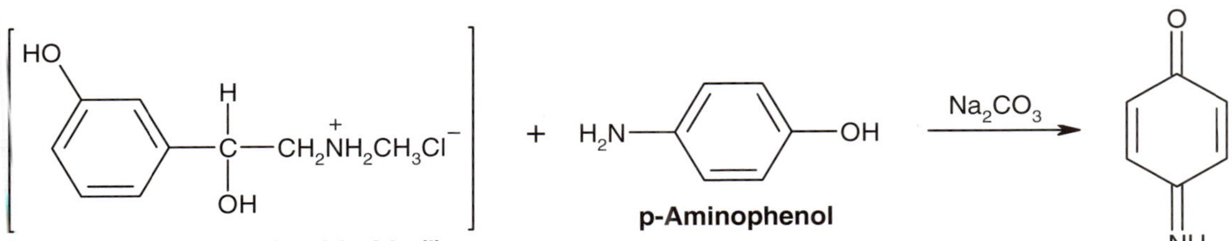

Phenylephrine hydrochloride (I) p-Aminophenol (II)

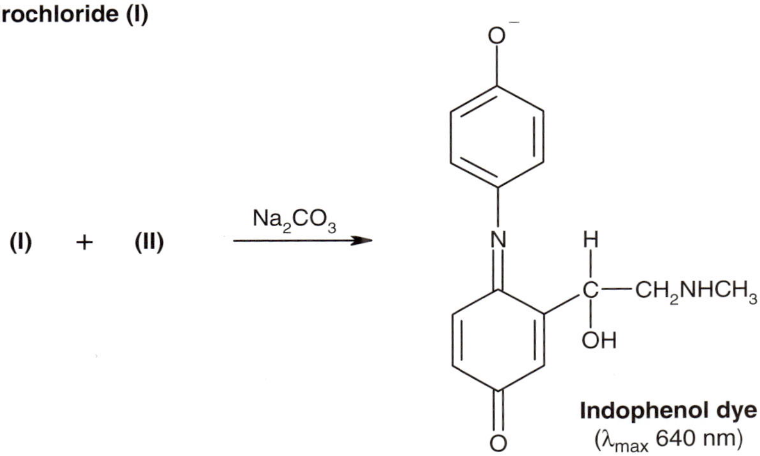

Indophenol dye (λ_{max} 640 nm)

Several reagents with primary aromatic amines are diazotized and coupled with phenylephrine at ortho position to the phenolic-OH as proposed by the authors. However, coupling at para position is often favoured.

1. Benzocaine (λ_{max} 460 nm)
2. Sulphanilamide (λ_{max} 445 nm)
3. Dapsone (λ_{max} 470 nm)
4. p-Aminoacetophenol (λ_{max} 475 nm)

Probable Reaction Mechanism

$$NaNO_2 + CCl_3COOH/H_2SO_4 \longrightarrow HNO_2$$

$$HNO_2 + \overset{+}{H_3}O \longrightarrow H_2O + \overset{+}{N}{=}O$$

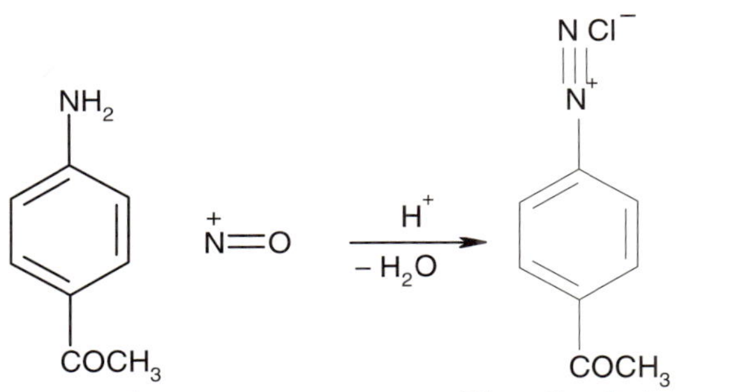

p-Aminoacetophenone Diazotized phenone

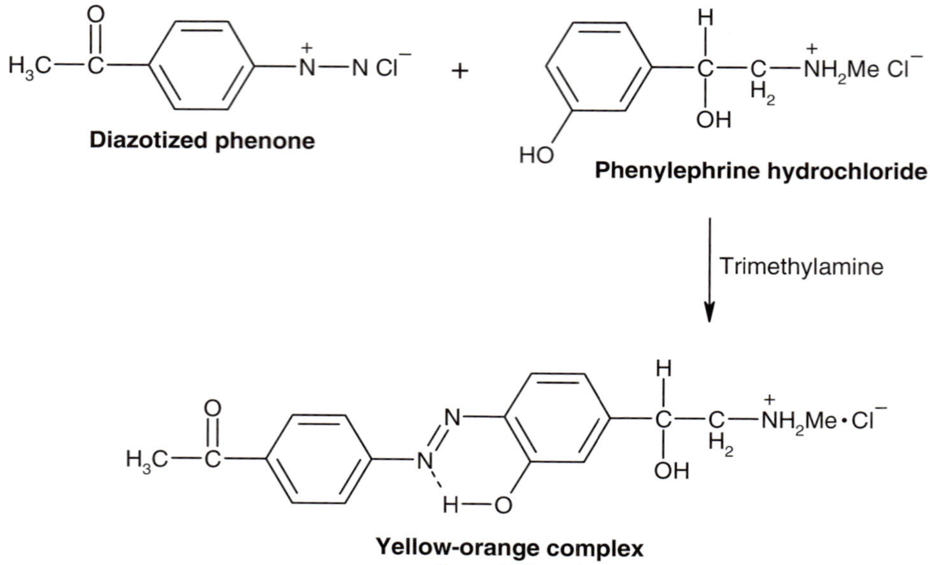

Yellow-orange complex
(λ_{max} 475 nm)

Probable Reaction Mechanism

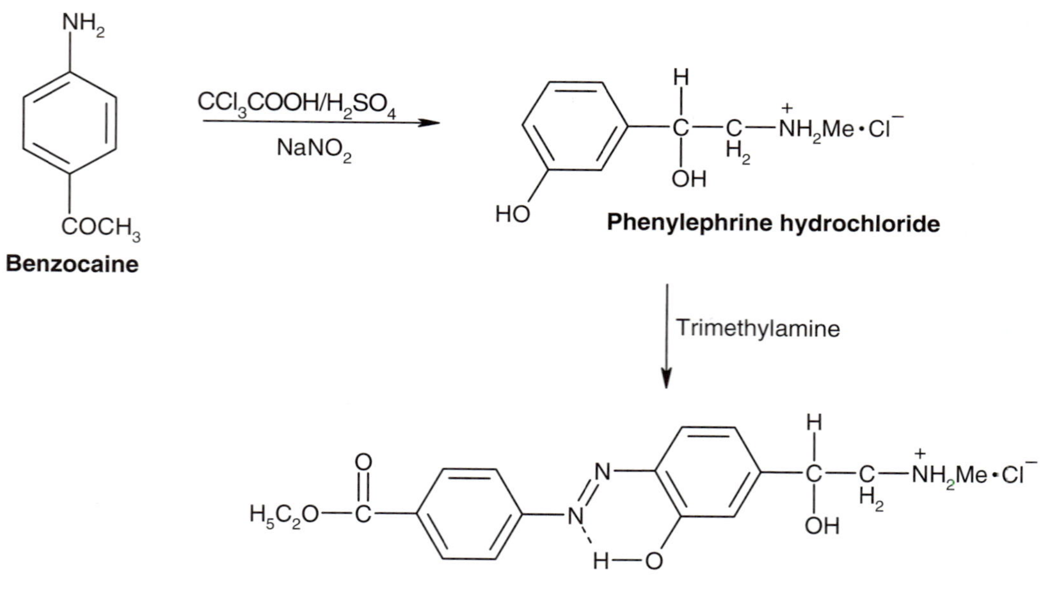

Yellow-orange complex
(λ_{max} 460 nm)

Probable Reaction Mechanism

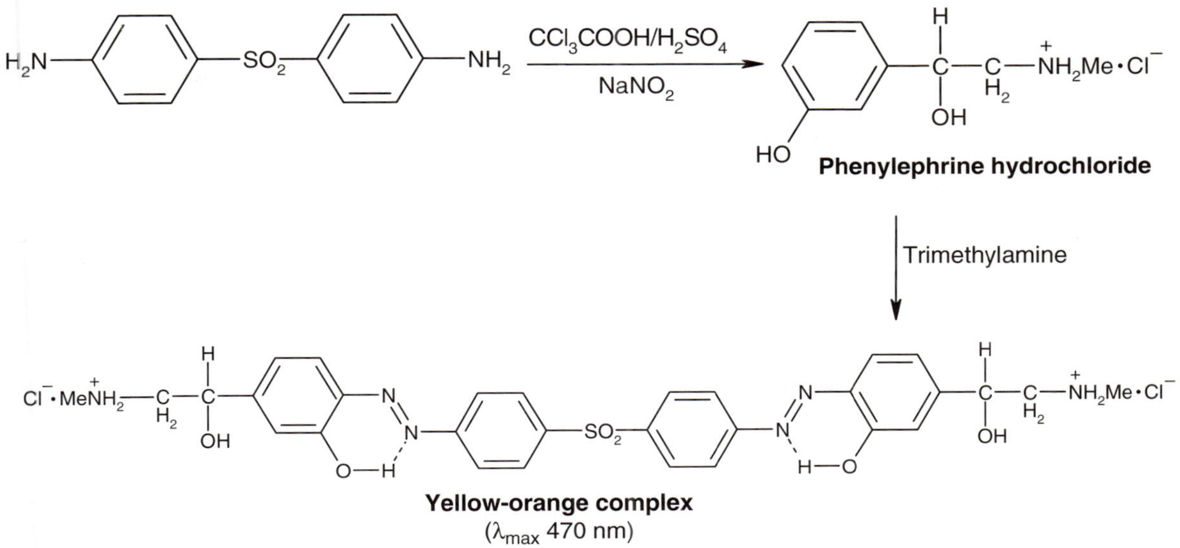

Note

The method is applicable to tablets, nasal drops and creams.

GENERAL METHOD

The reagents stated above were diazotized ($NaNO_2$ + HCl) and then ethyl alcohol was added to stabilize the nitroso derivative. To the diazotized reagent, appropriate quantity of sample/standard was added, followed by addition of trimethylamine (alkaline medium), diluted and absorbance measured as respective wavelengths.

Reference

R.T. Sane, A.D. Nadkarni, Swati Jukar, G.J. Bhonsale & M. Chakraborty, *Indian Drugs*, **20(8)**, 337-340, 1983.

Ephedrine hydrochloride

Follow the method described in formulation 8 of this chapter.

Formulation 12

Promethazine hydrochloride, Noscapine, Codeine phosphate, Ephedrine hydrochloride

ESTIMATION

Promethazine hydrochloride

Reagents

1. Stock solution of palladium chloride: To 500 mg of palladous chloride add 5 ml of conc. hydrochloric acid and warm the mixture on a steam-bath. Add 200 ml of hot water in small increments with continuous stirring until solution is complete. Dilute to 500 ml with water (1 mg/ml).
2. Buffered palladous chloride solution: To 25 ml of stock solution of Pd(II) chloride add 50 ml of 1 M sodium acetate solution and 48 ml of conc. hydrochloric acid, mix and dilute to 500 ml with water.
3. Conc. hydrochloric acid.
4. 1 M sodium acetate solution.
5. 0.1% aqueous solution of magnesium or sodium lauryl sulphate.

Procedure

To 3 ml of buffered $PdCl_2$ solution add 2 ml of sample/standard solution, mix, add 2 ml of lauryl sulphate solution, mix, dilute to 25 ml with water and measure the absorbance against reagent blank.

Note

Aspirin, caffeine, iodine, meprobamate, phenol and sulphur-containing antioxidants did not interfere. Higher concentration of acids, bases, salts and organic solvents should be avoided.

Probable Reaction Mechanism

$PdCl_2$ causes oxidative coupling of phenothiazine. This reaction was carried out in SLS micellar medium. Sodium lauryl sulphate (SLS), an anion surfactant like other surfactant benzalkonium chloride (a cationic) are reported to cause increase in reaction rate by means of micellar catalyst; also improves the analytical procedure as well stabilizes the coloured complex via surfactant association.

Since colour development was poor if the lauryl sulphate was added prior to addition of the sample/standard solution to $PdCl_2$ solution. This suggested the formation of Pd - lauryl sulphate complex which does not properly react with phenothiazine. Palladium - phenothiazine has λ_{max} 470 nm, however, when lauryl sulphate is added, there is two-fold increase in sensitivity with bathochromic shift (470 $\rightarrow$ 525 nm). If we add lauryl sulphate prior to addition of sample, we get Pd - lauryl sulphate complex and poor colour development. The above is explained as under.

$$Pd^{2+} + \underset{\textbf{Lauryl sulphate}}{CH_3(CH_2)_{10}SO_4^-} \longrightarrow \underset{\textbf{Pd - lauryl sulphate complex}}{Pd[CH_3(CH_2)_{10}SO]_2}$$

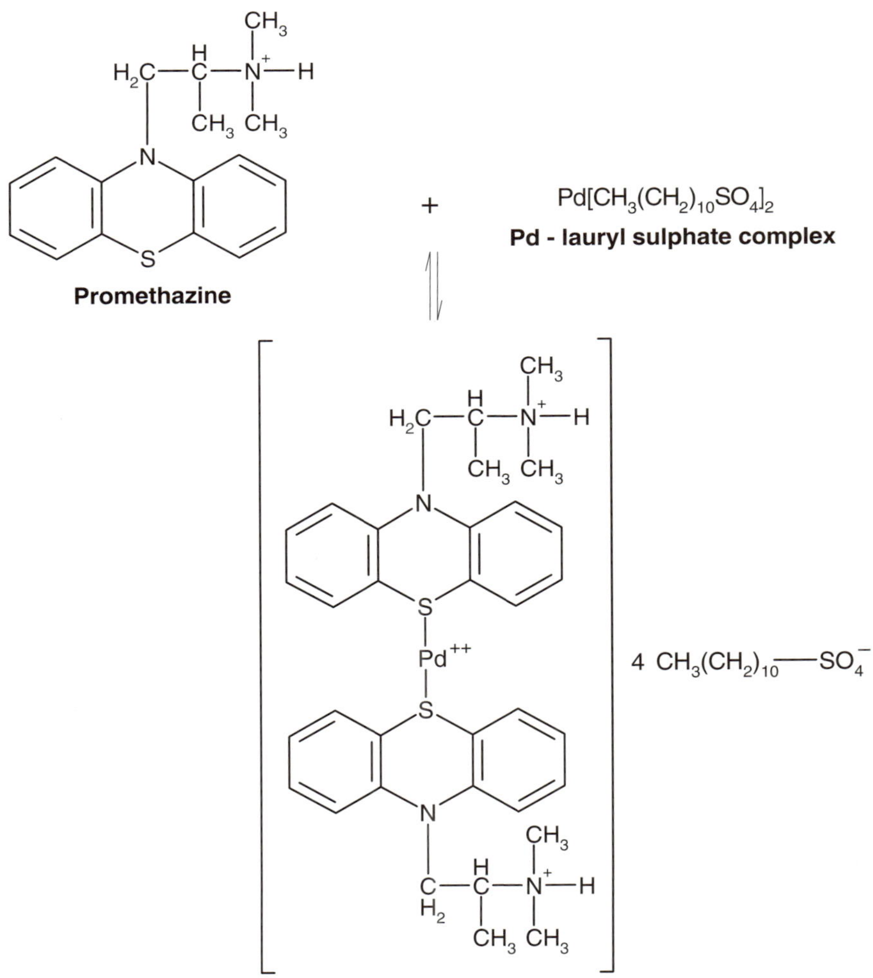

Poor complex formation
(Lauryl sulphate added to Pd(++) solution prior to drug)
Pd - phenothiazine complex

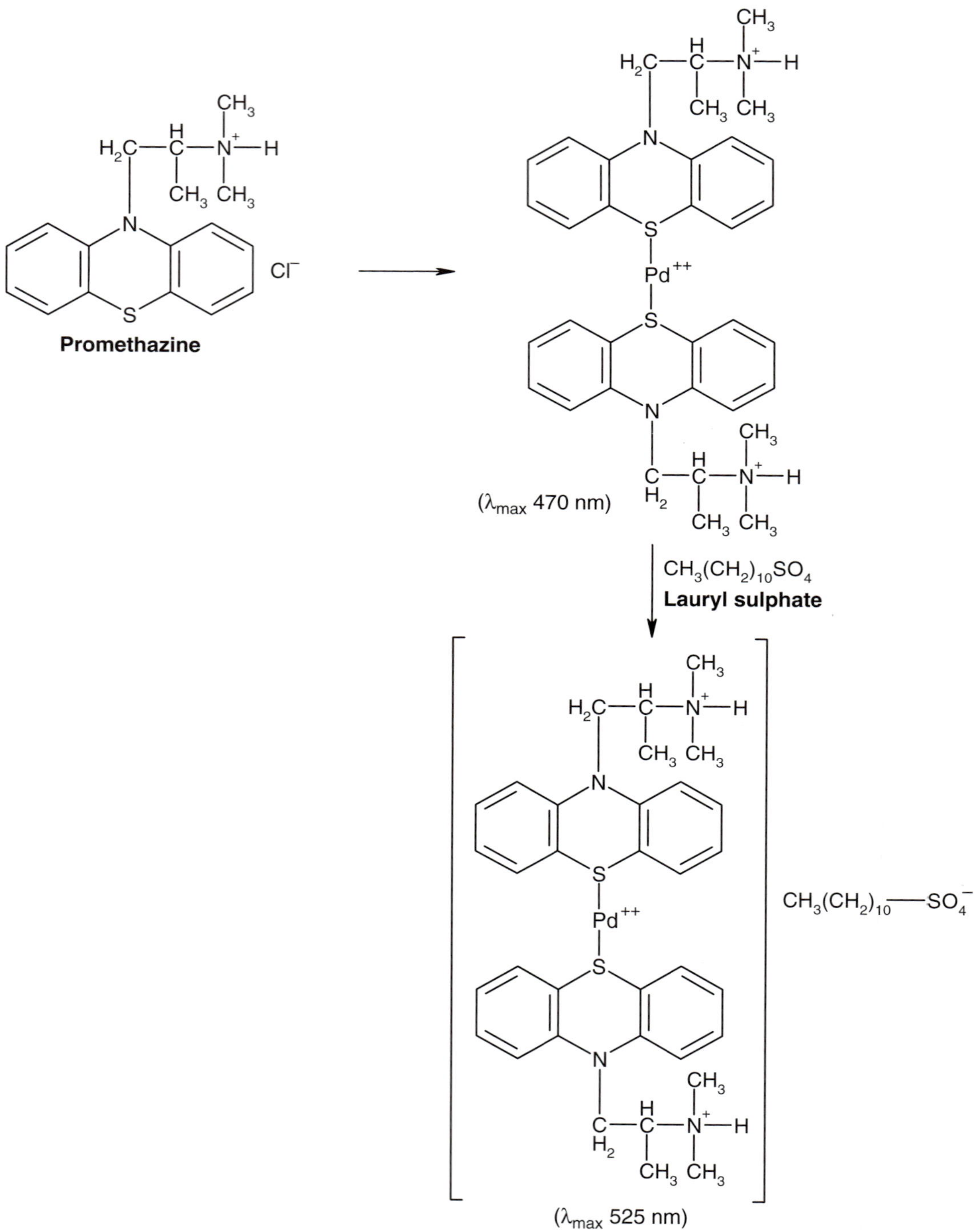

(Reaction when lauryl sulphate added after the drug)
Pd - phenothiazine - lauryl sulphate complex

Note

Details of the reaction provided by Dr. V.K. Kapoor, Inst. of Pharm. Sci., Punjab University, Chandigarh.

Reference

J.A. Ryan, Am. J. Pharm. Assoc. Sci. ed., **48**, 240, 1959.

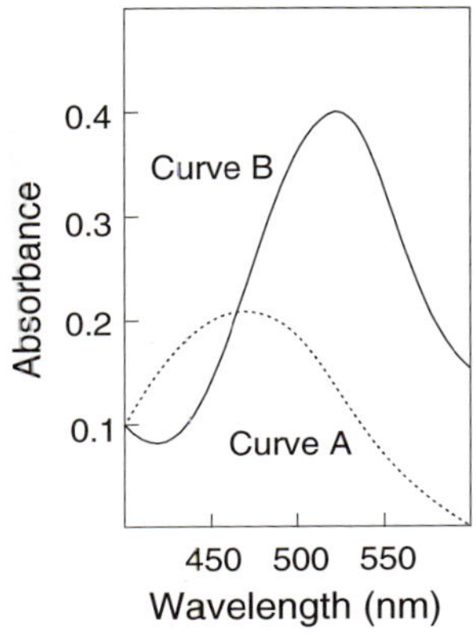

A. Spectra of Pd - phenothiazine complex (λ_{max} 470 nm)
B. Spectra of Pd - phenothiazine - lauryl sulphate complex (λ_{max} 525 nm)

Note

Spectra clearly shows increase in sensitivity and bathochromic shift (470 → 525 nm).

Noscapine

Reagents

1. Chloroform, water saturated.
2. Chloramine-T, 2% w/v solution in water.
3. 30% w/v solution of sodium sulphite in water, prepare fresh each day.
4. 5% w/v solution of sodium hydrogen phosphate in water.
5. 2.5 N hydrochloric acid, approximately.

Standard solution

0.3 mg/ml of pure noscapine in water saturated chloroform. 5 ml of this solution is transferred to a 50 ml graduated flask and evaporated to dryness on water-bath. Dissolve the residue in 5 ml of methanol.

Sample solution

Weigh/measure accurately, a quantity of the sample equivalent to 30 mg of noscapine, evaporate to dryness and dry at 105°C for 1 hour. Extract the residue with four 20 ml portions of anhydrous cyclohexane. Discard the cyclohexane layer and dry the residue in vacuum for 15 minutes to remove traces of cyclohexane. Extract the dried residue with four 20 ml portions of water saturated chloroform and adjust the volume with same solvent. Evaporate 5 ml of this solution on water-bath and dissolve residue in 5 ml of methanol.

Blank solution

To 5 ml of methanol, add 5 ml of 2.5 N hydrochloric acid, 5 ml of chloramine-T solution and 15 ml of sodium sulphite solutions, dilute to 50 ml with sodium hydrogen phosphate solution.

Procedure

Store sample, standard and blank solutions throughout colour development at 20°C. To 5 ml each of sample and standard solutions, add 5 ml of 2.5 N hydrochloric acid. Mix well and after 5 minutes, add 5 ml chloramine-T solution. Mix and after 15 minutes, add freshly prepared solution of sodium sulphite and finally adjust the volume to 50 ml with disodium hydrogen phosphate solution. Exactly after 5 minutes after the addition of sodium sulphite, measure the extinction of both the solutions at about 505 nm against blank solution as prepared above and calculate the results by comparison.

Probable Reaction Mechanism

C(1) - C(3) bond is labile; on treatment with dilute acid and on cleavage we get cortarnime and opionic acid.

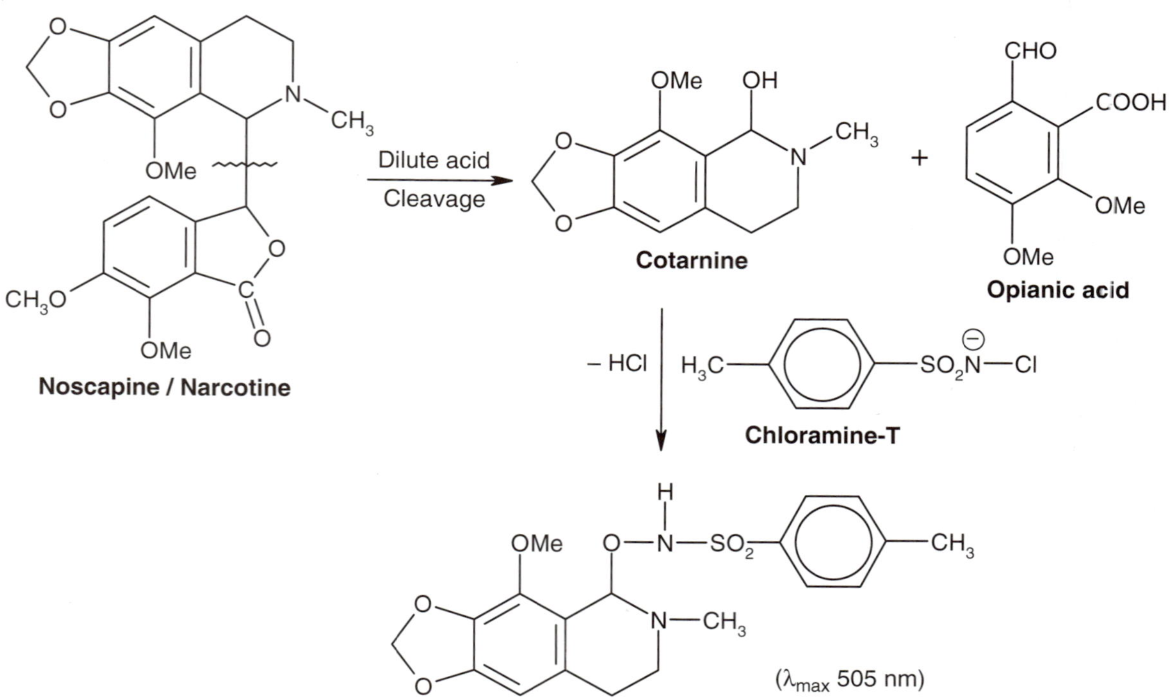

Note

Sodium sulphite is added to remove excess of chloramine T.

Reference

Pharmaceutical Chemistry (Vol. 2), H.J. Roth, p. 636.

Ephedrine hydrochloride

Follow the ammoniacal copper sulphate method as described in formulation 1 of the chapter on bronchospasm relaxants (anti-asthma). Alternatively, the method based on distillation of volatile base (ephedrine) as described in formulation 8 of the chapter on anti-asthma drugs.

Codeine phosphate

Reagents

1. Phosphate buffer, pH 5.7 : Dissolve 0.5 g of potassium dihydrogen phosphate in 50 ml of water and adjust the pH to 5.7 and make up volume to 100 ml with water.
2. Buffered dye solution : 0.0030% w/v solution of bromothymol blue in phosphate buffer, pH 5.7.
3. 0.05 N sodium hydroxide solution.

Standard solution

750 mcg/ml of codeine phosphate in water.

Sample solution

Extract accurately weighed quantity of the sample equivalent to 70 mg of the compound with water and adjust to 100 ml.

Procedure

Take 2 ml each of sample and standard solutions in a separator, add 10 ml of water and make alkaline with dilute solution of ammonia. Extract with three 25 ml portion of chloroform, washing each chloroform layer with the same 20 ml of water. Add 25 ml of buffered dye solution to chloroform layer and shake vigorously for 2 minutes. Allow the layers to separate and discard the aqueous layer. Filter chloroform layer through a filter paper moistened with chloroform. Shake the filtered chloroform layer with 40 ml of sodium hydroxide solution. Separate alkaline aqueous layer, filter and adjust to 100 ml with sodium hydroxide solution. Measure the extinction of both the solutions at 617 nm and calculate the results by comparison. The method is based on ion-pair complex formation, extractable into chloroform layer. However, to increase the sensitivity of the method, the chloroform-soluble complex is extracted into sodium hydroxide for final spectrophotometric measurements (λ_{max} 617 nm). the ion-pair complex in chloroform layer would have λ_{max} at about 410 nm.

Probable Reaction Mechanism

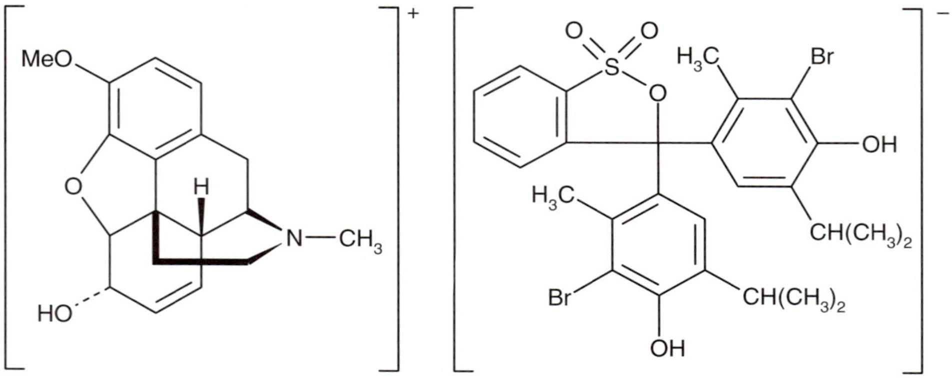

Codeine Bromothymol blue

Drug-dye ion-pair complex extractable into chloroform (λ_{max} about 410 nm), however, extracted back into alkaline layer, the λ_{max} is 617 nm. Extraction back into alkali improves the sensitivity of the method.

Caution: Ensure that there is no un-complexed dye in chloroform layer. Otherwise it will interfere in assay.

Formulation 13

Dextromethorphan hydrobromide, Ephedrine hydrochloride, Cetylpyridinium chloride, Benzocaine, Menthol

ESTIMATION

Dextromethorphan hydrobromide

Reagents

1. 0.2 N sodium hydroxide.
2. 25% w/v solution of sodium hydroxide in water.
3. 0.1 N hydrochloric acid.

Standard solution

100 mcg/ml of standard dextromethorphan hydrobromide in 0.1 N hydrochloric acid.

Sample solution

Weigh accurately, powdered lozenges equivalent to 10 mg of dextromethorphan, add 15 ml of 0.1 N sodium hydroxide and swirl to dissolve. Heat on a water-bath for 20 minutes. Cool and extract with five 35 ml portion of ether. Combine ether extract and wash the combined ether extract with 5 ml of 0.1 N sodium hydroxide. Extract ether layer with 20 ml, 15 ml, 10 ml portions of 0.1 N hydrochloric acid. Combine acid layer and make strongly alkaline with sodium hydroxide solution and extract with four 25 ml portions of n-hexane. Extract the combined hexane extract with 40, 20, 20 ml portions of 0.1 N hydrochloric acid and dilute the acid layer to 100 ml with 0.1 N hydrochloric acid.

Determine the extinction of sample and standard solutions at maximum at about 278 nm using 0.1 N hydrochloric acid as blank and deduce the results. Use 0.733 as factor to convert dextromethorphan hydrobromide to the base.

Note

Due to blocked phenolic group, there is no bathochromic shift in alkaline medium. In methanol, the compound exhibits the maxima i.e. at 280 nm and 287 nm. The compound is an example of phenolic ether similar to codeine or ethylmorphine. On heating in acidic medium (mineral acid), free phenolic group is librated which then forms nitroso derivative at position ortho to phenol which can be stabilized by addition of alkali. For reaction mechanism, see under paracetamol.

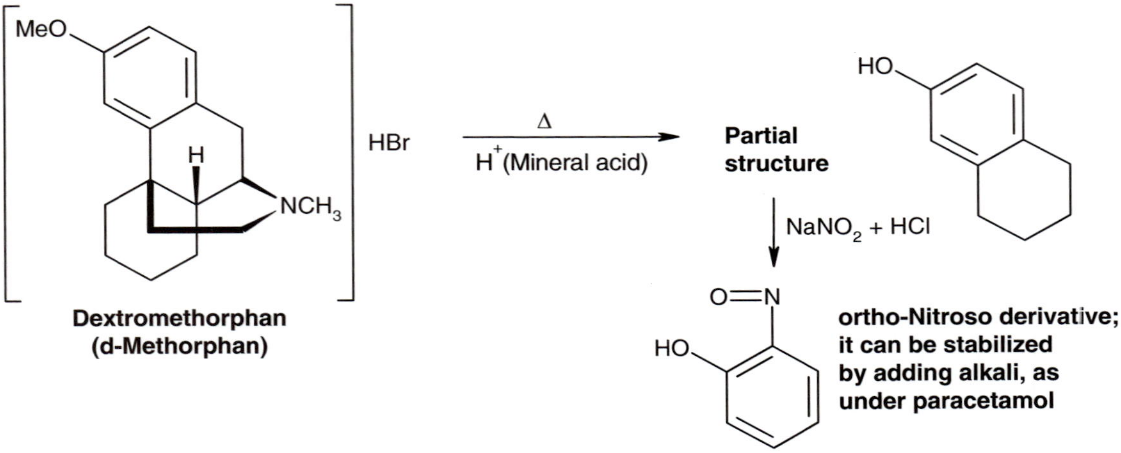

Cetylpyridinium chloride

Reagents

1. 2 N hydrochloric acid.
2. 0.1% w/v picric acid in water.
3. Sodium sulphate anhydrous, granular.
4. Ammonium hydroxide solution.

Standard solution

30 mcg/ml of cetylpyridinium chloride, in water.

Sample solution

Accurately weigh a quantity of the sample equivalent to 750 mcg of the compound, transfer to 125 ml separatory funnel containing 15 ml of 2 N hydrochloric acid. Stopper the funnel and shake to dissolve the sample, adjust the volume to 25 ml with water.

Procedure

Transfer 15 ml of the sample and standard solutions to a separatory funnel. Add 2 ml of picric acid solution and 2 ml of ammonium hydroxide solution. Swirl to mix the contents and extract with four 10 ml portions of chloroform. Pass the chloroform extract through a small pledget of cotton contained in a funnel into a 50 ml volumetric flask, dilute to the mark with chloroform, mix. Determine the absorbance of the sample and standard solutions at 365 nm using chloroform as blank.

Note

The chloroform solutions should be absolutely clear. If either of the chloroform solutions is hazy, the solutions should be rapidly filtered through 5 g of anhydrous sodium sulphate, supported in a funnel by a pledget of cotton, directly into a 5 ml glass stoppered flask. Both standard and sample solutions should be treated similarly. Calculate the contents by comparison.

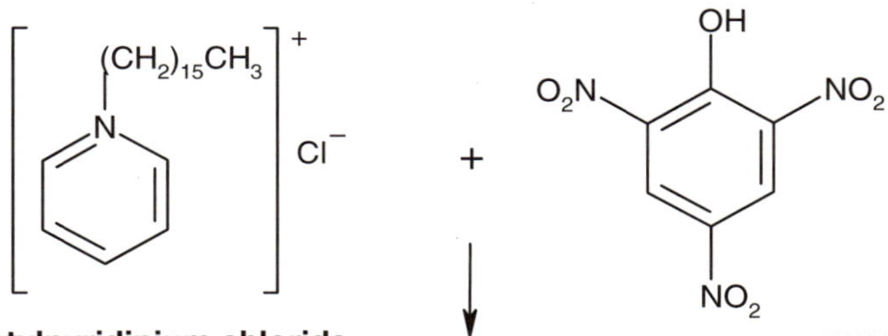

Cetylpyridinium chloride **Trinitrophenol (Picric acid)**

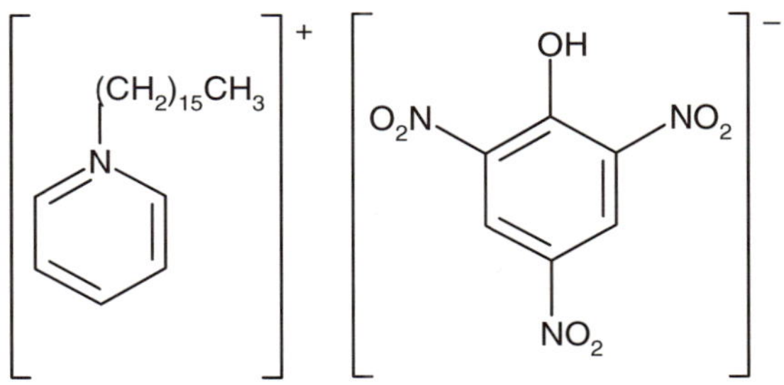

Drug - picric acid complex
(λ_{max} 365 nm)

It forms coloured complex with picric acid similar to the one described for ephedrine.

Note

The compound also forms lipophilic ion-pair complex with bromophenol blue.

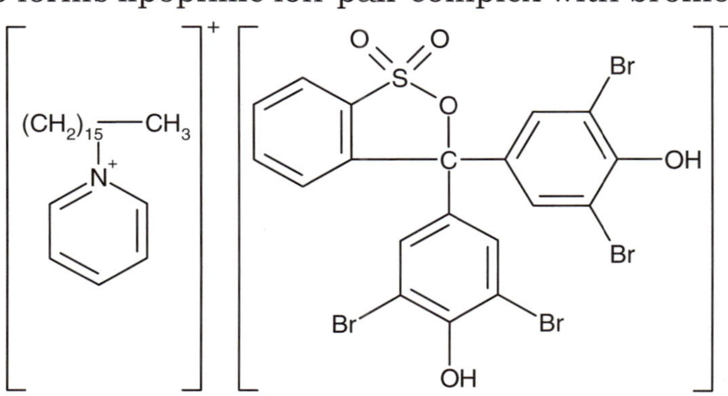

Cetylpyridinium **Bromophenol blue**
Drug-dye complex is extractable into chloroform

Reference

Pharmaceutical Chemistry (Vol. 2), H.J. Roth, p. 334.

Benzocaine

Reagents

1. 0.1 N hydrochloric acid.
2. Hydrochloric acid, dilute.
3. 0.1% w/v sodium nitrite solution in water, prepare weekly.
4. 0.5% w/v sulphamic acid solution in water, prepare weekly.
5. Bratton-Marshall reagent : Dissolve 100 mg of N-1-naphthyl-ethylenediamine dihydrochloride in 100 ml of water. Store the solution in a dark bottle, prepare weekly.
6. 10% v/v ammonium hydroxide solution.
7. Sodium sulphate anhydrous, granular.

Standard solution

10 mcg/ml of benzocaine in 0.1 hydrochloric acid.

Sample solution

To accurately weighed powdered sample equivalent to 1 mg of benzocaine, add about 10 ml of water and shake until the sample is dissolved. Make the solution alkaline to phenolphthalein, using ammonia solution. Without delay, extract the aqueous solution with four 25 ml portions of ether. Pass the ether extracts through 20 g of anhydrous sodium sulphate supported on a funnel by a pledget of cotton into a 400 ml beaker. Rinse the sodium sulphate layer with two 20 ml portions of ether. Add 35 ml of dilute hydrochloric acid, and several non-porous boiling chips. Heat on the water-bath until free from ether, cover with a watch glass and heat for an hour. Remove the beaker from the water-bath and cool to room temperature. Quantitatively transfer the solution to a 100 ml volumetric flask using water, dilute to volume with water and mix well.

Procedure

Transfer 5 ml each of standard and sample solutions to 50 ml flasks. Add 10 ml of dilute hydrochloric acid and heat on a water-bath for 1 hour. Cool the solution to room temperature. To each flask, add 5 ml of sodium nitrite solution, swirl to mix, and allow to stand for 3 minutes. Add 5 ml of sulphamic acid solution and swirl to mix. Stopper securely and shake to remove most of the gas bubbles. Add 5 ml of Bratton-Marshall reagent to each flask, dilute to volume with water and mix well. Determine the absorbance of the standard and sample solutions at about 550 nm using the reagent blank. Calculate the contents of benzocaine in each lozenge.

Probable Reaction Mechanism

The nitrosonium ion formed being electron deficient will attack the amino group of the drug resulting in the formation of diazotized product.

The diazotized product so formed will couple with the Bratton-Marshall reagent (i.e. N-1-naphthylethylene diamine dihydrochloride) at position 4 as shown below.

Step 1: $NaNO_2$ reacts with HCl to produce nitrous acid.

$$NaNO_2 + HCl \longrightarrow NaCl + HNO_2$$

Step 2: The nitrous acid so formed undergoes further reaction to form the nitrosonium ion.

$$HNO_2 + H_3\overset{+}{O} \longrightarrow H_2O + \overset{+}{N}{=}O$$

Nitrosonium ion

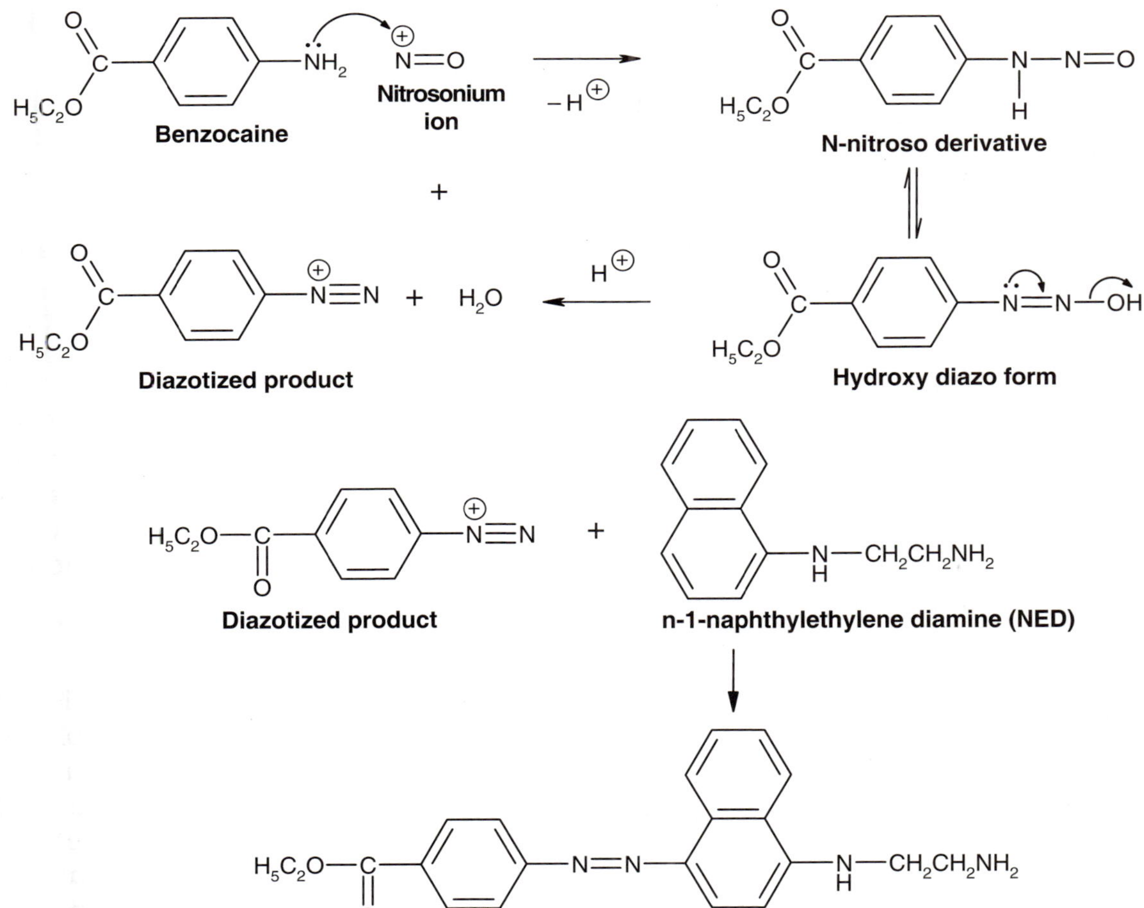

Coupled product
(λ_{max} 550 nm)

Sulfamic acid is added to destroy the excess of nitrous acid present.

$$HNO_2 + H_2NSO_3H \longrightarrow H_2SO_4 + N_2\uparrow + H_2O$$

Reference

R.T. Sane & P.P. Karkhanis, Indian Drugs, **18(6)**, 218-219, 1981.

After diazotization, the product can couple with different reagents i.e. like m-aminophenol, resorcinol, α-naphthylamine and 8-amino-1-naphthol.

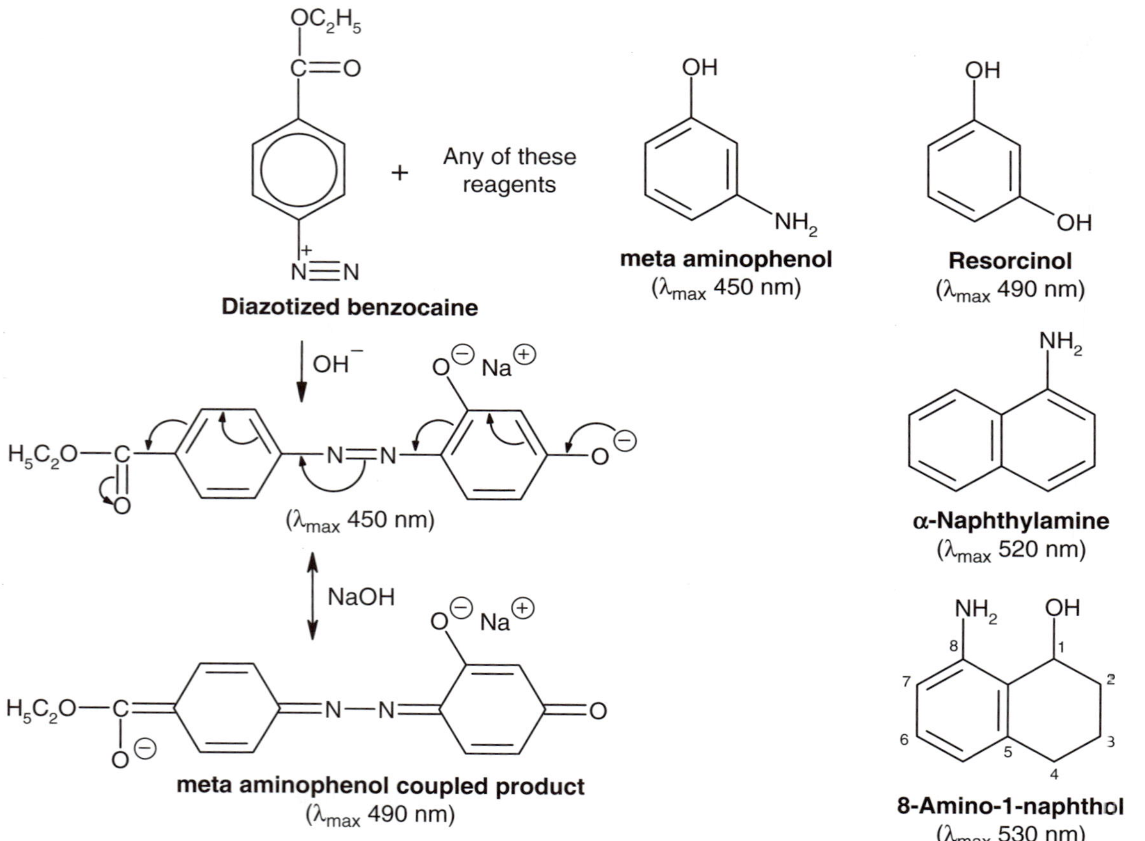

Reference

R.T. Sane & A.Y. Dhamankar, Indian Drugs, **19(2)**, 74-76, 1981.

Note

1. On acid hydrolysis, the compound gives 4-aminobenzoic acid.

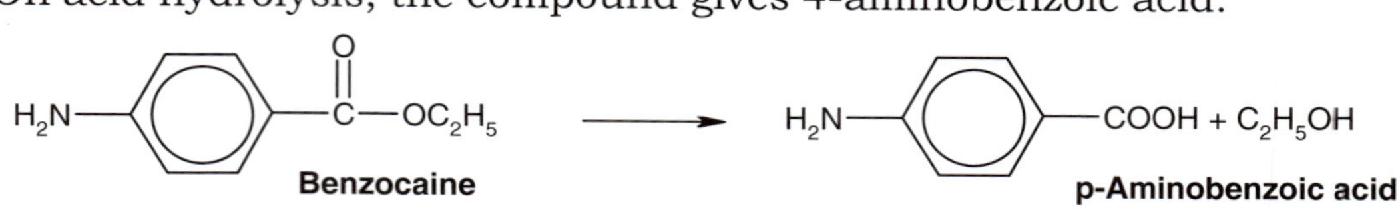

2. The compound can be directly estimated nitritometrically (titration with $NaNO_2$) because of the presence of free aromatic amino group.
3. It condenses with PDAB, PDAC and vanillin to give coloured Schiff's bases.
4. Diazotized product can couple with 2-naphthol.
5. The amino group can condense with furfural.
6. Bromometric determination also gives good results.

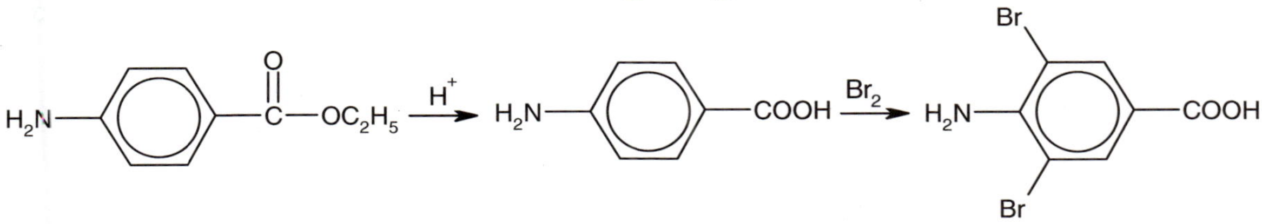

The compound forms coloured complex with 9-chloroacridine in acidic medium. The reaction mechanism as proposed by the author is as under.

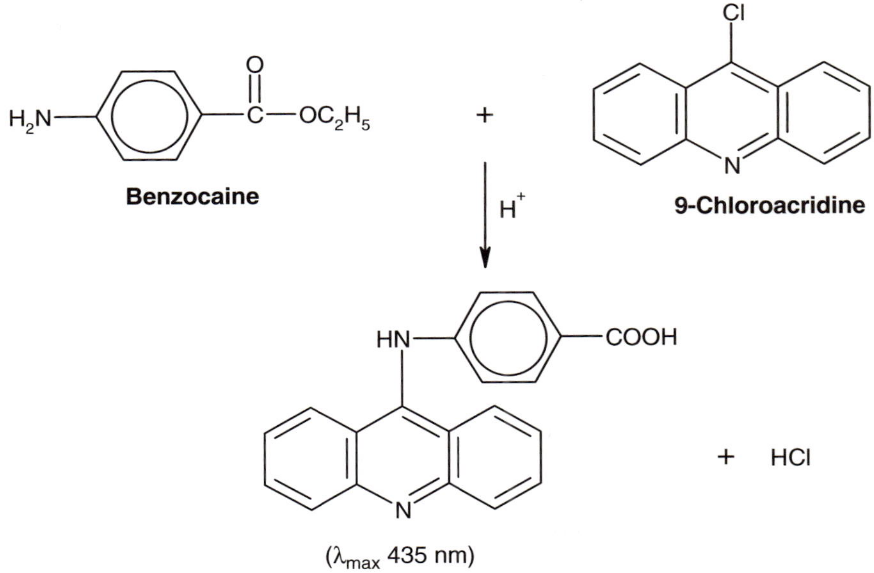

Note

The solution of acridine was prepared in DMF as ethanolic solution undergoes rapid ethanolysis.

Reference

J.T. Stewart & D.M. Lotti, *J. Pharm. Sci.*, **59(6)**, 838-840, 1970.

Benzocaine undergoes Michael addition with 1,2-naphthoquinone-4-sulphonic acid.

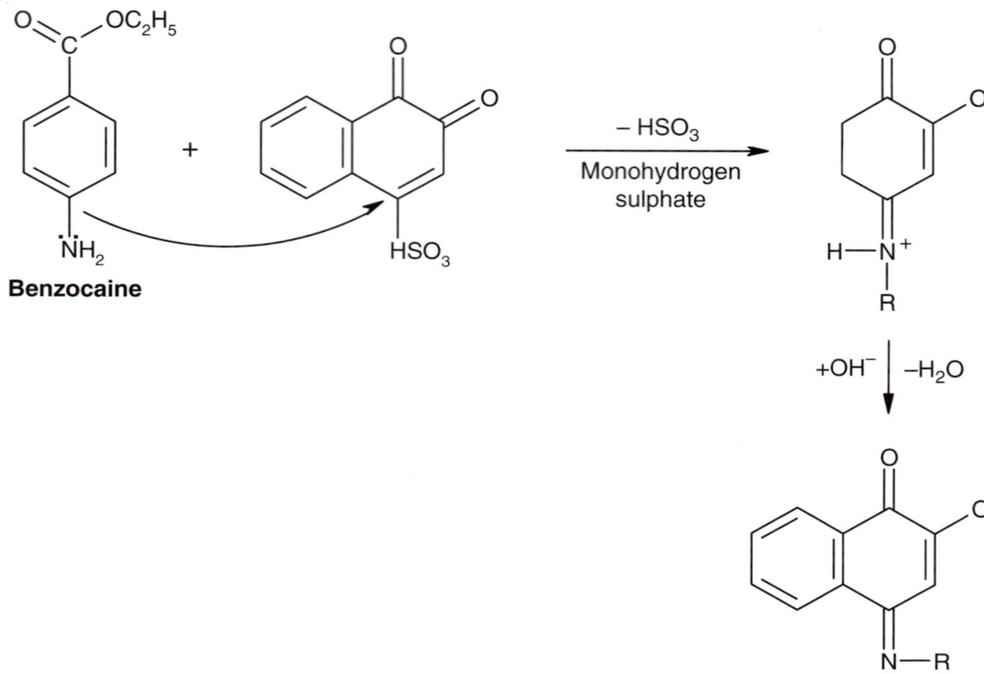

Pink-coloured quinonimine derivative
(λ_{max} 485 nm)

Menthol

Follow the method involving reaction with p-dimethylaminobenzaldehyde as described in formulation 5 of this chapter.

Ephedrine hydrochloride

Follow the ammoniacal copper sulphate method. For details refer to method under formulation of the chapter on anti-asthma drugs. Alternatively, follow the method described in formulation 1 of this chapter.

Formulation 14

Dextromethorphan hydrobromide, Ephedrine hydrochloride, Ammonium chloride, Liquid extract of ipecac

ESTIMATION

Dextromethorphan hydrobromide

Reagents

1. Buffer solution, pH 4.0: Dissolve 5.25 g of citric acid monohydrate in 50 ml of 1 N sodium hydroxide in a 250 ml volumetric flask, add water to volume and mix. On the day of the use, combine 55 ml of this solution with 45 ml of 0.1 N hydrochloric acid. Check pH and adjust with acid or alkali.
2. Bromocresol purple solution : Dissolve 150 mg of bromocresol purple and 150 mg of anhydrous sodium carbonate in water to make 100 ml.
3. Chloroform-butanol solution : Mix 1 ml of n-butanol with chloroform to make 100 ml.

Standard solution

7.5 mcg/ml of dextromethorphan hydrobromide in water.

Sample solution

Transfer volume of the sample equivalent to 100 mg of the compound into a 100 ml volumetric flask and make to volume with water and mix. Transfer 10 ml of this solution into a separator, add about 40 ml of 1 N hydrochloric acid and extract with six 15 ml portions of chloroform. Wash the combined chloroform extract with 20 ml of 1 N hydrochloric acid. Discard the wash and filter the chloroform extract through a pledget of glass wool overlaid with about 5 g of anhydrous sodium sulphate into a 100 ml volumetric flask. Dilute to volume with chloroform. Dilute 4 ml of the chloroform solution to 50 ml with chloroform-butanol solution (8 mcg/ml).

Procedure

Pipette 5 ml of the sample preparation into a 30 ml glass-stoppered centrifuge tube and add 5 ml of water. Pipette 5 ml of the standard preparation into a second centrifuge tube and 5 ml of water into a third centrifuge tube to serve as a blank. Add to these two tubes 15 ml of chloroform-butanol solution. Now treat the three tubes concurrently in the following manner:

Add 5 ml of pH 4.0 buffer solution and 1 ml of bromocresol purple solution. Stopper the tubes and shake vigorously for 2 minutes. Centrifuge, and remove the aqueous layer by aspiration. Determine the absorbance of the sample and standard solutions at 415 nm using reagent solution as blank and calculate the results.

The method is based on formation of ion-pair complex between basic drug and acidic dye at pH 4.0.

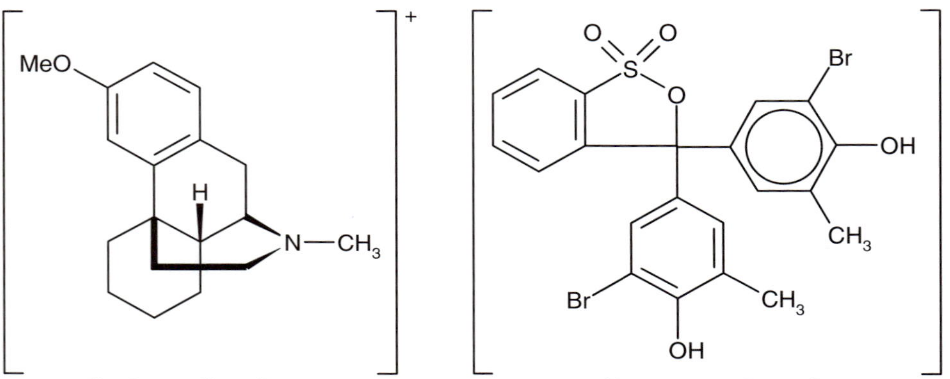

Dextromethorphan **Bromocresol purple**

Drug - dye ion-pair complex extractable into chloroform-butanol
(λ_{max} 415 nm)

Note

Phosphate buffer pH 5.3 is also suitable.

Ephedrine hydrochloride

Follow the ammoniacal copper sulphate method as described in formulation 1 of chapter on anti-asthma drugs.

Ammonium chloride

Follow the ammonia distillation method as described in formulation 7 of this chapter.

Ipecac liquid extract

Follow the method as described for tincture ipecac under formulation 4 of this chapter.

Formulation 15

Dextromethorphan hydrobromide, Pseudoephedrine hydrochloride, Chlorpheniramine maleate, Menthol

ESTIMATION

Dextromethorphan hydrobromide

Follow the method described in formulation 12 of this chapter.

Pseudoephedrine hydrochloride

Follow the method described in formulation 19 of this chapter.

Chlorpheniramine maleate (CPM)

Reagent

1% w/v solution of bromothymol blue.

Standard solution

1 mg/ml of CPM in water.

Sample solution

Directly take the sample (usually liquid) of standard solution. Add 1 ml of dye solution and extract with 25 ml of chloroform. Pass the chloroform layer through anhydrous sodium sulphate and measure the absorbance at about 420 nm using chloroform as blank.

Probable Reaction Mechanism

The method is based on ion-pair complex formation which is extractable into chloroform (λ_{max} 420 nm).

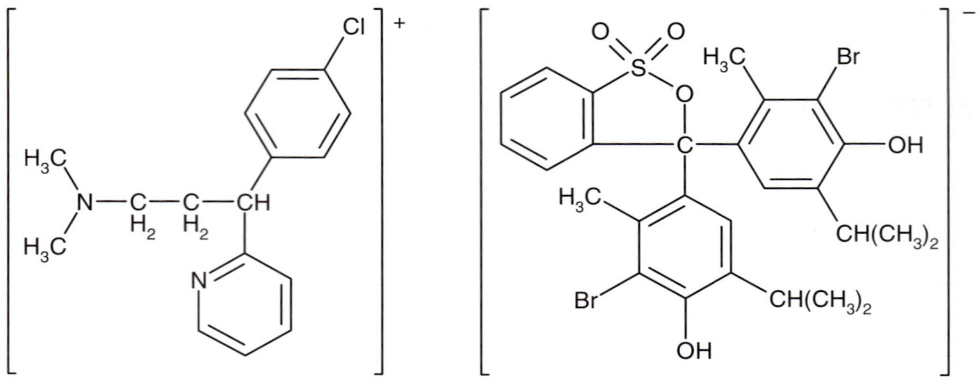

Chlorpheniramine **Bromothymol blue**

Drug - dye ion-pair complex
(λ_{max} 420 nm)

Menthol

Follow the method described in formulation 5 of this chapter.

Formulation 16

Dextromethorphan hydrobromide, Ephedrine hydrochloride, Paracetamol, Potassium guaiacolsulphonate

ESTIMATION

Dextromethorphan hydrobromide

METHOD 1

Follow the method for estimation of dextromethorphan described in formulation 12 of this chapter involving formation of ion-pair complex with bromocresol purple (λ_{max} 415 nm).

METHOD 2

Reagents

1. Bromothymol blue solution : Triturate 100 mg of bromothymol blue with 1.6 ml of 1 N sodium hydroxide, then dilute with about 200 ml of water. Boil, filter it after cooling and dilute to 250 ml with water.
2. Phosphate buffer solution, pH 7.5 : Dissolve 17 g of potassium dihydrogen phosphate in little water, add 105 ml of 1 N sodium hydroxide and dilute to 500 ml with water, check pH.

Standard stock solution

Weigh accurately 25 mg of dextromethorphan hydrobromide, monohydrate and dilute to 100 ml with water. This may be used as stock solution. If stored in refrigerator, it is stable for quite some time.

Working standard

Dilute 10 ml of the stock solution to 100 ml with water (25 mcg/ml).

Sample solution

Weigh accurately, appropriate quantity of the sample equivalent to 25 mg of dextromethorphan hydrobromide and transfer to a separating funnel. Add 5 ml of dilute sodium hydroxide and 30 ml of water. Extract with four 25 ml portions of chloroform. Wash combined chloroform extracts with 30 ml of dilute sodium hydroxide and evaporate chloroform layer. Dissolve the residue in 100 ml of water and 10 ml of the resultant solution is diluted to 100 ml with the same solvent to get sample solution (25 mcg/ml).

Procedure

Take 5 ml each of sample, standard and water (blank). To each tube, add 5 ml of buffer solution, 5 ml dye solution and 15 ml of chloroform. Shake for 15 min, centrifuge to separate the layers. Measure the absorbance of benzene layer at about 405 nm using chloroform layer of blank in reference cell and calculate the results.

Note

The method is based on formation of ion-pair complex with the dye i.e. bromothymol blue in pH 7.5 buffer. The complex can be extracted into chloroform for spectrophotometric measurements (λ_{max} 405 nm).

Paracetamol

Reagents

1. 10% w/v solution of α-naphthol in methanol, prepare fresh.
2. 4% w/v solution of sodium hydroxide in water.

Standard solution

0.5 mg/ml of paracetamol in water.

Sample solution

Accurately measured/weighed quantity of the sample is appropriately diluted with water to get 0.5 mg/ml concentration.

Procedure

To 2 ml each of sample, standard and water, add 15 ml of hydrochloric acid, 25 ml of water and heat on boiling water-bath for 2 hours. Cool to room temperature and dilute to 50 ml with water and proceed as under :

Take 5 ml each of hydrolysed sample and standard solutions in 25 ml volumetric flasks. To each, add 0.5 ml of a-naphthol solution and 5 ml of sodium hydroxide solution. Mix well after the addition of each reagent and dilute to 25 ml with methanol. After 30 min, measure the absorbance of both the solutions at 620 nm against the reagent blank. Calculate the contents of paracetamol by comparison.

Probable Reaction Mechanism

On acid hydrolysis, the compound is changed to p-aminophenol.

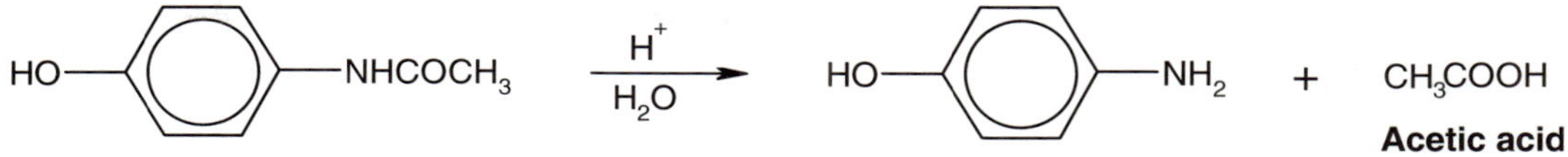

Paracetamol — p-Aminophenol — Acetic acid

In case of α-substituted naphthalene like α-naphthol the phenolic-OH being electron-donating group is ortho or para directing, with preference to substitution in para position.

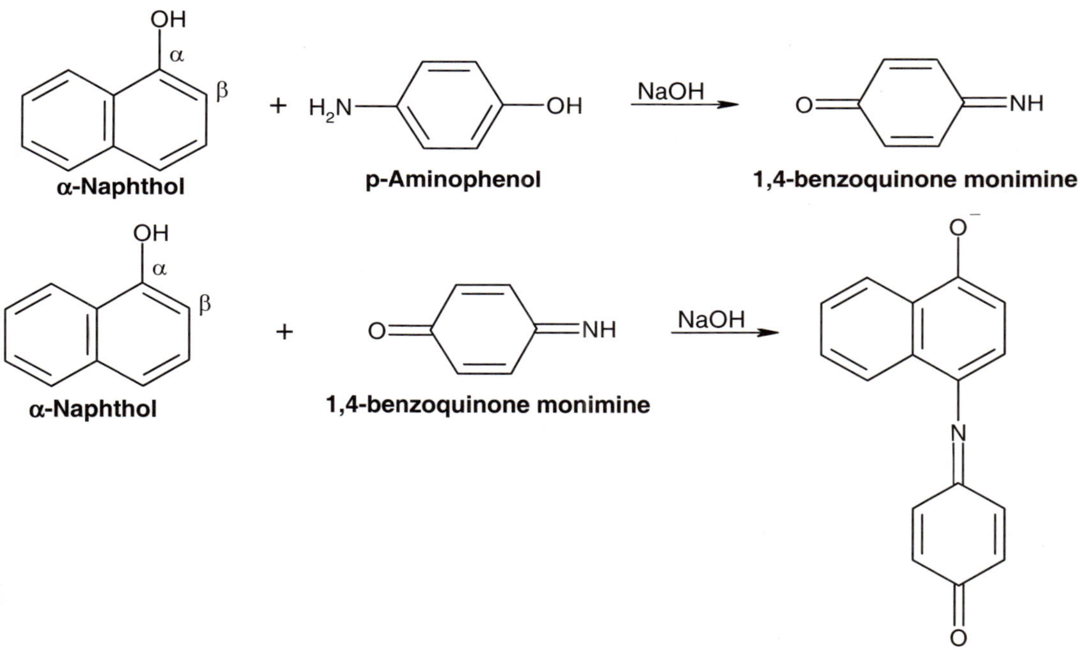

α-Naphthol — p-Aminophenol — 1,4-benzoquinone monimine

α-Naphthol — 1,4-benzoquinone monimine — Indophenol dye (λ_{max} 620 nm)

Potassium guaiacolsulphonate (PGS)

Reagents

1. 1% w/v solution of 4-aminoantipyrine in water.
2. 2% w/v solution of potassium ferricyanide in water.
3. Phosphate buffer solution : 11.88 g of disodium hydrogen phosphate dissolved in water to produce 1000 ml.

Standard solution

40 mcg/ml of potassium guaiacolsulphonate in water.

Sample solution

Weigh accurately sample equivalent to 40 mg of the compound and dilute appropriately with water to get 40 mcg/ml.

Procedure

To 10 ml each of the sample and standard solutions, add 15 ml of buffer solution and 2 ml of aminoantipyrine reagent. Shake to mix, add about 15 ml of water, 2 ml of potassium ferricyanide solution and dilute to 50 ml with water. After 10 min, measure the extinction of both the solutions at 550 nm against reagent blank.

Note

Codeine phosphate, promethazine, diphenhydramine and ammonium chloride do not interfere. Phenylephrine will interfere.

Potassium guaiasulphonate is a mixture of 3-hydroxy-4-methoxy benzene sulfonic acid monopotassium salt and 4-hydroxy-3-methoxy benzene sulfonic acid monopotassium salt.

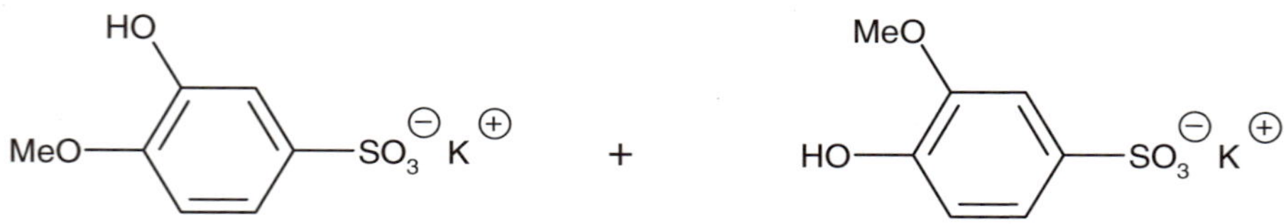

Potassium guaiacolsulphonate (PGS)

Explanatory Note

This reaction involves oxidative coupling at ortho position to the phenolic hydroxy group in the drug. The presence of an oxidizing agent i.e. $K_3Fe(CN)_6$ is necessary for the reaction. The reaction can be represented as:

Probable Reaction Mechanism

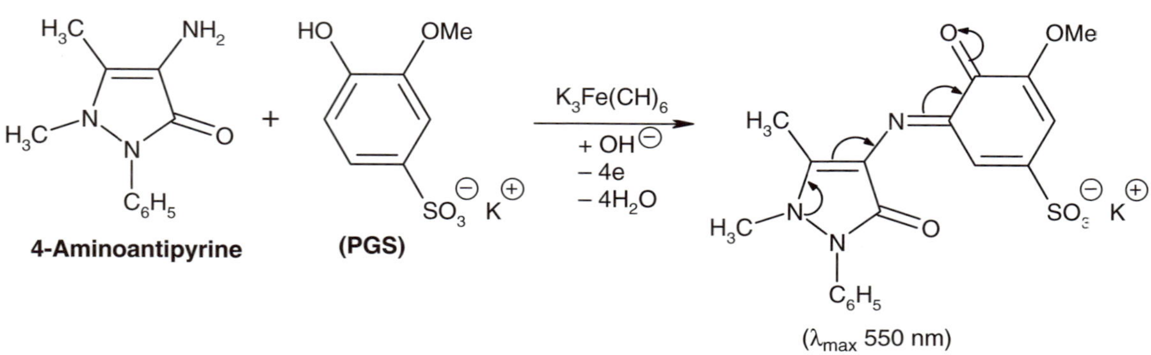

Ephedrine hydrochloride

Follow the method as described in formulation 8 of the chapter on broncho-spasm relaxants. Ephedrine, a volatile base is subjected to distillation and then estimated by acid-base titration; refer to chapter on bronchospasm relaxants.

Formulation 17

Pheniramine maleate, Ammonium chloride, Sodium citrate, Menthol

ESTIMATION

Pheniramine maleate

Reagents

1. 0.02 N perchloric acid.
2. 10% w/v solution of sodium hydroxide in water.

Procedure

Transfer equivalent to 60 mg of pheniramine maleate into a separating funnel. Dilute with 20 ml water. Make alkaline with sodium hydroxide solution and extract with three 20 ml portions of solvent ether. The combined ethereal extracts are dried over anhydrous sodium sulphate. Evaporate the ether extract carefully. The residue is dissolved in previously neutralised glacial acetic acid and titrated with 0.02 N perchloric acid, using crystal violet as indicator. Each ml of 0.02 N perchloric acid is equivalent to 0.003564 g of pheniramine maleate.

Ammonium chloride

Transfer the preparation equivalent to 100 mg of ammonium chloride into a conical flask, dilute with 20 ml water. Titrate with 0.1 N silver nitrate using solutions of fluorescein sodium as indicator. The end point is detected by the appearance of a pronounced pink tint of the precipitates. 1 ml of 0.1 N silver nitrate is equivalent to 0.00535 g of ammonium chloride.

Sodium citrate

Follow the calcium chloride precipitation method as described in formulation 7 of this chapter.

Menthol

Follow the method involving reaction with p-dimethylaminobenzaldehyde. For details refer to formulation 6 of this chapter.

Formulation 18

Ephedrine hydrochloride, Ethylmorphine hydrochloride

ESTIMATION

Total alkaloids

To accurately measured volume of the sample equivalent to 100 mg of ephedrine hydrochloride, add 50 ml of normal saline and 5 ml of 4% w/v aqueous solution of sodium hydroxide. Add sufficient sodium chloride powder to saturate. Extract with three 50 ml portions of ether. Wash ether layer with the same 10 ml of brine solution. Extract ether layer with exactly 20 ml of 0.1 N sulphuric acid. Warm the acid extract (A) to dispel dissolved ether and titrate excess acid with 0.1 N sodium hydroxide using bromothymol blue as indicator. Each ml of 0.1 N sulphuric acid is equivalent to 0.02017 g of total alkaloids calculated as ephedrine hydrochloride. For calculations, refer to formulation 2 of this chapter.

Ephedrine and Ethylmorphine hydrochloride

METHOD 1

Dilute part of the acid extract (A) as obtained above to 100 ml with 0.1 N sulphuric acid and measure the extinction (E_1) at 256 nm and (E_2) at 284 nm and calculate the results as under :

$$\%\ w/v\text{ of Ephedrine hydrochloride} = \frac{E_1 - 0.25}{8.4}$$

0.25 is E 1%, 1 cm of Ethylmorphine hydrochloride at 256 nm.
8.4 is E 1%, 1 cm of Ephedrine hydrochloride at 256 nm.

$$\%\ w/v\text{ of Ethylmorphine} = \frac{E_2 - 0.03}{42.5}$$

0.03 is E 1%, 1 cm of Ephedrine hydrochloride at 284 nm.
42.5 is E 1%, 1 cm of Ethylmorphine hydrochloride at 284 nm.
As may be seen, ephedrine has negligible absorption at 284 nm, hence ethyl morphine can be directly estimated at 284 nm.

METHOD 2

Ephedrine hydrochloride

As ephedrine (base) is volatile, follow the distillation method as described in formulation 13 of the chapter on bronchospasm relaxants. Alternatively, follow the general ammoniacal copper sulphate method.

Ethylmorphine hydrochloride

Follow the method described in formulation 29 of the chapter on analgesics and antipyretics.

Formulation 19

Pseudoephedrine hydrochloride, Diphenhydramine hydrochloride, Ammonium chloride, Menthol, Sodium citrate

ESTIMATION

Pseudoephedrine hydrochloride

METHOD 1

Reagents

1. Benzene-carbon disulphide (3 : 1) mixture.
2. 5% w/v solution of copper sulphate in water.

Standard solution

100 mcg/ml of pseudoephedrine hydrochloride in water.

Sample solution

Take appropriate quantity of the sample equivalent to 25 mg of pseudoephedrine hydrochloride and dilute to 250 ml with water to get 100 mcg/ml.

Procedure

Pipet out 2 ml each of standard, sample and water into respective tubes. Into each tube, add 2 ml strong ammonia solution, 2 ml copper sulphate solution and shake it gently. Then, to each tube, add 10 ml of mixture of benzene-carbon disulphide, stopper the tubes and shake it for one minute. Collect the organic phase, filter through filter paper and measure the absorption immediately against reagent blank at 440 nm and calculate the results.

Explanatory Note

The compound in basic conditions i.e. in the presence of ammonia rearranges itself so that the —OH group and secondary amine group are on the same side. Then the re-arranged molecule undergoes chelation with copper sulphate. This reaction is called 'Chen-Kao' reaction.

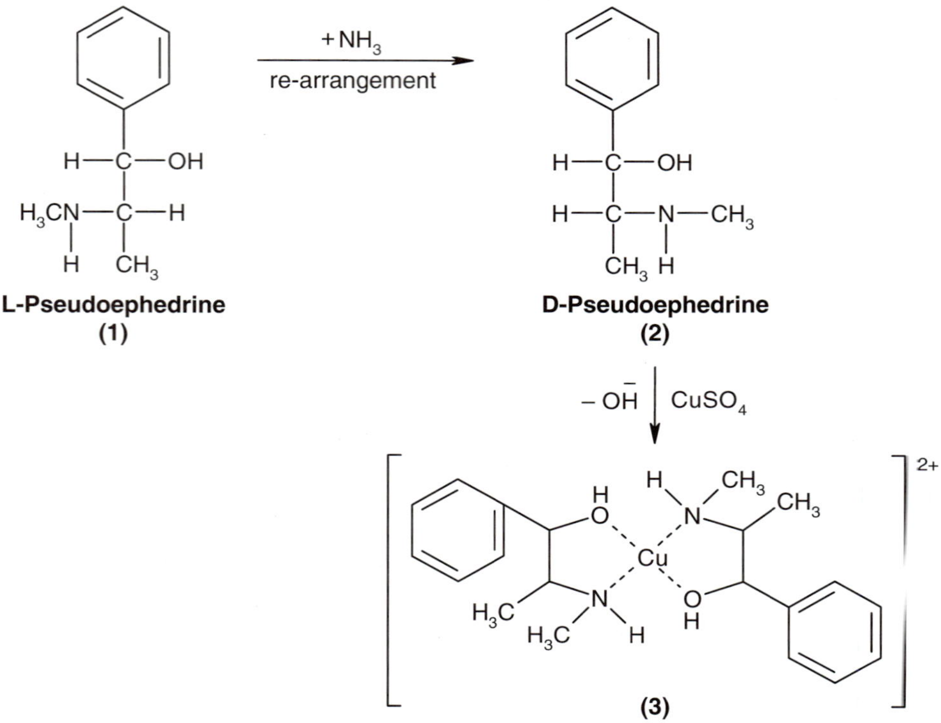

L-Pseudoephedrine (1)

D-Pseudoephedrine (2)

(3)

(λ_{max} 440 nm)

The copper complex is extracted into benzene-carbon disulphide mixture for spectrophotometric measurement (λ_{max} 440 nm).

Reference

Pharmaceutical Chemistry (Vol. 2), H.J. Roth, pp. 373, 374.

With alkaline sodium nitroprusside the compound is oxidized to benzaldehyde, CH_3CHO and methylamine.

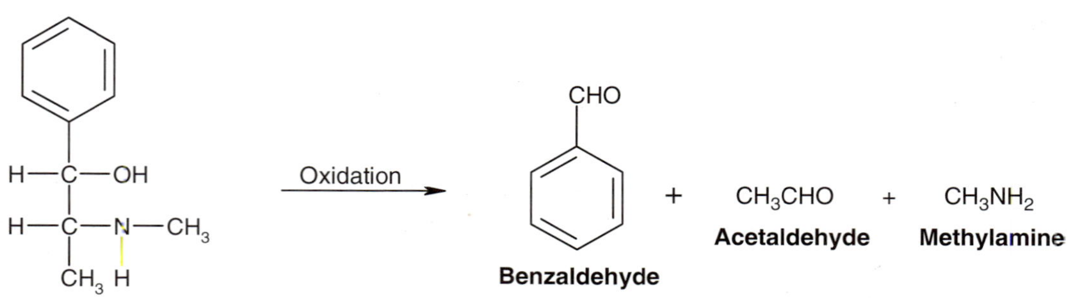

Benzaldehyde has λ_{max} 242 nm, which can be used for quantitative estimation as under ephedrine.

METHOD 2

Follow the method described under formulation of the chapter on bronchospasm relaxants.

Diphenhydramine hydrochloride

Follow the cobalt thiocyanate method as described in formulation 9 of this chapter. Alternatively, follow ammonium reineckate precipitation method as described in formulation of this chapter.

Sodium citrate

Follow any one of the four methods described in formulation 7 of this chapter.

Menthol

Follow the method as described in formulation 7 of this chapter involving reaction with p-dimethylaminobenzaldehydes.

Ammonium chloride

Follow any one of the three methods described in formulation 9 of this chapter.

Formulation 20

Dextromethorphan hydrobromide, Guaiphenesin, Phenylpropanolamine hydrochloride

ESTIMATION

Dextromethorphan hydrobromide

Follow the method described in formulations 13, 14 and 15 of this chapter.

Guaiphenesin

Standard solution

30 mcg/ml of guaiphenesin in chloroform.

Sample solution

To accurately weighed/measured aliquot of the sample equivalent to 75 mg of the compound, add 10 ml of saturated solution of sodium bicarbonate and extract with four 25 ml portions of chloroform. Wash the combined chloroform layer with 15 ml of 1 N hydrochloric acid. Combine the aqueous acidic layer and preserve for assay of phenylpropanolamine. Dilute the chloroform layer to 100 ml and carry out further dilution appropriately to get a solution of 30 mcg/ml.

Concomitantly measure the extinction of both the solutions at maxima at 276 nm with chloroform as blank.

Phenylpropanolamine hydrochloride

Reagents

1. Saturated solution of sodium bicarbonate in water.
2. 2.5% w/v solution of sodium carbonate in water.
3. 0.2% w/v solution of sodium metaperiodate in water.
4. Methylene chloride.
5. 1 N hydrochloric acid.

Standard solution

0.2 mg/ml of the compound in water. To 10 ml of above solution, add 10 ml of saturated solution of sodium bicarbonate and 45 ml of 1 N hydrochloric acid and dilute to 200 ml with water (10 mcg/ml).

Sample solution

Dilute the aqueous layer reserved during estimation of guaiphenesin to 200 ml with water.

Procedure

To 10 ml each of sample and standard solutions, add 10 ml of sodium carbonate solution and 10 ml of sodium metaperiodate solution. Allow to stand for 15 min, and extract with three 30 ml portions of methylene chloride. Dilute organic layer to 100 ml with the same solvent and measure the extinction at 242 nm using solvent as blank.

Probable Reaction Mechanism

The compound belongs to phenylalkylamine group similar to ephedrine.

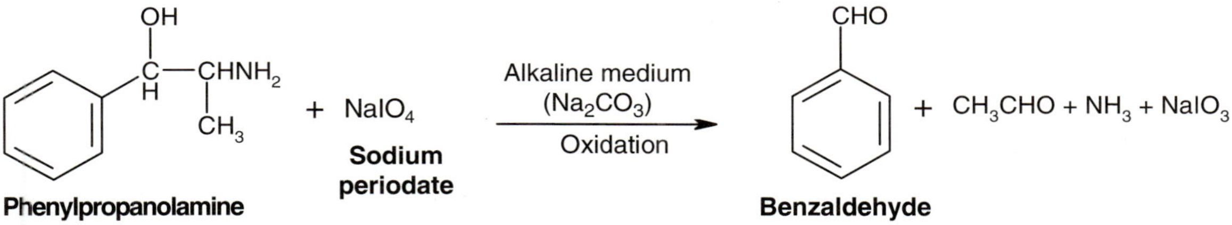

Note

For detailed reaction, see formulation 61 under analgesics.

Benzaldehyde is responsible for λ_{max} of 242 nm and can be extracted into dichloromethane for spectrophotometric measurement.

Because of the presence of amino group the compound undergoes condensation with 1,2-naphthoquinone-4-sulphonate sodium in alkaline medium giving a coloured product with the elimination of hydrogen sulphite (HSO_3^-).

Probable Reaction Mechanism

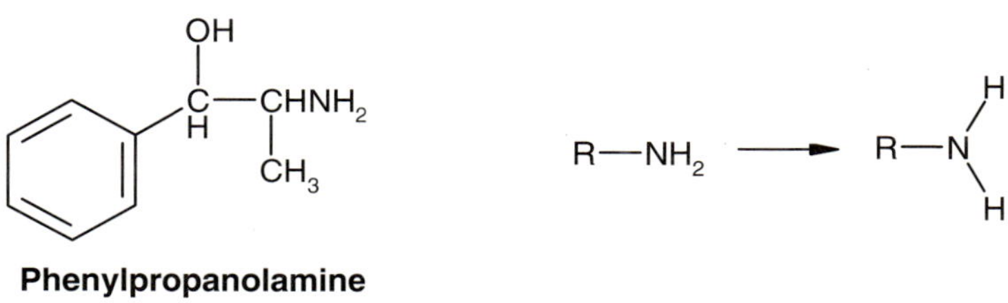

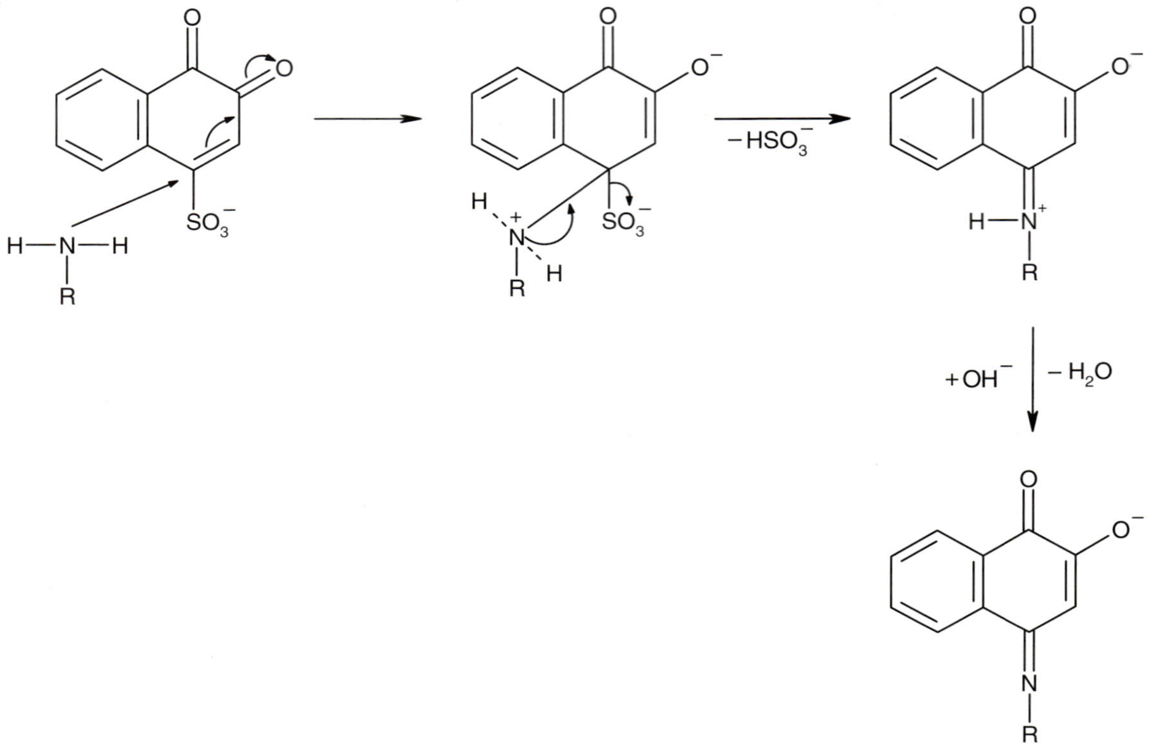

Orange-coloured quinonimine derivative

Reference

Pharmaceutical Chemistry (Vol. 2), H.J. Roth, p. 378.

Similar to ephedrine, the compound can form Cu(2) chelate in alkaline medium i.e. it answers Chen-Kao reaction. This can form the basis for analysis.

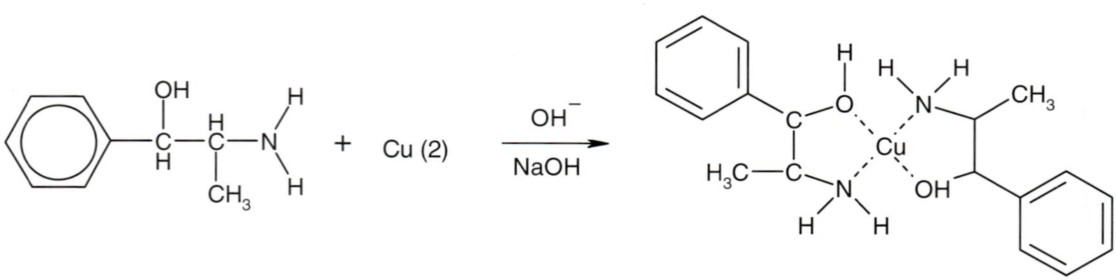

Coloured Cu(II) complex

The compound also forms coloured complex with picrolonic acid similar to ephedrine.

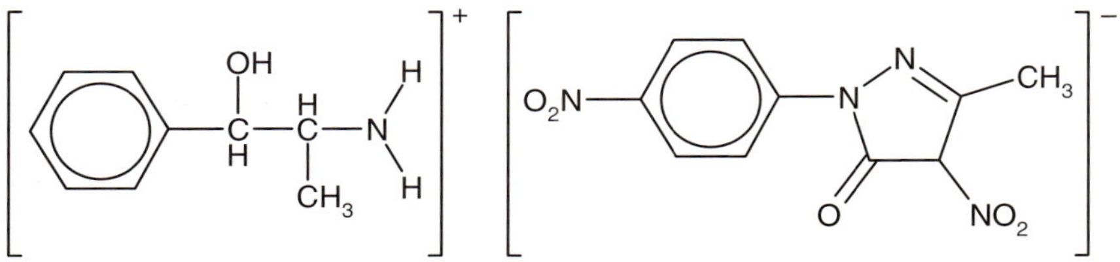

Phenylpropanolamine **Picrolonic acid**

The complex can be extracted into organic solvent for spectrophotometric analysis. The drug is a base whereas picrolonic acid is acidic in character, hence complex formation.

A spectrophotometric method was proposed by Burke et al. (1974) based on reaction with ninhydrin, the mechanism being similar to that for amino acids. This determination is dependent upon the continued presence of hydroxyl and primary amino moieties. It was postulated by the authors that primary amine having hydroxyl group on the same carbon chain reacts with ninhydrin to form Schiff's base diketohydrindylidene-diketohydrindamine or Ruhemann's purple. The maximum reaction occurs at pH 5.0.

The probable reaction mechanism as proposed by the author

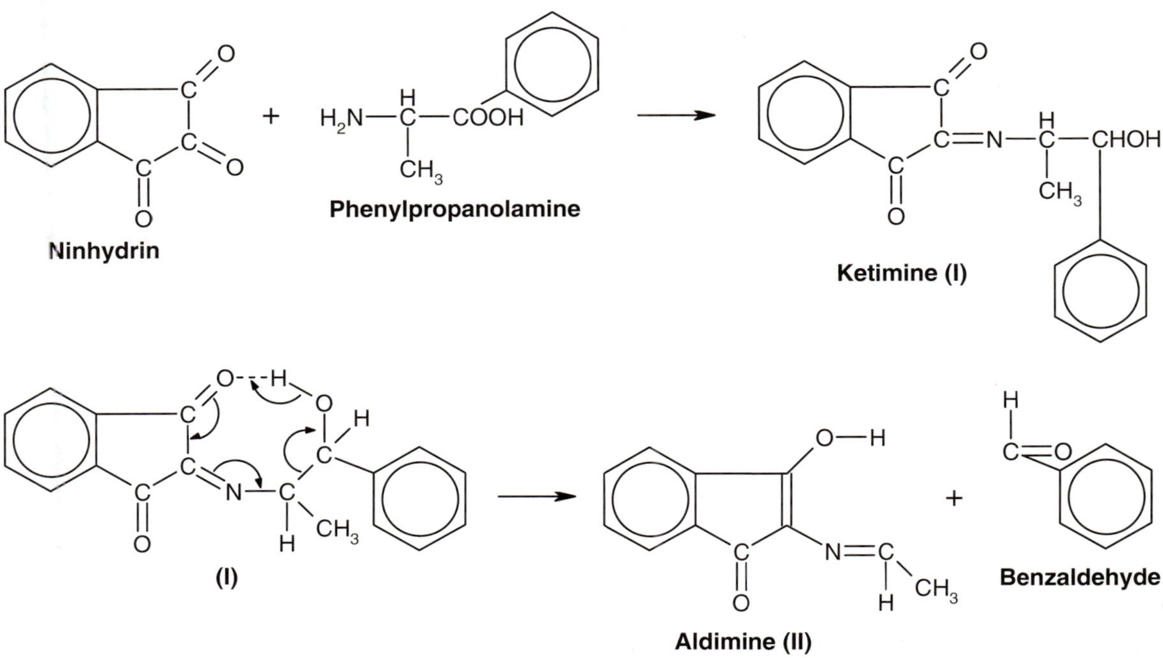

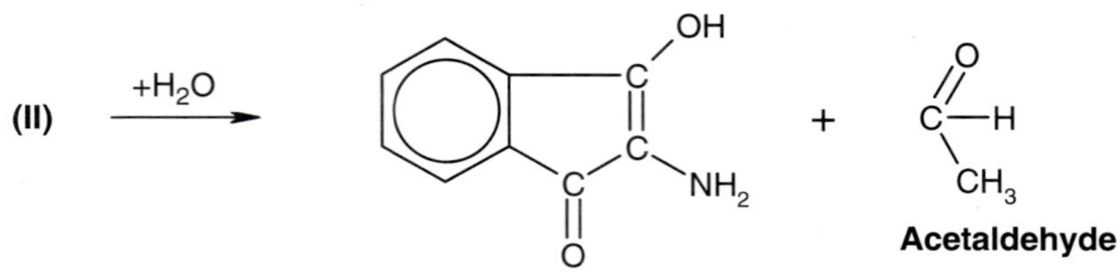

Acetaldehyde

Diketohydrindamine
(2-Amino-3-hydroxy-1,3-diketoindane)
(III)

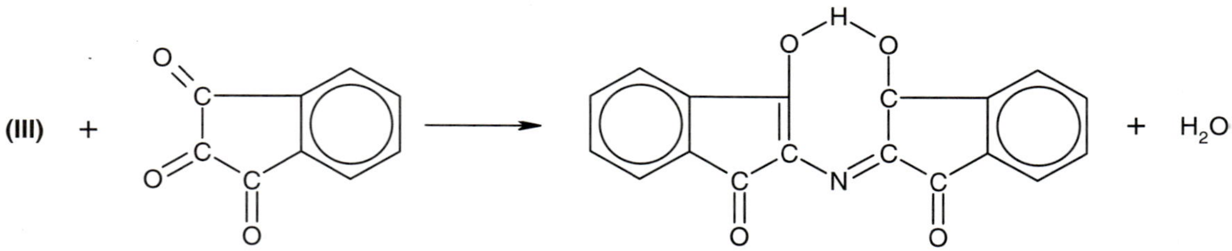

Ninhydrin

Ruhemann's purple (Schiff's base)
(λ_{max} 570 nm)

Reference

D. Burke, U.S. Venturella & B.S. Senkowski, *J. Pharm. Sci.*, **63(2)**, 69-273, 1974.

The authors did propose an alternative mechanism for amino alcohol i.e. the compound is first converted to imino derivative followed by formation of ammonia. The liberated ammonia reacts with ninhydrin to form III as explained above; further reaction step is as above to form Ruhemann's purple.

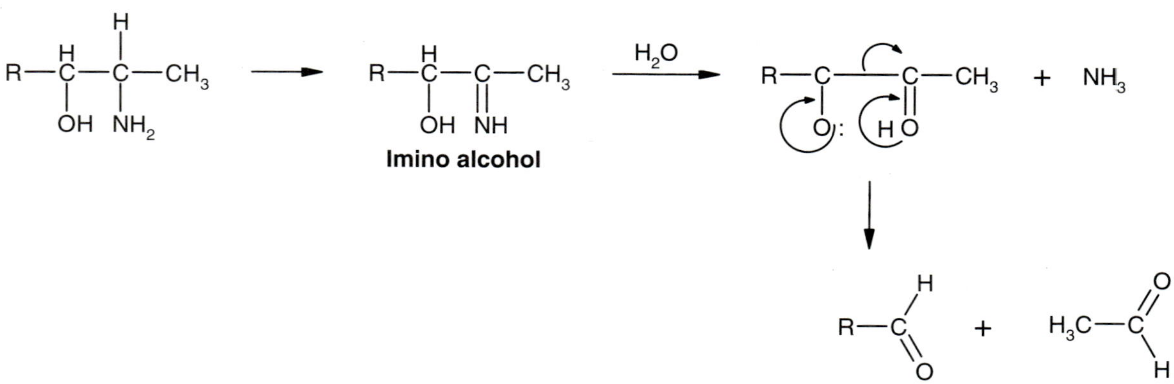

Imino alcohol

NH_3 + III ⟶ IV

Ruhemann's purple
(λ_{max} 570 nm)

Formulation 21

Diethylcarbamazine citrate, Glyceryl guaiacolate (Guaiphenesin), Chlorpheniramine maleate

ESTIMATION

Diethylcarbamazine citrate

Take sample accurately measured/weighed equivalent to 50 mg of the compound and carry out non-aqueous titration using thymol blue as indicator. Each ml of 0.1 N perchloric acid is equivalent to 0.03914 g of diethylcarbamazine citrate.

Note

The reaction based on citrate moiety of the molecule can be used for quantitative estimation of the compound. For details, refer to method 2 for estimation of sodium citrate described under formulation 6 of this chapter.

Guaiphenesin

Dissolve or dilute the sample with water to get a concentration of 15 mcg/ml. Measure the extinction at maxima at about 275 nm and calculate the result by comparing with the standard (15 mcg/ml).

A spectrophotometric method has been reported by Devani et al. (1994) based on oxidation with sodium periodate to liberate formaldehyde which reacts in situ with acetylacetone in the presence of ammonium acetate to give coloured product (λ_{max} 412 nm).

Probable Reaction Mechanism

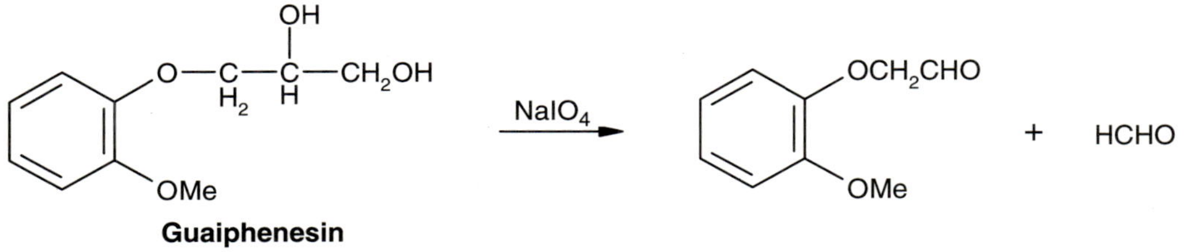

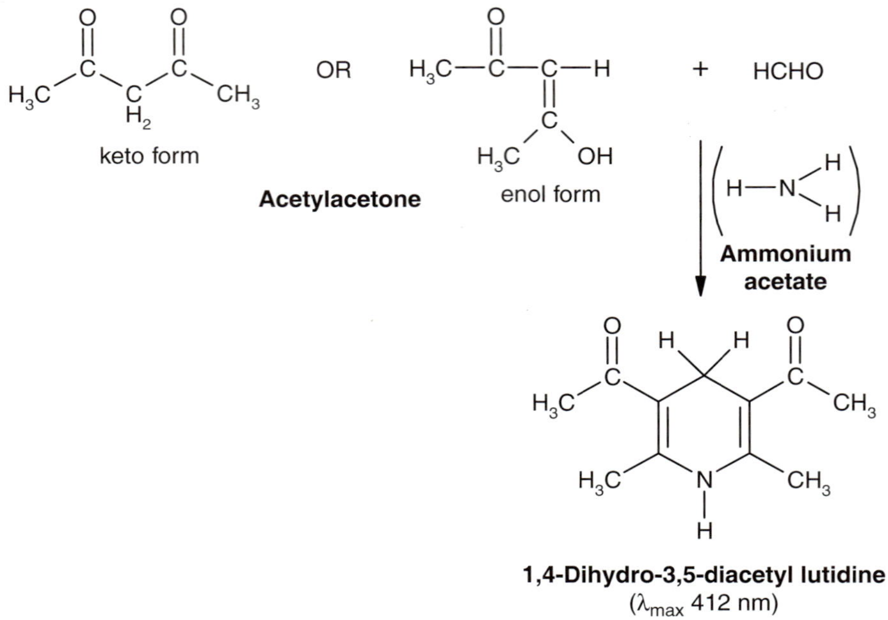

Reference

M.H. Devani, C.J. Shishoo, B.N. Suhagia & S.A. Shah, *Ind. J. Pharm. Sci.*, **56(2)**, 41-44, 1994.

The compound couples with diazotized dinitroaniline to give coloured product which can form the basis of quantitative analysis.

Probable Reaction Mechanism

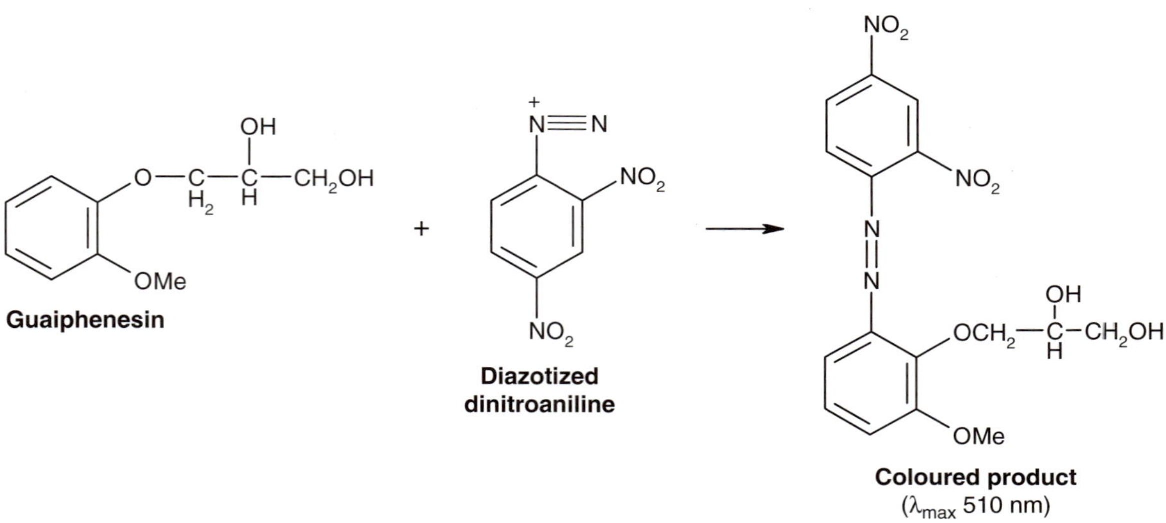

Reference

Vandana et al., *Indian Drugs*, **27(11)**, 581-582, 1994.

Chlorpheniramine maleate

Carry out the cyanogen bromide method as described in formulation 3 of this chapter.

Formulation 22

Mepyramine maleate, Pheniramine maleate, Phenylpropanolamine hydrochloride

ESTIMATION

Mepyramine maleate / Pyrilamine maleate

Standard solution

25 mcg/ml of mepyramine maleate in 0.1 N hydrochloric acid.

Sample solution

Measure appropriate portion of the sample equivalent to 5 mg of the compound. Make it alkaline with ammonia and extract with four 30 ml portions of solvent ether. Wash the combined ether layer with 20 ml of water and reject the aqueous layer. Extract the base back into acid from ether layer using four 25 ml portions of 0.1 N hydrochloric acid. Remove the traces of ether from acid layer by slight warming and make the volume to 250 ml.

Measure the extinction of both the sample and standard solutions at maximum at about 316 nm and calculate the results by comparison.

Pheniramine maleate

Follow the cyanogen bromide method as described in formulation 3 of this chapter under chlorpheniramine maleate. Use a solution of 25 mcg/ml and measure the chromogen at 480 nm. Both mepyramine and pheniramine have pyridine moiety, can be estimated by cyanogen bromide method. For details of reaction mechanism see under chapter on rubefacients.

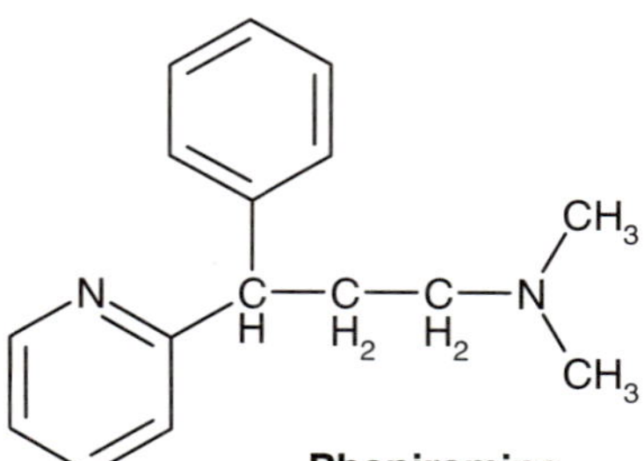

Pheniramine

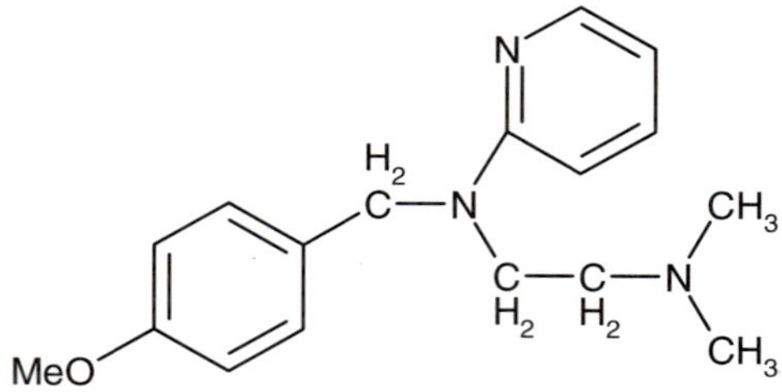

Mepyramine / Pyrilamine

Probable Reaction Mechanism

Both the drugs are pyridine derivative and have hydrogen adjacent to heterocyclic nitrogen, so answer 'König reaction'. As a result of action of Br—CN (cyanogen bromide) glutaconic acid derivative is produced which is stabilized by coupling with arylamine to yield polymethine dye.

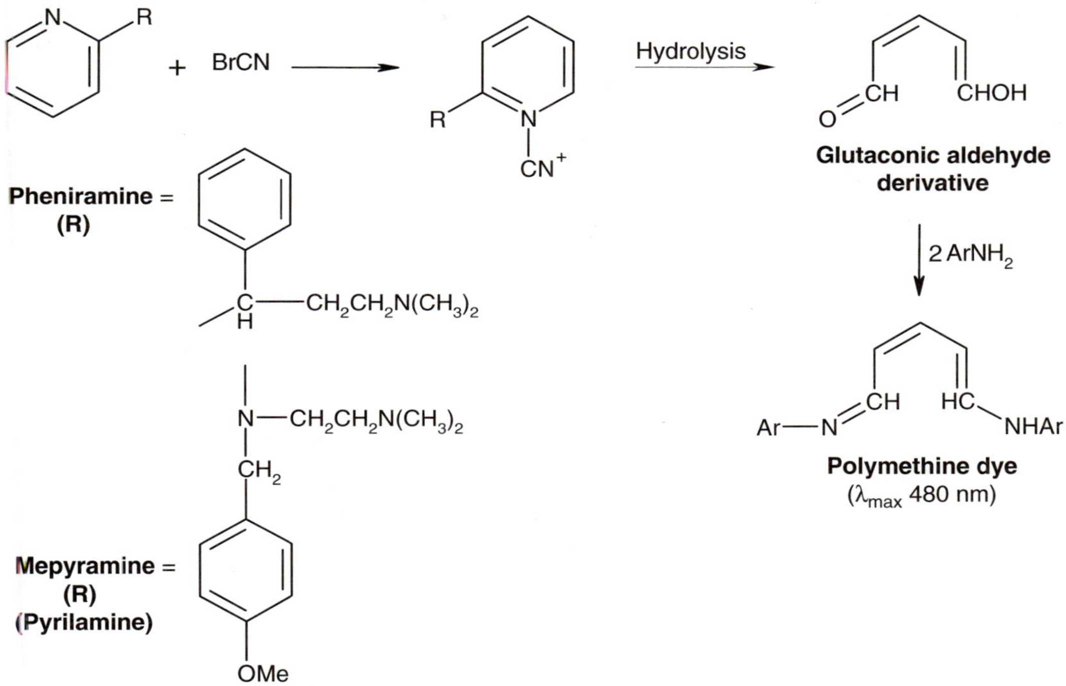

Note

Other coupling agents such as o-toluidine and anthranilic acid can also be used.

Mepyramine is reported to form ion-pair complex with several dyes in different pH buffers. All the yellow-coloured complexes have λ_{max} 420 nm. All the complexes are extractable into chloroform.

Dye	Buffer
Methyl orange (MO)	4.5
Bromocresol green (BCG)	3.5
Bromophenol blue (BPB)	2.5
Bromothymol blue	2.8
Bromocresol purple	6.0

Phenylpropanolamine hydrochloride

Measure appropriate portion of the sample equivalent to 60 mg of the compound. Make it alkaline with dilute ammonia and extract with four 25 ml portion of chloroform. Wash the combined chloroform extract with water and pass the organic layer through anhydrous sodium sulphate. Evaporate chloroform layer, dissolve the residue in glacial acetic acid and carry out the non-aqueous titration. From the total volume of perchloric acid consumed in the above titration, subtract the volume of the acid equivalent to the estimated contents of mepyramine maleate and pheniramine maleate and calculate the contents of phenylpropanolamine hydrochloride from the remaining volume using a factor of 0.003754 g for each ml of 0.02 N perchloric acid.

Formulation 23

Diphenhydramine hydrochloride, Ephedrine hydrochloride, Noscapine, Ammonium chloride, Sodium citrate

ESTIMATION

Diphenhydramine hydrochloride

Follow the cobalt thiocyanate method as described under formulation 6 of this chapter.

Ephedrine hydrochloride

Follow the ammoniacal copper sulphate method as described under formulation 1 of the chapter on bronchospasm relaxants.

Ammonium chloride

Follow the ammonia distillation, followed by acid-base titration as described under formulation 6 of this chapter.

Sodium citrate

Follow the method 4 involving colour with ferric chloride as described under formulation 7 of this chapter.

Noscapine

Measure 10 ml of the sample, basify with ammonia solution and extract with chloroform. Evaporate chloroform layer which contains all the three bases i.e. ephedrine, diphenhydramine and noscapine. Carry out non-aqueous titration with perchloric acid using crystal violet as indicator. This gives the total volume of perchloric acid required for three bases. Subtract the volume of perchloric acid equivalent to the amount of ephedrine and diphenhydramine as determined by the method described above. The remaining volume of perchloric acid is equivalent to the amount of noscapine present in 10 ml of the sample. This is best exemplified by working example given below.

Typical laboratory analysis

Each 10 ml of the sample is labelled to contain 21 mg of diphenhydramine hydrochloride, 11 mg of ephedrine hydrochloride and 20 mg of noscapine.

1. Total volume of 0.01102 N perchloric acid consumed by three bases in non-aqueous titration = 15.8 ml ...(A)
2. Volume of 0.01102 N perchloric acid equivalent to 21 mg of diphenhydramine hydrochloride = $(0.021 \times 0.01) \div (0.01102 \times 0.002918) = 6.5$ ml ...(a)
   (each ml of 0.01 N perchloric acid is equivalent to 0.002918 g of diphenhydramine hydrochloride)
3. Volume of 0.01102 N perchloric acid equivalent to 11 mg of ephedrine hydrochloride = $(0.011 \times 0.01) \div (0.01102 \times 0.002017) = 4.9$ ml ...(b)
   (each ml of 0.01 N perchloric acid is equivalent to 0.002017 g of ephedrine hydrochloride)
4. Volume of 0.01102 N perchloric acid consumed by noscapine present in 10 ml of the sample = A – (a + b) = 15.8 – (6.5 + 4.9) = 4.4 ml
   (each ml of 0.01 N perchloric acid is equivalent to 0.004134 g of noscapine)
   Total amount (mg) of Noscapine/10 ml = $(4.4 \times 0.01102 \times 0.004134 \times 1000) \div 0.01 = 20.04$ mg

   Claim = 20 mg

Formulation 24

Dextromethorphan hydrobromide, Pseudoephedrine hydrochloride, Azatadine maleate

ESTIMATION

Dextromethorphan hydrobromide

Follow the method described in formulation 15 or 16 of this chapter.

Pseudoephedrine hydrochloride

Follow the method described in formulation 19 of this chapter.

Azatadine maleate

Follow the method described in formulation 27 of the chapter on analgesics and antipyretics.

Formulation 25

Dextromethorphan hydrobromide, Bromhexine hydrochloride, Ammonium chloride, Menthol

ESTIMATION

Dextromethorphan hydrobromide

Follow the method described in formulation 15 or 16 of this chapter.

Menthol

Follow the method described in formulation 6 of this chapter. Use distillate for the colour development.

Bromhexine hydrochloride

Follow the method described in formulation 26 of this chapter.

Ammonium chloride

Follow the method described in formulation 7 of this chapter.

Formulation 26

Salbutamol sulphate, Bromhexine hydrochloride, Guaiphenesin

ESTIMATION

Salbutamol sulphate

METHOD 1

Follow the method 1 described in formulation 14 of the chapter on broncho-spasm relaxants.

METHOD 2

Reagents

1. 8% w/v solution of potassium ferricyanide in water.
2. 0.1% w/v solution of N,N-dimethyl-p-phenylene-diammonium sulphate.
3. 5% w/v solution of sodium carbonate in water.

Standard solution

40 mcg/ml of salbutamol as salbutamol sulphate in water.

Sample solution

Dilute sample equivalent to 2 mg of salbutamol to 50 ml with water.

Procedure

To 5 ml each of sample and standard solutions, add 50 ml of water, 5 ml of sodium bicarbonate solution and 4 ml of N,N-dimethyl reagent, shake to mix, add 4 ml of potassium ferricyanide solution. Allow to stand for 15 minutes and then extract with 10, 5, 5 ml portions of chloroform. Pass chloroform layer through a layer of anhydrous sodium sulphate and make up to 25 ml with chloroform. Measure the extinction of each solution at about 620 nm using chloroform as blank. Calculate the results by comparing with standard.

Explanatory Note

This is oxidative breakdown of side chain (ethanolamine) to aldehyde by alkaline $K_3Fe(CN)_6$ and then coupling with the reagent to give complex (λ_{max} 620 nm).

Probable Reaction Mechanism

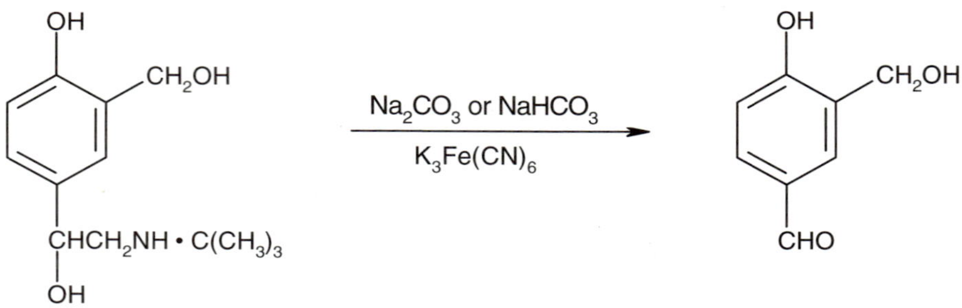

Salbutamol

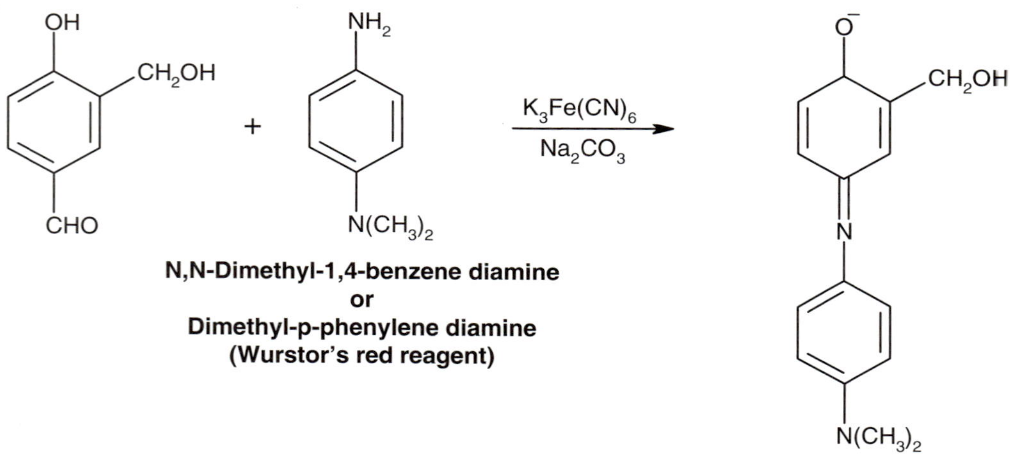

N,N-Dimethyl-1,4-benzene diamine
or
Dimethyl-p-phenylene diamine
(Wurstor's red reagent)

(λ_{max} 620 nm)

According to this reaction mechanism p-N,N-dimethyl phenylene diamine is oxidized by alkaline $K_3Fe(CN)_6$ to highly reactive and less stable p-benzoquinone diamine derivative which will react with salbutamol at para or ortho position. If para position is occupied then reaction will occur at ortho position to phenol-OH group. This is because phenolic-OH is para and ortho directing i.e. both ortho and para positions are richer in electrons and hence attack of the electron-deficient reagent occurs at these positions.

Probable Reaction Mechanism

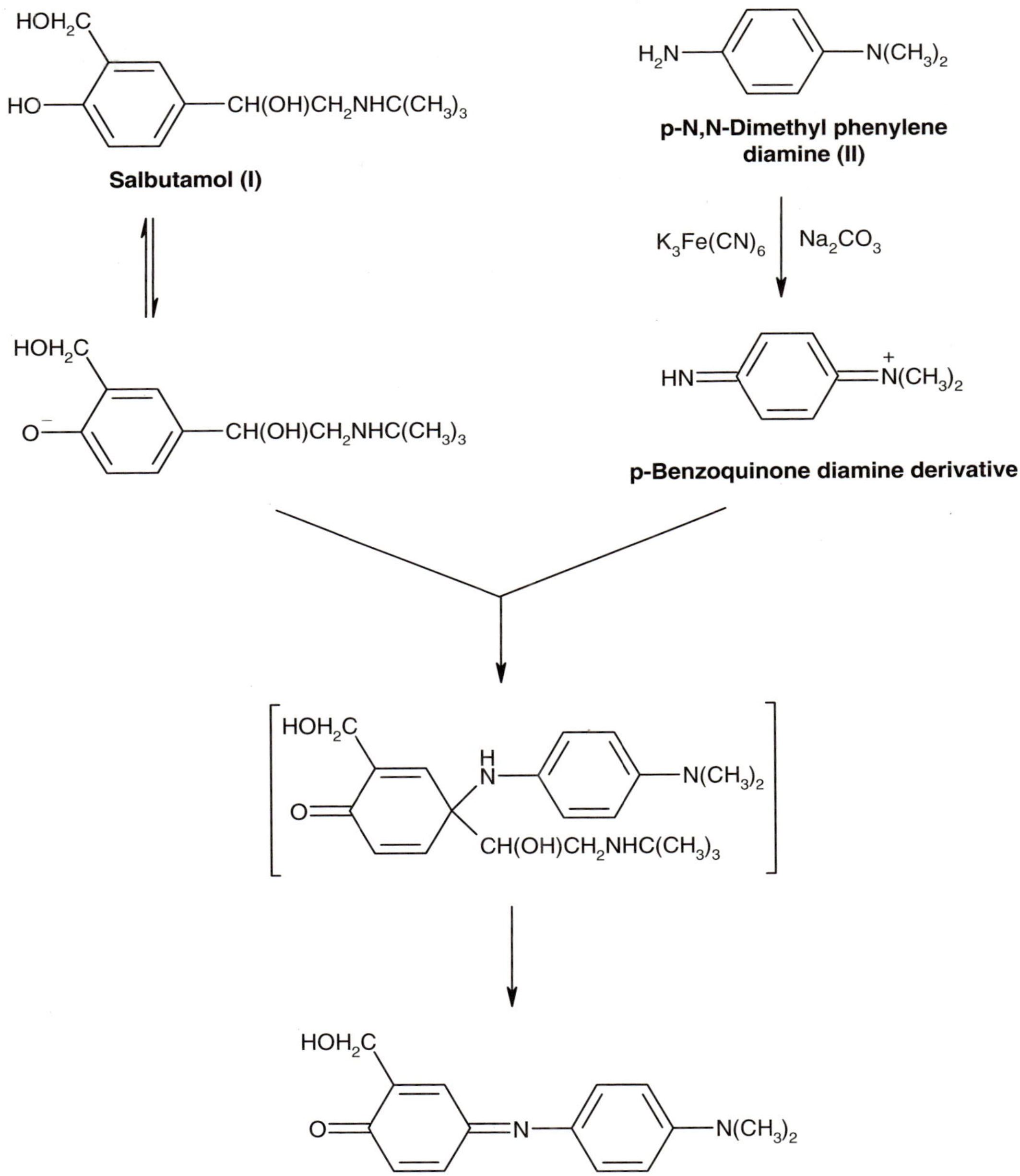

III

(λ_{max} 620 nm)

METHOD 3

Reagents

1. 0.1 M and 2 M sodium hydroxide.
2. 0.01 M sodium periodate.
3. Acetylacetone reagent.
4. 4 M hydrochloric acid.

Sample and standard solutions

200 μg/ml in water.

Procedure

To 2 ml each of sample and standard solutions add 1 ml of 0.1 M NaOH, 2 ml of 0.01 M periodate. Allow the reaction mixture to stand at room temperature for 10 min. Then to each add 5 ml of acetylacetone reagent, mix, keep in boiling water-bath for 10 min, cool, dilute and measure the absorbance at 412 nm against reagent blank.

Probable Reaction Mechanism

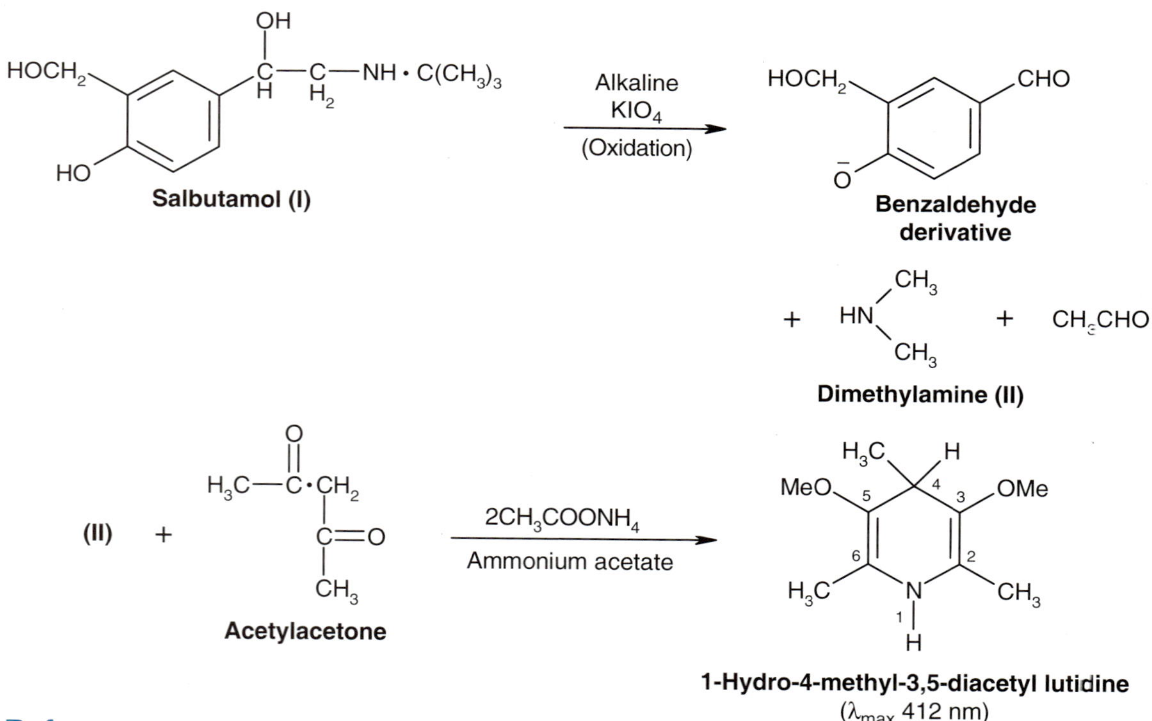

Reference

K.K. Bhatt, S.A. Shah & S.S. Pandya, Indian Drugs, **36(8)**, 524-528, 1999.

Bromhexine hydrochloride

Reagents

1. Dilute ammonia solution : Dilute 210 ml of ammonia solution to 500 ml with distilled water.
2. 0.1 N methanolic hydrochloric acid : To 20 ml of water, add 5 ml of hydrochloric acid and dilute to 500 ml with methanol.

Standard solution

Weigh accurately 4 mg of material, suspend in 5 ml of water, basify with ammonia and extract with 4×25 ml of dichloromethane, pass combined layer through light cotton plug, washing the cotton plug with 5 ml of methanol. Evaporate organic layer and take up the residue in 0.1 N methanolic hydrochloric acid to get 40 μg/ml.

Sample solution

Measure sample equivalent to 4 mg of the substance, add 25 ml of water, basify and proceed as under standard solution.

Measure the extinction of the standard and sample solutions at 317 nm using 0.1 N methanolic hydrochloric acid as blank. Calculate the results by comparison.

Alternatively, to 2 ml of standard and sample solutions prepared above, add 8 ml of p-dimethylaminobenzaldehyde solutions (10% w/v in methanol) and 5 ml of hydrochloric acid. Mix and allow to stand for 10 minutes and make up the volume to 25 ml with water. Measure the absorption at 425 nm against reagent blank and calculate the results by comparison with standard.

Guaiphenesin

Standard solution

Weigh accurately 100 mg of guaiphenesin, transfer to a separating funnel. Add 20 ml of water and 5 ml of sodium hydroxide solution (20% w/v). Extract with four 40 ml portions of petroleum ether (60-80°C). Discard ether layer, collect the aqueous layer and extract four 20 ml portions of chloroform. Pass combined chloroform layer through anhydrous sodium sulphate and make up to 100 ml with chloroform. Evaporate 5 ml of the above solution, take up the residue in methanol to produce 100 ml (50 mcg/ml).

Sample solution

Measure accurately sample equivalent to 100 mg of the substance, add 20 ml of water and continue the procedure as described under preparation of standard solution. Alternatively further dilute chloroform solution appropriately (50 mcg/ml) with chloroform and concomitantly determine the absorption of sample and standard solutions at 276 nm.

Measure the extinction of the standard and sample solutions at 275 nm using methanol as blank. Calculate the results by comparison.

Formulation 27

Bromhexine hydrochloride, Pseudoephedrine hydrochloride, Chlorpheniramine maleate

ESTIMATION

Bromhexine hydrochloride

METHOD 1

Reagents

1. Dilute ammonia solution : Dilute 15 ml of strong ammonia solution to 100 ml with water.
2. 0.1 N methanolic hydrochloric acid : Dilute 8 ml of hydrochloric acid to 1000 ml with methanol.

Standard solution

Prepare 30 mcg/ml solution of bromhexine hydrochloride in 0.1 N methanolic hydrochloric acid.

Sample solution

Take the sample equivalent to 8 mg of bromhexine hydrochloride in a 250 ml separating funnel, add 10 ml of water and 15 ml of dilute ammonia solution. Extract with four 20 ml portions of chloroform. Evaporate the chloroform layer, dissolve the residue in 0.1 N methanolic hydrochloric acid and make up the volume to 50 ml. Dilute 10 ml to 50 ml with the same solvent (32 mcg/ml).

Procedure

Measure the absorbance of both standard and sample solutions at the maximum at about 317 nm using 0.1 N methanolic hydrochloric acid as the blank and deduce the results by comparison.

METHOD 2

Follow the method described in formulation 29 of this chapter involving diazotization and coupling with n-naphthyl-ethylenediamine dihydrochloride (NED).

Pseudoephedrine hydrochloride

METHOD 1

Reagents

1. Saturated sodium carbonate solution.
2. 2% w/v solution of sodium metaperiodate in water.
3. n-Hexane or petroleum ether (40-60°C).

Standard solution

Prepare 30 mcg/ml solution of pseudoephedrine hydrochloride in water.

Sample solution

Weigh the sample accurately equivalent to 60 mg of pseudoephedrine hydrochloride and dilute to 100 ml with water. Further dilutions are made with water appropriately and step-wise to get a solution of 30 mcg/ml.

Procedure

To 5 ml each of standard and sample solutions add 4 ml of sodium carbonate solution and 2 ml of sodium metaperiodate solution. Mix, allow to stand for 10 minutes, add 20 ml of n-hexane or petroleum ether and shake for 30 seconds. Measure the absorbance of both standard and sample solutions (organic layer) at the maximum at about 242 nm. Deduce the results by comparison.

Explanatory Note

The compound undergoes alkaline oxidation with potassium periodate giving benzaldehyde, acetaldehyde and methylamine. Benzaldehyde is responsible for UV absorption at 242 nm and forms the basis for quantitative analysis. For reaction mechanism, see under ephedrine.

METHOD 2

Reagents

1. Phosphate buffer, pH 7.5: Mix 45 ml of 0.2 N sodium hydroxide and 50 ml of 0.2 N potassium dihydrogen phosphate, dilute to 200 ml with water.
2. Bromothymol blue solution: 1 mg/ml solution of dye in phosphate buffer, pH 7.5.

Standard solution

500 mcg/ml of pseudoephedrine hydrochloride in water.

Sample solution

Extract accurately weighed quantity of the powdered sample with water to produce concentration of 500 mcg/ml.

Procedure

To 10 ml each of sample and standard solutions, add 10 ml of phosphate buffer, 25 ml of bromothymol blue solution. Make it alkaline (litmus) with sodium hydroxide (20%). Extract with benzene (3 × 30 ml), pass combined benzene extract through anhydrous sodium sulphate and extract with 50% sodium hydroxide solution (4 × 25 ml). Combine the alkaline layer and dilute to 200 ml. Further, dilute 5 ml to 50 ml with 5% sodium hydroxide solution and measure the absorption of both sample and standard solutions at about 620 nm with 5% solution of sodium hydroxide as blank. Calculate the results by comparison. The method is based on ion-pair complex formation between the base and acidic dye.

Chlorpheniramine maleate

Reagents

1. 1% w/v solution of sodium dithionate in water.
2. 4% v/v solution of aniline (distilled) in methanol.
3. 10% w/v solution to potassium cyanide in water.
4. 10% w/v solution of cyanogen bromide in water.

Standard solution

Prepare 20 mcg/ml solution of chlorpheniramine maleate in water.

Sample solution

Dilute the sample appropriately with water to get 20 mcg/ml in water.

Procedure

To 10 ml each of standard and sample solutions, add one or two drops of dithionate solution, 5 ml of aniline and 2 ml of cyanogen bromide solution. Shake and allow to develop the golden-yellow colour. Measure the absorbance of standard and sample solutions at the maximum at about 430 nm using a blank prepared in the same manner omitting the substance to be analysed. Deduce the results by comparison.

The method is based on König reaction. Pyridine derivatives like nicotinic acid, nicotinamide with hydrogen in at least one of the positions adjacent to the heterocyclic nitrogen react with cyanogen bromide to produce a derivative of glutaconic aldehyde. Stability of this compound is very poor, but a stable polymethine dye can be obtained by coupling with arylamine. Several coupling reagents have been proposed such as anthranilic acid, sulphonic acid, o-toluidine etc. but aniline has been considered superior to others.

Probable Reaction Mechanism

Cyanogen bromide is used as hydrolysing agent.

$$Br_2 + \overline{C}N \longrightarrow Br{-}C{\equiv}N + Br^-$$

Bromocyanogen

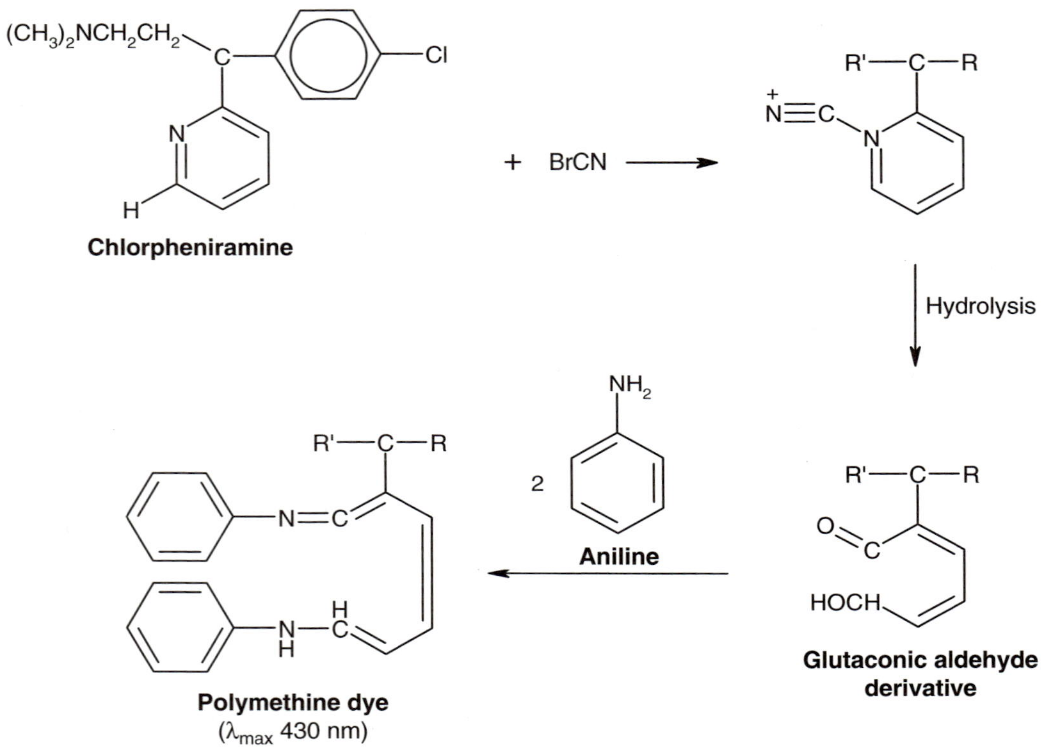

$R = C_6H_4Cl$

$R' = CH_2CH_2N(CH_3)_2$

Reference

W.J. König, *J. Prakt. Chem.*, **19**, 70, 1904.

Alternatively, chlorpheniramine can be estimated by ion-pair complex formation with bromocresol green. The ion-pair complex is extractable into chloroform (λ_{max} 420 nm).

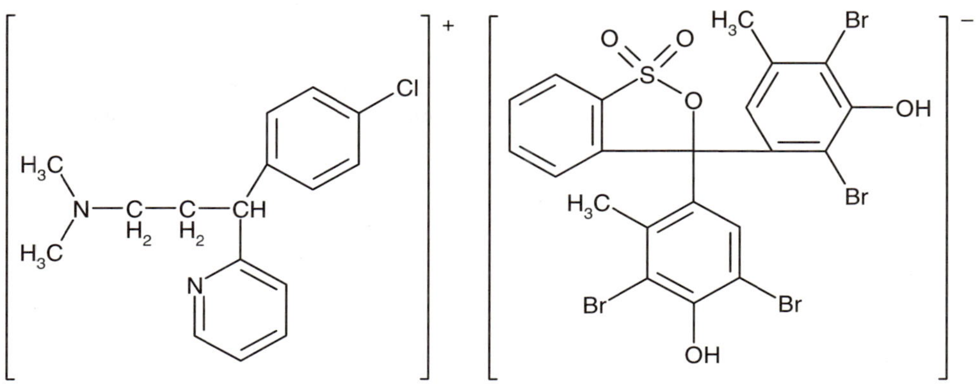

Chlorpheniramine **Bromocresol green**

Drug - dye ion-pair complex
(λ_{max} 420 nm)

Reference

Indian Drugs, **23(10)**, 577, 1986.

This method described below is based on oxidative hydramine cleavage with the help of potassium permanganate in acidic medium to give formaldehyde. Liberated aldehyde reacts with acetylacetone in the presence of ammonium acetate to give a coloured product having absorption maxima at 412 nm.

Reagents

1. 0.1 M sulphuric acid.
2. 0.2 M potassium permanganate.
3. Reacting solution: 30 g of ammonium acetate and 10 ml of acetylacetone were mixed and diluted to 100 ml with water.
4. 1% w/v solution of sodium thiosulphate.

Standard and sample solutions

200 μg/ml in water.

Procedure

To 2 ml each of sample/standard solutions add 1.5 ml of sulphuric acid and 1.25 ml of potassium permanganate solution. Shake and allow to stand for 10 min. Add sufficient sodium thiosulphate solution till the solution is colourless. Then add 5 ml of the reacting solution and keep in water-bath (37°C) for 30 min, dilute to 25 ml with water and measure the absorbance at 412 nm against reagent blank.

Probable Reaction Mechanism

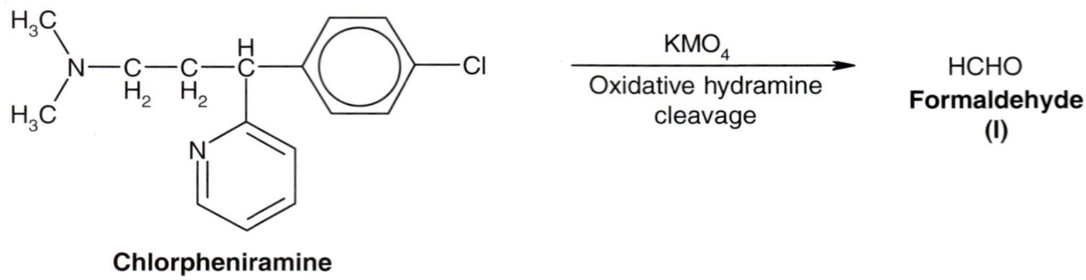

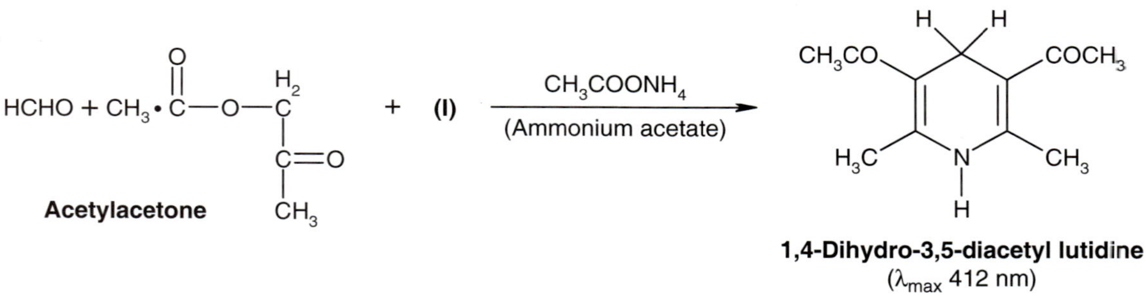

Reference

B.N. Suhagia & S.A. Shah, *Indian Drugs*, **36(1)**, 33-36, 1999.

Formulation 28

Bromhexine hydrochloride, Ambroxol hydrochloride

Bromhexine hydrochloride

Follow the different methods described in formulation 29 of this chapter.

Ambroxol hydrochloride

Reagents

1. Carbon disulphide - pyridine - isopropyl alcohol reagent (CPI): Mix 35 ml of carbon disulphide, 25 ml of pyridine and 65 ml of isopropyl alcohol, all measured accurately.
2. Cupric chloride solution: Dissolve 0.12 g of cupric chloride in 250 ml of water, dilute to 500 ml with pyridine.
3. 10% v/v acetic acid.

Standard solution

1 mg/ml solution of ambroxol hydrochloride in methanol.

Sample solution

Powdered sample equivalent to 50 mg of ambroxol hydrochloride suspended in methanol. Shake, dilute to 50 ml with methanol, filter through Whatman filter paper No. 42 and use the filtrate for estimation.

Procedure

1 ml each of sample and standard solutions taken in separating funnel, add 4 ml of CPI reagent, 2 ml of cupric chloride solution to each, shake to mix, add 3 ml of acetic acid solution and 3 ml of benzene, shake vigorously for 5 min, separate the organic layer (upper), dilute to 10 ml with isopropyl alcohol, allow to stand for 20 min and measure the absorbance of both the solutions at 448 nm.

Probable Reaction Mechanism

The compound forms complex with Cu^{2+} which is stabilized by pyridine.

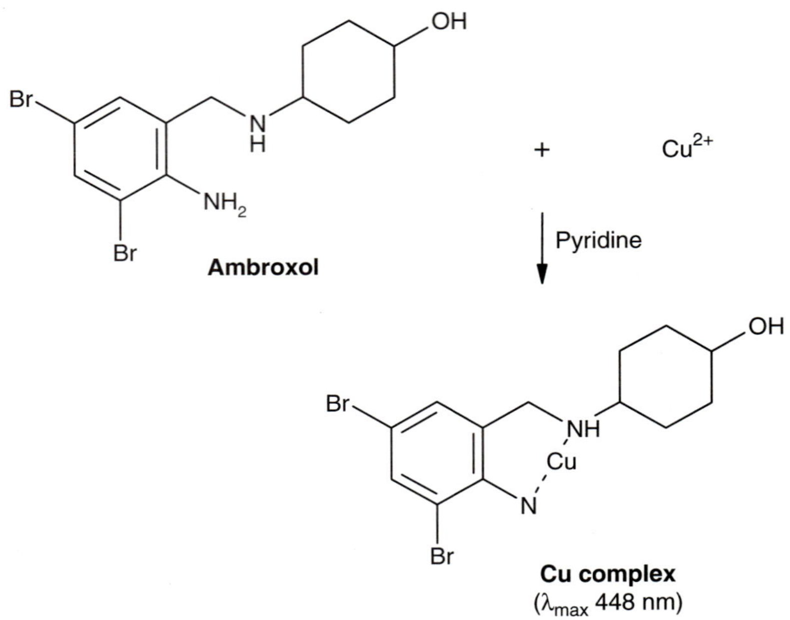

Formulation 29

Amoxycillin, Bromhexine hydrochloride

ESTIMATION

Amoxycillin

METHOD 1

Follow the method described under formulation 8 of the chapter on antibiotics. The method is based on alkaline oxidation of phenolic group and coupling with 4-aminoantipyrine.

METHOD 2

Follow the method described under formulation 8 of the chapter on antibiotics. Each ml of 0.1 N sodium hydroxide is equivalent to 0.03654 g of amoxycillin.

Note

The method official in Indian Pharmacopoeia based on reaction with imidazole mercury reagent can be used in such combinations.

Qureshi et al. described spectrophotometric and volumetric methods for the determination of amoxycillin, ampicillin and cloxacillin based on catalystic hydrolysis followed by oxidation with iodate.

Reagents

1. 0.1 M sodium hydroxide.
2. 1 M hydrochloric acid.
3. 0.1 M potassium iodate.

Standard solution

200 µg/ml in water.

Sample solution

Contents of tablets/capsules suspended in water, shaken for 30 min and diluted to get 200 µg/ml.

General procedure

To 2.5 ml of 0.1 M sodium hydroxide add sample equivalent to any of the penicillins (amoxycillin, ampicillin or cloxacillin), pH about 13.0, shake and keep in water-bath (80°C) for 10-15 min, cool, add 0.5 ml of 1.0 M hydrochloric acid and 5 ml of carbon tetrachloride, shake and titrate with iodate with intermittent shaking till the non-aqueous layer (CCl_4 layer) is deep red in colour i.e. end point. Further, separate organic layer and subject to spectrophotometric measurements (λ_{max} 520 nm). The compounds are first hydrolysed with 0.1 M sodium hydroxide by heating. Excess alkali is neutralized by 1 M hydrochloric acid so that the mixture attains pH 2.0. This provides conducive environment for quantitative titration of degraded penicillins with KIO_3. As a result of oxidation by KIO_3 thiol gets oxidized to sulphonic acid and iodate to ICl and finally to iodine, the visible end point.

General Reaction Mechanism as proposed by the authors

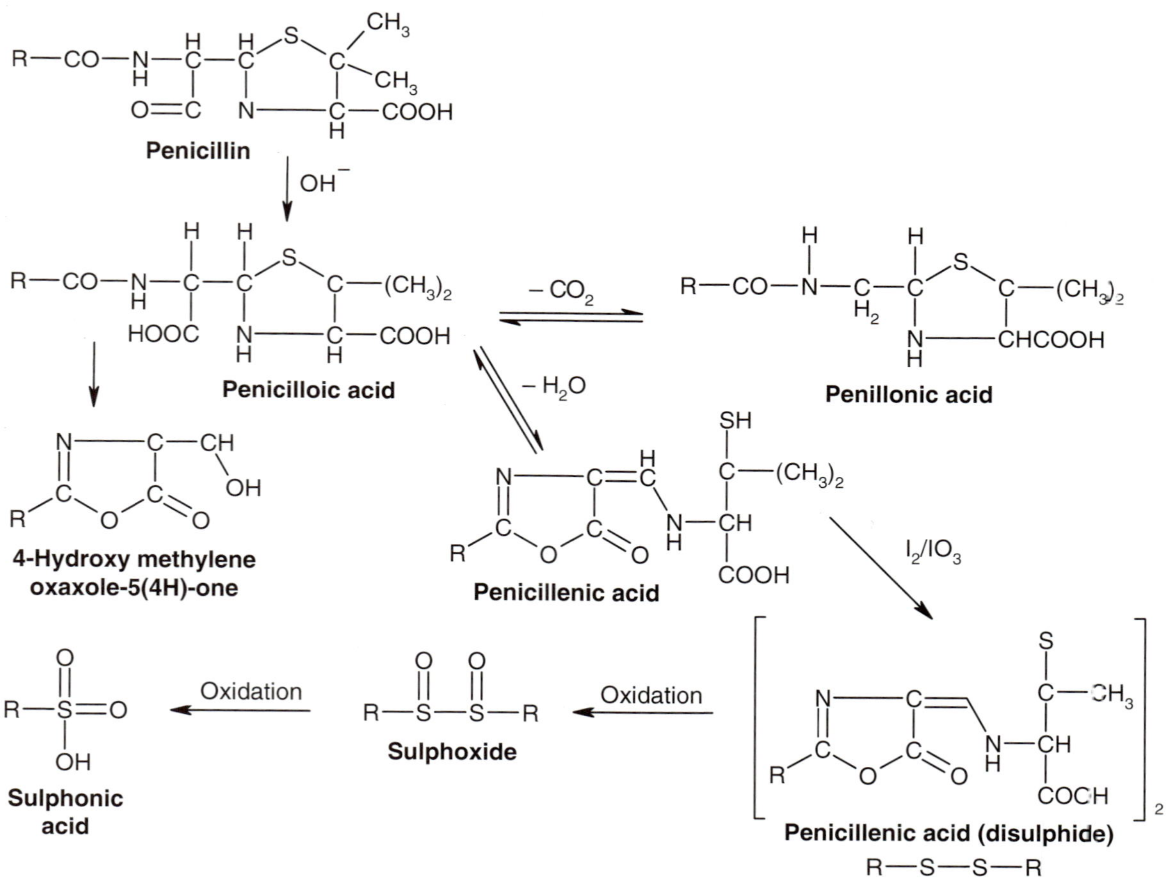

The possible degradation pathways of penicillin: followed by oxidation with iodate ions

Reference

Saidul Zafar Qureshi, Talat Qayoom & Marud I. Helalet, *J. Pharm. & Biomed. Analysis*, **21**, 473-482, 1999.

Bromhexine hydrochloride

METHOD 1

Standard solution

50 mcg/ml in 0.1 N methanolic hydrochloric acid.

Sample solution

Weigh accurately quantity of the sample equivalent to about 12 mg of substance and transfer to a separating funnel. Add about 15 ml of water; basify with dilute solution of ammonia and extract with three 25 ml portions of n-hexane. Combined organic layer is extracted with three 25 ml portions of 0.1 N hydrochloric acid ensuring complete separation of layers after each extraction. Dilute the acidic layer to 250 ml with 0.1 N methanolic hydrochloric acid.

Measure the extinction of both sample and standard solutions at 317 nm using 0.1 N methanolic hydrochloric acid as blank. Calculate the results by comparison.

METHOD 2

Reagents

1. 1 N hydrochloric acid.
2. 1% w/v solution of sodium nitrite in water.
3. 0.5% w/v solution of ammonium sulphamate in water.
4. 0.1% w/v solution of N-naphthyl ethylenediamine dihydrochloride (NED) in water.
5. 2% w/v solution of resorcinol in water.

Standard solution

Weigh accurately about 25 mg of bromhexine hydrochloride. Add about 40 ml of alcohol, shake for 5 minutes and dilute to volume with 1 N hydrochloric acid. Further dilution is done with 1 N hydrochloric acid to get a concentration of 40 mcg/ml.

Sample solution

Prepare the sample as under method 1 above. Filter, if necessary.

Procedure

Take 3 ml each of sample and standard solutions in 25 ml volumetric flask. Cool in ice-bath for about 10 minutes. Add 1 ml each of sodium nitrite solution, ammonium sulphamate solution and 'NED' reagent each at an interval of 2 minutes. Mix and dilute to 25 ml with water. Measure the absorbance of both sample and standard solutions at about 550 nm against reagent blank. Calculate the contents of bromhexine hydrochloride in the sample by comparison.

Note

Instead of 'NED' reagent, add 1.2 ml of resorcinol solution and dilute to 25 ml. The chromophore exhibits absorption maximum at about 435 nm.

Probable Reaction Mechanism

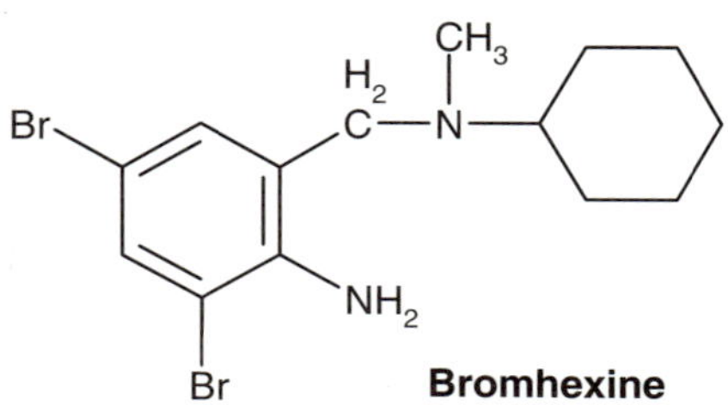

Bromhexine

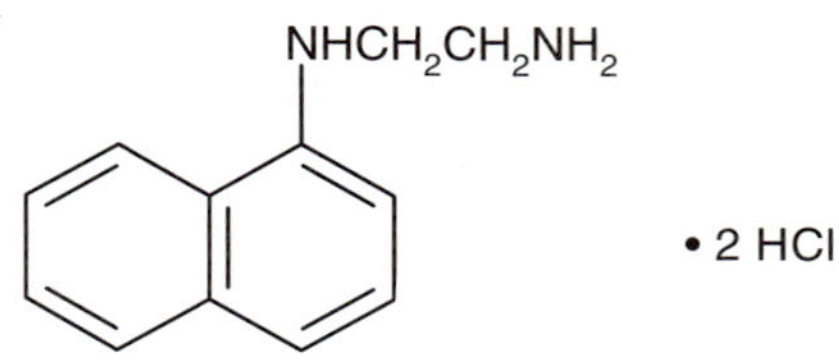

N-1-Naphthyl ethylene diamine dihydrochloride

Step 1: Reaction between $NaNO_2$ and HCl reasults in the formation of HNO_2.

$$NaNO_2 + HCl \longrightarrow NaCl + HNO_2$$

$$HNO_2 + H \longrightarrow H_2\overset{\oplus}{O}NO \xrightarrow{Cl^{\ominus}} H_2O + \overset{+}{N}{=}OCl^{-}$$

Nitrosonium ion

Step 2: The nitrosonium ion being electron deficient, it will attack the amino group of bromohexine resulting in the formation of diazotized product as shown.

Step 3:

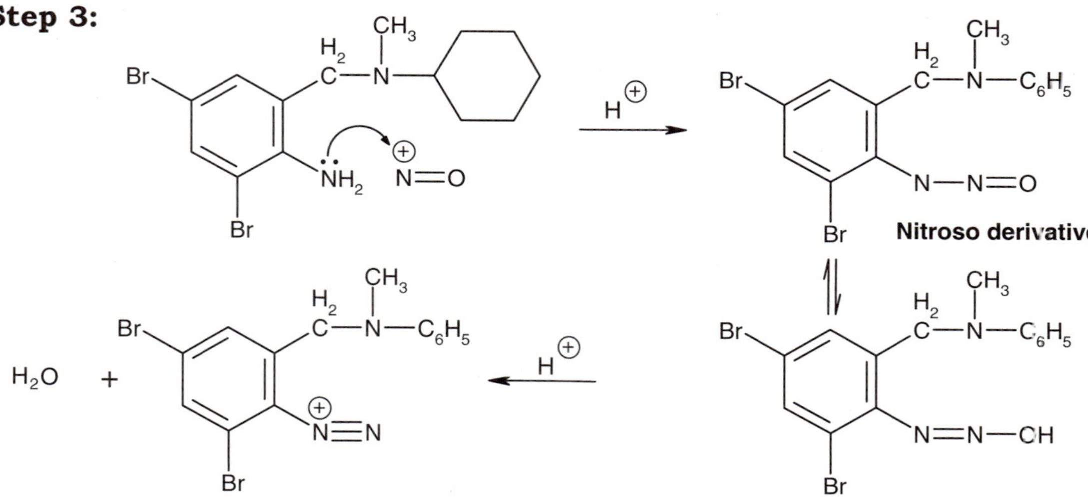

Dizonium ion **Hydroxy diazo form**

Step 4: This diazotized product couples at the para position of N-1-Naphthyl ethylene diamine (NED) as shown below:

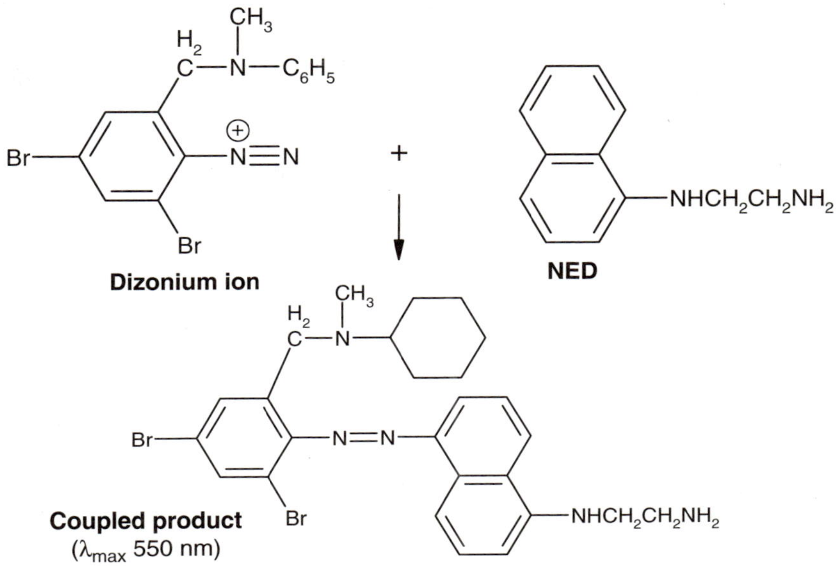

Ammonium sulphamate is added to destroy the excess of HNO_2 formed.

$$HNO_2 + \underset{\text{Sulphamic acid}}{H_2NSO_3H} \longrightarrow H_2SO_4 + N_2\uparrow + H_2O$$

Reference

D.M. Shingbal & V. Ramakrishna Rao, *Indian Drugs*, **22(5)**, 275, 19??.

Sanghvi et al. (1989) described a similar method using phloroglucinol as coupling reagent with diazotized bromhexine in alkaline medium. The reaction mechanism proposed by the authors is as under:

Reaction Mechanism as proposed by the authors

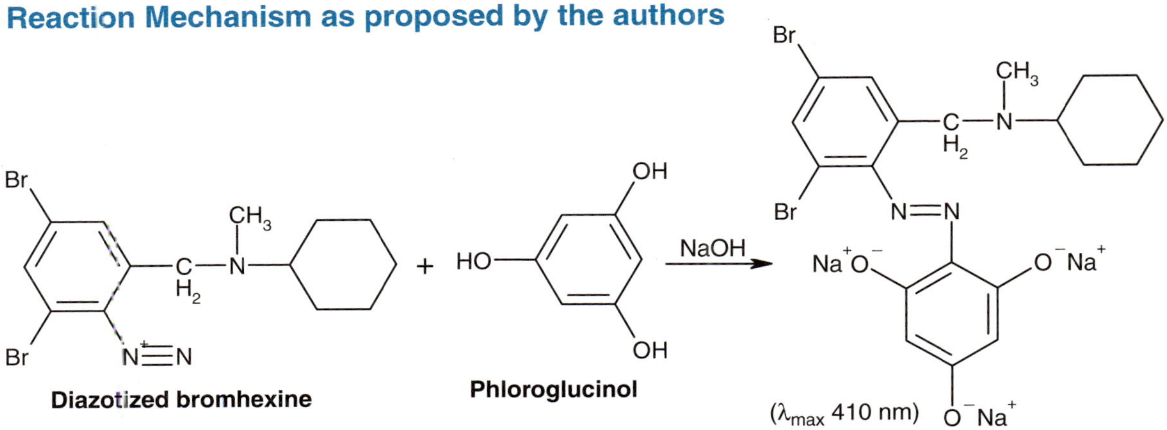

Reference

N.M. Sanghvi, M.M. Samarth, Rajender Singh & P.S. Matharu, Indian Drugs, **27(9)**, 486-488, 1989.

The diazotized bromhexine as under method 2 above can be coupled with orcinol or resorcinol or catechol and β-naphthol in alkaline medium. The reaction mechanism is given below.

Reagents

1. 10% acetic acid.
2. 0.1% each of sodium nitrite, resorcinol, β-naphthol and catechol.
3. 4% w/v solution of NaOH.

Standard solution

100 μg/ml in water.

Sample solution

Powdered sample extracted with water to get the desired concentration.

Procedure

To 1 ml of diazotized sample/standard add 1 ml of the respective reagent, dilute to volume and measure the absorbance at respective maximum.

Reference

S.S. Zarapkar, R.V. Rele & V.J. Doshi, Indian Drugs, **26(1)**, 38-41, 1987.

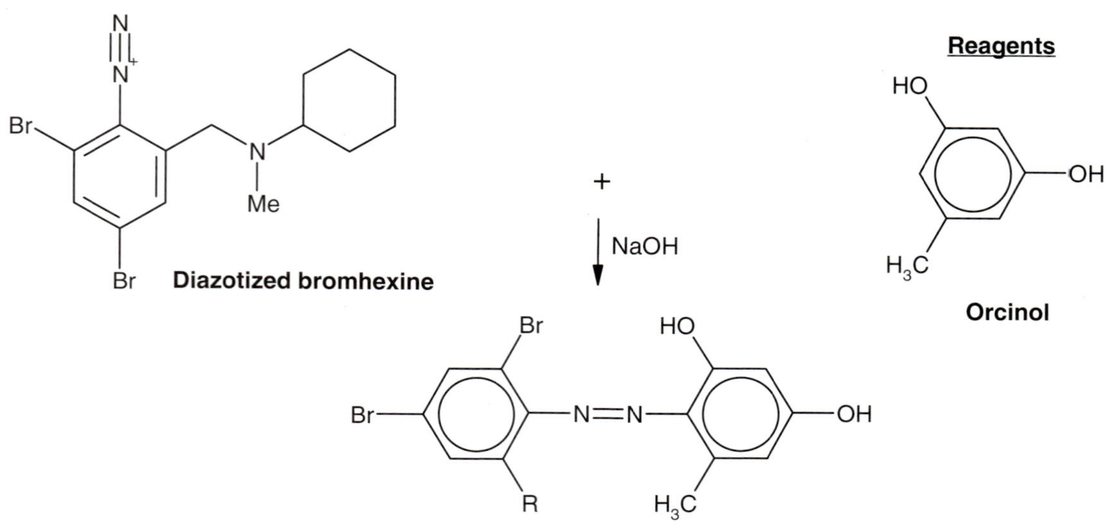

Orcinol coupled product
(λ_{max} 435 nm)

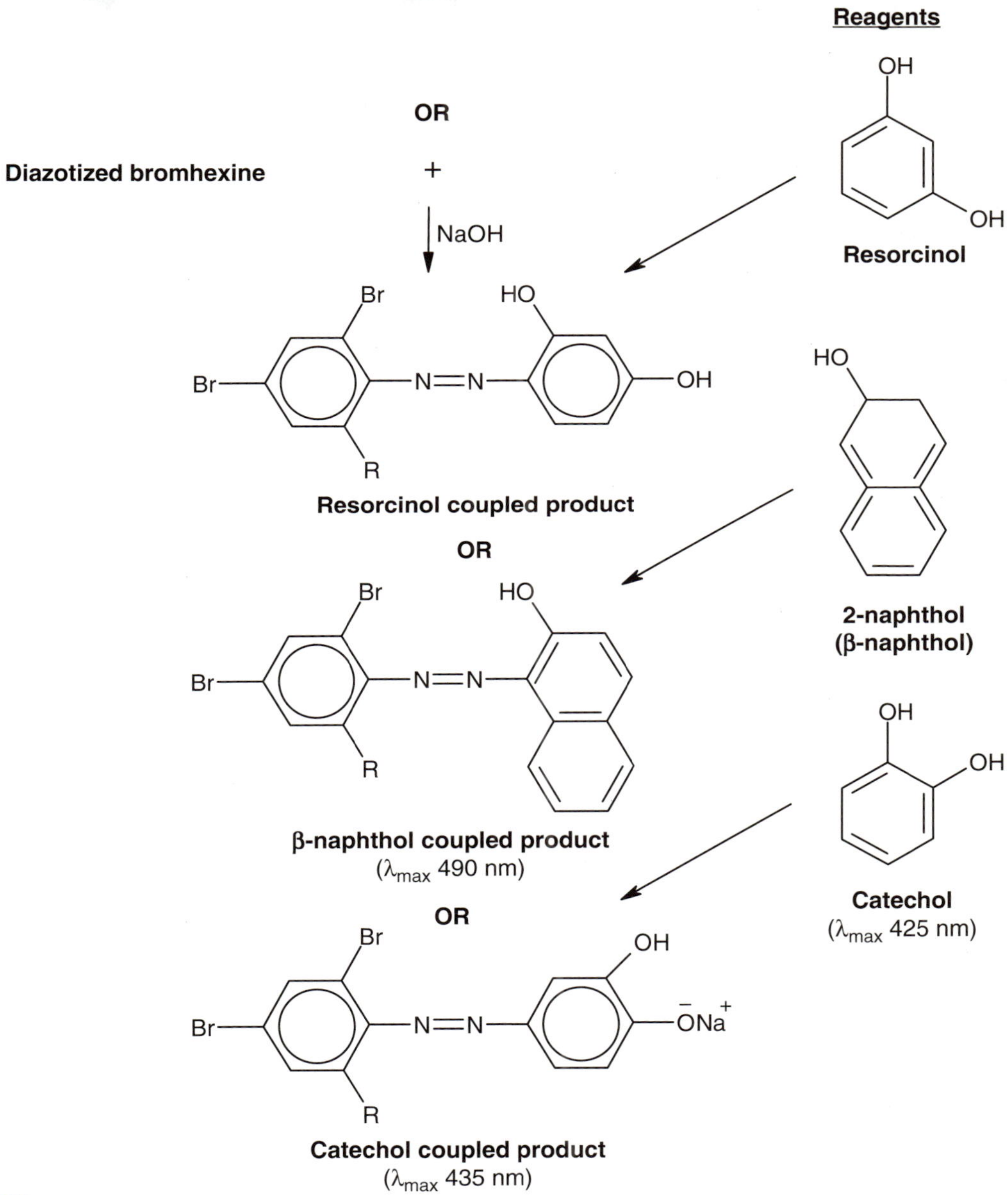

Reference

1. *Indian Drugs*, **22(7)**, 387, April 1985.
2. *Indian Drugs*, **24(8)**, 417, May 1987.
3. *Indian Drugs*, **24(6)**, 311, March 1987.
4. *Indian Drugs*, **22(6)**, 275, March 1985.
5. S.S. Zarapkar, R.V. Rele & V.J. Doshi, *Indian Drugs*, **26(1)**, 38, 1989.
6. Textbook of Practical Organic Chemistry by Vogel, pp. 920, 948.

It forms Schiff's base with PDAB or PDCA under acid conditions because of amino group present in the molecule.

Probable Reaction Mechanism

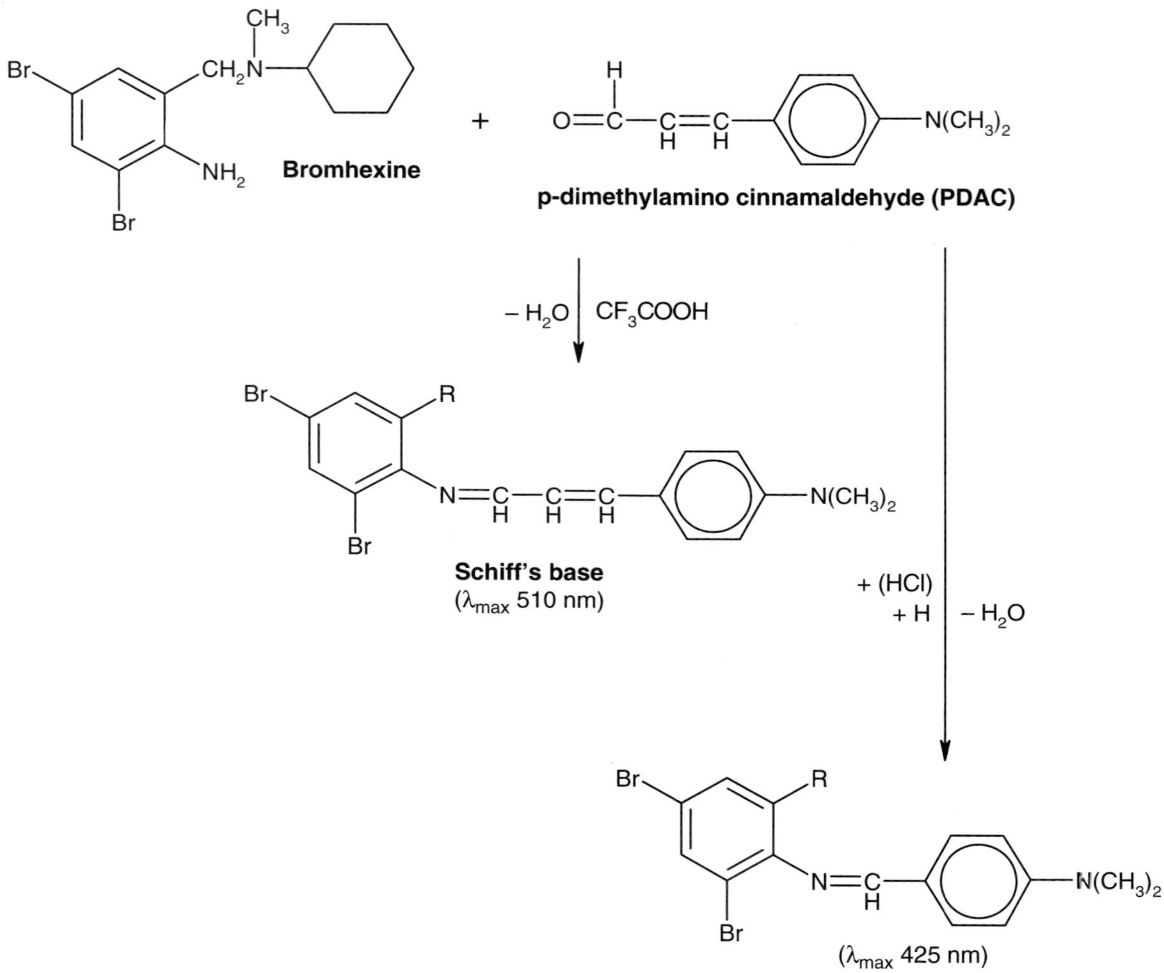

Reference

P. Parimoo & Surinder Kumar, *Indian Drugs*, **31(2)**, 41-43, 1994 & Indian Drugs, **24(1)**, 51, 1986.

The reaction proposed by K. Ramakrishnam Raju et al. involving the coupling of diazo derivative with ethyl acetoacetate with an active hydrogen atom. Diazotized bromhexine as obtained under method reported earlier can be made to react with ethyl acetoacetate in strong alkaline medium.

Probable Reaction Mechanism

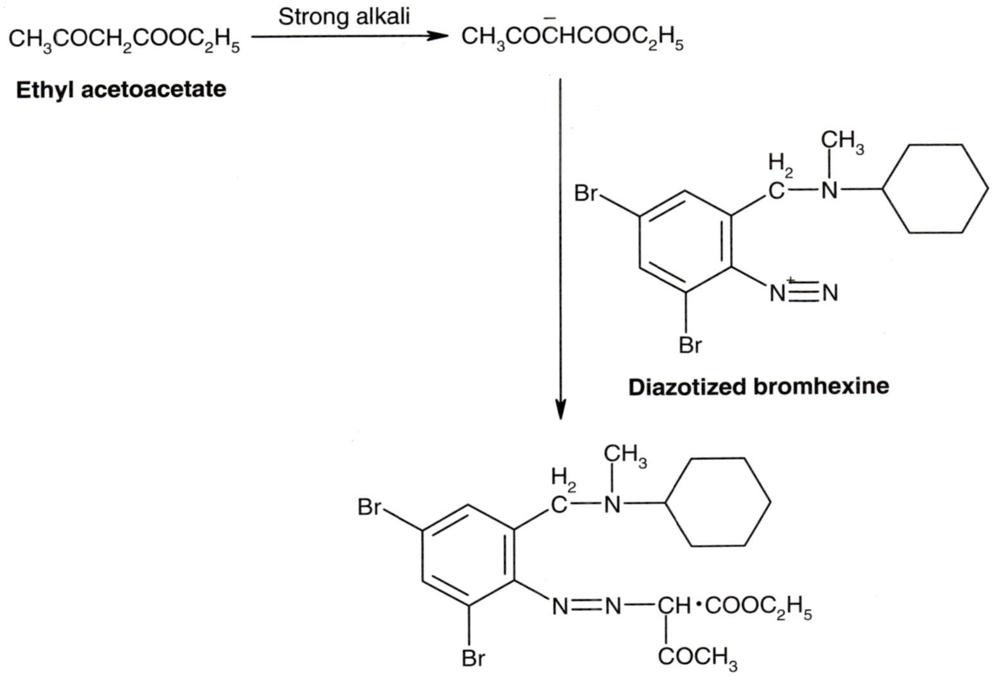

Coloured product

Reference

K. Ramakrishnam Raju, S.R.K.M. Aikella, J.V.S. Murthy & U.T. Bhalerao, *Talanta*, **43**, 577-581, 1996.

Formulation 30

Bromhexine hydrochloride, Cephalexin

ESTIMATION

Bromhexine hydrochloride

Accurately weighed quantity of the sample equivalent to 4 mg of bromhexine hydrochloride is suspended in 10 ml of 0.1 N hydrochloric acid and extracted with three 25 ml portions of chloroform (retain aqueous layer for estimation of cephalexin). The combined chloroform layer diluted to 100 ml with chloroform. Further dilutions are done appropriately and stepwise to get a concentration of 20 mcg/ml. Measure extinction of the solutions at maximum at about 317 nm. Calculate the results by comparing with the standard solution of bromhexine hydrochloride in chloroform (20 mcg/ml). Alternatively, evaporate appropriate volume of above solution and take up the residue in 0.1 N methanolic hydrochloric acid and measure the extinction at 317 nm. Alternatively, follow the method described in formulation 16 of the chapter on bronchospasm relaxants.

Cephalexin

The aqueous acidic extract retained during estimation of bromhexine hydrochloride is diluted appropriately with 0.1 N methanolic hydrochloric acid to get a concentration of 20 mcg/ml. Measure extinction of the solution at maxima at about 258 nm. Calculate the results by comparing with the standard (20 mcg/ml). Aqueous solution of the substance has λ_{max} 263 nm.

Note

Cephalexin and other antibiotics as tetracycline, oxytetracycline, phenoxymethyl penicillin exhibit maxima at about 260 nm, 280 nm and 340 nm. Bromhexine hydrochloride shows zero absorbance above 330 nm. It is therefore preferable to estimate cephalexin and other antibiotics at 340 nm instead of 258 nm as indicated above. This will eliminate the possibility of interference, if any, due to bromhexine hydrochloride.

Alternatively, sample equivalent to 250 mg of cephalexin is dissolved in 20 ml of neutral methanol and titrated with 0.1 N sodium hydroxide using bromothymol blue as indicator, perform blank for necessary correction. Each ml of 0.1 N sodium hydroxide is equivalent to 0.03474 g of cephalexin.

Cephalexin having free carboxylic group (—COOH), this method is based on titration of the acidic group with sodium hydroxide.

Follow the different methods involving reaction with 2,4-dinitrofluorobenzene in alkaline medium or reaction with p-dinitrobenzene as described in formulation of the chapter on antibiotics.

Another spectrophotometric method using imidazole reagent is described by Alwarthan et al. This method is similar to the one used for penicillins and had been official in several pharmacopoeias.

Reagents

1. Imidazole reagent: 1.2 M imidazole solution containing 0.001 M HgC12, adjust pH to 6.8.
2. Acetic anhydride (AA) solution: 0.2 M in acetonitrile.
3. Borate buffer, pH 11.5.
2. 0.1 M solution of sodium hydroxide.

Standard solution

100 μg/ml solution of cephalexin in water.

Sample solution

Powdered sample equivalent to 20 mg suspended in 50 ml of water, diluted to 100 ml with water, filtered and further diluted to get 100 μg/ml.

Procedure

To 1 ml each of sample and standard solutions, add 0.5 ml of borate buffer, 0.03 ml of AA solution and 2 ml of imidazole reagent, dilute to 25 ml with water. Heat in water-bath (60°C) for 55 min, cool immediately and measure the absorbance at 370 nm against reagent blank.

Probable Reaction Mechanism

The reaction depends on the catalytic effect of the imidazole base on the β-lactam bond and on the formation of an oxazolinone ring in the side chain. Binding of the mercury (II) to the thiol group which is freed by the cleavage of the dihydrothiazine ring stabilizes the product. The methoxyimino group present in the side chain becomes conjugated to the oxazolinone ring at the end of the reaction and is responsible for the colour (λ_{max} 370 nm).

Note

1. Heating at lower temperature takes longer time for the reaction to complete i.e. 60°C (55 min), 83°C (20 min).
2. If the reaction solution is left at high temperature there is fading of colour, hence immediate cooling to quench the reaction.

Probable Reaction Mechanism

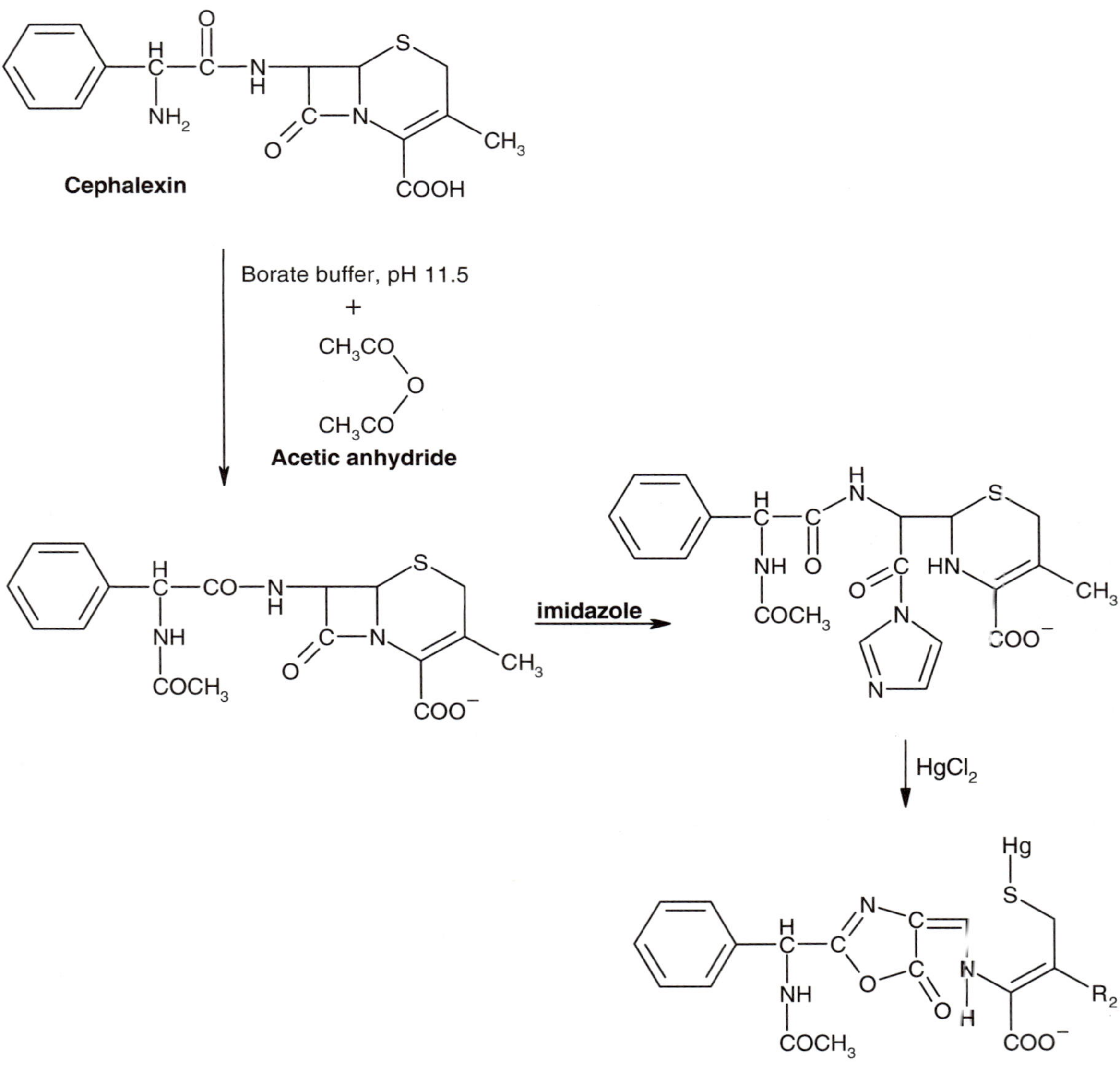

Cephalexin - imidazole complex
(λ_{max} 370 nm)

Reference

1. F. Inci Sengün & Kösal Ulas, *Talanta*, **33(4)**, 363-365, 1986.
2. A.A. Alwarthan, S. Abdel Fattah & N.M. Zahran, *Talanta*, **39(6)**, 703-707, 1992.

The authors (Sengün et al.) have described another analytical method based on reaction of the carboxylic (—COOH) moiety with hydroxylamine to yield hydroxamic acid which is then treated with iron (III) to give coloured complex using nickel (II) which catalyzes the hydroxamic acid formation of cephalosporins and also stabilize the colour formed with Fe (III).

Reagents

1. Hydroxylamine-nickel reagent: Dissolve 6.95 g of hydroxylamine hydrochloride and 7.9 g of nickel nitrite hexahydride in 30 ml of water, adjust to pH 6.2 with 10 M NaOH and finally dilute to 50 ml with water. This solution contains 2 M NH_2OH and 0.2 M Ni (II).
2. Iron (III) reagent: Dissolve 15 g of ammonium iron (III) sulphate dodecahydride in sufficient 0.5 M sulphuric acid to produce 100 ml.

Standard/sample solution

1 mg of cephalexin in 10% sodium bicarbonate solution.

Procedure

To 0.5 ml of sample/standard solution add 2 ml of hydroxylamine-nickel reagent. Allow to react at room temperature exactly for 20 min, then add 5 ml of iron (III) reagent. Allow to react exactly for 20 min, centrifuge and then measure the absorbance of the clear supernatant at 470 nm against reagent blank.

Basically, this reaction is based on the work of Bamberger (1999) involving reaction of hydroxylamine with carboxylic acid (—COOH) derivatives. However, Munson et al. (1979) have suggested the use of nickel (II) salt as catalyst for the formation of hydroxyamine acid before treating with Fe (III) to give coloured complex.

Probable Reaction Mechanism

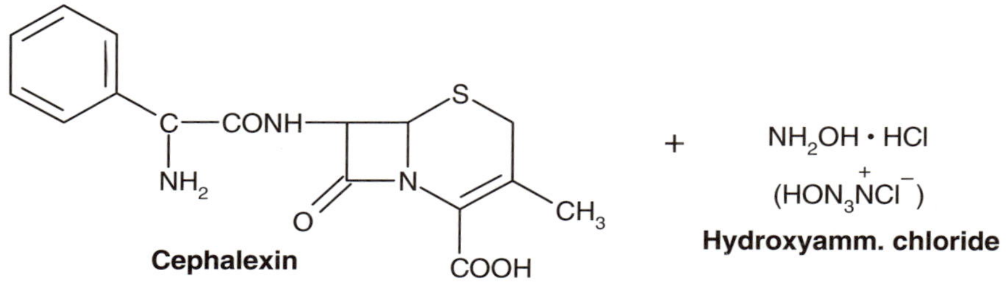

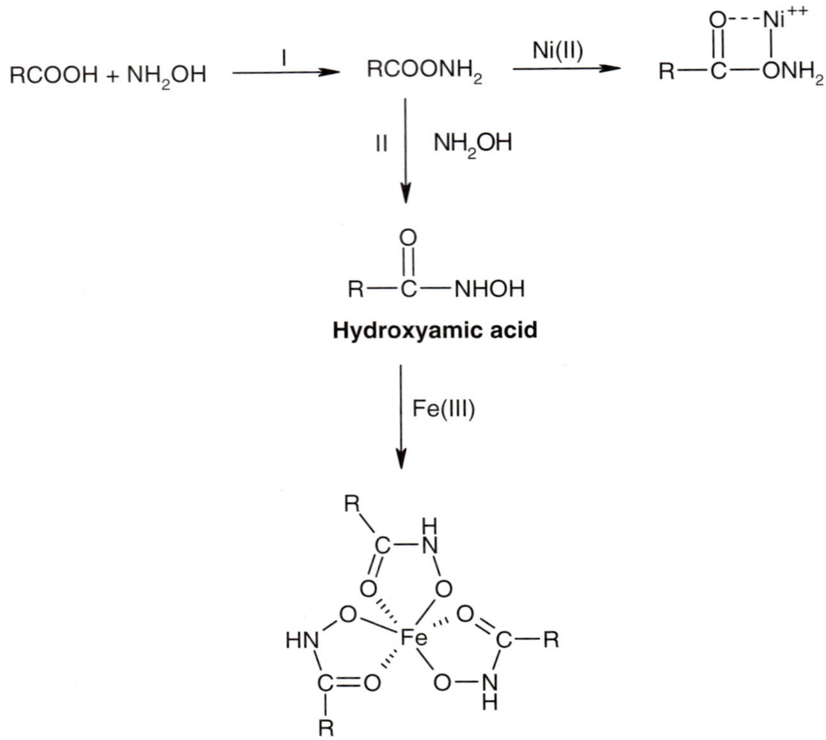

Hydroxyamic acid

Hydroxyamic acid - iron (III) chelate
(λ_{max} 470 nm)

Reference

1. E. Bamberger, *Ber.*, **32**, 1805, 1999.
2. J.W. Munson & K.A. Connors, *J. Amm. Chem. Soc.*, **94**, 1979, 1972 & J. Pharm. Sci., **61(2)**, 211-213, 1972.
3. F. Inci Sengün & Köksai Ulas, Talanta, **33(4)**, 365-367, 1986.
4. D.L. Mays, F.K. Bangert, W.C. Cantrell & W.G. Evans, *Analytical Chem.*, **47(13)**, 2229-2234, 1975.

Note

Ni^{++} acts as catalyst in the third step for the formation of hydroxyamic acid.

This is general reaction mechanism for different caphalosporins.

Another reaction mechanism for iron chelate formation is:

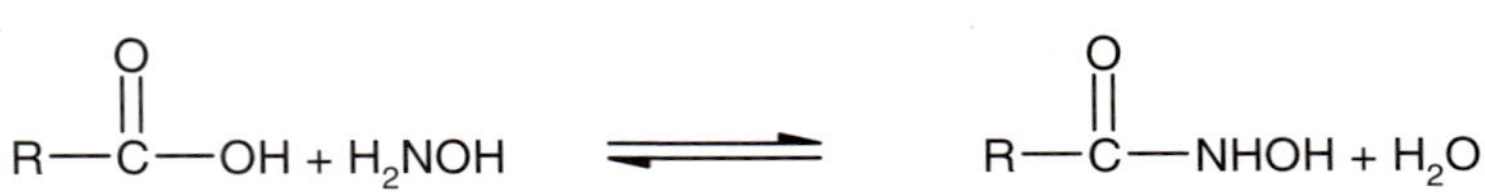

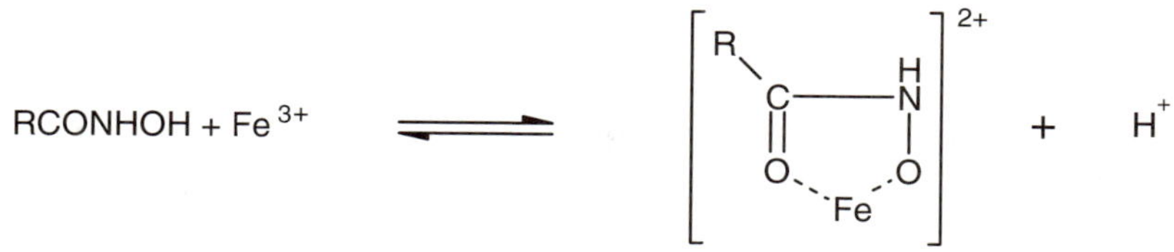

This reaction is based on 1 : 1 complex formation (Textbook of Pharmaceutical Analysis (3rd ed.) by Kenneth A. Connors, Wiley Interscience Publications, p. 530.

Connors et al. have reported the method for determination of several carboxylic acids by nickel (II) catalysed hydroxamic acid formation. The spectrophotometric method was based on general equation:

$$\underset{}{RCOX} + \underset{\textbf{Hydroxylamine}}{NH_2OH} \rightleftharpoons \underset{\textbf{Hydroxamic acid derivative}}{RCONH} + HX$$

This method is suitable for estimation of esters, amides, lactones, imides and anhydride.

Reference

K.A. Connors & James W. Munson, *Analytical Chemistry*, **44(2)**, 336-339, 1972.

Cephalexin reacts with Folin-Ciocalteu reagent in the presence of 20% sodium carbonate to give a blue-coloured chromogen (λ_{max} 753 nm).

Reference

S.A. Patel, N.M. Patel & M.M. Patel, *Ind. J. Pharm. Sci.*, **68(2)**, 278-280, 2006 & Ind. J. Pharm. Sci., **68(1)**, 101-103, 2006.

Note

Cefotaxime and ceftriaxone, the third generation broad-spectrum cephalosporins, also react with Folin-Ciocalteu reagent to give coloured chromogen (λ_{max} 750 nm).

Formulation 31

Bromhexine hydrochloride, Erythromycin estolate

ESTIMATION

Bromhexine hydrochloride

Follow the method described in formulation 29 of this chapter.

Erythromycin estolate

METHOD 1

Reagents

1. 0.4% w/w solution of o-nitrobenzaldehyde in glacial acetic acid.
2. Concentrated hydrochloric acid.

Standard solution

250 mcg/ml of erythromycin (base) in glacial acetic acid.

Sample solution

Accurately weighed quantity of powdered sample equivalent to 100 mg of erythromycin (base) is suspended in glacial acetic acid to make 100 ml. Filter and dilute appropriately to get solution of 250 mcg/ml.

Procedure

To 2 ml each of sample and standard solutions, add 2 ml of benzaldehyde reagent and 3 ml of concentrated hydrochloric acid. Keep at room temperature for 15 minutes and dilute to 25 ml with glacial acetic acid. Measure the absorbance of both sample and standard solutions within 10 min at 490 nm, and calculate the results by comparison.

METHOD 2

The hydroxy functions present in the molecule get oxidized by $FeCl_3$ and in return Fe(III) is reduced to Fe(II) which forms complex with 1,10-phenanthroline to produce a ferroin-coloured complex (λ_{max} 520 nm).

Probable Reaction Mechanism

$$\text{Erythromycin} + FeCl_3 \longrightarrow Fe(II)$$

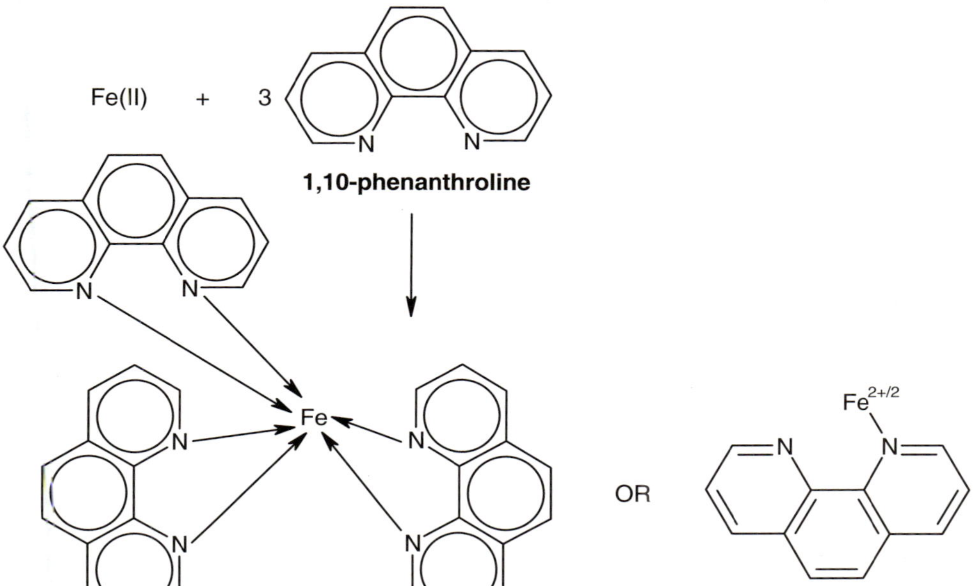

Ferroin complex
(λ_{max} 520 nm)

This reduction is similar to the one proposed by M.N. Reddy, T.K. Murthy, G.V.H. Raju, Murli Krishna, K. Seshukumar & D.G. Sankar, *Ind. J. Pharm. Sci.*, **64(2)**, 73-76, 2002 for roxithromycin and by Y.S. Rao, T.K. Murthy, K.P.R. Chowdary & J.V.L.N.S. Rao, *Indian Drugs*, **39(6)**, 348-349, 2002 for clarithromycin (6-methoxy erythromycin).

On oxidation, the amino alcohol moiety in the molecule liberates formaldehyde and the same is determined in-situ using acetylacetone in the presence of ammonium acetate which gives yellow-coloured chromogen (3,5-diacetyl-1,4-dihydrolutidine).

$$\text{Roxithromycin} \xrightarrow[\text{Oxidation}]{KMNO_4} \underset{\textbf{Formaldehyde}}{HCHO}$$

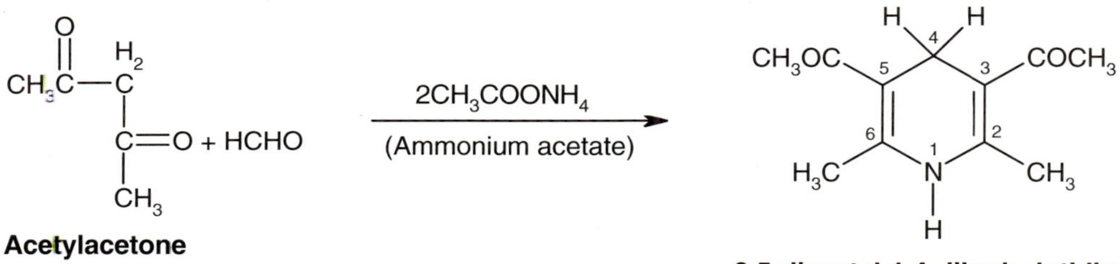

3,5-diacetyl-1,4-dihydrolutidine
(λ_{max} 412 nm)

Note

1. Oxalic acid is used to neutralize excess of $KMnO_4$.
2. This reaction is similar to the one described for guaiphenesin in formulation 2 of this chapter.

Reference

B.N. Suhagia, S.A. Shah, I.S. Rathod, H.M. Patel, K.R. Doshi & V.K. Parmar, *Ind. J. Pharm. Sci.*, **68(4)**, 543-546, 2006.

A spectrophotometric method based on interaction of 2,4-dinitrophenyl hydrazine with carbonyl function of the macrolide antibiotics (azithromycin, clarithromycin and roxithromycin) can be extended to erythromycin. The reaction takes place in the presence of acid which acts as catalyst. The hydrazone derivative so formed is converted to an intensely coloured quinoidal ion on addition of alkali.

General procedure

To an appropriate volume of the sample (1 mg/ml in methanol), add 2 ml of 0.005 M 2,4-DNPH followed by 0.05 ml of conc. HCl. Keep in boiling water-bath and evaporate to almost dryness. Add 3 ml of 1.786 M KOH, mix, allow to stand at room temperature and dilute to 10 ml with DMF. Measure the absorption at the maxima (490–520 nm) against reagent blank. The molar ratio of the complex is 1 : 1.

Probable Reaction Mechanism

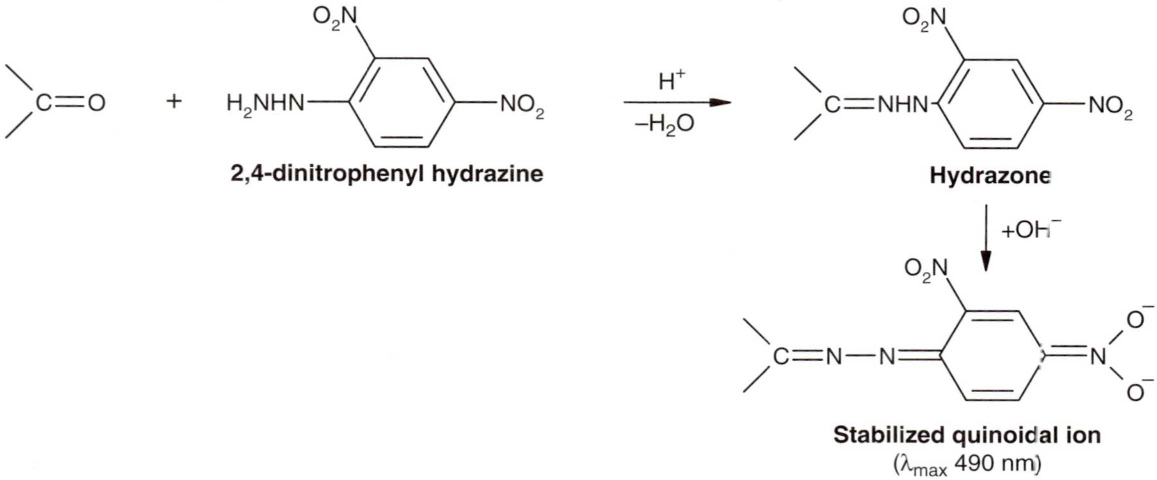

Reference

Osama H. Abdamageed, *JAoAc. Int.*, **90(2)**, 364-371, 2007.

Formulation 32

Betamethasone, Bromhexine hydrochloride, Salbutamol sulphate

ESTIMATION

Betamethasone

Reagents

1. 10% v/v solution of tetramethyl ammonium hydrochloride (TMAH) in methanol.
2. 0.5% w/v solution of tetrazolium blue in methanol.

Standard solution

10 mcg/ml of betamethasone in chloroform.

Sample solution

Accurately weighed quantity of the sample equivalent to 1 mg of the substance is extracted with 3 × 20 ml portions of chloroform and chloroform layer passed through anhydrous sodium sulphate kept on cotton plug and made up to 100 ml with chloroform (10 mcg/ml).

Procedure

To 10 ml each of sample and standard solutions, add 2 ml of tetrazolium blue solution and 2 ml of TMAH. Keep for 45 min at 37°C and dilute to 25 ml with chloroform. Measure absorbance of both the solutions at 525 nm using chloroform as blank and calculate the results by comparison. For reaction mechanism, see formulation 17 of the chapter on bronchospasm relaxants.

Bromhexine hydrochloride

Follow the method 2 described in formulation 29 of this chapter.

Salbutamol sulphate

Follow the method 2 described under formulation 14 of the chapter on bronchospasm relaxants.

Formulation 33

Bromhexine hydrochloride, Guaiphenesin, Pseudoephedrine hydrochloride

ESTIMATION

Bromhexine hydrochloride

Follow the method described in formulation 29 of this chapter.

Pseudoephedrine hydrochloride

Follow the method described in formulation 19 of this chapter.

Guaiphenesin

Reagents

1. Formaldehyde methanol reagent : Prepared by diluting 30 ml of formaldehyde solution (38-40% w/v) to 1000 ml with absolute methanol.
2. Solvent : Cautiously add 600 mg of concentrated sulphuric acid to 400 ml of methanol-water (1 + 1) mixture previously cooled in ice-bath.

Standard solution

80 mcg/ml of guaiphenesin in solvent.

Sample solution

To accurately measured quantity of sample equivalent to 100 mg of guaiphenesin, add 10 ml of water and 10 ml of 1 N sodium hydroxide, mix and extract with chloroform (3 ´ 25 ml). Combined chloroform layer is in turn extracted with the solvent (3 ´ 25 ml). The combined acidic layer is made up of 100 ml with the solvent and 2 ml of the resultant solution is further diluted to 25 ml with the solvent and used for analysis (80 mcg/ml).

Procedure

To 5 ml each of sample and standard solution, add 15 ml of solvent and 1 ml of formaldehyde methanol reagent, mixed and diluted to 25 ml with the solvent.

Measure absorbance of sample and standard solutions at maxima at about 550 nm against reagent blank and calculate the results by comparison.

Probable Reaction Mechanism

This reaction is based on 'Marquis' reaction. Two moles of the drug condense with 2 moles of HCHO in the presence of sulphuric acid. This reaction is similar to the one described for.

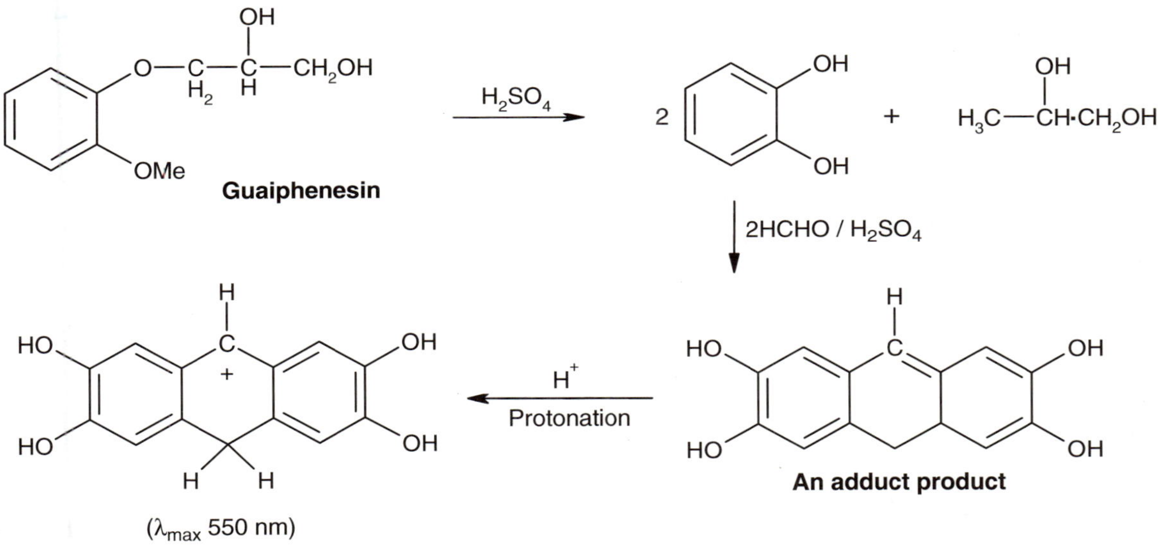

Reference

Pharmaceutical Chemistry (Vol. 2) by H.J. Roth, p. 623.

Formulation 34

Salbutamol sulphate, Bromhexine hydrochloride, Phenylephrine hydrochloride

ESTIMATION

Salbutamol sulphate

Follow the method described in formulation 14 of the chapter on bronchospasm relaxants.

Bromhexine hydrochloride

Follow the method described in formulation 29 of this chapter.

Phenylephrine hydrochloride

Follow the method 1 described in formulation 1 of the chapter on analgesics and antipyretics.

Formulation 35

Bromhexine hydrochloride, Diphenhydramine hydrochloride, Guaiphenesin, Ammonium chloride, Menthol

ESTIMATION

Bromhexine hydrochloride

Follow the method described in formulation 29 of this chapter. Sample and standard solution are prepared in methanol.

Ammonium chloride

Follow the method 2 described in formulation 7 of this chapter.

Diphenhydramine hydrochloride

Follow the method described in formulation 6 of this chapter based on coloured complex formation with cobalt thiocyanate.

Guaiphenesin

Follow the method described in formulation 26 of this chapter. Alternatively, follow the method given below :

This method is based on oxidation of terminal vicinal hydroxyl group, liberating formaldehyde which reacts with acetyl acetone in presence of ammonium acetate to give yellow coloured chromogen (λ_{max} 412 nm).

Reagents

1. 0.214% w/v solution of sodium periodate in water.
2. 30% w/v solution of ammonium acetate.
3. 1% v/v solution of acetyl acetone in ammonium acetate solution.
4. Saturated solution of sodium bicarbonate.
5. 1 N hydrochloric acid.

Standard solution

150 mcg/ml of guaiphenesin in 5% acetic acid.

Sample solution

To the sample equivalent to 100 mg of the add 10 ml of saturated solution of sodium bicarbonate and extract with 25 ml portions of chloroform, washing each layer with 5 ml of 1 N hydrochloric acid. Combine layer and make up to 100 ml with chloroform (1 mcg/ml). Evaporate 15 ml of chloroform by and take up the residue in 5 ml of glacial acetic acid and dilute to 100 ml with water (150 mcg/ml).

Procedure

To 2 ml each of sample and standard solutions, add 2 ml of sodium periodate solution and allow to stand at room temperature for 5 minutes with occasional stirring. Add 5 ml of acetyl acetone reagent and retain at room temperature for 30 min, dilute to 25 ml with water. Measure the absorbance of both the solution at 412 nm against reagent blank and calculate the results by comparison.

Probable Reaction Mechanism

Guaiphenesin has side chain containing terminal visinal hydroxyl group. Periodate oxidation liberates formaldehyde (HCHO) which reacts with acetylacetone in the presence of ammonium acetate giving a yellow-coloured product (λ_{max} 412 nm).

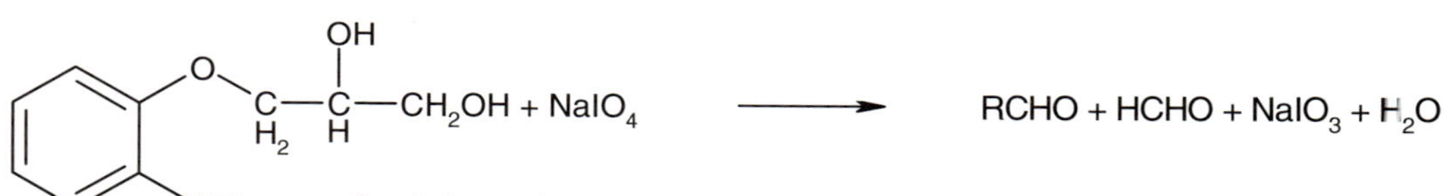

Guaiphenesin

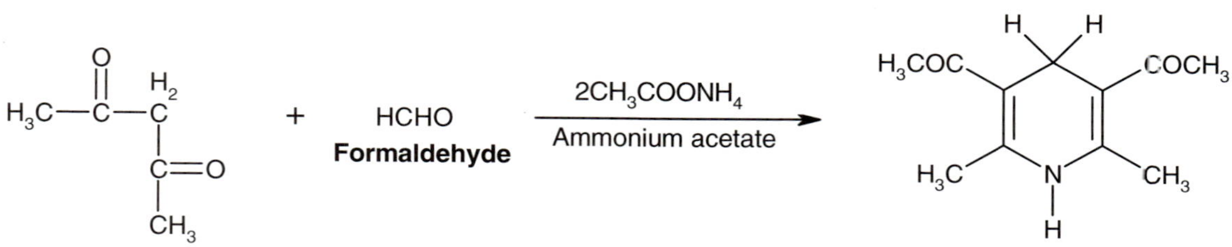

Acetylacetone **Formaldehyde**

1,4-dihydro-3,5-diacetyl lutidine
(λ_{max} 412 nm)

Formulation 36

Ibuprofen, Pseudoephedrine hydrochloride

ESTIMATION

Ibuprofen

To accurately weighed quantity of a sample equivalent to 150-200 mg of the substance, add 4-5 ml of water and acidify with 0.1 N hydrochloric acid. Extract with four 25 ml portions of chloroform. Pass the chloroform layer through anhydrous sodium sulphate, placed on a copper plate. Evaporate the chloroform extract till there is no precipitate smell of chloroform. Dissolve the entire residue in 50 ml of neutral (phenolphthalein) methanol and dilute with 0.1 N sodium hydroxide. Each ml of 0.1 N sodium hydroxide is equivalent to 0.020639 g of ibuprofen.

Explanatory Note

On acidification, ibuprofen is extracted into chloroform, whereas pseudoephedrine, being a salt, remains in acidic layer.

Pseudoephedrine hydrochloride

Pipette out appropriate volume of the uniformly suspended sample representing 90-100 mg of the substance, add 4-5 ml of water and basify distinctly with dilute solution of ammonia. Extract with four 25 ml portions of ether, passing each ether layer through cotton plug. Evaporate the combined ether extract till no precipitate smell of ether.

To the residue, add 40 ml of glacial acetic acid, 10 ml of acetic anhydrite and titrate with 0.1 N perchloric acid using crystal violet as indicator.

Each ml of 0.1 N perchloric acid is equivalent to 0.02017 g of pseudoephedrine hydrochloride.

Explanatory Note

On basification, ibuprofen being acidic in character remains in alkaline layer, whereas pseudoephedrine, the base, gets extracted into ether. Ether layer is evaporated and subjected to non-aqueous titration as usual.

Formulation 37

Amoxycillin, Carbocysteine (S-Carboxymethyl cysteine)

ESTIMATION

Amoxycillin and Carbocysteine

Reagents

1. Dimethyl sulphoxide (DMSO)
2. 1% w/v solution of nickel (II) nitrate in DMSO.

Standard solution

50 mcg/ml each drug in water.

Sample solution

Accurately weighed or measured aliquot of the sample equivalent to 5 mg of the drug was extracted with water to produce 100 ml. The filtrate was used for analysis.

Procedure

To 5 ml of sample and standard solutions, add 2 ml nickel nitrate solution, mix and after 30 min (optimum time for complete complexation) measure the absorbance of solutions at 259 nm (for carbocysteine) and 327 nm (for amoxycillin). The results were calculated by comparison. The method obeys Bear's law in the range of 5-50 mcg/ml. The complexes were stable for at least 3 hrs.

After complexation with nickel (II), significant improvement in spectral characteristics was observed with bathochromic and hyperchromic shift. Molar absorptivity increases by 3-4 folds for amoxycillin and 6-7 folds for carbocysteine.

Amino and ketonic functions present in the molecule appear to be responsible for complexation. DMSO plays important role as nickel formed complex only in DMSO and not in water by coordinate bond through ion-pairs of electrons on oxygen.

Probable Reaction Mechanism

Both the compounds form complex with Ni(II). $DMSO_4$ is used as solvent as the compound fails to form the complex in water. Amino and carboxyl groups are involved in both the cases.

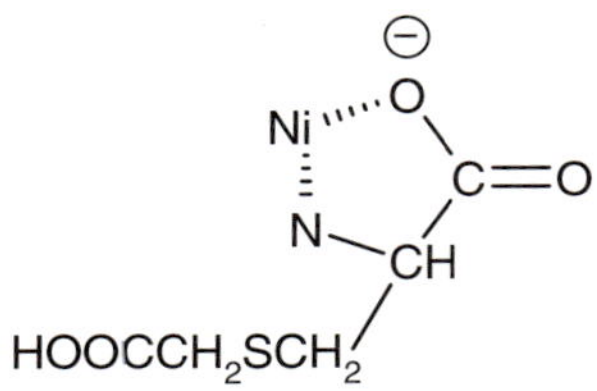

Ni(II) - carbocysteine complex
(λ_{max} 259 nm)

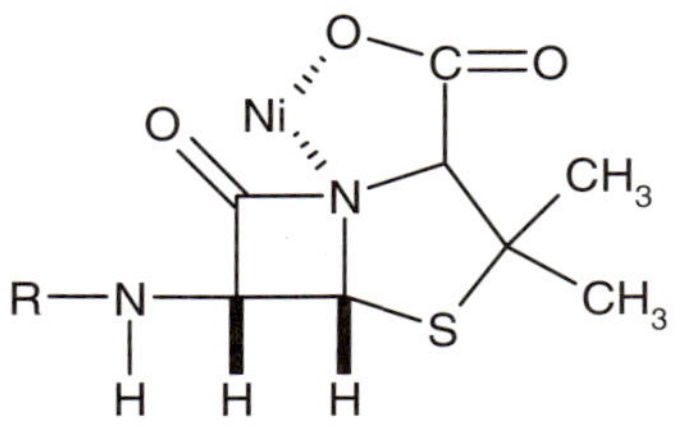

Ni(II) - amoxycillin complex
(λ_{max} 327 nm)

Note

Both the complexes show bathochromic and hyperchromic shifts.

Reference

G.G. Paragaonkar & S.G. Kashedikar, Indian Drugs, **31(12)**, 590-592, 1994.

METHOD 2

Reagents

1. 0.1 M p-benzoquinone (PBQ) in DMSO, stable for 5 days if stored in dark.
2. Na_2HPO_4 - NaH_2PO_4 phosphate buffer, pH 7.0.

Standard solution

100 μg/ml in phosphate buffer, pH 7.0.

Sample solution

Initial solution made in water, further dilutions made with phosphate buffer, pH 7.0.

Procedure

To 2 ml each of sample and standard solutions add 0.1 ml of the PBQ reagent, incubate at 37°C for 10 min, cool, dilute to volume and measure at 500 nm. This involves Michael addition of amino group at enone system.

Probable Reaction Mechanism

In reaction between cysteine and N-acetylcysteine, 'PBQ' reaction takes place through sulphahydryl (SH) group—N-acetylcysteine; amino group is blocked by acetyl, whereas in case of carbocysteine the reaction takes place between amino (NH_2) group of the compound and PBQ as sulphahydryl group is blocked by carboxy group. The reaction between cysteine and PBQ shows two absorption bands i.e. 352 nm and 500 nm as both —SH group and amino group are involved whereas in case of carbocysteine only one absorption band (500 nm) is observed due to involvement of amino group.

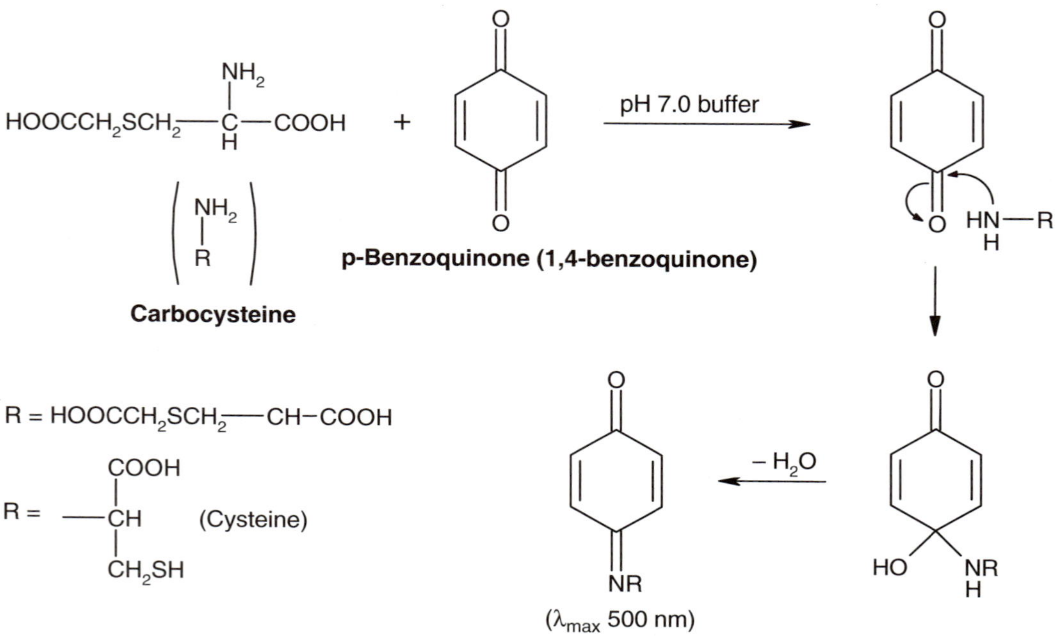

Note

The method is suitable for shampoo.

Reference

Dimas A.M. Zaia, Kelly C.L. Ribas & Cassla T.B.V. Zaia, *Talanta*, **50**, 1003-1010, 1999.

METHOD 2 (for carbocysteine)

Accurately weighed quantity of sample equivalent to 300 mg of carbocysteine is suspended in 25 ml of 0.1 N sodium hydroxide and stirred for 45 min (use magnet stirrer). Filter and wash the flask and filter paper with water (3 × 50 ml). Combine both the aqueous washings with the filtrate and titrate with 0.1 N hydrochloric acid (methyl red). Carry out the blank titration or carry out potentiometric titration.

Each ml of 0.1 N hydrochloric acid is equivalent to 17.92 mg of carbocysteine.

Note

1. Amoxycillin interference is in the range of 5-7.5%.
2. Though the compound has two carboxylic groups but only one carboxylic group (COOH) will react with sodium hydroxide. As the other COOH group has amino group so it will behave as zwitter ion and cannot react with NaOH as such unless subjected to formol titration; hence equivalent factor is 17.92, the molecular weight for the substance being 179.2 g.

METHOD 3 (for carbocysteine)

Dissolve the sample in 10 ml of formic acid (98-100%) and add further 50 ml of formic acid and titrate with 0.1 N perchloric acid using 0.05 ml of oracet blue B solution (0.5% solution of the dye in glacial acetic acid) as indicator (change from blue to clear purple). Each ml of 0.1 N perchloric acid is equivalent to 17.92 mg of carbocysteine.

A titrimetric method was reported by Krishna et al. treating the sample with 0.05 M potassium ferricyanide in pH 7.0 phosphate buffer. Then add excess of ascorbic acid and residual ascorbic acid titrated with iodine. Alternatively, residue $K_3Fe(CN)_6$ is titrated with 0.02 M ascorbic acid using 2,6-dichlorophenol indophenol as indicator, discharge of the colour of the dye being end point.

Reference

K.K. Verma & Sameer Bose, *Talanta*, **22**, 74-75, 1975.

A spectrophotometric method based on reaction of thio (—SH) with phenols in the presence of oxidant was proposed by C.S.P. Sastry et al. (1985). Metol (p-methyl aminophenol) and aminophenol were used as phenols and ferric chloride was used as oxidant. In addition to several compounds analysed, cysteine hydrochloride was of the pharmaceutical interest.

The following reaction mechanism was proposed by the authors. The oxidation products formed in-situ acted as chromogens.

Probable Reaction Mechanism

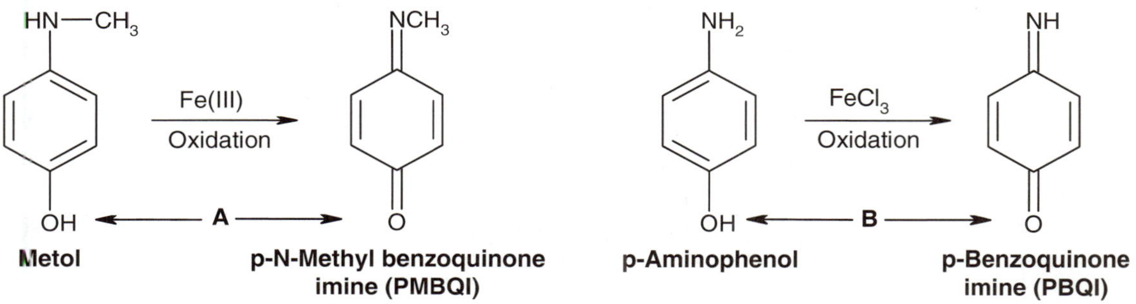

Note

N-bromosuccinimide could also be used as oxidizing agent. The coloured species formed between 'PMBQI' and 'PBQI' are similar. The final product can be extracted into n-butanol and measured at 580 nm.

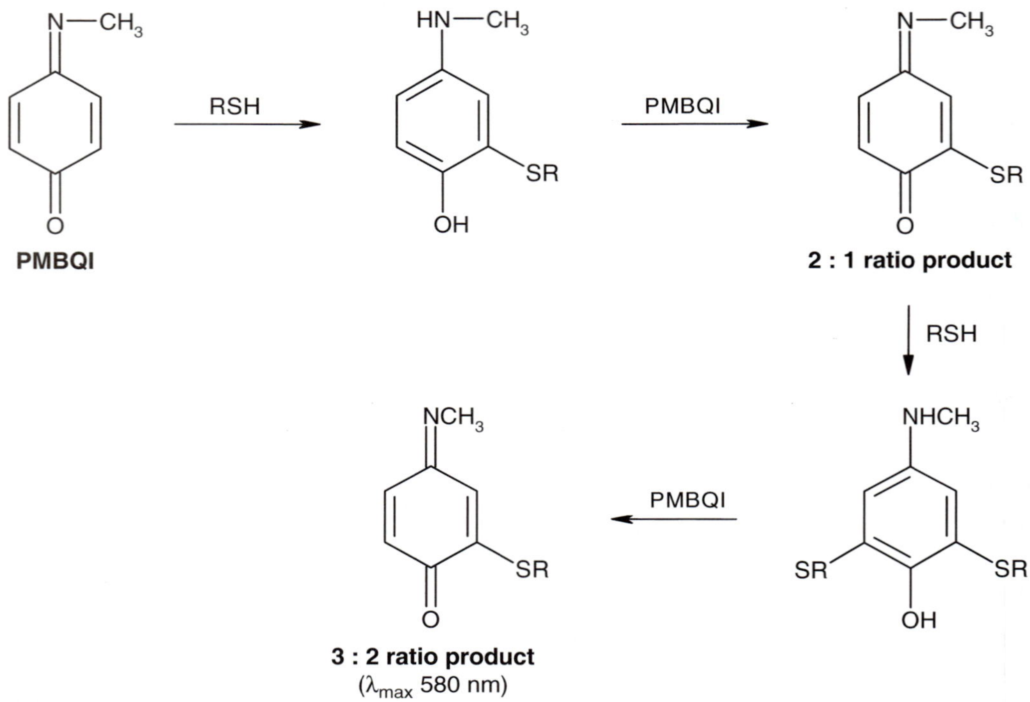

Reference

C.S.P. Sastry, P. Satyanarayana & Murli K. Tummru, *Analyst*, **110(2)**, 189-191, 1985.

Formulation 38

Chlorpheniramine maleate, Diphenhydramine hydrochloride, Pyrilamine maleate

ESTIMATION

Pyrilamine (Mepyramine) maleate

Standard solution

20 mcg/ml of pyrilamine maleate in 0.1 N sulphuric acid.

Sample solution

Shake accurately weighed quantity of the sample equivalent to 25 mg of pyrilamine maleate with 0.1 N sulphuric acid and dilute to produce 100 ml. Filter and dilute the resultant solution with 0.1 N sulphuric acid to get 20 mcg/ml concentration.

Determine the extinction of both the standard and sample solutions at 315 nm using 0.1 N sulphuric acid as blank and calculate the results.

Diphenhydramine hydrochloride

Follow the cobalt-thiocyanate method as described in formulation 7 of this chapter.

Chlorpheniramine maleate

Follow the cyanogen bromide method as described in formulation 3 of this chapter or formulation 1 of the chapter on rubefacients.

Note

For additional quality control, estimate the total salts/organic nitrogenous bases : "Accurately weighed quantity of the material equivalent to about 100-125 mg of the organic salts is extracted with chloroform to get about 2 mg/ml solution. 20 ml of chloroform solution is evaporated and residue dissolved in 30-40 ml of glacial acetic acid (warm if required). Add 10 ml of mercuric acetate solution (5% w/v in glacial acetic acid) and titrate with 0.02 N perchloric acid using crystal violet as indicator, perform blank."

% of total salts of organic nitrogenous bases =

$$\frac{(A - B) \times N \times F \times 100}{\text{Weight of sample (mg) present in 20 ml of chloroform layer}}$$

A = Volume of perchloric acid used in sample titration
B = Volume of perchloric acid used in blank titration
N = Actual normality of perchloric acid
F = Weight (mg) of salts of organic bases equal to 1 ml of 0.02 N perchloric acid. This factor (F) is calculated on the basis of molecular weight and amount of each salt present in the formulation as explained below.

Working example

Each dose contains :

1. Chlorpheniramine maleate—(CPM) 2.5 mg
2. Pyrilamine maleate—(Pm) 12.5 mg
3. Diphenhydramine hydrochloride (DPH) 12.5 mg

Each ml of 0.02 N perchloric acid is equivalent to :

1. 3.908 mg of 'CPM'
2. 4.0014 mg of 'Pm'
3. 5.836 mg of 'DPH'

Compound	Amount present (mg)	Volume (ml) of 0.02 N perchloric acid required
'CPM'	2.5	0.6937
'Pm'	12.5	3.1239
'DPH'	12.5	2.1418

27.5 mg of total organic salts require 5.905 ml of 0.02 N perchloric acid for titration.

1 ml of 0.02 N perchloric acid is equivalent to 4.657 mg of total organic nitrogenous salts.

Formulation 39

Aspirin, Caffeine, Noscapine, Chlorpheniramine maleate

ESTIMATION

Caffeine

Triturate accurately weighed quantity of powdered material equivalent to 100 mg of caffeine with 30-40 ml of 0.1 N hydrochloric acid. Extract the aqueous suspension with four 20 ml portions of chloroform, washing each extract with the same 10 ml of 0.1 N hydrochloric acid. Combine the acid washing with main acidic extract and reserve for estimation of chlorpheniramine maleate. Extract the chloroform layer with four 20 ml portions of 1 N sodium hydroxide and reserve alkaline layer for estimation of aspirin. Filter chloroform layer and evaporate on water-bath to dryness and then dry to a constant weight in an oven at 80°C. Weigh the material which represents caffeine only.

Chlorpheniramine maleate

The acidic extract reserved during estimation of caffeine above is diluted appropriately and contents of chlorpheniramine are estimated by cyanogen bromide method as described in formulation 3 of the chapter on Expectorants and Cough Suppressants.

Aspirin

Acidify the alkaline extract reserved during caffeine estimation with dilute hydrochloric acid. Extract with ether, dry ethereal layer over anhydrous sodium sulphate and evaporate at low temperature. Final drying is done under current of air. Dry the residue in a desiccator and weigh salicylic acid.

Each g of salicylic acid is equal to 1.305 g of aspirin.

Noscapine

Take powdered material, accurately weighed equivalent to 25 mg of noscapine. Add 5 ml of 1 N hydrochloric acid and extract with three 20 ml portions of ether. The combined ether extract is shaken with 10 ml of N/50 hydrochloric acid. The acidic extracts are combined, made alkaline and extracted with five 20 ml portions of ether. The acidic extracts are combined ethereal layers are extracted with N/50 hydrochloric acid to produce 50 mcg/ml solution. Measure the extinction of the sample solution at 312 nm and calculate the results by comparing with the standard (50 mcg/ml) solution of noscapine in N/50 hydrochloric acid.

Formulation 40

Dexchlorpheniramine maleate, Betamethasone

ESTIMATION

Dexchlorpheniramine maleate

Reagents

1. 0.1 N hydrochloric acid.
2. Sodium bicarbonate - sodium chloride solution: 5% w/v solution of sodium chloride in 0.1 N sodium bicarbonate.

Standard solution

0.5 mg/ml of pure dexchlorpheniramine maleate in 0.1 N hydrochloric acid (take 20 ml for assay).

Sample solution

Weigh accurately the sample equivalent to 10 mg of the compound. Add 25 ml of 0.1 N hydrochloric acid and shake.

Procedure

Adjust the pH to 8.0 of both the solutions by cautiously adding sodium bicarbonate-sodium chloride solution (be sure that the entire carbon dioxide has escaped before processing further). Add 30 ml of ethyl acetate and shake for 2-3 min. Separate organic layer and repeat above extraction step with two more 30 ml of ethyl acetate. Discard the aqueous layer. Wash the combined ethyl acetate layer with three 30 ml portions of sodium bicarbonate-sodium chloride solution. Discard the aqueous wash and extract the ethyl acetate layer with two 30-35 ml portions of 0.1 N hydrochloric acid. Collect the acidic extract and dilute to 100 ml with the acid. Retain ethyl acetate layer. Dilute 5 ml of the acidic solution of both sample and standard to 25 ml with 0.1 N hydrochloric acid and measure the absorbance of both the solutions at about 264 nm using 0.1 N acid as blank and calculate the results.

Betamethasone

Standard solution

0.25 mg/ml of betamethasone in ethyl acetate.

Sample solution

Ethyl acetate layer retained during assay of dexchlorpheniramine is diluted with ethyl acetate to get concentration of 25 mcg/ml in respect of betamethasone. Add 5 g of anhydrous sodium sulphate to both the solutions to remove traces of moisture in the organic layer.

Pipette 10 ml of the sample solution (25 mcg/ml) and 1 ml of standard solution (250 mcg/ml), evaporate carefully on water bath and proceed with isoniazid reagent method as described in formulation 4 of the chapter on antifungal and anti-infective preparations.

Formulation 41

Chlorpheniramine maleate, Trithioparamethoxyphenylpropene

ESTIMATION

Chlorpheniramine maleate

Standard solution

30 mcg/ml of chlorpheniramine maleate in water.

Sample solution

Transfer accurately weighed quantity of the powdered sample equivalent to 10 mg of chlorpheniramine maleate to 100 ml volumetric flask. Add about 50 ml of water, shake vigorously and make up the volume. Further dilutions are done appropriately with water to get a concentration of 30 mcg/ml.

Measure the extinction of both the solutions at maxima at about 262 nm and deduce the results by comparison. Alternatively, follow the cyanogen bromide method.

Trithio-p-methoxyphenylpropene

Standard solution

10 mcg/ml of trithioparamethoxyphenylpropene in methanol.

Sample solution

Remove the sugar coating (if coated) of the tablets with wet cotton. Dry the core and determine average weight of the core. Transfer accurately weighed quantity of the powdered sample equivalent to 10 mg of the substance to a dry 100 ml volumetric flask. Add about 50 ml of methanol and dissolve by slight warming in water-bath. Make up the volume and filter. The filtrate is appropriately diluted with methanol to get a final concentration of 10 mcg/ml.

Measure the absorption of both the sample and standard solutions at about 435 nm using methanol as blank and calculate the results by comparison.

Note

1. The compound is orange-coloured; can be directly estimated in visible range (λ_{max} 435 nm).
2. It is more soluble in chloroform, pyridine and dioxan.
3. Syn.: Anethol trithione, anethole dithiothione.

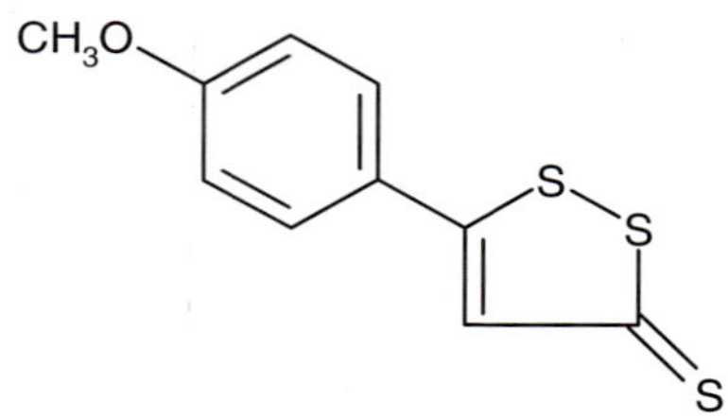

Trithio-p-methoxyphenylpropene

Note

The methoxyphenyl moiety of the molecule can undergo bromination, being electrophilic substitution, and simultaneously sulphur is oxidized to sulphate which can be estimated gravimetrically as barium sulphate.

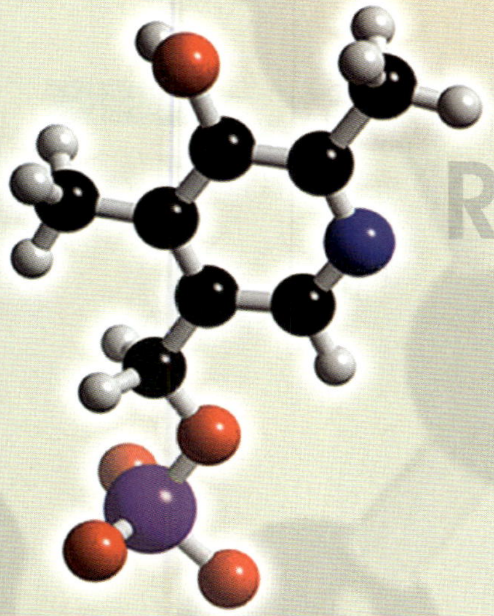

Reaction Mechanism

12

Bronchospasm Relaxants (Anti-Asthma)

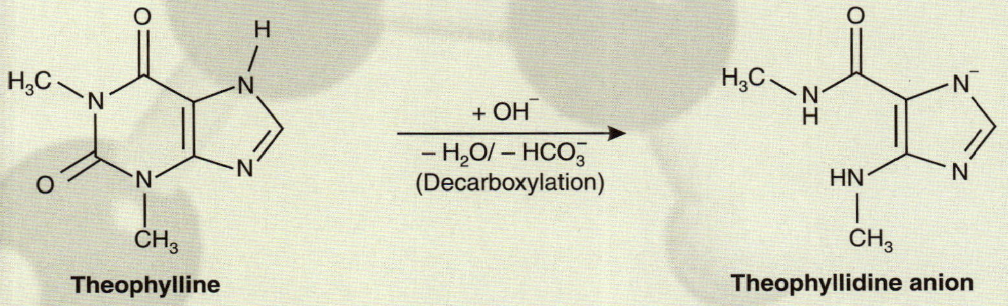

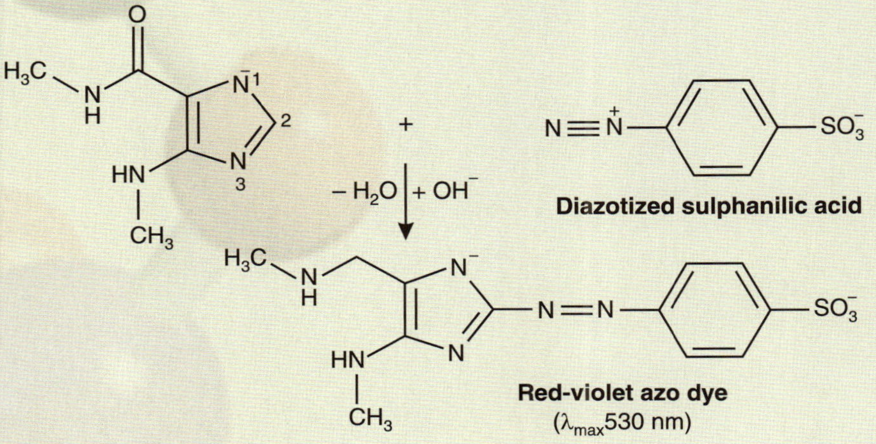

Formulation 1

Theophylline, Ephedrine hydrochloride, Phenobarbitone

ESTIMATION

METHOD A

Theophylline

METHOD 1

Standard solution

50 mcg/ml of theophylline in phosphate buffer pH 7 and 9 separately.

Sample solution

Weigh accurately a quantity of powdered tablets or capsule material equivalent to 50 mg of theophylline. Extract and adjust to 50 ml with water, filter.

(a) Transfer 5 ml of the filtrate and adjust to 100 ml with phosphate buffer pH 7.0.

(b) Transfer 5 ml of the filtrate and adjust to 100 ml with phosphate buffer pH 9.0.

Procedure

Measure the extinction of the sample and standard solutions in pH 9 buffer using corresponding solutions in pH 7.0 buffer as blank at 275 nm and calculate the results.

Note

Large amount of caffeine, if present, gives low recovery of the compound.

METHOD 2

Standard solution

Weigh accurately 60 mg of anhydrous theophylline, add 5 ml of 1 N hydrochloric acid and 25 ml of water. Shake well for 15 min and dilute to 100 ml with water. Dilute the resultant solution further to get 6 mcg/ml solution.

Sample solution

Weigh accurately a quantity of powdered tablets or capsule material equivalent to 60 mg of anhydrous theophylline and process as per standard solution.

Procedure

Measure the extinction of both the standard and sample solutions at absorption maximum at about 271 nm using water as blank. Calculate the results by comparison.

Ephedrine hydrochloride

METHOD 1

Reagents

1. Saturated solution of sodium bicarbonate in water.
2. 2% w/v solution of sodium metaperiodate in water.

Standard solution

40 mcg/ml of ephedrine hydrochloride in water.

Sample solution

Accurately weigh a quantity of the sample equivalent to 20 mg of ephedrine hydrochloride, extract and dilute with water to get 40 mcg/ml solution.

Procedure

To 3 ml each of the sample and standard solutions, add 1 ml of saturated solution of sodium bicarbonate. After evolution of carbon dioxide has stopped, add 1 ml of sodium metaperiodate solution. Allow to stand for 15 minutes, add 20 ml of n-hexane, shake well and allow the layers to separate. Measure the extinction of the organic layer at about 242 nm using n-hexane as blank. Calculate the results by comparison.

Probable Reaction Mechanism

Periodate has selective oxidizing action upon compounds having hydroxyl group and an amino group attached to adjacent carbon atoms i.e. they bring about the cleavage of the carbon-carbon bond. This is known as Malaprade reaction. Applying the above concept in case of ephedrine, the cleavage takes place resulting in the formation of benzaldehyde as shown below which is responsible for UV absorption at 242 nm.

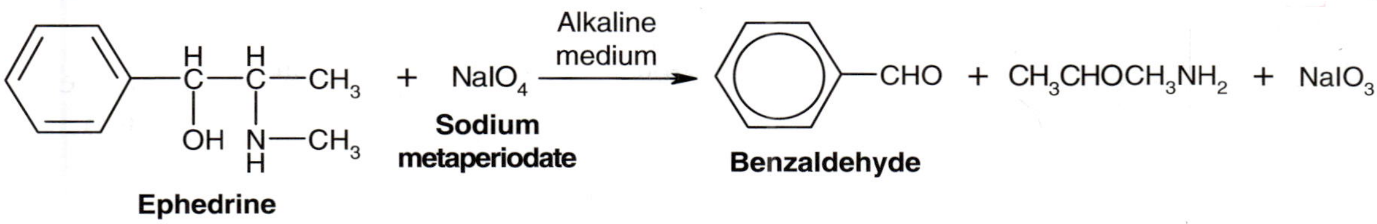

Note

Similar reaction is possible with oxidizing agents such as $K_3Fe(CN)_6$ or $KMnO_4$ leading to oxidative breakdown of side chain resulting in different fragments.

METHOD 2

Reagents

1. 0.2 N disodium acid phosphate adjusted to pH 9.5 with 0.5 N sodium hydroxide (buffer).
2. Picronolic acid: 26.5 mcg/ml in ethylene dichloride.

Standard solution

1 mg/ml of ephedrine (base) in water.

Sample solution

Weigh accurately appropriate quantity of the sample and extract with water to get 1 mg/ml of ephedrine (base).

Extraction

To 1 ml of standard and sample solutions add 5 ml of buffer solution, pH 9.5 and extract with the two 4 ml portions of ethylene dichloride, passing each separated organic layer through 2 g of anhydrous sodium sulphate supported in a funnel over a cotton plug. Dilute the filtrate to 10 ml with ethylene dichloride.

Procedure

Pipette 1 ml of above ethylene dichloride solutions standard and sample to a dry 5 ml volumetric flask, add 1 ml of picrolonic acid solution and dilute to volume with ethylene dichloride. Measure absorbance of both the solutions at maximum at about 362 nm. The method obeys Beer's law in the range of 2-20 mcg/ml. Phenobarbitone normally present in the formulation is eliminated during course of above alkaline extraction procedure.

Picronolic acid is a reagent for alkaloids. It forms salt with nitrogenous base such as ephedrine, the salt being soluble in ethylene dichloride. It behaves like picric acid. In higher concentrations of the alkaloid this can serve as a gravimetric method.

Probable Reaction Mechanism

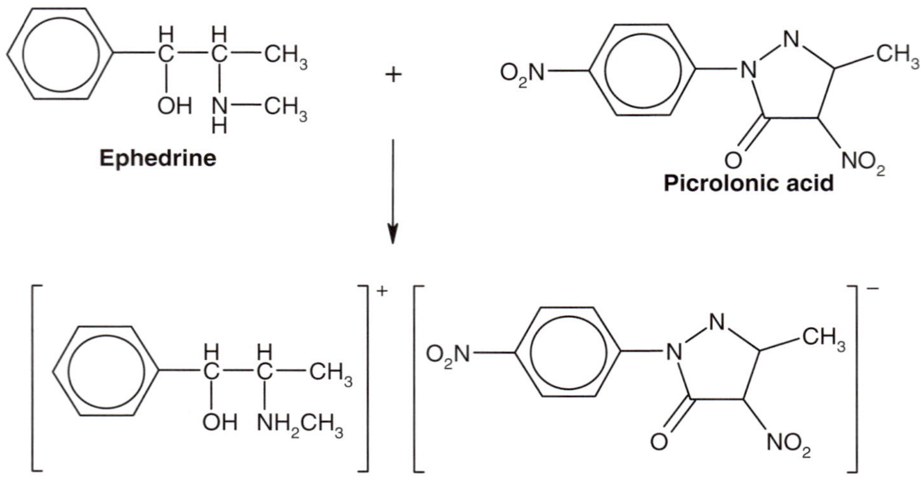

(λ_{max} 362 nm)

Note

As both picronolic acid, alkaloid (base) complex are soluble in organic solvent, hence the use of ethylene dichloride for colorimetric method.

Reference

1. Pharmaceutical Analysis by T. Higuchi & E. Brochmann-Hanssen, p. 378.
2. Pharmaceutical Chemistry (Vol. 2) by H.J. Roth, p. 334.

Theophylline

On heating theophylline with aqueous sodium hydroxide, sodium hydroxide being strong nucleophilic agent it attacks at C-2 of the pyrimidine ring causing ring opening followed by decarboxylation to yield theophyllidine which reacts with diazotized sulphanilic acid to give violet-red azo dye (Pauly reaction).

Probable Reaction Mechanism

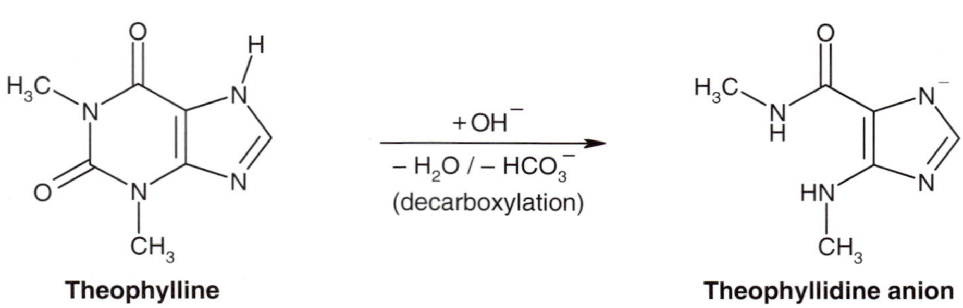

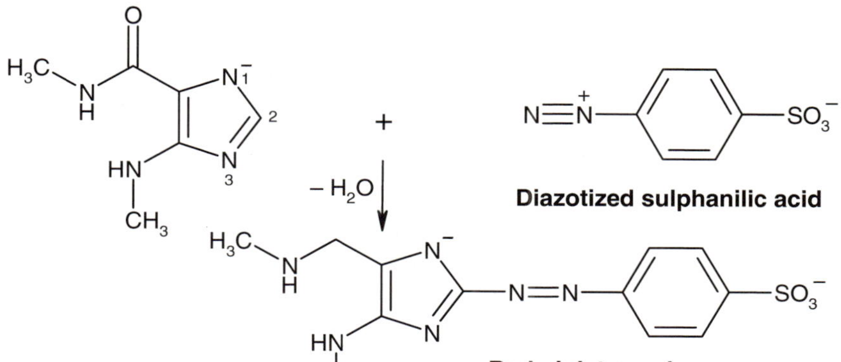

Red-violet azo dye
(λ_{max} 530 nm)

Note

Both theophylline and aminophylline give similar reaction.

Reference

Pharmaceutical Chemistry (Vol. 2) by H.J. Roth, p. 598.

Shabouri et al. (1989) have described spectrophotometric method based on their coupling with diazotized p-nitroaniline in alkaline medium giving yellow azo dye with λ_{max} 440 nm (theophylline) and 410 nm (aminophylline). In the proposed method, the authors have suggested to add alkali before addition of diazotized nitroaniline to replace the active hydrogen atom at position 7 with sodium, otherwise triazo derivative so formed is unstable.

Note

The diazonium salt directly couples with the compound without prior hydrolysis.

Probable Reaction Mechanism

The coupling involves proton-eliminating reaction of a diazonium salt with a compound having an active hydrogen atom. However, theophylline couples at position 2 with diazonium salt as it has pronounced nucleophilic character.

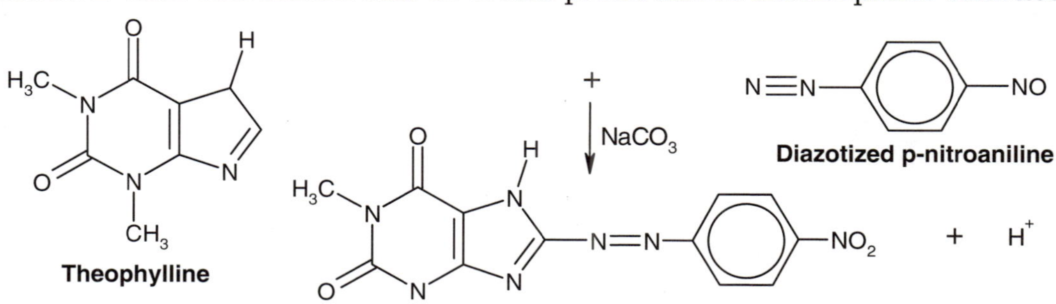

Coupled derivative of theophylline and aminophylline
(λ_{max} 440 and 410 nm)

Note

Ephedrine and phenobarbitone did not interfere.

Reference

S.R. El-Shabouri, S.A. Hussein & S.E. Emara, *Talanta*, **36(12)**, 1288-1290, 1989.

The compound also couples with 2,6-dichloroquinone chlorimide (Gibbs reagent) in alkaline medium to give deep blue merocyanine dye.

Probable Reaction Mechanism

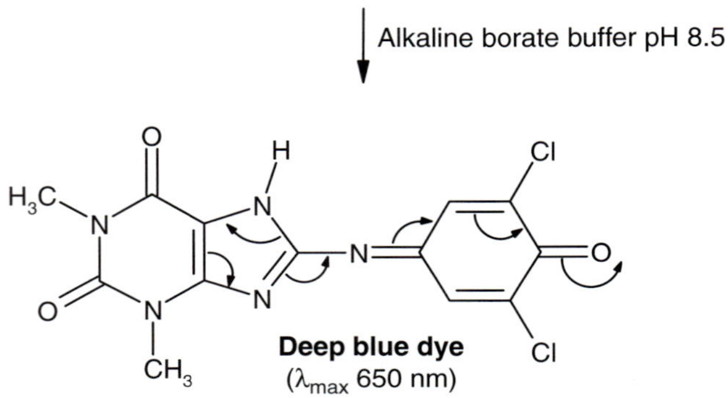

Note

1. Because of the instability of the reagent, this method is not preferred.
2. Theophylline can be directly titrated with NaOH in non-aqueous medium such as DMF, 'N' at position 1 imparting acidic character to the molecule. Xanthine derivatives such as theophylline is oxidized by chloramine-T in the presence of hydrochloric acid and then couples with ammonia to give purple-red salt of purpuric acid (murexide) which has fluorescence properties as well (λ_{ex} 313 nm; λ_{em} 390 nm).

Probable Reaction Mechanism

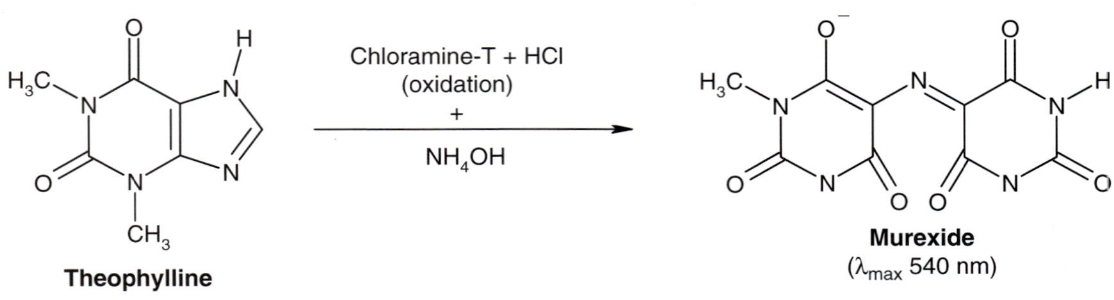

Reference

Thin Layer Chromatography: Reagents and Detection Methods (Vol. 1b), by Jork, Funk & Fischer, p. 174.

Saraswathi et al. have employed ferric chloride as oxidizing agent. Fe^{2+} so produced is coupled with 2,2′-bis-pyridine to give a coloured complex (λ_{max} 522 nm).

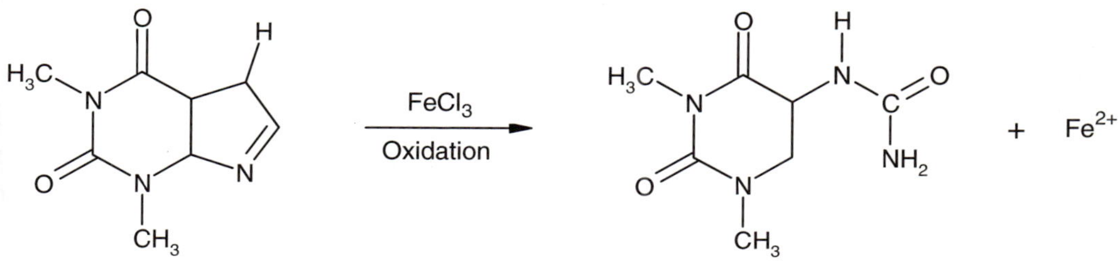

Theophylline

$$Fe^{2+} + 3\ 2,2'\text{-bis-pyridine} \longrightarrow \text{Fe - bis-pyridine complex } (\lambda_{max}\ 442\ \text{nm})$$

Note

For structures, see the text under different formulations.

Reference

D. Saraswathi, G.P. Gigsi, Aruna Ajithadas & A. Suresh Jerad, *J. Pharm. Research*, **9(1)**, 29-30, 2010.

METHOD B

Theophylline

Standard solution

Weigh accurately about 140 mg of pure theophylline (anhydrous), transfer into a 500 ml volumetric flask containing 200 ml of distilled water and mix. Add few drops of methyl red solution, acidify with 1 N sulphuric acid and heat in a steam bath to effect solution. Cool to room temperature and dilute to volume with water.

Sample solution

Weigh accurately a quantity of powdered sample equivalent to about 140 mg of theophylline. Add about 200 ml of water, few drops of methyl red solution and acidify with 1 N sulphuric acid. Place the flask in a steam bath until the tablet base has completely dissolved (about 1 h is required for waxy base).

Transfer the hot solution to a mechanical shaker and shake for 30 min. After shaking, allow the solution to cool to room temperature, dilute to 500 ml with water and mix well. Filter the mixture through a G_4 sintered glass funnel, discarding first 15 ml of the filtrate.

Note

Retain the remaining clear sample filtrate for the estimation of ephedrine hydrochloride.

Procedure

Dilute separately 15 ml of the clear sample filtrate and 20 ml of the standard solution to 100 ml water and mix well. Further dilute 10 ml of each solution to 100 ml with water. Concomitantly determine the absorbance of the sample and the standard solutions at the wavelength of maximum absorbance, at about 271 nm and calculate the results by comparison.

Ephedrine hydrochloride

Reagents

1. Ammoniacal copper sulphate solution : Weigh 50 g of ammonium acetate and 0.5 g of cupric sulphate, pentahydrate. Transfer to a 250 ml volumetric flask containing 75 ml of water and mix until solution is complete, cool. Dissolve 25 g of sodium hydroxide in 50 ml of water, cool, add this solution and 50 ml of ammonia solution to the above volumetric flask, mix. Dilute to volume with water and mix thoroughly (prepare fresh bi-weekly).
2. Carbon disulphide-benzene solution : Mix 5 ml of carbon disulphide with 95 ml of benzene, prepare fresh. Caution : Prepare solution in a well-ventilated area.
3. Acetic acid solution : Transfer 40 ml of glacial acetic acid into a 100 ml volumetric flask, carefully dilute to volume with water and mix thoroughly.

Standard solution

Weigh accurately, about 115 mg of ephedrine hydrochloride into a volumetric flask, add about 400 ml of water and mix. Add a few drops of methyl red solution, acidify with 1 N sulphuric acid, dilute to 1000 ml with distilled water and mix thoroughly, prepare fresh.

Procedure

Pipette 5 ml of the clear sample filtrate retained in estimation of theophylline under method B into a 100 ml volumetric flask and 5 ml of the standard solution into a second 100 ml volumetric flask. Add 15 ml of water to each flask, mix well, add 2 ml of the ammoniacal copper sulphate solution and 20 ml of the carbon disulphide-benzene solution into each flask. Mix well, stopper tightly and heat each flask in a water-bath at 45°C for 5 minutes. Remove from the bath and shake mechanically for 10 minutes. Add 2 ml of acetic acid and shake for another 5 minutes. Decant the benzene layers into separate small glass-stoppered flasks each containing a small amount of anhydrous sodium sulphate. Concomitantly determine the absorbance of benzene layer of the sample and standard solutions at about 430 nm using benzene as blank and calculate the results.

Note

In solid dosage formulations, if lactose is present, it is likely to interfere because of its reducing action on copper sulphate. In such case, the alkaloid should be first extracted with methylene chloride from ammoniacal solution. Further, while concentrating organic layer, to avoid loss of ephedrine, add 1 ml of 1% benzoic acid solution.

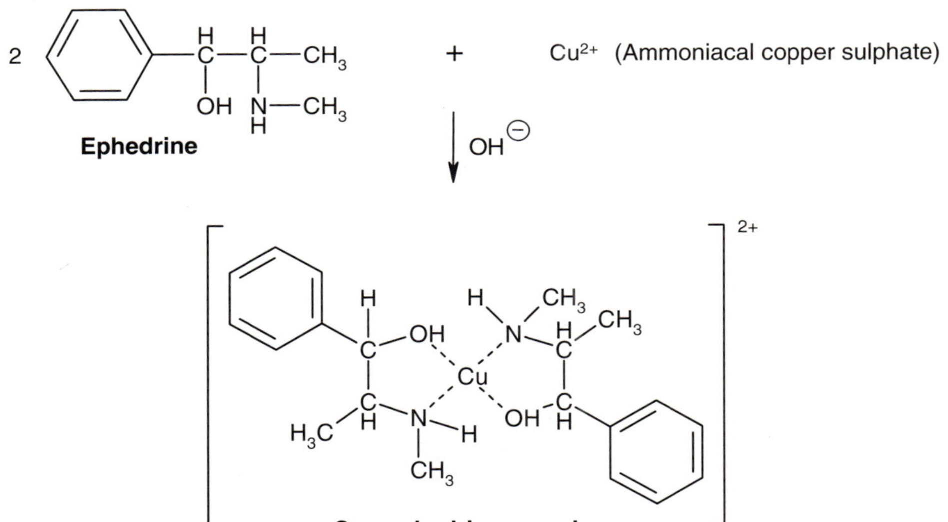

Cu - ephedrine complex
(λ_{max} 430 nm)

Probable Reaction Mechanism

Involves formation of coloured Cu chelates with ephedrine. The reaction is also known as Chen-Kao reaction. This reaction is specific for phenylalkylamines with neighbouring amino and hydroxy groups.

Reference

Pharmaceutical Chemistry (Vol. 2) by H.J. Roth, 1991, p. 374.

METHOD C

Estimation of Ephedrine hydrochloride

Reagents

Bromothymol blue solution: Dissolve 6.576 g of disodium hydrogen phosphate in about 200 ml of water, add 1.0 g of bromothymol blue and warm to dissolve. It is important to ensure that the solution is absolutely complete at this stage. Dissolve 1.814 g of potassium dihydrogen phosphate in about 50 ml of water and mix the two solutions. Dilute to 1000 ml with water.

Standard solution

10 mcg/ml of ephedrine hydrochloride in water.

Sample solution

Accurately weigh a quantity of the powdered sample on a filter paper, extract the powder with three 50 ml portions of hot methanol and three 50 ml portions of hot water. Wash the residue down into the cone of the filter paper with cold water and allow to drain. Pierce the filter paper and wash the solid into a 500 ml volumetric flask with 1 N hydrochloric acid. Ensure that no trace of the residue remains on the filter paper. Stopper the flask and keep for 4 h at room temperature with frequent shaking. After 4 h make up the volume to 500 ml with 1 N hydrochloric acid. Dilute 25 ml of the filtrate with water to 200 ml in a volumetric flask (10 mcg/ml of ephedrine).

Procedure

Pipette 10 ml aliquots of sample and standard solutions into 125 ml separating funnels. From this stage, all the separators receive identical treatment. To each separator add one drop of thymophthalein solution and sufficient sodium hydroxide solution (20% w/v) drop by drop to just produce the full blue colour of the indicator. Add exactly 20 ml of benzene and shake well for two minutes. Discard the aqueous layer. To the benzene layer add 2 ml of bromothymol blue solution and shake well for one minute. Allow to stand, discard the aqueous layer and centrifuge the benzene layer to clarify. Determine the optical density of clarified solution each of the test and standard solutions at 405 nm using benzene as blank and calculate the results. This method is based on air-pair complex.

Reference

P.B. Marshall & E.W. Rogers, *Biochemical J.*, **39**, 258, 1941.

Phenobarbitone

Reagents

1. Barium hydroxide saturated aqueous solution.

2. Buffer solution, pH 9.5: Dissolve 6.19 g boric acid and 7.46 g potassium chloride in water and dilute to 1000 ml. To 500 ml of this solution add from a buret 34.4 ml of 1 N sodium hydroxide, dilute to 1000 ml with water and mix well. If necessary, adjust the pH to 9.5 with 1 N sodium hydroxide or with the remaining boric acid - potassium chloride buffer.

Procedure

Weigh accurately a quantity of the powdered sample equivalent to 100 mg of phenobarbitone into a 100 ml volumetric flask. Weigh accurately about 160 mg of phenobarbitone standard into a 200 ml volumetric flask. Add 50 ml of saturated barium hydroxide solution to the flask containing the sample and 100 ml of saturated barium hydroxide solution to the flask containing the phenobarbitone standard. Shake each flask mechanically for 30 min, then dilute each to volume with water and mix well. Filter each solution separately through Whatman No. 40 filter paper, discarding first 20 ml of each filtrate. Pipette 20 ml of the clear sample and standard filtrate into a suitable separator. Cautiously, add 10 ml of hydrochloric acid to each separator and then extract each solution with three 50 ml portions of ether. Wash each ether extract with three 10 ml portions of water. Combined ether extracts of both sample and standard are evaporated to dryness on a steam-bath using small pieces of porcelain to avoid bumping. Dissolve the residue in 50 ml of buffer solution, pH 9.5, with heating. Cool the resulting solutions and transfer quantitatively into separate 200 ml volumetric flasks. Dilute each solution to volume with buffer solution, pH 9.5, mix well and filter, discarding first 20 ml of the filtrate from each. Dilute 10 ml of the clear sample and the standard filtrate to 100 ml with buffer solution, pH 9.5 and mix well. Concomitantly determine the absorbance of the sample and the standard solutions in a suitable spectrophotometer at the wavelength of maximum absorbance, about 240 nm, using buffer solution as blank.

Note

On acidification, phenobarbitone gets precipitated which is extracted into ether. The residue obtained on evaporation of ether layer is taken up in alkaline buffer and used for spectrophotometric measurements.

One of the best identification reactions for phenobarbitone was originally proposed by “Zwikker reaction”. This reaction is positive for barbiturates not substituted at the nitrogen. It forms coloured complex with Co(2) in alkaline medium and the complex is stabilized as diamino complex [(barbiturate)$_2$Co] by isopropylamine and excess of amine also helps in deprotonation of the barbituric acid.

Probable Reaction Mechanism

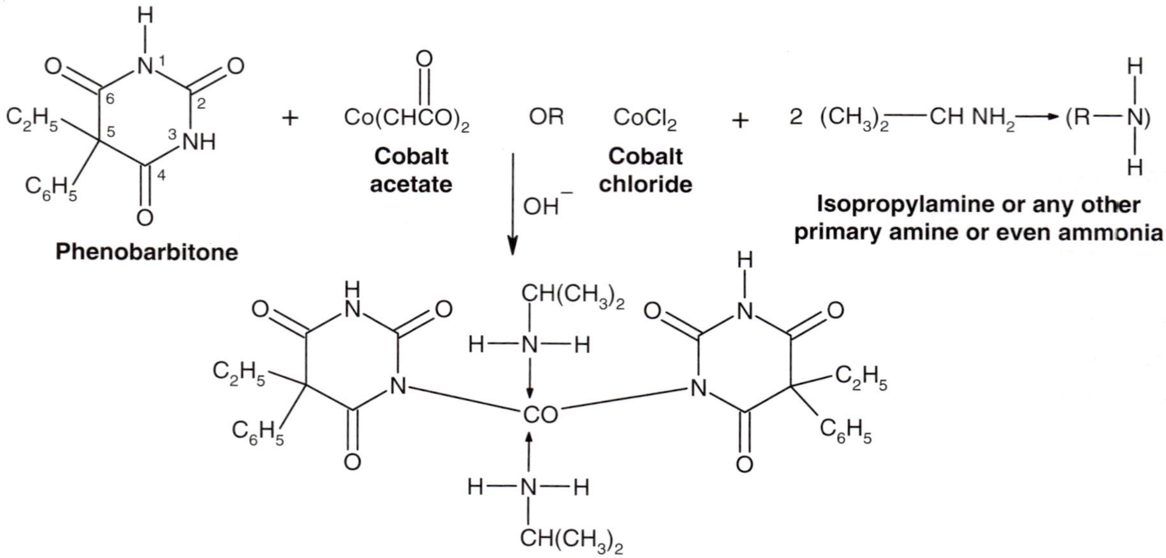

Diamino cobalt complex Co(barb)$_2$
(λ_{max} 570 nm)

Note

The reaction given below is more sensitive when tetrahedral Co(II) complex is formed due to greater molar extinction coefficient.

To 2 ml of each sample/standard solution (1 mg/ml in methanol) add 2 ml of isopropylamine and 2 ml of cobalt acetate solution (0.125% in methanol) and measure the absorbance at 570 nm against reagent blank. In the presence of pyridine, phenobarbitone forms coloured complex with $CuSO_4$ as under.

Probable Reaction Mechanism

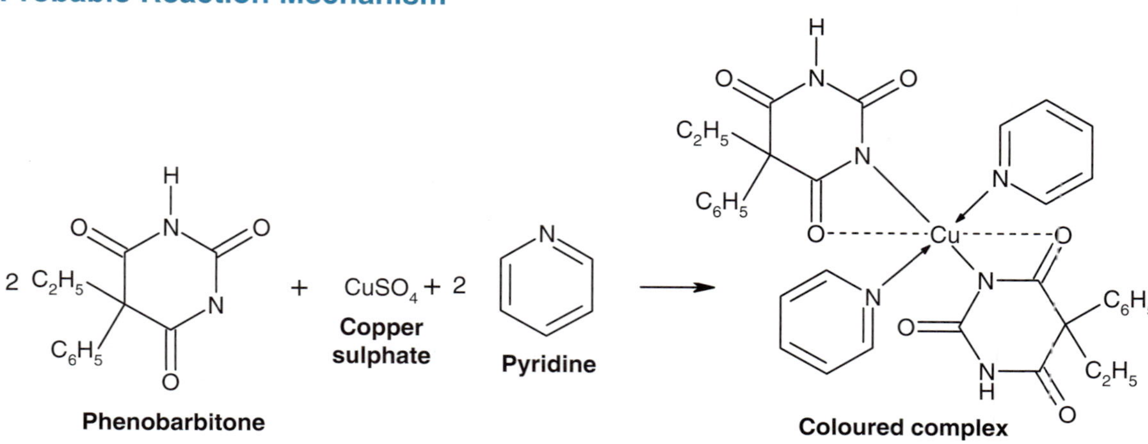

Note

Barbiturate complex is soluble in chloroform and not the blue copper - pyridine complex. So, for better sensitivity, the complex can be extracted into chloroform for spectrophotometric measurements.

Reference

Pharmaceutical Chemistry (Vol. 2) by H.J. Roth, p. 314.

Phenobarbitone, a barbituric derivative with N-1 and N-3 being unsubstituted, imparts acidic character and can be titrated with sodium hydroxide. The compound with phenyl ring at C-5 can give rise to orange-yellow nitroso derivative ($NaNO_2$ + H_2SO_4) and reaction with sulphuric acid/formaldehyde yields fluorescent derivative.

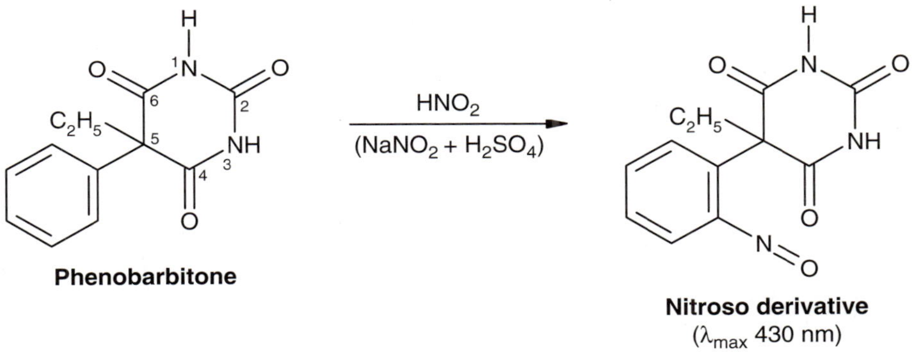

Formulation 2

Dihydroxypropyltheophylline, Phenobarbitone, Chlorpheniramine maleate, Ephedrine hydrochloride

ESTIMATION

Sample

Shake an accurately weighed quantity of powdered sample equivalent to 200 mg of theophylline with 50 ml of ether. Filter, repeat the process 6-7 times. The residue thus obtained is dissolved in water to make 100 ml. This solution A is used for estimation of various ingredients of the formulation.

Dihydroxypropyltheophylline

Transfer 0.5 ml of the sample solution (A) to a 100 ml volumetric flask and make up the volume to 100 ml with water. Measure the extinction at 273 nm and calculate the contents of dihydroxypropyltheophylline, taking 361 as the value of A 1%, 1 cm at the maximum at 273 nm.

Ephedrine hydrochloride

Reagents

1. Buffer solution, pH 10 : Dissolve 5.40 g of ammonium chloride in 50 ml water. Adjust the pH to 10.0 with ammonia solution and dilute to 100 ml with water.
2. 0.1% w/v solution of copper acetate in alcohol.
3. In a 50 ml volumetric flask, pipette out 10 ml of alcoholic solution of copper acetate, 5 ml carbon disulphide, 4 ml of glacial acetic acid and make up the volume to 50 ml with absolute alcohol.

Standard solution

80 mg of ephedrine hydrochloride is dissolved in 100 ml of distilled water.

Procedure

Appropriate volume of solution A containing 1.6 mg of ephedrine hydrochloride and 2 ml of standard solutions are taken in two separating funnels. To each, add 3 ml of 0.1 N hydrochloric acid, 10 ml buffer solution and 2 ml copper acetate solution. Mix well and allow to stand for 5 minutes. Add 15 ml chloroform and shake for one minute. Separate the chloroform layer, wash immediately with 20 ml of 0.1 N hydrochloric acid and filter through anhydrous sodium sulphate placed on filter paper into a 50 ml volumetric flask. Repeat the extraction with 15 ml, 10 ml and 10 ml portions of chloroform. Wash each chloroform extract with the same 20 ml 0.1 N hydrochloric acid and filter as described above. Adjust the combined extracts to 50 ml with chloroform. Measure the extinction of chloroform layer at 438 nm using chloroform as blank. Calculate the result by comparing with the standard. For reaction mechanism see formulation 1 of this chapter.

Phenobarbitone

Follow the method described under formulation 1 of this chapter using appropriate volume of solution A.

Chlorpheniramine maleate

Reagents

1. Dilute hydrochloric acid: Dilute 1 ml of hydrochloric acid to 20 ml with water.
2. 10% w/v silicotungstic acid solution in water, filter through G_4 sintered glass funnel before use.

Procedure

Shake an accurately weighed quantity of the powdered tablets equivalent to 20 mg of the substance with 50 ml of water and filter through filter paper. Repeat this process 3 to 4 times. To the filtrate, add 2 ml of dilute hydrochloric acid and boil. To the boiling solution, add 4 ml of silicotungstic acid solution. Boil for 5-10 minutes and filter through a tared G_4 sintered glass funnel. Wash the precipitate with boiling dilute hydrochloric acid and then twice with 5 ml of water. Dry the residue at 105°C to constant weight. Each g of the precipitate is equivalent to 0.2281 g of chlorpheniramine maleate.

Note

Silicotungstic acid ($SiO_2 \cdot 12WO_3 \cdot nH_2O$) is used as quantitative precipitant for alkaloids from acidic solutions. In general, acidic solution of the alkaloid is brought to boiling and silicotungstic acid is added to boiling solution, the precipitates are filtered and dried at 105-110°C and weighed. The experimentally determined gravimetric factor is taken for calculations. The general formula for calculations is:

$$(SiO_2 \cdot 12WO_3 \times \text{alkaloid} \cdot nH_2O)$$

This method is no longer favoured.

Formulation 3

Dried aluminium hydroxide gel, Ephedrine hydrochloride, Theophylline, Phenobarbitone

ESTIMATION

Aluminium hydroxide gel, as aluminium oxide

Sample solution

Weigh accurately powdered tablets equivalent to 0.2 g of aluminium hydroxide and transfer to 150 ml conical flask. Add approximately 2 ml of hydrochloric acid and 50 ml of water. Boil this solution for sometime, cool, make the volume to 100 ml with water, shake and filter.

Procedure

Pipette 25 ml of the above filtrate into a 250 ml conical flask and neutralise with sodium hydroxide solution. Follow the method 3 for estimation of aluminium hydroxide described under formulation 1 of the chapter on antacids.

Ephedrine hydrochloride

Reagent

1. 50% w/v solution of potassium carbonate in water.
2. 0.01 M H_2SO_4.
3. 0.05 M NaOH.

Procedure

Weigh accurately a quantity of sample equivalent to 50 mg of ephedrine in a dry 250 ml stoppered flask. Add 2 ml of potassium carbonate solution and 5 ml of water. Mix well and extract with five 30 ml portions of dichloromethane for fifteen minutes. Add approximately 2 g of gum tragacanth and again extract for five minutes. Filter the extract through cotton plug into a drug 250 ml conical flask. Wash the stoppered flask and funnel with sufficient dichloromethane. Add exactly 15 ml of 0.02 N sulphuric acid and separate the organic layer completely. Cool, add 2-3 drops of methyl red indicator and titrate against 0.05 N sodium hydroxide. Run a blank side by side. Each ml of 0.01 N sulphuric acid consumed is equivalent to 0.004033 g of ephedrine hydrochloride.

Note

On basification, the base is generated, extracted into organic layer and back extracted into acid. The method is based on acid-base titration i.e. on addition of sulphuric acid the generated base is converted to ephedrine sulphate. The excess acid is back titrated with sodium hydroxide to calculate the volume of acid consumed by the base.

Theophylline and phenobarbitone

Follow the method for estimation of theophylline and phenobarbitone described in formulation 1 of this chapter.

Formulation 4

Theophylline, Hydroxyzine hydrochloride, Ephedrine hydrochloride

ESTIMATION

Theophylline

Standard solution

7.5 mcg/ml of theophylline in 0.1 N sodium hydroxide.

Sample solution

Accurately weigh a quantity of powdered tablets or capsule material equivalent to 100 mg of theophylline. Add 100 ml of 0.1 N sodium hydroxide, shake for 5 min, and dilute to 200 ml with 0.1 N sodium hydroxide. Set aside for 10 min and filter through filter paper, discarding first 20-30 ml of the filtrate. Dilute 3 ml of the filtrate to 200 ml with 0.1 N sodium hydroxide.

Measure the extinction of both standard and sample solutions at the maxima at about 275 nm against 0.1 N sodium hydroxide as blank. Calculate the results by comparison (or calculate the results taking 650 as value of A 1%, 1 cm).

Hydroxyzine hydrochloride

Standard solution

15 mcg/ml of hydroxyzine hydrochloride in 0.1 N hydrochloric acid.

Sample solution

Weigh accurately a quantity of powdered material equivalent to 15 mg of hydroxyzine hydrochloride. Shake with 50 ml of chloroform for 60 min and dilute to 100 ml with chloroform. To 20 ml of the chloroform extract, add 20 ml of 1 N sodium hydroxide, shake, separate chloroform layer and pass through anhydrous sodium sulphate. Extract the alkaline layer with further 20 ml of chloroform. Combine chloroform layers and adjust to 50 ml with chloroform. Evaporate 10 ml of the chloroform layer to dryness, cool and dissolve in 0.1 N hydrochloric acid to produce 50 ml (12 mcg/ml).

Measure the extinction of standard and sample solutions at maximum at about 232 nm using 0.1 N hydrochloric acid as blank. Calculate the results by comparison.

The drug forms ion-pair complex with different dyes: bromophenol blue (pH 2.6—phthalate buffer), bromocresol green (pH 3.5—phthalate buffer), methyl orange (pH 4.5—acetate buffer). All the complexes are extractable into chloroform and have absorption maxima at about 420 nm.

Note

Vit. B_1, vit. B_6 and meclozine hydrochloride do not interfere in this method.

Reference

R.T. Sane, C.H. Thambare, P.G. Anaokar & A.D. Pandit, *Indian Drugs*, **18(8)**, 295-298, 1981.

Ephedrine hydrochloride

Reagents

1. 10% v/v methyl alcohol in water.
2. 10% v/v acetic acid in water.
3. 0.1% w/v solution of sodium bicarbonate in water.
4. Cupric chloride reagent : To 60 mg of cupric chloride, add 125 ml of water and adjust to 250 ml with pyridine.
5. Carbon disulphide-pyridine reagent : Mix 25 ml of pyridine with 65 ml of isopropyl alcohol. Immediately prior to use, add 35 ml of carbon disulphide to above mixture and mix well.

Standard solution

Weigh accurately 70 mg of pure ephedrine hydrochloride, anhydrous and dissolve in water to make 100 ml. Dilute 10 ml of this solution to 25 ml with sodium bicarbonate solution.

Sample solution

Weigh accurately a quantity of powdered material equivalent to 70 mg of ephedrine hydrochloride and shake for 15 minutes with 100 ml of 10% v/v methyl alcohol. Filter, discard first few ml and dilute 10 ml of the filtrate to 25 ml with sodium bicarbonate solution.

Procedure

To 3 ml each of sample and standard solutions, add 10 ml of carbon disulphide-pyridine reagent and then in succession, add to each 5 ml of cupric chloride reagent, 6 ml of 10% acetic acid, swirling gently after each addition. Then, add

10 ml of benzene and shake for 2-3 times. Collect benzene layer and dilute to 25 ml with isopropyl alcohol. After 35 minutes, read the absorbance of both standard and sample solutions at about 440 nm and calculate the results by comparison.

The compound forms chelate with Cu(II). For detailed reaction mechanism, see formulation 1 of this chapter.

Formulation 5

Meprobamate, Papaverine hydrochloride, Phenobarbitone

ESTIMATION

Meprobamate

Reagents

1. Acetone-glacial acetic acid mixture (3 : 1 v/v).
2. 1% w/v solution of p-dimethylaminobenzaldehyde (PDAB) in benzene.
3. Antimony trichloride-acetic anhydride reagent: 4 parts of antimony trichloride (25% w/v in chloroform) and one part of acetic anhydride are mixed.

Standard solution

50 mcg/ml of meprobamate in acetone.

Sample solution

Weigh accurately a quantity of powdered tablets equivalent to 100 mg of meprobamate. Add 50 ml acetone, shake for 2 minutes and dilute to 100 ml with acetone. Dilute the resulting solution appropriately with acetone to get 50 mcg/ml.

Procedure

Evaporate separately 1 ml each of sample and standard solutions on water bath, cool and add 0.5 ml of acetone-acetic acid reagent, 0.5 ml of p-dimethylaminobenzaldehyde solution and 4 ml of antimony reagent. Place the tubes in water bath maintained at 50°C for 10 minutes. Shake, cool in ice bath and dilute to 10 ml with benzene. Measure the absorbance of both the solutions at about 540 nm using benzene as blank. Deduce the results by comparison.

Probable Reaction Mechanism

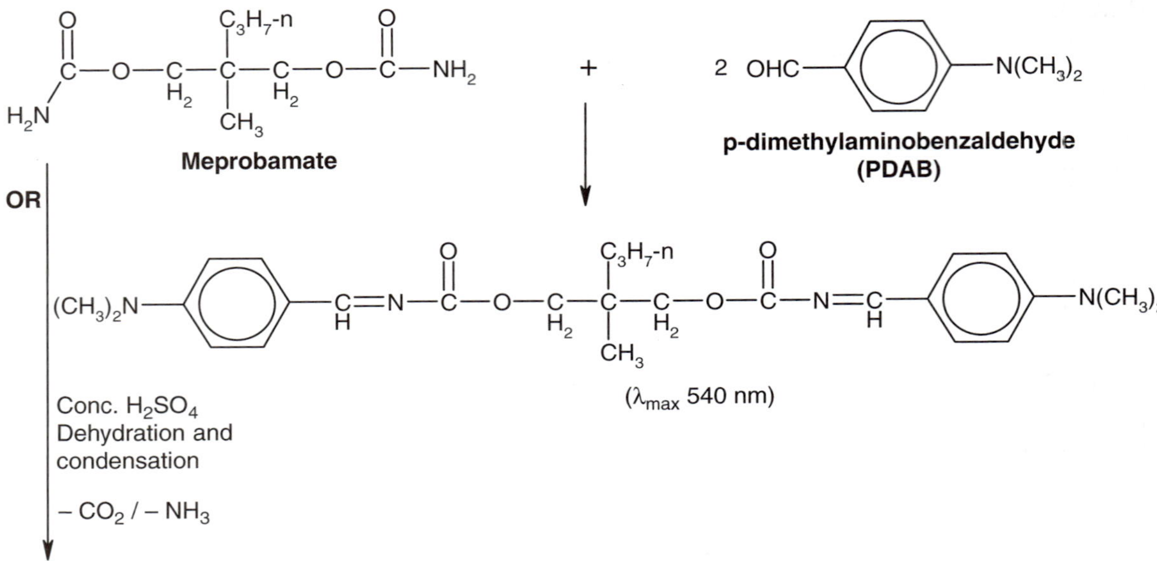

In the presence of sulphuric acid, there is dehydration leading to formation of cyclopentenyl carbenium ion which condenses with PDAB to give coloured product.

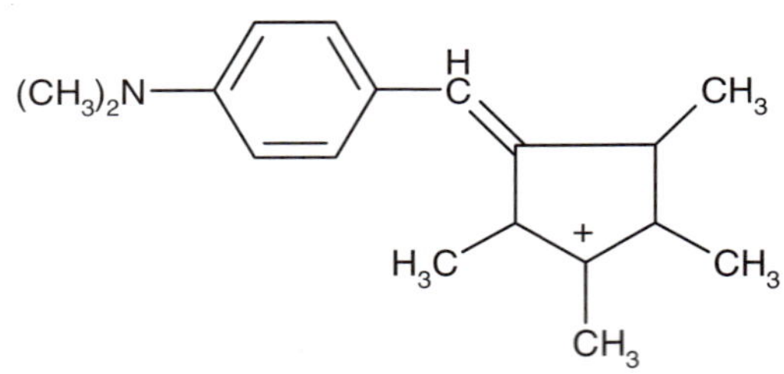

On heating with ethanolic potassium hydroxide, cyanate is formed which forms coloured complex with Co^{2+}.

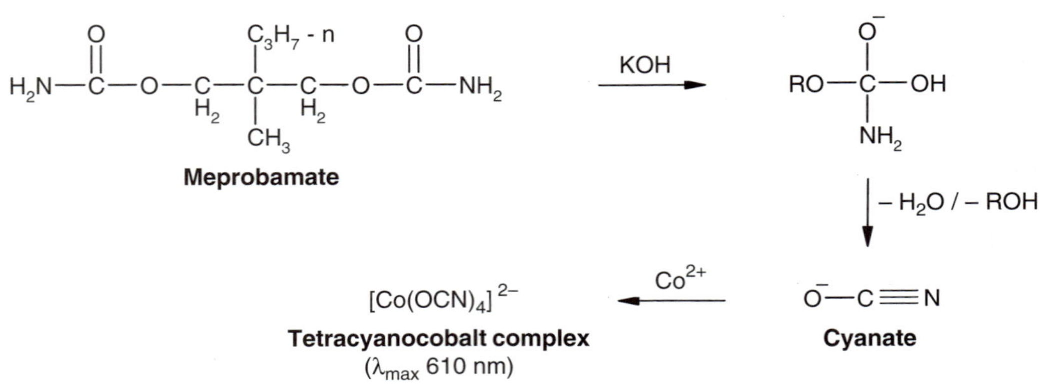

Reference

Pharmaceutical Chemistry (Vol. 2) by H.J. Roth, p. 294.

Papaverine hydrochloride

Weigh sample accurately equivalent to 50 mg of papaverine hydrochloride, add 40 ml of 1 N hydrochloric acid, shake and dilute to 50 ml with 1 N hydrochloric acid. Keep at room temperature for 60 min and filter. Dilute the filtrate appropriately with 1 N hydrochloric acid to get 15 mcg/ml solution. Measure the extinction at 310 nm and calculate the results using 228 as value of A 1%, 1 cm at 310 nm.

Alternatively, papaverine is first reduced by heating with zinc + HCl to give product with secondary amine which interacts with the reagent fluoranil (tetrafluoro-p-benzaquinone) as explained below.

Probable Reaction Mechanism

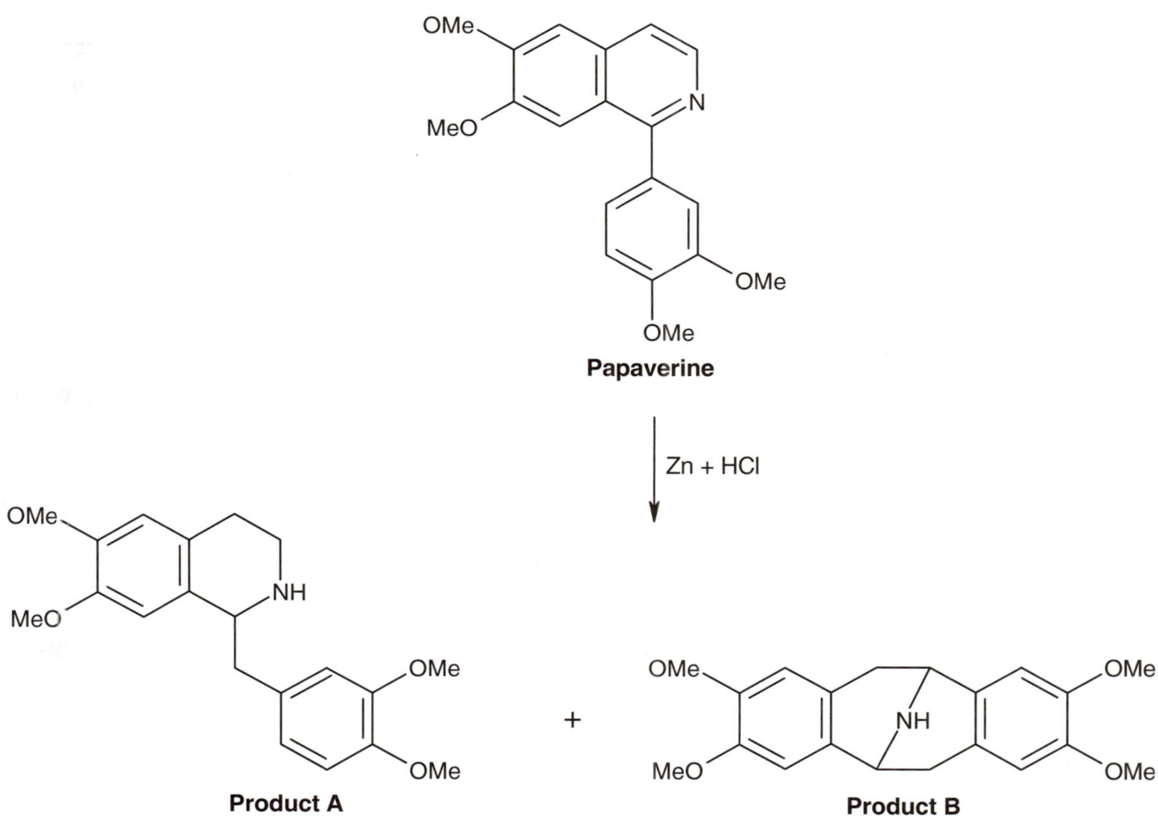

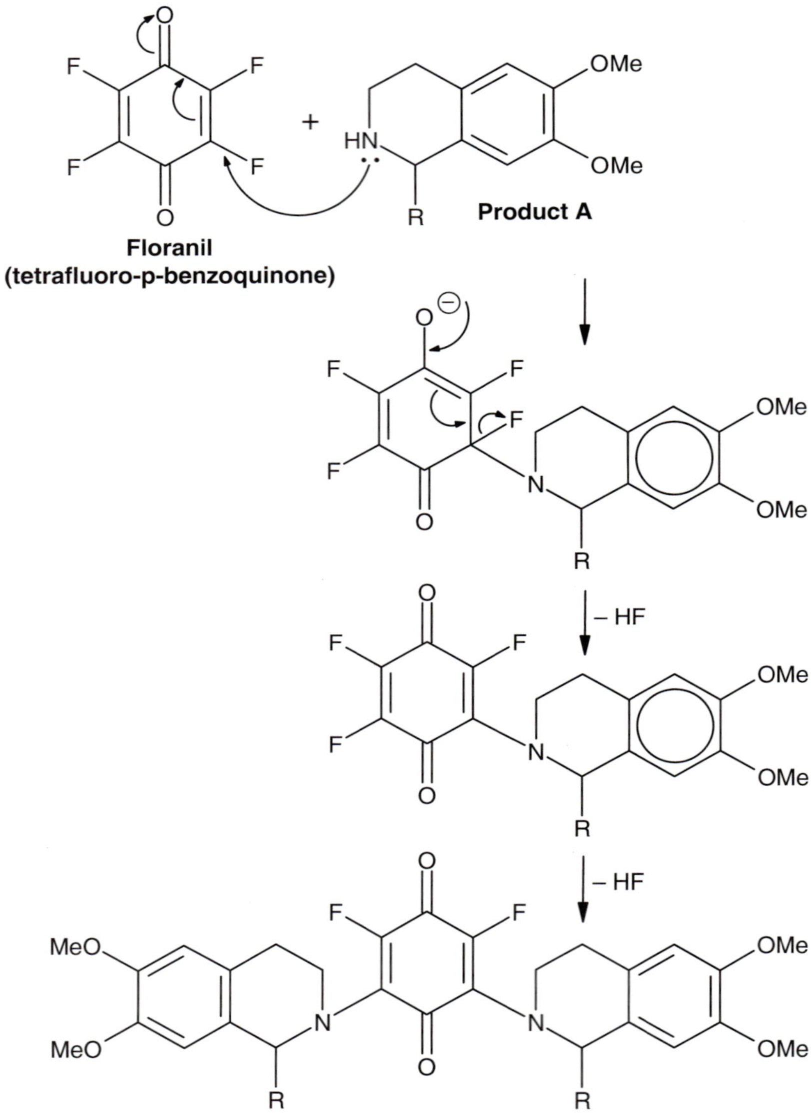

Reference

1. Organic Chemistry (Vol. 2) by I.L. Finar, p. 74.
2. Pharmaceutical Chemistry (Vol. 2) by H.J. Roth, 1991, p. 108.

By heating with concentrated sulphuric acid it gives pale violet colour. It is sulphonated at C-6 of the benzyl group due to action of sulphuric acid giving an intramolecular compound with violet colour. By further heating both —OCH_3 groups are demethylated and two phenolic —OH form dark green complex with Fe(III).

Probable Reaction Mechanism

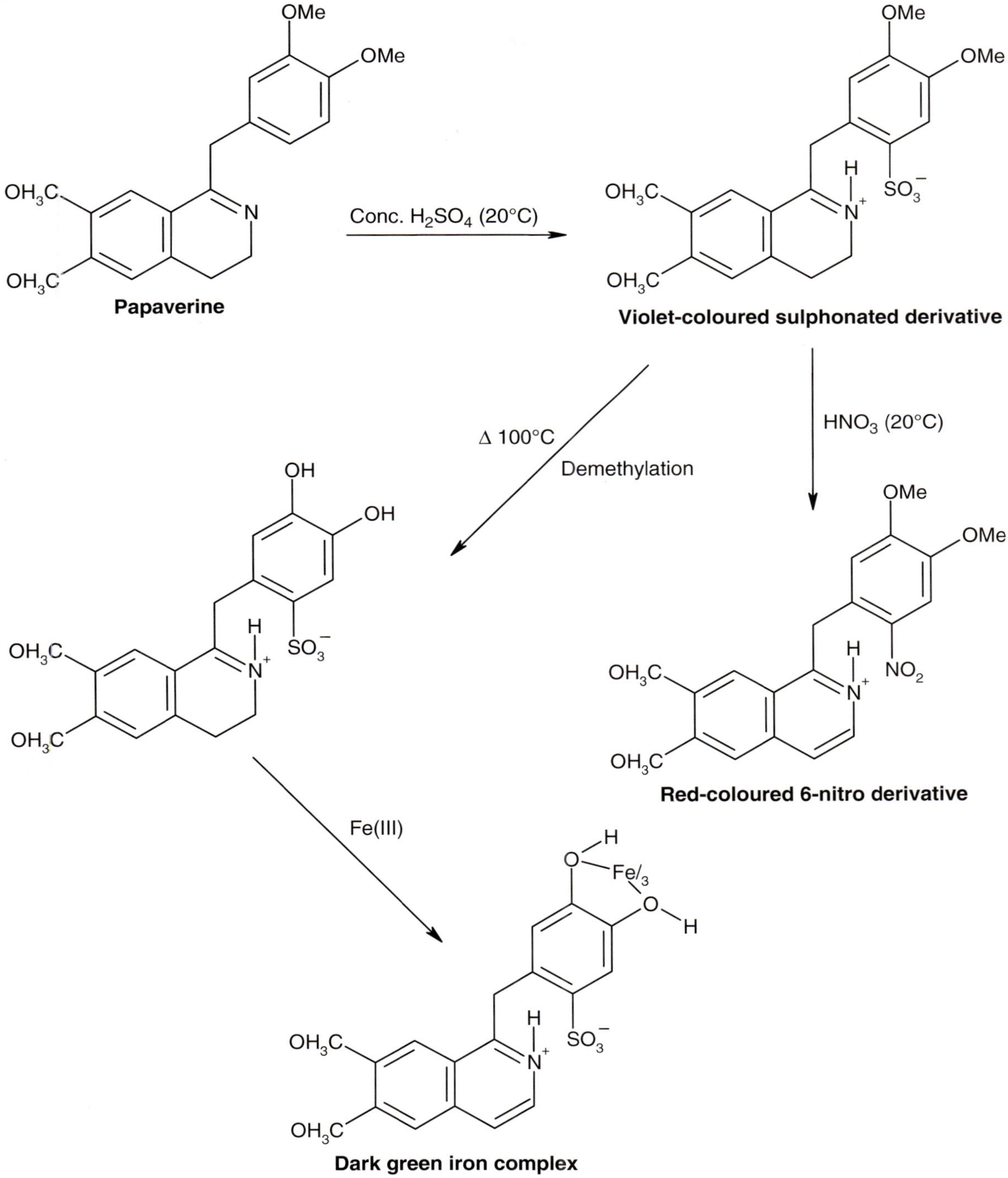

Reference

Pharmaceutical Chemistry (Vol. 2) by H.J. Roth, 1991, pp. 84 and 620.

Note

Two hydroxyl groups (OH) being ortho to each other react with Fe(III) giving dark green colour similar to the colour obtained with pyrocalechol, a polyhydric phenol with two phenolic functions being ortho to each other.

Phenobarbitone

Follow the method 1 for estimation of phenobarbitone, described under formulation 1 of this chapter.

Formulation 6

Papaverine hydrochloride, Caffeine citrate, Phenobarbitone

ESTIMATION

Papaverine hydrochloride and Caffeine citrate

Standard solution of papaverine and caffeine

Appropriate weight of each substance is dissolved in chloroform to get a concentration of 10 mcg/ml in respect of each substance.

Sample solution

Weigh accurately a quantity of powdered material, equivalent to 10 mg of papaverine hydrochloride. Suspend in water and basify with dilute ammonia solution. Extract with four 25 ml portions of chloroform (reserve aqueous ammonia layer for estimation of phenobarbitone). Pass each chloroform layer through anhydrous sodium sulphate and dilute with chloroform appropriately.

Measure the extinctions of both the solutions at 308 nm and 276 nm. The extinction values at 308 nm and 276 nm are used for calculations of papaverine and caffeine respectively by comparison. There is no mutual interference.

Phenobarbitone

Aqueous ammoniacal layer reserved during estimation of papaverine above can be used. The solution is diluted appropriately with dilute ammonia to get a concentration of 10 mcg/ml, having absorption maxima at about 240 nm or acidify the aqueous ammoniacal layer and proceed with the method A described under formulation 1 of this chapter.

Formulation 7

Papaverine hydrochloride, Ephedrine hydrochloride, Phenobarbitone, Theophylline / Aminophylline

ESTIMATION

Papaverine hydrochloride and Ephedrine hydrochloride (total alkaloids)

Transfer an accurately weighed quantity of the sample powder equivalent to 50 mg of total alkaloids to a 125 ml separator with the aid of 5 ml of water. Add 5 ml of 1 N sodium hydroxide solution and shake vigorously for 2 minutes. Extract with five quantities, each of 25 ml of chloroform. Wash the combined chloroform extracts with water till free from alkali. Add 5 g of anhydrous sodium sulphate to remove any dissolved water. Filter into a previously dried and weighed beaker through anhydrous sodium sulphate. Wash sodium sulphate with chloroform. Add 5 drops of hydrochloric acid and evaporate the chloroform. When the volume is reduced to about 5 ml, remove the beaker from the water-bath and dry residue in vacuum. Finally dry the residue at 105°C for 1 h and weigh (A). Calculate the contents of papaverine and ephedrine in each tablet.

Papaverine hydrochloride

Dissolve the above residue (A) in 1 N hydrochloric acid to get a concentration of 15 mcg/ml of papaverine hydrochloride. Measure the extinction at 310 nm and calculate the contents of papaverine hydrochloride using 228 as value of A 1%, 1 cm at 310 nm. Ephedrine hydrochloride does not interfere as it is poorly UV-absorbing compound.

Ephedrine hydrochloride

METHOD 1

Subtract the contents of papaverine as determined by the method above from the weight of residue (A) obtained in the method for total alkaloids. The difference gives the weigh of ephedrine present in the portion of the sample taken for analysis.

METHOD 2

Suspend the residue (A) obtained in the method 1 for total alkaloids in water, add 10 g of sodium chloride and 15 ml of 20% w/v solution of sodium hydroxide. Carry out the steam distillation into receiver containing 25 ml of 0.05 N sulphuric acid. Collect about 100 ml of the distillate. Titrate excess of the acid with 0.05 N sodium hydroxide using methyl red as indicator. Carry out the blank determination using same quantities of the reagents. Each ml of 0.025 N sulphuric acid neutralized by the volatile base is equivalent to 0.00826 g of anhydrous ephedrine. Multiply the results by 1.221 or 1.297 to get the contents of ephedrine hydrochloride or ephedrine sulphate respectively.

Note

Ephedrine (base) is volatile, hence can be subjected to steam distillation after basification and distillate received into acid.

Phenobarbitone

Follow the method A for estimation of phenobarbitone described under formulation 1 of this chapter.

Aminophylline

Follow the method 2 for determination of theophylline described under formulation 1 of this chapter. Calculate the contents of aminophylline by multiplying the contents of theophylline by 1.267.

Formulation 8

Papaverine hydrochloride, Ephedrine hydrochloride, Phenobarbitone, Theophylline, Prednisolone

ESTIMATION

Papaverine hydrochloride and Ephedrine hydrochloride (total alkaloids)

Transfer an accurately weighed quantity of the sample powder equivalent to 50 mg of total alkaloids to a 125 ml separator with the aid of 5 ml of water. Add 5 ml of 1 N sodium hydroxide solution and shake vigorously for 2 minutes. Extract with five quantities, each of 25 ml of chloroform. Wash the combined chloroform extracts with water till free from alkali. Add 5 g of anhydrous sodium sulphate to remove any dissolved water. Filter into a previously dried and weighed beaker through anhydrous sodium sulphate. Wash sodium sulphate with chloroform. Add 5 drops of hydrochloric acid and evaporate the chloroform. When the volume is reduced to about 5 ml, remove the beaker from the water-bath and dry residue in vacuum. Finally dry the residue at 105°C for 1 h and weigh (A). Calculate the contents of papaverine and ephedrine in each tablet.

Papaverine hydrochloride

Dissolve the above residue (A) in 1 N hydrochloric acid to get a concentration of 15 mcg/ml of papaverine hydrochloride. Measure the extinction at 310 nm and calculate the contents of papaverine hydrochloride using a value of 228 as E 1%, 1 cm.

Ephedrine hydrochloride

METHOD 1

Subtract the contents of papaverine as determined by the method above from the weight of residue (A) obtained in the method for total alkaloids. The difference gives the weigh of ephedrine.

METHOD 2

Suspend the residue (A) obtained in the method 1 for total alkaloids in water, add 10 g of sodium chloride and 15 ml of 20% w/v solution of sodium hydroxide. Carry out the steam distillation into receiver containing 25 ml of 0.05 N sulphuric acid. Collect about 100 ml of the distillate. Titrate excess of the acid with 0.05 N sodium hydroxide using methyl red as indicator. Carry out the blank determination using same quantities of the reagents. Each ml of 0.025 N sulphuric acid neutralized by the volatile base is equivalent to 0.00826 g of anhydrous ephedrine. Multiply the results by 1.221 or 1.297 to get the contents of ephedrine hydrochloride or ephedrine sulphate respectively.

This method is based on volatile nature of ephedrine (base) which is generated on adding sodium hydroxide.

Phenobarbitone

Follow the method A for estimation of phenobarbitone described under formulation 1 of this chapter.

Aminophylline

Follow the method for determination of theophylline described under formulation 1 of this chapter. Calculate the contents of aminophylline by multiplying the contents of theophylline by 1.267.

Prednisolone

Follow the isoniazid reagent method for estimation of betamethasone described in formulation 4 of the chapter on topical preparations.

Formulation 9

Caffeine, Phenobarbitone, Dihydroxypropyltheophylline, Adiphenine hydrochloride

ESTIMATION

Caffeine

Transfer an accurately weighed quantity of the powdered material equivalent to 200 mg of caffeine. Make it acidic with dilute hydrochloric acid and extract with successive portions each of 30 ml of chloroform until extraction is complete. Reserve the aqueous solution (A) for the determination of theophylline and adiphenine. Extract the combined chloroform extract with three successive portions each of 20 ml of 1 N sodium hydroxide and then, with 20 ml of water. Set aside the alkaline aqueous extracts (B) for estimation of phenobarbitone. Evaporate off chloroform and dry the residue of anhydrous caffeine to a constant weight at 105°C and calculate the total weight of anhydrous caffeine in the sample.

Phenobarbitone

Make acidic to litmus paper the alkaline layer (B) obtained in the estimation of caffeine by the addition of dilute sulphuric acid and extract with successive portions each of 30 ml of chloroform until extraction is complete. Wash combined chloroform layer with 20 ml of water and evaporate off chloroform. Dry the residue of phenobarbitone to constant weight at 105°C. From this weight calculate the amount of phenobarbitone in the sample. Alternatively, the residue may be dissolved in dilute ammonia. For details refer to formulation 1 of this chapter.

Adiphenine hydrochloride

Make alkaline to litmus paper the aqueous acidic solution (A) reserved in the determination of caffeine with sodium hydroxide solution and extract as under phenobarbitone. Evaporate off chloroform to 2 ml, add 2 drops of dilute hydrochloric acid and evaporate off completely. The residue weighs adiphenine.

Retain extracted aqueous layer (A) reserved in the determination of caffeine. Use combined aqueous layer for the estimation of theophylline as under.

Note

It is anti-cholinergic, hence used as anti-spasmodic. It is no longer used. Due to the presence of phenyl group it can undergo bromination. The tertiary nitrogen can easily form Co(II) complex.

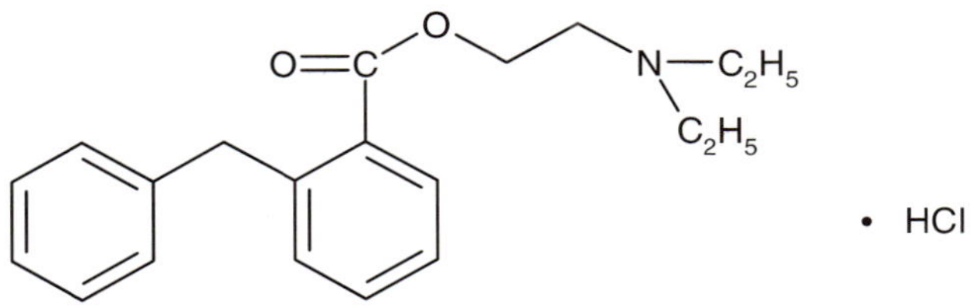

Adiphenine hydrochloride

Dihydroxypropyltheophylline

Make the aqueous layer (A) and aqueous layer obtained during extraction of adiphenine slightly acidic and heat on water-bath to remove chloroform. Cool and dilute to 250 ml with distilled water. Make further dilutions to get a concentration of 10 mcg/ml of dihydroxypropyltheophylline. Measure the extinction at the maximum at about 273 nm. For the purpose of calculation, use a value of 361 for E 1%, 1 cm.

It is more soluble derivative of theophylline. Its reactions are similar to theophylline.

Formulation 10

Pseudoephedrine hydrochloride, Triprolidine hydrochloride, Paracetamol

ESTIMATION

Sample solution

Weigh accurately a quantity of powdered tablets equivalent to 20 mg of triprolidine hydrochloride. Add 70 ml water, shake for 15 minutes and adjust to 100 ml with water (200 mcg/ml of triprolidine hydrochloride) Solution A.

Triprolidine hydrochloride

Standard solution

25 mcg/ml of triprolidine hydrochloride in 0.1 N hydrochloric acid.

Sample solution

Weigh accurately powdered sample equivalent to 2.5 mg of the substance, dissolve in 10-15 ml water, add 5 ml of copper sulphate solution and 5 ml of strong ammonia solution. Extract with two 25 ml portions of chloroform. Wash combined chloroform layer with water and extract with 0.1 N hydrochloric acid to produce 100 ml.

Measure the extinction of sample and standard solutions at 290 nm using acid as blank, calculate the results by comparison.

Paracetamol

Follow the nitroso-derivative method described under formulation of the chapter on analgesics and antipyretics diluting solution A above appropriately.

Pseudoephedrine hydrochloride

METHOD 1

Transfer 50 ml of solution A into a separator, add 5 g of sodium chloride, 3 ml of 1 N sodium hydroxide. Extract with four 100 ml portions of ether. Wash the combined ether extract with 10 ml of water. To the total ether extract, add 25 ml of 0.1 N hydrochloric acid and shake vigorously. Allow the two layers to separate and transfer the aqueous acidic layer to conical flask. Wash the ether layer with two 10 ml portions of water and combine the washings with the acidic layer. Warm the acid layer to remove trace of ether, cool and titrate with 0.1 N sodium hydroxide using methyl red as indicator.

Calculate the total volume of 0.1 N hydrochloric acid (A) consumed by pseudoephedrine and triprolidine hydrochloride. From the contents of triprolidine hydrochloride as determined above, calculate equivalent volume of 0.1 N hydrochloric acid (B) (33.29 mg of triprolidine hydrochloride is equivalent to 1 ml of 0.1 N hydrochloric acid.) Subtract the volume (ml) B from total volume A and calculate the contents of pseudoephedrine hydrochloride in the formulation by using the factor that each ml of 0.1 N hydrochloric acid is equivalent to 20.17 mg of pseudoephedrine hydrochloride.

The compound answers Chen-Kao reaction i.e. copper chelate in alkaline medium analogous to ephinephrine.

METHOD 2

This method is based on two phase acid-base titration.

Reagents

1. Mixed indicator solution

Chlorophenol red	0.30 g
Congo red	0.15 g
Alcohol	50 ml
0.1 N sodium hydroxide	12 ml
Water to produce	500 ml

Protect from light.

Sample solution

Weigh accurately a quantity of sample equivalent to 500 mg of pseudoephedrine, add 45 ml of water, 1 g of sodium sulphate and 5 ml of dilute sulphuric acid. Shake well and add 4 ml of 5 N sodium hydroxide. Extract with four portions of 40 ml each of chloroform, washing each extract with the same 10 ml of water. Combine chloroform layer and dilute to 200 ml with chloroform.

Procedure

Take 50 ml of the chloroform extract of the sample, add 50 ml of water and few drops of mixed indicator and titrate with 0.1 N hydrochloric acid shaking well between additions. The colour change in aqueous layer is red → colourless → yellow. The end point is taken as first appearance of yellow tinge. The colour change can be assessed without allowing the separation of phases. Each ml of 0.1 N hydrochloric acid is equivalent to 20.17 mg of pseudoephedrine hydrochloride. Or the chloroform extract may be evaporated and the residue dissolved in glacial acetic acid for non-aqueous titration (crystal violet).

Note

1. Addition of acid before basification and extraction ensures complete dissolution of the drug.
2. Sodium sulphate minimises formation of emulsion.
3. Ephedrine does not interfere in this method.

Formulation 11

Theophylline, Ephedrine hydrochloride, Chlordiazepoxide

ESTIMATION

Theophylline

Weigh accurately a quantity of the powdered tablets equivalent to 200 mg of theophylline, add 20 ml of water and 5 ml of dilute sulphuric acid. Extract with four 25 ml portions of chloroform-isopropyl alcohol (3 : 1 v/v) mixture. Wash the combined organic layer with 10 ml of dilute sulphuric acid. Pass organic layer through anhydrous sodium sulphate and evaporate. Find out the contents of theophylline gravimetrically. Retain the acid layer for estimation of chlordiazepoxide.

Ephedrine hydrochloride

METHOD 1

Reagents

1. 0.1% w/v solution of ninhydrin in ethyl alcohol.
2. 1% w/v potassium hydroxide solution in ethyl alcohol.

Standard solution

300 mcg/ml of ephedrine hydrochloride in water.

Sample solution

Weigh accurately a quantity of sample equivalent to 30 mg of ephedrine hydrochloride, shake with 100 ml of water and filter (300 mcg/ml).

Procedure

To 2 ml each of standard and sample solutions, add 2 ml ninhydrin solution and 0.1 ml of potassium hydroxide solution. Heat on a water bath for 30 minutes, cool and adjust the volume to 25 ml with isopropyl alcohol. Measure the absorbance of both the standard and sample solutions at about 560 nm and calculate the results by comparison.

Secondary aliphatic amine group of ephedrine reacts with ninhydrin resulting in the formation of semi-aminal and the aminal.

Probable Reaction Mechanism

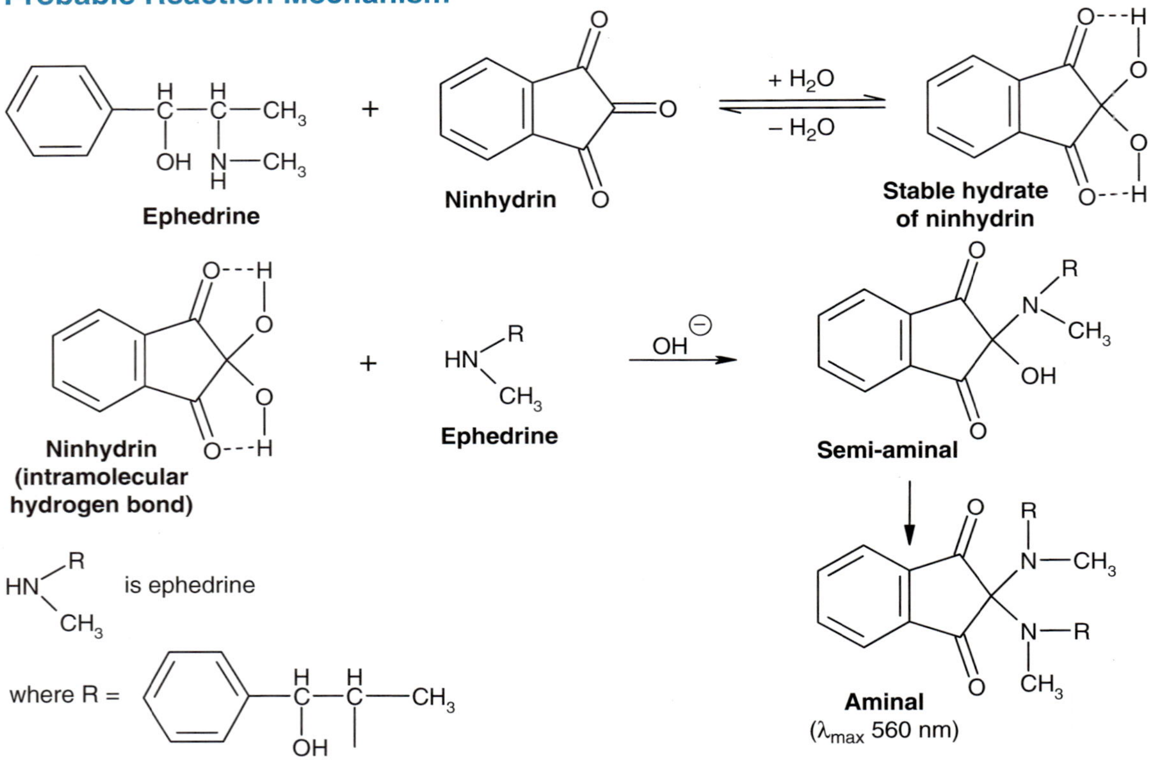

METHOD 2

Follow the method 2 for estimation of ephedrine hydrochloride described under formulation 8 of this chapter. This is based on volatile nature of ephedrine as base.

Chlordiazepoxide and Ephedrine hydrochloride

Make the acidic layer obtained in the estimation of theophylline alkaline with 20% w/v solution of sodium hydroxide and extract with four 25 ml portions of chloroform. Pass chloroform layer through anhydrous sodium sulphate. Evaporate and dissolve the residue in 20 ml of glacial acetic acid and titrate with 0.05 N perchloric acid using crystal violet as indicator. Subtract the volume of perchloric acid equivalent to ephedrine determined earlier. The remaining volume represents chlordiazepoxide.

Each ml of 0.05 N perchloric acid is equivalent to 0.01681 g of chlordiazepoxide.

Note

Before proceeding with extraction, the alkaline solution can be heated on water-bath to remove ephedrine (volatile base). The volume of 0.05 N perchloric acid consumed shall correspond to chlordiazepoxide only.

Alternatively chlordiazepoxide can be subjected to acid hydrolysis and yellow colour measured at 410 nm.

Probable Reaction Mechanism

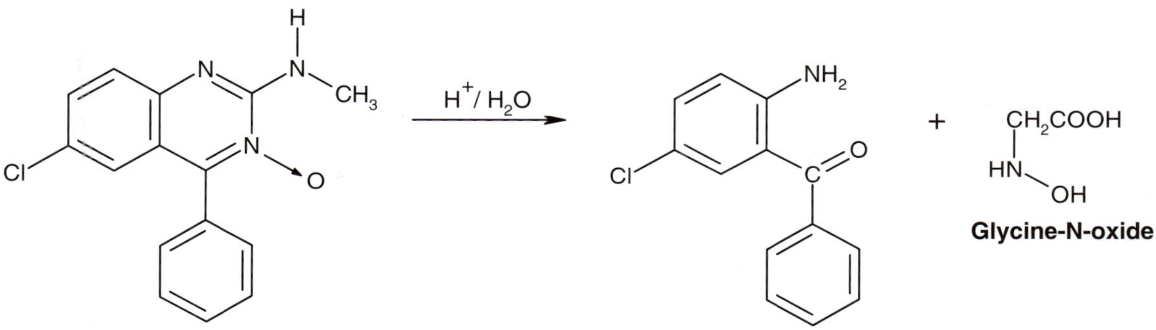

Chlordiazepoxide **2-amino-5-chlorobenzophenone**
(Coloured species λ_{max} 410 nm)

Note

1. In the analysis of benzodiazepines like diazepam, 2-aminophenone derivative plays the main role.
2. 2-aminophenone can be diazotized and forms azo dye with Bratton-Marshall reagent as under.

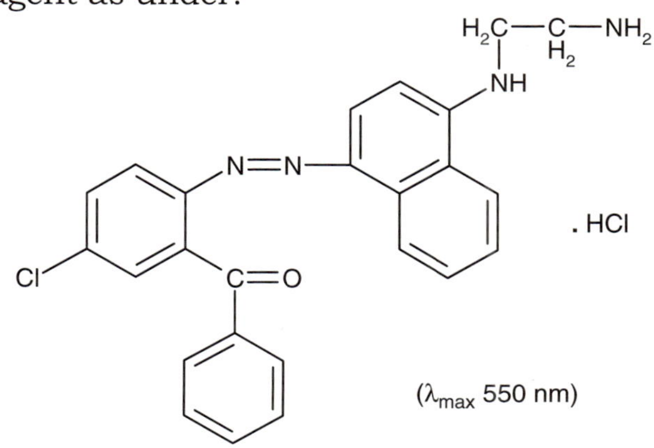

(λ_{max} 550 nm)

Reference

Pharmaceutical Chemistry (Vol. 2) by H.J. Roth, p. 664.

Formulation 12

Theophylline, Ephedrine hydrochloride, Dexamethasone, Chlordiazepoxide

ESTIMATION

Theophylline

Weigh accurately a quantity of the powdered tablets equivalent to 200 mg of theophylline, add 20 ml of water and 5 ml of dilute sulphuric acid. Extract with four 25 ml portions of chloroform : isopropyl alcohol (3 : 1 v/v) mixture. Wash the combined organic layer with 10 ml of dilute sulphuric acid. Pass organic layer through anhydrous sodium sulphate and evaporate. Find out the contents of theophylline gravimetrically. Retain the acid layer for estimation of chlordiazepoxide.

Ephedrine hydrochloride

Reagents

1. 0.1% w/v solution of ninhydrin in ethyl alcohol.
2. 1% w/v potassium hydroxide solution in ethyl alcohol.

Standard solution

300 mcg/ml of pure ephedrine hydrochloride in water.

Sample solution

Weigh accurately a quantity of powdered tablets equivalent to 30 mg of ephedrine hydrochloride, shake with 100 ml of water and filter (300 mcg/ml).

Procedure

To 2 ml of standard and sample solutions add 2 ml of ninhydrin solution and 0.1 ml of potassium hydroxide solution. Heat on a water-bath for 30 minutes, cool and adjust the volume to 25 ml with isopropyl alcohol. Measure the absorbance of both the standard and sample solutions at maximum at about 560 nm and calculate the results by comparison. For reaction mechanism see formulation 11 of this chapter.

Chlordiazepoxide and Ephedrine hydrochloride

Make the acidic layer obtained in the estimation of theophylline alkaline with 20% w/v solution of sodium hydroxide and extract with four 25 ml portions of chloroform. Pass chloroform layer through anhydrous sodium sulphate. Evaporate and dissolve the residue in 20 ml of glacial acetic acid and titrate with 0.05 N perchloric acid using crystal violet as indicator. Subtract the volume of perchloric acid equivalent to ephedrine determined earlier. The remaining volume represents chlordiazepoxide.

Each ml of 0.05 N perchloric acid is equivalent to 16.81 mg of chlordiazepoxide. Alternatively chlordiazepoxide can be subjected to acid hydrolysis and yellow colour measured at 410 nm. For details refer to formulation 11 of this chapter or chapter on sedatives and tranquillizers.

Note

Before chloroform extraction the solution may be heated on boiling water-bath to remove ephedrine (volatile base) and then volume of 0.05 N perchloric acid consumed shall be directly equivalent to chlordiazepoxide.

Dexamethasone

Weigh accurately a quantity of powdered tablets equivalent to 1 mg of dexamethasone, add 20 ml of water and extract with five 20 ml portions of chloroform. Pass chloroform extract through anhydrous sodium sulphate. Evaporate, take up the residue in 20 ml of methanol and follow isoniazid reagent method. For details, refer to formulation 4 of the chapter on topical preparations.

Formulation 13

Diethylcarbamazine citrate, Theophylline, Dried aluminium hydroxide gel

ESTIMATION

Diethylcarbamazine citrate

METHOD 1

Weigh a quantity of sample equivalent to 500 mg of the compound, add 50 ml of water, shake vigorously to dissolve and filter. Extract the residue with three more 50 ml portions of water and filter. Add 5 ml of 20% sodium hydroxide solution to the filtrate and extract with three 20 ml portions of chloroform. Combine chloroform layers and wash with water to get free of alkali. Extract chloroform layer with 25 ml of 0.1 N sulphuric acid and 20 ml of water. Combine acid and water extracts, warm slightly to remove traces of chloroform. Cool and titrate excess of the acid with 0.1 N sodium hydroxide using bromocresol green solution as indicator. Each ml of 0.1 N sulphuric acid is equivalent to 0.03914 g of diethylcarbamazine citrate.

METHOD 2

Reagent

Acetic anhydride-pyridine reagent: 57 ml of acetic anhydride is mixed with 13 ml of pyridine.

Standard solution

Prepare solution of diethylcarbamazine citrate in water (5 mg/ml). 5 ml of the resulting solution is diluted to 100 ml with glacial acetic acid (250 mcg/ml).

Sample solution

To an aliquot of composite (syrup, powder and tablets) sample equivalent to 25 mg of the compound, add 10 of water and sufficient glacial acetic acid to produce 100 ml, mix and filter (250 mcg/ml).

Procedure

To 2 ml each of sample and standard solutions, add 5 ml of the anhydride reagent. Keep at 37°C for 1 h and then allow it to come to room temperature. Measure the absorbance of both the solutions at about 480 nm and calculate the results. The method obeys Beer's law in the range of 10-100 mcg/ml. The colour of the complex is stable for 2 hours.

Note

1. As the method involves reaction with citrate ion, it may not be applicable in syrups where citric acid has been used for pH adjustment.
2. Chlorpheniramine maleate, if present, does not interfere.
3. Citric acid reacts with acetic anhydride to give acetyl citric acid anhydride which yields red colour with pyridine.

Aluminium hydroxide

Follow the method described in formulation 22 of the chapter on alimentary drugs.

Theophylline

Follow the method described in formulation 1 of this chapter.

Formulation 14

Theophylline, Ephedrine hydrochloride, Phenobarbitone, Caffeine citrate

ESTIMATION

METHOD 1

Theophylline

Weigh accurately a quantity of powder equivalent to 250 mg theophylline, add 50 ml of water and 8 ml of dilute ammonia solution. Keep on water bath, add 50 ml of 0.1 N silver nitrate solution and warm for 15 minutes. Cool to 5-10°C for 20 minutes, filter through G_4 sintered funnel and wash the precipitates silver theophyllinate (poorly soluble complex) with three 20 ml portions of water. Acidify the combined filtrate with concentrated nitric acid, adding 3 ml of acid in excess and titrate the excess silver nitrate with 0.1 N ammonium thiocyanate using ferric ammonium sulphate solution as indicator. Perform reagent blank. Each ml of 0.1 N silver nitrate is equivalent to 18.02 mcg of theophylline, anhydrous.

Probable Reaction Mechanism

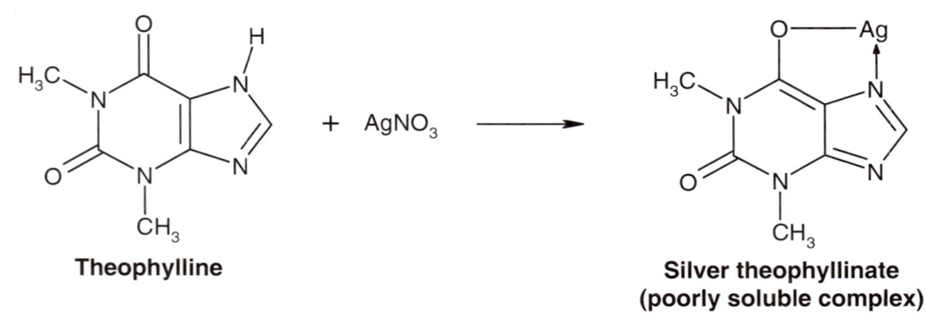

Reference

Pharmaceutical Chemistry (Vol. 2) by H.J. Roth, p. 601.

Phenobarbitone

Weigh sample accurately equivalent to about 80 mg of phenobarbitone, add 10 ml of 0.1 N sodium hydroxide, shake and saturate with sodium chloride. Acidify with hydrochloric acid and extract with three 30 ml portions of ether. Reserve aqueous layer for estimation of caffeine. Wash combined ether extracts with 10 ml of dilute hydrochloric acid (1 : 1) and then with two 20 ml water. Pass ether layer through anhydrous sodium sulphate (ether washed), evaporate ether layer and dissolve the residue in 0.5 N ammonium hydroxide or borate buffer, pH 9.6 to get 10 mcg/ml. Measure the extinction at 240.5 nm and calculate the results by comparing with the standard. For further details, refer to formulation 1 of this chapter.

Caffeine citrate

Aqueous layer reserved during extraction of phenobarbitone is basified and extracted with five 20 ml portions of chloroform. Wash combined chloroform layer with ammoniacal water for 3-4 times. Filter, dry at 80°C and weigh. Weight represents the amount of caffeine present in the sample taken for analysis. Alternatively, chloroform layer may be used for spectrophotometric analysis as described in formulation of the chapter on analgesics and antipyretics.

Ephedrine hydrochloride

Weigh accurately a quantity of powdered material equivalent to 100 mg of ephedrine. Suspend in water and basify with ammonia solution. Extract with four 25 ml portions of ether. Evaporate ether at low temperature and take the residue in 10 ml of 0.1 N sulphuric acid. Excess acid is titrated with 0.1 N sodium hydroxide using methyl red solution as indicator. Alternatively, wash ether layer with water till neutral. Add exactly 50 ml of 0.02 N sulphuric acid and evaporate ether layer completely. Cool, add 2-3 drops of methyl red solution and titrate with 0.02 N sodium hydroxide. Each ml of 0.02 N sulphuric acid is equivalent to 0.004033 g of ephedrine hydrochloride.

Note

Basification liberates ephedrine base which can be extracted into ether. Ether is to be evaporated at low temperature bacause ephedrine base is volatile and is likely to be lost on evaporation.

METHOD 2

Phenobarbitone

In a 150 ml separator containing about 5 ml 1 N hydrochloric acid, transfer quantity of powder accurately weighed equivalent to 100 mg of phenobarbitone and shake well. Extract with five 50 ml portions of solvent ether. Collect the ether layers. Wash the combined ether layer with 10 ml acidified water and then twice with 50 ml each of 1% w/v sodium acetate solution. Finally, wash the combined ether layer twice with 50 ml water, each. Filter the washed ether extracts into a 500 ml conical flask. Evaporate to dryness on water bath, cool, add 10 ml ethanol and 2 ml indicator (0.1% w/v thymolphthalein in ethanol). Titrate against 0.1 N alcoholic potassium hydroxide. Make the correction for blank containing 10 ml ethanol and 2 ml indicator solution. Each ml of 0.1 N alcoholic potassium hydroxide is equivalent to 0.02322 g of phenobarbitone.

Caffeine citrate

Transfer accurately weighed quantity of powdered material equivalent to 100 mg of caffeine to a separator having 15 ml water. Add about 10 ml of 1 N hydrochloric acid, shake well and extract with five 30 ml portions of chloroform. Combine the chloroform layers, add about 20 ml of 0.1 N sodium hydroxide and 15 ml of water to the combined chloroform layers. Shake well and reject aqueous layer. Then chloroform layer is washed twice with 20 ml water. Reject aqueous layer and filter chloroform layer through cotton plug into a dry 500 ml conical flask. Evaporate chloroform to dryness. Dissolve the residue in 2 ml of chloroform, add 10 ml of benzene and 10 ml of acetic anhydride. Then titrate with 0.1 N perchloric acid using 0.2 ml of solution of neutral red (0.2% w/v solution in acetic acid). Carry out the blank determination and make necessary correction.

Each ml of 0.1 N perchloric acid is equivalent to 0.01942 g of caffeine.

Aminophylline

This method is for estimation of theophylline component of aminophylline.

Reagents

1. Borate buffer
   (a) 0.5% w/v solution of boric acid in water.
   (b) 1% w/v solution of sodium borate in water.
   Mix solutions (a) and (b) (1 : 1) to prepare the buffer.
2. 0.04 w/v solution of 2,6-dichloroquinone chlorimide in isopropyl alcohol.

Standard solution

Weigh accurately about 97 mg of aminophylline, transfer to a 200 ml volumetric flask and make up the volume with water.

Sample solution

Transfer accurately weighed quantity of powder equivalent to 100 mg of the compound to a 200 ml volumetric flask. Shake well with 100 ml water, make up the volume with water and filter.

Procedure

To 1 ml each of sample and standard solutions, add 5 ml of borate buffer and 2 ml of 2,6-dichloroquinone chlorimide solution. Make up the volume to 50 ml with water and keep in a refrigerator for 90 minutes. Remove and after attaining the room temperature, transfer exactly 25 ml of each of sample and standard solutions into two separating funnels and extract blue colour formed with exactly 25 ml of amyl alcohol. Reject aqueous layer and measure the optical density of the alcoholic layer at 620 nm using amyl alcohol as blank. Deduce the results by comparison.

For detailed reaction mechanism, see formulation 1 of this chapter.

Ephedrine hydrochloride

Standard solution

160 mcg/ml of ephedrine hydrochloride in 1 N hydrochloric acid.

Sample solution

Weigh accurately a quantity of powdered tablets equivalent to 32 mg of ephedrine hydrochloride and transfer into a 200 ml volumetric flask. Add about 100 ml of 1 N hydrochloric acid, warm on a water bath for 15 minutes, cool, make up the volume to 200 ml with 1 N hydrochloric acid and mix.

Procedure

Follow ammoniacal copper sulphate method B described in formulation 1 of this chapter.

Formulation 15

Diethylcarbamazine citrate, Theophylline, Prednisolone, Dried aluminium hydroxide gel

ESTIMATION

Diethylcarbamazine citrate

METHOD 1

Weigh a quantity of sample powder equivalent to 500 mg of the compound, add 50 ml of water, shake vigorously to dissolve and filter. Extract the residue with three more 50 ml portions of water and filter. Add 5 ml of 20% sodium hydroxide solution to the filtrate and extract with three 20 ml portions of chloroform. Combine chloroform layers and wash with water to get free of alkali. Extract chloroform layer with 25 ml of 0.1 N sulphuric acid and 20 ml of water. Combine acid and water extracts, warm slightly to remove traces of chloroform. Cool and titrate excess of the acid with 0.1 N sodium hydroxide using bromocresol green solution as indicator. Each ml of 0.1 N sulphuric acid is equivalent to 0.03914 g of diethylcarbamazine citrate.

METHOD 2

Reagent

Acetic anhydride - pyridine reagent: 57 ml of acetic anhydride is mixed with 13 ml of pyridine.

Standard solution

Prepare solution of diethylcarbamazine citrate in water (5 mg/ml). 5 ml of the resulting solution is diluted to 100 ml with glacial acetic acid (250 mcg/ml).

Sample solution

To an aliquot of composite (syrup, powder and tablets) sample equivalent to 25 mg of the compound, add 10 of water and sufficient glacial acetic acid to produce 100 ml, mix and filter (250 mcg/ml).

Procedure

To 2 ml each of sample and standard solutions, add 5 ml of the anhydride reagent. Keep at 37°C for 1 h and then allow it to come to room temperature. Measure the absorbance of both the solutions at about 480 nm and calculate the results. The method obeys Beer's law in the range of 10-100 mcg/ml. The colour of the complex is stable for 2 hours.

Note

1. As the method involves reaction with citrate ion, it may not be applicable in syrups where citric acid has been used for pH adjustment.
2. Chlorpheniramine maleate, if present, does not interfere.

The compound forms C-T complex with picrolonic acid, which has λ_{max} 350 nm.

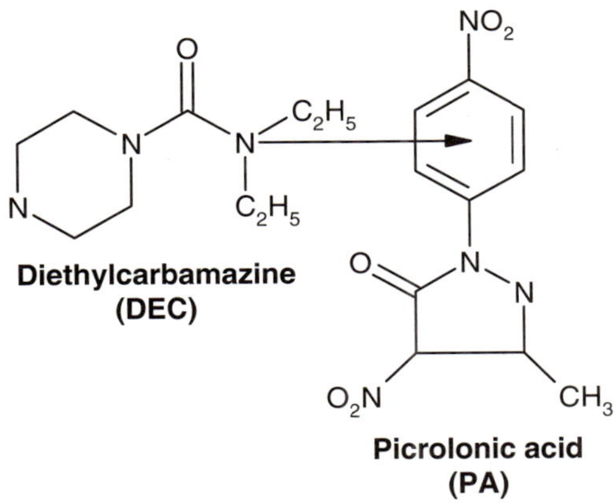

DEC - PA C-T complex
(λ_{max} 350 nm)

Reference

S.K. Baveja & K.V. Ranga Rao, *Analyst*, **106**, 726-728, 1981.

Aluminium hydroxide

Follow the method described in formulation 13 of this chapter.

Prednisolone

Follow the extraction procedure as described for dexamethasone in formulation of this chapter. For estimation, follow the isoniazid reagent method for determination of betamethasone described in formulation 4 of the chapter on topical preparations.

Formulation 16

Aminophylline, Phenobarbitone, Ephedrine hydrochloride, Codeine phosphate

ESTIMATION

METHOD 1

Aminophylline

(a) **Ethylenediamine :** Weigh accurately a quantity of powdered material equivalent to 100 mg of aminophylline. Dissolve in 30 ml of water and titrate with 0.1 N hydrochloric acid using bromocresol green solution as indicator (colour change from blue to green). Each ml of 0.1 N hydrochloric acid is equivalent to 0.003003 g of ethylenediamine.

(b) **Theophylline**

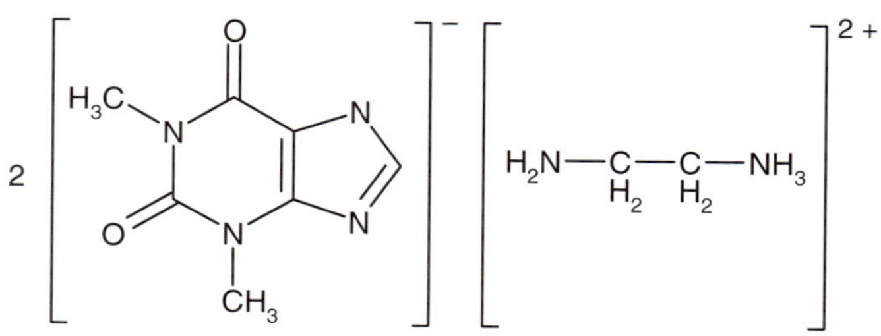

Theophylline component **Ethylenediamine component**

Reagents

1. 0.1 N silver nitrate.
2. 0.1 N ammonium thiocyanate.
3. Ferric ammonium sulphate solution (indicator).
4. Dilute solution of ammonia.

Procedure

Weigh accurately a quantity of powdered material equivalent to 150 mg of aminophylline, add 40-50 ml of water and 10 ml of dilute ammonia solution. Reflux on water bath to effect solution. Add 100 ml of 0.1 N silver nitrate, heat to boiling and boil for 5 min. Cool to 5°C for 30 minutes, dilute to 200 ml with water and filter (A). Acidify 20 ml of the filtrate (A) with nitric acid, add an excess of 3 ml of nitric acid. Cool, add 2 ml of ferric ammonium sulphate solution and titrate excess of silver nitrate with 0.1 N ammonium thiocyanate. Each ml of 0.1 N silver nitrate is equivalent to 0.01802 g of theophylline (anhydrous). From the volume of silver nitrate consumed, calculate the contents of theophylline.

Probable Reaction Mechanism

In hydroxide ions (OH^-) imidazole ring gets stabilized which reacts with $AgNO_3$ to form silver theophyllinate and excess silver nitrate titrated with ammonium thiocyanate.

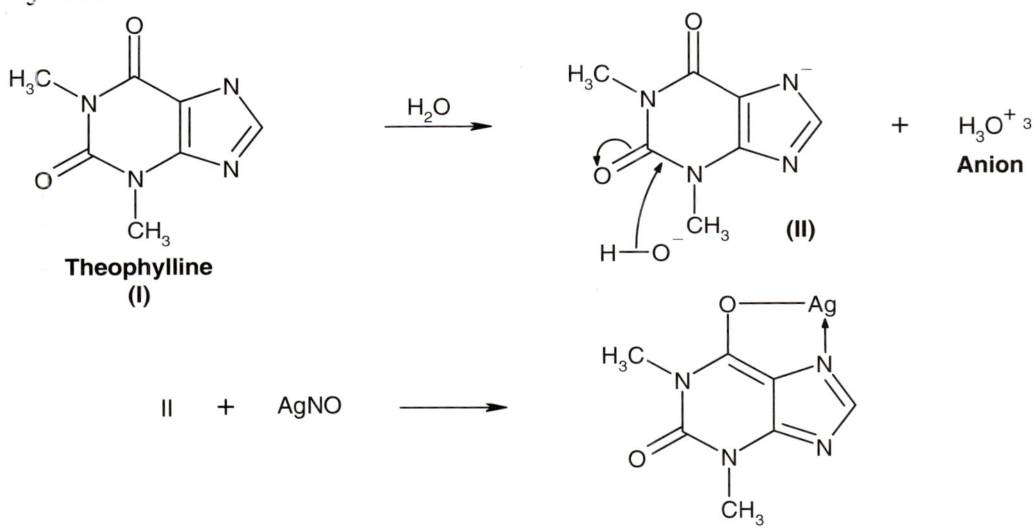

Theophylline (I)

(II)

Anion

Silver theophyllinate

Note

1. Argentometric titration is likely to give higher results as same silver is likely to be absorbed on voluminous silver theophyllinate precipitates.
2. Mercuric acetate $(CH_3COO)_2Hg$ can be used to precipitate theophylline as Hg(theophylline)$_2$ and excess Hg^{++} titrated with ammonium thiocyanate and on similar basis the compound can be precipitated as Cu(theophylline)$_2$ and excess copper estimated by EDTA titration.
3. This test is non-specific, both caffeine and theophylline, both xanthine derivatives give precipitates. Caffeine gives precipitates immediately whereas theophylline gives precipitates on standing.

Reference

1. Pharmaceutical Chemistry (Vol. 2) by H.J. Roth, p. 601.
2. Analytical Profile of Drug Substances by K. Florey.

Ethylenediamine component and theophylline component of aminophylline can be determined by a colorimetric method as well.

Estimation of Ethylenediamine component

Chloroform solution of the substance is extracted with 1 mM HCl coupled with 2% PDAB (in HCl) and absorption measured at 408 nm for quantitative estimation.

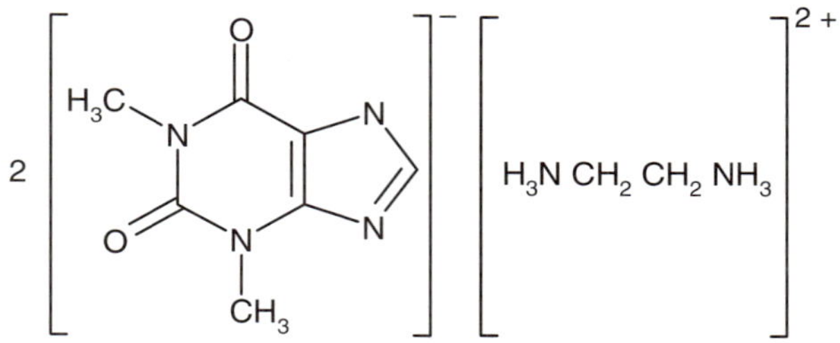

Composition: theophylline 85.7%, ethylenediamine 13%

Note

Water contents being variable.

Probable Reaction Mechanism

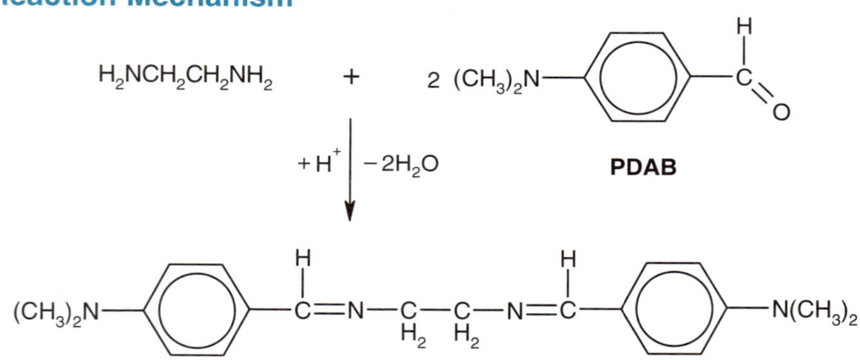

Schiff's base
(λ_{max} 408 nm)

Reference

R.H. Pryce-Jones & J.M. Megguffic, *J. Pharm. & Pharmacol.*, **32(Suppl.)**, 689, 1980.

This bifunctional amine reacts with 2,3-dichloro-1,4-naphthoquinone to form yellow quinonimine (λ_{max} 420 nm). On acidification, the colour of the quinonimine changes to violet-red (λ_{max} 525 nm). This is the most useful test for identifying this portion of the drug in aminophylline.

Probable Reaction Mechanism

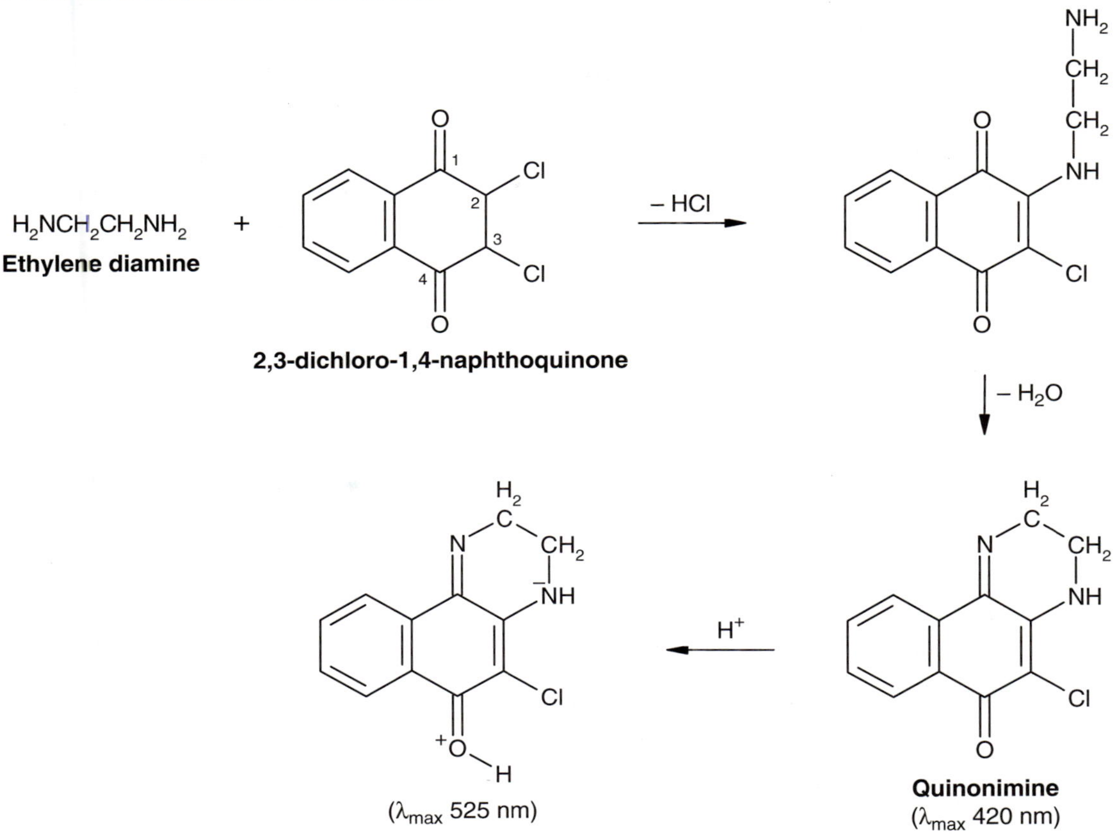

Reference

1. Pharmaceutical Chemistry (Vol. 2) by H.J. Roth, p. 344.
2. T. Datta Samanto & Subrata Laska, *J. Planar Chromatogr.*, **19(3)**, 252, 2006.

Note

1. It is a divalent base. It can be estimated by acid-base titration by adding excess of acid and then back titrating with alkali.
2. It is volatile in nature.

Ethylenediamine is non-chromophoric; hence no absorption in UV light. A chromophore group is introduced as thiourea derivative. Two molecules of 1-naphthyl isothiocyanate react with one mole of ethylenediamine in nitrogen with lone pair of electrons to give thiourea derivative of ethylenediamine which is UV active (λ_{max} 220 nm).

Probable Reaction Mechanism

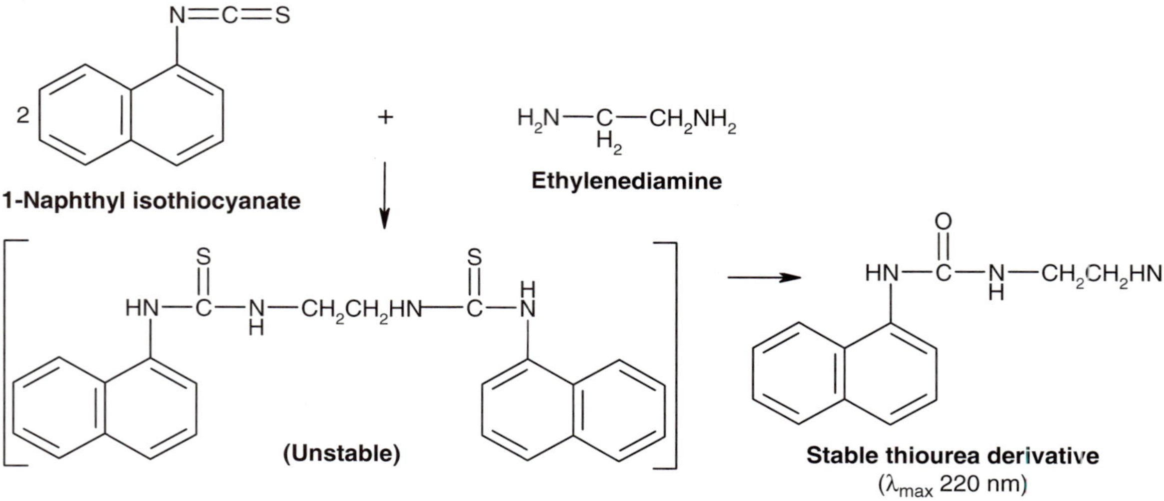

Reference

R.H. Pryce-Jones & J.M. Megguffic, *J. Pharm. & Pharmacol.*, **32(Suppl.)**, 689, 1980.

Estimation of Theophylline component

Probable Reaction Mechanism

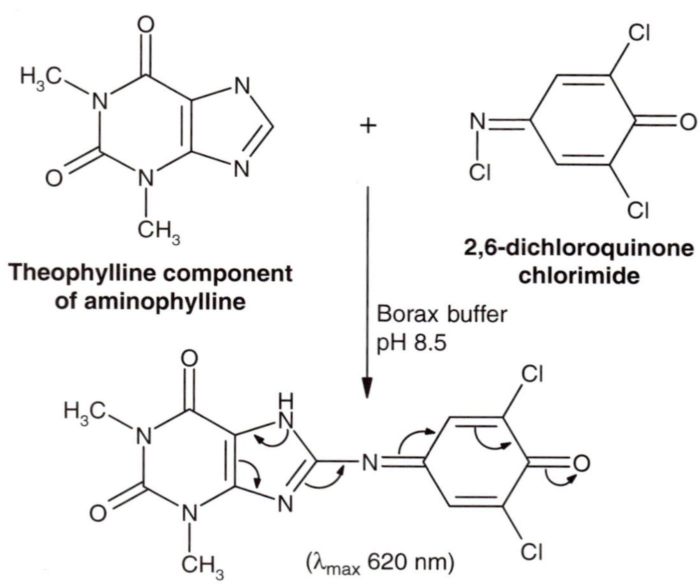

Reference

Pharmaceutical Chemistry (Vol. 2) by H.J. Roth, p. 600.

As a result of acid hydrolysis of the compound, 1,3-dimethyl-4-amino-5-nitroso-2,6-pyrimidione is formed which forms chelate with copper acetate.

Probable Reaction Mechanism

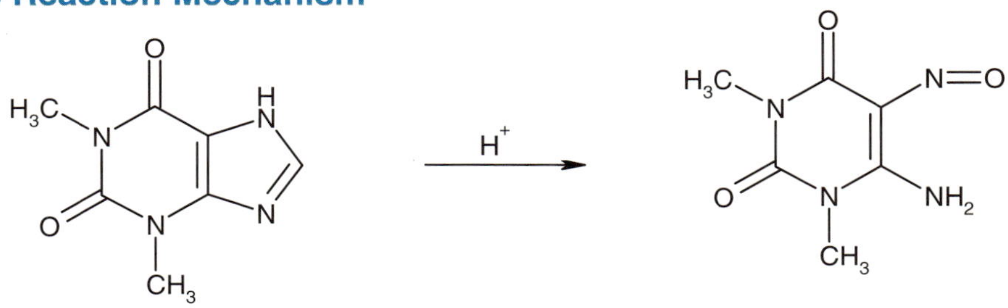

Theophylline → 1,3-dimethyl-4-amino-5-nitroso-2,6-pyrimidione

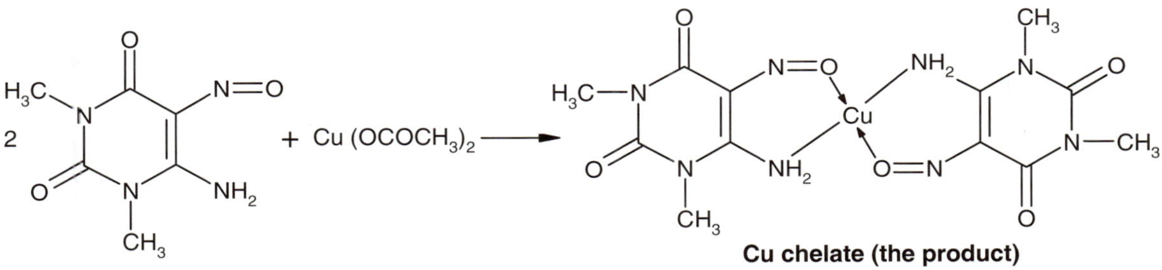

Cu chelate (the product)

METHOD 2

Phenobarbitone

Acidify 50 ml of the filtrate (A) obtained under estimation of theophylline with dilute hydrochloric acid. Add sodium chloride to saturate it. Extract with four 20 ml portions of chloroform, washing each chloroform layer with same 10 ml of water. Filter through filter paper previously moistened with chloroform into a tared flask. Evaporate on water bath, add 2 ml of alcohol and again evaporate. Dry the residue at 105°C in an oven for 3 hours, cool and weigh. The residue is only of phenobarbitone. The residue can be dissolved in 0.5 N ammonia solution and subjected to spectrophotometric solution described in formulation 1 of this chapter.

Ephedrine hydrochloride and Codeine phosphate (as total alkaloids)

METHOD 1

Weigh accurately a quantity of powdered material equivalent to 60 mg of ephedrine hydrochloride, add 10 ml of 0.1 N hydrochloric acid, shake to suspend. Filter through G_4 glass sintered funnel. Wash sintered funnel with water. Combine the filtrate, add 12 ml 0.1 N sodium hydroxide and extract with four 50 ml portions of ether. Wash ether layer with brine solution till washings are free from alkali (use litmus). Wash brine solution with two 25 ml of ether. Mix ether layers, add 50 ml of 0.02 N hydrochloric acid to ether layer. Shake for 2-3 minutes to bring alkaloid back into acid layer. Separate acid layer quantitatively. Wash ether layer with two 10 ml portions of water to ensure quantitative removal of the acid. Add water washings to the acid layer and titrate with 0.02 N sodium hydroxide using methyl red solution as indicator. Say "A" ml of 0.02 N hydrochloric acid is consumed for titration of total alkaloids. The above titrated sample is subjected to steam distillation after adding excess of sodium hydroxide and ephedrine is estimated in the distillate by acid-base titration. Say "B" ml of 0.02 N hydrochloric acid is consumed for ephedrine. Volume of 0.02 N hydrochloric acid consumed by codeine = (A – B). For calculations, see formulation 2 of the chapter on expectorants and cough suppressants.

METHOD 2

The combined filtrate after basification is subjected to steam distillation and the contents of ephedrine (base) are estimated in the filtrate by acid-base titration. For details, refer to method for estimation of ephedrine under formulation 8 of this chapter. The contents in the distillation flask are used for estimation of codeine phosphate as per method 1 above.

Codeine

Like morphine, codeine answers Marquis reaction i.e. treating the substance with formaldehyde/sulphonic acid a purple colour turning to white is produced. Here 2 moles of codeine condenses with 2 moles of formaldehyde and resulting condensation product.

Probable Reaction Mechanism

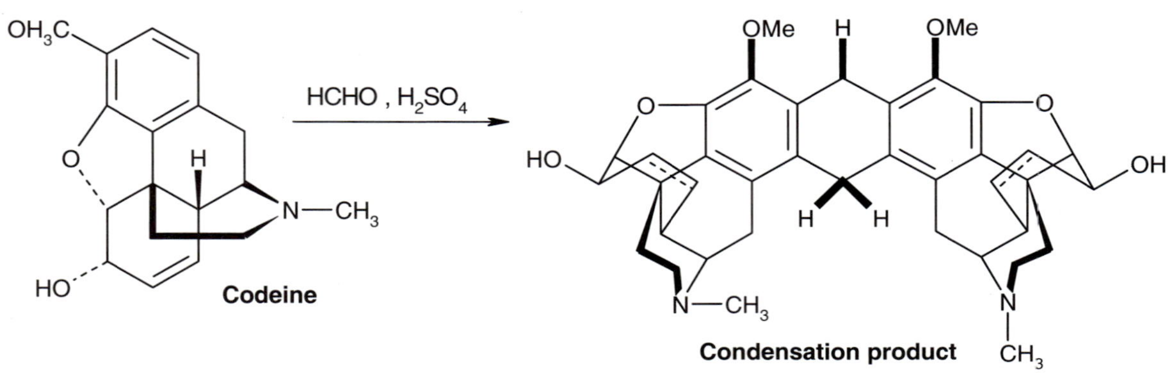

Reference

Pharmaceutical Chemistry (Vol. 2) by H.J. Roth, p. 624.

Due to absence of phenolic function, codeine does not form o-nitro derivative with HNO_3 nor it forms Cu(II) chelate.

Photometric method based on the work of Taha and Rücker [Taha G., Rücker G., Arch. Pharm. (Weinheim, Ger.), 310, 485, 1977 through Pharm. Chem. (Vol. 2) by H.J. Roth], the compound produces intensely coloured anion with polyhalogen quinone or polycyanoquinone such as 7,7,8,8-tetracyanoquinone methane, an electron acceptor.

Probable Reaction Mechanism

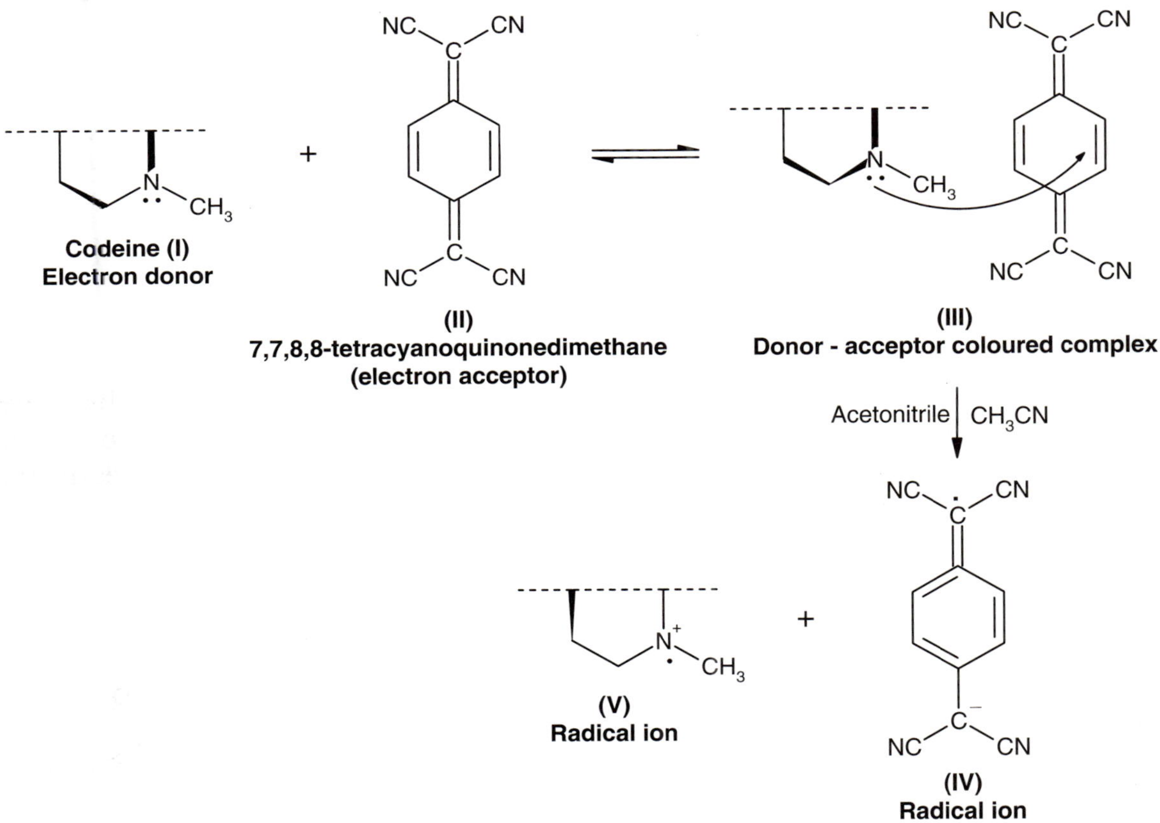

In acetonitrile the complex decomposes to radical ions (IV) and (V).

Formulation 17

Salbutamol sulphate

METHOD 1

Reagents

1. 0.2% w/v solution of p-aminophenol in ethyl alcohol.
2. 1 M solution of sodium carbonate in water.

Standard solution

100 mcg/ml of pure salbutamol sulphate in water.

Sample solution

Accurately weighed quantity of the sample is extracted with water to get 100 mcg/ml in respect of salbutamol sulphate.

Procedure

To 3 ml of standard and sample solutions add 3 ml of sodium carbonate solution, 0.2 ml of p-aminophenol reagent and volume is adjusted to 10 ml with water. After 25 min the absorbance of both the solutions is measured at maximum at about 635 nm against blank. The method obeys Beer's law over the concentration range of 5-60 mcg/ml.

Explanatory Note

p-Aminophenol in alkaline medium reacts at ortho or para to phenolic-OH of the compound to form indophenol.

Probable Reaction Mechanism

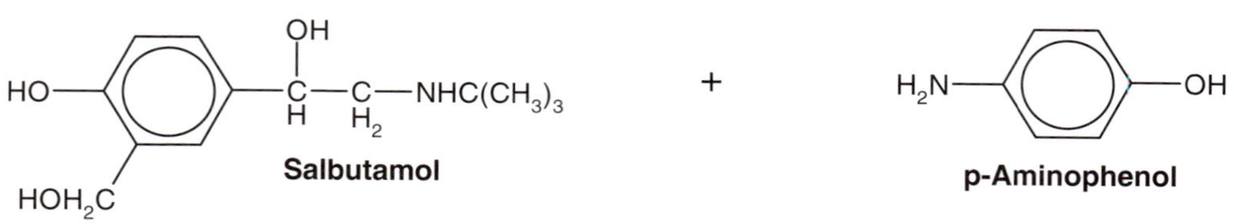

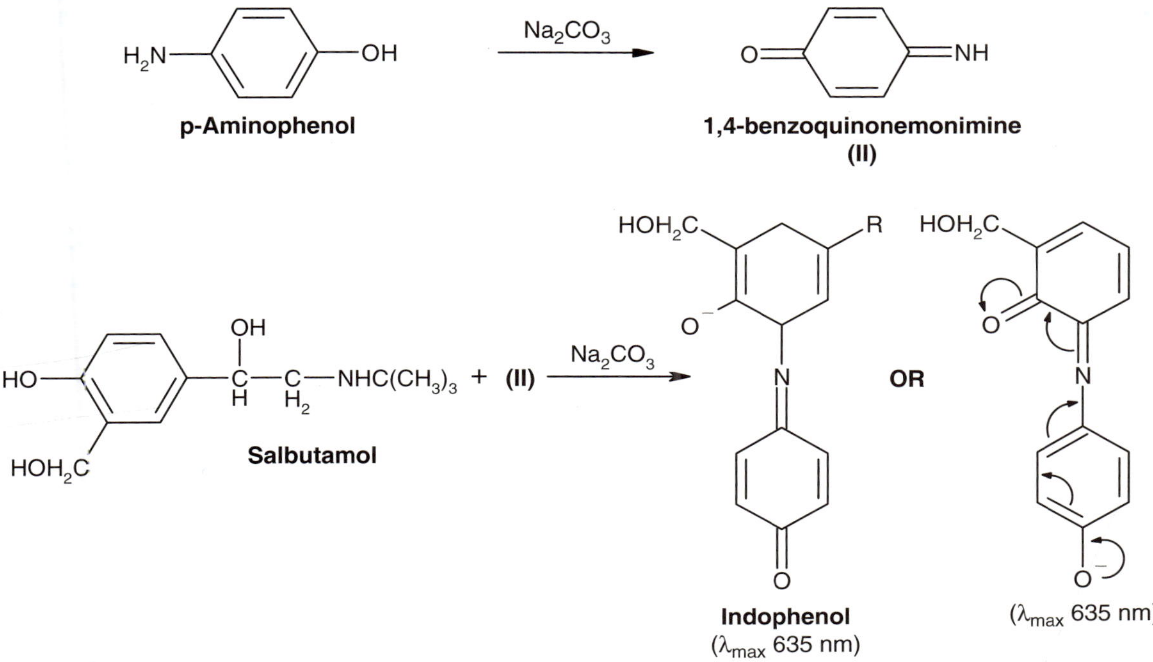

Reference

R.T. Sane, C.H. Thambre, A.B. Ambardekar & A.Y. Sathe, *Indian Drugs*, **19(5)**, 195-197, 1982.

METHOD 2

Reagents

1. Borate buffer, pH 8.2.
2. 0.04% w/v solution of 3,5-dichloro-p-benzoquinone chlorimide.

Sample and standard solutions

100 mcg/ml of the compound in water; see method 1 above.

Procedure

To 2 ml of standard and sample solutions add 1 ml of borate buffer, 1 ml of the reagent and dilute to 10 ml with water. After 25 mins measure the absorbance of both standard and sample solutions at maximum at about 610 nm against reagent blank. The method obeys Beer's law over the concentration range of 2-12 mcg/ml.

This method is based on oxidative coupling. Gibbs' reagent acts as oxidizing agent in alkaline medium (pH 8.2). The chlorimide reagent is first hydrolysed and then couples with the compound at para position.

Probable Reaction Mechanism

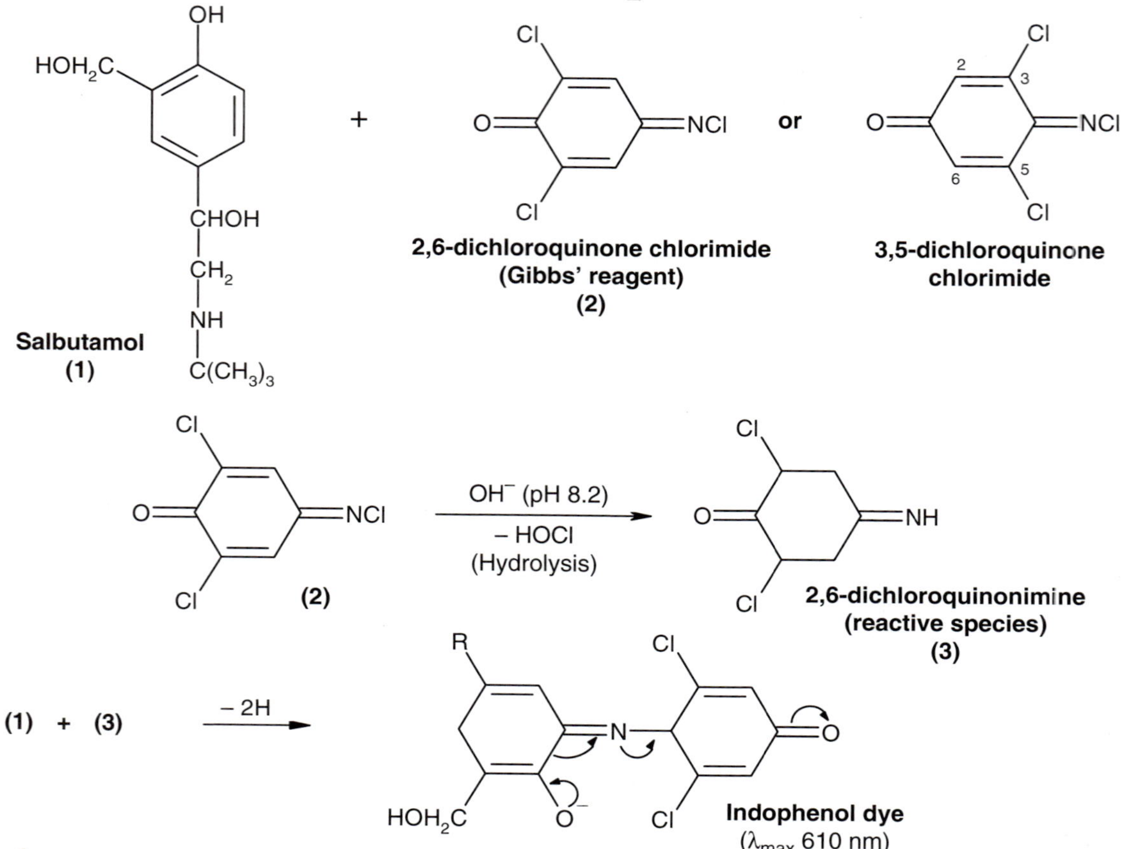

Reference

Shingba, D.M. & Naik S.D., *Canadian J. Pharm. Sci.*, **16(1)**, 65-67, 1981.

METHOD 3

Reagents

1. 5% w/v freshly prepared solution of sodium cobaltinitrite in water.
2. 20% w/v solution of sodium hydroxide in water.

Standard solution

0.5 mg/ml of pure salbutamol sulphate in water.

Sample solution

Weigh accurately a quantity of the sample equivalent to 10 mg of salbutamol sulphate and dissolve in 20 ml of water, shake, filter and discard first few ml of the filtrate.

Procedure

(A) Accurately measure 2 ml of sample and standard solutions, add 2 ml of glacial acetic acid and 2 ml of cobaltinitrite reagent. Heat on a water-bath for 15 min or till blank (reagents and 2 ml of water) turns bright pink. Cool and adjust to 50 ml with water. Measure the absorption of both the solutions at maximum at about 325 nm against blank. The method obeys Beer's law in the range of 8-35 mcg/ml.

(B) Follow procedure A. After heating the solutions for 15 min add 10 ml of water and 20 ml of sodium hydroxide solution, filter and adjust to 50 ml with water. Measure the absorbance of both the solutions at maximum at about 412 nm against reagent blank. The method obeys Beer's law in the range of 6-40 mcg/ml. The colour is stable for 5 h. In case of coated tablets, colour of the coating should be removed to avoid interference due to the dye.

Explanatory Note

Sodium cobaltinitrite $Na_3Co(NO_2)_6$ is the source of NO_2 ion for nitrosation reaction at ortho position to phenolic-OH. Nitroso derivative so formed is unstable in acid medium. It can be stabilized by adding alkali.

Probable Reaction Mechanism

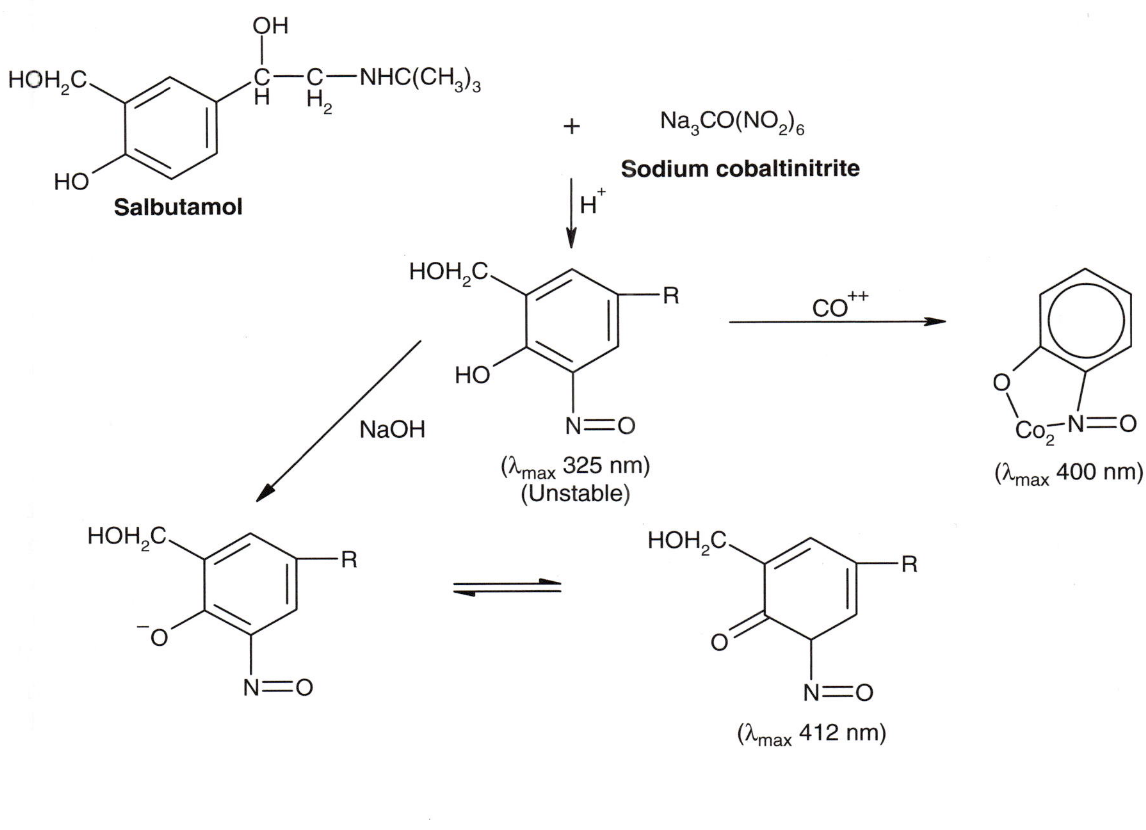

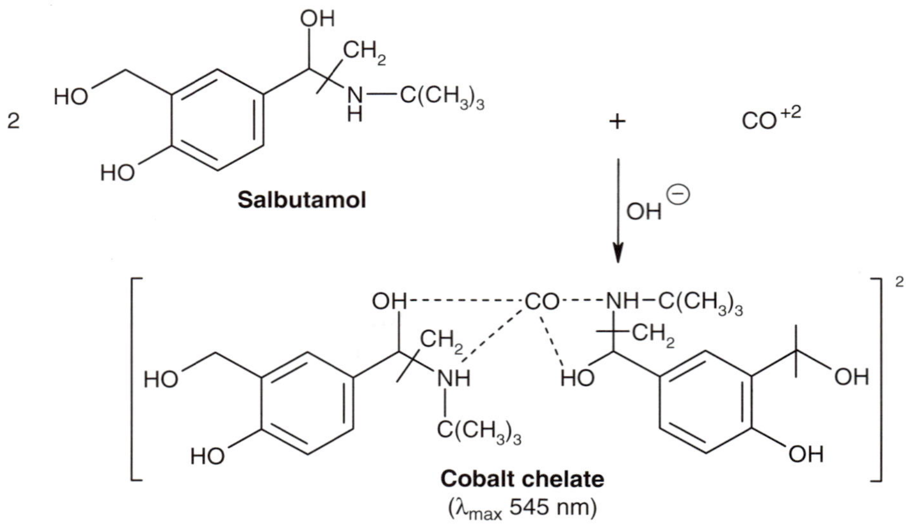

This is Chen-Kao reaction specific for phenylalkylamines with neighbouring amino and hydroxyl group.

METHOD 4

Reagents

1. 1 N hydrochloric acid.
2. 3% w/v solution of sodium nitrite in water.
3. 1 N sodium hydroxide.
4. 1% w/v solution of copper acetate in water.

Standard solution

0.1 mg/ml of salbutamol sulphate in water.

Sample solution

Sample accurately weighed is extracted with water to get 100 mcg/ml solution of the compound.

Procedure

(a) To 5 ml of sample and standard solutions add 3 ml of sodium nitrite solution and 1 ml of hydrochloric acid. Allow to stand for 5 min and render the solutions alkaline with 3 ml of sodium hydroxide solution. Mix and allow to stand for 5 min and measure the absorbance of both the solutions at maximum at about 425 nm against reagent blank. The method obeys Beer's law in the range of 2-20 mcg/ml.

(b) To 3 ml of sample and standard solutions add 2 ml of sodium nitrite solution and 0.1 ml of 1 N hydrochloric acid. Heat on a water-bath for 5 min, cool, add 1 ml of 1 N sodium hydroxide and adjust to 25 ml with water and measure the absorbance at about 425 nm. Procedure (b) is more sensitive than procedure (a). Beer's law is obeyed in the range of 1-10 mcg/ml.

(c) To 10 ml of sample and standard solutions add 2 ml of sodium nitrite solution and 2 ml of copper acetate solution. Mix and add 0.2 ml of 1 N hydrochloric acid. Heat on water-bath for 25 min, cool and dilute to 25 ml with water. Measure the extinction of both the solutions at maximum at about 525 nm. Beer's law is obeyed in the range of 40-400 mcg/ml.

Probable Reaction Mechanism

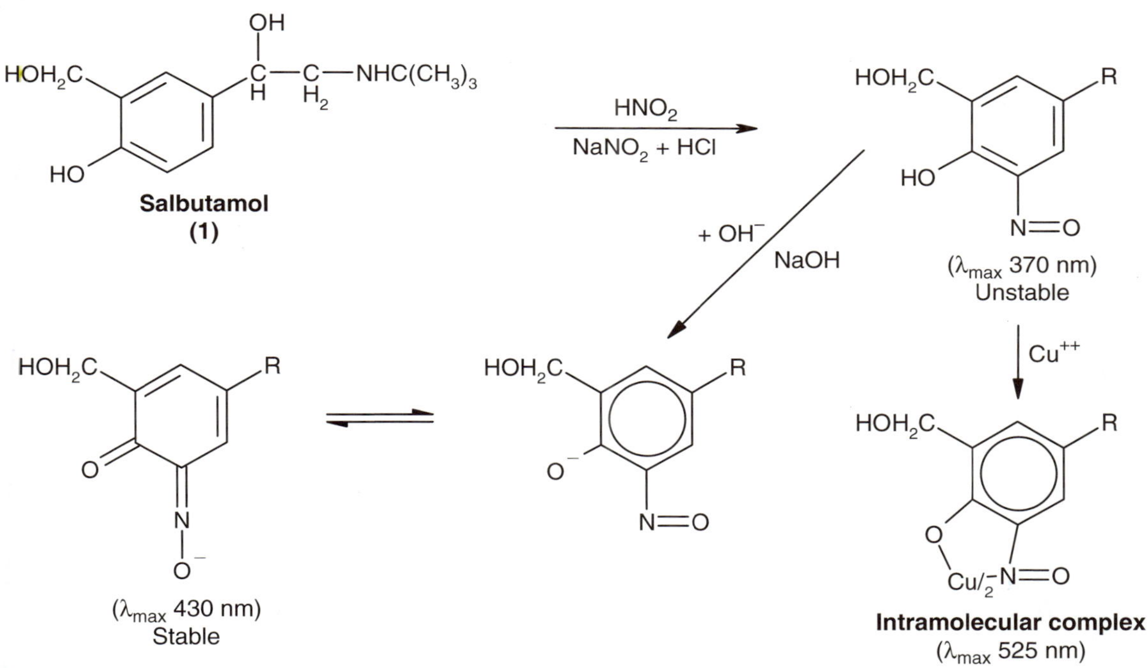

Explanatory Note

Salbutamol with aromatic hydroxyl group is capable of forming nitroso derivative (yellow chromogen) by reaction with sodium nitrite and hydrochloric acid. Nitrosation both at ortho or para position is possible, but since para is occupied, the compound forms nitroso derivative at ortho position. The nitroso derivative is unstable in acidic medium, but can be stabilized in NaOH with bathochromic shift and hyperchromic effect. This is probably due to the contribution of an extra pair of unshared electrons in the interaction with the aromatic nucleus.

Note

For intermolecular copper chelate, see next page.

Probable Reaction Mechanism

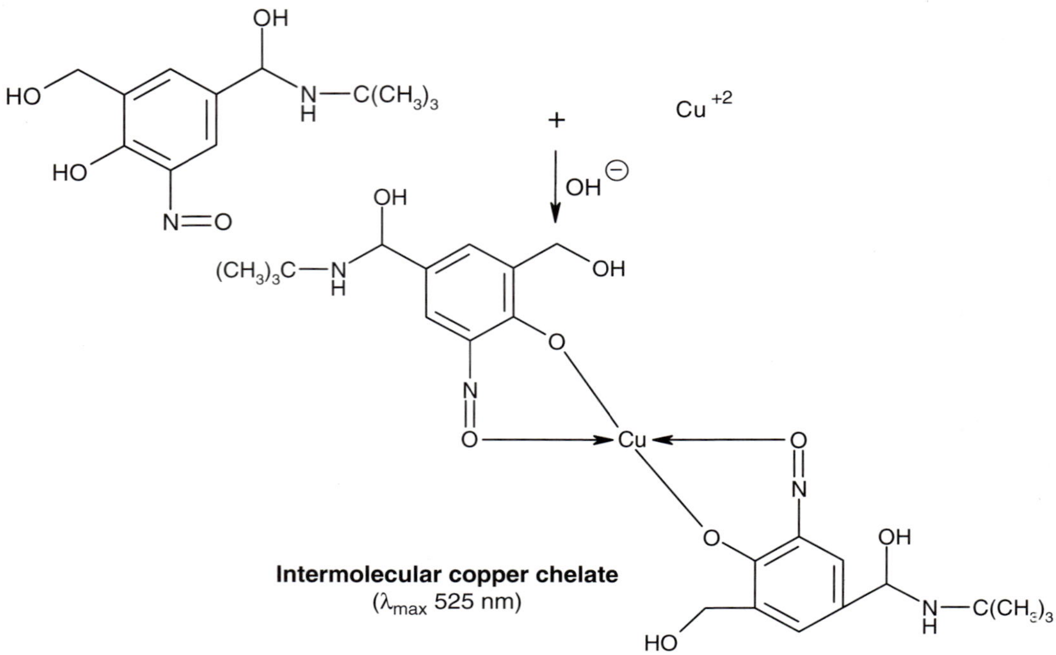

Intermolecular copper chelate
(λ_{max} 525 nm)

Reference

P.K. Chatterjee, C.L. Jain & P.D. Sethi, *Indian Drugs*, **23(11)**, 635, 1986.

METHOD 5

This method is based on the reaction of phenols with 4-aminoantipyrin after oxidation with alkaline potassium ferricyanide. The following alkaline media have been recommended.

Reagents

1. Alkaline solutions:
   (a) 8.4% w/v solution of sodium carbonate in water.
   (b) Buffer, pH 10: Boric acid - 2.370 g, potassium chloride - 14.910 g, water to produce 1000 ml. 250 ml of this solution is mixed with 44 ml of 1 N sodium hydroxide and diluted to 1000 ml with water.
   (c) Ammonia - ammonium chloride buffer: 67.5 g of ammonium chloride and 570 ml of strong ammonia solution are mixed and diluted with water to 1000 ml. 2 ml of this solution is diluted to 1000 ml with water. Any one of the alkaline solutions indicated above can be used, however, alkaline solutions (b) and (c) are reported to give better results.
2. 2% w/v solution of 4-aminoantipyrin in water, prepare fresh.
3. 8% w/v solution of potassium ferricyanide in water, prepare fresh.

Standard solution

0.4 mg/ml of the salbutamol (base) in water (40 mg of base is equivalent to 48.2 mg of salbutamol sulphate).

Sample solution

Accurate quantity of the sample is weighed and extracted with water to get 0.5 mg/ml of the base.

Procedure

To 2.5 ml of sample and standard solutions add 5 ml of antipyrin solution and 5 ml of ferricyanide solution. Shake and add 5 ml of either of alkaline solutions. Keep for 30 min and extract with three portions of 25 ml, 10 ml, 10 ml of chloroform. Pass each chloroform layer through anhydrous sodium sulphate previously washed with chloroform and dilute to 50 ml with chloroform. Measure the absorbance of both the solutions at maximum at about 470 nm against reagent blank.

Explanatory Note

This involves oxidative coupling. The oxidizing agent used is K3Fe(CN)6 in alkaline buffer, pH 8-10 and coupling reagent used is 4-aminoantipyrin. This is called Emerson reaction. The coupling usually occurs at para position to phenolic-OH, but since para position is occupied, there are two possibilities in case of salbutamol: (1) either an oxidative coupling occurs at ortho position or (2) oxidative breakdown of ethanolamine side chain followed by coupling at para position.

Probable Reaction Mechanism

(1)

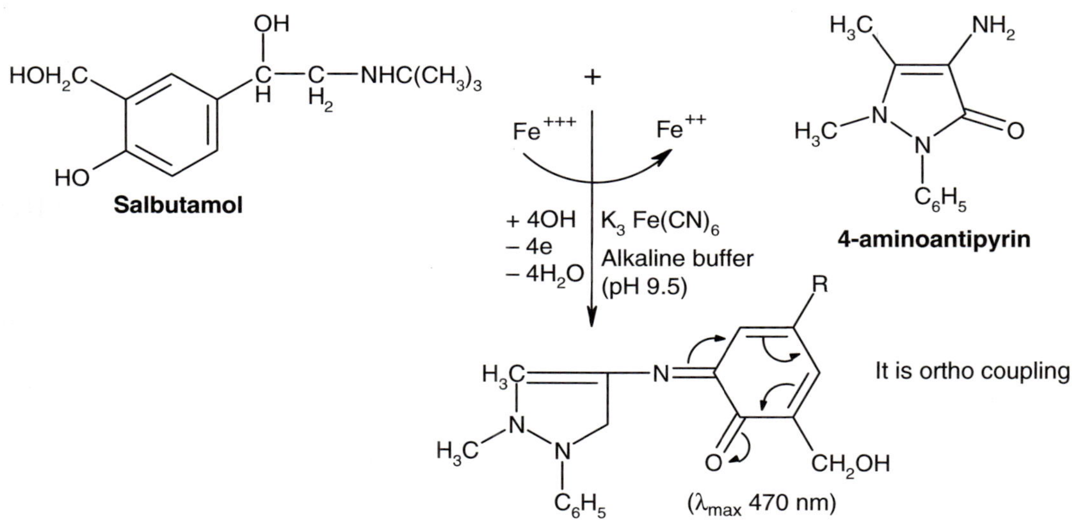

(2) Or an oxidative breakdown of ethanolamine side chain followed by para coupling.

Probable Reaction Mechanism

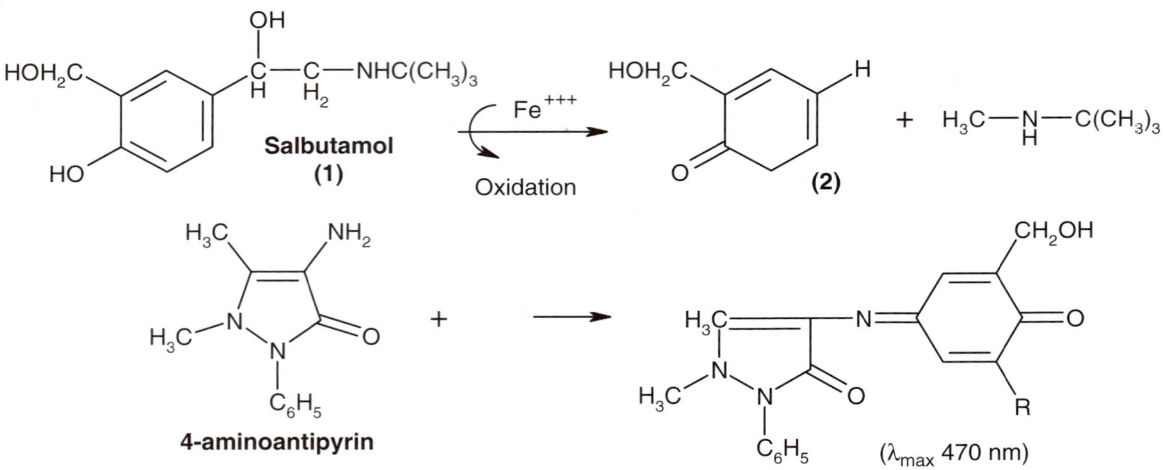

Reference

1. Pharmaceutical Chemistry (Vol. 2) by H.J. Roth, 1991, p. 76.
2. K. Shivaramchandra, S. Khanna & V.J. Dighe, *Indian Drugs*, **21(1)**, 32-33, 1983.
3. R.T. Sane, V.L. Nayak, V.B. Malkar, D.S. Sapre, A.D. Nadkarni, U.R. Pandit & V.J. Doshi, *Indian Drugs*, **21(2)**, 76-78, 1983.
4. M. Basu et al., *Indian Drugs*, **28(2)**, 109, 1990.

METHOD 6

This method is based on oxidation of salbutamol sulphate by ferric chloride in acidic medium and subsequent coupling of Fe(II) with 2,2′-bispyridyl to form red-coloured dye (λ_{max} 520 nm).

Reagents

1. 0.003 M ferric chloride solution in water.
2. 0.2 M o-phosphoric acid.
3. 0.01 M solution of 2,2′-bispyridyl.

Standard solution

200 μg/ml solution of salbutamol sulphate in water.

Sample solution

Powdered tablets or syrup extracted with water to appropriate concentration.

Procedure

To 2 ml each of sample and standard solutions add 1 ml of Fe(III) chloride solution and heat in boiling water-bath for 15 min, cool to room temperature, add 2 ml of 0.2 M o-phosphoric acid, dilute to 10 ml with water and measure the absorbance of red colour at 520 nm against reagent blank.

Probable Reaction Mechanism

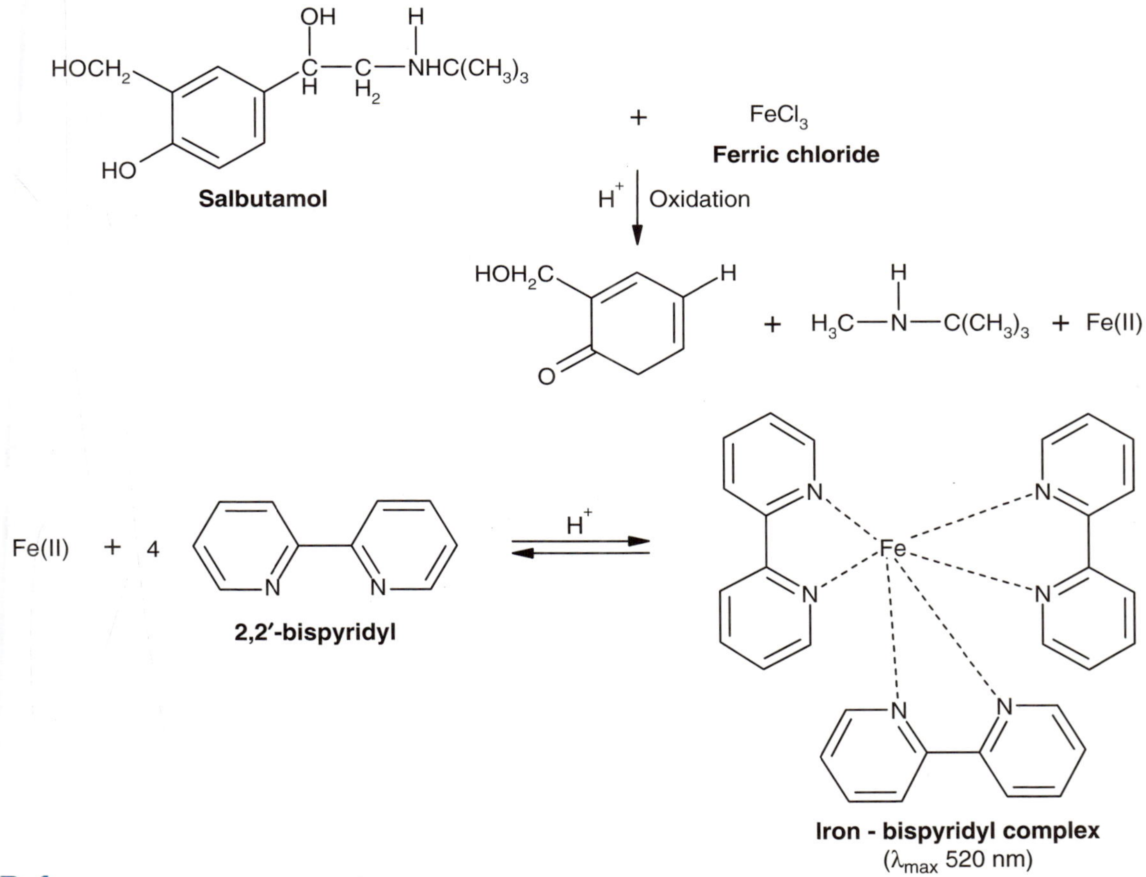

Reference

K.P.R. Chowdary & G. Devala Rao, *Indian Drugs*, **34(5)**, 283-285, 1997.

METHOD 7

Reagents

1. 3% w/v solution of sodium nitrite in water.
2. 0.5% sulphanilic acid in (1 : 9) in hydrochloric acid.
3. 5% sodium hydroxide.

Sample and standard solutions

100 μg/ml of salbutamol sulphate in water.

Procedure

To 1 ml each of sample and standard solutions add 5 ml of diazotized sulphanilic acid and 5 ml of sodium hydroxide solution, dilute to 25 ml with water and measure the absorbance at 445 nm against reagent blank.

Probable Reaction Mechanism

Diazotized sulphanilic acid (Pauly's reagent) couples with the compound at ortho position to phenolic-OH in alkaline medium. As para position is occupied, hence coupling at ortho.

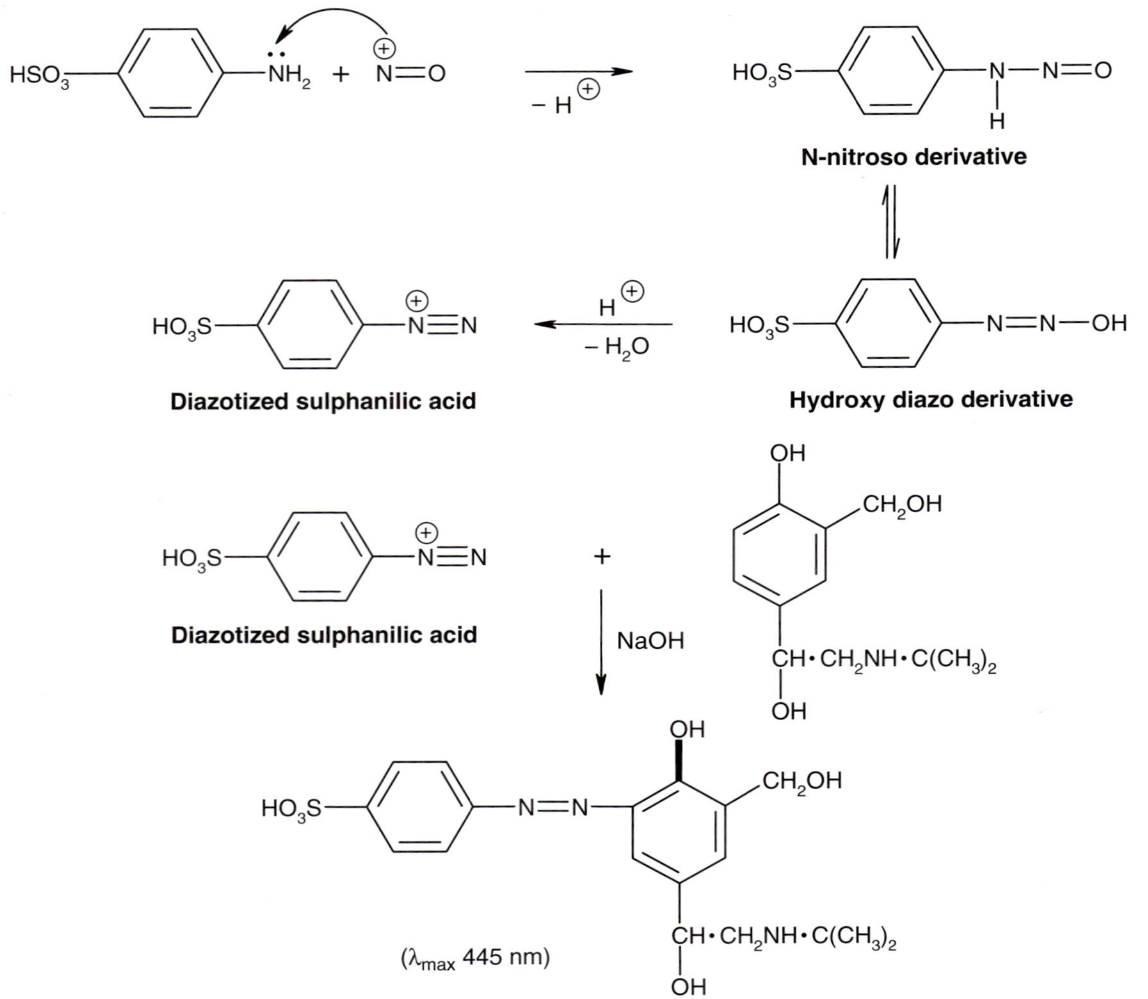

Reference

D.M. Shingbal & R.R. Naik, Indian Drugs, **22(5)**, 273-274, 1985.

METHOD 8

Reagents

1. 0.1% p-nitroaniline in 10% v/v HCl.
2. 0.5% w/v solution of $NaNO_2$.
3. 5% w/v aqueous solution of NaOH.

Sample and standard solutions

25 µg/ml in water.

Procedure

To 5 ml each of sample and standard solutions add 2.5 ml of p-nitroaniline, and then add 1 ml of $NaNO_2$ solution, mix and add 3 ml of NaOH solution, dilute to 25 ml with water and measure the absorbance at 485 nm against reagent blank.

Probable Reaction Mechanism

Nitrosonium ion formed will diazotize the amino group of p-nitroaniline to give diazotized product. Then coupling takes place between diazotized product and salbutamol to give orange-coloured coupled product (λ_{max} 485 nm).

$$NaNO_2 + HCl \longrightarrow NaCl + HNO_2$$

$$HNO_2 \xrightarrow{H^+} H_2O\,\overset{+}{N}O \xrightarrow[Cl^-]{} \overset{-}{Cl}\;\overset{+}{N}{=}O$$

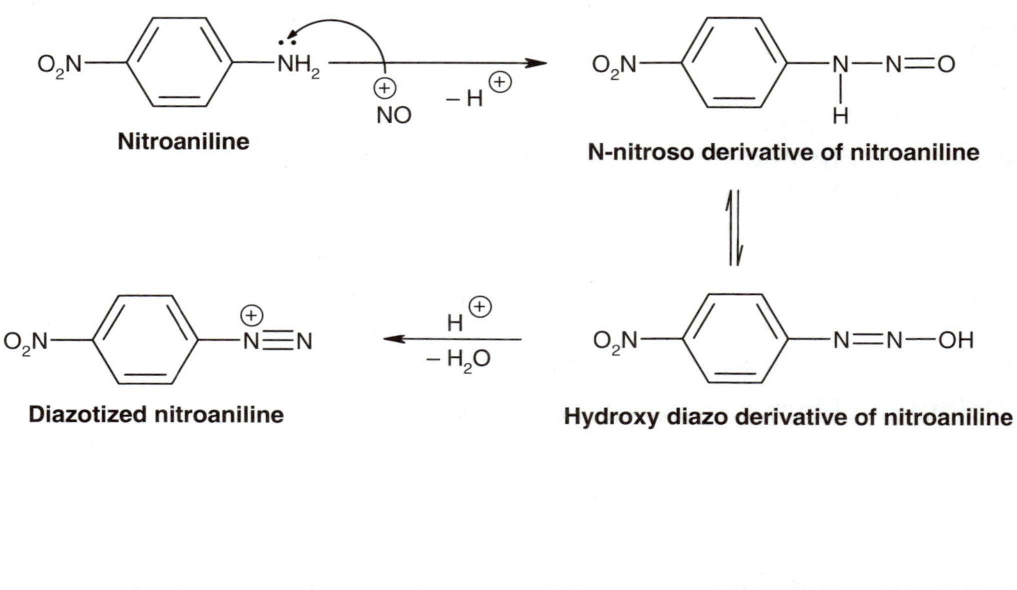

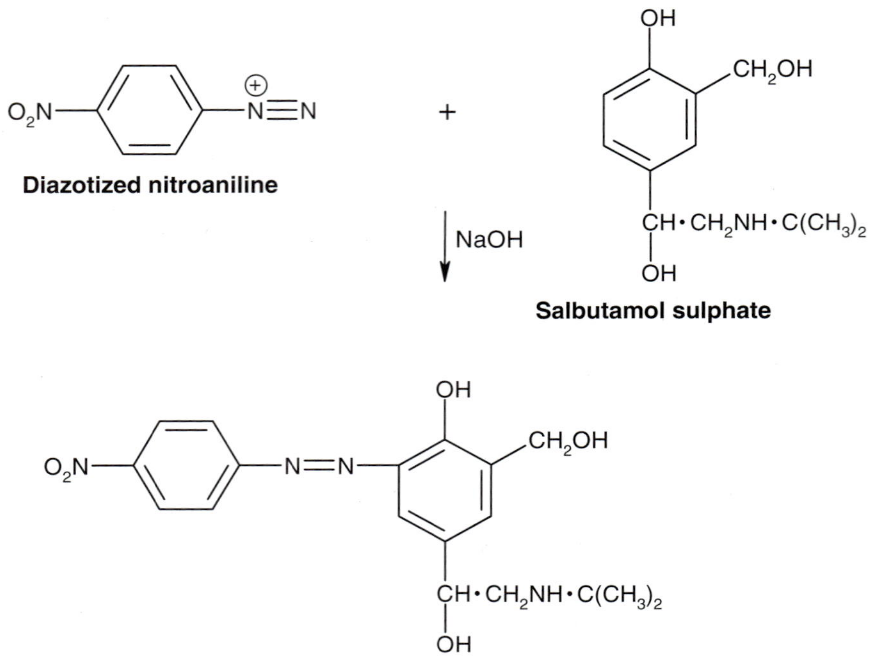

(λ_{max} 485 nm)

Reference

D.M. Shingbal & S.V. Joshi, *Indian Drugs*, **21(9)**, 398-399, 1984.

Note

1. On similar lines the drug reacts with diazotized dapsone to yield coloured complex (l_{max} 475 nm) in alkaline medium (trimethylamine).

Reference

R.T. Sane, N.R. Naik & S.S. Zarapkar, *J. of University of Bombay*, Vol. L_1-L_{11}, 78-79, 1983.

2. Salbutamol sulphate couples with diazotized benzocaine in triethylamine to give coloured chromogen (l_{max} 460 nm), the reaction mechanism being similar to the one described with p-nitroaniline.

Reference

R.T. Sane, V.G. Nayak & V.B. Malkar, *Talanta*, **32(1)**, 31-33, 1983.

The following reactions can be used for quantitative estimation.

(a) Salbutamol forms chelate with $FeCl_3$.

Probable Reaction Mechanism

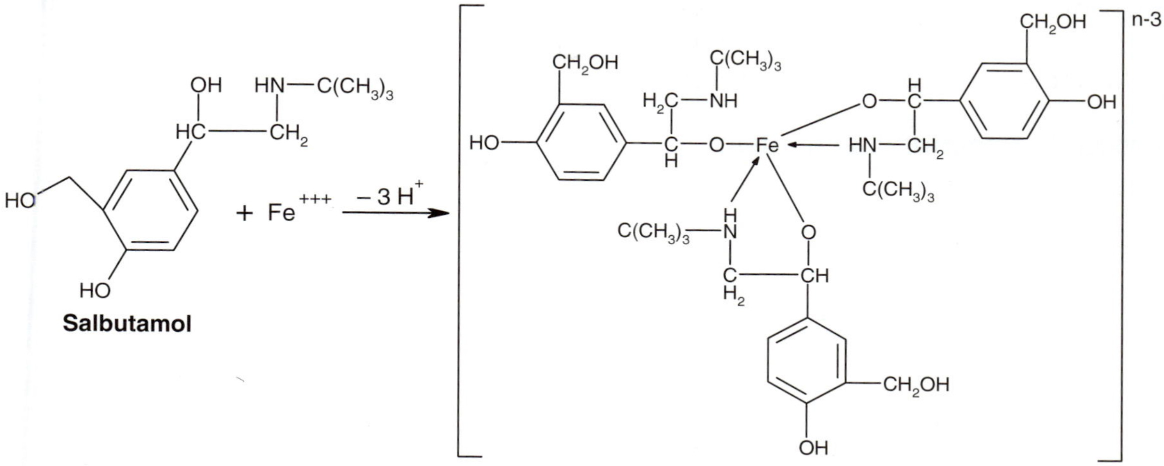

(b) On treatment of the drug with NaOH, first sodium salt is formed which is oxidized with sodium metaperiodate. The aldehyde so formed reacts with acetylacetone to give yellow-coloured product (λ_{max} 410 nm).

Probable Reaction Mechanism

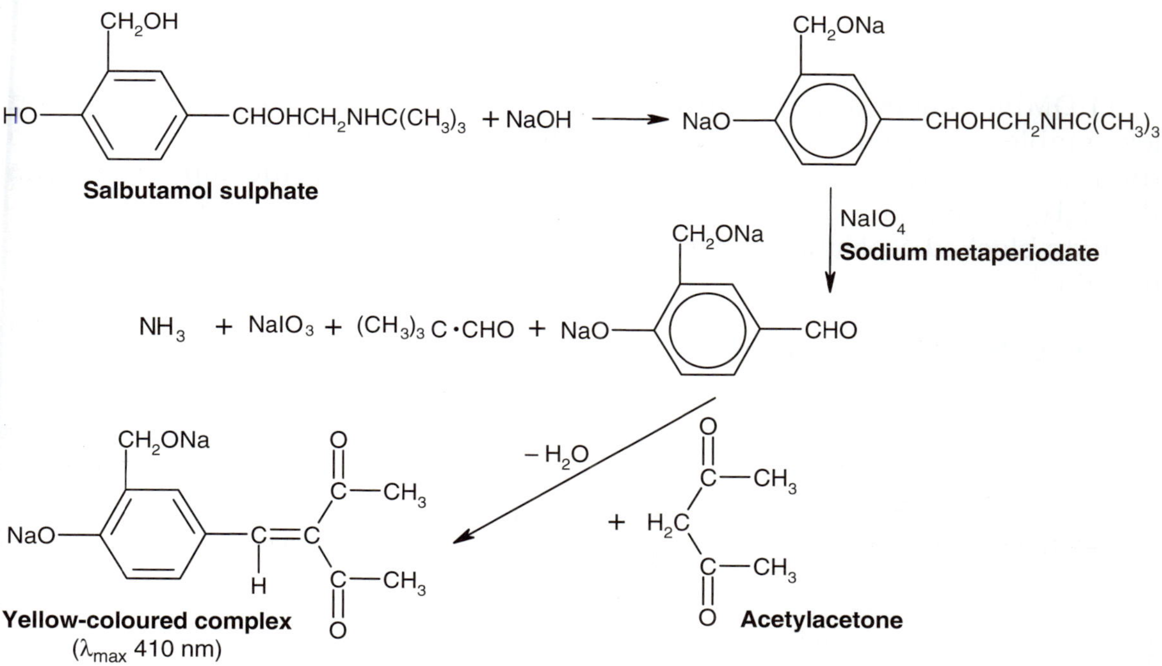

Reference

K.K. Bhatt, S.A. Shah & S.S. Pandya, Abstract No. C-4, IPC-1992.

(c) The compound reacts with HNO_3 in the presence of H_2SO_4. Initially nitronium ion is produced which being electron-deficient will attack at ortho position to the phenolic-OH (para being occupied) resulting in the formation of yellow-coloured nitro compound.

Probable Reaction Mechanism

$$HNO_3 + H_2SO_4 \longrightarrow H_3O^+ + NO_2^+ + 2HSO_4^-$$

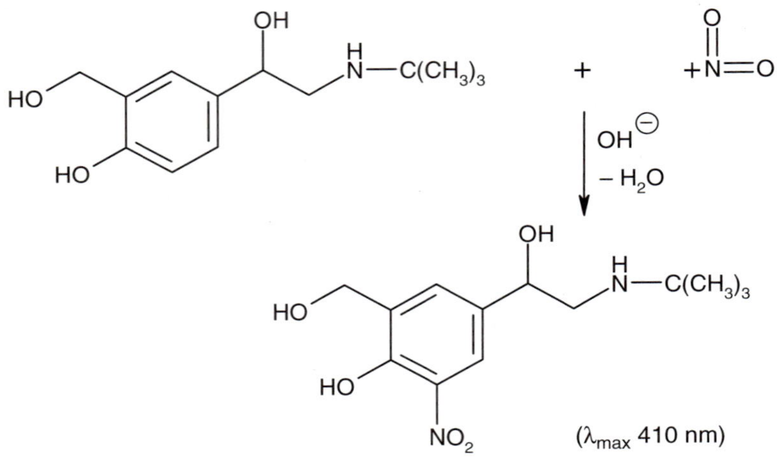

(c) DMPD reacts initially with CAT to produce highly reactive species but less stable p-benzoquinone diamine derivative which may further react with the phenolic coupler by electrophilic attack in the most nucleophilic site on the C_6H_6 ring of the coupler i.e. p-position to the phenolic hydroxyl or if p-position blocked o-position to the phenolic-OH. Resulting dye is further oxidized to indo dye.

Probable Reaction Mechanism

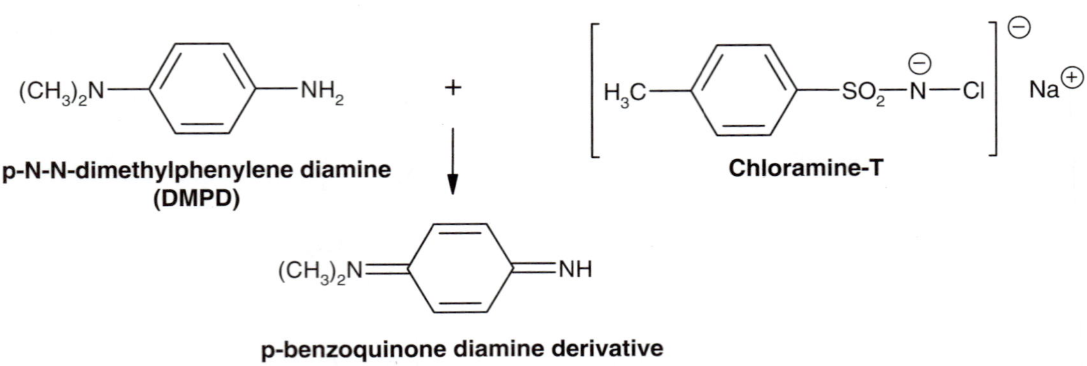

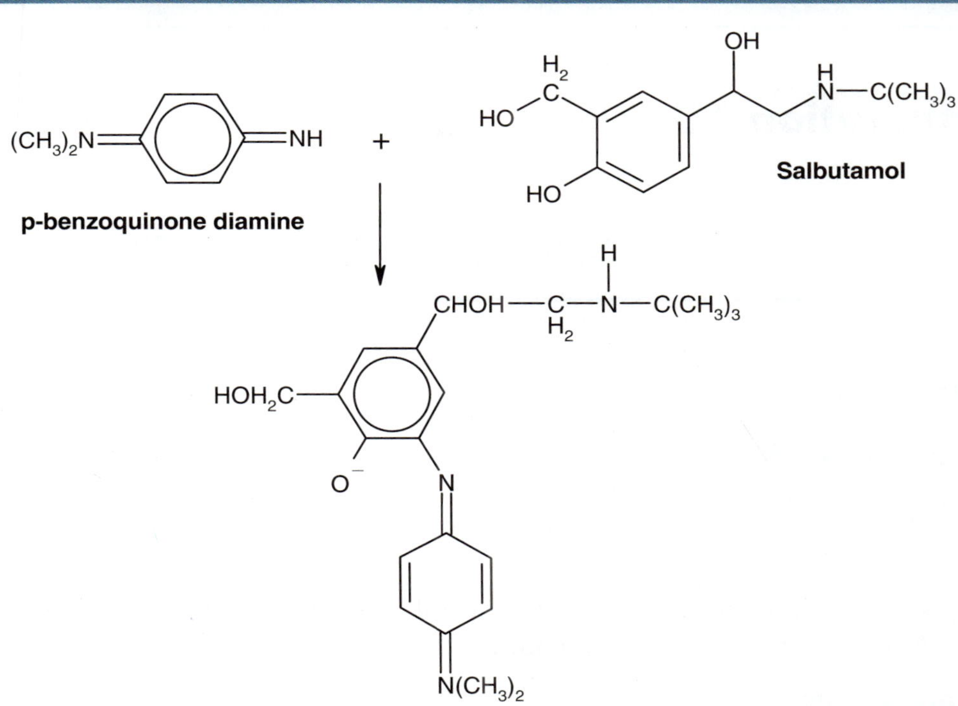

Indoaniline dye (extractable into isobutanol)
(λ_{max} 620 nm)

Reference

1. Gowri Sankar, C.S.P. Sastry, M.N. Reddy & Rajendra Prasad, *Indian Drugs*, **24(1)**, 410, 1986.
2. K.V. Colthup, F.A.A. Dallas, D.A. Saynov, P.F. Carey, L.F. Skimore & L.E. Martin, *J. Chromatography, Biomed. Application*, **346**, 111-118, 1985.

Formulation 18

Salbutamol sulphate, Theophylline

ESTIMATION

Salbutamol sulphate

METHOD 1

Reagents

1. 0.2% w/v solution of p-aminophenol in ethyl alcohol (prepare fresh).
2. 1 M solution of sodium carbonate in water.

Standard solution

100 mcg/ml of salbutamol sulphate in water.

Sample solution

Accurately weighed quantity of the sample is extracted with water to get 100 mcg/ml in respect of salbutamol sulphate.

Procedure

To 3 ml each of standard and sample solutions, add 3 ml of sodium carbonate solution, 0.2 ml of p-aminophenol reagent and volume is adjusted to 10 ml with water. After 25 min, the absorbance of both the solutions is measured at about 635 nm against blank. The method obeys Beer's law over the concentration range of 5-60 mcg/ml. For reaction mechanism, see method under formulation 17 of this chapter.

METHOD 2

Reagents

1. Borate buffer, pH 8.2.
2. 0.04% w/v solution of 3,5-dichloro-p-benzoquinone chlorimide.

Sample and standard solution

100 mcg/ml of the compound in water; see method 1 above.

Procedure

To 2 ml each of sample and standard solutions, add 1 ml of borate buffer and 1 ml of chlorimide reagent, dilute to 10 ml with water. After 20 minutes, measure the absorbance of both standard and sample solutions at about 610 nm against reagent blank. The method obeys Beer's law over the concentration range of 2-12 mcg/ml. For reaction mechanism, see formulation 17 of this chapter.

Theophylline

Follow the method 2 described under formulation 1 of this chapter.

Formulation 19

Salbutamol sulphate, Choline theophyllinate

ESTIMATION

Salbutamol sulphate

Follow the methods described under formulation 17 of this chapter.

Choline theophyllinate

Measure sample equivalent to about 100 mg of the substance, add 25 ml of water and few drops of bromocresol solution. Add 0.5 N hydrochloric acid till the colour changes to full yellow. Add 5 g of sodium chloride and extract with four 25 ml portions of chloroform : isopropanol (3 : 1) mixture. Wash each extract with the same 10 ml of water. Pass the combined organic layer through anhydrous sodium sulphate. Wash the sodium sulphate bed with solvent mixture. Evaporate the combined extract to dryness on water bath and dry the residue to constant weight at 150°C. Cool, weigh and calculate the results.

$$\% \text{ (w/v) of choline theophyllinate} = \frac{\text{Weight (mg) of the residue} \times 1.572 \times 100}{200}$$

Alternatively, the residue obtained above after evaporation of combined organic extract may be taken up in 0.1 N hydrochloric acid and measure the absorbance at maximum at about 275 nm. Calculate the results by measuring the absorbance of standard solution at 275 nm. Or, suspend the sample in 20 ml of water and 20 ml of 0.1 N sulphuric acid, extract with 2 ´ 50 ml portions of ether. Collect the acidic layer and dilute with 0.1 N sulphuric acid to give a concentration of 10 mcg/ml and measure the extinction of both sample and standard (10 mcg/ml) at about 275 nm using 0.1 N sulphuric acid as blank and calculate the results.

Note

The residue may be dissolved in 50 ml of hot water, cooled and 20 ml of 0.1 N silver nitrate added and titrated with 0.1 N sodium hydroxide using bromothymol blue as indicator. Each ml of 0.1 N sodium hydroxide is equivalent to 28.33 mg of choline theophyllinate.

Probable Reaction Mechanism

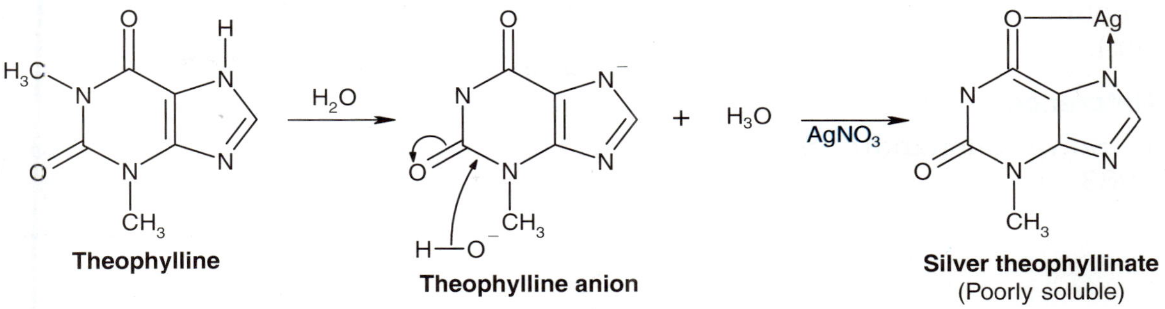

Note

Theophylline gives white precipitate with silver nitrate. Because of the acid strength of theophylline an equilibrium is set up in aqueous solution between dissociated and undissociated theophylline. The equilibrium gets shifted towards right by addition of $AgNO_3$. This poorly soluble silver theophyllinate is soluble in dilute alkali hydroxyl.

Reference

Pharmaceutical Chemistry (Vol. 2) by H.J. Roth, 1991, p. 604.

Theophylline can be directly titrated with aq. sodium hydroxide in certain non-aqueous solvents such as DMF. Among the different xanthine derivatives, theophylline is relatively the strongest acid. This acidity is explained by N-unsubstituted imidazole derivative structure. Further, the theophylline partial structure consisting of vinylogous acid amide leads to resonance stabilization of the anion and thus to the strength of the acid.

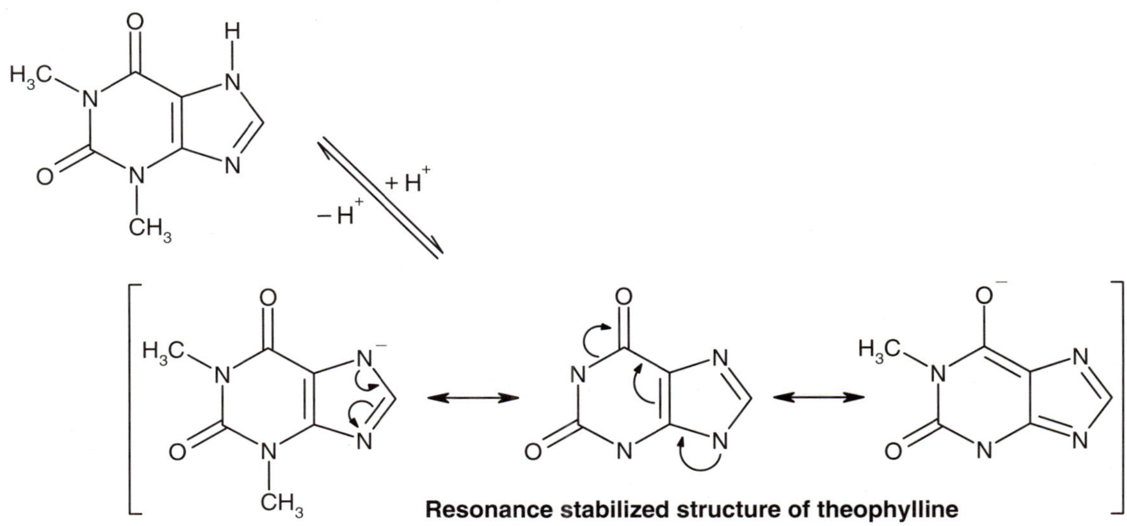

Resonance stabilized structure of theophylline

Note

Choline theophylline can be estimated by UV spectrophotometry (λ_{max} 275 nm).

Reference

K. Shivaramchandra, S. Khanna & V.J. Dighe, Indian Drugs, **21(2)**, 32-33, 1983.

Formulation 20

Salbutamol sulphate, Bromhexine hydrochloride, Hydroxyethyltheophylline

ESTIMATION

Salbutamol sulphate

Reagents

1. 5% w/v solution of sodium bicarbonate in water.
2. 1% w/v solution of 4-aminoantipyrine in alcohol.
3. 8% w/v solution of potassium ferricyanide in water.

Standard solution

20 mg/100 ml of salbutamol sulphate in water. Further dilute 10 ml of the solution to 50 ml with alcohol.

Sample solution

Weigh accurate quantity of sample equivalent to 20 mg of the substance. Add about 50 ml of water. Shake vigorously and make up to 100 ml with water. Filter and dilute 10 ml of the filtrate to 50 ml with alcohol.

Procedure

Transfer 10 ml each of the sample and standard solutions to 250 ml separator. Add 100 ml of water, 4 ml each of bicarbonate solution, antipyrine reagent and potassium ferricyanide solution. Mix and allow to stand in subdued light for 15 min. Extract with three 15 ml portions of chloroform. Pass the chloroform layer through pre-moistened anhydrous sodium sulphate layer. Make up the volume to 50 ml with chloroform and measure the absorption of both the solution at about 465 nm using chloroform as blank, deduce the results by comparison. For reaction mechanism, see formulation 17 of this chapter.

Hydroxyethyltheophylline (Etofylline)

Standard solution

10 mcg/ml of hydroxyethyltheophylline in water.

Sample solution

Weigh accurately quantity of sample equivalent to 200 mg of the substance and transfer to a 100 ml volumetric flask. Add about 70-80 ml of water, shake and dissolve and make up the volume. Filter and dilute the filtrate appropriately with water to get a concentration of 10 mcg/ml. Measure the extinction of both the solutions at maxima at about 273 nm using water as blank. Calculate the results by comparison.

Bromhexine hydrochloride

Reagents

1. 5 N hydrochloric acid.
2. 2% w/v sodium nitrite solution in water.
3. 5% w/v solution of ammonium sulphamate in water.
4. 0.1% w/v solution of N-1-naphthyl-ethylene-diamine dihydrochloride (NED).

Standard solution

40 mg/ml of bromhexine in methanol. Dilute 5 ml of this solution to 100 ml with water containing 2-3 drops of dilute hydrochloric acid.

Sample solution

Weigh accurately the sample equivalent to 40 mg of substance and prepare the final solution as described under standard solution.

Procedure

To 5 ml each of sample and standard solutions, add 1 ml of 5 N hydrochloric acid, 1 ml of sodium nitrite solution. Allow to stand for 5 min, add 1 ml of ammonium sulphamate solution, allow to stand for 3 min, followed by 1 ml of NED reagent. After 10 min measure the absorption of both the solutions at about 525 nm against reagent blank. Deduce the results by comparison.

Note

For quantitative estimation, extinction of the sample (40 mcg/ml) as obtained above can directly be measured at 317 nm and results calculated by using 87 as of A 1%, 1 cm at 317 nm.

For reaction mechanism, see formulation 29 of the chapter on expectorants.

Formulation 21

Hydroxyethyltheophylline (Etofylline), Theophylline

ESTIMATION

Hydroxyethyltheophylline (Etofylline)

Reagents

1. Formic acid, anhydrous.
2. 0.1 N perchloric acid.
3. Acetic anhydride.
4. Chloroform.
5. Crystal violet solution, indicator.

Procedure

Weigh sample accurately equivalent to about 250 mg of the substance, add about 75 ml of chloroform. Shake for about 15 min, filter into dry conical flask. Repeat extraction with further 25 ml of chloroform. Evaporate combined chloroform layer on water-bath. Dissolve the residue in 2 ml of formic acid, anhydrous, add 50 ml of acetic anhydride, few drops of indicator and titrate with 0.1 N perchloric acid to yellow end point. Each ml of 0.1 N perchloric acid is equivalent to 0.02242 g of etofylline.

Note

This derivative of theophylline has better solubility than the parent compound.

Because of alcoholic hydroxy group at position 7, it can be acetylated.

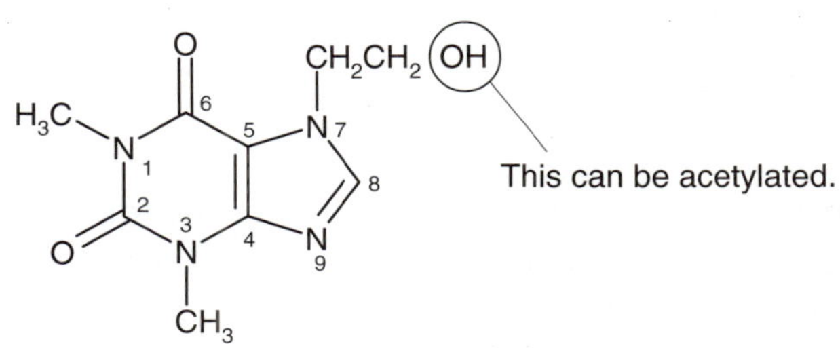

Theophylline

METHOD 1

Reagents

1. 0.1 N sodium hydroxide.
2. Bromothymol blue solution, indicator.

Procedure

Accurately weighed quantity of the sample equivalent to 200 mg of theophylline is dissolved in about 50 ml of water by gently heating on water-bath, filter, wash the residue with water, combine the filtrate. Add 25 ml of 0.1 N silver nitrate, 1 ml of bromothymol blue solution and titrate with 0.1 N sodium hydroxide to blue end point. Each ml of 0.1 N sodium hydroxide is equivalent to 18.02 mg of theophylline (anhydrous). For reaction mechanism, see formulation of this chapter.

METHOD 2

Reagents

1. 0.1 N silver nitrate.
2. 0.5% v/v solution of ammonium hydroxide in water.
3. 25% v/v nitric acid.
4. 0.1 N ammonium thiocyanate.
5. Ferric ammonium sulphate solution-indicator.
6. Ammonium acetate.

Procedure

Weigh accurately quantity of the sample equivalent to 200 mg of theophylline, add 50 ml of ammonia solution and shake vigorously for about 10-15 min. Centrifuge and to the clear solution, add 2 g of ammonium acetate and heat to boiling. Add 15 ml of silver nitrate solution drop-wise. Cool in ice-bath, filter, wash the precipitates with ice cold water. Dissolve the silver-theophylline precipitates in 20 ml of nitric acid (25%), cool, add 25 ml of water and 5-10 drops of indicator. Titrate with 0.1 N ammonium thiocyanate solution. Each ml of 0.1 N ammonium thiocyanate solution is equivalent to 0.0198 g of theophylline monohydrate (A).

Note

The precipitates of silver-theophylline complex should not be exposed to direct sunlight as reduction would occur. For structure of silver theophyllinate, see formulation of this chapter.

Theophylline and Etofylline (total)

Standard solution

10 mcg/ml of etofylline in 0.1 N hydrochloric acid.

Sample solution

Weigh sample accurately equivalent to 200 mg of etofylline, add 25-30 ml of 0.1 N hydrochloric acid, heat to boiling and cool. Dilute to 100 ml with acid, filter and dilute the filtrate appropriately and step-wise with 0.1 N hydrochloric acid to get a concentration of 10 mcg/ml.

Procedure

Measure the extinction of both sample and standard solutions at maxima at about 273 nm using 0.1 N hydrochloric acid as blank. Calculate the results by comparison. This will give total (theophylline monohydrate + etofylline) = (B).

$$\text{Contents of etofylline} = B - (A \times 1.31).$$

Formulation 22

Bromhexine hydrochloride, Salbutamol sulphate

ESTIMATION

Bromhexine hydrochloride

Follow the method described in formulation 29 of the chapter on expectorants and cough suppressants.

Salbutamol sulphate

The acidic extract obtained during estimation of bromhexine hydrochloride as described in formulation of the chapter on expectorants is diluted appropriately and subjected to analysis as per method described in formulation 17 of this chapter.

Formulation 23

Bromhexine hydrochloride, Salbutamol sulphate, Betamethasone

ESTIMATION

Bromhexine hydrochloride

Follow the method described in formulation 20 of this chapter.

Betamethasone

Reagents

1. 0.5% w/v solution of tetrazolium blue in methanol.
2. 10% w/v solution of tetramethyl ammonium hydroxide (TMAH) solution in methanol.

Standard solution

10 mcg/ml of betamethasone in chloroform.

Sample solution

Weigh powdered sample equivalent to 1 mg of betamethasone suspended in 10 ml of water and extract with chloroform (3 × 20 ml), passing each extract through anhydrous sodium sulphate, make up the final volume to 100 ml.

Procedure

To 10 ml each of sample and standard solutions add 2 ml of tetrazolium blue solution, followed by 2 ml of TMAH solution. Keep aside for 45 min at 37°C and measure the absorbance of both the solutions at 525 nm against reagent blank. Calculate the results by comparison.

This is one of the steroids with α-ketol group at C-17. These steroids are sensitive to oxidation because of substituents at ring D. They have β-position ketol structure at C-17 and with dihydroxy acetone structure. The compound reacts with triphenyltetrazolium salt (TTC) or tetrazolium blue (TZB) and gets oxidized to aldehyde and thereby TZB undergoes reductive opening of hetero-cyclic ring to give formazane derivative.

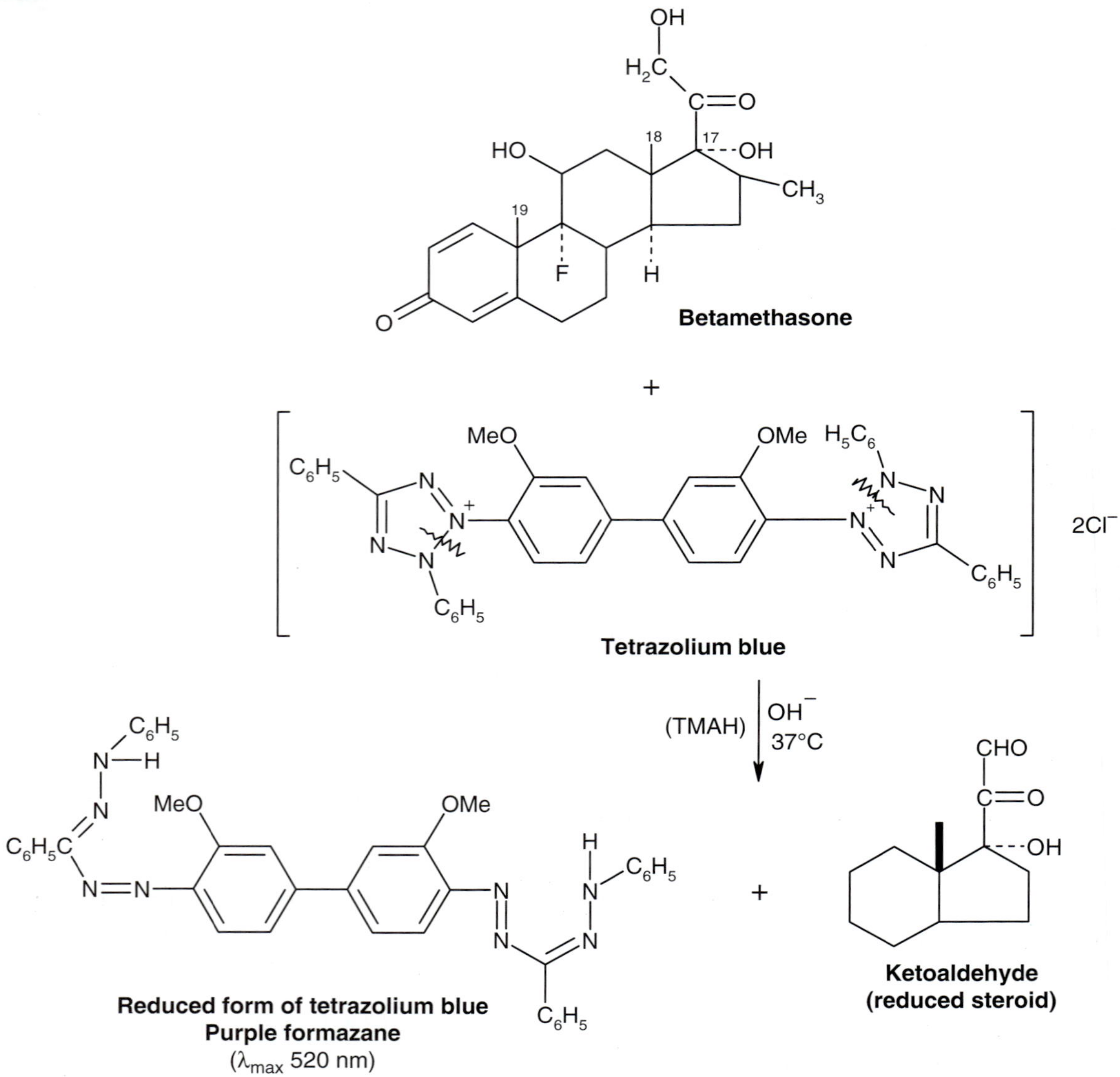

Note

Tetrazolium blue is less sensitive to light and more stable.

Salbutamol sulphate

Reagent

1. 0.1% w/v solution of 2,6-dichloroquinone chlorimide in isopropyl alcohol.
2. Dilute ammonia solution.
3. Isopropyl alcohol.

Standard solution

40 mcg/ml of salbutamol sulphate in water as sample solution.

Sample solution

Accurately weighed quantity of the powdered tablet equivalent to 4 mg of the substance is dissolved in water by sonication, diluted to 100 ml and filtered (40 mcg/ml).

Procedure

To 2 ml each of sample and standard solutions, add 2 ml of dilute ammonia solution, followed by 1 ml of chlorimide reagent. Make up to 25 ml with isopropyl alcohol and measure absorbance of both the solutions at 650 nm against reagent blank. To calculate amount of salbutamol (base), multiply by the factor 239.3/288.4.

Note

In case of liquid formulations (syrups) prior extraction with ether may be necessary to remove interference due to excipients.

For reaction mechanism, see formulation 17 of this chapter.

Formulation 24

Bromhexine hydrochloride, Salbutamol sulphate, Theophylline

ESTIMATION

Bromhexine hydrochloride

METHOD 1

Follow the method described in formulation 29 of the chapter on expectorants and cough suppressants.

METHOD 2

Reagents

1. 0.04% w/v solution of p-dimethylaminocinnamaldehyde (PDAC) in methanol.
2. Trifluoracetic acid (TFA).

Standard solution

200 mcg/ml solution of bromhexine hydrochloride in methanol.

Sample solution

Accurately weighed quantity of powdered sample equivalent to 100 mg of the substance was dissolved in methanol, filtered (for removal of the colour in coated tablets, boiling with activated charcoal is necessary) and appropriately diluted to get final concentration of 200 mcg/ml.

Procedure

To 2 ml of sample and standard solutions, add 2 ml of PDAC solution followed by 1 ml of TFA. Both the solutions were allowed to stand at room temperature for 10 min and absorbance of reddish colour was measured at 510 nm against reagent blank and results calculated by comparison.

Note

1. The method obeys Beer's law in the concentration range of 100-1000 mcg.
2. The red colour so developed in stable for more than 60 min.

Probable Reaction Mechanism

The compound having free amino group forms Schiff's base with PDAC.

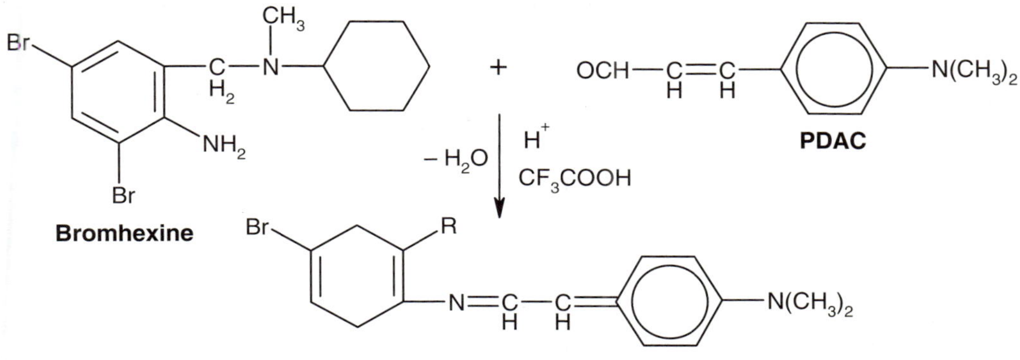

Red-coloured Schiff's base
(λ_{max} 510 nm)

Note

It also forms Schiff's base with PDAB in acidic medium.

Salbutamol sulphate

The acidic extract obtained during estimation of bromhexine hydrochloride as described in formulation 29 of the chapter on expectorants is diluted appropriately and subjected to analysis as per method described in formulation 17 of this chapter.

It has been reported that theophylline can couple with certain diazonium salts in alkaline medium. On alkaline hydrolysis, theophylline is converted to theophyllidine which can couple with diazotized sulphanilic acid at carbon-2 of the imidazole ring as shown below. This reaction is of analytical interest.

Probable Reaction Mechanism

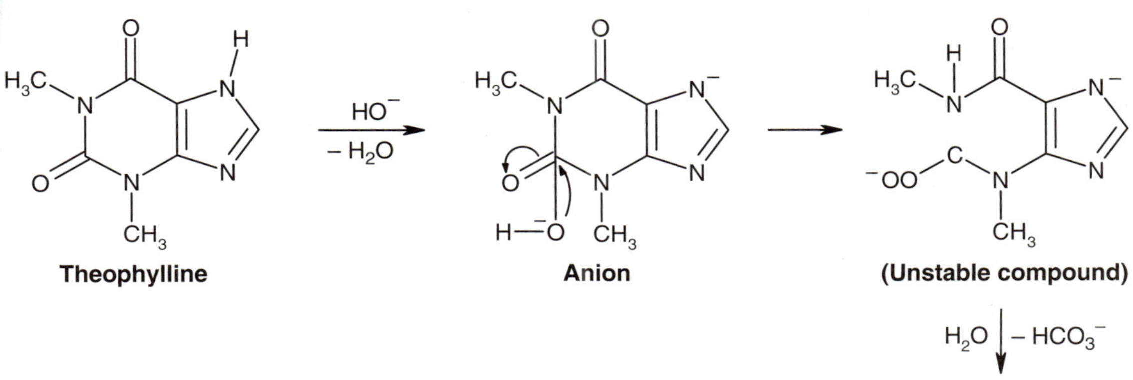

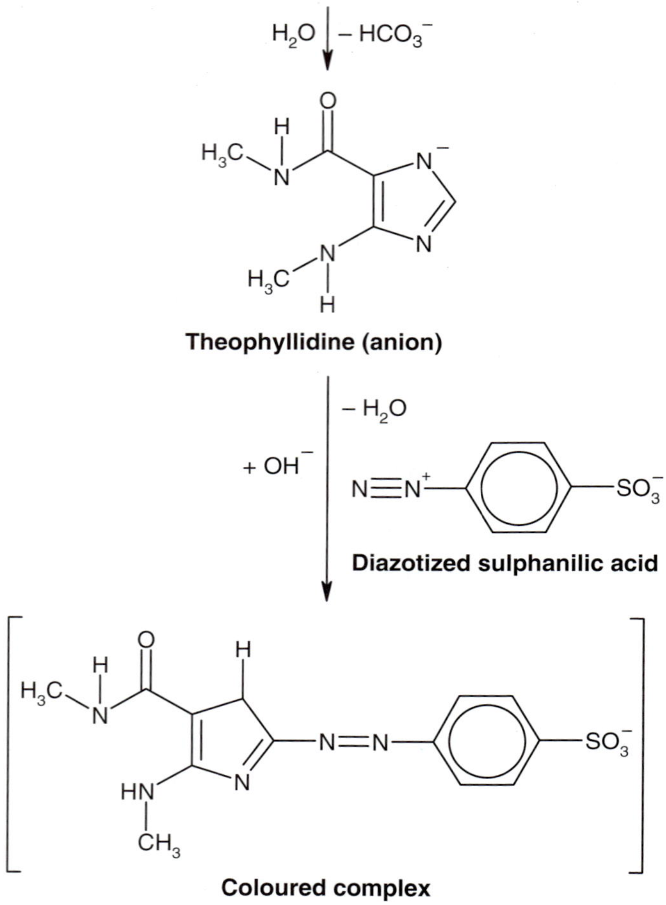

Reference

Pharmaceutical Chemistry (Vol. 2) by H.J. Roth, p. 597.

Formulation 25

Bromhexine hydrochloride, Terbutaline sulphate, Guaiphenesin

ESTIMATION

METHOD 1

Terbutaline sulphate

Follow the method described in formulation of this chapter based on alkaline oxidation and coupling with 4-aminoantipyrine.

Bromhexine hydrochloride

Standard solution

50 mcg/ml of bromhexine hydrochloride in 0.1 N hydrochloric acid.

Sample solution

Suspend accurately weighed quantity of sample equivalent to 5 mg of the substance in 10 ml of water, basify with dilute ammonia solution and extract with n-hexane (4 × 25 ml). Combine the organic layer and extract with 0.1 N hydrochloric acid (4 × 20 ml). Combine the acidic layer and dilute to 100 ml. Measure the absorbance of both sample and standard solutions at 317 nm using 0.1 N hydrochloric acid as blank. Calculate the results by comparison.

Guaiphenesin

Standard solution

Dissolve 50 mg of guaiphenesin in 50 ml of water containing 1 ml of hydrochloric acid and dilute with water to produce 100 ml. Further dilutions are done with water to get working standard solution of 50 mcg/ml.

Sample solution

Accurately weighed quantity of sample is diluted as described under standard solution.

Procedure

25 ml each of sample and standard solutions are extracted with petroleum ether. The absorbance of aqueous layers is measured at 273 nm using 0.1 N hydrochloric acid as blank and results calculated by comparison.

Typical laboratory analysis

Bromhexine hydrochloride

Weight of the standard = 0.0453 g
Volume of sample = 5 ml
Absorbance (standard) = 0.848
Absorbance (sample) = 0.775
Concentration of Bromhexine HCl/10 ml

$$= \frac{0.775}{0.843} \times \frac{\text{Weight of standard}}{\text{Volume of sample}} \times d_f$$

$$= \frac{0.495}{0.490} \times \frac{0.0496}{10} \times \frac{5}{50} \times \frac{25}{50} \times \frac{10}{1}$$

= 0.828 mg

Claim = 8 mg
% claim = 103.50%

Guaiphenesin

Weight of standard = 0.0511 g
Volume of the sample = 10 ml
Absorbance (Std.) = 0.677
Absorbance (Sample) = 0.655
Concentration of Guaiphenesin (mg/10 ml)

$$= \frac{0.655}{0.677} \times \frac{\text{Weight of standard}}{\text{Weight of sample}} \times d_f$$

$$= \frac{0.655}{0.677} \times \frac{0.0511}{10} \times \frac{1}{5} \times \frac{5}{100} \times \frac{100}{10} \times \frac{100}{5}$$

= 98.88 mg

Claim = 100 mg
% claim = 98.88

Terbutaline sulphate

Weight of the standard = 0.0496 g
Volume of the sample = 10 ml

Absorbance (std.) = 0.490
Absorbance (sample) = 0.495
Concentration of Terbutaline sulphate (mg/10 ml)

$$= \frac{A_u}{A_s} \times \frac{\text{Weight of standard}}{\text{Weight of sample}} \times d_f$$

$$= \frac{0.495}{0.490} \times \frac{0.0496}{10} \times \frac{5}{50} \times \frac{25}{50} \times \frac{10}{1}$$

$$= 2.505 \text{ mg}$$

Claim = 2.5 mg
% claim = 100.20

METHOD 2

Reagents

1. 0.003 M ferric chloride solution in water.
2. 0.2 M ortho-phosphoric acid.
3. 0.01 M solution of 2,2′-bispyridyl.

Sample and standard solutions

200 µg/ml.

Procedure

Transfer sample/standard equivalent to 200 µg, add to each 1 ml each of ferric chloride solution and 2,2′-bispyridyl solution, heat in boiling water-bath for 15 min, cool, add 2 ml of o-phosphoric acid, dilute to 10 ml with water and measure the absorbance at 520 nm against reagent blank.

Probable Reaction Mechanism

Fe(III) oxidizes terbutaline and itself gets reduced to Fe(II). Since two nitrogen atoms in 2,2′-bispyridyl have one unshared pair of electrons which it can share with iron(II) obtained as a result of the reaction.

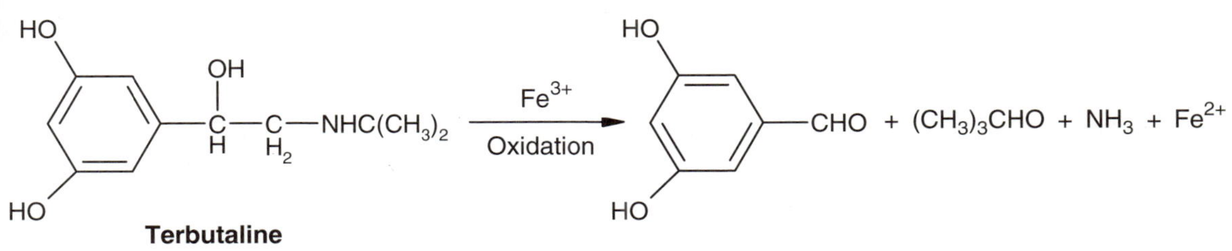

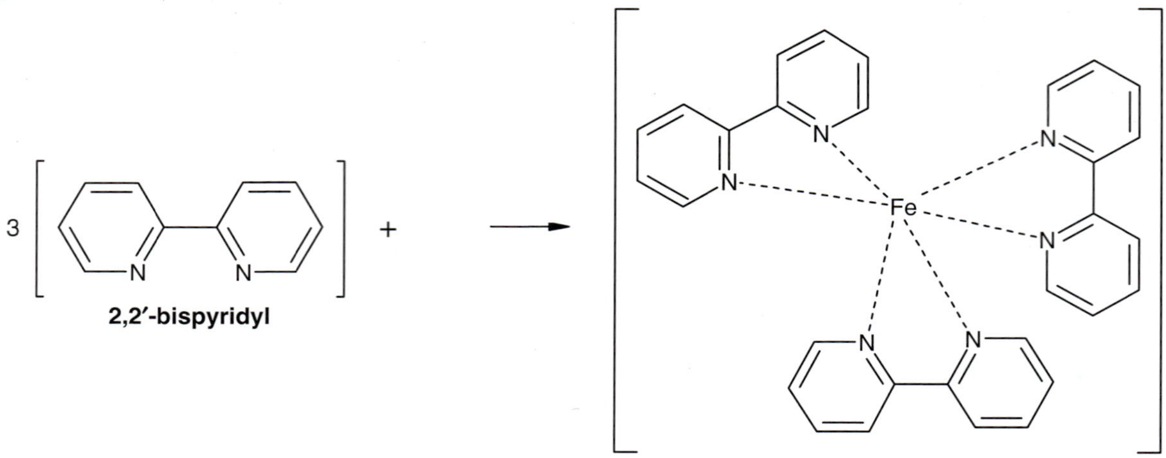

Iron (II) - bispyridyl complex
(λ_{max} 520 nm)

Reference

1. K.P.R. Chowdary & G. Devala Rao, *Indian Drugs*, **34(5)**, 283-285, 1997.
2. R.T. Sane et al., *Indian Drugs*, **21(2)**, 76-78, 1983.

Formulation 26

Theophylline or Etofylline, Terbutaline sulphate, Bromhexine hydrochloride

ESTIMATION

Terbutaline sulphate

METHOD 1

The method is based on alkaline oxidation of terbutaline (a phenol) by ferricyanide and coupling with 4-aminoantipyrine.

Reagents

1. 0.3 M tris (hydroxymethyl) amino methane buffer pH 9.5.
2. 2% w/v solution of 4-aminoantipyrine in water (prepare fresh).
3. 8% w/v solution of potassium ferricyanide in water.

Standard solution

100 mcg/ml of terbutaline sulphate in water.

Sample solution

Accurately weighed quantity of the sample equivalent to 10 mg of terbutaline sulphate is suspended in 5 ml of 0.1 N hydrochloric acid and 25 ml of water. Shake for 10-15 min and dilute to 25 ml with water. Filter and use the filtrate for analysis.

Procedure

To 5 ml each of sample, standard and blank, add 35 ml of tris buffer, 1 ml of antipyrine reagent, followed by 1 ml of ferricyanide solution. Mix and make up of the volume to 50 ml with tris buffer. Immediately measure the absorbance at 520 nm.

Note

1. The colour is not stable but reproducible results can be obtained if time from addition of reagent and measurement of absorption is kept constant (1 min).

2. Theophylline gives slight colour with this reagent, it is preferable if the 'BLANK' contains appropriate quantity of theophylline.

Probable Reaction Mechanism

This reaction is known as Emerson reaction. This is based on oxidative coupling at ortho position to phenolic group in the presence of oxidizing agent i.e. $K_3Fe(CN)_6$.

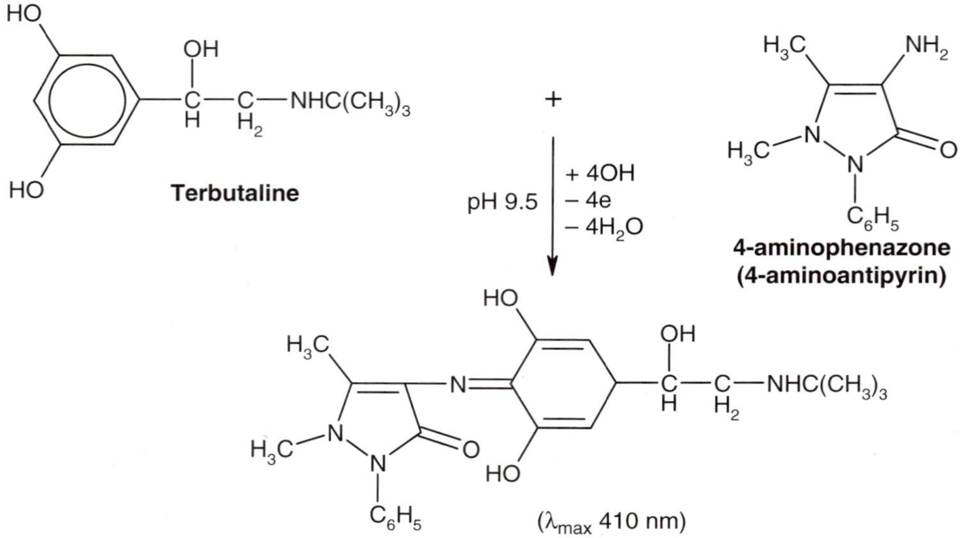

Reference

R.T. Sane, V.L. Nayak, V.B. Malkar, D.S. Sapre, A.D. Nadkarni, U.R. Pandit & V.J. Doshi, *Indian Drugs*, **21(2)**, 76-78, 1983.

METHOD 2

Reagents

1. 2% w/v solution of sodium metaperiodate in water.
2. Ammonium acetate solution : Dissolve 30 g of ammonium acetate in small volume of water, add 1 ml of freshly distilled acetyl acetone and dilute to 100 ml with water (pH 4.7).

Standard solution

2 mg/ml of terbutaline sulphate in water.

Sample solution

Dilute the sample appropriately with water to get solution of 2 mcg/ml.

Procedure

To 1 ml each of sample and standard solutions, add 2 ml of periodate solution and heat in water-bath (50°C) for 10 min. Then add 5 ml of ammonium acetate reagent and again heat in boiling water-bath for 10 min, cool and dilute to 100 ml with water. Measure the absorbance of both the solutions at 412 nm against reagent blank and calculate the results by comparison. The method obeys Beer's law in the concentration range of 20-160 mcg/ml.

Probable Reaction Mechanism

Sodium metaperiodate causes selective oxidation of compounds like terbutaline which contain a hydroxyl and an amino group attached to adjacent carbon atom which is characterised by the cleavage of the carbon-carbon bond. Reaction is known as Malaprade reaction. The aromatic aldehyde so formed will undergo condensation reaction with acetylacetone resulting in the formartion of coloured chromogen. This is Malaprade reaction.

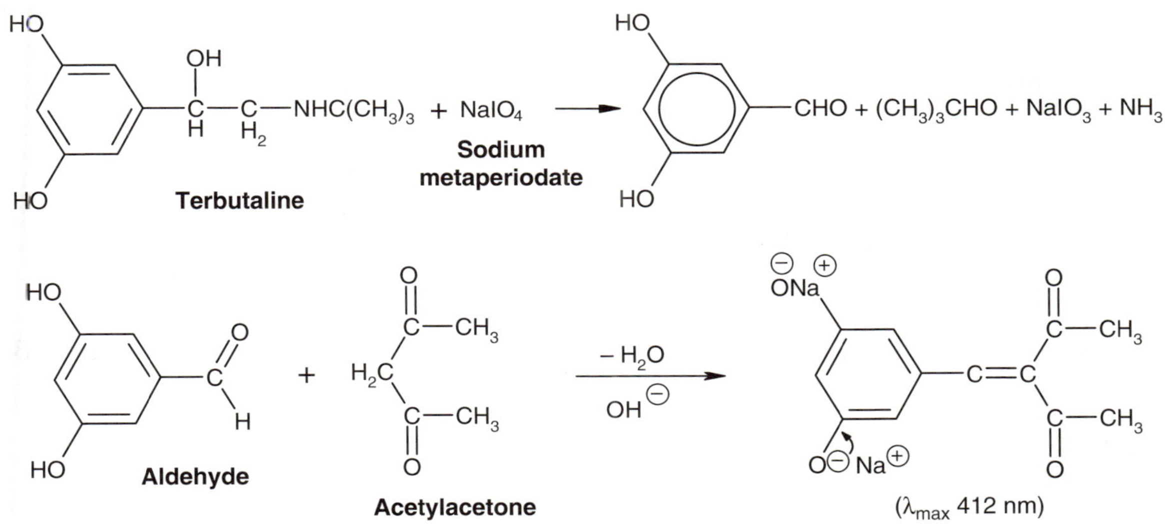

Reference

45th IPC, Abstract No. P-29.

METHOD 3

Reagents

1. 0.04% p-aminophenol (PAP) solution.
2. 1 M sodium hydroxide solution.
3. Ethyl alcohol.

Sample and standard solutions

100 μg/ml of terbutaline sulphate in water.

Procedure

To 1 ml each of sample and standard solutions add 1.4 ml of 'PAP' reagent and 2 ml of sodium hydroxide solution. Allow to stand for 5 min and dilute to 10 ml with ethyl alcohol and measure the absorbance at 600 nm against reagent blank.

Probable Reaction Mechanism

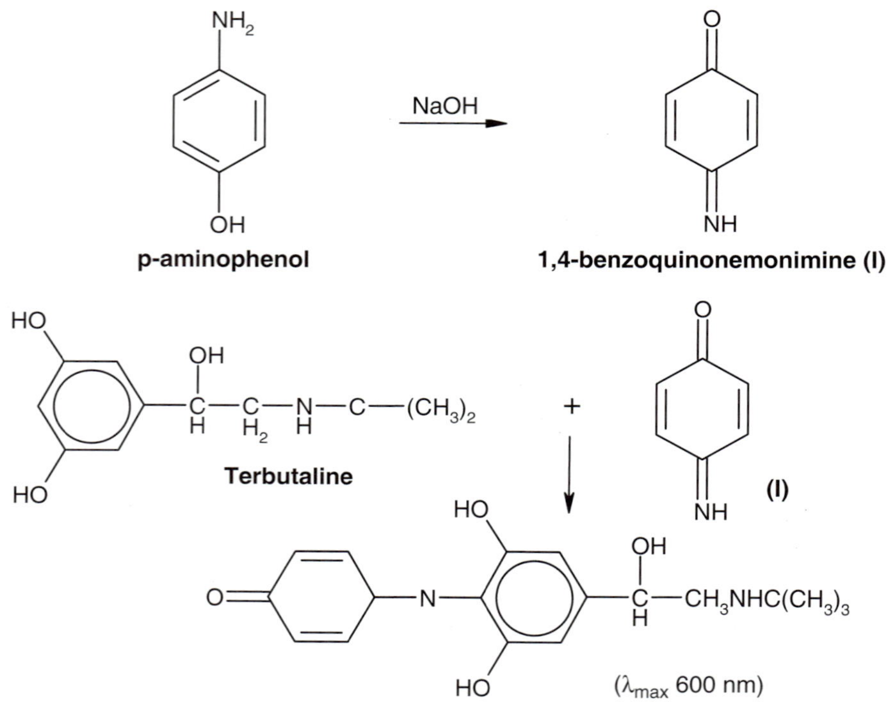

Reference

R.T. Sane, V.L. Nayak, V.B. Malkar & A.D. Nadkarni, *Indian Drugs*, 34-35, Oct. 1983.

Most of the colour reactions used for the estimation of salbutamol are applicable to terbutaline as well.

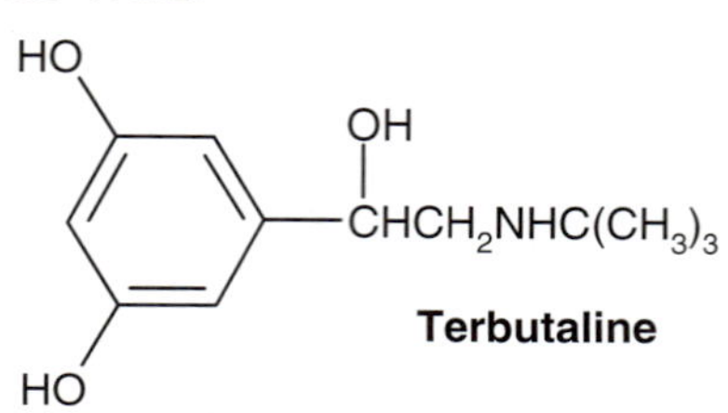

Probable Reaction Mechanism

(a) It forms nitroso derivative.

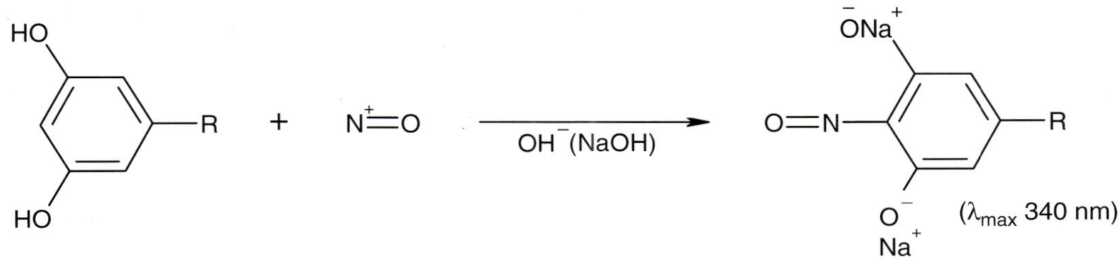

Note

Shingbal et al. have reported λ_{max} 385 nm.

Reference

1. D.M. Shingbal & R.M. Agni, *Indian Drugs*, **19**, 167-168, 1983.
2. J. Emmanuel & Arun R. Shelly, *Indian Drugs*, **21(9)**, 402-403, 1984.

(b) It couples with PDAB and PDAC at ortho position to phenolic-OH under acidic conditions.

Probable Reaction Mechanism

Under acidic conditions the aldehyde group present in PDAC or PDAB interacts with the most electron-rich position in the benzene skeletal of the drug i.e. position between the two phenolic-OH groups resulting in the formation of the products shown.

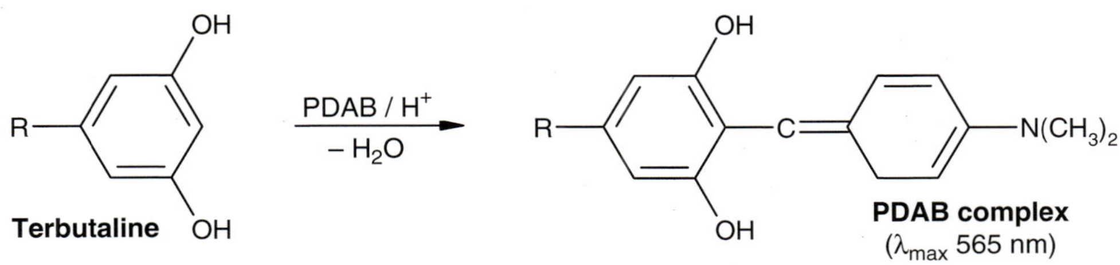

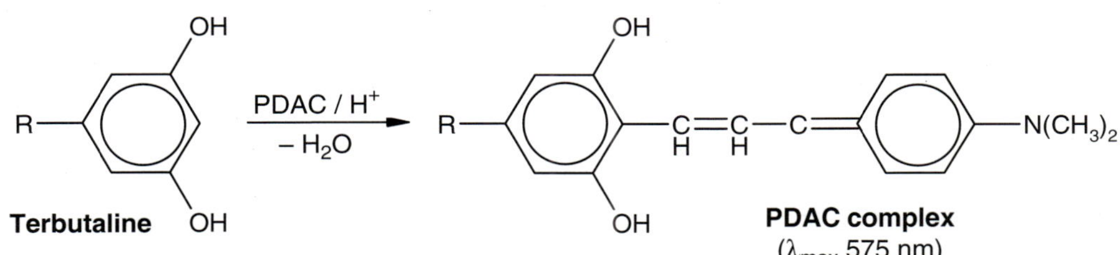

R = $CHOHCH_2NHC(CH_3)_3$

Reference

Gowri Sarla, C.S.P. Sastry & M.N. Reddy, *Indian Drugs*, **28(6)**, 269, 1991.

The compound reacts with diazotized sulphanilic acid to give coloured product (λ_{max} 425 nm). To appropriate quantity of the drug, add NaOH solution and 1 ml of solution of diazotized sulphanilic acid, followed by 1 ml of 20% w/v solution of hydroxylamine hydrochloride (used to adjust the pH).

Probable Reaction Mechanism

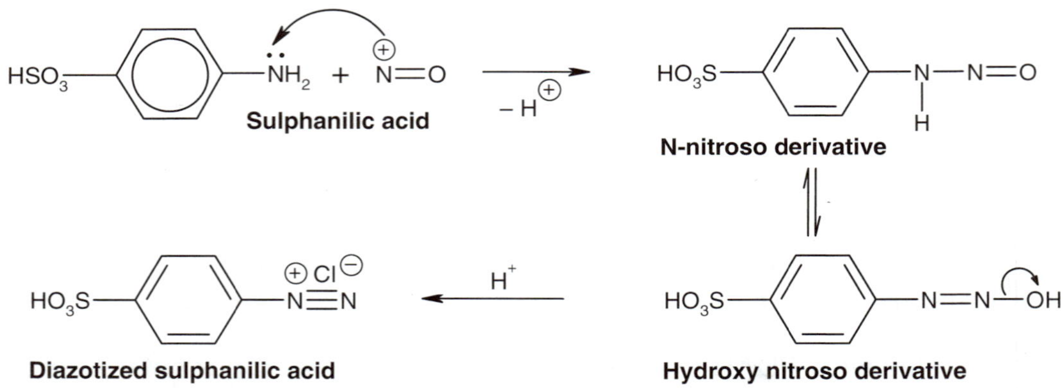

This diazotized product will couple with the drug at the ortho position to the phenolic-OH group as the position is electron-rich resulting in the formation of the product. Hydroxyl amine solution is added to maintain the pH of the solution.

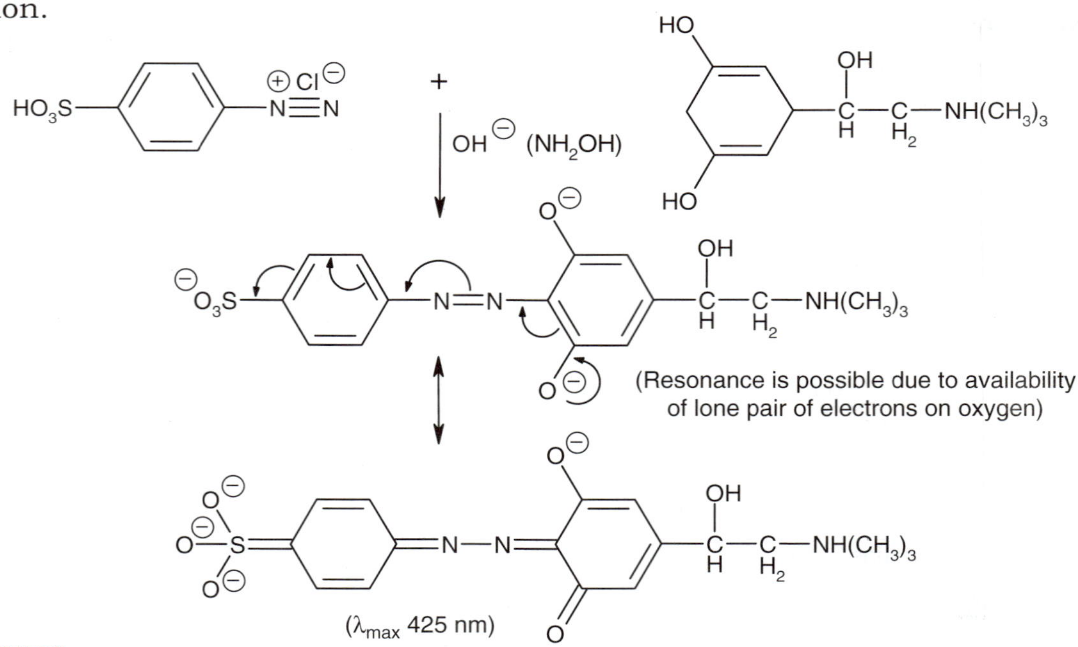

Reference

Indian Drugs, **20(8)**, 324, 1983.

Note

The nitroso derivative so formed can chelate with Co (II) or Cu (II) to yield coloured chelates as shown below.

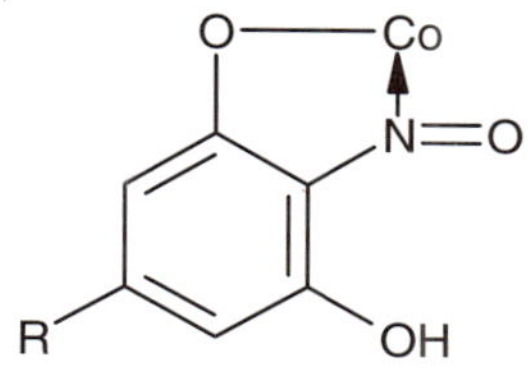

Co (II) or Cu (II) chelate
λ_{max} 410 nm (Co^{2+})
λ_{max} 406 nm (Cu^{2+})

Reference

Y.K.S. Rathor et al., *Indian Drugs*, **29(9)**, 416, 1992.

Similarly Sane at al. have reported a spectrophotometric method based on coupling of diazotized dapsone and p-nitroaniline with the drug at room temperature leading to the formation of coloured azo dye (λ_{max} 420 nm).

Probable Reaction Mechanism

WITH DAPSONE

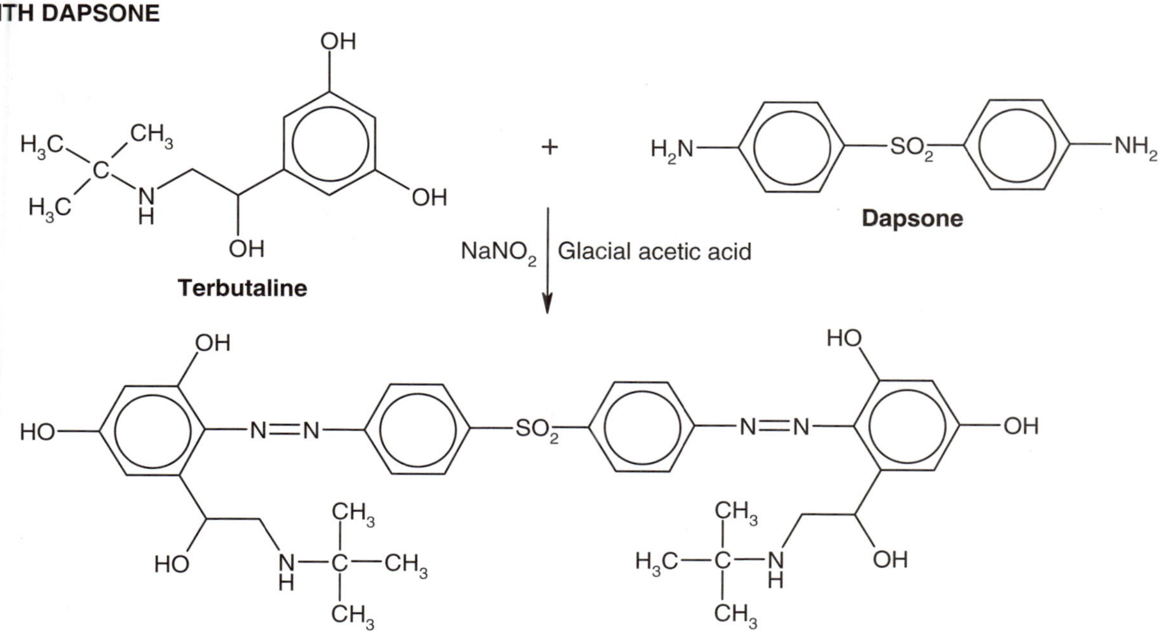

(λ_{max} 420 nm)

WITH p-NITROANILINE

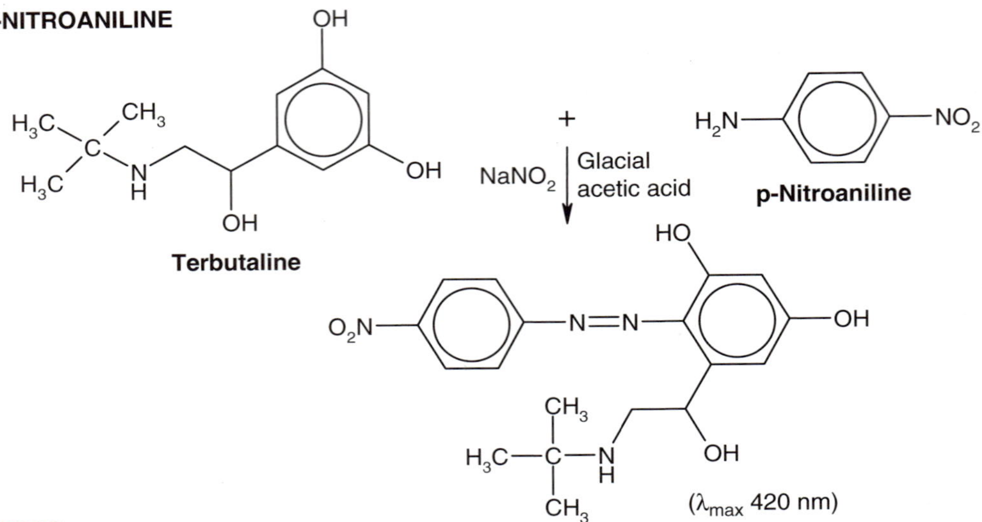

Reference

R.T. Sane, V.B. Malkar, V.G. Nayak & D.S. Sapre, Personal communication.

According to this reaction mechanism suggested, p-N-N-dimethylphenylene diamine reacts initially with chloramine-T to produce highly reactive and less stable p-benzoquinone diamine derivative which may further react with the mentioned drugs at the para position or ortho position to the phenolic-OH group of the drug. Resulting leuco dye is oxidized to indo dye.

Probable Reaction Mechanism

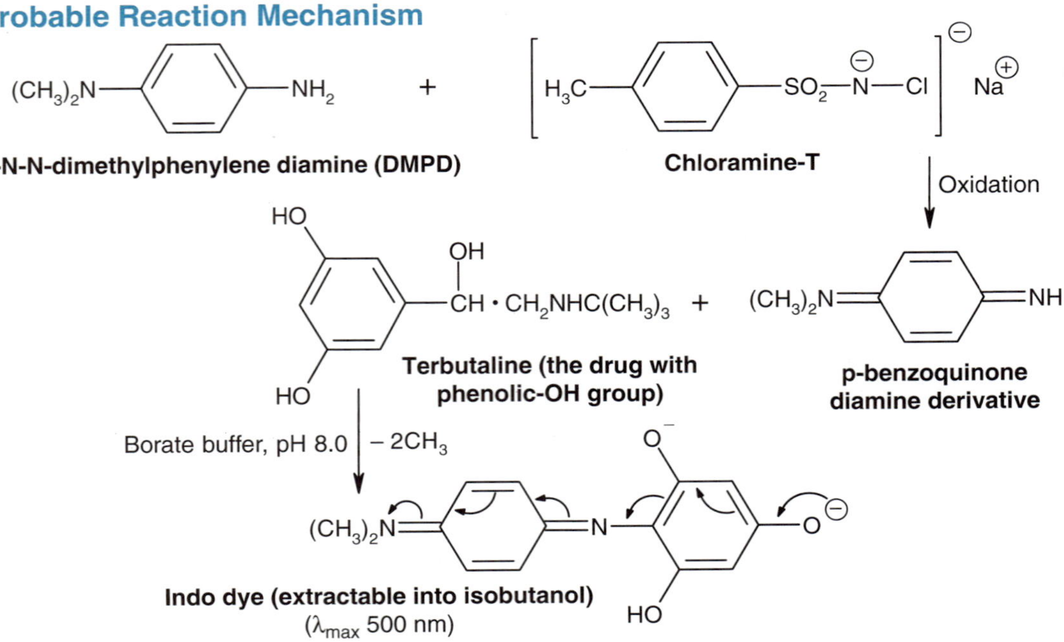

If the para position is not available the reaction will occur at the ortho position to the phenolic-OH group. This is because the phenolic-OH group is ortho and para directing i.e. the ortho and para postions are richer in electrons and hence attack of the electron-deficient agent occurs at these positions.

Theophylline

Follow the method described in formulation of this chapter. Alternatively, the sample may be extracted with 0.1 N hydrochloric acid (10 mcg/ml) and measure the extinction at 271 nm. Calculate the results by comparing with the standard (10 mcg/ml in 0.1 N hydrochloric acid).

Bromhexine hydrochloride

Follow the method described in formulation 20 of this chapter.

Reaction Mechanism

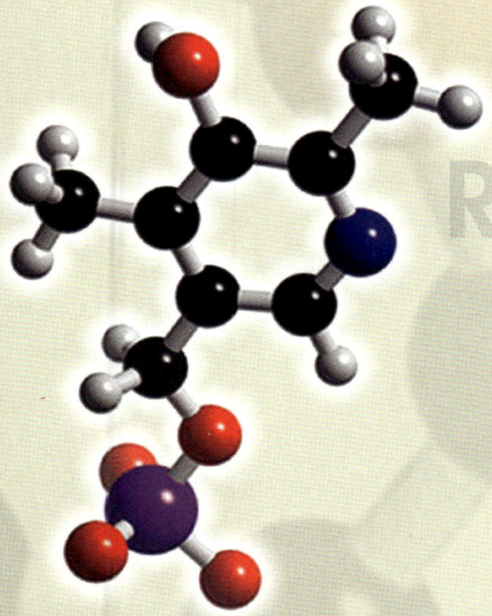

13

Alimentary Drugs

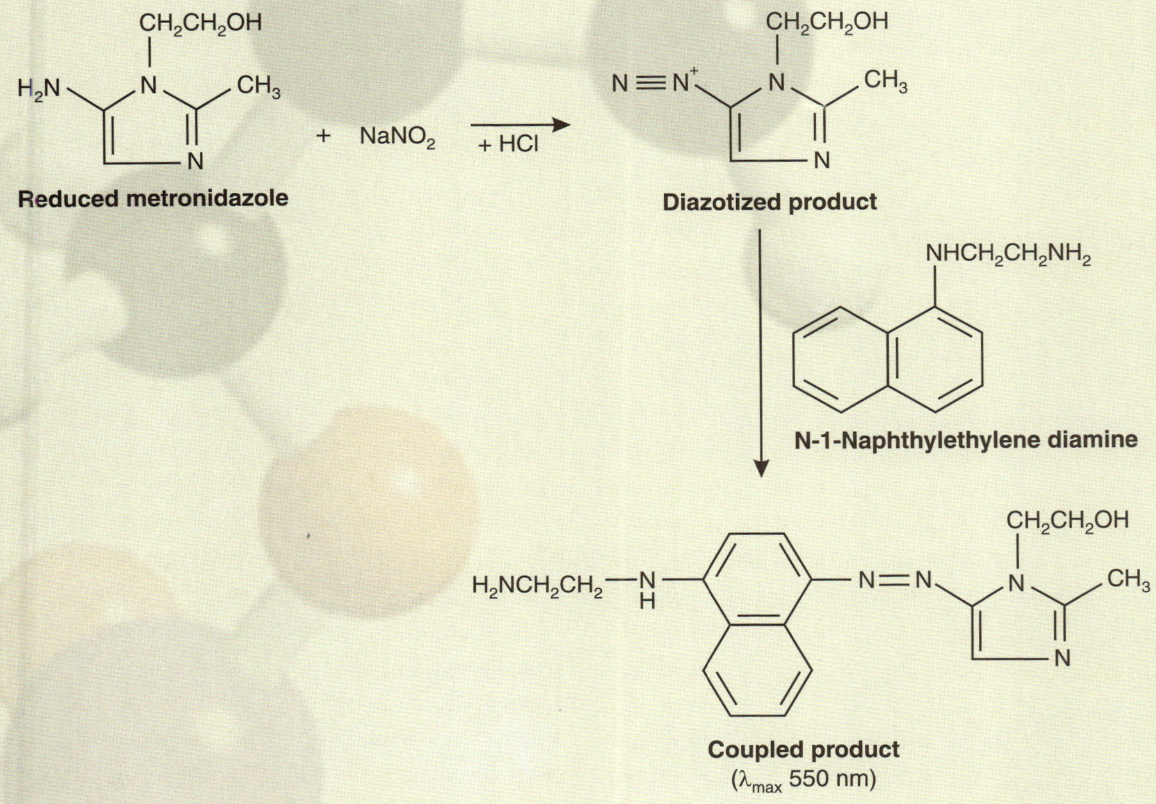

Formulation 1

Di-iodohydroxyquinoline, Metronidazole, Chloroquine phosphate, Belladonna dry extract

ESTIMATION

Di-iodohydroxyquinoline

METHOD 1

Standard solution

2.5 mcg/ml of di-iodohydroxyquinoline in absolute alcohol.

Sample solution

Weigh sample accurately equivalent to 50 mg of di-iodohydroxyquinoline in a 200 ml volumetric flask, add absolute alcohol to make up the volume. Dilute appropriately with absolute alcohol to get 2.5 mcg/ml. Measure the absorbance of both standard and sample solutions at 253 nm using methanol as blank and calculate the results by comparison.

METHOD 2

Reagents

1. 0.1% v/v acetone in dimethylformamide (DMF).
2. 25% v/v benzyl trimethylammonium hydroxide (BTAH) in distilled water.

Standard solution

10 mcg/ml of the substance in dimethylformamide (DMF).

Sample solution

Weigh accurately powdered sample equivalent to 100 mg of the compound and add 'DMF' to produce 100 ml, shake and filter. The filtrate is suitably diluted with 'DMF' to get concentration of 10 mcg/ml.

Procedure

To 0.5 ml each of standard and sample solutions, add 0.2 ml of acetone solution and 0.1 ml of 'BTAH' reagent and make up the volume to 5 ml with 'DMF'. Measure the absorbance after 10 minutes at 360 nm against reagent blank. The method obeys Beer's law in the range of 2-14 mcg/ml. The yellow complex is stable for 20 minutes.

METHOD 3

Reagents

1. 0.02% w/v vanadyl sulphate in ethyl alcohol.
2. Hydrochloric acid, dilute.
3. Cyclohexane.

Standard solution

200 mcg/ml of di-iodohydroxyquinoline in dilute hydrochloric acid.

Sample solution

Weigh accurately powdered sample equivalent to about 20 mg of the compound, add 75 ml of dilute hydrochloric acid, shake and make up to 100 ml with the acid (200 mcg/ml).

Procedure

To 2.5 ml each of standard and sample solutions, add 7 ml of vanadyl reagent and 10 ml of cyclohexane. Shake for 2 minutes, allow to separate the cyclohexane layer. Measure absorbance of the organic layer at 415 nm against reagent blank. The method obeys Beer's law in the range of 10-100 mcg/ml. The yellow colour is stable for 45 minutes.

METHOD 4

Reagents

1. 0.1% w/v p-aminophenol solution in 0.2 N hydrochloric acid (freshly prepared).
2. 0.5 N sodium carbonate.
3. 1,4-dioxane.

Standard solution

100 mg of the compound is dissolved in 1,4-dioxane to produce 100 ml (1 mg/ml).

Sample solution

Powdered sample accurately weighed equivalent to 25 mg of the compound is shaken with 20 ml of dioxane and filtered. The final volume is adjusted to 25 ml with dioxane (1 mg/ml).

Procedure

To 0.4 ml each of the sample and standard solutions, add 3 ml of sodium carbonate solution and 0.4 ml of p-aminophenol reagent. Keep at room temperature for 5 minutes and then dilute to 10 ml with water. The absorbance of the resultant solution is measured at 570 nm after 15 minutes against reagent blank. The contents of di-iodohydroxyquinoline are calculated by comparison with the standard. The method obeys Beer's law in the concentration range of 15-500 mcg/ml.

For detailed reaction mechanism, see under formulation 2 of this chapter.

Note

1. The colour attains maximum intensity after 15 minutes and is stable for 50 minutes.
2. Metronidazole, chloramphenicol, chloroquine, brobenzoxalidine, hyoscine and hyoscyamine do not interfere.

Metronidazole

METHOD 1

Transfer a quantity of the sample accurately weighed equivalent to 200 mg of metronidazole in a 125 ml separating funnel. Extract with six 30 ml portions of warm acetone. Collect the acetone extracts, cool and pass through a pledget of cotton and collect in a beaker. Add to the beaker, 50 ml of acetic anhydride and 2 drops of 1% w/v solution of brilliant green in glacial acetic acid. Titrate this solution with 0.1 N perchloric acid to a yellowish green end point. Repeat the operation without the sample (blank) and subtract the blank reading from the main reading. Each ml of 0.1 N perchloric acid consumed is equivalent to 0.01712 g of metronidazole.

METHOD 2

Weigh accurately a quantity of the sample equivalent to about 50 mg of metronidazole, add 80-90 ml 0.1 N hydrochloric acid, shake for 15 minutes, add sufficient 0.1 N hydrochloric acid to produce 200 ml. Filter and dilute 5 ml of the filtrate to 100 ml with 0.1 N hydrochloric acid. Measure the extinction of the resulting solution at the maximum at about 277 nm and calculate the content of metronidazole taking 380 as the value of A 1%, 1 cm at 277 nm. However, when measured in methanol, λ_{max} is at 310 nm.

METHOD 3

Standard solution

1 mg/ml of metronidazole in water.

Sample solution

(a) Tablets: Weigh accurately powdered sample equivalent to about 100 mg of metronidazole, and 60-70 ml of water, shake and make up the volume to 100 ml with water. Filter and use for colour development.

(b) Syrups/suspensions: Measure sample equivalent to about 100 mg of substance, extract with three 30 ml portions of chloroform. Combine chloroform layer and evaporate on water-bath. Dissolve the residue in water to produce 100 ml and use appropriate volume for colour development.

Procedure

To 2 ml each of the standard and sample solutions, add 3 ml of 20% w/v sodium hydroxide solution and keep at room temperature for 8 minutes (this is the optimum time for completion of the reaction). Adjust to 10 ml with water and read at 500 nm within 12 minutes against reagent blank. The colour is stable for 13 minutes and starts fading after that. The method obeys Beer's law in the concentration range of (100-150 mcg/ml).

Probable Reaction Mechanism

On alkaline hydrolysis of the heterocyclically bonded nitro group gives the heterocyclic phenol and nitrite. Phenol is responsible for colour in alkaline medium.

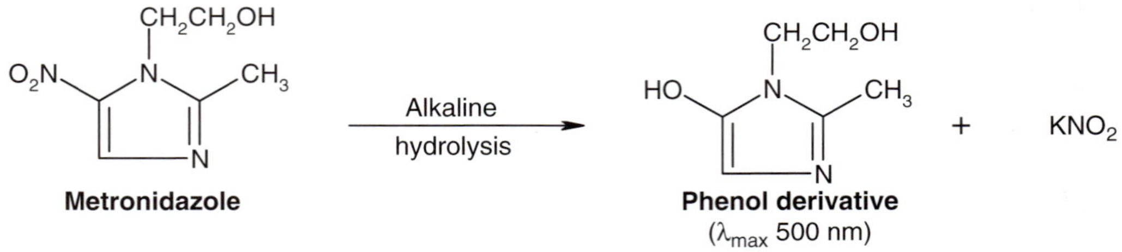

Note

On alkaline hydrolysis, the NO_2 group present in the molecule produces KNO_2. This will diazotize sulphanilamide in acidic medium to produce diazonium salt which can be coupled with Bratton-Marshall reagent to give coloured compound. Sodium nitrite is used as standard. This method can be used for anlaysis of the substance. It also couples with β-naphthol to give azo dye.

$$KNO_2 + HCl \longrightarrow HNO_2 + KCl$$

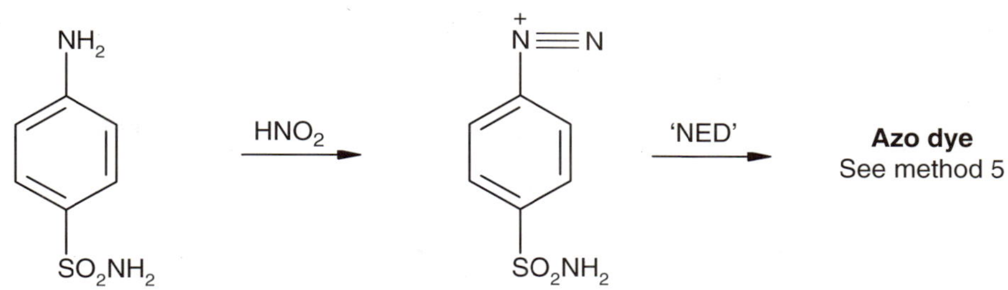

Sulphanilamide **Diazotized sulphanilamide**

Reference

Lau, E., Yao, C. & Lewis M.J., *J. Pharm. Sci.*, **58(1)**, 55, 1969.

METHOD 4

Reagents

1. Hydrochloric acid.
2. Zinc dust.
3. 1% w/v solution of vanillin in water.

Standard solution

Weigh accurately about 100 mg of metronidazole and dissolve in 25 ml of water. Add 10 ml of hydrochloric acid and 3 g of zinc dust. Keep in water-bath for 15 minutes for completion of the reaction. Cool, filter and wash the residue with water till filtrate is free of acidity. Washings and main filtrate are combined and adjusted to 100 ml. 10 ml is further diluted to 100 ml with water.

Sample solution

Prepare the initial sample (tablets, syrups and suspensions) solutions as per procedure described under method 3 under sample solution. These solutions are further treated and diluted as described under standard solution in this method.

Procedure

To 2.5 ml each of the standard and sample solutions, 1 ml of vanillin solution is added and heated on water-bath for 20 minutes. Cool to room temperature, adjust the volume to 10 ml with water and read at about 410 nm. The yellow complex thus produced is quite stable. The method obeys Beer's law in the concentration range of 10-50 mcg/ml.

Explanatory Note

The nitro group present in the molecule is first reduced with zinc and hydrochloric acid. The amino group so produced is coupled with vanillin to produce Schiff's base (λ_{max} 410 nm).

Probable Reaction Mechanism

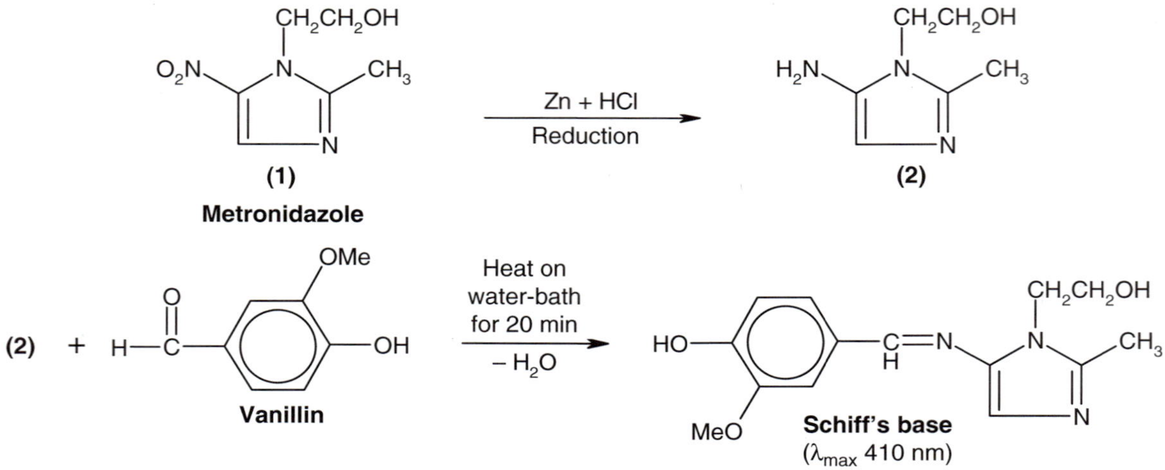

Reference

Textbook of Practical Organic Chemistry by Vogel, p. 891.

Note

The above reduced product can also react with furfuraldehyde to form Schiff's base.

Probable Reaction Mechanism

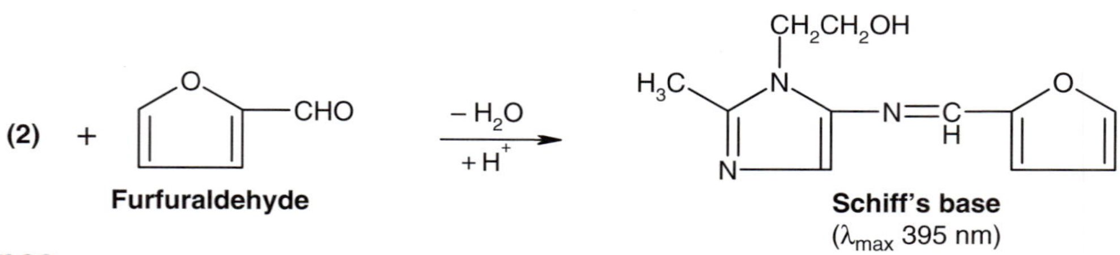

Reference

Indian Drugs, **20(9)**, 391, 1983.

METHOD 5

The final standard and sample solutions obtained after zinc and acid treatment as described under method 4 above are used in this method.

Reagents

1. 1% w/v solution of sodium nitrite in water.
2. 0.5% w/v solution of ammonium sulphamate in water.
3. 0.1% w/v solution of N-1-naphthyl-ethylenediamine dihydrochloride in water.

Procedure

To 2.5 ml each of sample and standard solutions as indicated above, 0.5 ml of sodium nitrite solution is added. Keep for 3 minutes, neutralize excess of nitrous acid by adding 0.5 ml of ammonium sulphamate solution. Again leave the solution for 3 minutes and finally add 0.5 ml of naphthyl-ethylenediamine dihydrochloride solution. Determine the absorption of resulting solutions at about 550 nm against reagent blank and calculate the results by comparison.

After reduction with zinc and HCl the product is diazotized and coupled with N-1-naphthyl ethylene diamine.

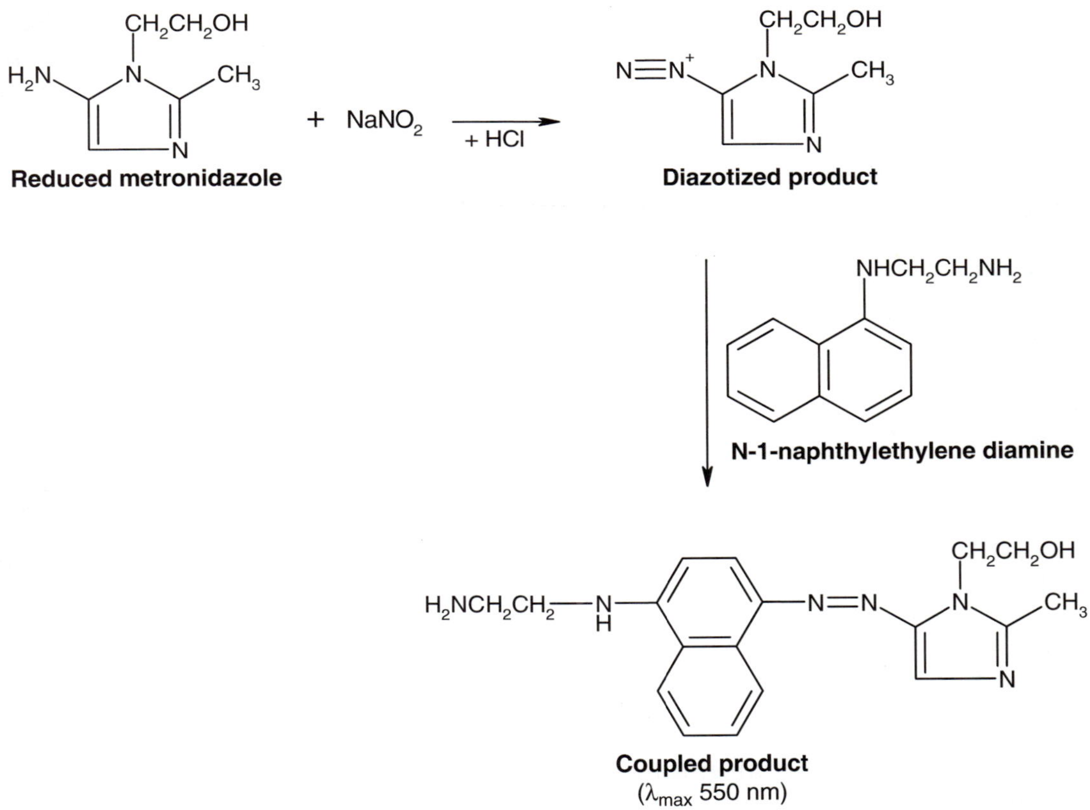

$$HNO_2 + H_2NSO_3H \longrightarrow H_2SO_4 + N_2\uparrow + H_2O$$

Ammonium sulphamate

Reference

Bratton, A., Marshall, E., et al., *J. Biol. Chem.*, **128**, 537, 1939.

METHOD 6

Reagents

1. 0.2% w/v aqueous solution of metol, freshly prepared.
2. 0.01 M potassium dichromate solution in water.
3. 0.2 M potassium hydrogen phthalate buffer.

Standard solution

20 mg of metronidazole was treated with 10 ml of 1 M HCl and 250 mg of zinc. Allow to stand for 20 min for complete reduction of the molecule. Filter, wash the residue with water. Neutralize the filtrate with sodium hydroxide solution and dilute to 100 ml with water.

Sample solution

Extract appropriate quantity of the powdered sample with 3 × 5 ml acetone. Evaporate the combined extract on steam-bath and residue treated as under standard solution.

Procedure

To 1 ml each of sample and standard solutions add 15 ml of pH 2.5 buffer, 1 ml of metol reagent and 1 ml of 0.01 M potassium dichromate solution, dilute to 25 ml with water and measure the absorbance at 720 nm against reagent blank.

Note

1. Other active components commonly present in combined dosage forms such as diloxanide furoate, di-iodohydroxyquinolone, furazolidone along with common excipients do not interfere.
2. Tinidazole, benzoyl metronidazole and niclosamide can be estimated by above method.

Probable Reaction Mechanism

The nitro compound is first reduced to corresponding amino derivative. p-N-methylbenzoquinone monoimine formed in-situ from metol - chromium (VI) couples with the drug at ortho position to the amino group present in the drug resulting in the formation of a coloured product (λ_{max} 720 nm).

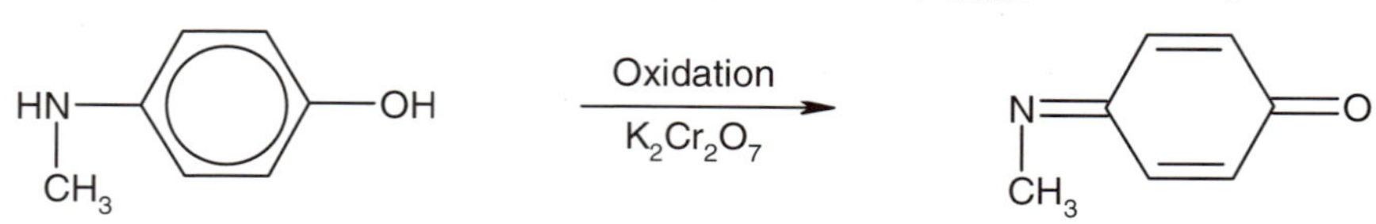

p-N-methylaminophenol (Metol) **Benzoquinone monoimine**

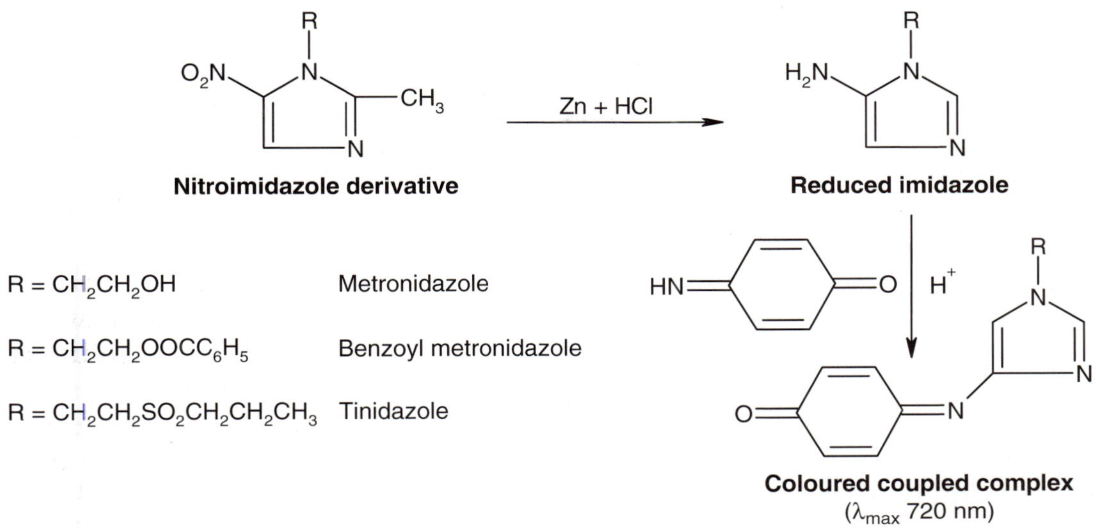

Reference

C.S.P. Sastry, M. Aruna & A. Rama Mohana Rao, Talanta, **35(1)**, 23-26, 1988.

A simple spectrophotometric method has been described by A.K. Sanyal (1992) for the estimation of benzoyl metronidazole in oral suspension.

Probable Reaction Mechanism

On treating with sodium hydroxide, benzoyl metronidazole undergoes hydrolysis to yield 2-(2-methyl imidazol-1-yl) ethyl benzoate and sodium nitrite. It is imidazol derivative which shows λ_{max} 276 nm for quantitative analysis.

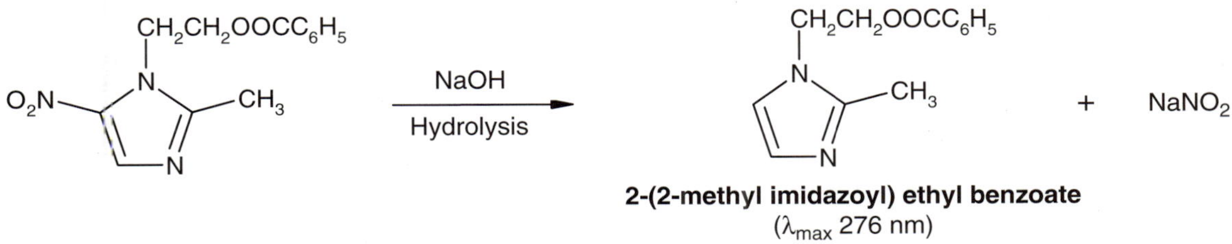

Reference

1. A.K. Sanyal, *Analyst*, **117**, 93-95, 1992.
2. Pharmaceutical Chemistry (Vol. 2) by H.J. Roth, p. 331.

Chloroquine phosphate

Standard solution

10 mcg/ml of chloroquine phosphate in water.

Sample solution

Weigh accurately a portion of the sample equivalent to about 200 mg of chloroquine phosphate and dissolve in 20 ml of water. Filter the solution to 250 ml separator, wash any undissolved residue with several small portions of water, add 5 ml of ammonia, agitate, and extract the liberated base with five 25 ml portions of chloroform. Wash the combined chloroform extract with 10 ml of water, then extract the water washing with 10 ml of chloroform. Evaporate the combined chloroform extracts on a steam-bath to about 10 ml, add 50 ml of dilute hydrochloric acid and continue heating in the steam-bath until the odour of chloroform is no longer perceptible. Transfer the aqueous acidic solutions to a 200 ml volumetric flask, wash the evaporating dish with portion of dilute acid, adding the washings to the volumetric flask and dilute to volume. Dilute the solution further quantitatively and step-wise with dilute acid to give a concentration of about 10 mcg per ml.

Determine the absorbance of both the solutions at maximum at about 343 nm in a suitable spectrophotometer. Calculate the contents of chloroquine phosphate by comparison or use A 1%, 1 cm value of 360 for calculations.

The drug is reported to form ion-pair complex with different dyes i.e. bromothymol blue (phthalate buffer, pH 2.5), bromocresol green (phthalate buffer, pH 8.5), bromocresol purple (phthalate buffer, pH 6.0) and methyl orange (phthalate buffer, pH 4.7). All the ion-pair complexes are extracted into chloroform and subjected to spectrophotometric measurements (λ_{max} 420 nm).

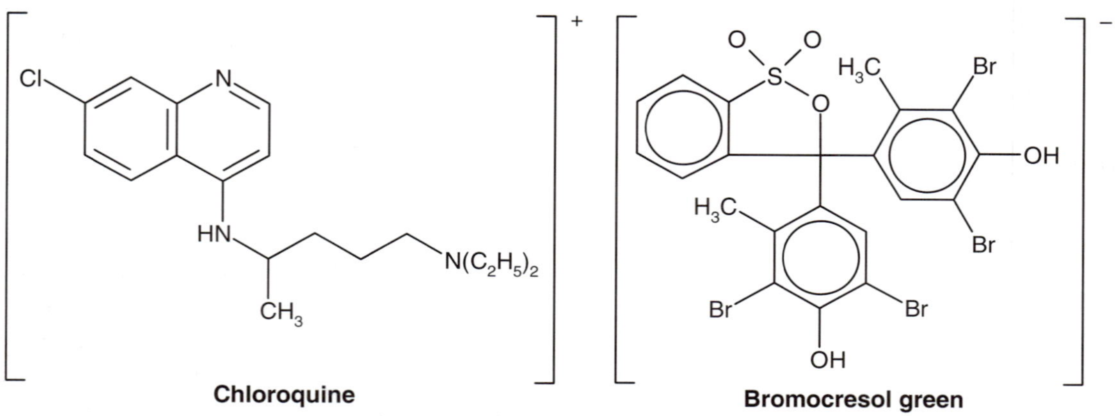

Drug - dye ion-pair complex
(λ_{max} 420 nm)

Reference

R.T. Sane, P.G. Anaokar & B.S. Narkar, J. of University of Bombay, Vol. L_I-L_{II}, No. 78-79, 1982-83.

Total belladonna alkaloids calculated as atropine

Reagents

1. Chloroform.
2. Acetone (water contents not more than 0.02% v/v).
3. Anhydrous sodium sulphate, granular.
4. Phosphoric acid (88% w/w).
5. Solvent (6% v/v of acetic acid in 5% v/v alcohol): Take 6 ml of the glacial acetic acid and 5 ml of dehydrated alcohol in a 250 ml conical flask. Add 89 ml of distilled water and shake well.
6. Dehydrated alcohol.
7. Fuming nitric acid (it is highly corrosive; handle with care).
8. Potassium hydroxide (pellets).
9. Methyl alcohol.
10. 50% v/v alcohol.

Standard stock solution

Take about 80 mg of atropine sulphate accurately weighed in 100 ml volumetric flask and dissolve in solvent. Make up the volume to 100 ml with the solvent. Prepare this solution once every month and store in a refrigerator to serve as stock solution.

Dilute standard solution

Dilute 10 ml of the standard stock solution to 100 ml with the solvent (80 mcg/ml). Prepare this solution freshly before use.

Calculate the contents of atropine (base) in mg/ml in the diluted standard solution as follows:

$$\text{Weight of atropine sulphate taken} = \frac{578.76 \times 10}{694.86 \times 100 \times 100}$$

Sample solution

Take sample accurately weighed in a 250 ml stoppered conical flask. Extract the alkaloids by shaking the sample twice, each with 50 ml of a mixture of 2 ml of phosphoric acid and 48 ml of 50% v/v alcohol in a mechanical shaker. Filter both the extracts through the same Whatman filter paper No. 4 into 500 ml beaker and wash the residue with a further 50 ml of mixture of 0.5 ml of phosphoric acid and 49.5 ml of ethyl alcohol. Add the washings to the filtrate and reduce the volume of the combined filtrate and the washings on a water-bath to about 50 ml. Transfer to a separator with the aid of little alcohol. Wash the container with chloroform and add the washings to the separator. Make distinctly alkaline with dilute solution of ammonia and extract with four 30 ml portions of chloroform. Wash each chloroform layer with same 10 ml of water. Filter organic layer through anhydrous sodium sulphate and evaporate just to dryness. Add 2 ml of ethyl alcohol and finally dry at 105°C for 3 h. Dissolve the residue in 9 ml of chloroform and transfer into stoppered 25 ml cylinder. Wash the flask with 15 ml of solvent and add to the cylinder. Shake vigorously for 2 minutes and allow to settle till the aqueous portion is distinctly clear. Transfer 5 ml of the aqueous layer into a porcelain dish and completely evaporate off the liquid to dryness. Add 5 drops of fuming nitric acid, keep on water-bath for 3 minutes and transfer quickly to a 10 ml volumetric flask with the aid of acetone. Make up the volume with acetone and mark the flask as 'sample'.

Take 1 ml of standard solution and 1 ml of water in two 25 ml porcelain dishes and proceed according to preceding para beginning with "completely evaporate off the liquid to dryness". Mark these flasks as 'standard' and 'blank' respectively.

Procedure

Dissolve one pellet of sodium hydroxide in 5 ml of methyl alcohol and add 0.1 ml of this solution to each of three 10 ml volumetric flasks marked as 'standard', 'sample' and 'blank'. Shake and allow to stand for 3 minutes. Measure immediately the optical densities of the standard and sample at 550 nm in a spectrophotometer against the blank. Calculate the total belladonna alkaloids as hyoscyamine by comparison.

Note

If morphine is also present, it should be oxidized with ferric chloride as described below and then tropane alkaloids extracted as usual.

Take sample equivalent to 1 mg of the alkaloids, add 0.5 ml of ferric chloride solution (5%), allow to stand for 2 minutes, add 2 g of sodium citrate and shake until dissolved. Make alkaline with ammonium hydroxide and then follow general extraction procedure and colour development for belladonna alkaloids.

Explanatory Note

This test is based on "Vitali Morin" reaction. For this, the substance is boiled to dryness with fuming nitric acid and the residue treated with acetone and alcoholic potassium hydroxide which gives violet colour (λ_{max} 550 nm). Boiling with fuming HNO_3 produces nitration of aromatic ring at position 4 and esterification of alcoholic-OH group by nitric acid at the same time. Alcoholic ester being very unstable it dissociates to nitro atropic acid ester. In alkaline medium nitro atropic acid takes up —OH ion to form a new compound as Michael addition. For this reaction to proceed a sufficiently activated methylene or methine group is a pre-requisite.

Tropic acid itself does not answer Vitali reaction. For this reason, the oxidative destruction of the molecule by nitric acid is necessary. If Vitali reaction is used without addition of acetone, positive reaction will be given by all compounds which have methylene or methine group as element of their structure, which is activated by C=O group and is on phenyl ring nitrable in o- or p-postion. However, as per Moris (with acetone), the reaction is positive for all compounds which contain nitrable aromatic ring and which can also react with acetone as —CH— acid component to form Meisenheimer complex

Note

The compound should have methylene group which is activated by carbonyl group and is on phenyl ring nitrable in "o" or "p" position.

Probable Reaction Mechanism

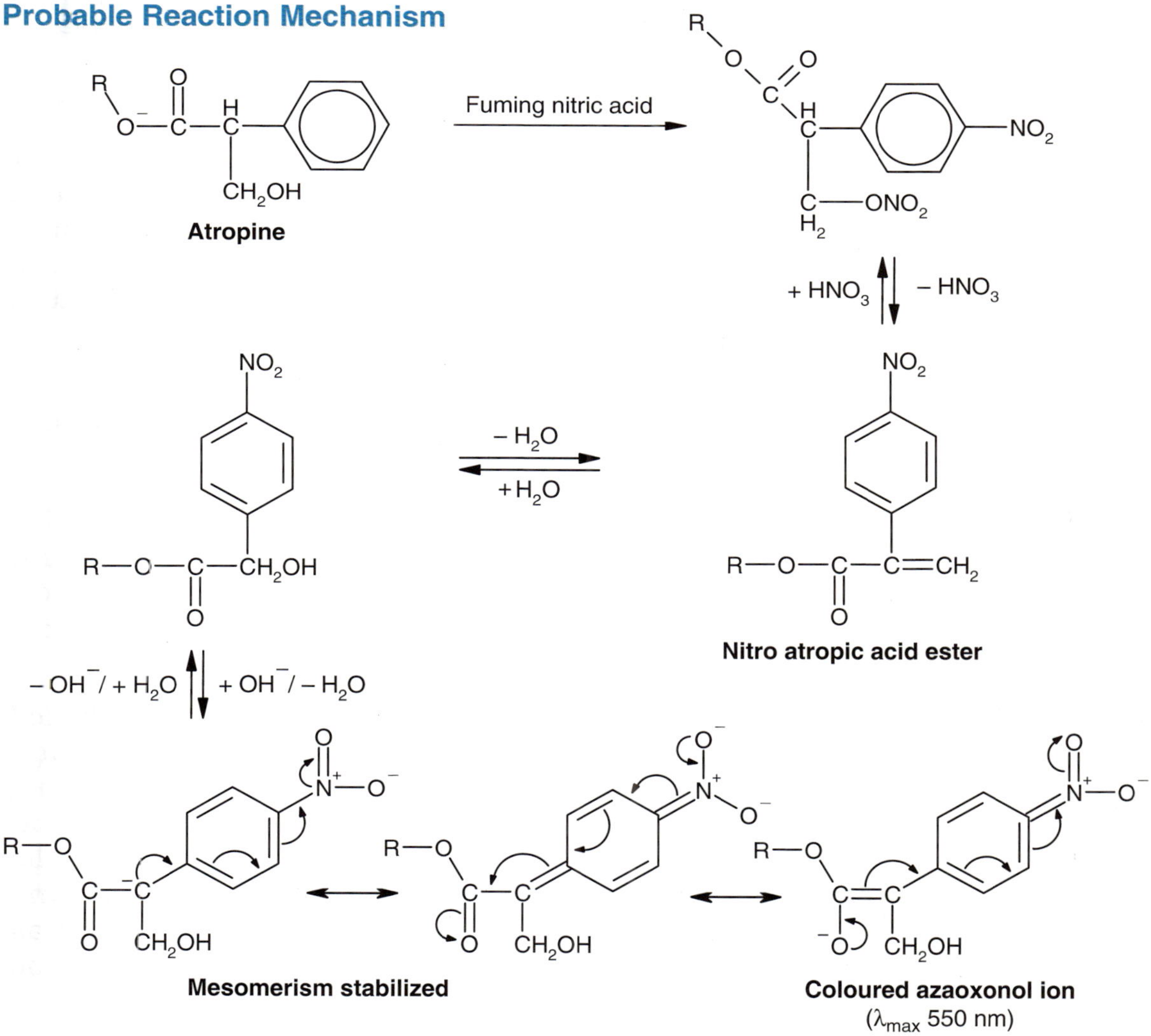

Atropine

Nitro atropic acid ester

Mesomerism stabilized

Coloured azaoxonol ion (λ_{max} 550 nm)

Reference

Pharmaceutical Chemistry (Vol. 2) by H.J. Roth, pp. 185-186.

Reaction mechanism with acetone (Morin variant)

Compounds with nitrable phenyl ring can react with acetone as 'CH' acid component or having methylene group to form Meisenheimer complex based on Janovsky reaction.

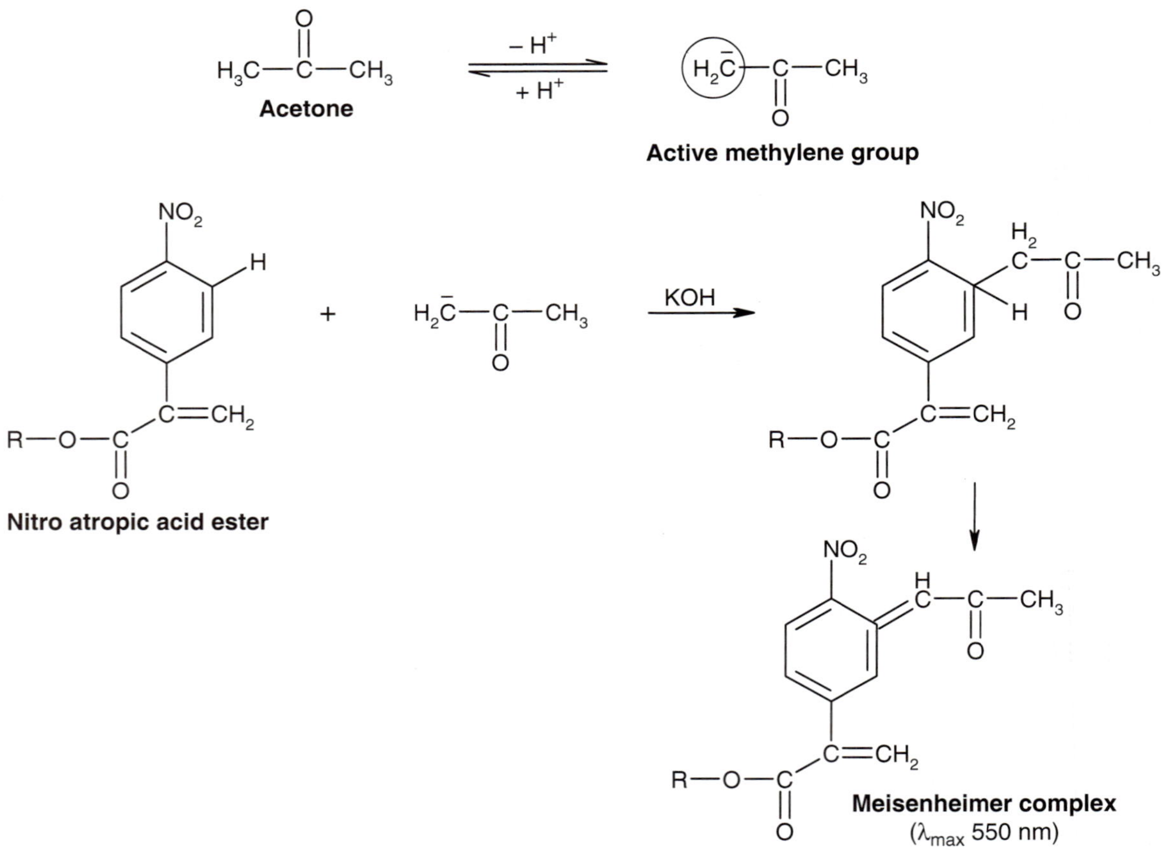

Reference

Modern Methods of Pharmaceutical Analysis by Schirmer E. Roger, 2nd ed., (Vol. I).

Note

Other compounds which can be analysed with this method after nitration are ephedrine phenobarbitone, etc.

Formulation 2

Di-iodohydroxyquinoline, Bismuth glycolyl arsanilate, Chloroquine phosphate, Niacinamide

ESTIMATION

Chloroquine phosphate

METHOD 1

Weigh accurately crushed tablets equivalent to 125 mg of chloroquine phosphate, dissolve in warm water to produce 200 ml and filter. Dilute 4 ml of the filtrate to 100 ml with water. 4 ml of this solution is further diluted to 100 ml with water (10 mcg/ml). Measure optical density of this solution at 343 nm and calculate the contents of chloroquine phosphate taking 360 as valus of E 1%, 1 cm at 343 nm.

METHOD 2

Reagents

1. Dilute hydrochloric acid.
2. Hydrochloric acid.
3. 10% w/v silicotungstic acid solution in water.

Procedure

Crush 20 tablets and weigh accurately a quantity of the powder equivalent to 200 mg of chloroquine phosphate and dissolve in water to produce 250 ml. Filter and reject first few ml of the filtrate. To 5 ml of the filtrate add 2 ml of hydrochloric acid and heat to boiling. Add 4 ml of silicotungstic acid solution, boil for 2 min, filter while hot in a tared sintered glass cricible G_4. Wash the precipitate with three 10 ml portions of nearly boiling hydrochloric acid, dry to constant weight at 100-105°. From weight of the residue, calculate the weight of chloroquine phosphate per tablet. Each g of the residue is equivalent to 0.2932 g of chloroquine phosphate.

Explanatory Note

Chloroquine forms complex with silicotungstic acid as chloroquine - silica tungstate $[SiO_2 - 12WO_3 \cdot 2(C_{18}H_6N_3Cl)2H_2O]$ in acidic medium which is estimated gravimetrically.

Reference

P.M. Parikh & S.P. Mukherji, *Ind. J. Pharm.*, **25**, 269, 1963.

Phosphate contents of the substance react with ammonium molybdate resulting in the formation of phosphomolybdate which gets reduced to molybdenium blue by stannous chloride. The complex is extracted into isobutyl alcohol (λ_{max} 720 nm).

Reference

Indian Drugs, **21(8)**, 338, 1984.

The drug also forms insoluble complex with ammonium reinckate which can be used for gravimetric estimation of the drug or can be dissolved in acetone for colorimetric method (λ_{max} 520 nm).

Di-iodohydroxyquinoline

8-hydroxyquinoline derivatives can be benzoylated, nitrosated and give characteristic phenolic reaction with $FeCl_3$.

METHOD 1

Reagents

1% w/v solution of ferric chloride in acetone.

Standard solution

Weigh accurately about 40 mg of standard sample of di-iodohydroxyquinoline in a dry 100 ml volumetric flask and dissolve it in acetone by shaking thoroughly for 15 to 20 min. Keep aside for at least an hour and make up the final volume with acetone.

Sample solution

Weigh accurately powdered tablets equivalent to about 40 mg of di-iodohydroxyquinoline in a dry 100 ml volumetric flask. Add about 75 ml of acetone, shake thoroughly well for 10 to 15 min. Keep aside for at least an hour and make up the volume with acetone.

Procedure

Take 5 ml of sample and standard solutions in a 25 ml dry volumetric flask, add 1 ml of ferric chloride solution and make up to the mark with acetone. Shake well and measure the absorbance of the stable green colour at 575 nm against reagent blank prepared by diluting 1 ml of ferric chloride solution to 25 ml with acetone.

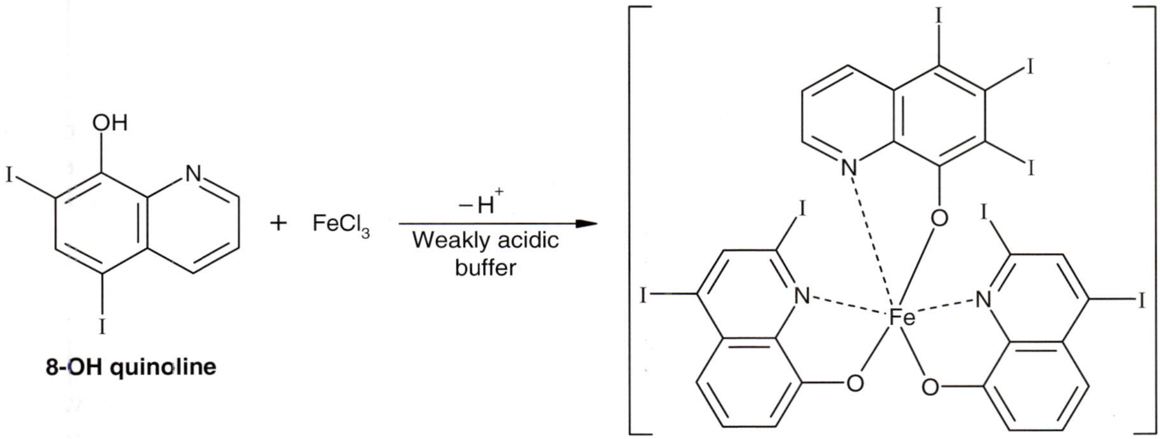

8-OH quinoline

Coloured Fe(III) neutral chelate formation
(λ_{max} 575 nm)

Reference

Pharmaceutical Chemistry (Vol. 2) by H.J. Roth, p. 608.

Note

All trivalent metal ions give similar complex.

Hydroxyquinoline yields chelates with monovalent, divalent and trivalent metal ions. With Cu(II) positively charged complex is formed which further reacts with 1 mole of the compound to give neutral chelate. With trivalent ions like Al(III) and Fe(III) neutral chelates are formed as shown.

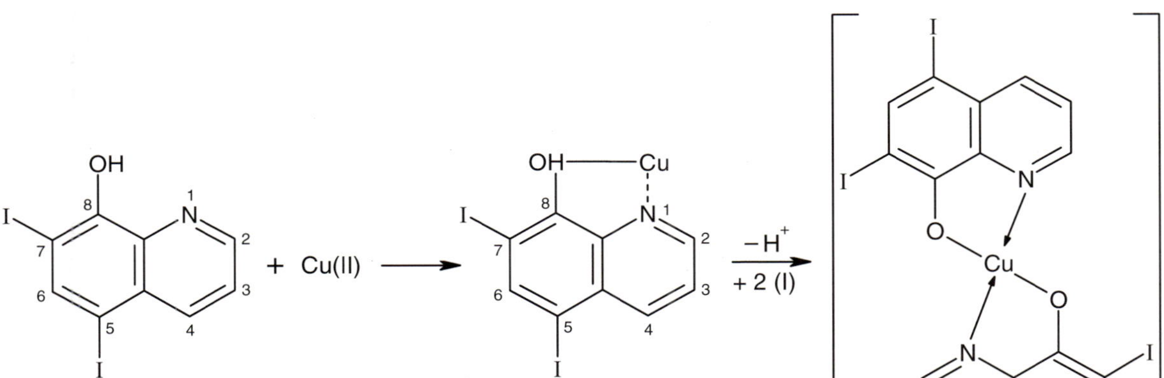

(I)

(II)
Positively charged copper complex

Neutral Cu(II) complex
(λ_{max} 403 nm)

Other metal complexes

Fe(II) Purple
Co(II) Yellow
Mg(II) Red

Reference

S.C. Mathur, C.L. Jain & P.D. Sethi, Indian Drugs, **26(1)**, 42-43, 1988.

A method based on formation of chelate with Co^{++} by hydroxyquinoline derivatives has been reported by Sen et al. (1989). The yellow-coloured chelate was measured at 410 nm.

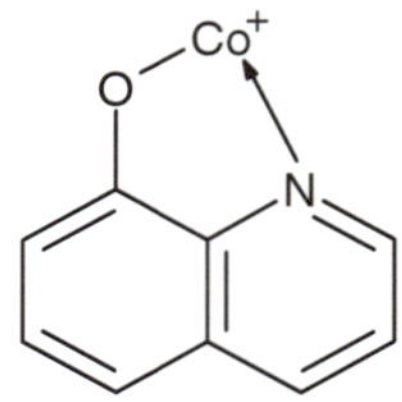

Cobalt chelate of hydroxyquinoline
(λ_{max} 410 nm)

Reference

A.K. Sen & T.K. Das, Indian Drugs, **27(2)**, 124-128, 1989.

General structures of monovalent, divalent and trivalent metal complexes

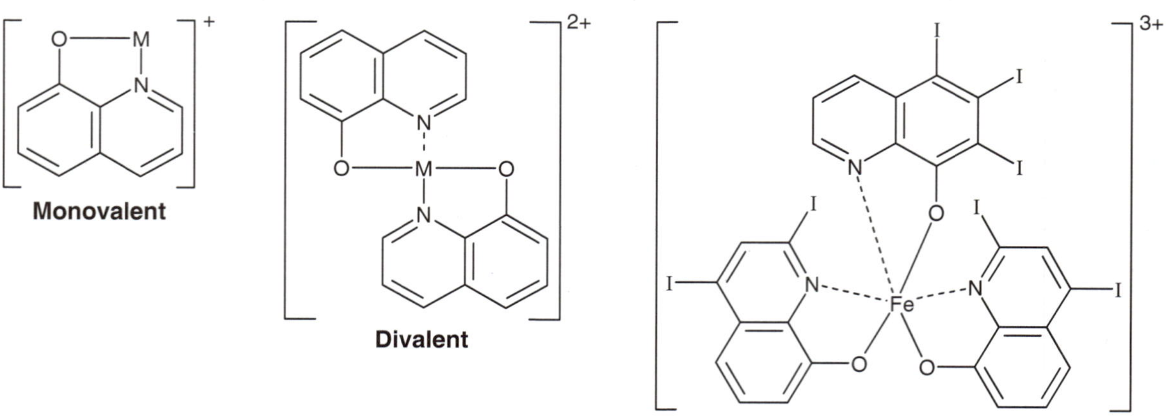

Monovalent **Divalent** **Trivalent**

METHOD 2

This method is based on the formation of colour complex of the compound with p-aminophenol in alkaline conditions.

Reagents

1. 0.1% w/v p-aminophenol solution in 0.2 M hydrochloric acid.
2. 0.5 N sodium carbonate.
3. 1,4-dioxan.

Standard solution

100 mg of the compound is dissolved in 1,4-dioxan to produce 100 ml (1 mg/ml).

Sample solution

Powdered tablets are accurately weighed equivalent to 25 mg of the compound, shaken with 20 ml of dioxan and filtered. The final volume is adjusted to 25 ml with dioxan (1 mg/ml).

Procedure

To 0.4 ml of the sample and standard solutions add 3 ml of sodium carbonate solution and 0.4 ml of p-aminophenol reagent. Keep at room temperature for 5 minutes and then dilute to 10 ml with water. The absorbance of the resultant solution is read at 570 nm after 15 minutes against reagent blank. The contents of di-iodohydroxyquinoline are calculated by comparison with the standard. The method obeys Beer's law in the concentration range of 15-500 mcg/ml.

Note

1. The colour attains maximum intensity after 15 minutes and is stable for 50 minutes.
2. Metronidazole, chloramphenicol, brobenzoxalidine, hyoscine and hyoscyamine do not interfere.

Probable Reaction Mechanism

This reaction is carried out in alkaline medium. p-Aminophenol is spontaneously oxidized to p-benzoquinone monimine in alkaline medium which in the presence of phenol forms indophenol. Based on this analogy, hydroxy-quinoline derivatives containing phenolic-OH group couples with oxidized aminophenol as shown below.

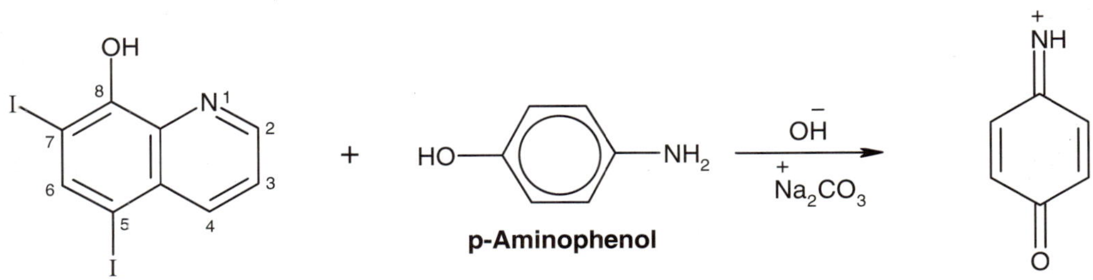

Diiodohydroxyquinoline (5,7-diiodohydroxyquinoline)

p-Aminophenol

p-Benzoquinone monimine (I)

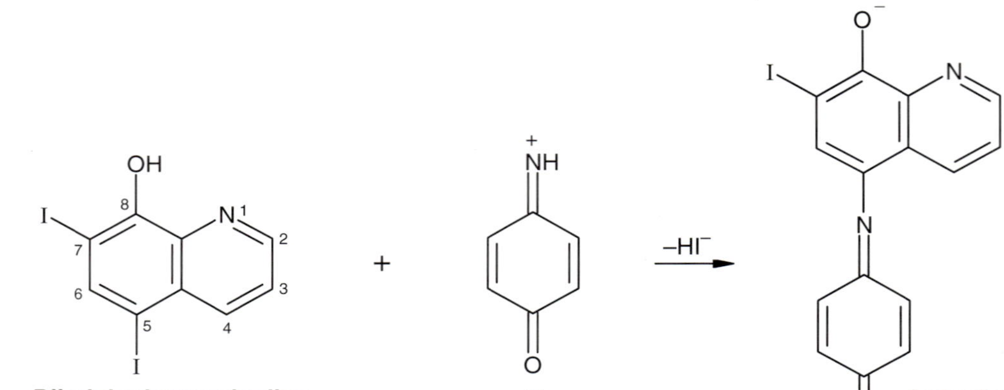

Diiodohydroxyquinoline (5,7-diiodohydroxyquinoline) — (I) — Indophenol (λ_{max} 570 nm)

Note

Iodochlorhydroxyquinoline (ICHQ) and dibromohydroxyquinoline (DBHQ) also answer similar reaction.

Reference

R.T. Sane, A.B. Ambardekar & V.K. Shastri, Indian Drugs, **18(8)**, 290-294, 1981.

METHOD 3

This method is suitable both for iodo- and di-iodohydroxyquinolines.

Reagents

1. 2% w/v solution of potassium ferricyanide in water.
2. 1% w/v solution of 4-aminoantipyrin in water.
3. Borate buffer solution: 2 g of sodium borate and 0.4 g of 'Tris' are dissolved in water to produce 100 ml.
4. Dimethylformamide (DMF).

Standard solution

25 mg of the accurately weighed compound is dissolved in 3 ml of 'DMF' and 80 ml of isopropanol. The mixture is diluted to 100 ml with isopropanol.

Sample solution

Accurately weighed amount of the powdered tablets equivalent to 25 mg of the compound is treated as under standard solution.

Procedure

To 1 ml of the sample and standard solutions add 9 ml of isopropanol, 0.5 ml of potassium ferricyanide solution, 10 ml of buffer solution and 1.5 ml of antipyrin reagent. Allow the reaction flask to stand at room temperature for 90 min, and measure the extinction of both the solutions at 500 nm against reagent blank. The method obeys Beer's law in the concentration range of 50-500 mcg/ml.

Note

Chloroquine phosphate, furazolidone and streptomycin do not interfere.

This reaction is known as Emerson reaction. The reaction proceeds via oxidative coupling at para position or ortho position if the para position is occupied with respect to phenolic-OH group. The presence of oxidizing agent i.e. κ-hexacyanoferrate is necessary for the reaction. If the p-position is substituted by a halogen as in the above drug, it is easily oxidatively dissociated by the oxidizing agent. Optimal reaction medium required is pH 8 which is achieved by the buffer solution.

Probable Reaction Mechanism

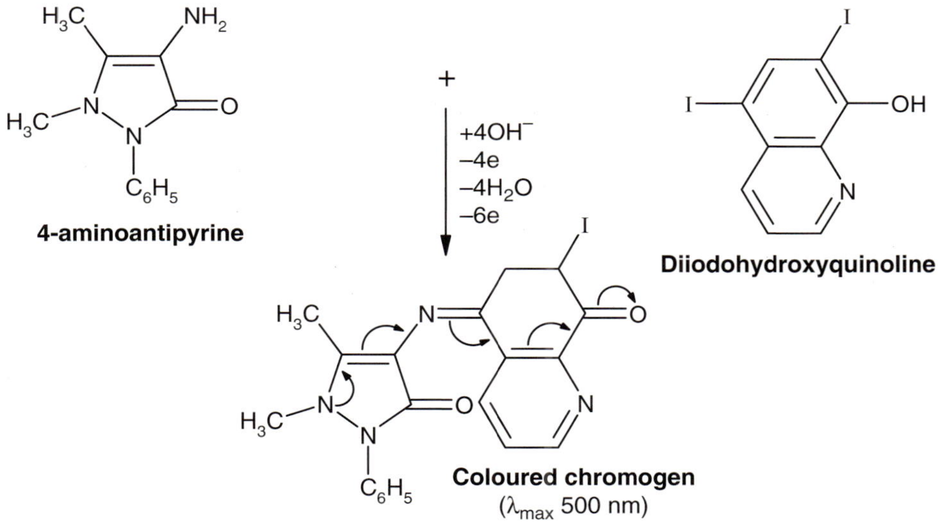

The 2,6-dichlorochlorimide reagent (Gibbs' reagent) oxidatively couples at the para-position to the phenolic hydroxy group in the drug resulting in the formation of desired product. For the reaction to occur, a pH of 8.5 is required which is achieved by the phosphate buffer.

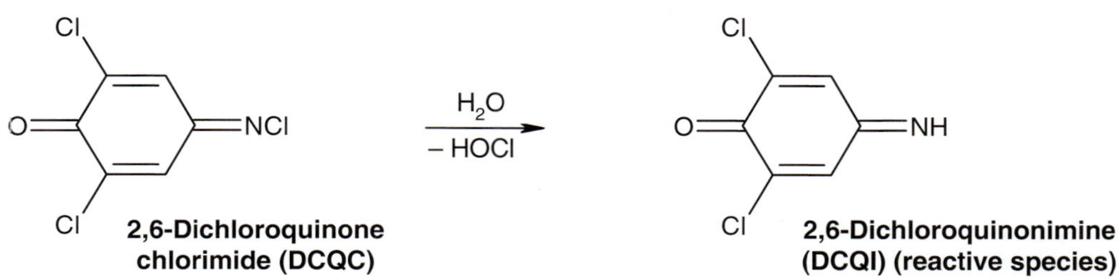

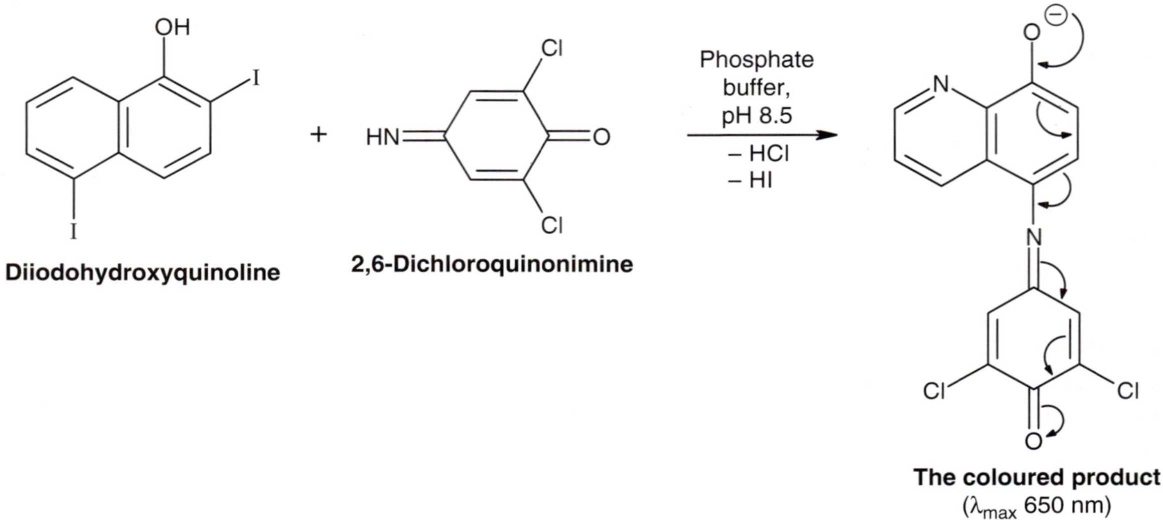

Reference

Vinay Navrekar, Indian Drugs, **19**, 102-103, 1982.

Diazotized benzocaine can couple with halogenated 8-hydroxyquinoline to give coloured products in alkaline medium.

Probable Reaction Mechanism

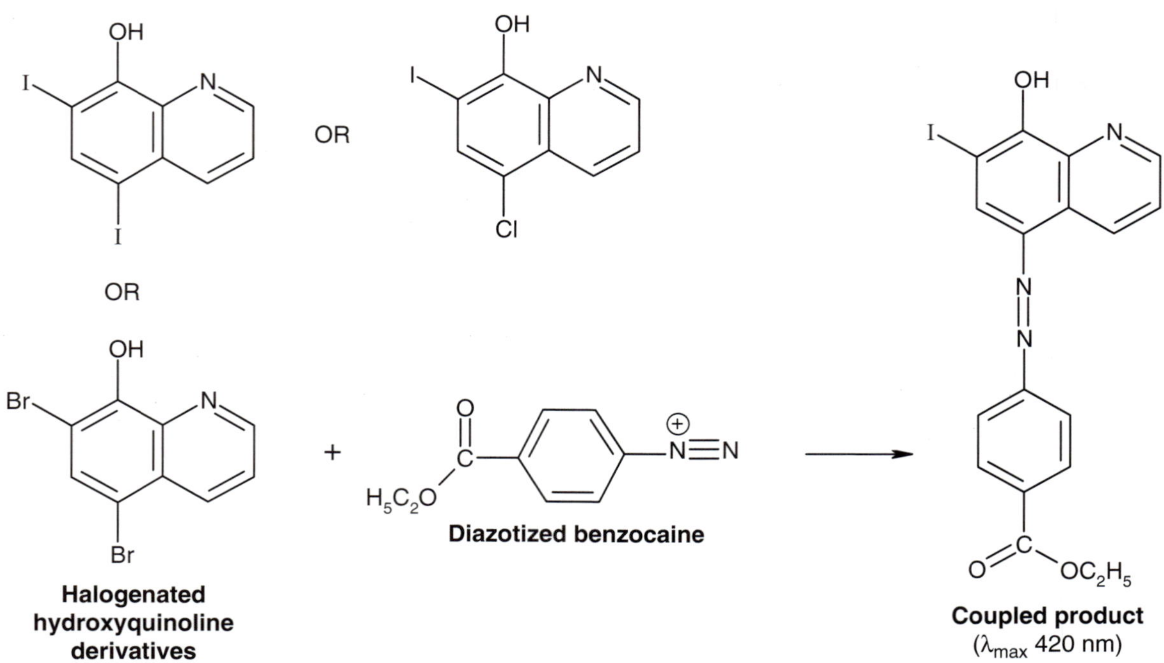

Reference

R.T. Sane, V.B. Malkar & V.G. Nayak, Indian Drugs, **19(12)**, 487-492, 1982.

An analytical method has been reported for the estimation of DIHQ and ICHQ involving reaction with diazotized dapsone (4,4′-sulphoyl dianiline) in alkaline medium (triethylamine) giving an orange-coloured complex (λ_{max} 430 nm).

Probable Reaction Mechanism

As usual, coupling reaction shall take place at the para-position to the phenolic-OH group. If the para position is not free, then coupling can also occur at the ortho position to the phenolic-OH. Coupling at both para or ortho positions is explained below.

Ortho coupling

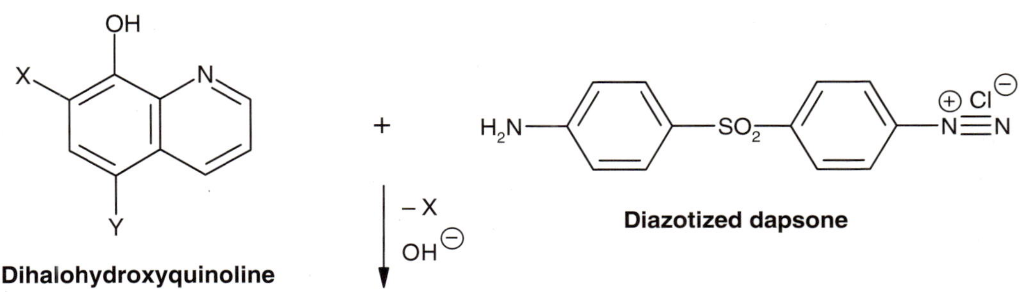

Dihalohydroxyquinoline **Diazotized dapsone**

where X and Y are halogens

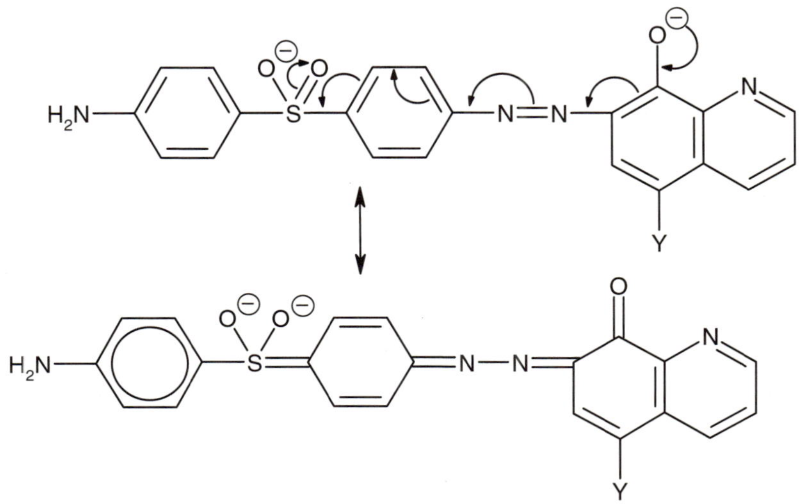

(λ_{max} 430 nm or λ_{max} 530 nm)

Para coupling

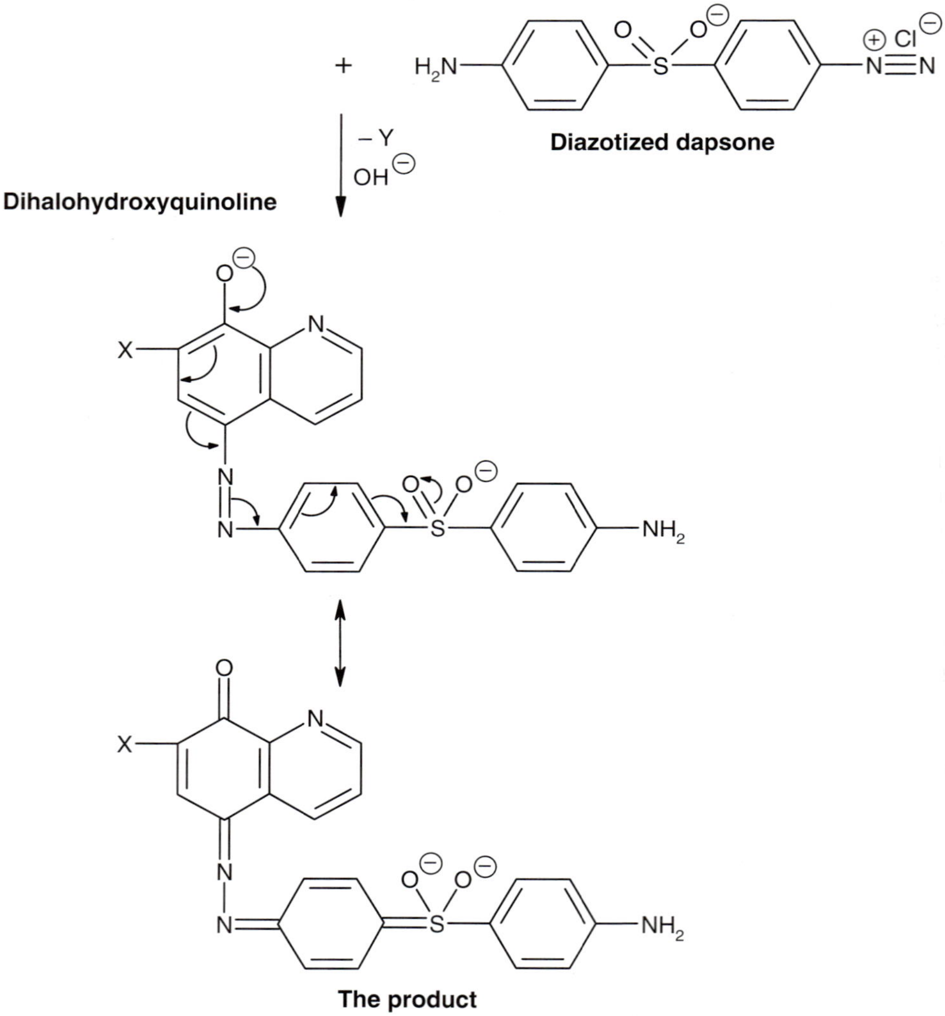

Note

Sastry et al. have reported λ_{max} 430 nm whereas Sane et al. have reported 530 nm.

Reference

1. C.P.S. Sastry & M. Aruna, Indian Drugs, **26(10)**, 567, 1988.
2. R.T. Sane, N.R. Naik & S.S. Zarapkar, J. University of Bombay, Science Vol. L_I-L_{II}, No. 78-79, 1982-1983.

Bismuth N-glycolyl arsanilate (Glycobiarsol)

METHOD 1

Reagents

1. 12% w/v solution of dibasic ammonium phosphate in water.
2. 3% w/v solution of ammonium nitrate in water.
3. Nitric acid.

Procedure

Powder 20 tablets and transfer a powdered material accurately weighed equivalent to 200 mg of the substance into 500 ml Kjeldahl's flask. Add 50 ml of nitric acid and heat till solution is colourless. Cool and transfer the acid solution to a 250 ml volumetric flask. Dilute to volume with water and mix. Transfer 100 ml to a beaker, add ammonia solution dropwise until a faint precipitate is permanent. Then add 2 ml of nitric acid and heat to boiling. To the boiling solution add 5 ml solution of dibasic ammonium phosphate dropwise and with continuous stirring until bismuth is precipitated. Then add the remaining solution more rapidly. Allow to stand on a water-bath until the supernatant liquid is practically clear. Then filter through G_4 sintered crucible and wash with ammonium nitrate solution till free from phosphate. Dry the precipitate at 105° to constant weight. Each g of the precipitate is equivalent to 1.642 g of glycobiarsol.

Note

The bismuth is precipitated as phosphate and estimated gravimetrically.

METHOD 2

Reagents

1. 0.05 M Edetate disodium salt.
2. 0.25 M Zinc sulphate.
3. Acetic acid - ammonium acetate buffer.
4. Dithizone test solution.

Procedure

Weigh accurately a quantity of crushed tablets equivalent to 250 mg of glycobiarsol, add 10 ml of edetate solution and warm till dissolved. Cool to room temperature, add 10 ml of acetate buffer solution, 25 ml of ethyl alcohol and 2 ml of dithizone solution. Titrate excess of edetate with zinc sulphate solution to a clear rose pink colour. Each ml of 0.05 M edetate is equivalent to 24.95 mg of glycobiarsol.

Note

EDTA acts as chelating agent for bismuth and excess EDTA is back-titrated.

Niacinamide

Reagents

1. 50% w/v solution of sodium hydroxide in water.
2. 4% w/v solution of boric acid in water.
3. 0.1 N Hydrochloric acid.

Procedure

Weigh accurately a quantity of the sample powder equivalent to about 150 mg of the substance and transfer to a 500 ml Kjeldahl's flask. Add about 100 ml water and warm for 30 minutes on a water-bath with occasional shaking. Fix the flask to a Kjeldahl's distillation apparatus. Add 10 ml of sodium hydroxide solution, distil and collect the distillate in a 250 ml conical flask containing 25 ml of boric acid solution and 2-3 drops of methyl red and titrate with 0.1 N hydrochloric acid. Carry out a blank determination exactly as above but without the sample and note the difference in the two titrations to calculate the volume of 0.1 N acid consumed by the compound. Each ml of 0.1 N hydrochloric acid is equivalent to 12.21 mg of niacinamide.

As a result of alkaline hydrolysis, the ammonia generated is distilled and estimated by titrating with 0.1 M HCl.

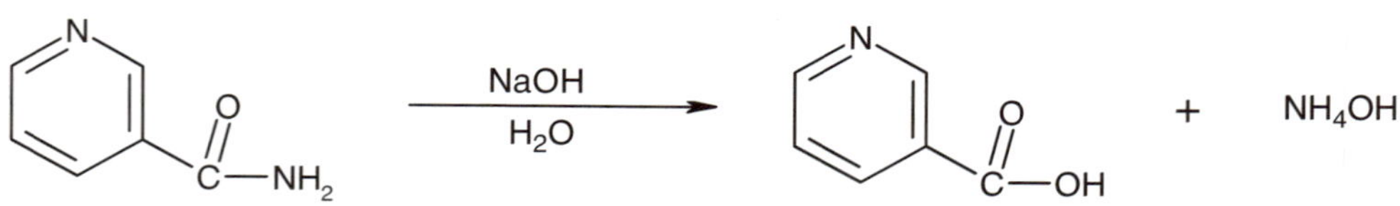

Note

This method often yields higher results due to the presence of volatile basic compounds in the sample.

Boric acid is used to fix ammonia as ammonium borate, which can be directly titrated as a base with standard HCl. This titration involves displacement of the weak acid (boric acid) by the strong acid (hydrochloric acid). The advantage of the method over the routine method is the use of only one standard solution instead of two standard solutions.

Formulation 3

Di-iodohydroxyquinoline, Phthalylsulphathiazole

ESTIMATION

Di-iodohydroxyquinoline

METHOD 1

Reagents

1. Dilute hydrochloric acid.
2. Dimethylformamide (DMF).

Standard solution

Weigh accurately 100 mg of pure compound, add 10 ml of 'DMF' and shake vigorously for 5 minutes. Further make appropriate dilution with dilute hydrochloric acid to obtain a concentration of 50 mcg/ml.

Sample solution

Weigh accurately a quantity of powdered sample equivalent to 100 mg of the compound, add 10 ml of 'DMF' and treat as per standard solution. Concomitantly determine the extinctions of both the standard and sample solutions at absorption maximum at about 390 nm and calculate the results by comparison.

METHOD 2

Follow the method 4 described for estimation of diiodohydroxyquinoline under formulation 1 of this chapter.

METHOD 3

Reagents

1. 0.4% w/v solution of 2,6-dichloroquinone chlorimide in isopropyl alcohol (Gibbs' reagent).
2. Buffer solution: 3.3% w/v solution of dipotassium hydrogen phosphate in water.
3. 1,4-dioxane.

Standard solution

100 mcg/ml of the compound in 1,4-dioxane.

Sample solution

Weigh accurately powdered sample or measure aliquot equivalent to 25 mg of the compound and extract with 1,4-dioxane to get 100 mcg/ml solution.

Procedure

To 1 ml each of the sample and standard solutions, add 2 ml buffer and 5 ml chlorimide reagent and dilute to 10 ml with water. After 5 minutes, measure the absorbance of both the solutions at 650 nm against reagent as blank. The method obeys Beer's law in the range of 1-16 mcg/ml. Metronidazole, metronidazole benzoate and tetracycline hydrochloride do not interfere.

Probable Reaction Mechanism

This reaction involving Gibbs' reagent is applicable for 8-hydroxyquinolines and its halogenated derivatives such as iodochlorhydroxyquinolines. The reaction is carried out in buffer of alkaline pH. The molar ratio is 2 : 1 for 8-hydroxyquinoline and 1 : 1 for halogenated derivatives.

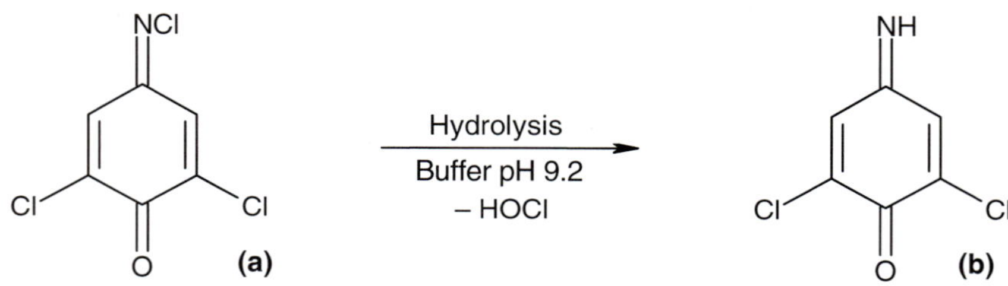

2,6-Dichloroquinone chlorimide (Gibbs' reagent)

Active species (II) 2,6-Dichloroquinonimine

(A)

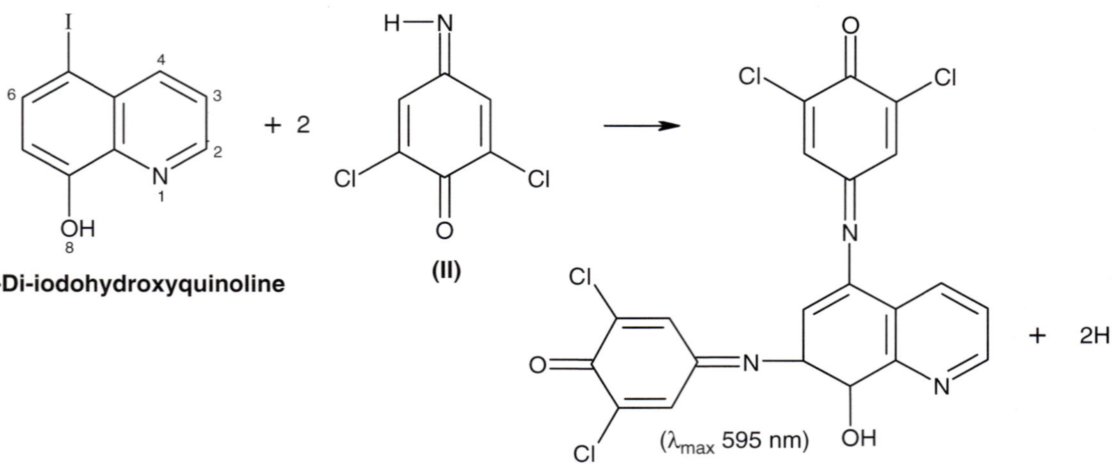

5,7-Di-iodohydroxyquinoline

(B)

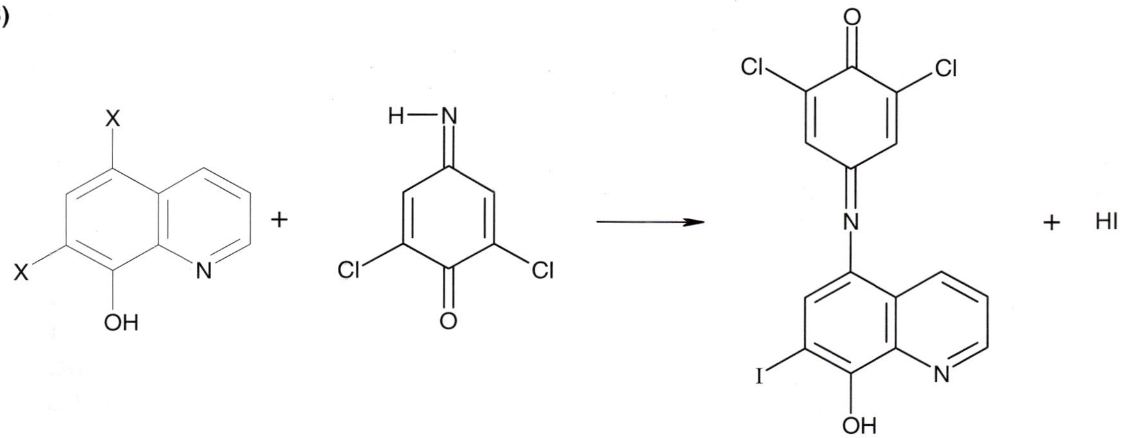

Blue complex
(λ_{max} 650 nm)

Proposed reaction pathway between 2,6-dichloroquinone chlorimide and (A) 8-hydroxyquinoline and (B) substituted derivatives.

Note

The chlorimide reagent is first converted to active species i.e. 2,6-dichloroquinonimine which ultimately reacts with quinoline derivative.

Reference

Fathalla Belal, Analyst, **109**, 615-618, 1984.

Phthalylsulphathiazole

METHOD 1

Weigh accurately a quantity of sample equivalent to about 0.25 g of phthalylsulphathiazole. Add 100 ml of 25% w/v sodium hydroxide solution and reflux for four hours. Cool, filter through cotton, wash with water and acidify with hydrochloric acid. Cool below 15°C and titrate against 0.1 M sodium nitrite with constant shaking using starch iodide paste as an external indicator. Each ml of 0.1 M sodium nitrite is equivalent to 0.04034 g of phthalylsulphathiazole.

METHOD 2

Transfer a quantity of powder equivalent to about 400 mg of phthalylsulphathiazole in a dry beaker. Add 30-40 ml of ethyl acetate, boil on water-bath, stir and decant the solution through filter paper. Repeat the extraction 4-5 times with boiling ethyl acetate and filter while hot. Iodochlorhydroxyquinoline, soluble in hot ethyl acetate, gets removed by above extraction procedure. Collect the residue, dry and reflux for 30 minutes with water and 20 ml of hydrochloric acid. Cool to 15°C and proceed for estimation as under method 1 above.

Probable Reaction Mechanism (Methods 1 and 2)

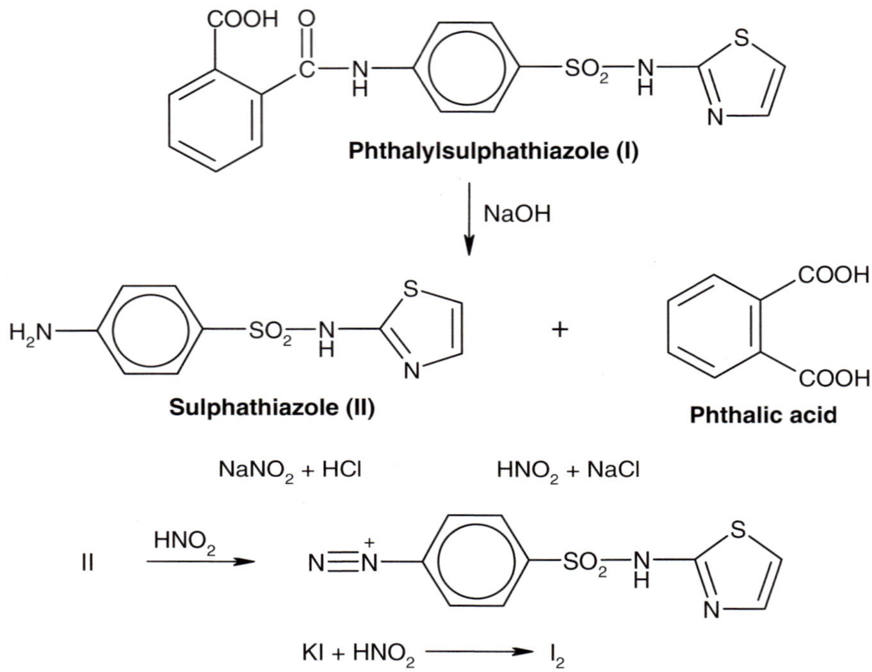

I_2 forms blue inclusion complex with starch, the end point.

Formulation 4

Chloroquine phosphate, Di-iodohydroxy-quinoline, Phthalylsulphathiazole

ESTIMATION

Chloroquine phosphate

METHOD 1

Follow the method 2 for estimation of chloroquine phosphate described under formulation 1 of this chapter.

METHOD 2

Reagents

1. 0.4% w/v solution of bromothymol blue in water.
2. Chloroform.
3. Buffer solution, pH 5.6: Weigh 41.5 g of disodium hydrogen phosphate and 8.72 g of citric acid and dissolve in water to produce 1000 ml.

Standard solution

Weigh chloroquine phosphate or sulphate equivalent to 40 mg of the chloroquine base and dissolve in water to produce a solution of 10 mcg/ml (base).

Sample solution

Weigh accurately powdered sample equivalent to 40 mg of chloroquine base, shake with water and adjust the volume to 100 ml with water. Filter and dilute the filtrate appropriately to get a sample solution of 10 mcg/ml (base).

Procedure

To 5 ml each of the sample and standard solutions, add 5 ml of the buffer solution, pH 5.6, and 5 ml of the dye solution. Shake and add 10 ml of chloroform. Shake vigorously for 1 minute and allow the chloroform layer to separate. Measure absorption of chloroform layer of both the solutions at about 410 nm and calculate the contents of chloroquine phosphate by comparison.

Note

It is an ion-pair complex.

Reference

P.D. Shirsat, Ind. J. Pharm. Sci., **38**, 77, 1976.

METHOD 3

1. Cobalt thiocyanate reagent: Dissolve 1.33 g of $CoCl_2$ and 3.33 g of potassium thiocyanate to make 100 ml.
2. Universal buffer, pH 1.98.
3. Isobutylmethylketone (IBMK).

Sample and standard solutions

100 µg/ml in water.

Procedure

To 4 ml each of sample and standard solutions add 1.5 ml of cobalt reagent, 1 ml of buffer and 3.5 ml of water, shake well and extract with 4 × 10 ml of IBMK, filter each extract through cotton plug, dilute to 50 ml and measure the absorbance at 625 nm.

Probable Reaction Mechanism

As tertiary aliphatic amine it forms complex with Co(II).

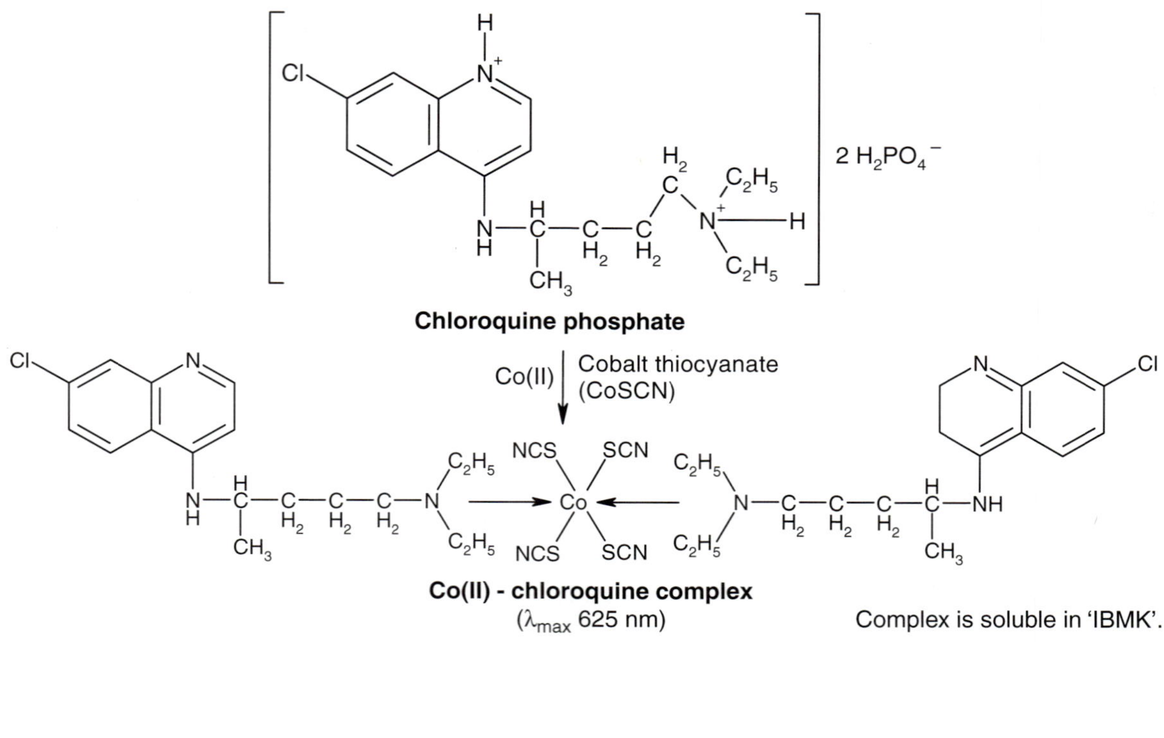

Reference

G. Rama Rao, Y. Pulla Rao & I.R.K. Raju, Indian Drugs, **19(4)**, 162-164, 1982.

Phthalylsulphathiazole

METHOD 1

Reagents

1. 10% w/v solution of sodium bicarbonate in water.
2. 0.1 M sodium nitrite solution.
3. Hydrochloric acid.

Procedure

To accurately weighed quantity of the sample equivalent to 500 mg of the substance, add 50 ml of sodium bicarbonate solution and allow the mixture to stand for 30 minutes with occasional stirring. After the suspended matter has settled down, the supernatant liquid is filtered through G_4 sintered crucible. Extract the residue with further three successive 25, 15, 10 ml portions of bicarbonate solution, filtering each through the same crucible. Neutralize the combined filtrate with hydrochloric acid and add 10 ml of the acid in excess. Reflux for 1 hour, cool to 15°C and slowly titrate with 0.1 M sodium nitrite. Each ml of 0.1 M sodium nitrite is equivalent to 0.04034 g of phthalylsulphathiazole.

METHOD 2

Follow the method described under formulation 4 of this chapter.

Diiodohydroxyquinoline

Follow the method described under formulation 4 of this chapter.

Formulation 5

Phthalylsulphacetamide/Phthalylsulphathiazole, Iodochlorhydroxyquinoline, Diiodohydroxyquinoline, Sulphaguanidine

ESTIMATION

METHOD A

Iodochlorhydroxyquinoline and Diiodohydroxyquinoline

Total iodine from iodochlorhydroxyquinoline and diiodohydroxyquinoline

Reagents

1. 0.1 N Hydrochloric acid.
2. 0.1 N Sodium hydroxide.
3. 20% w/v solution of sodium hydroxide in water.
4. M/20 Potassium iodate solution.
5. 10% w/v solution of potassium cyanide in water.
6. Concentrated sulphuric acid.

Procedure

Transfer accurately weighed amount of the powdered sample to a conical flask and add 20 ml of cold (8°C or below) 0.1 N hydrochloric acid to dissolve sulphaguanidine present in the sample. Filter the mixture and preserve the acidic filtrate for the determination of sulphaguanidine (A). Continue the process of extraction with 10 ml portions of cold 0.1 N acid until a little portion of the solution, made alkaline with 5 ml of sodium hydroxide solution and boiled, does not evolve ammonia. Generally 80 to 100 ml of cold acid are required for complete extraction of sulphaguanidine.

Transfer the residue left after acid extraction to a beaker with the help of water and treat the insoluble residue with 5 ml portions of cold (8°C or below) 0.1 N sodium hydroxide to dissolve phthalylsulphacetamide present in it. Filter the mixture, and preserve the alkaline filtrate for the determination of phthalylsulphacetamide (B). The process is continued until a little portion, when heated with 5 ml of dehydrated alcohol and 5 ml of concentrated sulphuric acid, fails to produce any odour of ethyl acetate. Generally 25-30 ml of cold alkali are sufficient for complete extraction.

Note

If at any stage of extraction, with either cold acid or alkali, there is any production of colour of iodine, the whole process should be repeated to obtain almost colourless solution. The residue left after alkali extraction is then dried at 80°C and transferred to a small nickel crucible containing anhydrous sodium carbonate. The crucible is strongly heated to convert the mass to sodium iodide. Cool the crucible and transfer to a beaker containing distilled water. Boil, cool, remove the crucible carefully and wash it thoroughly with distilled water so that any adhering material (sodium iodide) may be quantitatively transferred to the beaker containing the extract. Filter the extracted mass, acidify the filtrate with hydrochloric acid and cool to 15°C. Transfer the acidified solution to a stoppered flask, add 15 ml of hydrochloric acid and cool well. Titrate the liquid with M/20 potassium iodate solution using 5 ml of potassium cyanide solution and adding mucilage of starch as indicator towards the end of titration. Perform a blank omitting the sample. Each ml of M/20 potassium iodate consumed is equivalent to 0.01269 g of iodine. Calculate the content of total iodine per tablet of average weight. Iodochlorhydroxyquinoline and diiodohydroxyquinoline contain 63.5% and 41.2% w/w of iodine respectively.

Explanatory Note

As iodine liberated by action of IO_3 as NaI is also coloured a simple visual detection of end point is not possible, hence KCN is added as it reacts with iodine to give iodine cyanide.

$$IO_3^- + 5I^- + 6H^+ \rightleftharpoons 3I_2 + 3H_2O$$

$$I + KCN + H^+ \longrightarrow ICN + H^+ + 2e$$

Sulphaguanidine

To the acidic filtrate (A) preserved during estimation of hydroxyquinolines, add 25 ml of dilute hydrochloric acid, cool the mixture to 15°C and add crushed ice. Titrate the liquid with M/10 sodium nitrite solution using starch iodide paper as external indicator until instant blue ring produced is reproducible after 2 min. Each ml of M/10 sodium nitrite is equivalent to 0.02142 g of sulphaguanidine.

Phthalylsulphacetamide/Phthalylsulphathiazole

To the alkaline filtrate (B) preserved during estimation of hydroxyquinolines, add 15 ml of hydrochloric acid. Reflux the acidic solution for 2 hours, cool the solution to 15°C and add crushed ice. Titrate the liquid with M/10 sodium nitrite as under sulphaguanidine. Each ml of M/10 sodium nitrite is equivalent to 0.03624 g of phthalylsulphacetamide or 0.04034 g of phthalylsulphathiazole.

Note

After hydrolysis the free amino group so liberated is titrated with sodium nitrite as usual.

METHOD B

Iodochlorhydroxyquinoline and Diiodohydroxyquinoline

METHOD 1

Follow the method for estimation of total iodine as described under method A.

METHOD 2

To the powdered material equivalent to 100 mg of hydroxyquinolines, add 10 ml of dimethylformamide, shake for 5 min, and dilute with 3 N hydrochloric acid to obtain a concentration of 50 mcg/ml. Prepare the standard solution of the compound similarly and measure the extinction at 390 nm against solvent blank. Calculate the results by comparison.

Sulphaguanidine

Reagents

1. 10% w/v zinc sulphate solution in water.
2. 0.1 N Hydrochloric acid.
3. 0.5% w/v ammonium sulphamate solution in water.
4. 0.1% w/v N-1-naphthyl ethylenediamine dihydrochloride in water (NED).
5. 0.1% w/v sodium nitrite solution in water.

Standard solution

Weigh accurately 100 mg of pure sulphaguanidine, dissolve in water and make up the volume to 100 ml. Filter and to 10 ml of the filtrate add 10 ml of zinc sulphate solution and adjust the volume to 100 ml with 0.1 N hydrochloric acid (100 mcg/ml).

Sample solution

Weigh accurately a quantity of the powdered tablets equivalent to 200 mg of sulphaguanidine, add 20 ml of water, warm and shake well. Filter and make up the filtrate to 200 ml. Reserve the residue for assay of phthalylsulphacetamide. 10 ml of the filtrate is treated as per standard to get sample solution (100 mcg/ml).

Procedure

To 2 ml of standard and sample solutions, add 1 ml of sodium nitrite solution, keep for 2 minutes and then add 1 ml of ammonium sulphamate solution. Wait for 2 minutes for complete neutralization of nitrous acid, then add 1 ml of 'NED' reagent. After 10 minutes, read both the solutions at 525 nm against reagent blank and calculate the results.

Phthalylsulphacetamide//Phthalylsulphathiazole

Sample solution

Transfer the residue obtained above in the sample preparation for estimation of sulphaguanidine to 250 ml flask. Add 20 ml of hydrochloric acid and reflux for 1 hr, cool and dilute with water appropriately to get 100 mcg/ml.

Standard solution

Standard solution of phthalylsulphacetamide is hydrolysed with hydrochloric acid and diluted to get 100 mcg/ml solution as described under the preparation of sample solution.

Procedure

2 ml each of standard and sample solutions are taken and colour is developed as in the case of sulphaguanidine. The maximum absorption in this case is also observed at about 525 nm. Results are computed by comparison.

Note

Preparation of sample and standard solutions involves hydrolysis to liberate free amino group which is used for analysis as per method described.

Formulation 6

Broxyquinoline, Brobenzoxalidine, Hyoscyamine, Hyoscine

ESTIMATION

Broxyquinoline and Brobenzoxalidine as Broxyquinoline

METHOD 1

Reagents

1. Glacial acetic acid.
2. Acetic anhydride.
3. Methylene chloride.
4. 0.1 N perchloric acid in glacial acetic acid.
5. Crystal violet solution, indicator.

Procedure

Weigh accurately quantity of the sample equivalent to 250 mg of both the ingredients. Transfer to sintered glass funnel (G_4) and percolate ten times 10 ml portions of methylene chloride. Evaporate the organic layer under reduced pressure to dryness below 40°C. Dissolve the residue thus obtained in 100 ml of mixture of glacial acetic acid and acetic anhydride (1: 1) and titrate with 0.1 N perchloric acid using crystal violet as indicator. Each 1 ml of 0.1 N perchloric acid is equivalent to 0.0303 g of broxyquinoline.

METHOD 2

This method is specific for broxyquinoline.

Reagents

1. 0.5 N sodium carbonate.
2. 0.1% w/v solution of p-aminophenol in 0.2 N hydrochloric acid (freshly prepared).
3. 1,4-Dioxane.

Standard solution

500 mcg/ml of the substance in dioxane.

Sample solution

Weigh accurately quantity of the sample equivalent to about 25 mg of substance. Shake with 30 ml of dioxane, filter, adjust the final volume to 50 ml with dioxane (500 mcg/ml).

Procedure

To 0.5 ml each of the sample and standard solutions, add 4 ml of sodium carbonate solution and 0.5 ml of p-aminophenol reagent. Keep at room temperature for 10 minutes and then dilute to 10 ml with water and shake to mix. The absorbance of solutions is measured after 20 minutes at 570 nm against reagent blank. The method obeys Beer's law in the concentration range of 5-40 mcg/ml. The colour attains maximum intensity after 20 minutes and is stable for 45 minutes. Calculate the contents of broxyquinoline per tablets/ capsule by comparison.

From the weight of broxyquinoline thus found, calculate equivalent volume of 0.1 N perchloric acid. Each ml of 0.1 N perchloric acid is equivalent to 0.0303 g of broxyquinoline.

Subtract the volume of 0.1 N perchloric acid thus calculated from the total volume of 0.1 N perchloric acid used in the titration for determination of both broxyquinoline and Brobenzoxalidine (see method 1). This will give the net volume of 0.1 N perchloric acid required for brobenzoxalidine.

Note

While estimating broxyquinoline and brobenzoxalidine in suspension, add 10 g of silica gel (column chromatography grade) to the accurately weighed quantity of the suspension, mix to get homogeneous free flowing powder. Extract the powder with methylene chloride for further determination as per details discussed above under method 1 and 2. To calculate the contents in each 5 ml, specific gravity of the sample is required to be determined.

Probable Reaction Mechanism

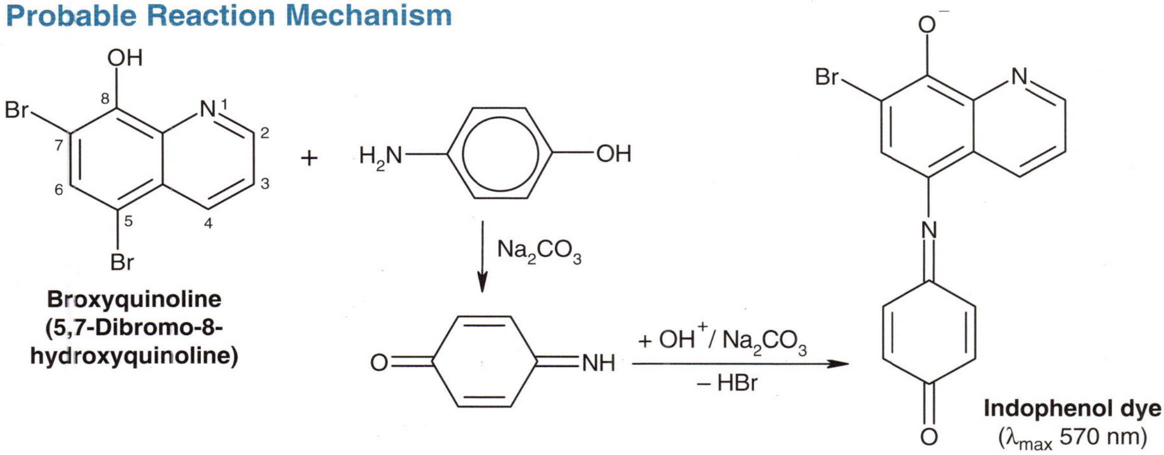

Note

Similarly, the compound reacts with metol (N-methylaminophenol) to give indophenol derivative.

Reference

1. R.T. Sane, A.B. Ambardekar & V.K. Shastri, Indian Drugs, **18(8)**, 290-294, 1981.
2. R.T. Sane, V.B. Malkar & V.G. Nayak, Indian Drugs, **19(12)**, 487-492, 1982.
3. S.S. Zarapker & V.J. Doshi, *Indian Drugs*, **25(9)**, 374-379, 1992.

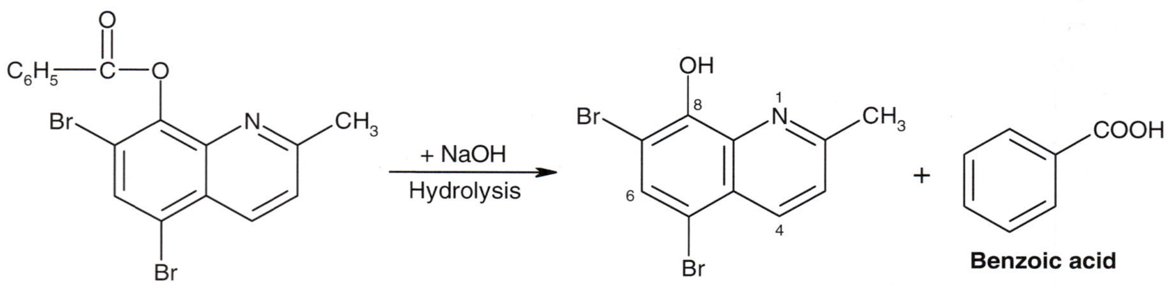

Brobenzoxalidine (5,7-dibromo-2-methyl-8-quinolylbenzoate) — **5,7-dibromo-2-methyl-8-OH-quinoline** — **Benzoic acid**

This will answer all the reactions of broxyquinoline.

Hyoscyamine and Hyoscine (total alkaloids)

METHOD 1

Follow the method described in formulation 1 of this chapter.

METHOD 2

Reagents

1. 0.1 M citric acid.
2. 0.2 M disodium hydrogen phosphate, dihydrate.
3. Citric acid-phosphate buffer, pH 7.5: Dilute 7.5 ml each of 0.1 M citric acid and 0.2 M disodium hydrogen phosphate to 100 ml with water.
4. Bromothymol blue solution: Dissolve 0.15 g bromothymol blue and 0.15 g of anhydrous sodium carbonate in 100 ml of water.
5. Alcoholic solution of boric acid: Dissolve 20 g of boric acid in 800 ml of ethanol and 80 ml of water and then make up to 1000 ml with ethanol.

Standard solution

100 mcg/ml of the substance in water.

Sample solution

Quantity of the sample equivalent to 5 mg of the substance is accurately weighed and dissolved in water to produce 50 ml (100 mcg/ml).

Procedure

Pipette 5 ml each of the sample and standard solutions and 0.5 ml of 0.1 N sodium hydroxide into separate 100 ml separating funnels. To each separating funnel, add 2 ml of bromothymol blue solution and 20 ml of buffer solution. Extract by shaking for about one minute with exactly 30 ml of chloroform. Separate chloroform layer and make up to 50 ml with alcoholic boric acid solution to clear the chloroform phase. Determine the extinctions of the sample and standard solutions at about 420 nm against chloroform as a blank. Compute the results by comparison.

METHOD 3

Reagents

Solution 1: Phosphate buffer solution of pH 2.5. To 55 ml of 7.8% w/v solution of potassium phosphate dibasic, add 20 ml of 9.6% w/v solution of citric acid and dilute to 100 ml with water.

Solution 2: Bromocresol purple: To 400 mg of bromocresol purple, add 6.5 ml of 0.1 N sodium hydroxide and make up to 500 ml with water.

Dye solution: Mix equal volumes of solution 1 and solution 2, extract with chloroform and reject chloroform layer. This step reduces the blank value.

Standard solution

50 mcg/ml of L-hyoscyamine in 0.1 N hydrochloric acid.

Sample solution

Weigh accurately a quantity of the sample equivalent to 5 mg of substance and shake with 0. N hydrochloric acid to produce 100 ml.

Procedure

To 10 ml each of the sample and standard solutions, add 10 ml of dye solution and exactly 25 ml chloroform. Shake for 2 minutes, and allow the layers to separate out. Filter the chloroform layer through cotton plug. Read extinction of sample and standard solutions at about 440 nm against chloroform as blank and calculate the results by comparison.

METHOD 4

Reagents

1. Bromothymol blue solution: 2×10^{-4} solution in chloroform.
2. McIvaine's buffer, pH 5.6.
3. Chloroform.

Standard solution

Evaporate appropriate volume of the standard solution as given under method 1 and dissolve the residue in buffer, pH 5.6, to get a solution of 50 mcg/ml.

Sample solution

Evaporate appropriate quantity of the main chloroform extract obtained during the extraction procedure described under method 1 above for determination of total alkaloids. Dissolve the residue in buffer solution, pH 5.6, to get a solution of 0.05 mg/ml in respect of hyoscyamine or hyoscine.

Procedure

Follow the method 2 for determination of atropine sulphate described under formulation of this chapter except that buffer of pH 5.6 may be used instead of pH 6.6. This will give total tropane alkaloids present. Determine the net contents of hyoscyamine by the method described for determination of atropine sulphate under formulation 14 of this chapter. Substract the amount of hyoscyamine thus determined from the total alkaloids (hyoscyamine and hyoscine) as determined above to give the net content of hyoscine.

Note

All the three methods (2, 3 and 4) are based on formation of ion-pair complex formation extractable into chloroform.

1. Bromothymol blue, pH 7.5 buffer λ_{max} 420 nm
2. Bromocresol purple, pH 2.5 buffer λ_{max} 440 nm
3. Bromothymol blue, pH 5.6 buffer λ_{max} 410 nm

Formulation 7

Chloramphenicol, Broxyquinoline, Brobenzoxalidine

ESTIMATION

Chloramphenicol

Standard solution

150 mg of chloramphenicol is shaken with water to dissolve and adjusted to 100 ml. 5 ml is further diluted to 50 ml with methanol.

Sample solution

Weigh accurately a quantity of powdered tablets or capsule material equivalent to about 150 mg chloramphenicol. Add 50 ml of distilled water, shake for 15-20 minutes and make up the volume to 100 ml with water. Filter and dilute 5 ml of the filtrate to 50 ml with methyl alcohol.

Procedure

Measure the extinction of both the solutions at maxima at about 278 nm which coincides with p-nitrophenyl chromophore. Use 90% methyl alcohol as blank and deduce the results by comparison.

The compound gives purple colour with methanolic tetraethyl ammonium hydroxide (TEAH). This may be due to electron attracting character of nitro (NO_2) group, which also is the cause of increase in —NH activity.

Broxyquinoline and Brobenzoxalidine

For estimation follow the methods given under formulation 6 of this chapter. Detailed reaction mechanism given under method 2.

Formulation 8

Streptomycin sulphate, Phthalylsulphathiazole, Iodochlorhydroxyquinoline

ESTIMATION

Streptomycin sulphate

METHOD 1

Weigh accurately a quantity of the powdered tablets equivalent to 250 mg of streptomycin base. Shake thrice each with 50 ml of ethyl acetate (this step will remove iodochlorhydroxyquinoline). Discard the supernatant liquid and dissolve the residue in water to produce 250 ml (1 mg/ml, base). Filter and estimate the streptomycin contents by method 2 described for determination of streptomycin sulphate under formulation 10 of this chapter.

METHOD 2

The above sample solution containing 1 mg/ml of the base is appropriately diluted further to produce a 15 mcg/ml solution. Proceed with colour development by method 1 described for estimation of streptomycin sulphate under formulation 10 of this chapter.

Iodochlorhydroxyquinoline

METHOD 1

Weigh accurately a quantity of the sample equivalent to 0.125 g of iodochlorhydroxyquinoline, add 50 ml ethyl acetate, boil and filter. Repeat the extraction three times with hot ethyl acetate. Evaporate ethyl acetate extract to dryness and dissolve the residue in 40 ml acetone. Add 2 ml acetic acid and 20 ml saturated solution of cupric acetate in methanol. Keep for 10 minutes, filter through a sintered glass crucible. Wash the precipitate two to three times with acetone and then with n-hexane. Dry at 105°C for one hour and weigh. Each g of the residue is equivalent to 0.975 g of iodochlorhydroxyquinoline.

Note

Ethyl acetate extract obtained under estimation of streptomycin can also be used for estimation of iodochlorhydroxyquinoline by the above method.

METHOD 2

Reagents

1. 0.1% w/v p-aminophenol solution in 0.2 N hydrochloric acid.
2. 0.2 N sodium carbonate solution.
3. Absolute alcohol.

Standard solution

40 mg of pure iodochlorhydroxyquinoline is dissolved in alcohol to produce 100 ml (0.4 mg/ml).

Sample solution

Weigh accurately a quantity of powdered tablets equivalent to 10 mg of the compound and shake with 15 ml of alcohol. Boil and filter. The final volume is adjusted to 25 ml with alcohol (0.4 mg/ml).

Procedure

Take 0.5 ml of standard and sample solutions and follow the method 2 described for determination of diiodohydroxyquinoline under formulation 1 of this chapter along with detailed reaction mechanism.

METHOD 3

As the drug contains both 'O' as well as 'N' atoms which are capable of donating or sharing electrons hence the drug forms coloured complex with Cu(II) in alkaline medium.

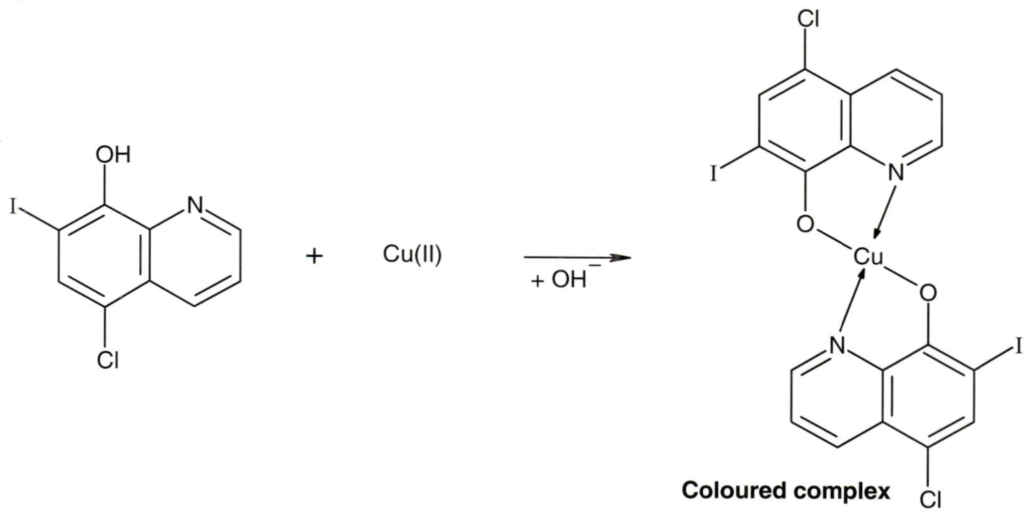

Coloured complex

Reference

Pharmaceutical Chemistry (Vol. 2) by H.J. Roth, p. 608.

Phthalylsulphathiazole

METHOD 1

Weigh accurately a quantity of powder equivalent to 0.25 g of phthalylsulphathiazole. Add 100 ml of 25% w/v sodium hydroxide solution anf reflux for four hours. Cool, filter through cotton, wash with water and acidity with hydrochloric acid. Cool below 10°C and titrate against 0.1 M sodium nitrite with constant shaking using starch iodide paste as an external indicator. Each ml of 0.1 M sodium nitrite is equivalent to 0.04034 g of phthalylsulphathiazole (nitritometric titration).

Note

Phthalylsulphathiazole must be hydrolysed before titration. Excess of HNO_2 shall oxidize KI to I_2 which will form blue coloured inclusion complex with starch.

METHOD 2

Transfer a quantity of powder equivalent to about 400 mg of phthalylsulphathiazole in a dry beaker. Add 30-40 ml ethyl acetate, boil on water-bath, stir and decant the solution through filter paper. Repeat the extraction 4-5 times with boiled ethyl acetate and filter while hot. Iodochlorhydroxyquinoline, soluble in hot ethyl acetate, gets removed by above extraction procedure. Collect the residue, dry and reflux for 30 min with water and 20 ml of hydrochloric acid. Cool to 10°C and proceed with estimation as under method 1 above.

Probable Reaction Mechanism

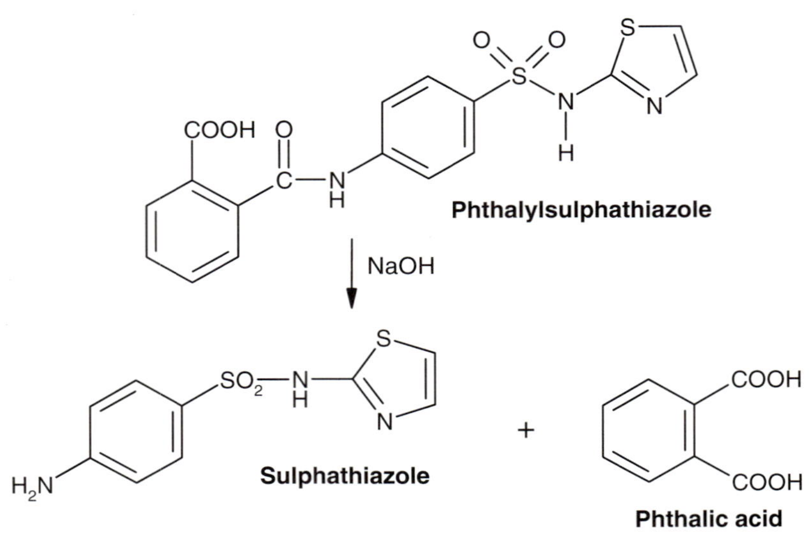

Sulphathiazole so liberated having free 'NH$_2$' group can be titrated with $NaNO_2$ leading to diazotization.

Alternatively, amino group forms condensation product with xanthydrol.

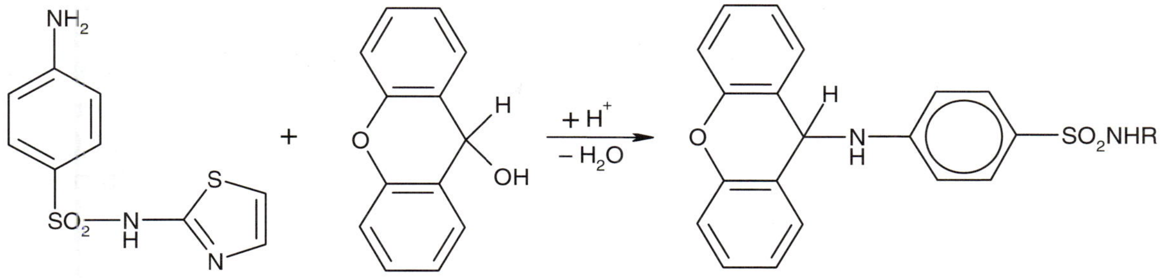

Sulphathiazole Xanthydrol

Note

If the other 'NH$_2$' is not substituted one more mol of xanthydrol shall react.

Heating the compound with sulphuric acid and then adding resorcinol followed by making the solution alkaline produces intense green fluorescence. This can be used for analytical methodology.

Probable Reaction Mechanism

Phthalic acid produced after acid treatment gets further dehydrated to produce anhydride.

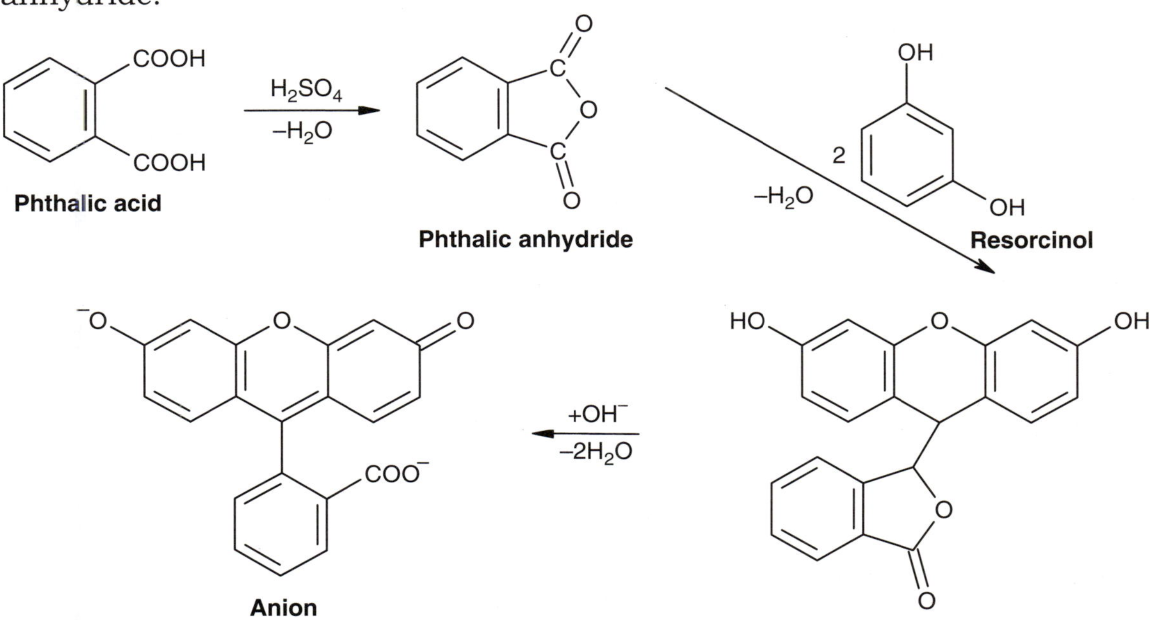

Anion
(Intense green fluorescent compound)

Formulation 9

Diiodohydroxyquinoline, Sulphaguanidine, Phthalylsulphathiazole

ESTIMATION

Diiodohydroxyquinoline

METHOD 1

Reagents

1. Dilute hydrochloric acid.
2. Dimethylformamide (DMF).

Standard solution

Weigh accurately 100 mg of pure compound, add 10 ml of 'DMF' and shake vigorously for 5 minutes. Further make appropriate dilution with dilute hydrochloric acid to obtain a solution of 50 mcg/ml.

Sample solution

Weigh accurately a quantity of powdered tablets equivalent to 100 mg of the compound, add 10 ml of 'DMF' and treat as per standard solution.

Concomitantly determine the extinctions of both the standard and sample solutions at absorption maximum at about 390 nm and calculate the results.

METHOD 2

Follow the method 2 described for determination of diiodohydroxyquinoline under formulation 1 of this chapter.

METHOD 3

Reagents

1. 0.4% w/v solution of 2,6-dichloroquinone chlorimide in isopropyl alcohol.
2. Buffer solution: 33.3% w/v aqueous solution of dipotassium hydrogen phosphate.

Standard solution

100 mcg/ml of pure compound in 1,4-dioxan.

Sample solution

Weigh accurately powdered tablet or measure aliquot equivalent to 20 mg of the compound and extract with 1,4-dioxan to get 100 mcg/ml solution.

Procedure

To 1 ml of the sample and standard solutions, add 2 ml buffer, 2 ml water and 5 ml chlorimide reagent, dilute to 10 ml with water. After 5 minutes, measure the absorbance of both the solutions at 650 nm against water as blank. The method obeys Beer's law in the range of 1-16 mcg/ml.

Metronidazale, metronidazole benzoate and tetracyclin hydrochloride do not interfere.

For detailed reaction mechanism, refer to formulation 2 of this chapter.

Sulphaguanidine

Follow the method described for determination of sulphaguanidine under formulation of this chapter.

The compound undergoes diazotization and coupling with NED. On heating of aqueous solution ammonia is liberated. It answers "Sakaguchi reaction" i.e. on treating with α-naphthol in the presence of hypobromite solution it forms a complex i.e. presence of guanidine structure.

Probable Reaction Mechanism

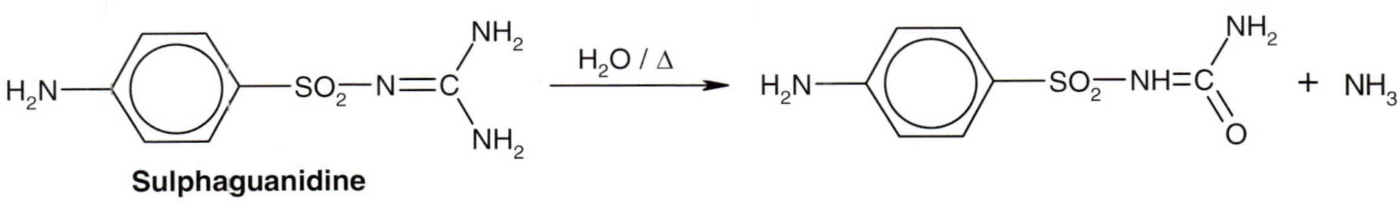

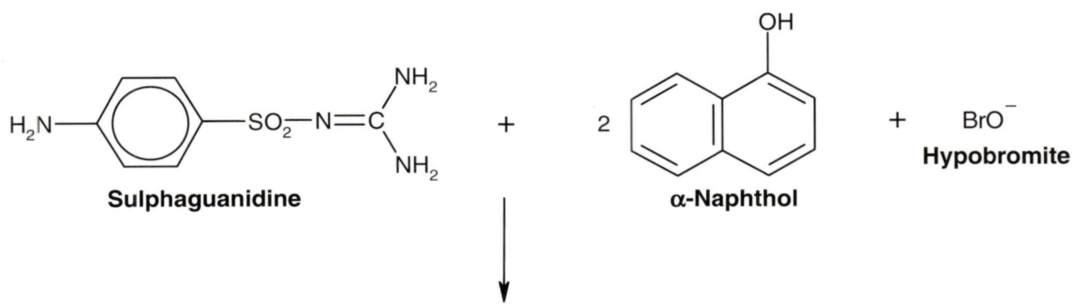

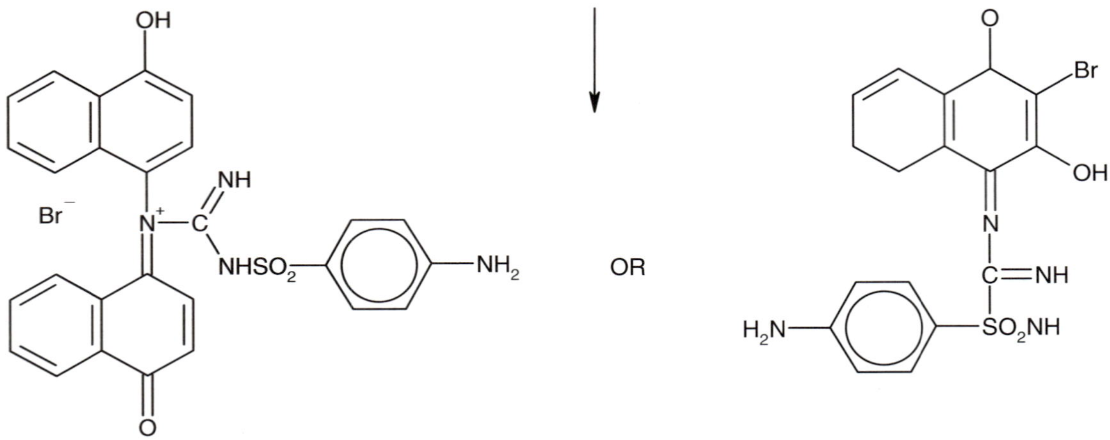

Reference

Pharmaceutical Chemistry (Vol. 2) by H.J. Roth, p. 437.

Phthalylsulphathiazole

Follow any one of the methods described for determination of phthalylsulphathiazole under formulation 8 of this chapter.

Note

To separate sulphaguanidine and phthalylsulphathiazole, follow the procedure described in formulation 5 of this chapter and then carry out the estimation.

Formulation 10

Streptomycin sulphate, Chloramphenicol, Diloxanide furoate

ESTIMATION

Diloxanide furoate

METHOD 1

Standard solution

10 mcg/ml of diloxanide furoate in chloroform.

Sample solution

Transfer an accurately weighed quantity of the mixed contents of capsules equivalent to 0.2 g of diloxanide furoate to a separating funnel containing 25 ml of water. Shake well and acidify with 1 N sulphuric acid. Shake well and extract with three quantities each of 40 ml of chloroform. Wash each chloroform extract in succession with same 15 ml of 0.1 N sulphuric acid and 15 ml of water, contained in two different separators. Collect the washed chloroform extracts into a dry, 200 ml volumetric flask after passing through anhydrous sodium sulphate held over a plug of cotton wool. Dilute the combined extracts to volume with chloroform and mix. Dilute further appropriately with chloroform to get a concentration of 10 mcg/ml.

Procedure

Concomitantly determine the extinctions of the standard and sample solutions at the absorption maximum at about 260 nm using chloroform as blank. Calculate average net content per capsule using a value of 690 for A 1%, 1 cm at 260 nm.

METHOD 2

Diloxanide furoate on acid hydrolysis gives blue colour with sodium nitroprusside in alkaline medium.

Reagents

1. 4 N hydrochloric acid.

2. Ethyl alcohol.
3. 0.2% w/v solution of sodium nitroprusside in water.
4. 1 N sodium hydroxide.

Standard solution

100 mg of pure diloxanide furoate is dissolved in ethyl alcohol to get 1 mg/ml solution. To 10 ml of this solution, add 10 ml of 4 N hydrochloric acid, boil on water-bath for 60 minutes, cool and dilute to 100 ml with water. 10 ml of the resultant solution is further diluted with water to 100 ml.

Sample solution

Accurately weigh sample equivalent to 100 mg of diloxanide furoate, add 50 ml of ethyl alcohol, warm at 50°C for few minutes to ensure extraction. Filter and wash the residue with three 15 ml portions of ethyl alcohol previously warmed to 50°C. Adjust combined filtrate to 100 ml with ethyl alcohol. Subject 10 ml of solution to acid hydrolysis as described under standard solution.

Procedure

To 5 ml each of the hydrolysed sample and standard solutions, add 0.3 ml of sodium nitroprusside solution and dilute to 10 ml with 1 N sodium hydroxide. Shake and keep at room temperature for 30 minutes and measure the absorbance of both the solutions at 690 nm and calculate the results. The method obeys Beer's law in the range of 10-50 mcg/ml.

Note

Streptomycin, chloroquine, chloramphenicol and common excipients do not interfere.

Explanatory Note

On acid hydrolysis the compound is converted to furoic acid and 4-aminophenol. 4-Aminophenol is oxidized by sodium nitroprusside and on basification we get a coloured complex (λ_{max} 690 nm).

Probable Reaction Mechanism

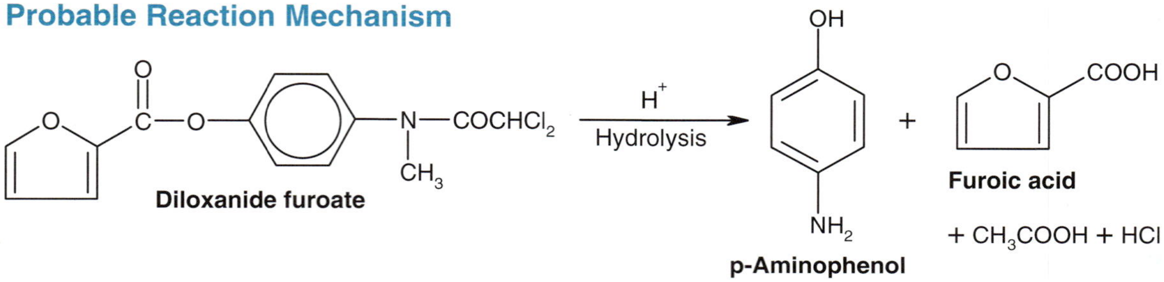

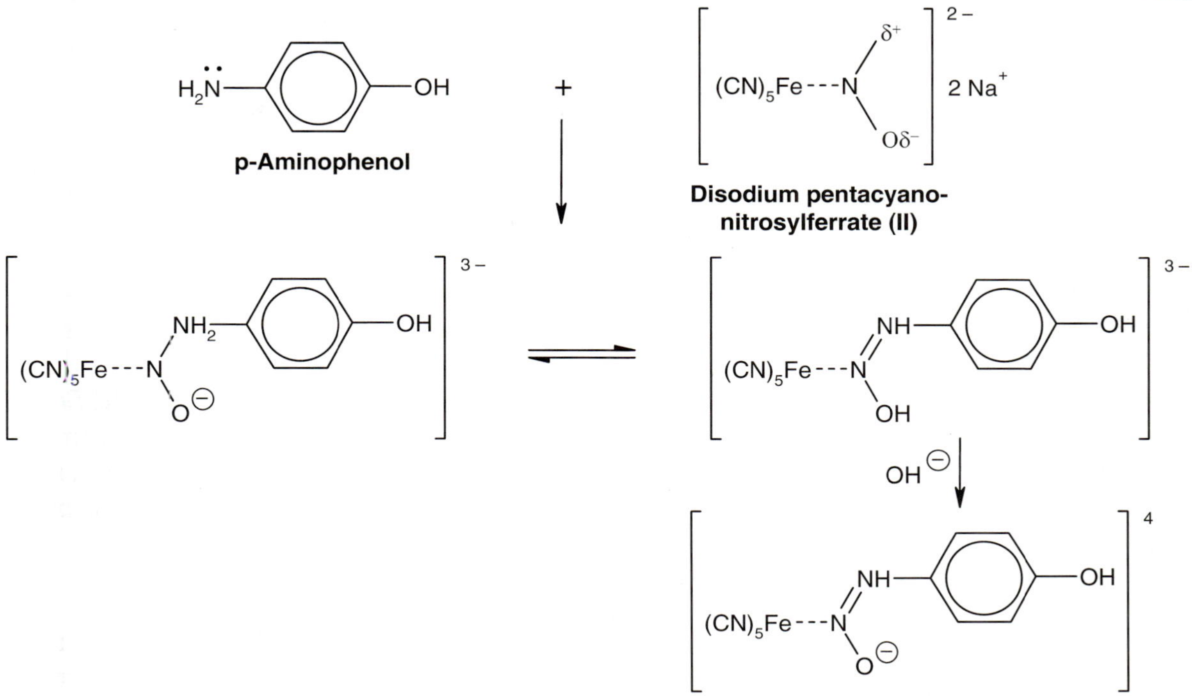

Note

Hydrolysed product also gives blue colour with Folin's reagent as well.

Reference

R.T. Sane, S.V. Desai & R.S. Samant, Indian Drugs, **23**, 369-370, 1986.

METHOD 3

Furohydroxamic acid formed combines with ferric (Fe^{+++}) ion to form purple coloured chromophore. Free furoic acid does not interfere, only intact moiety reacts with this reagent.

Reagents

1. Ethyl alcohol (aldehyde free).
2. 10% w/v solution of hydroxylamine sulphate in water.
3. 4 N sodium hydroxide.
4. 4 N hydrochloric acid.
5. 10% w/v ferric chloride solution in 0.1 N hydrochloric acid.

Standard solution

Transfer accurately weighed about 50 mg of pure diloxanide furoate to a volumetric flask, add 40 ml of 60% v/v alcohol (aldehyde free). Heat on water-bath for 10 minutes, cool and adjust the volume to 50 ml with 60% alcohol.

Sample solution

Transfer sample of powdered tablets, capsule or suspension accurately weighed/ measured equivalent to about 50 mg of diloxanide furoate to a volumetric flask, add 40 ml of 60% alcohol and treat the sample as per standard.

Procedure

Transfer 2 ml each of standard and sample solutions to a volumetric flask of 25 ml. To each flask, add 1 ml of hydroxylamine reagent and 1 ml of 4 N sodium hydroxide. Mix and leave aside for 1 hour at room temperature. Add 1 ml of hydrochloric acid, followed by 1 ml of iron solution. Shake vigorously and adjust the volume with water. Concomitantly determine within 5 minutes, the absorption of the resulting solutions at about 530 nm against reagent blank and calculate the results. The method obeys Beer's law in the concentration range of 1-4 mg/ml.

Note

Neomycin, chloroquine phosphate and other usual excipients used in tablets and suspension do not interfere.

Explanatory Note

After acid hydrolysis the furoic acid so produced reacts with hydroxylamine in alkaline medium to give furohydroxamic acid. On acidification it forms complex with Fe(3).

Probable Reaction Mechanism

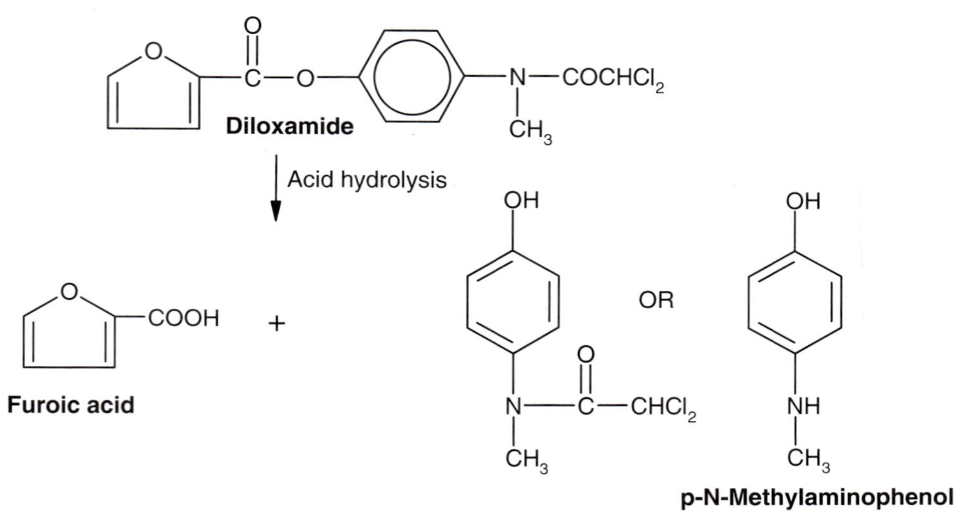

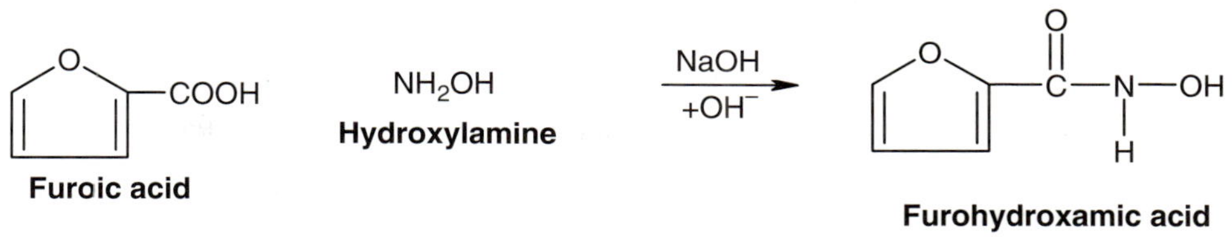

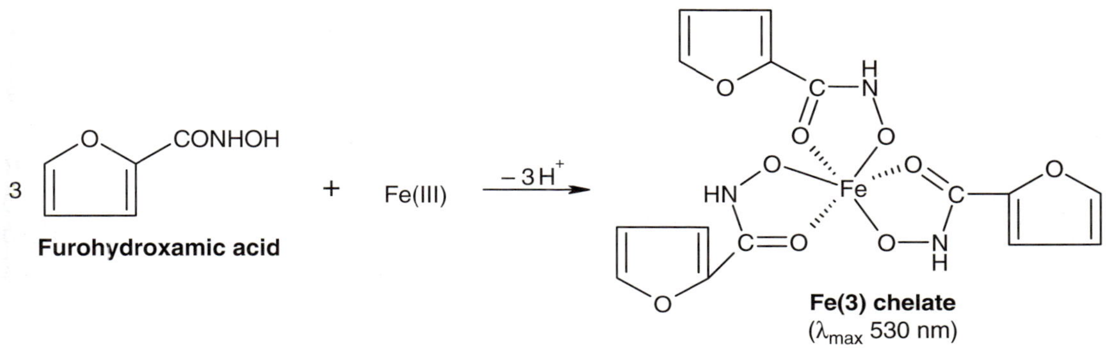

Reference

1. P.P. Shah & R.C. Mehta, *Ind. J. Pharm. Sci.*, **43(4)**, 147-149, 1981.
2. Pharmaceutical Chemistry (Vol. 2) by H.J. Roth, p. 156.

METHOD 4

Reagents

1. 2 N sodium hydroxide.
2. 6% w/v phenol in water.
3. 5 N hydrochloric acid.

Standard solution

1 mg/ml of diloxanide furoate in alcohol.

Sample solution

Accurately weighed or measured aliquot of the sample equivalent to 50 mg of the compound is extracted with alcohol at 45°C, filtered and the residue washed and filtrate adjusted to 50 ml with alcohol (1 mg/ml).

Treatment of sample and standard solutions

10 ml each of the sample and standard solutions, prepared above, is heated with 20 ml of 5 N hydrochloric acid on water-bath for 1 h. The excess acid is expelled under suction and the resultant solutions are diluted to 200 ml with water (50 mcg/ml).

Procedure

To 5 ml each of the above treated sample and standard solutions, add 1 ml of sodium hydroxide solution, 2 ml of phenol solution and dilute to 25 ml with water. After 10 minute, measure the absorbance of both the solutions at 630 nm against reagent blank.

Note

Streptomycin, chloroquine, chloramphenicol and neomycin do not interfere in this method.

Probable Reaction Mechanism

Diloxanide furoate on heating with HCl yields p-N-methylaminophenol and furoic acid. The p-N-methylaminophenol so formed undergoes oxidative coupling with phenol in the presence of NaOH resulting in the formation of coloured indophenol.

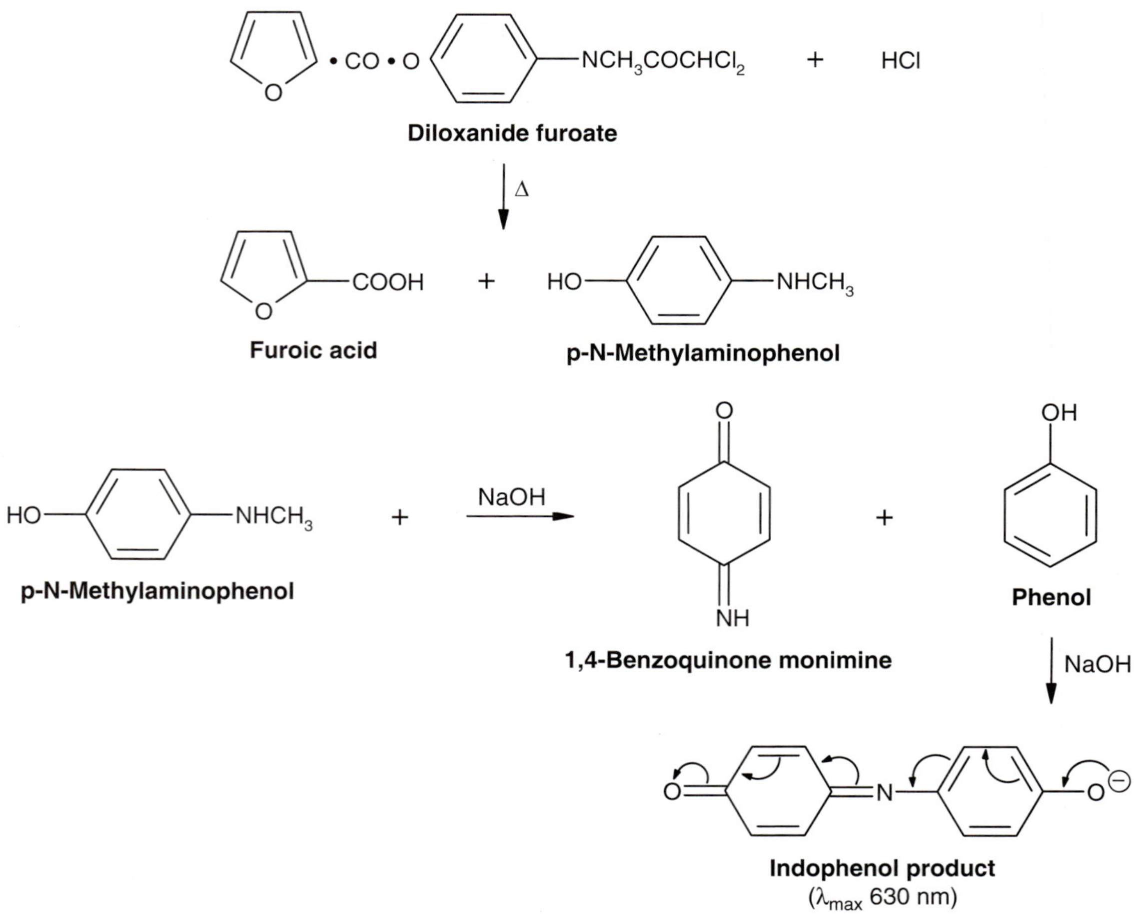

Note

The above-mentioned product can exhibit resonance structure due to the lone pair of electron available on oxygen atom.

Reference

1. C.T.H. Ellcock & A.G. Fogg, Analyst, **16**, 100, 1975.
2. C.S.P. Sastry, B.G. Rao & B.S. Reddy, Indian Drugs, **20(7)**, 294, 1983.

METHOD 5

Reagents

1. 0.1% w/v solution of isoniazid (INH).
2. 0.1 M phosphate buffer, pH 3.0.
3. 1% iodine solution.

Procedure

To acid hydrolysed product add 1.5 ml of I_2 solution and 1 ml of INH solution, dilute and measure the colour.

Diloxanide furoate is made to undergo acid hydrolysis where p-N-methylaminophenol is obtained as product. Excess of I_2 was allowed to react with p-N-methylaminophenol causing the oxidation of latter and resulting in the formation of p-N-methylbenzoquinone monoimine in the reaction medium. p-N-Methylbenzoquinone monoimine then interacts with isoniazid, the reagent used. The reaction is represented as under.

Probable Reaction Mechanism

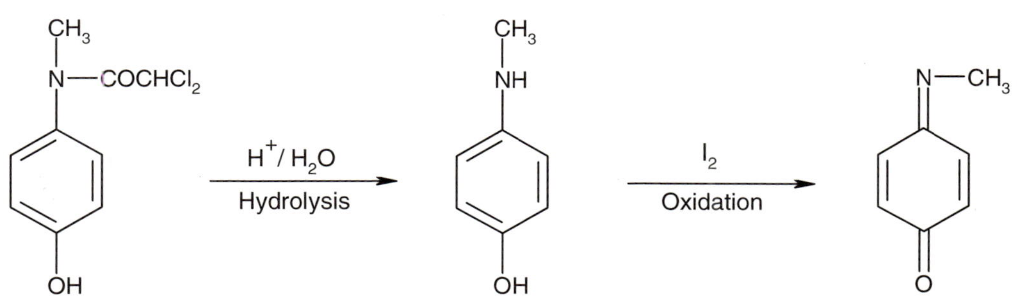

p-N-Methylaminophenol p-N-Methylbenzoquinone monimine

p-N-Methylbenzoquinone monoimine forms a coloured 2 : 1 charge transfer complex with isoniazid.

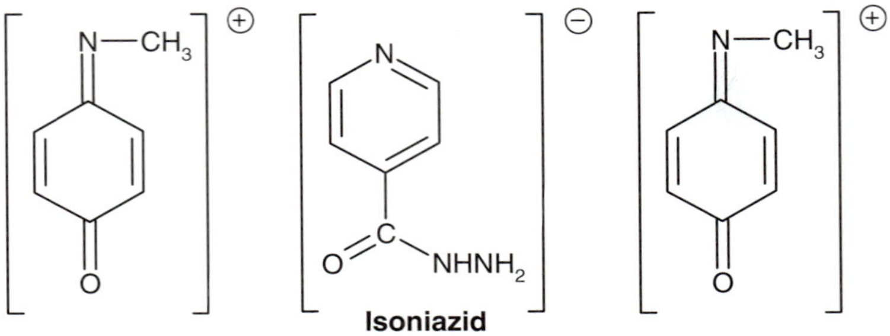

Isoniazid

Charge transfer complex
(λ_{max} 630 nm)

Reference

C.S.P. Sastry, M. Arun & A.R.S. Prasad, *Indian Drugs*, **26(10)**, 581-582, 1989.

Sastry et al. (1988) have described oxidative coupling of hydrolysed product p-aminophenol with 'MBTH' leading to coupling at o-position giving a coloured product (λ_{max} 500 nm).

Reference

C.S.P. Sastry & M. Arun, Pharmazic, **43**, 361, 1988.

Streptomycin sulphate

METHOD 1

Reagents

1. 10% w/v solution of sodium nitroprusside in water.
2. 10% w/v solution of potassium ferricyanide in water.
3. 10% solution of sodium hydroxide in water.
   (All these solutions are stable at least for 2 months if stored in amber coloured bottle).
4. Oxidised nitroprusside solution: Equal volumes of solution of sodium nitroprusside, solution of potassium ferricyanide and solution of sodium hydroxide, are combined in the order given. After the solution becomes yellowish green (it takes 15-30 minutes), 1 ml aliquot of the mixture is diluted to 100 ml with water. The mixture and the final solution is prepared fresh daily.

Standard solution

Weigh accurately 150 mg of streptomycin sulphate which has been previously assayed for streptomycin (base content) and dissolve in water to produce 100 ml. 10 ml aliquot of this solution is further diluted to 100 ml with water. Each

10 ml of this final solution contains 0.015 × 'A' mg of streptomycin sulphate used as standard. This solution should be made fresh. 'A' is the percentage of base in streptomycin sulphate.

Sample solution

Transfer accurately weighed quantity of the sample equivalent to about 100 mg of streptomycin (base) into a separating funnel containing about 80 ml of solvent ether. Shake well and extract with four successive quantities each of 20 ml of water. Wash each aqueous extract separately with same 50 ml quantity of solvent ether contained in another separating funnel. Collect the aqueous extracts, filter through a plug of cotton, make up the volume to 100 ml with water and mix.

Procedure

To 10 ml each of sample and standard solutions in 25 ml volumetric flasks, add 10 ml of oxidised nitroprusside solution, after 3 minutes dilute to volume with water. Measure the extinctions of standard and sample at about 490 nm using blank similarly prepared but replacing sample solution/standard solution by water. Calculate the results by comparison. Or to 5 ml of aqueous sample/standard solution add 1 ml of sodium nitroprusside solution and 0.1 ml of 3% H_2O_2 solution, heat at 55 ± 5°C for 4 min, scarlet red colour appears, cool and after 20 min.

Probable Reaction Mechanism

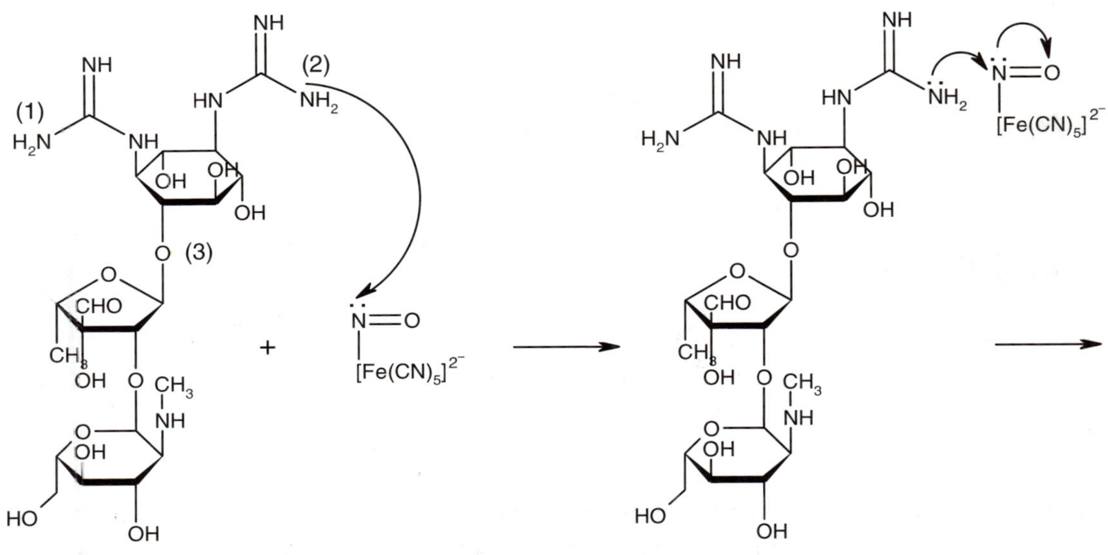

Streptomycin

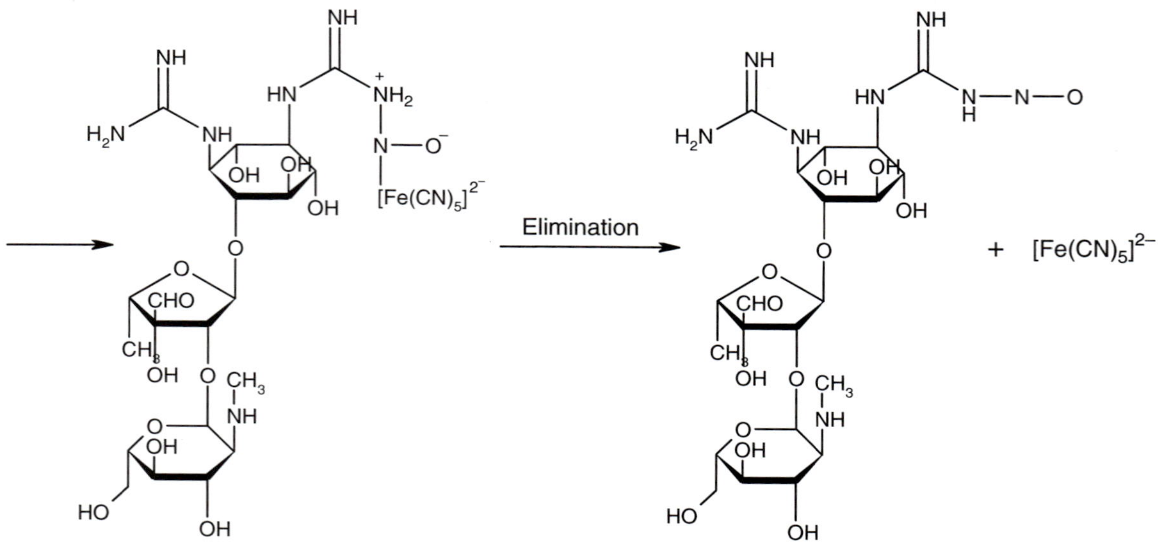

Product
(λ_{max} 490 nm)

METHOD 2

Reagents

1. 0.25% ferric chloride solution: Dissolve 5 g of ferric chloride in 50 ml of 0.1 N hydrochloric acid. Dilute 2.5 ml of the solution to 100 ml with 0.01 N hydrochloric acid.
2. 1 N sodium hydroxide.
3. 1 N hydrochloric acid.

Standard solution

1 mg/ml of streptomycin (base) as streptomycin sulphate in water.

Sample solution

Weigh accurately, a quantity of the sample equivalent to about 100 mg of streptomycin (base) and prepare the sample solution (1 mg/ml base) as described under method 1 above.

Procedure

To 10 ml each of sample and standard solutions, add 2 ml of sodium hydroxide solution. Heat in boiling water-bath for 10 minutes and cool in ice water for 3 minutes. Acidify with 2.5 ml of 1 N hydrochloric acid. Add 5 ml of iron reagent and dilute to 25 ml with water. Measure the absorbance of sample and standard solutions at about 530 nm against reagent blank and calculate the results by comparison.

Explanatory Note

Streptose part of the molecule is detected by maltol reaction in which it is hydrolysed with sodium hydroxide solution and then heated with hydrochloric acid and iron(III). This involves rearrangement of the furanoid streptose to a pyranose form which gets converted to maltol by stripping off the streptidine residue and N-methylglucosamine. Maltol is a bidenate chelate former and complexes with iron(III) to give a complex (λ_{max} 525 nm). Streptose is unstable in acid medium and decomposes to form maltol.

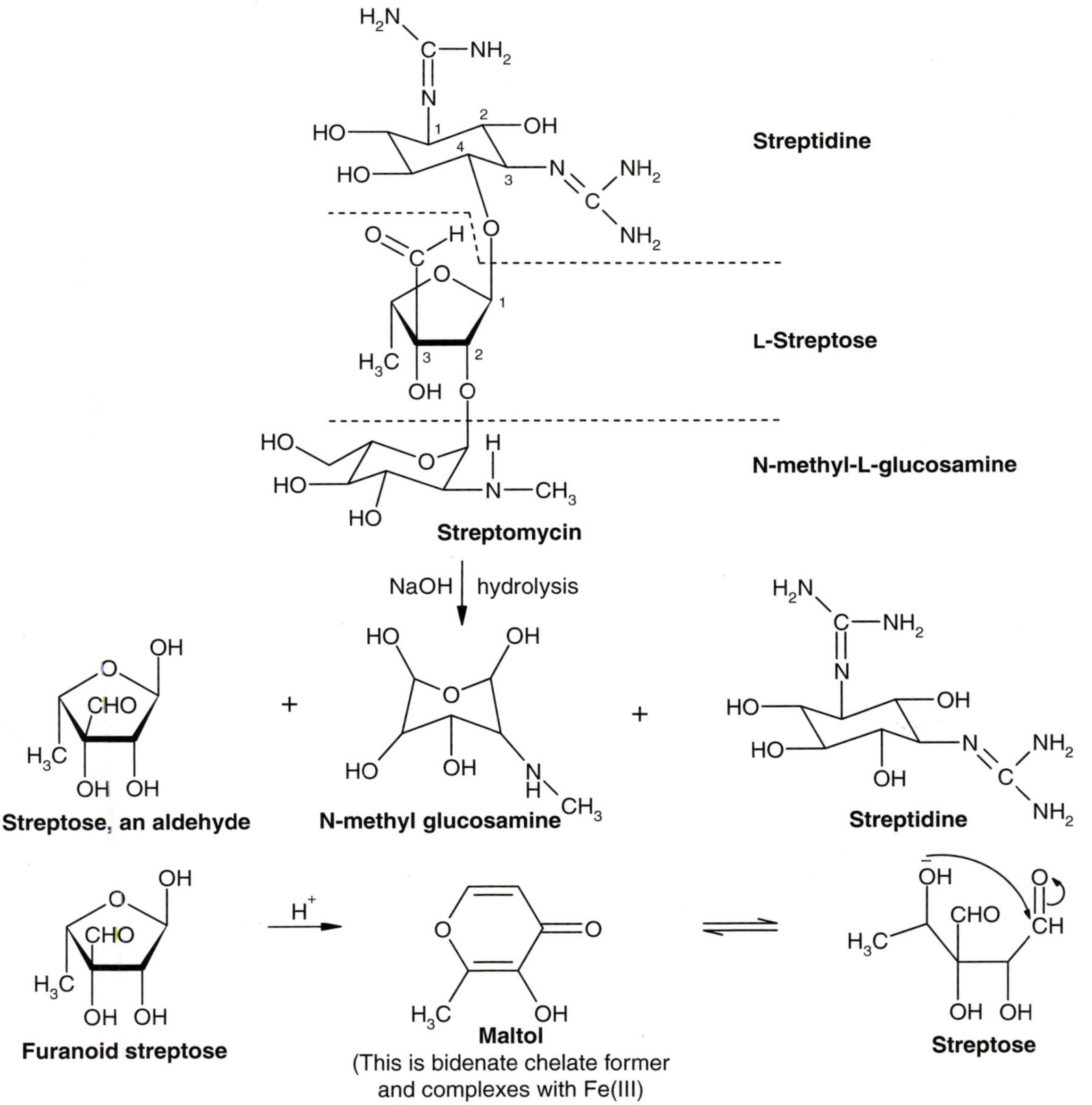

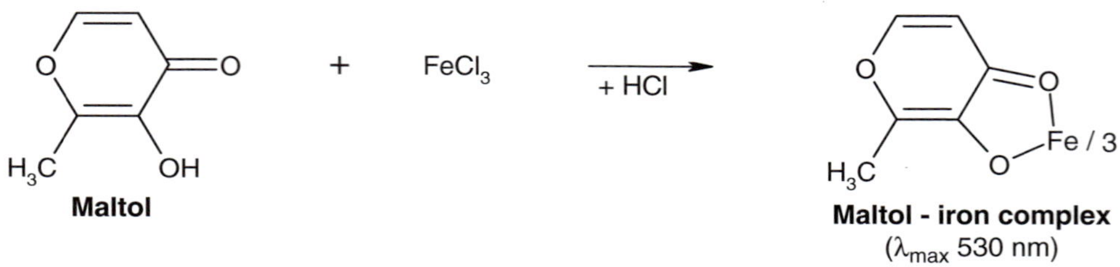

Because of two guanidine groups and one methyl amino group streptomycin is a trivalent base.

Reference

Pharmaceutical Chemistry (Vol. 2) by H.J. Roth, pp. 357-359.

Note

1. Maltol generated as a result of alkaline hydrolysis has λ_{max} 322 nm (Edward Titus & Josef Priod, J. Biol. Chem., **174**, 57, 1948).
2. Guanidine structures present in the molecule shall answer Sakaguchi reaction i.e. reaction with 1-naphthol and hypobromite (BrO^-) yielding red colour. (For reaction mechanism, refer to formulation 9 of this chapter under sulphaguidine.)
3. Because of the aldehyde group present in the molecule it can react with 2,4-dinitrophenylhydrazine or isoniazid giving corresponding hydrazone.

Note

A similar fluorometric method is described involving aldehyde function of the molecule with 9-hydrazinoacridine hydrochloride yielding a fluorescent hydrazone.

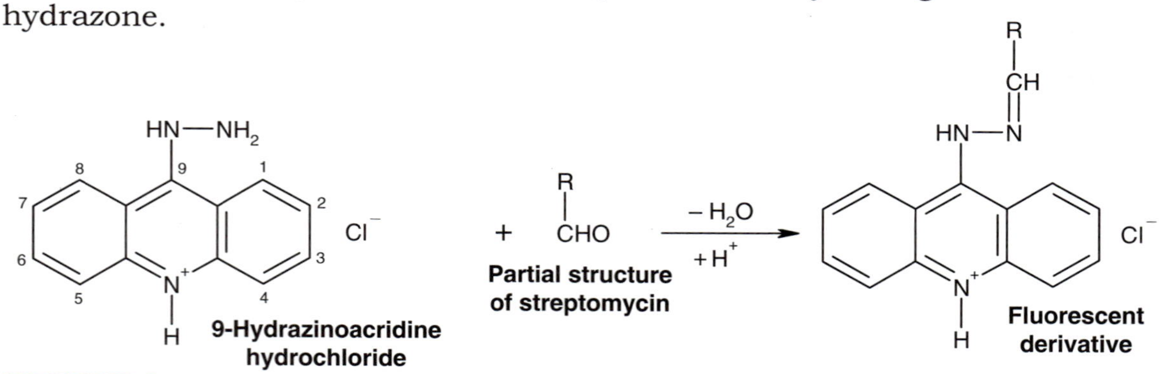

METHOD 3

This method is based on spectrophotofluorometric measurement.

Reagents

1. 1 M NaOH.
2. 10 M HCl.
3. 1% w/v solution of 9,10-phenanthroquinone in DMF.

Standard solution

10 µg/ml in distilled water.

Sample solution

The sample suspended in water, filtered and used for assay. In case of suspension first extract with chloroform discarding the organic layer and using aqueous layer for estimation.

Procedure

To 2 ml each of sample/standard solutions, add 2 ml of phenanthroquinone reagent and 0.25 ml of NaOH solution. Leave for 30 min at room temperature and then add 0.1 ml of 10 M HCl, adjust to volume and then measure the fluorescence (Exc: 310; Em: 395 nm).

Probable Reaction Mechanism

Phenanthroquinone forms highly fluorescent product with guanidine moiety of the molecule.

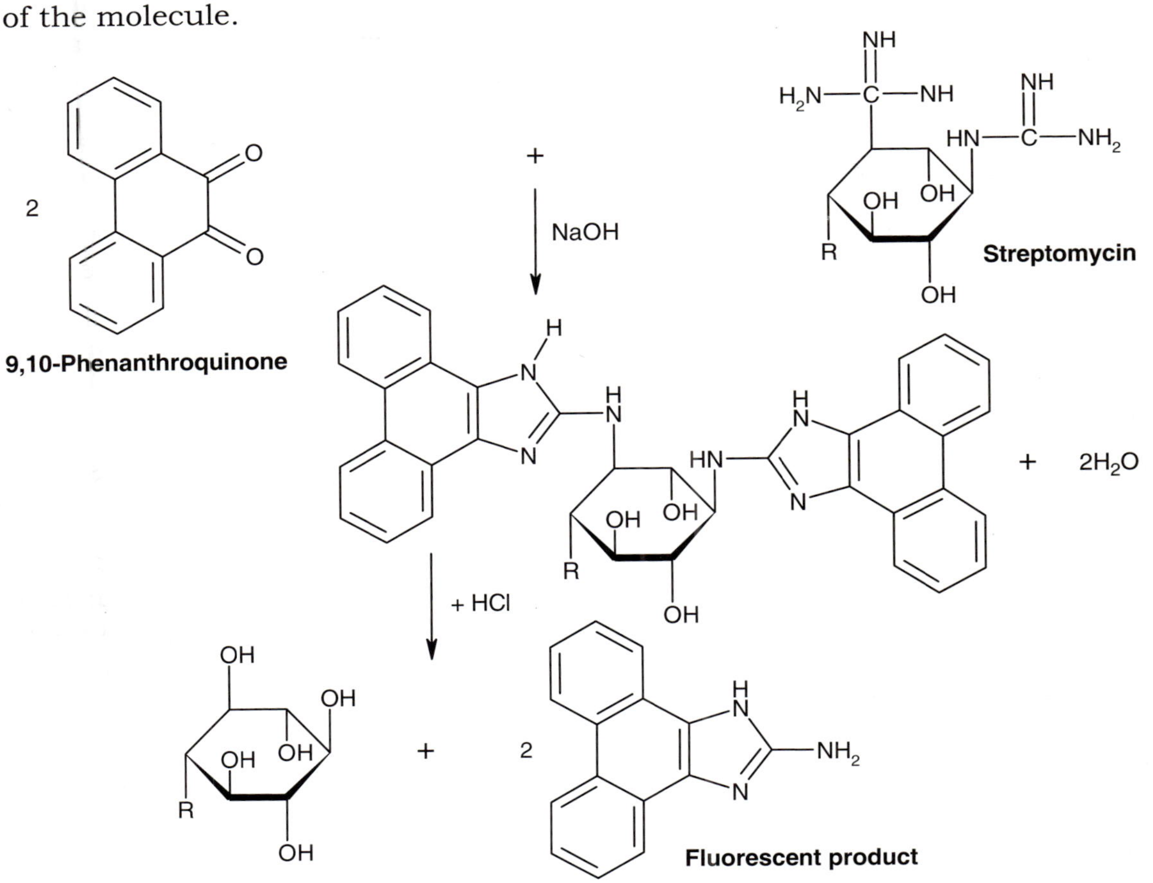

Reference

F. Belal, S.M. El-Ashry, M.M. El Kerdawy & D.R. El Wasseef, J. Pharm. Biomed. Analysis, **26**, 435-44, 2001.

Chloramphenicol

METHOD 1

Reagents

1. 5% w/v solution of sodium nitrite in water.
2. 5% w/v solution of sulphamic acid in water.
3. 0.5% w/v solution of N-1-naphthyl-ethylenediamine dihydrochloride in water.
4. Metallic aluminium wire.

Standard solution

Accurately weigh 250 mg of pure chloramphenicol and transfer quantitatively into a 100 ml volumetric flask with the aid of alcohol. Dissolve and make up the volume with alcohol.

Sample solution

Transfer an accurately weighed quantity of the mixed contents of 20 capsules equivalent to 25 mg of chloramphenicol to a 100 ml round bottom flask, add 10 ml of alcohol. To another round bottom flask, transfer 10 ml of standard solution. To each flask, add 30 ml of 1 N hydrochloric acid and 1.5 g of small pieces of metallic aluminium wire. Reflux on a water-bath the contents of each flask for one hour. Cool and with the help of water, transfer quantitatively the contents of each flask into separate 100 ml volumetric flasks, make up the volume with water and filter.

Procedure

To 1 ml each of reduced standard and sample solutions and water (to serve as blank) add 1 ml of solution of sodium nitrite and 5 to 10 drops of hydrochloric acid. Shake and leave for 2 minutes. Add 5 ml of solution of sulphamic acid, shake well and remove any nitrous acid fumes present in the flask under mild suction. Add 1 ml of n-naphthyl ethylenediamine solution. Dilute the solutions to 50 ml with water and read the extinction of both the solutions at about 558 nm using blank in the reference cuvette. Calculate the results by comparison.

Probable Reaction Mechanism

The reduced products answer Bratton-Marshall reaction.

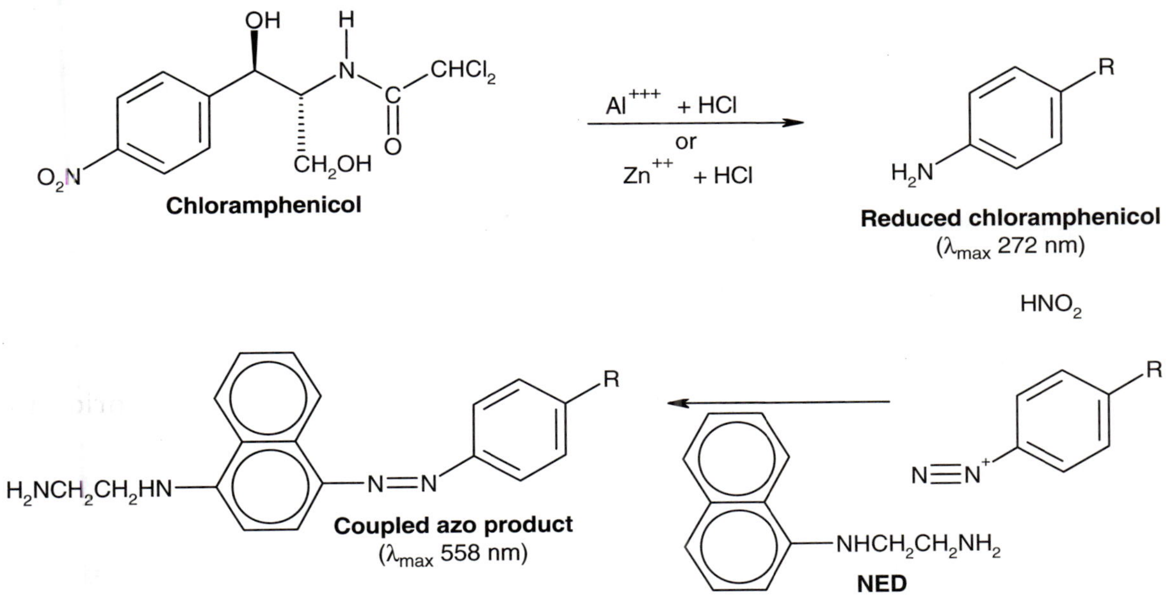

$$NaNO_2 + HCl \longrightarrow HNO_2 + NaCl$$

For removing excess of HNO_2 sulphamic acid is added.

$$HNO_2 + H_2NSO_3H \longrightarrow H_2SO_4 + N_2\uparrow + H_2O$$

Reference

1. A.C. Bratton & E.K. Marshall, *J. Biol. Chem.*, **128**, 537, 1939.
2. Textbook of Chemistry by A. Kenneth, p. 225.

After hydrolysis in alkaline medium the compound undergoes Malapride cleavage to produce 4-nitrobenzaldehyde, formic acid, formaldehyde and ammonia.

Probable Reaction Mechanism

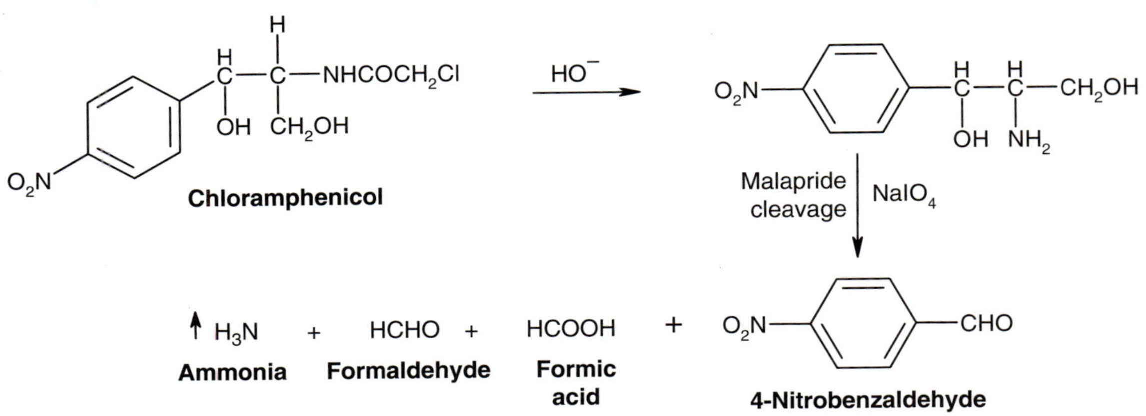

Reference

Pharmaceutical Chemistry (Vol. 2) by H.J. Roth, p. 324.

METHOD 2

Reagents

1. 0.05% solution of sodium nitrite in water.
2. Sulphamic acid solution
3. 5% w/v solution of ethylacetoacetate in methanol.
4. 50% w/v solution of sodium hydroxide in water.

After the product is diazotized and excess HNO_2 removed with the addition of sulphamic acid or ammonium sulphamate as under method 1 allow the reaction mixture to stand for 5 min, then add 1.5 ml of ethylacetoacetate solution followed by 3 ml of sodium hydroxide solution, dilute to volume and measure the absorbance at 345 nm against reagent blank.

Probable Reaction Mechanism

Diazotized product can react with ethylacetoacetate reagent in the presence of base. In the presence of base, ethylacetoacetate forms carbonium ion which couples with diazotized product to form coloured complex. The base (sodium hydroxide) is required for full colour development.

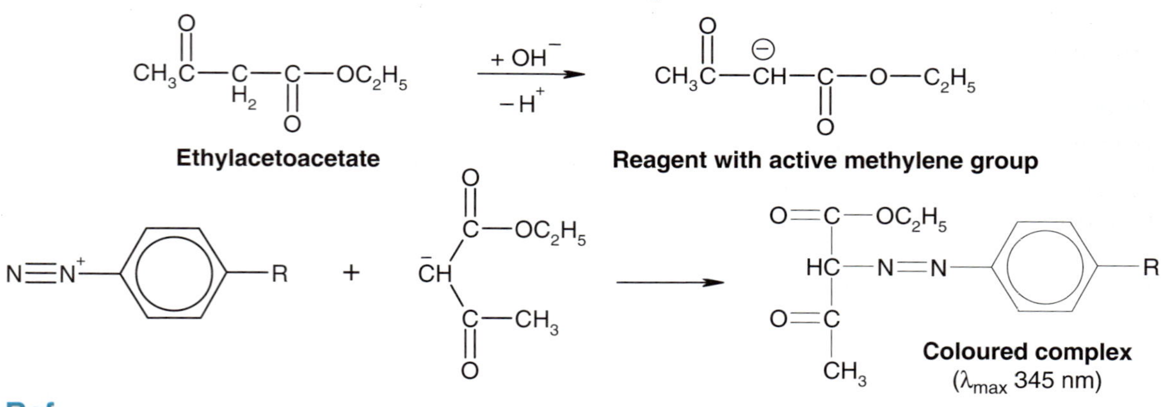

Reference

S.M. Hassan, F. Belal, M. Sharaf El Din & M. Sullan, Analyst, **113**, 1087-1089, 1988.

Note

1. This reaction is not specific and is answered by hydrolysis product.
2. λ_{max} at 278 nm is due to nitrophenylchromophore, hence not specific.
3. Other substances such as nitrazepam having nitro group also answer similar reaction.

Nitro group can oxidize Fe(II) to Fe(III) giving red-brown colour/precipitate.

$$R \bullet NO_2 + 6Fe(OH)_2 + 4H_2O \longrightarrow R \bullet NH_2 + Fe(OH)_3$$

Earlier pharmaceutical method of assay was based on the work of Crooks & Rebstock. Reduction with 'Zn' in the presence of $CaCl_2$ yields hydroxylamine derivative which gives violet colour with $FeCl_3$ in the presence of benzoylchloride.

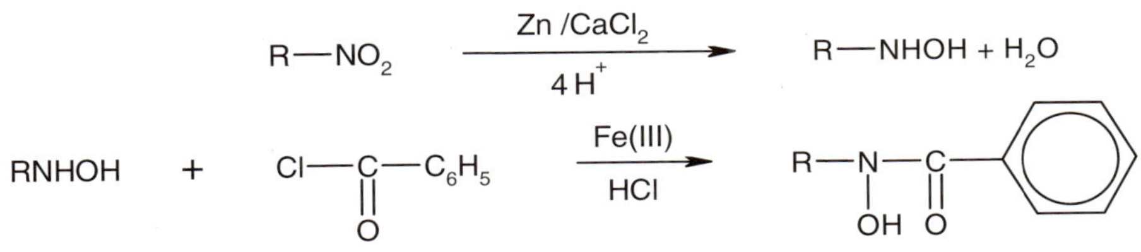

Violet-coloured product

Jayaram et al. (1983) have described a titrimetric method for the estimation of the compound in capsules, eye drops, eye ointments, etc. The method is based on reaction between chloramphenicol and chloramine-T, chloramine-B and bromamine-B or bromamine-T —(N—haloamines) in alkaline medium. Since diresct titration was not feasible as oxidation was not instantaneous so a back titration procedure was followed i.e. excessive volume of oxidant was added to known quantity of the sample and excess oxidant estimated by adding sulphuric acid, potassium iodide and titrating the liberated iodine with thiosulphate.

Note

Benzocaine, phenylmercuric nitrate, phenol interfere and have to be removed by extracting with ethylacetate or diethylether and cyclohexane in case of eye ointment.

Probable Reaction Mechanism

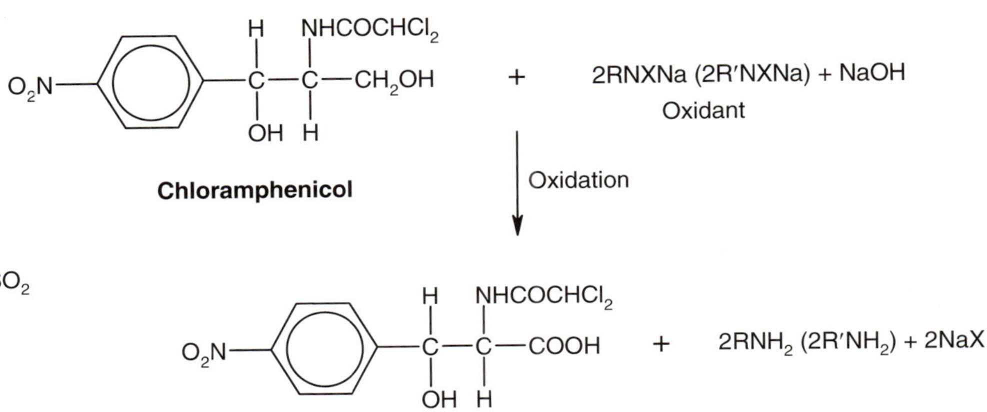

$R = CH_3C_6H_4SO_2$
$R' = C_6H_5SO_2$
X = Cl or Br

Note

The oxidant (N—haloamines) undergo four-electron reduction to sulphonamides.

Reference

B. Jayaram & S.M. Mayanna, *Talanta*, **30(10)**, 798-800, 1983.

Formulation 11

Chloroquine phosphate, Iodochlorohydroxy-quinoline, Diiodohydroxyquinoline

ESTIMATION

Chloroquine phosphate

Follow method 1 for the determination of chloroquine phosphate as described under formulation 1 of this chapter. Alternatively, follow method 2 for the determination of chloroquine phosphate as described under formulation 6 of this chapter.

Diiodohydroxyquinoline and Iodochlorohydroxyquinoline

Accurately weighed powdered material equivalent to 2 tablets is fused with anhydrous sodium carbonate in a nickel crucible to convert into respective halides. The mass is then taken in boiling water and filtered to free it from carbonaceous matter and the volume is adjusted to 250 ml with water (solution A).

Total Iodine

Take 50 ml aliquot from solution A in a 500 ml conical flask, keep in an ice-bath, add 50 ml of hydrochloric acid and 15 ml of chloroform. The solution is titrated against 0.05 M potassium iodate. Say (X) ml of 0.05 M iodate solution is consumed in this titration.

Total Halides

Take 50 ml aliquot from solution A in a beaker, cool in ice-bath. Add 25 ml of 0.1 N silver nitrate solution, acidify with concentrated nitric acid and titrate against 0.1 N ammonium thiocyanate solution using ferric alum solution as indicator. Say (Y) ml of ammonium thiocyanate solution is consumed. From the above titre values, the contents of iodochlorhydroxyquinoline per tablet are calculated as under:

Volume of 0.1 N silver nitrate used for total halides (iodide and chloride) present in 50 ml of the aliquot = (25 – Y) ml.

Volume of 0.1 N silver nitrate used for 250 ml aliquot (2 tablets) = 5(25 – Y) ml.

Volume of 0.1 N silver nitrate used for one tablet = 5/2 (25 – Y) ml.

Volume of 0.05 M iodate used for 250 ml (2 tablets) = 5 (X) ml.

100 mg of chloroquine phosphate contains 6.87 mg of chloride.

1 ml of 0.1 N silver nitrate is equivalent to 3.572 mg of chloride (Cl^-).

Volume of 0.1 N silver nitrate required for chloride (from chloroquine phosphate) present in 50 ml of aliquot = X′ ml.

Volume of 0.1 N silver nitrate for 250 ml (2 tablets) = 5 (X′) ml.

Actual volume of 0.1 N silver nitrate consumed for chloride due to iodochlorhydroxyquinoline in 2 tablets = 5 (25 – Y) – 5 (X) – 5 (X′) ml.

For 1 tablet = $\left\{\frac{5}{2}(25-Y)-5(X)-5X'\right\}$ ml

Working example

Each tablet contains chloroquine phosphate - 120 mg, iodochlorohydroxyquinoline - 300 mg, diiodohydroxyquinoline - 400 mg. The above material was carbonized and dissolved in 250 ml. 20 ml aliquot was titrated but the calculations are for 250 ml.

Volume of 0.05 M silver nitrate consumed (for total halides) = 40.10 ml.

Volume of 0.1 N silver nitrate consumed (for total chloride) = (40.10 – 28.25) = 11.85 ml.

(A) Volume of 0.1 N silver nitrate equivalent to chloride present in 120 mg of chloroquine phosphate = 2.33 ml.

Volume of 0.1 N silver nitrate equivalent to amount of iodochlorohydroxyquinoline = (11.85 – 2.33) = 9.52 ml.

Each ml of 0.1 N silver nitrate is equivalent to 30.55 mg of iodochlorohydroxyquinoline.

Total iodochlorohydroxyquinoline = 30.55 × 9.52 = 290.83 mg.

Claim = 300 mg; 96.94% of the claim.

(B) Volume of 0.05 M iodate equivalent to 290.83 mg (as found above) of iodochlorohydroxyquinoline = 9.52 ml.

Volume of 0.05 M iodate consumed by diiodohydroxyquinoline = (28.25 – 9.52) = 18.73 ml.

Each ml of 0.05 M iodate is equivalent to 19.8 mg of diiodohydroxyquinoline (DIHQ)

Total 'DIHQ' = 19.8 × 18.73 ml = 370.85 mg.

Claim = 400 mg; 92.7% of the claim.

Formulation 12

Diloxanide furoate, Chloroquine phosphate, Streptomycin sulphate

ESTIMATION

Diloxanide furoate

Follow any one of the methods described for estimation of diloxanide furoate under formulation 10 of this chapter.

Streptomycin sulphate

Follow the method 1 for estimation of streptomycin as described under formulation 10 of this chapter.

Chloroquine phosphate

Standard solution

25 mcg/ml of chloroquine phosphate in water.

Sample solution

Weigh accurately a quantity of powdered tablets equivalent to about 100 mg of chloroquine phosphate, add 150 ml of water and shake for 30 minutes. Adjust the volume to 200 ml and filter. Reject the first 25 ml and dilute 5 ml of the filtrate to 100 ml with water.

Concomitantly measure the extinction of standard and sample solutions at the absorption maxima at about 343 nm or use 360 as value of A 1%, 1 cm at 343 nm for calculation of the results.

Formulation 13

Chloroquine phosphate, Cloquinate (neutral salt of one mole of chloroquine and 2 moles of iodohydroxyquinoline), Diiodohydroxyquinoline

ESTIMATION

Chloroquine phosphate

The method is applicable only to phosphate salt of the compound.

Reagents

1. 10 N sulphuric acid.
2. Ammonium molybdate solution: 6.4 g of ammonium molybdate is dissolved in 40 ml of water. 50 ml of 10 N sulphuric acid is added, shaken and diluted to 100 ml with water.
3. Stannous chloride solution: 1 g of stannous chloride is dissolved in 5 ml hydrochloric acid. Dilute 1 ml with water to 100 ml just before use.

Standard solution

200 mg of chloroquine phosphate is dissolved and made to 100 ml with water. 25 ml of this solution is taken in 100 ml volumetric flask. To this, 10 ml 10 N sulphuric acid, 10 ml of ammonium molybdate solution are added. Wait for 5 minutes and adjust to volume. Shake and wait for 10 minutes. The solution is filtered and 10 ml of the filtrate is diluted to 100 ml with water. 10 ml of the resulting solution is taken for colour development.

Sample solution

The powder equivalent to 200 mg of the substance is shaken with 50 ml of water and made to 100 ml with water. This is filtered and to 25 ml of the filtrate add 10 ml of 10 N sulphuric acid, 10 ml of ammonium molybdate solution and wait for 5 minutes. The volume is made to 100 ml with water and wait for 10 minutes. The solution is filtered and 10 ml of the filtrate is diluted to 100 ml with water. 10 ml is taken for colour development.

Colour development

10 ml each of the standard and sample solutions are taken in 100 ml volumetric

flask containing 50 ml of water. 10 ml of 10 N sulphuric acid, 10 ml of ammonium molybdate solution and 10 ml of water are added to both the flasks. After each addition, the flask should be shaken vigorously. Slowly, while shaking, 5 ml of stannous chloride solution is added and shaken. The solution is kept for 45 minutes and made to volume. The solutions are read at 675 nm and results calculated by comparison.

Explanatory Note

Phosphate contents of the molecule are involved in reaction with ammonium molybdate in acidic medium resulting in the formation of phosphomolybdate and its subsequent reduction with stannous chloride to molybdenum blue. The absorption of the blue complex can be measured as such as this complex can be extracted into isobutyl alcohol and absorption of organic layer measured.

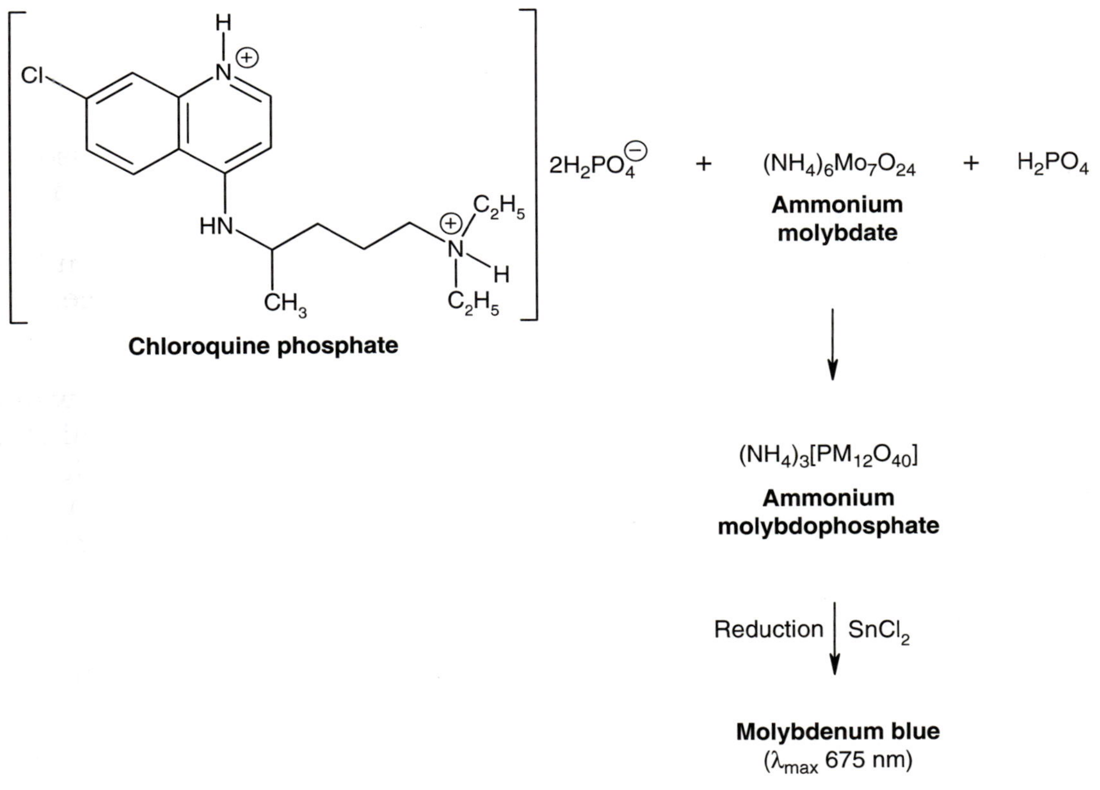

Chloroquine forms complex (2 : 1) with cobalt thiocyanate which can be used for quantitative estimation. The complexation occurs at pH 2.0 and the complex can be extracted into isobutyl alcohol.

Probable Reaction Mechanism

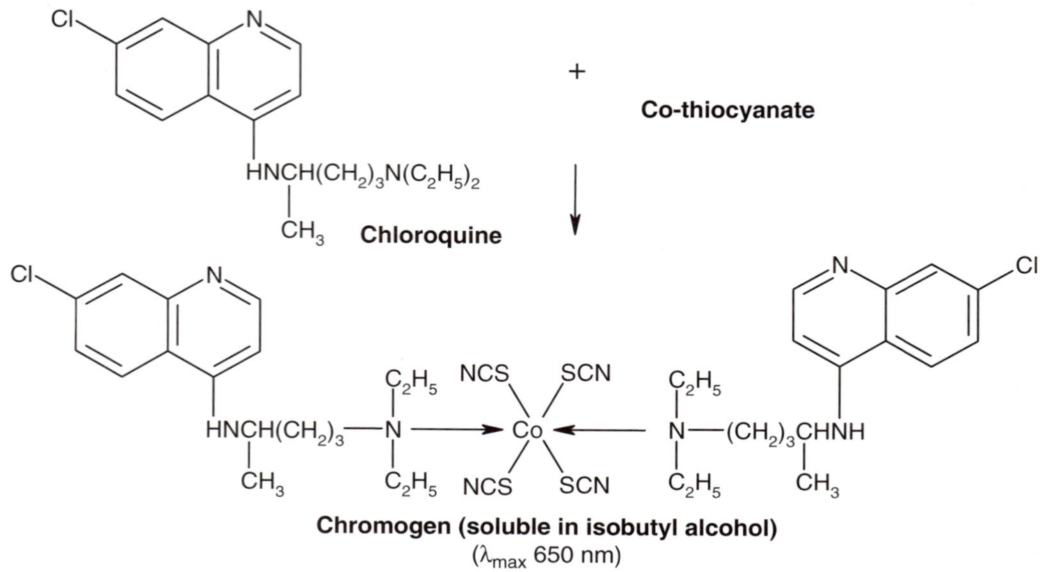

Diiodohydroxyquinoline

About 0.5 g of the powdered tablet, accurately weighed, is shaken with a mixture of 50 ml methyl alcohol and 5 ml 1 N sodium hydroxide until a grey sediment has disappeared. If necessary, use gentle heating. The solution is filtered into 250 ml beaker, the residue is washed with a little methyl alcohol. To the clear solution add 100 ml of water and 10 ml of 1 N hydrochloric acid. The diiodohydroxyquinoline separates as a voluminous precipitate. This is filtered through G_4 porosity sintered glass funnel, washed and dried at 100°C to constant weight which represents diiodohydroxyquinoline.

Note

If powdered sample is shaken with acetic acid (5% v/v), chloroquine phosphate and cloquinate remain in the filtrate, while the insoluble residue is diiodohydroxyquinoline which can be quantitatively estimated by suitable method.

Cloquinate (Iodochlorohydroxyquinoline)/Chinoform

Reagents

1. Hydrochloric acid - potassium chloride buffer solution: 25 ml of 0.2 N hydrochloric acid and 50 ml of 0.2 M potassium chloride are diluted to 100 ml with water, pH 1.5 approximately.

2. Ferric chloride solution: 5.5 g ferric chloride hexahydrate and 2.5 ml of hydrochloric acid are mixed and diluted to 100 ml with water.
3. 1 N Sodium hydroxide.

Procedure

Accurately weighed material of both sample and standard are heated with 100 ml of water and 1.5 ml hydrochloric acid for one hour on a water-bath. After cooling, the volume is made to 250 ml with water. 20 ml each of standard and sample are taken in 50 ml volumetric flask and neutralized with 1 N sodium hydroxide. 10 ml of acid - potassium chloride buffer solution and 1 ml of ferric chloride solution are added and the volume is made to 50 ml. The absorbance of both the solutions is measured at 633 nm. Blank is prepared without ferric chloride solution.

Probable Reaction Mechanism

8-Hydroxyquinoline forms chelates with monovalent, divalent and trivalent metal ions; hence forms chelate with Fe(III).

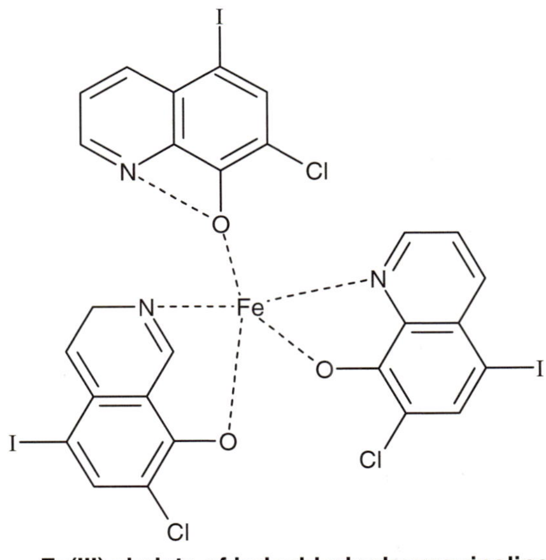

Fe(III) chelate of iodochlorhydroxyquinoline

Formulation 14

Diloxanide furoate, Metronidazole

ESTIMATION

Diloxanide furoate

Weigh accurately a quantity of powdered sample equivalent to 200 mg of diloxanide furoate. Add 25 ml of 0.1 N hydrochloric acid, shake well and extract with four 25 ml portions of chloroform, washing each chloroform layer with the same 10 ml of 0.1 N hydrochloric acid (preserve aqueous acidic layer for estimation of metronidazole). Evaporate chloroform layer, dry at 105°C and weigh which represents amount of diloxanide present in the portion of the sample taken for analysis.

Alternatively, the combined chloroform layer is quantitatively diluted with chloroform to get 10 mcg/ml concentration of diloxanide furoate. Measure the extinction at 260 nm and calculate the results taking 690 as value of A 1%, 1 cm at 260 nm.

Metronidazole

Dilute aqueous acidic layer, obtained above, appropriately with distilled water to get a solution of 0.5 mg/ml in respect of metronidazole. Dilute 5 ml of resultant solution with 0.1 N hydrochloric acid to 200 ml and measure the extinction at absorption maximum at about 277 nm. Calculate the results using 380 as value of A 1%, 1 cm at 277 nm.

Alternatively, follow the method described under formulation 1 of this chapter.

Note

Extraction with chloroform can be eliminated if the finely powdered sample is directly extracted with 0.1 N hydrochloric acid and filtered through G_4 sintered glass funnel. The residue is used for analysing of diloxanide furoate by either dissolving it in water or methanol with absorption maximum at 258 nm.

Formulation 15

Metronidazole, Iodo-chlorhydroxyquinoline

ESTIMATION

Metronidazole

METHOD 1

Measure the sample accurately equivalent to about 100 mg of metronidazole, add 10 ml of 0.1 N hydrochloric acid. Extract with four 25 ml portions of chloroform. Evaporate chloroform layer and take up the residue in water to get 1 mg/ml solution. Follow any one of the methods described for estimation of metronidazole under formulation 1 of this chapter. Spectrophotometric method described under formulation 8 of this chapter can also be followed using 380 as value of A 1%, 1 cm at 277 nm.

METHOD 2

Reagents

1. 0.04% w/v solution of bromothymol blue in water.
2. Citrate-phosphate buffer, pH 4.4.

Standard solution

1 mg/ml of metronidazole in chloroform.

Sample solution (tablets, capsules, syrups and suspensions)

Weigh or measure accurately sample equivalent to about 100 mg of metronidazole. Extract with four 20 ml portions of chloroform. Pass each chloroform layer through cotton plug and adjust the volume with chloroform to 100 ml (1 mg/ml).

Procedure

To 2 ml each of sample and standard solutions, add 4 ml of buffer solution, 5 ml of the dye and 10 ml of the chloroform. Shake for 2 minutes, allow the chloroform layer to separate and read the absorbance of organic layer at about 430 nm.

Note

Metronidazole benzoyloxylate when subjected to above method, gives absorption maximum at about 418 nm.

The method is based on ion-pair complex.

Iodochlorhydroxyquinoline

METHOD 1

Follow the method 2 for estimation of iodo-chlorhydroxyquinoline described under formulation 1 of this chapter.

METHOD 2

Weigh accurately sample equivalent to about 100 mg of iodochlorhydroxyquinoline, add 50 ml of ethyl acetate and heat to boiling. Decant the hot ethyl acetate through filter paper. Repeat extraction with further three 50 ml portions of ethyl acetate. Evaporate the total ethyl acetate extract, dissolve the residue in 40 ml of acetone. Add 2 ml of glacial acetic acid and 20 ml of 1% methanolic copper acetate solution. Keep for 5 minutes and filter through G_4 glass sintered funnel, wash the residue with five 5 ml portions of n-hexane and dry at 105°C. Each g of the residue is equivalent to 0.975 g of iodo-chlorhydroxyquinoline.

For detailed reaction mechanism, see formulation 2 of this chapter.

Formulation 16

Di-iodohydroxyquinoline, Metronidazole

ESTIMATION

Diiodohydroxyquinoline

Standard solution

5 mcg/ml of di-iodohydroxyquinoline (DIHQ) in absolute alcohol.

Sample solution

Weigh sample accurately equivalent to 50 mg of substance, add sufficient absolute alcohol to produce 200 ml. Dilute appropriately with absolute alcohol to get 5 mcg/ml. Measure the extinction of both sample and standard solutions at 253 nm using alcohol as blank and calculate the results by comparison.

Iodochlorhydroxyquinoline / Diiodohydroxyquinoline

Since both iodochlor and diiodochlor contain "N" as well as "O" which can donate or share a lone pair of electrons, hence form complex with uranylacetate which can be used for quantitative estimation. DMF is used as solvent because of its powerful solvating power.

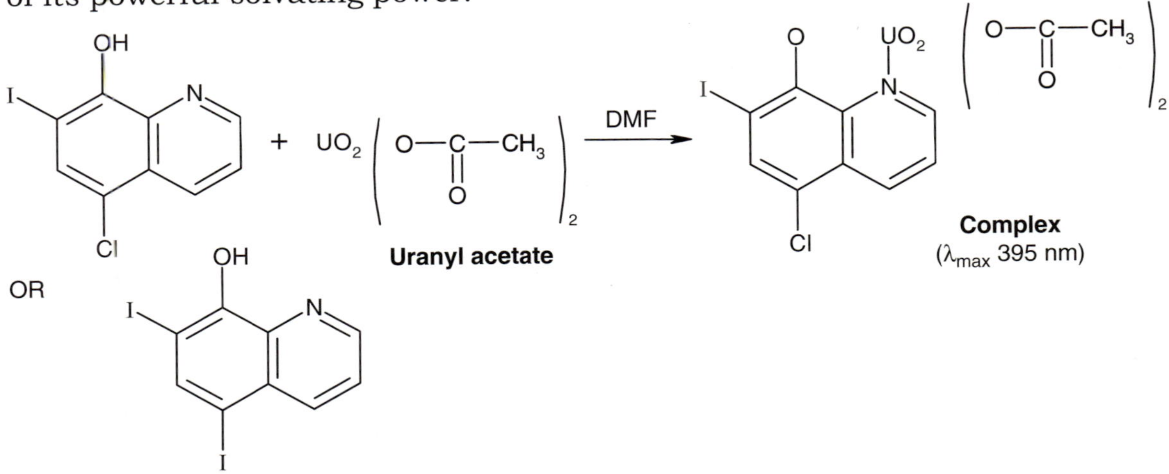

Note

1. DMF is used as solvent.
2. Metronidazole, furazolidone, chloroquine, berberine, sulphonamides, papain and streptomycin do not interfere.

Reference

J. Saha, A.K. Sen & T.K. Das, *Analyst*, **113**, 1653-1655, 1988.

Metronidazole

METHOD 1

Weigh accurately a quantity of the sample equivalent to 50 mg of the substance, add 80-90 ml of 0.1 N hydrochloric acid, shake for 15 min and add sufficient 0.1 N hydrochloric acid to produce 200 ml. Filter and dilute 5 ml to 100 ml with 0.1 N hydrochloric acid. Measure the extinction of the resultant solution at maxima at about 277 nm and calculate the results taking 380 as value of A 1%, 1 cm at the maxima.

Note

The residue obtained during estimation of metronidazole is dissolved in alcohol and used for estimation of 'DIHQ' as described above.

Alternatively, methods described in formulation 1 and 9 of this chapter may be used. Extraction with ethyl acetate will separate both the compounds.

METHOD 2

Reagents

1. 0.2% w/v solution of benzocaine in methanol.
2. 0.1% w/v solution of sodium nitrite in water.
3. Acid mixture: To 85 ml of trichloroacetic acid (15%) add 20 ml of 2 M sulphuric acid and dilute to 200 ml with water.

Standard solution

1 mg/ml in 1,4-dioxan.

Sample solution

Extract the powdered sample with dioxan by slight warming, cool, dilute to get solution of 1 mg/ml.

Procedure

To 1.5 ml of benzocaine solution taken in 2 different 25 ml volumetric flasks add 1 ml of acid mixture and 2 ml of sodium nitrite solution. Allow to stand for at least 15 min to ensure complete diazotization, then add 2.5 ml of methanol and 1 ml each of sample and standard solutions, 3 ml of triethylamine and allow the colour to develop (20 min). Dilute to 25 ml with methanol and measure the absorbance of both the solutions at about 510 nm against reagent blank and calculate the results by comparison.

Probable Reaction Mechanism

Imidazole anion reacts with the diazonium cation (diazotized benzocaine). Formation of anion is pre-requisite because of low chlorophilic nature of diazonium salt. Diazotized benzocaine being a weak electophilic reagent preferably couples at postion 2 of heteroaromatic ring, but since position 2 is occupied, it couples at position 4 of the molecule to give coloured couple products. This is based on 'Pauly reaction'.

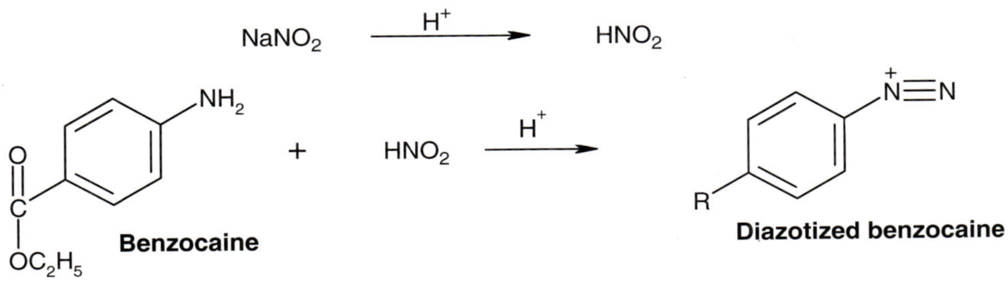

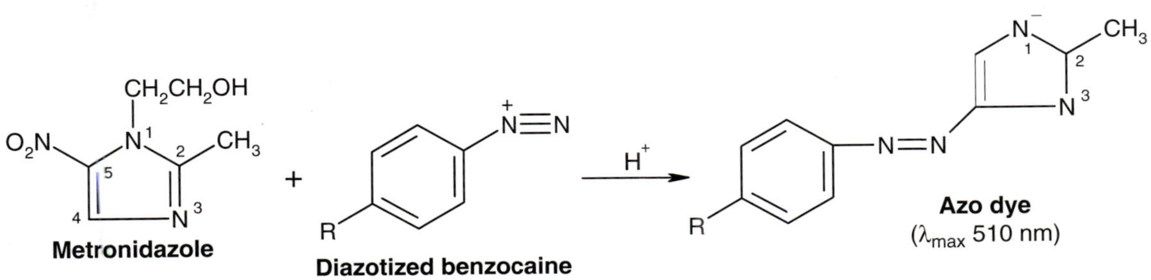

Note

p-Nitroaniline instead of benzocaine is preferred to prepare diazonium salt as the final product can be extracted into organic solvent.

Reference

Pharmaceutical Chemistry (Vol. 2) by H.J. Roth, p. 519 under histamine.

Formulation 17

Metronidazole as benzoate or benzoyloxylate, Furazolidone

METHOD A

This is based on simultaneous spectrophotometric determination of both the components without prior separation.

Standard solution

In 25 ml volumetric flask separately dissolve 25 mg accurately weighed amount of metronidazole and of furazolidone in dimethylformamide (1 mg/ml). Dilute resulting solutions appropriately with distilled water to get 10 mcg/ml solutions. Record the absorption spectra of both the compounds in the spectral range of 200 to 360 nm using 1% aqueous dimethylformamide as blank. Furazolidone exhibits absorption maxima at 262 and 367 nm whereas metronidazole had absorption maximum at 320 nm. Note the absorption values of both the standard solutions at all the three maximas (262, 320 and 367 nm).

Sample solution

Extract an accurately weighed/measured quantity of the sample equivalent to about 50 mg of the either compound with three 15 ml portions of dimethylformamide. Filter and adjust the volume to 50 ml with dimethylformamide. Dilute 1 ml of the resulting solution to 100 ml with distilled water. Measure the absorption at 320 and 367 nm. Calculate the concentration of either component of the mixture from the following equations based on modified Vierordt's method.

$$C_x = \frac{A_1}{\alpha_1} \times [(b-m)/(b-a)]$$

$$C_y = \frac{A_2}{\beta_2} \times b \times (m-a)/m \times (b-a)$$

C_x = Concentration (g/100 ml) of metronidazole
C_y = Concentration (g/100 ml) of furazolidone

A = Absorbance of 1 cm layer of solution
β = E (1%, 1 cm) for metronidazole and furazolidone at 320 and 367 nm
1, 2 = Subscripts refer to the wavelengths of maximum absorption for metronidazole (320 nm) and furazolidone (367 nm)
m = A_2/A_1 (ratio of absorbance of mixture at 367 nm and 320 nm)
a = α_2/α_1 (ratio of E (1%, 1 cm) for metronidazole at 367 nm and 320 nm)
b = β_2/β_1 (ratio of E (1%, 1 cm) for furazolidone at 367 nm and 320 nm)

The values of A at 320 and 367 nm are determined for pure compounds and are used as constant values in the above equations for calculating individual components.

Although furazolidone has two absorption maxima (262 and 367 nm) but for calculation purposes only one wavelength (367 nm) is considered as degradation product (nitrofurfural) of furazolidone would interfere at 262 nm and may lead to erroneous results.

The observed absorption values of standard solutions of metronidazole and furazolidone (10 mcg/ml) at 320 and 367 nm are given below. These values are mean of 5 observations.

	320 nm	367 nm
Metronidazole	0.527	0.088
Furazolidone	0.254	0.740

These values are required to be determined with each instrument. From the above values, various standard factors are calculated and substituted in equations (i) and (ii) above.

Method B

Metronidazole

Follow the method 2 described for estimation of metronidazole in formulation 1 of this chapter.

Furazolidone

Standard solution

1 mg/ml of pure furazolidone in dimethylformamide (DMF).

Sample solution

Weigh accurately powdered tablets equivalent to about 50 mg of furazolidone and extract with 25 ml of DMF. Filter and adjust the volume to 50 ml with DMF (1 mg/ml).

Procedure

To 10 ml of the sample and standard solutions add 1 drop of 0.1 N alcoholic potassium hydroxide and concomitantly read both the solutions at absorption maximum at about 550 nm against solvent blank. Calculate the results by comparison.

Probable Reaction Mechanism

The shift of absorption maximum (bathochromic shift) from the UV to the visible region is brought about by electron attracting character of 5-nitro group. Thus furazolidone gives rise to coloured stabilized anion (λ_{max} 550 nm).

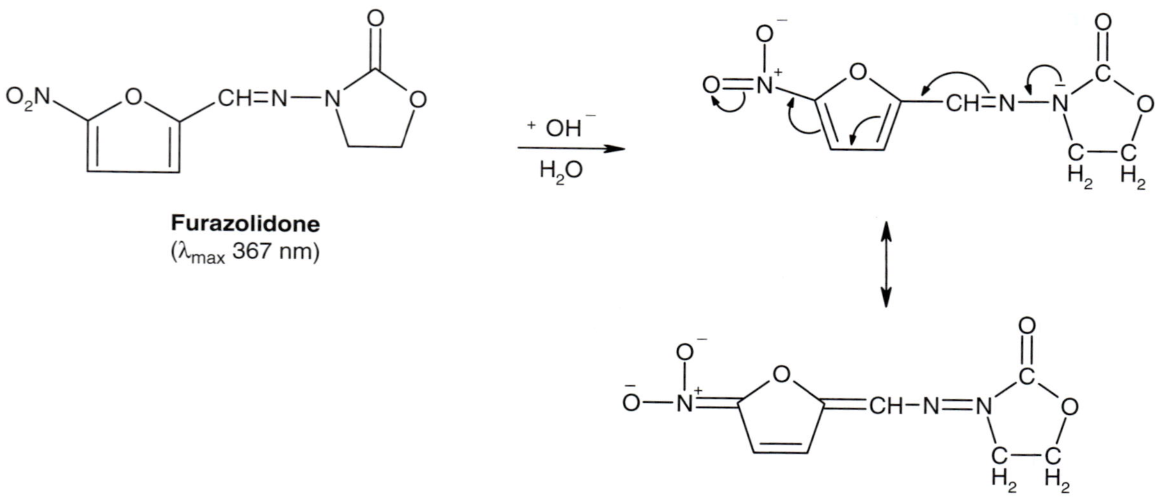

Furazolidone
(λ_{max} 367 nm)

(λ_{max} 550 nm)

Note

This reaction is analogous to the one described for furazolidone.

Reference

1. Pharmaceutical Chemistry (Vol. 2) by H.J. Roth, p. 329 under nitrofural.
2. G. Rama Rao, S. Raghuveer, S.S.N. Murthy & B. Bajirangrao, *Indian Drugs*, **17(2)**, 50-51, 1979.

METHOD

Reagents

1. 1.5% w/v solution ofi phenyil hydrazine in water.
2. Hydrochloric acid : water mixture (3 : 1, v/v).
3. Toluene.

Sample and standard solutions

10 μg/ml of the substance prepared by suspending the substance in acetic acid - pyridine (25 : 2.5, v/v) mixture. Keep in water-bath for 30 min, cool and dilute with water to get final concentration of 10 μg/ml.

Procedure

To 5 ml each of sample and standard solutions add 1 ml each of reagents (1) and (2), keep in water-bath (70°C) for 30 min, cool, add 20 ml of toluene, shake, separate organic layer and pass through anhydrous sodium sulphate and measure the absorbance at 440 nm against reagent blank.

Probable Reaction Mechanism

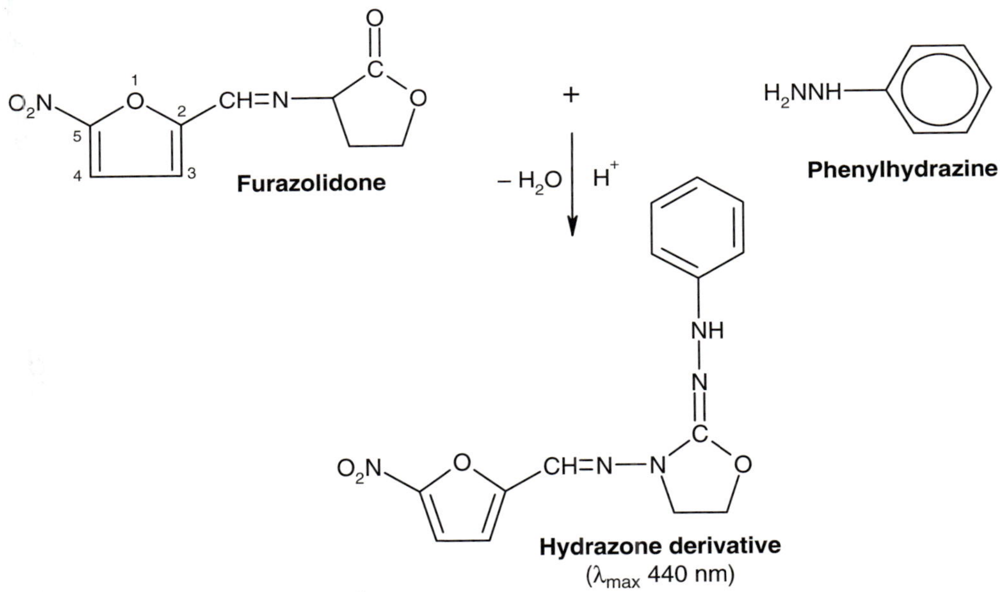

Metronidazole benzoyloxylate

This compound is normally used in suspension.

Reagents

1. Chloroform-acetone mixture (7: 3 v/v).
2. Glacial acetic acid.
3. 0.1 N perchloric acid.
4. 2% α-naphtholbenzeine in glacial acetic acid, indicator.

Procedure

Shake the suspension mechanically for 10 minutes for uniform mixing and then weigh accurately the sample equivalent to 200 mg of the compound.

Transfer into 125 ml separating funnel and extract with eight 40 ml portions of chloroform-acetone mixture. Collect the clear chloroform-acetone layer and pass through anhydrous sodium sulphate. Add 2-3 glass beads and evaporate carefully on warm water-bath to about 10 to 15 ml. To it, add 25 ml glacial acetic acid and again evaporate further for 10 minutes on warm water-bath to remove chloroform/acetone. Cool it to room temperature, add 1 ml indicator and titrate it against 0.1 N perchloric acid.

Each ml of 0.1 N perchloric acid is equivalent to 17.12 mg of metronidazole. Calculate the contents in each 5 ml, taking into consideration weigh per ml of the sample preparation.

Note

1. Since metronidazole is only slightly soluble in chloroform, alcohol and ether, several successive extractions are required for complete extraction of the compound into organic layer.
2. As metronidazole is more soluble in water than organic solvent, further addition of water is to be avoided.
3. Extraction procedure is necessary to eliminate water for non-aqueous titration.

The hydrolysis of 5-nitroimidazole takes place as C—N bond as position 5 is susceptible to alkaline hydrolysis particularly when position 1 in the heterocyclic ring is substituted. The hydrolysis liberates nitrite ion (NO_2) with the formation of 2-(2-methylimidazol-1-yl)ethyl benzoate. The nitrite so produced can be used for diazotization of sulphanilic acid and coupling with b-naphthol to give an azo dye.

Probable Reaction Mechanism

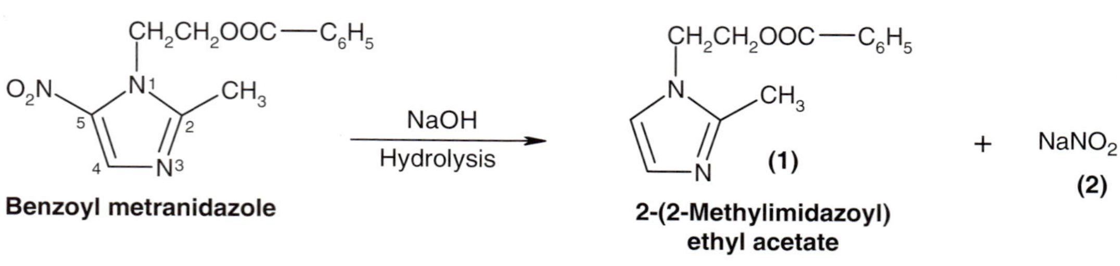

Note

1. The compound has no λ_{max} at 277 nm typical of metronidazole molecule. The change in absorption has linear relationship with concentration; hence can be used for analytical purpose.
2. Can be used for diazotization reaction for quantification.

Reference

A.K. Sanyal, Analyst, **117**, 93-95, 1992.

METHOD C

Metronidazole

Reagent

1 N hydrochloric acid.

Procedure

Shake the preparation mechanically for 10 minutes for uniform mixing and pipette out 5 ml of the preparation into 100 ml volumetric flask containing 70 ml 1 N hydrochloric acid. Rinse the pipette with acid. Shake it mechanically for 15 minutes and make the volume to 100 ml with 1 N acid. Shake well and filter through No. 1 filter paper, discard first 10-15 ml of the filtrate. Reserve insoluble material for assay of furazolidone. Dilute 10 ml of the clear filtrate to 100 ml with 1 N acid. Further dilution is done with water to get a concentration of 10 mcg/ml of metronidazole. Measure the extinction of the solution at 277 nm against 0.1 N acid as blank. A value of 390 as E 1%, 1 cm at 277 nm can be used for calculations of the contents.

Furazolidone

Dissolve the insoluble material as obtained above in 1% v/v DMF (aqueous) to produce 10 mcg/ml. Record the absorbance at 367 nm against 1% DMF and calculate the results by comparison with the standard.

METHOD D

This method has been found to give excellent results in solid dosage forms (capsules and tablets).

Furazolidone

Standard solution

0.5 mg/ml of pure furazolidone in dimethylformamide (DMF). Dilute 2 ml of the solution to 100 ml with water (10 mcg/ml).

Sample solution

Weigh accurately a quantity of powdered material equivalent to 50 mg of furazolidone. Add 50 ml of water and warm on a water-bath. Shake vigorously and filter through G_4 glass sintered funnel. Repeat the above process thrice.

Combine the filtrate and adjust to 250 ml with water and reserve for estimation of metronidazole. Dissolve the residue obtained above in DMF to get a concentration of 1 mg/ml. 2 ml of the resultant solution is further diluted to 100 ml with water (10 mcg/ml).

Measure the extinction of both the solutions at maxima at about 367 nm using 2% v/v DMF solution in water as blank and calculate the results.

Metronidazole

Standard solution

10 mcg/ml in water.

Sample solution

Dilute the filtrate obtained in the estimation of furazolidone appropriately to get a concentration of 10 mcg/ml with water. Measure the absorbance of both the solutions at 320 nm against water as blank. Calculate the contents by comparing with the standard.

Formulation 18

Iodochlorhydroxyquinoline, Berberine hydrochloride

ESTIMATION

Iodochlorhydroxyquinoline

Reagents

1. 1 N sodium hydroxide.
2. 0.1% w/v copper sulphate in water.
3. 3 N hydrochloric acid.

Standard solution

Weigh accurately 250 mg of pure substance, add 35-40 ml of 3 N hydrochloric acid, digest for 30 minutes, cool and adjust to 100 ml with 3 N hydrochloric acid.

Sample solution

Weigh accurately powdered tablets equivalent to 250 mg of the compound, digest with 3 N acid and dilute to 100 ml as per standard.

Procedure

To 1.5 ml of sample and standard solutions add 50 ml of 1 N sodium hydroxide and 1 ml of copper sulphate solution. Mix and extract each with four 20 ml portions of chloroform. Pass each chloroform layer through cotton plug and adjust to 100 ml with chloroform. Measure the absorption of both the solutions against reagent blank at maximum at about 430 nm.

Probable Reaction Mechanism

The compound has “N” and “O”, can share lone pair of electrons, can form complex with Cu(2).

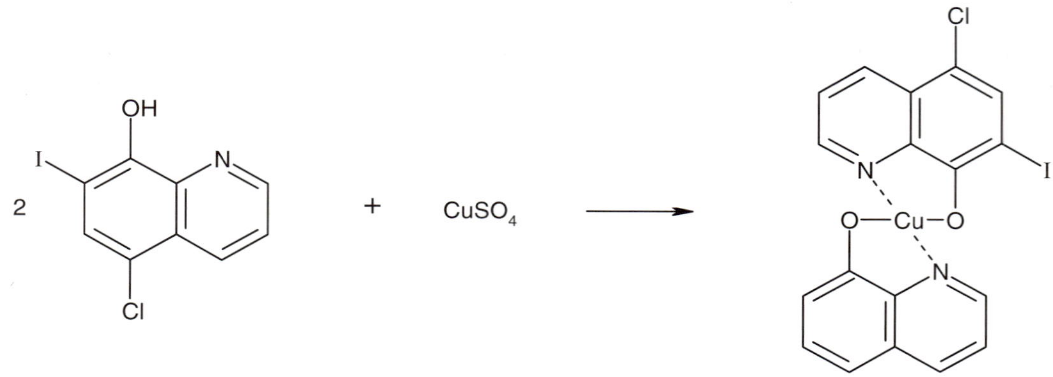

Coloured copper complex
(λ_{max} 430 nm)

Berberine hydrochloride

METHOD 1

Reagents

1. Acetone.
2. Ethyl alcohol.
3. Saturated solution of ammonium reineckate in water.

Standard solution

Weigh accurately 50 mg of berberine hydrochloride and dissolve in ethyl alcohol to produce 100 ml. 4 ml of the resultant solution is diluted to 100 ml with acetone.

Sample solution

Weigh accurately a quantity of powdered tablets equivalent to 50 mg of berberine hydrochloride. Add 50 ml of ethyl alcohol and warm on water-bath for 10 minutes, stir for 1 hour and adjust with ethyl alcohol to 100 ml. Filter and dilute further with acetone as under standard solution.

Procedure

To 4 ml of the sample filtrate and standard solutions add 2-3 ml of strong ammonia solution and 15 ml of reineckate solution. Keep in ice-bath for 2 hours to get complete precipitation. Filter the precipitate through G_4 sintered funnel, wash the precipitate with distilled water till the filtrate is colourless. Dry at 105°C for 1 hour and at 50°C for 3 hours. Cool and dissolve the residue in acetone to produce 100 ml. Measure the intensity of the resultant complex solution at absorption maximum at about 420 nm.

Note

Berberine, an alkaloid, is precipitated as reineckate; the precipitates are dissolved in acetone to yield a yellow-coloured solution (λ_{max} 420 nm).

METHOD 2

Reagents

1. Phosphate buffer, pH 8.0.
2. 4 mM picric acid solution in water.
3. 1,2-dichloroethane.

Standard solution

Weigh accurately pure berberine hydrochloride equivalent to 5 mM and dissolve in water to produce 100 ml.

Sample solution

Weigh accurately powdered tablets equivalent to 5 mM of berberine hydrochloride and shake with 30-35 ml of water, filter and wash the residue with water and adjust to 100 ml.

Procedure

To 5 ml of standard and sample solutions add 5 ml of picric acid solution and shake vigorously. Add 10 ml of dichloroethane and again shake vigorously for 3 minutes. Read absorption of the organic layer at maximum at about 360 nm against water as reagent blank.

Note

The alkaloid precipitated as picrate which is soluble in dichloromethane.

METHOD 3

Reagents

1. 0.1% Tetrabromophenolphthalein ethylester in ethyl alcohol.
2. Borate buffer solution, pH 8.5.

Standard solution

A stock solution of pure berberine hydrochloride (dried at 105°C) is prepared in water to contain 0.4 mg/ml. The solution is further diluted with water to get 10 mcg/ml solution.

Sample solution

Weigh accurately powdered tablets equivalent to 40 mg of berberine hydrochloride. Extract with water and appropriately dilute with water to produce 10 mcg/ml solution.

Procedure

To 2.5 ml of sample and standard solutions add 2 ml of the dye solution and 5 ml of borate-phosphate buffer. Dilute to 50 ml with water and shake with 10 ml of ethylene dichloride for 5 minutes. The absorbance of the organic layer is first mesured at about 610 nm at about 25°C against reagent blank. The temperature of the organic layer is then raised to 60°C and absorbance measured again at 610 nm. The difference in absorption values at 25°C and 60°C is related to berberine contents. The results are calculated by comparison. The method is based on ion-pair complex.

Note

1. At 60°C, the absorbance due to secondary and tertiary amines and alkaloids is decreased to zero and thus do not interfere in the estimation of berberine hydrochloride.
2. Diphenhydramine hydrochloride (0.3 : 1), thiamine hydrochloride (1 : 1), papaverine (10 : 1) do not interfere in the estimation in the molar ratio indicated.

METHOD 4

Reagents

1. Hydrochloric acid.
2. Dilute hydrochloric acid.
3. Bromine water: Dilute 5 ml of saturated solution of bromine (aqueous) to 100 ml with water.

Standard solution

200 mcg/ml of berberine hydrochloride in water.

Sample solution

Accurately weighed quantity of powdered tablets equivalent to 50 mg of the substance was suspended in 200 ml of water and digested on boiling water-bath for 30 min, cooled and adjusted to 250 ml with water.

Procedure

To 2.5 ml each of sample and standard solutions add 41 ml of dilute hydrochloric acid and 1 ml of bromine water. Mix and allow to stand for 10 min. Subsequently add 1 ml of hydrochloric acid and dilute to 50 ml with dilute hydrochloric acid. Measure the absorbance of the resulting solution at 485 nm against reagent blank and calculate the results by comparison. The method obeys Beer's law in the concentration range of 4-24 mcg/ml. Sulphadiazine usually present in the combination does not interfere.

Probable Reaction Mechanism

Br_2 causes oxidation of ring C of the molecule resulting in the formation of two double bonds. As a result there is extension of conjugation, hence bathochromic shift from 425 nm to 485 nm.

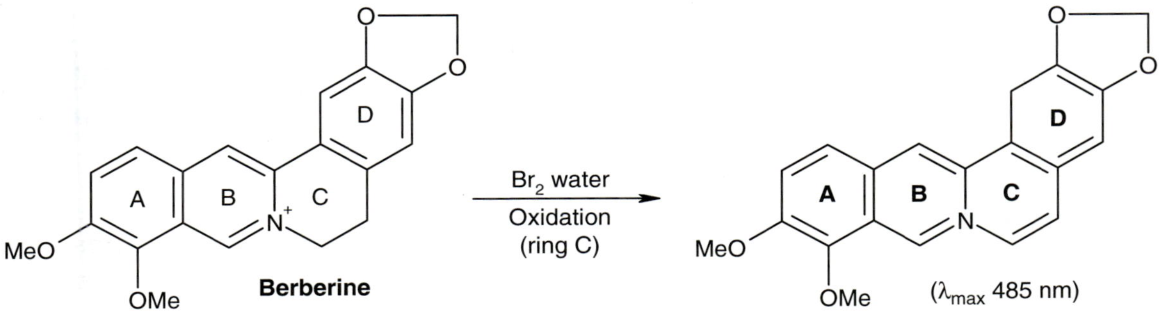

Reference

D.K. Desai, S.P. Kurani & A.G. Sesharinathan, *Indian Drugs*, **25(12)**, 533-534, 1988.

A spectrophotometric method for estimation of berberine in formulations has been reported by Prasanna et al. The drug is dissolved in aqueous solution of 20% propylene glycol and the absorption is measured at 425 nm. The method obeys Beer's law in the range of 2-8 μg/ml and was fully validated.

Note

The method is based on measurement of absorption of inherent colour of the compound.

Reference

S.M. Prasanna, G.S. Kumar & V. Madhavan, 54th IPC, Abstract No. GP-19.

Formulation 19

Tinidazole

ESTIMATION

METHOD 1

Accurately weigh a quantity of the finely powdered tablets equivalent to 450 mg of tinidazole and transfer to 500 ml volumetric flask. Make up the volume with methanol and stir for 30 minutes. Filter the resulting suspension through a Whatman No. 1 filter paper, rejecting the first 20 ml and dilute 5 ml of the filtrate to 500 ml with methanol. Measure the absorbance of this final solution on a suitable spectrophotometer at 310 nm against methanol and calculate the result by using 355 as value of E 1%, 1 cm. The method obeys Beer's law in the range of 5-25 mcg/ml.

Note

1. Tinidazole is light sensitive. Therefore, all solutions must be protected from light either by using amber glassware or by covering the glassware with opaque material.
2. Several other solvents can be used for extraction and spectrophotometric determination. The absorption maxima and values of E 1%, 1 cm in different solvents are given as under:

Solvent	λ_{max} (nm)	E 1%, 1 cm	Range of Beer's law
Chloroform	315	400	
Ethyl alcohol	310	355	
Methyl alcohol	310	355	5-25 mcg/ml
Benzene	322	380	
0.1 N hydrochloric acid	277	244	0.5-4 mcg/ml

METHOD 2

Standard solution

10 mg/ml of pure tinidazole is dissolved in methyl alcohol to produce 100 ml (100 mcg/ml).

Sample solution

Weigh accurately powdered tablets equivalent to 10 mg of tinidazole. Add 70-80 ml methyl alcohol, shake, filter, wash the residue with methyl alcohol and adjust the filtrate to 100 ml with methanol (100 mcg/ml).

Procedure

2 ml of sample and standard solutions are evaporated on boiling water-bath. Cool and add 2.5 ml of 20% w/v aqueous sodium hydroxide solution and dilute to 10 ml with water. Measure the absorbance of standard and sample solutions at maximum at about 368 nm and calculate the result. The method obeys Beer's law in the range of 5-25 mcg/ml.

Probable Reaction Mechanism

The drug in alkaline solution generates additional non-bonded electron that interacts with imidazole ring π electrons to produce bathochrome shift from 277 nm to 368 nm with hyperchromic shift.

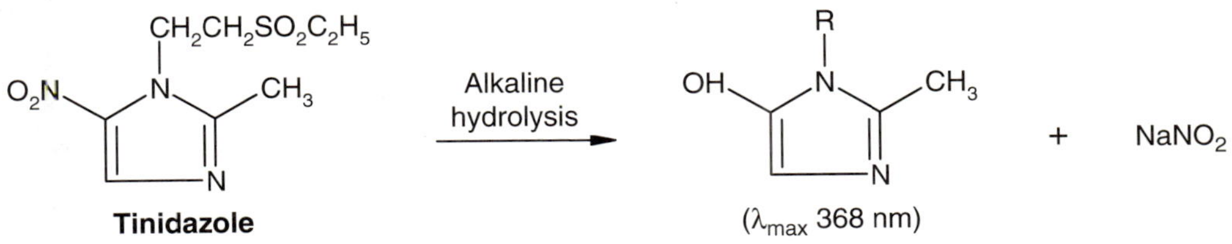

Reference

S.J. Dahawal et al., *J. Pharm. Res.*, **6(2)**, 51-53, 2007.

METHOD 3

Reagents

1. 0.1 N hydrochloric acid.
2. Hydrochloric acid.
3. Zinc dust.
4. 1.0% w/v solution of vanillin in water.

Standard solution

1 mg/ml of tinidazole in 0.1 N hydrochloric acid.

Sample solution

Weigh accurately powdered tablets equivalent to 100 mg of tinidazole, add 50 ml of 0.1 N acid, shake and filter through G_4 glass sintered funnel. Wash the residue with 0.1 N acid and adjust to 100 ml with the acid.

Procedure

To 25 ml of the standard and sample solutions, add 2.5 ml of 0.1 N hydrochloric acid, 5 g zinc dust and 4 ml of hydrochloric acid. Keep aside for 30 minutes to ensure complete reaction (reduction). Dilute both sample and standard reduced solutions to get 100 mcg/ml. To 2.5 ml each of standard and sample solutions add 1 ml of vanillin reagent and heat on water-bath for 20 minutes, cool and dilute to 10 ml with water. Measure the extinction of solutions at absorption maximum at about 410 nm against reagent blank and calculate the results. The method obeys Beer's law in the range of 10-50 mcg/ml. The coloured complex is stable for 6 hours.

Probable Reaction Mechanism

The treatment of tinidazole with Zn-HCl results in the reduction of —NO_2 group to amino group. The reduced —NO_2 group i.e. —NH_2 group couples with vanillin resulting in the formation of Schiff's base.

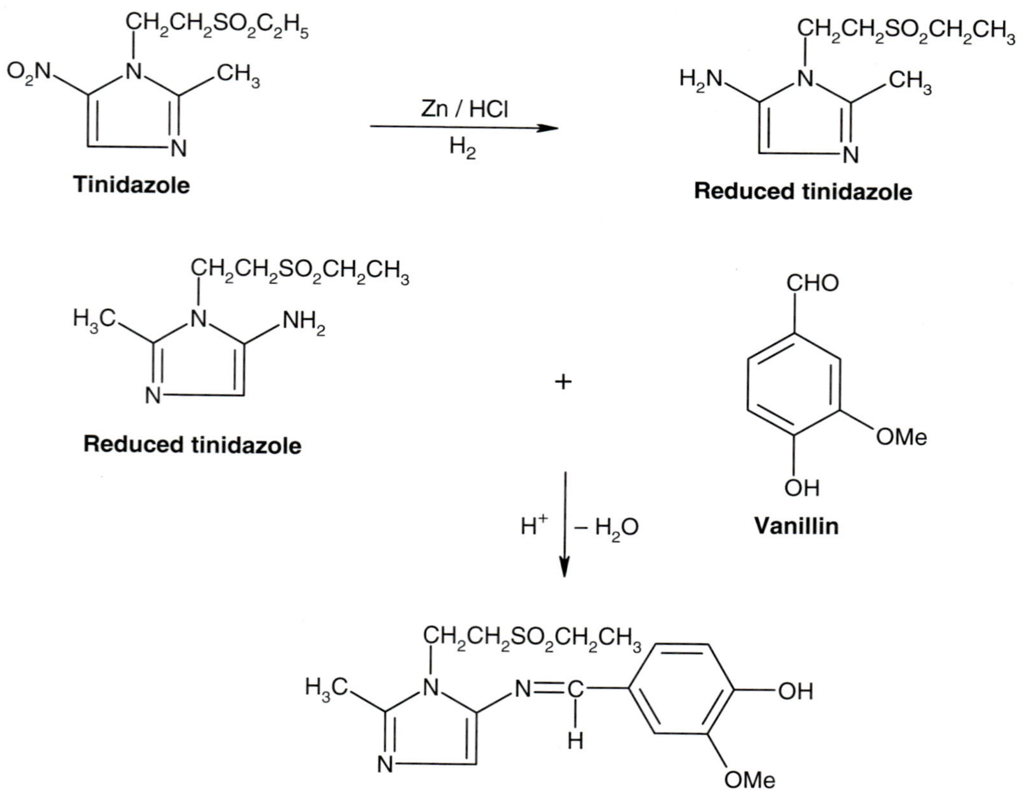

Schiff's base, coloured product
(λ_{max} 410 nm)

METHOD 4

Reagents

1. 0.1% w/v solution of potassium ferricyanide in water.
2. 0.1% w/v solution of sodium nitroprusside in water.
3. 0.1% w/v solution of sodium hydroxide in water.
4. Methyl alcohol.

Standard solution

Weigh accurately 100 mg of pure tinidazole, add 50 ml of methyl alcohol, shake to dissolve and dilute to 100 ml with methanol. Suitable quantity of above methanolic solution (1 mg/ml) is diluted with water to produce solution of 40 mcg/ml.

Sample solution

Weigh accurately a quantity of powdered tablets equivalent to 100 mg of tinidazole and extract with methanol as described under method 1 above. 5 ml of the resultant solution (1 mg/ml) is diluted with water to produce 25 ml.

Procedure

To 25 ml of the standard and sample solutions add 3 ml each of sodium hydroxide, sodium nitroprusside and potassium ferricyanide solutions in turn. Keep aside for 30 minutes for colour to develop. Adjust the volume to 10 ml with distilled water. Measure the absorption of standard and sample solutions at absorption maximum at about 460 nm against reagent blank and calculate the contents of tinidazole in the formulation. The method obeys Beer's law in the range of 8-80 mcg/ml.

METHOD 5

Reagents

1. 1% phosphomolybdic acid.
2. 2 N hydrochloric acid.

Procedure

Accurately weigh powdered tablets equivalent to 100 mg of tinidazole, extract with methanol, filter and reduce the volume of methanol to 5 ml. Add 5 ml of phosphomolybdic acid reagent, shake for 5 minutes, add 30 ml of 1 N hydrochloric acid and keep for 60 minutes. Collect the precipitates on G_4 glass sintered cricible. Wash the precipitates with distilled water and dry at 110-115°C till constant weight. Each g of the residue is equivalent to 0.521 g of tinidazole.

Note

The compounds answer most of the reactions as explained under metronidazole such as (a) liberation of nitrite (NO_2) on alkaline hydrolysis, (b) after reduction it can be diazotized and undergo Bratton-Marshall reaction, and (c) after reduction it forms Schiff's base with vanillin, furfural, PDAB and PDAC, the aldehydes.

Formulation 20

Diloxanide furoate, Tinidazole

ESTIMATION

Diloxanide furoate

Weigh accurately a quantity of powdered tablets equivalent to 200 mg of diloxanide furoate. Add 25 ml of 0.1 N hydrochloric acid, shake well and extract with four 25 ml portions of chloroform washing each chloroform layer with the same 10 ml of 0.1 N hydrochloric acid. Preserve acidic layer for determination of tinidazole. Evaporate chloroform layer, dry at 105°C and weigh which represents the amount of diloxanide furoate present in the sample taken for analysis.

Alternatively, the combined chloroform extract may be diluted quantitatively with chloroform and subjected to spectrophotometric analysis. For details, refer to method 1 for estimation of diloxanide furoate under formulation 10 of this chapter.

Tinidazole

METHOD 1

Dilute acidic layer obtained above appropriately with 0.1 N hydrochloric acid to get a concentration of 500 mcg/ml in respect of tinidazole. Dilute 5 ml of resultant solution with 0.1 N hydrochloric acid to 200 ml and measure the extinction at absorption maximum at 277 nm. Calculate the results using 244 as value of E 1%, 1 cm at 277 nm. Alternatively, other methods described in formulation 19 of this chapter may be employed.

METHOD 2

Standard solution

10 mcg/ml of tinidazole in methanol.

Sample solution

An accurately weighed quantity of the powdered sample equivalent to 25 mg of tinidazole was shaken with about 60 ml of methanol, filtered through G_4 sintered funnel. The residue was washed with methanol, filtrate adjusted to 100 ml. 2 ml of the filtrate was further diluted to 50 ml with methanol.

The absorbance of both sample and standard solutions was measured at about 311 nm and results calculated by comparison. Diloxanide furoate showing zero absorbance at 311 nm, the absorption maximum for tinidazole. The method obeys Beer's law in the concentration range of 5-15 mcg/ml.

Formulation 21

Diloxanide furoate, Tinidazole, Methylpolysiloxane

ESTIMATION

Diloxanide furoate

Weigh accurately a quantity of powdered tablets equivalent to 200 mg of diloxanide furoate. Add 25 ml of 0.1 N hydrochloric acid, shake well and extract with four 25 ml portions of chloroform washing each chloroform layer with the same 10 ml of 0.1 N hydrochloric acid. Preserve acidic layer for determination of tinidazole. Evaporate chloroform layer, dry at 105°C and weigh which represents the amount of diloxanide furoate present in the sample taken for analysis.

Alternatively, the combined chloroform extract may be diluted quantitatively with chloroform and subjected to spectrophotometric analysis. For details, refer to method 1 for estimation of diloxanide furoate under formulation 10 or 12 of this chapter.

Tinidazole

METHOD 1

Dilute acidic layer obtained above appropriately with 0.1 N hydrochloric acid to get a concentration of 500 mcg/ml in respect of tinidazole. Dilute 5 ml of resultant solution with 0.1 N hydrochloric acid to 200 ml and measure the extinction at absorption maximum at 277 nm. Calculate the results using 244 as value of A 1%, 1 cm at 277 nm. Alternatively, other methods described in formulation 19 of this chapter may be employed.

METHOD 2

Standard solution

10 mcg/ml of tinidazole in methanol.

Sample solution

An accurately weighed quantity of the powdered sample equivalent to 25 mg of tinidazole was shaken with about 60 ml of methanol, filtered through G_4 sintered funnel. The residue was washed with methanol, filtrate adjusted to 100 ml. 2 ml of the filtrate was further diluted to 50 ml with methanol.

The absorbance of both sample and standard solutions was measured at about 311 nm and results calculated by comparison. Diloxanide furoate showing zero absorbance at 311 nm, the absorption maximum for tinidazole. The method obeys Beer's law in the concentration range of 5-15 mcg/ml.

METHOD 3

Transfer accurately weighed powdered sample equivalent to 300 mg of tinidazole, add 50 ml of glacial acetic acid, shake well and add 2-3 ml of acetic anhydride and titrate against 0.1 N perchloric acid (crystal violet). Each ml of 0.1 N perchloric acid is equivalent to 0.02473 g of tinidazole.

Estimation of Tinidazole and Diloxanide furoate

Standard solution

Prepare mixed standard by dissolving 40 mg of tinidazole and 50 mg of diloxanide furoate in 50 ml of DMF, keep aside for 15 min and dilute to 100 ml with water. 1 ml of resultant solution is diluted to 50 ml with water.

Sample solution

To accurately weighed quantity of the sample equivalent to 40 mg of tinidazole add 50 ml of DMF, stir to dissolve and dilute to 100 ml with water. Filter and dilute 1 ml to 50 ml with water.

Measure the absorption of both the sample and standard solutions at 262 nm (diloxanide furoate) and 318 nm (tinidazole) and calculate the results by comparison.

Activated methylpolysiloxane (MPS)

METHOD 1

Suspend a quantity of powdered tablets equivalent to 50 mg of activated methylpolysiloxane in 25 ml of dilute hydrochloric acid. Extract with four 40 ml of petroleum ether (40 to 60°C), wash the organic layer with two 10 ml portions of water, filter the organic layer through anhydrous sodium sulphate, collect the filtrate in a pre-dried, weighed beaker and dry it on a water-bath and then in air oven at 105°C for one hour.

The difference in weight is the amount of activated methylpolysiloxane present in the weighed quantity of the sample taken for analysis.

METHOD 2

Silicates give yellow colour with ammonium molybdate in acidic medium.

Reagent

1. Ammonium molybdate solution: Dissolve 8.0 g of ammonium molybdate monohydrate in 9 ml of concentrated sulphuric acid, dilute to 100 ml with water.

Standard solution

Weigh accurately 50 mg of MPS, add 20 ml of carbon tetrachloride and 15 ml of dilute hydrochloric acid. Heat to boiling, cool and separate organic layer. Pass the organic layer through anhydrous sodium sulphate placed over a plug of cotton.

Sample solution

Weigh accurately the sample equivalent to 50 mg of MPS and proceed as under standard solution.

Procedure

Evaporate 5 ml each of sample and standard solutions in platinum dish. Add 1 g of sodium carbonate, anhydrous, ignite, cool and dissolve the residue in 20 ml of water.

Wash the crucible with 10 ml of water, mix with main aqueous extract. Adjust the pH to 5.0 (± 0.5) with dilute sulphuric acid and dilute to 50 ml with water (use for estimation).

To 5 ml each of the above solutions, add 2 ml of ammonium molybdate solution. Set aside for 10 min. Measure the absorption of both the solutions at about 400 nm using water instead of sample solution for blank. Calculate the results by comparison.

Formulation 22

Kaolin, Pectin, Sodium lactate, Potassium chloride, Sodium chloride, Neomycin, Tincture belladonna

Determination of total Tropane alkaloids and Tincture Belladonna

Carry out the general alkaloidal extraction and purification as described for determination of total belladonna alkaloids under formulation 1 of the chapter on antacids to obtain the total alkaloids in chloroform layer. Evaporate appropriate quantity of the chloroform layer representing 0.2 ml of tincture belladonna and carry out the method 2 described for total belladonna alkaloids under formulation 9 of this chapter.

Determination of Total Chlorides

Follow the method for determination of total chlorides as described in formulation 1 of the chapter on oral rehydration salts.

Differential determination of Potassium chloride and Sodium chloride

Follow the methods described in formulation 1 of the chapter on oral rehydration salts.

Determination of Kaolin

Weigh accurately 5 ml of the suspension, dilute with water and filter through G_4 sintered funnel. Wash the residue with water, ignite and weigh, which represents contents of kaolin.

Determination of Neomycin

Microbiological method using *Bacillus pumilus* as test organism is the most reliable method. However, a chemical method based on hydrolysis of neomycin to ribose and amino group also gives satisfactory results. The amino group thus liberated is reacted with ninhydrin to give violet-coloured complex.

Method

Reagents

1. Alcohol (50%, v/v), ammonia-free.
2. Alkaline water, pH 8: prepared by adding dilute sodium hydroxide solution to water.
3. Ninhydrin reagent.
   (a) Ninhydrin solution: Dissolve 4.5 g of ninhydrin in methoxyethanol. When stored in amber-coloured bottle and in a refrigerator the solution is stable for one month.
   (b) Acetate - methoxyethanol buffer: To 20 ml of water add 24.48 g of sodium acetate and heat to dissolve. Cool it to room temperature, add 4.5 ml of glacial acetic acid and dilute to 90 ml with water. Check its pH (it should be 5.5) and add 10 ml of methoxyethanol. The solution is stable for one month at room temperature.
   On the day of experiment, 100 g of stannous chloride is dissolved in 50 ml of acetate - methoxy buffer (b) and mixed with ninhydrin solution (a) in the ratio of 10 : 8 to give ninhydrin reagent.

Standard solution

Neomycin sulphate equivalent to 24 mg of neomycin base is dissolved in 12 ml of alkaline water. It is appropriately diluted with alkaline water to get a solution of 50 mcg/ml neomycin (base). Neomycin (base) = 0.676 × water-free neomycin sulphate.

Sample solution

Dilute the sample suspension appropriately with alkaline water to get a concentration of 50 mcg/ml neomycin base, and filter.

Procedure

To 0.5 ml aliquots of the standard and sample solutions add 1 ml of ninhydrin reagent and heat in a water-bath for 15 minutes. Cool to room temperature and add 5 ml of ammonia-free alcohol (50%, v/v). Concomitantly measure the absorbance of violet-coloured complex at absorption maximum at about 570 nm. The violet complex is stable for 1 hr and method obeys Beer's law in the concentration range of 0.75 to 5 mcg/ml of neomycin.

Probable Reaction Mechanism

Ninhydrin can react with a variety of primary and secondary amines resulting in a so-called Ruhemann purple colour (diketohydrindamine - diketohydrindylidene).

On heating the solution, the amino group reacts with ninhydrin and then the formed amine reacts with one molecule of ninhydrin to give purple-coloured product (λ_{max} 570 nm).

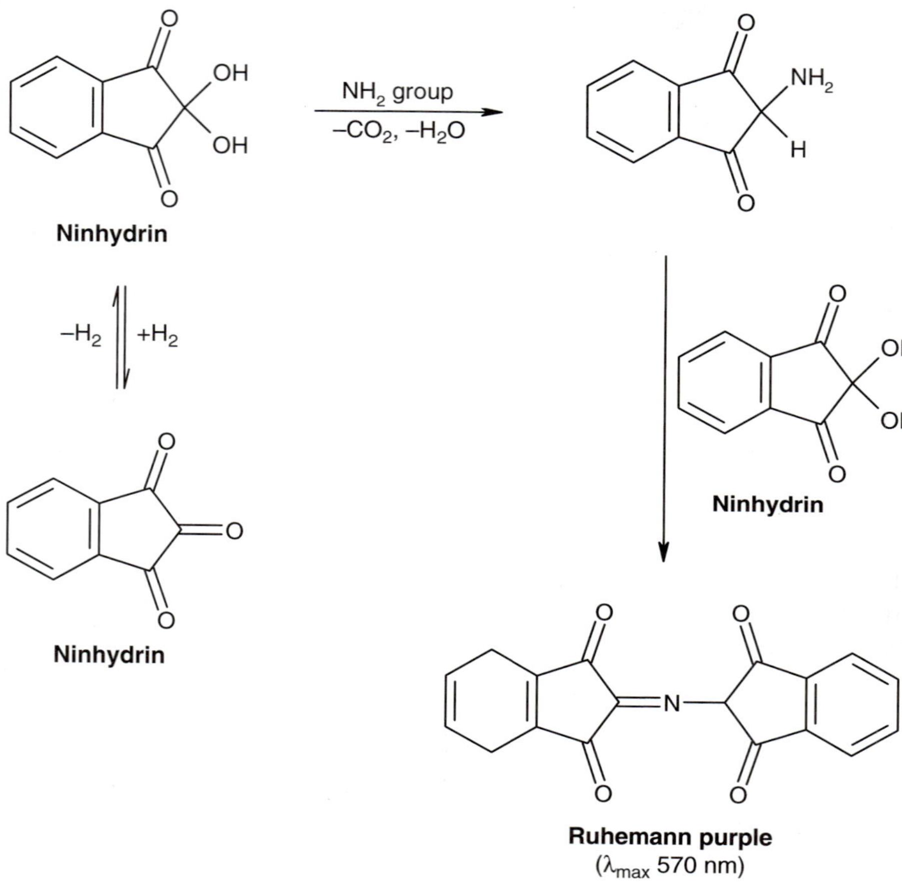

Reference

Yunqi Wu, Munir Hussain & Reza Fassihi, *J. Pharm. & Biomed. Analysis*, **38**, 263-269, 2005.

Formulation 23

Loperamide hydrochloride, Furazolidone

ESTIMATION

Loperamide hydrochloride

Reagents

1. Tropeolin reagents: Weigh accurately 50 mg of tropeolin-00 (acid orange) in a 50 ml volumetric flask, dissolve and make up the volume with water.
2. Acidified methanol: Dilute 1 ml of concentrated sulphuric acid to 100 ml with methanol.
3. Buffer, pH 3.0: Dissolve 11 g of dibasic sodium phosphate and 18.3 g of citric acid monohydrate in 800 ml of distilled water. Adjust the pH to 3.0 with citric acid or dibasic sodium phosphate and make up the volume to 1000 ml with water.

Standard solution

20 mcg per ml of loperamide hydrochloride in chloroform.

Sample solution

Extract the powdered sample equivalent to 2 mg of loperamide hydrochloride with 100 ml of chloroform.

Procedure

Pipette out 20 ml each of standard and sample solutions in separate stoppered centrifuge tube. Add 10 ml of buffer pH 3.0 and 3 ml of tropeolin reagent to each tube. Shake the tubes for five minutes and centrifuge. Pipette out 10 ml of chloroform, add 3 ml of acidified methanol. Measure the extinctions of both standard and sample solutions at about 540 nm using chloroform as the blank and deduce the results by comparison. The method is based on ion-pair complex. The method was official in earlier edition of USP (1985).

Furazolidone

Sample solution

Dissolve the powdered sample equivalent to 20 mg of furazolidone in 25 ml of dimethylformamide in a 100 ml volumetric flask. Shake well and make up the volume with water. Dilute 25 ml with distilled water.

Procedure

Measure the extinction of sample solution at the maximum at about 367 nm against blank prepared by diluting 1.5 ml of dimethyl formamide to 25 ml with water. Calculate the contents of furazolidone using 750 as value of the A 1%, 1 cm at 367 nm.

Formulation 24

Loperamide hydrochloride, Streptomycin sulphate

ESTIMATION

Loperamide hydrochloride

Follow the colour reaction with tropeolin-00 (acid orange) as described in formulation 15 of this chapter.

The compound also forms ion-pair complex with bromocresol purple in buffer pH 5.3. The complex can be extracted into chloroform and measured at 408 nm.

The drug has two main centres i.e. amide and basic piperidine nitrogen. The drug is relatively basic in character. In addition to ion-pair complex formation with bromocresol purple other dyes have also been used such as bromothymol blue, bromophenol blue and naphthol blue black B in different buffers.

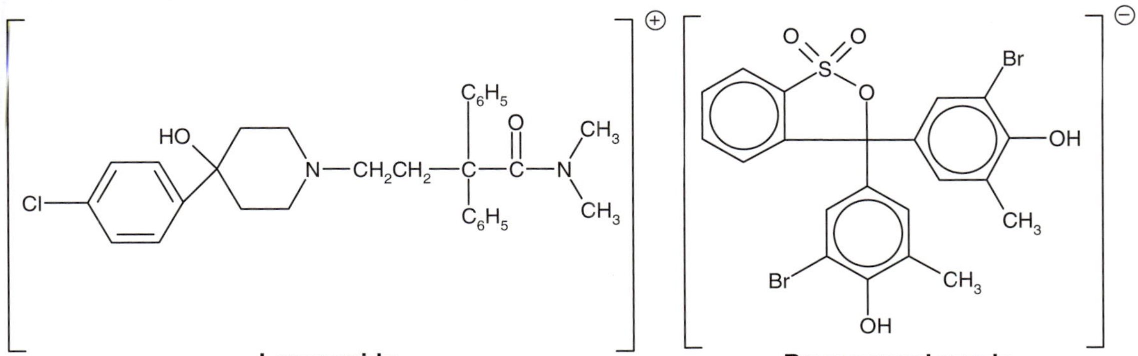

Loperamide **Bromocresol purple**

Drug-dye ion-pair complex
(λ_{max} 408 nm)

Reference

K.M. Thomas, *Indian Drugs*, **27(11)**, 586, 1990.

Earlier Khashaba et al. have described ion-pair complex formation with methyl orange claiming that degradation products of the compounds did not interfere [P.Y. Khoshaba & O.H. Abdalmageed, *J. Anal. Chem.*, **4(1)**, 41, 1995].

The ion-pair complex formation (1 : 1) with above-mentioned dyes was proposed by Sherifel. All the coloured complexes are extractable into chloroform, bromothymol blue (414 nm), bromophenol blue (415 nm) and naphthol blue black B (627 nm).

Reference

Z.A. El Sherif, A.O. Mohamed, M.I. Walash & F.M. Tarras, J. Pharm. & Biomed. Analysis, **22**, 13-23, 2000.

Note

1. The authors have claimed that degradation products generated by alkaline potassium permanganate oxidation did not interfere in acid-dye method.
2. The authors also proposed a charge-transfer (CT) method using iodine and measuring the absorbance of the resulting solution at 295 nm.

Streptomycin sulphate

Follow the method 1 (reaction with oxidised sodium nitroprusside) for estimation of streptomycin sulphate described in formulation 10 of this chapter.

Formulation 25

Furazolidone, Diphenoxylate hydrochloride, Atropine sulphate

ESTIMATION

Furazolidone

Follow the method described under formulation 17 of this chapter.

Diphenoxylate hydrochloride

Transfer accurately weighed quantity of the sample equivalent to 100 mg of the substance to a separating funnel. Add 25 ml of water and 2 ml of 10 N sodium hydroxide solution. Extract with five 25 ml portions of chloroform. Wash the combined chloroform layer with water and pass through anhydrous sodium sulphate placed over cotton plug (pre-moistened). Evaporate chloroform layer to dryness and take up the residue in 50 ml of glacial acetic acid. Titrate with 0.05 N perchloric acid using crystal violet solution as indicator. Each ml of 0.05 N perchloric acid is equivalent to 0.02445 g of diphenoxylate hydrochloride. The compound has λ_{max} 258 nm in 0.01 N methanolic hydrochloric acid as well.

Atropine sulphate

Reagents

1. 88% sulphuric acid (44 ml of concentrated sulphuric acid and 6 ml of water).
2. Acetic anhydride.
3. 16.0% w/v solution of p-dimethylaminobenzaldehyde (PDAB) in 88% sulphuric acid.

Standard solution

50 mcg/ml of atropine sulphate in methanol.

Sample solution

Accurately weigh the sample equivalent to 1 mg of atropine sulphate. Add about 100 ml of water, boil on water-bath for 15 min, cool and make up to 200 ml with water. Acidify 100 ml of the resultant solution with 0.1 N sulphuric acid and extract with four 25 ml portions of chloroform. Discard the chloroform layer. Basify the acidic layer with 5 N ammonium hydroxide and extract with five 25 ml portions of chloroform, washing each separated layer with the same 20 ml water. Shake the combined chloroform layer with 25 ml of 0.1 N sulphuric acid, discard the organic layer. Repeat the process of basification and extraction into chloroform as described above. The final chloroform extract is passed through anhydrous sodium sulphate and evaporated to dryness. The residue is taken in methanol to get a concentration of 50 mcg/ml.

Procedure

Evaporate 2 ml each of sample and standard solutions on water-bath. Add 0.5 ml of 'PDAB' solution and allow to stand for 2 minutes. Heat on water-bath exactly for 5 minutes, cool, add 5 ml of acetic anhydride, mix and allow to stand for 30 minutes. Measure the absorption of both the solutions at about 515 nm against reagent blank. Calculate the results by comparison.

Probable Reaction Mechanism

'PDAB' will condense at methylamino ($NHCH_3$) site of the molecule to give coloured product.

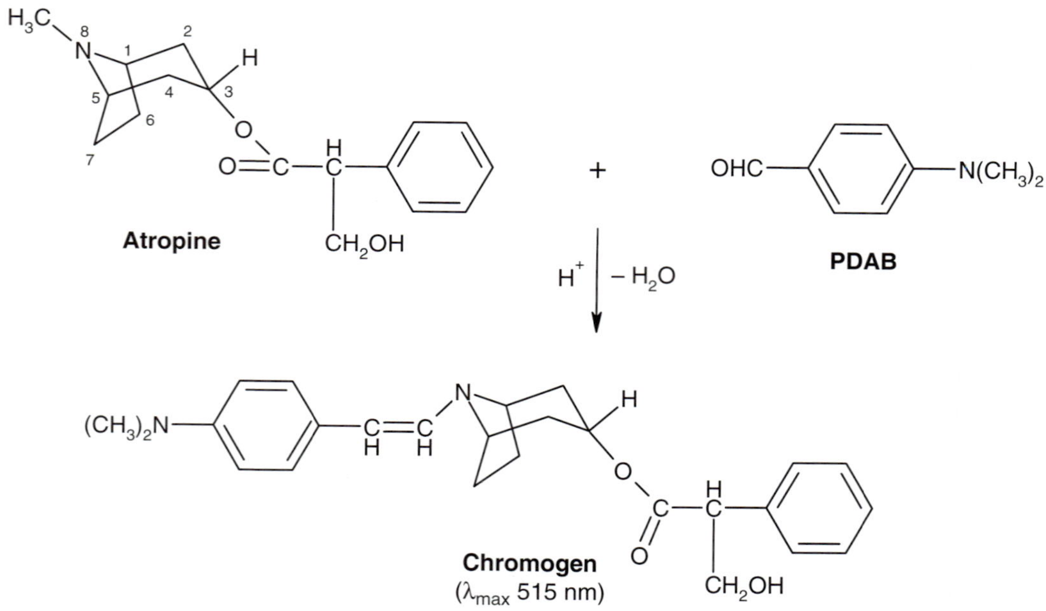

Reference

Pharmaceutical Chemistry (Vol. 2) by H.J. Roth, pp. 507, 508.

The final chromogen extract of atropine (base) as obtained may be used for forming charge-transfer (C-T) complex with chloranilic acid (CA). The alkaloid acts as donor whereas chloranilic acid acts as acceptor. 2% solution of chloranilic acid is used for complex formation with λ_{max} 535 nm.

To appropriate quantity of the atropine (base) solution in chloroform add 15 ml of chloranilic acid solution, mix, add 20 ml of dioxan and measure the absorbance of resulting purple-coloured solution at 535 nm.

In dioxan-chloroform medium, atropine reacts instantaneously with 'CA'. In non-aqueous medium, 'CA' exists as HA which acts as acceptor. By experimental studies the author confirmed it to be 1 : 1 C-T complex. It is similar to the one for amino acid C-T complex with CA. The linearity range was 0.03-0.25 mg/ml (as free base). As acceptor, chloranilic acid is superior to chloranil in that the reaction is instantaneous and colour stable for 24 hr whereas with chloranil the complex formation is slow and colour is stable for 2 hr only.

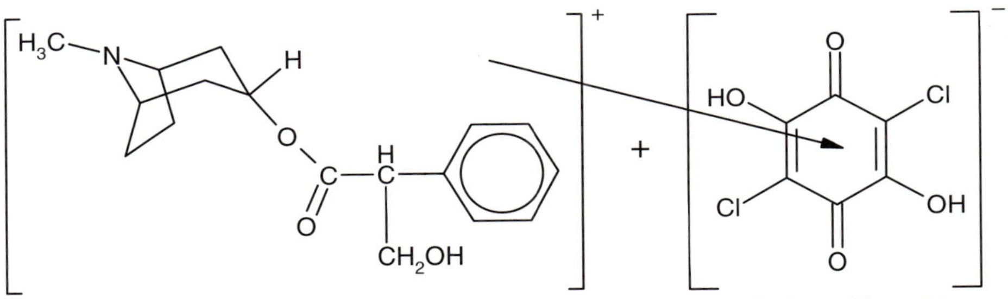

Chloranilic acid

Atropine - CA C-T complex
(λ_{max} 535 nm)

Reference

M. Abdel-Hady Elsayed & Suraj P. Agarwal, *Talanta*, **29**, 535-537, 1982.

Formulation 26

Furazolidone, Iodochlorhydroxyquinoline, Homatropine methyl bromide

ESTIMATION

Furazolidone

Standard solution

Transfer accurately weighed 25 mg of furazolidone to a 50 ml volumetric flask, add 25 ml of dimethylformamide, heat to dissolve and make up the volume with dimethyl formamide. Dilute 2 ml of the resultant solution to 200 ml with water (5 mcg/ml).

Sample solution

Transfer accurately weighed quantity of the sample equivalent to 25 mg of furazolidone to a 50 ml volumetric flask, add 25 ml of dimethylformamide, heat to dissolve and make up the volume. Filter and dilute 2 ml of the filtrate to 200 ml with water (5 mcg/ml).

Measure the absorption of both the solutions at 367 nm using dimethylformamide as blank. Deduce the results by comparison or by using 750 as value of A 1%, 1 cm at 367 nm.

Iodochlorhydroxyquinoline

Reagents

1. 1% w/v solution of ferric chloride in water.
2. Acetone.

Standard solution

Dissolve accurately weighed quantity of iodochlorhydroxyquinoline in acetone with slight warming to get a concentration of 500 mcg/ml.

Sample solution

Extract accurately weighed quantity of sample with acetone by slight warming to produce 500 mcg/ml of iodochlorhydroxyquinoline.

Procedure

To 2 ml each of sample and standard solutions, add 1 ml of ferric chloride solution and make up the volume to 25 ml with acetone. Measure the absorption of both the solutions at about 650 nm against reagent blank. Calculate the results by comparison.

Probable Reaction Mechanism

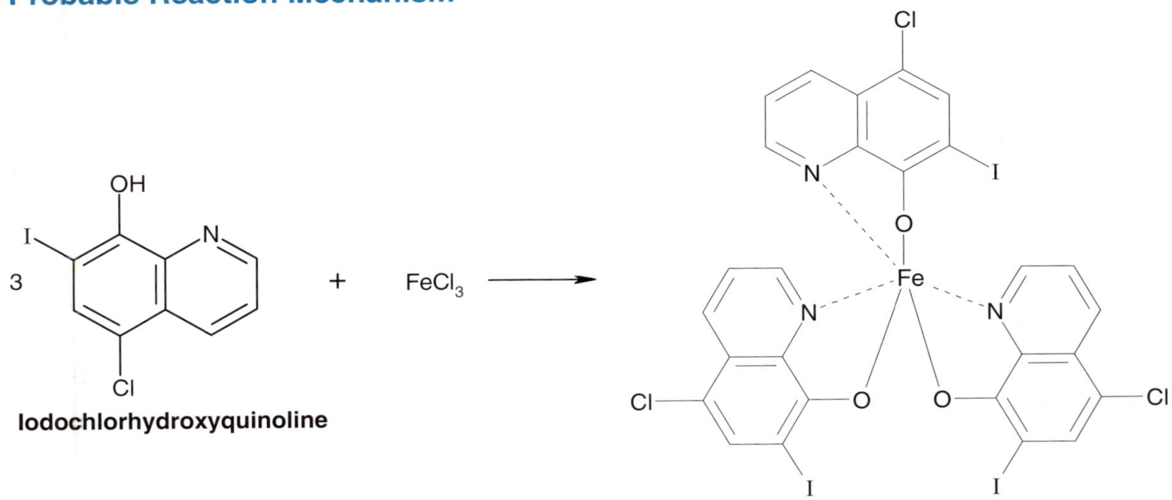

Iodochlorhydroxyquinoline

3 : 1 Drug - Fe^{3+} deep green-coloured complex
(λ_{max} 650 nm)

Note

1. When DMF was used as solvent, λ_{max} was observed at 635 nm.
2. Metronidazole, sulphonamides, chloroquine, berberine and papaverine did not interfere.

Reference

1. A.K. Sen & T.K. Das, Indian Drugs, **26(10)**, 583-585, 1989.
2. L. Ramadevi & K. Sriraman, Indian Drugs, **34(2)**, 81-84, 1992.

Homatropine methyl bromide

Reagents

1. 0.2 M cerric ammonium sulphate.
2. 1 N sodium hydroxide.
3. Anion-exchange resin-1R-400 (Cl^-).
4. Glass column 50 cm × 1.5 cm (ID) fitted with G_2 sintered disc.

Column preparation

Place a small quantity of fine glass wool on the base of the column. Suspend the resin in water and pour over the column to an height of 25 cm. Cover the tip of the column with a glass wool plug. Wash the column with 150-200 ml of water. The column is ready for use.

Sample solution

Transfer accurately weighed quantity of the sample equivalent to 5 mg of the substance to a 100 ml volumetric flask, add 40-50 ml of water. Shake well and make up the volume with water. Filter and add the entire filtrate to the prepared column. Wash the column first with 30 ml of water and discard the eluate. Collect subsequent eluates and make up to 100 ml with water.

Standard solution

Equivalent to 5 mg of the substance is treated as sample solution.

Procedure

Transfer 10 ml each of sample and standard solutions to a stoppered flask. To each add 20 ml of sodium hydroxide solution and heat in a water-bath at 80°C for 15 min. Cool, add 8 ml of 0.2 M cerric ammonium sulphate and mix, add 25 ml of n-hexane and shake for 15 min. Decant the organic layer and concomitantly determine the absorbance of both the solutions at about 242 nm using n-hexane as blank. Calculate the results by comparison.

Note

Separation through column is not often required. Directly basify the sample, standard solutions and follow the procedure as described above.

The compound being cation, it forms insoluble salts with different anions such as reineckate, silicotungstate followed by spectrophotometric determination. Hanna et al. (1977) have reported a spectrophotometric method based on formation of a picric acid - quaternary amm. complex, adsorbed on acid-washed diatomaceous earth and column eluted with chloroform and absorbance of yellow complex measured at 365 nm.

Note

The method is stability indicating as hydrolytic degradation product of homatropine methyl bromide did not form complex with picric acid.

Reference

S. Hanna, M. Rosen, L. Rasero & H. Lachman, *J. Pharm. Sci.*, **66(1)**, 123-124, 1977.

Formulation 27

Norfloxacin / Ciprofloxacin, Tinidazole

ESTIMATION

Norfloxacin/Ciprofloxacin

METHOD 1

Reagents

1. 0.1 M hydrochloric acid.
2. 1% w/v solution of ferric chloride in 0.1 M hydrochloric acid to prevent hydrolysis.

Standard solution

100 mcg/ml of norfloxacin in 0.1 N hydrochloric acid.

Sample solution

Weigh accurately powdered sample equivalent to 100 mg of the substance, add 60-70 ml of 0.1 N hydrochloric acid, shake for 10 min and make up to 100 ml with the acid. Further dilution is done with the acid to get final concentration of 100 mcg/ml.

Procedure

To 5 ml each of sample and standard solutions, add 1 ml of freshly prepared ferric chloride solution and make up to 50 ml with 0.1 N hydrochloric acid. Measure the absorption of both the solutions at a maximum at about 438 nm against reagent blank (1 ml of ferric chloride solution diluted to 50 ml with the acid) and calculate the contents of norfloxacin by comparison.

As the ring has both ketocarbonyl as well as carboxylic acid functions, oxygen can donate or share a lone pair of electrons with iron (Fe^3) to form a complex. The compound may form 2 : 1 complex.

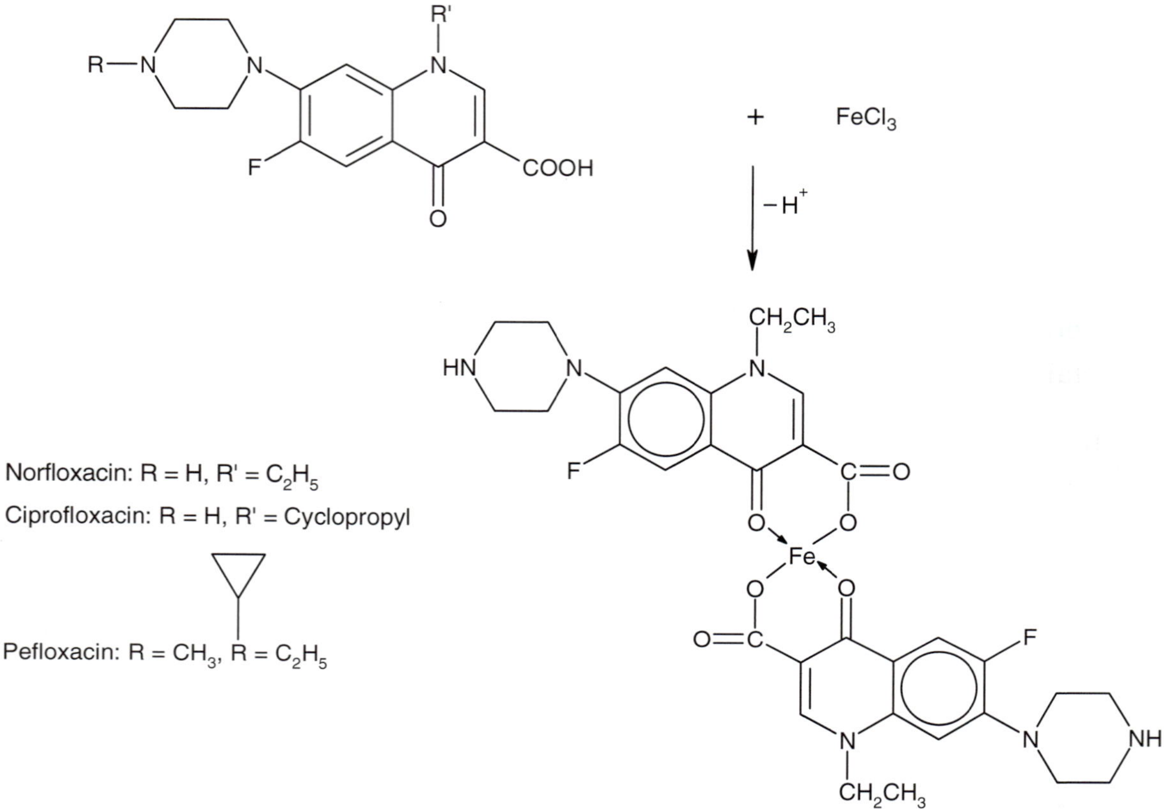

Probable structure of the iron(III) - NRF chelate yellow orange
(λ_{max} 438 nm)

Reference

1. Avadhanulu & Pantulu, *Indian Drugs*, **31(6)**, 258-262, 1993.
2. K.P.R. Chowdary & A. Annapurna, *Indian Drugs*, **29(13)**, 612-615, 1992.
3. Lorena Fratini & Elfrides E.S. Schapoval, *International J. Pharmaceutics*, **127**, 279-282, 1996.
4. Sangeeta Gaba et al., *The Eastern Pharmacist*, p. 115, 1998.
5. R.C. Mashru et al., *The Eastern Pharmacist*, pp. 113-114, 1997.

Note

Other quinoline derivatives produce similar iron chelate.

Belal et al. have given comprehensive review of analytical methods for analysis of 4-quinoline derivatives. While describing the method based on reaction with ferric chloride, the following reaction product was proposed.

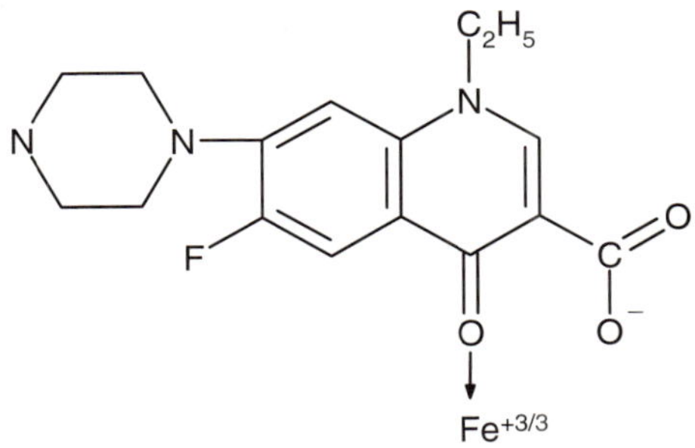

Reference

F. Belal, A.A. Al-Majed & A.M. Al-Obaid, *Talanta*, **50**, 765-786, 1999.

The same reaction based on 1 : 1 complex was proposed by G. Rama Rao (1990) and Shanbag (1991).

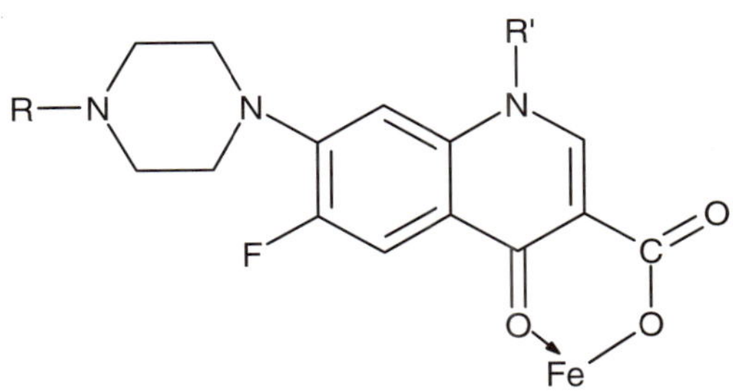

Ciprofloxacin and other quinoline derivatives shall react similarly.

Reference

1. G. Rama Rao et al., *Indian Drugs*, **27(10)**, 532, 1990.
2. S.G. Shanbag, P.P. Thampi & C. Sarla Thampi, *Indian Drugs*, **28(6)**, 279-280, 1991.

Other authors who have reported methods with different quinoline derivatives based on complexation with Fe^{3+} are: S.C. Mathur, Y. Kumar, N. Murgesan & Y.K.S. Rathor, *Indian Drugs*, **27(7)**, 398, 1990; **29(8)**, 376, 1992; *Eastern Pharmacist*, **35**, 117-118, 1992.

Norfloxacin - iron(III) complex was studied in detail by Issopoulos, 1989, while estimating trace amount of iron. Complexation was carried out at pH 3 with ionic strength of about 0.3 M (maintained with 0.1 M ammonium sulphate). By mole ratio method and continuous method the author established the composition of norfloxacin - Fe(III) as 2 : 1. It was also observed by the author that at lower pH values i.e. 0.5-2 the complex was yellowish-orange whereas at pH 3.0 and above the colour of the complex was yellow (λ_{max} 377 nm).

Note

Structure of the complex (2 : 1) is the same as under method 1.

Reference

Prodromos B. Issopoulos, *Analyst*, **114**, 627-630, 1989.

M.E. El-Konmnos et al. have described the general structure of several fluoroquinoline derivatives (ciprofloxacin, norfloxacin, difloxacin, amifloxacin, lomefloxacin, ofloxacin, pefloxacin, nalidixic acid) - metal (M) chelate.

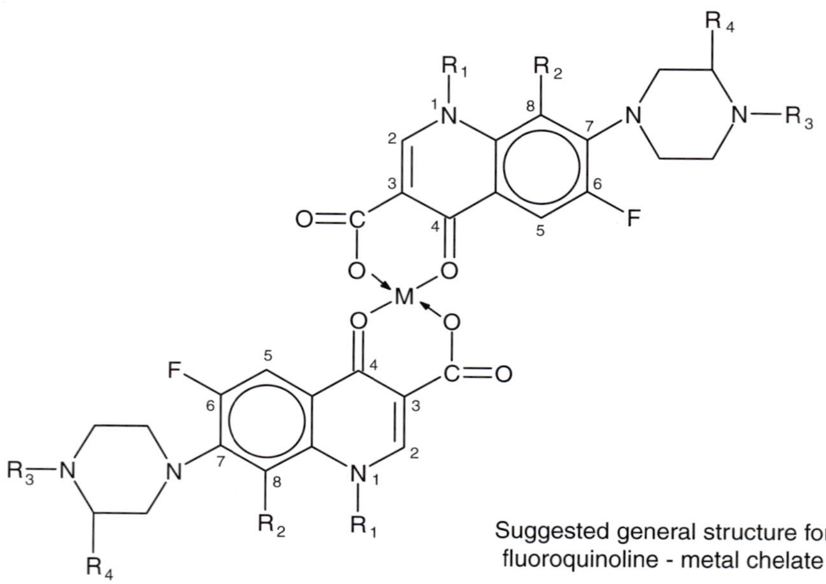

Suggested general structure for fluoroquinoline - metal chelate

Reference

M.E. El-Konmnos et al., *Talanta*, **60**, 1044-1054, 2003.

METHOD 2

Reagents

1. 0.005 M solution of p-chloranil (Cl) in acetonitrite.
2. 0.005 M solution of chloranilic acid (CLA) in acetonitrite.

Standard solution

500 mcg/ml of norfloxacin in acetonitrite.

Sample solution

An accurately weighed quantity of the sample equivalent to 50 mg of the substance was extracted with acetonitrite to produce 100 ml (500 mcg/ml).

Procedure

To 2 ml each of the sample and standard solutions, add 2.5 ml of either of the reagents and heat on water-bath at 60°C for 10 min, cool and make up to 25 ml with acetonitrite. Measure the absorption of the sample and standard solutions against reagent blank at 550 nm (Cl) and 531 nm (CLA). The method obeys Beer's law in the concentration range of 10-230 mcg/ml (Cl) and 20-250 mcg/ml (CLA) and the colour is stable for about 2 hrs. The reaction is based on exchange of p electrons, norfloxacin being the donor and p-chloranil/chloranilic acid being the π electron acceptors.

Note

While analysing the eye drops, sample is required to be extracted with chloroform after basification and chloroform solution was used for analysis.

Probable Reaction Mechanism

The secondary amine group (less sterically hindered and most basic) present in the ring of the drug being nucleophilic will attack the benzene skeletal of the chloranil or chloranilic acid (π acceptor) and add to the enone system of the reagent as Michael addition.

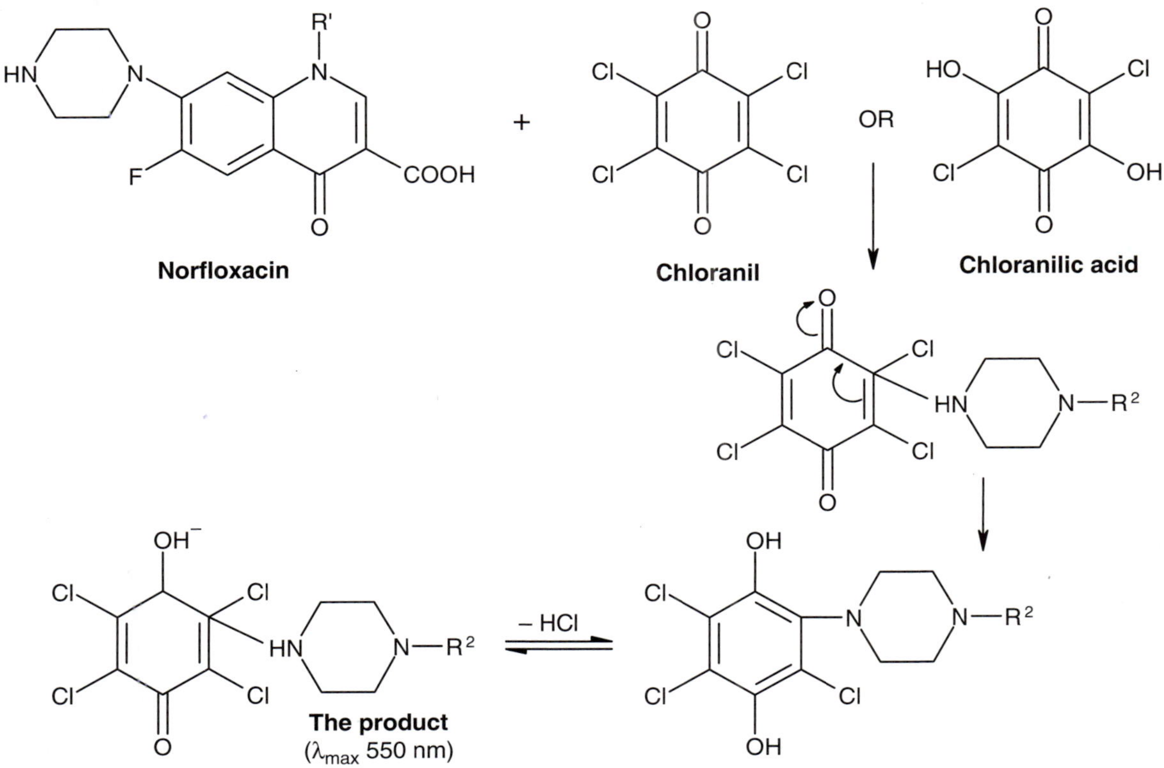

The complex with chloranilic acid is represented as under:

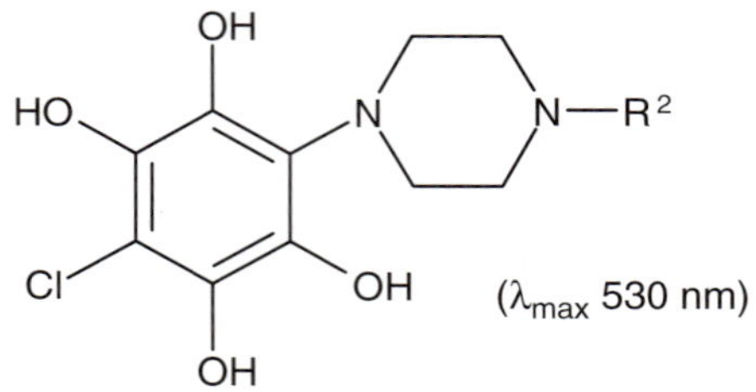

This reaction is answered by other fluoroquinolones such as enoxacin and lomefloxacin as well.

Note

Charge transfer complexation with tetracyanoethylene (TCNE) and 2,3-dichloro-5,6-dicyano-p-benzoquinone (DDQ) has been reported for quantity analysis of different quinoline derivatives by different authors.

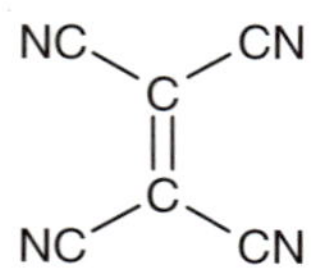

TCNE

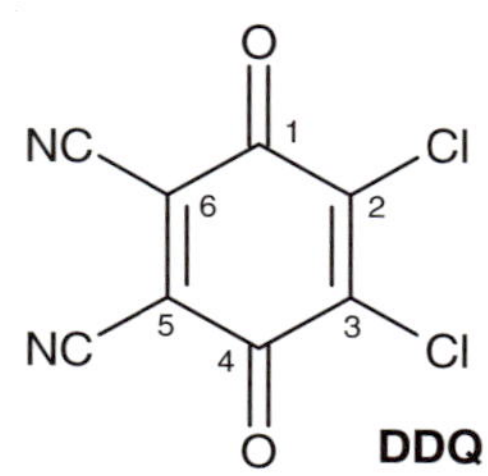

DDQ

The complex is represented as under:

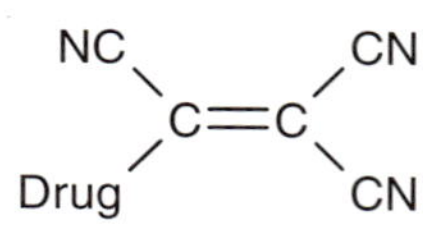

Tricyanovinyl derivatives

Reference

1. S.P. Agarwal & Sanjula Baboola, *Ind. J. Pharm. Sci.*, **63(1)**, 345-347, 2001.
2. Sania Mostafa et al., *J. Pharm. & Biomed. Anal.*, **27**, 133, 2002.

METHOD 3

This method is based on charge transfer between the reagent, electron acceptor and the drug. The N-atom with lone electron pair is predominantly involved due to spacial structure resulting in the formation of a π-π^* CT complex. This reaction is also answered by analgin and cinnarizine whereas benzene ring of analgin is the most electron-rich.

Reagent

0.2% solution of 7,7,8,8-tetrachlorocyanoquinodimethane in acetone (TCNQ).

Sample and standard solutions

100 μg/ml in acetone.

Procedure

To 1 ml each of sample and standard solutions add 2 ml of TCNQ reagent, keep at 35°C for 30 min and measure the absorbance at λ_{max} 740 nm against reagent blank.

Probable Reaction Mechanism

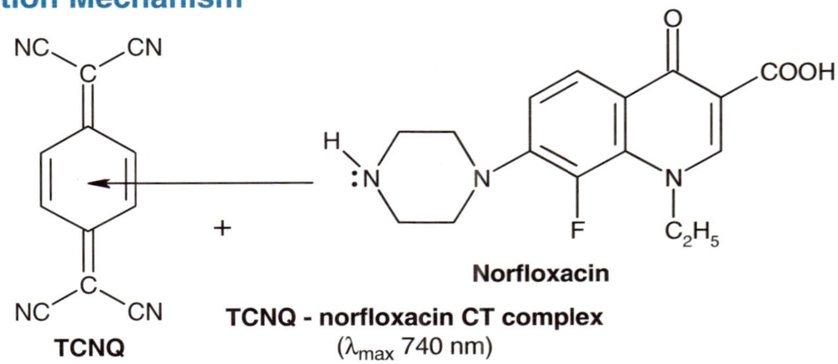

Reference

Zhao Feng-hin, Xu Bian-zhen, Zhang Zhi-quan & Tong Shen-yang, *J. Pharm. & Biomed. Analysis*, **21**, 355-360, 1999.

METHOD 4

It forms coloured Meisenheimer complex with Sanger's reagent.

Reagents

1. 1.3% w/v solution of 2,4-dinitrofluorobenzene (DNFB) in acetone.
2. Borate buffer, pH 8.0.
3. 0.2% w/v solution of 'DNFB' in DMSO.
4. Acidified dioxan: Saturate dioxan with HCl gas and then prepare 0.5 M acidified dioxan.

Procedure

(a) To 1 ml each of sample/standard solution (500 μg/ml), prepared in acetone, add 0.6 ml of the reagent (1.3%), keep in water-bath (60°C) for 20 min, cool, add acidic dioxan to produce 25 ml. Measure the absorbance at 365 nm against reagent blank.

Note

To remove excess of reagent, which interferes in measurement, it was hydrolysed by HCl.

(b) To 0.5 ml of sample/standard solution (100 µg/ml), prepared in $DMSO_4$, add 'DNFB' reagent prepared in DMSO, dilute to 25 ml with DMSO and measure the absorbance at 410 nm against reagent blank.

Probable Reaction Mechanism

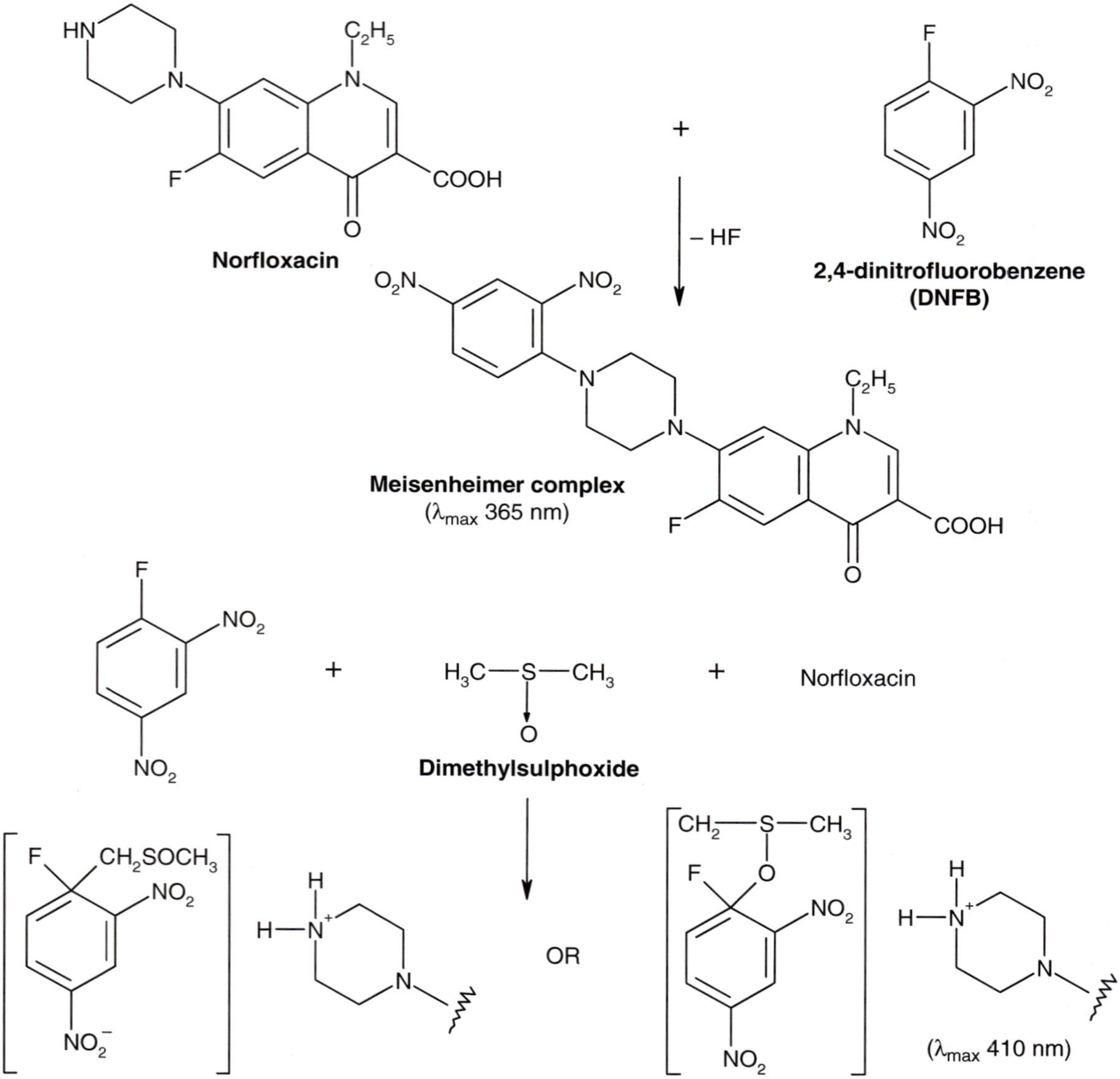

Note

1. DMSO being bipolar aprotic solvent it stabilizes the conjugate base of polynitro derivative.

2. While using DMSO, the colour development was instantaneous and no heating required due to better solvation power.
3. In method (a), in slightly alkaline medium (pH 8.0), 'DNFB' reagent is hydrolysed to dinitrophenolate which is coloured (λ_{max} 365 nm). Hence, it interferes in the analysis of the compound. However, after completion of the reaction, on addition of acidic dioxane, dinitrophenolate gets converted to phenol which is colourless, hence no interference.

Probable Reaction Mechanism

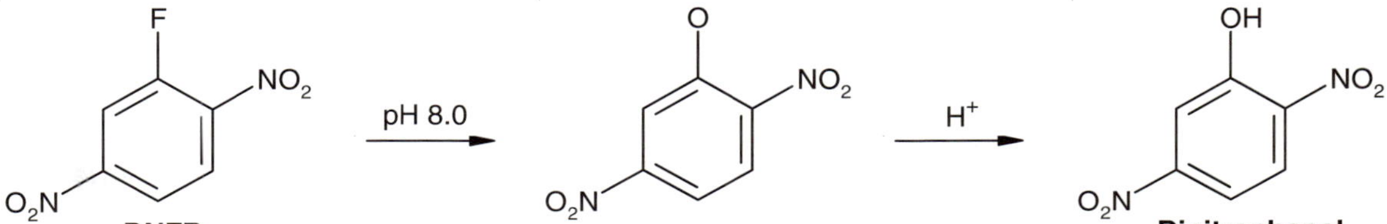

DNFB **Phenolate (coloured)** (λ_{max} 365 nm) **Dinitrophenol**

Note

Other quinoline derivatives also undergo similar reaction.

Reference

1. Abdel Fattah, M. El-Walily Omayma, Abdel Razak, S.F. Belal & Ranias Bakry, *J. Pharm. & Biomed. Analysis*, **21**, 1069-76, 1999.
2. K.P.R. Chowdary & N. Ravikumar, *Indian Drugs*, **37(9)**, 448-450, 2000.

METHOD 5

Reagents

1. 0.1 M cerric ammonium sulphate in 1 M sulphuric acid.
2. 0.1 M sodium hydroxide.

Sample and standard solutions

500 μg/ml in 0.1 M sodium hydroxide.

Procedure

To 0.5 ml of the sample or standard solution add 1 ml of cerric(IV) solution and make up the volume to 10 ml with 0.1 M NaOH and measure the absorption at 484 nm.

Probable Reaction Mechanism

Secondary amines are oxidized initially to secondary amine oxides and then tautomerize to N,N-dialkylhydroxylamines. Another reaction mechanism is proposed by other authors.

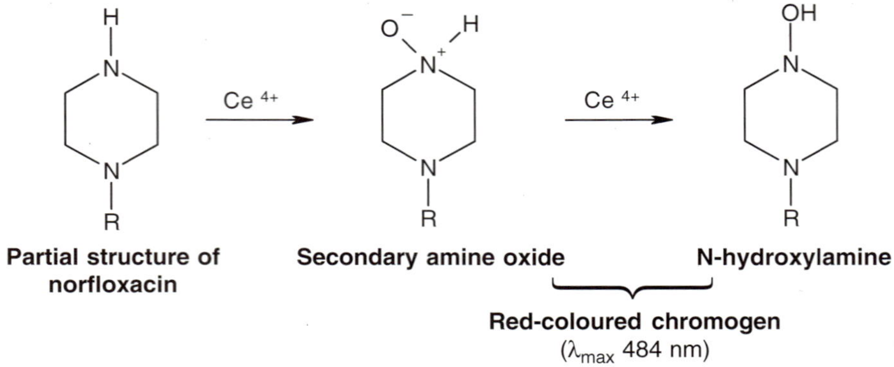

OR

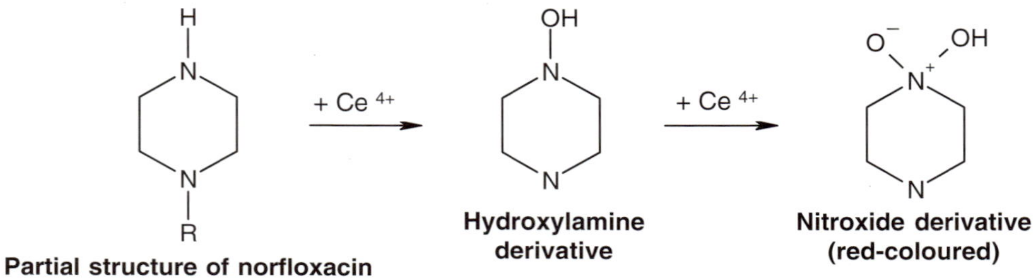

Reference

Organic Chemistry by Norman Allinger et al., Worth Publishers Inc., 1971, p. 576.

The detailed experimental conditions have been described by S.N. Mayyanathan, Manoj Sebastian & B. Suresh, Indian Drugs, 35(6), 344-347, 1998; and V.B. Patel & Rajani Giridhar, *Indian Drugs*, **34(2)**, 78-80, 1997.

Note

1. V.B. Patel et al. have recommended the use of ammonium sulphamate to increase the stability of chromogen by reducing the cerric(IV) ammonium sulphate thereby maintaining the integrity of the structure by preventing excess oxidation of the drug.
2. Patel et al. in their work have reported that the oxidative product is stable for 24 hrs and extractable into chloroform and have reported that chromogen has λ_{max} 350 nm and no NaOH was used in the method.

The compound reacts with croton aldehyde and 2,3-dichloro-1,4-naphthoquinone in DMF at 60°C to give blue chromogen (λ_{max} 640 nm). In this case first 1,4-naphthoquinone, being oxidizing agent, oxidizes croton aldehyde into corresponding acid which in turn condenses with piperazinyl function of the drug to give blue chromogen.

Probable Reaction Mechanism

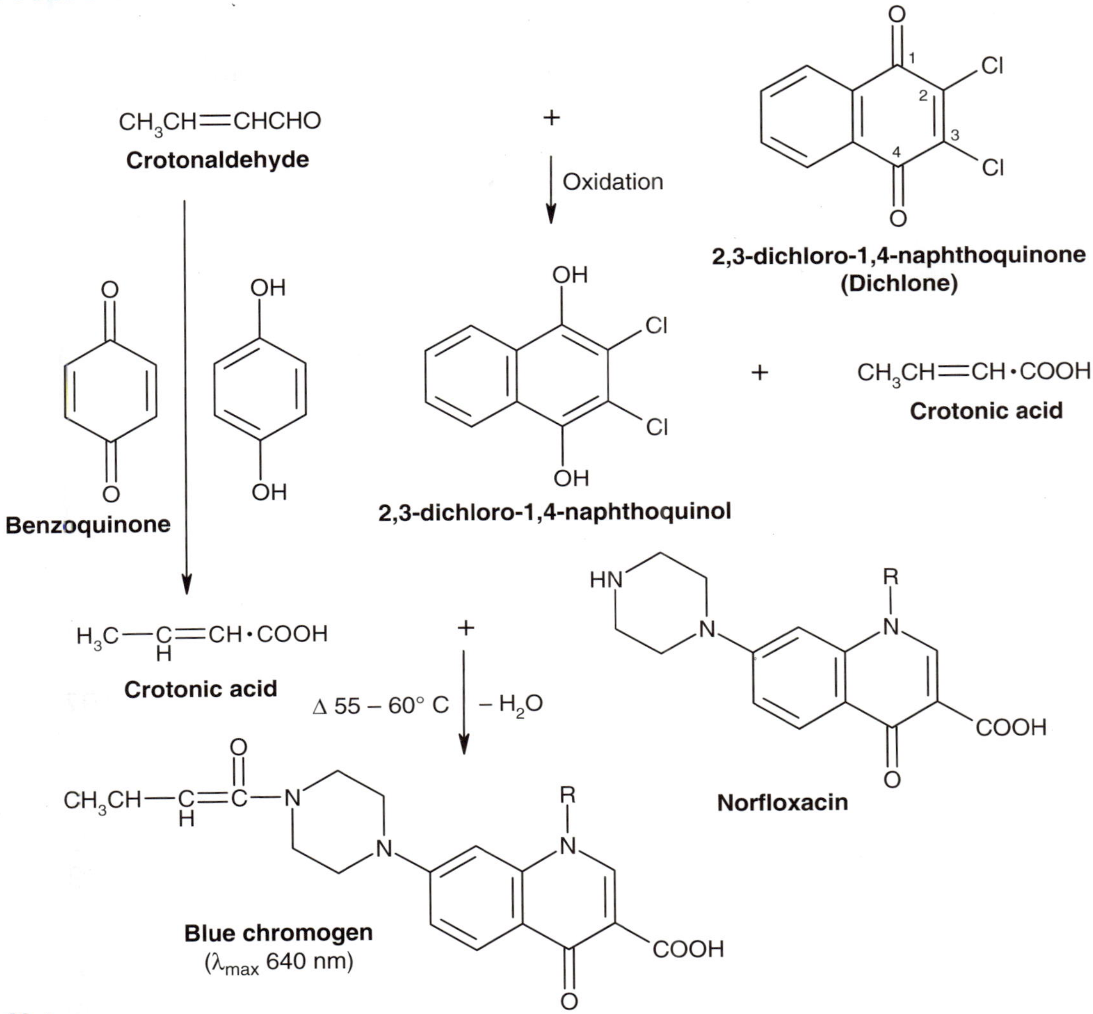

Note

1,4-Benzoquinone can also be used as oxidizing agent.

Reference

1. B.N. Suhagia, S.A. Shah, I.S. Rathod, H.M. Patel & Y.M. Rao, *Ind. J. Pharm. Sci.*, **68(2)**, 247-249, 2006.
2. Shaik Miftah Ahmed et al., *The Eastern Pharmacist*, pp. 145-146, 1997.

Note

This reaction is analogous to the one described by Buckly et al. (J. Chem. Soc., 3032, 1957), i.e. crotonaldehyde reacts with dichlone and diethylamine to give blue chromogen.

G. Rama Rao et al. (1989) have described spectrophotometric method for the estimation of norfloxacin based on oxidative coupling of MBTH with carbonyl (—C=O) group of the molecule to yield a chromogen (λ_{max} 630 nm).

To appropriate quantity of the sample and standard add 'MBTH' reagent followed by solution of cerric ammonium sulphate. The solution is allowed to stand for 20 min and then absorbance measured at 630 nm against reagent blank.

Probable Reaction Mechanism

This method is based on oxidative coupling of MBTH with carbonyl (C—O) group present in the molecule. On oxidation MBTH loses two electrons and one proton (H^+) to give intermediate nucleophilic species and attacks on the most nucleophilic site of the molecule.

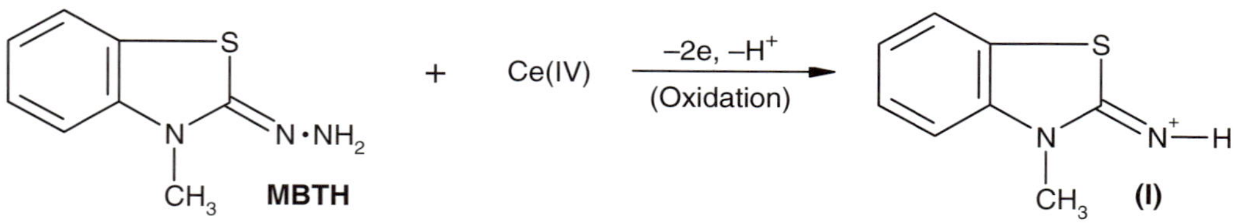

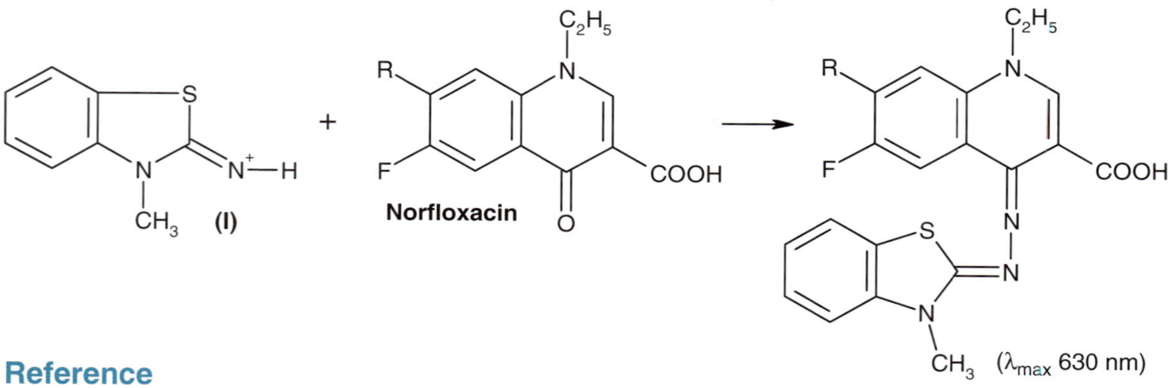

Reference

1. G. Rama Rao & A.B. Avadhanulu, *Indian Drugs*, **26(10)**, 580-581, 1989.
2. M. Gandhimathi, T.K. Ravi & J.V. Susheel, *Ind. J. Pharm. Sci.*, **67(8)**, 759-764, 2005.
3. P.G. Panzade et al., *The Eastern Pharmacist*, pp. 115-116, April 1997.
4. V. Phani Sekhar et al., *The Eastern Pharmacist*, pp. 113-114, Nov. 2001.
5. K.P.R. Chowdary et al., *The Eastern Pharmacist*, pp. 119-121, 1998.
6. V.K. Chakravarthy et al., *The Eastern Pharmacist*, pp. 121-122, 2000.

Recently Ilango et al. have reported estimation of gatifloxacin, another fluoroquinolone derivative, based on reaction involving oxidative coupling with MBTH using Fe(III) chloride as oxidizing agent. The authors have proposed different reaction mechanisms.

Probable Reaction Mechanism

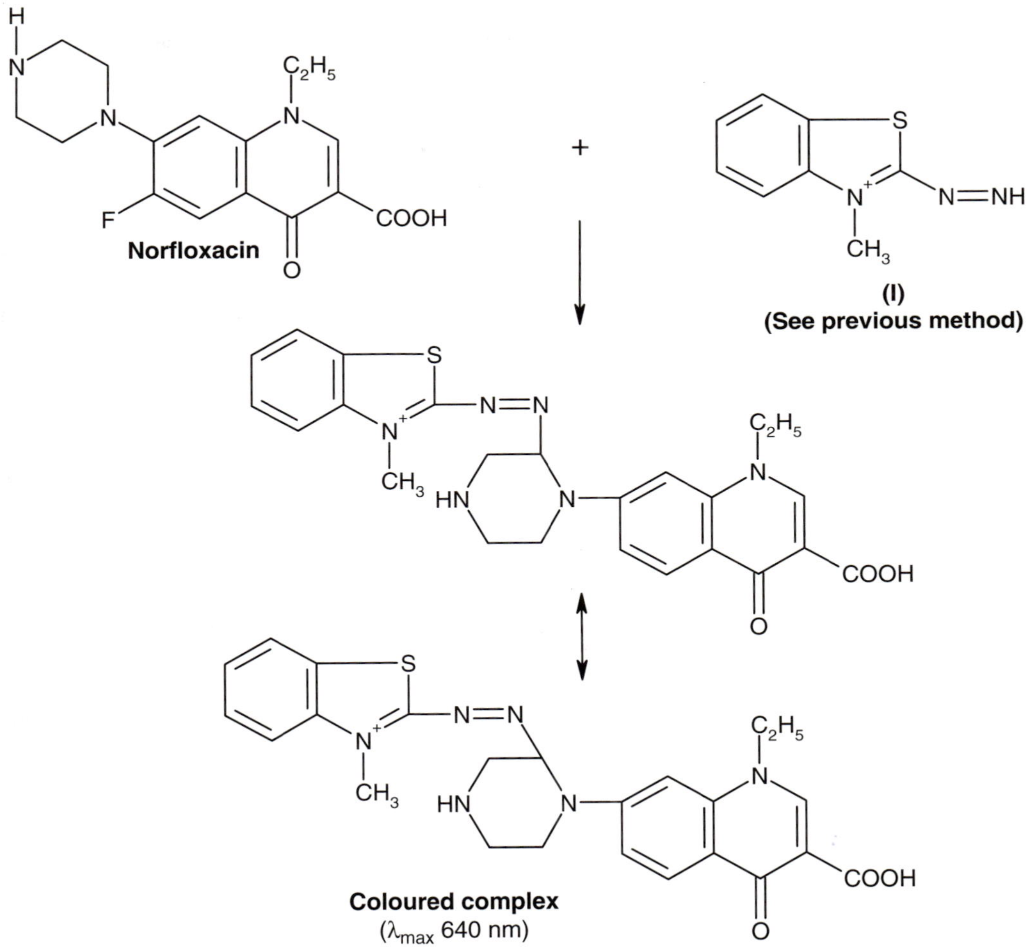

Reference

K. Ilango, P. Valentina, K.S. Lakshmi, Arvind Canhea, Sapana Rachel Abraham, V. Bhaskar Raju & A. Kiran Kumar, *Ind. J. Pharm. Sci.*, **68(2)**, 273-275, 2006.

Note

This reaction is similar to the one proposed by Murthy et al. for oxidative coupling of MBTH with trimetazidine (T.K. Murthy, Sankar Gowry & Y.S. Rao, *Indian Drugs*, **39(4)**, 230-233, 2002).

The secondary piperazine function of norfloxacin gets oxidized in alkaline medium and couples with resorcinol to give coloured complex.

Probable Reaction Mechanism

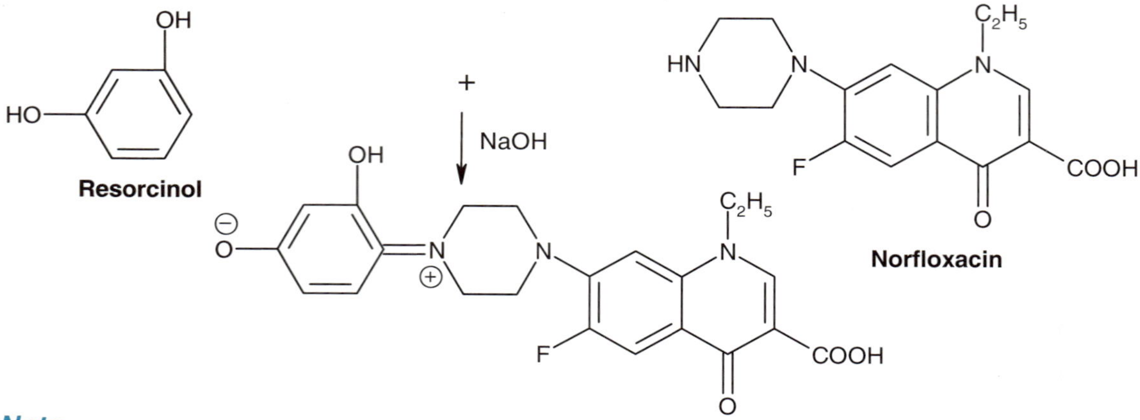

Note

This method was presented at 45th IPC.

The carbonyl group of quinoline 'derivatives' (norfloxacin, ciprofloxacin, ofloxacin, pefloxacin) condense with dinitrophenylhydrazine to give coloured condensation product.

Probable Reaction Mechanism

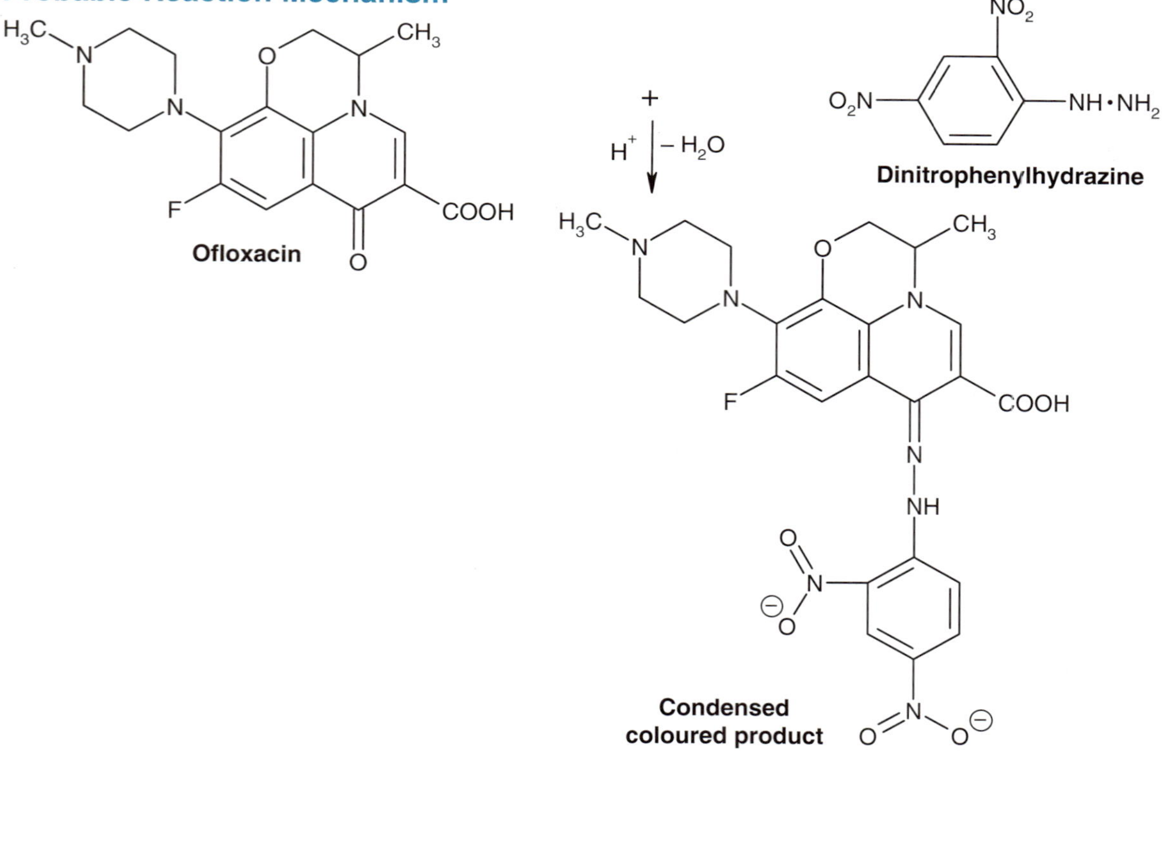

Reference

M.S. Nagar, K.R. Mahadik, N.N. Moore & S.S. Kadam, Abstract No. E-16, 45th IPC.

Norfloxacin gets oxidized on treatment with 5 M H_2SO_4 and cerric ammonium sulphate (CAS) to give product having λ_{max} 365 nm. The ethyl group at N-1 gets oxidized to corresponding aldehyde.

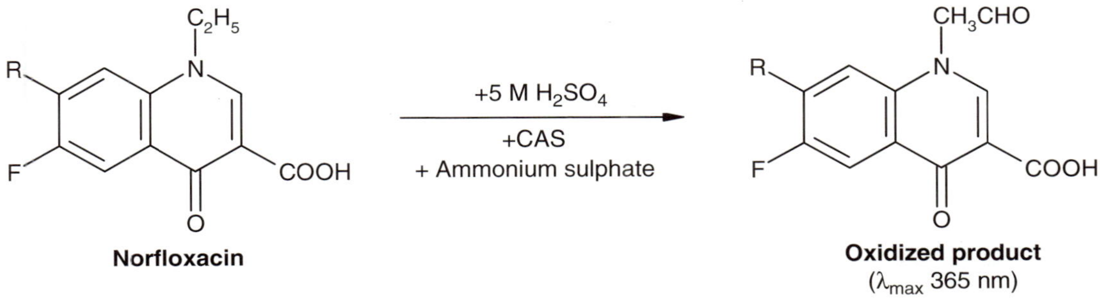

Note

Ammonium sulphate is added to increase stability of the colour by reducing excess of 'CAS' thereby preventing excessive oxidation of the compound.

Reference

1. Vandana B. Patel, *Indian Drugs*, **34(9)**, 497, 1997.
2. Analytical Profile of Drug Substances by K. Florey, Vol. 20, p. 590, 1991.
3. S.P. Hiremath et al., *The Eastern Pharmacist*, pp. 119-120, 1995.

Another oxidation product which is major metabolite of norfloxacin is:

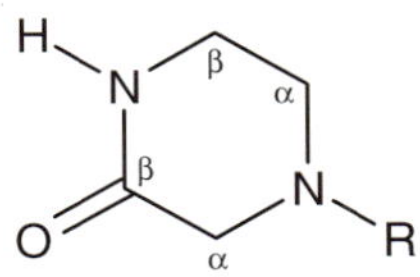

METHOD 6

Reagents

1. 0.2% solution of SV 3B in water.
2. 0.2% solution of TP 000 in water.
3. 0.1 M HCl.
4. Glycine - HCl buffer, pH 1.3.

Sample and standard solutions

1 mg/ml of substance in 0.01 M HCl, further dilute to get 100 μg/ml.

Procedure

(a) To 0.4 ml each of sample/standard solution add 6 ml of glycine buffer, pH 1.3 and 2 ml of the dye (SV 3B), dilute to 15 ml with water, add 10 ml of chloroform, shake for 2 min, separate organic layer and measure its absorbance at 575 nm against reagent blank.

(b) To appropriate quantity of the sample/standard solution add 6 ml of 0.1 M HCl and 2 ml of TP 000 and proceed further as under method (a).

Measure the absorbance of the sample and standard solutions at 485 nm against reagent blank.

Probable Reaction Mechanism

Method (a)

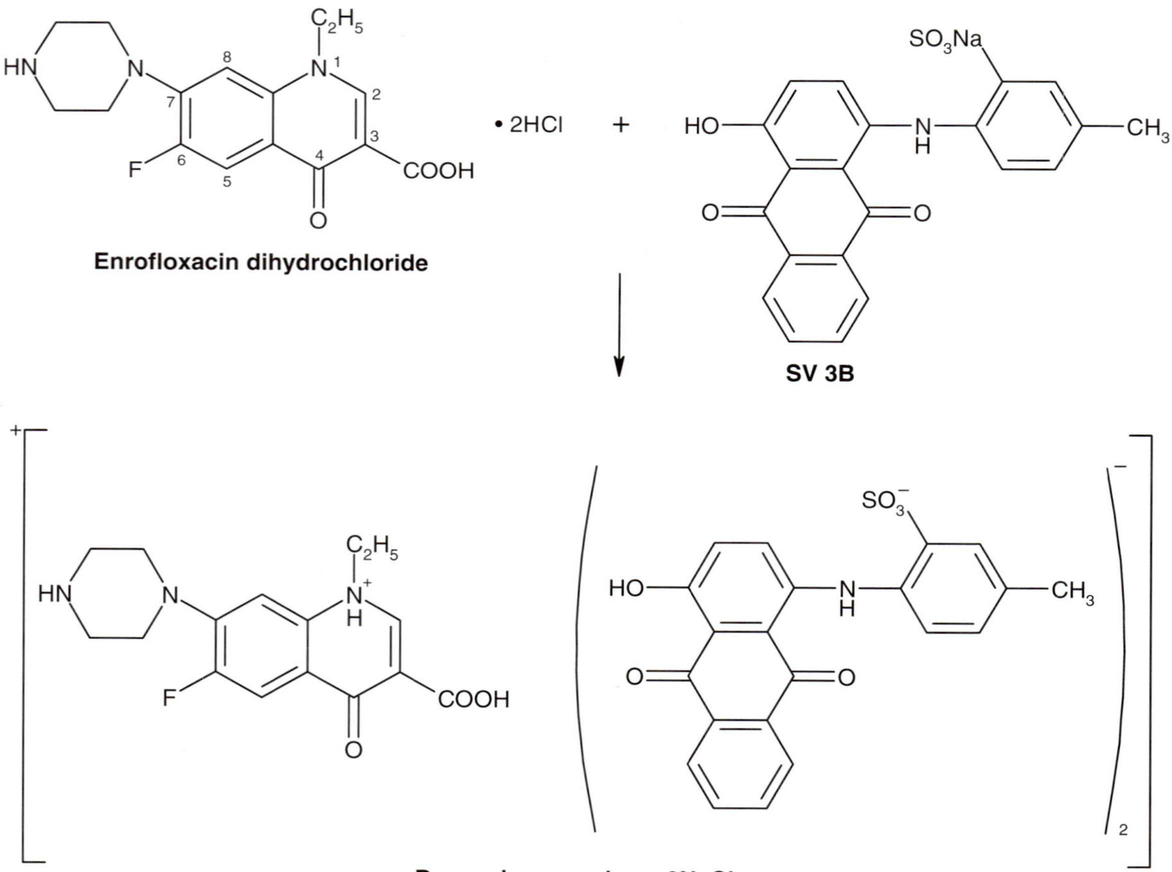

Drug - dye complex + 2NaCl
(λ_{max} 575 nm)

Method (b)

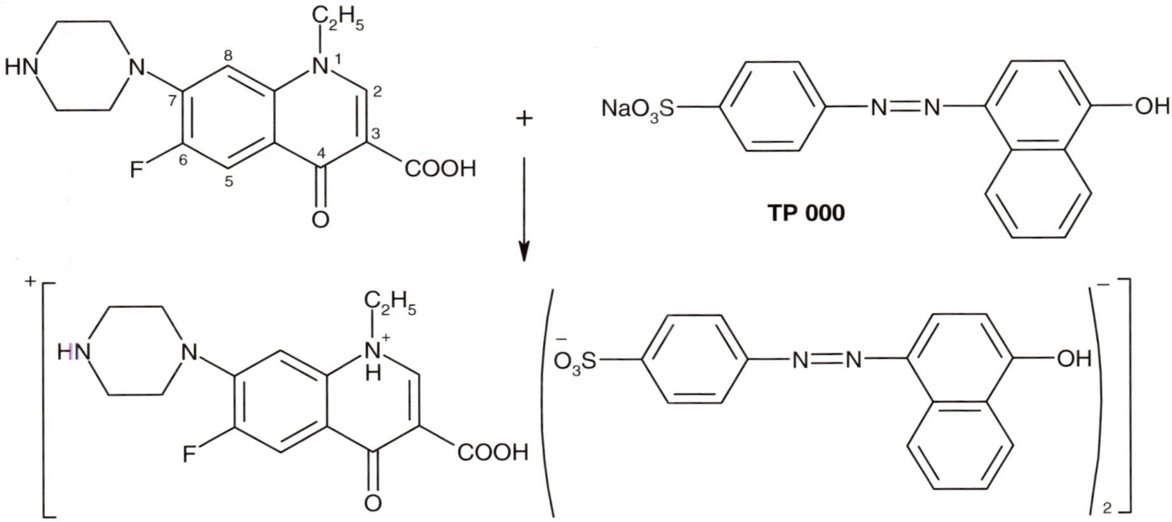

Drug - dye complex + 2NaCl
(λ_{max} 485 nm)

Note

Other fluoroquinolines such as ciprofloxacin and ofloxacin form coloured complexes with these dyes.

Reference

C.P.S. Sastry, Kolli Rama Rao & D. Shiva Prasad, *Talanta*, **42(3)**, 311-316, 1995.

Norfloxacin and ciprofloxacin are reported to form complex with eosin and palladium(II) for analysis.

Reagents

1. Conc. hydrochloric acid.
2. 0.5% solution of methylcellulose (1500 CP).
3. 0.2 M acetic acid.
4. 0.2 M sodium acetate.
5. Eosin solution 2×10^{-3} in water.
6. Palladium chloride solution: Dissolve 35.5 mg of $PdCl_2$ in 1 ml of conc. HCl with the aid of heat, add 50 ml of boiling water and then dilute to 100 ml.
7. Acetic acid - acetate buffer pH 4.0.

Sample and standard solutions

250 µg/ml in water.

Procedure

To 0.5 ml each of sample and standard solutions add 1.5 ml of methylcellulose solution, 2 ml of acetate buffer, 0.75 ml of eosin solution and 0.75 ml of $PdCl_2$ solution in this order, shake to mix and keep in water-bath (60°C) for 20 min, cool and measure the absorbance of the resulting solution at 545 nm.

Note

For spectrofluorometric measurements dilute 0.5 ml of the above solution to 100 ml with water and measure the fluorescence (exc: 310 nm; em: 540 nm).

Probable Reaction Mechanism

This method is based on chelate forming ability of the carboxylic and carbonyl groups present in quinolone derivatives with Pd^{++} with the subsequent formation of a ternary complex with eosin (sodium salt of 2,4,5,7-tetrabromofluorescein) in the presence of methylcellulose. Methylcellulose being non-ionic surfactant and helps to increase the reaction rate and also stabilizes the coloured complex.

Note

Other surfactants such as benzalkonium chloride (cationic), sodium laurylsulphate (anionic) and tween-80 were not found suitable.

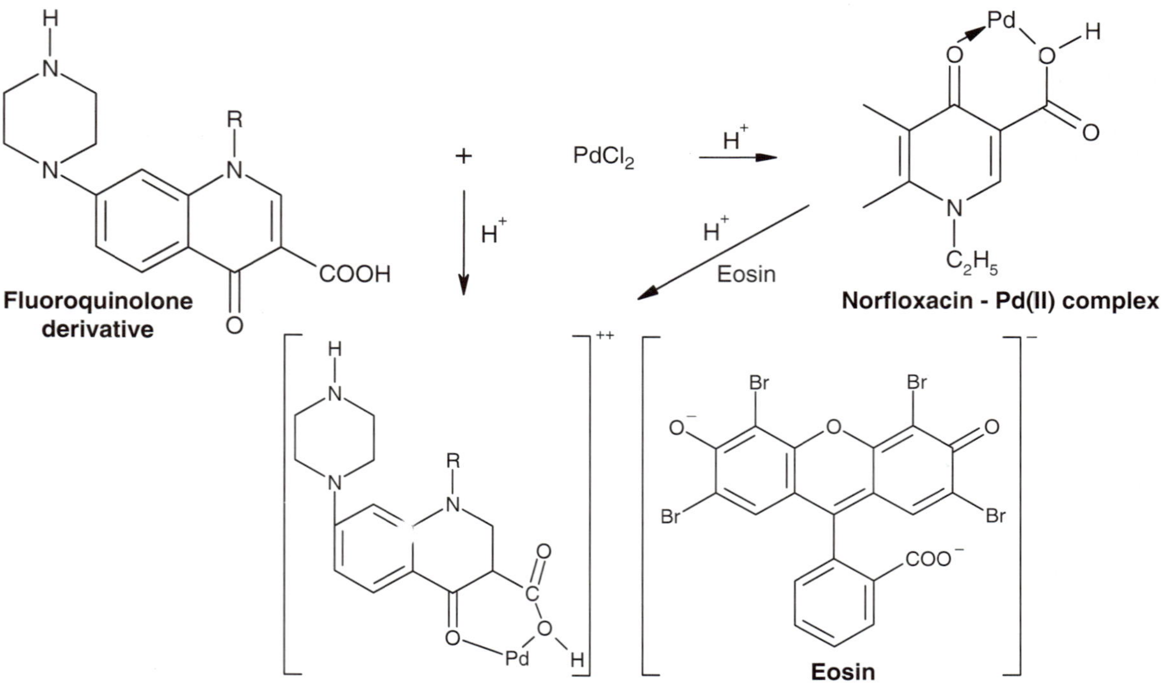

Ternary complex of fluoroquinoline Pd(II) and eosin
(λ_{max} 545 nm)

Reference

Abdel Fattah M. El-Walily, Said F. Belal & Rania S. Bakry, J. Pharm. & Biomed. Analysis, **14**, 561-569, 1996.

A similar method has been reported by Akram et al. (2007) with the proposed reaction mechanism which is similar to the one given above.

Probable explanation

The drug has 2 active groups i.e. —COOH and —C=O in the molecule. They have strong tendency to form coordinate compounds with transition metal ions. The drug reacts with Pd(II) ion and eosin to form ternary complex. First the drug forms chelate with Pd(II), being a transition element, through carbonyl and carboxylic group. Addition of eosin, a xanthine dye, to the drug - Pd chelate, an ion-pair complex sparingly soluble in water is formed in acetate buffer, pH 4.2. The presence of surfactant solubilizes the ternary complex so formed, hence extraction of the complex into organic solvent was not required. The composition of the ternary complex was 1 : 1 : 1.

Reference

Akram M. et al., *Analytical Letters*, **40**, 2708-2720, 2007.

Norfloxacin/ciprofloxacin has been reported to form charge-transfer (C-T) coloured complex with β-naphthol in acidic medium with λ_{max} 365 nm. β-nephthol acts as electron donor whereas fluoroquinolone acts as electron acceptor.

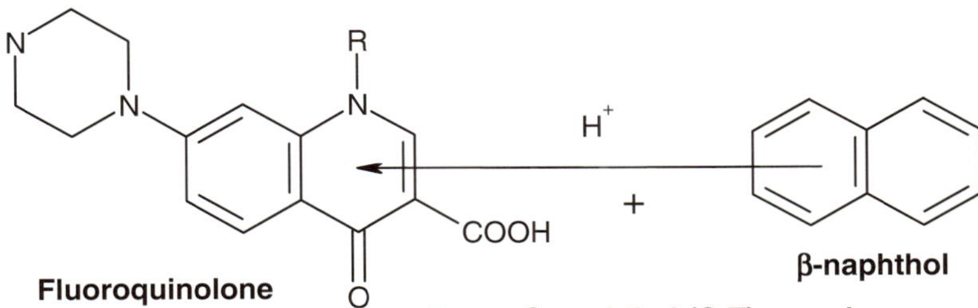

Drug - β-naphthol (C-T) complex
(λ_{max} 365 nm)

Reference

Varsha Jatav, S.K. Kashaw & P. Mishra, Indian J. Pharm. Sci., **67(4)**, 482-484, 2005.

A spectrophotometric method based on ion-pair complex formation with methyl orange (pH 3.5-3.7) and bromophenol blue (pH 2.4-2.6) has been reported as analytical method for the estimation of fluoroquinolones in tablets and solutions by Mostafa et al. (2002). Coloured complex has λ_{max} 420-425 nm.

Reference

Samia Mostafa, Mohamed El-Sadek & Esmail Awad Alla, *J. Pharm. & Biomed. Analysis*, **28**, 173-180, 2002.

An extractive colorimetric method described for lomefloxacin by R.T. Sane et al. could be applied to norfloxacin with suitable pH buffer. Four acidic dyes (BCP, BCG, BTB and BPB) form complexes at pH between 2.4–3.4 with λ_{max} at 412–422 nm.

Probable Reaction Mechanism

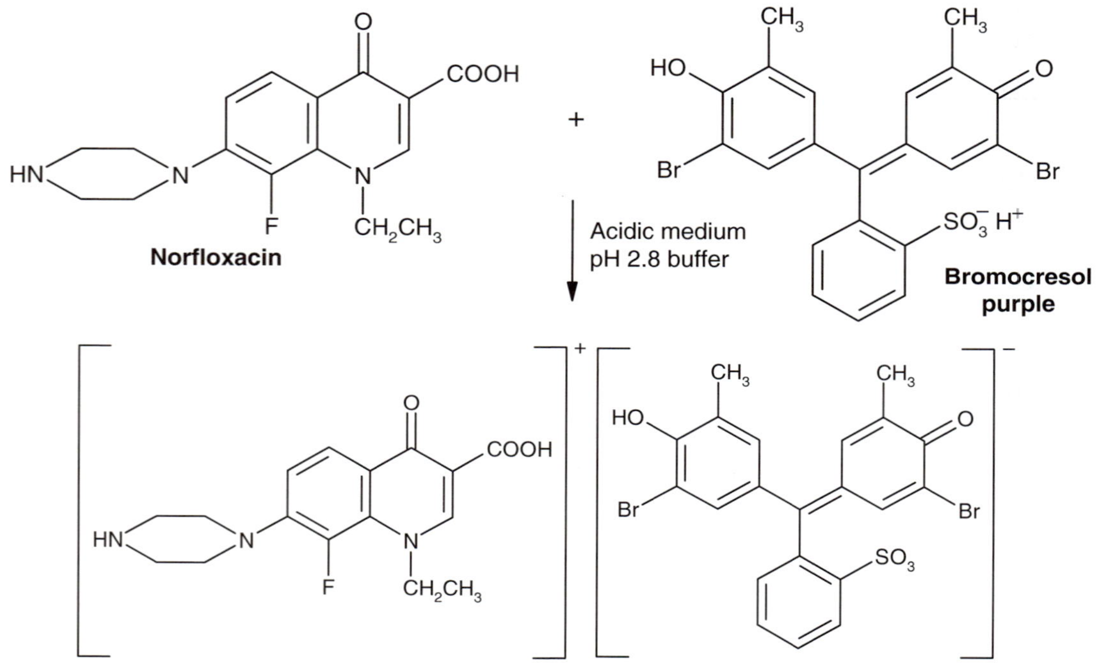

Ion-pair extracted in chloroform
(λ_{max} 416 nm)

Reference

Renu A. Sodhi, Jyoti L. Chawla & R.T. Sane, *Indian Drugs*, **34(9)**, 512, 1997.

A spectrophotometric method based on ion-pair complex formation has been described by Alaa S. Amin et al. (2008). The method is based on formation of complex between fluoroquinolines (norfloxacin, ciprofloxacin and ofloxacin) and the dyes (Sudan II, Congo red and Gentian violet). The stoichiometry of complex formation between the drugs and the dyes is 1 : 3. This does not need extraction to halogenated organic solvents such as chloroform.

Dye	Drugs		
	Norfloxacin	Ciprofloxacin	Ofloxacin
1. Sudan-II			
Universal buffer pH	3.5	5.5	6.0
λ_{max} (nm)	550	550	560
2. Congo-red			
Universal buffer pH	8.5	2.5	8.5
λ_{max} (nm)	520	517	530
3. Gentian violet			
Universal buffer pH	10.5	2.5	11.0
λ_{max} (nm)	591	585	590

Note

Decarboxylated/degradation products do not interfere.

Reference

Alaa S. Amin, Moustafa E. Moustafa & Rehman M.S. El-Dosoky, *Analytical Letters*, **41**, 837-852, 2008.

Tinidazole

Reagents

1. Dimethyl formamide (DMF).
2. 1% v/v tetramethyl ammonium hydroxide (TMAH) in methanol.

Standard solution

100 mg of the substance accurately weighed and dissolved in 20 ml of DMF and diluted to 100 ml with water. Further dilutions are done with water to get final concentration of 100 mcg/ml.

Sample solution

To accurately weighed quantity of powdered sample, add 20 ml of DMF and 20 ml of water. Shake for 15 min to effect solution and dilute to 100 ml with water. Filter and further dilute appropriately with water to get final concentration of 100 mcg/ml.

Procedure

To 5 ml each of sample and standard solutions, add 5 ml of TMAH solution. Allow it to stand for 60 min at room temperature and dilute to 50 ml with water.

Measure extinction of both sample and standard solutions at about 370 nm against reagent blank and calculate the contents of tinidazole by comparison.

Note

The bathochromic effect i.e. shift of maximum from 310 nm to 370 nm in alkaline medium is brought about by electron attracting character of nitro group present in the molecule. Alternatively, if the sample solution is treated with 0.1 M NaOH in boiling water-bath for 15 min, due to bathochromic shift, the λ_{max} is observed at 400 nm and ciprofloxacin/norfloxacin have insignificant absorption at 400 nm, hence no interference.

Reference

1. D.N. Tipre & A.V. Kasture, 56th IPC, Abstract No. GP-31, p. 107.
2. Sangeeta Gaba et al., *Eastern Pharmacist*, p. 115, 1998.

Typical laboratory analysis

Each tablet contains 400 mg of norfloxacin and 600 mg of tinidazole.
Average weight of tablet = 1201 mg

Norfloxacin

Weight of standard (S) = 99.6 mg
Weight of sample (U) = 300.8 mg

$$\text{Norfloxacin (mg)/tablet} = \frac{A_u}{A_s} \times \frac{S}{U} \times \text{dilution factor} \times 1201$$

$$= \frac{0.587}{0.584} \times \frac{99.6}{300.8} \times \text{dilution factor} \times 1201$$

$$= 389.38 \text{ mg}$$

% claim = 97.35

Tinidazole

Weight of standard (S) = 101.4 mg
Weight of sample (U) = 200.7 mg

$$\text{Tinidazole (mg)/tablet} = \frac{A_u}{A_s} \times \frac{S}{U} \times \text{dilution factor} \times 1201$$

$$= \frac{0.884}{0.892} \times \frac{101.4}{200.7} \times \text{dilution factor} \times 1201$$

$$= 601.34 \text{ mg}$$

% claim = 100.20

Formulation 28

Doxycycline hydrochloride, Tinidazole

ESTIMATION

Doxycycline

To the solutions of standard/sample (10 μg/ml) add glacial acetic acid followed by reagent (5% aqueous solution of sodium cobaltinitrile), heat in water-bath for 15 min, cool, dilute appropriately with water and measure the absorbance at 407 nm.

Probable Reaction Mechanism

Since doxycycline has large number of oxygen atoms with lone pair of electrons, chelate formation takes place with divalent and trivalent metals like Co^{++}, Cu^{++}, Fe^{+++} as shown below leading to coloured complexes.

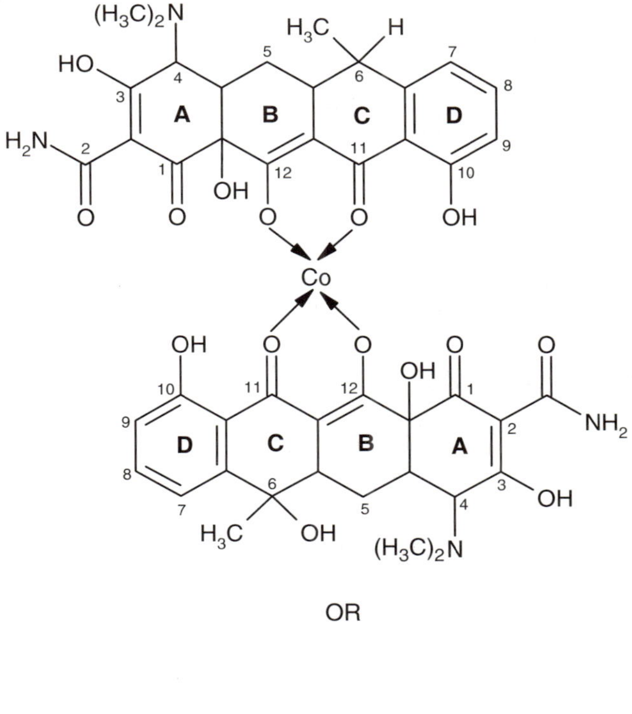

OR

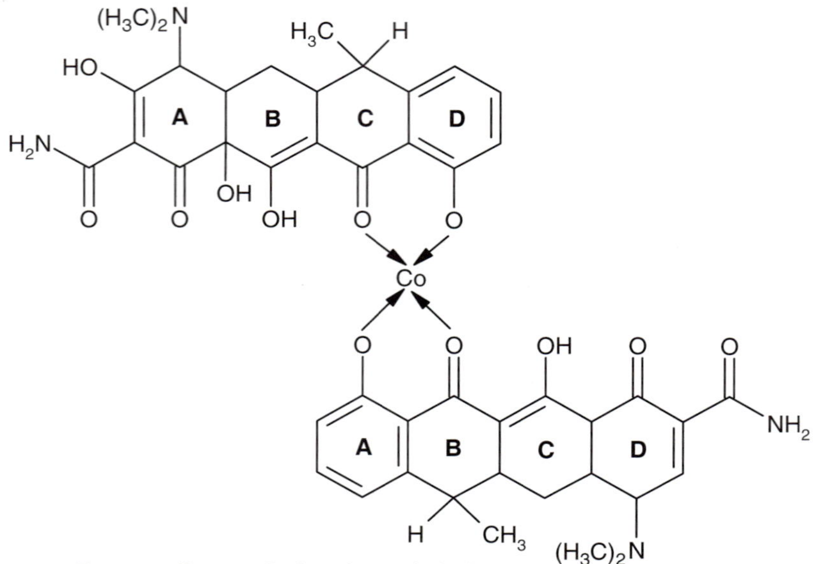

Doxycycline - cobalt coloured chelate
(λ_{max} 400 nm)

Reference

1. Pharmaceutical Chemistry (Vol. 2) by H.J. Roth, p. 455.
2. *Indian Drugs*, **20(9)**, 389, June 1983.

The compound undergoes Emerson reaction based on oxidative coupling in weakly alkaline medium (pH 8.0) at para position.

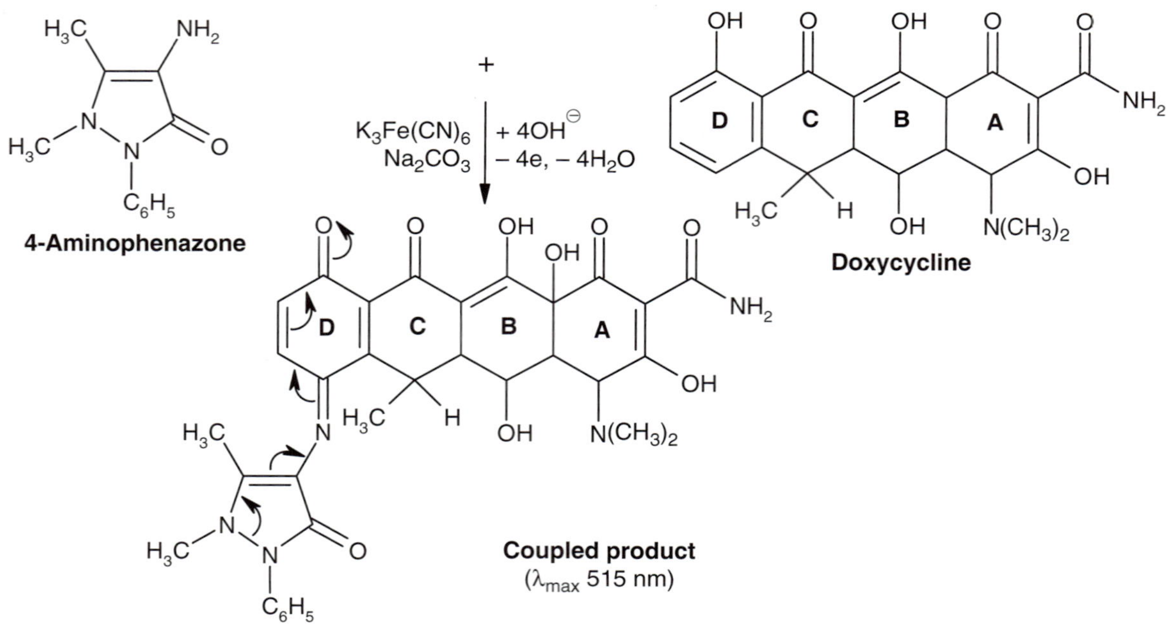

4-Aminophenazone + **Doxycycline** $\xrightarrow[Na_2CO_3 \;|\; -4e, -4H_2O]{K_3Fe(CN)_6 \;|\; +4OH^{\ominus}}$

Coupled product
(λ_{max} 515 nm)

Reference

1. Pharmaceutical Chemistry (Vol. 2) by H.J. Roth, p. 75.
2. *Indian Drugs*, **21(4)**, 167, June 1984.

Formation of chelate with Cu^{++} was used as analytical method for estimation of doxycycline by G. Rama Rao et al. (1981).

Probable Reaction Mechanism

It is similar to one described under complex formation with Co^{++}.

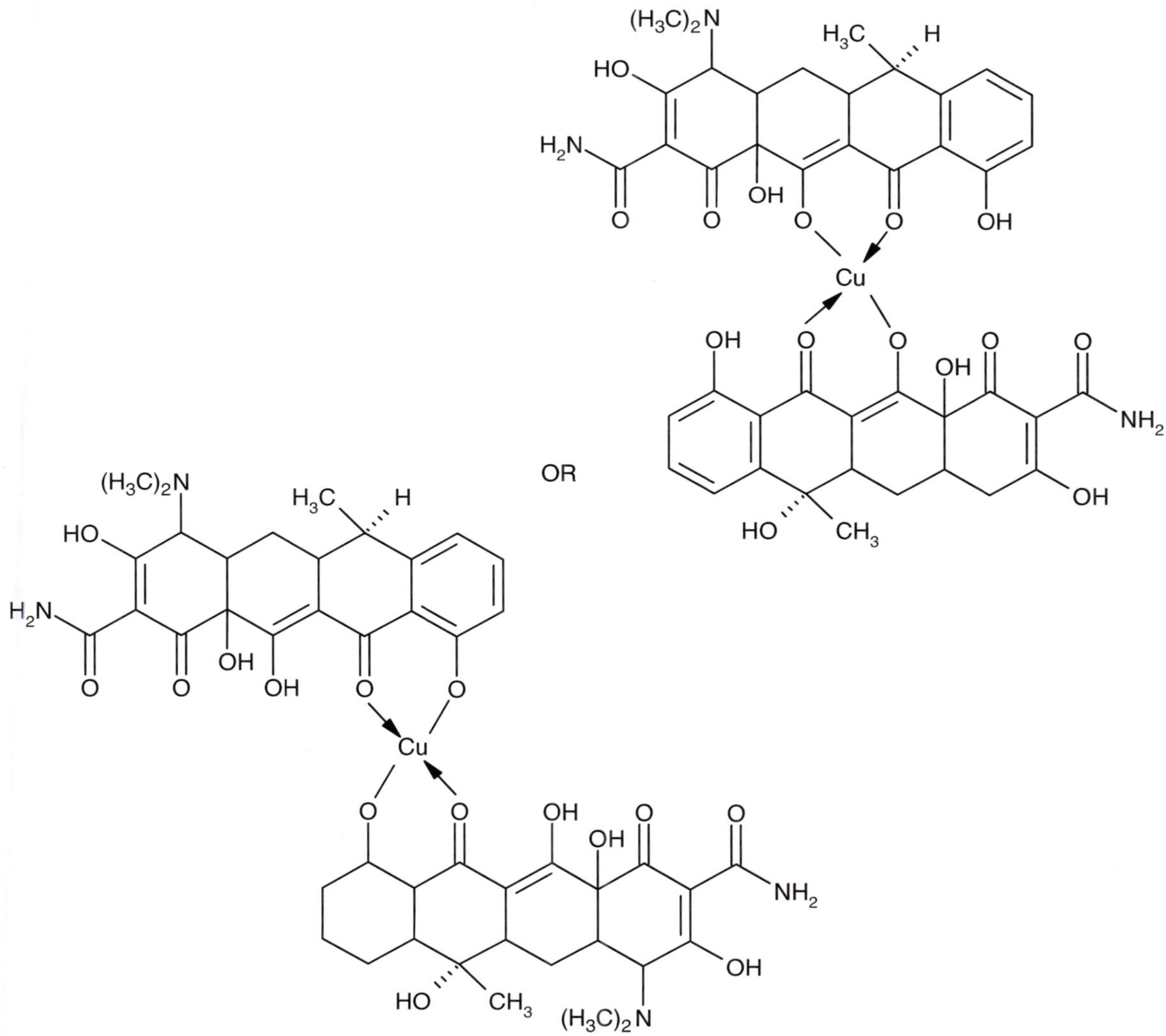

Doxycycline - Cu^{++} chelate
(λ_{max} 450 nm)

Note

1. Although tetracyclines have fluorescent, however metal chelates show more intense fluorescence than the compound.
2. Chemical method of assay of tetracyclines have disadvantage that it will include inactive compounds as well.

Reference

G. Rama Rao, S.S.N. Murty & B. Bajrangrao, *Eastern Pharmacist*, **24**, 121, Oct. 1981.

Formulation 29

Tetracycline hydrochloride, Metronidazole

ESTIMATION

Tetracycline

The compound forms chelate with sodium tungstate to give yellow-coloured product (λ_{max} 386 nm). The complex is formed in the ratio of 1 : 2.

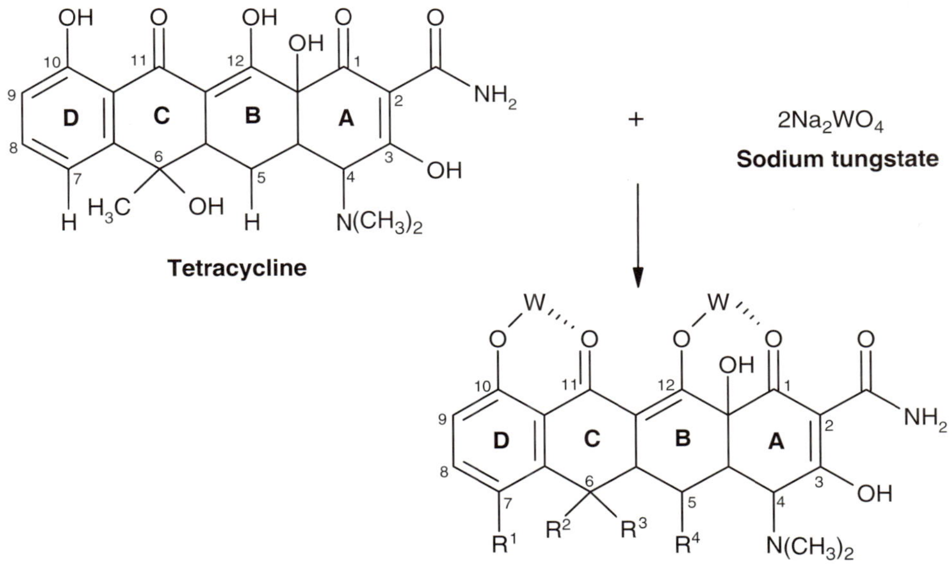

Tetracycline - metal (1 : 2) complex
(λ_{max} 386 nm)

Metronidazole

See formulation 1 of this chapter.

Note

Tetracyclines shall also form metal chelate with Co^{2+} and Cu^{2+}. For details refer to estimation of doxycycline.

Formulation 30

Doxycycline hydrochloride, Serratiopeptidase

ESTIMATION

Doxycycline hydrochloride

See formulation 28 of this chapter.

Serratiopeptidase

See under chapter on analgesics.

Weigh powdered sample equivalent to 100 mg of doxycycline and shake the dry powder with 1 ml of analyte methanol, filter, wash the residue with 1 ml of methanol under suction. The residue was taken up for analysis of enzyme as described under chapter on analgesics.

Formulation 31

Furazolidone, Berberine hydrochloride

ESTIMATION

Furazolidone

Standard solution

40 mcg/ml of furazolidone in DMF.

Sample solution

Weigh accurately finely powdered sample equivalent to 100 mg of furazolidone, add 60-70 ml of dimethyl formamide (DMF) and warm on water-bath for 15-20 min, cool and dilute to 100 ml with DMF. Filter through G_4 sintered funnel rejecting 15-20 ml of the filtrate. Dilute 2 ml of the filtrate to 50 ml with DMF—40 mcg/ml. All the apparatus should be absolutely dry.

Procedure

To 2 ml each of sample and standard solutions, add 2 ml of 0.1 N tetrabutyl ammonium hydroxide (TBAH) and dilute to 25 ml with DMF. Measure the absorption of both sample and standard solutions at 570 nm against reagent blank and calculate the results by comparison.

Probable Reaction Mechanism

This method is based on the work of G. Rama Rao et al. for the estimation of nitrofurazone. In alkaline medium (TBAH) there is shift from UV region (367 nm) to visible region (550 nm). For detailed reaction mechanism see under formulation 17 of this chapter.

Reference

G. Rama Rao, S. Raghuveer, S.S.N. Murthy & B. Bajrangrau, *Indian Drugs*, **17(2)**, 50-51, 1979; and *Ind. J. Pharm.*, **39(4)**, 83-85, 1977.

Berberine hydrochloride

Follow the method described in formulation 18 of this chapter.

Formulation 32

Tinidazole, Diloxanide furoate, Dicyclomine hydrochloride

ESTIMATION

Tinidazole and Diloxanide furoate

Follow the method described in formulation 20 of this chapter.

Dicyclomine hydrochloride

Reagents

1. Sulphuric acid: Add 3 ml of concentrated sulphuric acid to 100 ml of water.
2. Methyl orange solution: Dissolve 300 mg of methyl orange in 800 ml of water, add 30 ml of sulphuric acid. Stir and filter to get clear solution.
3. Sodium acetate solution: Dissolve 2 g of sodium acetate in 400 ml of methanol, filter to get clear filtrate.
4. Hydrochloric acid: 1 ml of concentrated hydrochloric acid is diluted to 100 ml with water.

Standard solution

(a) 250 mcg/ml in hydrochloric acid.
(b) 10 ml of (a) diluted to 100 ml with methanol—25 mcg/ml.

Sample solution

Accurately weighed quantity of the sample equivalent to 2.5 mg of the substance is suspended in 10 ml of hydrochloric acid and heated at 80°C with stirring for dissolving the substance. Dilute to 100 ml with methanol and filter.

Procedure

To 10 ml of sample and standard solutions, add 50 ml of methyl orange solution. Mix and extract with 3 × 15 ml portions of chloroform. Combine the organic layers and dilute to 100 ml with sodium acetate solution. Measure the absorption of both the solutions at 420 nm against blank. Repeat the experiment without the substance and calculate the results by comparison.

Note

The method is based on formation of ion-pair complex between the drug (dicyclomine) and the dye (methyl orange).

Formulation 33

Kaolin, Dried aluminium hydroxide gel, Magnesium carbonate, Calcium carbonate, Sodium bicarbonate, Belladonna alkaloids

ESTIMATION

Kaolin

Procedure

Weigh and powder 20 tablets in a dry pestle mortar. Take about 3 g of the powder accurately weighed in a 100 ml beaker and boil with 20 ml of 1 N hydrochloric acid for 5 minutes. Filter through Whatman filter paper into a 250 ml volumetric flask. Wash the filter paper several times with water collecting the washings in the volumetric flask till the volume is made upto the mark. Reserve the filtrate-A for the estimation of aluminium hydroxide.

Put the filter paper together with the residue in crucible and another similar filter paper in a second crucible and dry both at 105°C to a constant weight and weigh. From the difference in two weights, determine the weight of the dried residue which represents the weight of kaolin in sample taken for analysis.

Aluminium hydroxide (as Aluminium oxide)

METHOD 1

Reagents

1. Ammonium chloride.
2. Dilute ammonia solution.
3. 2% wv solution of ammonium chloride in water.

Procedure

Take 20 ml of the filtrate-A obtained in the estimation of kaolin in a 100 ml beaker, saturate the solution with ammonium chloride and heat to boiling. Add 40 ml of dilute ammonia solution dropwise, while the solution is boiling. Continue boiling for another 20 minutes and filter while hot through a Whatman filter paper (No. 1) into a 250 ml beaker. Wash the precipitates six times, each with 5 ml of hot (60-80°C) ammonium chloride solution. Add the washings to the filtrate and reserve the filtrate-B for the estimation of calcium carbonate. Ignite the precipitate along with filter paper in a muffle furnace at a temperature of about 1000°C to a constant weight. Aluminium hydroxide contains 47% w/w of aluminium oxide.

METHOD 2

Reagents

1. 0.01 M disodium edetate solution in water.
2. 30% w/v sodium hydroxide solution in water.
3. Congo red paper (indicator).
4. 2 M Monochloroacetic acid solution.
5. 1 M sodium acetate solution.
6. Alizarin-S indicator, 0.1% w/v in water.
7. 0.01 M thorium nitrate solution.

Procedure

Transfer 25 ml of the filtrate-A obtained in the estimation of kaolin to a 500 ml conical flask. Add 80 ml of water and 50 ml of 0.01 M sodium edetate solution. Neutralize the solution with sodium hydroxide solution using conge red paper. Add 5 ml of monochloroacetic acid, 10 ml of sodium acetate solution, 1.5 ml of alizarin-S indicator and shake thoroughly. Titrate the solution against 0.01 M thorium nitrate solution until the colour changes to cherry-red. Take the blank reading simultaneously using above reagents except the sample solution.

Each ml of 0.01 M thorium nitrate solution is equivalent to 0.0002698 × 3.81 g of aluminium hydroxide gel calculated as aluminium oxide.

METHOD 3

5 g of the sample is taken in 3 ml of concentrated hydrochloric acid, diluted to 100 ml with water, warmed on water-bath and cooled. To 20 ml of the above sample solution add 80 ml water and 40 ml 0.05 M disodium edetate. Adjust the pH to below 6.0 with 1 N sodium hydroxide using methyl red solution as indicator. Warm on a water-bath for 30 minutes, add 3 g hexamine and titrate with 0.05 M lead nitrate using xylenol orange solution as indicator. Each ml of 0.05 M disodium edetate is equivalent to 0.002549 g of aluminium oxide.

Magnesium carbonate

METHOD 1

Reagents

1. 2% w/v solution of ammonium chloride in water.

2. 0.05 M disodium edetate solution.
3. Ammonia - ammonium chloride buffer solution: Dissolve 13.5 g of ammonium chloride in 130 ml of strong ammonia solution and dilute to 200 ml with water.
4. Solochrome black indicator solution: 0.5 w/v solution in 95% ethyl alcohol.

Procedure

Take 20 ml of the filtrate-A reserved in the estimation of kaolin and separate out aluminium hydroxide by precipitating in the same way as described in the estimation of aluminium hydroxide (method 1) above. Filter the precipitates through a Whatman filter paper (No. 1) collecting the filtrate in a 500 ml conical flask. Wash the precipitates six time, each with 15 ml of hot (60-80°C) ammonium chloride solution and collect the washings in the same conical flask. To the combined filtrate and washings, add 10 ml of ammonium chloride - ammonia buffer and solochrome black indicator solution and titrate with 0.05 M disodium edetate solution to a blue end point.

Calculation

Content of magnesium carbonate as $3MgCO_3(OH)_3 \cdot 4H_2O$ mg/tab.

$$\frac{(X_1 \times F_1 - X \times F) \times 0.004789 \times \text{average weight of tab (g)}}{\text{Weight of the sample (g) taken in the estimation of kaolin}}$$

where X_1 = Titre value of 0.05 M disodium edetate.
F_1 = Factor of 0.05 M disodium edetate.
X = Titre value of 0.1 N potassium permanganate solution used in the estimation of calcium carbonate.
F = Factor of 0.1 N potassium permanganate solution.

Calcium carbonate

METHOD 1

Reagents

1. 2.5% w/v ammonium oxalate solution in water.
2. 0.1 N potassium permanganate solution.
3. Dilute sulphuric acid 10% w/v.

Procedure

To the filtrate-B, reserved in the estimation of aluminium hydroxide (method 1), add sufficient water to make up the volume to about 100 ml. Add 10 ml of ammonium oxalate solution and heat on a water-bath for 2 hours. Filter through a Whatman filter paper (No. 42). Wash the precipitates with hot water until the washings are free from oxalate ion (test with calcium chloride solution). Dissolve the precipitate on the filter paper in hot dilute sulphuric acid, collecting the solution in a 250 ml conical flask. Dilute with water to about 100 ml and then titrate, while hot, rapidly with 0.1 N potassium permanganate solution until a faint pink colour persists for 15 seconds. Each ml of 0.1 N potassium permanganate is equivalent to 0.005008 g of calcium carbonate. From the total volume of titrant required, calculate the amount of calcium carbonate in the sample.

METHOD 2

Reagents

1. 30% w/v triethanolamine solution in water.
2. 30% w/v sodium hydroxide solution in water.
3. Murexide indicator : Grind 0.2 g of indicator with 100 g of sodium chloride.
4. 0.01 M disodium edetate solution.

Procedure

To 10 ml of the filtrate-B, reserved in the estimation of aluminium hydroxide (method-1) taken in a 500 ml conical flask, add 25 ml of triethanolamine solution and mix thoroughly. Add 200 ml of water, 2.5 ml of sodium hydroxide solution, and shake thoroughly. Add 0.1 g murexide indicator and titrate against 0.01 M disodium edetate solution. Each ml of 0.01 M disodium edetate is equivalent to 0.001002 g of calcium carbonate.

Sodium bicarbonate

METHOD 1

Reagents

1. 1 N hydrochloric acid.
2. 1 N sodium hydroxide.
3. 0.05 M disodium edetate solution.
4. Methyl orange—indicator solution.
5. Solochrome black indicator solution, 0.5% w/v solution in alcohol.
6. Ammonia - ammonium chloride buffer solution: For the preparation of this buffer, see under estimation of magnesium carbonate.

Procedure

Take about 3 g of the sample (W1) accurately weighed in a 250 ml glass-stoppered conical flask and add 150 ml of water. Shake the flask in a mechanical shaker for 1 hour and filter through Whatman filter paper (No. 1). Wash the filter paper with 50 ml of water and add the washings to the filtrate. Add 20 ml of 1 N hydrochloric acid to the filtrate, warm slightly to expel carbon dioxide and titrate the excess acid with 1 N sodium hydroxide using methyl orange as indicator until the colour changes from pink to orange.

Take another 3 g of the sample (W2) accurately weighed in another 250 ml glass-stoppered conical flask and proceed in the same manner. Neutralize the filtrate with dilute hydrochloric acid, add 10 ml of ammonia - ammonium chloride buffer and solochrome black indicator solution and titrate with 0.05 M disodium edetate to a blue end point.

Calculations

Content of disodium bicarbonate (mg)/tablet

$$\frac{10 \times F_3 - V_1 \times F_1}{W1} - \frac{V_2 \times F_2}{10 \times W2} \times 0.084 \times 1000 \times 5 \times a$$

where V_1 = Volume of 1 N sodium hydroxide consumed in the back titration.
V_2 = Volume of 0.05 M disodium edetate required.
F_1 = Volumetric factor of 1 N sodium hydroxide.
F_2 = Volumetric factor of 0.05 M disodium edetate.
F_3 = Volumetric factor of 1 N hydrochloric acid.
W_1 = Weight (g) of sample taken in the first titration.
W_2 = Weight (g) of sample taken in the second titration.
a = Average weight (mg) of the tablet.

Note

First titration takes care of sodium bicarbonate contents, whereas volume of 'EDTA' required in second titration is about estimation of 'calcium' as calcium carbonate.

Total belladonna alkaloids as Hyoscyamine

Reagents

1. Chloroform.
2. Acetone, water content not more than 0.02% v/v.
3. Anhydrous sodium sulphate, granular.
4. Phosphoric acid (88% w/w).
5. Solvent: 6% v/v of acetic acid in 5% v/v alcohol : Take 6 ml of the glacial acetic acid and 5 ml of dehydrated alcohol in a 250 ml conical flask. Add 89 ml of distilled water and shake well.
6. Dehydrated alcohol.

7. Fuming nitric acid. It is highly corrosive, handle with extreme care.
8. Potassium hydroxide, pellets.
9. Methyl alcohol.
10. 50% v/v alcohol.

Standard stock solution

Take about 80 mg of atropine sulphate accurately weighed in 100 ml volumetric flask and dissolve in solvent. Make up the volume to 100 ml with the solvent. Prepare this solution once in every month and store in a refrigerator to serve as stock solution.

Dilute standard solution

Dilute 10 ml of the stock standard solution to 100 ml with the solvent (80 mcg/ml). Prepare this solution freshly before use.

Calculate the content of atropine (base) in mg/ml in the diluted standard solution as follows :

$$\frac{\text{Weight of atropine sulphate taken}}{100} \times \frac{578.76 \times 10}{694.86 \times 100}$$

Sample solution

Take sample accurately weighed in a 250 ml stoppered conical flask. Extract the alkaloids by shaking the sample twice, each with 50 ml of a mixture of 2 ml of phosphoric acid and 48 ml of 50% v/v alcohol in a mechanical shaker. Filter both the extracts through the same Whatman filter paper No. 4 into 500 ml beaker and wash the residue with a further 50 ml of mixture of 0.5 ml of phosphoric acid and 49.5 ml of ethyl alcohol. Add the washings to the filtrate and reduce the volume of the combined filtrate and the washings on a water-bath to about 50 ml. Transfer to a separator with the aid of little alcohol. Wash the container with chloroform and add the washings to the separator. Make distinctly alkaline with dilute solution of ammonia and extract with four 30 ml portions of chloroform. Wash each chloroform layer with same 10 ml of water. Filter organic layer through anhydrous sodium sulphate and evaporate just to dryness. Add 2 ml of ethyl alcohol and finally dry at 105°C for 3 h. Dissolve the residue in 9 ml of chloroform and transfer into stoppered 25 ml cylinder. Wash the flask with 15 ml of solvent and add to the cylinder. Shake vigorously for 2 minutes and allow to settle till the aqueous portion is distinctly clear. Transfer 5 ml of the aqueous layer into a porcelain dish and completely evaporate off the liquid to dryness. Add 5 drops of fuming nitric acid, keep on water-bath for 3 minutes and transfer quickly to a 10 ml volumetric flask with the aid of acetone. Make up the volume with acetone and mark the flask as ‘sample’.

Take 1 ml standard solution and 1 ml of water in two 25 ml porcelain dishes and proceed according to preceding para beginning with “completely evaporate off the liquid to dryness”. Mark these flasks as ‘standard’ and ‘blank’ respectively.

Procedure

Dissolve one pellet of potassium hydroxide in 5 ml of methyl alcohol and add 0.1 ml of this solution to each of three 10 ml volumetric flasks marked as ‘standard’, ‘sample’ and ‘blank’. Shake and allow to stand for 3 minutes. Measure immediately the optical densities of the standard and sample at 550 nm in a spectrophotometer against the blank. Calculate the total belladonna alkaloids as hyoscyamine by comparison.

Formulation 34

Dried aluminium hydroxide gel, Magnesium hydroxide, Dimethylpolysiloxane

ESTIMATION

Aluminium hydroxide

Follow any one of the methods for estimation of aluminium hydroxide described under formulation 1 of this chapter.

Magnesium hydroxide

Follow the method for estimation of magnesium carbonate described under formulation 1 of this chapter. Each ml of 0.05 M sodium edetate is equivalent to 0.002016 g of magnesium oxide.

Dimethylpolysiloxane (DMP)

METHOD 1

This method is based on defoaming activity of the compound. The foam is generated by dissolving 200 mg of sodium lauryl sulphate or ordinary detergent in 100 ml of purified water at 37°C in a 250 ml graduated cylinder. Adust pH of the foam solution to 1.2 with 0.1 N hydrochloric acid.

Sample solution

Transfer powdered tablets corresponding to 200 mg of the compound in 150 ml dried conical flask. Extract 4 times with 30 ml portions of boiling benzene. Concentrate total benzene extract to exactly 10 ml in a 10 ml volumetric flask.

Procedure

Transfer 1 ml of the sample solution to 250 ml graduated cylinder containing 100 ml of foam solution. The cylinder is then stoppered and shaken till slightly more than 150 ml of foam is generated. When foam level comes to 150 ml, the reading in the cylinder will be 250 ml. Counting of time is started and at every 15 second interval, the volume of remaining foam is noted. Not less than 80% of the foam should disappear within 5 minutes. Alternatively, the time required for complete disappearance of the foam is noted and co-related with the standard solution of polysiloxane in benzene.

METHOD 2

This method is based on the estimation of silicone dioxide (SiO_2) contents of the compound. To the sample equivalent to 100 mg of the compound, add 10 ml of 1 N sulphuric acid and heat on water-bath for ninety minutes. Filter through an ashless filter paper. The residue is washed with hot water and transferred to a platinum crucible. Heat to dryness, incinerate and ignite at 1000°C, cool and weigh (a). The residue is moistened with water and then add 5 ml of hydrofluoric acid and few drops of sulphuric acid. Evaporate to dryness and ignite at 1000°C, cool and weigh (b). The difference between weights (a) and (b) represent the weight of silicone dioxide.

Note

Silicone dioxide forms volatile complex (silicone tetrafluoride) with hydrofluoric acid.

METHOD 3

Measure 10 ml of suspension or weigh powdered tablets equivalent to 200 mg of the compound and transfer to a separating funnel. Add 50 ml of 5 N hydrochloric acid and 50 ml of saturated solution of sodium chloride. Shake well and extract with four 50 ml portions of ether. Wash the combined ethereal extract with 20 ml of saturated solution of sodium chloride. In turn, wash the saline layer with 20 ml of ether, combine the latter ether extract with the main ether extract. Filter through anhydrous sodium sulphate placed over cotton plug. Rinse the sodium sulphate with two 10 ml portions of ether. Evaporate combined ether layer on steam-bath to about 2-3 ml. Transfer to a tared 30 ml Kjeldahl flask. Wash the flask 3-4 times each with 4 ml of ether. Evaporate the oily liquid to dryness on steam-bath using nitrogen gas to prevent bumping. Add 2 ml of concentrated sulphuric acid and 0.5 ml concentrated nitric acid. Place the Kjeldahl flask on a sand-bath equipped with a thermometer (0-360°C). Heat slowly to 140°C and maintain at this temperature for 30 minutes. Increase temperature to 280°C and maintain the sample again at this temperature for 30 minutes. Draw back the flask and place on direct flame slowly at the beginning to prevent bumping, then strongly heat to constant weight which represents silicone dioxide present in the sample.

METHOD 4

Take sample accurately weighed equivalent to 50 mg of the compound, add 50 ml water and extract with four 50 ml portions of chloroform. Pool chloroform layer, evaporate on rotary evaporator and proceed as per method 1 or 2 above.

Note

Use ground glass joint apparatus and separating funnel free of silicone greese. Alternatively, the sample is neutralized with 1 N hydrochloric acid (amount of acid required can be calculated from acid consuming capacity) and neutralized sample solution is used directly for defoaming actively. Aqueous sample solution gives more satisfactory results.

METHOD 5

Silicates give yellow colour with ammonium molybdate in acidic medium. For details refer to method described in formulation of the chapter on anti-diarrhoeals.

Formulation 35

Dried aluminium hydroxide gel, Magnesium hydroxide, Deglycyrrhizinated liquorice, Dimethylpolysiloxane

ESTIMATION

Aluminium hydroxide

Reagents

1. Concentrated hydrochloric acid.
2. 0.05 M EDTA solution.
3. 0.05 M zinc sulphate solution.
4. Acetic acid - ammonium acetate buffer: Dissolve 7.71 g of ammonium acetate in water, add 5.7 ml of glacial acetic acid and dilute to 100 ml with water.
5. Dithizone solution: Dissolve 25.6 mg of dithizone in 100 ml of methanol. Stable for 2 months if stored in cold place.

Sample preparation

Weigh powdered sample equivalent to 500 mg of aluminium hydroxide, add 20 ml of concentrated hydrochloric acid and boil for 5 min, cool and make up to 250 ml with water. Filter and use this solution for assay. To 25 ml of the sample solution, add 25 ml of 0.05 M EDTA solution, 25 ml of buffer solution with constant stirring. Add 20 ml of methanol and 1 ml of dithizone solution and titrate with 0.05 M zinc sulphate solution to a bright rose pink colour. Perform blank. Each ml of 0.05 M EDTA is equivalent to 2.549 mg of aluminium oxide (Al_2O_3).

Magnesium hydroxide

Reagents

1. Triethanolamine.
2. Ammonia - ammonium chloride buffer.
3. 0.05 M EDTA.

Procedure

To 25 ml of sample solution as prepared under estimation of aluminium hydroxide, add 25 ml of triethanolamine and 10 ml of ammonia-ammonium chloride buffer solution and titrate with 0.05 M EDTA using eriochrome black T as indicator. Each ml of 0.05 M EDTA is equivalent to 2.916 mg magnesium hydroxide $Mg(OH)_2$.

Glycyrrhizic acid

Follow the method described in formulation 1 of the chapter on urinary anti-infectives. Deglycyrrhizinated liquorice usually contains not more than 3% of the acid.

Dimethicone in creams such as Triamcinolone acetonide

Mix the cream with 5 g of anhydrous sodium sulphate in a beaker till uniform mixture is obtained. Extract with warm toluene (6 ´ 15 ml), filtering each extract through G_3 sintered funnel, make up to 50 ml with toluene. Record the IR in 4% liquid paraffin in toluene and compare with standard.

Note

Anhydrous sodium sulphate abstracts water from cream as decahydrate, leaving readily filtered organic layer.

Dimethylpolysiloxane (DMP)

METHOD 1

This method is based on defoaming activity of the compound. The foam is generated by dissolving 200 mg of sodium lauryl sulphate or ordinary detergent in 100 ml of purified water at 37°C in a 250 ml graduated cylinder. Adjust pH of the foam solution to 1.2 with 0.1 N hydrochloric acid.

Sample solution

Transfer powdered tablets corresponding to 200 mg of the compound in 150 ml dried conical flask. Extract 4 times with 30 ml portions of boiling benzene. Concentrate total benzene extract to exactly 10 ml in a 10 ml volumetric flask.

Procedure

Transfer 1 ml of the sample solution to 250 ml graduated cylinder containing 100 ml of foam solution. The cylinder is then stoppered and shaken till slightly more than 150 ml of foam is generated. When foam level comes to 150 ml, the reading in the cylinder will be 250 ml. Counting of time is started and at every 15 second interval, the volume of remaining foam is noted. Not less than 80% of the foam should disappear within 5 minutes. Alternatively, the time required for complete disappearance of the foam is noted and co-related with the standard solution of polysiloxane in benzene.

METHOD 2

This method is based on the estimation of silicone dioxide contents of the compound. To the sample equivalent to 100 mg of the compound, add 10 ml of 1 N sulphuric acid and heat on water-bath for ninety minutes. Filter through an ashless filter paper. The residue is washed with hot water and transferred to a platinum crucible. Heat to dryness, incinerate and ignite at 1000°C, cool and weigh (a). The residue is moistened with water and then add 5 ml of hydrofluoric acid and few drops of sulphuric acid. Evaporate to dryness and ignite at 1000°C, cool and weigh (b). The difference between weights (a) and (b) represents the weight of silicone dioxide.

Note

Silicone dioxide forms volatile complex (silicone tetrafluoride) with hydrofluoric acid.

METHOD 3

Measure 10 ml of suspension or weigh powdered tablets equivalent to 200 mg of the compound and transfer to a separating funnel. Add 50 ml of 5 N hydrochloric acid and 50 ml of saturated solution of sodium chloride. Shake well and extract with four 50 ml portions of ether. Wash the combined ethereal extract with 20 ml of saturated solution of sodium chloride. In turn, wash the saline layer with 20 ml of ether, combine the latter ether extract with the main ether extract. Filter through anhydrous sodium sulphate placed over cotton plug. Rinse the sodium sulphate with two 10 ml portions of ether. Evaporate combined ether layer on steam-bath to about 2-3 ml. Transfer to a tared 30 ml Kjeldahl flask. Wash the flask 3-4 times each with 4 ml of ether. Evaporate the oily liquid to dryness on steam-bath using nitrogen gas to prevent bumping. Add 2 ml of concentrated sulphuric acid and 0.5 ml concentrated nitric acid. Place the Kjeldahl flask on a sand-bath equipped with a thermometer (0-360°C). Heat slowly to 140°C and maintain at this temperature for 30 minutes. Draw back the flash and place on direct flame slowly at the beginning to prevent bumping, then strongly heat to constant weight which represents silicone dioxide present in the sample.

METHOD 4

Take sample accurately weighed equivalent to 50 mg of the compound, add 50 ml water and extract with four 50 ml portions of chloroform. Pool chloroform layer, evaporate on rotary evaporator and proceed as per method 1 or 2 above.

Note

Use ground glass joint apparatus and separating funnel free of silicone. Alternatively the sample is neutralized with 1 N hydrochloric acid (amount of acid required can be calculated from acid consuming capacity) and neutralized sample solution is used directly for defoaming actively. Aqueous sample solution gives more satisfactory results.

METHOD 5

Silicates give yellow colour with ammonium molybdate in acidic medium. For details refer to method described in formulation of this chapter.

Formulation 36

Aluminium hydroxide, Magnesium trisilicate, Sodium bicarbonate, Alginic acid

ESTIMATION

Aluminium hydroxide and Magnesium trisilicate

Sample preparation

Weigh accurately, powdered sample equivalent to 200 mg of aluminium hydroxide, add 10 ml of water, mix, allow to stand and then add 30 ml of 6 N hydrochloric acid, allow to stand at room temperature for 45 min. Add 30 ml of water and heat on a water-bath for 40-45 min with continuous stirring to prevent charring. Cool and filter, wash filter paper with water and adjust the volume of filtrate to 250 ml with water. Use this solution for estimation of aluminium hydroxide and magnesium trisilicate (if the solution is coloured, treat with acid-washed charcoal and filter).

Aluminium hydroxide

Neutralise 20 ml of the sample solution with dilute ammonia solution (Congo red paper) and proceed as per method described in formulation 1 of this chapter.

Magnesium trisilicate

50 ml of the sample solution is made alkaline with ammonia (litmus paper) and then follow the method described in formulation 1 of this chapter.

Alginic acid

Accurately weighed quantity of sample equivalent to 250 mg of alginic acid is transferred to a stoppered flask. Add 60 ml of acetone and 40 ml of dilute hydrochloric acid (10% w/v). Stopper the flask and shake occasionally for 30 min. Filter through Whatman No. 4 filter paper transferring as much of the precipitate as possible to a filter paper. Transfer precipitates and filter paper to a flask. Ensure that all the precipitates/residue sticking to the funnel are also removed to the flask. Add 25 ml of 0.1 N sodium hydroxide and shake for 15 min. Titrate excess of the alkali with 0.1 N hydrochloric acid using phenolphthalein as indicator. Treat 250 mg of working standard of alginic acid simultaneously. Carry out the blank determination and calculate by comparison.

Formulation 37

Isopropamide iodide, Trifluoperazine

ESTIMATION

Isopropamide iodide

Reagents

1. Buffer solution, pH 10.2: Dissolve 43.5 g of potassium phosphate, dibasic, and 21 g of sodium bicarbonate, anhydrous, in 1000 ml of water. Adjust the pH to 10.2 with phosphoric acid.
2. Methyl orange solution: Add 0.2 g of methyl orange to about 190 ml of pH 10.2 buffer in a 500 ml conical flask and stir on a steam-bath for 30 min. Dilute to 200 ml with pH 10.2 buffer while hot. Stir mechanically until cold and then continue to stir overnight. Filter through a Whatman No. 1 filter paper and extract the filtrate with successive 20 ml of chloroform until the chloroform extracts are colourless and do not yield a red colour on shaking with 2% hydrochloric acid.
3. 1% w/v solution of sodium sulphite in water.

Standard solution

Accurately weigh about 200 mg of isopropamide iodide in a 100 ml volumetric flask. Add 0.1 N sulphuric acid to dissolve and to make up to 100 ml. Pipette 10 ml into a 250 ml volumetric flask, add 0.1 N sulphuric acid to about 200 ml. Add 2 ml of sodium sulphite solution and shake for 20 minutes. Dilute to 250 ml with 0.1 N sulphuric acid and mix well.

Sample solution

Powder tablets finely and weigh accurately powder equivalent to 15 mg of isopropamide into a 250 ml volumetric flask washing with 0.1 N sulphuric acid to about 200 ml. Add 2 ml of sodium sulphite solution and shake for 20 minutes. Dilute to 250 ml with 0.1 N sulphuric acid and mix well. Filter through a No. 1 Whatman paper discarding the first 20 ml of the filtrate.

Procedure

Place 50 ml of chloroform and 30 ml of methyl orange solution in a separator. Pipette 5 ml of the standard and sample solutions into the separators, shake well and allow to stand for 3 to 4 minutes or until the layers are completely separated. Slowly run the chloroform layer into another separator through a pledget of cotton moistened with chloroform. Repeat the extraction with two more 50 ml portions of chloroform and wash the cotton pledget with 25 ml of chloroform. Extract the combined chloroform layer with 20 ml of dilute hydrochloric acid and 30 ml of water. Discard the chloroform layer and run the acid phase into a 100 ml volumetric flask. Rinse the separator and dilute to 100 ml with water. Measure the absorbance of the final solutions at 510 nm using 1% v/v hydrochloric acid as blank. Calculate results by comparison. The method is based on ion-pair complex formation. Though chloroform layer is yellow in colour (λ_{max} 410 nm) but by extracting with HCl the aqueous layer is red (λ_{max} 510 nm) thus increasing the sensitivity of the method.

The iodide component of the molecule can be subjected to argentimetric titration. The sample is dissolved in the mixture of water : methanol : glacial acetic acid (5 : 5 : 1) and titrated with 0.1 M $AgNO_3$ using eosin Y as indicator till the precipitate becomes red rose. Each ml of 0.1 M $AgNO_3$ is equivalent to 0.04804 g of isopropamide.

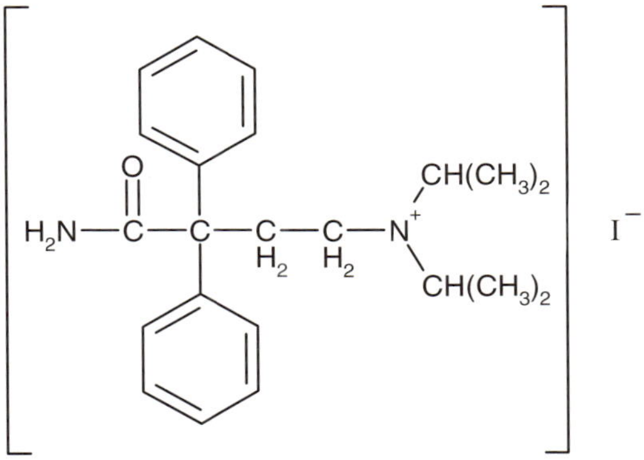

Isopropamide iodide

Trifluoperazine

Powder tablets finely and weigh accurately quantity of the powder equivalent to 5 mg of trifluoperazine into 500 ml volumetric flask. Shake for 15 min with 400 ml of a mixture of one volume of hydrochloric acid and 19 volumes of water. Dilute to 500 ml with the same solvent mixture, mix and filter. Measure the extinction of the filtrate at maxima at about 256 nm and calculate the results by taking 743 as value of E 1%, 1 cm.

The compound forms coloured nitroso derivative with sodium nitrite in acidic medium. The nitrosonium ion so formed being electron deficient attacks the aromatic ring of the drug at C-2 and results in the formation of nitroso derivative. Conc. sulphuric acid present in the reaction is a strong oxidizing agent and the molecule gets oxidized as well.

$$NaNO_2 + H_2SO_4 \longrightarrow HNO_2 + NaHSO_4$$

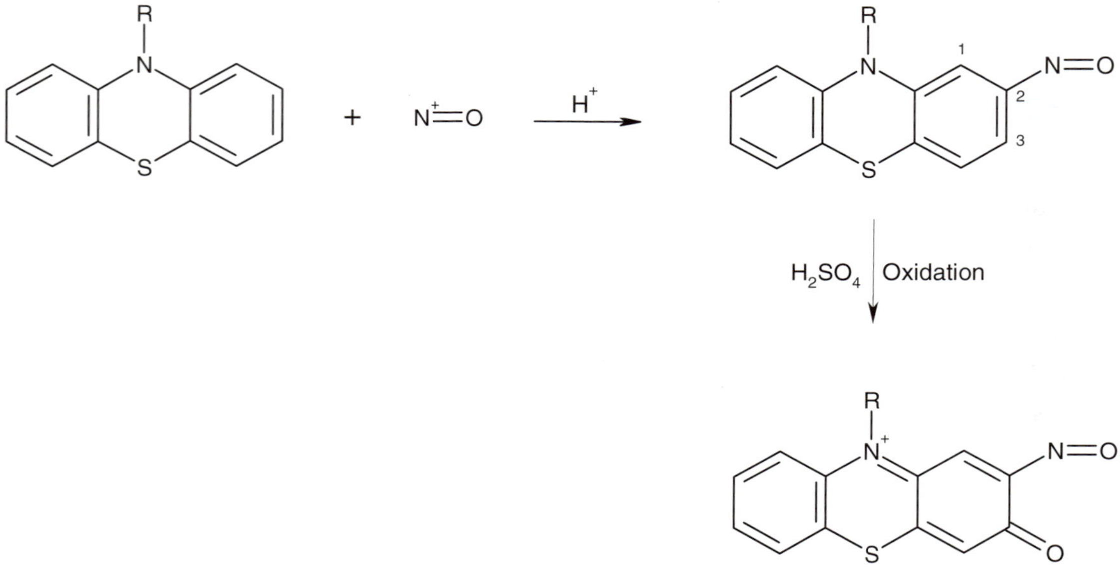

Oxidized coloured species

Reference

R.T. Sane et al., Indian Drugs, **18(1)**, 19-22, 1980.

Formulation 38

Cimetidine

METHOD 1

Reagents

1. Isopropyl alcohol - water mixture (1 : 1) v/v.
2. Ninhydrin reagent.

Standard solution

Weigh accurately 200 mg of cimetidine and dissolve in water to produce 100 ml. Take 10 ml of the resulting solution, adjust to pH 7.0 and dilute to 50 ml with isopropanol - water mixture.

Sample solution

Weigh accurately powdered tablets equivalent to 20 mg of cimetidine, extract with 10 ml of water, adjust to pH 7.0 and dilute to 50 ml with isopropyl - water mixture.

Procedure

Take 2.5 ml each of standard and sample solutions separately and to each add 6.5 ml of ninhydrin reagent. Heat in water-bath for 40 minutes, cool and dilute to 25 ml with isopropyl alcohol - water mixture. Measure the absorbance of both the solutions at about 570 nm against reagent blank and calculate the results by comparison.

Probable Reaction Mechanism

There are three secondary amino groups present in cimetidine for reaction with ninhydrin resulting in the formation of coloured compound (λ_{max} 570 nm)

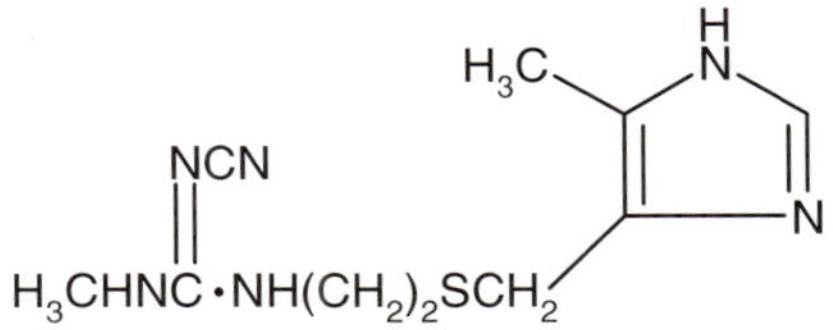

Cimetidine

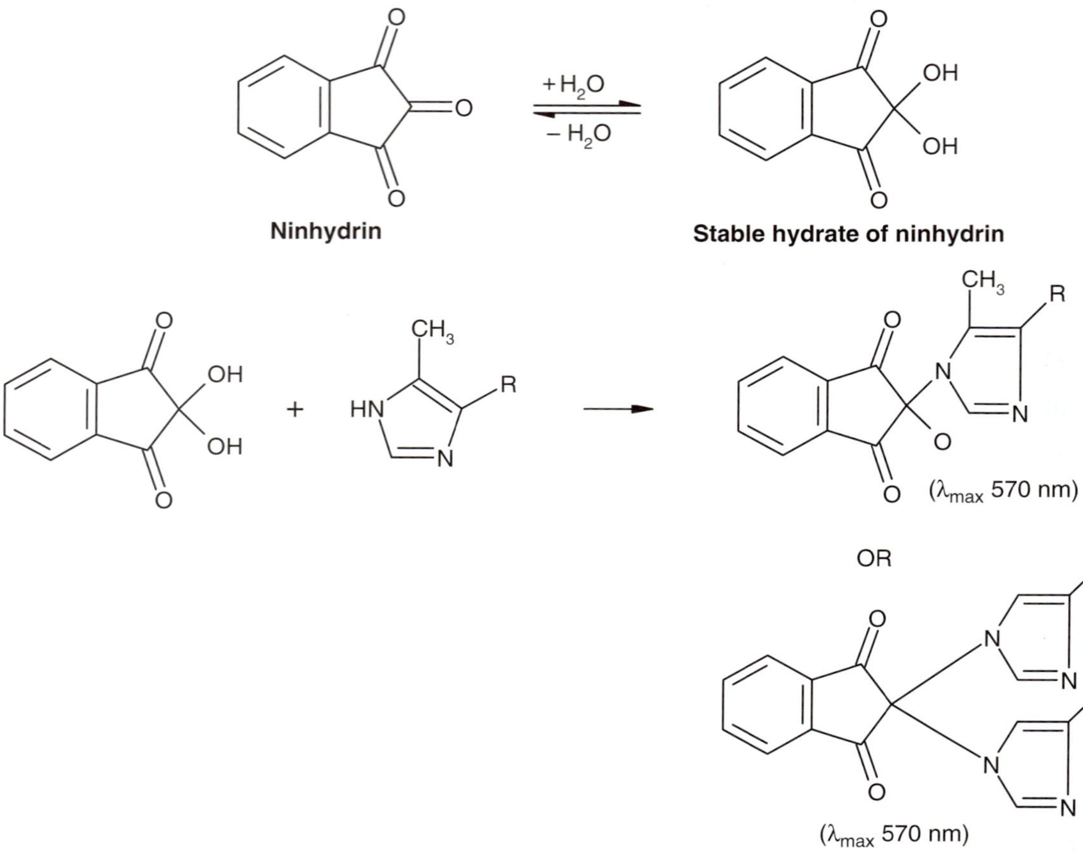

Reference

1. Pharmaceutical Chemistry (Vol. 2) by H.J. Roth, p. 214.
2. G. Rama Rao & S. Raghuveer, *Indian Drugs*, **18(11)**, 408, 1981.

METHOD 2

Weigh accurately a quantity of powdered tablets equivalent to about 60 mg of cimetidine, shake and make up to 20 ml with 0.1 N sulphuric acid. 5 ml of this solution is further diluted to 200 ml with acid.

Measure the extinction of both the solutions at 218 nm and 260 nm using 0.1 N sulphuric acid as blank. Calculate the difference between the extinctions at 218 and 260 nm (A).

Calculation

$$\% \text{ of cimetidine} = \frac{\text{'A'} \times 0.01212 \times \text{dilution factor} \times 100}{\text{weight of sample taken (corrected for isopropyl alcohol)}}$$

0.01212 = mg of cimetidine per ml per unit. This absorptivity factor (A) is experimentally determined with pure sample of cimetidine. The factor is likely to vary with the instrument used.

METHOD 3

Reagents

1. 0.5% w/v solution of cupric acetate in water.

Standard solution

1 mg/ml of pure cimetidine in water.

Sample solution

Weigh accurately a quantity of powdered tablets equivalent to 50 mg of cimetidine, dissolve and make up to 50 ml with water (1 mg/ml).

Procedure

Transfer 1 ml each of standard and sample solutions to two separate 10 ml volumetric flasks, add 0.2 ml of cupric acetate reagent and adjust the volume with water. Allow to stand for 10 minutes and measure the absorbance at about 640 nm. The method obeys Beer's law in the concentration range of 10-700 mcg/ml.

Probable Reaction Mechanism

The compound forms complex with Cu^{++}.

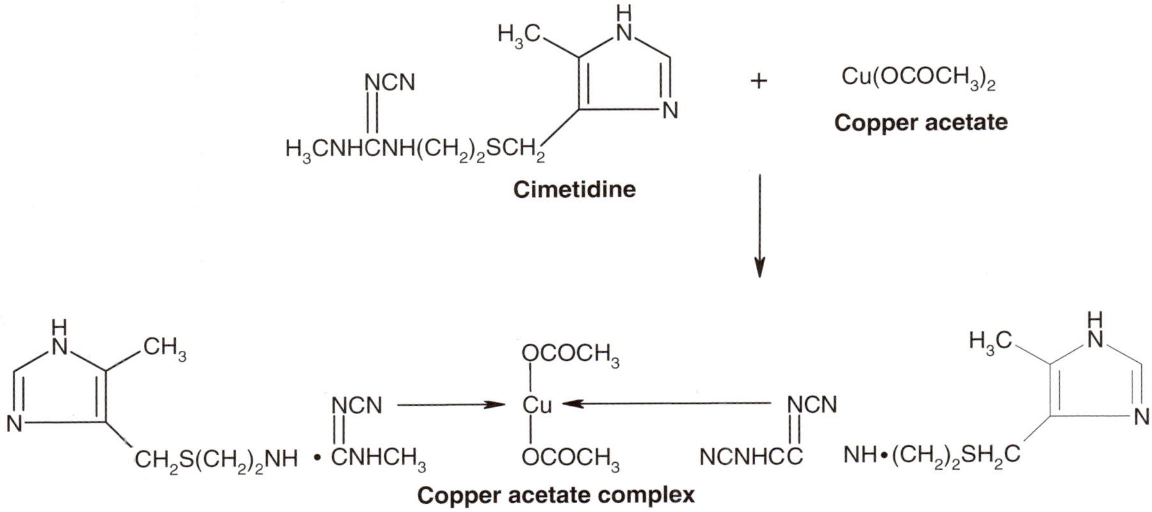

OR

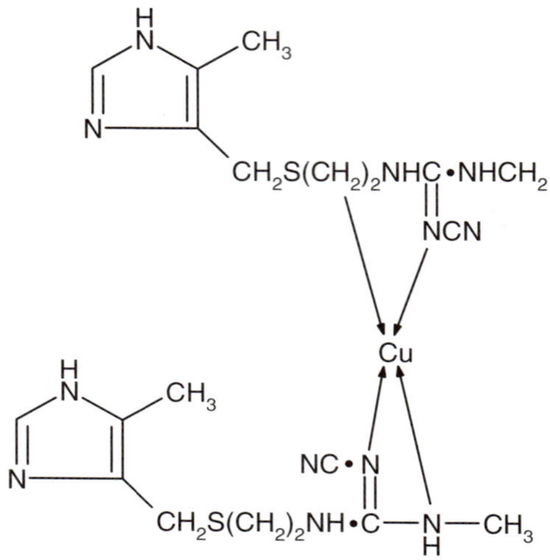

Copper acetate complex
(λ_{max} 640 nm)

Reference

R.B. Patel, T.P. Gandhi, G.F. Shah, P.R. Patel, M.R. Patel, V.C. Patel & R.N. Gilbert, *Indian Drugs*, **18(5)**, 177-179, Feb. 1981.

METHOD 4

Reagents

1. 1% w/v solution of sulphanilic acid in 0.5 N hydrochloric acid.
2. 1% w/v solution of sodium nitrite in water.
3. 1% w/v solution of sodium bicarbonate in water.

Standard solution

1 mg/ml of pure cimetidine in 0.1 N hydrochloric acid. Further dilution is done with water to produce 50 mcg/ml solution.

Sample solution

Tablets/capsules: Weigh accurately powdered tablets equivalent to 100 mg of cimetidine and dissolve in 0.1 N hydrochloric acid to produce 100 ml and filter. 5 ml of the filtrate is further diluted to 100 ml with water (50 mcg/ml).

Procedure

1 ml of sulphanilic acid solution taken in two separate test tubes is allowed to remain in crushed ice for 10 minutes. Add 1 ml of sodium nitrite solution, previously chilled, to each tube, shake and keep in ice-bath for another 10 minutes. Then to each tube add 1 ml each of standard and sample solutions

(50 mcg), shake vigorously and keep in ice-bath for 30 minutes with shaking at an interval of 5 minutes. Add 5 ml of water followed by 2 ml of sodium bicarbonate solution to each tube. Shake vigorously and again keep in ice-bath for 10 minutes and measure the absorbance of both the solutions at about 405 nm against reagent blank. The method obeys Beer's law in a concentration range of 1-10 mcg/ml.

Diazotized sulphanilic acid couples at position 2 of the imidazole ring of the drug resulting in the formation of coloured compound. $NaHCO_3$ is added to maintain weakly alkaline conditions required for coupling.

Probable Reaction Mechanism

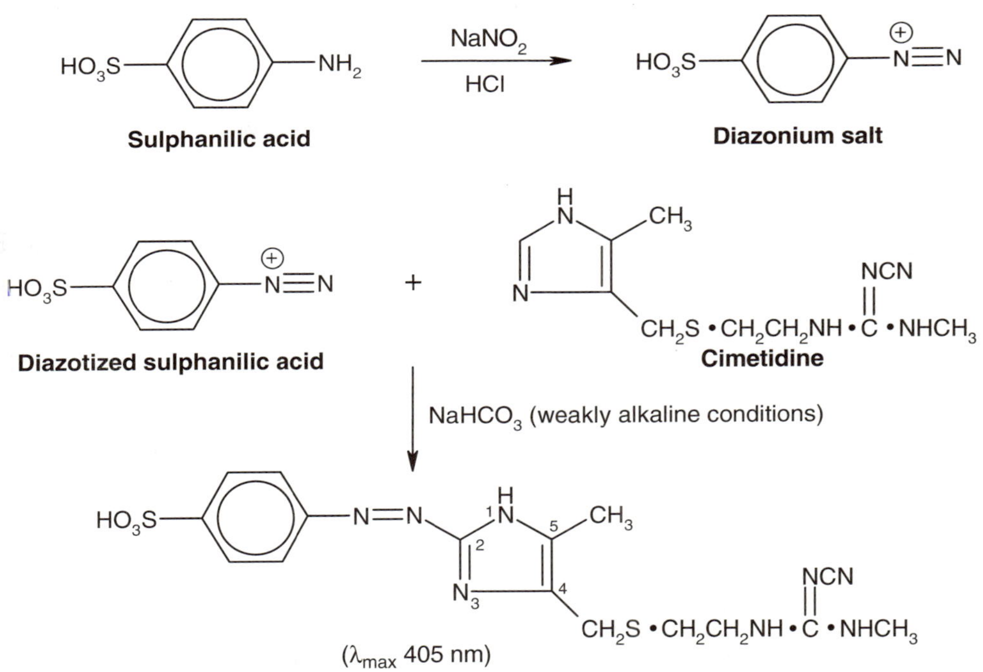

Reference

H.K. Mehta & M.L. Chainani, *Ind. J. Pharm. Sci.*, **42(2)**, 58-60, 1980.

METHOD 5

Reagents

1. 0.5% w/v solution of 2,6-dichloroquinone chlorimide in isopropyl alcohol. The reagent should always be freshly prepared.

Standard solution

200 mcg/ml of pure cimetidine in water. Dissolve by slight warming.

Sample solution

Weigh accurately powdered tablets equivalent to 20 mg of cimetidine and extract with sufficient water to produce a solution of 200 mcg/ml.

Procedure

To 5 ml of the standard and sample solutions add 1.25 ml chlorimide reagent and heat on a water-bath for 20 minutes. Cool to room temperature, add 1 ml of hydrochloric acid and make up to 25 ml with water. Measure the absorbance of both the solutions at about 440 nm against a reagent blank run concomitantly. The method obeys Beer's law in the range of 6-60 mcg/ml and the orange-coloured complex is stable for over 6 hours. Commonly encountered excipients do not interfere in this method.

Probable Reaction Mechanism

2,6-dichloroquinone chlorimide reagent in H_2O is converted into dichloroquinonimine which is the reacting agent. Oxidative coupling occurs between dichloroquinonimine and the drug. In the drug, the attack of dichloroquinonimine occurs at position 2 of the imidazole ring.

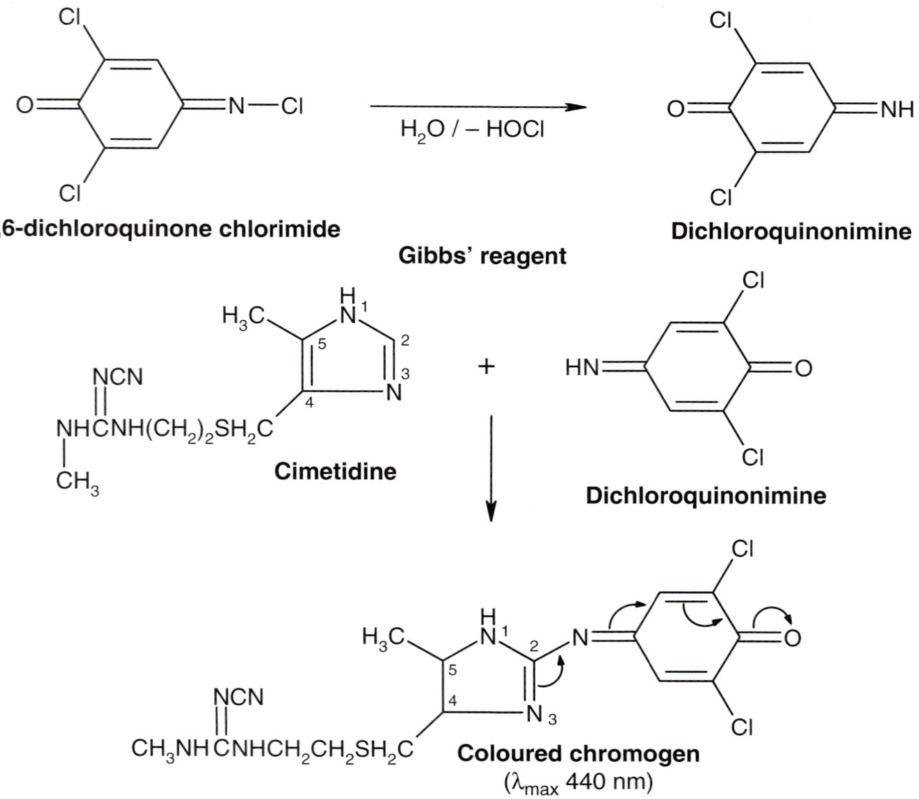

METHOD 6

Reagents

1. 0.1 M citric acid, monohydrate.
2. 0.2 M disodium phosphate.
3. 0.04% w/v solution of bromothymol blue in water.
4. Citrate - phosphate buffer, pH 5.5: 30 ml of 0.2 M disodium phosphate and 20 ml of 0.1 M citric acid are mixed together and diluted with water to 100 ml. Check pH and adjust with 0.2 M phosphate or 0.1 M citric acid.

Standard solution

Weigh accurately 25 mg of pure cimetidine and dilute to 100 ml with the buffer. 20 ml of the resultant solution is further diluted with the buffer to get 50 mcg/ml solution.

Sample solution

Weigh accurately a quantity of the powdered tablets equivalent to 20 mg of cimetidine, add 80 ml of buffer solution and shake for few minutes. Dilute to 100 ml with buffer solution and filter. Dilute the filtrate with buffer appropriately to produce 50 mcg/ml solution.

Procedure

To 2.5 ml each of standard and sample solutions add 5 ml of buffer solution, 5 ml of dye solution and 20 ml of chloroform. Shake and allow the chloroform layer to separate. Measure the absorbance of the chloroform layer at maxima at about 420 nm using chloroform as blank. The method obeys Beer's law in the concentration range of 1-15 mcg/ml. The coloured complex is stable for more than 1 h.

Note

The method is based on ion-pair complex formation. The colouring matter and common excipients do not interfere.

METHOD 7

Reagents

1. Cobalt - thiocyanate reagent: Dissolve 1.33 g of cobaltous chloride and 3.33 g of potassium thiocyanate in water to produce 100 ml.
2. Universal buffer, pH 7.96.
3. Isobutyl methyl ketone.

4. 0.4% w/v solution of 1,2-naphthoquinone-4-sulphonic acid (sodium salt) in water (Folin's reagent).
5. 1 N sodium hydroxide.

Standard solution

250 mcg/ml of pure cimetidine in water dissolved by slight warming.

Sample solution

Weigh powder accurately equivalent to 20 mg of cimetidine and extract with water by gentle warming to produce 250 mcg/ml.

Procedure

A. Cobalt - thiocyanate method: To 3 ml each of sample and standard solutions add 1 ml of buffer solution, 1.5 ml of cobalt reagent and 4.5 ml of water. Extract the coloured complex with four 10 ml portions of isobutyl methyl ketone. Combine organic extract and dilute to 50 ml and measure the absorbance at about 625 nm against reagent blank. The method obeys Beer's law in the concentration range of 80-140 mcg/ml.
Note: The blue colour of the complex in organic layer is stable for 24 hours. For detailed reaction mechanism, refer to method 3 based on complexation with Cu^{2+}.

B. Naphthoquinone - sulphonic acid method: To 5 ml each of sample and standard solutions add 4 ml of naphthoquinone reagent and 2 ml of 1 N sodium hydroxide. Mix and dilute to 50 ml with water. Set aside for 10 min at room temperature and read absorbance at about 435 nm against reagent blank. The method obeys Beer's law in the range of 10-40 mcg/ml.

Probable Reaction Mechanism

There are two secondary aliphatic amino groups (1) and (2) in the side chain of the drug. Out of these two, the first aliphatic amino group has less steric hindrance and hence can be the first to attack and undergoes Michael addition eliminating the monohydrogen sulphite radical.

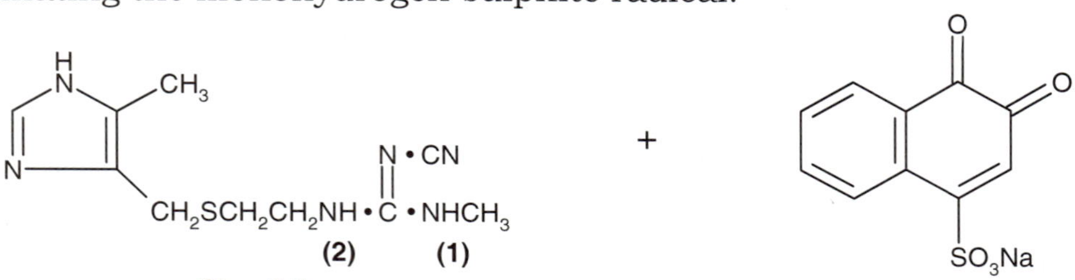

Cimetidine

1,2-naphthaquinone-4-sulphonic acid
(reagent used as sodium salt)

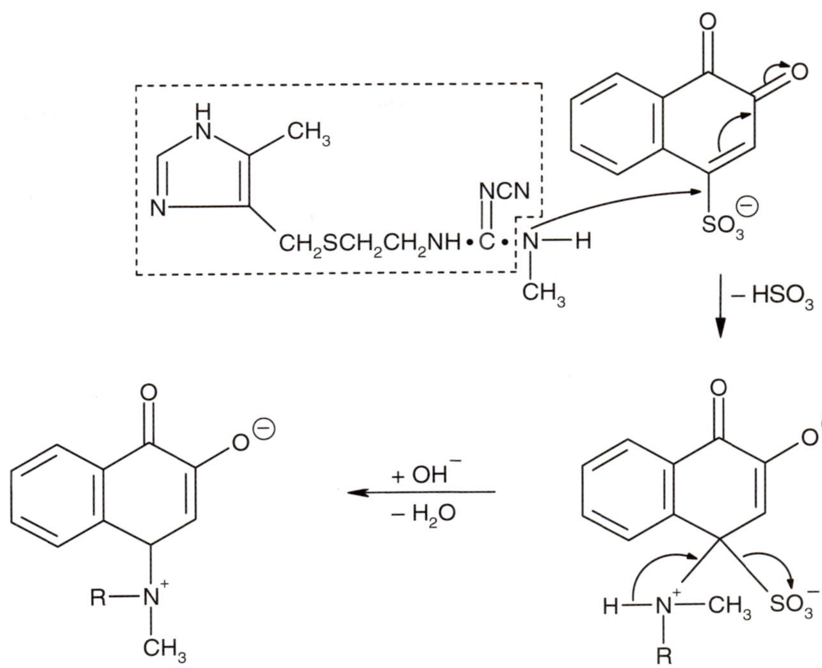

Yellow-coloured quinonimine
(λ_{max} 435 nm)

Reference

1. Pharmaceutical Chemistry (Vol. 2) by H.J. Roth, p. 378.
2. G. Rama Rao, S. Raghuveer & Y. Pulla Rao, *J. Inst. Chem.*, **54**, 146, May 1982 (methods A & B).

Formulation 39

Propantheline bromide, Meprobamate, Dried aluminium hydroxide gel

ESTIMATION

Propantheline bromide

Weigh accurately quantity of the powdered tablets equivalent to 50 mg of the substance and transfer to a 250 ml conical flask. Add 20 ml of water and 5 ml of dilute nitric acid. Boil, cool and add 25 ml of 0.01 N silver nitrate solution. Shake and titrate excess silver nitrate with 0.01 N ammonium thiocyanate using ferric alum as indicator. Run a blank with 25 ml of 0.01 N silver nitrate, 5 ml of dilute nitric acid and 20 ml of water. Difference in titration values gives the amount of 0.01 N silver nitrate consumed by the sample. Each ml of 0.01 silver nitrate is equivalent to 0.00448 g of propantheline bromide. The method is based on estimation of halogen (Br^-) with $AgNO_3$.

Meprobamate

This method is based on formol titration.

Extract the powdered tablets equivalent to 100 mg of meprobamate accurately weighed with three 50 ml portions of acetone and filter. Evaporate the solvent on a water-bath. To the residue, add 40 ml of hydrochloric acid (1: 1) and reflux on a burner for 90 minutes. Remove the condenser and boil until the volume is reduced to about 8 ml. Cool the flask in ice, add 50 ml of water, 1 drop of methyl red indicator and neutralise with 10 N sodium hydroxide, until the colour is just changed. If necessary, add 1 N hydrochloric acid to restore the pink colour. Then carefully neutralise with 0.1 N sodium hydroxide. Add a mixture of 15 ml of formaldehyde solution and 15 ml of water previously neutralised to phenolphthalein with 0.1 N sodium hydroxide. Titrate with 0.1 N sodium hydroxide until the solution becomes yellow. Add 0.2 ml of phenolphthalein and continue to titrate with 0.1 N sodium hydroxide to a distinct pink colour. Each ml of 0.1 N sodium hydroxide is equivalent to 0.01091 g of meprobamate.

Method 2

Standard solution

1 mg/ml of meprobamate in acetone.

Sample solution

Extract accurately weighed quantity of powdered sample with acetone to get sample concentration of 1 mg/ml.

Procedure

To 1 ml each of sample and standard solutions add 0.5 ml of furfuraldehyde (0.5% in glacial acetic acid) and 10 ml of hydrochloric acid. Mix and measure the absorbance at 580 nm after 45 seconds.

Probable Reaction Mechanism

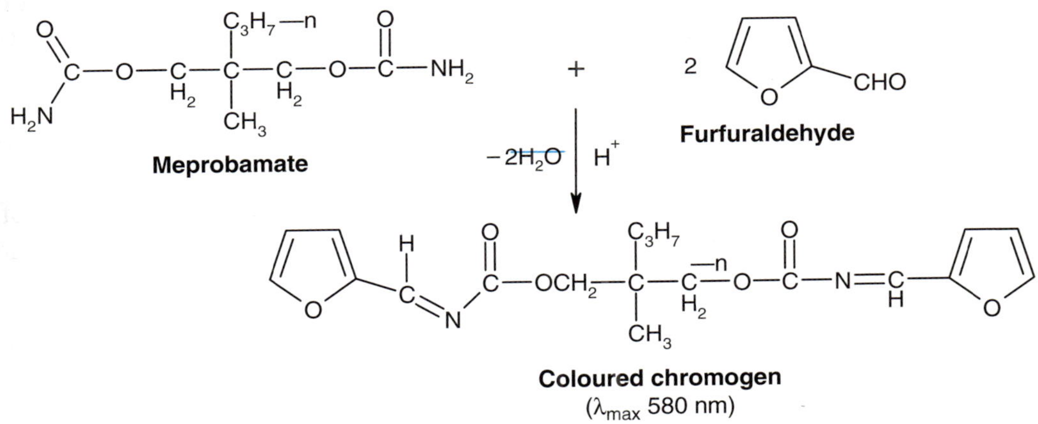

Explanatory Note

Condensation reaction occurs between meprobamate and furfuraldehyde. This is known as Schiff's base formation or imine formation. Here two molecules of furfuraldehyde can react at both ends of the drug under acidic conditions to give the coloured product.

On similar analogy PDAB also forms condensation product with meprobamate.

A titrimetric method under anhydrous conditions as well as gravimetric method had been described in literature. The substance is dissolved in pyridine and refluxed with excess of 0.1 M sodium methoxide in benzene - methanol for 60 min and excess sodium methoxide determined by titration with 0.1 M benzoic acid using thymol blue as indicator. Sodium cyanate formed as reaction product being insoluble can be used for gravimetric assay.

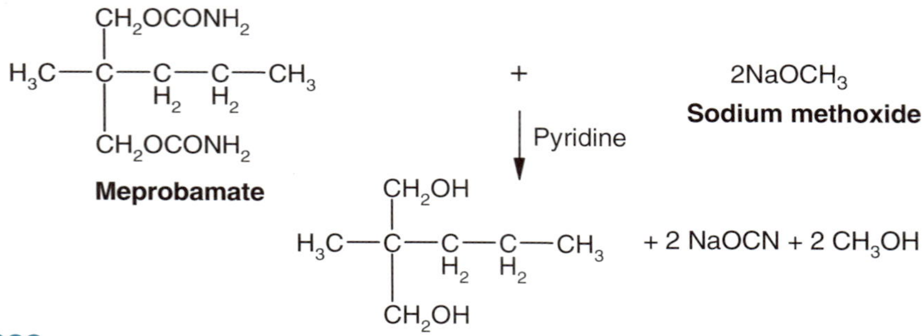

Reference

Pharmaceutical Analysis by T. Higuchi et al., CBS Publishers & Distributors, New Delhi, 1997.

In case of formol titration, formaldehyde forms imine on reaction with amino group. The imine is a weaker base than amine, so acid titration proceeds smoothly.

$$NH_2RCOOH + HCHO \rightleftharpoons H_2C{=}NRCOOH + H_2O$$

In case of meprobamate, on hydrolysis we get acid and ammonia; on addition of formaldehyde it forms a compound with ammonia (hexamethylene tetramine - methamine rather than imine). This product is much weaker than ammonia, so the titration reaction proceeds favourably.

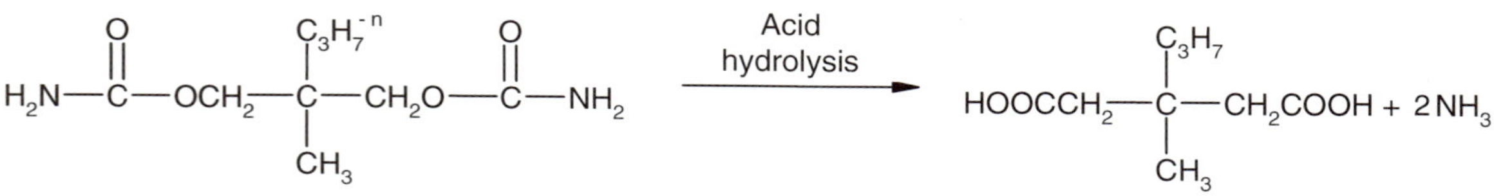

$$HCHO + NH_3 \longrightarrow H_2C{=}NH + H_2O$$

Formaldimine

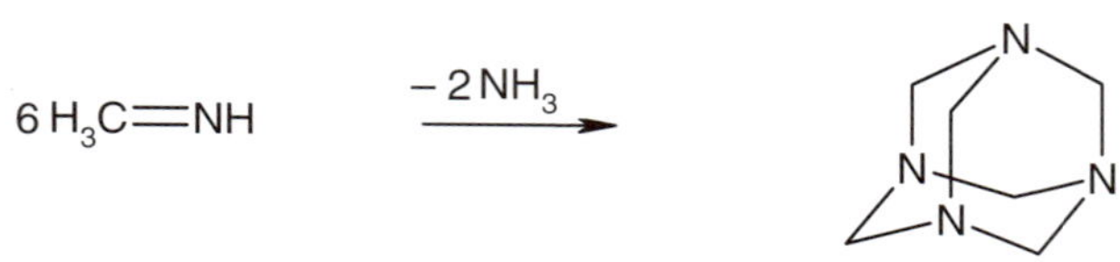

Hexamethylene tetramine (methamine)

Hexamethylene tetramine is also called methamine, an aliphatic amine. On acid hydrolysis it gives formaldehyde and ammonia.

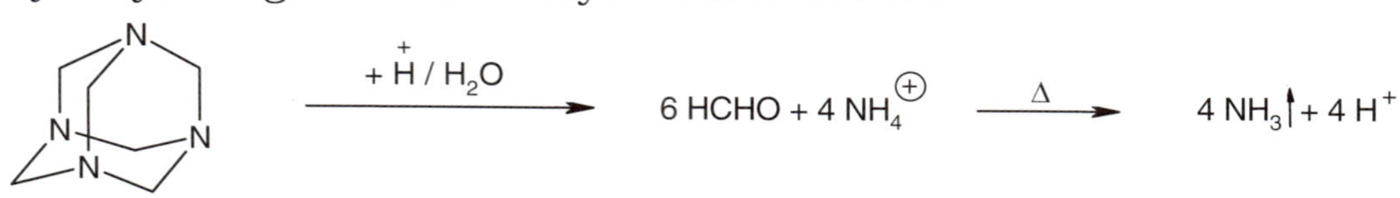

Hexamethylene tetramine

Note

Formaldimine rapidly undergoes self-condensation. With loss of ammonia it gives an unusual compound known as hexamethylene tetramine.

Reference

Textbook of Pharmaceutical Analysis, 3rd ed., by K.A. Connors, John Wiley & Sons, p. 548.

On heating with ethanolic potassium hydroxide, cyanate is produced which forms blue-coloured complex with $Co(2)^+$. This forms the basis for quantitative estimation.

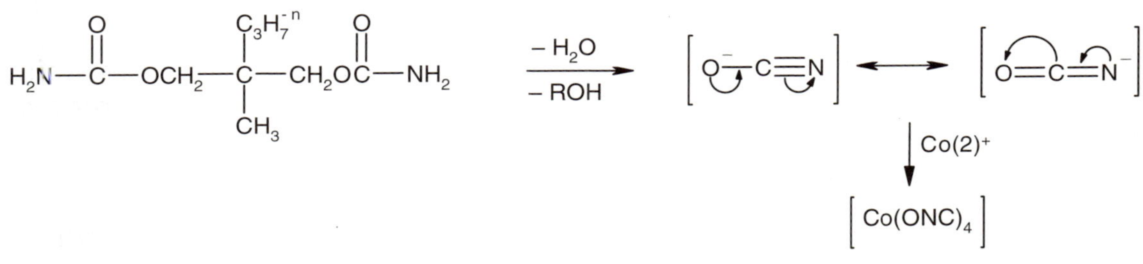

Tetracyano-cobalt complex
(λ_{max} 610 nm)

Reference

Pharmaceutical Chemistry (Vol. 2) by H.J. Roth, 1991, pp. 293-294 & 347.

(a) On hydrolysis in acidic medium, ammonia is liberated.
(b) On alkaline hydrolysis:

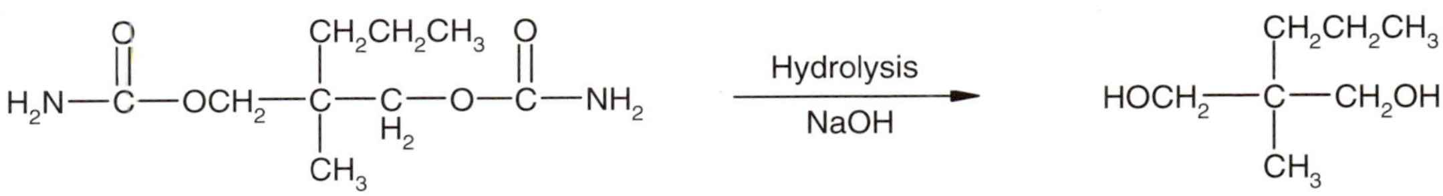

2-methyl-2-propyl-1,3-propanolol

This can be converted into benzoyl ester for HPLC analysis.

Reference

Analytical Profile of Drug Substances (Vol. 2) by Klaus Florey, p. 587.

Total aluminium calculated as aluminium oxide

Transfer an accurately weighed powder of the sample equivalent to 100 mg of the gel. Add 30 ml of dilute hydrochloric acid and warm on a water-bath for 30 minutes and cool. Add 40 ml of 0.05 N disodium edetate and neutralise with sodium hydroxide solution (10% w/v) using methyl red as indicator and keep on water-bath for 30 minutes. Cool, add 6 g of hexamine and titration with 0.05 M lead nitrate solution using xylenol orange as indicator. Run a blank omitting the sample. Each ml of 0.05 M disodium edetate consumed is equivalent to 0.002549 g aluminium oxide.

Formulation 40

Meprobamate, Ethoheptazine citrate, Aspirin

ESTIMATION

Meprobamate

Weigh accurately powdered tablets equivalent to 100 mg of meprobamate and follow the method described for meprobamate under formulation 39 of this chapter.

Ethoheptazine citrate

Reagents

1. 0.1 N perchloric acid in glacial acetic acid.
2. 1% w/v crystal violet solution.
3. Carbon tetrachloride.
4. Alkaline salt solution: 100 ml of saturated ammonium chloride solution in water containing 2 g of sodium hydroxide.

Procedure

Weigh sample equivalent to about 200 mg of ethoheptazine. Add 20 ml of alkaline salt solution, shake vigorously for 5 minutes and extract with four 30 ml portions of carbon tetrachloride. Pass organic layer through anhydrous sodium sulphate, add 20 ml of glacial acetic acid, 2 drops of crystal violet solution and titrate with 0.1 N perchloric acid to blue colour. Each ml of 0.1 N perchloric acid is equivalent to 0.04535 g of ethoheptazine citrate. From the total volume of the acid consumed in the above titration, calculate the amount of ethoheptazine citrate present in the sample.

Note

Addition of alkaline salt solution will generate ethoheptazine base which can be extracted into organic solvent and finally subjected to non-aqueous titration.

Aspirin

Weigh accurately quantity of powdered tablets equivalent to 500 mg of aspirin, add 25 ml of 0.5 N sodium hydroxide, boil gently for ten minutes and titrate excess of alkali with 0.5 N hydrochloric acid using phenol red as indicator. Each ml of 0.5 N sodium hydroxide is equivalent to 0.04507 g of aspirin.

Note

Each mol of aspirin will consume 2 mols of sodium hydroxide, hence equivalent factor is ½.

Probable Reaction Mechanism

Based on intramolecular mechanism

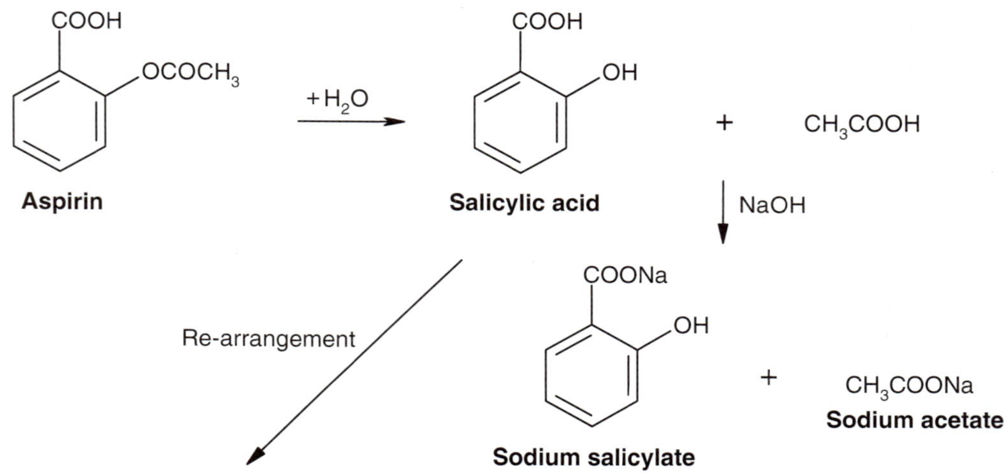

Mechanism of alkaline hydrolysis (based on intramolecular mechanism)

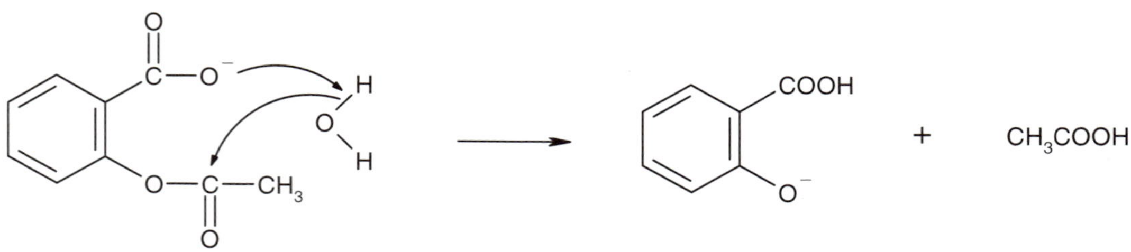

Aspirin

Reference

Organic Chemistry (Vol. 1), 6th ed., by I.L. Finar, p. 767.

Formulation 41

Analgin, Diazepam, Papaverine hydrochloride, Homatropine sulphate

ESTIMATION

Analgin

Follow the colorimetric method using p-dimethylaminobenzaldehyde reagent as described in formulation of the chapter on analgesics and antipyretics along with detailed reaction mechanism.

Diazepam

Suspend accurately weighed quantity of the sample equivalent to 2 mg of the compound in phosphate buffer, pH 7. Extract into ether (peroxide free) and follow the method as described in formulation of the chapter on analgesics and antipyretics along with detailed reaction mechanism.

Homatropine sulphate

Reagents

1. 1 N sodium hydroxide.
2. 0.2 M cerric ammonium sulphate in 6 N sulphuric acid.

Standard preparation

Weigh accurately 50 mg of homatropine sulphate into a 100 ml volumetric flask, dissolve and make up to 100 ml with water. 10 ml of this solution is further diluted to 100 ml with water (50 mcg/ml).

Sample preparation

Weigh accurately the sample equivalent to 5 mg of homatropine into a 100 ml volumetric flask and add 50 ml of water. Shake well and make up with water (50 mcg/ml).

Procedure

Transfer 10 ml each of the standard and sample preparations to separate glass-stoppered 100 ml flasks. To each flask, add 20 ml of 1 N sodium hydroxide and heat in a water-bath at 80°C for 15 minutes. Cool to room temperature, wash the solution with two 25 ml portions of chloroform before addition of cerric reagent. Add 8 ml of 0.2 M cerric ammonium sulphate and mix. To each flask add 25 ml of iso-octane and shake for 15 minutes. Decant the organic layer and concomitantly determine the absorbance of both the solutions, at the maximum at about 242 nm, on a suitable spectrophotometer using iso-octane as the blank.

Probable Reaction Mechanism

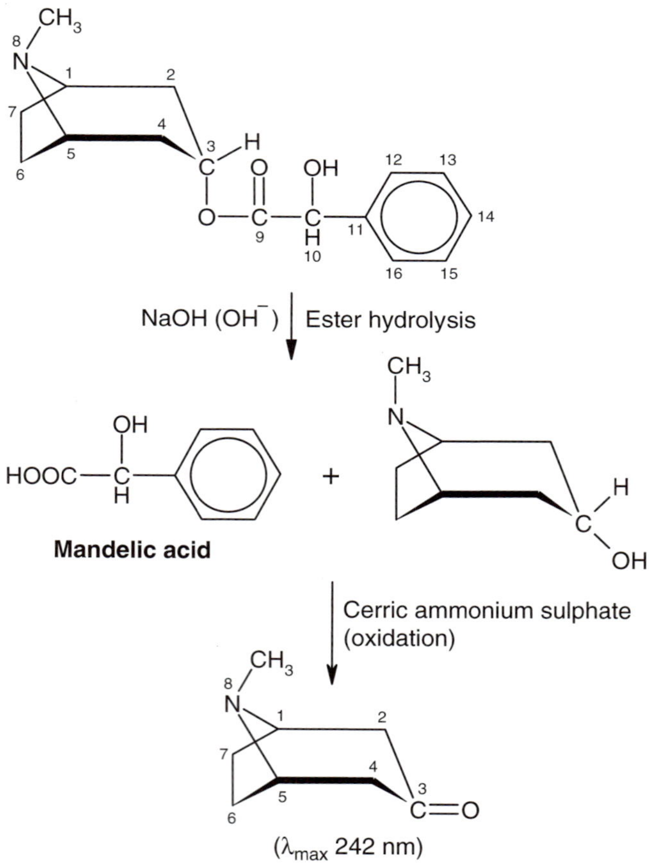

Note

Due to oxidation of mandelic acid, nitration in para position is not possible due to loss of 'CH' activity, only meta nitration is possible in phenyl ring of the molecule.

However, if the drug is first acetylated, then p-nitration is possible leading to formation of coloured product in alkaline medium.

Probable Reaction Mechanism

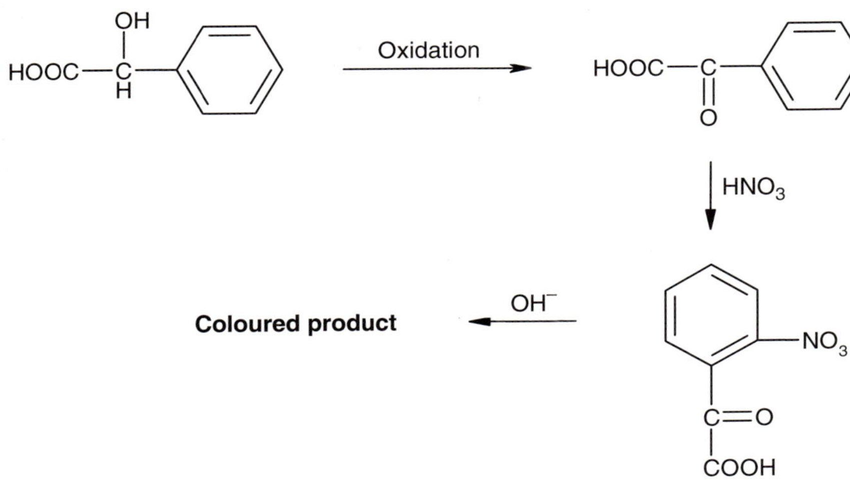

Reference

Organic Chemistry (Vol. 1), 6th ed., by I.L. Finar, p. 189.

- Homatropine reacts with Folin's reagent to give blue colour.
- Homatropine forms ion-pair complex with bromocresol purple in pH 4.0 buffer extractable into chloroform (λ_{max} 405 nm). Hydrolysis products do not interfere.

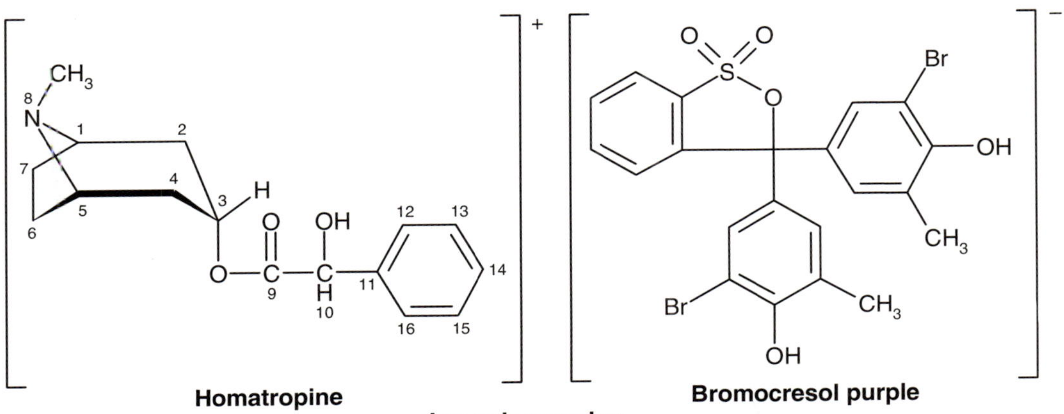

Ion-pair complex
(λ_{max} 405 nm)

Papaverine hydrochloride

Reagents

1. 1% w/v ammonium molybdate solution in water.
2. 10% w/v solution of catechol in water.
3. 0.1 N hydrochloric acid.

Standard solution

To 50 mg of pure papaverine, add 10 ml of 1 N hydrochloric acid and 50 ml of water. Boil on water-bath for 10 min, cool and dilute to 100 ml with water (0.5 mg/ml).

Sample solution

Weigh accurately a quantity of the powdered tablets equivalent to 50 mg of papaverine and proceed as per standard (0.5 mg/ml) solution.

Procedure

To 2 ml each of standard and sample solutions, add 1 ml of ammonium molybdate solution and 3 ml of catechol solution. Mix and extract with three 15 ml portions of chloroform. Pass chloroform layer through dry filter paper (do not use anhydrous sodium sulphate) and adjust to 50 ml with chloroform. Measure the absorbance of both the solutions at about 635 nm and calculate the results by comparison.

Note

Catechol is a powerful reducing agent. After papaverine - molybdate is formed it is reduced to molybdenium blue (λ_{max} 635 nm) by catechol and catechol gets oxidized to o-benzoquinone.

Probable Reaction Mechanism

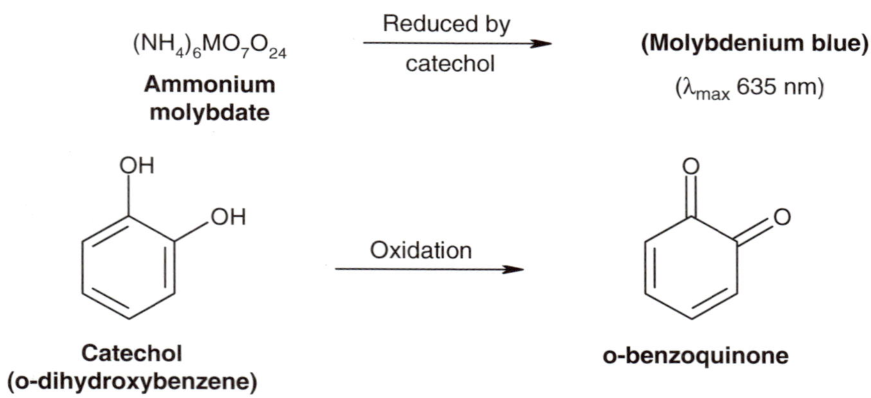

Formulation 42

Analgin, Baralgan ketone (Pitofenone hydrochloride), Baralgan amide (Diphenyl-piperidinoethyl acetamide methobromide)

Preparation of test solution

Powdered sample accurately weighed equivalent to 25 mg of baralgan ketone is extracted with four 10 ml portions of 0.1 N hydrochloric acid, diluted to 50 ml with acid.

ESTIMATION

Analgin

Standard solution

10 mcg/ml of analgin in 0.01 N hydrochloric acid.

Sample solution

2 ml of the test solution is diluted to 100 ml with water. Further dilutions are done with 0.01 N hydrochloric acid to get a solution of 10 mcg/ml.

Measure the extinction of standard and sample solutions at maxima at about 257 nm using 0.01 N hydrochloric acid as blank. Calculate the results by comparison.

Baralgan ketone (p-piperidionethoxy-o-carbomethoxy benzophenone hydrochloride)

Reagents

1. 30% w/v solution of sodium hydroxide in water.
2. 0.1 N hydrochloric acid.
3. 0.2% w/v solution of sodium hydroxide in water (dilute sodium hydroxide solution).
4. n-hexane.

Standard solution

10 mcg/ml of baralgan ketone in water.

Sample solution

To 10 ml of test solution prepared above, add 5 ml of sodium hydroxide solution. Extract with three 20 ml portions of n-hexane (reserve the alkaline extract for estimation of baralgan amide). Combine the organic layer and shake vigorously with 40 ml of dilute sodium hydroxide solution and allow complete separation of layers. Reject the alkaline layer. The organic layer is extracted with three 20 ml portions of 0.1 N hydrochloric acid, the acidic extract is combined and diluted to 500 ml with water (10 mcg/ml).

The extinction of both sample and standard solutions is measured at maximum at about 290 nm and results calculated by comparison.

Baralgan amide

Reagents

1. 5% w/v solution of EDTA (disodium) in water.
2. 0.12% w/v solution of dithizone in chloroform.
3. 1 N hydrochloric acid.
4. Dithizone reagent: To 5 g of potassium cyanide and 11 g of sodium hydroxide add 30 ml water, shake to dissolve and dilute to 100 ml with water. Add 8 ml each of EDTA solution and dithizone solution. Wash the above solution twice with 25 ml of chloroform, rejecting organic layer. The alkaline aqueous solution is the dithizone reagent. (The reagent is to be freshly prepared.)
5. Saturated solution of sodium sulphate in water.

Standard solution

100 mcg/ml of baralgan amide in water.

Sample solution

The entire alkaline solution reserved during estimation of baralgan ketone is used for estimation of amide contents in the sample.

Procedure

Transfer 10 ml of standard solution and the entire sample solution to separating funnel containing 10 ml of freshly prepared ice cold dithizone reagent. Add 20 ml of chloroform and shake vigorously for about 2 minutes. Allow the layers to separate. The chloroform layer is shaken with 5 ml of 1 N hydrochloric acid. The separated chloroform layer is passed through a layer of anhydrous sodium sulphate placed over the plug of cotton.

The absorption of sample and standard solutions is measured at about 605 nm and results calculated by comparison.

Formulation 43

Ibuprofen/Ketoprofen, Baralgan ketone, Baralgan amide

ESTIMATION

Ibuprofen/Ketoprofen

Weigh accurately quantity of powdered sample equivalent to about 500 mg of ibuprofen/ketoprofen and dry extract with 20 ml of chloroform. Filter chloroform extract through cotton plug and wash the powder and cotton plug with three more 10 ml portions of chloroform. Evaporate the combined filtrate to dryness by gentle heating with the aid of current of air. Dissolve the residue in 100 ml of methanol previously neutralized to phenol red and titrate with 0.1 N sodium hydroxide solution using phenol red solution as indicator. Each ml of 0.1 N sodium hydroxide solution is equivalent to 0.02063 g of ibuprofen or 0.02543 g of ketoprofen.

Note

Do not employ filter paper for filtration as lower assay values are often obtained. Instead of dry extraction, suspend in 0.1 N hydrochloric acid and extract with chloroform. This procedure will give more consistent results.

Baralgan ketone and amide

Preparation of test solution

Weigh accurately powdered sample equivalent to 2.5 mg of baralgan ketone and extract with four 10 ml portions of 0.1 N hydrochloric acid, dilute to 50 ml with acid.

Estimate both baralgan ketone and amide by the methods described in formulation 30 of this chapter.

Alternatively, sample equivalent to 500 mg of ibuprofen is suspended in 20 ml of 0.1 N hydrochloric acid and extracted with chloroform as described above under ibuprofen. The acidic extract may be used for estimation of baralgan amide and ketone as per methods described in formulation 30 of this chapter.

Formulation 44

Propyphenazone, Pitofenone hydrochloride, Baralgan amide

ESTIMATION

Propyphenazone

Weigh accurately powdered sample equivalent to 300 mg of the substance and dry extract with four 30 ml portions of dry ether. Evaporate the combined ether layer to remove water completely adding few drops of methanol during last stages of evaporation to ensure complete removal of moisture. Add 40 ml of glacial acetic acid and 10 ml of acetic anhydride and titrate with 0.1 N perchloric acid using crystal violet as indicator. Each ml of 0.1 N perchloric acid is equivalent to 0.023031 g of propyphenazone.

Pitofenone hydrochloride (baralgan ketone)

Accurately weighed quantity of the sample equivalent to 50 mg of the substance is extracted thrice (3×50 ml) with boiling water. The combined aqueous extract is cooled. Add 10 ml of 0.05 N hydrochloric acid and back titrate with 0.05 N sodium hydroxide (phenolphthalein). Carry out blank titration. Each ml of 0.05 N hydrochloric acid is equivalent to 20.175 mg of ketone.

Baralgan amide

Standard solution

5 mcg/ml of baralgan amide in water.

Sample solution

Dry extract the powdered sample equivalent to 0.2 mg of the substance with chloroform (3×25 ml), filter through G_4 sintered funnel. Evaporate the combined organic layer and take up the residue in 40 ml of water.

Procedure

To 40 ml of the standard solution and entire sample solution add 5 ml of 1 N sodium hydroxide and 5 ml of tropeolin OO solution (0.1%). Extract with chloroform (3 × 40 ml), and extract combined organic layer with dilute hydrochloric acid (3 × 30 ml). Make up the volume to 100 ml and measure the absorbance of both sample and standard solutions at about 535 nm against blank prepared by using 40 ml of water. Calculate the results by comparison.

Note

The compound forms ion-pair complex with the dye extractable into chloroform.

Formulation 45

Analgin, Papaverine hydrochloride, Phenobarbitone

ESTIMATION

Analgin

Weigh sample accurately equivalent to 200 mg of analgin, add 100 ml of water and 35 ml of 0.1 N iodine solution, stir and allow to stand for 30 minutes. Then add 10 ml of hydrochloric acid. Heat the solution on a burner till it becomes clear and pale yellow. Filter while hot through G_4 sintered funnel. To the filtrate add 20 ml of 15% w/v solution of barium chloride and digest on steam-bath for 1 hr. Filter through G_4 sintered funnel, wash the precipitates with water till the filtrate is free of chloride. Dry the precipitate at 105°C for 2 hours and weigh the residue.

$$\text{Analgin} = \text{Weight of precipitate (g)} \times 351.30/233.80$$

Probable Reaction Mechanism

On oxidation with I_2 in acidic conditions we get hydroxymethylamine derivative and $NaHSO_4$. $BaCl_2$ is used to estimate SO_4^- as $BaSO_4$.

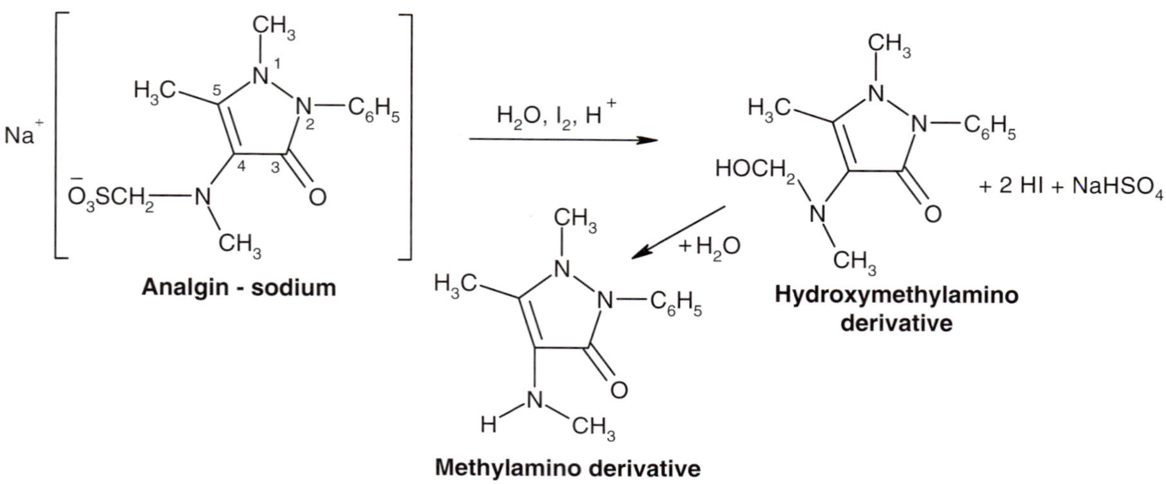

The sulphate can be precipitated as $BaSO_4$ by using $BaCl_2$ and this forms the basis for gravimetric assay.

$$NaHSO_4 + BaCl_2 \longrightarrow BaSO_4 + NaCl + HCl$$

With $FeCl_3$ reddish colour is produced due to complex formation.

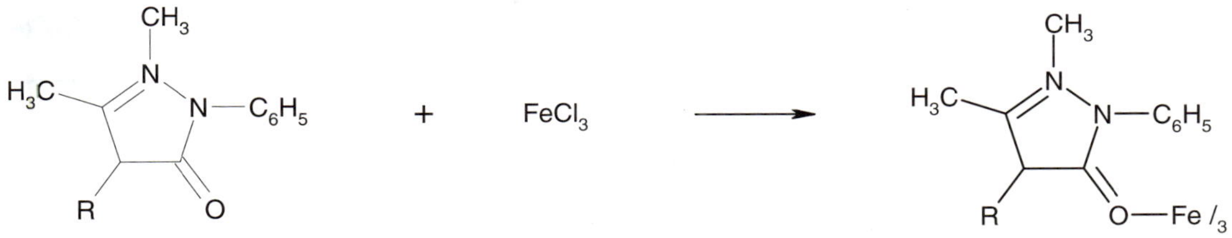

Phenobarbitone

Weigh accurately powdered tablets equivalent to 40 mg of phenobarbitone, suspend in water and acidify with dilute hydrochloric acid. Extract with four 25 ml portions of ether. Retain aqueous layer for estimation of papaverine. Evaporate ether layer and dissolve the residue in dilute ammonia solution to get 10 mcg/ml. Measure the extinction at 240.5 nm and compare the results with the standard solution (10 mcg/ml).

Papaverine hydrochloride

The aqueous layer retained during determination of phenobarbitone is made alkaline with 0.1 N sodium hydroxide and extracted with four 20 ml portions of ether. The ether layer is extracted with 0.1 N hydrochloric acid and the extinction of acidic layer is read at maxima at about 310 nm. Calculate the results from E 1%, 1 cm value of 228.

Formulation 46

Pipenzolate methyl bromide, Paracetamol, Phenobarbitone

ESTIMATION

Pipenzolate methyl bromide

METHOD 1

Reagents

1. 10% w/v solution of silicotungstic acid in water.
2. Acidic sodium lauryl sulphate: Dissolve about 5 mg of sodium lauryl sulphate in 100 ml of 0.1 N hydrochloric acid.

Procedure

Add 20 ml of sample to each of two 200 ml beakers. Add 60 ml of water, 1 ml of hydrochloric acid and 5 ml of silicotungstic acid solution. Mix and heat for 5 minutes in a water-bath. Remove the beaker from the water-bath and allow it to stand at room temperature for 30-40 minutes, then keep in ice-bath for at least 30 minutes. Filter the solution on a tared gouch crucible using the acidic lauryl sulphate solution to aid the quantitative transfer of the precipitates. Wash the precipitates in the crucible three times with acidic lauryl sulphate solution. Dry at 110°C for 2-3 hours or until constant weight is attained.

$$\text{Weight of pipenzolate} = \frac{\text{Weight of the residue (g)}}{2.41} \times \text{dilution factor} \times 100$$

METHOD 2

Reagent

Cobalt nitrate solution: Dissolve 3.75 g of $Co(NO_3)_2$ in 5 ml of water, add 15 g of amm. hydrochloride solution and dilute to 100 ml with water.

Sample and standard solutions

250 µg/ml in 0.1 M HCl.

Procedure

Take 5 ml of each of dilution standard, test and N/10 hydrochloride as blank in separate separating flasks, add 20 ml of reagent to each flask and allow to stand for 2 minutes, then extract with 4 × 5 ml of chloroform passing organic layer through sodium sulphate anhydrous in a 25 ml volumetric flask and make up the volume with chloroform and take reading at 610 nm.

Probable Reaction Mechanism

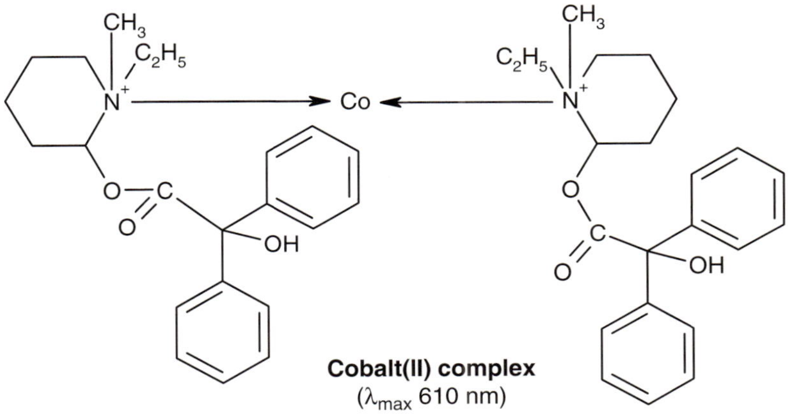

Cobalt(II) complex
(λ_{max} 610 nm)

Paracetamol

Reagents

1. Hydrochloric acid, dilute.
2. 10% w/v solution of sodium nitrite in water.
3. Ethyl alcohol.
4. Methanol.

Standard solution

2 mg/ml of paracetamol in methanol.

Sample solution

Take accurately measured volume of the syrup equivalent to 100 mg of paracetamol in a dry 50 ml volumetric flask, make up the volume with methanol.

Procedure

Take 1 ml aliquot of standard as well as sample solutions in two different 100 ml volumetric flasks. To each flask add 10 ml of water, then add 1 ml each of dilute hydrochloric acid and sodium nitrite solution. Allow the solutions to stand for 10 minutes, then add 5 ml of dilute hydrochloric acid, 5 ml ethyl alcohol and make up the volume with water. Measure the absorbance of both the solutions at 395 nm against water as blank. Calculate the results by comparison.

Probable Reaction Mechanism

Owing to the presence of aromatic hydroxyl group, the compound is capable of forming nitroso derivative—yellow chromogen (λ_{max} 370 nm).

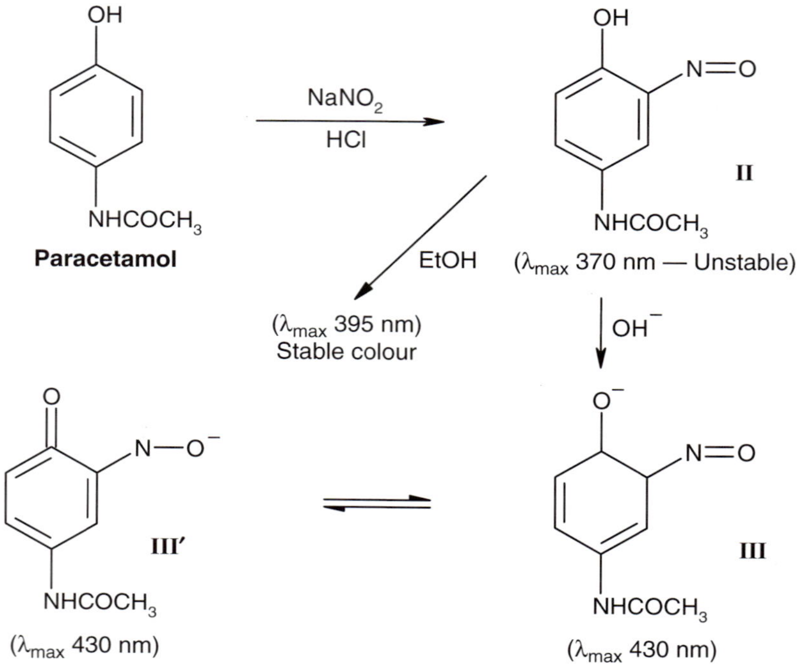

$$HNO_2 + C_2H_5OH \xrightarrow{-H_2O} C_2H_5NO_2$$

Note

1. Unreacted HNO_2 causes variation in colour measurements, hence destroyed by adding ethyl alcohol. The derivative has two maxima i.e. 370 and 395 nm but 395 nm is more stable. Aspirin, analgin, caffeine, phenylephrine, CPM, codeine, doxylamine succinate, dicyclomine, phenobarbitone and ascorbic acid do not interfere.
2. In alkaline medium, the derivatives (III and III′) are highly stable both with bathochromic and hyperchromic shift. This is due to contribution of an extra pair of unshared electrons in the interaction with the aromatic nucleus.

Reference

1. S.F. Belal, M. Abdel-Hady El Sayed, A. El Walily & H. Abdine, *Analyst*, **104**, 919-927, 1979.
2. M.C. Inamdar & N.N. Kadji, *Ind. J. Pharm.*, **31**, 79, 1969.

In order to increase the sensitivity of the nitrosation reaction, the nitroso derivative was chelated with cobalt(II) ion. The OH group with easily replacable proton ortho to N==O group, which offers lone pair of electrons to Co^{++}. The coloured Co(2) chelate so formed is extractable into chloroform (λ_{max} 400 nm).

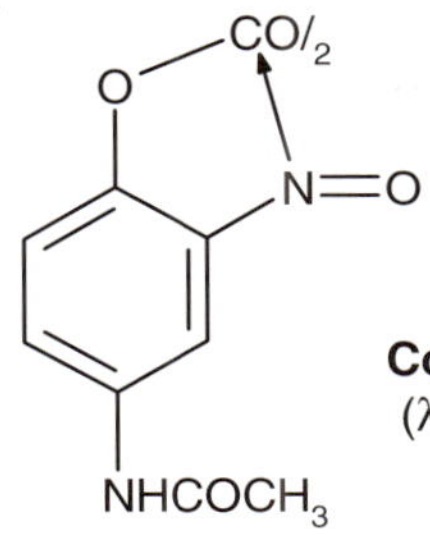

Cobalt chelate
(λ_{max} 400 nm)

Note

Salicylamide does not form chelate with Co(2) as nitrosation favourably occurs at para position to phenolic-OH instead of ortho position.

Phenobarbitone

Reagents

1. Chloroform.
2. Methanol, absolute.
3. 1% v/v hydrochloric acid in water.
4. Isopropylamine solution: 25% v/v in ethyl alcohol. Prepare fresh each day.
5. Cobaltous acetate solution (0.125%): Dissolve 32 mg of anhydrous cobaltous acetate in 25 ml methanol. Prepare fresh each day.

Standard solution

Weigh exactly 50 mg of phenobarbitone in 50 ml volumetric flask. Add 20 ml methonol, shake and make up the volume with methanol.

Sample solution

Pipette sample equivalent to 50 mg of phenobarbitone into a separatory funnel, add about 25 ml of 1% hydrochloric acid and extract with four 40 ml portions of chloroform. Collect the chloroform extracts in a dry beaker. Evaporate the chloroform extracts and dry the residue by keeping in an oven (105°C) for about 2 hours. Add about 20 ml methanol and dissolve the residue by warming on a water-bath. Cool and transfer it to the 50 ml volumetric flask. Make up the volume with methanol and filter.

Procedure

To 2 ml of the sample solution add 2 ml of isopropylamine solution and 2 ml of cobalt acetate solution and measure the absorbance immediately at 570 nm against reagent blank. For comparison, run standard separately.

Note

Treat the sample and standard solutions with the reagents one at a time as the colour fades of very quickly. It is important to keep the time between addition of reagent and reading constant to get reproducible results. This is based on experimental observation by the author.

The complex is formed between the drug and cobalt acetate in the presence of isopropylamine (λ_{max} 570 nm). The excess amine causes deprotonation of the acid. This is called "Zwikker" reaction.

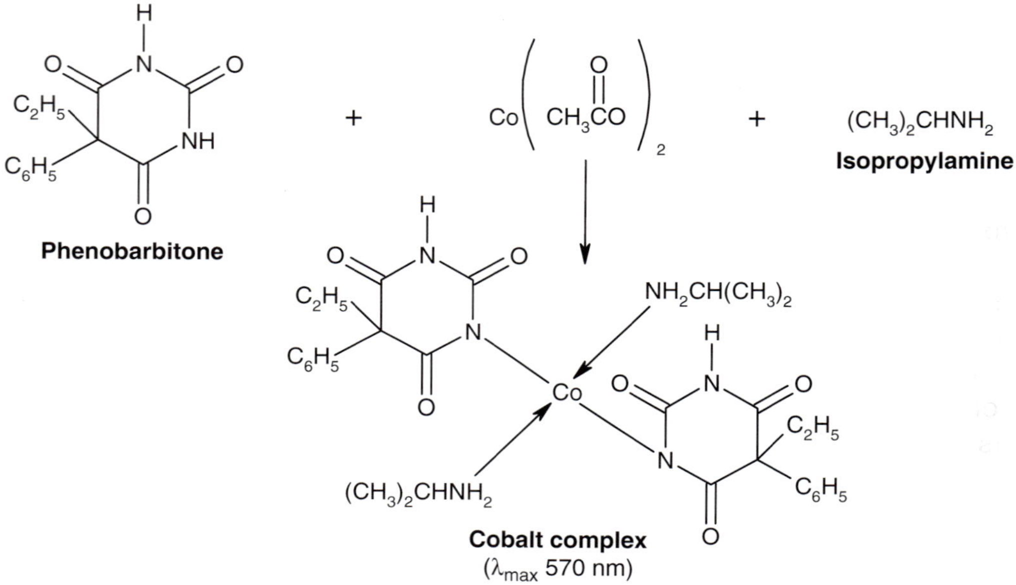

An alternative Zwikker-like reaction is possible using pyridine and copper sulphate. The pale white precipitates are soluble in chloroform.

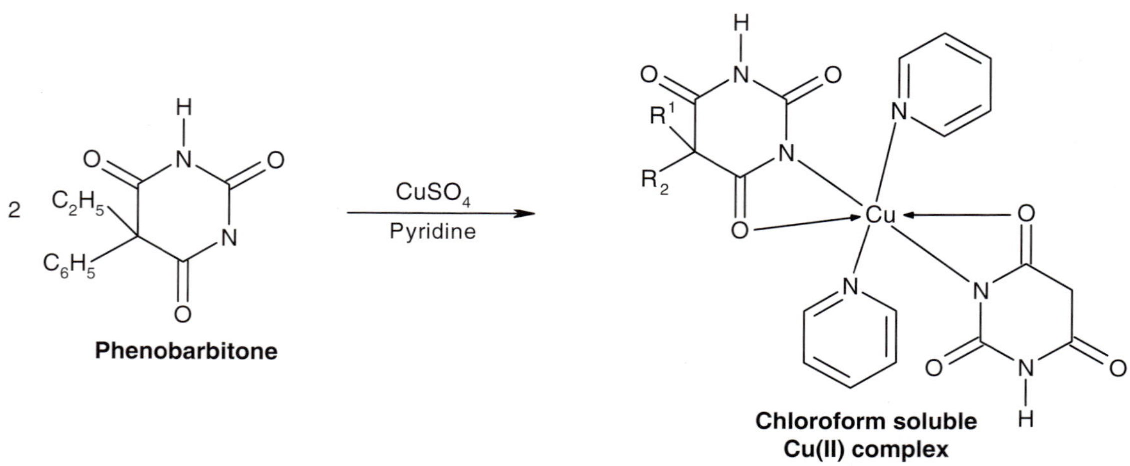

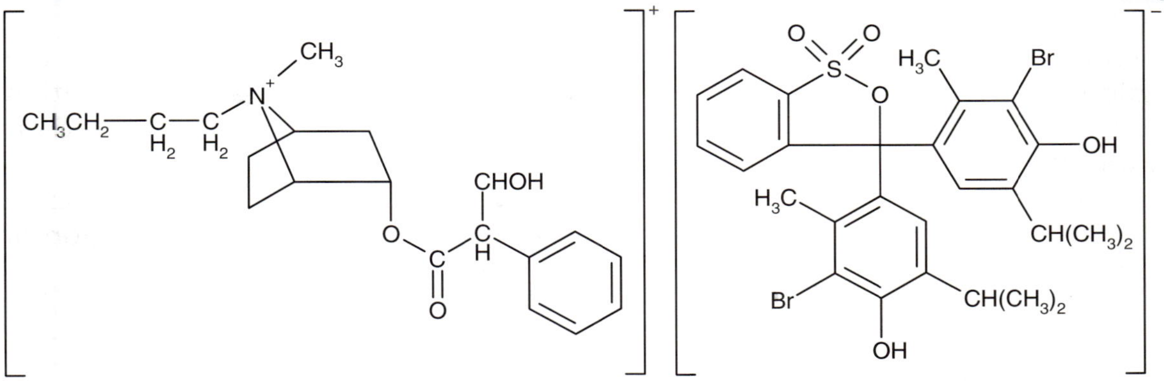

Hyoscyamine-N-butyl bromide **Bromothymol blue**

Ion-pair complex (chloroform soluble)
(λ_{max} 420 nm)

Thomas et al. have reported that the compound forms ion-pair complex with bromocresol purple as well in pH 5.3 phosphate buffer. Other drugs commonly present in the combination do not interfere. The complex is extractable into chloroform and has λ_{max} 408 nm.

The drug reacts with diphenylpicrylamine in alkaline medoum and on shaking with chloroform the organic layer turns yellow owing to ion-pair formation. This is general identification test.

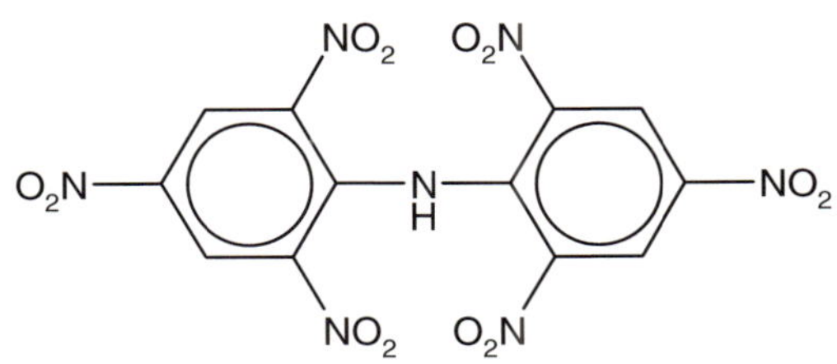

Diphenylpicrylamine, 'NH' - acid part of the reagent, is involved in reaction with the alkaloids.

Reference

Pharmaceutical Chemistry (Vol. 2) by H.J. Roth, p. 189.

Formulation 47

Hyoscyamine-N-butyl bromide, Analgin

ESTIMATION

METHOD 1

Reagents

1. 0.1 M citric acid.
2. 0.2 M disodium hydrogen phosphate, dihydrate.
3. Citric acid - phosphate buffer, pH 7.5: Dilute 7.5 ml each of 0.1 M citric acid and 0.2 M disodium hydrogen phosphate to 100 ml with water.
4. Bromothymol blue solution: Dissolve 0.15 g bromothymol blue and 0.15 g of anhydrous sodium carbonate in 100 ml of water.
5. Alcoholic solution of boric acid: Dissolve 20 g of boric acid in 800 ml of ethanol and 80 ml of water and then make up to 1000 ml with ethanol.

Standard solution

Transfer about 25 mg of standard substance accurately weighed to a 250 ml volumetric flask and make up to volume with water (100 mcg/ml).

Sample solution

Quantity of the sample equivalent to 5 mg of the substance is accurately weighed and dissolved in water to produce 50 ml (100 mcg/ml).

Procedure

Pipette 5 ml each of the sample and standard solutions and 0.5 ml of 0.1 N sodium hydroxide into separate 100 ml separating funnels. To each separating funnel, add 2 ml of bromothymol blue solution and 20 ml of buffer solution. Extract by shaking for about one minute with exactly 30 ml of chloroform. Separate chloroform layer and make up to 50 ml with alcoholic boric acid solution to clear the chloroform phase. Determine the extinctions of the sample and standard solutions at about 420 nm against chloroform as a blank. Compute the results by comparison. The method is based on ion-pair complex extractable into chloroform (λ_{max} 420 nm).

METHOD 2

Reagents

1. Iodine solution: 0.255 mg/ml in ethylene dichloride.
2. Phosphate buffer, pH 9.0.

Standard solution

Dissolve the pure compound in water to get concentration of 500 mcg/ml. To 1 ml of standard solution, add 5 ml of buffer solution and 10 ml of ethylene dichloride. Shake vigorously for 5 minutes and allow the layers to separate. Pass organic layer through anhydrous sodium sulphate and dilute to 10 ml with ethylene dichloride (50 mcg/ml).

Sample solution

Weigh accurately sample equivalent to 0.5 mg of hyoscyamine N-butyl bromide. Add 5 ml of buffer solution, 10 ml of ethylene dichloride and proceed as described under standard solution.

Procedure

To 1 ml each of standard and sample solutions, add 1 ml of iodine solution and 10 ml of ethylene dichloride. Shake and measure the extinction at maxima at about 280 nm (atropine, homatropine and scopolamine exhibit maxima at about 295 nm).

Probable Reaction Mechanism

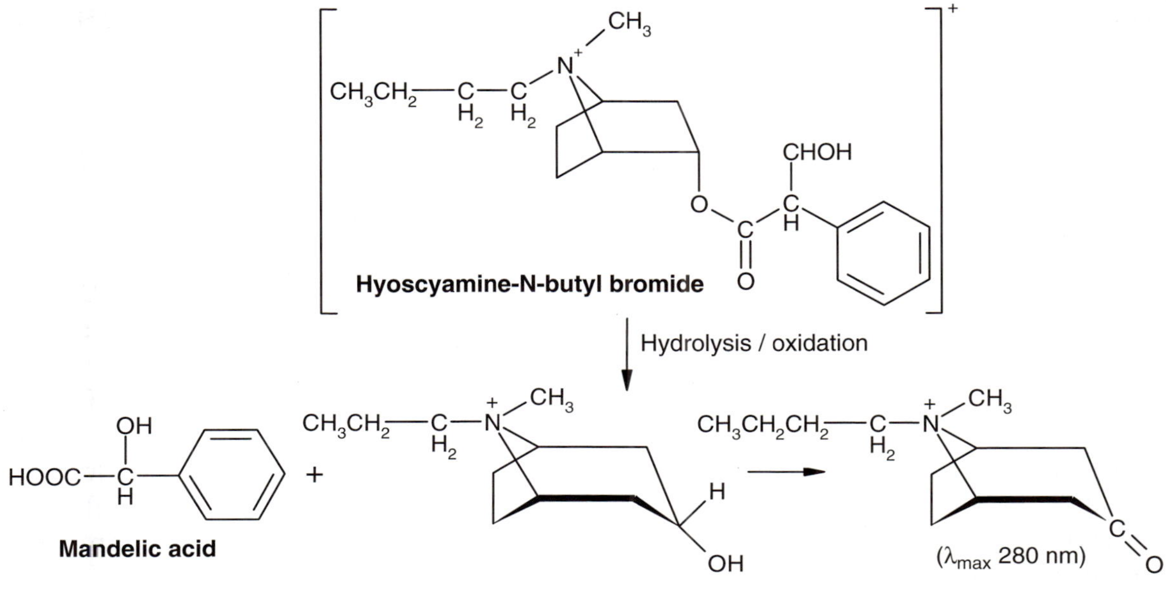

Analgin (Dipyrone)

METHOD 1

Standard solution

In a 100 ml volumetric flask dissolve about 250 mg of dipyrone standard substance, accurately weighed, in sufficient 0.01 N hydrochloric acid to produce 100 ml. Pipette 5 ml of this solution into a 500 ml volumetric flask and make up to volume with 0.01 N hydrochloric acid.

Test solution

In a 100 ml volumetric flask shake up powdered tablets accurately weighed equivalent to 250 mg of analgin with about 80 ml of 0.01 N hydrochloric acid for 15 minutes and then make up to volume with 0.01 N hydrochloric acid. Pipette 5 ml of the filtrate into a 500 ml volumetric flask and make up the volume with 0.01 N hydrochloric acid.

Determine the extinctions of the test and standard solutions at the maximum at about 257 nm against 0.01 N acid as blank. Deduce results by comparison.

METHOD 2

Weigh accurately, powdered sample equivalent to 0.5 g of analgin, add 10 ml of water and shake for one minute. Immediately add 25 ml of methyl alcohol, shake and make up the volume to 50 ml with methyl alcohol. Filter immediately and to 25 ml of the filtrate, add 5 ml of 0.01 N hydrochloric acid and titrate with 0.1 N iodine till pale yellow colour persists for 30 seconds. Each ml of 0.1 N iodine is equivalent to 0.01757 g of analgin.

Probable Reaction Mechanism

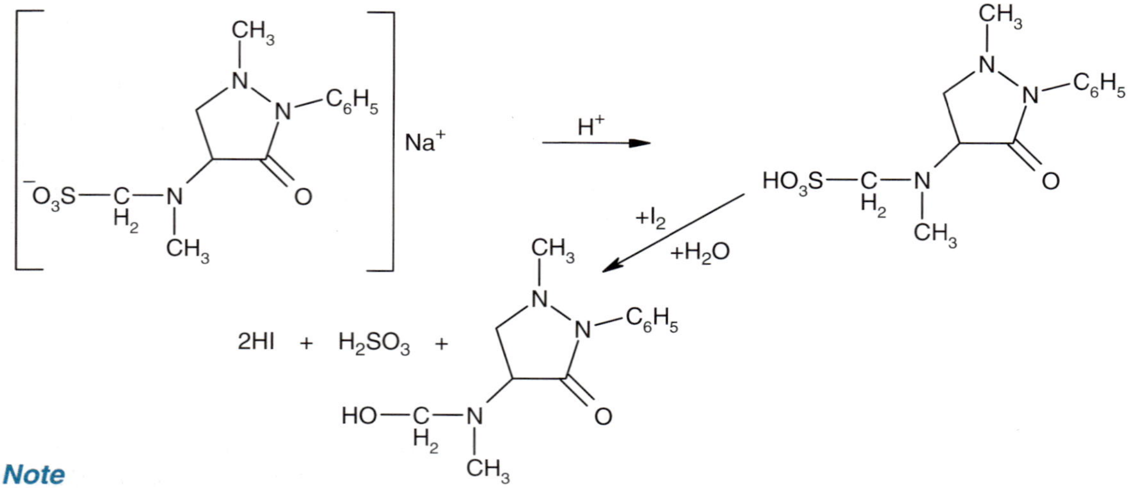

Note

Pale yellow colour, the end point, is due to excess of iodine.

Formulation 48

Diazepam, L-Hyoscyamine

ESTIMATION

Diazepam

Standard solution

50 mcg/ml of diazepam in alcoholic sulphuric acid.

Sample solution

Weigh accurately powdered sample equivalent to 10 mg of diazepam, add 10 ml of water, 20 ml of borate buffer, pH 9.0 or phosphate buffer, pH 7.0 and extract with four 25 ml portions of solvent ether. For further details, refer to formulation 25 of the chapter on analgesics and antipyretics.

Note

Diazepam usually contains a hydrolytic decomposition product, 2-methylamino-5-chlorobenzophenone which interferes in the above assay as its absorbance overlaps at 368 nm and 285 nm. To eliminate the interference due to decomposition product, the following procedure is usually recommended:

(a) Process the sample as above.

(b) Follow the ether extraction procedure as above, however, reconstitute the residue with alcohol instead of acidified alcohol and read the resultant solution at 405 nm. This absorbance is multiplied by 19.314 to get amount (mg) of the diazepam present as decomposition product in the sample. This amount is subtracted from the amount of diazepam determined by the main method.

L-Hyoscyamine

Reagents

1. Solution 1: Phosphate buffer solution, pH 2.5: To 55 ml of 7.8% w/v solution of potassium phosphate dibasic, add 20 ml of 9.6% w/v solution of citric acid and dilute to 100 ml with water.

2. Solution 2: Bromocresol purple: To 400 mg of bromocresol purple, add 6.5 ml of 0.1 N sodium hydroxide and make up to 500 ml with water.
3. Dye solution: Mix equal volumes of solution 1 and solution 2, extract with chloroform and reject chloroform layer. This step reduces the blank value.

Standard solution

50 mcg/ml of L-hyoscyamine in 0.1 N hydrochloric acid.

Sample solution

Weigh accurately a quantity of the sample equivalent to 5 mg of substance and shake with 0.1 N hydrochloric acid to produce 100 ml (50 mcg/ml).

Procedure

To 10 ml each of the sample and standard solutions, add 10 ml of dye solution and exactly 25 ml chloroform. Shake for two minutes, and allow the layers to separate out. Filter the chloroform layer through cotton plug. Read extinction of sample and standard solution at about 440 nm against chloroform as blank and calculate the results by comparison. The method is based on formation of ion-pair complex extractable into chloroform.

Formulation 49

Analgin, Phenobarbitone, Homatropine methyl bromide

ESTIMATION

Analgin

Transfer an accurately weighed portion of tablet powder equivalent to 0.5 g of analgin to a 250 ml conical flask. Add 10 ml of water, shake and immediately add 25 ml of ethyl alcohol. Make up to volume with alcohol, mix thoroughly and filter. Take 25 ml of the filtrate in a conical flask, add 5 ml of 0.01 N hydrochloric acid and titrate with 0.1 N iodine solution until a pale yellow colour persists for thirty seconds. Each ml of 0.1 N iodine is equivalent to 0.01757 g of analgin. For reaction mechanism refer to formulation of this chapter.

Phenobarbitone

Transfer an accurately weighed portion of tablet powder equivalent to 100 mg of phenobarbitone to a 150 ml round botton flask and extract with 100 ml of ether for three hours using a sauxhlet apparatus. Evaporate the ether and dissolve the residue in 20 ml of 0.1 N sodium hydroxide. Transfer to a separating funnel and extract the alkaline solution with two 25 ml portions of ether. Wash the combined ether extracts with 2 × 5 ml of water and add the water washings to the alkaline solution. Reject the ether. Make the aqueous extract acidic with hydrochloric acid (litmus paper), add about 10 g of sodium chloride for saturation and again extract with four 25 ml portions of ether. Combine the ether extracts and evaporate the ether in a tared flask. Dry at 105°C for 1 hour and weigh the residue. Calculate the content of phenobarbitone per tablet from the weight obtained. We can also perform the identification test with this residue.

Homatropine methyl bromide

Reagents

1. Anion-exchange resin—IR-400 (Cl^-).

2. 1 N sodium hydroxide.
3. 0.2 M cerric ammonium sulphate in 6 N sulphuric acid.

Column preparation

Place a small quantity of fine glass wool in the base of a 50 ml burette. Add strong anion-exchange resin in the chloride form (IR-400) to form a uniform column of 25 cm. Cover the top of the column with a plug of fine glass wool and wash by eluting with six 20 ml portions of water. The column is ready for use.

Standard preparation

Weigh accurately 50 mg of homatropine methyl bromide into a 100 ml volumetric flask, dissolve and make up to 100 ml with water. 10 ml of this solution is further diluted to 100 ml with water.

Sample preparation

Weigh and powder 20 tablets. Weigh accurately the powder equivalent to 5 mg of homatropine methyl bromide into a 100 ml volumetric flask and add 50 ml of water. Shake well and make up with water, mix, filter and add entire volume to the column. Wash column with 30 ml water and discard eluate. Collect subsequent eluates and dilute to 50 ml with water.

Procedure

Transfer 10 ml each of standard and sample preparations in a separate glass-stoppered 100 ml flasks. To each flask add 20 ml of 1 N sodium hydroxide and heat in a water-bath at 80°C for 15 min. Cool to room temperature, wash the solution with 2×25 ml of chloroform before addition of cerric reagent. Add 8 ml of 0.2 M cerric ammonium sulphate and mix. To each flask add 25 ml of iso-octane and shake for 15 min. Decant the iso-octane layers and concomitantly determine the absorbance of both the solutions at the maximum at about 242 nm with a suitable spectrophotometer using iso-octane as the blank. For reaction mechanism, see under homatropine sulphate involving oxidation of the molecule and extraction into iso-octane.

Formulation 50

Diacetoxy-diphenyl-pyridyl-methane, Casanthranol

ESTIMATION

Diacetoxy-diphenyl-pyridyl-methane

Reagents

1. Chloroform.
2. Activated charcoal.
3. N/10 Perchloric acid in glacial acetic acid.
4. 0.2% w/v 1-naphthol benzein in glacial acetic acid.

Procedure

To an accurately weighed quantity of the powder equivalent to 100 mg of the compound add about 50 ml of chloroform and shake vigorously for 15 minutes. Filter through cotton into a dry 250 ml conical flask. Further, extract twice each with 50 ml of chloroform and filter. Add 10 g of activated charcoal to the combined chloroform layer. Shake and filter through anhydrous sodium sulphate. Chloroform extract is then evaporated to complete dryness. The residue is then dissolved in 25 ml of glacial acetic acid and titrated against N/10 perchloric acid using 1-naphthol benzein solution as indicator. Change in colour is from orange to dark green. Each ml of N/10 perchloric acid is equivalent to 36.14 mg of diacetoxy-diphenyl-pyridyl-methane.

Casanthranol

Standard solution

50 mcg/ml of casanthranol in water.

Sample solution

Accurately weighed quantity of the sample equivalent to 100 mg of casanthranol is extracted with water by vigorous shaking for 30 min. The solution is appropriately diluted with water to get 50 mcg/ml. Measure the extinction of both the solutions at 268 nm using water as blank and calculate the results.

Formulation 51

Milk of magnesia, Liquid paraffin

ESTIMATION

Magnesium hydroxide

Shake the preparation for few minutes in its original container and transfer about 5 g into a tared flask, stopper the flask and weigh accurately. Add 30 ml of 1 N sulphuric acid and after solution is complete titrate the excess acid with 1 N sodium hydroxide using methyl red as indicator.

Each ml of 1 N sulphuric acid is equivalent to 0.02916 g of magnesium hydroxide.

Milk of magnesia (ml) per 5 ml of the sample =

$$\frac{A \times f \times 0.02916 \times \text{specific gravity of the sample} \times 5 \times 100}{\text{weight of the sample taken} \times 7.75 \times 1.106}$$

A = nett volume of 1 N sulphuric acid consumed
f = exact strength of the acid
1.106 = average specific gravity of milk of magnesia I.P.
7.75 = average percentage of magnesium hydroxide w/w present in milk of magnesia

Liquid paraffin

After the above titration for magnesium hydroxide is complete transfer the entire contents of the flask to a separating funnel. Extract twice each with 40 ml of alcohol - ether mixture (1 : 3). Extract the aqueous layer with further 30 ml solvent ether. Mix this ether extract with the main ether - alcoholic extract. Evaporate the combined extract in a tared china dish. Add 5 ml of acetone just before drying and evaporate completely. Dry at 105°C for 15 min, cool and weigh the oily liquid. Calculate the contents of liquid paraffin (ml) for 5 ml of the sample. 0.88 is the specific gravity of liquid paraffin.

$$\frac{\text{Weight of the oily liquid} \times \text{specific gravity of the sample} \times 5}{\text{Weight of the sample taken} \times 0.88}$$

Note

Extraction with chloroform (3 × 50 ml) instead of alcohol - ether mixture also gives satisfactory results.

Formulation 52

Liquid paraffin, Phenolphthalein

ESTIMATION

Liquid paraffin

Transfer about 5 g of the sample accurately weighed to a separator. Add 10 ml of water and extract twice each with 40 ml of alcohol - ether mixture (1 : 3). Extract again the aqueous layer with 30 ml of solvent ether. Wash the combined extracts with 15 ml of 0.5 N sodium hydroxide and then with 15 ml of water. Retain the aqueous washing for the assay of phenolphthalein. Evaporate the ether extract in a tared glass basin. Add 5 ml of acetone just before drying and evaporate completely. Dry at 105°C for 15 min, cool and weigh the oil and calculate the results by the formula described in formulation 51 of this chapter.

Phenolphthalein

METHOD 1

To the aqueous washing obtained in the estimation of liquid paraffin above, add dilute hydrochloric acid drop by drop till pink colour disappears. Extract with three successive quantities, each of 20 ml of solvent ether. Wash the mixed ethereal extract with two successive quantities each of 10 ml of water. Transfer the ether extract into a tared glas basin and evaporate adding 5 ml of acetone just before drying. Evaporate completely and dry at 100°C for one hour, cool and weigh as phenolphthalein.

Explanatory Note

Phenolphthalein is a weak acid. On adding hydrochloric acid it remains undissociated, hence easily soluble in ether. The method involves gravimetric assay.

METHOD 2

Reagent

Aminoacetate buffer solution, pH 11.0-11.5: A solution containing 0.75% w/v of glycin (aminoacetic acid) and 0.58% w/v of sodium chloride is diluted with 0.1 N sodium hydroxide. The pH of the buffer should be between 11.0 and 11.5.

Procedure

Take sample equivalent to 50 mg of phenolphthalein and extract with two 40 ml portions of alcohol. Make up the volume to 100 ml. Dilute 5 ml of this to 50 ml with alcohol. Evaporate 5 ml of the resultant solution to dryness on boiling water-bath. Dissolve the residue in the buffer to produce 100 ml, mix and measure the absorbance at the maximum at about 550 nm. Use 1055 as the value of E 1%, 1 cm for calculations.

Phenolphthalein is a weak acid and can be represented as HPh. In its undissociated form it is colourless; Ph^- ion has pink colour. In acid medium, due to common ion effect, its dissociation is suppressed, so solution remains colourless; whereas in alkaline medium OH^- ions combine with H^+ from the indicator to form water and thus compound dissociates, so the solution becomes pink. In this method, the buffer has pH > 10.0, hence pink colour due to dissociation radical of phenolphthalein (Ph^-).

$$\underset{\textbf{Phenolphthalein}}{HPh} \rightleftharpoons H^+ + \underset{\textbf{(Pink)}}{Ph^-}$$

$$HPh + OH^- \longrightarrow H_2O + Ph^-$$

(Pink)
(λ_{max} 550 nm)

In the alkaline medium (pH 11.0-11.5) the lactone ring in phenolphthalein opens to yield triphenylcarbinol structure which with loss of water produces resonating structure.

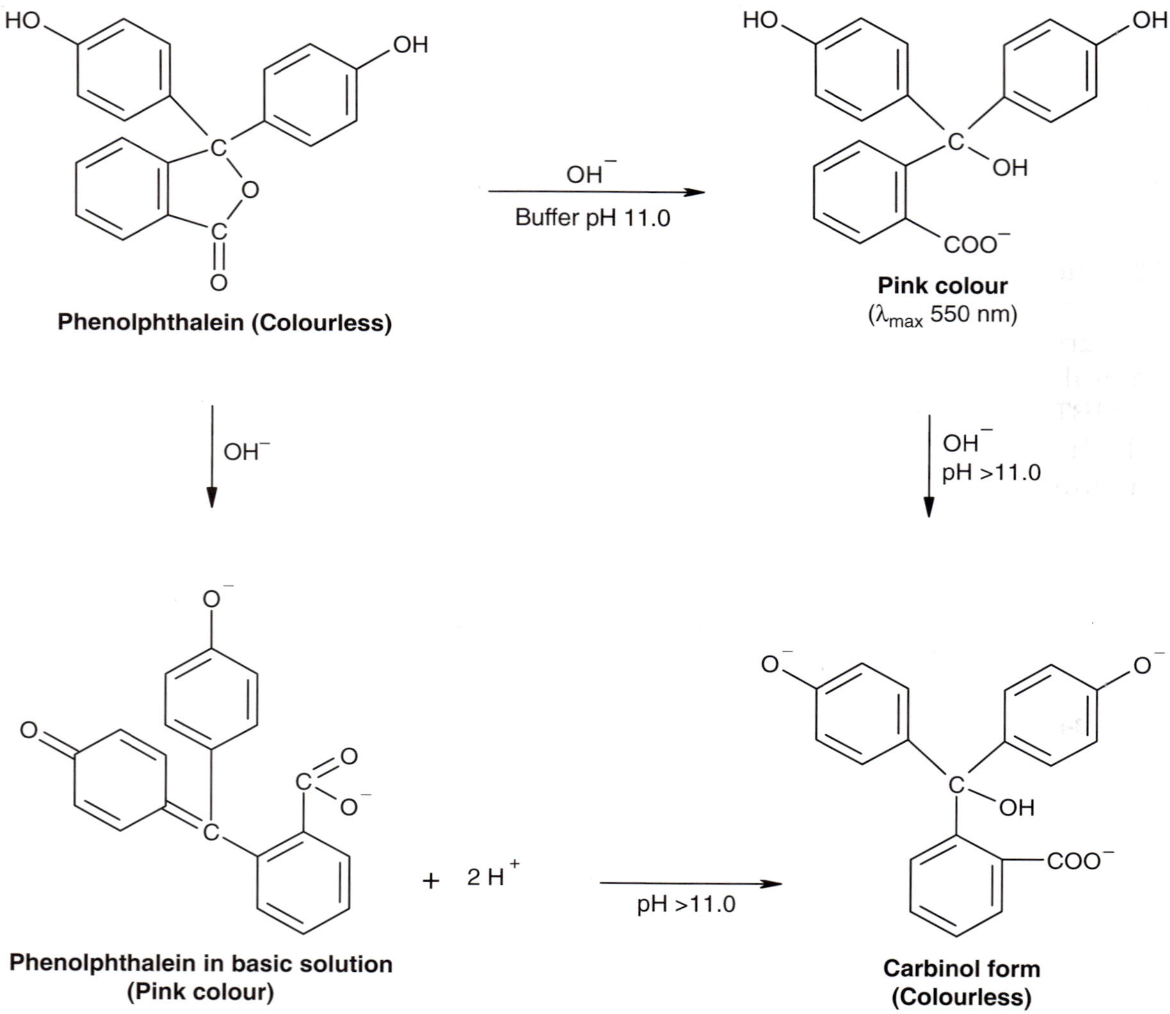

Note

Below pH 8.0 the compound exists in lactone form.

Method 3

Reagents

1. 0.002 M MBTH solution in water.
2. 0.003 M cerric ammonium sulphate (CAS) solution in 0.07 M sulphuric acid.
3. Buffer solution: Dissolve 0.96 g of sodium hydroxide, 0.4 g of EDTA (Na^+) and 1.6 g of boric acid in 100 ml of water.

Procedure

To 1 ml of standard and sample solutions add 10 ml of MBTH reagent and after 5 min add 10 ml of CAS solution, allow to stand and then add 20 ml of buffer. Extract the coloured complex with chloroform, adjust volume and measure at 545 nm.

Explanatory Note

The method involves oxidative coupling of MBTH with phenolphthalein in the presence of cerric ammonium sulphate as an oxidizing agent to yield magenta-coloured complex (λ_{max} 545 nm). Liquid paraffin and other excipients present in oral emulsion formulation do not interfere.

MBTH loses one proton and two electrons to form electrophilic intermediate which is the coupling species. It couples ortho or para or both to phenolic function.

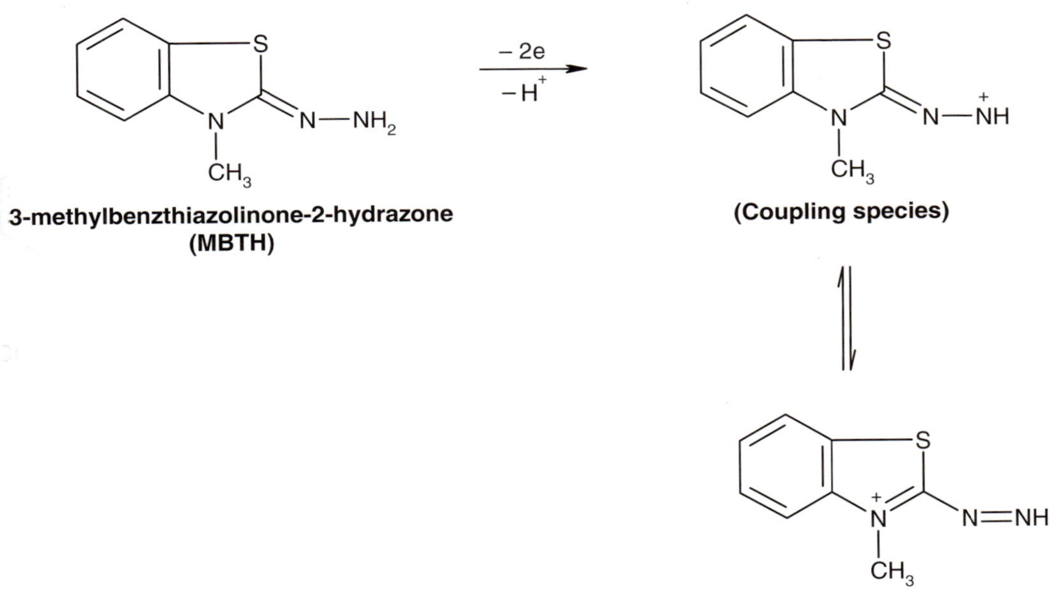

Note

Three reaction products are possible as a result of oxidative coupling with MBTH reagent as explained below.

Probable Reaction Mechanism

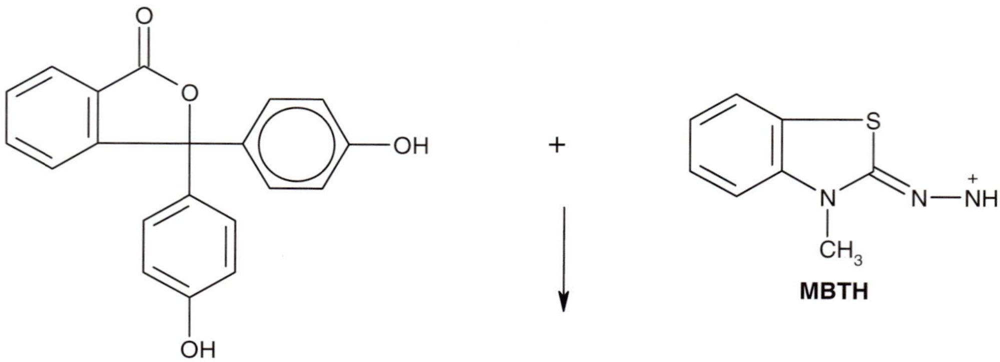

Phenolphthalein

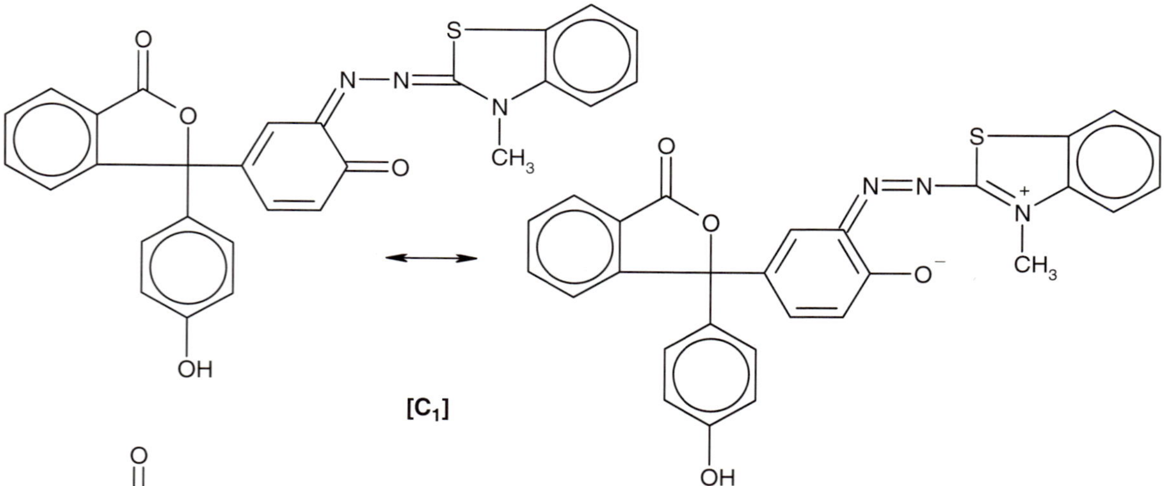

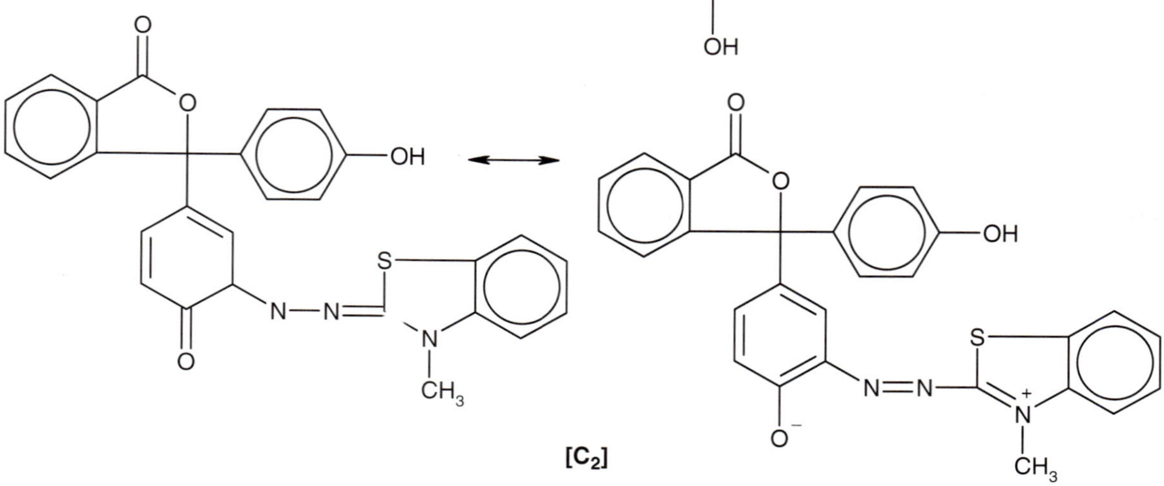

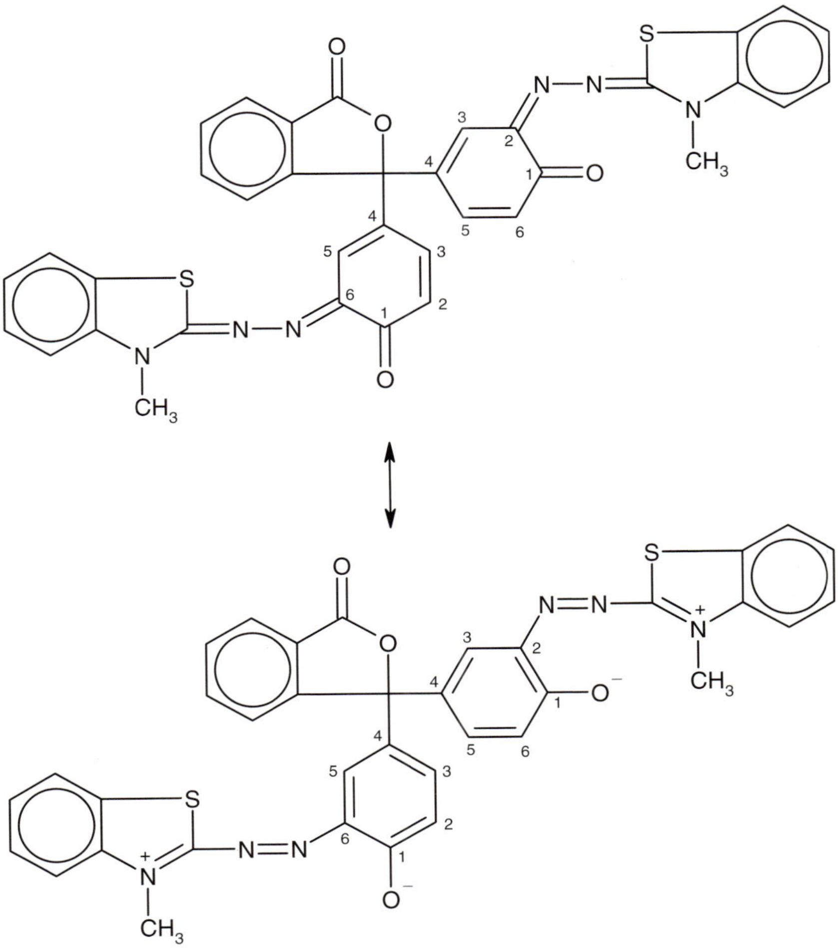

[C_3]

C_1, C_2 and C_3 are the three possible reaction products.

Reference

N. Geeta, A.P. Veena & T.R. Baggi, *Microchemical Journal*, **40**, 304-310, 1989.

Formulation 53

Sodium chloride, Potassium chloride, Sodium bicarbonate, Sodium citrate, Dextrose

ESTIMATION

Sodium bicarbonate

Weigh accurately sample equivalent to about 300 mg of sodium bicarbonate, add 25 ml of water and shake to dissolve. Titrate with 0.5 N hydrochloric acid using methyl orange as indicator. Each ml of 0.5 N hydrochloric acid is equivalent to 0.042 g of sodium bicarbonate.

Dextrose

Weigh accurately powder equivalent to 10 g of dextrose, add 80 ml of water and 0.2 ml of ammonia solution. Shake and dilute to 100 ml with water. Determine the angular rotation in a 0.2 metre tube at 25°C and calculate the result as under:

$$n \text{ (g \% of glucose)} = \frac{a \times 100}{l \times 53}$$

a = angle of rotation observed;
l = length of tube in metres;
n = % w/v of glucose present in the solution under test;
53 = claimed optical rotation of 10% w/v solution of glucose.

Note

If the powder contains colouring material and flavouring agents (flavouring agents produce opalescence on dilution), they will interfere in the assay of glucose by the above method. It is, therefore, desirable to add 0.5 g of activated charcoal to the glucose solution. Shake for 5 minutes and filter. This treatment will yield a clear solution.

Total chlorides

METHOD 1

Weigh powder accurately equivalent to 10 mg of total chlorides, add 25 ml of distilled water and 3 ml of nitric acid. While agitating, add 50 ml of 0.1 N silver nitrate and 5 ml of nitrobenzene. Shake vigorously for 1 minute and add 2 ml of ferric ammonium sulphate solution (indicator) and titrate excess of silver nitrate with 0.1 N ammonium thiocyanate. Each ml of 0.1 N silver nitrate is equivalent to 3.545 mg of chloride.

METHOD 2

Weigh accurately powder equivalent to 100 mg of total chloride. Add 20 ml of water, 10 ml of dilute nitric acid, 50 ml of water and boil the solution. Add 50 ml of 0.1 N silver nitrite solution to the boiling liquid. Digest the precipitate for 30 minutes on a water-bath. Filter, wash the precipitate with water for 4-5 times and titrate the combined washing with 0.1 N ammonium thiocyanate, using ferric alum solution as indicator. Each ml of 0.1 N silver nitrate equivalent to 0.003545 g of chloride. Carry out a blank titration side by side.

Potassium chloride

Take powder equivalent to 5 mg of potassium chloride, add 5 ml of water and 1.5 ml alcohol. Then, add drop-wise and with continuous shaking, 2 ml of solution of sodium cobaltinitrite (30% w/v in water). Allow to stand at room temperature for 1 hr, centrifuge till precipitates are firmly packed at the bottom. Decant and drain for 5 min. Wash the precipitates with 5 ml of 70% alcohol. Centrifuge for 5 minutes and again drain. Dry at 80°C for 1 hr. Add 25 ml of 0.02 N cerric sulphate and 1 ml of sulphuric acid (50% v/v) and heat in water-bath till precipitates disappear. Cool to room temperature and add a drop of orthophenanthroline - ferrous complex and titrate excess cerric sulphate with 0.02 N ferrous ammonium sulphate. Each ml of 0.02 N cerric sulphate is equivalent to 0.2485 mg of potassium chloride.

Sodium chloride

From the total chlorides determined above, subtract the amount of chloride corresponding to the amount of potassium chloride determined above (1 g of potassium chloride contains 478 mg of chloride (Cl^-). The remaining amount of chloride corresponds to the amount of sodium chloride present in the sample. Convert this to sodium chloride (1 g of sodium chloride contains 607 mg of chloride Cl^-).

Working example

Each 35 g of sample contains:

Sodium chloride	3.5 g
Sodium bicarbonate	2.5 g
Potassium chloride	1.5 g
Dextrose	20 g

Total chlorides in 35 g

(a) From sodium chloride	2.124 g
(b) From potassium chloride	0.715 g
Total	2.839 g of chloride (Cl^-)

$$\text{Total chlorides per g of the material} = \frac{2.839}{35} = 0.081 \text{ g (81 mg)}$$

(a) Chloride per g of the powder corresponding to sodium chloride = 60.6 mg
(b) Chloride per g of the powder corresponding to potassium chloride = 20.4 mg

Sodium bicarbonate

Quantity of the sample powder taken for analysis = 5.0 g
Volume of 0.5 N hydrochloric acid used for titration = 8.3 ml

$$\text{Amount of sodium bicarbonate (\%)} = 8.3 \times 0.042 \times \frac{2.5}{35} \times 5 \times 100$$

$$= 97.7\% \text{ w/w of the claim.}$$

Total chlorides

Weight of the sample powder taken for analysis = 1 g
Net volume of 0.1 N silver nitrate used in titrating halides = 23.7 ml

$$\text{Total chloride (\%)} = \frac{23.7 \times 3.545 \times 1}{81} \times 100$$

$$= 103.53\% \text{ of the claim.}$$

Note

Sodium bicarbonate causes decomposition of glucose to 5 hydroxymethyl furfural which on polymerisation imparts yellow colour to the preparation. To overcome this problem, sodium bicarbonate has been replaced by trisodium citrate. With this salt, no decomposition of glucose has been observed. In such formulations, trisodium citrate can be estimated by method 4 described in formulation 7 of the chapter on expectorants.

Formulation 54

Calcium chloride, Potassium chloride, Sodium lactate, Dextrose

All the electrolytes can be estimated without separation by flame photometric method.

Reagents

1. Calcium carbonate: Dry at 285°C for 2 hrs, cool in desiccator and use for preparation of standard solutions.
2. Potassium chloride: Dry at 500-600°C for 2 hrs, cool in desiccator and use.
3. Sodium chloride: Dry at 500-600°C for 2 hrs, cool in desiccator and use.

Note

All solutions are prepared in glass distilled water.

(a) **Standard solution of calcium carbonate (10 mg/ml):** Take 24.975 g of dried calcium carbonate accurately weighed, add 150 ml of distilled water, acidify gradually with 45 ml of hydrochloric acid. Cool to room temperature and dilute to 100 ml with distilled water. Dilute 10 ml further to 200 ml with distilled water.

(b) **Standard solution of potassium chloride (1 mg/ml):** Transfer 1.907 g accurately weighed of dried potassium chloride and dilute to 1000 ml with distilled water.

(c) **Standard solution of sodium chloride:** Dissolve 25.240 g of dried sodium chloride accurately weighed in distilled water and adjust the volume to 1000 ml with distilled water.

Mixed cationic standard solution: Take 10 ml of solution (a), 10 ml of solution (b) and 20 ml of solution (c), and dilute to 200 ml with distilled water.

Note

1. Store the mixed standard solution in a clear polyethylene bottle. This is stable for more than 1 month.
2. The readings on the instrument with the standard solutions should be adjusted between 20% and 95% of the scale.
3. Prepare median range of standards for different cations from standard solution of mixed cations.

The sample should be appropriately diluted with distilled water to give ionic concentrations close to the standard solution for better comparison. For calcium (Ca^{++}), read at 422.7 nm; for potassium (K^{+}) at 766.5 nm and for sodium (Na^{+}) at 589.0 nm.

Dextrose

Weigh sample accurately equivalent to about 100 mg of dextrose, dissolve in 5 ml of distilled water, add 25 ml of buffer solution containing 14.3% w/w of sodium carbonate and 4% w/v of potassium iodide and 25 ml of 0.1 N iodine. Stopper and allow to stand exactly for 30 minutes at 20°C. Add 30 ml of dilute hydrochloric acid and titrate immediately the excess iodine with 0.1 N sodium thiosulphate. Repeat the entire procedure with 5 ml of distilled water. The difference between the titrations represent the amount of iodine required to oxidize dextrose. Each ml of 0.1 N iodine is equivalent to 0.00901 g of dextrose. Alternatively, follow the method described in formulation 1 of this chapter.

Formulation 55

Sodium chloride, Potassium chloride, Sodium citrate, Dextrose

ESTIMATION

Dextrose

Weigh accurately powder equivalent to 10 g of dextrose, add 80 ml of water and 0.2 ml of ammonia solution. Shake and dilute to 100 ml with water. Determine the angular rotation in a 0.2 metre tube at 25°C and calculate the result as under:

$$x \text{ (g \% of glucose)} = \frac{a \times 100}{l \times 53}$$

a = angle of rotation observed;
l = length of tube in metres;
x = % w/v of glucose present in the solution under test;
53 = claimed optical rotation of 10% w/v solution of glucose.

Note

If the powder contains colouring material and flavouring agents (flavouring agents produce opalescence on dilution), they will interfere in the assay of glucose by the above method. It is, therefore, desirable to add 0.5 g of activated charcoal to the glucose solution. Shake for 5 minutes and filter. This treatment will yield a clear solution. Alternatively method described under formulation 2 of this chapter may be used.

Total chlorides

METHOD 1

Weigh powder accurately equivalent to 10 mg of total chlorides, add 25 ml of distilled water and 3 ml of nitric acid. While agitating, add 50 ml of 0.1 N silver nitrate and 5 ml of nitrobenzene. Shake vigorously for 1 minute and add 2 ml of ferric ammonium sulphate solution (indicator) and titrate excess of silver nitrate with 0.1 N ammonium thiocyanate. Each ml of 0.1 N silver nitrate is equivalent to 0.003545 g of chloride.

METHOD 2

Weigh accurately powder equivalent to 100 mg of total chloride. Add 20 ml of water, 10 ml of dilute nitric acid, 50 ml of water and boil the solution. Add 50 ml of 0.1 N silver nitrite solution to the boiling liquid. Digest the precipitate for 30 minutes on a water-bath. Filter, wash the precipitate with water for 4-5 times and titrate the combined washing with 0.1 N ammonium thiocyanate, using ferric alum solution as indicator. Each ml of 0.1 N silver nitrate equivalent to 0.003545 g of chloride. Carry out a blank titration side by side.

Potassium chloride

Take powder equivalent to 5 mg of potassium chloride, add 5 ml of water and 1.5 ml alcohol. Then, add drop-wise and with continuous shaking, 2 ml of solution of sodium cobaltinitrite (30% w/v in water). Allow to stand at room temperature for 1 hr, centrifuge till precipitates are firmly packed at the bottom. Decant and drain for 5 min. Wash the precipitates with 5 ml of 70% alcohol. Centrifuge for 5 minutes and again drain. Dry at 80°C for 1 hr. Add 25 ml of 0.02 N cerric sulphate and 1 ml of sulphuric acid (50% v/v) and heat in water-bath till precipitates disappear. Cool to room temperature and add a drop of orthophenanthroline - ferrous complex and titrate excess cerric sulphate with 0.02 N ferrous ammonium sulphate. Each ml of 0.02 N cerric sulphate is equivalent to 0.2485 mg of potassium chloride.

Sodium chloride

From the total chlorides determined above, subtract the amount of chloride corresponding to the amount of potassium chloride determined above (1 g of potassium chloride contains 478 mg of chloride (Cl^-). The remaining amount of chloride corresponds to the amount of sodium chloride present in the sample. Convert this to sodium chloride (1 g of sodium chloride contains 607 mg of chloride Cl^-).

Formulation 56

Calcium lactate, Potassium chloride, Sodium chloride, Magnesium sulphate, Sodium acid phosphate, Dextrose, Sodium citrate

ESTIMATION

Dextrose

Follow the methods described for determination of glucose under formulation 33 or 34 of this chapter.

Electrolytes

Weigh accurately appropriate quantity of the sample powder and dissolve in water. Use this solution (A) for determination of various electrolytes present in the formulation as under:

Magnesium sulphate

Magnesium sulphate is estimated gravimetrically by precipitating with barium chloride as barium sulphate. Take 100 ml of aliquot (A) in a 250 ml beaker and add 50 ml of dilute hydrochloric acid. Boil the solution and add 5 ml of 10% w/v aqueous solution of barium chloride. Keep it overnight after digestion. Filter through a weighed G_4 sintered glass crucible under vacuum. Give washings with water until free from chloride. Dry the precipitate to a constant weight at 105°C and calculate the percentage of magnesium sulphate as follows:

$$\frac{\text{Weight of barium sulphate precipitate} \times 1.056 \times 250 \times 100}{100 \times \text{Weight of the powder taken for analysis}}$$

Calcium lactate

Take 100 ml of aliquot (A) in a 250 ml beaker, add 5 ml of hydrochloric acid and boil. To the hot solution, add 15 ml of saturated solution of ammonium oxalate. Add with constant stirring, dilute ammonia solution until the solution is alkaline to litmus paper. Acidify with glacial acetic acid and digest on a water-bath for 30 minutes. Filter, wash the precipitate with water until free from oxalate. Puncture the filter paper and transfer the precipitates along with the filter paper to 500 ml conical flask. Dissolve the precipitates in about 5 ml of hydrochloric acid, add 5 ml of 0.02 M magnesium sulphate and 10 ml of strong ammonia - ammonium chloride buffer and titrate with 0.02 M disodium edetate using solochrome black as indicator. From the volume of 0.02 M disodium edetate required, subtract the volume of 0.02 M magnesium sulphate equivalent to disodium edetate. Each ml of 0.02 M disodium edetate is equivalent to 0.006168 g of calcium lactate.

Note

Conventional methods of combined estimation of calcium and magnesium using solochrome black as indicator by EDTA titration is not possible because in the presence of phosphates both calcium and magnesium get precipitated out with ammonia.

Sodium acid phosphate

This is based on estimation of phosphate moiety of the salt.

Reagents

1. Molybdate reagent: 5 g of ammonium molybdate is dissolved in about 80 ml of water. Add slowly 10 ml of sulphuric acid to dissolve the powder, cool, make up the volume to 100 ml with water.
2. Metol reagent: Dissolve 100 mg of p-N-methyl aminophenol sulphate in about 50 ml of distilled water in a 100 ml volumetric flask. Add 20 g of sodium metabisulphite and 1 g of sodium sulphite. Dissolve adding more water and make up to 100 ml.

Stock standard solution of sodium acid phosphate

Dissolve 20 mg of sodium acid phosphate in 50 ml water and dilute to make up 100 ml with water.

Working standard solution

Dilute 10 ml of stock solution to 100 with water (200 mcg/ml).

Sample solution

10 ml aliquot of solution (A) is diluted appropriately with water to get a concentration of 200 mcg/ml.

Procedure

Transfer 5 ml each of the sample and standard solutions to 50 ml volumetric flasks. To each of the flasks, add 1 ml of dilute sulphuric acid and about 20 ml of distilled water. Then, add 5 ml of molybdate reagent, mix and add 2 ml of the metol reagent, mix and allow to stand for 10 minutes. Make up the volume to 50 ml with distilled water and shake well. Measure the absorption of both the solutions at about 650 nm against blank and calculate the results by comparison.

Total chlorides

Follow the method described for total chlorides under formulation 33 of this chapter.

Calcium lactate, Sodium chloride and Potassium chloride

Follow the flame photometric method described for calcium lactate, sodium chloride and potassium chloride under formulation 33 of this chapter.

Sodium citrate

Follow the method 4, based on colour reaction with ferric chloride, as described for estimation of sodium citrate under formulation 6 of the chapter on expectorants and cough suppressants.

Typical calculations for various ions and ingredients (mEq/L, mmol/L, total osmolarity) in ORS-A (I.P.)

I.P. formula (ORS-A) g/L

Sodium chloride	1.25 g
Potassium chloride	1.50 g
Sodium citrate	2.90 g
Dextrose anhydrous	36.40 g

Calculations

1 g of sodium chloride = 0.3934 g of Na^+; 0.6066 g of Cl^-

1 g of sodium citrate = 0.2345 g of Na^+; 0.6430 g of citrate ion

1 g of potassium chloride = 0.5245 g of K^+; 0.4756 g of Cl^-

$$\text{mEq/L} = \frac{\text{mg/L}}{\text{Equivalent wt.}} \qquad \text{mmol} = \frac{\text{mEq/L}}{\text{Valency}}$$

1250 mg of sodium chloride contains 491.75 mg of Na^+

$$= 21.38 \text{ mEq/L or mmol/L} \qquad \left(\frac{491.75}{23}\right)$$

Sodium in sodium citrate

100 mg of sodium citrate contains 234.5 mg of Na^+

2900 mg of sodium citrate will contain $\dfrac{234.5 \times 2900}{1000} = 680.05$ mg of Na^+

or $\dfrac{680.05}{23} = 29.5$ mEq/L or mmol/L

Total sodium in ORS-A = 21.38 + 29.5 = 50.88 or 51 mEq/L (mmol/L)

Chloride in sodium chloride

1000 mg of sodium chloride contains 606.6 mg of Cl^-

1250 mg of sodium chloride will contain $\dfrac{606.6 \times 1250}{1000} = 758.25$ mg of Cl^-

or $\dfrac{758.25}{35.453} = 21.39$ mEq/L (mmol/L)

Chloride in potassium chloride

1000 mg of KCl contains 475.6 mg of Cl^-

1500 mg of KCl will contain $\dfrac{475.6 \times 1500}{1000} = 713.4$ mg of Cl^-

or $\dfrac{713.4}{35.453} = 20.12$ mEq/L (mmol/L)

Total chloride in ORS-A = 21.39 + 20.12 = 41.50 mEq/L or 41.00 mEq/L

Potassium in potassium chloride

1000 mg of potassium chloride contains 524.5 mg of K^+

1500 mg of potassium chloride will contain $\dfrac{524.5 \times 1500}{1000} = 786.75$ mg of K^+

or $\dfrac{786.75}{39} = 20.12$ mEq/L (mmol/L)

Citrate in sodium citrate

1000 mg of sodium citrate contains 643 mg of citrate

2900 mg of sodium citrate will contain $\dfrac{643 \times 2900}{1000} = 1864.7$ mg of citrate

= 29.60 mEq/L or 30 mEq/L or 10 mmol/L of citrate (valency of citrate ion = 3)

mEq of glucose/L

Amount of glucose per litre = 27.0 g or 27000 mg
Mol. wt./Eq. wt. of glucose = 180

$$\text{mEq of glucose/L} = \frac{27000}{180} = 150$$

Total osmolarity of ORS-A (total ions or ingredients in mmol/L)

Na^+	51	Citrate[3]	10
K^+	20	Glucose	150
Cl^-	41	Total osmolarity	272

Drug Index

A

B

C

N

P

S

T

SETHI'S
Quantitative Analysis *of* Pharmaceutical Formulations

SETHI'S

Quantitative Analysis *of* Pharmaceutical Formulations

Methods With Reaction Mechanism

Fourth Edition

Volume 4

Dr. P.D. Sethi
M.Pharm., Ph.D.

CBS

CBS PUBLISHERS & DISTRIBUTORS PVT. LTD.

NEW DELHI • BENGALURU • PUNE • KOCHI • CHENNAI

ISBN : 978-81-239-2187-7

Third Edition : 1997
Reprint : 2003, 2004, 2005, 2008, 2010, 2011
Fourth Edition : 2012

Published by:
Satish K. Jain and produced by Vinod K. Jain for CBS Publishers & Distributors Pvt. Ltd.,
4819/XI Prahlad Street, 24 Ansari Road, Daryaganj, New Delhi - 110002 (India)
E-mail: cbspubs@airtelmail.com, delhi@cbspd.com • www.cbspd.com

Branches:
- ***Bengaluru:*** 2975, 17th Cross, K.R. Road, Bansankari 2nd Stage, Bengaluru - 560070
  Ph.: +91-80-26771678/79
  E-mail: cbsbng@gmail.com, bangalore@cbspd.com
- ***Pune:*** Bhuruk Prestige, Sr. No. 52/12/2+1+3/2, Narhe, Haveli (Near Katraj-Dehu Road By-pass), Pune - 411051
  Ph.: +91-20-64704058/59, 32342277 • E-mail: pune@cbspd.com
- ***Kochi:*** 36/14, Kalluvilakam, Lissie Hospital Road, Kochi - 682018, Kerala
  Ph.: +91-484-4059061-65 • Fax: +91-484-4059065
  E-mail: cochin@cbspd.com
- ***Chennai:*** 20, West Park Road, Shenoy Nagar, Chennai - 600030
  Ph.: +91-44-26260666, 26208620 E-mail: chennai@cbspd.com

Printed at :
Aegean Offset Printers, Greater Noida (UP)

To

Usha, my wife

Although no one is ever born talented nor talent obtained
as a gift or lucky coincidence, it is a resource acquired
through one's own endeavour,
but without her active support and inspiration,
I would never have been an author.

Dedicated to Fellow Analysts, Students, Teachers, Professionals and Mentors

I am quite aware that this compilation may not be flawless, but if I would have waited till it could be done without any error, probably this would never have been possible considering the fact that incompleteness is inevitable feature of any book. I do hope that this compilation will provide adequate stimulus for you to be a sound professional. I would like to appeal the fellow analysts, students, teaching fraternity and professionals to evaluate my efforts in proper perspective. It took me almost 15 years to scan most of the old analytical journals from 1950 onward, the period when analytical methods based on chromogenic reactions were most prevalent. I would like to express my gratitude to fellow analysts, teachers and the mentors in the profession who helped me to shape my ideas for compiling this text. The wide popularity of my books on spectrophotometric analysis, TLC, HPTLC and HPLC among pharmaceutical analysts, students and teachers has been gratifying and encouraging. My aim has never been to use my knowledge as a vehicle but only as a means of sharing my experience with prefessional fraternity.

P.D. Sethi
Pharmaceutical Analyst

"There is no barrier to acquisition of knowledge. Nobody owns it, everybody partakes it and the world becomes richer."

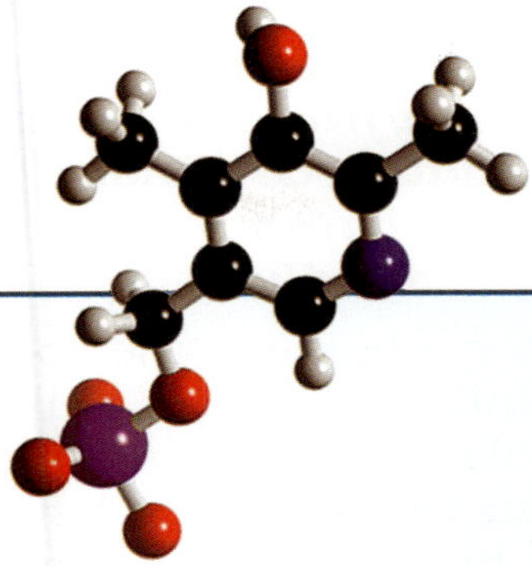

Preface to the Fourth Edition

After the first edition this book appeared in 1985, analytical and teaching fraternity have been of the considered opinion that for professional competency the knowledge of the chemistry involved in the analytical methods i.e. "Reaction Mechanism" needs to be provided, even though not legally mandated, to enable the analysts to perceive the methodology in proper perspective since all aspects of different methods are ultimately founded on chemistry. This is how the idea for contents of this book originated.

Although I had conceptualized the project in 1992 but being busy in compiling books on other subjects of current importance i.e. TLC, HPTLC, HPLC including revision of this title, I could not take up this project due to paucity of time and resources. Further, in view of complexity of the project, I did harbour serious doubts regarding its ultimate completion if and when taken up. If anyone feels that the books can be written by setting an author on his or her way and then waiting for the manuscript to appear, they are delusioned. It needs constant adaptation, definite level of discipline and hunger to keep going. I had been exploring the possibility of associating some teachers with sound knowledge of basic organic chemistry, but met with no success. It has been my ultimate **desire** to complete the project before I close my shop forever.

Knowing fully well that nothing can be achieved without enthusiasm and dedication, being **SCORPIO** decided to accept the challenge with the **SELF BELIEF** and complete the project by myself. I sincerely hope that this series shall find permanent place in every analytical laboratory and teaching institutions with the assurance that such an exhaustive compilation on the subject may never be available.

"Desire is perhaps the starting point of achieving something."

"Belief is the knowledge that we can do something. It is the inner feeling that what we undertake, we can accomplish."

"Scorpio have creative mind with sharp memory, truly explorer of new intelligent horizon, have great stamina and never shy away from challenges, extremely introspective with analytical mind, highly intuitive, determined in pursuit of their goal, passionate about every thing they do, have strong sense of purpose in life with determination to do nothing half-heartedly."

For practical consideration, in addition to introductory chapters, the book has been arranged in 13 principal chapters each containing different multi-component formulations. Analytical methods for each ingredient in a formulation have been described on the pattern similar to 3rd edition using mainly UV-Vis spectroscopy as principal analytical tool. However, as clear from the title, uniqueness of 4th edition is that with each method "probable reaction mechanism" has been described for proper understanding of the methodology as describing methods while ignoring chemistry was considered to be an incomplete endeavour. This should help analysts to integrate fully the analytical methods with the chemistry involved and enable them to transmit the knowledge to others who want to learn. Majority of the reactions included in the text are of the type – addition, elimination, substitution, condensation, rearrangement or oxidation-reduction invariably resulting in the formation of a coloured end product, which could easily be quantified spectrophotometrically in visible region (400-800 nm). This once again established the importance of UV-Vis spectroscopy as an indispensable, reliable and well established analytical tool in spite of steep increase in the use of other physical methods of analysis (HPLC, HPLC/MS, GC, GC/MS, HPTLC, etc.). Analytical methods based on chromogenic reactions have stood the test of time and are still recommended for the fledgling analysts.

Understanding the reaction mechanism allows us to know its specificity and the reaction with the drug being analysed. For drugs having more than one functional group, the methods have been designed depending on the specificity of a particular functional group. With selective chemical reactions, the analyst can manipulate the sample to reveal the desired information and increase the selectivity of the analyte eliminating the possible interference due to other substances present in the formulation while analyzing. It is not

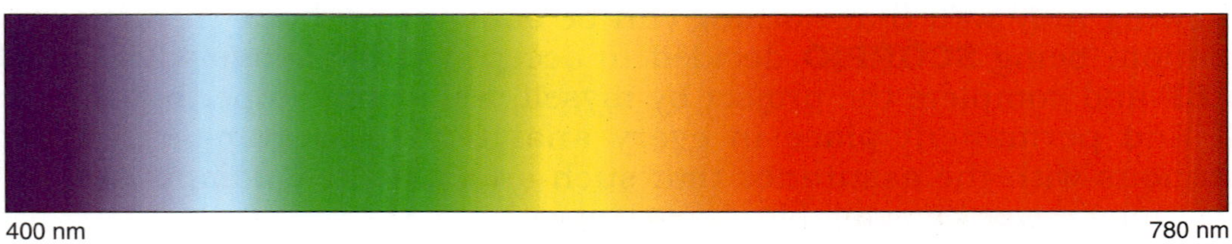

The light that human eye can perceive ranges from deep-violet (short wavelength) through blue, green, yellow and orange to deep red (long wavelength).

"One who never made a mistake never learnt anything."

necessary to learn thousands of individual reactions, instead we can learn few common reactions really well and apply the knowledge to similar cases.

Based on the functional group present in a molecule, the following reagents have been most commonly employed for quantification of the drug molecule: Gibbs' reagent, Bratton-Marshall reagent, Emerson's reagent, Ehrlich's reagent, Pauly's reagent, INH reagent, MBTH reagent, Besthorn's reagent, Folin's reagent, Van Urk's reagent, Wurster's Red reagent, Sanger's reagent, Chromotropic acid reagent, N-Bromosuccinimide reagent and DNPH reagent.

Most of the reaction mechanisms described in the text are as reported by the authors for which relative references have been cited under each reaction. However, the book "Pharmaceutical Chemistry, Vol. 2" by H.J. Roth et al. has been extensively referred to and has been extremely helpful in visualizing the reaction mechanism of several drug substances. Other textbooks of organic chemistry and analytical chemistry invariably consulted have been added under references at the end of introduction.

I am confident that 'Reaction Mechanism' described in this book along with method of analysis shall provide the most stimulating learning experience and will enable you to appreciate the excitement of this fascinating field.

Since newer molecules are invariably chemical modifications of existing drug substances, this compilation should be of help to the analysts in developing suitable method of analysis for newer drug molecules and also understand the chemistry involved and the confidence to tackle newer situations.

Over the years it was observed that at postgraduate level several practical exercises in pharmaceutical analysis were based on the methods described in 1st, 2nd and 3rd editions of this book. The students were invariably keen to know the detailed chemistry involved in methods. I do hope, my attempt in this direction will help students to perform practicals with better understanding. I expect this four-volume book on pharmaceutical analysis with reaction mechanism should make analytical science easier to understand for students, analysts and educators.

The icon representing structure of codeine with "Reaction Mechanism" reflects the underlying concept of this book.

Although I have exerted all my efforts to ensure that the text is free from errors, but it is quite possible that methodology details, certain structures and reaction mechanism may be inaccurate. I hope my efforts shall be evaluated in proper perspective.

It is the analyst who is consistently if not constantly involved with all the aspects of analysis. His/her interest necessarily is not of a curious bystander. This book does not purport to make analysts out of its readers, although it is hoped that some will be "turned on" to such a pursuit.

New Delhi, India

P.D. Sethi, M.Pharm., Ph.D.
Pharmaceutical Analyst

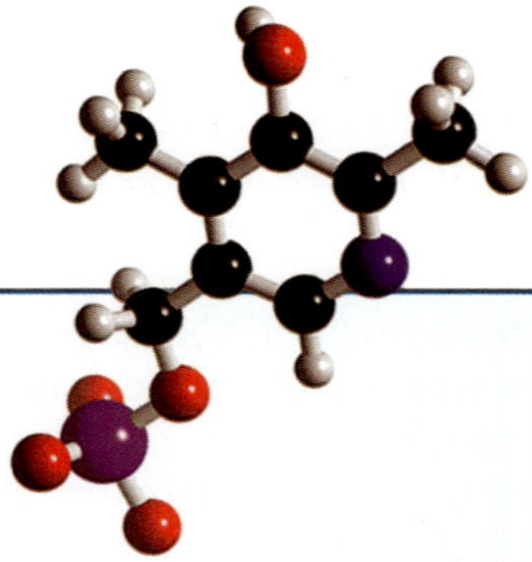

Acknowledgement

I would like to express my most sincere gratitude to analysts, students, teachers and professionals for their continuous support and encouragement and shaping my analytical career and ideas for compiling this book. The support extended by Professor Vijay K. Kapoor, University Institute of Pharmaceutical Sciences, Panjab University, Chandigarh in explaining and correcting several reactions included in the text is sincerely acknowledged. I am deeply indebted to Mr. Dilip Charegaonkar, Managing Director, M/s Anchrom Enterprises (I) Pvt. Ltd., Mumbai for supporting my scientific activities. I would like to convey my appreciation to the management of M/s Anchrom Enterprises (I) Pvt. Ltd., Mumbai and Kongposh Publications Pvt. Ltd., New Delhi for independently establishing life-time annual awards for Best Research Papers in "HPTLC Analysis" and "Pharmaceutical Analysis" respectively in recognition of my contribution in the field of Pharmaceutical Analysis. I am confident, their gesture shall provide impetus to young analysts for their interest in pharmaceutical analysis, currently the most creative and challenging field.

Without the support and untiring efforts of Mr. Dharmvir of 'CBS' my hand-written text particularly the reactions would never have been converted into book, thanks for his dedication and commitment for completing the assignment meticulously. I am thankful to Mr. Satish K. Jain, Managing Director, CBS, for accepting the hand-written manuscript of most challenging project and providing all the required facilities to bring this series to fruition.

New Delhi, India

P.D. Sethi, M.Pharm., Ph.D.
Pharmaceutical Analyst

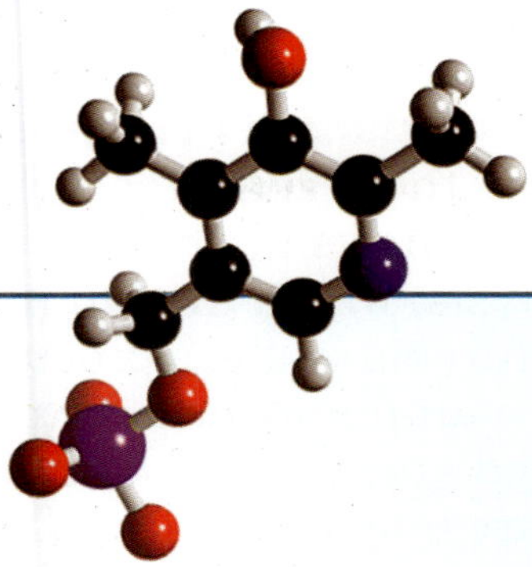

Preface to the First Edition

Devising accurate assay procedures for each ingredient of complex dosage formulations containing several therapeutically and chemically compatible drugs with very similar chemical nature is a monumental undertaking. The very idea of separation, identification and estimation of each ingredient in such complex formulations would make the analyst's hair stand on end. Not only are the multiple active constituents present but they are usually there in widely divergent concentrations depending upon their relative potency and therapeutic need of the patient. The presence of additives, excipients and decomposition products further complicates the development of analytical procedures. Many of the classical tests long regarded as specific for certain substances are now answered by many more compounds. Nevertheless, the therapeutic advantage of such complex drug combinations should take precedence over any potential analytical problem which is ultimately the concern of the analyst. The increasing complexities of pharmaceutical preparations and the marked emphasis on quality control by the ethical manufacturers have placed greater load on the ingenuity of the quality control chemist.

An analyst who is in the need of an analytical method may be obliged to survey tremendous amount of literature in order to select one procedure which may appear to suit his need and facilities available, but when he subjects the selected procedure to actual test, he may find that he cannot reproduce the method. It is, therefore, essential that the practising analyst should have access to analytical procedures which are simple, reliable and workable under routine laboratory conditions.

"No one is ever born talented nor talent obtained as a gift or lucky coincidence. It is a resource acquired through one's own endeavour. In this process, others may provide some help and inspiration, but it is a quality earned by one's own hard endeavour."

Modern analytical techniques rely increasingly on complex techniques of analysis that require expensive equipments and highly specialized personnel. Such methods are not of much help in countries lacking these resources. For the most part, modern analytical techniques merely permit analysis to be carried out more rapidly than the conventional method of analysis, which though not bad are tedious and time-consuming. Even if a manufacturer is ready to procure and install modern instruments/equipments, their maintenance in fittest condition is a herculean task. Non-availability of trained analytical personnel and precise, simple and suitable methods of analysis are major handicaps for pharmaceutical manufacturers in developing countries.

Taking into consideration the technical and economic constraints, it is necessary that the recommended methods should permit their use by drug laboratories located in developing countries. It is significant to stress that even simple instruments like colorimeter and spectrophotometer result in sensitive and accurate measurements with clear advantage of speed, simplicity and easy maintenance. The large volume of literature devoted to their application in almost every field of scientific research constitutes irrefutable evidence of their utility. It is, therefore, reasonable to assume that the analytical procedures involving the use of such simple instruments will find greater application. Selection of analytical method is a very critical point. The method must be accurate, sensitive, selective, reproducible and convenient.

In view of rapid advance during the last several years in the field of pharmaceutical analysis and marketing of ever increasing multi-component formulations, the available texts dealing in pharmaceutical analysis that have been written so far do not in general deal with the analysis of each component in wide range of complex pharmaceutical dosage formulations, particularly in presence of interfering substances. The official compendias are rarely of help in such formulations. To fill the existing gap in literature and keeping in view the economic and technical limitations of drug manufacturers, particularly in medium and small scale sector, it was felt that there exists a need to have a compilation of a simple, suitable and reliable methods for analysis of each ingredient of multi-component drug formulations.

This text, a maiden attempt, is meant to fulfill these needs. Analytical procedures for more than 200 drug formulations of divergent combinations have been compiled to serve as a convenient source of information for analysts and scientists engaged in the field. The focal point for this compilation is the presentation of practical aspect of the methodology using colorimeter and spectrophotometer as the main analytical tools.

For practical considerations, the drug formulations have been classified into 23 different categories based upon their common therapeutic uses as under:

1. Analgesics and antipyretics
2. Antacids and other ulcer healing drugs
3. Antacids, sedatives, antispasmodics
4. Anthelmintics
5. Anti-allergic drugs
6. Antibiotics
7. Anti-diarrhoeals
8. Anti-inflammatory drugs
9. Antimalarials
10. Anti-tuberculous drugs
11. Bronchospasm relaxants (anti-asthma)
12. Enzymes and digestives
13. Expectorants and cough suppressants
14. Eye, ear preparations
15. Keratolytics and cleansers
16. Laxatives, purgatives and lubricants
17. Nasal preparations
18. Oral rehydration salts
19. Rubefacients
20. Sedatives and tranquillisers
21. Topical antifungal, anti-infective preparations
22. Urinary anti-infective preparations
23. Vitamins, minerals and other nutritional additives.

For most of the formulations, several alternative methods have been described for a particular substance so that the analyst can intelligently select and apply the method to suit his need and the laboratory facilities available. Preliminary treatment of the sample for analysis utilizing conventional isolation and extraction procedures have been applied wherever necessary to eliminate the presence of potentially interfering substances. In other cases, the methods are sufficiently specific to permit the analysis of individual ingredients without pre-treatment. The procedures have been described in sufficient details highlighting the important steps in methodology so that these can be reproduced without much difficulty. Merits and demerits of each method and possibility of its application to other formulations have been discussed. To help the analyst and to enhance the book's usefulness, several worked out examples based on actual experimental data have been included. For drug manufacturers, who are interested to set up their independent quality control division, chapter on the profile of a quality control laboratory has been included giving brief outline of different sections.

Its importance for pharmaceutical teachers, students and institutions imparting special course in drug analysis cannot be overestimated. Science graduates interested in pursuing career as analytical chemist will find this compilation invaluable for daily use which will provide ready answers to most of their analytical problems. It is earnest feeling of the author that knowledge of the basic inorganic and organic chemistry tempered by judicious changes and the special skill needed in pharmaceutical analysis and the information included in this text will enable the analyst to overcome most specific problems and he will be able to analyse any viable combination of drug formulations he may encounter in future. It is pertinent to mention that analyst should cautiously choose the method and interpret the results carefully before certifying the product. It is hoped that this text will enable the analyst to take their rightful place in the pharmaceutical industry and in government laboratories concerned with the quality control of medicinal preparations.

The author is indebted to his wife, Usha for her moral support throughout his career.

The author wishes to express his sincere appreciation to Dr. O.P. Ghai, Professor and Head, Department of Pediatrics, All India Institute of Medical Sciences, New Delhi, for his helpful suggestions and guidance.

How far I have succeeded in my attempt, the decision is left to my fellow pharmacists and analysts.

New Delhi, India
1985

P.D. Sethi

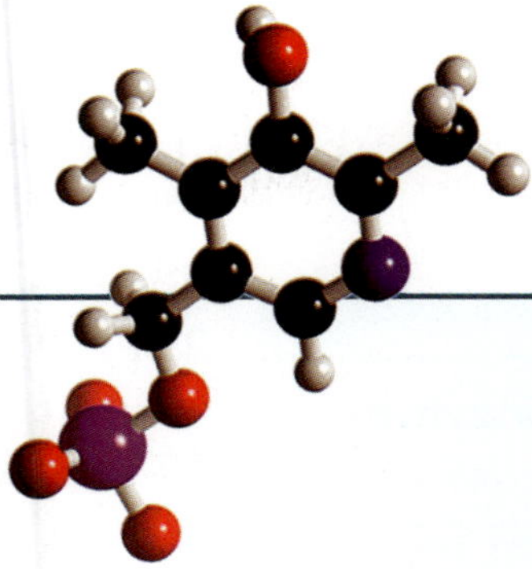

Brief Contents
Volumes I – IV

VOLUME 1

VOLUME 2

VOLUME 3

VOLUME 4

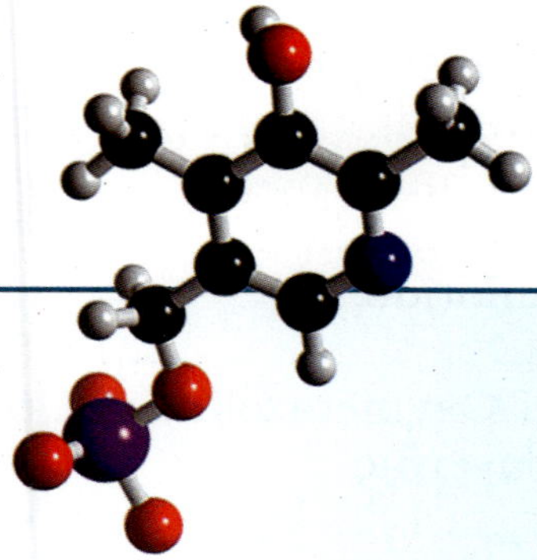

Contents

CHAPTER 15

Formulation No. and Name

CHAPTER 18

Miscellaneous (Vitamins, Minerals and Digestive Enzyme Preparations) 271–458

Formulation No. and Name

Reaction Mechanism

14

Eye, Ear and Nose Preparations

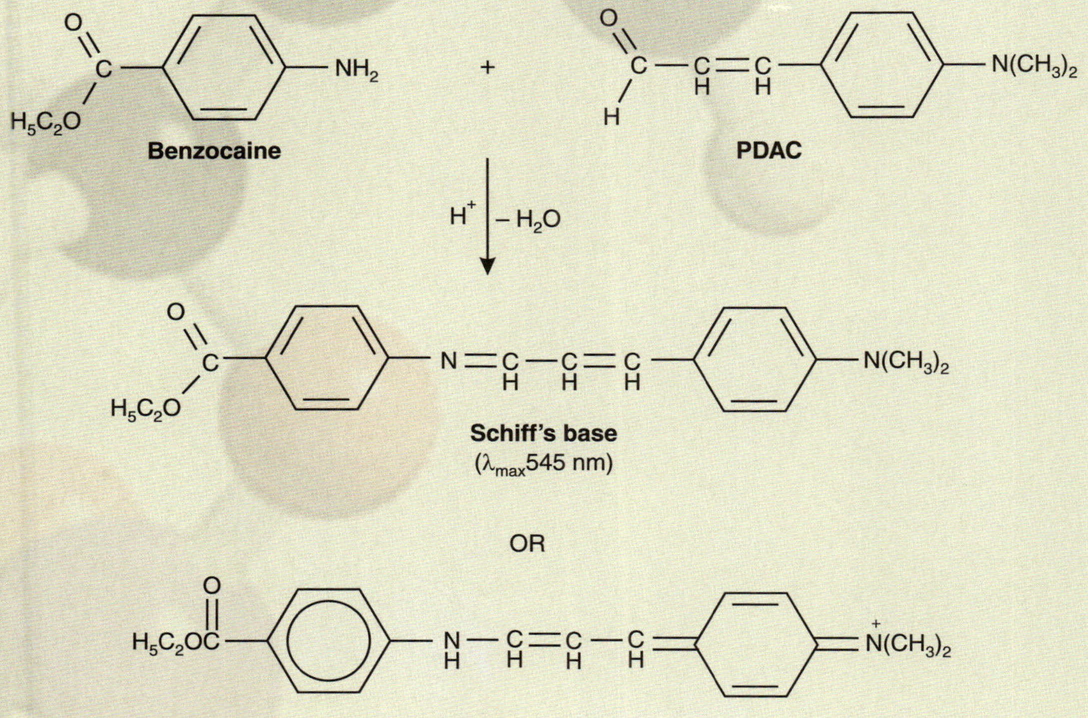

Formulation 1

Domiphen bromide, Boric acid, Borax, Salicylic acid, Zinc sulphate, Allantoin, Chlorbutol

ESTIMATION

Domiphen bromide

Reagents

1. Sodium lauryl sulphate solution, 0.00025 M: Dissolve 360 mg of pure sodium lauryl sulphate which has been previously dried at 105°C and cooled, in 100 ml of water. Dilute 10 ml of this to 500 ml. Standardise this solution against dicyclomine hydrochloride.
2. 0.003% w/v solution of methylene blue in water.

Procedure

Transfer sample equivalent to 2 mg of domiphen bromide into dry separating funnel and extract with three 10 ml portions of chloroform, allowing each extract to separate fully before proceeding with the next. Combine the chloroform extract in a 250 ml stoppered measuring cylinder and to this, add 25 ml of methylene blue solution and 50 ml of water. Stopper and shake the cylinder. The colour remains in the aqueous phase. Titrate with small addition of 0.00025 M sodium lauryl sulphate shaking after each addition until the colour is of equal intensity in both the phases. Each ml of 0.00025 M sodium lauryl sulphate is equivalent to 0.000208 g of domiphen bromide.

Salicylic acid

Reagents

1. Ammonium ferric sulphate solution: Dissolve 8 g of ferric ammonium sulphate in 100 ml of water and warm on a water-bath. Filter, if necessary, to remove any precipitate that might have formed.
2. Acidic ammonium ferric sulphate solution: To 2 ml of ammonium ferric sulphate solution, add 1 ml of 1 N hydrochloric acid and make up the volume to 100 ml with distilled water, solution to be freshly prepared.

Standard solution

25 mcg/ml of salicylic acid in water.

Sample solution

Dilute sample equivalent to 2.5 mg of salicylic acid with water to produce 100 ml (25 mcg/ml).

Procedure

Take 5 ml each of sample and standard solutions in two test tubes, add 2 ml of acidic ferric ammonium sulphate solution and mix thoroughly. Measure the absorption of both the solutions against water as blank at about 540 nm and calculate the results by comparison. The method is based on formation of iron complex in acidic medium. For detailed reaction mechanism, see chapter on analgesics.

Zinc sulphate

Reagents

1. Zincon reagent: Dissolve 60 mg of 'Zincon' in 2 ml of 0.2 N sodium hydroxide and 10 ml distilled water. Dilute to 50 ml with water, stable only for 2 days at room temperature.
2. Buffer solution, pH 9.2: Dissolve 12.4 g of boric acid and 15 g of potassium chloride in 86 ml of 1 N sodium hydroxide. Dilute to 1000 ml with water.

Standard solution

40 mcg/ml of zinc sulphate in water.

Procedure

To accurately measured volume of sample containing 200 mcg of zinc sulphate and 5 ml of standard solution, add 50 ml of buffer solution, 2 ml of zincon reagent and dilute to 100 ml with buffer. Mix and measure the absorbance of sample and standard solutions at about 625 nm against reagent blank and compare the results.

Borax

Measure accurately aliquot of the sample equivalent to 100 mg of borax and titrate with 0.1 N hydrochloric acid using methyl orange or methyl red as indicator. Each ml of 0.1 N hydrochloric acid is equivalent to 0.09536 g of borax.

Total boric acid

Transfer the sample equivalent to 100 mg of boric acid into 250 ml conical flask, and neutralise it with 0.1 N sulphuric acid using methyl orange as indicator to a faint pink colour. Add about 10 g of mannitol, warm to dissolve and titrate against 0.1 N sodium hydroxide solution using phenolphthalein as indicator. Each ml of 0.1 N sodium hydroxide is equivalent to 0.006183 g of boric acid.

Note

Although glycerol is widely used as organic polyhydroxy compound, mannitol and sorbitol are more effective and have advantage of being solid. They do not increase the volume of solution being titrated.

Borax and Boric acid

First carry out titration with hydrochloric acid using methyl red as indicator for estimation of borax. Then add mannitol or glycerine and carry out the titration with sodium hydroxide. It forms 1 : 1 or 1 : 2 mole ratio complex.

Note

The boric acid liberated while estimating borax will also get titrated.

1.

$$\underset{\textbf{Borax}}{Na_2B_4O_7} + 2H^+(HCl) + H_2O \longrightarrow \underset{\textbf{Boric acid}}{4H_3BO_3} + 2NaCl$$

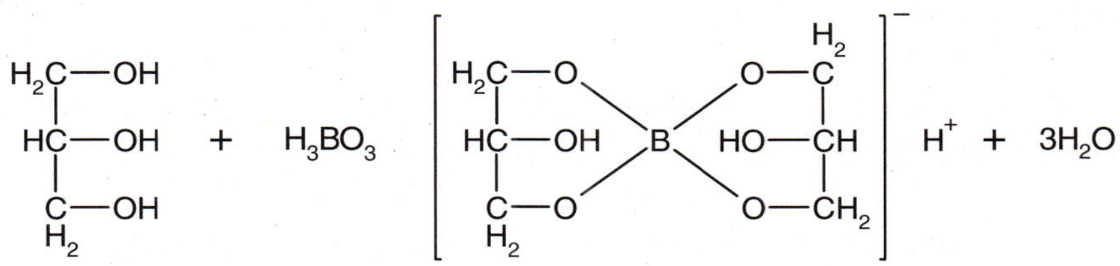

Glycerin

$$H^+ + NaOH \longrightarrow (\text{Na-boric acid complex}) + H_2O$$

Estimation of Boric acid and Borax

(A) Take 5-10 ml of the sample (containing 0.2-1 mEq of boric acid) in 100 ml of iodine flask, add 1.5 g of mannitol, swirl the flask for 2 min. Add 1 g each of potassium iodate and potassium iodide and again swirl for 5 min. Titrate the librated iodine with 0.02 M sodium thiosulphate using starch as indicator. Each ml of 0.1 M thiosulphate ≡ 6.18 mg of boric acid.

(B) Take another 5-10 ml of sample (containing 0.025-0.1 mmol of borax) in 100 ml of iodine flask. Add known and excessive volume of hydrochloric acid, followed by 0.5 g of KI and 5 ml of 5% KIO_3 solution, swirl and titrate the librated iodine with 0.1 M thiosulphate using starch as indicator. Each ml of 0.1 M thiosulphate ≡ 10.07 mg of borax ($Na_2B_4O_7$).

Analysis of mixture

(a) Determine the borax in a portion of sample as described above. Calculate the volume (*x* ml) of hydrochloric acid consumed, the quantity of borax and amount (A) of boric acid produced during the reaction between borax and boric acid.

To an equal volume of sample add the volume (*x* ml) of hydrochloric acid as calculated under experiment (a), then determine the total boric acid (original plus that produced from borax). From the total amount (B) subtract the amount of boric acid librated from borax reaction to obtain the net quantity of boric acid present in the sample.

Note

1. During titration of boric acid with alkali in the presence of mannitol, carbon dioxide is likely to interfere and further phenolphthalein end point is not very sharp.
2. In the above iodometric method quantitative titration of iodine was complete within 5 min.
3. For direct titration of borax with hydrochloric acid, there is likelihood of interference by boric acid librated during reaction between borax and acid.
4. Consecutive titration of both the components in the same solution i.e. first borax and then total boric acid by this method appears to be feasible in principle, but is not satisfying in practice as starch as indicator shall be present from the start of titration which is against the recommended practice.
5. Titration of borax with acid using methyl orange as indicator is not suitable on micro scale.

Reference

R. Saxena & R.M. Verma. *Talanta*, 30(5), 365-367, 1983.

Chlorbutol (Chlorobutanol)

Reagents

1. 0.1 N silver nitrate.
2. 0.1 N ammonium thiocyanate.
3. 10% w/v solution of ferric ammonium sulphate in water.
4. 10% w/v solution of sodium hydroxide in water.

Procedure

Transfer sample equivalent to 30 mg of chlorbutol into a distillation flask. Add 5 ml of sodium hydroxide solution. Reflux for 30 minutes and cool. Add 5 ml of concentrated nitric acid, 2 ml of nitrobenzene and 10 ml of 0.1 N silver nitrate solution. Shake the contents vigorously for one minute. Add 1 ml of ferric ammonium sulphate solution and titrate excess of silver nitrate with 0.1 N ammonium thiocyanate to a pale red end point. Carry out the blank. Each ml of 0.1 N ammonium thiocyanate is equivalent to 0.003108 g of chlorbutol.

Explanatory Note

The method is based on Volhard titration. After hydrolysis with alkaline medium (NaOH) we get NaCl which is subjected to Volhard titration.

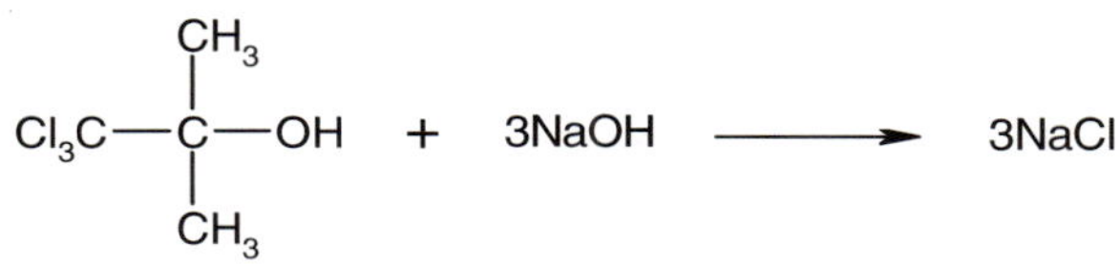

$$AgNO_3 + NaCl \longrightarrow AgCl$$

$$Ag^+ + SCN^- \rightleftharpoons AgSCN + Cl^-$$

First silver thiocyanate is precipitated. Ferric ion present as indicator reacts with excess thiocyanate to yield reddish-brown ferric thiocyanate; so this acts as indicator.

Note

During titration, some silver is likely to be adsorbed by the precipitates, so frequent, vigorous shaking may be required to desorb unreacted silver from precipitate. Nitrobenzene is added to coat the silver chloride particles making them inaccessible for reaction. Otherwise, one may get higher results.

Chlorbutol answers 'Guareschi-Lustgarten' reaction with resorcinol in alkaline medium to give red colour (λ_{max} 490 nm).

Probable Reaction Mechanism

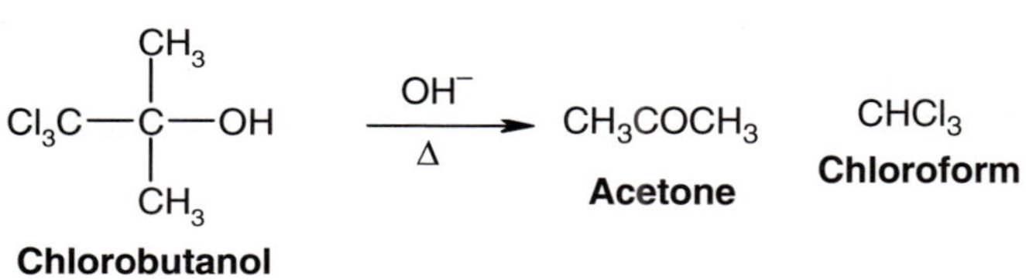

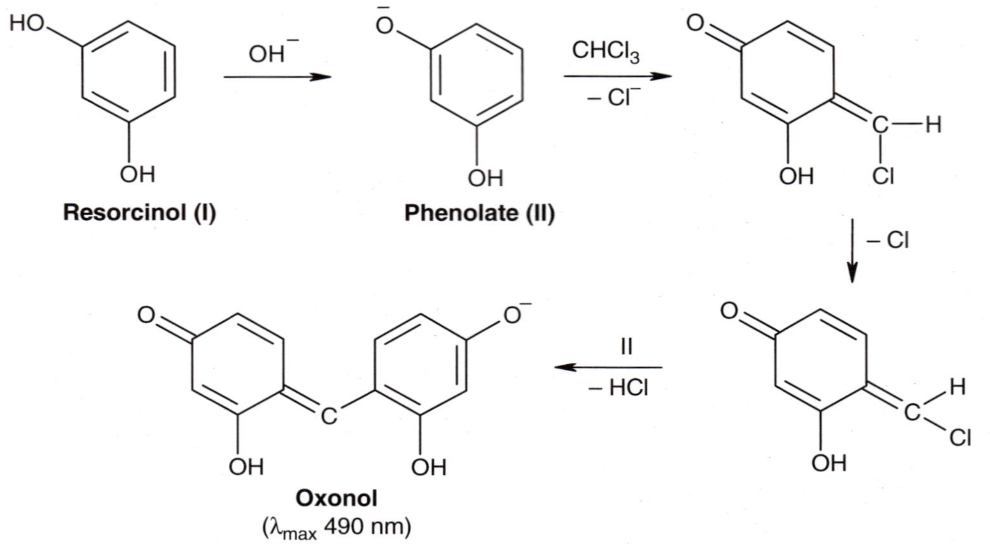

Allantoin

In alkaline medium, allantoin is hydrolysed to allantoic acid, then in acidic medium to glyoxylic acid and urea. Glyoxylic acid reacts with phenylhydrazine to give hydrazone which is converted to coloured chromophore (λ_{max} 520 nm) on oxidation with potassium ferricyanide.

Reagents

1. 1% w/v solution of phenylhydrazine hydrochloride in water.
2. 1% w/v solution of potassium ferricyanide in water, stable for 1 day only.
3. 12.5% w/v solution of oxalic acid in water.

Standard solution

2.5 mcg/ml of allantoin in water.

Sample solution

Dilute sample appropriately with water to get 2.5 mcg/ml.

Procedure

Transfer 5 ml each of sample and standard solutions, and 5 ml of distilled water in 25 ml boiling tubes. To each tube, add 1 ml of 0.5 N sodium hydroxide and heat in boiling water-bath for exactly 5 minutes. Remove from heat and add 2 ml of oxalic acid solution and 1 ml of phenylhydrazine solution. Heat the tubes in boiling water for exactly 2 minutes. Cool, add 4 ml of hydrochloric acid, boil for 2 min, cool and add 0.5 ml of potassium ferricyanide solution. Mix well and measure the extinction of the solutions after 5 minutes against water as blank at about 520 nm and calculate the results by comparison.

Probable Reaction Mechanism

Heating the compound with NaOH probably cleaves the side chain and results in the formation of a compound as shown below.

Step 1

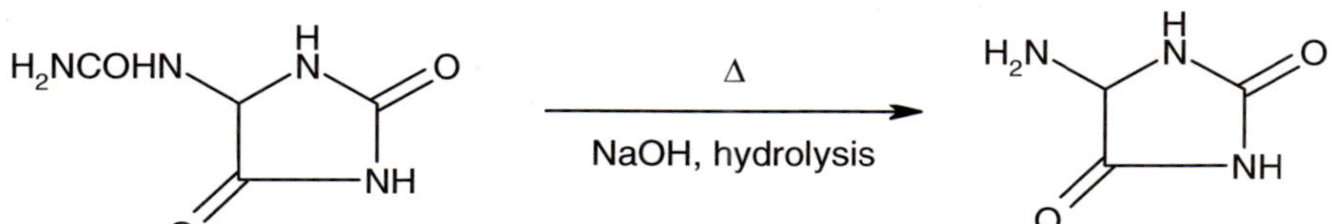

Allantoin

Step 2

The resultant compound is then heated with phenylhydrazine.

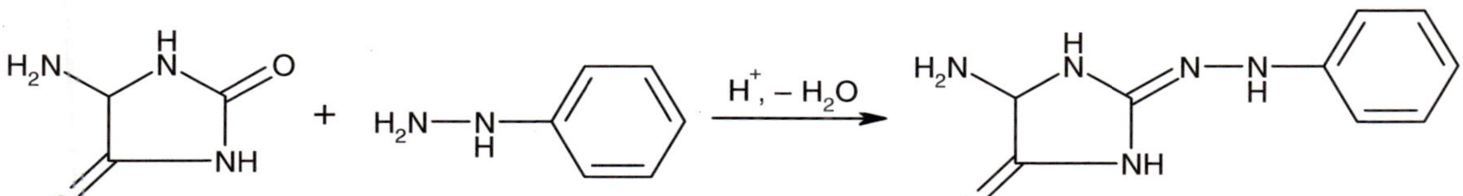

Phenylhydrazine

Step 3

The product formed is treated with $K_3Fe(CN)_6$ and HCl which functions as oxidising agent.

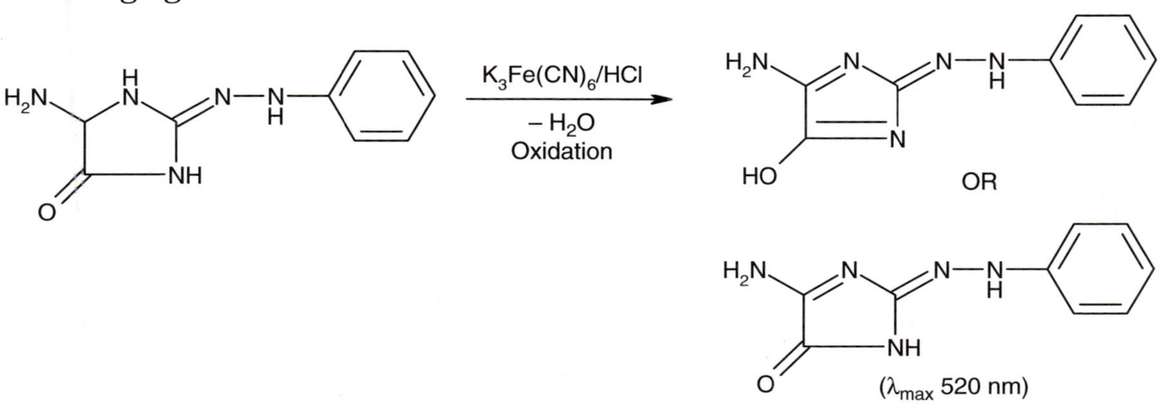

Another reaction mechanism is proposed which appears to be more probable.

In alkaline medium, there is ring opening due to 3,4 cleavage as a result of nucleophilic attack by hydroxide ion on the carbonyl group to form an acid i.e. allantoic acid (diureidoacetic acid), finally leading to formation of glyoxylic acid and urea. Glyoxylic acid shall react with phenylhydrazine to give hydrazone which is converted to a chromophore on oxidation with $K_3Fe(CN)_3$.

Probable Reaction Mechanism

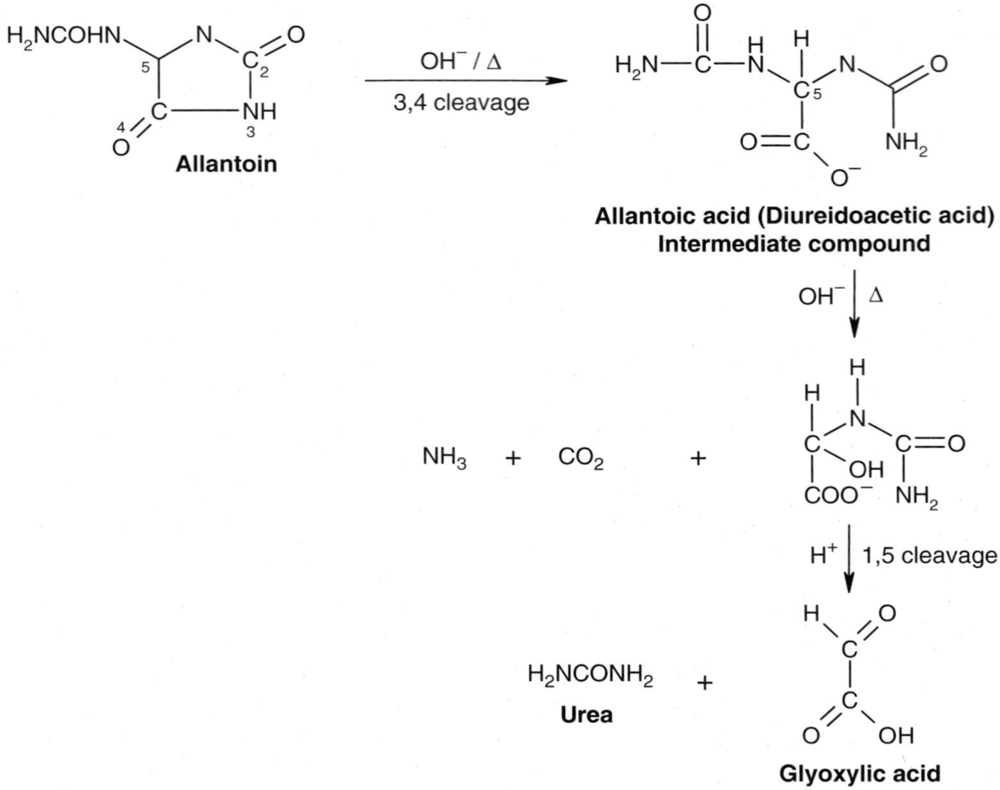

As C-5 is activated for nucleophilic attack by alkali (OH^-) it leads to formation of carbonyl compound (glyoxylic acid) through keto-enol tautomerism. There are two possibilities:

(A) Either glyoxylic acid on heating in acidic medium loses CO_2 to give formaldehyde which ultimately reacts with phenylhydrazine to give hydrazone.

OR

(B) Glyoxylic acid with carbonyl (C==O) function reacts with phenylhydrazine to give phenylhydrazone. In phenylhydrazine the 'N' atom which is not directly bonded to aromatic ring is more nucleophilic and reacts with (C==O) group. This reaction is catalysed by oxalic acid (acetic acid can also be used).

Note

For similar reaction with 2,4-dinitrophenylbutazine, stronger acid (H_2SO_4) is required as catalyst.

On addition of $K_3Fe(CN)_6$, excess of the reagent (phenylhydrazine) is oxidized to give diazonium salt which in turn couples with hydrazone to give intense coloured formazone (λ_{max} 520 nm).

Probable Reaction Mechanism

(A)

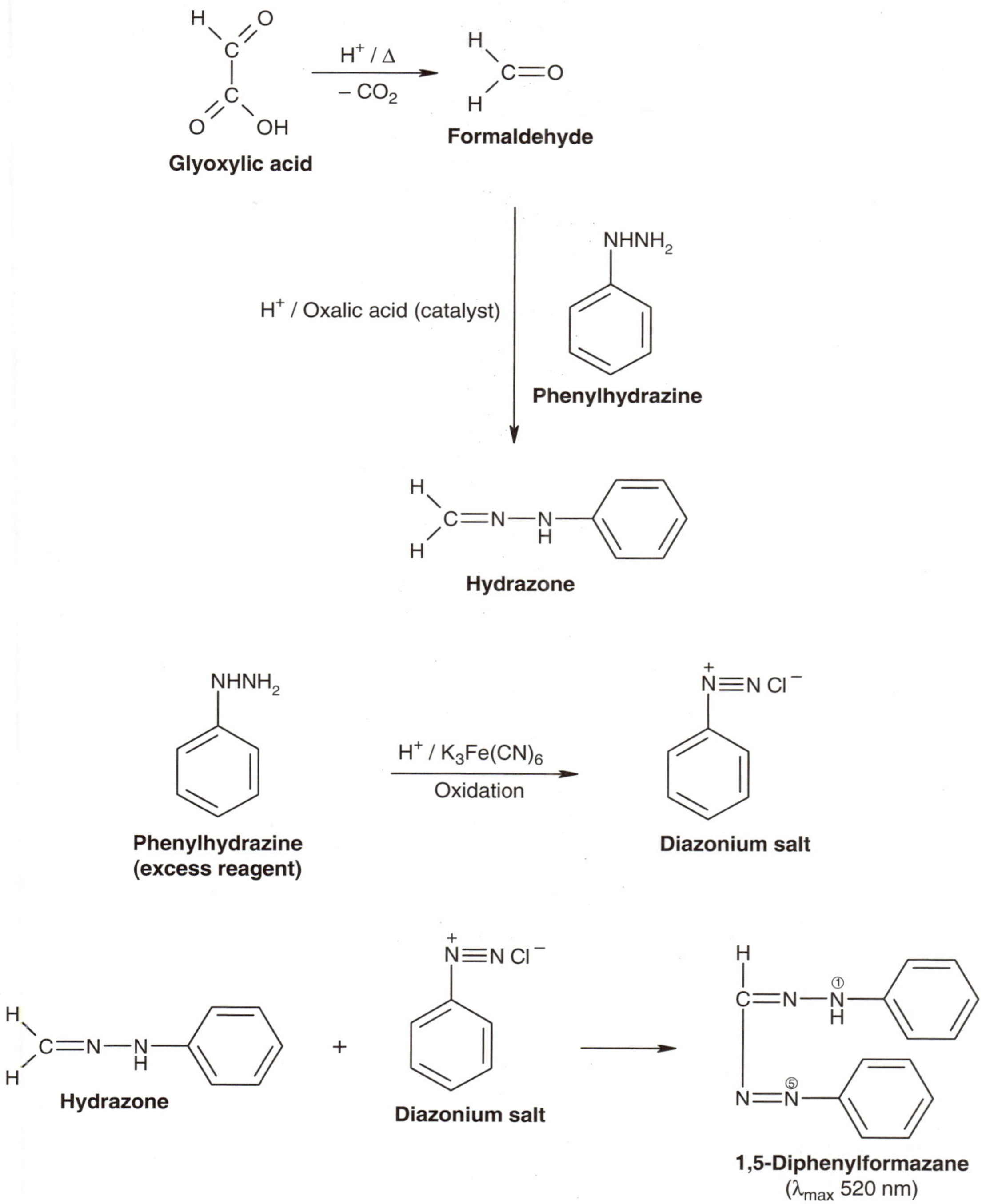

(B)

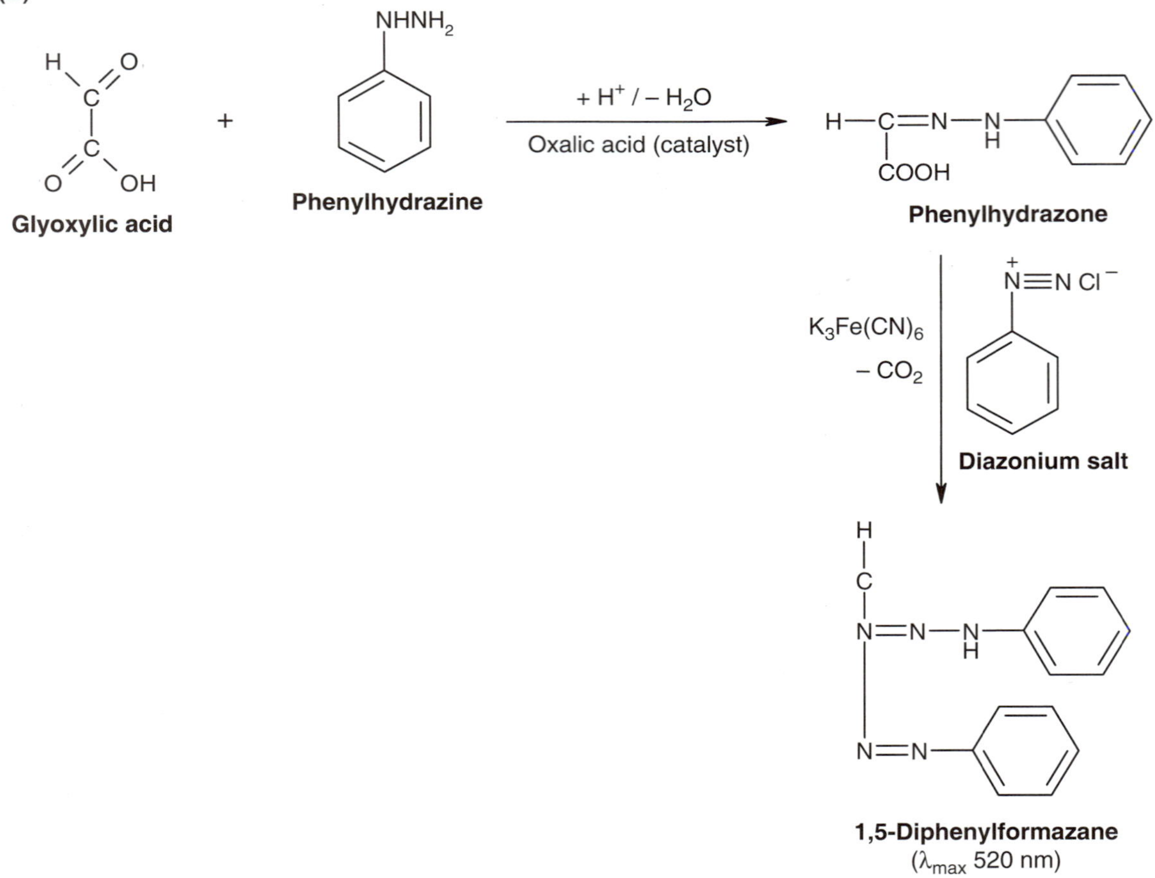

Reference

1. Pharmaceutical Chemistry (Vol. 2) by H.J. Roth, pp. 122, 160, 178.
2. Organic Chemistry (2nd ed.) by Sehan N. ege, pp. 506-508, 1989.

Formulation 2

Benzocaine, Antipyrine, Hexylresorcinol

ESTIMATION

Benzocaine

METHOD 1

Take 5 ml each of sample and standard solutions (15 mcg/ml in water) and follow the method described in formulation 13 of the chapter on expectorants and cough suppressants.

METHOD 2

Reagents

1. 0.1% w/v solution of p-dimethylaminocinnamaldehyde in methanol.
2. 50% w/v solution of trichloroacetic acid in methanol.
3. Methyl alcohol, acetone free.

Standard solution

10 mcg/ml of benzocaine in methyl alcohol.

Sample solution

(a) Ear drops, creams and ointments (water soluble bases): Weigh or measure accurately sample equivalent to 10 mg of benzocaine, suspend or dissolve in methanol and dilute to 100 ml with methyl alcohol. Filter through dry filter paper and discard first 5 ml of the filtrate. Dilute 1 ml of the filtrate to 50 ml with methyl alcohol.

(b) Ointment (water insoluble bases): Dissolve accurately weighed or measured quantity of the sample equivalent to 10 mg of substance in 15 ml of cyclohexane. Transfer to 100 ml volumetric flask, rinse the beaker thrice with 2 ml portions of cyclohexane and transfer to the flask. Shake vigorously for 2-3 minutes and make up the volume with methyl alcohol. Filter through dry filter paper and carry out further dilutions for preparation of sample solutions as under (a) above.

(c) Lozenges: Powder finely and weigh accurately equivalent to 10 mg of benzocaine. Add 75 ml of methyl alcohol and shake for 30 minutes, dilute to 100 ml with methyl alcohol. Carry out further dilutions with methanol as described under (a) above for preparation of sample solution.

Procedure

To 2 ml each of the sample and standard solutions, add 4 ml of p-dimethylaminocinnamaldehyde reagent, followed by 2 ml of trichloroacetic acid solution. Keep at room temperature for 10 minutes and record the absorbance of both the solutions at about 545 nm against reagent blank.

Note

1. The red Schiff's base produced in anhydrous medium is stable for 2 h. This reaction is more sensitive than the reaction with p-dimethylaminobenzaldehyde (yellow colour).
2. Menthol, camphor, benzalkonium chloride do not interfere.
3. Pink dye, usually present in lozenges, does not interfere.
4. Method is suitable for ointments, suppositories and lozenges.
5. The use of PDAC as aldehyde is more advantageous as the Schiff's base is red in colour.

Explanatory Note

Condensation reaction occurs between benzocaine and p-dimethylaminocinnamaldehyde (PDAC) in the presence of trichloroacetic acid resulting in the formation of Schiff's base (λ_{max} 545 nm).

Probable Reaction Mechanism

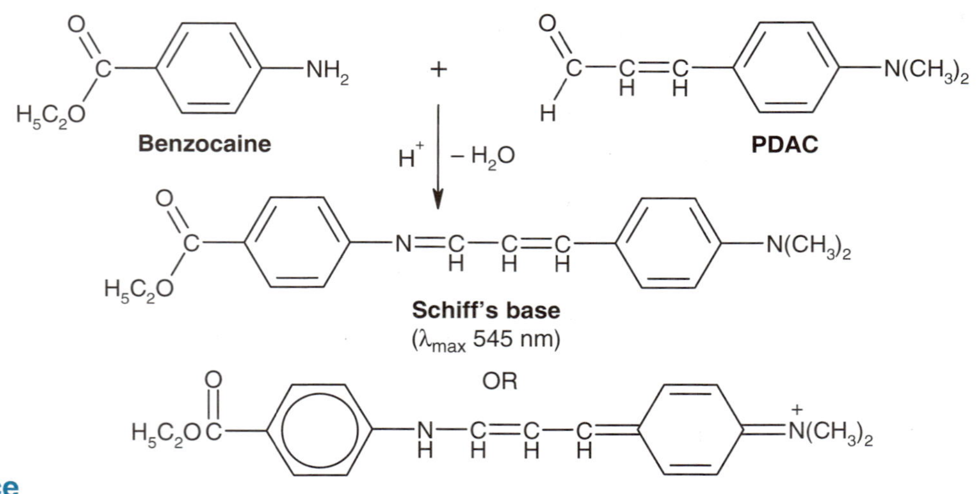

Reference

Henry, S.L. et al. J. Pharm. Sci., **66(7)**, 1037-1038, 1977.

Similarly, the compound will form Schiff's base with 'PDAB', vanillin and other aromatic aldehydes in acidic medium (CCl_3COOH) analogous to above reaction mechanism giving yellow-coloured Schiff's base.

Diazotized benzocaine ($NaNO_2$ + CCl_3COOH) couples with following reagents to give respective coloured complexes. The coupling takes place at position ortho to phenolic-OH function.

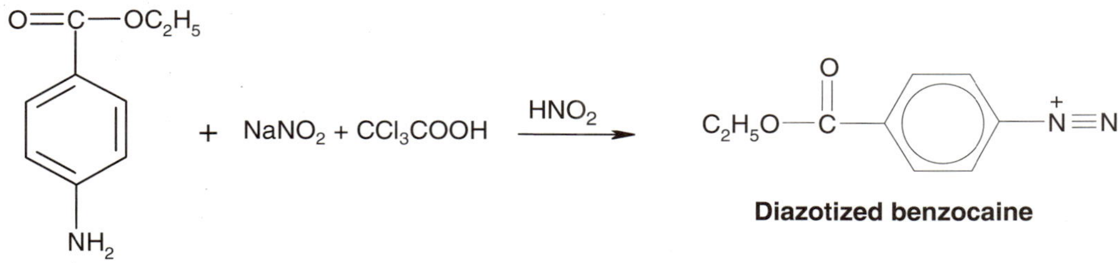

Benzocaine **Diazotized benzocaine**

Coupling reagent		λ_{max}
1. Meta-amiphenol	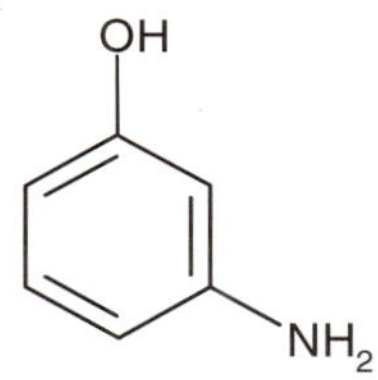	Yellow 450 nm
2. Resorcinol	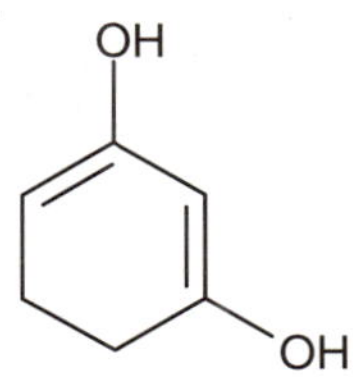	Red 490 nm
3. α-naphthylamine + NaOH	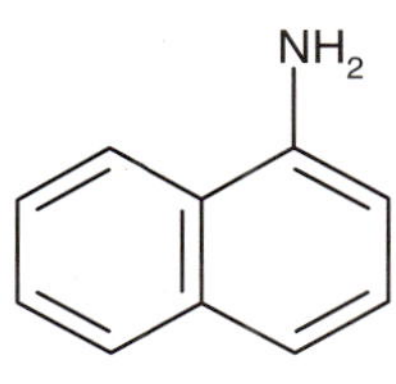	Violet 520 nm
4. 8-amino-1-naphthol	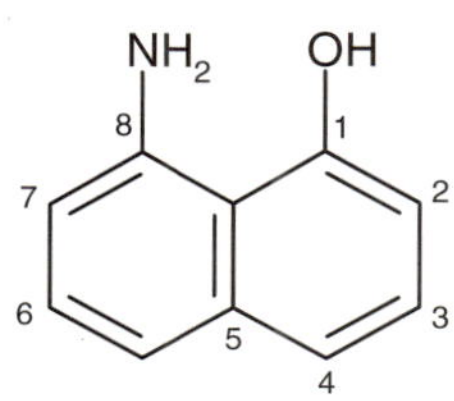	Violet 530 nm

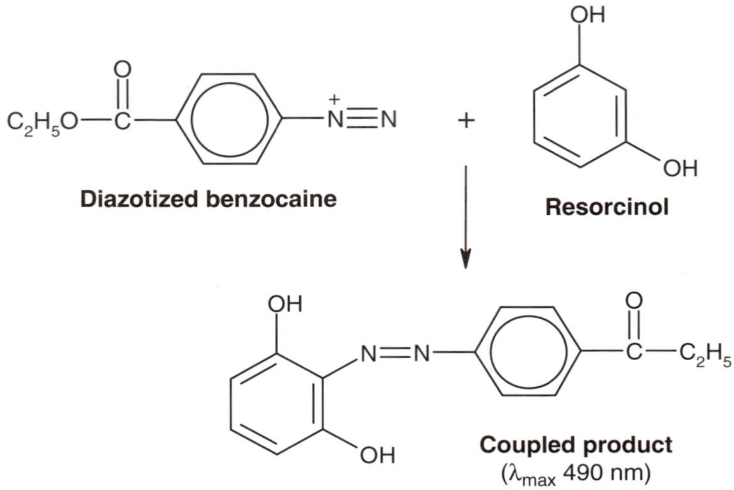

Reference

R.T. Sane & A.Y. Dhamankar. *Indian Drugs*, **19(2)**, 74-76, 1981.

R. Rama Krishna et al. (1979) have described a general method for determination of primary amine. The method was extended to drugs containing a free primary aromatic amine or released through hydrolysis/reduction. Drugs like folic acid, chloramphenicol, chlordiazepoxide, benzocaine, sulphonamide were taken up for studies. The method is based on oxidation of metol with potassium dichromate at pH 3 to give p-N-methylbenzoquinone-imine which couples at position ortho to amino group. The primary aromatic amine with electron acceptor groups (—SO_3H, —SO_2NH_2, —SO_2NHR, —COOH, —COOR and $COCH_3$) para to amino groups produce similar colour reaction.

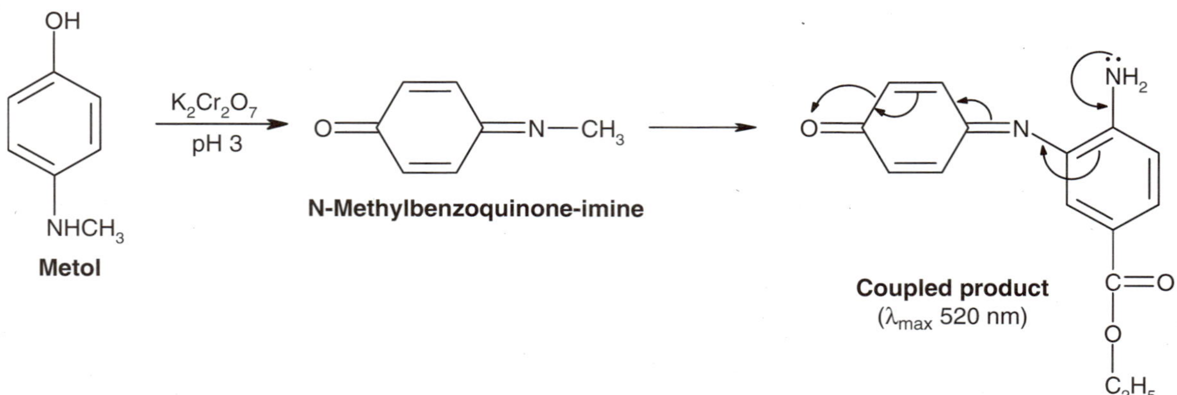

Reference

R. Rama Krishna & C.P.S. Sastry. *Talanta*, 861-865, 1979.

Diazotized benzocaine may also undergo electrophilic substitution with carbanions associated with active hydrogen such as ethylacetoacetate in alkaline medium to give a coloured product (λ_{max} 405 nm).

Probable reaction mechanism as proposed by the author

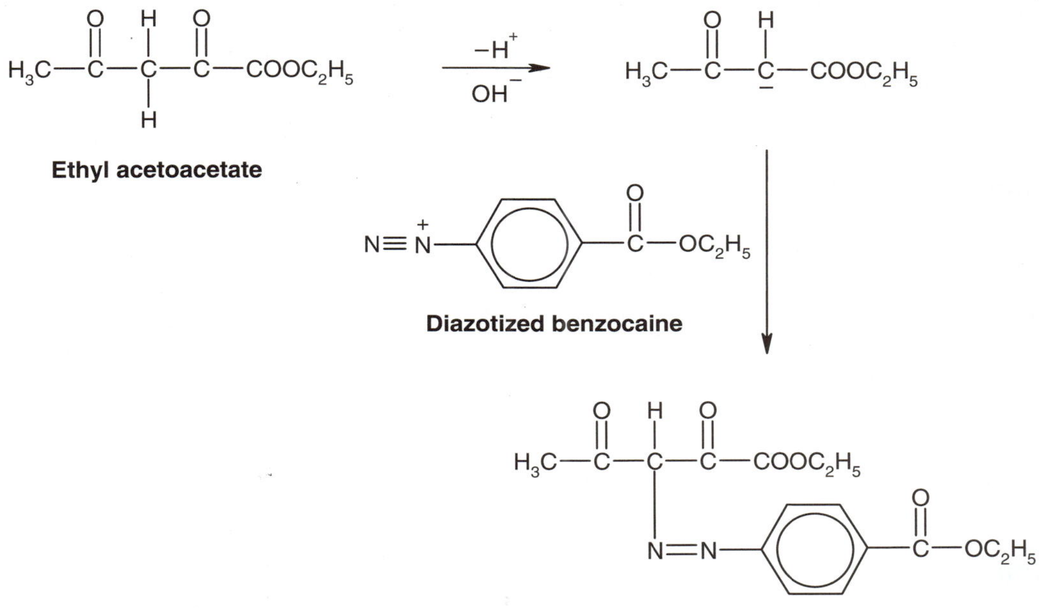

(λ_{max} 405 nm)

Hexylresorcinol

METHOD 1

Reagents

1. Dilute hydrochloric acid.
2. Molybdophosphotungstate solution.
3. 10% w/v solution of sodium carbonate in water.

Standard solution

Weigh accurately 250 mg of standard hexylresorcinol and transfer to a 250 ml volumetric flask. Add 10 ml of alcohol to dissolve and dilute to volume with water. Dilute 10 ml of this solution to 100 ml with water (100 mcg/ml).

Sample solution

Accurately weigh, a quantity of the sample equivalent to 5 mg of hexylresorcinol and transfer to 50 ml volumetric flask. Dilute to volume with water and filter.

Procedure

Transfer 10 ml each of standard, water and sample solutions into separate 100 ml volumetric flasks. Add 2 ml of dilute hydrochloric acid, 1 ml of molybdophosphotungstate solution, about 60 ml of water and allow to stand for 10 minutes. Add 25 ml of sodium carbonate solution and dilute to volume with water. Mix thoroughly and allow to stand for 1 hr. Filter through a dry filter paper, rejecting the first portion of the filtrate. Determine the absorbance of the standard and the sample at about 640 nm using blank in the reference cell. Calculate the contents of hexylresorcinol by comparison.

This method is based on reducing property of the compound wherein the compound itself gets oxidized.

METHOD 2

Reagents

1. 0.5 N ammonium hydroxide.
2. 0.5% w/v solution of 1,2-naphthoquinone-4-sulphonic acid (sodium salt) in water.

Standard solution

7.5 mcg/ml of hexylresorcinol in water.

Sample solution

Weigh accurately, a quantity of the sample equivalent to about 7.5 mg of hexylresorcinol, extract with water and make up to 100 ml with water. Further dilution is done with water to obtain solution of 7.5 mcg/ml.

Procedure

To 1 ml each of the standard and sample solution, add 0.5 ml of naphthoquinone reagent, 1.5 ml of 0.5 N ammonium hydroxide and dilute to 10 ml with water. Mix and read immediately (within 5 minutes) at 580 nm against reagent blank. Calculate the results by comparison. The method obeys Beer's law in the range of 2.5 to 7.5 mcg/ml.

Note

1. The colour of the complex is stable for 5 minutes.
2. The method can be directly applied to lozenges without isolation.

Probable Reaction Mechanism

Like resorcinol and orcinol it is prone to oxidation. 1,2-naphthoquinone-4-sulphonic acid acts as oxidizing agent in alkaline medium.

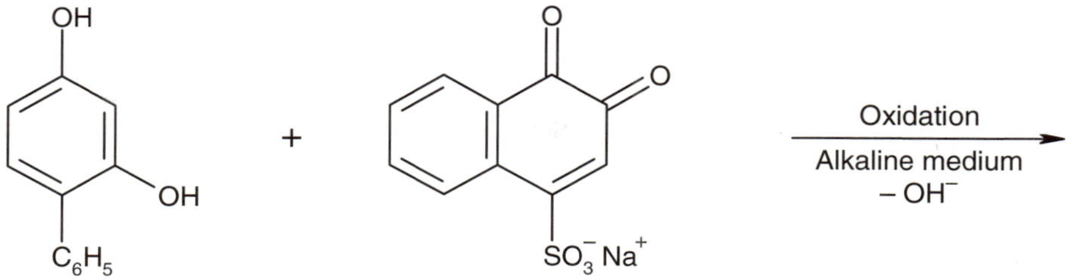

Hexylresorcinol **1,2-naphthoquinone-4-sulphonate**

Reaction sequence

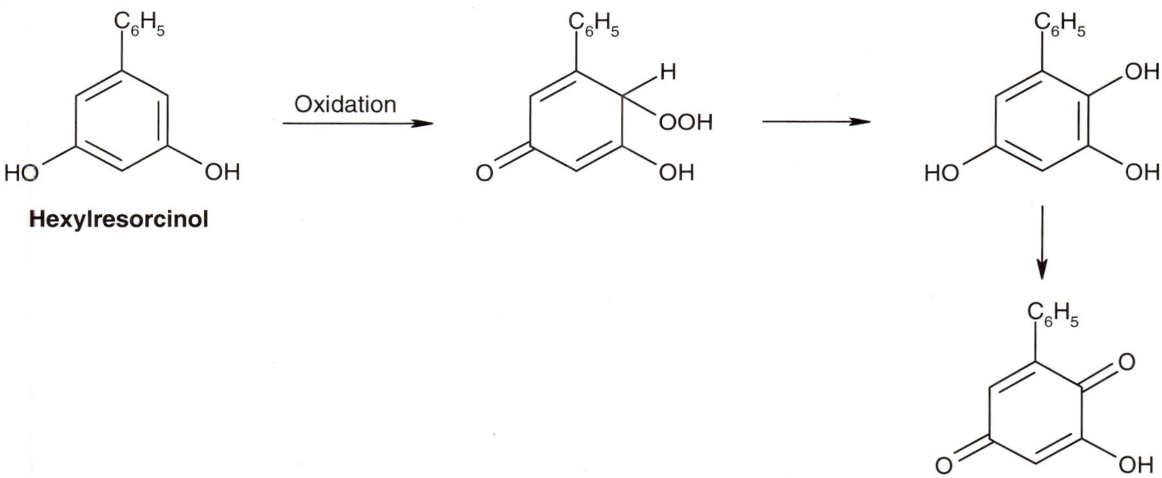

Coloured species
(λ_{max} 580 nm)

The above reaction is analogous to the oxidation of orcinol as described (Pharmaceutical Chemistry, Vol. 2 by H.J. Roth, p. 84).

Naphthoquinone is being reduced to hydroxy derivative (1,2-hydroxynaphthoquinol).

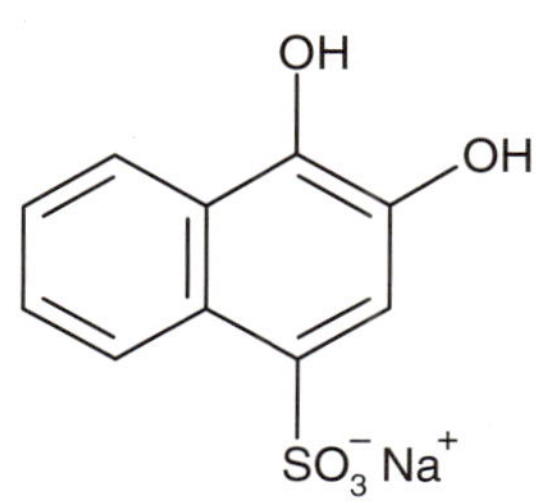

Reference

R.T. Sane & Medha Mainkar. *Indian Drugs*, 265-266, April 1979.

Antipyrine

Reagent

5% w/v solution of ferric chloride in water.

Standard solution

1 mg/ml of antipyrine in water.

Sample solution

Dilute an accurately weighed quantity of the sample equivalent to 100 mg of antipyrine to 100 ml with water.

Procedure

Transfer 1 ml each of the standard, sample and water into three separate test tubes. Add 5 ml of water into each tube followed by 1 ml of ferric chloride solution and mix well. Determine the absorbance of the sample and standard solutions at 540 nm using the blank in the reference cell and calculate the results by comparison.

Explanatory Note

Fe(3) forms a complex with antipyrin resulting in the formation of a coloured complex (λ_{max} 540 nm).

Probable Reaction Mechanism

The compound exists in Zwitterionic form due to vinylogous acid amide structure between N-1 and C=O. Nitrogen at position 2 is not basic as it is flanked by phenyl ring and C=O ring which take up free electron pair.

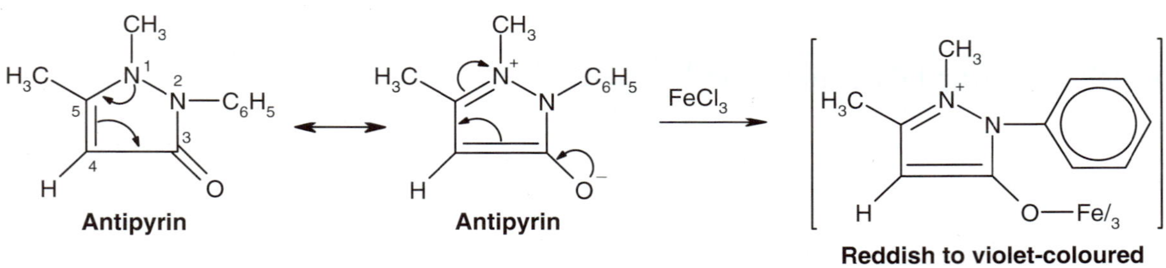

Reddish to violet-coloured iron complex
(λ_{max} 540 nm)

Note

Colour disappears on addition of H_2SO_4 indicating pH dependent stability of the colour. This is similar to iron (III) complexes of enols.

Reference

Pharmaceutical Chemistry (Vol. 2) by H.J. Roth, p. 499.

Owing to reactive enamine group present in the compound, it condenses with 'PDAB' or any other suitable aldehyde to give coloured complex.

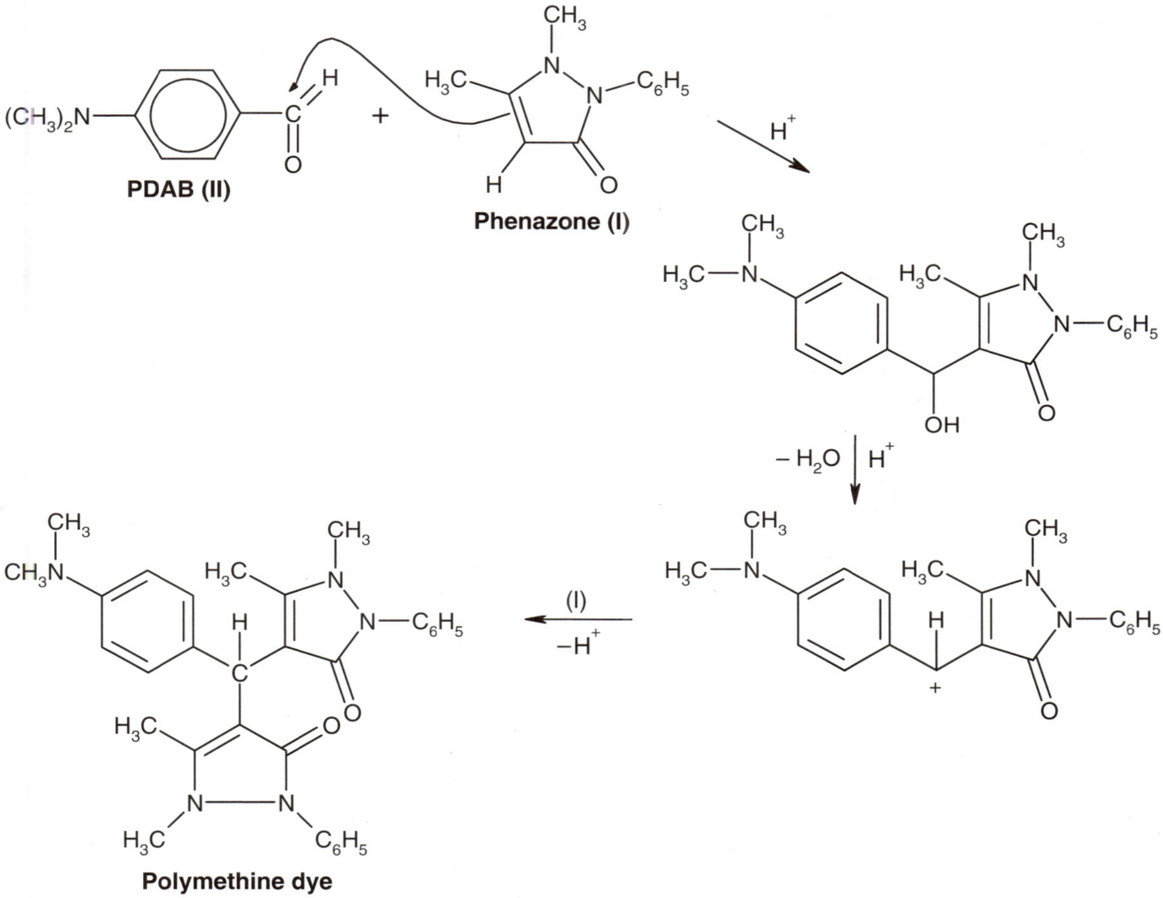

Phenazone and related compounds which are substituted at N-1, N-2 and C-5 react with electrophilic reagents such as NO_2^+, NO^+, Cl^+, Br^+, I^+ to give 4 substituted derivatives stabilized by elimination of a proton to form stable compound such as nitrophenazone.

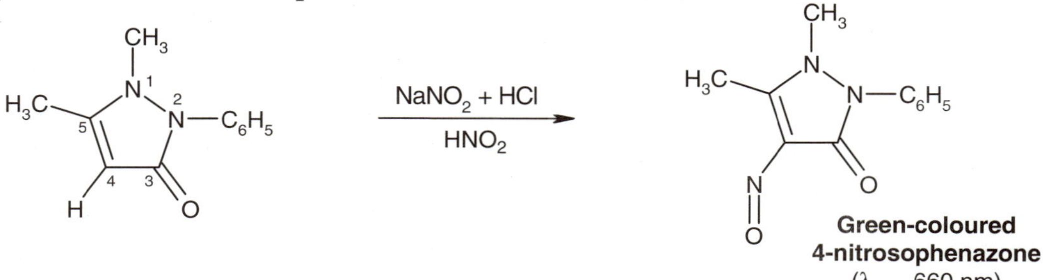

Hydrolysis with hydrochloric acid produces hydrazine derivative which can be diazotized and coupled with 1-naphthylamine to produce azo dye (λ_{max} 520 nm).

Probable Reaction Mechanism

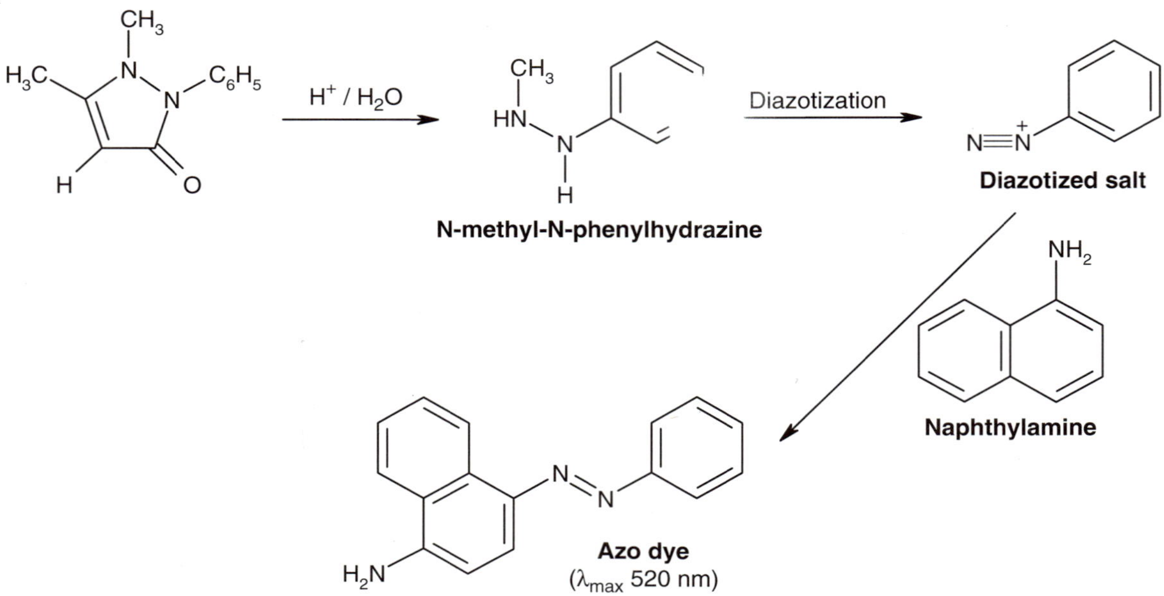

Reference

Pharmaceutical Chemistry (Vol. 2) by H.J. Roth, p. 501.

Formulation 3

Pilocarpine nitrate, Benzalkonium chloride, Potassium chloride, Boric acid, Polyvinyl alcohol

ESTIMATION

Pilocarpine nitrate

METHOD 1

Reagents

1. McLivaine's buffer solution, pH 6.0: 36.85 ml of 0.1 M citric acid and 63.15 ml of disodium hydrogen phosphate are mixed and adjusted to pH 6.0.
2. Bromocresol purple solution: It is prepared by dissolving 30 mg of bromocresol purple in 500 ml of chloroform.

Standard solution

1 mg/ml of pilocarpine nitrate in buffer, pH 6.0.

Sample solution

The sample is appropriately diluted with pH 6.0 buffer to get 1 mg/ml concentration of pilocarpine nitrate.

Procedure

To 1 ml each of sample and standard solutions, add 10 ml of dye solution and 10 ml of buffer, pH 6.0. Shake for 2 minutes and allow the layers to separate. Transfer the chloroform layer to a separator containing 10 ml of 0.1 N sodium hydroxide and shake for 15 seconds to liberate the dye. Dilute the alkaline layer to 10 ml with water or 0.1 N sodium hydroxide and measure the absorption of standard and sample solutions at about 580 nm against reagent blank. The method is based on ion pair transfer.

Note

This method is quite suitable for estimation of pilocarpine in presence of its degradation product, pilocarpinic acid.

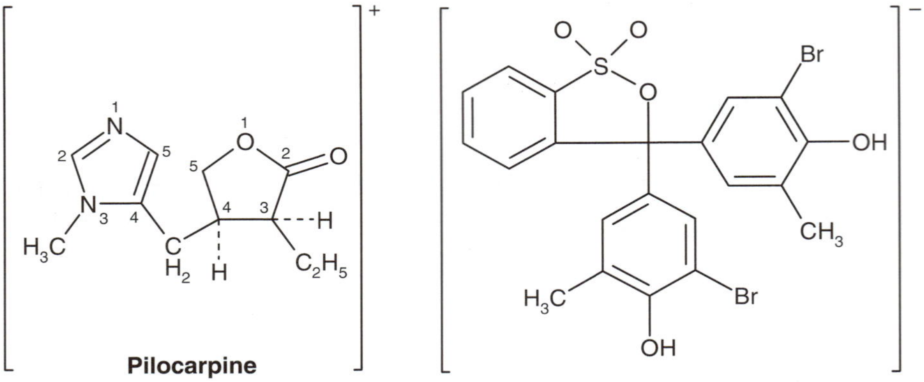

Drug-bromocresol purple ion pair complex in pH 6.0 buffer
(λ_{max} 580 nm)

Note

When the ion pair complex is extracted with chloroform, it has λ_{max} 405 nm, however for increased sensitivity the chloroform layer is extracted with NaOH to get violet colour as coupled dye gets librated and goes into alkaline phase.

The compound can undergo Pauly reaction i.e. diazotized sulphanilic acid couples at position 2 of the heteroaromatic ring, while other electrophilic reagents such as nitric acid or sulphuric acid will attack at position 5, position 4 being occupied.

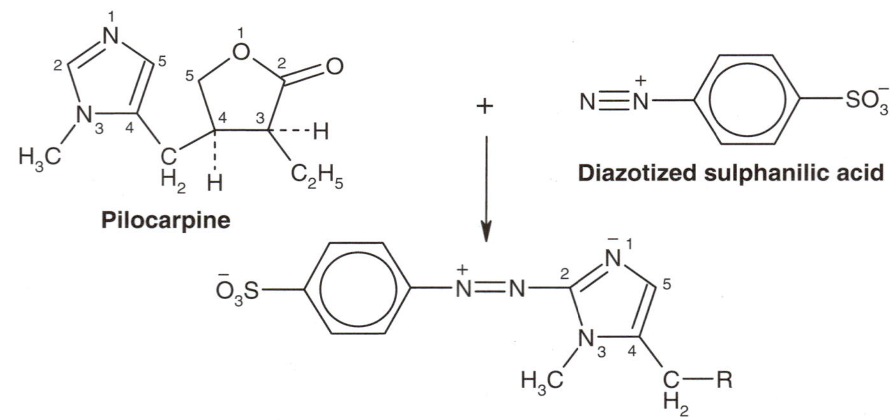

This reaction is analogous to that of histamine.

METHOD 2

Reagents

1. 1 M hydroxylamine HCl.
2. 5 M hydrochloric acid.

3. Alkaline phosphate buffer prepared by mixing 7% trisodium phosphate and 3.5 M sodium hydroxide (10 : 2).
4. 0.3 M ferric chloride solution in 0.1 M hydrochloric acid.

Procedure

To appropriate quantity of sample/standard solutions add 1 ml of hydroxylamine hydrochloride and 3 ml of alkaline buffer, mix, keep for 10 min and then add 1 ml of 5 M hydrochloric acid followed by 1 ml of ferric chloride. After 10 min dilute to 25 ml with water and measure the absorbance at 480 nm against reagent blank.

Probable Reaction Mechanism

In alkaline medium, by the attack of OH^- on the carbonyl (C==O) group resulting in the formation of pilocarpinic acid anion which reacts with hydroxylamine to give hydroxamic acid. Hydroxamic acid so formed couples with Fe(III) ion to form coloured complex (λ_{max} 480 nm).

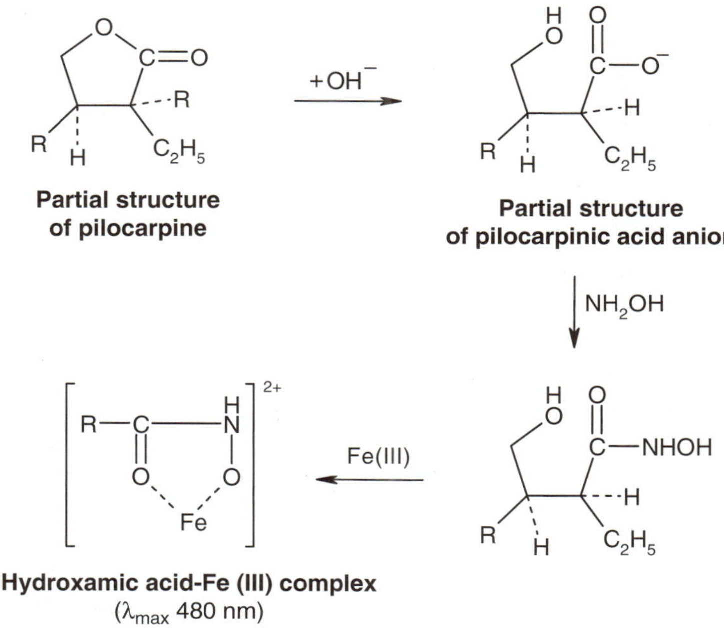

Partial structure of pilocarpine

Partial structure of pilocarpinic acid anion

Hydroxamic acid-Fe (III) complex
(λ_{max} 480 nm)

Reference

I.S. Gibbs & Murray M. Tuckerman. *J. Pharm. Sci.*, **59(3)**, 395-396, 1970.

Note

The structure of hydroxamic acid-iron (III) is as described in Textbook of Pharmaceutical Analysis by Kenneth A. Connors, p. 530.

Benzalkonium chloride

METHOD 1

Reagents

1. Dye solution: 0.06 w/v solution of bromothymol blue in ethyl alcohol.
2. Buffer solution, 0.05 M and 0.25 M, pH 7.5: 0.05 M and 0.25 M solutions of dibasic and monobasic potassium phosphate are mixed to get buffer solutions of pH 7.5 with different molarity.

Standard solution

100 mcg/ml of benzalkonium chloride in water.

Sample solution

Dilute sample approximately with water to get concentration of 100 mcg/ml of the compound.

Procedure

To 3 ml each of the sample and standard solutions, add 25 mg of sodium chloride and 10 ml of 0.05 M buffer solution and 5 ml of dye solution. Shake and then extract the complex with chloroform (3 × 15 ml), make up the volume to 50 ml and measure the absorption of sample and standard at 610 nm against reagent blank.

Note

1. When pilocarpine hydrochloride or epinephrine bitartrate are present in the formulation, 0.25 M buffer should be used as these salts are more acidic and buffer of higher buffering capacity is required to maintain pH at 7.5 as pH of the medium is very critical for complex formation.
2. The above method is suitable for estimation of chlorhexidine gluconate.

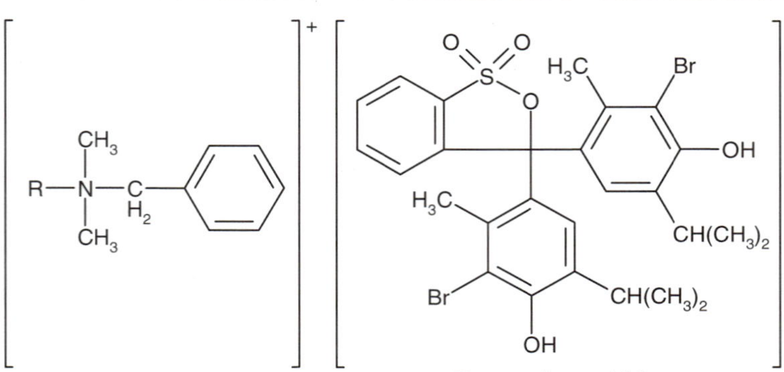

Bromothymol blue

R = Homologues of C_{12}, C_{14} and C_{16} straight chain alkyls.

Drug-dye ion pair complex
(λ_{max} 610 nm)

METHOD 2

Follow the method as described under formulation 15 of this chapter.

It forms coloured ion pair complex with bromophenol blue or bromothymol blue in alkaline medium.

Reaction mechanism as proposed by Lowry

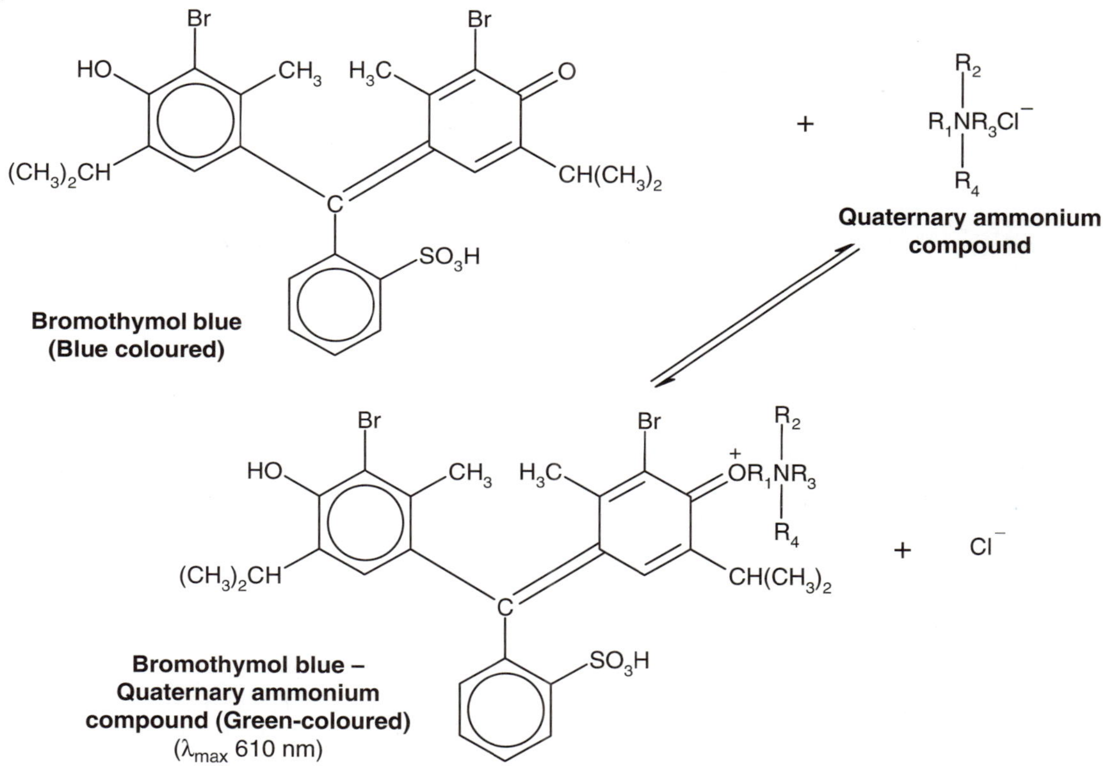

Reference

J.B. Lowry. *J. Pharm. Sci.*, **68(1)**, 110-111, 1979.

The method based on formation of ion-pair complex between BZC and the dye orange-II (RSO_3Na) is also reported by Afshar et al. The complexation between the drug and the dyes (methyl red and methyl orange) was carried out in pH 9.0 buffer and the coloured complex ($BZ + RSO_3^-$) was extracted into chloroform and organic layer has λ_{max} 487 nm.

Reference

Z.GH. Afshar & H. Parham. *Asian J. Chem.*, **23(10)**, 4464-4466, 2011.

Although the undermentioned method has no practical utility for estimation in formulations and only suitable raw material, it is being included as it involves interesting analytical aspect which may be useful for general knowledge of the analytical community and students.

Reagents

1. 0.1 M NaOH (sodium hydroxide).
2. 5% w/w of potassium iodide.
3. 0.05 M potassium iodate.
4. Concentrated hydrochloric acid.
5. Chloroform.

Procedure

Dissolve 4 g in sufficient water to produce 100 ml, transfer 25 ml to a separating funnel and add 25 ml $CHCl_3$ and 10 ml N/10 NaOH, 10 ml 5% w/w KI solution. Shake well and allow to separate and discard the chloroform layer. Now extract with three further quantities of $CHCl_3$ and discard the chloroform layer.

Now in aqueous solution add 4 ml of concentrated hydrochloric acid and 10 ml of $CHCl_3$, cool and titrate with 0.05 M KIO_3 until the chloroform layer becomes colourless.

Perform a blank 20 ml water + 10 ml 5% of KI + 40 ml conc. HCl and titrate with it manner is test. Each ml of 0.05 M KIO_3 is equivalent to 0.354 g of the compound.

Explanatory Note

Addition of KI gives rise to ion-pair trimethylammonium iodate complex which is removed from aqueous layer quantitatively by repeated chloroform extraction. Further any non-quaternary amine present along with the quaternary ammonium salt is converted into free amine by addition of sodium hydroxide and is also extracted with chloroform.

While titrating with KIO_3, KI is first converted into free iodine and then in the presence of HCl to iodomonochloride. Since I_2 is soluble in chloroform, it imparts its yellow colour whereas iodomonochloride which is dissociated in strong acid solution is not soluble in chloroform. Hence chloroform layer becomes colourless when entire I_2 is converted to ICl.

$$2I^- + IO_3^- + 6H^+ + 3Cl^- \rightarrow 3ICl + 3H_2O$$

The above method is applicable for other quaternary ammonium compounds as well like cetylpyridinium chloride.

Polyvinyl alcohol

Reagents

1. 3.5 M sodium hydroxide solution.
2. 2.5 M hydrochloric acid.
3. 0.5 N ferric chloride solution in 0.1 N hydrochloric acid.
4. 1% w/v hydroxylammonium chloride solution, to be prepared fresh every day.

Standard solution

Dissolve 200 mg of the compound in 50 ml of water by warming at 70-80°, cool and dilute with water to 100 ml (2 mg/ml).

Sample solution

Dilute appropriate volume of the eye drops with water to get 2 mg/ml solution.

Procedure

To 5 ml each of the sample and standard solutions, add 1 ml of hydroxylammonium chloride solution and 1 ml of the sodium hydroxide solution. Allow to stand for 10 minutes, acidify with 2 ml of 2.5 N hydrochloric acid and add 1 ml of ferric chloride solution. After a period of minimum of 10 minutes, measure the absorbance at about 500 nm against a reagent blank. The method obeys Beer's law in the range of 1-20 mcg/ml.

Note

Preservatives (chlorhexidine salts, benzalkonium chloride, mercury salts), surface active agents, electrolytes, buffering agents, acetic acid and its salts, viscosity-binders (polyvinyl pyrrolidine and cellulose derivatives) do not modify the absorption of the chromophore. Homatropine hydrobromide, chloramphenicol and sulphacetamide do not interfere. The potential interference by pilocarpine and other alkaloidal salts, local anaesthetics (benzocaine) often used in eye drops can be eliminated by extraction with chloroform prior to analysis by the above method.

Alternatively, polyvinyl alcohol is quantitatively precipitated by using 4% w/v aqueous solution of boric acid and the precipitates are taken up in water and analysed by above method.

Boric acid

Follow the method as described in formulation 1 of this chapter.

Formulation 4

Chlorpheniramine maleate, Naphazoline hydrochloride, Boric acid, Zinc sulphate, Chlorbutol

ESTIMATION

Chlorpheniramine maleate

Follow the method described in formulation of the chapter on rubefacients.

Naphazoline hydrochloride

Follow the method described in formulation 16 of this chapter.

Boric acid

Follow the method described in formulation 1 of this chapter.

Chlorbutol

Follow the method described in formulation 1 of this chapter.

Zinc sulphate

Take sample equivalent to 100 mg of zinc sulphate, add 2 ml of strong ammonia-ammonium chloride buffer solution and 2 drops of eviochrome black solution and dilute with 0.05 M EDTA to a deep blue end point. Each ml of 0.05 M EDTA is equivalent to 0.01438 g of zinc sulphate ($ZnSO_4 \cdot 2H_2O$). Perform blank.

Estimation of zinc sulphate is based on complexometric titration. Many ligands are capable of bonding to metal ions. In this case, EDTA (ethylene-diamine tetraacetic acid) is a bidentate ligand. This type of ligand complexes are also called chelates and ligand may be called chelating agent or chelons. In EDTA, effective complexing groups are amino and carboxylate components. EDTA possesses six groups—two amino and four carboxylate—capable of complexing with metal. It forms chelate with about all metal ions and serves as general analytical method.

Probable Reaction Mechanism

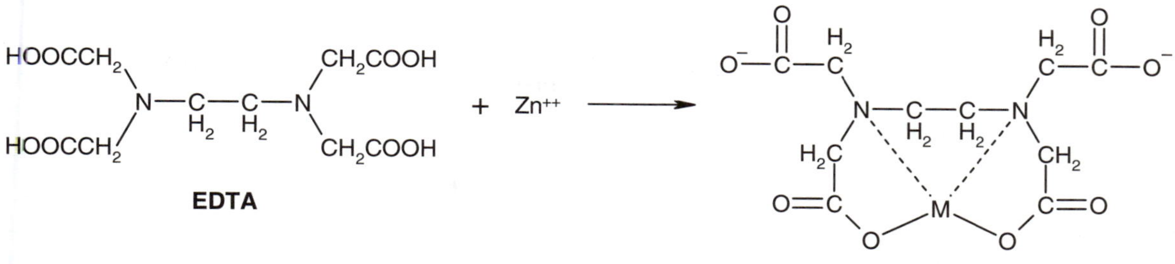

Metal - EDTA chelate

Reference

Pharmaceutical Analysis by T. Higuchi et al., John Wiley & Sons, p. 732.

A spectrophotometric method based on reaction of Zn (II) with di-2-pyridyl ketone benzoylhydrazone (DPKBH) at pH 5.5 was recently described by L.E.M. Vieira et al. (2008). The method does not require any extraction and can be directly applied to pharmaceutical formulations such as antiseptic powders, creams and eye drops. The sample containing 20 µg of zinc (II) is mixed with pH 5.5 acetate buffer and 'DPKBH' reagent and absorption of the yellow-coloured ligand measured at 378 nm. The optimum ligand-metal ratio was 20 : 1. The method was linear in the range of 0.02-2.0 µg/ml of Zn (II).

Probable Reaction Mechanism

Both the hetero-nitrogens with reagent have electron pair, hence donor, but both cannot be involved in ligand formation as they are quite apart. The complex is coloured due to presence of auxochromic group i.e. —N=O. Ring with amino-H is formed after enolization of carbonyl group.

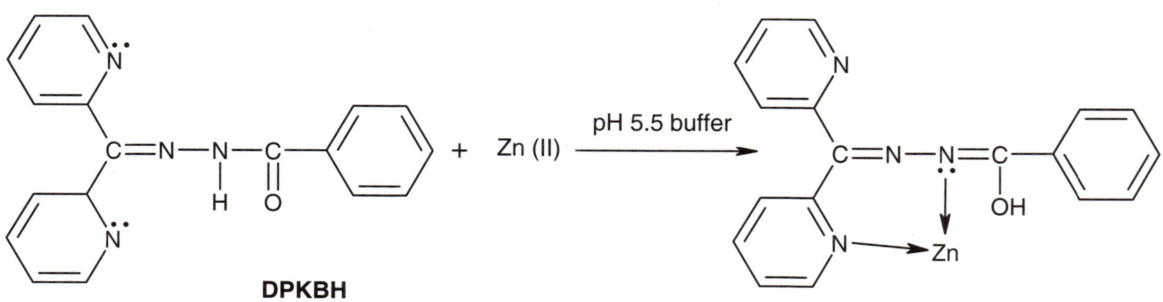

Six-membered DPKBH - Zn (II) chelate
(λ_{max} 378 nm)

Reference

L.E.M. Vieira et al. *Analytical Letters*, **41**, 779-788, 2008.

Typical laboratory analysis

Chlorpheniramine maleate

(Follow the cyanogen bromide method, see formulation of the chapter on expectorants)

Weight of the standard = 0.106 g

Volume of the sample = 4 ml of 0.01%

$$\text{Contents of naphazoline hydrochloride} = \frac{A_u}{A_s} \times \frac{0.103}{100} \times \frac{2}{100} \times \frac{100}{3.6} \times 100$$

$$= \frac{0.194}{0.199} \times \frac{0.106}{10}$$

$$= 0.01035$$

$$\%\ \text{claim} = \frac{0.01035}{0.01} \times 100 = 103.5$$

Naphazoline hydrochloride

Weight of the standard = 0.103 g

Volume of the sample = 3.6 ml of 0.056%

$$\text{Contents of naphazoline hydrochloride} = \frac{A_u}{A_s} \times \frac{0.103}{100} \times \frac{2}{100} \times \frac{100}{3.6} \times 100$$

$$= 0.0538$$

$$\%\ \text{claim} = \frac{0.0538}{0.056} \times 100 = 95.99$$

Formulation 5

Choline salicylate, Benzalkonium chloride

ESTIMATION

Benzalkonium chloride

Follow the ion-pair complex method described in formulation 3 of this chapter.

Choline salicylate

Follow the method described under formulation of this chapter and chapter on miscellaneous formulations for choline dihydrogen citrate. Each g of the residue (as reineckate) is equivalent to 0.241 g of choline salicylate ($C_{12}H_{19}NO_4$).

On acidification of aqueous solution, free salicylic acid is produced. This can be quantitatively estimated. For details refer to estimation of salicylic acid under formulation 1 of this chapter.

Probable Reaction Mechanism

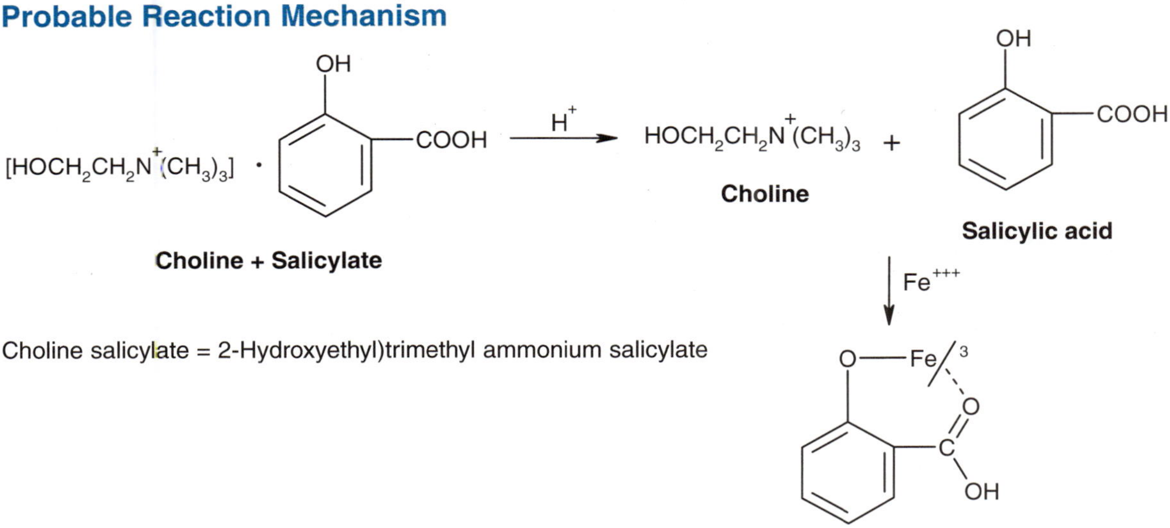

Choline salicylate = 2-Hydroxyethyl)trimethyl ammonium salicylate

Violet-coloured iron complex
(λ_{max} 525 nm)

Formulation 6

Phenazone, Benzocaine, Potassium hydroxyquinoline sulphate, Chlorbutol

ESTIMATION

Phenazone

Procedure

Transfer the sample solution equivalent to 200 mg of phenazone to a 250 ml separating funnel, add 100 ml water and extract the solution with three 30 ml portions of chloroform. Transfer the chloroform extracts to a 250 ml conical flask and evaporate the chloroform. Add to the residue, 20 ml sodium acetate solution, 40 ml 0.1 N iodine and leave the solution for 20 minutes in a cool dark place. Then, add 10 ml chloroform and shake vigorously. Titrate the excess of iodine with 0.1 N sodium thiosulphate using starch solution as indicator. Repeat the procedure omitting the sample (blank titration). Each ml of 0.1 N iodine is equivalent to 0.09412 g of phenazone.

In weakly buffered solution, phenazone reacts with iodine to form 4-iodo-phenazone. Titrating solution is taken up in chloroform to dissolve iodo-phenazone. The excess iodine is determined by back titration with sodium thiosulphate. Without buffer (sodium acetate) the reaction is not quantitative.

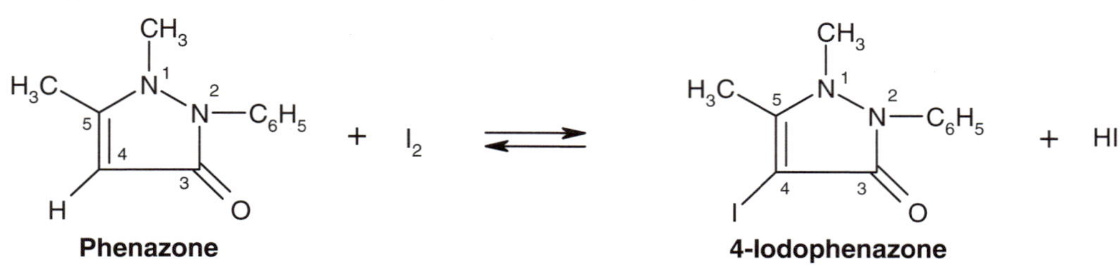

Note

Bromination of the compound (Br_2 | KBr or $KBrO_3$ | KBr) also takes place at C-4, making it a quantitative method of analysis.

Alternatively, iodophenazone so formed can be extracted with chloroform and then heated with hydrochloric acid which librates iodine. The librated iodine can then be estimated by titration with thiosulphate.

Potassium hydroxyquinoline sulphate

The substance is suspended in methanol and titrated with 0.1 M sodium hydroxide. Each ml of 0.1 M sodium hydroxide is equivalent to 0.03884 mg of $(C_9H_7NO)_2 \cdot H_2SO_4$. The compound forms chelate with monovalent, divalent and trivalent metal ions.

Similarly, it can form chelate with Fe(III). See under other quinoline derivatives described in the text.

Probable Reaction Mechanism

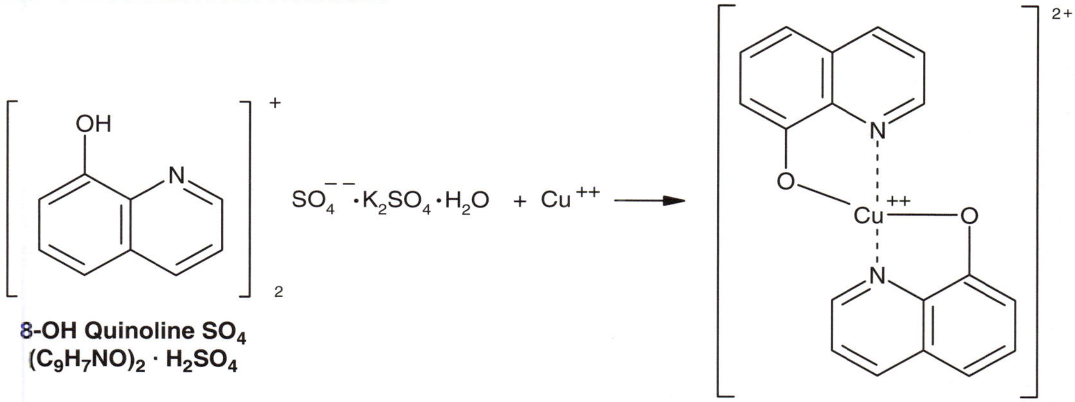

8-OH Quinoline SO_4
$(C_9H_7NO)_2 \cdot H_2SO_4$

Coloured chelate of divalent metal

Reference

Pharmaceutical Chemistry (Vol. 2) by H.J. Roth, p. 609.

Benzocaine

Transfer sample solution equivalent to 100 mg of benzocaine to a 100 ml separating funnel, add 20 ml water and extract with three 25 ml portions of ether. Wash the combined ether extracts thrice with 30 ml water each. Evaporate the combined ether extracts to dryness. Add 30 ml water and 10 ml hydrochloric acid to the residue. Titrate the solution with 0.1 M sodium nitrite at temperature not exceeding 15°C till a blue colour is produced using starch iodide paper as indicator. The titration is complete when the end point is reproducible after leaving the titrated solution for one minute. Repeat the procedure omitting the sample for blank titration.

Each ml of 0.1 M sodium nitrite is equivalent to 0.01652 g of benzocaine.

Chlorbutol

Follow the method described in formulation 1 of this chapter. Each ml of 0.1 N silver nitrate is equivalent to 0.005917 g of chlorbutol.

Formulation 7

Sulphacetamide sodium, Phenylephrine hydrochloride, Boric acid

ESTIMATION

Sodium sulphacetamide

METHOD 1

Reagents

1. 3% w/v solution of sodium nitrite in water.
2. 2% w/v solution of urea in water.
3. 3% ethanolic solution of ethyl aceto-acetate.
4. 20% w/v solution of sodium hydroxide in water.

Standard solution

15 mcg/ml of sodium sulphacetamide in water.

Sample solution

Dilute appropriate volume of the sample with water to get 15 mcg/ml of sodium sulphacetamide.

Procedure

To 1 ml each of the sample and standard solutions, add 1 ml of 1 N hydrochloric acid and 1 ml of sodium nitrite solution. Cool in ice-bath and allow to stand for 2 minutes. Add 2 ml of urea solution, shake and allow to stand for 2 minutes. Then, add 1 ml of ethyl aceto-acetate solution, 2 ml of sodium hydroxide solution and dilute to 25 ml with water. Measure the absorbance of both the solutions at about 420 nm against reagent blank. Calculate the results by comparison.

Probable Reaction Mechanism

Diazotized sulphonamide couples with compound having active methylene (CH_2) group such as ethylacetoacetate or acetylacetone in strong alkaline solution to give azo dye.

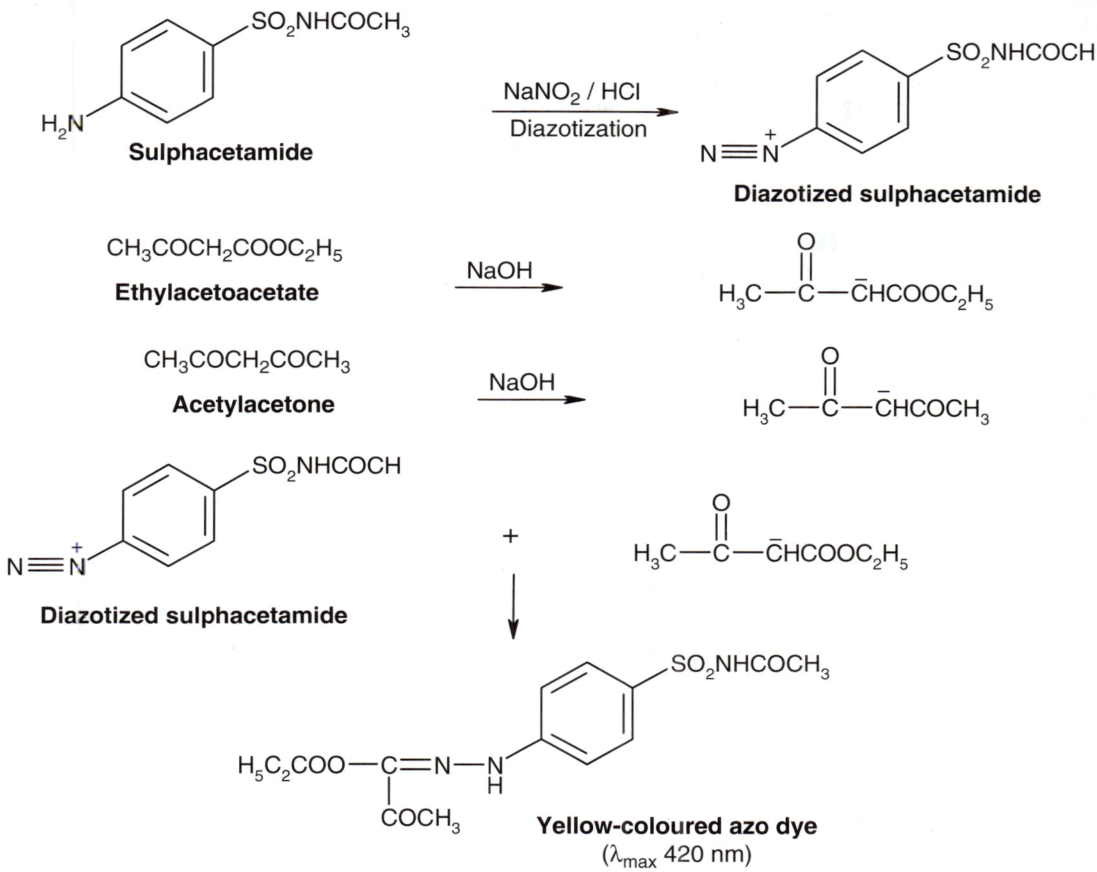

Note

Similar reaction is possible with ethyl malonate $\left(C_2H_5-O-\overset{O}{\overset{\|}{C}}-\underset{H_2}{C}-\overset{O}{\overset{\|}{C}}-O-C_2H_5\right)$

Reference

1. Finar I.L. Organic Chemistry, 6th ed. (Vol. 1), 2003.
2. Organic Chemistry by Morrison & Boyd, 6th ed., 2002.
3. Ajay Gaur, R.K. Gupta & B. Shrivastava. *Ind. J. Pharm. Sci.*, **69(3)**, 464-467, 2007.

METHOD 2

Take sample equivalent to 250 mg of the compound and carry out general sodium nitrite titration for sulphonamides. Each ml of sodium nitrite is equivalent to 0.02362 g of sulphacetamide sodium. Excess HNO_2 ($NaNO_2$ + HCl) will librate iodine from starch-iodide paper and iodine forming blue inclusion complex with starch, the end point.

Phenylephrine hydrochloride

Follow the method involving alkaline oxidation with potassium ferricyanide, followed by coupling with 4-aminophenazone. For details, refer to method described in chapter on analgesics and antipyretics.

Boric acid

Follow the method described in formulation 1 of this chapter. Each ml of 0.1 N sodium hydroxide is equivalent to 0.006183 g of boric acid.

Formulation 8

Dexamethasone sodium phosphate, Bacitracin, Benzalkonium chloride

ESTIMATION

Dexamethasone sodium phosphate

Reagents

1. Phenylhydrazine reagent: Dissolve 65 mg of phenylhydrazine hydrochloride in 40 ml of water. Add 60 ml of phosphoric acid and 50 ml of isopropyl alcohol, prepare fresh.
2. 1 N sodium hydroxide.
3. 10% w/v sodium chloride solution in water.
4. Methylene chloride.

Standard solution

Weigh accurately 100 mg of dexamethasone sodium phosphate, add 1 ml of 1 N sodium hydroxide and dilute to 100 ml with water. 10 ml of the resulting solution is further diluted with water to 100 ml (100 mcg/ml).

Sample solution

Weigh or measure accurately, a portion of ointment, cream or solution equivalent to 1 mg of the compound. Add 10 ml of sodium chloride solution and 25 ml of methylene chloride. Agitate to disperse the cream. Allow the organic layer to separate and discard it. Extract with further 25 ml of methylene chloride and discard organic layer. Dilute aqueous layer to 10 ml with water (100 mcg/ml).

Procedure

To 2 ml each of the sample and standard solutions, add 5 ml of freshly prepared phenylhydrazine reagent. Insert the stopper loosely and maintain at 60°C for 2 h. Cool and measure the absorbance of both the solutions at about 410 nm and calculate the results by comparison.

Probable Reaction Mechanism

This is based on reaction of phenylhydrazine with keto group present in the molecule at C-3. This is called Porter-Silber reaction.

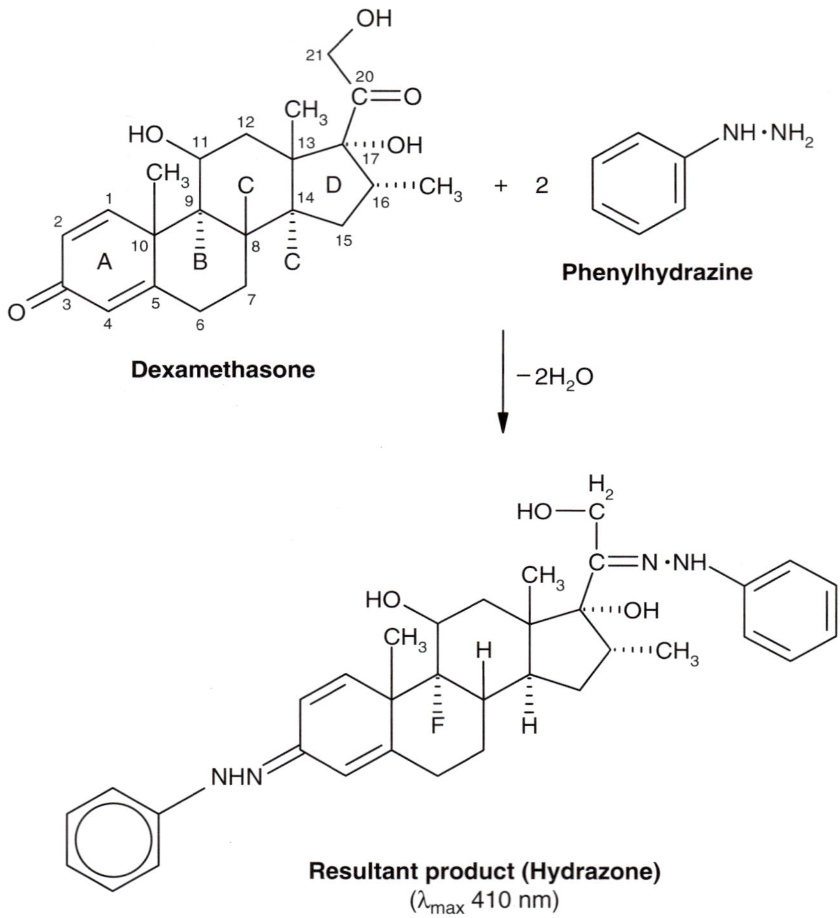

An alternative reaction mechanism is proposed.

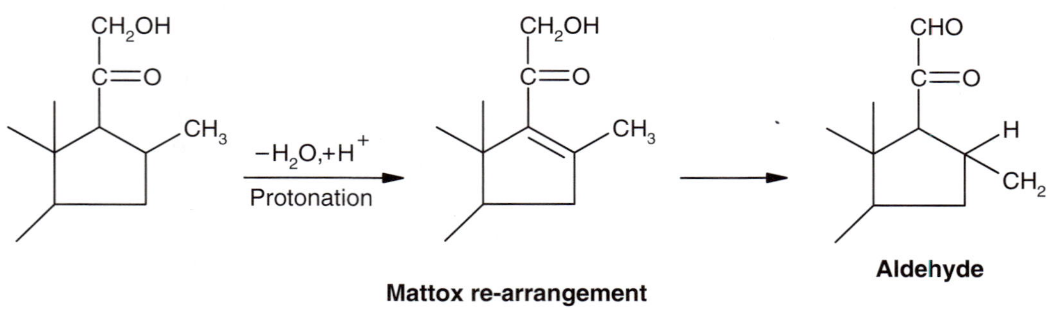

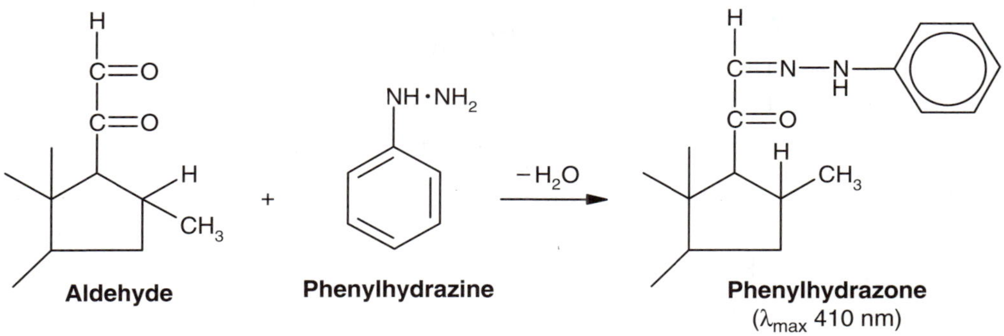

Reference

Pharmaceutical Chemistry (Vol. 2) by H.J. Roth, p. 609.

Benzalkonium chloride

Follow the method described in formulation 3 or 15 of this chapter.

Bacitracin

Reagents

1. Sodium hypobromite solution: Dissolve 2 g of bromide in 100 ml volumetric flask which has been previously half-filled with 1 N sodium hydroxide solution. Dilute to volume with the same solvent.
2. Phloroglucinol reagent: Dissolve 0.5 g of phloroglucinol in 15 ml of distilled water by warming in hot water and shaking. Dilute to 50 ml with concentrated hydrochloric acid (37%).

Standard solution

200 mcg/ml of bacitracin in water.

Sample solution

Weigh accurately, a quantity of the sample of the ointment, equivalent to approximately 10 mg (650 units) of bacitracin into a 50 ml centrifuge tube with ground glass joint. Add 2 ml of petroleum ether (40-60°), warm slightly in a water-bath at 40°C, and shake briefly until the contents of the tube become a homogenous viscous mass. Add 4 ml of distilled water and shake mechanically for one hour. To assist solution of the active compounds, interrupt the shaking two or three times for 1 minute intervals and place the tube briefly in the water-bath each time. Finally, centrifuge for 5 minutes at 4000 rpm. Remove the aqueous (lower phase) layer with the help of a pipette, and filter it through a filter paper previously washed with distilled water and dried. Dilute the filtrate appropriately with water to get 200 mcg/ml.

Procedure

Transfer 4 ml of above aqueous solutions of both sample and standard into 20 ml test tubes and add 1 ml of sodium hypobromite solution. Place the tubes in a boiling water-bath for 5 minutes and then add 3 ml of phloroglucinol reagent. Stir and again place the tubes in the bath for a further 10 minutes, a stable pink colour is developed. Cool the tube in cold water (20°C) for about 10 minutes. Add 2 ml of 25% aqueous ethanol into each tube (occasionally an opalescence develops which disappears when ethanol is added and shaken well). Determine the absorbance of both the solutions at about 505 nm against a reagent blank. Calculate the amount (mg) of bacitracin. To convert the weight into units, multiply by the factor (i), microbiological potency of standard bacitracin in units per mg.

Probable Reaction Mechanism

This method takes advantage of the liability of the aminocarboxylic groups towards oxidation. These groups are oxidized to the aldehyde by alkali sodium hypobromite fairly readily and further condensed with phloroglucinol in an acidic medium to give coloured product (λ_{max} 505 nm).

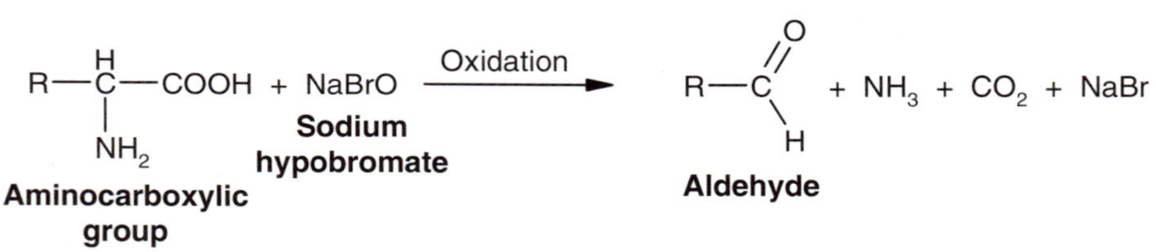

α-aminocarboxylic acids are both deaminated and decarboxylated on treatment with alkali hypobromite. An aldehyde with one carbon atom less than the original amino acid results. The resulting aldehyde is then coupled with phloroglucinol in concentrated hydrochloric acid to yield pink-coloured monomethine chloride (λ_{max} 505 nm).

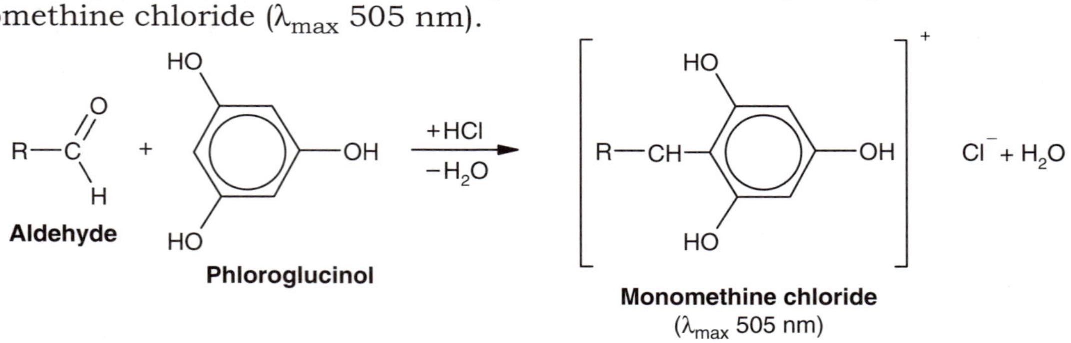

Reference

J. Doulakas. *J. Pharm. Sci.*, **64(2)**, 307-310, 1975.

Formulation 9

Pilocarpine nitrate, Phenylephrine hydrochloride

ESTIMATION

Pilocarpine nitrate

METHOD 1

Reagent

1% w/v solution of chromotropic acid in sulphuric acid.

Standard solution

2 mg/ml of pilocarpine nitrate in water.

Sample solution

Eye drops: Transfer sample equivalent to 20 mg of pilocarpine nitrate, basify with 1 N sodium hydroxide and extract with four 10 ml portions of chloroform. Wash combined chloroform layer with 1 ml of water and evaporate chloroform to dryness. Dissolve the residue in acidified water to produce 10 ml (2 mg/ml).

Eye ointment: Weigh accurately ointment equivalent to 20 mg of the substance, add 20 ml of chloroform-water (1 : 1) mixture, shake and separate chloroform layer. Extract water layer with further quantities of chloroform till fatty base is completely removed. Wash the combined chloroform layer with 5 ml of water and add this aqueous wash to the original aqueous liquid. Make the aqueous layer alkaline and extract with four 10 ml portions of chloroform. Evaporate the combined chloroform layer and take up the residue in 10 ml of acidified water.

Procedure

Transfer accurately measured volume of the sample and standard solutions equivalent to 4 mg of pilocarpine nitrate to 250 ml distillation flask. Add 20 ml of water, 25 g of sodium chloride and 5 g of purified sand, previously pulverized and mixed. Start distillation by rapidly heating to boiling. Collect 20 ml of the distillate and adjust to 25 ml with water. To 2 ml distillate of the sample and standard solutions, add with caution 3 ml of chromotropic acid reagent by letting the reagent run down the side of the tubes and mix thoroughly by gentle swirling. Allow to stand for 10 minutes at room temperature and then measure the absorbance of both the solutions at about 545 nm against reagent blank. The method obeys Beer's law in the concentration range of 20-100 mcg/ml.

Probable Reaction Mechanism

The carbonyl group present in the furan ring of pilocarpine will condense with the aromatic system of chromotropic acid in the o-position to the phenolic hydroxy group in the presence of H_2SO_4 and forms the product which is further acted upon by H_2SO_4 as an oxidizing agent.

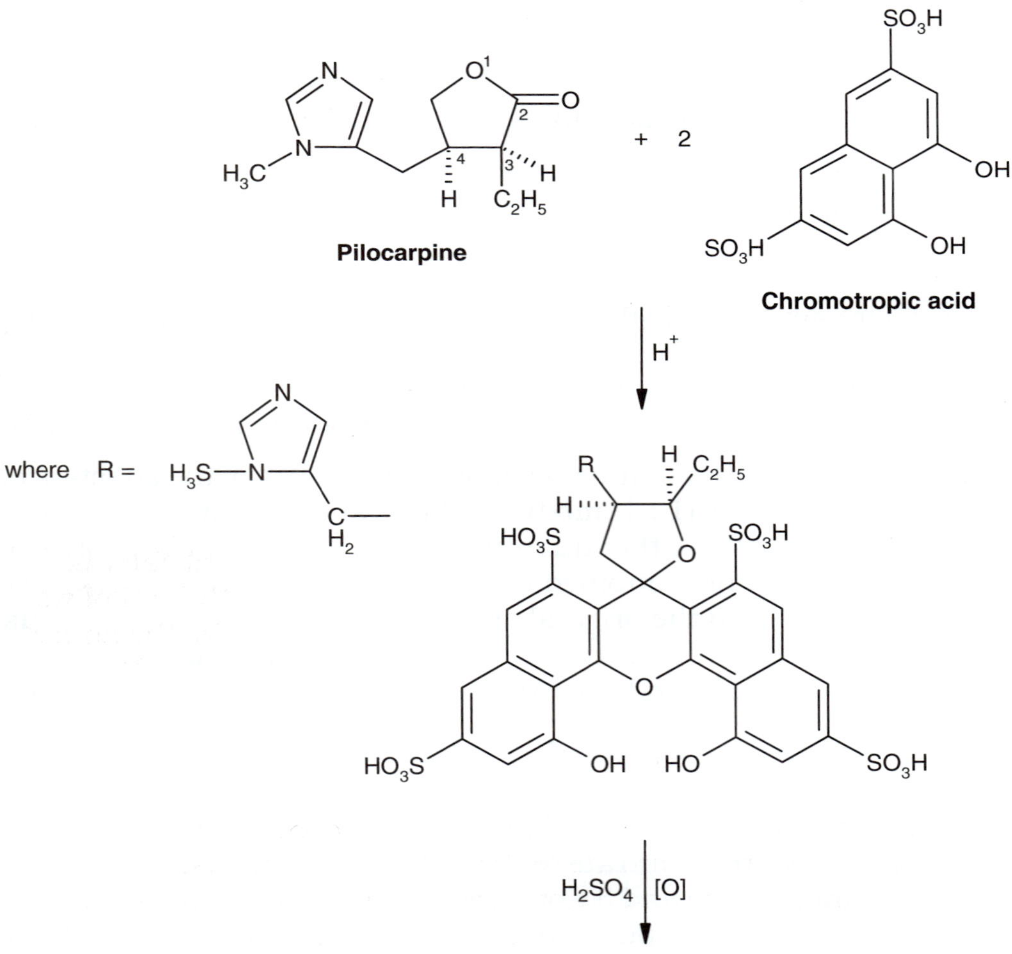

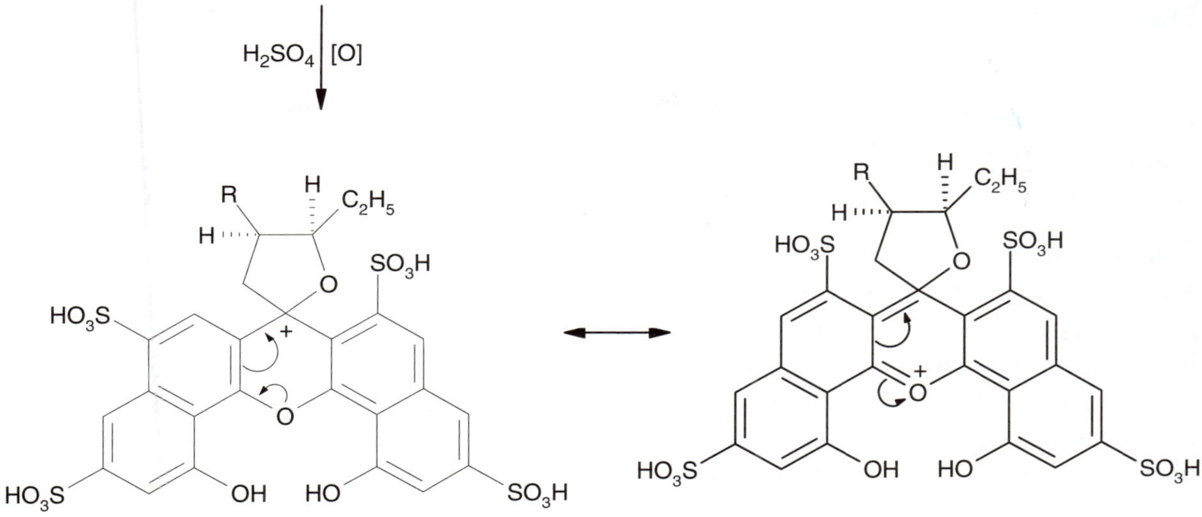

(λ_{max} 545 nm)

Note

It is reported that on oxidation with benzyl peroxide, formaldehyde (HCHO) is librated which reacts with chromotropic acid to give coloured complex (λ_{max} 545 nm). For reaction mechanism of HCHO with chromotropic acid, refer to method of analysis for analgin in chapter on analgesics.

Reference

Pharmaceutical Chemistry (Vol. 2) by H.J. Roth, p. 121.

The compound forms metallic complexes with $[Co(CNS)_4]$ (λ_{max} 420 nm), reineckate salt (λ_{max} 533 nm in acetone) and picric acid (λ_{max} 420 nm in alcohol). The complexes can be used as spectrophotometric or gravimetric analytical procedures.

Reference

Analytical Profile of Drug Substances (Vol. 12) by Klaus Florey, p. 419.

METHOD 2

Reagents

1. 0.1 N sulphuric acid.
2. 2% w/v sodium nitroprusside in water.
3. 1 N sodium hydroxide.
4. 0.01 N solution of potassium permanganate.
5. Dilute sulphuric acid.

Standard solution

800 mcg/ml of pilocarpine nitrate in water.

Sample solution

Take sample preparation equivalent to 20 mg of pilocarpine nitrate in 25 ml volumetric flask and dilute to volume with 0.1 N sulphuric acid (800 mcg/ml).

Procedure

To 5 ml each of sample and standard solutions, add 1 ml each of sodium nitroprusside solution and 0.1 N sodium hydroxide solution. Allow to stand for 5 minutes, then add 5 ml of 0.01 N potassium permanganate, followed immediately by 3 ml of dilute sulphuric acid. Dilute to volume (25 ml) and measure the absorbance of both the solutions at about 520 nm against reagent blank. The absorbance should be measured within 5 minutes.

Note

1. The reaction with sodium nitroprusside in alkaline medium is answered by other imidazoline derivative such as tolazoline.
2. The compound forms ion-pair complexes with bromocresol green (pH 3.4 buffer), bromophenol blue (pH 2.5 buffer), bromothymol blue (pH 6.0 buffer) and methyl orange (pH 6.0 buffer). All the complexes are extracted into chloroform (λ_{max} 420 nm).

Reference

R.T. Sane & Sandhya Sane. *Indian Drugs*, **16(10)**, 239-241, 1979.

METHOD 3

Pilocarpine forms 1 : 1 molecular complex with chloranilic acid based on charge-transfer (C-T) complex formation.

Reagent

1. 0.2% p-chloranilic acid solution in 1,4-dioxan.

Sample and standard solutions

Both sample and standard solutions were basified with ammonia and extracted with chloroform to get solution of free base.

Procedure

To appropriate volume of the sample/standard in chloroform, add 15 ml of 0.2% solution of the reagent, mix and dilute to 20 ml with dioxan and measure the absorbance of the purple colour at λ_{max} 515 nm against reagent blank.

Note

1. Chloranilic acid has golden-yellow colour (λ_{max} 428 nm) in dioxan-chloroform.
2. As the reaction is carried out in non-aqueous medium, HA form of chloranilic acid is involved in complexation.
3. The experimental data confirmed 1 : 1 complex C-T formation.
4. The linearity range was 0.01-0.08 mg/ml.
5. Phenylmercuric nitrate up to 0.002% did not interfere.
6. As an acceptor chloranilic acid is superior to chloranil as reaction with chloranil is slow and the colour is stable for 2 hrs whereas with chloranilic acid the reaction is immediate and the colour is stable for 24 hrs.

Probable Reaction Mechanism

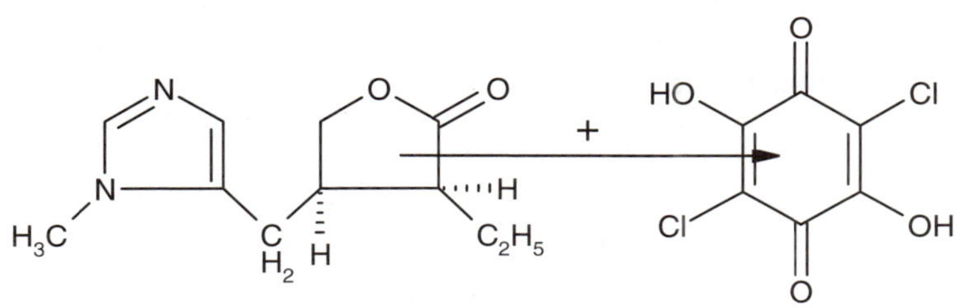

Pilocarpine (donor)

Chloranilic acid (acceptor)
(λ_{max} 515 nm)

Reference

M. Abdel-Hady-Elsayed & Suraj P. Agarwal. Talanta, **29**, 535-537, 1982.

METHOD 4

Reagents

1. 'MAA' reagent: 10% solution of malonic acid in acetic anhydride prepared by dissolving the acid with heating. This malonic acid/acetic anhydride mixed anhydride system is known as 'MAA'.

Procedure

To appropriate quantity of the sample/standard (base) solutions add 3 ml of 'MAA' reagent, heat in water-bath at 80°C for 15 min, cool and dilute to volume with alcohol and measure the absorbance at 334 nm.

Probable Reaction Mechanism

Acetic anhydride is used as dehydrating agent; it may dehydrate malonic acid to give malonic anhydride with an active methylene (CH_2) group.

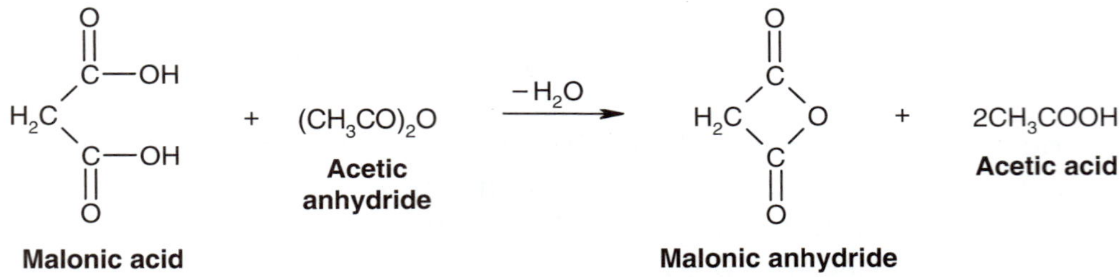

Malonic anhydride reacts with ternary amine yielding an alcohol-soluble complex.

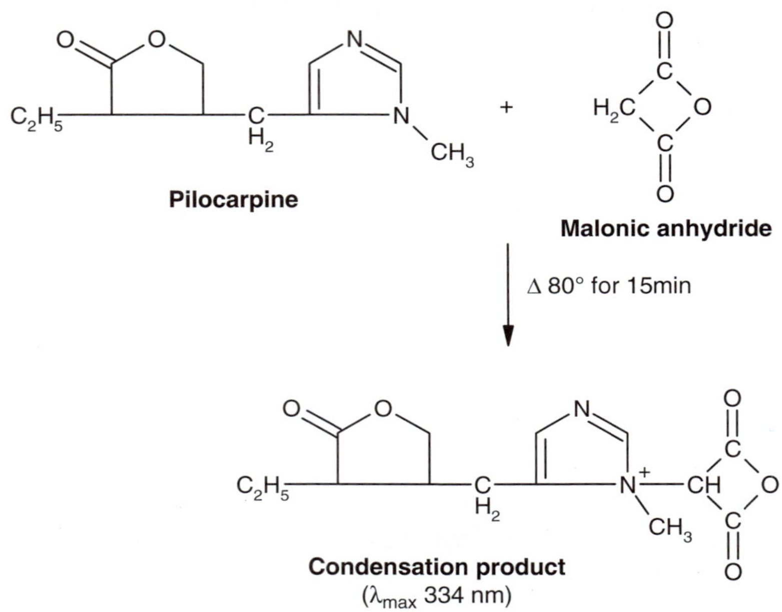

The complex has also fluorescence property (Exc: 395 nm; Em: 450 nm).

It is a base-catalysed condensation of mixed anhydride of an organic acid with ternary amine which functions as basic catalyst resulting in the formation of a coloured complex. This reaction is specific for ternary amines as they retain their basic properties in an acetylating medium such as acetic anhydride.

Reference

A.D. Thomas. *Talanta*, 22, 865-869, 1975.

A spectrophotometric method is based on oxidative hydrolysis of pilocarpine to pilocarpinic acid and then reacting with hydroxylamine to give hydroxamic acid which in turn couples with Fe^{3+} to form red-violet complex (λ_{max} 530 nm).

Probable Reaction Mechanism

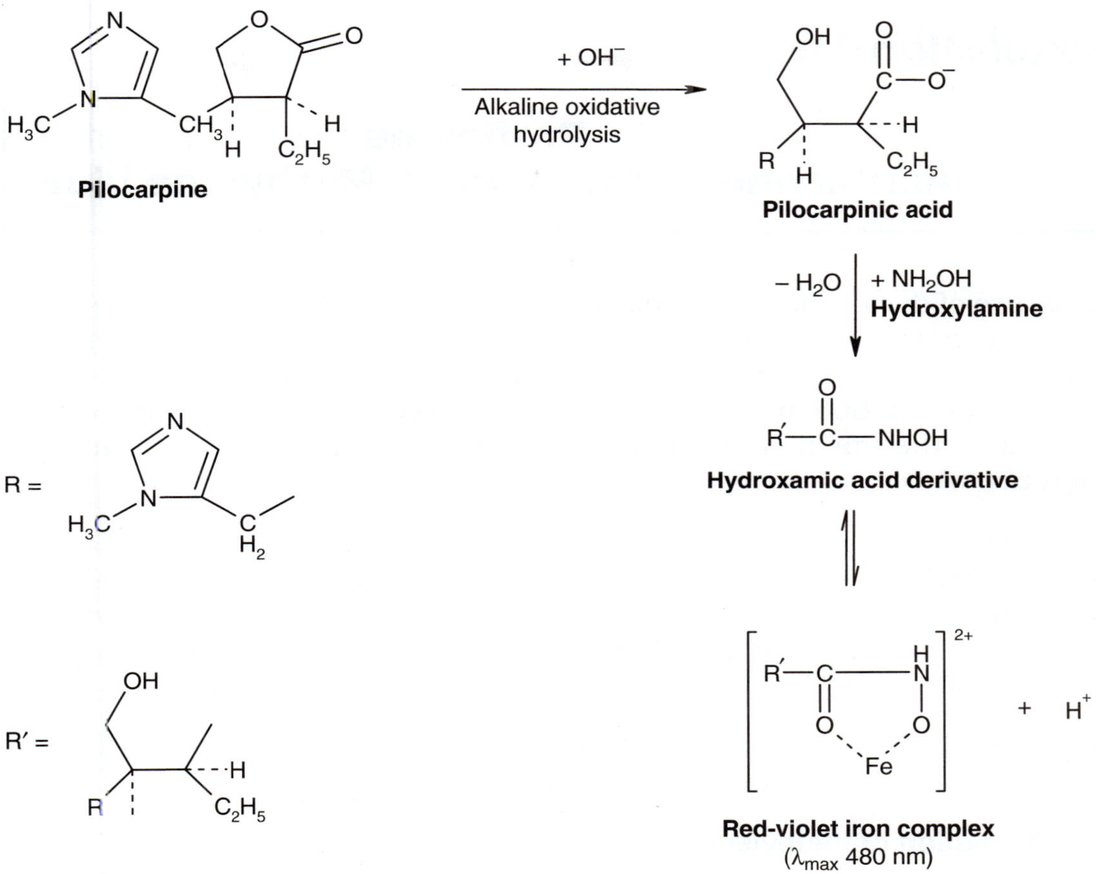

Reference

I.S. Gio, M. Murray Tuckerman. *J. Pharm. Sci.*, 59(3), 395-396, 1970.

Note

The reaction mechanism as described in Textbook of Pharmaceutical Analysis by Kenneth A. Connor, 3rd ed., pp. 530 and 537 has been included.

Phenylephrine hydrochloride

Follow the methods as described in the chapter on analgesics and antipyretics.

Formulation 10

Proflavine hemisulphate, Acriflavine hydrochloride, Methylene blue

In a mixture of dyes, whenever their absorption spectra is well separated, it is one of the convenient methods for analysis of individual dye. Proflavine and acriflavine exhibit maxima at about 450 nm, whereas methylene blue shows maxima at about 665 nm. It has been observed that absorbance of one compound at the maxima of other is almost nil, hence there is no mutual interference while estimating the above compounds in combination.

Total acridines

As both acriflavine and proflavine exhibit maxima at about the same wavelength i.e. 450 nm, it is only possible to estimate total acridines whenever they are in combination. Proflavine is usually the major component, hence is used for preparation of standard solution.

Standard solution of proflavine hemisulphate

5 mcg/ml of proflavine hemisulphate in water.

Standard solution of methylene blue

5 mcg/ml of methylene blue in water.

Sample solution

The sample is appropriately diluted with water to get a concentration of 5 mcg/ml of each substance.

Procedure

For total acridines, the absorbance of one part of the sample solution is measured at 450 nm and results calculated by measuring the absorbance of the respective standard solution at the same wavelength. For methylene blue, measure the absorbance of both sample and standard solutions at 665 nm.

Note

Buffering agents and plant extracts, usually present in such formulation, do not interfere.

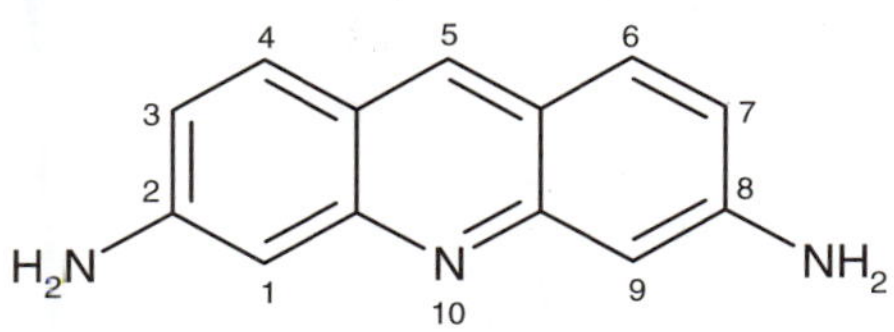

Acridine
2,8-diaminoacridine

OR

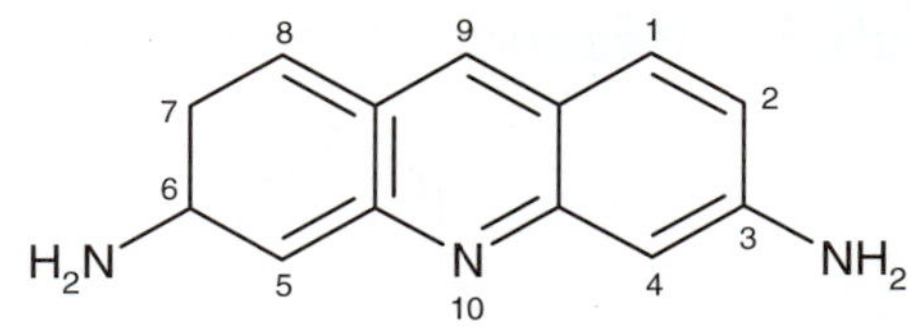

3,6-diaminoacridine

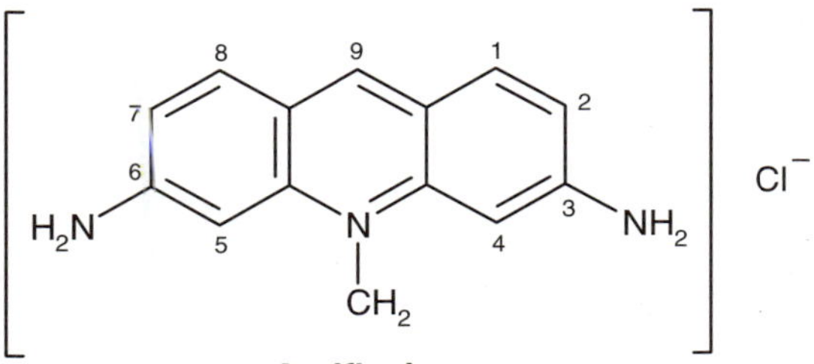

Acriflavin
3,6-diamino-10-methylacridinium chloride

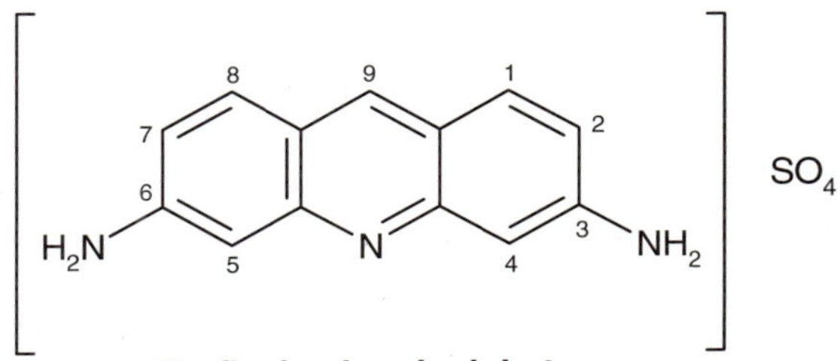

Proflavine hemisulphate
($C_{13}H_{11}N_3H_2SO_4$)

Acriflavine is a mixture of 3,6-diaminoacridine derivative (35%) and 3,6-diamino-10-methylacridine derivative (65%).

Both acridine derivatives are coloured having λ_{max} 450 nm and can be estimated spectrophotometrically. Being basic, both form hydrochlorides and sulphates. Both compounds answer general reactions of primary aromatic amines i.e. can be diazotized to form diazonium salt which can couple with phenols to form azo dyes.

Probable Reaction Mechanism

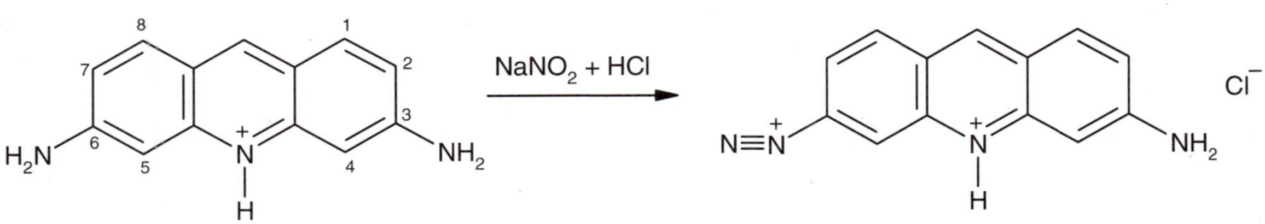

Violet diazonium salt

Both compounds condense with aromatic aldehydes to form Schiff's base i.e. both diazotization and Schiff's base can form the basis for quantitative analysis.

Note

For reaction with HNO_2 to give diazonium salt, amino group at position-6 is diazotized.

Probable Reaction Mechanism

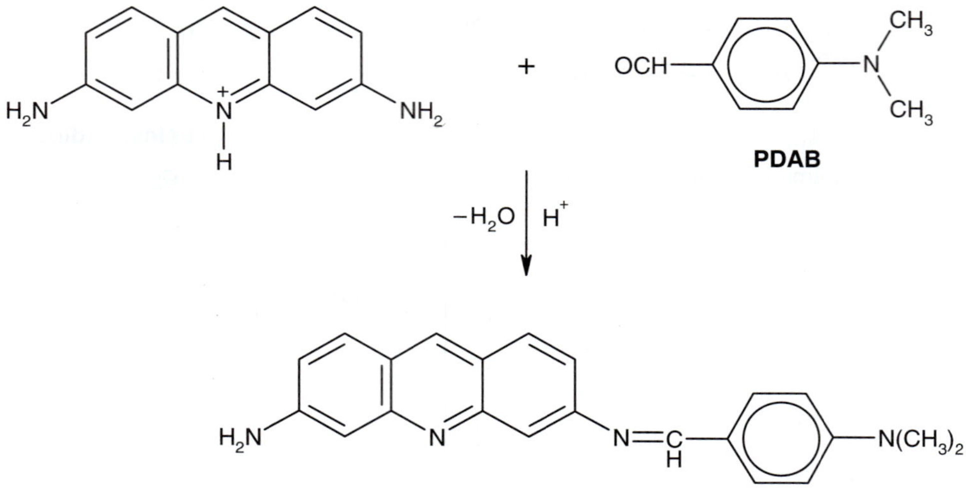

Coloured Schiff's base

Note

In aqueous ethanolic solution, acridines exhibit strong fluorescence which is due to acridinium ion. However, in acidic (HCl) or alkaline solution (NaOH), no fluorescence is observed.

Formulation 11

Naphazoline nitrate (Privine nitrate), Antazoline sulphate (Antistine sulphate)

ESTIMATION

Naphazoline nitrate

Reagents

1. 0.5% w/v solution of chloranil in chloroform (chloranil may be purified by crystallization from double distilled benzene before use).
2. 10% w/v solution of sodium carbonate in water.

Standard solutions

Solutions of both the pure compounds (as their salts) are separately basified with dilute ammonia solution and extracted with chloroform. Pooled chloroform layer is dried over anhydrous sodium sulphate and diluted to get required concentrations (10 mcg/ml for naphazoline nitrate and 100 mcg/ml for antazoline sulphate).

Sample solution

An accurately measured aliquot of the sample equivalent to 0.25 mg of naphazoline nitrate is taken and to this add about 10 ml of water, add slowly and with stirring 5 ml of solution of sodium carbonate. Allow to stand for 10 minutes and filter. Wash the precipitate with three 10 ml portions of water. Extract the combined filtrate with two 10 ml portions of chloroform and final volume is adjusted to 25 ml with chloroform.

Procedure

Take 4 ml each of chloroform extract of sample and standard solutions, add 5 ml of solution of chloranil. Maintain at 40°C in a water-bath for 45 minutes, cool and adjust to 10 ml with chloroform. Measure the absorbance of both the solutions at about 515 nm against blank prepared by diluting 5 ml of chloranil solution to 10 ml with chloroform. The above colour is stable for 1 h. The method obeys Beer's law in the concentration range of 16-50 mcg/ml.

Note

1. After precipitation with sodium carbonate, some amount of antazoline salt still remains in assay solution with no loss of naphazoline. This residual antazoline forms no complex with chloranil in chloroform due to basicity.
2. Substances present as preservatives, antioxidants or buffering agents exhibit no interference during assay procedure as it is based on the extraction of free base prior to complexation.

Probable Reaction Mechanism

Naphazoline, having a secondary amine, adds at the enone system of the chloranil in alkaline medium resulting in the formation of a coloured product (λ_{max} 515 nm).

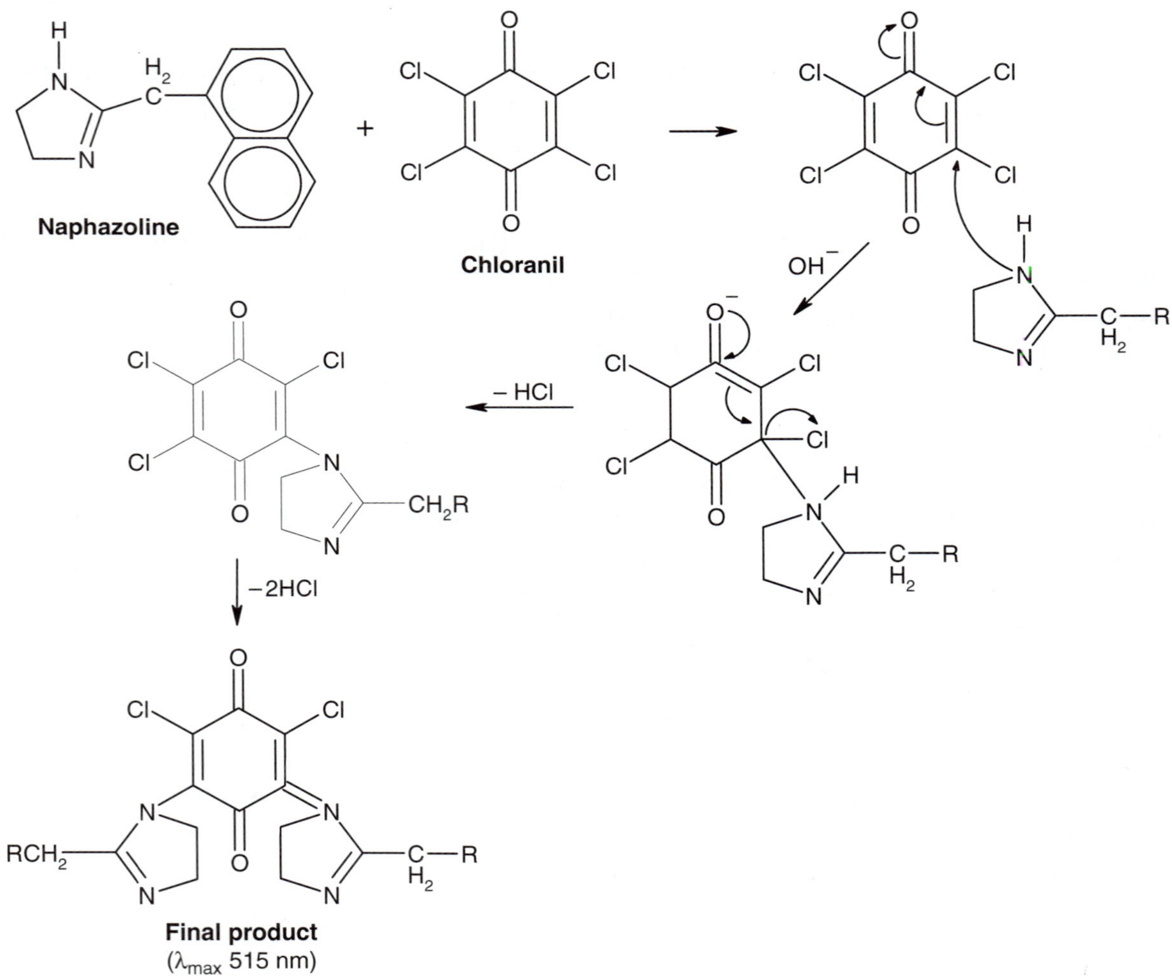

Note

Other electrophilic reagents like Cl^-, Br^-, NO_2 will attack at position 4 or 5 of the heteroaromatic moiety (see under antazoline).

Naphazoline forms ion-pair complex with bromocresol green (pH 3.4 buffer), bromophenol blue (pH 2.5 buffer), bromothymol blue and methyl orange (pH 6.0 buffer). All the complexes are extractable in chloroform and subjected to spectrophotometric measurements (λ_{max} 420 nm) for quantification.

Antazoline sulphate

METHOD 1

Reagent

1. 0.001 M iodine solution in chloroform.

Standard solution

100 mcg/ml; for preparation, refer to the method under naphazoline nitrate.

Sample solution

Portion of the sample equivalent to 10 mg of antazoline sulphate is processed for preparation of sample solution as described for naphazoline nitrate.

Procedure

To 5 ml each of sample and standard solutions, add 2 ml of iodine solution, mix and dilute to 25 ml with chloroform. Allow to stand at room temperature for 30 minutes and measure the extinction at 300 nm and 365 nm against a blank prepared by diluting 2 ml of iodine solution to 25 ml with chloroform. Calculate the absorbance value at 300 nm and 365 nm. Compare with the standard and calculate by subtracting extinction value at 365 nm from that at 300 nm.

Probable Reaction Mechanism

Most of the electrophilic reagents such as Br^-, Cl^-, I^-, NO_2 preferably attack at position 4 or 5 of heteroaromatic nucleus. Iodine can attack at C-4 or C-5 or both; the complex is soluble in chloroform (λ_{max} 365 nm).

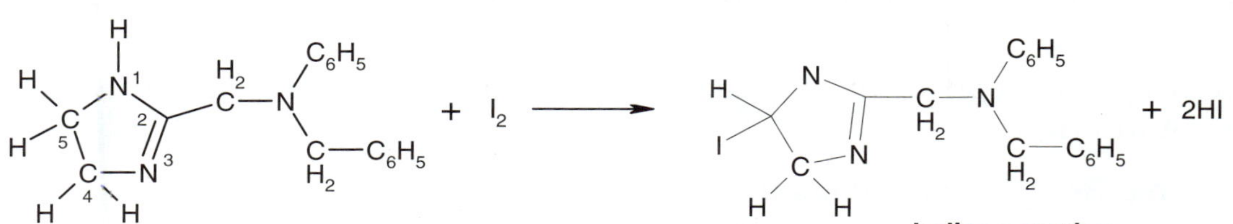

Antazoline **Iodine complex** (λ_{max} 365 nm)

METHOD 2

Reagents

1. Cerric sulphate reagent: Dissolve by slight warming 50 mg of dried cerric sulphate in 50 ml of concentrated sulphuric acid, cool and dilute to 100 ml with formate free acetic acid. The reagent is quite stable at room temperature.
2. Acetic acid, formate free.
3. Perchloric acid, 70%.

Standard solution

50 mcg/ml of antazoline sulphate in acetic acid.

Sample solution

Accurately measured aliquot of the sample is approximately diluted with acetic acid to get 50 mcg/ml.

Procedure

To 1 ml of the cerric sulphate solution, add 2 ml of perchloric acid, mix and then add 1 ml each of sample and standard solution and dilute to 10 ml with acetic acid. Measure the absorbance of both the solutions at about 505 nm against acetic acid as blank. Naphazoline and tolazoline do not interfere. Deduce the results by comparison.

METHOD 3

Reagents

1. 7.5% w/v solution of sodium nitrite in concentrated sulphuric acid.
2. 15% w/v solution of sodium acetate in water.

Procedure

To portion of the sample and standard solutions equivalent to 10 mg of antazoline, add 0.4 ml of sodium nitrite solution, mix and allow to stand for five minutes and then dilute to 50 ml with sodium acetate solution. Measure the absorbance of both the sample and standard solutions at about 416 nm against reagent blank. Calculate the results by comparison.

Note

Phenylephrine, ephedrine, naphazoline, chlorbutol, and benzalkonium chloride do not interfere.

Probable Reaction Mechanism

$$NaNO_2 + H_2SO_4 \longrightarrow HNO_2\ (HO{-}N{=}O) \xrightarrow{H_3O^+} H_2O + N{=}O^+$$

Nitrosonium ion

$N^{+}{=}O$ being electron deficient will attack at position 4 of the compound yielding coloured nitroso derivative.

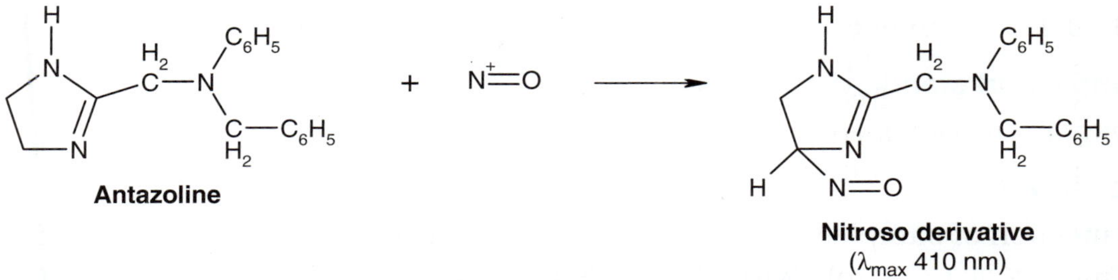

Note

1. Although naphazoline shall answer similar reactions, but while sample preparation both the compounds have been separated on basification with Na_2CO_3.
2. Both naphazoline and antazoline react with bromine, an electrophilic reagent, at position 4 giving bromo derivative of heteroaromatic moiety. For reaction mechanism refer to method 1.
3. Both naphazoline and antazoline condense with PDAB at C-4 as under.

Probable Reaction Mechanism

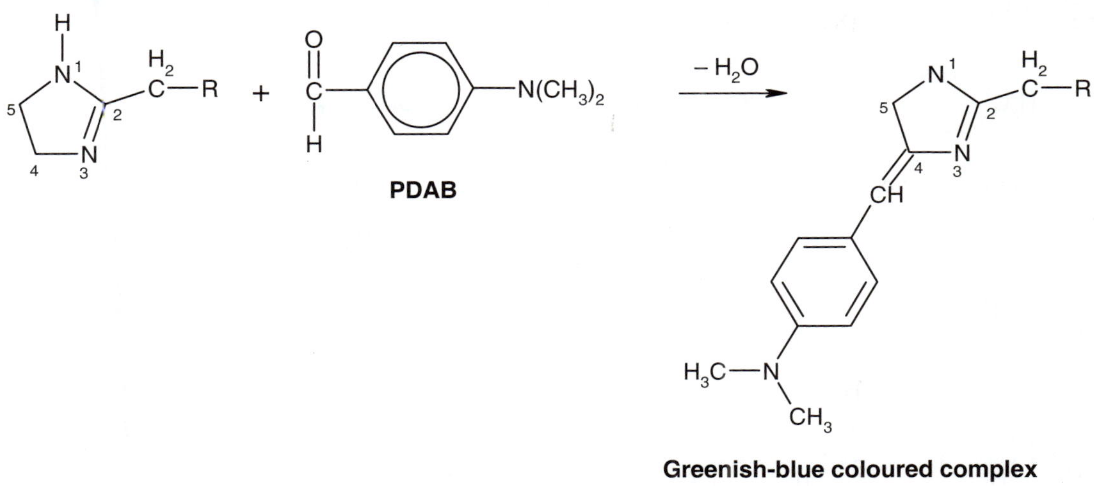

Reference

Pharmaceutical Chemistry (Vol. 2) by H.J. Roth, p. 525.

Note

The compound forms ion-pair complex with bromothymol blue, bromocresol green and bromophenol blue similar to naphthazoline nitrate.

METHOD 4

Reagents

1. 10% v/v malonic acid in acetic anhydride (MAA).

Sample and standard solutions

10 µg/ml in water.

Procedure

10 ml each of sample and standard is basified with 1 M sodium hydroxide, the titrated base extracted with ether, organic layer evaporated and to the residue add 3 ml of 'MAA' reagent. Heat in water-bath (80°C) for 20 min and then dilute to 25 ml with methanol. Measure the absorbance at 334 nm against reagent blank.

Probable Reaction Mechanism

Acetic anhydride acts as dehydrating agent; so it dehydrates malonic acid to give malonic anhydride. Malonic acid in acetic anhydride yields a highly coloured alcohol-soluble complex which has λ_{max} 334 nm. It is a base-catalyzed condensation of anhydride of an organic acid, ternary amine acting as catalyst leading to formation of a coloured complex.

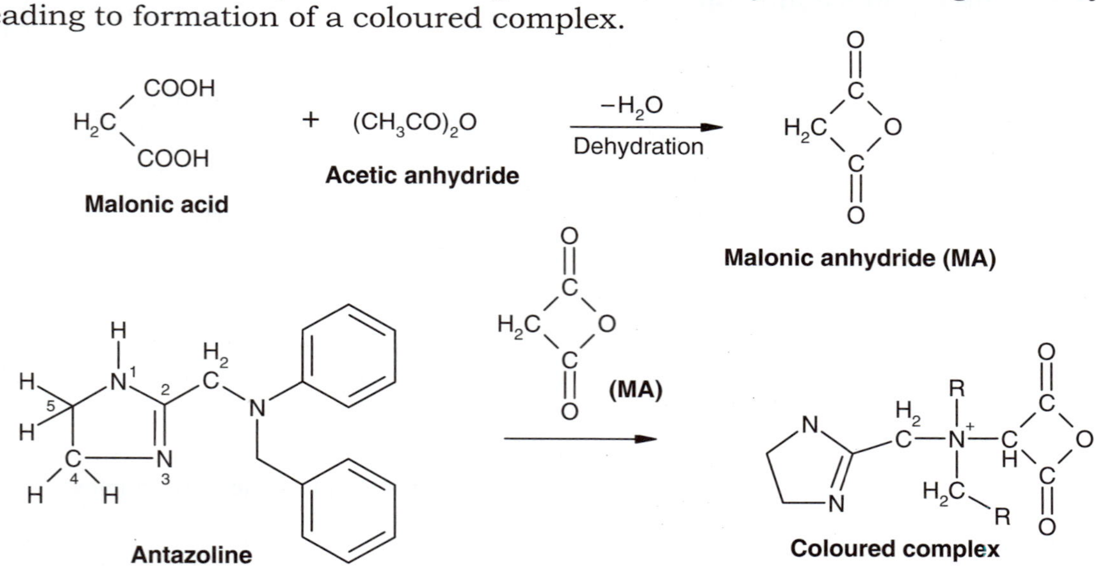

Note

Similar reaction with diphenhydramine.

Reference

A.V. Kasture, M.V. Bulbule & M.R. Tajne. *Indian Drugs*, **22(1)**, 42, 1984.

Formulation 12

Phenylephrine hydrochloride, Naphazoline hydrochloride, Diphenhydramine hydrochloride

ESTIMATION

Phenylephrine hydrochloride

Follow the method described in formulation 1 of the chapter on analgesics and antipyretics.

Naphazoline hydrochloride

METHOD 1

Reagents

1. 4.0% w/v solution of sodium hydroxide in water.
2. 5.0% w/v solution of sodium nitroprusside in water, freshly prepared.
3. 8.4% w/v solution of sodium bicarbonate in water.

Standard solution

Dissolve 0.025 g of naphazoline hydrochloride, 0.25 g of phenylephrine hydrochloride and 0.1 g of diphenhydramine hydrochloride, 0.25 g phenylephrine hydrochloride and 0.1 g of diphenhydramine hydrochloride in a 100 ml volumetric flask and dilute with water up to the mark. 5 ml of the solution is treated in the same way as the sample according to the following procedure.

Procedure

Take 5 ml of standard and 5 ml of sample containing 1.25 mg of the substance, add 1 ml of sodium hydroxide solution to each, followed by 1 ml sodium nitroprusside solution. After 10 minutes, add 2 ml of solution of sodium bicarbonate and shake. Dilute with water up to 50 ml and after 30 min, determine the absorption of both the solutions at about 575 nm against the reagent blank. Calculate the percentage of naphazoline hydrochloride in the sample by comparison.

Sodium nitroprusside or sodium pentacyanonitrosylferrate

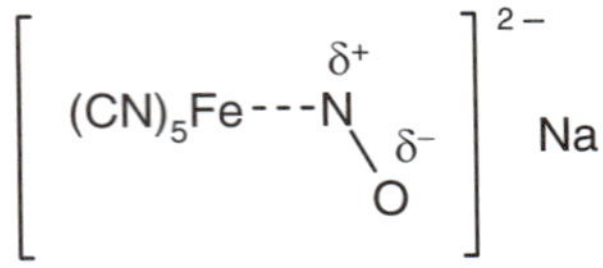

in alkaline medium forms complex with imidazoline ring giving violet colour. The exact structure of the complex is not known.

Naphazoline forms ion-pair complex with fast-green and orange-II in pH 5 phosphate buffer.

Probable Reaction Mechanism

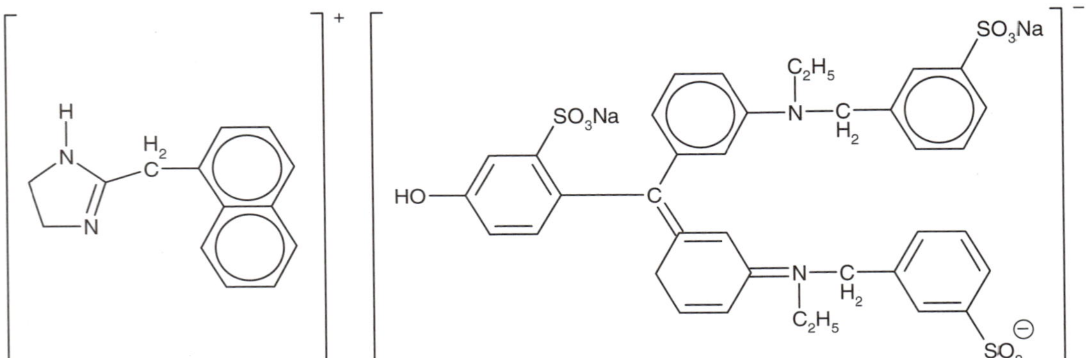

Naphazoline

Drug - Fast-green ion-pair complex
(λ_{max} 630 nm)

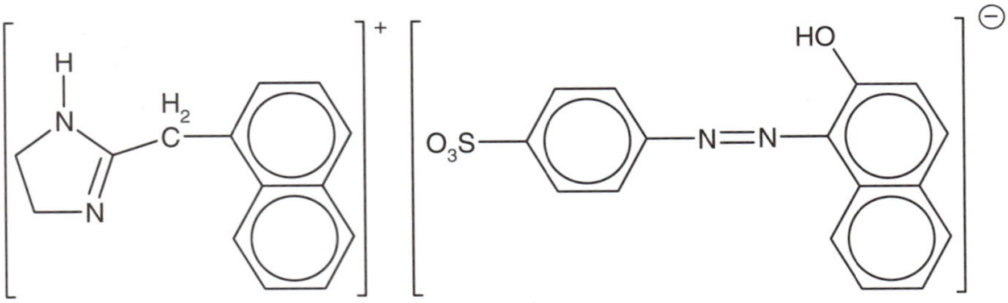

Naphazoline

Drug - Orange-II ion-pair complex
(λ_{max} 495 nm)

METHOD 2

Follow the method described in formulation 11 of this chapter.

Diphenhydramine hydrochloride

Follow the method described in chapter on expectorants and cough suppressants.

Formulation 13

Domiphen bromide, Xylometazoline hydrochloride/ Oxymetazoline

ESTIMATION

Domiphen bromide

Reagents

1. 2 N ammonia solution.
2. 0.1% w/v solution of bromocresol purple in ethanol.
3. Titrating solution: Dissolve 0.5 g sodium lauryl sulphate in water to make 1000 ml. Dilute 20 ml to 100 ml with water.

Standard solution

100 mcg/ml of domiphen bromide in water.

Procedure

Use stoppered test tube of 30 ml capacity as titrating vessel. Introduce sample aliquot equivalent to 0.4 mg of domiphen bromide into titrating vessel, add 10 ml water, 5 ml chloroform and 4 drops of bromocresol purple solution. Then add 1 ml of 2 N ammonia solution, thus causing the indicator to turn violet. Shake and titrate by adding the titrating solution from a 10 ml microburette and shaking slowly for 1 minute after each addition and waiting until the phases have separated.

The end-point is reached when the chloroform phase is colourless. In the vicinity of the end-point, add titrating solution slowly in portions of 0.1 ml. 4 ml of standard solution is titrated under similar conditions with sodium lauryl sulphate. From the volume of sodium lauryl sulphate used for sample and standard solutions, calculate the amount of domiphen bromide in the sample.

Xylometazoline hydrochloride

Reagents

1. 1 N sulphuric acid.
2. 2 N sodium acetate.

3. Benzene or chloroform.
4. 0.1% w/v solution of sodium lauryl sulphate in water.
5. Potassium cobalt thiocyanate reagent: Dissolve 10 g of cobalt (II) nitrate hexahydrate and 13.5 g of potassium thiocyanate in water to produce 100 ml.

Standard solution

1 mg/ml of xylometazoline hydrochloride in water.

Sample solution

The sample is appropriately diluted with water to get 1 mg/ml concentration of the substance.

Procedure

Transfer 5 ml each of sample and standard solutions into two separatory funnels. To each, add 5 ml sodium lauryl sulphate solution, and 20 ml of potassium cobalt thiocyanate reagent. Extract twice each with 20 ml of benzene and one with 10 ml of benzene. Combine benzene extract and dilute to 50 ml with benzene. Clear the solution by adding about 2 g anhydrous sodium sulphate, filter if necessary. Measure the absorption of clear sample and standard solutions at about 620 nm against solvent blank and calculate the results.

Probable Reaction Mechanism

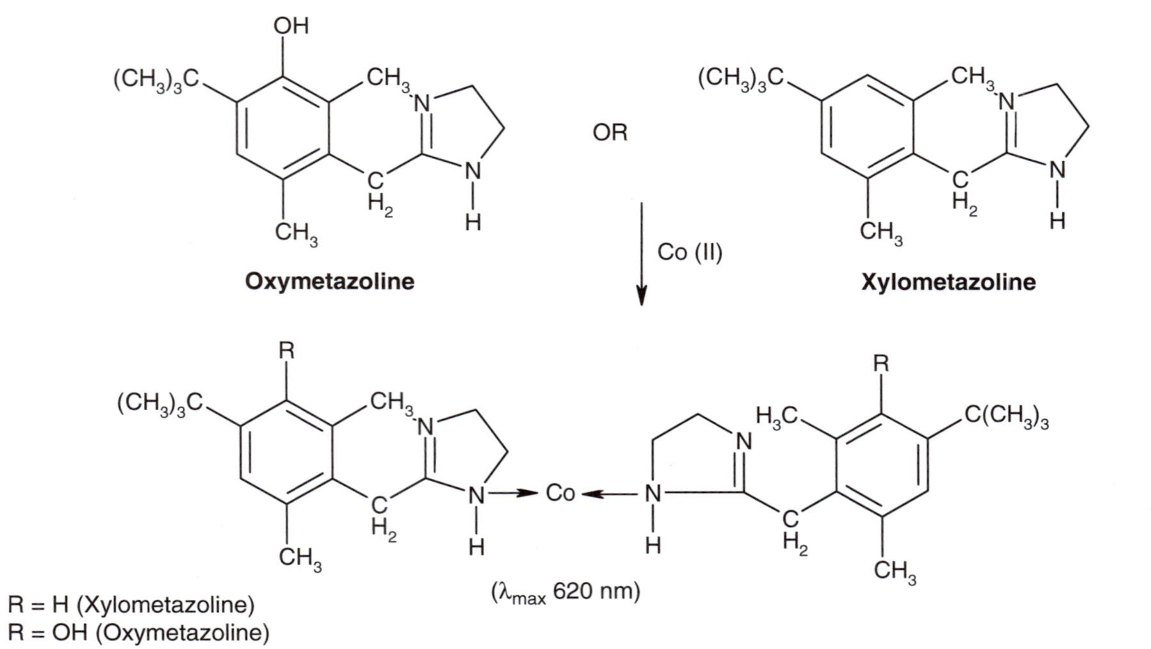

Alternative reaction with Co^{++} using sodium cobaltinitrate as reagent has been used for quantitative analysis.

Probable Reaction Mechanism

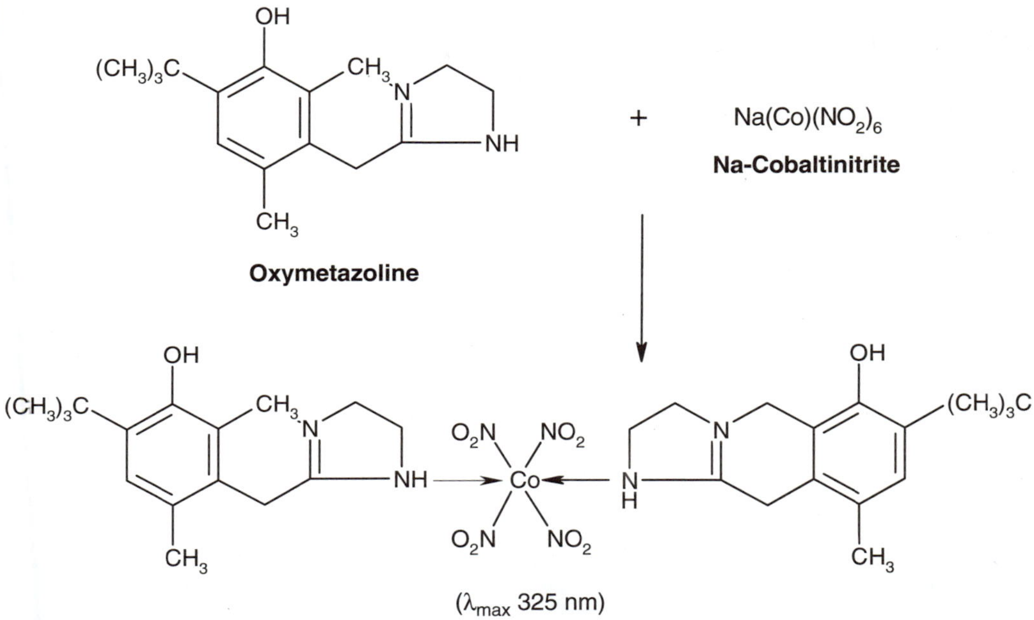

Reference

D.M. Shingbal & S.D. Naik. *Eastern Pharmacist*, **26(308)**, 201-202, 1983.

Zarapkar & Athalye (1990) have described a titrimetric method for analysis of several quaternary ammonium drugs such as antazoline, cetrimide, xylometazoline, naphazoline, oxyphenonium bromide and domiphen bromide using sodium lauryl sulphate or sodium lauryl ether sulphate as titrant and cobalt thiocyanate as indicator when quaternary ammonium compounds with long alkyl chain or a bulky aryl group is titrated with anion surfactant having a long alkyl chain (SLS), it forms an ion-pair complex with cobalt thiocyanate and goes into chloroform layer. Since the complex is blue in colour, so chloroform layer becomes blue. The remaining amine then complexes with surfactant as this titration progresses. Excess of surfactant then attacks the blue complex making chloroform layer colourless (end point).

Reference

S.S. Zarapkar & Kishore Athalye. *Indian Drugs*, **27(3)**, 195-197, 1990.

Both oxymetazoline and xylometazoline form ion-pair complex with Fast Green and orange II (dyes) in phosphate buffer, pH 5.0. Both dye complexes are exctractable into chloroform. For Fast Green λ_{max} 630 nm and for orange II λ_{max} 495 nm.

Probable Reaction Mechanism

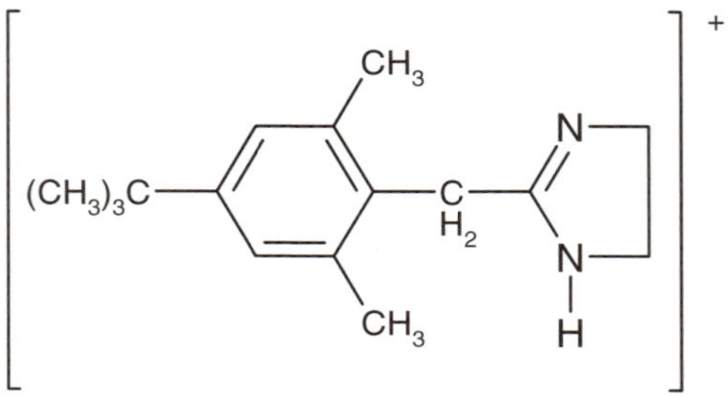

Xylometazoline

OR

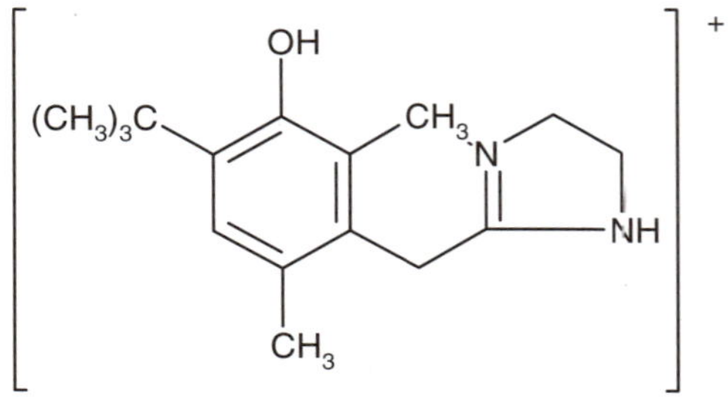

Oxymetazoline

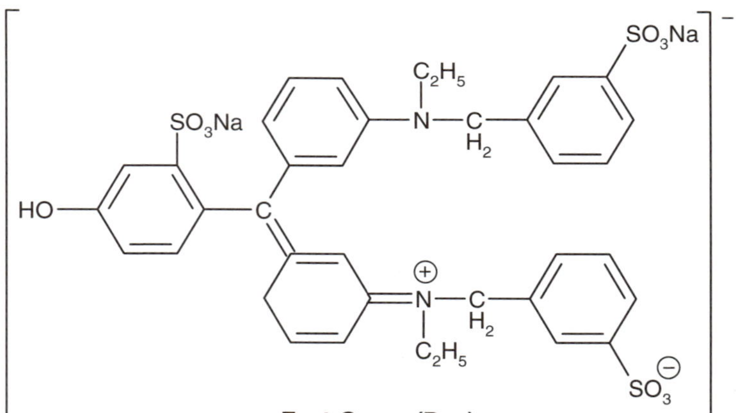

Fast-Green (Dye)
(λ_{max} 630 nm)

OR

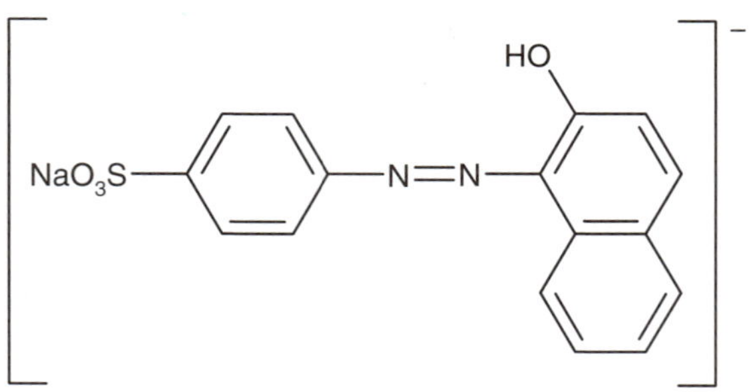

Orange-II (Dye used)
(λ_{max} 495 nm)

Reference

Indian Drugs, **26(7)**, 348, 1989.

Note

Naphazoline also forms similar ion-pair complex.

Oxymetazoline/xylometazoline also form ion-pair complex with bromocresol green (pH 3.4 buffer), bromophenol blue (pH 2.5 buffer), bromothymol blue (pH 3.8) and methyl orange (pH 6.0). All the complexes are extractable into chloroform and have λ_{max} 420 nm.

Reference

R.T. Sane, U.M. Vaidya & Sandhya Sane. *Curr. Sci.*, **47(22)**, 853-854, 1978; and *Indian Drugs*, **16(10)**, 239-241, 1979.

Note

The compound being imidazole derivative shall answer all the reactions as described under antazoline and naphazoline in the chapter.

Shingbal & Samant (1982) have described a spectrophotometric method of analysis using chlorimide reagent yielding an indophenol derivative (λ_{max} 420 nm).

Reagents

1. Chlorimide reagent (Gibbs reagent): 0.04% of w/v solution of isopropanol.
2. Alkaline borate buffer pH 7.2.

Sample/standard solutions

200 μg/ml of oxymetazoline/xylometazoline hydrochloride in water.

Procedure

To 2 ml each of sample/standard solutions add 2 ml of borate buffer followed by 1 ml of chlorimide reagent, dilute to 20 ml with water and measure the absorbance of sample and standard solutions at 420 nm against reagent blank.

Probable reaction mechanism as proposed by the authors

The compound being imidazole derivative shall answer all the reactions as described for antazoline and naphazoline in this chapoter. The chlorimide reagent shall couple at position 5 of the heteroaromatic ring as following.

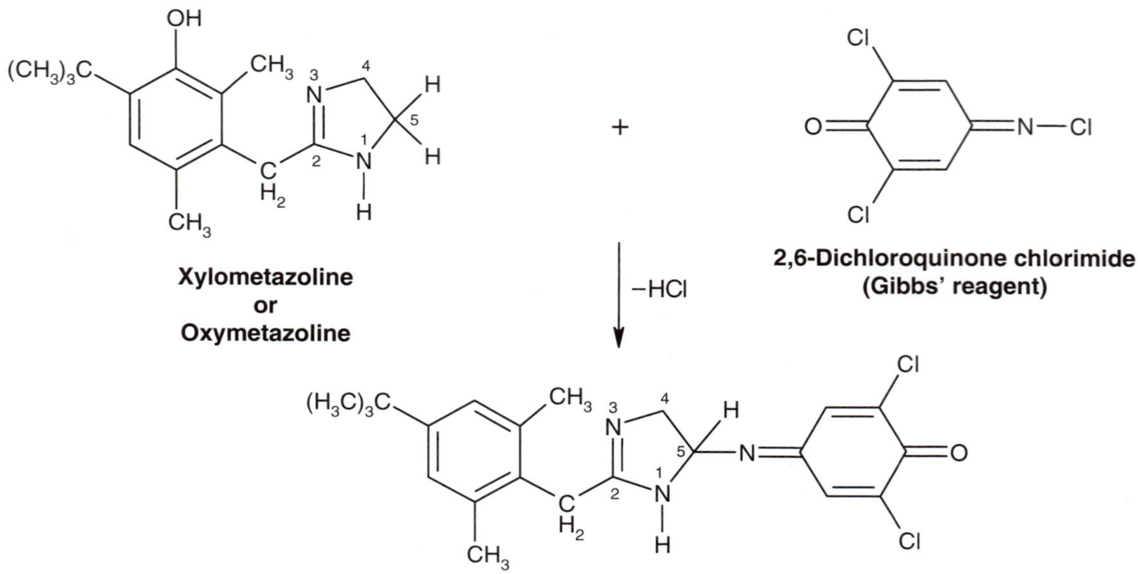

Indophenol derivative
(λ_{max} 430 nm)

Reference

D.M. Shingbal & K.V. Samant. *Indian Drugs*, **19(2)**, 106-107, 1982.

Note

Kamalapurkar & Priolkar have reported a quantitative method based on reaction with Folin-Ciocalteu reagent in alkaline medium yielding a blue-coloured molybdenum complex (λ_{max} 680 nm).

Reference

O.S. Kamalapurkar & Sanjay R.S. Priolkar. *Indian Drugs*, **20**, 164-166, Jan. 1983.

Formulation 14

Isoprenaline sulphate, Atropine methonitrate, Papaverine hydrochloride, Sodium metabisulphite

ESTIMATION

Isoprenaline sulphate

Reagents

1. 20% w/v solution of sodium hydroxide in water.
2. Sodium phosphate-tungstate reagent: Boil gently under reflux for 90 minutes 10 g of sodium tungstate with 75 ml of water and 8 ml of phosphoric acid (88% w/w), cool and dilute to 100 ml with water.

Standard stock solution of isoprenaline sulphate

Dissolve 0.1 g of isoprenaline sulphate, accurately weighed, and 0.515 g of sodium metabisulphite in water in a 100 ml volumetric flask, dilute to volume with water and mix.

Working standard solution

Immediately before use, dilute 5 ml of stock standard isoprenaline sulphate solution to 100 ml with water (50 mcg/ml).

Sample solution

Dilute appropriate volume of the sample with water to get 50 mcg/ml.

Procedure

Transfer 5 ml each of sample and standard solutions to a 100 ml volumetric flasks. To both the flasks, add the following reagents in the order given below:

1 ml of sodium phosphotungstate reagent, 30 ml of water and 1 ml of sodium hydroxide solution. Dilute the contents of both the flasks to volume with water and mix well. Immediately measure the absorption of both the solutions at about 730 nm using water in the reference cell and calculate the results by comparison.

Alternatively, the following reactions can be used for estimation of the compound in the formulations.

Probable Reaction Mechanism

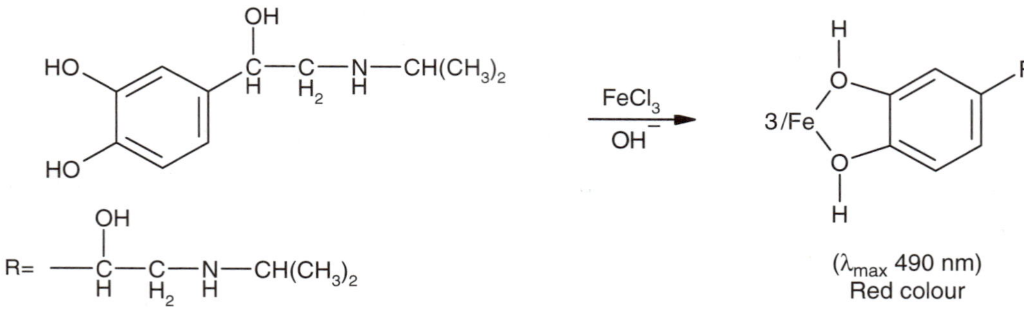

This is indicative of pyrocatechol derivative.

In alkaline solution the compound is oxidized to adrenochrome analogue and further oxidized to oxoadrenochrome analogue.

Probable Reaction Mechanism

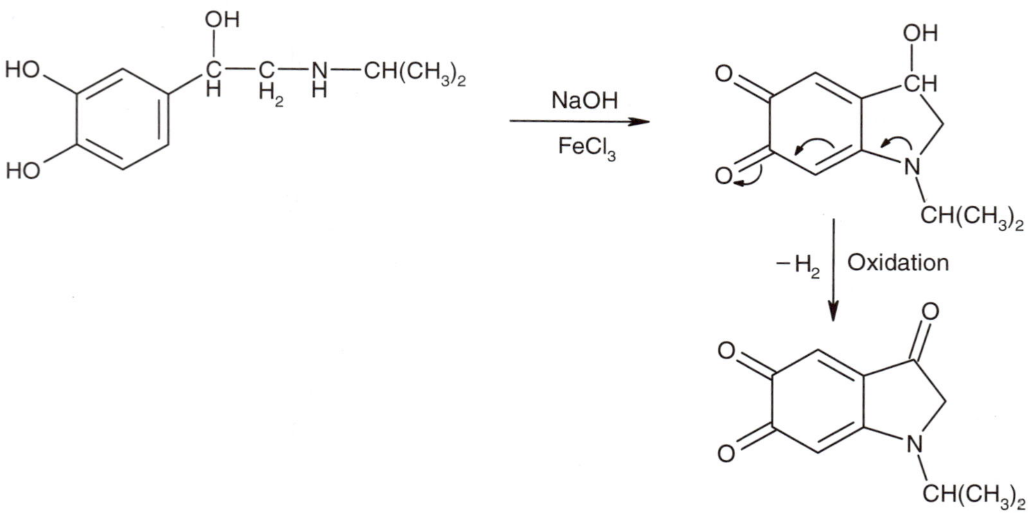

Further, due to the presence of pyrocatechol structure (orthodiphenolic character), it can reduce silver nitrate and itself get oxidized to o-quinone.

Probable Reaction Mechanism

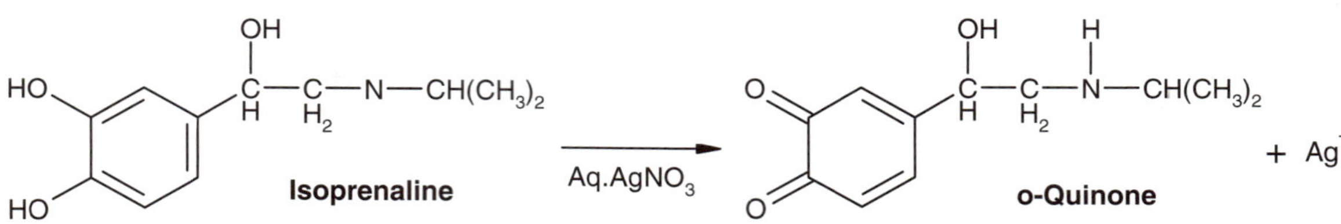

Atropine methonitrate

Reagent

Atropine methoreineckate wash solution: Mix equal volumes of 1% w/v solution of atropine methonitrate and solution of ammonium reineckate and acidify with dilute sulphuric acid. Wash the precipitates with water till washings are free from sulphate. Shake the precipitates with water to get saturated solution, filter and use as wash solution.

Procedure

Transfer sample solution equivalent to about 10 mg of the substance into a 150 ml separator; add 2 ml of dilute sulphuric acid. Extract with three 50 ml portions of chloroform, washing each extract with the same 10 ml portions of 0.1 N sulphuric acid. Discard the chloroform layer. Combine the aqueous acidic solutions, rinse the separator with 25 ml of dilute sulphuric acid and add the rinsing to the main aqueous solution. Add 30 ml of a freshly prepared and filtered solution of ammonium reineckate. Allow to stand for 30 minutes and filter through a weighed G_4 porosity sintered glass crucible. Wash the residue with four 5 ml quantities of atropine methoreineckate wash solution, followed by 3 ml of water. Dry the residue to a constant weight. Each g of the residue is equivalent to 0.5884 g of atropine methonitrate.

Alternatively, reineckate precipitate can be dissolved in acetone and estimation carried out spectrophotometrically.

Papaverine hydrochloride

Dilute sample solution equivalent to 100 mg of papaverine hydrochloride to 100 ml with water. Dilute further 10 ml of this solution to 100 ml with water. Transfer 20 ml of this solution into a 100 ml volumetric flask, add 1 ml of hydrochloric acid and dilute to volume with water (20 mcg/ml of papaverine hydrochloride). Measure the extinction of this solution at 310 nm using 0.1 N hydrochloric acid in the reference cell. Calculate using 228 as value of E 1%, 1 cm of papaverine hydrochloride at 310 nm.

Sodium metabisulphite

Transfer the sample solution equivalent to about 25 mg of the compound to a 150 ml conical flask. Add approximately 10 ml of chloroform and titrate with 0.05 N iodine till both layers have the same pale yellow colour. During the titration, stopper the flask and shake vigorously intermittently.

Each ml of 0.05 N iodine is equivalent to 0.002376 g of sodium metabisulphite.

Explanatory Note

This method is based on iodometric titration. Sodium metabisulphate is a reductant, hence I_2 is reduced to iodide whereas I_2 is an oxidant and shall oxidize metabisulphite to metabisulphate.

$$I_2 + 2e \longrightarrow 2I^-$$

$$S_2O_3^{--} + I_2 \longrightarrow S_4O_6^{--} + 2I^-$$

Formulation 15

Triamcinolone acetonide, Thimerosal, Phenylephrine hydrochloride, Neomycin sulphate, Benzalkonium chloride

ESTIMATION

Triamcinolone acetonide

Reagent

Isoniazid reagent: Dissolve 500 mg of isoniazid in 250 ml of methanol, add 0.63 ml of hydrochloric acid and adjust to 500 ml with methanol.

Standard solution

40 mcg/ml of triamcinolone acetonide in chloroform.

Sample solution

Accurately weigh the sample equivalent to 1 mg of triamcinolone acetonide in a 25 ml volumetric flask. Add about 15 ml of chloroform and shake well for about 10 minutes. Make up to the mark with chloroform. Filter, if necessary, through a No. 42 Whatman paper.

Procedure

Transfer 5 ml each of sample and standard solutions into 25 ml volumetric flasks. To each of two flasks, add 10 ml of isoniazid reagent. Place the flasks in a water-bath at 55°C (± 2°C) for 45 minutes. Cool the flasks to room temperature and make up to volume with chloroform and mix. Measure the absorbance of both the solutions at 415 nm and calculate the results.

Note

1. Prevent incorporation of moisture as it reduces the intensity of the final colour.
2. Addition of hydrochloric acid (0.63 ml) to the isoniazid reagent should be accurate as excessive acid reduces the sensitivity of the method.
3. Instead of heating, the solution after addition of isoniazid reagent can be kept at room temperature for 45 min and then made up the volume.

Primary amino group of isoniazid reacts with carbonyl group of the compound present in ring (A) at C-3 resulting in the formation of a complex (λ_{max} 415 nm).

Probable Reaction Mechanism

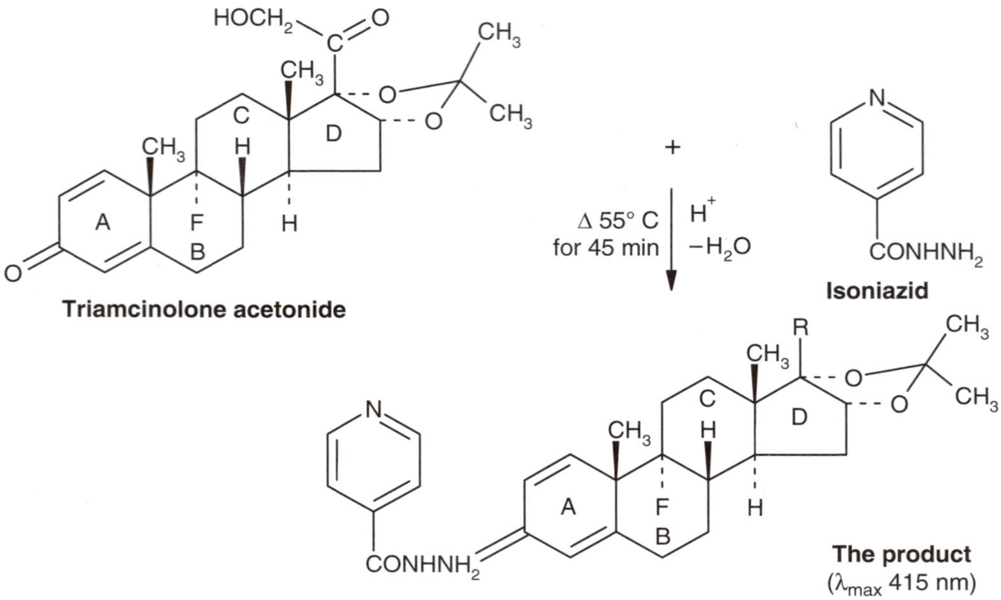

Triamcinolone interacts with 4-aminoantipyrin. The method is based not on oxidative coupling but simply amino group of antipyrin reacting with carbonyl group present in ring "A" of the molecule.

Probable Reaction Mechanism

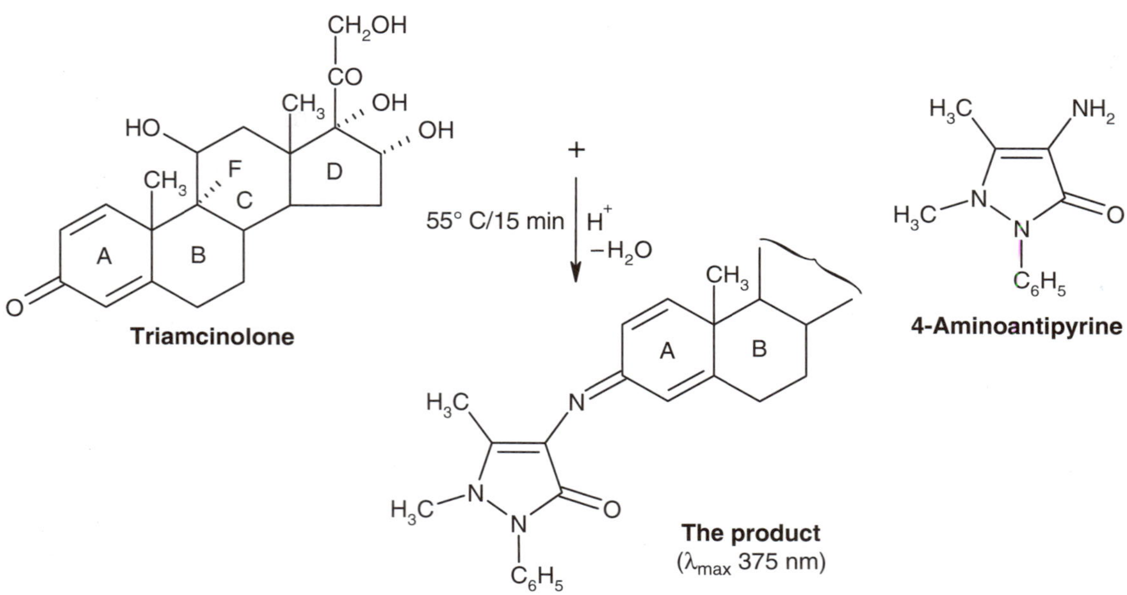

Reference

R.V. Gaitonde & G.J. Kamat. *Indian Drugs*, **23(9)**, 516, 1986.

The drug interacts with 2,4-dinitrophenyl hydrazine, thiosemicarbazide and N,N,dimethyl p-phenylene diamine giving respective derivative. In all these reactions, carbonyl group (C==O) at C-3 is involved. All these reactions have been reported to be of analytical interest.

Probable Reaction Mechanism

(A)

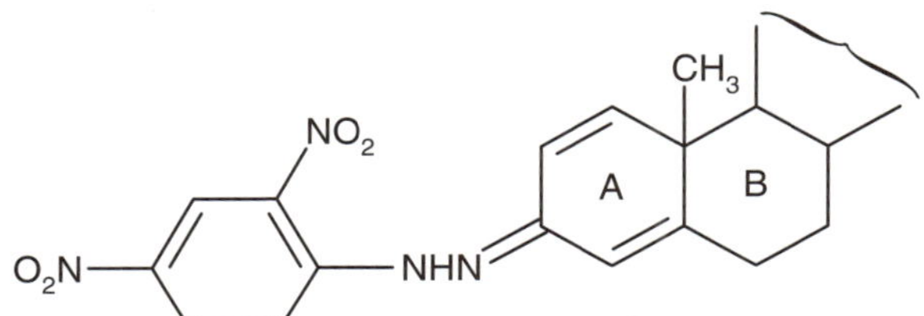

The product
(λ_{max} 370 nm)

2,4-Dinitrophenylhydrazone complex

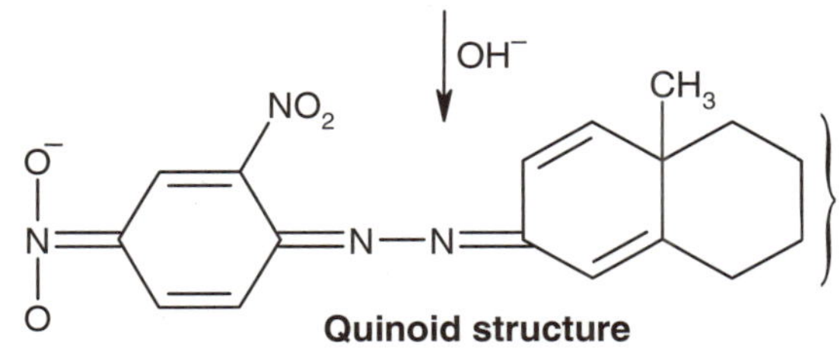

Quinoid structure
(λ_{max} 490 nm)

This complexation requires heating at 75°C for 10 min for colour development. In alkaline medium, quinoid structure is stabilized by removal of proton.

Reference

Gornall A.G. et al., *J. Biol. Chem.*, **201**, 279, 1953.

(B)

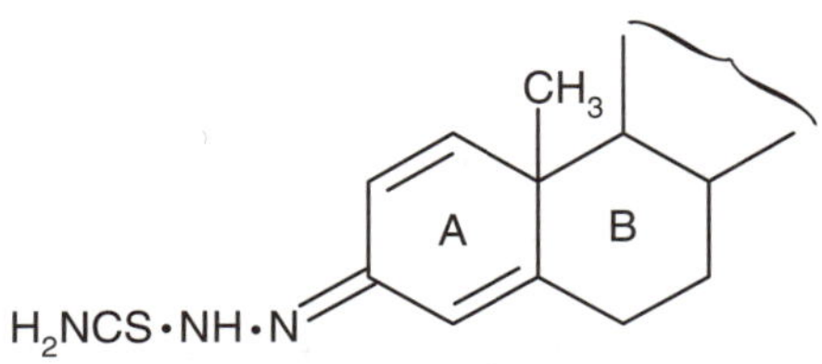

The product
(λ_{max} 382 nm)

Thiosemicarbazide complex

This requires heating at 75°C for 30 min for colour development.

(C)

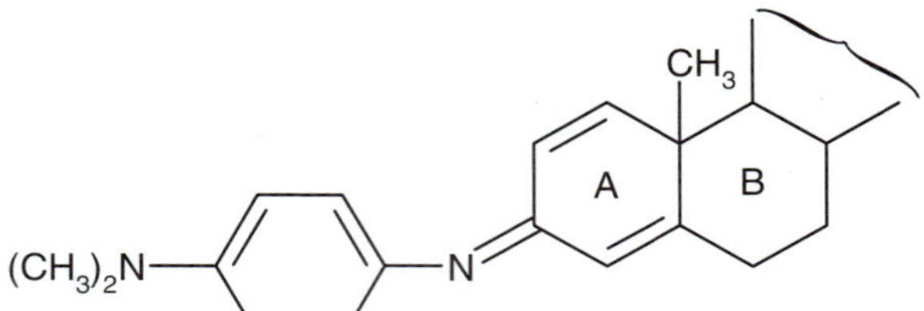

The product
(λ_{max} 460 nm)

N,N-Dimethyl-p-phenylene complex

This requires heating at 70°C for 40 min for colour development.

Reference

1. Indian Drugs, 22(9), 489, 1985; *Indian Drugs*, **24(1)**, 59, 1986; *Indian Drugs*, 24(9), 451, 1987.
2. E. Ryan et al., *J. Am. Chem. Soc.*, **71**, 2000, 1949.

Note

Steroid molecules with C-20 keto group shall also react with above reagents.

Thimerosal

Note

All glassware must be rinsed with warm dilute nitric acid (1: 2) and then rinsed with distilled water before using. The titration must be performed in one continuous operation.

Reagents

1. Dilute hydrochloric acid.
2. Strong dithizone solution: Dissolve 50 mg of dithizone (diphenylthio-carbizone) in 100 ml of chloroform.
3. Dilute dithizone solution: Transfer 25 ml of strong dithizone solution to a 250 ml volumetric flask, dilute to volume with chloroform and mix well.
4. 30% hydrogen peroxide.
5. Acidic potassium permanganate solution. Add 3 ml of sulphuric acid to 100 ml of 0.1 N potassium permanganate.
6. Dilute nitric acid: Dilute 3 ml of nitric acid to 100 ml with distilled water.
7. 1% w/v solution of hydroxylamine hydrochloride in water.

Standard mercury solution

Accurately weigh 80 mg of reagent grade mercuric oxide and transfer to a 250 ml volumetric flask, add sufficient dilute nitric acid to dissolve the powder.

Dilute to volume with distilled water and mix well. Dilute 10 ml to 500 ml with distilled water and mix well. Calculate the amount of mercury.

$$\text{Mercury, mcg/ml)} = \frac{A \times 0.9261 \times 1000 \times 10}{250 \times 500} = A \times 0.0741$$

where A = weight (mg) of sample taken for analysis; 0.9261 is factor to convert mercuric oxide to mercury.

Procedure

Transfer 10 ml of the sample and 15 ml of standard mercury solution into 500 ml standard joint flasks, add 40 ml of dilute hydrochloric acid, 2 ml of hydrogen peroxide and a few glass beads to each flask. Insert a reflux condenser and reflux on a hot plate for 2 h. Raise the temperature gradually as the sample solution may form foam as it starts to boil. Allow to cool to room temperature, then wash the condensers with distilled water, collecting the washings in the flasks. Quantitatively, transfer the contents to 125 ml separatory funnels with the aid of distilled water. Add 10 ml of dithizone solution to each and shake vigorously for 3 min. Allow the layers to separate, then transfer the chloroform layer to a 100 ml separatory funnel. Add 10 ml of acid potassium permanganate and 10 ml of distilled water. Shake vigorously for 3 minutes and allow the layers to separate. Drain off the chloroform layer and discard. Add 3 ml of hydroxylamine hydrochloride solution and shake until the solution is completely colourless. If an emulsion persists, add 1 ml more of hydroxylamine solution and mix well. Combine the resultant aqueous phase with the main. Add dilute dithizone solution from a burette in small volumes with shaking until the green colour turns to orange colour. Draw off each portion of dithizone before adding the next one. When a green tinge appears in the orange, use 0.2 ml at a time until completely green colour persists. Perform blank, not more than 1 ml should be required for the blank. Calculate thiomersal as under:

$$\text{Thimerosal (mg/ml)} = \frac{A \times C \times 15 \times 2.018}{B \times 10} = \frac{A \times C \times 3.027}{B}$$

where

A = volume (ml) of dithizone required for the sample (corrected for blank);
B = volume (ml) of dithizone required for the standard, corrected for the blank;
C = amount of mercury (mcg/ml) in standard solution.

We can follow colorimetric method i.e. after addition of dithizone solution and shaking vigorously, separate organic layer. Again, shake with 10 ml of chloroform till chloroform layer is colourless, combine chloroform layers and dilute to 25 ml with chloroform. Measure the absorbance of the sample and standard at about 500 nm.

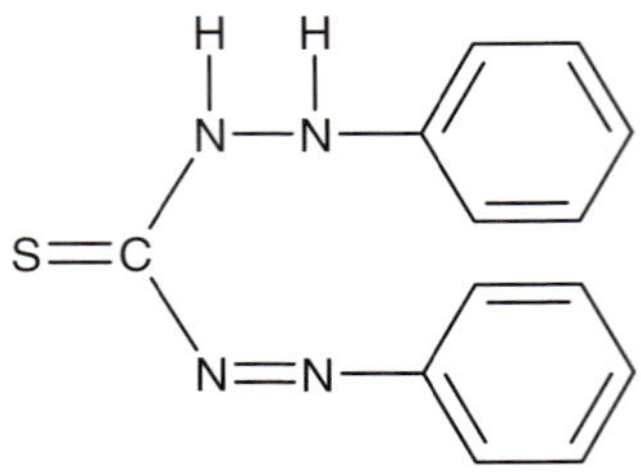

Dithizone (Diphenylthiocarbazone)

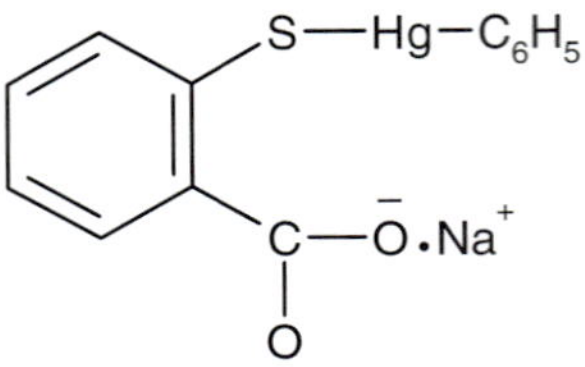

Thimerosal

It exists in keto and enol forms in acid and alkali.

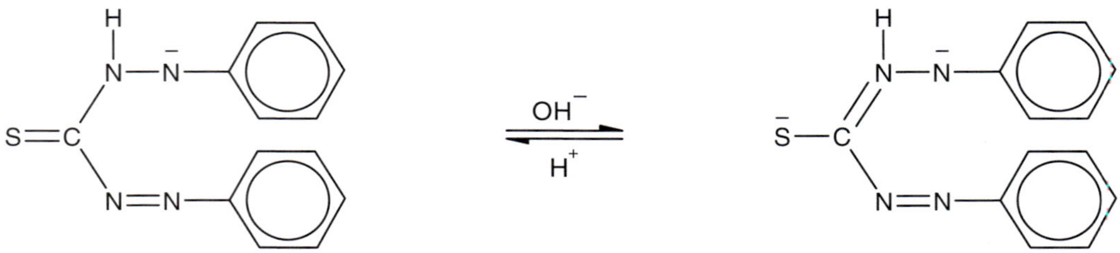

Keto form Enol form

The colour of keto complex is different from enol complex, so only one form of dithizone should be present during analysis. The Hg(2)-dithizone (metal ion - dithizonate) complex being soluble in chloroform is extractable into organic solvent for measurement.

Note

To remove excess of free organic layer containing mercuric-dithizonate complex, shake slightly with 5 ml of hydroxylamine solution before spectrophotometric readings.
A titrimetric method was reported by Verma involving titration with iodine trichloride (ICl_3).

Reagents

1. 0.02 M iodine trichloride (ICl_3) in dilute hydrochloric acid, standardized iodometrically.
2. Carbon tetrachloride and 3.6 M hydrochloric acid.

Sample and standard solutions

100 μg/ml in water.

Procedure

Mix 1 ml of sample/standard solution with 20 ml of water and 5 ml of carbon tetrachloride. The mixture is titrated with ICl_3 solution until the colour of organic layer has attained maximum intensity. Stopper the flask, shake well, add 20 ml of 6 M hydrochloric acid and shake well again, continue titration till organic layer is colourless.

Probable Reaction Mechanism

This method is based on reduction of ICl_3 to I_2 (oxidation of mercapto compounds).

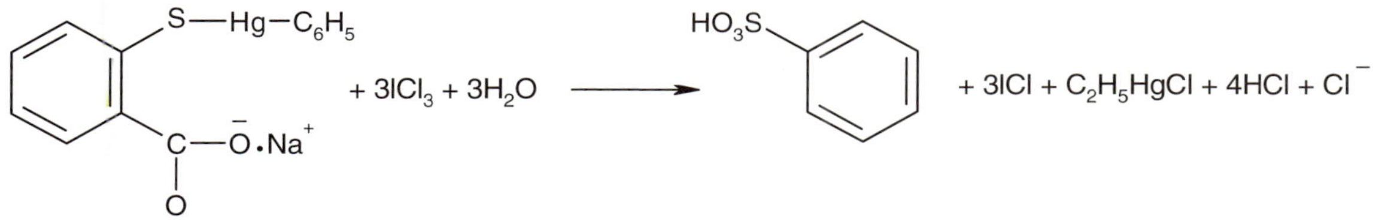

Thimerosal

Reference

K.K. Verma. *Talanta*, 27, 541-544, 1980.

Phenylephrine hydrochloride

Follow the method for estimation of phenylephrine described in the chapter on analgesics and antipyretics.

Benzalkonium chloride

Reagents

1. Acidified methanol.
2. Buffer solution, pH 10: Dissolve 3.09 g of boric acid, 3.725 g of potassium chloride and 1.75 g of sodium hydroxide in water to produce 1000 ml.
3. Methyl orange solution.

Standard solution

12.5 mcg/ml of benzalkonium chloride in water.

Sample solution

Transfer sample equivalent to 1.25 mg of the substance into 100 ml volumetric flask and dilute to volume with water (12.5 mcg/ml).

Procedure

Add 15 ml of pH 10 buffer and 1 ml methyl orange solution to two separating funnel. Shake well and let stand for two minutes. Pipette 3 ml of each sample, standard and water into separating funnels. Add 20 ml chloroform to each funnel and shake for two minutes. Separate chloroform layer and repeat the extraction procedure with another 10 ml portion of chloroform. Combine the two chloroform layers, dilute to 50 ml with chloroform. To 10 ml of chloroform layer, add 1 ml of acidified (HCl) methanol and measure the absorbance of sample and standard at 510 nm against reagent blank. The method is based on ion-pair complex formation.

Note

Before adding acidified methanol the chloroform layer shows λ_{max} 380 nm.

METHOD 2

Alternatively, we can use titration with sodium lauryl sulphate using dimethyl yellow as indicator.

Reagents

1. Dilute sulphuric acid.
2. 0.01% dimethyl yellow in methanol.
3. 0.1% sodium lauryl sulphate (SLS).

Sample and standard solutions

0.04% in water.

Procedure

Transfer 10 ml each of sample and standard solutions to two separating funnels, add 40 ml of water to each, shake. Then to each add 5 ml of dilute sulphuric acid and 1 ml of indicator (dimethyl yellow) and 20 ml of chloroform. Shake vigorously till chloroform layer is bright yellow. Then titrate with 'SLS' solution with vigorous shaking between two additions till chloroform layer changes to pink, the end point and calculate the results by calculation.

Neomycin sulphate

Follow the method described under formulation of the chapter on topical antifungal drugs involving the use of ninhydrin reagent; detailed reaction mechanism described.

Formulation 16

Naphazoline hydrochloride, Phenylephrine hydrochloride, Sulphacetamide sodium, Boric acid

ESTIMATION

Phenylephrine hydrochloride

Follow the method as described in the chapter on analgesics and antipyretics.

Naphazoline hydrochloride

Follow the method as described in formulation 11 of this chapter. Alternatively, method described in formulation 12 of this chapter may be used.

Sulphacetamide sodium

Transfer accurately measured aliquot of the sample equivalent to 250 mg of sulphacetamide sodium, add 10 ml of hydrochloric acid and about 50 ml of water. Shake and cool to 15°C. Titrate against 0.1 M sodium nitrite. Each ml of 1 M sodium nitrite is equivalent to 0.02362 g of sulphacetamide sodium.

Boric acid

Follow the method described in formulation 1 of this chapter.

Formulation 17

Naphazoline nitrate, Betamethasone sodium phosphate, Neomycin sulphate

ESTIMATION

Naphazoline nitrate

The following method is suitable for routine quality control.

Reagents

1. Dye solution: Dissolve 200 mg of bromophenol blue in 100 ml of distilled water and 6 ml of 0.1 N sodium hydroxide. Dilute to 250 ml with water.
2. Buffer solution: Dissolve 10.93 g of anhydrous disodium hydrogen phosphate and 10.93 g of anhydrous citric acid in water to make 1000 ml, adjust to pH 4.0.

Standard solution

50 mcg/ml of naphazoline nitrate in water.

Sample solution

Dilute accurately measured aliquot of the sample equivalent to 2.5 mg of the substance to 50 ml with water (50 mcg/ml).

Procedure

Into each of the three separating funnels, add 20 ml of buffer solution and 5 ml of dye solution. Add 5 ml of standard naphazoline nitrate solution, 5 ml aliquot of the sample solution and 5 ml of water (blank). To each separator, add 25 ml of chloroform and shake gently for one minute. Allow the layers to separate and collect the chloroform into 50 ml volumetric flasks. Repeat the extraction using 20 ml and 5 ml of chloroform. Adjust the volume to 50 ml with chloroform. Measure the absorption of the sample and standard solutions (405 nm) against the blank and calculate the naphazoline nitrate content in the sample by comparison.

The method is based on formation of ion-pair complex.

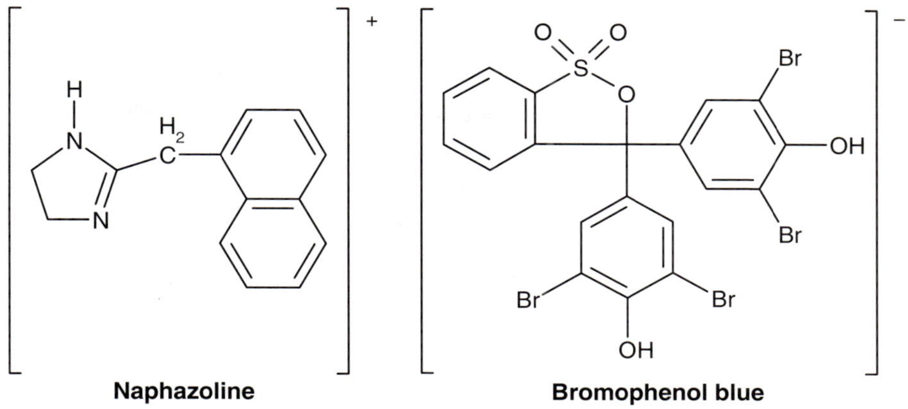

(λ_{max} 405 nm)

Reference

R.T. Sane & Sandhya Sane. *Indian Drugs*, **16(10)**, 239-241, 1979.

Betamethasone sodium phosphate

Follow the method described for estimation of dexamethasone sodium phosphate in formulation 8 of this chapter. Method is based on 'Porter-Silber' reaction i.e. reaction with phenyl hydrazine. Both reactions (a) and (b) are possible.

Neomycin sulphate

Follow the method described in formulation 15 of this chapter involving colour development with ninhydrin reagent.

Reaction Mechanism

15

Topical Antifungal and Anti-Infective Preparations

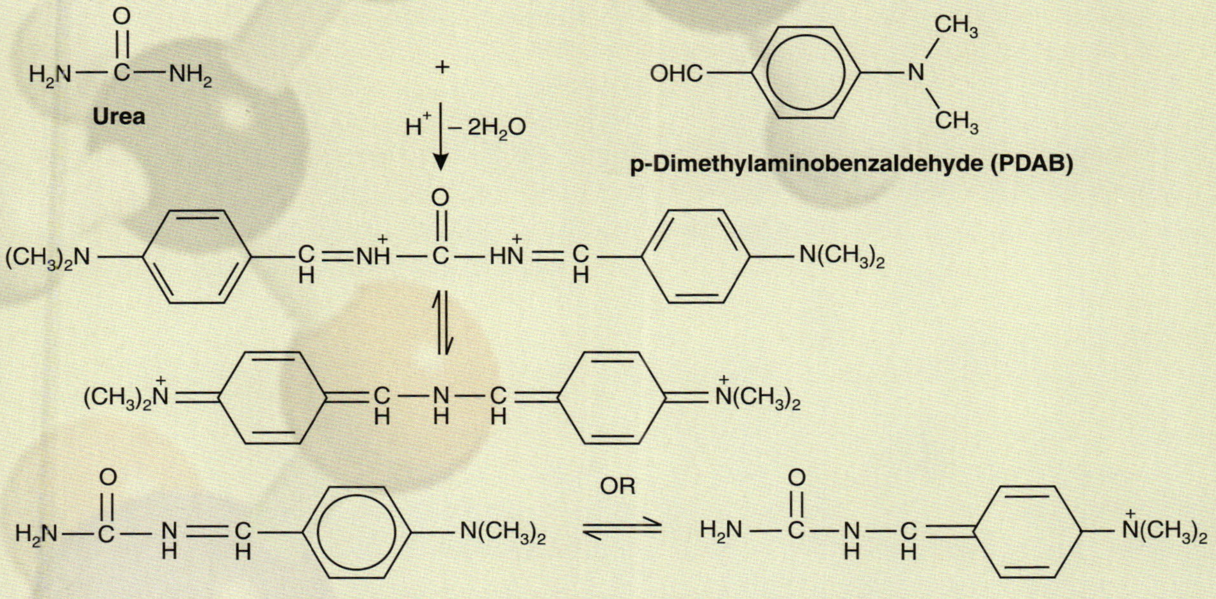

Yellow-coloured quinoid resonating Schiff's base
(λ_{max} 420 nm)

Formulation 1

Boric acid, Sulphanilamide, Acriflavine or Euflavine

ESTIMATION

Boric acid

Follow the method described in formulation 1 of the chapter on eye, ear & nasal preparations.

Sulphanilamide

Weigh accurately a quantity of the sample equivalent to 200 mg of sulphanilamide and dissolve in 75 ml of water and 10 ml of hydrochloric acid. Cool and titrate slowly with 0.1 M sodium nitrite at a temperature not above 15°C. The titration is complete when the end point is reproducible after the titrated solution has been allowed to stand for one min. Each ml of 0.1 M sodium nitrite is equivalent to 0.01722 g of sulphanilamide. Starch - iodide paste is used as external indicator.

Note

The method involves diazotization of aromatic amino group present in the drug.

Acriflavine

METHOD 1

Standard solution

10 mcg/ml of acriflavine in methyl alcohol.

Sample solution

Weigh accurate quantity of the aliquot equivalent to 2.5 mg of acriflavine, add 10 ml of methyl alcohol (in case of ointments and creams, heat on a boiling water-bath till base fully melts, cool) and dilute to 25 ml with methyl alcohol. An appropriate quantity of the above solution is further diluted with methyl alcohol to produce a concentration of 10 mcg/ml.

Procedure

Measure the absorption of the solutions at maximum at about 450 nm against methyl alcohol as blank. Calculate the results by comparing with the standard.

Note

The method is based on the spectrophotometric measurement of the inherent colour of the drug at 450 nm.

METHOD 2

Reagents

1. 1 N hydrochloric acid.
2. 0.05 M sodium nitrite in water.

Sample solution

100 mcg/ml of pure acriflavine in water.

Sample solution

Accurately weighed quantity of the sample is either diluted (in case of liquid preparation) or extracted with water by warming on water-bath to produce 100 mcg/ml concentration.

Procedure

To 2.5 ml each of the sample and standard solutions add 5 ml of 1 N hydrochloric acid and 1.5 ml of 0.05 M sodium nitrite and dilute to 25 ml with water. Measure the extinction at maximum at about 580 nm and deduce the results by comparison.

Acriflavine is a mixture of 3,6-diaminoacridine chloride (I) – 35% and 3,6-diamino-10-methyl acridinium chloride (II) – 65%. This method is based on the diazotization of aromatic amino group giving diazonium salt. With HNO_2, amino group at only position-6 is diazotized.

Probable Reaction Mechanism

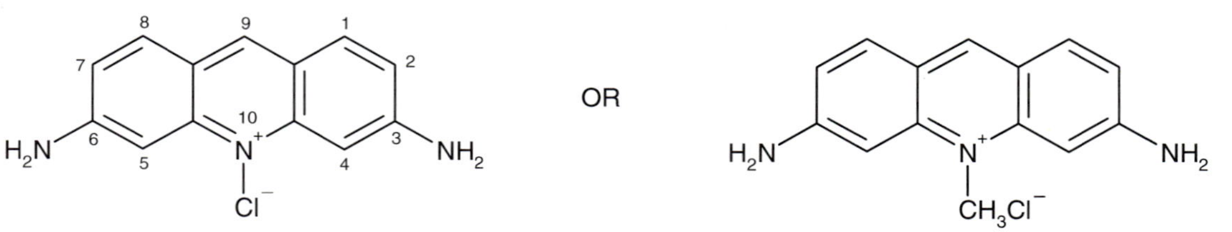

Acriflavine (3,6-diaminoacridine chloride (I)) OR **3,6-diamino-10-methyl acridinium chloride (II)**

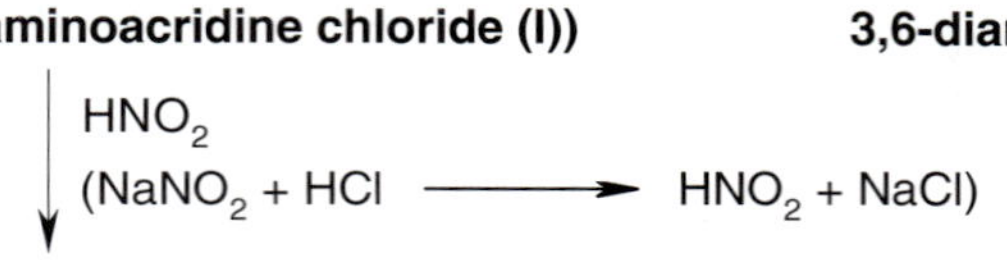

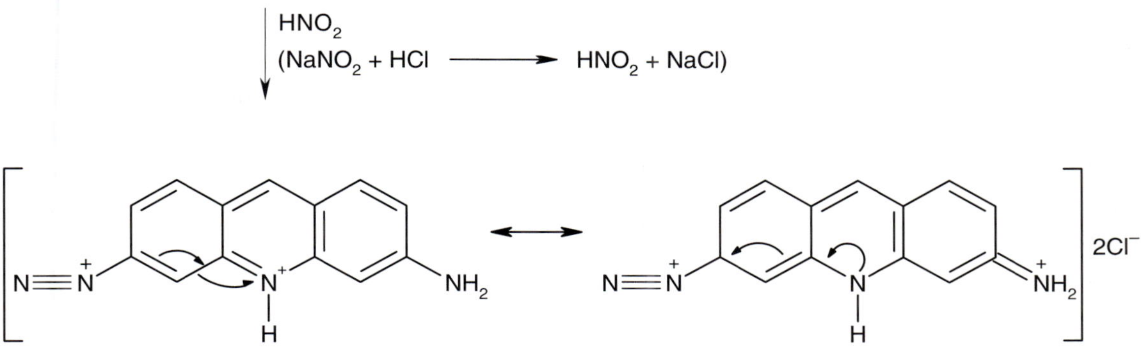

Vinylogous amidinium structure

Violet-coloured diazonium salt
(λ_{max} 580 nm)

Reference

Pharmaceutical Chemistry (Vol. 2) by H.J. Roth, p. 678.

The diazonium salt as usual can couple with phenols to form azo dyes and with aromatic aldehydes to form Schiff's bases.

Euflavine

Reagent

Methanolic hydrochloric acid: Dilute 100 ml of 0.5 N hydrochloric acid to 500 ml with methanol.

Standard solution

Dissolve about 25 mg of the euflavine accurately weighed (it is preferable to use the same batch of euflavine which is used to prepare the formulation) in 250 ml methanolic hydrochloric acid. Dilute 10 ml of the solution to 100 ml with the same solvents (10 mcg/ml).

Sample solution

Disperse accurate weight of the sample equivalent to 2.5 mg of euflavine in 50 ml of light petroleum ether (40-60°C). Extract the euflavine by shaking the mixture with 50, 20 and 20 ml volumes of methanolic hydrochloric acid, washing each extract with the same 20 ml of light petroleum and filtering it through a cotton wool plug into a 100 ml volumetric flask. Dilute the extracts to volume with methanolic hydrochloric acid. Dilute further with the solvent to get 10 mcg/ml concentration.

Procedure

Transfer 5 ml each of the sample and standard solutions into 50 ml volumetric flasks, dilute to 50 ml with methanolic hydrochloric acid. Measure the absorption of the solutions at about 462 nm with methanolic hydrochloric acid as blank. Calculate the results by comparison. This method is based on measurement of intrinsic colour of the compound spectrophotometrically (λ_{max} 460 nm).

Formulation 2

Benzocaine, Benzyl benzoate, Dicophane (DDT)

ESTIMATION

Benzocaine

Take accurately weighed quantity of the sample equivalent to 200 mg of benzocaine in beaker. Add 10 ml of water and 15 ml of hydrochloric acid. Heat to dissolve the benzocaine, cool the solution in an ice-bath to about 10°C and titrate with 0.1 M sodium nitrite until a blue colour is produced immediately, with starch iodide paste as an external indicator. Each ml of 0.1 N sodium nitrite is equivalent to 0.01652 g of benzocaine. Calculate the results from the volume of 0.1 M sodium nitrite consumed in the titration using the above factor. This method is based on diazotization of the primary amino group present in the drug. This is called nitrometric method.

Benzocaine can also be determined by UV visible spectrophotometry. In acidic medium, the NH_2 group is protonated and as a result there is no free pair of electrons available on the 'N' atom to exhibit resonance; hence decrease in absorption maxima.

Probable Reaction Mechanism

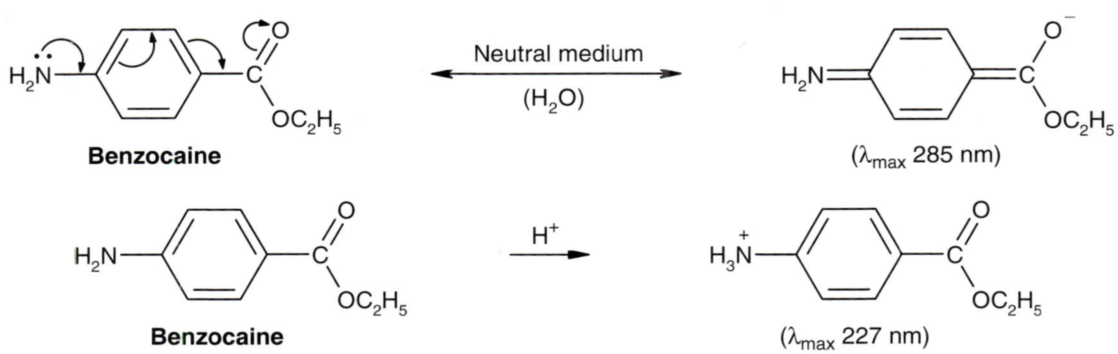

Note

The amino group is protonated, hence decrease in absorbance.

Reference

Indian Drugs, **25(3)**, 128, Dec. 1987.

Other methods involving diazotization and coupling with 'NED' reagent or β-naphthol, reaction with aromatic aldehyde (PDAB) involving reactions of primary amino group present in the molecule are described in different chapters of the book.

In stronger acid, the compound is hydrolysed to p-aminobenzoic acid.

Probable Reaction Mechanism

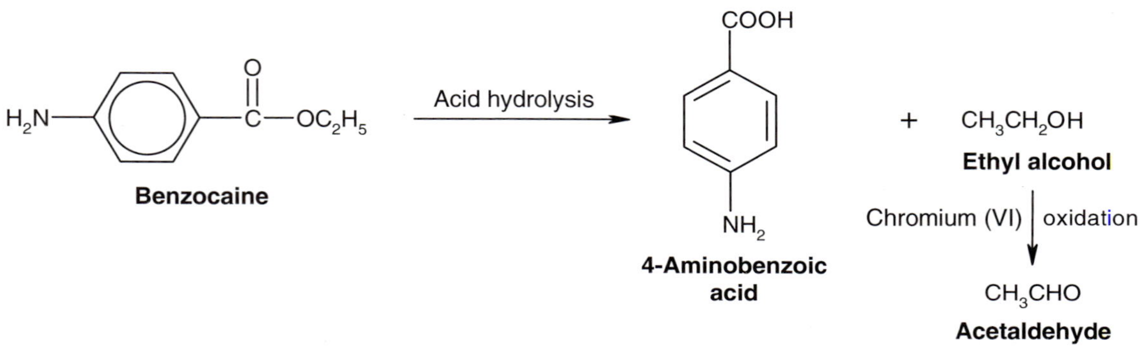

Acetaldehyde so formed answers Simon's reaction to give

$Na_3[Fe(CN)_5NO—CH_2CHO]$ – Coloured species

a blue-coloured complex based on reaction of aldehyde with disodium pentacyanonitrosyl ferrate (II) and piperidine (playing an intermediate role). It reacts with carbonyl (C==O) component to give an anamine, thus increasing nucleophilic activity.

Reference

Pharmaceutical Chemistry (Vol. 2) by H.J. Roth, p. 65.

The compound having primary —NH_2 group can be diazotized (HNO_2) coupled with β-naphthol and NED to give azo dyes. Further, the amino group gives condensation product with 'PDAB'.

Benzyl benzoate

Weigh accurately quantity of the sample equivalent to 2 g of benzyl benzoate and dissolve in 10 ml of neutralised alcohol. Neutralise the free acid with 0.1 N alcoholic potassium hydroxide using 0.2 ml solution of phenolphthalein as indicator. Add 50 ml of 0.5 N alcoholic potassium hydroxide, attach the flask to a reflux condenser, boil on water-bath for one hour. Add 20 ml of water and titrate the excess of alkali with 0.5 N sulphuric acid, using a further 0.2 ml of solution of phenolphthalein as indicator. Repeat the experiment with the same quantities of the reagents omitting the sample. The difference between the two titrations is equivalent to the alkali required to saponify benzyl benzoate. Each ml of 0.5 N alcoholic potassium hydroxide is equivalent to 0.1061 g of benzyl benzoate. Results are deduced by applying the above factor.

Explanatory Note

On refluxing with alcoholic potassium hydroxide, a saponification process, the compound is hydrolysed to give benzoic acid/potassium benzoate and excess alkali is back titrated with sulphuric acid. The amount of alkali actually used to saponify the compound is used for calculations.

Probable Reaction Mechanism

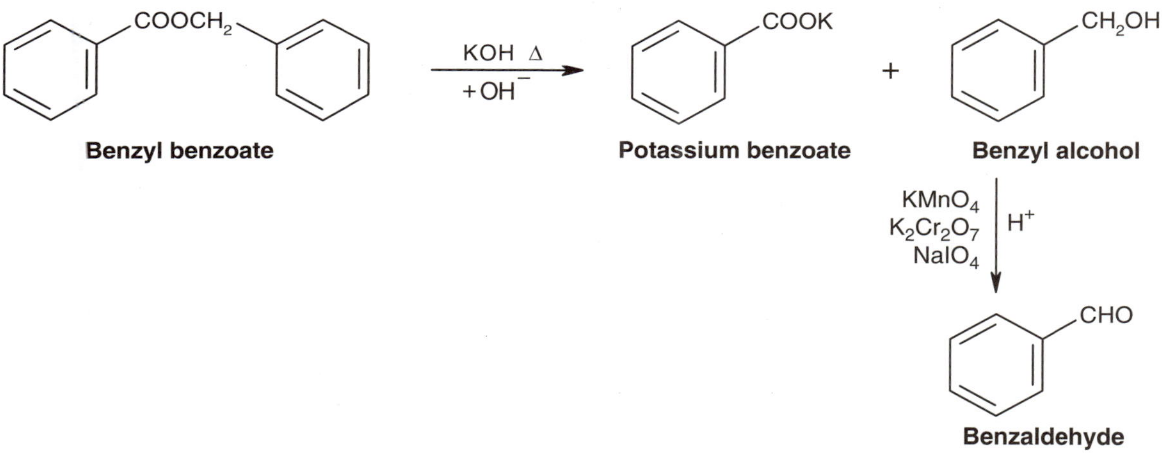

$$2\ KOH + H_2SO_4 \longrightarrow K_2SO_4 + 2\ H_2O$$

Note

In acidic medium, benzyl alcohol is oxidized to benzaldehyde.

DDT (Dicophane) - Dichlorodiphenyltrichloroethane

Weigh accurately sample equivalent to 250 mg of DDT and boil under a reflux condenser for thirty minutes with 20 ml of alcohol and 1 g of sodium hydroxide. Add 20 ml of water, 15 ml of dilute nitric acid and 20 ml of 0.1 N silver nitrate, shake vigorously and titrate with 0.1 N ammonium thiocyanate using ferric alum as indicator. Perform the blank experiment with the same quantities of the reagents omitting the sample. Each ml of 0.1 N silver nitrate is equivalent to 0.00709 g of DDT. On alkaline hydrolysis, the compound yields five chlorides (5 Cl^-); hence the equivalent

Formulation 3

Urea, Glycine, Ammonium chloride, Sodium chloride, Potassium chloride, Magnesium chloride, Sodium acid phosphate, Calcium lactate, Lactic acid, Hydrocortisone acetate

ESTIMATION

Urea

METHOD 1

Weigh accurately a quantity of the sample equivalent to 0.5 g of urea, add about 50 ml of water and extract with four 30 ml portions of chloroform. Wash the combined chloroform layer with 20 ml of water and add the water washing to the aqueous extract. Dilute aqueous extract to 250 ml with water (solution A).

To 20 ml of the solution A, add 90 ml of glacial acetic acid and 10 ml of xanthydrol solution (10% w/v in methanol). Mix and allow to stand at room temperature for 60 minutes. Filter through previously weighed G_3 sintered glass crucible. Wash the precipitates with 20-25 ml methanol and dry at 105°C to constant weight. Each g of the residue is equivalent to 0.1425 g of the urea.

Explanatory Note

The gravimetric assay method is based on reaction of urea with xanthydrol in acidic medium, the complex being insoluble in methanol and water is estimated gravimetrically.

End-position NH_2 group is reactive. Xanthydrol is a non-specific reagent for urea derivatives, imides, sulphonamides, amines and compounds with activated methylene group. In acid medium, xanthydrol produces carbenium ion which is nucleophilically substituted by urea to give insoluble precipitates, insoluble in methanol, the basis for gravimetric assay method.

Probable Reaction Mechanism

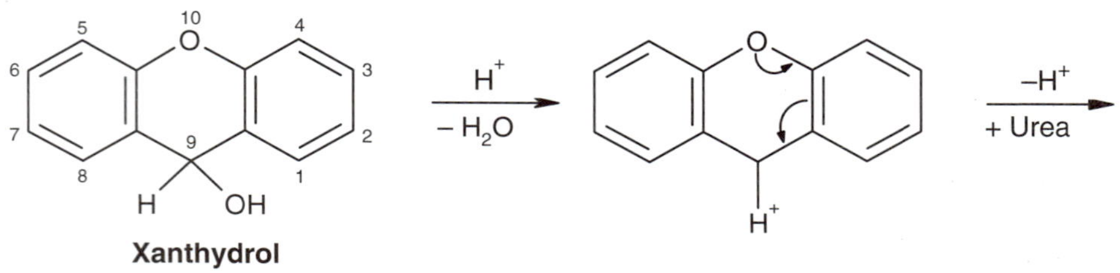

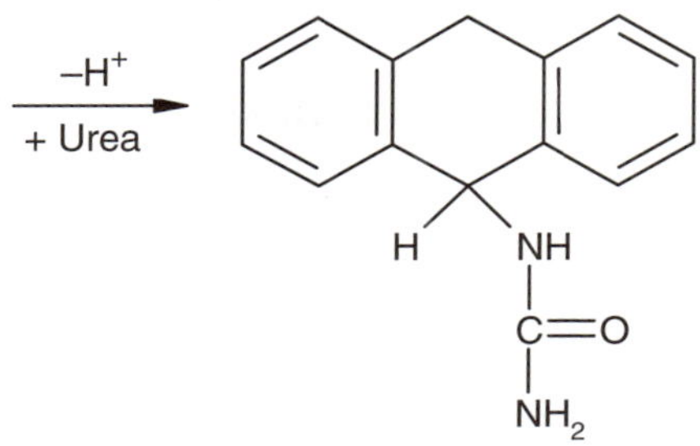

Xanthydrol - urea insoluble complex

Note

Urea can be estimated by Kjeldahl method involving estimation of evolved ammonia.

On dry heating urea, it produces ammonia along with biuret and cyanuric acid. Biuret complexes with copper(II) in alkaline medium to give violet-coloured complex.

Probable Reaction Mechanism

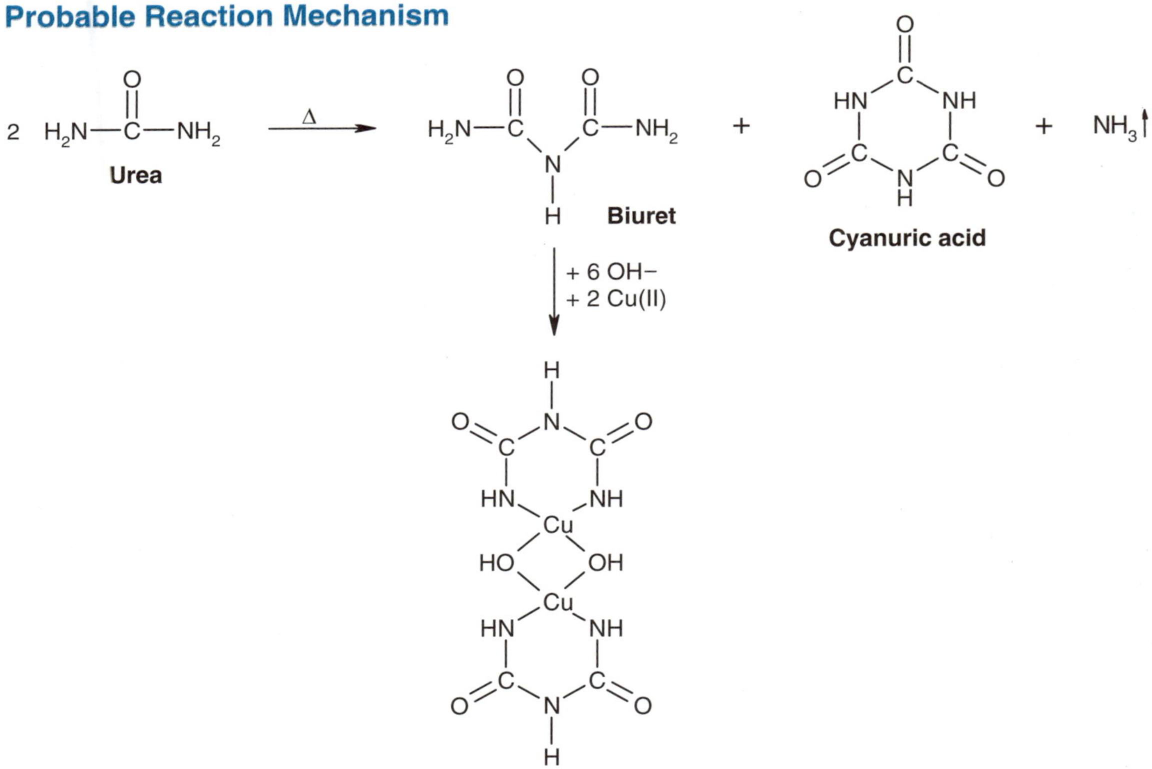

Violet-coloured copper complex
(λ_{max} 545 nm)

Note

Biuret forms three different Cu(II) complexes depending on the pH and ratio of NH-functions to Cu(II) ions.

Reference

Pharmaceutical Chemistry (Vol. 2) by H.J. Roth, pp. 240 & 294.

METHOD 2

Reagents

1. Urease.
2. 1 N sodium hydroxide.
3. Nessler's reagent.
4. 0.05 M zinc sulphate.

Standard solution

2 mg/ml of urea in water.

Sample solution

Weigh accurately sample equivalent to 500 mg of urea and suspend in 100-150 ml of water, warm gently in water-bath till uniform suspension is obtained. Cool and dilute to 250 ml with water, filter and use the filtrate as sample solution for analysis.

Procedure

To 7.5 ml each of sample and standard solutions, add 200 mg of urease dissolved in 50 ml of water and incubate at 37°C for 45 min. Run individual blanks (sample and standard) adding 50 ml of water instead of urease solution. Cool all the four flasks to room temperature and add to each 2 ml of 0.05 M zinc sulphate solution and 1 ml of 1 N sodium hydroxide solution and finally dilute to 250 ml with water, mix and filter. To 2 ml each of the four filtrates add 30 ml of water and 2 ml of Nessler's reagent and dilute to 50 ml. Keep at room temperature for 10 min and measure the absorbance of both sample and standard solutions at 400 nm against respective blanks and calculate the results by comparison.

Probable Reaction Mechanism

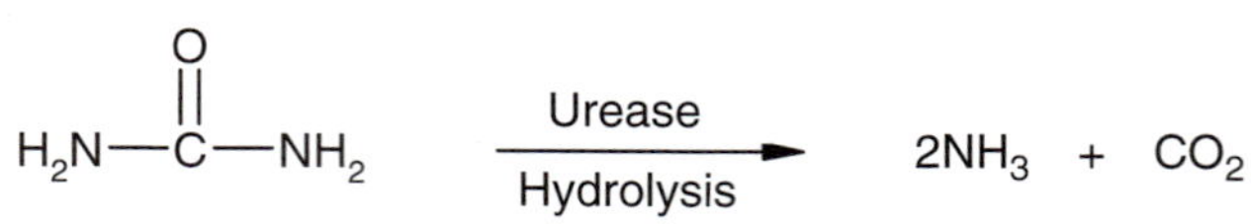

Ammonia is estimated by Nessler's reagent.

Note

Zinc sulphate is added to remove excess urease as it will interfere with colour development. Sodium tungstate can also be used for this purpose.

METHOD 3

Reagents

1. 4% w/v solution of PDAB in methanol.
2. 4% solution of sulphuric acid in methanol.

Standard solution

500 μg/ml in methanol.

Sample solution

Suspend sample equivalent to 25 mg of the sample in 20 ml of methanol, heat on water-bath to disperse the sample, shake for 30 min and dilute to 50 ml with methanol. Filter through Whatman No. 42 filter paper and use the filtrate for analysis.

Procedure

To 1 ml each of the reagents (1) and (2) add 2 ml of the sample and standard solutions. After 10 min measure the absorbance at 420 nm against reagent blank.

Note

The method is regularly used by laboratories while analysing moisture creams.

Explanatory Note

The method involves formation of Schiff's base with quinoid resonating structure (λ_{max} 420 nm).

Probable Reaction Mechanism

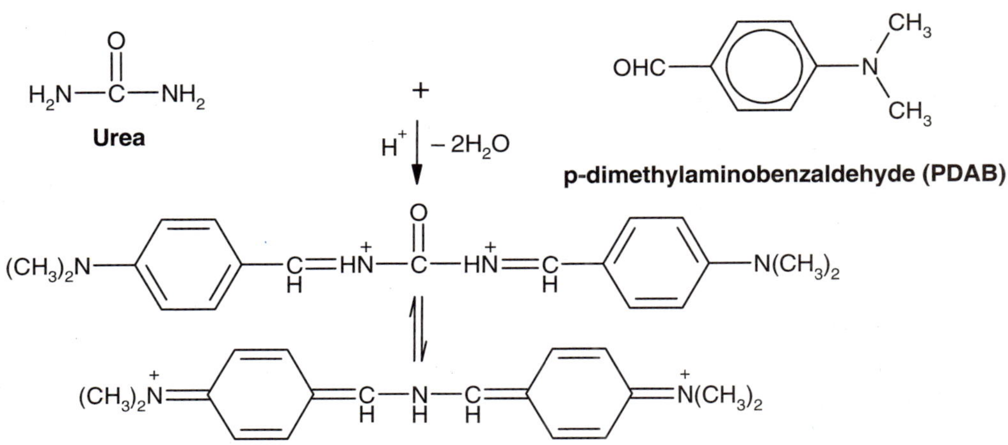

OR

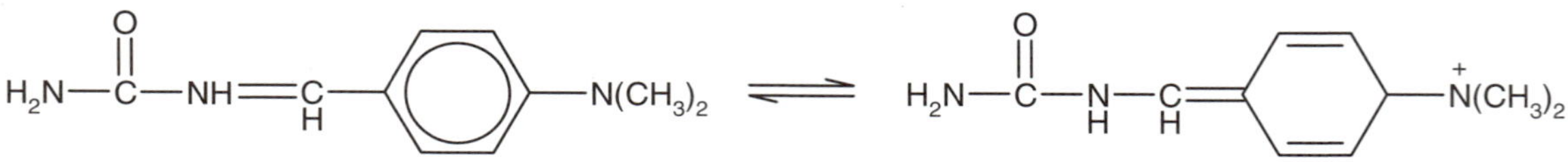

Yellow-coloured quinoid resonating Schiff's base
(λ_{max} 420 nm)

Note

The author also described HPTLC method and the results were comparable by both the methods.

Reference

Miriam T. Knorst, Reinhard Neubert & Wolfgang Wohlrab, *J. Pharm. & Biomed. Analysis*, **15(11)**, 1627-1632, 1997.

Total chlorides

Take 100 ml of the solution A, add 10 ml of nitric acid and boil. Add 25 ml of 0.1 N silver nitrate to the boiling solution. Digest the precipitates for 30 minutes on water-bath. Filter and wash the precipitates 4-5 times with water. The combined filtrate is titrated with 0.1 N ammonium thiocyanate using 2 ml solution of ferric alum as indicator, run blank. Each ml of 0.1 N silver nitrate is equivalent to 0.003545 g of chloride.

Total nitrogen

Take 10 ml of solution A in 500 ml Kjeldahl flask, add about 10 g of anhydrous potassium sulphate, 0.5 g of copper sulphate and 20 ml of sulphuric acid. Heat till the solution is green or blue. Cool and attach to ammonia distillation apparatus. The receiving flask should contain 50 ml of 1% boric acid. Add 100 ml of 3% w/v sodium hydroxide solution and heat. Collect about 125 ml of distillate and titrate the distillate with 0.1 N hydrochloric acid. Calculate nitrogen contents as under:

$$\text{\% of total nitrogen} = \frac{\text{Titre value (ml)} \times 0.001402 \times 100 \times \text{dilution factor}}{\text{Weight of the sample (g) taken for analysis}}$$

Hydrocortisone acetate

Follow the method described in formulation 2 of the chapter on keratolytics and cleansers.

Glycine (Aminoacetic acid)

Reagent

Indicator solution: 75 mg of phenolphthalein and 25 mg of thymol blue are dissolved in sufficient alcohol (50% v/v) to produce 100 ml.

Procedure

Weigh accurately a quantity of the sample equivalent to 100 ml of glycine, add 50 ml of water and shake. Filter, add 10 ml of formaldehyde previously neutralised to pH 9.0 and 4-5 drops of indicator solution. Titrate with 0.1 N sodium hydroxide until the yellow colour disappears and a faint violet colour appears. Each ml of 0.1 N sodium hydroxide consumed is equivalent to 0.007507 g of glycine.

Note

The method is based on formol titration of the carboxylic group present in the drug.

The amino acids are usually neutral as both basic (NH2 group) and acidic (carboxyl group) are present. In aqueous solution, protonation of the amino group and ionization of carboxyl function occurs — "Zwitterions".

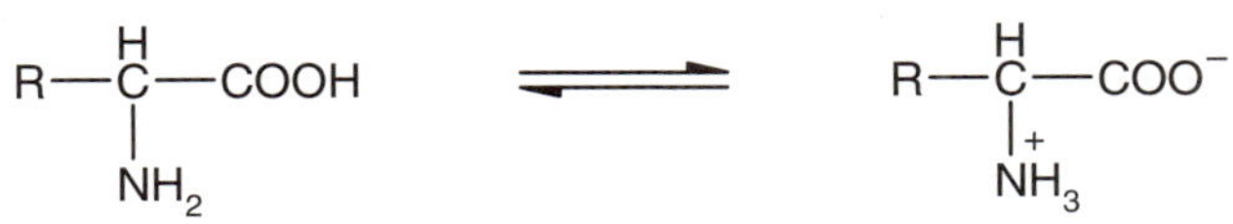

However, as suggested by Schiff (Schiff, H. Annalon, 319, 59, 1901 & 325, 348, 1902 — through Pharmaceutical Analysis by T. Higuchi, p. 269) that the presence of formaldehyde permitted titration of amino acids as acids. Different authors have proposed the reaction between NH_2 and formaldehyde in different ways.

Probable Reaction Mechanism

(a)

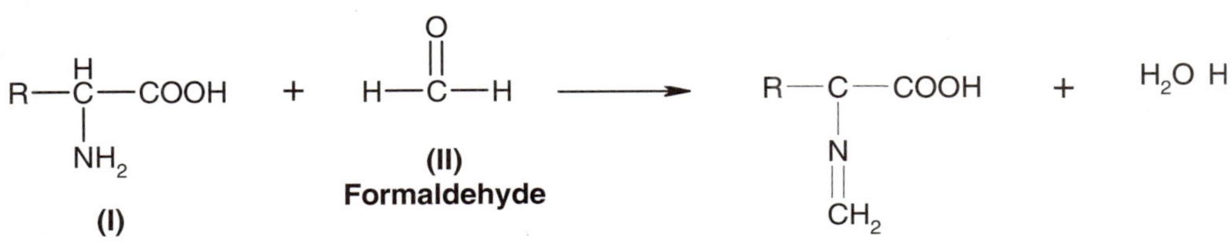

Reference

Sørensen, S.P.L., Pharmaceutical Analysis, T. Higuchi et al., p. 269.

(b)

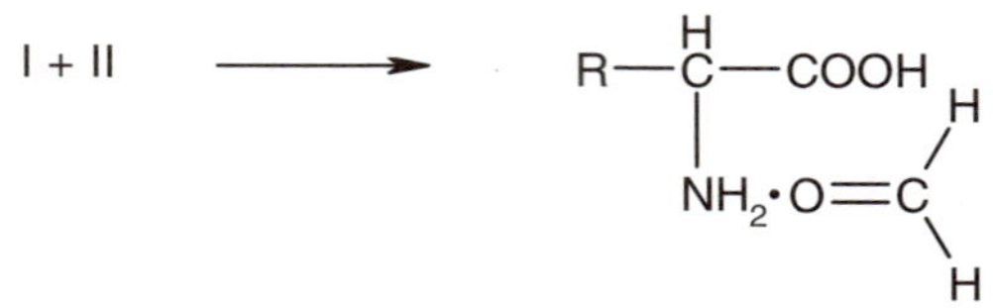

Reference

L.J. Harris, *Biochem. J.*, **24**, 1080, 1930.

(c)

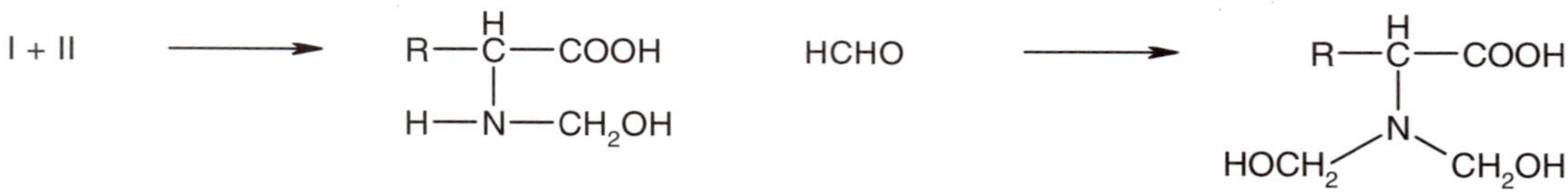

Reference

M. Levy, *J. Biol. Chem.*, 99767, 1973.

This reaction of amino group with formaldehyde destroys the zwitterion properties of the molecule in relation to carboxyl functions and allows the titration of carboxyl group (COOH) exhibiting usual properties of an organic acid which can be titrated with alkali. This is called formol titration.

Glycine, like other α-amino acid, is a chelate former. With Cu(II) it forms a coloured chelate in alkaline medium. This reaction is often used for analytical purposes.

Probable Reaction Mechanism

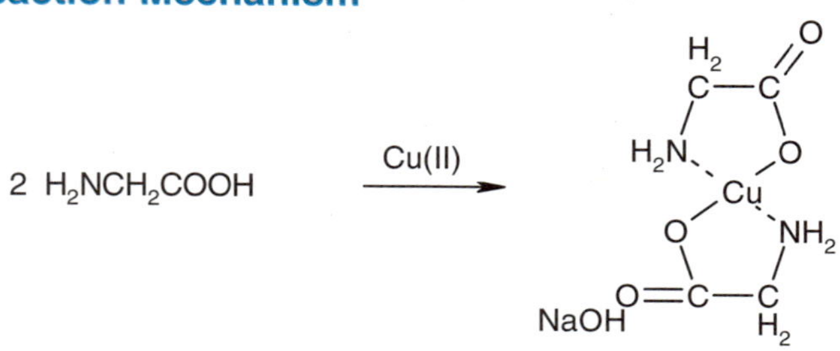

Blue-coloured copper chelate

In addition to its reaction with ninhydrin, other reactions of analytical interest are:

(1) Reaction with 2,4-dinitrofluorobenzene involving attack by amino acid on activated aromatic moiety.

(2) Condensation with dansyl chloride and fluorescamine to give fluorescent derivatives.

Probable Reaction Mechanism

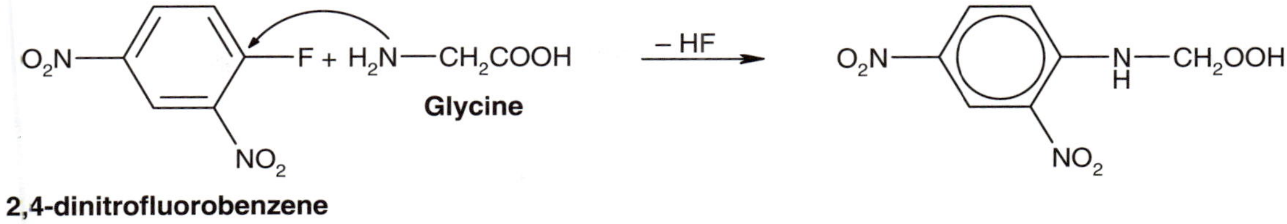

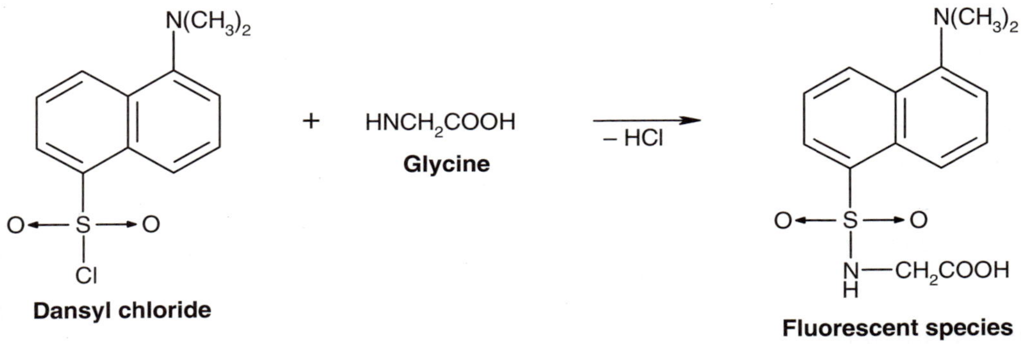

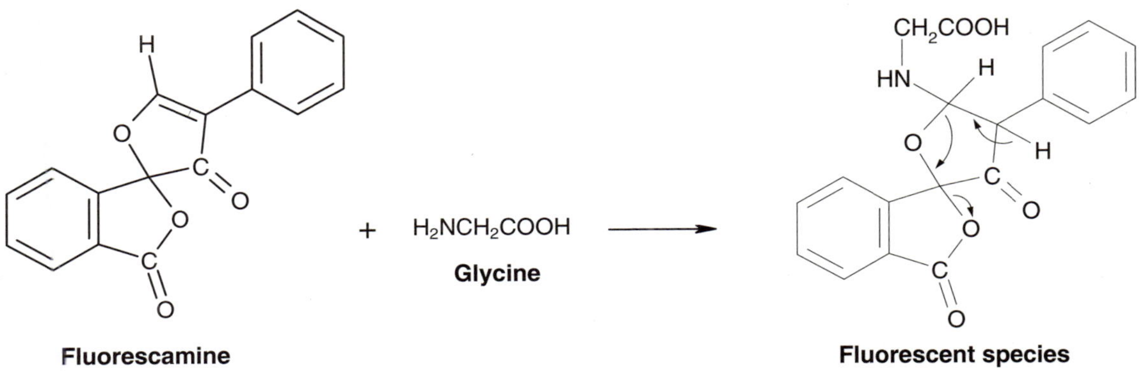

Reference

Pharmaceutical Chemistry (Vol. 2) by H.J. Roth, pp. 215-216.

S.A. Shah et al. and others have described a spectrophotometric method for primary aliphatic amines by reaction of dichlone with glycine or alanine in sodium bicarbonate medium to produce orange-coloured derivative (λ_{max} 470 nm).

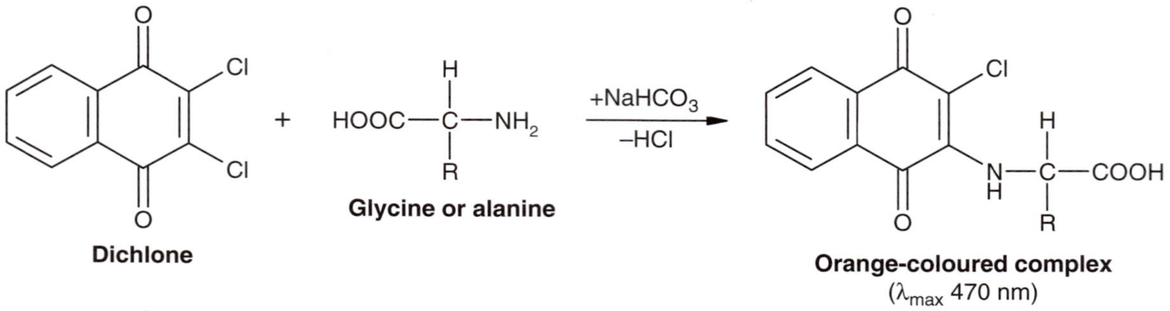

Reference

1. Abou-Ouf A.A., Taha A.M. & Saidhom M.B., *J. Pharm. Sci.*, **62**, 1700-1704, 1973.
2. S.A. Shah et al., *Ind. J. Pharm. Sci.*, **69(3)**, 462-464, 2007.

Sodium acid phosphate, Calcium lactate, Magnesium chloride

Follow the method described in chapter on alimentary drugs.

Note

Conventional method of estimation by EDTA titration is not possible in the presence of phosphate as both calcium and magnesium get precipitated out with ammonia.

Formulation 4

Clotrimazole/Econazole nitrate, Betamethasone dipropionate, Gentamycin sulphate

ESTIMATION

Clotrimazole

METHOD 1

Suspend accurately weighed quantity of sample in 100 ml of warm water, cool and extract with chloroform (3 × 25 ml), passing each extract through anhydrous sodium sulphate. Evaporate combined chloroform extract to dryness at 105°C. Dissolve the residue in previously neutralized glacial acetic acid (0.02 M perchloric acid). Carry out non-aqueous titration with 0.02 M perchloric acid using α-naphtholbenzein solution as indicator. Each ml of 0.02 M perchloric acid is equivalent to 6.896 mg of clotrimazole or 8.894 mg of econazole nitrate.

METHOD 2

Reagents

1. 0.1 N citric acid in water.
2. 0.1% w/v solution of acid orange 4S in 40% aqueous methanol (dye).

Standard solution

100 mcg/ml in 0.1 N hydrochloric acid.

Sample solution

100 mcg/ml in 0.1 N hydrochloric acid (see formulation 5 of this chapter).

Procedure

To 1 ml each of sample and standard solutions add 3 ml of citric acid solution and 2 ml of dye solution. Extract the colour with three 8 ml portions of chloroform. Make up the volume to 25 ml and pass through anhydrous sodium sulphate. The solution has absorption maxima at 422 nm. It follows Beer's law in the range of 2-14 mcg/ml, with detection limit of 0.05 μg/ml.

Note

Hydrolytic product of clotrimazole, betamethasone and lignocaine do not interfere. The method was found to be suitable for vaginal tablets, creams and optical solutions.

METHOD 3

Another method based on ion-pair complex formation was described by Sane et al. (1981).

Probable Reaction Mechanism

Ion pair complex formation takes place between the drug and the dye which is extracted with $CHCl_3$.

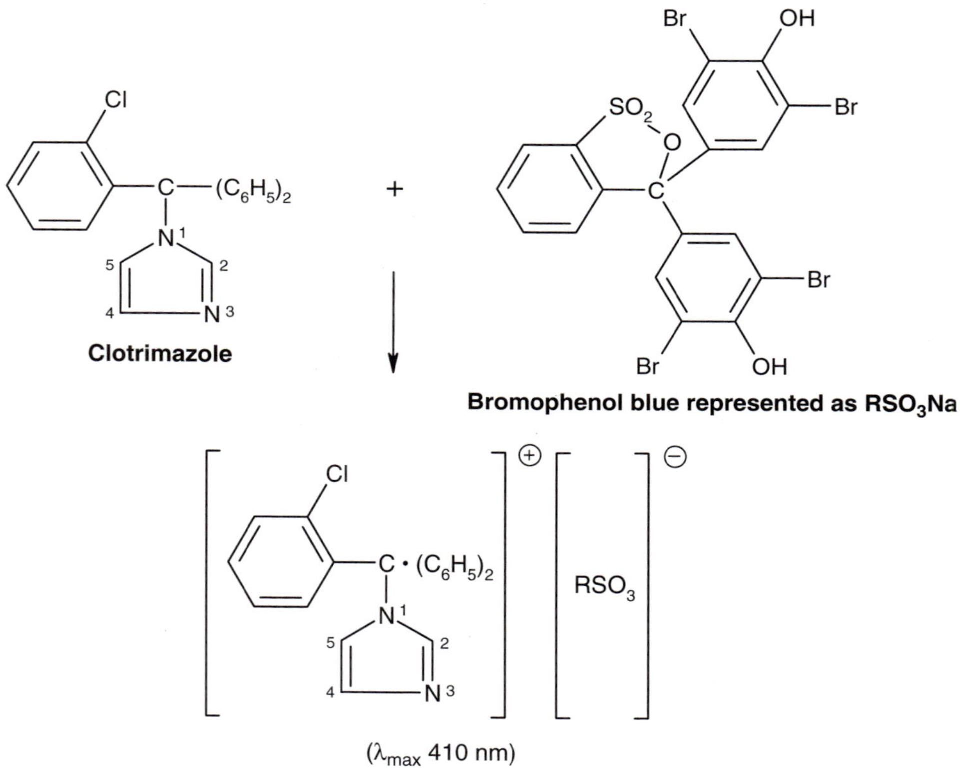

Reference

R.T. Sane et al., *Indian Drugs*, **18(11)**, 405, 1981.

In acidic medium (cerric ammonium sulphate) the drug will couple with MBTH reagent at electron-rich site in the drug. This reaction is similar to the one described for miconazole/econazole.

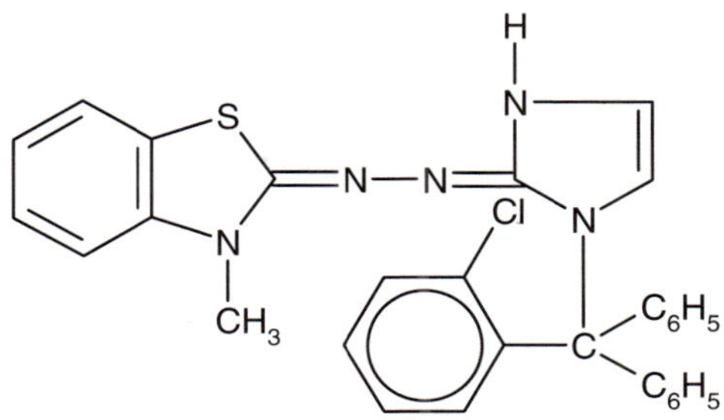

Clotrimazole, an imidazole derivative, will also react with Pauly reagent i.e. reaction with diazotized sulphanilic acid. The coupling takes place at position 2 of the heteroaromatic ring to produce azo dye. This reaction is similar to the one described for histamine.

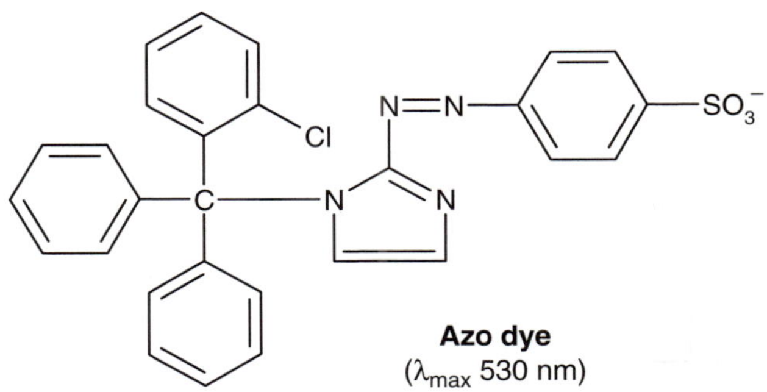

Azo dye
(λ_{max} 530 nm)

Note

Other electrophilic reagents preferably attack positions 4 and 5.

Reference

Pharmaceutical Chemistry (Vol. 2) by H.J. Roth, p. 520.

Betamethasone dipropionate

METHOD 1

Follow the method described in this chapter for beclomethasone dipropionate.

METHOD 2

Reagents

1. Acidic methanol: Dilute 1.2 ml of hydrochloric acid to 1000 ml with methanol.
2. 0.5 M sodium chloride solution in water.
3. INH reagent: Dissolve 50 mg of isonicotinic acid hydrazide in 200 ml of acidic methanol.

Standard solution

20 mcg/ml of betamethasone dipropionate in chloroform.

Sample solution

Suspend accurately weighed quantity of the sample (cream) equivalent to 2 mg of betamethasone dipropionate in 30 ml of methanol (90%) and 50 ml of n-hexane, shake till cream is completely dispersed. Transfer the contents to a separating funnel and shake vigorously. Separate lower layer (methanol-water), extract organic layer with quantity of acid - methanol (2 × 20 ml). Combine the aqueous layer and discard the n-hexane layer. Add 100 ml of 0.5 M sodium chloride solution and extract with chloroform (3 × 30 ml), passing each extract through a bed of anhydrous sodium sulphate. Make up the volume to 100 ml with chloroform (20 mcg/ml).

Procedure

Evaporate 20 ml each of sample and standard solutions to dryness in water-bath at 60°C, cool and add 25 ml of INH reagent to each and keep in water-bath (50°C) for 90 min. Cool and measure the absorbance of both the solutions at 405 nm against reagent blank and calculate the results by comparison.

Note

The reaction is similar to the one described under method 3 involving phenyl-hydrazine.

METHOD 3

Porter & Silber have described method for analysis of steroids with 17,21-dihydroxy-20 keto group based on reaction with phenylhydrazine - sulphuric acid to give a coloured chromogen.

Probable Reaction Mechanism

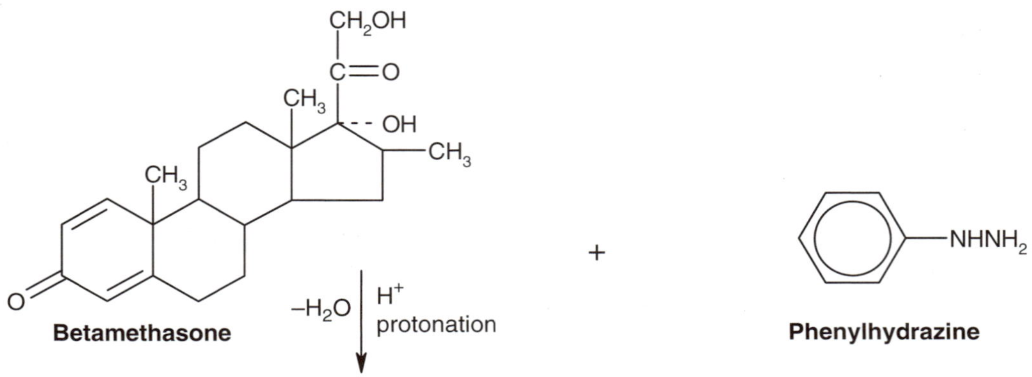

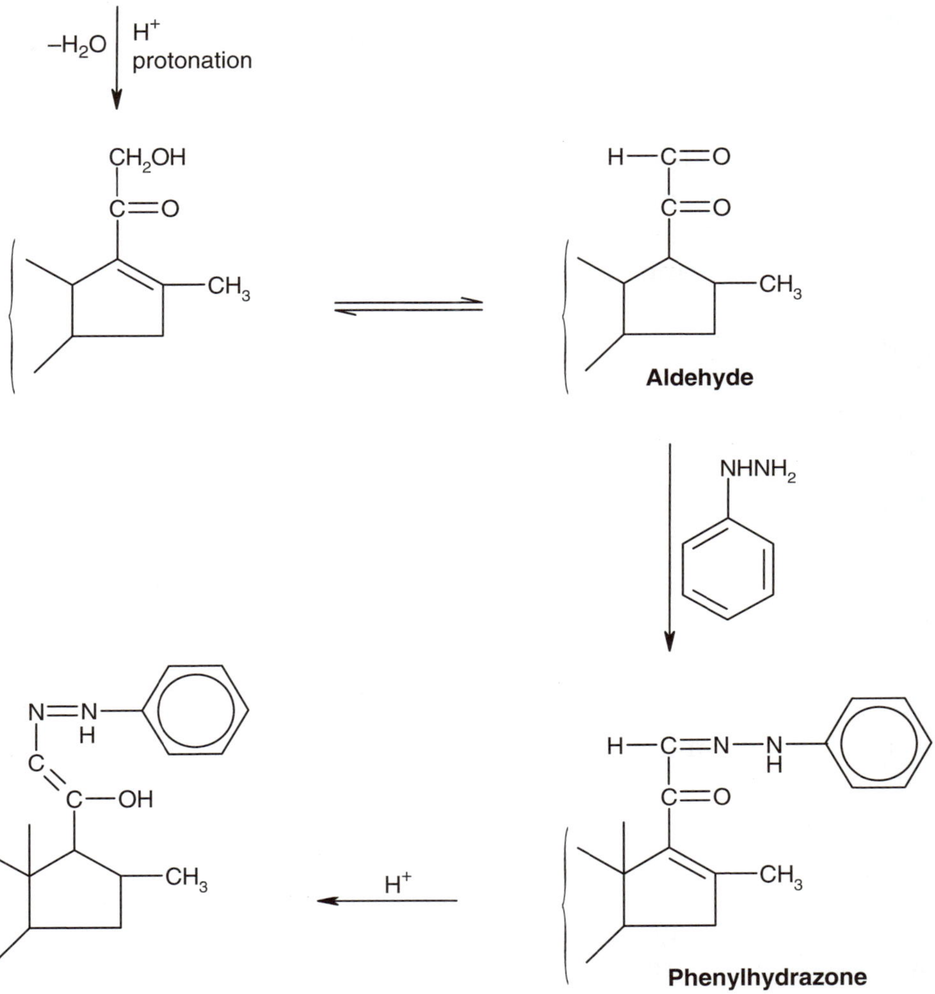

Stabilized phenylhydrazone
(λ_{max} 450 nm)

Reference

1. R.H. Silber & C.C. Porter, *J. Biol. Chem.*, **210**, 923, 1954.
2. C.C. Porter & R.H. Silber, *J. Biol. Chem.*, **185**, 201, 1950.

Depending on the reaction conditions, Cornall & MacDonald (1953) have reported that 2,4-dinitrophenylhydrazine shall react with α,β-unsaturated carbonyl (C==O) group at C-3 of ring 'A' to produce yellow-coloured product which is converted into deep red by addition of alkali by forming a stabilized quinoid structure due to removal of a proton.

Probable Reaction Mechanism

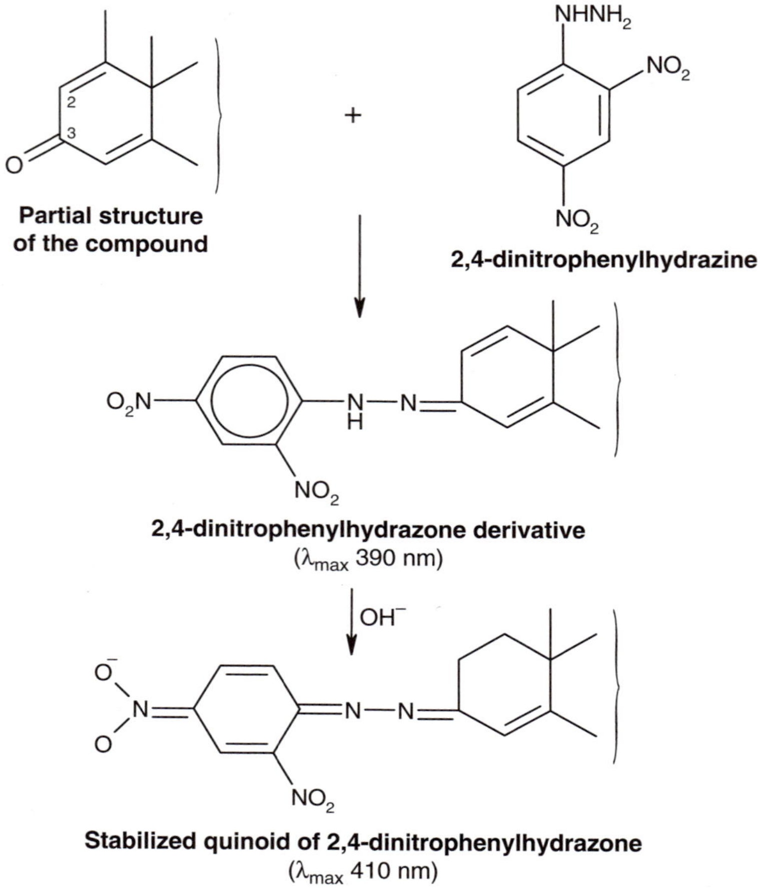

Reference

A.G. Cornall & M.P. MacDonald, *J. Biol. Chem.*, **210**, 279, 1953.

A spectrophotometric method based on reduction of C-3 carbonyl group in conjugated keto steroids (prednisolone) with sodium borohydrate followed by decrease in UV absorbance was reported by S. Görög (1968).

Reference

S. Görög, *J. Pharm. Sci.*, **57(10)**, 1737-1741, 1968.

Gentamycin

Reagents

1. 1.25% w/v aqueous solution of ninhydrin.

2. Phosphate buffer, pH 7.4: Mix 50 ml of 0.2 M potassium acid phosphate solution with 39.1 ml of 0.2 M sodium hydroxide solution, dilute to 200 ml with water.

Standard solution

200 µg/ml in pH 7.4 phosphate buffer.

Sample solution

200 µg/ml in pH 7.4 phosphate buffer.

Procedure

To 5 ml each of sample and standard solutions add 1 ml of ninhydrin reagent and dilute to 10 ml with pH 7.4 buffer, heat at 95°C for 15 min, cool in ice water bath and measure the absorbance of both sample and standard at 400 nm against blank prepared by adding 1 ml of ninhydrin reagent to 10 ml of phosphate buffer and proceeding as above.

Note

The chromogen was stable for 4 hrs. when stored in ice water and protected from light. However, it is preferable to take measurements within 1 hr.

Probable Reaction Mechanism

On heating the solution of drug with ninhydrin, the formed amine reacts with another mole of ninhydrin to give coloured complex (λ_{max} 400 nm).

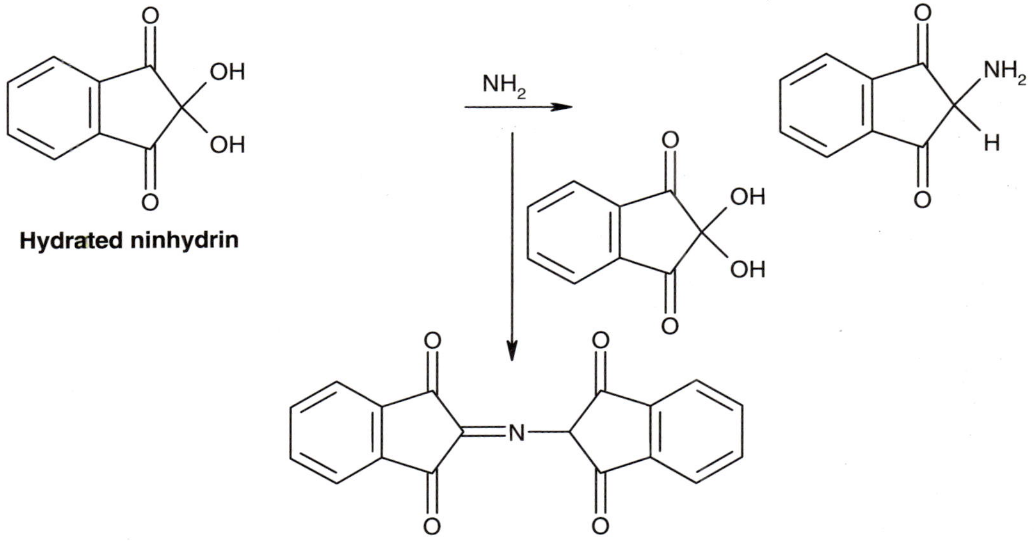

Coloured complex
(λ_{max} 400 nm)

Reference

P. Frutos, Susana Torrado, M.E. Perez-Lorenzo & G. Frutos, *J. Pharm. & Biomed. Analysis*, **21**, 1149-1159, 2000.

Earlier Wang et al. have reported a sensitive method for the estimation of gentamycin. 'PDAB' solution (1%) was prepared in acetic acid and adjusted to pH 4.1 with acetic acid/sodium acetate buffer. Coloured Schiff's base has λ_{max} 405 nm.

In both the methods 'PDAB' forms Schiff's base with amino group present in the substance. For detailed reaction mechanism, refer to the above method.

Probable Reaction Mechanism

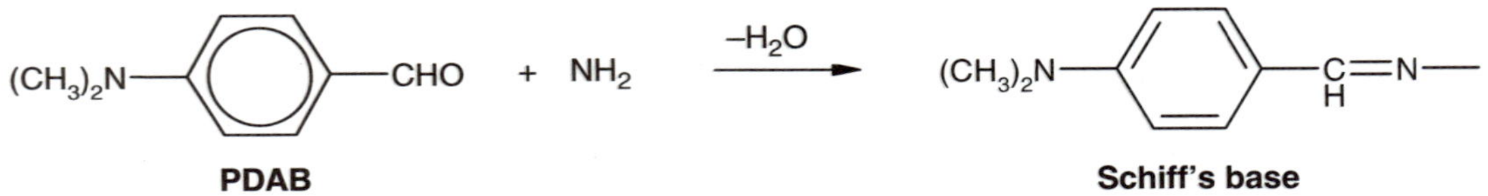

Reference

Huaiyou Wang, Jiancheng Ren & Yiu Zhang, *Talanta*, **40(6)**, 851-853, 1993.

Formulation 5

Miconazole nitrite, Neomycin sulphate, Betamethasone valerate

ESTIMATION

Miconazole nitrite

Reagents

1. Bromothymol blue solution (BTB): Dissolve 50 mg of water in 2 ml of 0.05 N sodium hydroxide and dilute to 500 ml with potassium biphthalate buffer, pH 3.5.
2. Potassium biphthalate buffer, pH 3.5.

Standard solution

400 mcg/ml of miconazole nitrate in chloroform.

Sample solution

Use chloroform extract reserved during estimation of neomycin sulphate.

Procedure

To 2 ml each of sample and standard solutions add 10 ml of bromothymol blue solution and 50 ml of chloroform. Shake and transfer the chloroform layer to a 100 ml volumetric flask through a layer of anhydrous sodium sulphate. Make up the volume and measure the absorbance of both sample and standard solutions at 410 nm against reagent blank and calculate the results by comparison.

Note

The method is based on formation of ion-pair complex with BTB in pH 3.5 buffer. The complex is extractable into chloroform.

Neomycin sulphate

Reagents

1. Phosphate buffer, pH 8.0: Dissolve 16.73 g of dipotassium hydrogen phosphate (anhydrous) and 0.523 g of potassium dihydrogen phosphate (anhydrous) in water to produce 1000 ml, adjust pH to 8.0.

2. Citrate buffer, pH 5.0: Dissolve 2.94 g of sodium citrate, monohydrate in 100 ml of water, add 2.10 g of citric acid, dilute to 200 ml, adjust pH to 5.0.
3. Ninhydrin reagent:
   (a) 80 mg of sodium chloride is dissolved in citrate buffer to produce 50 ml (heating may be required to dissolve).
   (b) 4.0% w/v solution of ninhydrin in water or methanol. Mix equal volumes of (a) and (b) just before estimation.

Standard solution

100 mcg/ml of neomycin sulphate in phosphate buffer, pH 8.0.

Sample solution

Weigh sample (cream) equivalent to 10.0 mg of neomycin sulphate, suspend in 25 ml of phosphate buffer and extract with chloroform (3 × 30 ml). Collect chloroform in a dry 100 ml volumetric flask filtering each layer through same anhydrous sodium sulphate bed. Rinse sodium sulphate layer with chloroform, the combined chloroform layer is made up to volume (reserve chloroform layer for estimation of miconazole nitrate and betamethasone valerate). Aqueous buffered layer, heated in water-bath till no perceptible smell of chloroform, is diluted to 100 ml with phosphate buffer and used for estimation of neomycin sulphate.

Procedure

To 5 ml each of sample, standard and buffer solutions add 5 ml of freshly prepared ninhydrin reagent and heat in water-bath for 20 min, cool, add 2 ml of methanol and dilute to 50 ml with phosphate buffer. Measure the absorbance of sample and standard against reagent blank at 570 nm and calculate the results by comparison.

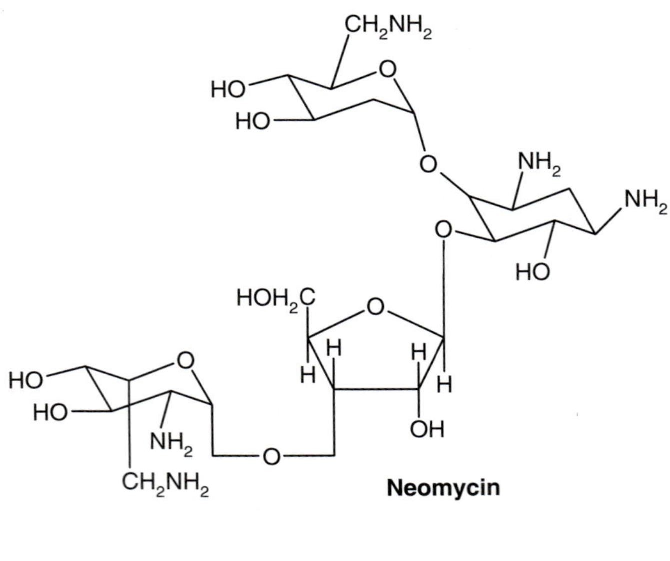

Neomycin

Explanatory Note

There are five amino groups in neomycin. Any one of these can react with ninhydrin resulting in the formation of a semi-aminal structure. It may so happen that under the given reaction condition all of them can react with the ninhydrin reagent.

Probable Reaction Mechanism

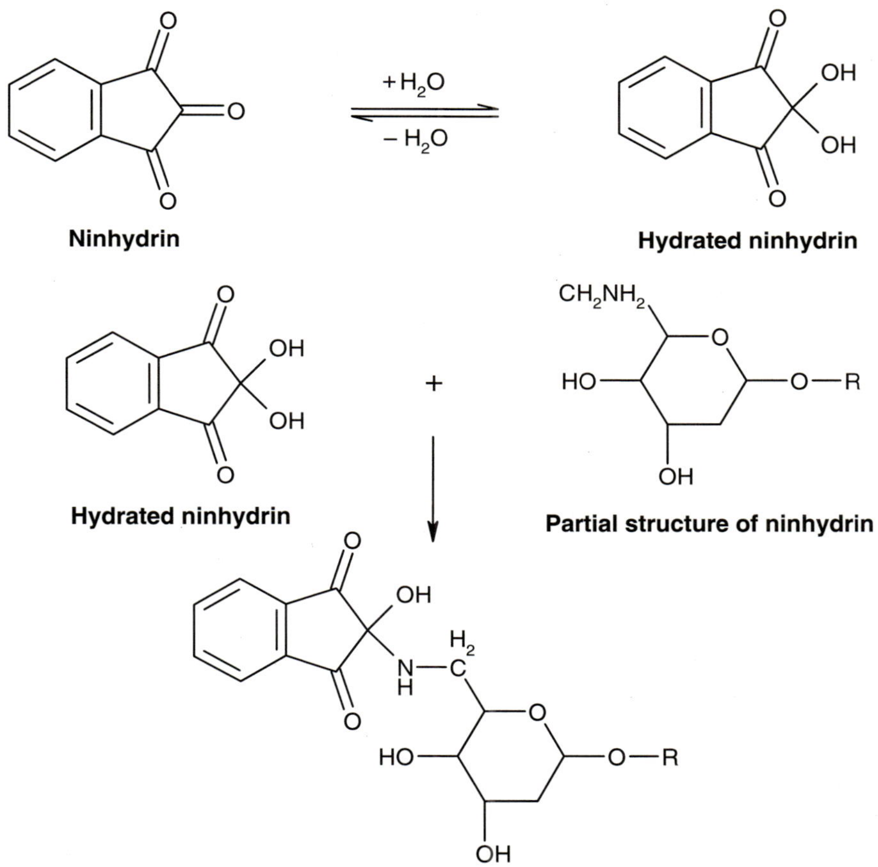

Semi-aminal like structure
(λ_{max} 570 nm)

Reference

A. Pradhan & M.K. Majumdar, *Indian Drugs*, 358-360, June 1982.

Neomycin on acid hydrolysis gives α-amino aldehyde. As a result, CH-acidic component on heating with acetylacetone at pH 9.5 (90°C) gives 2-methyl pyrrole derivatives. The secondary amine in pyrrole derivative reacts with PDAB in the presence of hydrochloric acid to form polymethine dye. The aldehyde (PDAB) reacts with nucleophilic pyrrole derivative to give colourless carbinol derivative which on losing water gives cyanine.

Probable Reaction Mechanism

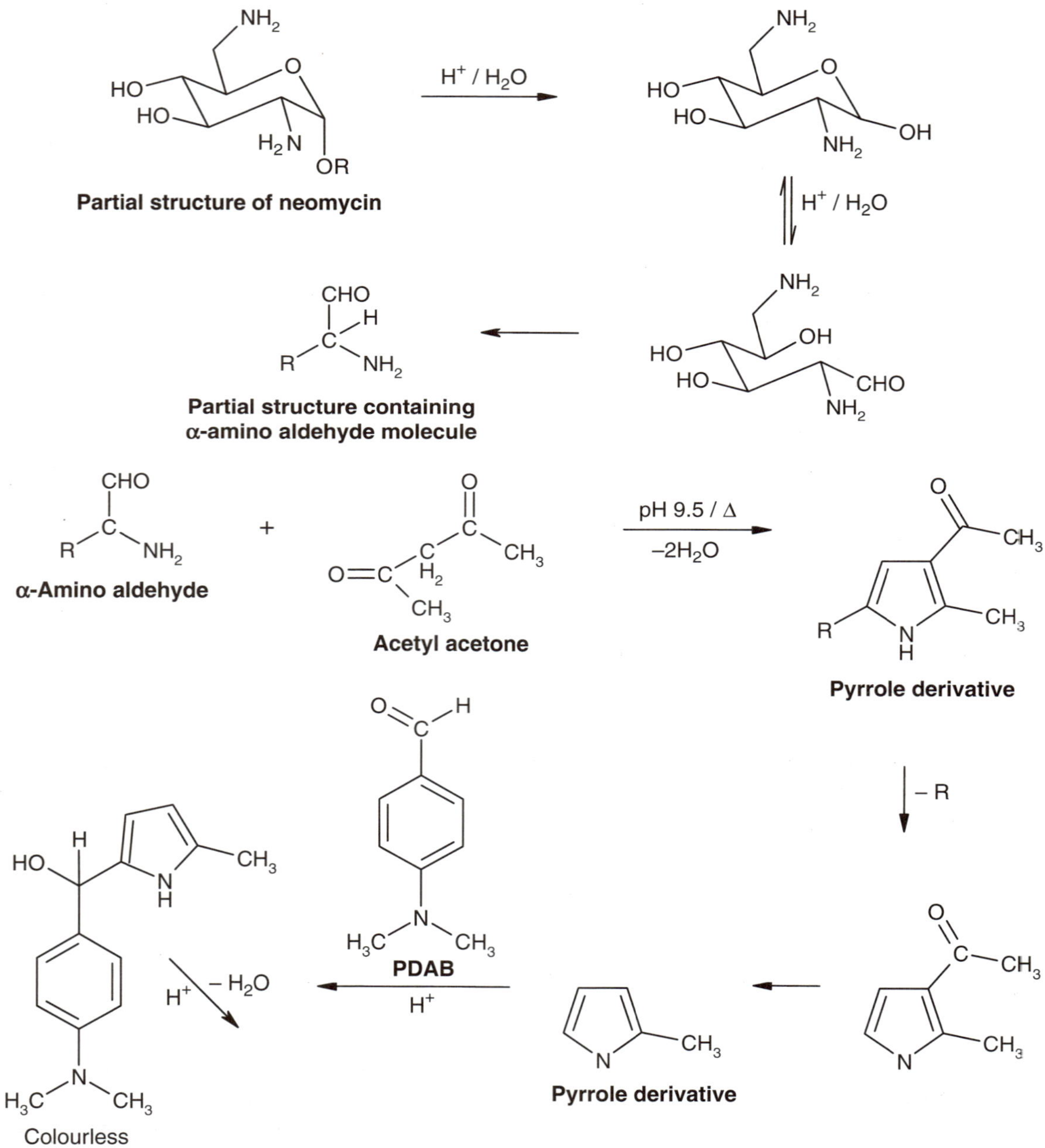

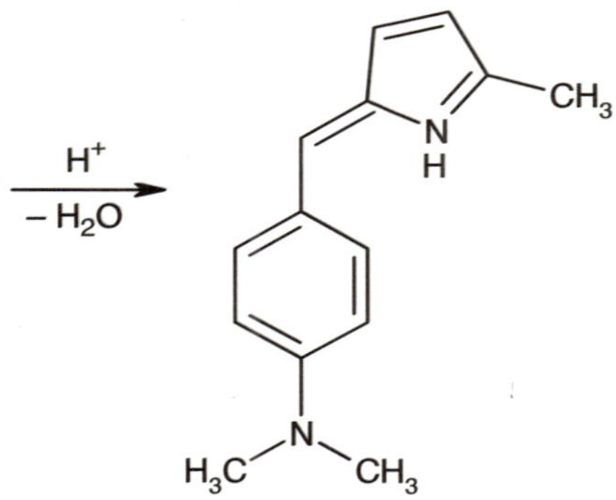

Coloured cyanine derivative

Reference

Pharmaceutical Chemistry (Vol. 2) by H.J. Roth, p. 365.

Betamethasone valerate

Follow the general method for assay of steroids based on reaction with tetrazolium blue. Colour development may be carried out in chloroform. For details, refer to formulation 6 of this chapter.

Formulation 6

Miconazole nitrate, Beclomethasone dipropionate

ESTIMATION

Miconazole nitrate

METHOD 1

Reagents

1. Solochrome dark blue: 0.1% w/v solution of the dye in distilled water. The dye solution should be prepared immediately before use.
2. Buffer, pH 4.0: Weigh and dissolve 5.1 g of potassium hydrogen phthalate in distilled water to make 500 ml.

Standard solution

Transfer, accurately weighed, about 50 mg of miconazole nitrate to volumetric flask containing about 50 ml of chloroform, warm in hot water-bath till a clear solution is obtained. Cool and dilute to 100 ml with chloroform. Further dilution of the standard solution may be done appropriately with chloroform to get a working standard of 100 mcg per ml.

Sample solution

Transfer accurately weighed quantity of the sample (cream) containing about 10 mg of the miconazole nitrate to a beaker, add about 50 ml of chloroform, warm for dissolving the substance. Transfer the contents to a 100 ml volumetric flask and dilute to the mark with chloroform.

Procedure

Transfer 10 ml each of the sample and standard solutions to 125 ml separating funnels. To each funnel, add 50 ml of chloroform, 5 ml of buffer solution and 5 ml of dye solution, shake gently and allow the layers to separate. Pass the chloroform layer through a bed of anhydrous sodium sulphate into dry flask. Measure the absorption of the coloured complex at about 513 nm against reagent blank prepared simultaneously. Calculate the results by comparison. The method is based on formation of ion-pair complex with the dye.

Probable Reaction Mechanism

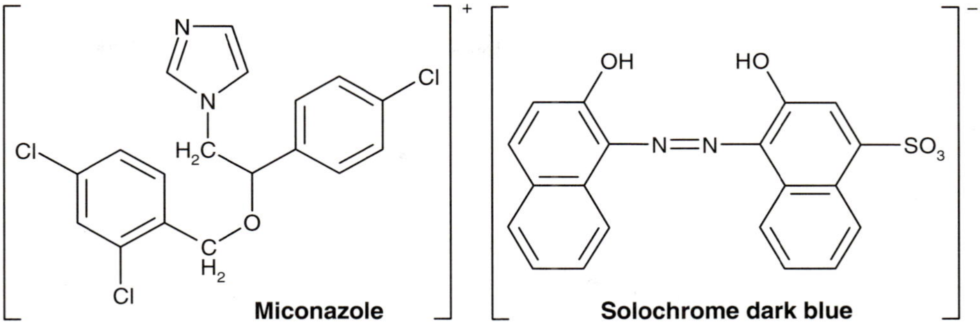

Drug - dye ion-pair complex in phosphate buffer, pH 4.0
(λ_{max} 530 nm)

METHOD 2

Miconazole, Econazole (oral gel, cream, vaginal suppositories)

Sample preparation

For miconazole the sample was prepared in methanol, whereas for econazole after basification with ammonium hydroxide, extracted into chloroform, organic layer evaporated and then sample taken up in methanol or acetonitrile. The method is based on interaction of tetracyanamine moiety of the drug with the reagents to yield coloured species which is used for quantitative estimation.

Reagents

1. Dichloro-dicyano-1,4-benzoquinone (DCQ): 4 mg/ml in methanol.
2. p-chloranilic acid (p-CA): 3.5 mg/ml in acetonitrile.

Procedure

To 1 ml of sample/standard solution (10 µg/ml) add 1 ml of DDQ reagent or 1 ml of p-CA reagent, allow to stand for 7 min at room temperature and then dilute with methanol (DCQ method) or acetonitrile (p-CA method) and measure the absorbance at 460 nm or 520 nm.

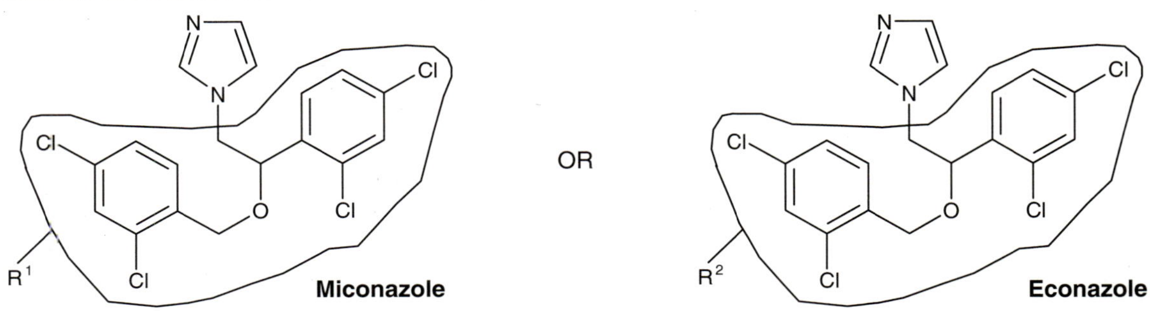

Probable Reaction Mechanism

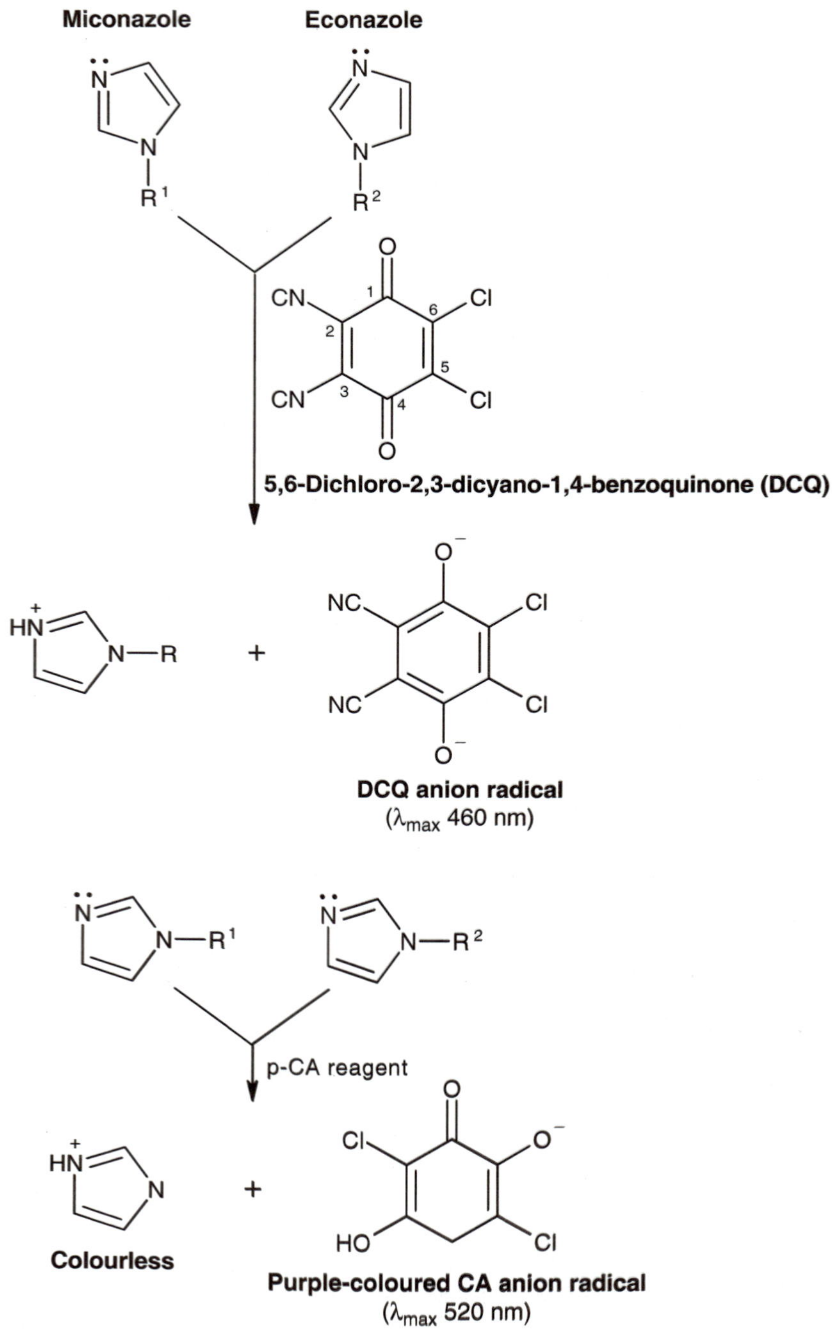

Both the drugs react with MBTH in acidic medium.

Probable Reaction Mechanism

In the presence of an oxidising agent i.e. cerric ammonium sulphate, MBTH loses two electrons and a proton. The cation formed now attacks electron-rich site in the drug resulting in the formation of coupled product. The reaction is represented as follows:

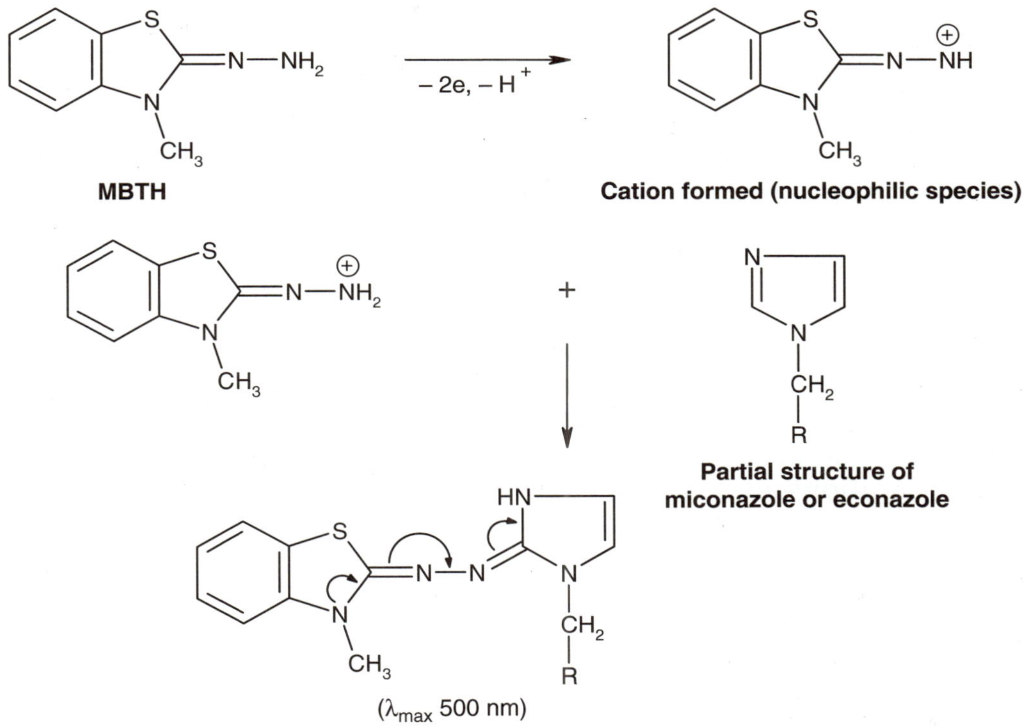

Note

Ketoconazole also gives similar reaction.

Reference

Pharmaceutical Chemistry (Vol. 2) by H.J. Roth, pp. 73, 74, 600.

Beclomethasone dipropionate

Reagents

1. Tetrazolium blue: 0.5% w/v solution in methanol.
2. Tetramethyl ammonium hydroxide solution: 10% v/v solution in methanol.

Standard solution

20 mcg/ml of beclomethasone dipropionate in methanol.

Sample solution

Weigh accurately the quantity of the sample (cream) equivalent to 2.5 mg of beclomethasone dipropionate and transfer to a separating funnel containing 50 ml methanol, shake for few minutes, add 100 ml of cyclohexane and shake vigorously. Allow the layers to separate and transfer the lower layer to a separating funnel containing about 50 ml of brine solution. Extract the cyclohexane layer with further two 10 ml portions of brine solution. Extract the cyclohexane layer with further 2 × 10 ml portions of methanol and collect the methanol layer into a separating funnel containing brine solution. Shake vigorously to mix the contents, separate chloroform layer. The aqueous layer is further extracted with 100 ml (2 × 50) of chloroform. The combined chloroform extract is evaporated and the residue is taken in methanol. Filter through cotton if necessary and make up the volume to 50 ml. Further dilution of the sample solution may be carried out with methanol to get a solution of 20 mcg/ml.

Procedure

10 ml each of standard and sample solutions is taken in 25 ml volumetric flask. Add 2 ml of tetrazolium blue solution and 2 ml of tetramethyl ammonium hydroxide, shake gently and allow to stand in water-bath at 37°C for two hours. Cool to 20°C and dilute to volume with methanol. Measure the absorption of resulting solutions at 525 nm against the reagent blank and calculate the results by comparing with standard.

The compound is oxidized by tetrazolium blue in the presence of alkali (tetramethyl ammonium hydroxide—a strong base) resulting in the formation of formazon—a coloured product (λ_{max} 525 nm).

Probable Reaction Mechanism

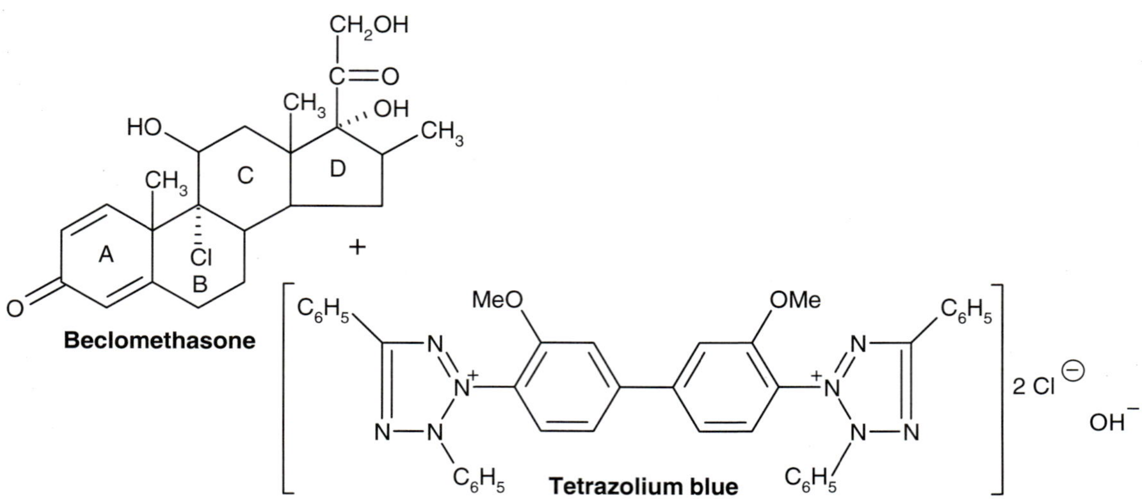

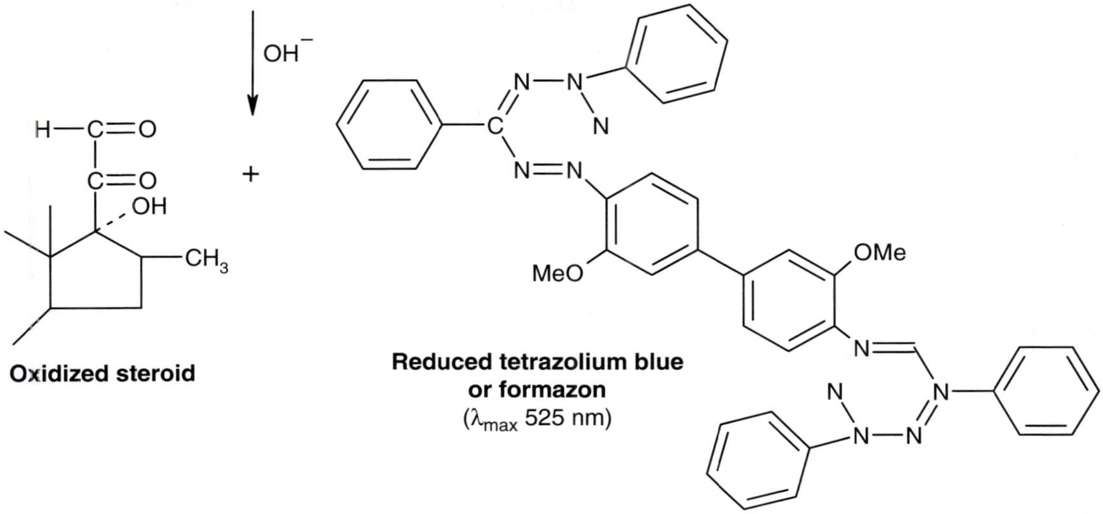

Oxidized steroid

Reduced tetrazolium blue or formazon
(λ_{max} 525 nm)

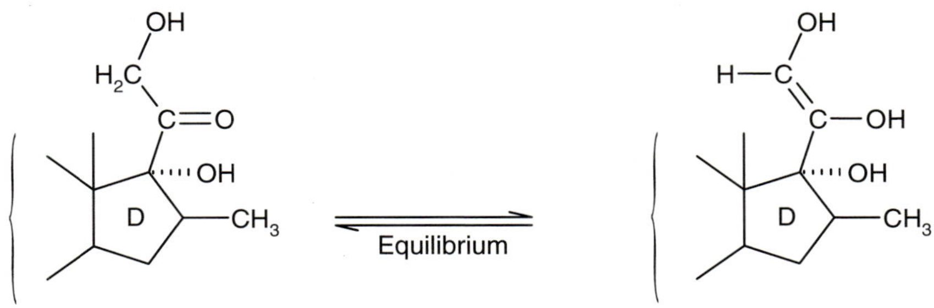

Ring D of steroid (A) **(B)**

Reference

N.M. Sanghavi & Subrata Mitra, *Indian Drugs*, **30(3)**, 129-131, 1993.

Note

Tetrazolium blue, triphenyltetrazolium chloride and phenylhydrazine react with corticosteroids with side chain at C-17 or their derivatives which are easily hydrolysed in acidic medium.

Reference

R.H. Silber & C.C. Porter, *J. Biol. Chem.*, **185**, 201, 1950 and **210**, 923, 1954.

Formulation 7

Miconazole nitrate, Beclomethasone dipropionate or Hydrocortisone acetate, Chlorocresol

ESTIMATION

Miconazole nitrate

Reagents

1. Solochrome dark blue: 0.1% w/v solution of the dye in distilled water. The dye solution should be prepared immediately before use.
2. Buffer, pH 4.0: Weigh and dissolve 5.1 g of potassium hydrogen phthalate in distilled water to make 500 ml.

Standard solution

Transfer, accurately weighed, about 50 mg of miconazole nitrate to volumetric flask containing about 50 ml of chloroform, warm in hot water-bath till a clear solution is obtained. Cool and dilute to 100 ml with chloroform. Further dilution of the standard solution may be done appropriately with chloroform to get a working standard of 100 mcg/ml.

Sample solution

Transfer accurately weighed quantity of the sample (cream) containing about 10 mg of miconazole nitrate to a beaker, add about 50 ml of chloroform, warm for dissolving the substance. Transfer the contents to a 100 ml volumetric flask and dilute to the mark with chloroform.

Procedure

Transfer 10 ml each of the sample and standard solutions to 125 ml separating funnels. To each funnel add 50 ml of chloroform, 5 ml of buffer solution and 5 ml of dye solution, shake gently and allow the layers to separate. Pass the chloroform layer through a bed of anhydrous sodium sulphate into dry flask. Measure the absorption of the coloured complex at about 513 nm against reagent blank prepared simultaneously. Calculate the results by comparison.

Beclomethasone dipropionate

METHOD 1

Reagents

1. Tetrazolium blue: 0.5% w/v solution in alcohol.
2. Tetramethyl ammonium hydroxide solution: 10% v/v solution in ethanol.

Standard solution

10 mcg/ml beclomethasone dipropionate in (TMAH) alcohol.

Sample solution

Weigh accurately the quantity of the sample (cream) equivalent to 2.5 mg of beclomethasone dipropionate and transfer to a separating funnel containing 50 ml methanol, shake for few minutes, add 100 ml cyclohexane and shake vigorously. Allow the layers to separate and transfer the lower layer (methanolic) to a separating funnel containing about 50 ml of brine solution. Extract the cyclohexane layer with further two 10 ml portions of brine solution. Extract the cyclohexane layer with further 2 × 10 ml portions of alcohol and collect the alcohol layer into a separating funnel containing brine solution. Shake vigorously to mix the contents. The aqueous layer is extracted with four 20 ml portions of chloroform. The combined chloroform extract is evaporated and the residue is taken in alcohol. Filter through cotton plug if necessary and make up the volume to 50 ml. Further dilution of the sample solution may be carried out with alcohol to get a solution of 20 mcg/ml.

Procedure

10 ml each of standard and sample solutions is taken in 25 ml volumetric flask. Add 2 ml of tetrazolium blue solution and 2 ml of tetramethyl ammonium hydroxide, shake gently and allow to stand in water-bath at 25-35°C for 90 min and measure the absorption of resulting solutions at 525 nm against the reagent blank (chloroform + both the reagents) and calculate the results by comparing with standard.

Note

It is always preferable to carry out the above procedure using aldehyde-free ethyl alcohol. As ethyl alcohol is not easily available, the following alternative methods based on practical experience are suggested to give excellent reproducible results.

- The standard solution should be initially prepared in methanol and further diluted appropriately with chloroform to get working standard (10 mcg/ml).

- The chloroform extract of the sample need not be evaporated, instead can be further diluted to get appropriate final concentration (comparable with standard—10-20 mcg/ml).
- Solutions of TMAH and tetrazolium blue may be prepared in methanol.

This modified procedure is suitable for most of the steroidal compounds.

METHOD 2

Reagents

1. 0.05% w/v solution of tetrazolium blue (BTZ) in methanol (stable for 7 days).
2. 0.1 N tetrabutyl ammonium hydroxide (TBAH) in methanol.
3. Glacial acetic acid.
4. Methanol.

Standard solution

10 mcg/ml of beclomethasone dipropionate in methanol.

Sample solution

Suspend an accurately weighed quantity of the sample (cream) containing 0.5 mg of the substance in 20 ml of methanol, dissolve by gentle stirring and filter through G_3 sintered glass funnel, wash the residue on funnel with methanol and adjust the filtrate to 25 ml with methanol. Further dilutions are made to get solution of 10 mcg/ml.

Procedure

To 1 ml each of sample and standard solutions, add 6 ml of TBAH reagent and 2 ml of BTZ solution. Heat on water-bath at 70°C for 15 min, cool to room temperature and dilute to 10 ml with glacial acetic acid. Measure the absorbance of both the solutions at 515 nm against reagent blank and calculate the results by comparison.

Note

1. The method obeys Beer's law in the concentration range of 2-50 mcg/ml.
2. Clotrimazole and neomycin commonly present in antifungal formulations do not interfere.
3. As the reaction is specific for α-ketol group, other non-steroidal drugs do not interfere.
4. Rate and extent of formazan formation bears inverse relationship with dielectric constant of the solvent used in the reaction; the formazan formation is faster in methanol than in ethanol (solvent in official method). In chloroform, though the reaction is faster, but has lower sensitivity.

For reaction mechanism in respect of methods 1 & 2, refer to this chapter.

Chlorocresol

Reagents

1. 4-aminoantipyrin reagent: 2% w/v solution in distilled water. Protect from light. It is stable only for 2-3 days.
2. Strong ammonia buffer: Dissolve 67.5 g of ammonium chloride in 570 ml of strong ammonia and dilute to 1000 ml with distilled water.
3. Dilute ammonia buffer: 2 ml of strong ammonia buffer is diluted to 1000 ml with distilled water.
4. 8% w/v potassium ferricyanide solution in water.

Procedure

Volume of the sample and standard solutions equivalent to 0.2 mg of chlorocresol is taken. To this add 1 ml of antipyrin reagent, followed by 1 ml of potassium ferricyanide solution and 1 ml of dilute ammonia buffer. The coloured complex is extracted with three 15 ml portions of chloroform and final volume is adjusted to 50 ml with chloroform. Measure the absorption at about 490 nm and calculate the contents of chlorocresol from the standard.

Probable Reaction Mechanism

This is based on Emerson's reaction. The reaction proceeds by an oxidative coupling in the p-position. Since p-position is occupied by a halogen radical, it is dehalogenated by oxidizing agent [$K_3Fe(CN)_6$] and then undergoes coupling.

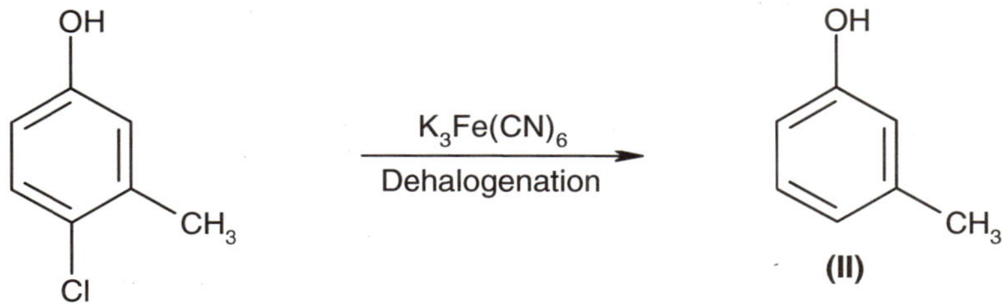

Chlorocresol (I)

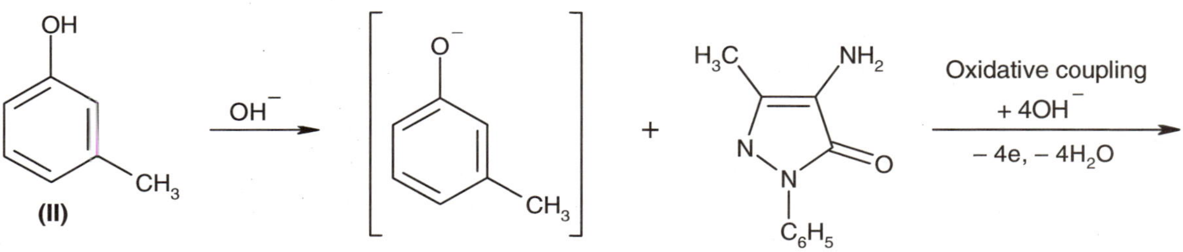

4-aminoantipyrin

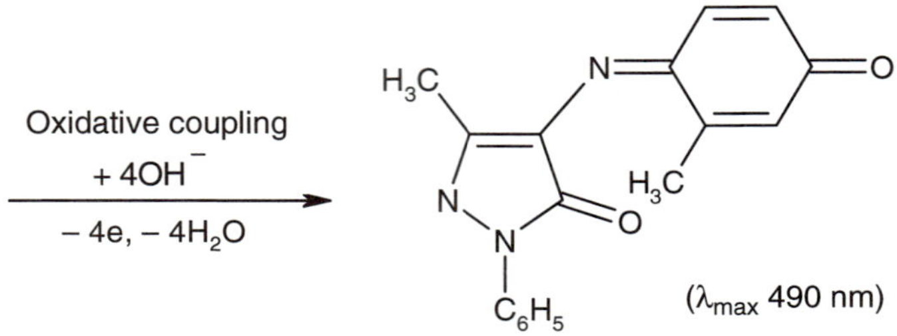

Note

4-Dimethylaminophenazone has similar reaction mechanism as in vivo; it undergoes demethylation due to oxidation resulting in formation of 4-aminophenazone.

It is a halogenated monohydric phenol. It can be estimated by Koppesschaar titration i.e. bromination of phenol. It gives 2,6-dibromo-4-chloro-3-methyl phenol. It answers "Emerson" reaction as well as it reacts with "Gibbs" reagent and MBTH reagent.

Probable Reaction Mechanism

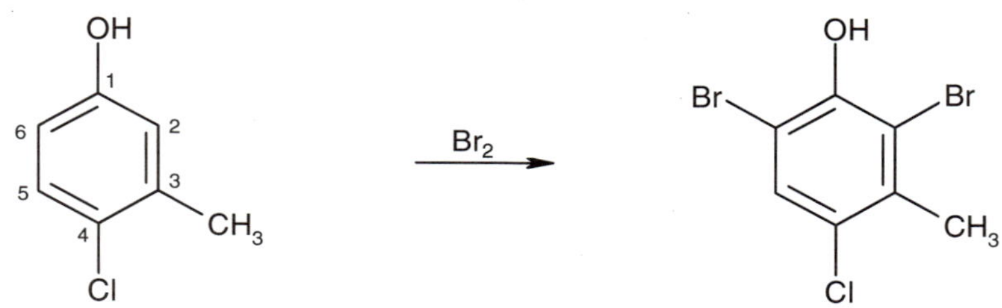

Chlorocresol **2,6-dibromo derivative**

(a)

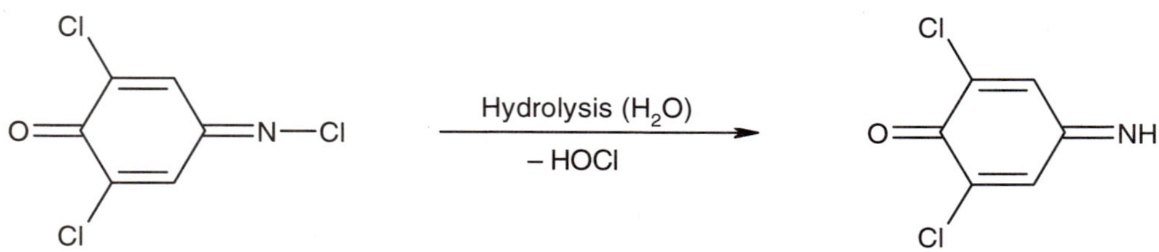

2,6-dichloroquinone chlorimide (Gibbs reagent) (I)

2,6-dichloroquinonimine (hydrolysed active species) (II)

Note

pH should be around 8.5.

Gibbs reagent is a strong oxidizing agent. In alkaline medium, in vivo, it dehalogenates the compound and then couples with the phenols as under.

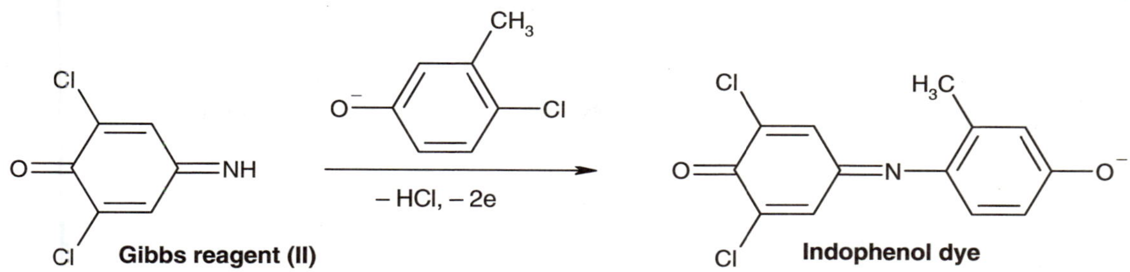

(b)

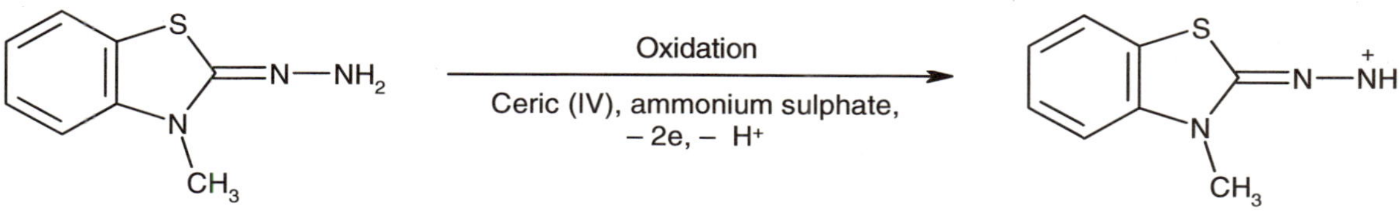

3-methylbenzthiazoline-2-one-hydrazone (MBTH)

The oxidizing agent causes in vivo oxidation of chlorocresol resulting in dehalogenation as explained earlier.

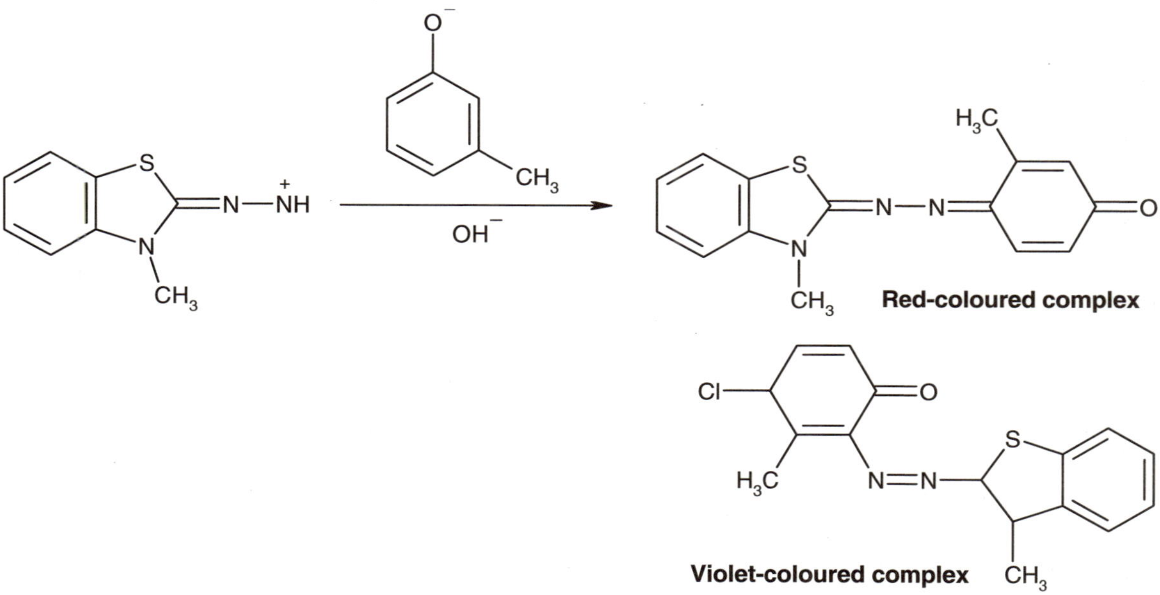

Note

Ortho substitution is also possible without dehalogenation of the compound.

Reference

R.T. Sane, M.L. Kubal & V.G. Nayak, *Indian Drugs*, **23(8)**, 466-468, 1986.

Formulation 8

Miconazole nitrate, Fluocinolone acetonide

ESTIMATION

Miconazole nitrate

METHOD 1

Follow the methanol described in formulation 4 of this chapter or titration with sodium lauryl sulphate using dimethyl yellow as indicator (see formulation of the chapter on analgesics and antipyretics under dicyclomine HCl).

Note

Sodium lauryl sulphate is used as titrant for quartenary and tertiary amines. These amines form slightly dissociated salt with SLS in acidic medium.

Reference

K. Marcali, *Analytical Letters*, **27**, 1586, 1955.

METHOD 2

Follow the non-aqueous titration method for determining the end point potentiometrically or using crystal violet as indicator. Each ml of 0.01 M perchloric acid is equivalent to 0.004792 g of miconazole nitrate.

METHOD 3

Reagents

1. 1 mg/ml of tropaeolin OO in water: Dissolve the dye in water by slight warming. Wash the dye solution with chloroform (1 × 25 ml), discard chloroform layer.
2. pH 3.0 phosphate buffer: Dissolve 1.67 g of citric acid monohydrate and 1 g of sodium phosphate, dibasic, in 100 ml of water.
3. Acidified methanol: 1 ml of sulphuric acid in 100 ml of methanol.

Standard solution

400 mcg/ml of miconazole nitrate in chloroform.

Sample preparation

Disperse accurately weighed quantity of sample (cream, ointment) equivalent to 4 mg of miconazole nitrate in water and extract with chloroform (3 × 25 ml), passing each extract through anhydrous sulphate placed in a funnel over cotton plug and make up the volume.

Procedure

To 15 ml each of sample and standard solutions add 3 ml of dye solution, 10 ml of phosphate buffer, pH 3.0, and 15 ml of chloroform. Shake for about 2-3 min and allow the layers to separate. Collect chloroform layer and repeat the extraction with chloroform (2 × 30 ml). Combine the chloroform layers, add 3 ml of acidified methanol and dilute to 100 ml with chloroform. Concomitantly measure the absorbance of solutions at about 540 nm and calculate the results by comparison.

The method is based on formation of ion-pair complex with the dye. The complex is first extracted with chloroform and then acidified to increase the sensitivity of the method with hyperchromic shift from 410 to 540 nm.

Probable Reaction Mechanism

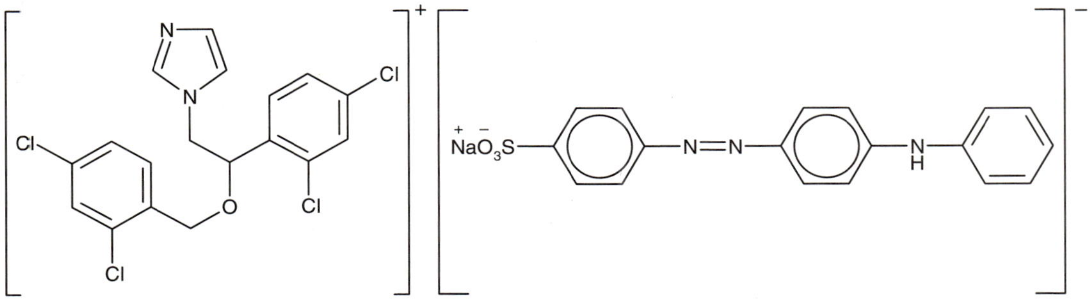

Miconazole **Tropaeolin OO (acid yellow/fast yellow)**

Drug - dye ion-pair complex in acidified methanol
(λ_{max} 540 nm)

Fluocinolone acetonide

Follow the method described in formulation 9 of this chapter.

Formulation 9

Fluocinolone acetonide, Iodochlorhydroxyquinoline (Chinoform), Tolnaftate

ESTIMATION

Fluocinolone acetonide

Reagent

1. Dehydrated alcohol, aldehyde-free.
2. Methanolic sodium chloride: Dilute 20 mg of 10% sodium chloride solution (aqueous) to 100 ml with methanol.
3. Tetrazolium blue solution: 0.5% w/v solution in aldehyde-free alcohol.
4. Dilute tetramethyl ammonium hydroxide solution (TMAH): Dilute 1 ml of 10% sodium to 10 ml with aldehyde-free alcohol.
5. Saturated solution of sodium chloride in water.
6. 5% w/v solution of aluminium potassium sulphate in water.

Standard solution

20 mcg/ml of fluocinolone acetonide in aldehyde-free alcohol.

Sample solution

To accurately weighed quantity of sample (cream, ointment) equivalent to 0.5 g of fluocinolone acetonide add 50 ml of cyclohexane, 25 ml of methanol and 1 ml of saturated solution of sodium chloride. Shake and allow the layers to separate. Cyclohexane layer is extracted with 10-15 ml of methanolic sodium chloride solution and aqueous layer is combined with the first extract. Dilute the combined methanolic extract to 100 ml with aluminium potassium sulphate solution and extract with chloroform (4 × 20 ml), passing each chloroform extract through anhydrous sodium phosphate. Evaporate combined chloroform layer and dissolve the residue in aldehyde-free alcohol to get solution of 20 mcg/ml.

Procedure

To each 10 ml of sample and standard solutions add 10 ml of aldehyde-free alcohol, 2 ml of tetrazolium blue solution and 2 ml of dilute TMAH solution. Keep in dark for 60 min and measure the absorbance of both the solutions at maximum at about 525 nm against reagent blank and calculate the results by comparison. For reaction mechanism, see under clobetasol propionate in this chapter.

Note

If aldehyde-free alcohol is not easily available then colour development of both standard and sample can be carried out with chloroform solution. For reaction mechanism see under beclomethasone.

Iodochlorhydroxyquinoline (Chinoform)

Reagent

10% w/v solution of copper sulphate in water.

Standard solution

100 mcg/ml of chinoform in chloroform.

Sample solution

To accurately weighed quantity of the sample equivalent to 100 mg of iodo-chlorhydroxyquinoline, add 50 ml of ethyl acetate, keep on water-bath and dissolve the residue obtained in chloroform to get a solution of 100 mcg/ml.

Procedure

To 10 ml each of sample and standard solutions add 10 ml of copper sulphate solution, shake vigorously and allow the layers to separate. Pass chloroform layer through anhydrous sulphate and measure the absorbance of both sample and standard solutions at 430 nm against reagent blank and calculate the results by comparison.

Probable Reaction Mechanism

The compound forms orange-coloured chelate with Cu^{2+}.

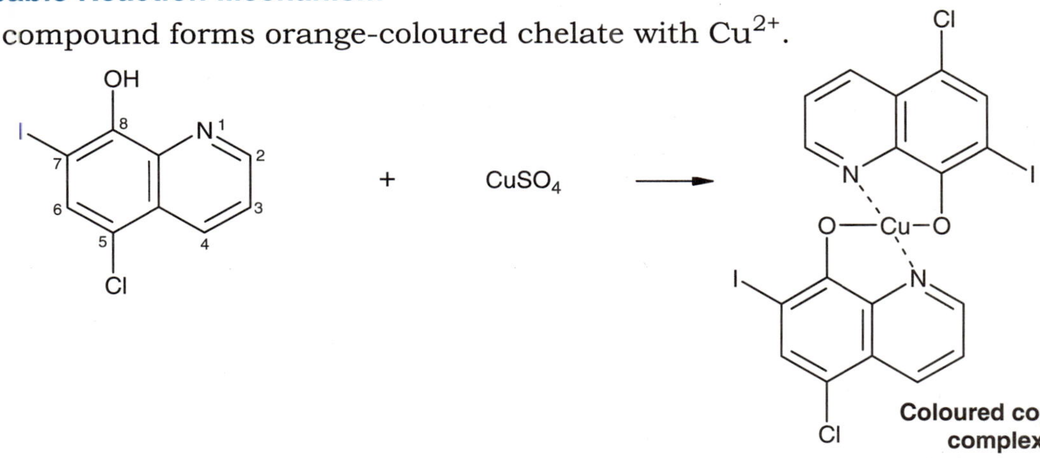

Coloured copper complex
(λ_{max} 430 nm)

Note

1. On heating, iodine is given off as violet vapours.
2. The compound forms chelate with monovalent and trivalent metal ions as shown below.

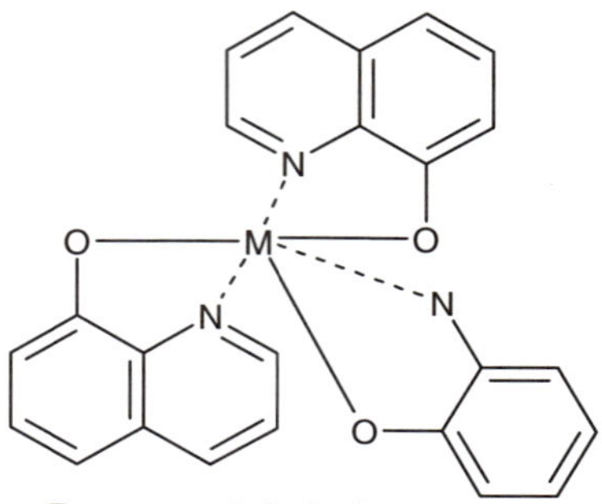

Drug - metal chelate

Reference

Pharmaceutical Chemistry (Vol. 2) by H.J. Roth, p. 610.

Tolnaftate

METHOD 1

Transfer portion of the sample (semi-solid) equivalent to 10 mg of the substance to a separator, add 70-80 ml of chloroform and wash successively with 0.1 N sodium hydroxide (2 × 25 ml) and 0.1 N hydrochloric acid (2 × 25 ml). Dilute chloroform layer to 100 ml (10 mcg/ml). Measure the absorbance at maximum at about 250 nm and compare the results with standard solution (10 mcg/ml in chloroform); OR wash the chloroform layer as obtained in the above method with water, evaporate to dryness and the residue taken up in methanol to obtain 2 μg/ml.

To 2 ml of sample/standard solution add 1 ml of 5 M NaOH, allow to stand in water-bath at 95°C ± 5°C for 40 min, cool to room temperature and dilute to 10 ml with 66% methanol and measure the fluorescence λ_{ex} 344 nm, λ_{em} 420 nm against reagent blank.

Probable Reaction Mechanism

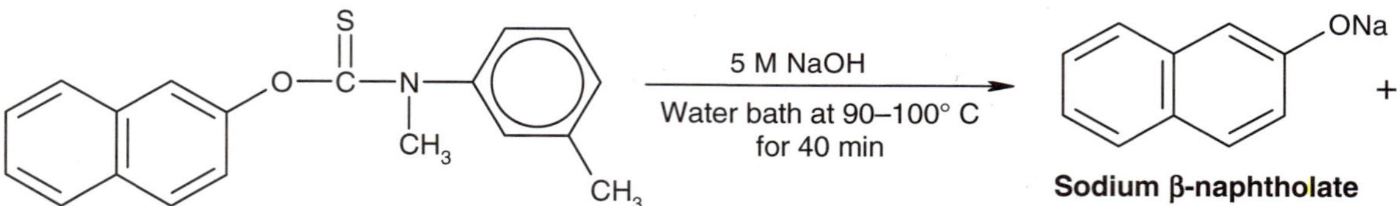

Sodium β-naphtholate (highly fluorescent species)
(λ_{ex}: 344 nm, λ_{em}: 420 nm)

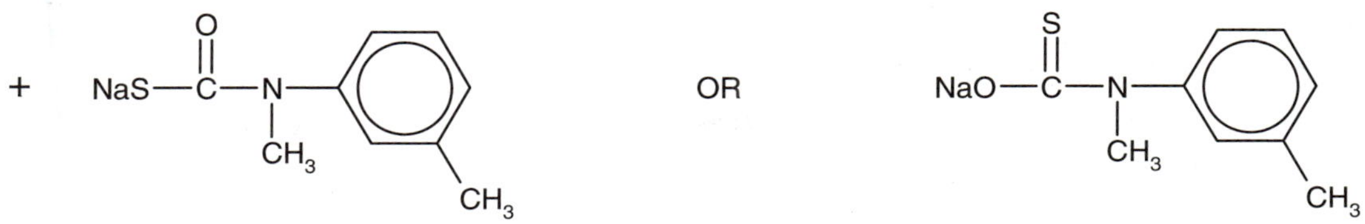

Reference

P.Y. Khashaba, S.R. El-Shabouri, K.M. Emara & A.M. Mohamed, *J. Pharm. Biomed. Analysis*, **22**, 363-376, 2000.

Alternatively, the compound reacts with Gibbs reagent (2,6-dichloroquinone-4-chlorimide) and Wurster's red reagent (p-N,N-dimethylphenylene diamine) to give coloured product. This forms the basis of spectroscopic methods of analysis.

METHOD 2

Reagents

1. 0.1% w/v solution of 2,6-dichloroquinone-4-chlorimide (DCQC—Gibbs reagent) in isopropanol.
2. 0.067 M Na_2HPO_4/KH_2PO_4 buffer, pH 7.0.
3. 0.1% w/v solution of chloramine-T (CAT).
4. 1% w/v solution of p-N,N-dimethylphenylene diamine (DMPD) in water.

Standard solution

500 μg/ml of tolnaftate in methanol. Further dilutions were made (40 μg/ml for method A and 100 μg/ml for method B).

Sample solution

Sample equivalent to 20 mg of TNF dissolved in 50 ml of chloroform. Organic layer shaken with 0.1 N NaOH (2 × 25 ml) and distilled water (1 × 25 ml). The aqueous layer extracted with chloroform (2 × 25 ml). Total chloroform extract combined, filtered, evaporated and residue taken up in methanol to get 200 μg/ml. Further dilutions made to get 40 μg/ml (method A) and 100 μg/ml (method B).

Procedure

Method A: To 1 ml each of sample and standard solutions add 3 ml of methanol and then 1 ml of DCQC reagent. Heated in water-bath (80°C) until entire solvent gets evaporated, cooled and residue taken up in isopropanol to produce 10 ml. Measure the absorbance of red-coloured solution at 490 nm and calculate the results.

Method B: To 1 ml each of sample and standard solutions add 3 ml of methanol, 9 ml of buffer, pH 7.0, followed by 0.5 ml of DMPD solution and 1 ml of CAT solution. Make up to 20 ml with water, mix well and allow to stand for 1 hr. Measure the absorbance at 530 nm within 60 min against reagent blank and calculate the results.

Explanatory Note

TNF possesses both substituted toluidine and substituted naphthol moieties. Based on reaction of amines and phenols with halo-substituted quinonimines to give coloured product, it is expected that TNF will undergo similar reaction. Although there are two possible sites for coupling in case of TNF such as C-4 of N-methyl-m-toluidine moiety or position 1 of naphthol moiety which is ortho to substituted OH-group. By reacting Gibbs reagent with β-naphthol and N-methyl aniline, the author could establish that coupling shall take place at position 1 of naphthyl moiety of TNF leading to formation of coloured product (λ_{max} 490 nm). Reaction of TNF with 'DMPD' requires presence of oxidant like CAT. Initially, by reaction of DMPD with CAT we get N-chloroquinone diimine (NCQDI) with substituent coupling with TNF. Like method A, coupling was at position 1 of naphthyl moiety of TNF leading to formation of coloured product (λ_{max} 530 nm).

Probable Reaction Mechanism

(Method A)

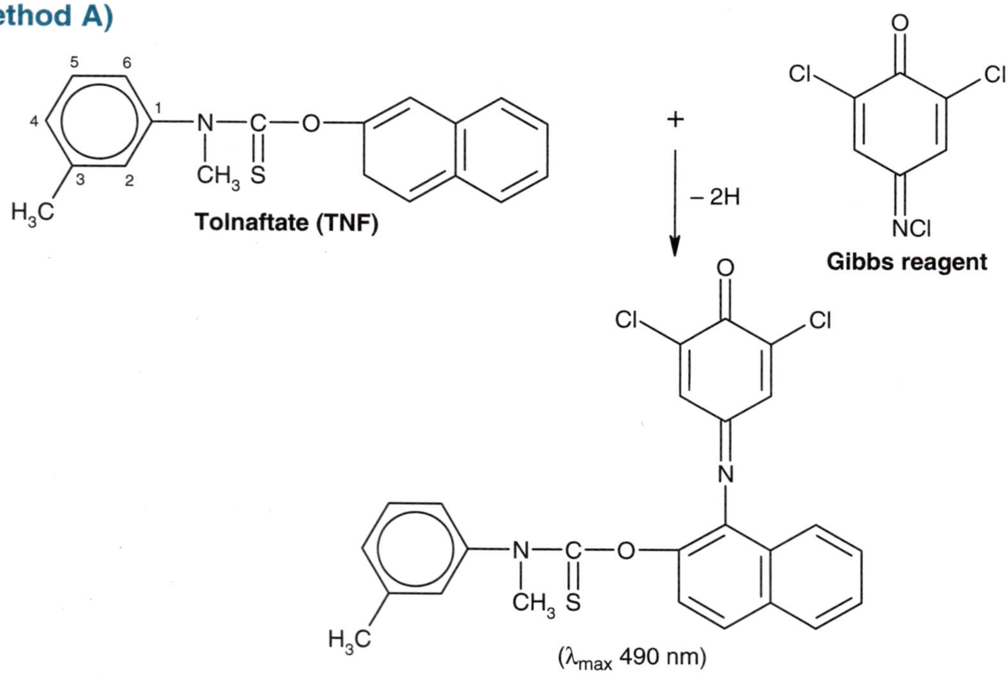

(Method B)

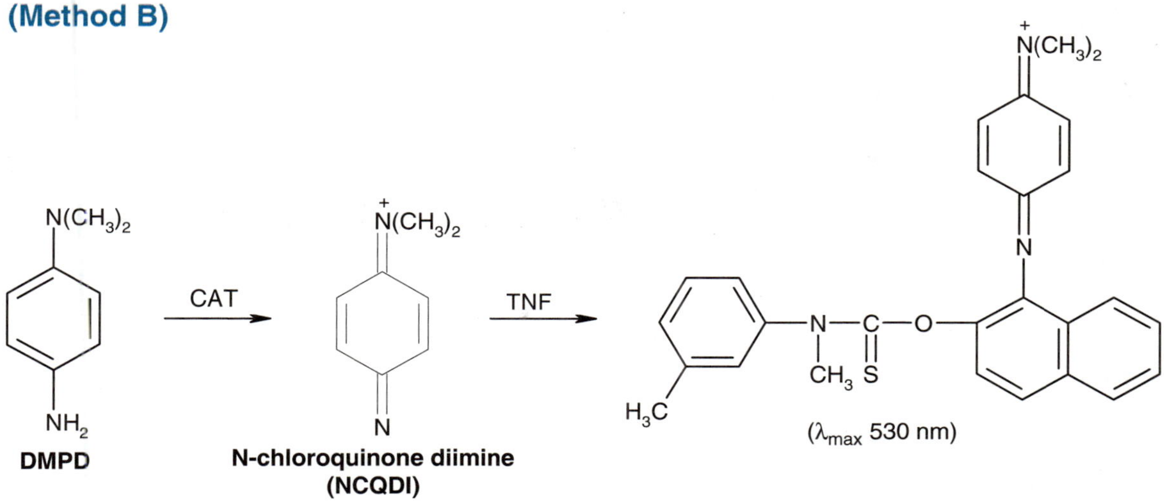

Reference

C.P.S. Sastry, B.S. Sastry, J. Venkateshwara Rao & R. Rama Krishna, *Talanta*, **40(4)**, 571-576, 1993.

Formulation 10

Clobetasol propionate, Miconazole nitrate

ESTIMATION

Clobetasol propionate

METHOD 1

Follow the method described in formulation 7 of this chapter.

METHOD 2

Reagents

1. 0.05% w/v solution of blue tetrazolium (BTZ) in methanol. The solution is stable for 7 days.
2. 0.1 N tetrabutyl ammonium hydroxide (TBAH).
3. Glacial acetic acid.
4. Methanol.
5. Toluene.

Standard solution

50 mcg/ml of clobetasol propionate in methanol.

Sample solution

Suspend accurately weighed quantity of the sample equivalent to 50 mg of the substance in 25 ml of methanol, filter and use the filtrate for analysis.

Procedure

To 1 ml each of sample and standard solutions add 2 ml of tetrazolium blue reagent and 6.5 ml of TBAH reagent. Heat on water-bath (80°C) for 5 min, cool to room temperature and dilute to 10 ml with glacial acetic acid. Measure the absorbance of red-coloured complex at 513 nm against reagent blank and calculate the results by comparison. The method obeys Beer's law in the concentration range of 5-40 mcg/ml and red-coloured complex is stable up to 2 hrs.

α-ketol group on C-17 side chain is oxidized by tetrazolium blue in the presence of strong base (TMAH) whereas tetrazolium blue is reduced and formazon so formed is measured at 513 nm.

Probable Reaction Mechanism

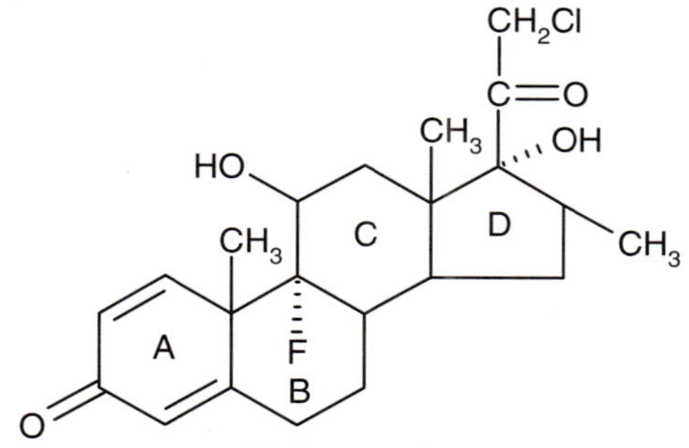

Clobetasol

+

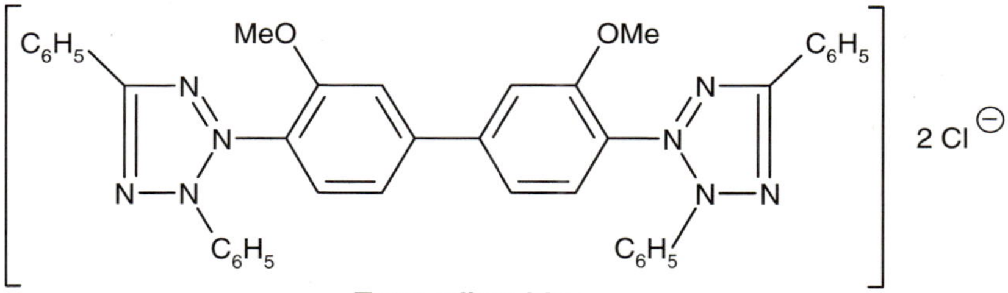

Tetrazolium blue

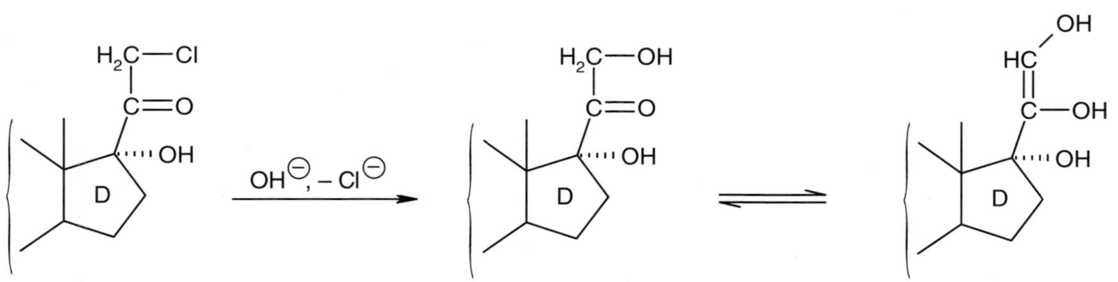

Ring D of steroid | Structure B | Structure A

Structure is then oxidized by tetrazolium blue in the presence of a strong base.

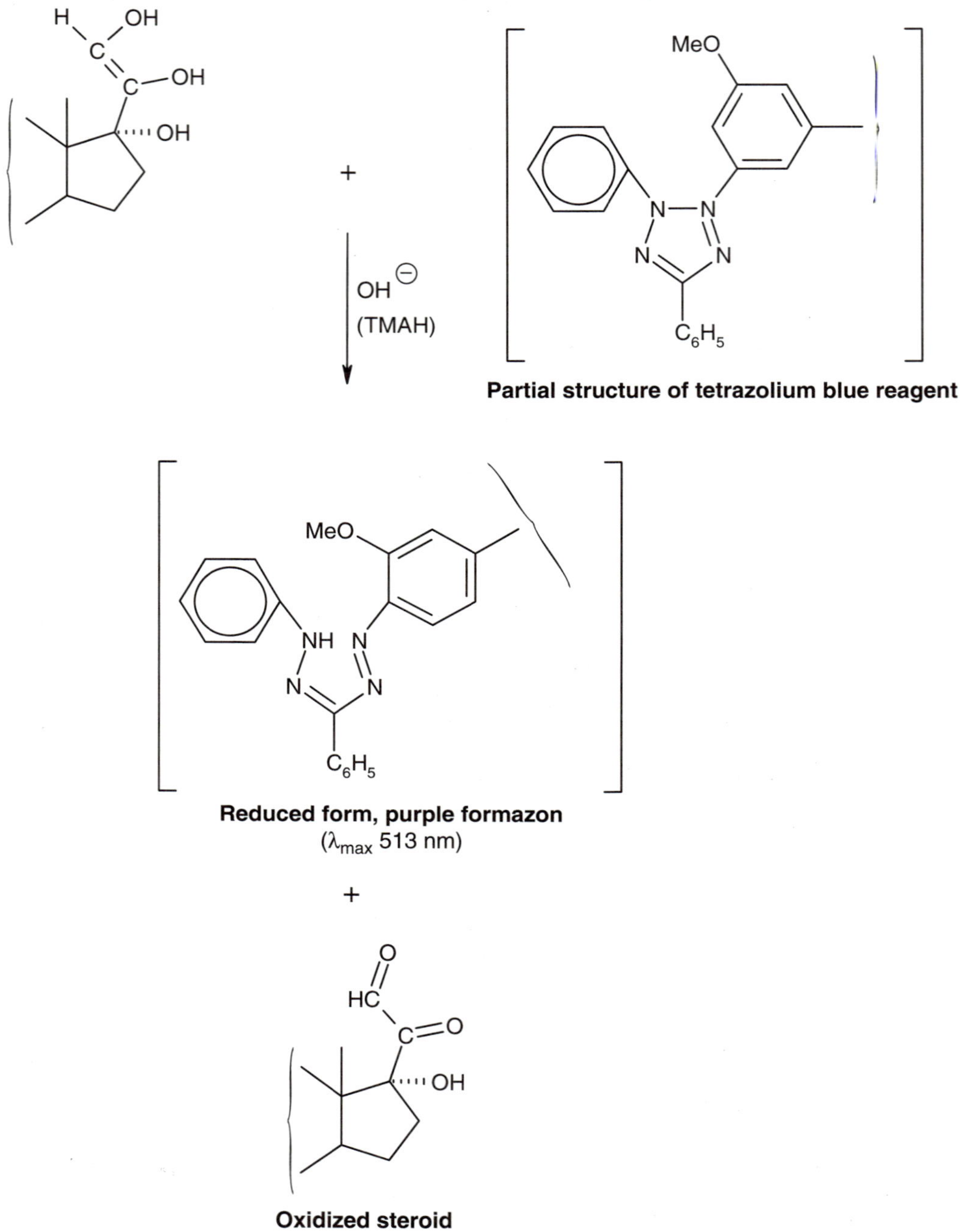

Reference

N.M. Sanghavi & D. Mahalaxmi, *Indian Drugs*, **30(7)**, 348-350, 1993 & **28(7)**, 334-335, 1991.

The primary amino (NH_2) group of isoniazid reacts with α,β-unsaturated carbonyl group (C==O) present in the molecule at C-3 to form a Schiff's base (λ_{max} 405 nm).

Probable Reaction Mechanism

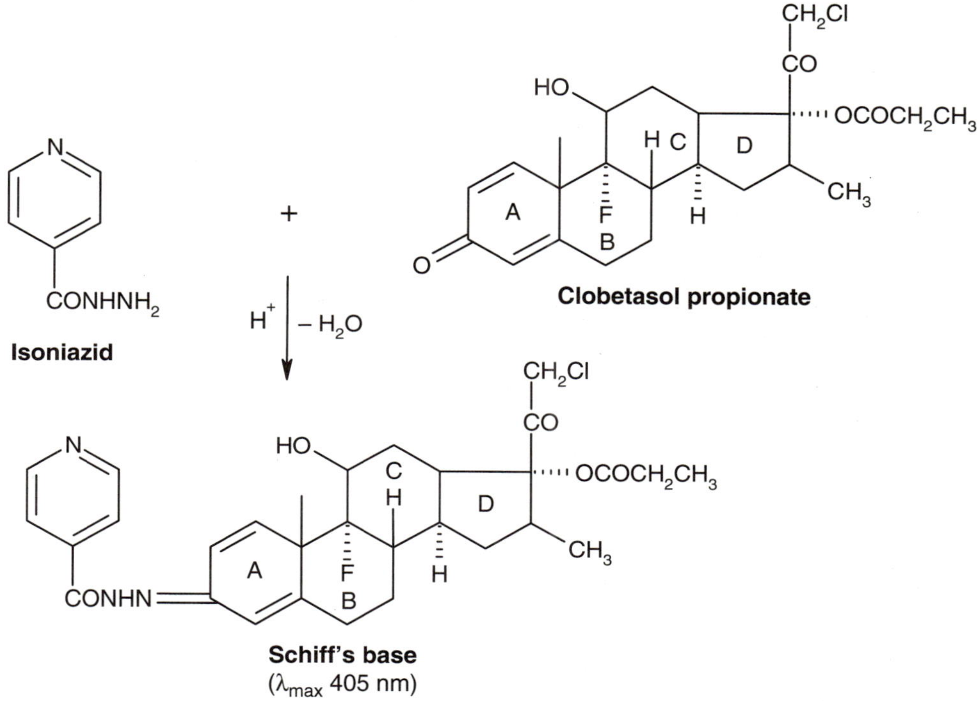

Note

INH method is called Umberger reaction.

Reference

G.S. Sadana & A.J. Potdar, *Indian Drugs*, **26(11)**, 635, 1989.

Note

Other compounds reacting with this reagent are betamethasone diloxanide furoate, nitrofurantoin, spironolactone and propanolol.

For steroids with carbonyl group at C-3 (ring A) and double band at position 4 (cortisone, hydrocortisone), this reaction is quantitative at room temperature, however for steroids with carbonyl group at C-3 and double bond at positions 1 and 4 (clobetasol, beclomethasone, dexamethasone, betamethasone, triamcinolone), the reaction is slow and requires heating at 55°C or use of high concentration of reagent and HCl to ensure quantitative reaction.

Suresh B. Patil et al. (1992) have described a method based on coupling of 4-aminoantipyrin with the drug having carbonyl group at C-3. This reaction is similar to the one with isoniazid as described above.

Probable Reaction Mechanism

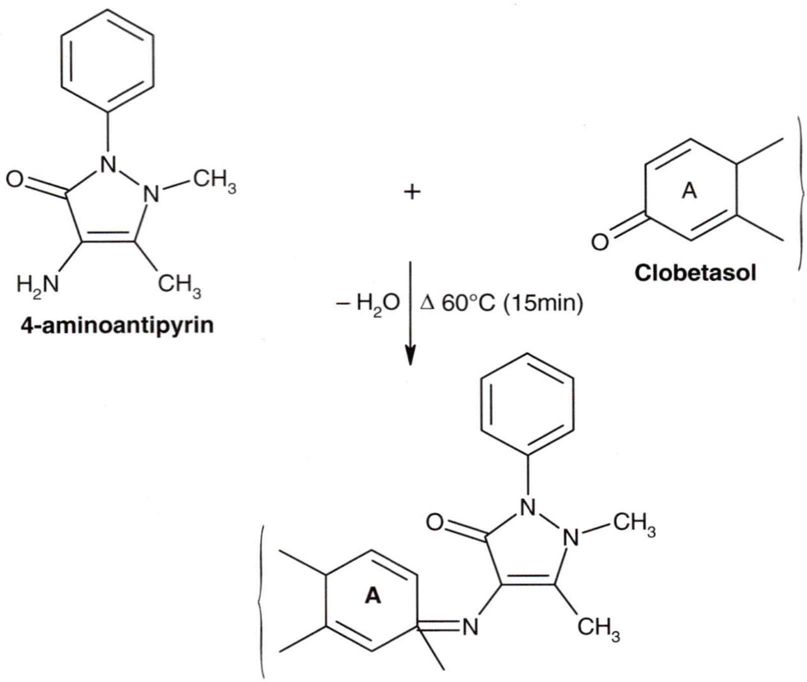

Schiff's base
(λ_{max} 385 nm)

Reference

Suresh B. Patil, G.N. Chaudhari & H.V. Kolte, *Indian Drugs*, **29(8)**, 367-368, 1992.

Miconazole nitrate

Follow the method 2 (non-aqueous titration) described in formulation 8 of this chapter.

Formulation 11

Halcinonide, Econazole nitrate

ESTIMATION

Halcinonide

Standard solution

30 mcg/ml of halcinonide in chloroform.

Sample solution

Weigh accurately sample (cream) equivalent to 30 mg of halcinonide, add 60 ml of chloroform, warm to disperse the sample, cool and make up to 100 ml with chloroform, pass through anhydrous sodium sulphate and use for estimation.

Procedure

To 10 ml each of sample and standard solutions in chloroform, add 10 ml of isoniazid reagent, shake and keep in water-bath (55 + 1°C) for 30 min, cool and dilute to 25 ml with chloroform. Measure the absorbance of sample and standard solutions at about 390 nm against reagent blank and calculate the results by comparison.

Condensation reaction occurs between the carbonyl group at C-3 position of the steroid and the primary amino group of isoniazide to form the resultant Schiff's base.

Note

This reaction is specific for corticosteroids with C-3 carbonyl (C=O) group such as hydrocortisone and prednisolone.

Reference

1. E.J. Umberger, *Anal. Chem.*, **27**, 768, 1955.
2. S. Görög & Fresenius Z., *Anal. Chem.*, **309**, 97, 1981.

Probable Reaction Mechanism

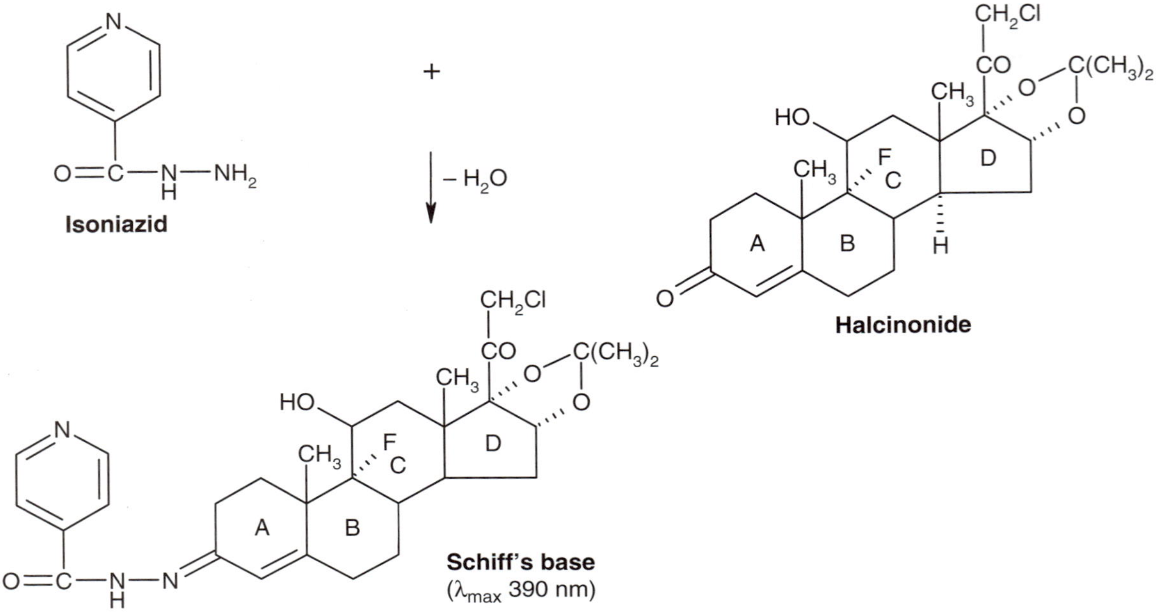

Hydrocortisone acetate

α-ketol group 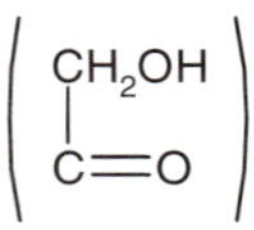 possesses reducing properties. It reduces alkaline triphenyltetrazolium chloride (TPTZ) to the corresponding red formazon (λ_{max} 490 nm).

Probable Reaction Mechanism

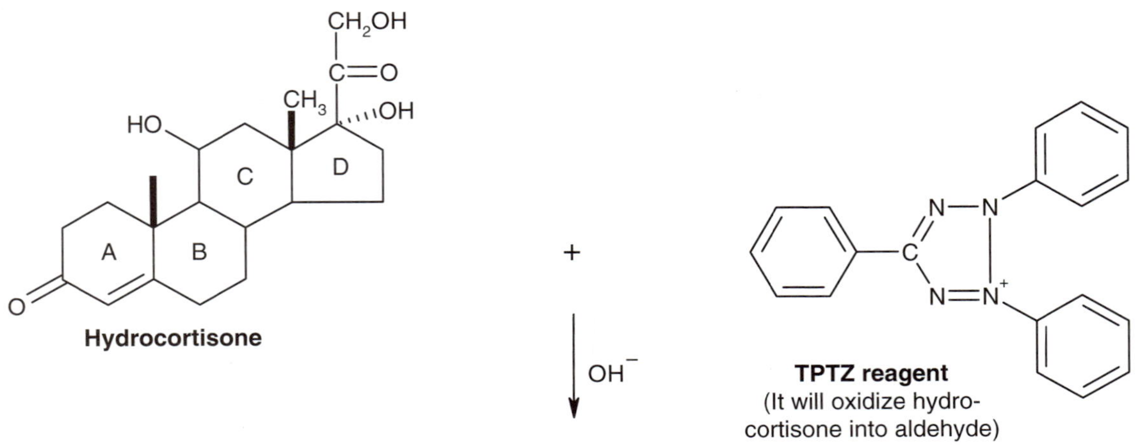

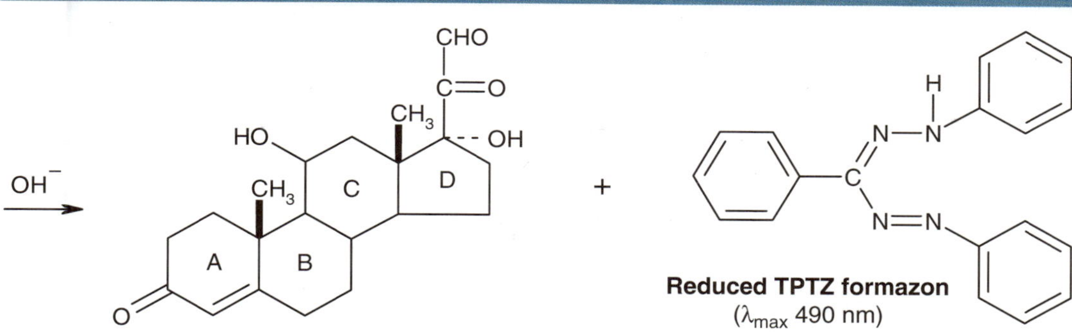

Oxidized hydrocortisone

Reduced TPTZ formazon (λ_{max} 490 nm)

Prednisolone

A carbanion is formed in the steroid when the steroid is treated with NaOH. The loss of hydrogen atom is from the above shown position because the proton here is very acidic in nature due to the presence of carbonyl group at the adjacent C atom. This cabanion will now react with o-dinitrobenzene resulting in the formation of a coloured complex (i.e. Meisenheimer salt-like formation).

Probable Reaction Mechanism

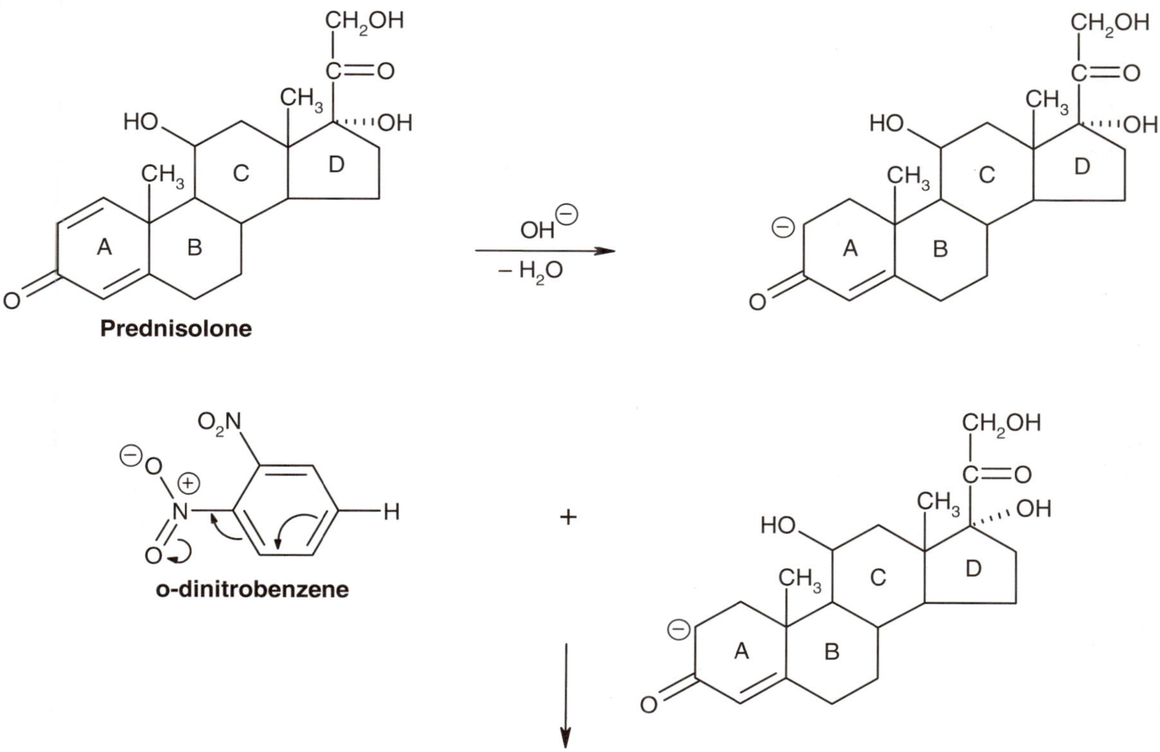

Prednisolone

o-dinitrobenzene

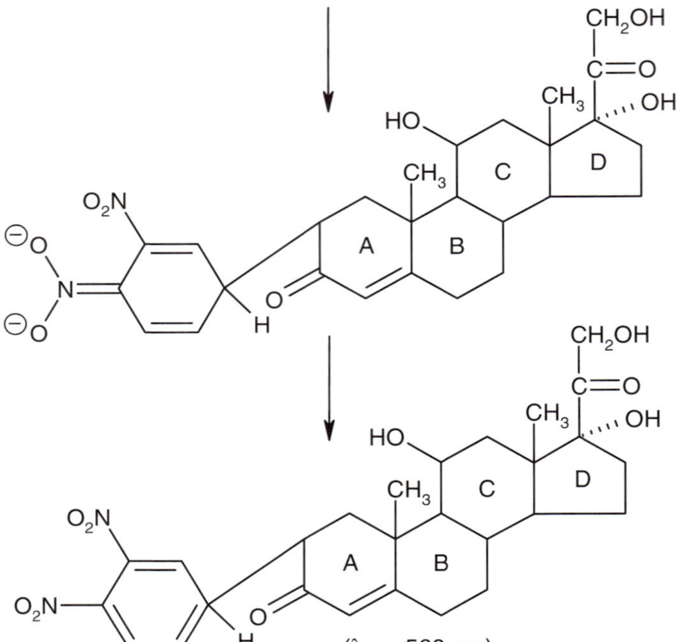

Note

A spectrophotometric method was described by Narurkar et al. (1981) involving reaction with Porter & Silber reagent. This reaction is specific for steroids with 17,21-dihydroxy-20-keto group. For detailed reaction mechanism, see under betamethasone in formulation of this chapter.

Reference

M.N. Narurkar & C.I. Jarowski, *J. Pharm. Sci.*, **70(7)**, 810-811, 1981.

Econazole nitrate

Weigh accurately sample (cream) equivalent to 50 mg of econazole nitrate acid and extract with chloroform (3 × 30 ml), passing each extract through same bed of anhydrous sodium sulphate. Dry the combined chloroform extract in vacuum oven at 60°C. Cool and take up the residue in 50 ml of glacial acetic acid by slight warming. Titrate with 0.01 N perchloric acid (violet). Carry out the blank titration for final calculations. Each ml of 0.01 N perchloric acid is equivalent to 4.447 mg of econazole nitrate.

Formulation 12

Tinidazole, Miconazole nitrate

ESTIMATION

Tinidazole

Follow the method described in formulation 13 of this chapter.

Miconazole nitrate

Reagent

Cobalt thiocyanate reagent: To 20 g of ammonium thiocyanate in 100 ml of water, add 5 g of cobalt nitrate, shake to dissolve. Add sufficient sodium chloride to saturate the solution.

Standard solution

Treat 40 mg of miconazole nitrate as described under preparation of sample solution.

Sample solution

An accurately weighed quantity of powdered sample equivalent to 50 mg of miconazole nitrate is suspended in 10 ml of water, basify with ammonia solution and extract with chloroform (4 × 50 ml). Combined chloroform layer is shaken with 15-20 ml of saturated solution of sodium chloride, separated, passed through anhydrous sodium sulphate, concentrated to about 60-70 ml and then finally adjusted to 100 ml.

Procedure

To 25 ml each of sample and standard solutions add 10 ml of cobalt thiocyanate reagent, shake for 5 min. Separate organic layer, pass through anhydrous sodium sulphate, measure the absorbance at about 620 nm against regent blank processed similarly.

Note

1. Solutions may sometime develop haziness if the laboratory working temperature is below 20°C.
2. Both the components can be identified by TLC by applying methanolic solution and n-hexane-chloroform-methanol-ammonia (60 + 30 + 10 + 1) as mobile phase, detection by exposing to iodine vapours.

Probable Reaction Mechanism

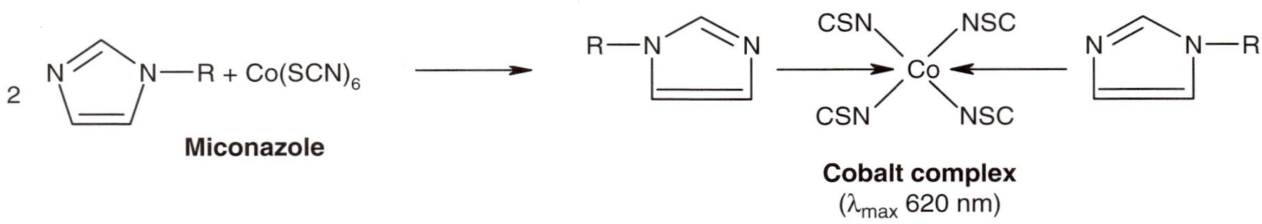

Note

The drug also forms complex with Cu(2) as well similar to Co^{++} complex.

Note

Cations of transition metals are electron acceptor that are capable of complexing with organic compounds having electron donor properties. Most important of these metals forming chelates are Cu^{+2}, Fe^{+3} and Co^{+2}. They have the greatest affinity for compounds containing oxygen and nitrogen.

Formulation 13

Tinidazole, Clotrimazole

ESTIMATION

Tinidazole

Standard solution

20 mcg/ml of tinidazole in water (slight warming may be necessary to aid the solution).

Sample solution

Accurately weighed quantity of the finely powdered sample equivalent to 50 mg of tinidazole is suspended in 70-80 ml of water and heated in a water-bath for about 15 min, cooled, filtered and diluted to 100 ml with water/methanol. 2 ml of the filtrate is further diluted with water/methanol to 100 ml (20 mcg/ml).

Measure the extinction of both sample and standard solutions at about 310 nm and calculate to results by comparison.

Clotrimazole

Suspend accurately weighed quantity of powdered sample equivalent to 100 mg of the substance in 10-15 ml of water. Add 10 ml of 1 N sulphuric acid and shake to obtain a uniform suspension. Add 30 ml of chloroform, 0.2 ml of indicator solution (dimethyl yellow), shake vigorously and titrate with 0.02 N sodium lauryl sulphate (SLS), shaking vigorously after each addition.

Each ml of 0.02 M SLS is equivalent to 6.987 mg of clotrimazole.

Formulation 14

Hydrocortisone acetate, Lidocaine (Lignocaine), Allantoin, Zinc oxide

ESTIMATION

Hydrocortisone acetate

Follow the method for estimation of steroids using tetrazolium blue or triphenyl tetrazolium chloride. The absorption of the resulting coloured solution is measured at 550 nm or 490 nm depending on nature of tetrazolium salt used.

For reaction mechanism, refer to formulation 13 of this chapter.

Lidocaine

Accurately weighed quantity of the sample (ointment) is suspended in water with slight warming. Extract with chloroform (3 × 50 ml). Wash the combined chloroform layer with 25 ml of water (discard the aqueous layer). Evaporate chloroform layer to dryness and carry non-aqueous titration by titrating with 0.1 N perchloric acid (crystal violet or brilliant green). Each ml of 0.1 N perchloric acid is equivalent to 23.43 mg of lidocaine.

Note

Its reaction with Cu^{2+} in alkaline medium giving blue-coloured complex has been adopted for quantitative estimation.

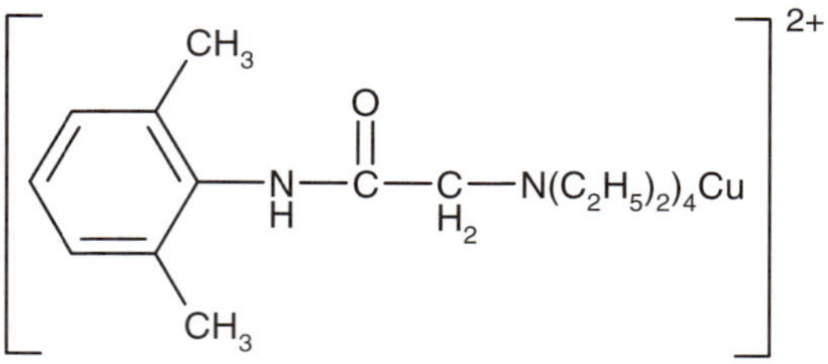

Lidocaine - copper complex

The compound is hydrolysed when treated with 80% sulphuric acid to give dimethylaniline. The hydrolytic product with primary aromatic amino group can be exploited for different analytical methods such as diazo reaction or condensation with 'PDAB'.

Allantoin

Reagents

(a) 2.5 w/v solution of dimethylglycoxime in concentrated hydrochloric acid.
(b) To 1 g of thiosemicarbazide add 100 ml of hydrochloric acid (1 : 1), heat in water-bath for 15 min, cool and filter.

Mix 10 ml each of solution (a) and (b), add sufficient hydrochloric acid (1 : 1) and produce 100 ml. Prepare the reagent fresh on the day of use.

Standard solution

50 mcg/ml of allantoin in 0.1 N hydrochloric acid, gentle warming may be necessary to effect the solution.

Sample solution

Accurately weighed quantity of sample (ointment) equivalent to 15 mg of the substance is suspended in 50 ml of 0.1 N hydrochloric acid with the aid of heating in a water-bath. Cool and shake with 20 ml of chloroform. Reject organic layer and dilute the acid layer to 100 ml. Filter and dilute appropriately to get final concentration of 30 mcg/ml for analysis.

Procedure

To 5 ml each of sample, standard and blank solutions add 10 ml of the dimethylglycoxime - thiosemicarbazide reagent. Heat on a water-bath at 90°C for 30 min, cool and dilute to 50 ml with hydrochloric acid (1 : 1). Measure the absorbance of both test and standard solutions at about 525 nm against reagent blank and calculate the results by comparison.

Note

Entire procedure is carried out in actinic liquid (use of amber-coloured flasks).

Probable Reaction Mechanism

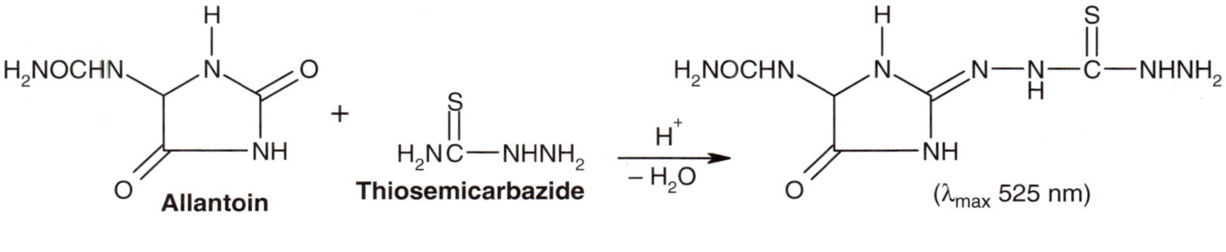

Due to deprotonation at N-3, the substance can be titrated with tetrabutyl-ammonium hydroxide in DMF i.e. in anhydrous medium.

Some pharmacopoeias include silver nitrate/pyridine in aqueous medium.

Probable Reaction Mechanism

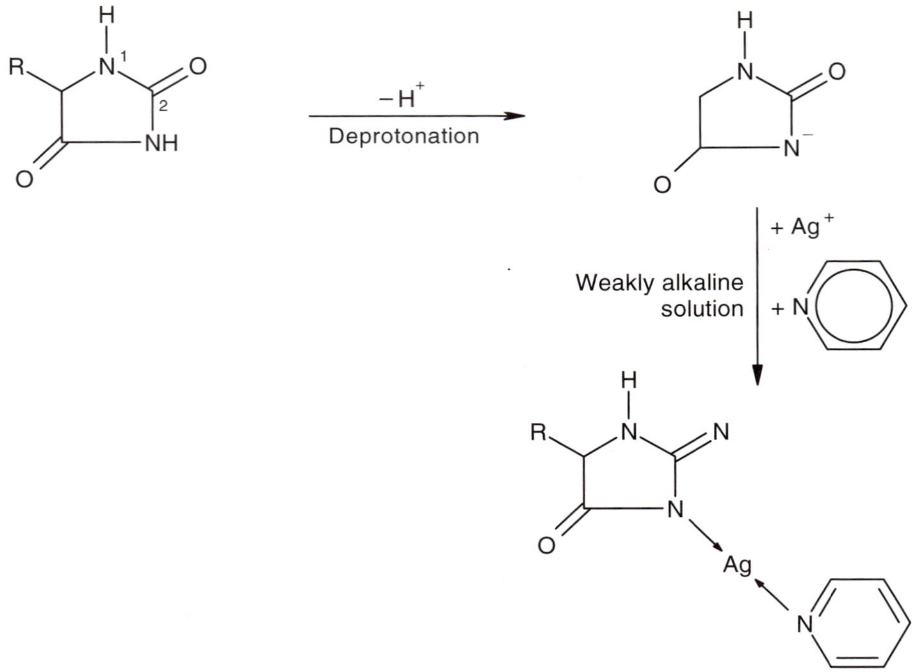

Poorly soluble silver complex

Pyridine serves two purposes: (a) inhibit precipitation of silver nitrate as Ag_2O from weakly alkaline medium; (b) it forms very poorly soluble silver complex, hence allow the reaction to proceed smoothly for a good end-point.

Zinc oxide

Ignite sample equivalent to about 150 mg of zinc oxide in a platinum crucible at 700°C. Cool, add few drops of concentrated sulphuric acid and 20 ml of water, warm to dissolve and transfer the contents to a conical flask. Wash the crucible with water and transfer the washings to the conical flask. Adjust the pH to 10.5 with ammonia - ammonium chloride buffer and titrate with 0.05 M EDTA (eriochrome black T). Each ml of 0.05 M EDTA is equivalent to 4.069 mg of zinc oxide.

Formulation 15

Clotrimazole, Lignocaine (Lidocaine/Xylocaine) hydrochloride

ESTIMATION

Clotrimazole

Transfer accurately weighed sample (ear drops) equivalent to 100 mg of clotrimazole to a separating funnel containing about 20 ml of water. Extract with solvent ether (3 × 40 ml). Wash the combined ethereal layer with 20 ml of water and pass through anhydrous sodium sulphate (preserve the combined aqueous layer for estimation of lignocaine hydrochloride). Evaporate ether layer on water-bath, cool and add 5 ml of acetic anhydride and 15-20 ml of dioxane. Carry out the non-aqueous titration using α-naphtholbenzein indicator (end point, pink to green). Each ml of 0.02 N perchloric acid is equivalent to 6.896 g clotrimazole.

Lignocaine (Lidocaine/Xylocaine) hydrochloride

Titrate the entire aqueous layer preserved during estimation of clotrimazole with 0.1 N silver nitrate using potassium chromate as indicator. Each ml of 0.1 N silver nitrate is equivalent to 28.88 mg of lignocaine hydrochloride. The method involves the estimation of hydrochloride moiety of the molecule.

Lignocaine complexes with Cu(II) and Co(II) in alkaline medium to give green-coloured complex. This colour reaction can be used for quantitative estimation of the drug.

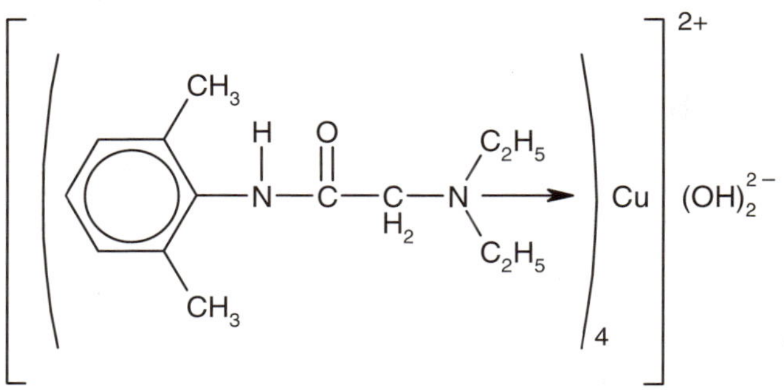

Green-coloured copper complex

Usually the amide group of the compound does not get easily hydrolysed by acid due to shielding effect of methyl group in o-position but on heating in 80% sulphuric acid it is hydrolysed to dimethylaniline. The aromatic amine can be diazotized and coupled with suitable reagent for quantitative work or can couple with PDAB/PDAC to form Schiff's base.

Probable Reaction Mechanism

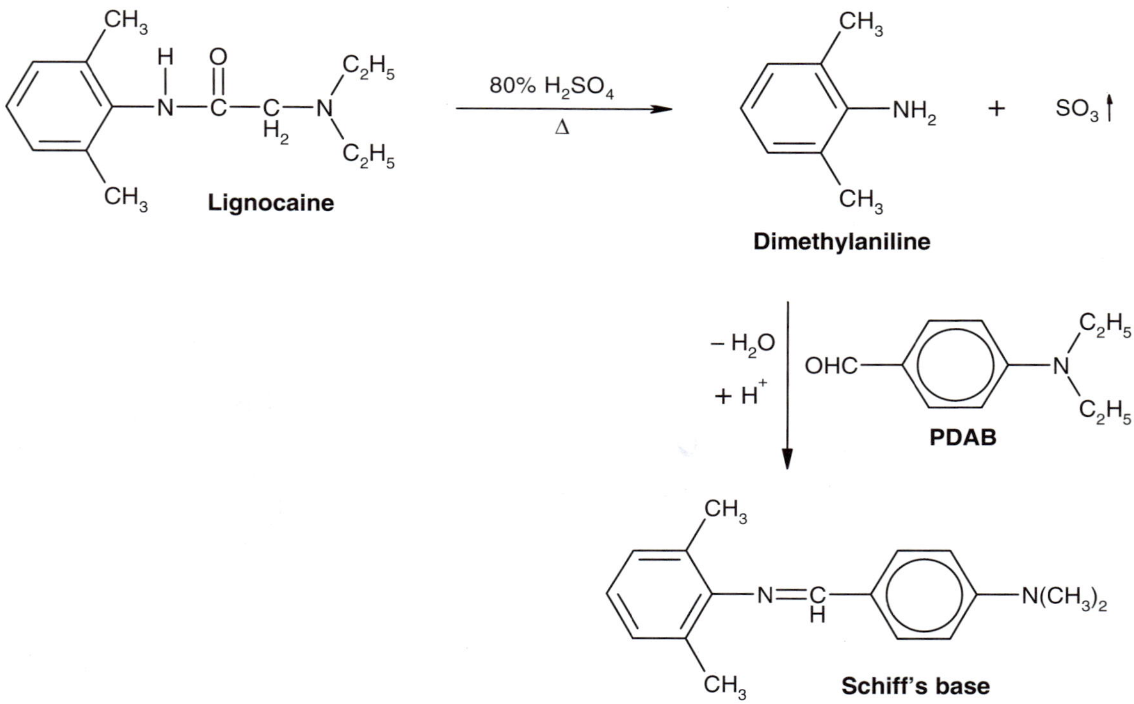

The compound undergoes nitration reaction at benzene moiety of the molecule to give dinitro derivative which ultimately forms Meisenheimer salt with acetone/ potassium hydroxide.

Probable Reaction Mechanism

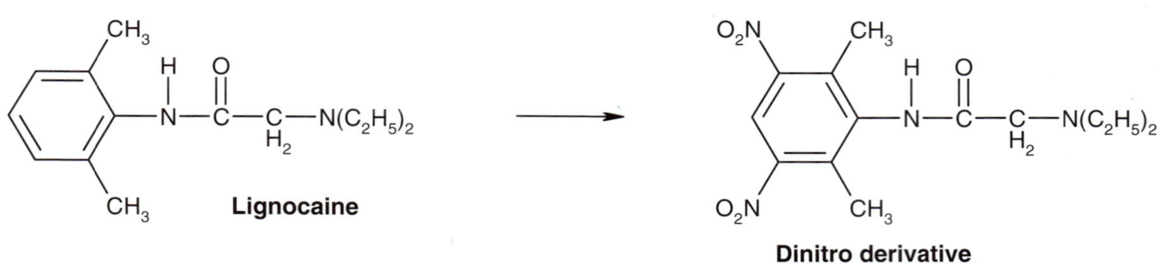

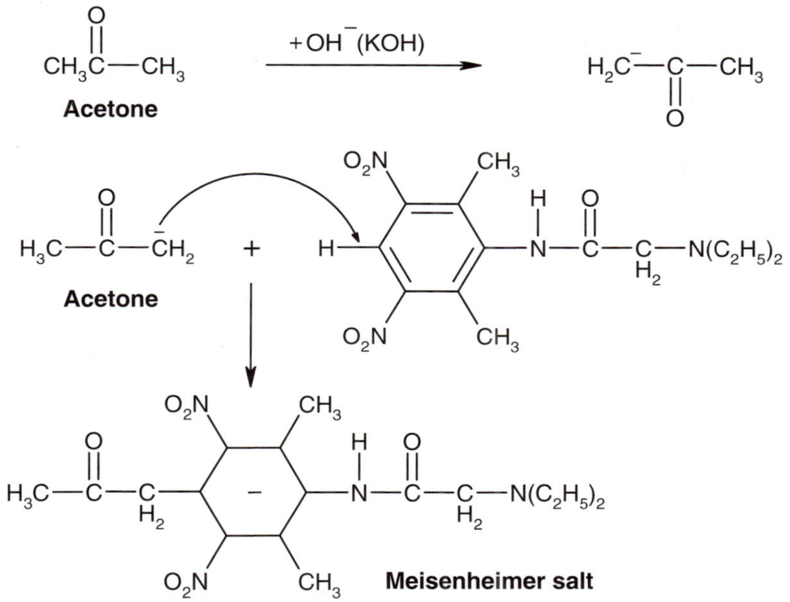

Note

1. Since Meisenheimer salt gives different colour, this test is used to distinguish lignocaine from tetracaine.
2. It has been reported that by using dimsyl anion instead of acetonyl anion as nucleophile, there is improvement in colour reaction.

Probable Reaction Mechanism

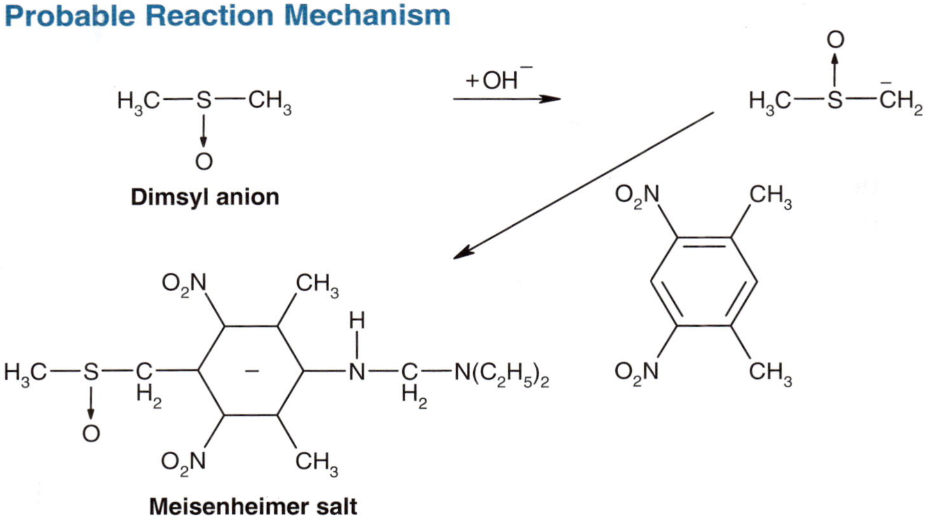

Reference

Pharmaceutical Chemistry (Vol. 2) by H.J. Roth, pp. 134-396.

Stewart & Lotti (1970) described a spectrophotometric method for estimation of lignocaine (lidocaine) based on reaction of primary aromatic amine with 9-chloroacridine yielding a coloured complex (λ_{max} 435 nm). The method is analogous to the one described for estimation of isoniazid. However, the solution of 9-chloroacridine was prepared in tetrahydrofuran as the solution of the reagent in ethanol was stable only for 30 min due to rapid ethanolysis of ethanolic 9-chloroacridine solution due to reaction between the two. The reaction was carried out at pH 5 resulting in first hydrolysis of the compound and then reaction with chloroacridine.

Probable Reaction Mechanism

As proposed by the author, the reaction mechanism is as under.

The dimethylaniline formed as a result of acidic hydrolysis reacts with chloroacridine.

Probable Reaction Mechanism

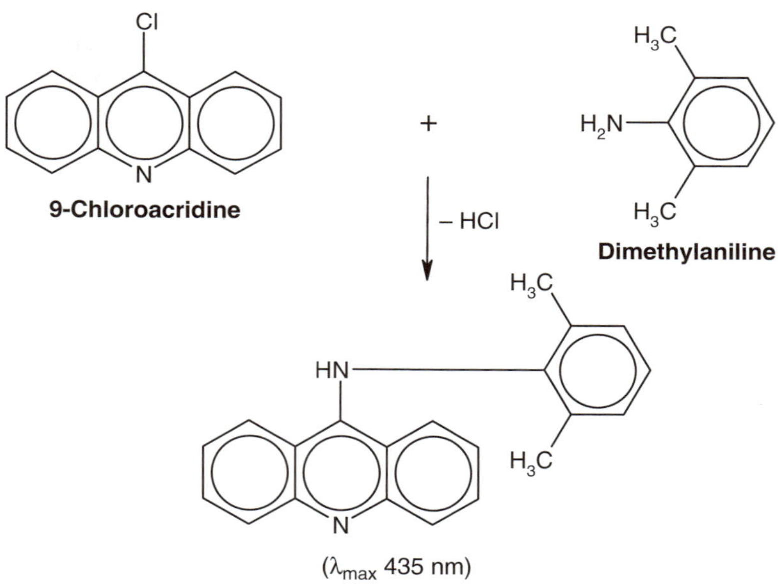

Note

Other local anaesthetics such as procaine, tetracaine and benzocaine undergo similar reaction.

Reference

J.T. Stewart & D.M. Lotti, *J. Pharm. Sci.*, **59(6)**, 838-840, 1970.

Formulation 16

Clotrimazole, Sulphamethoxazole

ESTIMATION

Clotrimazole

Standard solution

100 mcg/ml of clotrimazole in 0.1 N hydrochloric acid.

Sample solution

Accurately weighed quantity of the sample equivalent to 100 mg of the substance was shaken with 50-60 ml of 0.1 N hydrochloric acid and placed in a shaker at 37°C for 2 hrs. The volume was adjusted to 100 ml with acid and filtered through G_3 sintered funnel.

Procedure

To 2 ml each of sample and standard solutions add 8 ml of perchloric acid (70%), mix and place in boiling water-bath for 5 min. The orange yellow colour formed was measured at about 440 nm after cooling to room temperature against reagent blank. Deduce the results by comparison.

Clotrimazole in the formulation can be estimated by titration with sodium lauryl sulphate. Equivalent factor for sodium lauryl sulphate can be determined by titration with clotrimazole of known purity using methyl yellow as indicator. Refer to the procedure for dicyclomine in formulation 10 of the chapter on analgesics and antipyretics.

Sulphamethoxazole

METHOD 1

Weigh accurate quantity of the sample equivalent to 500 mg of the sample, add 20 ml of glacial acetic acid, 40 ml water and 15 ml hydrochloric acid. Shake to dissolve and carry out sodium nitrite titration. Each ml of 0.1 M sodium nitrite is equivalent to 0.02533 g of sulphamethoxazole. Excess HNO_2 reacts with iodide to produce iodine which gives colour with starch.

$$2I^- + 2HNO_2 + 2H \longrightarrow I_2 + 2NO\uparrow + 2H_2O$$

METHOD 2

Reagents

1. 0.1% w/v solution of p-dimethylaminocinnamaldehyde (PDAC).
2. 50% v/v methanolic phosphoric acid.

Sample and standard solutions

100 μg/ml of sulphamethoxazole in methanol.

Procedure

To 3 ml each of sample and standard solutions add 5 ml each of PDAC reagent and phosphoric acid solution, keep at room temperature for 15 min, make up the volume to 25 ml with methanol and measure the absorbance at 545 nm against reagent blank.

Probable Reaction Mechanism

The amino group of the drug will react with carbonyl group of the aldehyde reagent resulting in the formation of Schiff's base with loss of water.

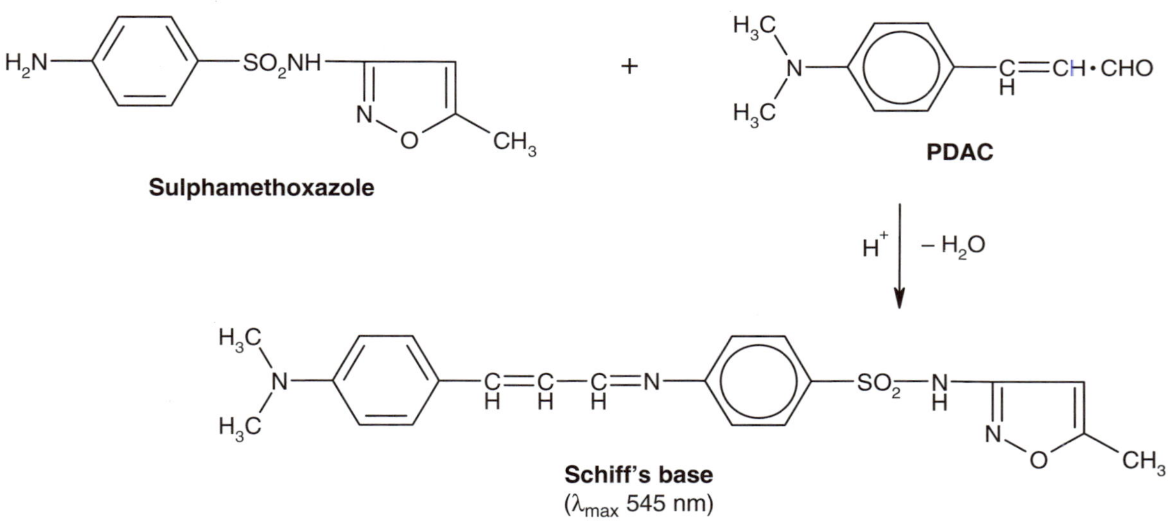

Reference

S. Raghuveer, I.R.K. Raju, D.K. Valsa & C.M.R. Srivastva, *Indian Drugs*, **30(3)**, 132-136, 1992.

Similarly, the drug can form Schiff's base with salicyldehyde in acidic medium to give yellow-coloured complex.

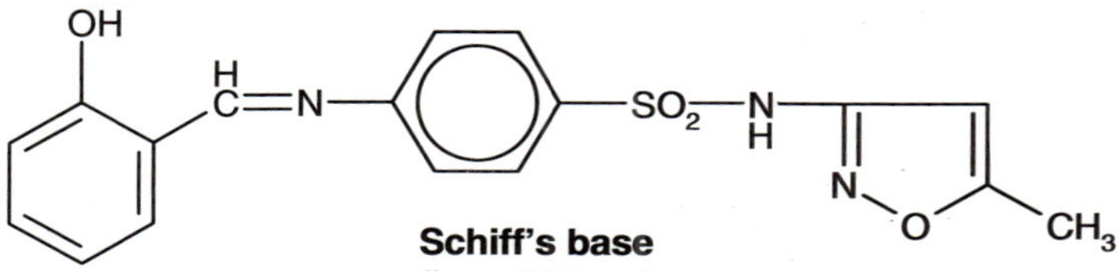

Schiff's base
(λ_{max} 380 nm)

Reference

O.S. Kamalapukar & G.L. Kamat, *Indian Drugs*, **22(2)**, 95-96, 1984.

Note

The drug can be diazotized and coupled with various reagents (see under general reactions of sulphonamides).

Formulation 17

Cetrimide, Chlorhexidine gluconate

ESTIMATION

Cetrimide

Reagents

1. Bromophenol blue solution: Prepare a 0.04% w/v solution of bromophenol blue in 20% v/v isopropyl alcohol in distilled water.
2. 0.001 M sodium lauryl sulphate solution: Dissolve about 0.3 g of sodium lauryl sulphate in 1000 ml of water. To stabilize the solution, see formulation 10 of the chapter on analgesics and antipyretics.
3. 0.001 M cetrimide solution: Dissolve 0.35 g of cetrimide of known strength in a small amount of warm distilled water, cool and dilute to 1000 ml.
4. 10% sodium carbonate solution in water.

Sample solution

Dilute the sample equivalent to 0.3 g of cetrimide to 100 ml with distilled water. Further dilute 10.0 ml of the above solution to 100 ml with distilled water.

Procedure

Pipette a 25.0 ml aliquot of the sample solution into a tall, narrow-necked, glass-stoppered bottle of 250 ml, add 50 ml of chloroform, 50 ml of 0.001 M sodium lauryl sulphate solution and 5-10 drops of bromophenol blue solution. Make the contents of the bottle alkaline with sodium carbonate solution. Prepare a blank in the same manner omitting the substance to be analysed.

Titrate both blank and sample solutions with 0.001 M cetrimide solution shaking after each addition of titrant. The end-point is indicated by the appearance of the permanent blue colour in the chloroform layer.

Note

The solution should remain alkaline during titration. The method utilises the stochiometric reaction between cetrimide and sodium lauryl sulphate. An excess of the reactant is added to the diluted sample followed by back titration of the excess sodium lauryl sulphate with a standard cetrimide solution.

Chlorhexidine gluconate

METHOD 1

Reagents

1. Alkaline sodium hypobromite solution: Dissolve 10 g of sodium hydroxide in 400 ml of distilled water and add, in small portions, 2.75 ml of bromine until the bromine is completely dissolved. Adjust the volume of the solution to 500 ml and standardize the solution as follows:

   Pipette 10.0 ml of the solution into a 250 ml conical flask and add 25 ml of distilled water, 2 g of potassium iodide and 10 ml of glacial acetic acid. Titrate the liberated iodine with 0.1 N sodium thiosulphate solution. Each ml of 0.1 N sodium thiosulphate solution is equal to 0.0080 g of bromine. Accordingly adjust the sodium hypobromite solution with water to contain 1.5% w/v of available bromine. The reagent is finally prepared by mixing 66 ml of hypobromite solution with 33 ml of 3 M sodium hydroxide solution.
2. 1 M hydrochloric acid.
3. 1 M sodium hydroxide acid.
4. 20% w/v solution of cetrimide.
5. Chloroform.
6. 1.0% solution of 1-naphthol in alcohol.

Standard solution

To 10 mg of chlorhexidine gluconate add 20 ml of water and 10 ml of 1 N HCl and extract with 3 × 25 ml of $CHCl_3$. Wash the combined extract with 10 ml of water and dilute the aqueous solution to 100 ml with water.

Sample solution

Take sample equivalent to 10 mg of chlorhexidine gluconate, add 20 ml of water and 10 ml of 1 N HCl and extract with 3 × 25 ml of $CHCl_3$. Wash the combined extract with 10 ml of water and dilute the aqueous solution to 100 ml with water.

Procedure

To 5 ml each of sample and standard solutions add 70 ml of water, 5 ml of cetrimide solution and 1 ml of 1-naphthol solution. Mix and add 2 ml of hypobromite solution, dilute to 25 ml with water and measure the absorbance at 480 nm against reagent blank.

Probable Reaction Mechanism

This method is based on Sakaguchi reaction i.e. reaction of biguanidine derivative with 1-naphthol in the presence of hypobromite. Cetrimide, a quaternary compound, facilitates the reaction and also stabilizes the final colour of quinonimine derivative.

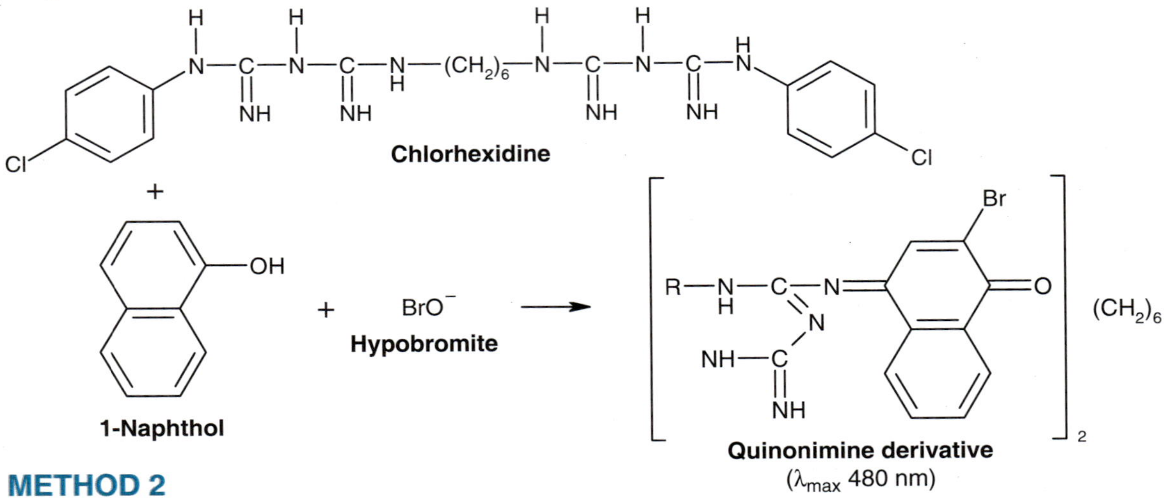

METHOD 2

Reagents

1. Phosphate buffer, pH 5.7: 100 ml of 0.1 M citric acid and 140 ml of 0.2 M disodium hydrogen phosphate are mixed to get the buffer of pH 5.7.
2. Bromocresol green solution: 0.03% solution in phosphate buffer, pH 5.7.

Standard solution

50 mcg/ml of chlorhexidine in water.

Sample solution

Accurately measured volume of the sample (lotions, shampoos, viscous solutions) equivalent to 10 mg of the substance is basified with 10 N sodium hydroxide and extracted with chloroform (2 × 20 ml), combine chloroform layer and dilute to 50 ml.

Procedure

To 1 ml each of sample and standard solutions add 3 ml of dye solution and 5 ml of chloroform. Shake for 3 min and centrifuge. Measure the absorbance of chloroform layer at 410 nm against reagent blank and calculate the results by comparison.

Explanatory Note

This method is based on formation of ion-pair complex between the drug and the dye in phosphate buffer, pH 5.7.

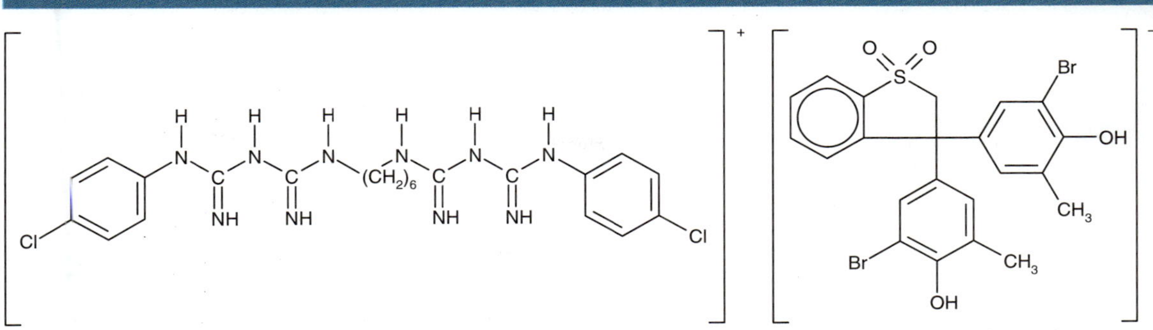

Chlorhexidine **Bromocresol purple**

Chlorhexidine - bromocresol purple complex

Drug - dye complex is extractable into chloroform and has λ_{max} 410 nm.

Note

The colour is stable for 8 hrs.

Reference

G. Andermann, M.O. Buhler & M. Erhart, *J. Pharm. Sci.*, **69(2)**, 215-217, 1980.

Lowry (1979) has proposed ion-pair complex formation with bromothymol blue in 0.2 M phosphate buffer, pH 7.5, with quaternary ammonium compounds.

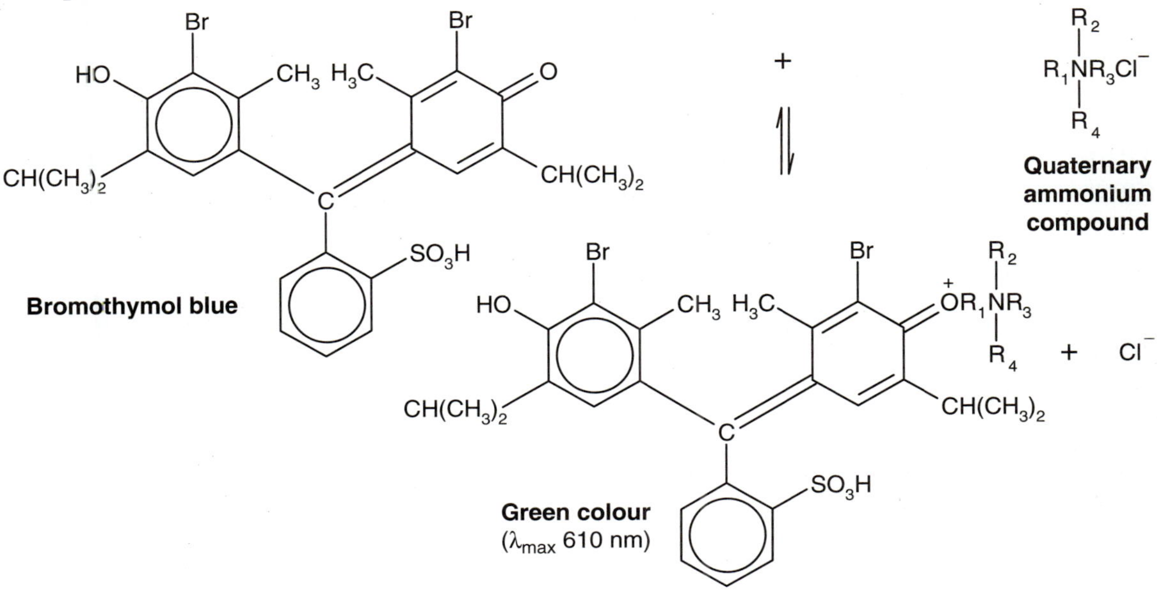

Reference

J.B. Lowry, *J. Pharm. Sci.*, **68(1)**, 110-111, 1979.

Formulation 18

Silver sulphadiazine, Chlorhexidine gluconate

ESTIMATION

Silver sulphadiazine

Standard solution

To 50 mg of silver sulphadiazine add 100 ml of water and 25 ml of concentrated hydrochloric acid, shake well, heat in water-bath for 10 min, cool and dilute to 250 ml. Filter and dilute to 10 ml of the filtrate to 100 ml with water (20 mcg/ml). This shall liberate free sulphadiazine.

Sample solution

Accurately weighed amount of sample (cream) equivalent to 50 mg of the substance is heated as under standard solution.

Procedure

Take 10 ml each of sample and standard solutions and proceed with diazotization and colour development as described for sulphonamides.

Chlorhexidine gluconate

Suspend the sample in 20 ml of water, add 10 ml of 1 N hydrochloric acid and shake with chloroform (3×25 ml), reject the chloroform layer and dilute the aqueous layer to get 300 mcg/ml.

Procedure

Follow the method described in formulation 17 of this chapter.

Formulation 19

Paraformaldehyde, Formaldehyde

ESTIMATION

Paraformaldehyde in tooth paste

Reagents

1. 0.01 N sodium hydroxide.
2. 0.002 N sodium hydroxide.
3. 2 N sodium hydroxide.
4. 1% w/v phenylhydrazinium hydrochloride solution.
5. 5% w/v potassium ferricyanide solution, to be prepared just before use.
6. Hydrochloric acid, concentrated.

Standard solution

Dissolve 100 mg of paraformaldehyde in 10 ml of 2 N sodium hydroxide and dilute to 100 ml with distilled water. Dilute suitably with distilled water to get 25 mcg/ml solution of paraformaldehyde.

To series of 50 ml volumetric flasks, transfer accurately 0.5, 1.0, 1.5, 2.0, 3.0, 4.0, 5.0, 6.0, 7.0 and 8.0 ml of standard solution. Add appropriate amount of 0.002 N sodium hydroxide to produce 10 ml of total volume in each flask. Add 5 ml of phenylhydrazinium hydrochloride reagent to each flask followed by 5 ml of 0.5 N hydrochloric acid and 1 ml of potassium ferricyanide reagent. Mix well and add 10 ml of hydrochloric acid to each flask, keep aside for 30 minutes. Measure the absorption of the resulting solutions at about 520 nm using a reagent blank prepared in the same manner omitting the substance (paraformaldehyde). Draw the standard curve to check the linearity.

Sample solution

Dissolve 1 g of the paste in 5 ml of 0.1 N sodium hydroxide, dilute to 100 ml with distilled water. Centrifuge in stoppered centrifuge tube for 20 minutes at 3000 rpm.

Take 5.0 ml each of standard (25 mcg/ml solution as prepared under linearity studies) and sample solution and proceed with colour development as described under general procedure for linearity studies.

The method obeys Beer's law in the range of 25-200 mcg/ml.

Formaldehyde in tooth paste

Standard solution

Dilute 5 ml of formaldehyde solution (40% w/v) to 100 ml with water. Further dilutions are done with 0.2 N sodium hydroxide to get a concentration of 25 mcg/ml. For sample preparation and procedure for estimation, refer to the method described above for paraformaldehyde.

Paraformaldehyde in the presence of H_2O liberates formaldehyde. In the presence of oxidizing agents, such as k-ferricyanide, formaldehyde reacts with the hydrazine to form an intense coloured formazone.

Excess of phenylhydrazine present is then oxidized to the dizonium salt which couples with hydrozone to give 1,5-diphenylformazone.

$$(CH_2O)_n \text{ ; n = 30 to 100} \xrightarrow[\text{Water (cold)}]{\text{Water (hot)}} HCHO$$

Paraformaldehyde **Formaldehyde**

Probable Reaction Mechanism

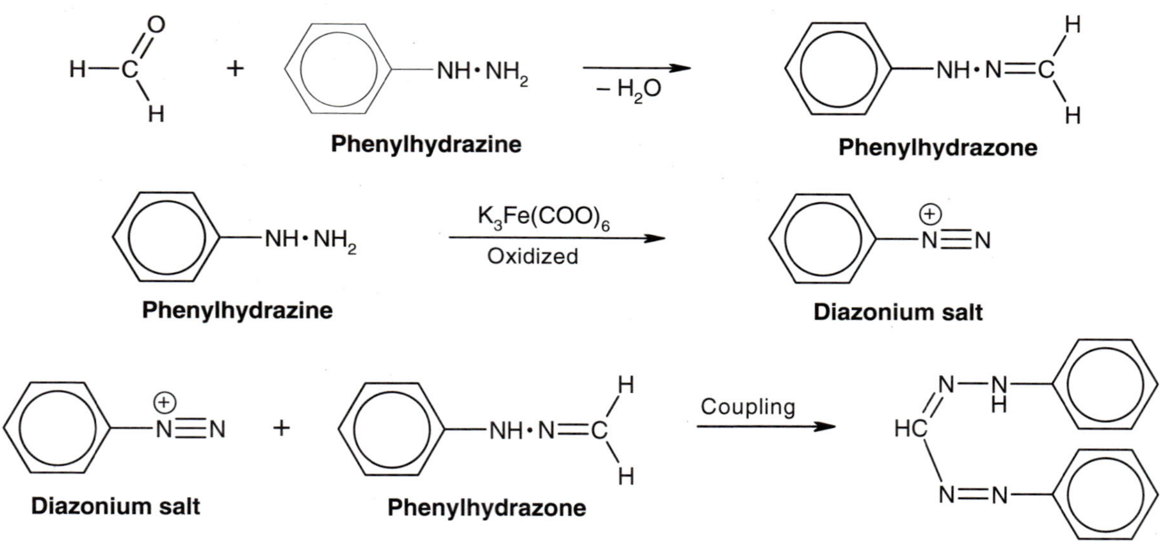

1,5-diphenylformazone
(coloured product)
(λ_{max} 520 nm)

Note

Other aldehydes similarly react producing formazone with varying colours.

HCHO condenses with the aromatic system of chromotropic acid in the ortho position to the phenolic hydroxy group in the presence of H_2SO_4 and forms an intermediate. H_2SO_4 acts as an oxidizing agent in the next step. Finally a mesomerically stabilized 3,4,5,6-dibenzoxanthylium cation is formed which is responsible for the colour.

Sulphuric acid acts both as dehydrating agent in first step and as an oxidizing agent in the second step.

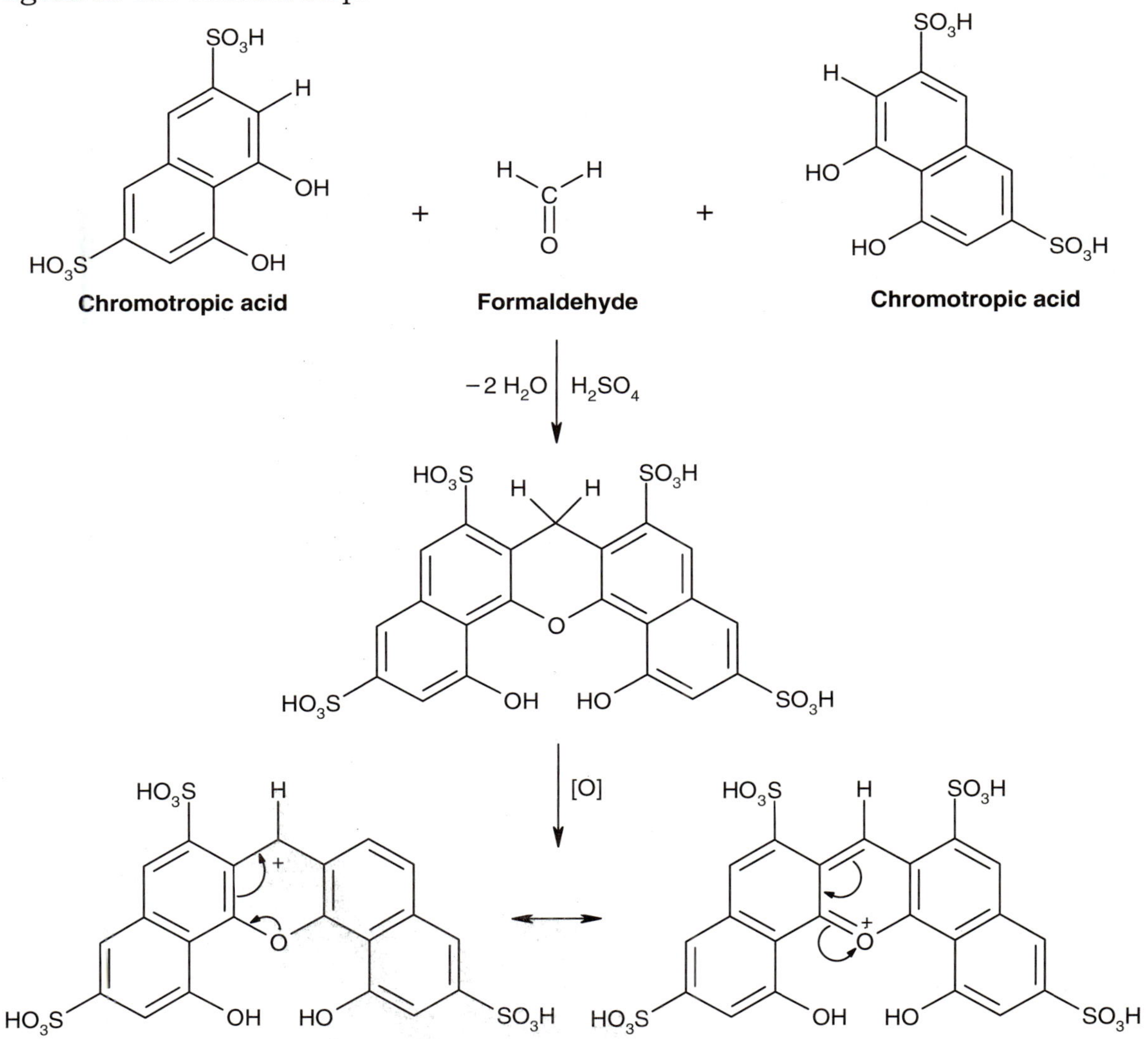

Mesomerically stabilized 3,4,5,6-dibenzoxanthylium cation

Reference

Pharmaceutical Chemistry (Vol. 2) by H.J. Roth, p. 122.

A direct oxidometric determination is possible by reaction with iodine in alkaline medium. Formaldehyde is oxidized to formic acid and iodine produced on acidification can be titrated with sodium thiosulphate.

$$I_2 + 2OH^- \longrightarrow \underset{\textbf{Hypoiodite}}{IO^-} + I^- + H_2O$$

$$HO^- + HCHO + IO^- \longrightarrow \underset{\textbf{Formate}}{HCOO^-} + I^- + H_2O$$

$$IO^- + I^- + 2H^+ \longrightarrow I_2 + H_2O$$

Iodine so formed is titrated with $Na_2S_2O_3$.

Note

Formaldehyde answers Nash reaction i.e. reaction with acetylacetone in the presence of conc. sulphuric acid leading to formation of coloured compound dihydrolutidine derivative.

Formulation 20

Clotrimazole, Selenium disulfide

ESTIMATION

Clotrimazole

METHOD 1

Follow the method described in formulation 4 of this chapter.

METHOD 2

Reagents

1. Phthalate buffer, pH 2.5.
2. 0.1% w/v solution of bromocresol in water.

Standard solution

200 mcg/ml of clotrimazole in isopropyl alcohol.

Sample solution

Weigh accurately sample equivalent to 25 mg of the substance, add 25 ml of isopropyl alcohol, slightly warm, vortex for 2 min and make up the volume to 100 ml.

Procedure

To 5 ml each of sample and standard solutions add 5 ml of buffer solution and 2.5 ml of the dye and 10 ml of chloroform. Shake vigorously and allow the layers to separate. Measure the absorption of chloroform layer at 430 nm and calculate the results by comparison.

METHOD 3 (Topical solution, cream, powder, vaginal tablets)

The method is based on interaction of tertiary amine moiety of the drug with the reagent giving coloured species (λ_{max} 475 nm).

Reagents

1. 1% w/v solution of p-chloranil in 1,4-dioxane or p-chloranilic acid in acetonitrile.
2. 1,4-dioxane.
3. 0.1 N hydrochloric acid.

Standard and sample solutions

As described under method 2.

Procedure

To 5 ml each of sample and standard solutions add 2 ml of chloranil reagent and keep in boiling water-bath for 60 min, cool, add 15 ml of dioxane to dissolve the residue completely. Add 2 ml of 0.1 N hydrochloric acid, shake well and dilute to 25 ml with isopropyl alcohol. Concomitantly measure the absorbance of both sample and standard solutions at 475 nm against reagent blank prepared by taking 5 ml of isopropyl alcohol and calculate the results by comparison.

Probable Reaction Mechanism

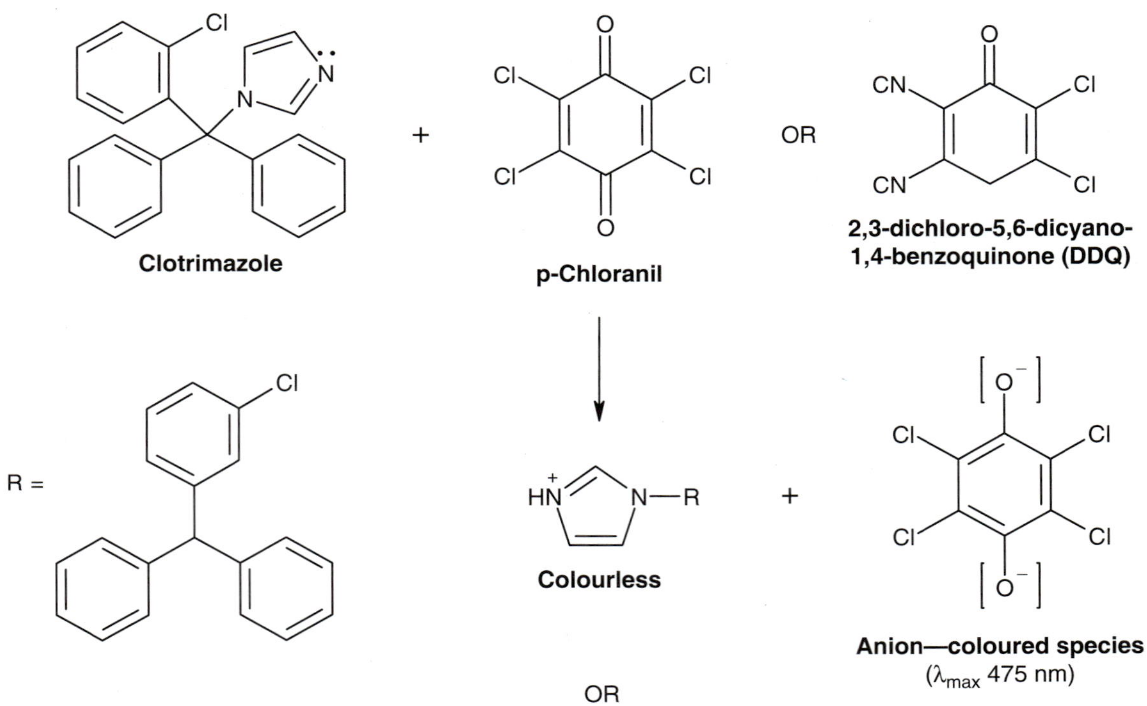

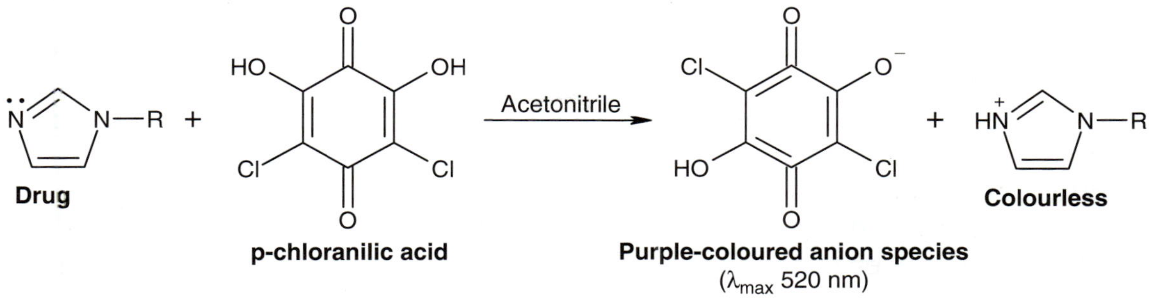

Reference

1. P.Y. Khashaba, S.R. El-Shabouri, K.M. Emara & A.M. Mohamed, *J. Pharm. & Biomed. Analysis*, **22**, 363-376, 2000.
2. D.M. Shingbal & H.S. Kudehadkar, *Indian Drugs*, **24(8)**, 408-410, 1986.

An alternative method based on formation of ion-pair complex with methyl orange (MO) has been described by Abdelmageed et al. (1993). To the sample and standard solutions (50-350 µg/ml in methanol) add 3 ml of 0.1 M citric acid, 2 ml of MO solution (0.1% in 40% aqueous methanol) followed by shaking and addition of 8 ml of chloroform. The organic layer diluted to 25 ml and passed through anhydrous sodium sulphate and absorption measured at 422 nm for quantitative evaluation.

Note

1. Acid hydrolysis products i.e. imidazole and o-chlorophenyl diphenyl methanol did not interfere.
2. Betamethasone/dexamethasone did not interfere.
3. The method was appropriate for analysis of powder, vaginal tablets, topical solution and cream.

Reference

Osama H. Abdelmageed & Pakinaz Y. Khashaba, *Talanta*, **40(8)**, 1289-1294, 1993.

Selenium disulfide

Reagent

Fuming nitric acid: To 250 ml concentrated nitric acid add slowly and carefully 3 ml of formaldehyde. When the reaction is completed, close it properly. This addition should be done in fuming chamber.

Procedure

Accurately weighed quantity of the sample (semi-solid) equivalent to 100 mg of the substance is digested with 25 ml of nitric acid for 2 hours at hot plate, cool and dilute to 250 ml with water. To 50 ml of this solution add 20 ml water, 10 g urea and heat to boiling till volume is reduced to almost half. Cool, add 10 ml of dilute sulphuric acid and 10 ml of potassium iodide (10%) and titrate with 0.02 N sodium thiosulphate using starch as indicator. End point is reddish brown. Each ml of 0.05 N sodium thiosulphate is equivalent to 987 μg of selenium (Se) or 1.789 mg of selenium sulfide (SeS_2).

Probable Reaction Mechanism

By treating with nitric acid, SeS_2 gets oxidized to selenious acid (H_2SeO_3). Selenious acid so formed oxidizes potassium iodide to iodine which is titrated with sodium thiosulphate. This method is not suitable for microdetermination.

Bodini et al. (1983) have described a spectrophotometric method for estimation of selenium at micro level. The method is based on reaction of oxidized selenium with 4,5,6-triaminopyrimidine. The reaction is analogous to the one described by Murashova et al. (1969) and J. Hoste & Gillis (1955). The reactions described by these authors involve reaction of the element (Se) with o-diamine to yield corresponding piazselnol with λ_{max} 420 nm. Since reagents (aminobenzidine derivatives) being banned, Bodini et al. have described the method using 4,5,6-triaminopyrimidine (TAP), the compound having three vicinal amino groups. The reaction was carried out in 0.3 M hydrochloric acid or 3.5 M phosphoric acid, phosphoric acid being preferred.

The reaction was carried out at 40°C and maximum absorbance (362 nm) reached after 90°C.

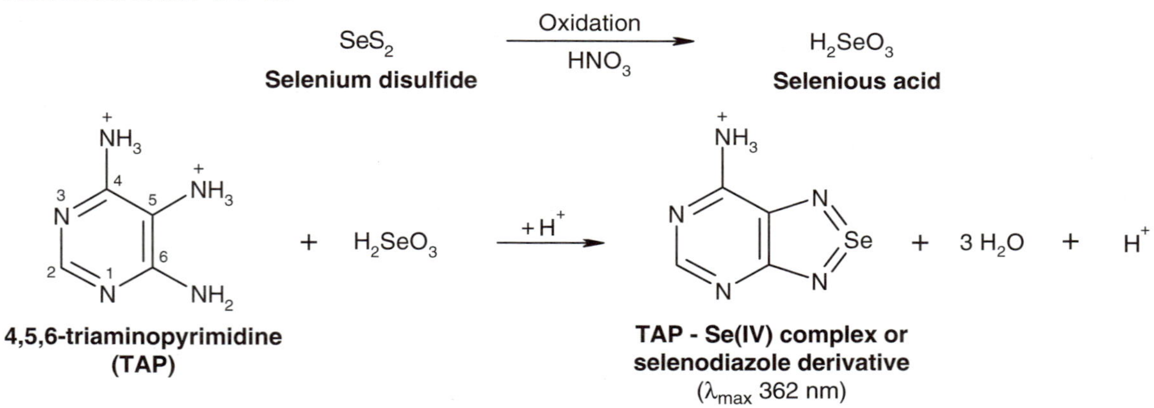

Note

1. LOQ for Se is 5 ppm, LOD 0.1 ppm, linearity range 5-20 ppm.

2. The reaction product is not extractable into non-polar solvents (toluene, chloroform, ether, carbon tetrachloride) due to the presence of third amino group in 'TAP' being protonated under experimental conditions.
3. Aromatic amines with two vicinal groups can be used as a reagent.

As per method proposed by Joste & Gillis (1955) and Murashova et al. (1969) the following mechanism was suggested which is similar to the one explained above.

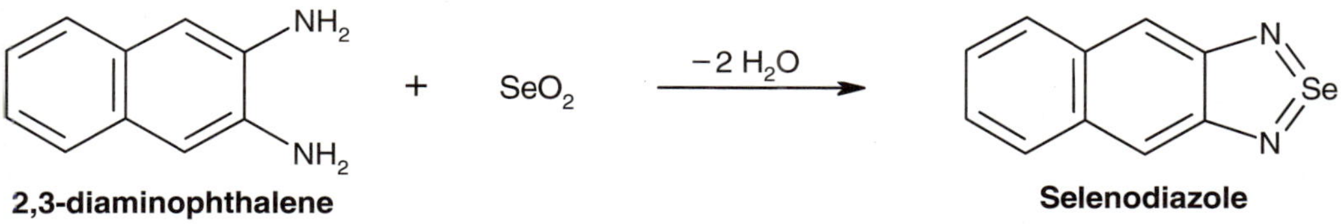

Note

2,3-diaminophthalene is banned.

Reference

1. Mario E. Bodini & Omar Alzamora E., *Talanta*, **30(6)**, 409-412, 1983.
2. J. Hoste & J. Gillis, *Anal. Chim Acta*, **12**,
3. V.I. Murashova & S.G. Sushkova, *J. Anal. Chem.* (USSR), **24**, 729, 1969.

Formulation 21

Cetrimide, Calcium pantothenate

ESTIMATION

Cetrimide

Reagents

1. 0.1 N sodium hydroxide.
2. 5% w/v solution of potassium iodide in water.
3. 0.05 M potassium iodate.

Procedure

Measure accurately quantity of the sample containing about 2.0 g of cetrimide, dilute to 100 ml with water. To 25 ml of the solution add 10 ml of 0.1 N sodium hydroxide and 10 ml of freshly prepared solution of potassium iodide. Extract with four 20 ml portions of chloroform. Discard the chloroform layer. To the aqueous layer add 50 ml of hydrochloric acid and titrate with 0.05 M potassium iodate till the solution is pale brown, add 2 ml of chloroform and continue titration, shaking well between each addition, until the chloroform layer is colourless. Carry out blank titration with 25 ml of water, 10 ml of potassium iodide. Difference between the two titrations represents the volume of 0.05 M potassium iodate consumed by the sample actually taken for analysis. Each ml of 0.05 M potassium iodate is equivalent to 0.03364 g of cetrimide.

Explanatory Note

Addition of KI gives rise to the ionic pair tetradecyltrimethylammonium iodide which gets extracted into chloroform layer quantitatively. Any non-quaternary ammonium salt gets converted into free amine by the addition of NaOH and is extracted into chloroform layer. Excess KI is estimated by titration with potassium iodate (KIO_3). Iodide is first converted into iodine and then in strong acid solution to iodomonochloride. By adding chloroform near the end point titration is continued till chloroform layer is colourless. Since aqueous layer is yellow in colour due to iodomonochloride which is dissociated in strong acidic solution and does not get extracted into chloroform layer.

$$2I^- + IO_3 + 6H^+ + 3Cl^- \longrightarrow 3ICl + 3H_2O$$

Calcium pantothenate

Follow the method 1 for estimation of calcium pantothenate under chapter on vitamins.

Typical laboratory analysis

Cetrimide

Volume of the sample taken for analysis = 25 ml
Volume of 0.05 M potassium iodate consumed by the sample = 16.1 ml
Volume of 0.05 M potassium iodate consumed in blank titration = 30.3 ml
Net volume of potassium iodate consumed by the sample = 14.2 ml
Each ml of 0.05 M potassium iodate is equivalent to 0.03364 g of cetrimide.

$$\text{Contents of cetrimide (\%)} = \frac{14.2 \times 0.03364 \times 100 \times 100}{25 \times 40}$$

$$= 4.78 \text{ g}$$

$$\text{Claim} = 5.0 \text{ g}$$

$$\text{\% claim} = 95.54$$

Calcium pantothenate

Weight of standard taken = 0.151 g
Volume of the sample taken = 7.5 ml (wt./ml = 1.02)

$$\text{Contents of calcium pantothenate (\%)} = \frac{A_u}{A_s} \times \frac{0.151}{100} \times \frac{5}{50} \times \frac{100}{7.5} \times \frac{50}{5} \times \frac{1.02}{1} \times 100$$

$$= \frac{0.286}{0.298} \times \frac{0.151}{7.5} \times \frac{1.02}{1} \times \frac{100}{1}$$

$$= 98.55\% \text{ of claim (2\%)}$$

Formulation 22

Zinc pyrithione, Ketoconazole

Ketoconazole

METHOD 1

Reagents

1. 0.2% w/v solution of 'MBTH' in water.
2. 0.2% w/v solution of ceric ammonium sulphate in sulphuric acid.

Standard solution

250 μg/ml solution of ketoconazole in methanol.

Sample solution

After thoroughly shaking the sample take sample equivalent to 25 mg of ketoconazole, add 50 ml of methanol. Shake for 10 min and make up the volume to 100 ml with methanol.

Procedure

To 1 ml each of sample and standard solutions add 2.5 ml of ceric ammonium sulphate solution, set aside for 10 min and then add 2 ml of MBTH solution. After 40 min dilute the reaction mixture to 25 ml with water and measure the absorbance of red-coloured chromogen at 500 nm against reagent blank. The developed colour is stable for 30 min.

Probable Reaction Mechanism

In the presence of oxidizing agent, MBTH loses two electrons and a proton. The cation so formed now attacks electron-rich site in the drug i.e. position 2 of imidazole structure resulting in the formation of coupled product. The reaction is as under.

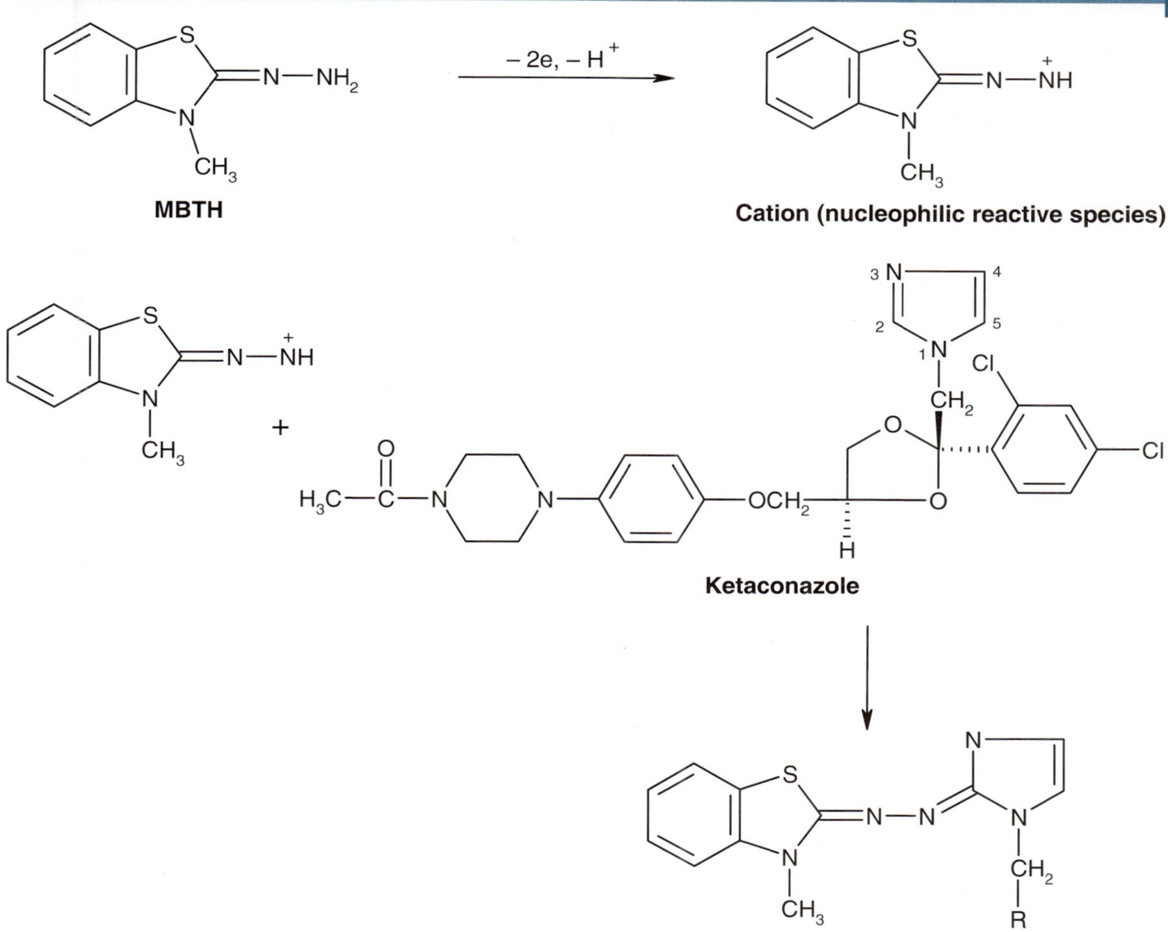

Coupled product
(λ_{max} 500 nm)

Reference

G. Ramana Rao, P. Jagannadha Rao & S.S.N. Murty, *Indian Drugs*, **26(3)**, 119-120, 1987.

METHOD 2

Reagents

1. 0.05 M solution of ferric chloride in water.
2. 0.1 M solution of 1,10-phenanthroline.
3. Ortho-phosphoric acid.

Standard solution

100 µg/ml of ketoconazole in methanol.

Sample solution

Shake the sample vigorously. Transfer appropriate quantity of the sample equivalent to 20 mg of the substance, dilute to 100 ml with methanol. Further dilution is made (1 : 1) with methanol to get 100 µg/ml.

Procedure

To 2 ml each of sample and standard solutions add 2 ml each of ferric chloride and phenanthroline solution, heat at 60°C in water-bath for 10 min, cool, add 1 ml of ortho-phosphoric acid (0.02 M) and dilute to 25 ml with water and measure the absorbance at 505 nm against reagent blank.

Note

As Fe(III) interferes even to a limited extent especially in lower range of linearity in determination of iron (Fe^{++}), the reactivity of Fe(III) is made insignificant by coupling with o-phosphoric acid.

Probable Reaction Mechanism

Iron (Fe^{+++}) oxidizes ketoconazole and in return Fe(III) itself gets reduced to Fe(II) which forms stoichiometric chelates with 1,10-phenanthroline or 2,2′-bispyridyl (λ_{max} 505 nm).

2,2′-bipyridine - Fe(III) chloride reagent is called "Emmerie-Engel reagent".

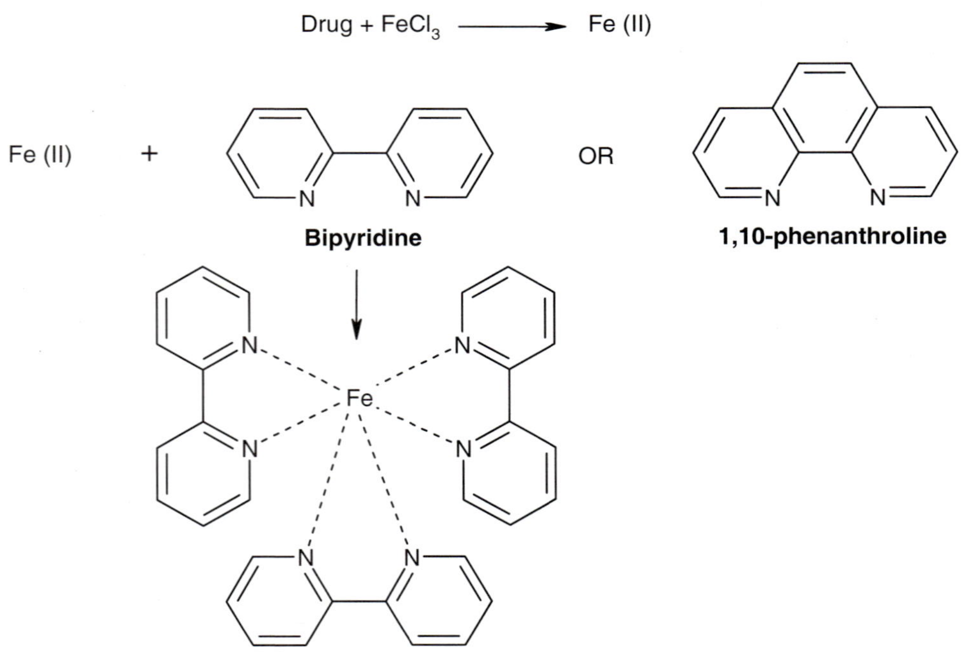

Bipyridine - Fe(II) chelate

Two nitrogen atoms in 2,2′-bipyridine have one unshared pair of electrons which can be shared by Fe(II).

Note

Other drugs which react with reagent to give similar chelates are salbutamol, U/E, ascorbic acid, terbutaline and phenols.

Reference

Thin Layer Chromatography: Reagents and Detection Methods (Vol. 1a) by Jork Funk, Fischer & Wimmer, p. 216.

Zarapkar et al. (1991) have reported method for estimation of ketoconazole based on formation of ion-pair complex with several acidic dyes in phthalate buffer solutions of different pH as under:

Dye	**pH**	λ_{max}
Bromocresol green	2.5	420 nm
Bromocresol purple	2.5	420 nm
Bromophenol blue	1.5	415 nm
Methyl orange	2.75	430 nm

Reference

S.S. Zarapkar, *Indian Drugs*, **28(6)**, 265, 1991.

A method based on 1 : 1 ion-pair complex formation with picric acid at pH 2.5 has been described for estimation of ketoconazole in tablets and creams by Sadeghi & Shamsipur (1998).

Standard solution

100 μg/ml of ketoconazole in water containing few drops of 0.04 M hydrochloric acid.

Sample solution

Powdered sample equivalent to 25 mg of the substance shaken with acidified water as under standard solution, dilute appropriately to get 100 μg/ml, filter and use for analysis. The sample of cream was dissolved in ethanol with slight warming and then further diluting with ethanol.

Procedure

To 1 ml each of sample and standard solutions add 3 ml of picric acid solution (0.1%) and 1 ml of 0.2 M citrate buffer pH 2.5, shake, add 5 ml of chloroform, shake for 10 min, allow to stand for clear separation of two phases and then measure the absorbance of organic layer at 410 nm against reagent blank.

Ketoconazole - picric acid complexation

Ketoconazole has maximum absorption at 245 and 300 nm, picric acid 336 nm, whereas ketoconazole - picric acid complex has absorption maximum 245, 344 and 410 nm. This pronounced spectral change after complex formation is presumably due to the occurrence of both charge-transfer (C-T) and proton-transfer during formation of molecular complex (1 : 1). Polynitrophenol derivatives such as picrate ion are known versatile chelating counter ions and form wide range of molecular complexes with variety of electron donor molecule. Reaction depends on the presence of imidazole ring which contains two types of nitrogen i.e. pyridine and pyrrole types. The two electrons of the pyrrole type are involved in the aromaticity of the ring whereas two electrons of the pyridine type are available as electron donor. Therefore, tertiary amine moiety of the ring (pyridine type nitrogen) acts as electron donor whereas polyphenol as electron acceptor and hence the formation of complex.

Ketoconazole is electron donor whereas picric acid, a polynitrophenol, is an electron acceptor.

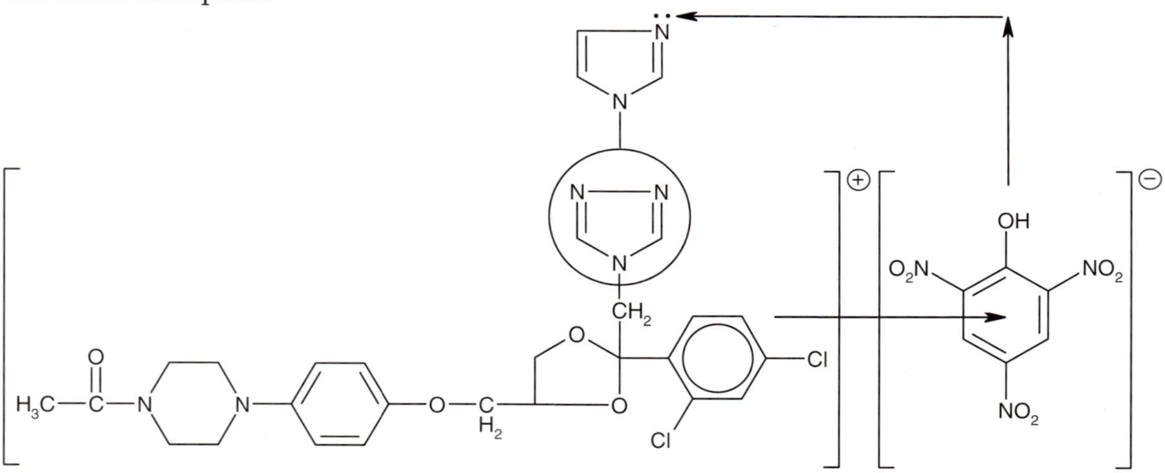

Note

This method has been found suitable for biological samples.

Reference

Susan Sadeghi & Mojtaba Shamsipur, *Analytical Letters*, **31(5)**, 2691-2705, 1998.

A spectrophotometric method has been reported for analysis of several antifungal agents containing imidazole ring i.e. clotrimazole, econazole, miconazole and ketoconazole. The method is based on formation of a charge-transfer (C-T) complex between the drug, the π-electron donor, and iodine as δ-acceptor.

Reagents

1. 0.01 M iodine solution in 1,2-dichloromethane; solution is stable for 7 days at 4°C; protect from light.
2. 1 M sulphuric acid.
3. 20% ammonium hydroxide.

Standard solution

1 mg/ml solution of each antifungal agent in 1,2-dichloromethane: 100-600 µg/ml (clotrimazole), 10-100 µg/ml (ketoconazole), 50-400 µg/ml (miconazole).

Econazole nitrate: Dissolved in 20% ethanol : water (1 : 1), basified with ammonium hydroxide, extracted with chloroform, chloroform layer evaporated and residue taken up in 1,2-dichloromethane to get 1 mg/ml. Further diluted to get 100-500 µg/ml.

Sample solution

Powder (clotrimazole and miconazole), tablets, vaginal tablets, topical solution, oral gel, cream, vaginal suppositories, all processed as under standard solution.

Procedure

To 1 ml each of sample and standard solutions add 1.5 ml of 0.01 M iodine solution, mix well, dilute to 10 ml with 1,2-dichloromethane, allow to stand for 50 min at room temperature, measure the absorbance at 290 nm against reagent blank.

Probable Reaction Mechanism as proposed by the author

The absorption spectrum of iodine in 1,2-dichloromethane shows only one peak with maximum absorption at 500 nm. Immediate change of the iodine colour in the solvent from violet to lemon-yellow upon reaction with above-mentioned antifungal agent is due to C-T complexation reaction which shows two absorption maxima i.e. 290 and 377 nm, the first is more intense than the second, hence measurement made at 290 nm. The mechanism of reaction depends on the presence of imidazole ring which contains two types of nitrogen, pyridine and pyrrole types. Two electrons of pyrrole type are involved in the aromaticity of the ring while two electrons of pyridine type are available as π-electron donor. Consequently the method is based on interaction between tertiary amine moiety of the drug (pyridine type nitrogen) as π-electron donor and iodine as δ-acceptor to form stable C-T complex. It is 1 : 1 complex with other drugs except ketoconazole where it is 2 : 1 complex. This is because one basic π-electron donating tertiary amine moiety (pyridine type nitrogen in the imidazole ring) whereas in ketoconazole another basic π-electron donating tertiary amine moiety besides the imidazole ring in the amide chain as shown below.

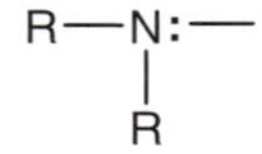

Normal tertiary amine moiety

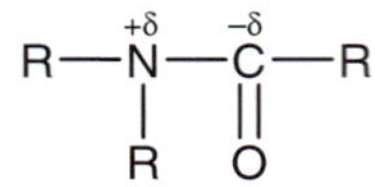

Tertiary nitrogen atom in amide moiety

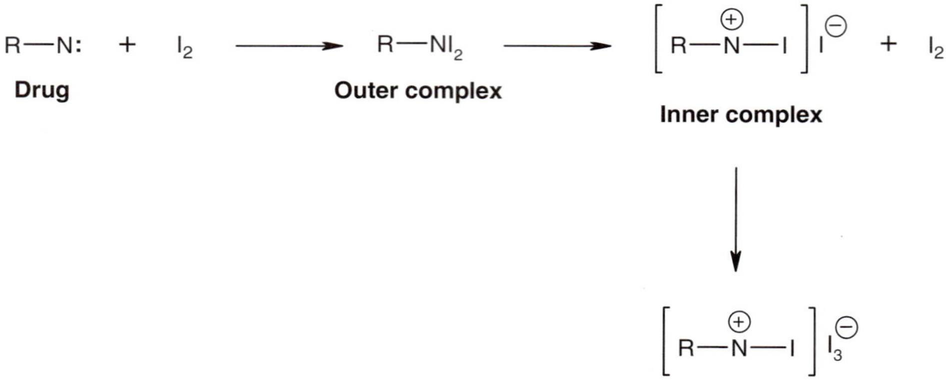

Tri-iodide ion-pair complex
(λ_{max} 290 nm)

The formation of tri-iodide ion-pair complex, the final measurable moiety, is due to transformation of the outer complex to an inner complex liberating iodide ion which reacts with free molecular iodine to give tri-iodide.

Reference

Salwa R. El-Shabouri, Kamla M. Emara, Pakinaz Y. Khashaba & Ashraf M. Mohamed, *Analytical Letters*, **31(8)**, 1367-1385, 1998.

Another method based on C-T complex formation has been described by Kelani et al. (1992) for estimation of ketoconazole and clotrimazole. The method involves interaction of these compounds, π-electron donors with 2,3-dichloro-5,6-dicyano-p-benzoquinone (DDQ) as π-acceptor to form highly coloured 1 : 1 reaction product (λ_{max} 588 nm). The method was applied to different dosage forms (tablets, capsules, powder and solution). C-T complex had three maxima i.e. 588 nm, 548 nm and 455 nm. At 588 nm it has the highest absorbance.

General method

To the sample/standard solution containing 20-100 μg/ml of the drug add 2 ml of DDQ (2×10^{-3}) solution, dilute to 5 ml with acetonitrile and measure the absorbance of sample/standard solution at 588 nm against reagent blank.

Probable Reaction Mechanism

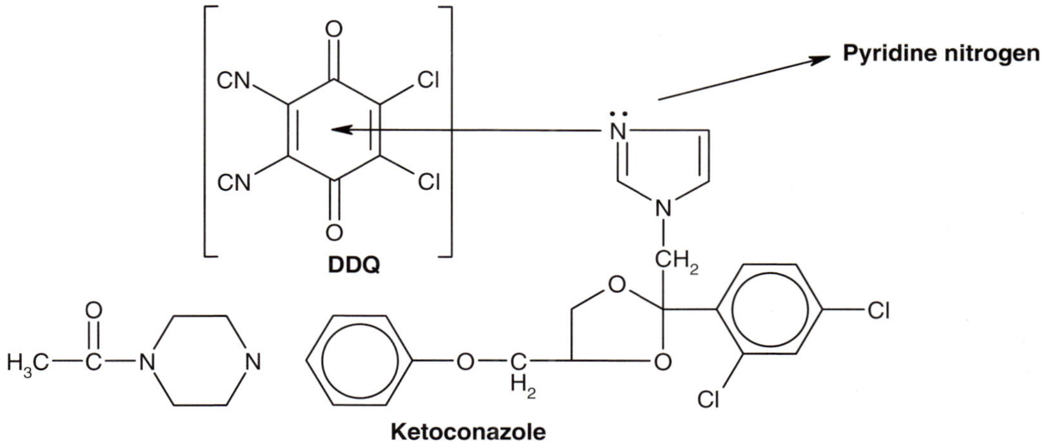

Ketoconazole - DDQ C-T complex
(λ_{max} 588 nm)

Reference

Khadiga Kelani, Lories I. Bebawy, Laila Abdel-Fattah & Abdel-Kader S. Ahmad, *Analytical Letters*, **30(10)**, 1843-1860, 1997.

Abdel-Gawad (1997) has reported two methods of analysis i.e. based on charge-transfer and ion-pair complexation. For 'C-T' method, 2,3-dichloro-5,6-dicyano-p-benzoquinone (DDQ) in acetonitrile was used as electron acceptor to yield intense orange-red product, a complex (λ_{max} 460 nm, 550 nm and 590 nm). These bands may be attributed to the formation of 'DDQ' radical anion resulting from dissociation of an original 'C-T' complex promoted by high dielectric constant of solvent (acetonitrile). Whereas for ion-pair complexation, bromophenol blue was used as acidic dye and the complex so formed was extractd with chloroform (λ_{max} 410 nm).

Reference

Fatma M. Abdel-Gawad, *J. Pharm. & Biomed. Analysis*, **15**, 1679-1685, 1992.

Zinc pyrithione (ZPT)

Reagents

1. 1 : 1 v/v aqueous hydrochloric acid.
2. 0.1 M iodine solution: Standardized against arsenious trioxide.

Procedure

Weigh sample equivalent to 0.2 g of zinc pyrithione in 10 mg of zinc, add 20 ml of hydrochloric acid (1 : 1), add 75 ml of water and titrate with 0.1 M iodine solution using starch as indicator and calculate the contents of ZPT as under:

$$\%\text{ZPT} = \frac{(V_2 - V_1) \times M \times 15.88}{S}$$

V_1 = Volume (ml) of blank
V_2 = Volume (ml) of the titrant for sample
M = Molarity of the titrant
S = Weight of sample taken
15.88 = Equivalent factor

Note

Zinc pyrithione is available as aqueous slurry/dispersion containing about 48.0% of 'ZPT'.

Probable Reaction Mechanism

The titrimetric method is based on oxidation of ZPT by iodine as follows:

$$2\,RSH + I_2 \xrightarrow{\text{Oxidation}} R{-}S{-}S{-}R + 2\,HI$$

OR

$$\underset{\textbf{ZPT}}{(RS)_2Zn} + I_2 \xrightarrow[\text{Oxidation}]{} R{-}S{-}S{-}R + ZnI_2$$

Zinc pyrithione has very poor UV-absorbing property. However, pyrithione also forms complexes with other metals such as Fe(III), Sn(II), Co(III), Ni(II) and Cu(II). The Cu(II) complex has the highest absorption at 335 nm.

Probable Reaction Mechanism

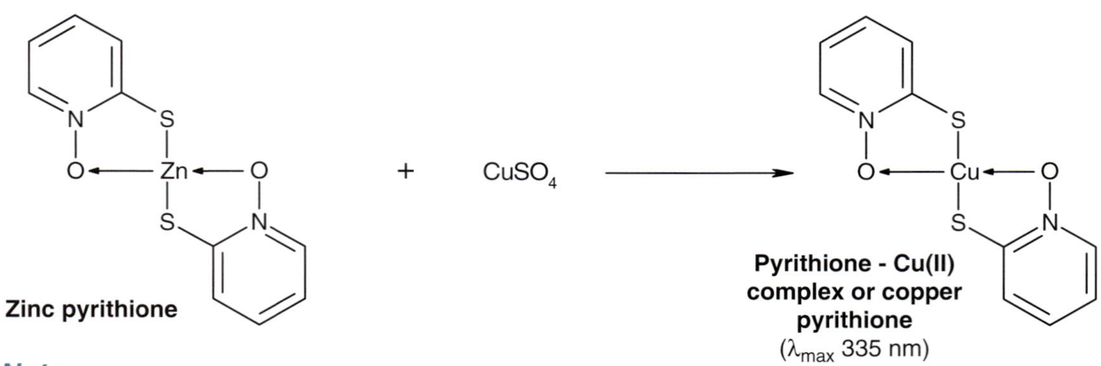

Note

The Cu(II) complex has been employed for HPLC determination of the molecule.

Reaction Mechanism

16

Rubefacients

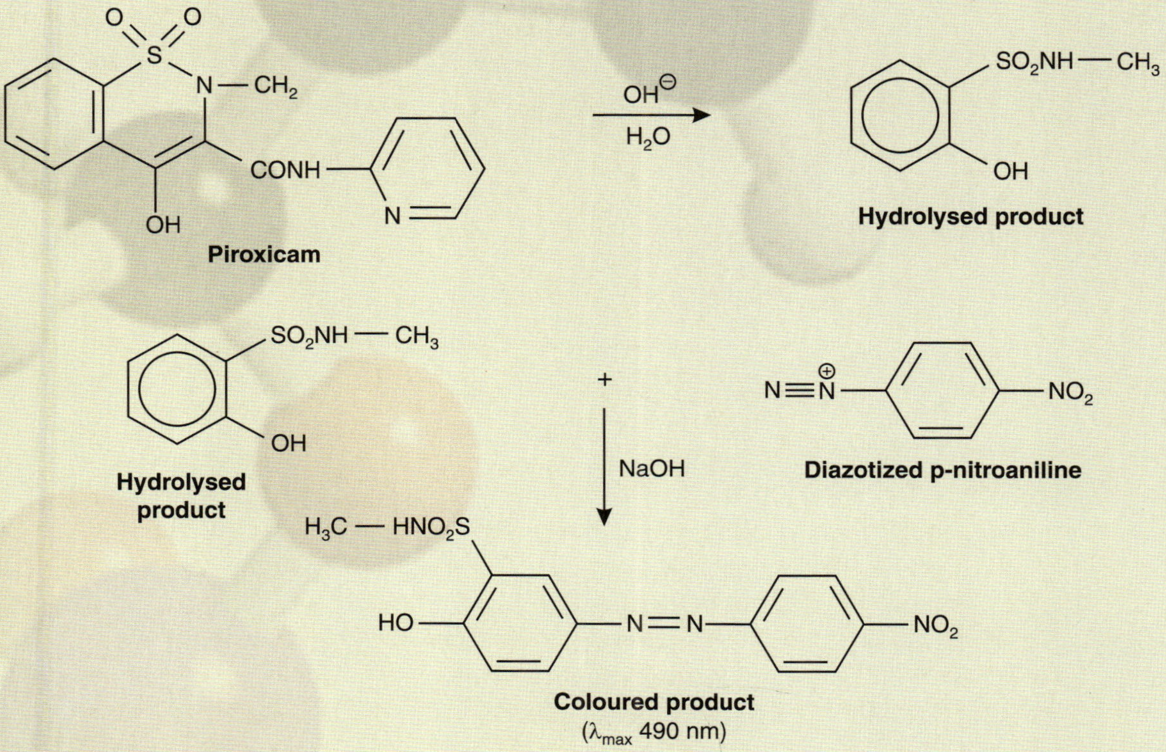

Formulation 1

Chlorpheniramine maleate, Methyl nicotinate, Methyl salicylate, Mephenesin, Menthol, Turpentine oil

ESTIMATION

Chlorpheniramine maleate

Reagents

1. 0.2 M phosphate buffer, pH 7.0.
2. Saturated solution of cyanogen bromide in water (prepare fresh).
3. 4% w/v solution of sulphanilic acid in freshly distilled methanol.

Standard solution

Prepare a 40 mcg/ml solution of chlorpheniramine maleate in water.

Sample solution

Weigh accurately sample equivalent to 4 mg of chlorpheniramine maleate in a 100 ml dry beaker. Add 20 ml of phosphate buffer, stir well and transfer to a 100 ml volumetric flask and make up the volume with phosphate buffer and filter.

Procedure

Take 5 ml each of sample and standard solutions in two separate 50 ml volumetric flasks. To each flask add 20 ml of phosphate buffer, 2 ml of sulphanilic acid solution and 3 ml of cyanogen bromide solution. Measure the absorbance of both the solutions, exactly at 5th minute after the addition of cyanogen bromide solution to each flask, against water.

Note

Colour of the solutions reaches maximum in about five minutes after the addition of cyanogen bromide solution and then fades away slowly. Prepare the blank in a similar manner except addition of cyanogen bromide solution. The solution exhibits absorption maximum at about 430 nm. Deduce the results by comparison.

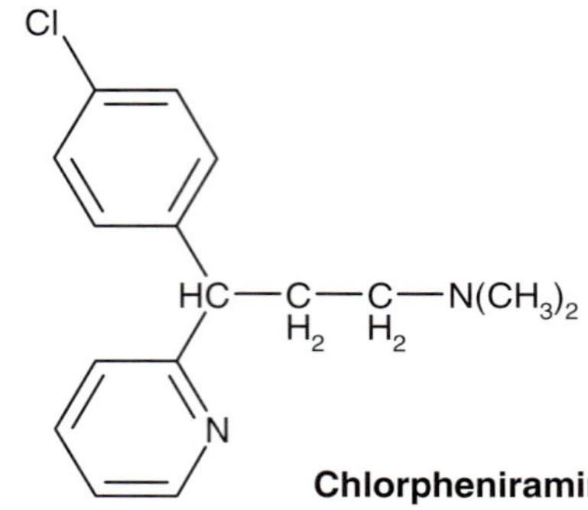

Chlorpheniramine

$$Br—C\equiv N$$

Bromocyanogen (reagent used)

Probable Reaction Mechanism

The above reagent is used to identify the pyridine ring which is identified by the formation of orange-yellow polymethine dye (cyanine) by the reaction with bromocyanogen/sulphanilic acid.

Step 1: Formation of bromocyanogen (by reacting KCN and Br_2).

$$Br_2 + CN^{\ominus} \longrightarrow Br—C\equiv N + Br^{\ominus}$$

Bromocyanogen

Step 2: The pyridine ring in the drug now reacts with bromocyanogen to produce N-cyanopyridinium bromide.

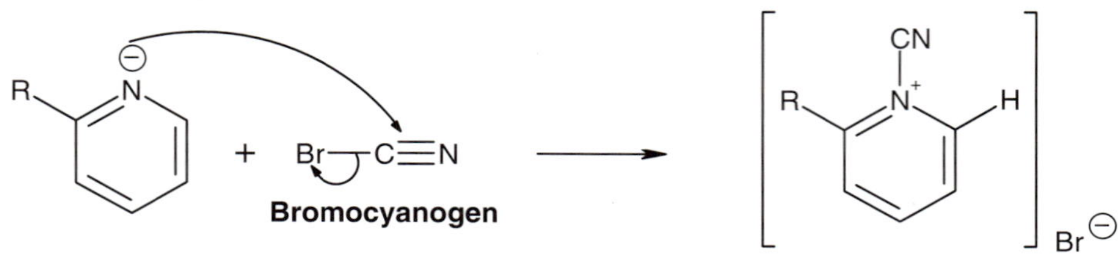

N-cyanopyridinium bromide

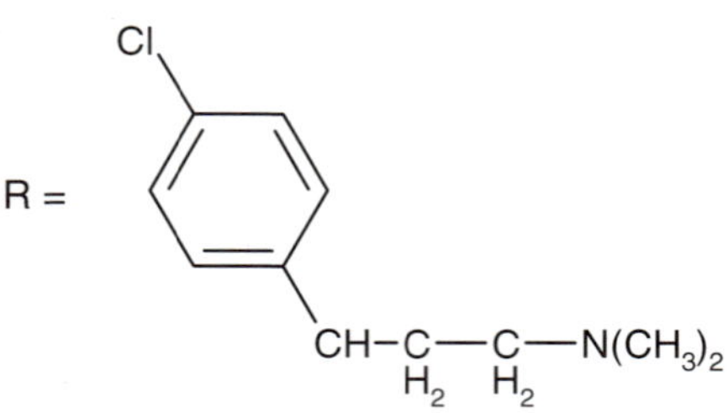

Step 3: Sulphanilic acid reacts nucleophilically with N-cyanopyridinium salt to form an adduct.

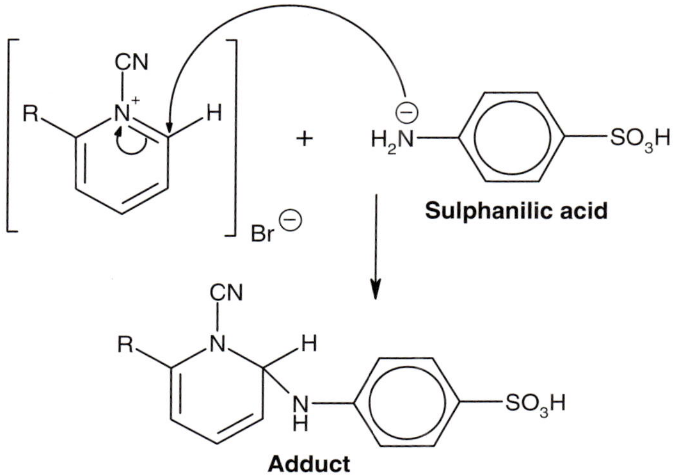

Step 4: The adduct then undergoes ring opening to form the following product.

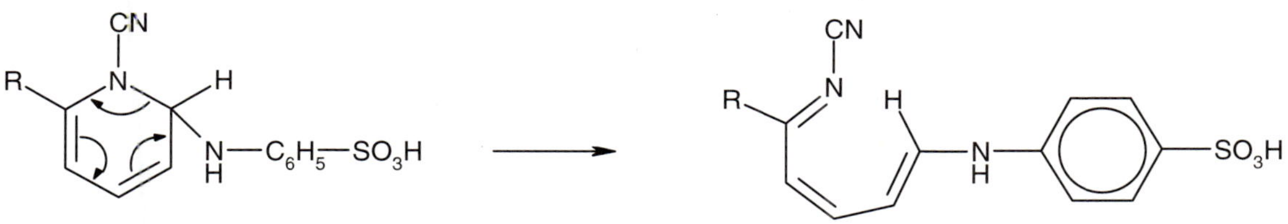

Step 5: Another molecule of sulphanilic acid reacts with the above formed product to give a new product by a carbonyl reaction.

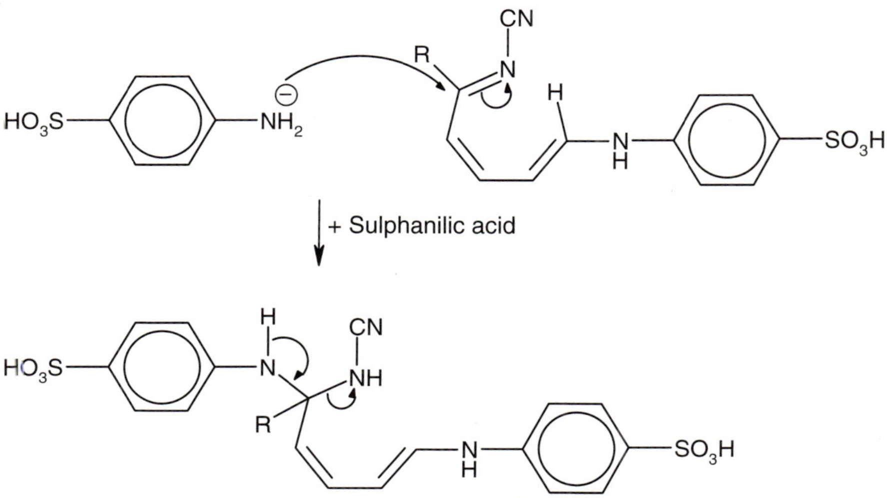

Step 6: The above product now eliminates cyanamide and is converted into amidine.

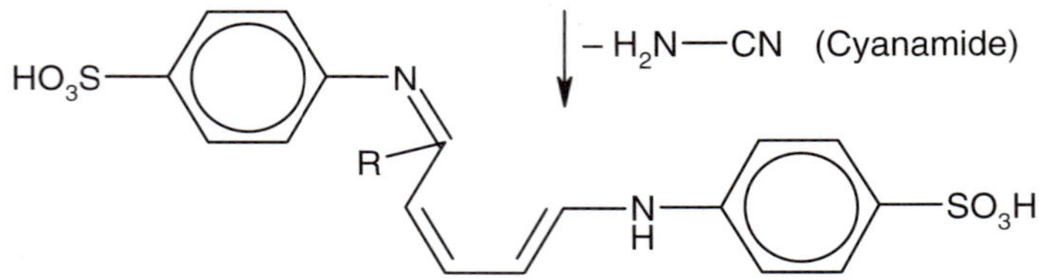

Amidine derivative

Step 7: The amidine is readily protonated and forms the resonance stabilized cyanine.

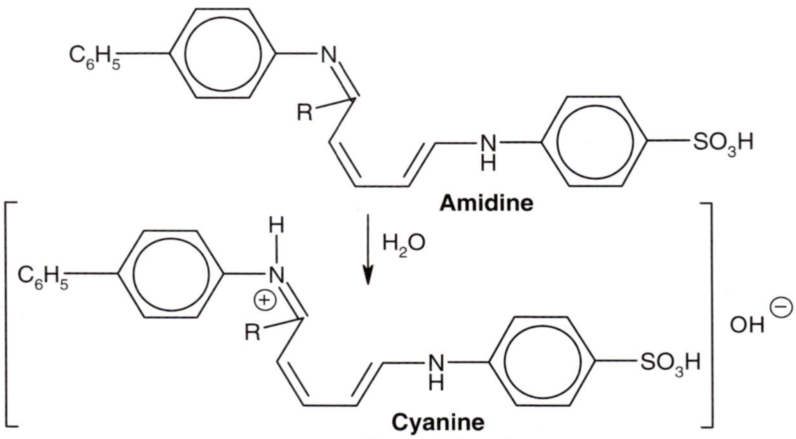

Cyanine
(λ_{max} 430 nm)

Reference

Pharmaceutical Chemistry (Vol. 2) by H.J. Roth, pp. 529-530.

Note

1. Use of aniline instead of sulphanilic acid gives better results.
2. Chlorocyanogen can be used instead of bromocyanogen which can be produced by reaction of chloramine T and potassium cyanide.

Methyl nicotinate

Reagents

1. Cyanogen bromide solution: Prepare as mentioned above in the determination of chlorpheniramine maleate.
2. Buffer solution, pH 6.6: Mix 2.5 ml of phosphoric acid (85%), 87.5 ml of methanol with 350 ml of water and sufficient 20% sodium hydroxide to give a pH of 6.6 and dilute to 500 ml with water. Check the final pH.
3. 10% procaine hydrochloride: Dissolve 10 g of procaine hydrochloride in 30 ml of hydrochloric acid and make up to 100 ml with water.
4. Concentrated hydrochloric acid.

Standard solution

Prepare 1 mg/ml solution of methyl nicotinate in distilled water.

Sample solution

Weigh accurately about 2 g of sample in 100 ml dry beaker. Add 2 ml of hydrochloric acid and about 20 ml of distilled water and warm. Transfer this to a 100 ml volumetric flask and sufficient washings to make up the volume with distilled water and filter.

Procedure

Take sample and standard solutions equivalent to 1 mg of methyl nicotinate in two different test tubes and adjust the volume to 10 ml. To each test tube, add 2 ml of hydrochloric acid and water. Keep the test tubes in a boiling water-bath for one hour. Adjust the pH of the standard and sample preparations to 6.5 ± 0.1 and dilute to 100 ml with water. Prepare a set of four test tubes marked S, SB, T and TB. To the tubes marked S and SB, add 5 ml of hydrolysed standard preparation and to the tubes marked T and TB, add 5 ml of hydrolysed sample preparation. Add to each tube, 5 ml of buffer. Then to S and T tubes add 5 ml of cyanogen bromide solution and to tubes marked SB and TB, add 5 ml of water. After 20 minutes, add 1 ml of procaine hydrochloride solution to each tube. After further 5 minutes measure the absorbance at about 430 nm. Deduce the results by comparison.

On acid hydrolysis, nicotinic acid is formed. The nicotinic acid formed can be estimated by cyanogen bromide method by Kōnig's method.

Probable Reaction Mechanism

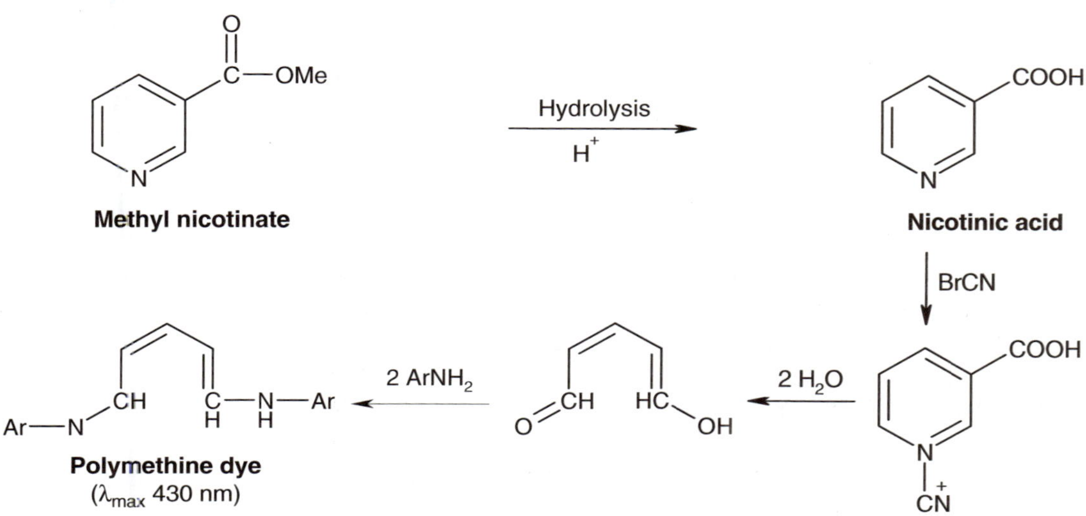

Reference

W.J. Kõnig, *J. Prakt. Chem.*, **70**, 19, 1904.

Mephenesin

METHOD 1

Reagents

1. Periodic-acetic acid solution: Dissolve 0.215 g of sodium metaperiodate in 25 ml of water in a 250 ml volumetric flask, make up to the mark with glacial acetic acid and mix well.
2. 0.01 N sodium thiosulphate solution.
3. Starch mucilage as indicator.
4. Chloroform.
5. Glacial acetic acid.
6. Saturated sodium chloride solution.
7. 1% w/v solution of potassium iodide in water.

Sample preparation

Weigh accurately about 0.2 g of sample in a dry 100 ml beaker. Add 10 ml of water and stir well with a glass-rod to disperse the sample in water. Transfer the solution, carefully, to a separating funnel. Rinse the beaker twice with 5 ml portions of water and transfer to the separating funnel. Rinse the beaker with 50 ml of chloroform and add to the separating funnel. Shake well for two minutes and allow the layers to separate. Extract the sample with further 50 ml of chloroform. Combine chloroform layers, add 10 ml of saturated solution of sodium chloride. Shake well and allow the layers to separate. Transfer the chloroform layer to 500 ml iodine flask through funnel fitted with cotton-plug (sodium chloride layer may be extracted with 10 ml of chloroform and after separation, transfer the chloroform layer to iodine flask).

Add exactly 15 ml of periodic-acetic acid solution to the chloroform in the iodine flask, mix and add sufficient glacial acetic acid to get clear solution. Keep aside for 30 minutes. Add 100 ml of potassium iodide solution and titrate the liberated iodine with 0.01 N sodium thiosulphate using starch mucilage as indicator to be added towards the end of the titration. Continue titration till both the aqueous and chloroform layers become colourless. Shake the flask vigorously towards the end of the titration and carry out the blank titration with the sample. Each ml of 0.01 N sodium thiosulphate is equivalent to 0.00912 g of mephenesin.

Probable Reaction Mechanism

$$NaIO_4 + H + K_9 \longrightarrow I_2 + H_2O$$

$$2\,S_2O_3^{--} + I_2 \longrightarrow S_4O_6^{--} + 2I^-$$

Note

Bromometric method involves addition of excess of $KBrO_3$ and Br and unreacted reagent is estimated bromometrically.

$$BrO_3^- + 6e + 6H^+ \longrightarrow Br^- + 3H_2O$$

$$BrO_3^- + 10e + 12H^+ \longrightarrow Br_2 + H_2O$$

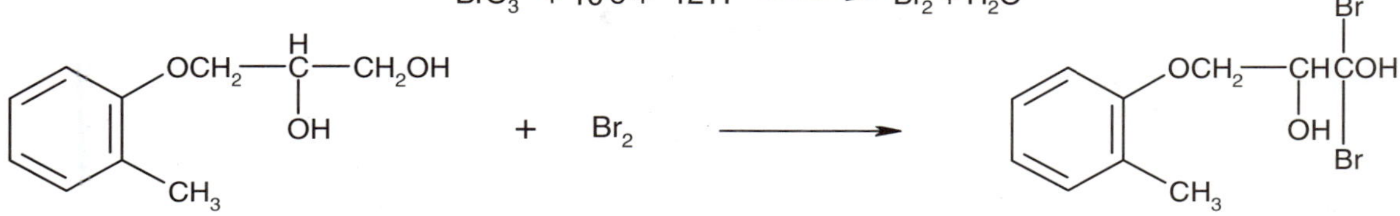

Mephenesin

Dibromo derivative of mephenesin

METHOD 2

Weigh the cream equivalent to 100 mg of mephenesin. Suspend in water by slight warming and add 5 ml of ammonia solution. Extract with 4 × 25 ml portions of chloroform. Wash the combined extract with 10 ml each of 0.02 N sodium hydroxide and water. Pass the extract through anhydrous sodium sulphate. Evaporate the combined chloroform extract and dissolve in water to get a volume of 200 ml. Dilute 5 ml of the solution to 100 ml with water to get a final concentration of 25 mcg/ml. Measure the absorbance of the resulting solution at about 270 nm. Calculate the content of mephenesin using 80 as value of A 1%, 1 cm at 270 nm.

METHOD 3

Reagents

1. Phosphate buffer, pH 7.4: Dissolve 6.805 g of potassium dihydrogen phosphate in 250 ml of water, add 195.5 ml of 0.2 N sodium hydroxide and dilute to 1000 ml. Check the final pH.
2. Diazotised 2,4-dinitroaniline: Dissolve 1 g of dinitroaniline in 5 ml of concentrated sulphuric acid by gentle warming on water-bath. Cool to 0°C in ice-bath (A). Separately dissolved 0.5 g of sodium nitrite in 5 ml of concentrated sulphuric acid and cooled to 0°C (B). Mix solutions (A) and (B) and to this add some of phosphoric acid (85%). Just before use, dilute 1 : 1 with phosphoric acid.

Standard solution

To 100 mg of the working standard of mephenesin, add 2 ml of methanol and dilute to 100 ml with buffer solution. 25 ml of this further diluted to 100 ml with buffer (250 mcg/ml).

Sample solution

Accurately weighed quantity of cream or any other semisolid preparation equivalent to 100 mg of substance is extracted and diluted as under standard solution.

Procedure

To 2 ml each of sample and standard solutions, add 5 ml of phosphoric acid and 1 ml of diluted reagent. Heat on boiling water-bath for 20 min, cool in ice-bath and dilute to 50 ml with phosphoric acid (85%). Measure the absorption of both sample and standard solutions at about 510 nm using phosphoric acid as blank. Calculate the results by comparison.

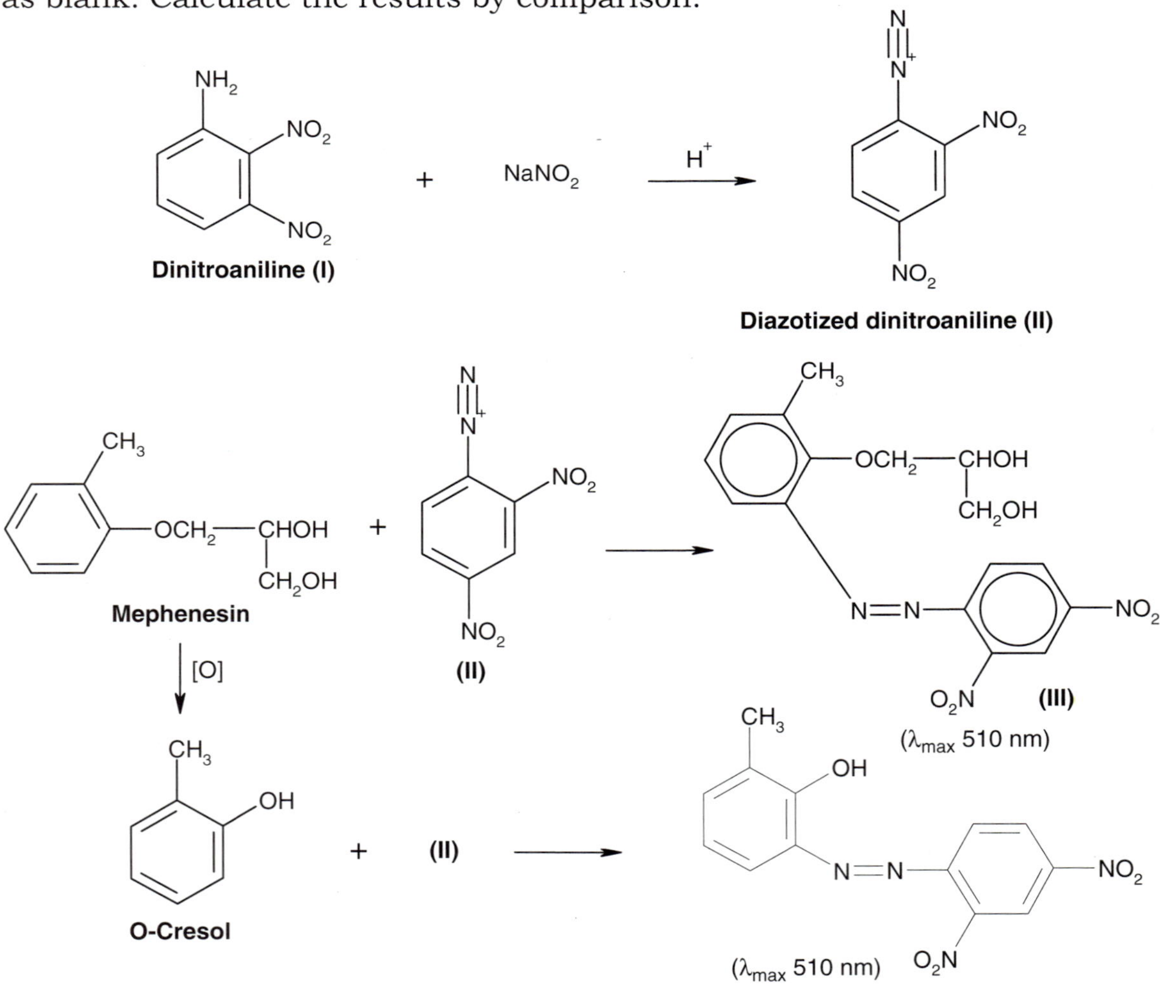

Note

The coupling can take place at ortho or para position.

Reference

1. Elwood Tikis, Stanley Ulick & Arthur P. Richardson, *J. Pharmacol. Expt. Therapeutics*, **93**, 129-134, 1948.
2. Vandana H. Bhalla et al., *Ind. Drugs*, **27(11)**, 581, 1990.

Note

O-cresol formed as a result of oxidation of mephenesin shall also couple with diazotized nitroaniline to give similar orange-red coloured complex.

METHOD 4

Standard solution

150 mcg/ml of mephenesin in water.

Sample solution

Suspend the sample (ointment, cream) in 20 ml of water by warming and extract with six 15 ml portions of chloroform. Wash the combined chloroform layer with 2 × 10 ml portions of water and dilute the organic layer to 100 ml. Evaporate 15 ml of chloroform layer to dryness on water-bath, take up the residue in 20 ml of ethanol and dilute to 100 ml with water.

Procedure

Follow the method described for guaiphenesin under formulation of the chapter on expectorants.

Note

The method is based on oxidation of terminal vicinal hydroxyl group with sodium periodate to liberate formaldehyde, followed by coupling with acetyl acetone in presence of ammonia.

Probable Reaction Mechanism

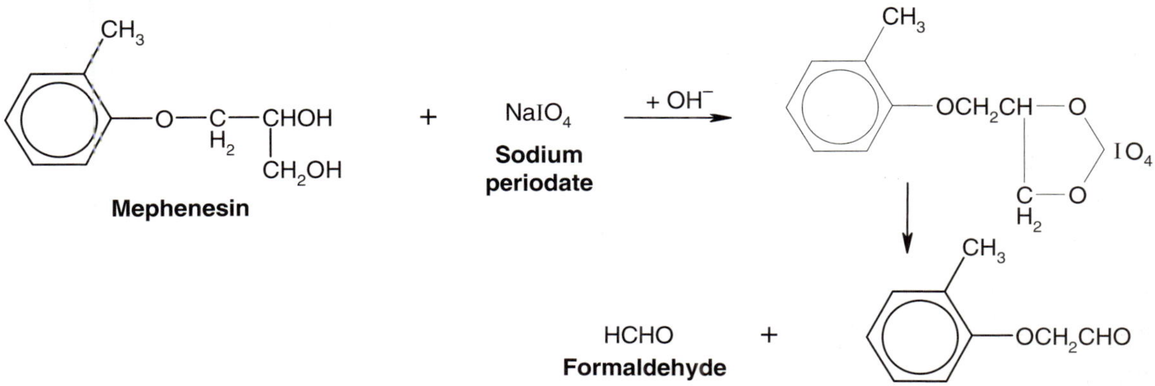

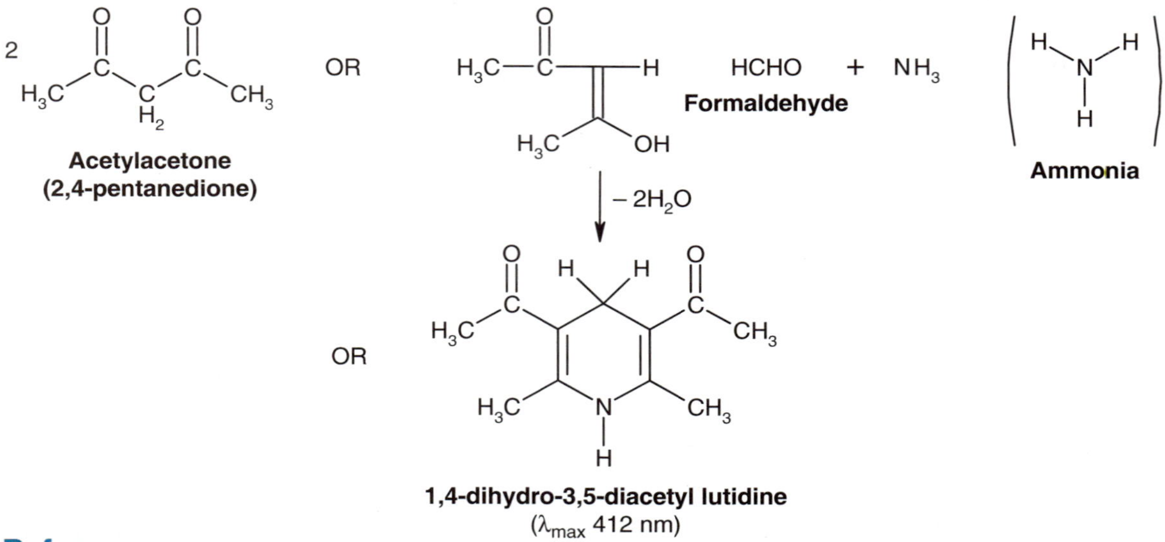

Reference

M.B. Devani, C.J. Shishoo, B.N. Suhagia & S.A. Shah, *Ind. J. Pharm. Sci.*, **56(2)**, 41-44, 1994.

A spectrophotometric method has been described by Morgan et al. (1967) based on reaction of formaldehyde (HCHO) formed as a result of alkaline hydrolysis followed by periodate oxidation with chromotropic acid. This method has also been applied for analysis of guaicolglyceryl ether, methocarbamol and mephenesin carbamate.

Reference

A.M. Morgan, Edward B. Truitt & J. Maxwell Little, J. Amm. Pharm. Assoc. (Scientific edition), **46**, 374-377, 1987.

METHOD 5

Reagent

Sulphuric acid : formaldehyde (90 : 10): Prepared by adding cooled formaldehyde to ice cold sulphuric acid.

Standard solution

Prepare 1 mg/ml solution in water. Extract 10 ml with 4 × 25 ml chloroform, adjust volume to 100 ml (100 μg/ml).

Sample solution

Take sample equivalent to 10 mg, suspend in water by slight warming, cool, extract with chloroform (4 × 25 ml), adjust volume to 100 ml (100 μg/ml).

Procedure

5 ml each of sample/standard is evaporated on water-bath to dryness, add 10 ml of the reagent, allow the colour to develop. Measure its absorbance at 550 nm against reagent blank and calculate the results.

Probable Reaction Mechanism

Aromatic ring of the compound is attacked by formaldehyde resulting in condensation reaction. Sulphuric acid acts as oxidizing agent resulting in the formation of quinoid structure which is coloured.

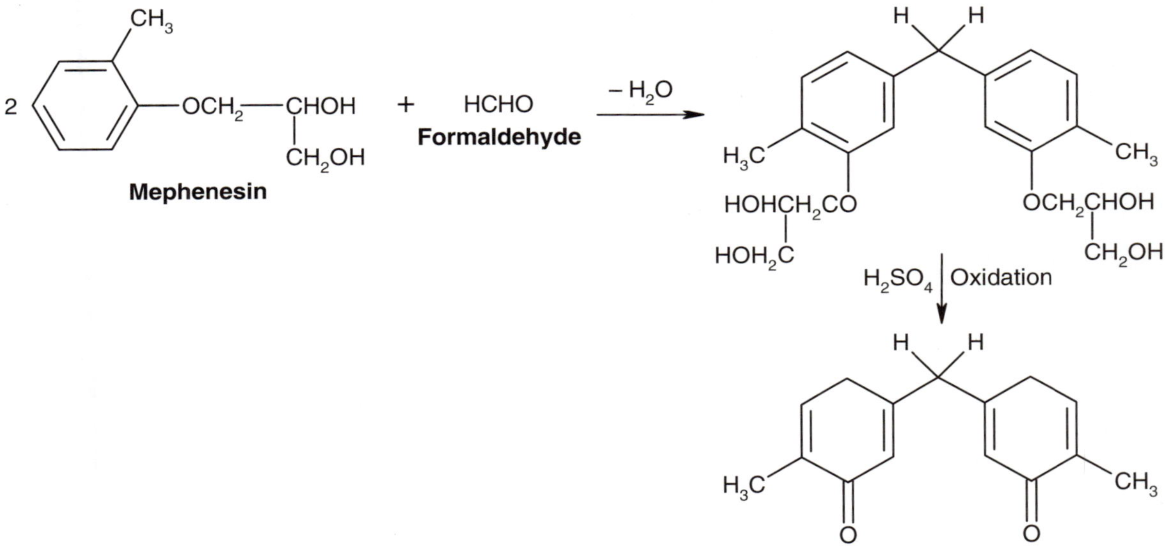

Quinoid coloured complex
(λ_{max} 550 nm)

METHOD 6

Reagents

1. 0.2% solution of sodium periodate.
2. 0.2% solution of 3-methyl-2-benzothiazoline hydrazone (MBTH) in water.

Sample/standard solution

As under method 4.

Procedure

To 1 ml each of sample and standard solutions add 3 ml of 'MBTH' reagent, after 2 min add 3 ml of periodate reagent, set aside for 30 min, dilute to 25 ml with water and measure the absorbance of the resulting solution at 635 nm against reagent blank.

Probable Reaction Mechanism

Mephenesin is oxidized by periodate to give two moieties as under method 4. The HCHO so produced reacts with 'MBTH' to give coloured species (λ_{max} 635 nm).

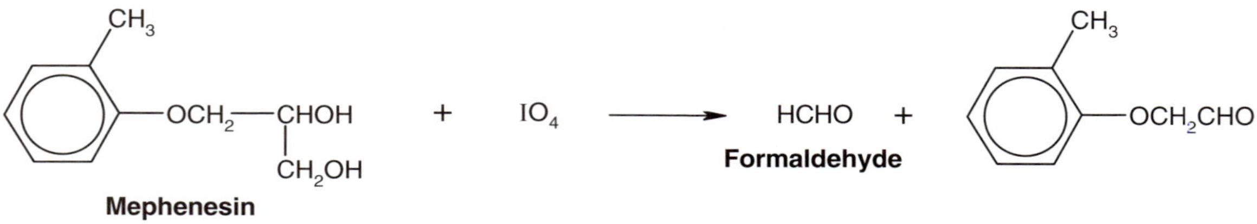

This reaction is similar to the one proposed by Fred and Sawicki involving reaction of aliphatic aldehydes with MBTH which on further oxidation gives coloured product.

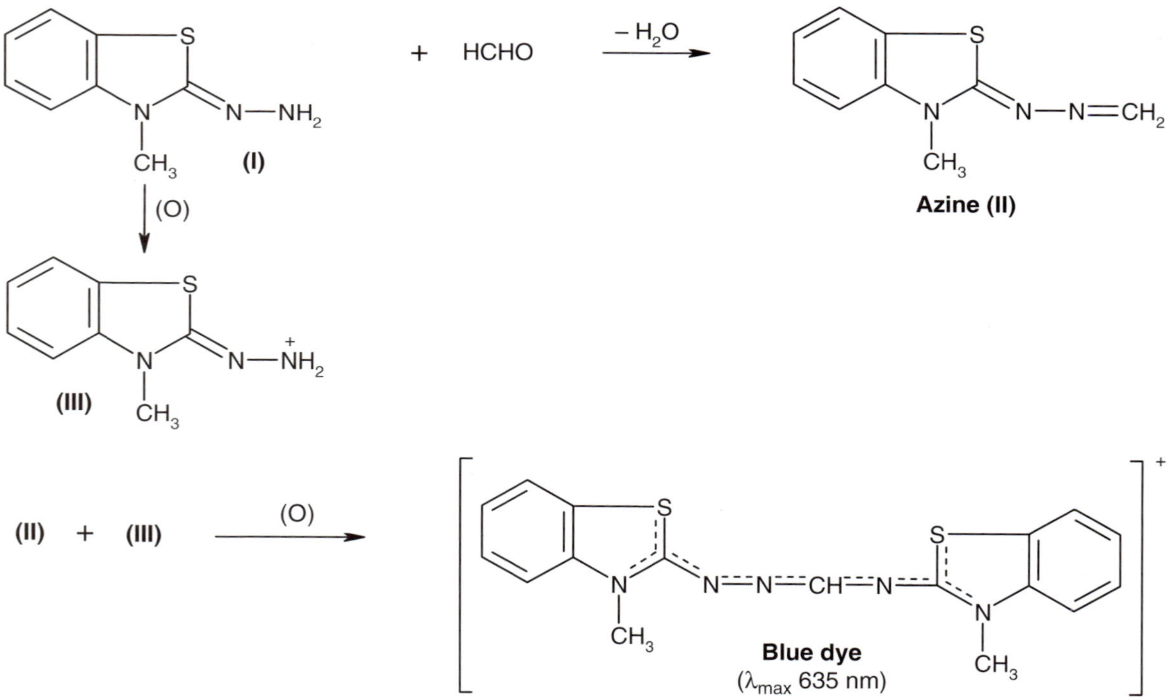

Reference

1. G. Rama Rao, A.B. Avadhanulu & R. Giridhar, *Indian Drugs*, **25(9)**, 418-420, 1988.
2. W.N. Fred, *Anal. Chem.*, **41**, 2077, 1969.
3. E. Sawicki, T. Hauser, T. Stanley & T. Elbert, *Anal. Chem.*, **33**, 93, 1961.

Methyl salicylate

METHOD 1

Reagents

1. Ferric ammonium sulphate solution.
4. 1 N and 0.02 N hydrochloric acid.

Standard solution

150 mcg/ml solution of salicylic acid in 0.02 N hydrochloric acid.

Sample solution

Take sample accurately weighed equivalent to 2 mg of total salicylate, add 30 ml of 0.5 N sodium hydroxide and 20 ml of methyl alcohol, mix and reflux for one hour on steam-bath to saponify and hydrolyse. Cool, add 20 ml of hydrochloric acid (resulting solution should be distinctly acidic) and dilute to 250 ml with water and filter.

Procedure

Take 15 ml of sample filtrate and 15 ml of standard solution. Extract each with 25 ml of chloroform, separate chloroform layer. To 5 ml of chloroform layer add 10 ml of ferric ammonium sulphate reagent. Centrifuge and separate the aqueous layer. Measure the extinction of aqueous layers at the maximum at about 530 nm. Deduce the results by comparison.

Probable Reaction Mechanism

The compound is hydrolysed by refluxing with methanolic sodium hydroxide. Salicylic acid so generated is coupled with ferric(III) ammonium sulphate in acidic medium to give a coloured iron complex (λ_{max} 530 nm).

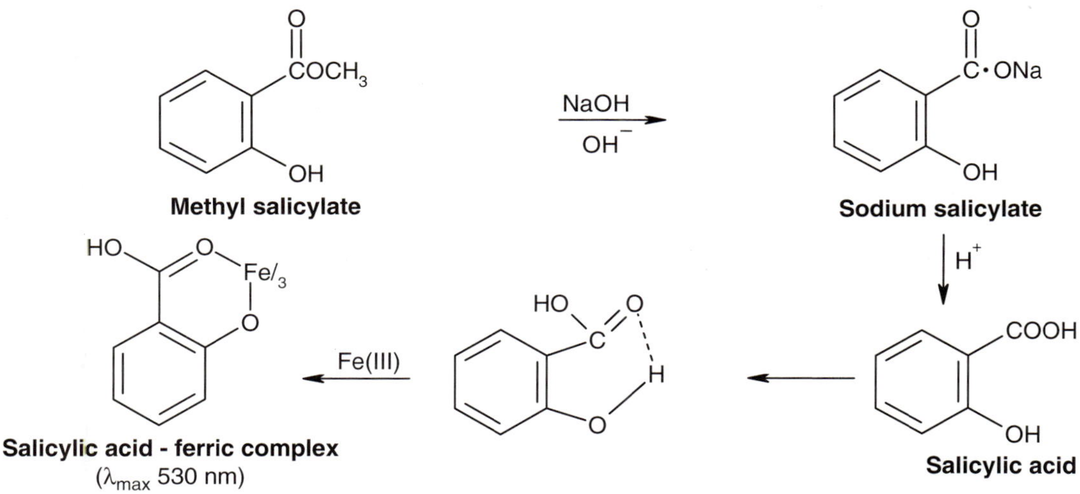

METHOD 2

This is based on the extraction of intact molecule (methyl salicylate) with cyclohexane. The λ_{max} (308 nm) corresponds to salicylic acid moiety of the molecule.

Weigh sample accurately equivalent to about 100 mg of the substance in a beaker, add about 15-20 ml of cyclohexane. Stir to dissolve the substance. Make up the volume to 100 ml with cyclohexane. 1 ml of the resulting solution is further diluted with cyclohexane to 100 ml. Measure the extinction of the solution at the maximum at about 308 nm. To convert methyl salicylate (v/v) to w/w, multiply by the factor 1.182. For calculations use 357 as value of A 1%, 1 cm at 308 nm.

Note

Since p-position to the phenolic —OH is unoccupied, Emerson reaction i.e. reaction with 4-aminophenazone can also be used for analytical purpose. Hydroxyethyl salicylate, often used in place of methyl salicylate, gives reactions similar to methyl salicylate.

Methyl salicylate

Reagents

1. Dilute sulphuric acid: Prepared by mixing 61 parts of sulphuric acid with 39 parts of water (v/v).
2. 0.5% w/v solution of paradimethylaminobenzaldehyde (PDAB) in dilute sulphuric acid.
3. 5% w/v solution of sodium hydroxide.
4. Methyl alcohol.

Standard solution

50 mcg/ml of menthol in methyl alcohol.

Sample solution

Suspend an accurately weighed quantity of sample (ointment) equivalent to 5 mg of menthol in 100 ml of sodium hydroxide solution. Distil and collect about 50 ml of distillate, cool and extract the distillate with ether. Pass ether extract through sodium sulphate (anhydrous). Evaporate ether layer to dryness at a very low temperature and dissolve the residue in methanol to get 50 mcg/ml solution.

Procedure

To 5 ml each of sample and standard solutions, add 2 ml of ice cold 'PDAB' reagent, dilute to 10 ml with methanol. Keep in boiling water-bath for 2-3 min, cool and measure the absorbance of both the solutions at the maximum at about 545 nm against reagent blank within 15 min.

Note

This test will serve as identification test for menthol as well.

Probable Reaction Mechanism

It is a cyclohexanol derivative. In acidic medium, it is first dehydrogenated to acetone derivative and then condenses with PDAB at position 2 to give coloured compound (λ_{max} 545 nm).

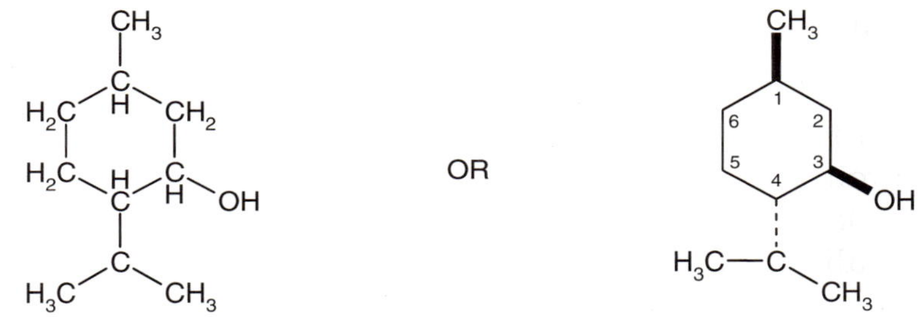

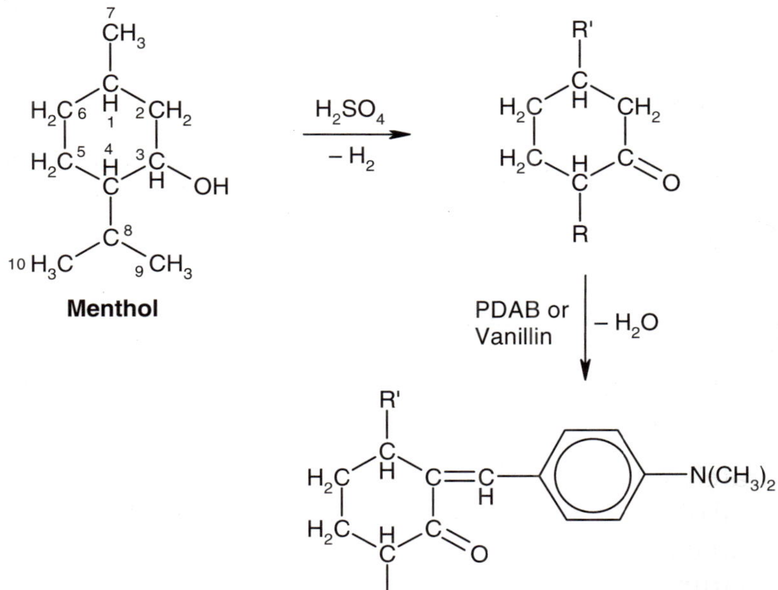

Benzalacetone derivative
(λ_{max} 545 nm)

Total volatile contents (Menthol, Methyl salicylate, Oil of turpentine)

For details, refer to formulation 4 of this chapter.

Formulation 2

Glycol monosalicylate, Histamine dihydrochloride, Methyl nicotinate, Capsaicin

ESTIMATION

Glycol monosalicylate

Reagents

1. Alcohol.
2. Potassium hydroxide.
3. Ferric ammonium sulphate solution.
4. Dilute acetic acid.

Standard solution

20 mcg/ml of salicylic acid in alcohol.

Sample solution

Take sample equivalent to 5 mg of the substance, add 25 ml of alcohol and 2 g of potassium hydroxide. Reflux for 1 h to saponify the material, cool and dilute to 250 ml with alcohol.

Procedure

To 2.5 ml each of sample and standard solutions, add 1 ml of dilute acetic acid, 15 ml of ferric ammonium sulphate solution and dilute to 100 ml with distilled water. Measure the absorption of both the solutions at about 530 nm. Compare the results for calculations.

Formation of an Fe-chelate with 3 molecules of salicylic acid is obtained as a result of saponification of glycol monosalicylate with KOH.

Probable Reaction Mechanism

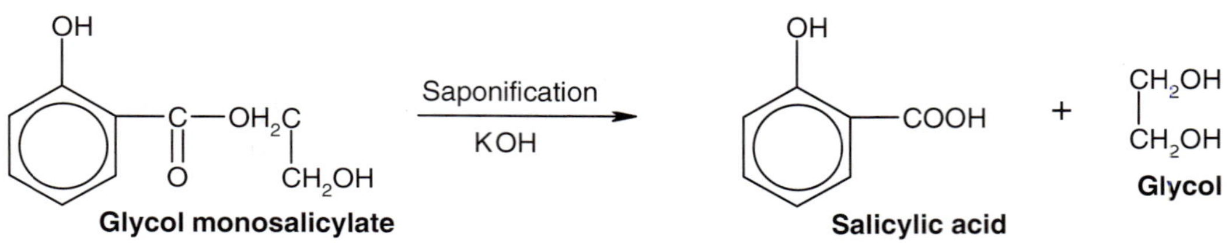

The salicylic acid so formed forms chelate with Fe^{+3} ions as shown below.

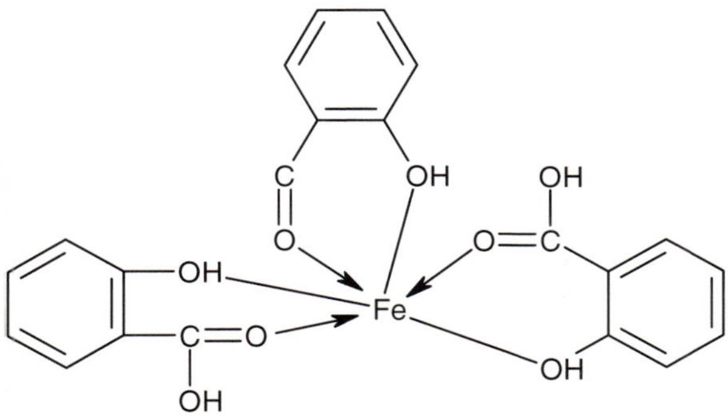

Fe-chelate
(λ_{max} 530 nm)

Or

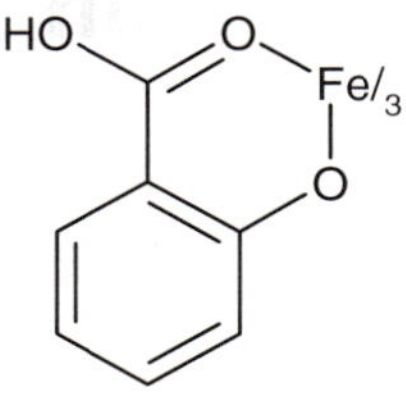

Histamine dihydrochloride

Reagents

1. 0.1% w/v sodium nitrite solution in water.
2. Sulphanilic acid solution: To 300 mg of sulphanilic acid, add 2.5 ml hydrochloric acid and dilute to 100 ml with water.
3. 4% w/v sodium hydroxide solution in water.

Standard solution

15 mcg/ml of histamine dihydrochloride in water.

Sample solution

Take sample accurately weighed equivalent to about 12.5 mg of the compound, add 30 ml of distilled water, 50 ml of alcohol and 5 g of potassium hydroxide. Reflux on boiling water-bath for about 1 h. Cool and transfer the contents to a volumetric flask with the aid of 50 ml of alcohol and dilute to 500 ml. Add 10 ml of hydrochloric acid, mix and make up the volume to 1000 ml with distilled water and filter (A). 50 ml of the filtrate is extracted with four 25 ml portions of chloroform. Discard chloroform layer, filter aqueous layer and use as sample for estimation of histamine.

Procedure

To 2 ml each of sample and standard solutions, add 2 ml of sodium nitrite solution. Wait for 2 min, add 4 ml of sulphanilic acid solution. After 3 min, add 4 ml of sodium hydroxide solution and dilute to 25 ml with water. Measure the absorption of both the solutions at 420 nm against reagent blank. Deduce the results by comparison.

Probable Reaction Mechanism

It involves coupling of diazotized sulphanilic acid with histamine. This is based on 'Pauly reaction'.

$$NaNO_2 + HCl \longrightarrow NaCl + HNO_2$$

The nitrous acid so generated results in the formation of nitrosonium ions under acidic conditions.

$$HNO_2 \xrightarrow[H^+]{} H_2O\overset{\oplus}{N}{=}O \xrightarrow[Cl^\ominus]{} H_2O + Cl^\ominus\underset{\oplus}{N}{=}O$$

These nitrosonium ions being electron-deficient will attack the primary amino group resulting in the formation of diazotized product.

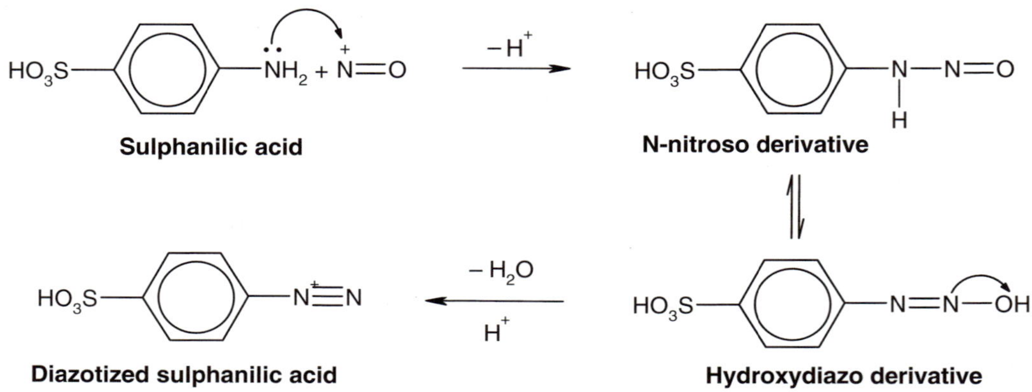

Diazotized sulphanilic acid couples at position-2 of the heteroaromatic ring. Imidazole anion reacts with diazonium cation. The formation of anion is pre-requisite because of low electrophilic nature of diazonium salt because sulphanilic acid group exists as anion whereas other electrophilic reagents such as nitric acid or sulphuric acid preferentially attack at position 4 or 5 of the molecule.

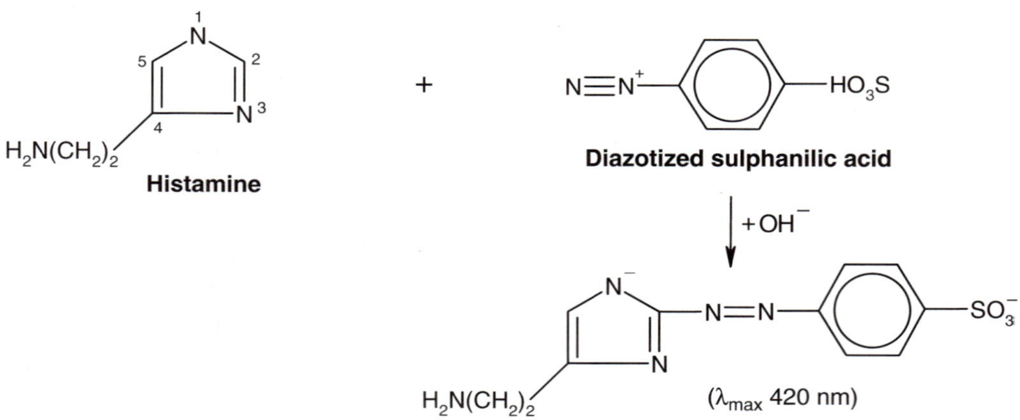

Reference

1. Textbook of Practical Organic Chemistry by Vogel, p. 920.
2. Pharmaceutical Chemistry (Vol. 2) by H.J. Roth, pp. 519 and 520.
3. K.K. Vishwanath, A.S. Rao & M.V. Sivaramakrishna, *Indian Drugs*, **24**, 453, 1987.

Note

Diazotized p-nitroaniline is preferred as the azo dye so formed can be extracted into organic solvent for measurements.

A method based on formation of chelate with Cu(II), followed by ion-associate with tetrabromophenolphthalein ethyl ester (TBPE) has been described by Sakai et al. (1984).

Reagents

1. 0.005 M solution of Cu(II) chloride.
2. 0.004 M TBPE solution in alcohol.
3. pH 9.5 borate buffer, prepared by mixing equal volume of 0.3 M potassium dihydrogen phosphate and 0.1 M sodium tetraborate, pH adjusted with 1 M sodium hydroxide.

Sample and standard solutions

1 mg/ml of histamine acid phosphate in water. Further dilution made to get solution of 5 μg/ml.

Procedure

To 3 ml each of sample and standard solutions add 1 ml of Cu(II) chloride solution and 15 ml of pH 9.5 buffer, allow to stand the mixture for 5 min, then add 2 ml of 'TBPE' solution, dilute to 50 ml with water. Shake the entire aqueous layer with 10 ml of dichloromethane till the entire red colour is passed on to organic layer. Centrifuge for 10 min, collect organic layer and measure the absorbance of both the solutions at 515 nm against reagent blank.

Note

1. Histamine (HA) forms complex with transition metal ions such as copper, zinc, cobalt, nickel and iron, but complex with Cu(II) was the most stable. These cationic complexes react with monoprotic dyes such as picric acid, 2,6-dichlorophenol indophenol and TBPE to form coloured ion-associates. Since 'TBPE' dye is hydrophobic, it has best extractability into organic phase. The reaction for formation of Cu(II) - histamine chelate and histamine - Cu(II) - TBPE ion-associate as proposed by the authors is as under.

Probable Reaction Mechanism

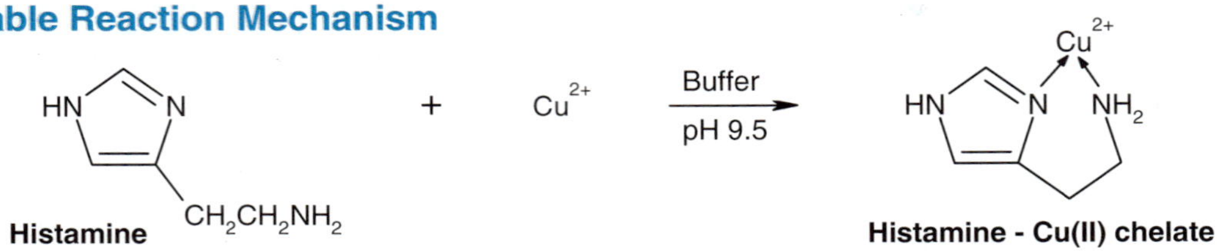

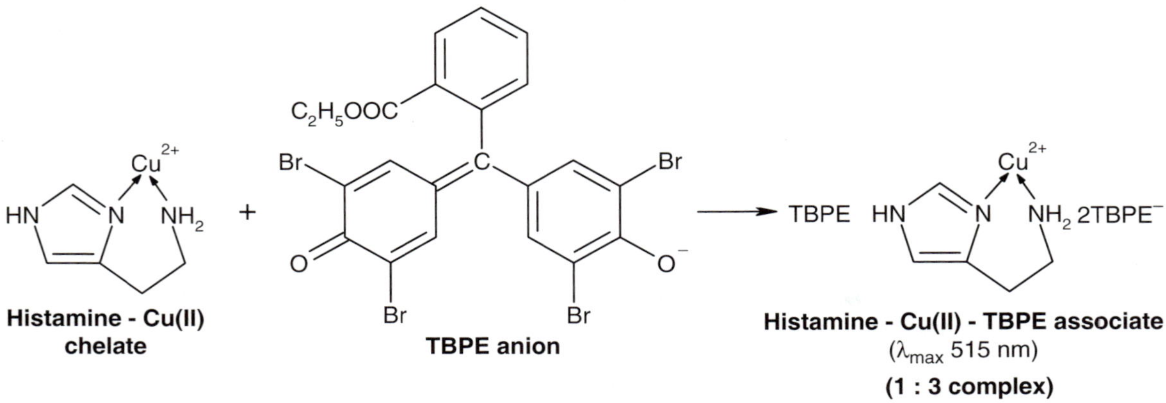

2. The molar ratio of Cu(II) to HA was 1 : 1 whereas HA to TBPE was 1 : 3 suggesting the final species as HA - Cu(II) - TBPE.

Reference

Tadao Sakai, Noriko Ohno, Masaya Tanaka & Toyohiko Okada, *Analyst*, **109(12)**, 1569-1572, 1984.

Histamine, an imidazole derivative, is more susceptible to electrophilic attack than pyrazole or furan derivative. Therefore, it undergoes nitration (NO_2), sulphonation (HSO_3), bromination and iodination. These reactions can form the basis of quantitative analysis.

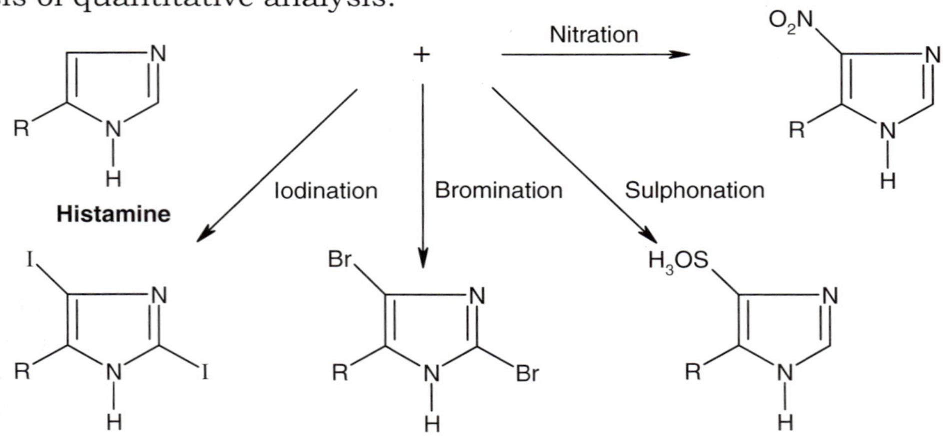

Note

Pilocarpine and metronidazole can undergo similar nucleophilic substitution reactions.

Methyl nicotinate

Take 10 ml of the filtrate (A) obtained during estimation of histamine and dilute to 100 ml. Proceed as per method described for this compound under formulation 1 of this chapter.

Capsaicin

METHOD 1

Reagent

0.5% w/v vanadium oxytrichloride solution in ethyl acetate.

Standard solution

100 mcg/ml of capsaicin in ethyl acetate.

Sample solution

Take sample accurately weighed equivalent to 10 mg of capsaicin, extract the material with ethyl acetate for 24 h in cold or reflux for 2 h and filter. Dilute to 50 ml with ethyl acetate.

Procedure

Take 5 ml each of the sample and standard solutions and just before absorption measurement, add 0.5 ml of vanadium oxytrichloride solution. Shake to mix and immediately measure the absorption at about 720 nm. Run the blank prepared by using 0.5 ml of the reagent and 5 ml of ethyl acetate.

Note

1. Although the colour fades away in 1 to 1.5 min, but 30 seconds elapse between the time the reagent is added and the absorbance is measured.
2. Use of acetone as extracting solvent is not recommended as due to its hygroscopic nature, it produces turbid solution.

METHOD 2

To accurately weighed quantity of sample equivalent to 2 mg of capsaicin (oleoresin capsicum containing about 8% of capsaicin), add 2 ml of anaesthetic ether and dilute to 50 ml with methanol. Add 2-3 g of sodium chloride, 10 ml of water and basify with 5 ml of 0.1 N sodium hydroxide. Extract with petroleum ether 80-100°C (4 × 10 ml). Combine the ether extract and wash with 60% methanol (3 × 25 ml). The combined hydroalcoholic layer is evaporated to about 5 ml. Add 30-40 ml water and adjust to pH 7.2 ± 0.2 (phenol red) with 0.1 N sodium hydroxide or 0.1 N hydrochloric acid as the case may be. The entire solution in turn is extracted with anaesthetic ether (4 × 50 ml). The combined ethereal layer is evaporated and residue taken up in 50 ml of methanol (decolourise with charcoal if the solution is coloured). To one 10 ml portion of alcoholic solution, add 5 ml of 0.1 N sodium hydroxide, cool and dilute to 25 ml with methanol, whereas to another 10 ml portion, add 5 ml of 0.05 N hydrochloric acid, cool and dilute to 25 ml with methanol. Measure extinction of alkaline solution at 248 nm against reagent blank. Calculate the results using 313 as value of A 1%, 1 cm for capsaicin.

Note

1. Addition of alkali or acid and subsequent spectrophotometric reading should be made very fast and first instrumental reading should be taken for calculations.
2. From the contents of capsaicin so estimated, calculate the amount of oleoresin capsicum present in the sample (oleoresin capsicum containing about 8% of capsaicin).

Typical laboratory analysis (based on assay value of 8.0% of raw material)

Weight of the sample taken for analysis = 12.75 g

A_s at 248 nm = 0.298

A_u at 248 nm = 0.245

$$\text{Capsaicin (contents) \%} = \frac{A_u}{A_s} \times \frac{d_f \times 100}{\text{Weight of the sample taken}}$$

$$= \frac{245}{298} \times \frac{1.25 \times 100}{12.75 \times 8}$$

% claim = 100.75

Formulation 3

Benzyl nicotinate, Salicylamide, Methyl salicylate, Camphor, Oil of turpentine

ESTIMATION

Benzyl nicotinate

Reagents

1. Saturated solution of cyanogen bromide in water (prepare fresh).
2. Aniline solution: 4.0% v/v solution of aniline (freshly distilled) in methanol.

Standard solution

100 µg/ml in methanol.

Sample solution

2 ml of liniment is boiled with about 30 ml of methanol for 5 minutes. Cool and filter into 100 ml volumetric flask. Wash the filter paper with methanol and make up the volume to 100 ml with methanol. 2.5 ml of this solution is further diluted to 50 ml with methanol.

Procedure

2 ml of the above solution is taken into 50 ml conical flask, add 10 ml of methanol and 5 ml of cyanogen bromide solution. Allow the solution to stand for 5 minutes, then add 5 ml of alcoholic aniline solution and keep aside for further 5 minutes. The extinction of yellow colour is measured at 436 nm using alcohol as a blank. The quantity of benzyl nicotinate in the sample is calculated by comparing with the standard processed similarly.

On hydrolysis, nicotinic acid is liberated which can be estimated by cyanogen bromide method. For details, see under methyl nicotinate.

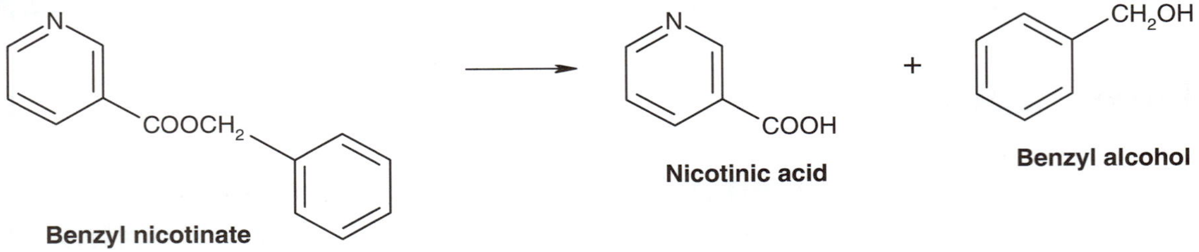

Salicylamide and Methyl salicylate (Total salicylic acid)

Reagents

1. Dilute hydrochloric acid (10% v/v).
2. 1% and 10% w/v solution of sodium hydroxide in water.
3. 2% w/v solution of ferric chloride in water.

Standard solution

20 mcg/ml of salicylic acid in water.

Sample solution

An accurately weighed amount of the sample equivalent to 5 mg of total salicylates is heated with 10 ml of dilute hydrochloric acid for 30 minutes on a boiling water-bath in order to destroy the emulsion. Add 30 ml of 10% sodium hydroxide solution and saponify for one hour while boiling under reflux. Transfer the solution into a separating funnel and shake twice with 50 ml solvent ether. The ether extract is discarded. The aqueous phase is acidified with hydrochloric acid and extracted with five 20 ml portions of ether. The combined ether extracts are shaken four time with 30 ml of 1% sodium hydroxide solution and 50 ml of water each. Slightly acidify the alkaline solution, make up the volume to 250 ml with water and filter.

Procedure

1 ml each of sample and standard solutions are taken in 10 ml volumetric flask, two drops of dilute hydrochloric acid and 0.2 ml of ferric chloric solution are added and the solution is made up to the volume with water. Measure the absorption of both solutions at about 550 nm against solution of 0.2 ml of ferric chloride solution in 10 ml water as blank. The amount of total salicylic acid is calculated by comparing with the standard.

For reaction mechanism see under salicylic acid, aspirin or salicylamide under chapter on analgesics & antipyretics.

Alternatively, follow the method for estimation of total salicylic acid described in formulation 1 of this chapter.

Formulation 4

Menthol, Thymol, Camphor, Methyl salicylate, Oil of turpentine, Oil of eucalyptus, Oil of lemon-grass

ESTIMATION

Total volatile contents

Procedure

1. Place in a one litre round bottom flask about 70 g of the sample accurately weighed and add 300-400 ml of water, add few pieces of pumice stone to avoid bumping. Connect the flask to a special reflux still fitted with oil-trap. Heat the contents to boiling in a heating mantle. Continue distillation for about 2 h. Cool the distillate (volatile contents) collected in the trap and measure the volume. Calculate the volume in terms of ml/100 g (% v/w) of the sample.
2. In a previously dried and weighed china dish, take an accurately weighed quantity of the sample, keep the china dish on a boiling water-bath for 30 minutes or till there is no aromatic odour. Then transfer the china dish to an oven and dry it to a constant weight at 105°C for 4 h. Transfer to desiccator to cool and weigh the residue. Calculate the total volatile matter from the loss in weight of the sample.

Thymol

METHOD 1

Reagents

1. Para-aminophenol solution, 0.1% w/v: Dissolve 10 mg of pure and freshly sublimed p-aminophenol in 10 ml of alcohol, prepare fresh.
2. 2 M ammonia solution.

Standard solution

100 mg of pure thymol, accurately weighed, is dissolved in 100 ml of alcohol. 5 ml of this solution is further diluted to 100 ml distilled water to give a solution of 50 mcg/ml.

General procedure for preparation of standard curve

An aliquot of standard solution ranging from 1 to 5 ml is taken in graduated stoppered 10 ml centrifuge tubes. Add 2.5 ml of 2 N ammonium hydroxide solution and 0.3 ml of p-aminophenol solution to each tube and dilute to 10 ml with distilled water. Shake and keep for 5 minutes and read the absorbance of blue complex at 600 nm against reagent blank. The standard curve against concentration of thymol is prepared.

Formulations

Generally three different types of formulations containing thymol are available in the market:

1. Creams and ointments.
2. Solutions (such as gum paints, mouth wash).
3. Powders and tablets (lozenges).

Creams and ointments: Accurately weighed quantity of the preparation is mixed with 10 ml of 10% sodium hydroxide solution and the mixture is heated on water-bath to melt. The wax is separated by cooling. Neutralise the solution with dilute hydrochloric acid and dilute to produce a solution of 50 mcg/ml. Take 1 ml of this solution and follow the general procedure and calculate the amount from the standard curve.

Solutions: Known volume of the sample solution is diluted with distilled water to produce a solution of 50 mcg/ml. Use 1 ml of this solution for estimation of thymol by the general method. If the sample contains iodine, it should be removed with sodium thiosulphate before proceeding with the estimation by general method.

Tablets or powders: Extract the powder or powdered tablets with 50 ml of alcohol and dilute with water to produce a solution containing 50 mcg/ml. Take 1 ml of the solution and proceed with the estimation by general method.

Note

1. The method obeys Beer's law over a concentration of 1.8 mcg/ml of the final solution.
2. Menthol, camphor, turpentine oil, cinnamon oil, methyl salicylate, salicylic acid, benzoic acid and boric acid do not interfere in this method.

Note

Chlorothymol, an antiseptic, can be analysed by the above method i.e. reaction with p-aminophenol in alkaline (NH_4OH) medium and reaction mechanism as under thymol.

Reference

R.T. Sane, P.P. Karkhanis & A.Y. Sathe, *Indian Drugs*, **18(4)**, 149-151, 1981.

p-Aminophenol is simultaneously oxidized to benzoquinone in an alkaline medium in the presence of phenol to form indophenol. Based on the above statement, thymol, a phenol, and alkaline condition maintained, indophenol-like product must be formed. The reaction is as shown below.

Probable Reaction Mechanism

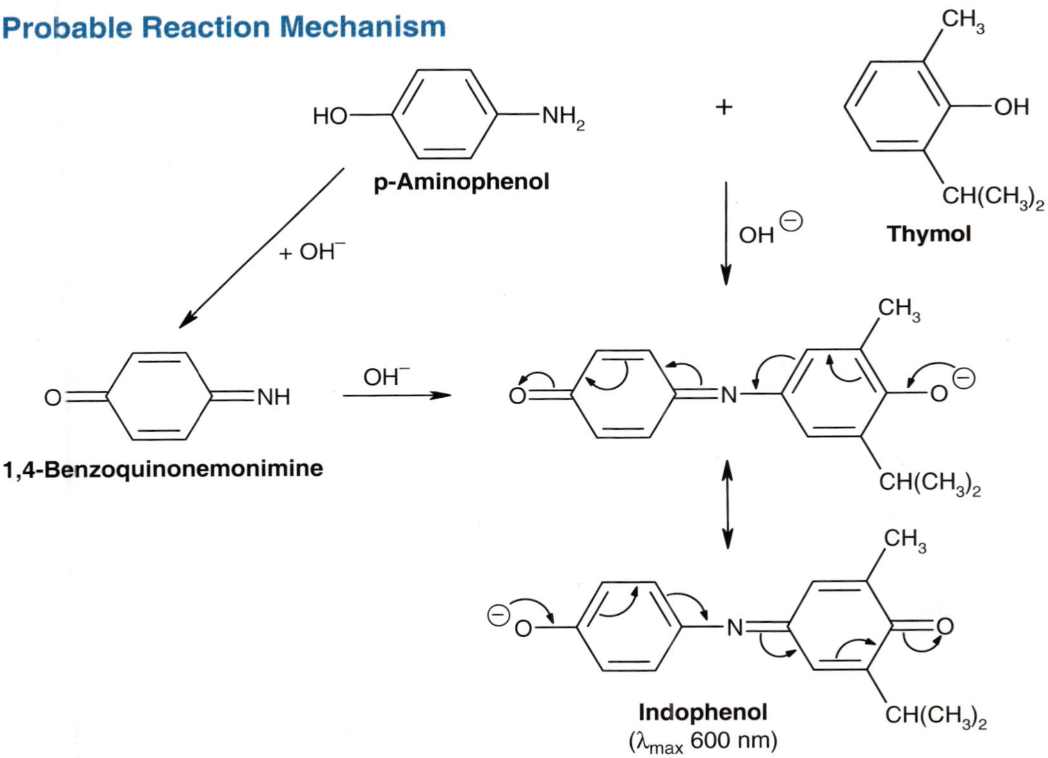

Reference

1. R.T. Sane, V.S. Narkar & U.M. Vaidya, *Indian Drugs*, **17(3)**, 82-83, 1979.
2. E. Ucock, C.T.H. & A.G. Fogg, Analyst, **16**, 100, 1975.

METHOD 2

A simple colorimetric method by coupling thymol with chlorimide reagent (Gibbs' reagent) is described.

Reagents

1. 0.4% w/v solution of 2,6-dichloroquinone chlorimide in methanol.
2. Alkaline borate buffer, pH 9.4.

Stock solution of thymol

1 mg/ml of thymol in methanol.

Working solution of thymol

1 ml of stock solution is diluted to 100 ml water (10 mcg/ml).

Preparation of standard curve

Take aliquot containing 10-70 mcg of thymol and dilute each of them to 10 ml with water. Add 2 ml of buffer solution and 0.1 ml of chlorimide reagent. Mix and measure the absorbance at 600 nm within 15 minutes. Prepare standard curve against concentration of thymol. The sample solutions of different types of formulations are prepared as described under method 1 and subjected to analysis as per method described under preparation of standard curve. Amount of thymol in the sample is calculated from the standard curve.

Note

1. The colour is stable for 15 minutes; measure the extinction as quickly as possible.
2. The method obeys Beer's law in the range of 10-70 mcg/ml of thymol. Menthol, camphor, salicylic acid, benzoic acid, methyl salicylate, cinnamon oil, turpentine oil, lemon grass oil, borax, sodium bicarbonate, iodine, potassium iodide, tannic acid and oleoresin capsicum in the concentration of 1 mg/ml do not give colour with this reagent. However, eucalyptus oil gives green and clove oil produces blue colour with this reagent.

Probable Reaction Mechanism

Oxidative coupling reaction occurs at the para position to the phenolic hydroxyl group in thymol by the reagent dichloroquinone chlorimide.

Initially the dichloroquinone chlorimide reacts with H_2O resulting in the formation of dichloroquinonimine. The dichloroquinonimine now acts as the oxidizing agent and attacks the para position of the phenol. The reaction is carried out at pH 9.4 using alkaline borate buffer.

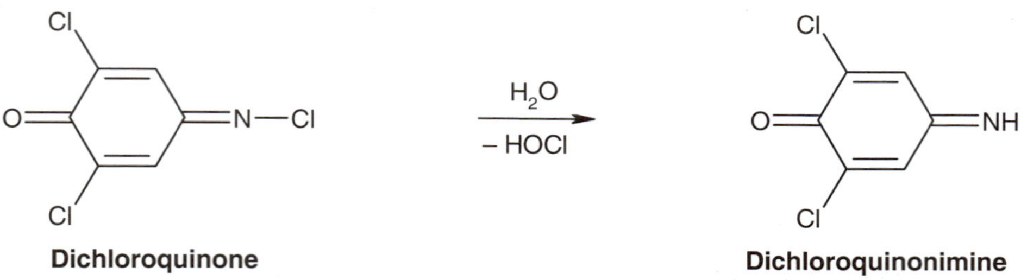

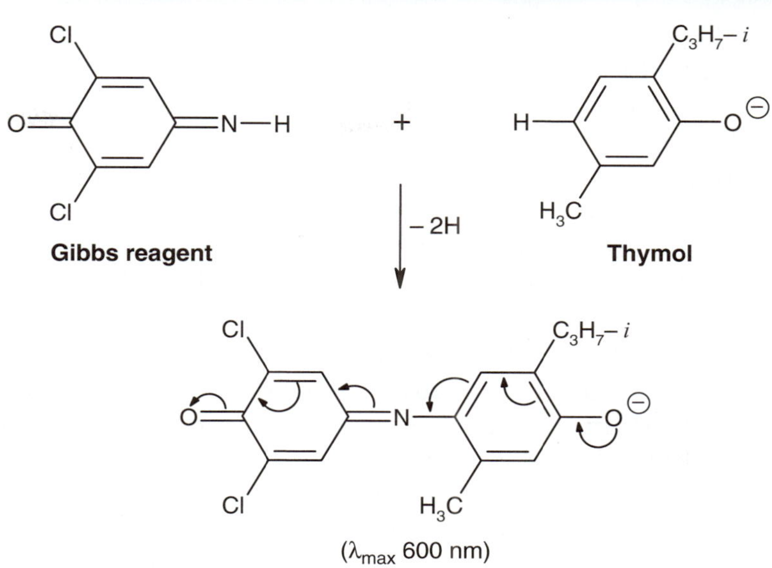

METHOD 3

A colorimetric method involving reaction of thymol with diazotised 4-nitroaniline-2-sulphonic acid is described.

Reagents

1. 4-nitroaniline-2-sulphonic acid solution: 0.158 g of the compound is dissolved and made up to 100 ml with dilute hydrochloric acid.
2. 0.2% w/v sodium nitrite solution in water.
3. Diazotised reagent: 18 ml of solution (1) is cooled to 5°C and completely diazotised with solution (2) using starch-iodide paste as external indicator. The final solution should be clear and colourless. It should be kept in cold and protected from light. Diazotised reagent should always be freshly prepared. Usually 1 ml of solution (2) is required for 4.5 ml of solution (1) for complete diazotization.
4. Alkaline borate buffer, pH 10.0.

Stock solution of thymol

1 mg/ml of thymol in ethyl alcohol.

Working solution of thymol

Stock solution is approximately diluted with water to obtain a concentration of 100 mcg/ml of thymol.

Standard curve

Take aliquot containing 10 to 60 mcg of thymol. Add 10 ml of water, 1 ml of 0.1 N sodium hydroxide and 6 ml of alkaline borate buffer solution to each and cool to about 5°C. Then, add 0.5 ml of freshly prepared diazotised reagent and dilute the contents to 25 ml with water and set aside for 15 minutes. The absorbance of the coloured product is measured at 520 nm and standard curve against the concentration of thymol is prepared. For estimation of thymol in analgesic balms, the following procedure is recommended for preparation of sample solution:

About 0.5 g of the balm is accurately weighed in a 50 ml capacity platinum dish containing 10 ml of 10 per cent sodium hydroxide solution and 25 ml distilled water. To this, add 5 mg thymol in alcoholic solution and mix. The dish is heated on a boiling water-bath and heating is continued till there is no easily perceptible camphoracious odour. The solution in the dish is not allowed to evaporate to less than 20 ml. The water lost is replaced from time to time. The solution is then chilled and the clear liquid is filtered into a 100 ml volumetric flask. The residue left in the dish is heated with about 25 ml of water three times on a water-bath and the extractives filtered into the volumetric flask. The solution in the flask is made up to volume with distilled water. One ml of this solution is taken for analysis. The amount of thymol is calculated from the standard curve.

Note

1. The method obeys Beer's law in the range of 10-60 mcg/ml.
2. Colour of the complex is stable for 24 hrs.

Probable Reaction Mechanism

Thymol **4-nitroaniline-2-sulphonic acid**

The $NaNO_2$ solution and 4-nitroaniline-2-sulphonic acid react resulting in the diazotization of the acid as shown below. 4-nitroaniline-2-sulphonic acid is diluted with HCl.

$$NaNO_2 + HCl \longrightarrow HNO_2 + NaCl$$

$$HNO_2 \xrightarrow[H^+]{} H_2O + \overset{+}{N}O \xrightarrow[Cl^{\ominus}]{} \overset{\ominus}{Cl}\ \overset{\oplus}{NO}$$

The nitrosonium ion being electron-deficient attacks the amino group of the acid resulting in the formation of diazonium ion.

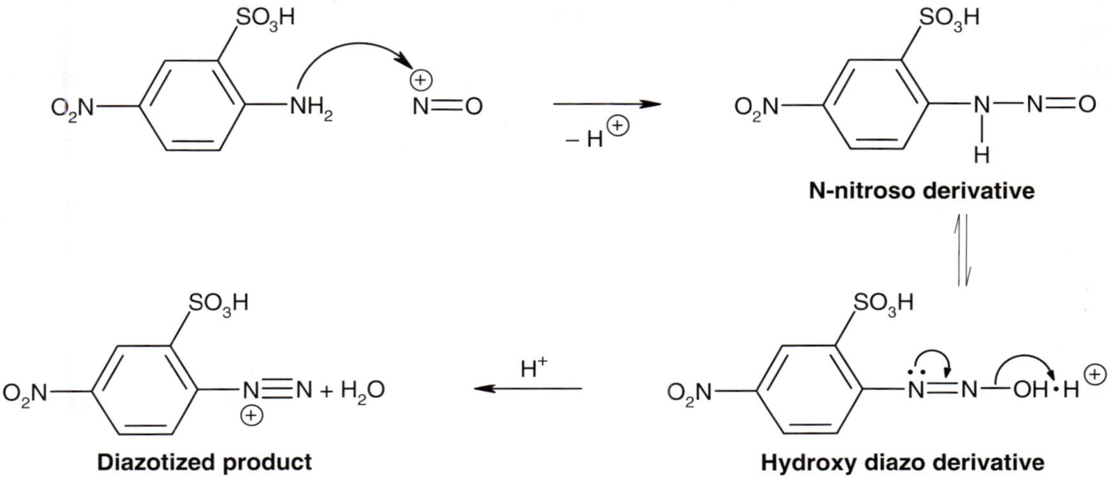

The diazotized product will couple at para position to the phenolic —OH group in the drug resulting in the formation of the product.

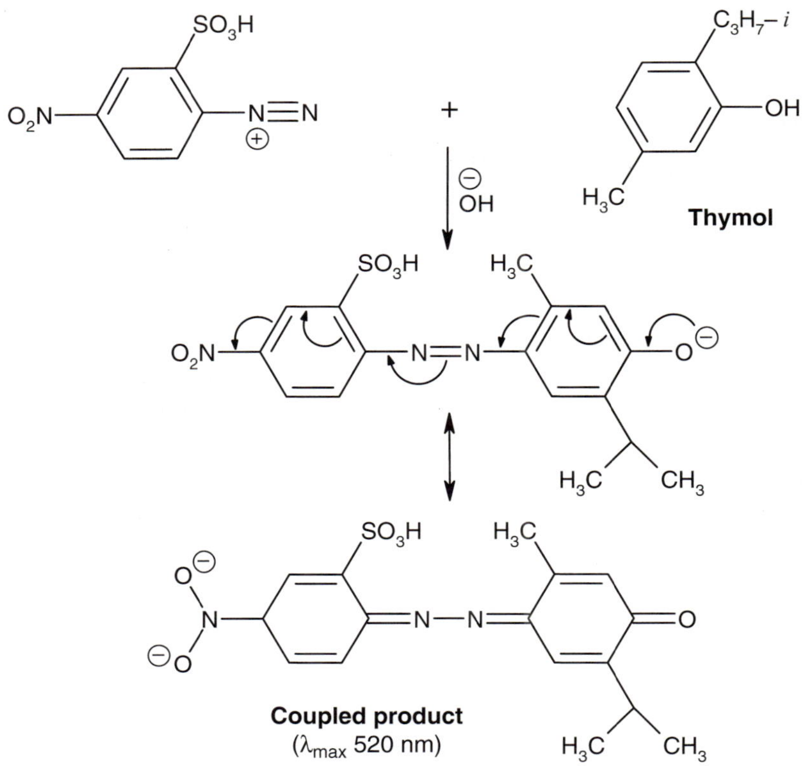

Reference

1. R.G. Tamhane & S.S. Rao. *Ind. J. Pharm.*, **33(4)**, 70-71, 1971.
2. Practical Oraganic Chemistry by Vogel, p. 920.

Conc. nitric acid acts both as oxidizing agent as well as nitrating agent; both are colouring compounds and are of analytical interest.

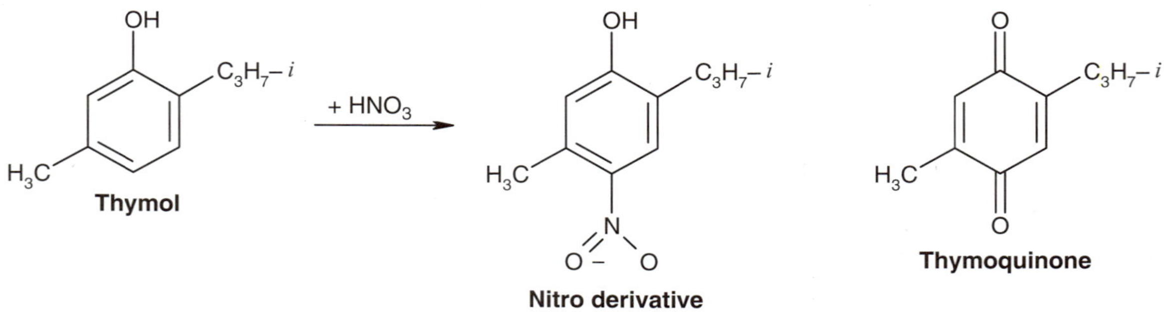

Reference

Pharmaceutical Chemistry (Vol. 2) by H.J. Roth, p. 79.

Methyl salicylate

METHOD 1

Take 2 g of the sample accurately weighed and suspend in 10 ml dilute hydrochloric acid by warming for about 15 minutes. Add 30 ml of 1 N sodium hydroxide and saponify by refluxing for 1 h. Carry out the extraction and colour development as described in formulation 3 of this chapter.

METHOD 2

Weigh accurately sample equivalent to 100 mg of methyl salicylate in a 100 ml beaker and add about 10 ml of cyclohexane. Stir the mixture thoroughly to effect the solution and then transfer quantitatively into 100 ml dry volumetric flask with the aid of cyclohexane. Finally make up the volume. Filter and dilute 1 ml of the filtrate to 100 ml with cyclohexane. Measure the extinction of the resulting solution at the maxima at 308 nm. Calculate the percentage of methyl salicylate (v/v) taking 357 as the value of E (1 per cent, 1 cm) v/v. To convert the so obtained percentage of methyl salicylate in v/v into w/w, multiply by 1.182 which is weight per ml of methyl salicylate.

Menthol

Follow the method described in formulation 1 of this chapter.

Formulation 5

Oxyphenbutazone, Phenylbutazone, Methyl salicylate, Mephenesin, Menthol

ESTIMATION

Oxyphenbutazone/Phenylbutazone

Follow the method described in chapter on anti-inflammatory drugs.

Methyl salicylate

Weigh the sample (cream) accurately equivalent to about 100 mg methyl salicylate, transfer to a volumetric flask, add about 25 ml of cyclohexane. Heat on a water-bath to effect solution. Cool and make up to 100 ml with cyclohexane. Further dilutions may be done with cyclohexane to get final concentration of 10 mcg/ml. Measure the extinction at 308 nm using cyclohexane as blank. Calculate the results using 357 as value of A 1%, 1 cm, at 308 nm. Also refer to formulation 3 of this chapter.

Mephenesin

Weigh the sample (cream) accurately equivalent to 100 mg of mephenesin. Suspend in water by slight warming and add 5 ml of ammonia solution. Extract with four 25 ml portions of chloroform. Wash the combined chloroform layer with 10 mg each of 0.02 N sodium hydroxide and water and then pass through a layer of anhydrous sodium sulphate. Evaporate the combined chloroform layer and take up the residue in water to get volume of 200 ml. Dilute further appropriately with water to get final concentration of 25 mcg/ml. Measure the absorbance of the resulting solution at maximum at about 270 nm. Calculate the contents of mephenesin taking 80 as value of A 1%, 1 cm at 270 nm. Alternately, the chloroform layer can be directly used for estimation by using a standard (25 mcg/ml) in chloroform for comparison.

As a result of periodate reaction, the formaldehyde so produced reacts with MBTH, as explained below, to give red colour. In the first step, iodate ions from sodium periodate interact with the diol system present in the drug resulting in the formation of formaldehyde as one of the products as shown below.

The formaldehyde so formed reacts with MBTH resulting in the formation of two products A and B. A and B react among themselves resulting in the formation of the final product.

Probable Reaction Mechanism

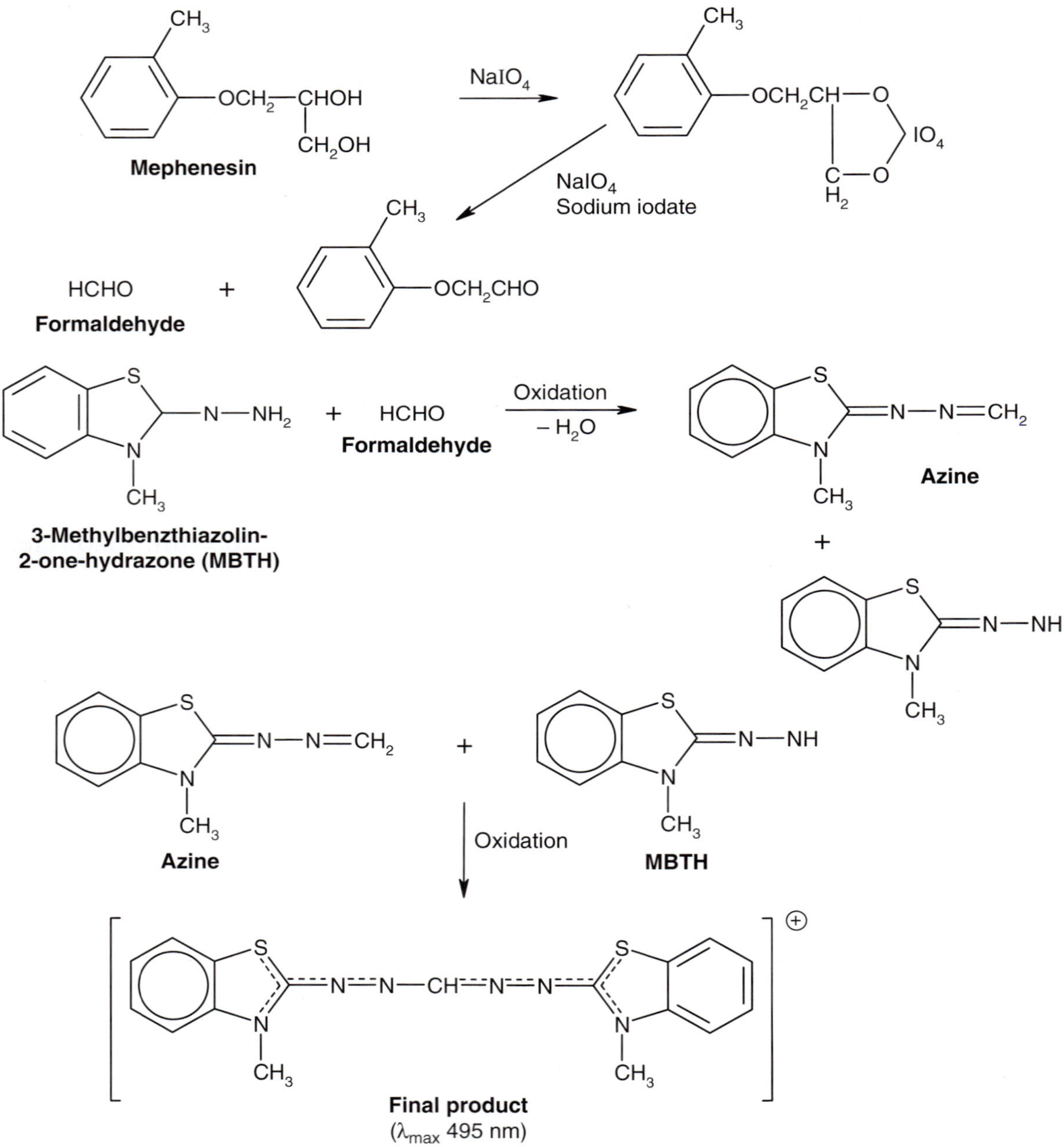

Menthol

Suspend adequate quantity of the sample equivalent to 1 mg of menthol in water and distil. For details, refer to the method described under formulation 1 of this chapter.

Formulation 6

Ibuprofen, Ketoprofen, Methyl salicylate, Mephenesin, Menthol

ESTIMATION

Ibuprofen

Follow the method described in formulation 34 of the chapter on analgesics and antipyretics. Each ml of 0.1 N sodium hydroxide is equivalent to 0.02063 g of ibuprofen or 0.02543 g of ketoprofen. Alternatively, suspend accurately weighed quantity of the sample in water by slight warming, add 1 ml of dilute HCl and extract the precipitated ibuprofen with n-hexane (3 × 25 ml), passing each extract through anhydrous sodium sulphate. Evaporate the combined chloroform layer in water-bath and take up the residue in 0.1 N sodium hydroxide to produce 100 ml (50 mcg/ml). Measure the absorbance of sample and standard solutions (processed as per sample) at 264 nm and calculate the results by comparison.

Explanatory Note

Both ibuprofen and ketoprofen have free carboxylic acid (—COOH) group which shall react with sodium hydroxide.

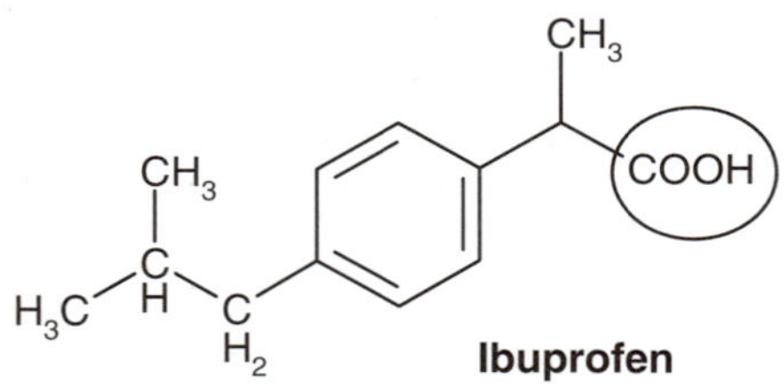

Ibuprofen

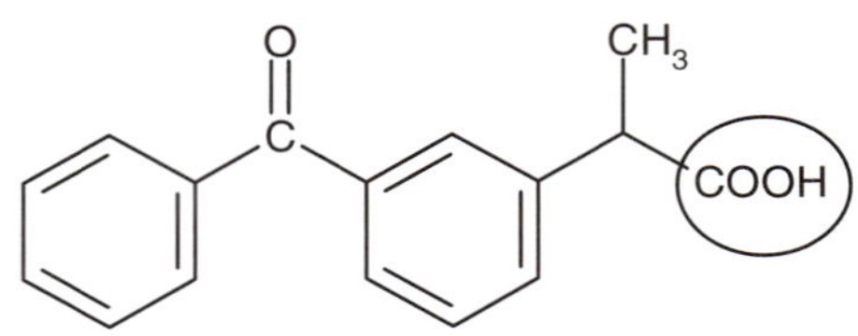

Ketoprofen

Methyl salicylate

Follow the method described in formulation 1 and 4 of this chapter.

Menthol

Follow the method described in formulation 1 of this chapter.

Mephenesin

Follow the method described in formulation 1 and 5 of this chapter.

Formulation 7

Diethylamine salicylate, Methyl nicotinate

ESTIMATION

Diethylamine salicylate

Reagent

Ferric chloride solution: To 5.5 g of ferric chloride, add 2.5 ml of concentrated hydrochloric acid and dilute to 100 ml with water.

Standard solution

80 mcg/ml of diethylamine salicylate in water.

Sample solution

The sample is extracted with water by slight warming, subsequently cooled and filtered. Further dilutions are done with water and kept cool while filtering.

Procedure

To 4 ml each of sample and standard solutions, add 0.5 ml of ferric chloride solution, mix and make up to 50 ml with water.

Measure the absorbance of both sample and standard solutions at about 540 nm against reagent blank and calculate the results by comparison.

Probable Reaction Mechanism

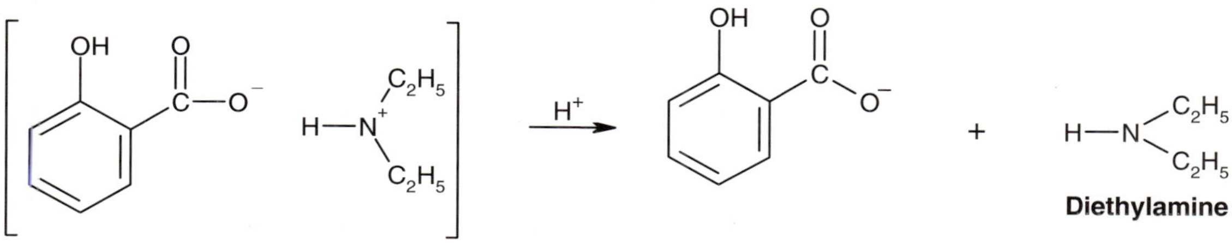

Diethylamine

Diethylamine salicylate

It is ester of strong base (diethylamine and acid).

As the ferric chloride reagent is acidic in character, we get

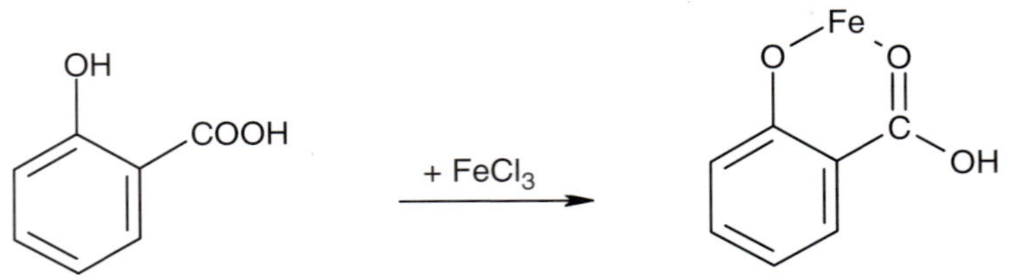

Salicylic acid

Violet-coloured iron complex (λ_{max} 540 nm)

The compound shall answer other reactions of salicylic acid. Diethylamine, a secondary aliphatic amine, shall react with nitrous acid (HNO_2) to give nitrosamine and shall also react with 1,2-naphthoquinone-4-sulphonate sodium. These reactions can be used for quantitative purpose.

A spectrophotometric method has been reported by Hassan et al. (1985). The method involves reaction of primary and secondary aliphatic amines with excess of p-benzoquinone in ethanol whereas 1 : 1 (amine : quinone) is formed with λ_{max} of 510 nm.

Probable Reaction Mechanism

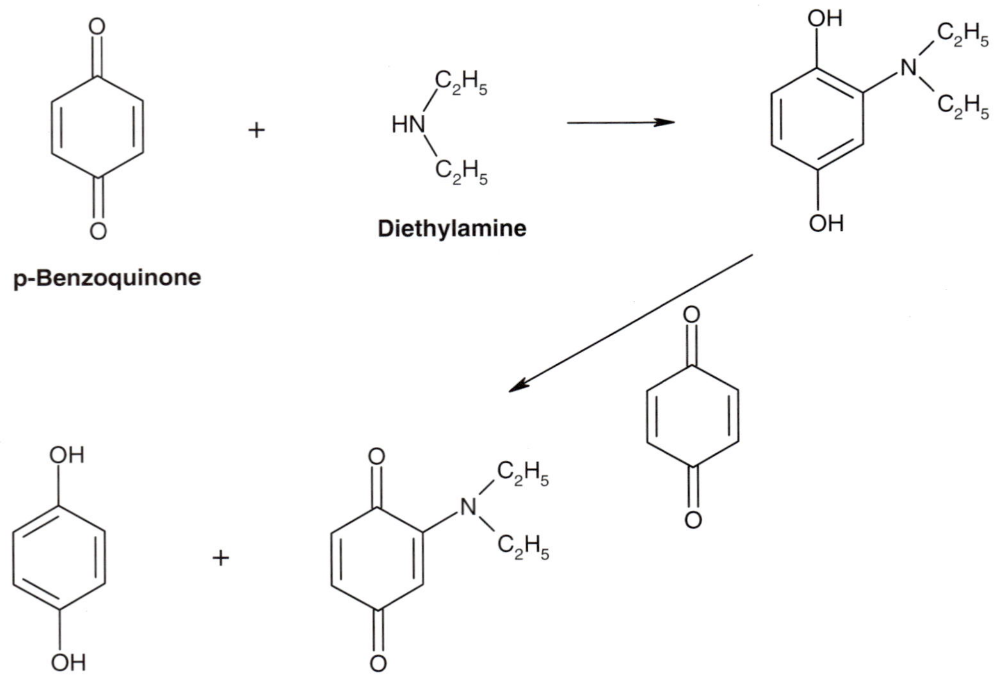

p-Benzoquinone

Diethylamine

1,4-Benzenediol

Amine - quinone complex (λ_{max} 510 nm)

Reference

Saad S.M. Hassan, M.L. Iskander & N.E. Nashed, *Talanta*, **32(4)**, 301-305, 1985.

Note

Other primary or secondary amines which can react with this reagent are propranolol, piperazine and ethylenediamine.

Methyl nicotinate

Follow the method described in formulation 1 of this chapter.

Formulation 8

Piroxicam, Capsaicin, Methylsalicylate, Menthol

ESTIMATION

Piroxicam

The method is based on differential spectroscopy.

Reagents

1. 0.01 N methanolic hydrochloric acid.
2. 0.01 N methanolic sodium hydroxide.

Standard solution

10 mcg/ml of piroxicam in 0.01 N methanolic hydrochloric acid and methanolic sodium hydroxide.

Sample solution

Accurately weighed quantity of the sample equivalent to 10 mg of the substance was extracted with methanol to get solution of 100 mcg/ml. Further dilutions were done as given under standard solution.

Procedure

Measure the absorbance of acidic solutions of both sample and standard at 326 nm using respective alkaline solutions as blank and calculate the results by comparison. The method obeys Beer's law in the concentration range of 4-22 mcg/ml.

Note

The following are reactions of analytical interest:

(a) Piroxicam can be estimated by reaction with 4-aminoantipyrin (Emerson reaction) i.e. oxidative coupling in the ortho position to phenolic —OH group present in the molecule in alkaline medium to give coloured product (λ_{max} 495 nm).

(b) After heating the drug with NaOH, the ring opens and resulting product couples with diazotized p-nitroaniline to yield coloured product (λ_{max} 490 nm).

(c) The compound reacts with Gibbs reagent by oxidative coupling to yield coloured product (λ_{max} 540 nm).

(d) The drug forms chelate with Fe(III) chloride in acidic medium to give coloured complex (λ_{max} 540 nm).

(e) The compound is oxidized by ferric ammonium sulphate and Fe^{++} forms complex with 1,10-phenanthroline (λ_{max} 510 nm).

(f) Fe^{++} also forms complex with 2,2-bispyridine (Emmerie-Engel reagent) to form complex (λ_{max} 522 nm).

Probable Reaction Mechanism

(a)

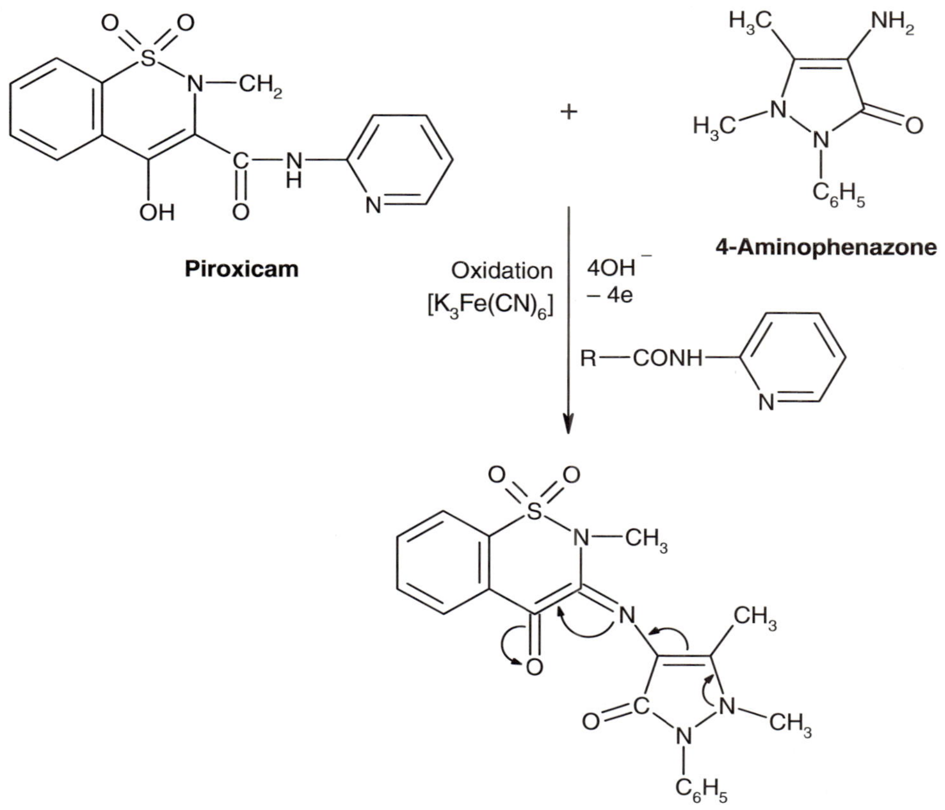

Coloured product
(λ_{max} 495 nm)

Reference

Indian Drugs, **25(6)**, 247, March 1988.

(b)

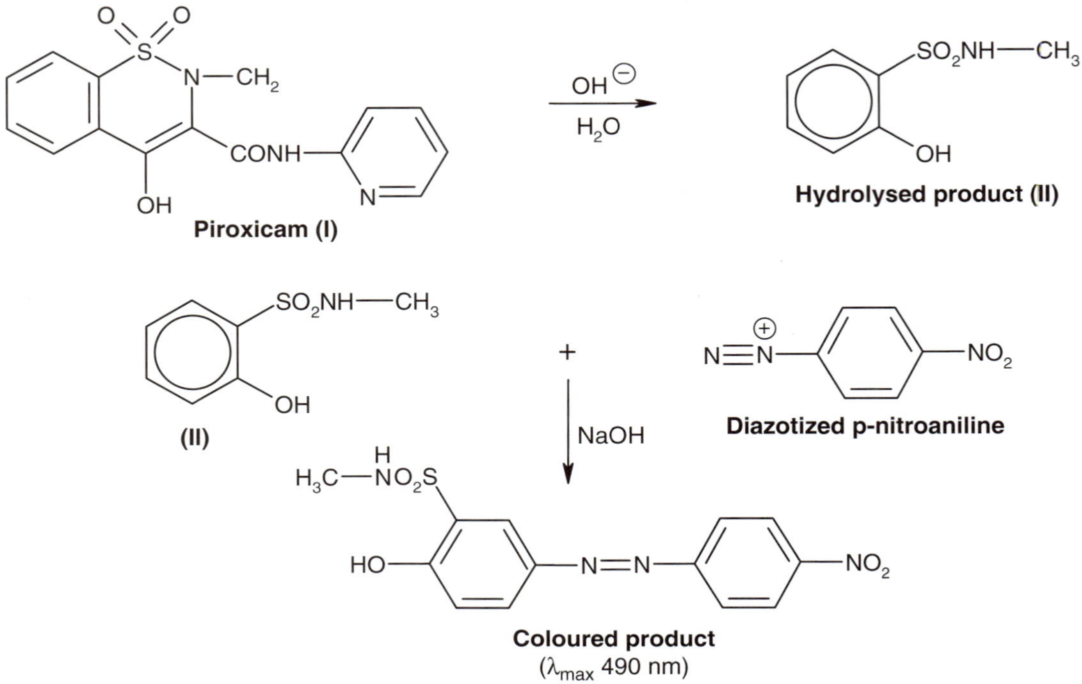

Reference

K.P.R. Chowdhary & A.S.R. Murthy, *Indian Drugs*, **26(2)**, 89, Nov. 1988.

(c)

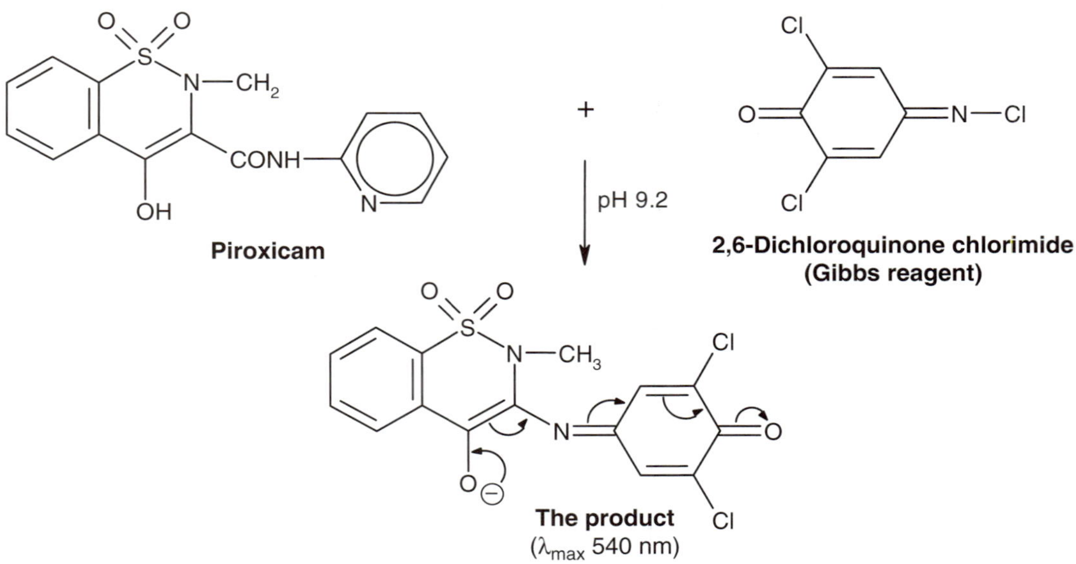

Reference

J. Emmanuel & S.D. Haldankar, *Indian Drugs*, **26(6)**, 320, March 1989.

(d)

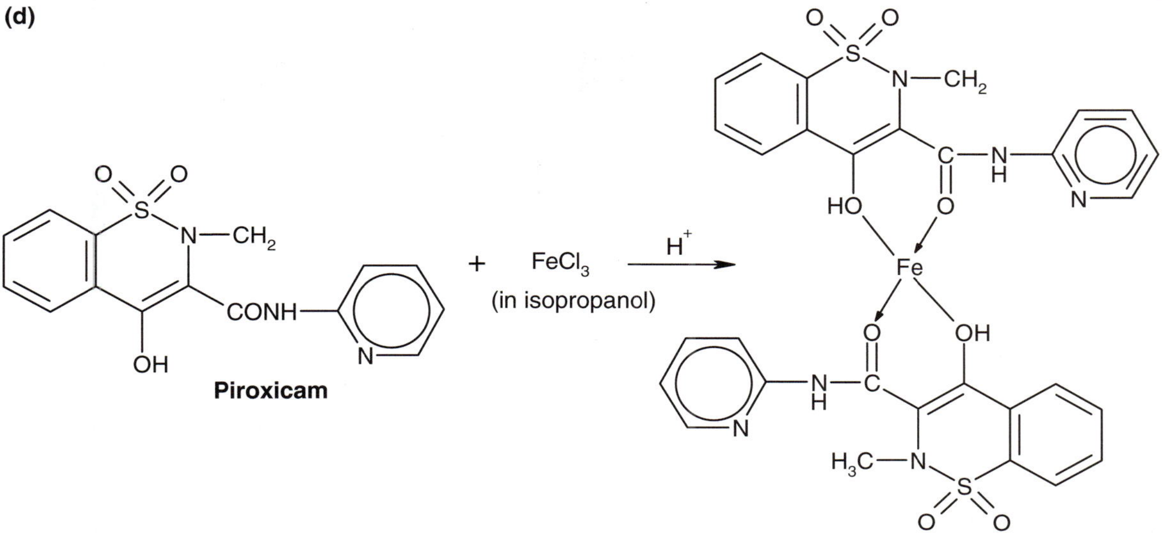

Piroxicam - Fe(III) chelate
(λ_{max} 530 nm)

Reference

D.M. Shingbal & Sangita Sarjyotishi, *Indian Drugs*, **25(12)**, 531-532, 1988.

(e)

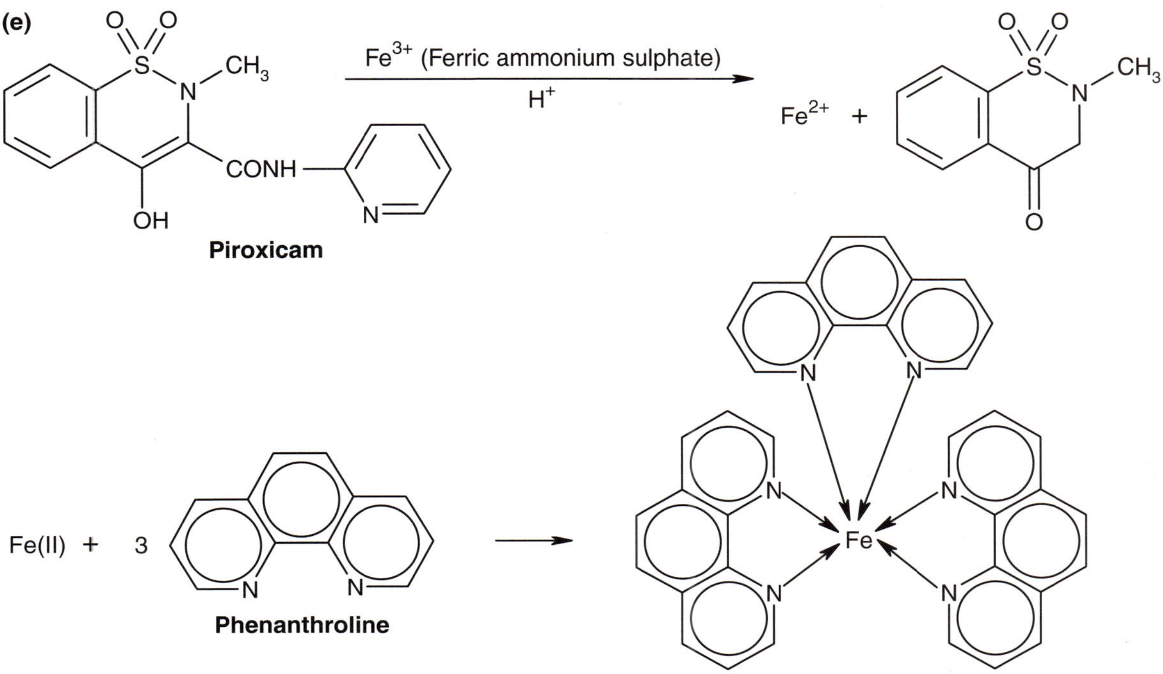

Fe - phenanthroline complex
(λ_{max} 510 nm)

(f)

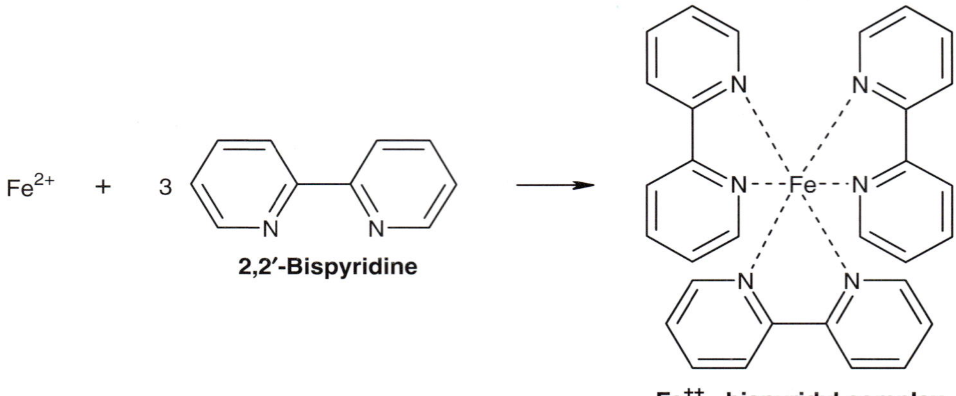

Fe^{++} - bispyridyl complex
(λ_{max} 522 nm)

Compound is also reported to form coloured chelate with Co^{++} and Cu^{++}. The chromopohore can be extracted into chloroform for spectrophotometric analysis: Cu^{++} chelate (378 nm) and Co^{++} chelate (495 nm). The following structure of the chelate was proposed by the authors.

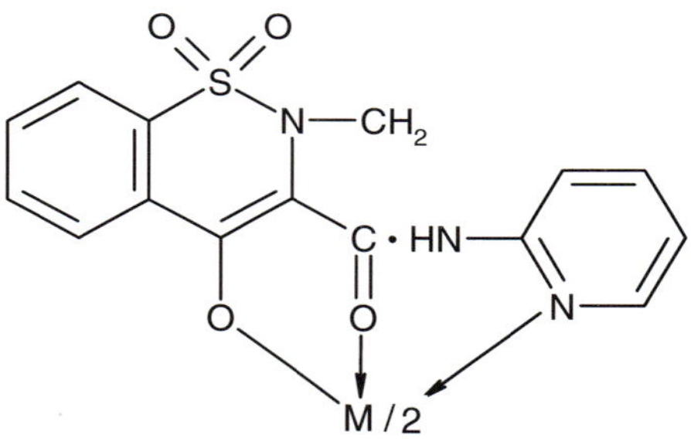

Metal - drug chelate

Reference

Y. Kumar, S.K. Talwar, Y.K.S. Rathor, P.D. Sethi & C.L. Jain, *Indian Drugs*, **28(3)**, 139-141, 1991.

Capsaicin

Follow the method described in formulation 2 of this chapter.

Methylsalicylate

Follow the method described in formulation 3 of this chapter.

Menthol

Follow the method described in formulation 1 of this chapter.

Reaction Mechanism

17

Keratolytics and Cleansers

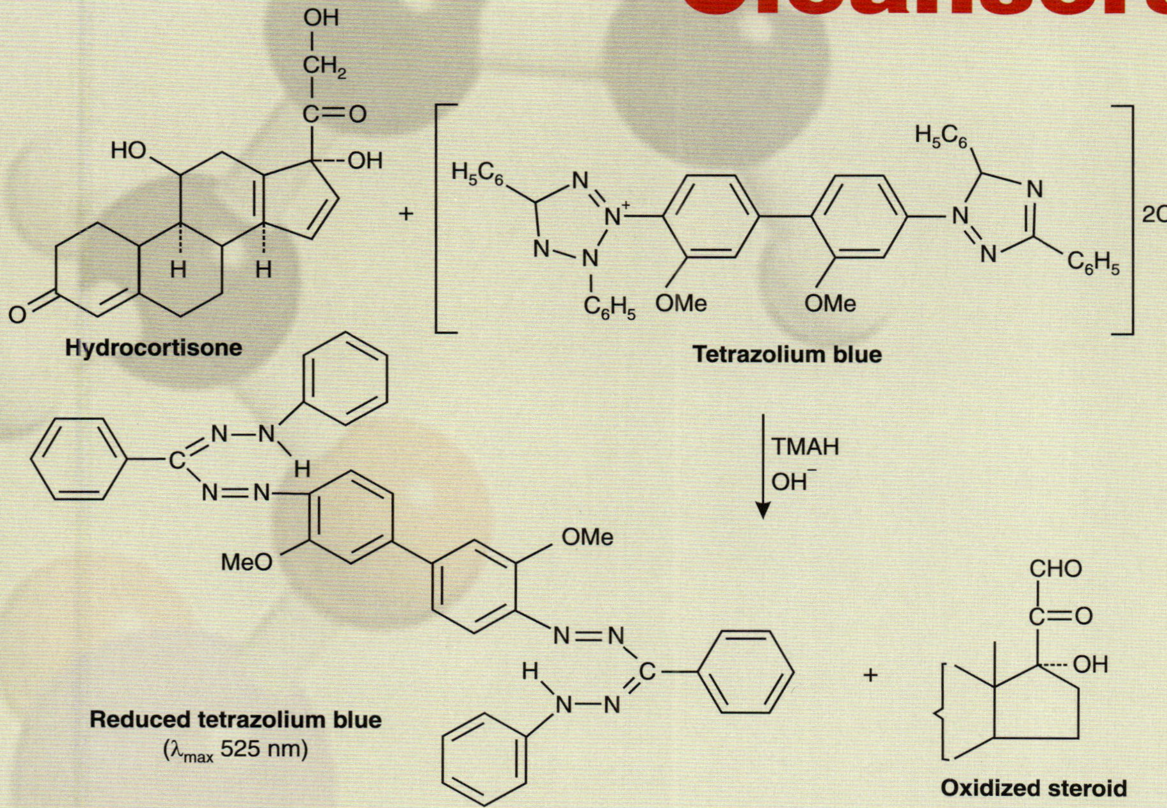

Formulation 1

Resorcinol (Resorcin), Sulphur, Alcohol base

ESTIMATION

Resorcinol

METHOD 1

Reagents

1. 0.1 N hydrochloric acid.
2. Chloroform.

Standard solution

25 mcg/ml resorcinol in 0.1 N hydrochloric acid.

Sample solution

Weigh into a stoppered conical flask sample equivalent to 10 mg of resorcinol and add 100 ml of chloroform. Add 50 ml of 0.1 N hydrochloric acid to the above flask. Shake the mixture thoroughly for at least one minute. After the sample is well shaken, decant the acid layer and filter. Transfer 5 ml of the clear filtrate to a 50 ml volumetric flask and dilute to volume with 0.1 N hydrochloric acid.

Procedure

Determine the extinction of the standard and sample solutions at about 273 nm using 0.1 N hydrochloric acid as reference solvent and calculate the results by comparison.

METHOD 2

The method is based on the formation of indophenol by reacting resorcinol with 2,6-dibromoquinone-4-chlorimide in alkaline medium (Gibbs reagent).

Reagents

1. 1% w/v sodium borate solution in water, prepare daily.
2. Borate buffer, pH 9.4.
3. 2,6-dibromoquinone-4-chlorimide solution: This solution is prepared daily by dissolving 40 mcg/ml of chlorimide in 10 ml of methanol.

Standard solution

10 mcg/ml of resorcinol in water, prepare weekly.

Sample solution

The sample equivalent to 25 mg of resorcinol is accurately weighed and dissolved in water to produce 25 ml and filtered. 1 ml of this solution is further diluted with water to produce 100 ml.

Procedure

To 2.5 ml each of the standard and sample solutions add 2 ml of borate buffer and dilute to 10 ml with water. Then add 0.1 ml of chlorimide solution, mix and measure the absorbance after 50 seconds but before 100 seconds at 530 nm against a reagent blank.

Note

1. Full resorcinol colour develops in about 50 seconds and after that phenol and salicylic acid begin to react with the chlorimide reagent and will cause positive interference after 120 seconds as with compounds having one phenolic group the reaction is delayed and this will not interfere if the colour is measured well within 120 seconds.
2. The method obeys Beer's law in the concentration range of 20-25 mcg/ml.
3. Boric acid, phenol and salicylic acid do not interfere in the proposed method.

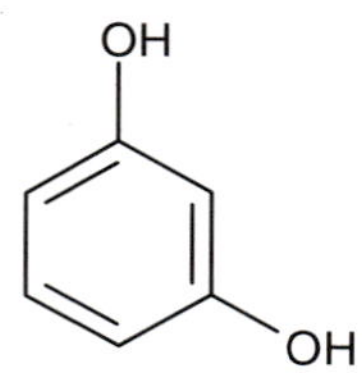

Resorcinol

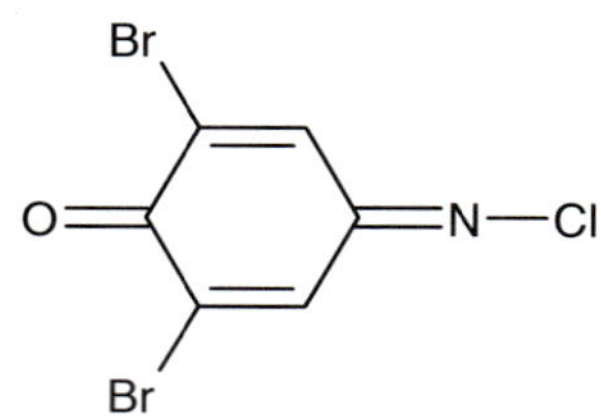

2,6-Dibromoquinone-4-chlorimide

Probable Reaction Mechanism

Here, in the presence of water, 2,6-dibromoquinone-4-chlorimide is hydrolysed into 2,6-dibromoquinonimine.

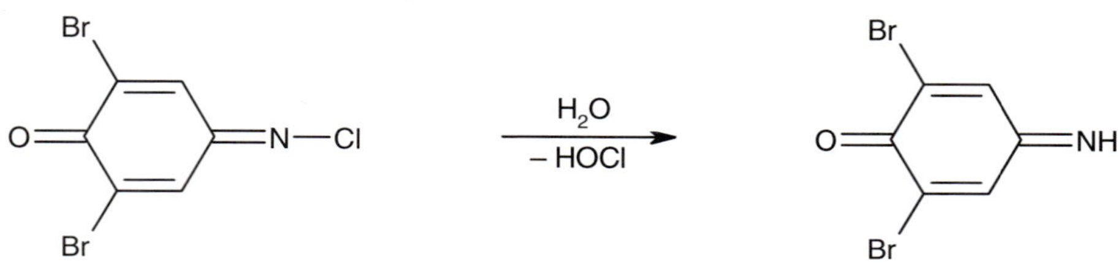

2,6-Dibromoquinone-4-chlorimide **2,6-Dibromoquinonimine**

Further reaction involves oxidative coupling at the para position to the phenolic hydroxyl group in the drug in which the quinonimine formed acts as the oxidizing agent. The pH for the reaction is maintained using borate buffer.

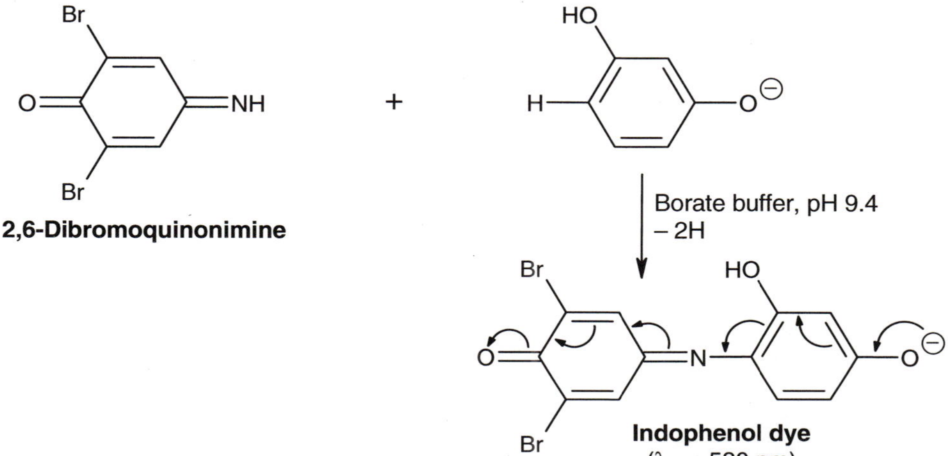

2,6-Dibromoquinonimine

Indophenol dye
(λ_{max} 530 nm)

Reference

1. V.D. Gupta & L.A. Cates, *J. Pharm. Sci.*, **63(1)**, 93, 1974.
2. V. Das Gupta, *J. Pharm. Sci.*, **65(1)**, 144-145, 1976.
3. H.D. Gibbs, *J. Biol. Chem.*, **72**, 649, 1927.

Resorcinol reacts with 'MBTH' reagent in the presence of an oxidizing agent $K_3[Fe(CN)_6]$. The reaction is possible both in acidic and alkaline medium.

First, 'MBTH' loses two electrons and one proton to give cation. The cation (II) attacks the phenol in an electrophilic substitution reaction and subsequent oxidation giving a red-coloured product.

Probable Reaction Mechanism

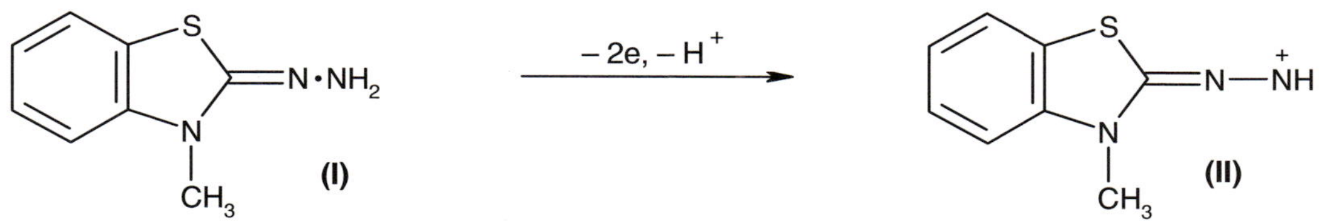

3-Methylbenzthiazolin-2-one hydrazone (MBTH) **Cation**

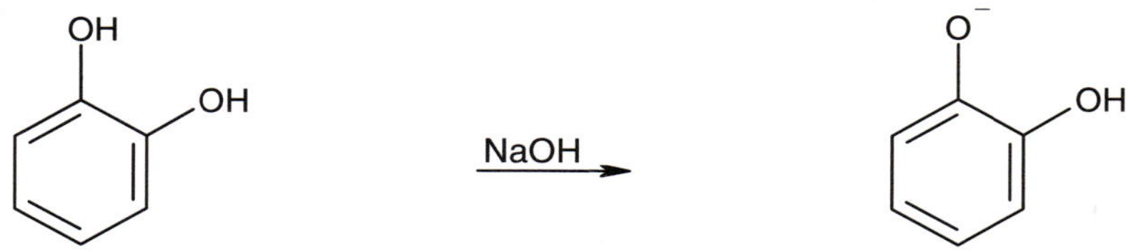

Resorcinol (III) **Phenolate (IV)**

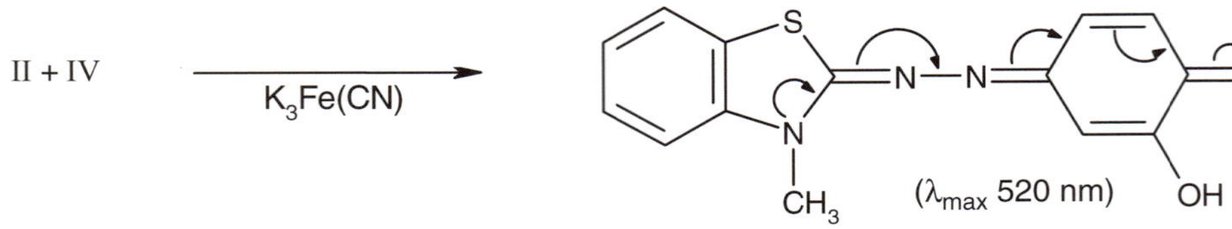

Note

Ceric (IV) ammonium sulphate can also be used as oxidizing agent.

METHOD 3

Reagents

1. 0.1 M sodium hydroxide.
2. 5% disodium tartrate in water.
3. 2% w/v solution of Cu(2) chloride in water.

Procedure

To 1 ml each of sample/standard solution (1 mg/ml), add 1 ml each of solutions (2) and (3), dilute to 20 ml with 0.1 M sodium hydroxide and measure the absorbance of green colour at 660 nm.

Note

Disodium tartrate is added to avoid turbidity formed due to addition of sodium hydroxide $Cu(OH)_2$.

Reference

Indian Drugs, **26(6)**, 306, March 1989.

Probably formation of chelate occurs with the use of $CuCl_2$ as reagent. The structure of the chelate is as shown below.

Probable Reaction Mechanism

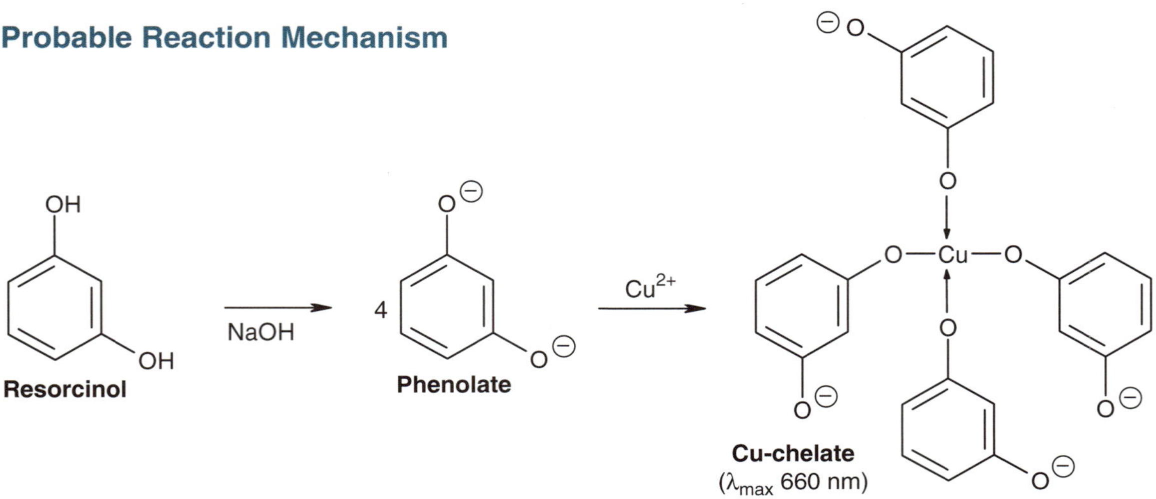

Sane et al. have reported that resorcinol couples with pyrocatechol to give pink to violet-red coloured complex in alkaline medium.

Probable Reaction Mechanism

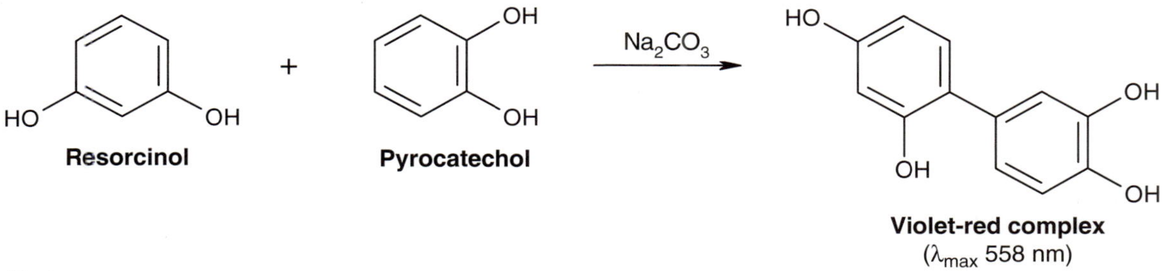

Note

Method is applicable for lotions, creams and ointments.

Reference

R.T. Sane, *J. Ind. Chem. Soc.*, **LX**, 381-382, April 1983.

The identification test as described for thymol based on "Guareschi-Lustgarten reaction" is answered by resorcinol and can be used for quantitative analysis i.e. when the substance is warmed with sodium hydroxide in the presence of chloroform it produces red colour turning to yellow on the addition of acetic acid.

Probable Reaction Mechanism

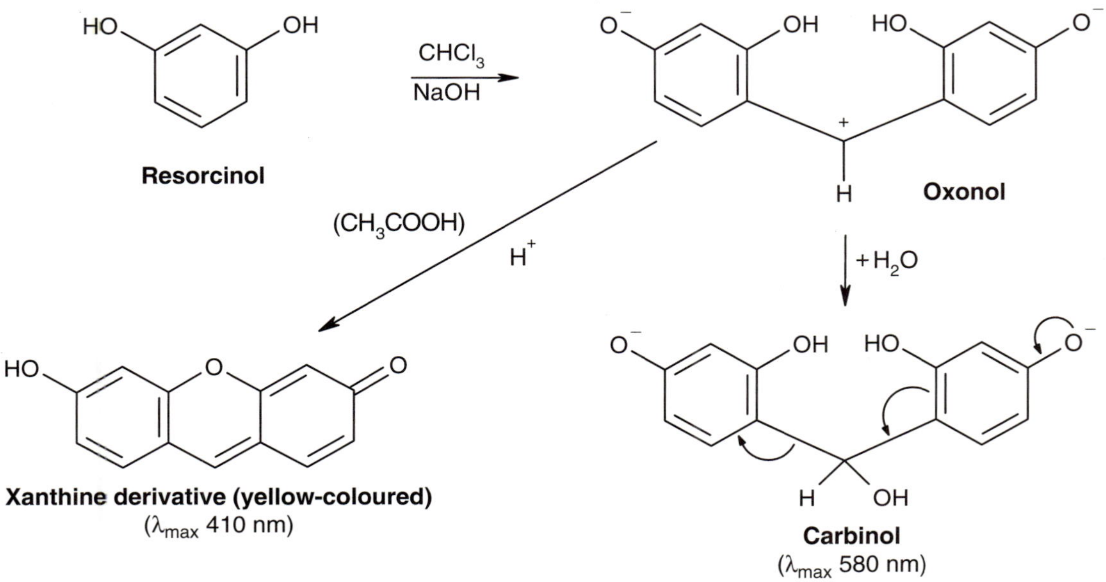

Resorcinol also forms violet colour with $FeCl_3$ similar to phenols. The composition of the complex is pH dependent which may correspond to the formulae $[Fe(OR)_6]^{-3}$. Gupta et al. have reported that reaction with ferric chloride is based on oxidation-reduction leading to formation of quinone.

Probable Reaction Mechanism

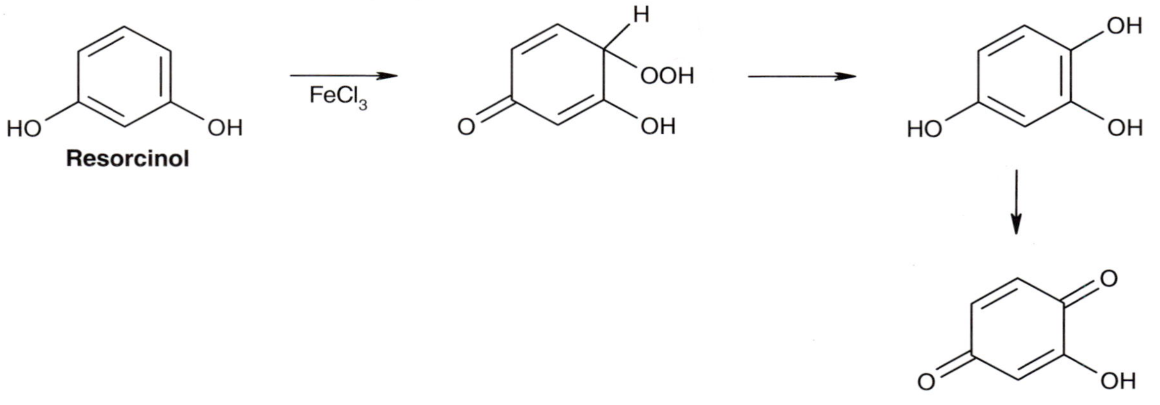

Violet-coloured quinone
(λ_{max} 442 nm)

Reference

1. Pharmaceutical Chemistry (Vol. 2) by H.J. Roth, pp. 72 and 83.
2. V. Das Gupta & K.A. Bomer, *J. Pharm. Sci.*, **64(7)**, 1199-1200, 1975.

Resorcinol when treated with potassium hydrogen phthalate gives yellow-coloured compound which gives intense green fluorescence on addition of potassium hydroxide.

Resorcinol forms dinitroso derivative with nitrous acid to give yellow-coloured product which is of analytical interest.

Probable Reaction Mechanism

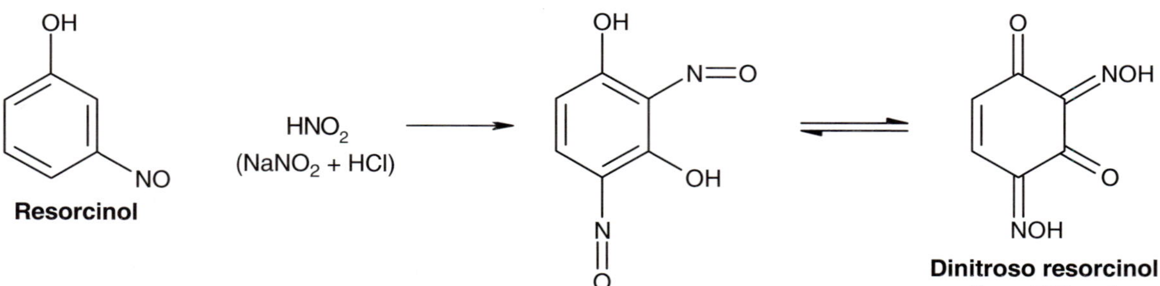

Dinitroso resorcinol
(λ_{max} 390 nm)

Note

Resorcinol reduces silver nitrate and Fehling solution on warming which can be exploited for analytical method development.

Reference

Organic Chemistry (Vol. 1) by I.L. Finar, 1973, p. 715.

The compound undergoes nitration to give 2,4,6-trinitro resorcinol.

Probable Reaction Mechanism

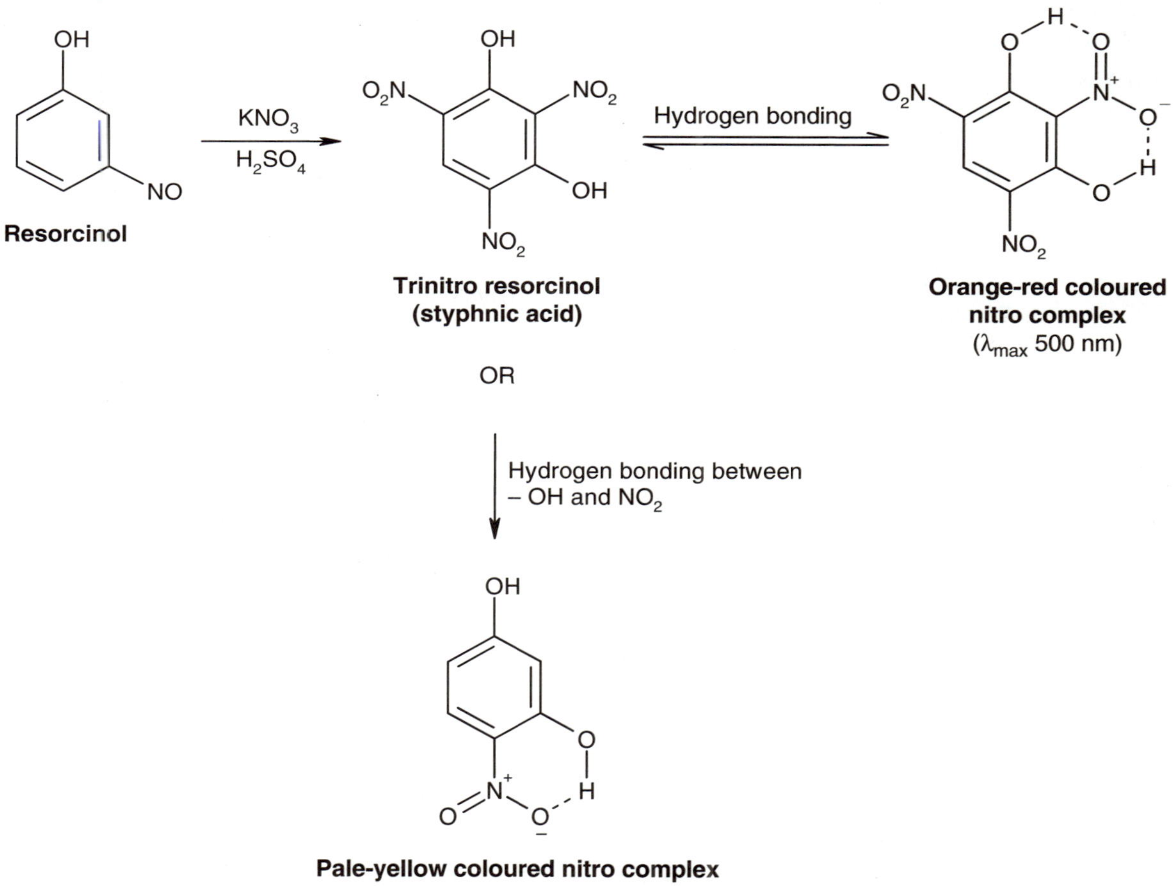

Reference

Pharmaceutical Chemistry (Vol. 2) by H.J. Roth, p. 70.

Bromometric method can be used for analytical purpose. Normally, tribromo derivative is formed.

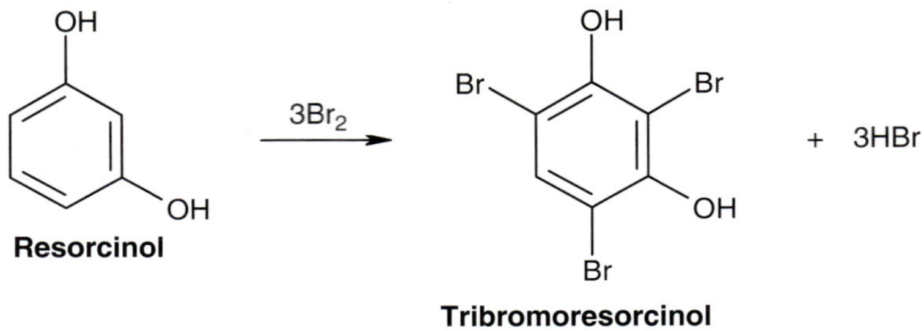

Resorcinol on treatment with tartaric acid and conc. sulphuric acid gives violet-red-coloured compound.

First, tartaric acid as a result of dehydration and oxidation yields glyoxylic acid which condenses with 2 moles of resorcinol to give oxonium coloured salt.

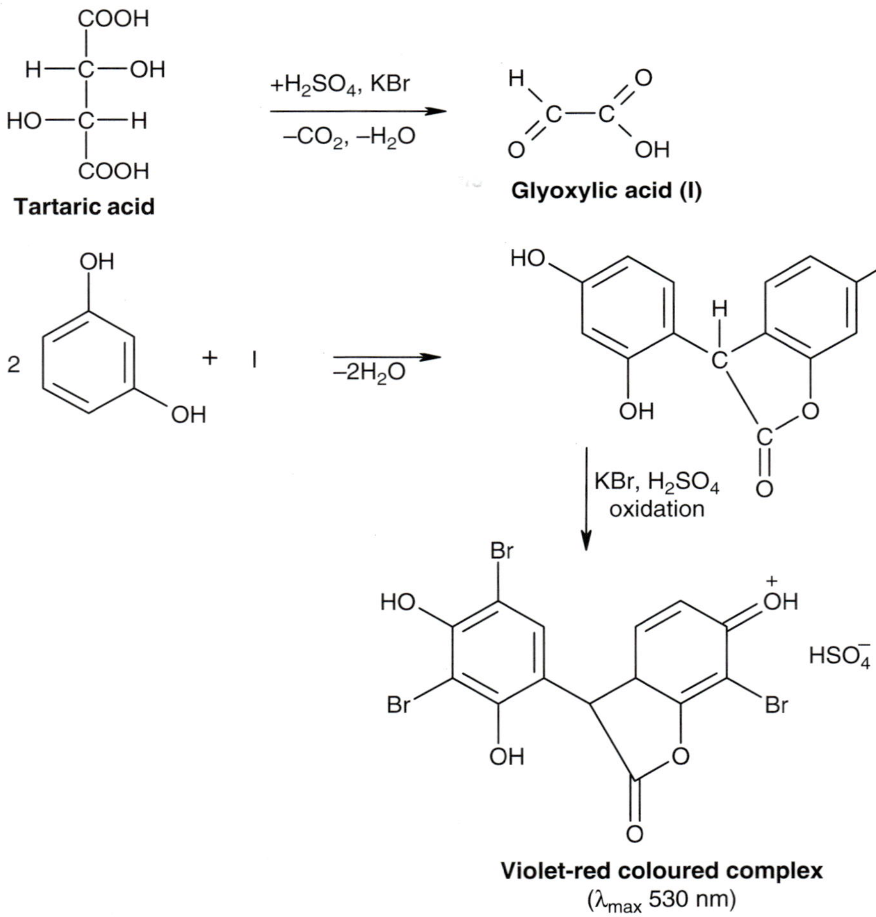

Reference

Pharmaceutical Chemistry (Vol. 2) by H.J. Roth, p. 163.

For resorcinol, a dihydric phenol, a titrimetric method using sodium methoxide in DMF medium and brilliant orange as indicator was described by the authors. The compound quantitatively consumes one mole of methoxide per mole. The authors have established that in compound with two —OH groups in the same benzene ring such as catechol/resorcinol, one of the two hydroxyl groups is active and the other is too weak to be titrated quantitatively with titrant in DMF medium as there is marked difference in their ionization i.e. one —OH group is 10^4 times more acidic than the other.

Reference

S.S.M. Hassan & M.T.M. Zaki, *Talanta*, **22**, 843-847, 1975.

Sulphur

Reagents

1. 5% w/v sodium sulfite solution, freshly prepared.
2. Formaldehyde solution.
3. 0.1 N iodine solution.
4. Silicone oil, defoamer.

Procedure

Weigh and transfer sample equivalent to approximately 50 mg of sulphur into a 250 ml round bottom flask. Add 40 ml solution of sodium sulphite, small piece of paraffin and few drops of silicone oil, defoamer. Stopper the flask and shake well to disperse the sample. Remove the stopper, rinse with several small portions of distilled water. Attach the flask to a reflux condenser and reflux until the sulphur is completely dissolved. Cool the solution and rinse inside of condenser with a small quantity of water. Add 10 ml of formaldehyde solution and 6 ml of glacial acetic acid. Titrate the solution immediately with freshly standardized 0.1 N iodine solution using starch solution as the indicator. Prepare blank in the same manner using all ingredients except sample. Each ml of 0.1 iodine is equivalent to 0.003207 g of sulphur.

Alcohol

Transfer appropriate volume of the sample into 500 ml round bottom flask. Add about 200 ml of distilled water and shake well. Attach to a condenser and distil slowly. Collect distillate in a 100 ml volumetric flask, collecting slightly less than 100 ml. Bring distillate to a temperature of 25°C and dilute to volume with distilled water. Determine the specific gravity at 25°C and calculate per cent alcohol by weight or in terms of % v/v by referring to alcohol table.

Formulation 2

Buclosamide, Hydrocortisone acetate, Salicylic acid

ESTIMATION

Chlorohydroxybenzoic acid butylamide (Buclosamide)

Reagents

1. 5% w/v solution of sodium bicarbonate in water.
2. 1 N sodium hydroxide.

Procedure

Ointment is extracted with methanol in the centrifuge, using 25 ml at a time. The ointment is brought into contact with the alcohol in the centrifuge tube, by cautious warming on the steam-bath while stirring, and subsequently resolidifying in ice-water. The combined alcoholic extract is made up to 100 ml with alcohol (use appropriate volume for estimation of hydrocortisone acetate). 20 ml of the alcoholic extract is cautiously dried on the steam-bath at low temperature. The residue is transferred into a separating funnel, using 50 ml of ether and is shaken with five 20 ml portions of sodium bicarbonate solution. The combined aqueous extract is made up to 100 ml with sodium bicarbonate solution and retained for assay of salicylic acid. The ethereal layer remaining in the separating funnel is extracted with five 20 ml portions of 1 N sodium hydroxide solution. The alkaline extracts are combined and made up to 100 ml with 1 N sodium hydroxide solution. 20 ml is further diluted to 100 ml with water.

Maximum absorption of alkaline solution is observed at 325 nm which is characteristic of chlorohydroxybenzoic acid butylamide. Results are calculated by comparing with the standard.

Explanatory Note

Because of the free carboxylic (—COOH group) salicylic acid gets extracted into sodium bicarbonate layer whereas the buclosamide remains in ether layer. On extracting the organic layer with strong alkali (sodium hydroxide) the amide is passed on to aqueous layer.

Buclosamide answers typical reactions of phenols, i.e., it gives red colour with Millon's reagent. The compound due to presence of phenolic function forms nitroso derivative as explained below.

Probable Reaction Mechanism

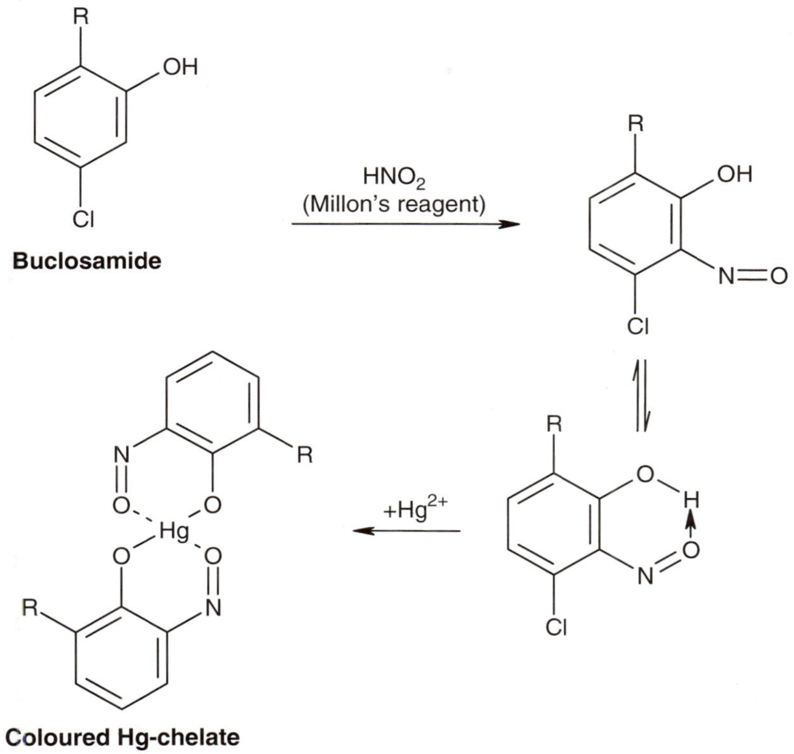

On treatment with alkali/acid the substance is hydrolysed giving butylamine and chlorohydroxy benzoic acid which gives colour with $FeCl_3$.

Probable Reaction Mechanism

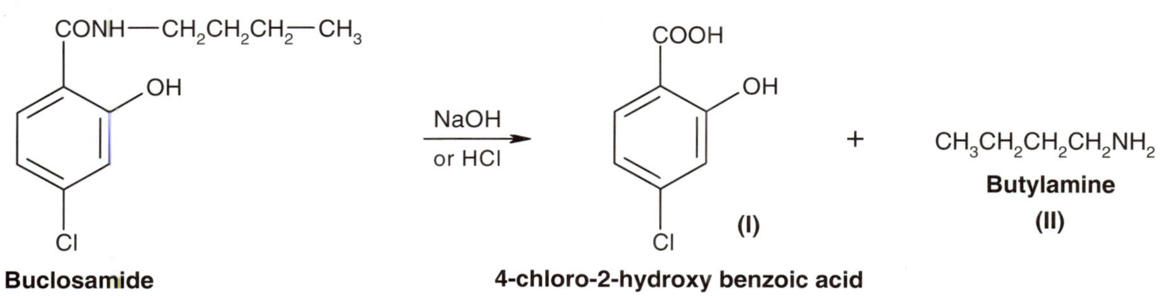

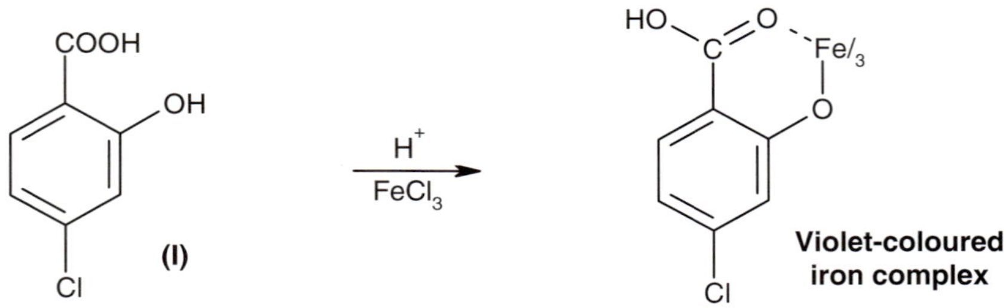

Butylamine liberated as a result of hydrolysis can form the basis for quantitative estimation by reacting with fluoroscamine giving intensely fluorescent pyrolidone derivative.

Probable Reaction Mechanism

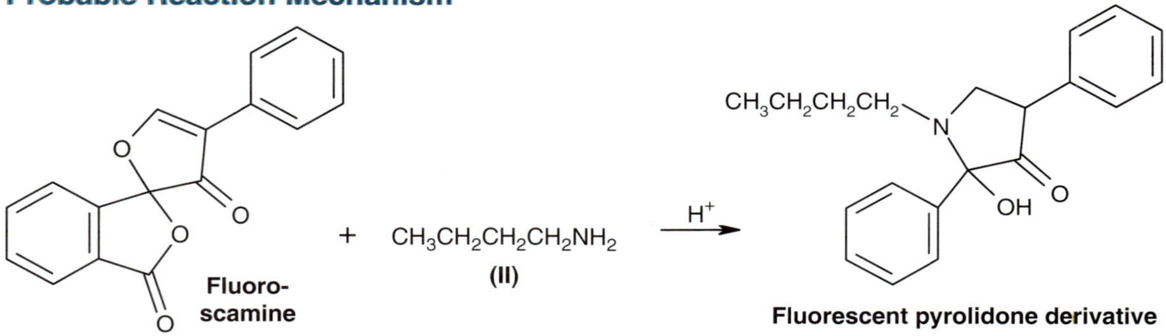

Butylamine, being primary aliphatic amine, will answer other general reactions such as reaction with ninhydrin, nitrous acid, 1,2-naphthoquinone-4-sulphonate sodium, etc. forming Schiff's base with PDAB. Mostly Schiff's bases with primary aliphatic amines are yellow in colour. These reactions of amine moiety can form the basis of quantitative estimation of the compound.

Probable Reaction Mechanism

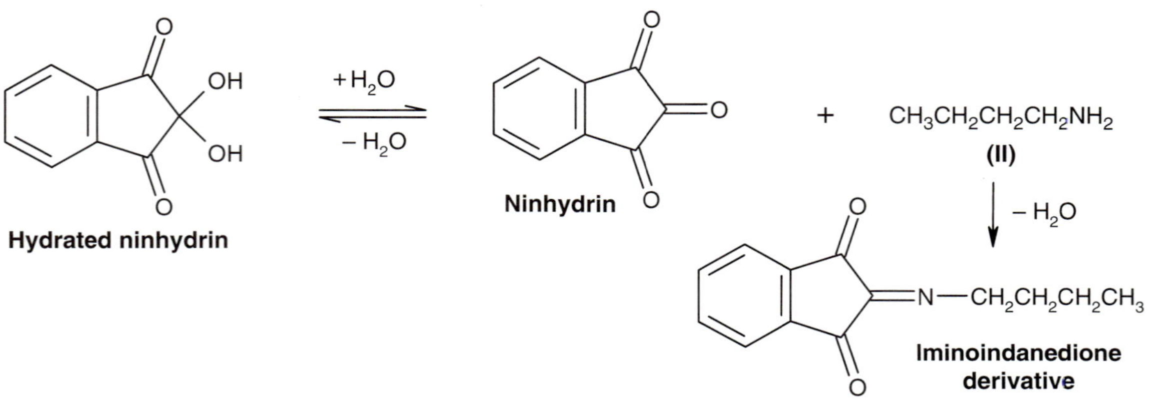

Another reported reaction with benzoquinone can be exploited for estimation.

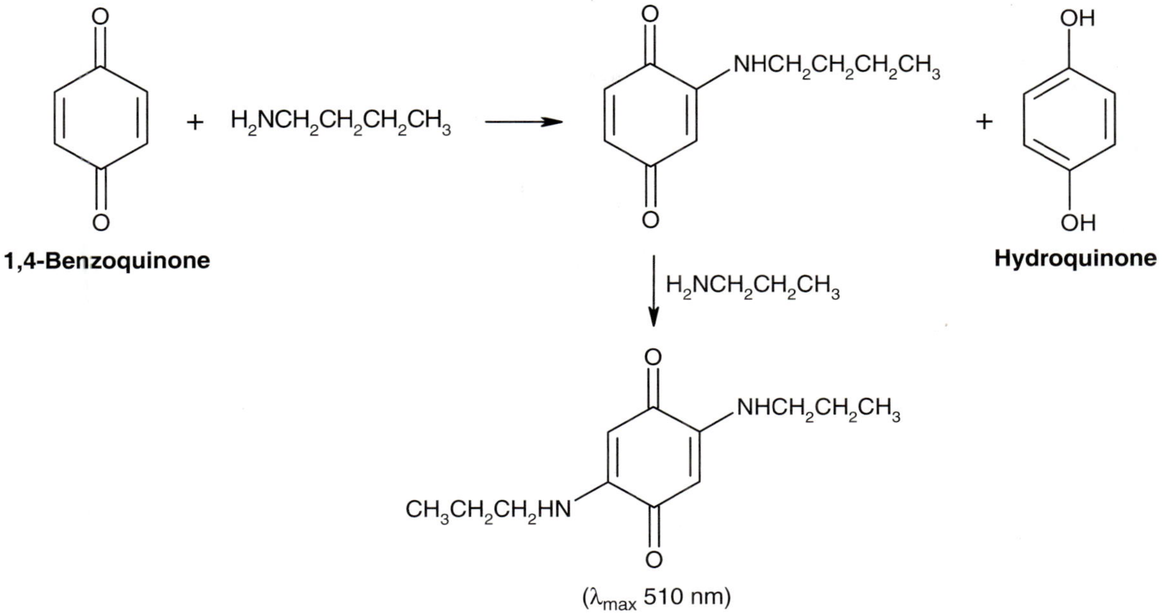

Note

Tertiary amines, ammonia, amide, imide, analides, hydrazines do not interfere.

Reference

Saad S.M. Hassan, M.L. Iskander & N.E. Nashed, *Talanta*, **32(4)**, 301-305, 1985.

Salicylic acid

10 ml of sodium bicarbonate extract obtained during estimation of buclosamide is made up to 100 ml with water. This solution exhibits maximum absorption at 295 nm which is characteristic for salicylic acid in sodium bicarbonate solution. Salicylic acid contents can be determined by comparison with standard solution of salicylic acid.

Hydrocortisone acetate

Reagents

1. 0.5% w/v solution of tetrazolium blue (TZB) in alcohol.
2. Tetramethylammonium hydroxide (TMAH)-alcohol (1 : 9) mixture.

Standard solution

Weigh accurately 10 mg of hydrocortisone acetate in a dry 100 ml volumetric flask, dissolve in methanol and make to 100 ml with methanol.

Sample solution

25 ml of alcoholic solution obtained in assay of buclosamide is passed through aluminium oxide (6 g) column. Collect the eluate in a dry 25 ml volumetric flask for estimation.

Procedure

To 2 ml each of sample and standard solutions, add 2 ml of tetrazolium blue solution and mix. Then to each flask, add 2 ml of tetramethyl ammonium hydroxide-alcohol mixture, mix and allow to stand in the dark for 90 minutes. Without delay, make up the volume with methanol and measure the absorbance of the assay and standard solutions at about 525 nm against the blank. Calculate the results by comparison.

Probable Reaction Mechanism

Hydrocortisone, a steroid with α,β-unsaturated carbonyl function and α-ketol group at C-17 is oxidized by TZB to aldehyde whereas TZB undergoes reductive opening of heterocyclic ring to give coloured formazone (λ_{max} 525 nm) forming the basis of above colorimetric method.

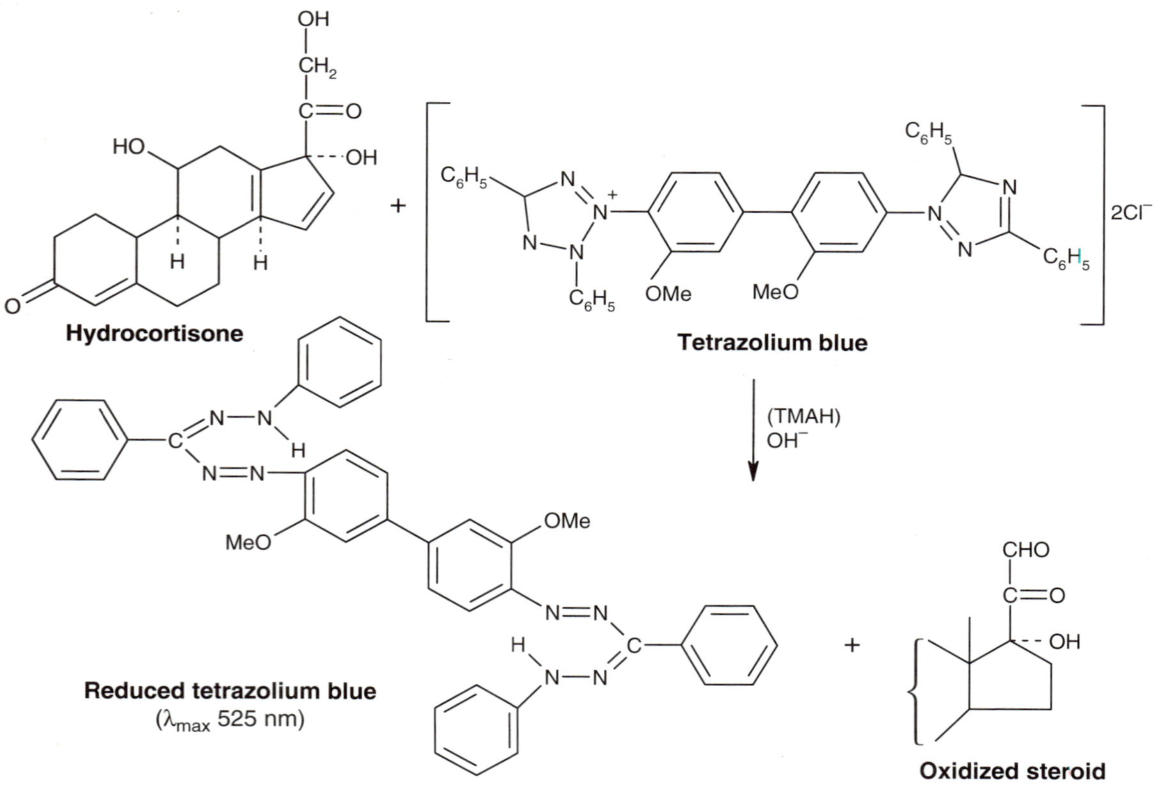

Salicylic acid and Benzoic acid

Suspend 5 ml of the sample in 100 ml of ether and extract the ethereal layer with four 20 ml portions of 0.5 N sodium hydroxide. Combine the alkaline extract and shake with 10 ml of ether, make up the volume to 100 ml. Carry out the subsequent dilutions with 0.5 N sodium hydroxide to get a solution of 20 mcg/ml in respect of salicylic acid. Carry out the quantitative determination by iso-absorption method as described in formulation 5 of this chapter.

Formulation 5

Salicylic acid, Benzoic acid, Menthol, Thymol, Camphor, Dusting powder base

ESTIMATION

METHOD 1

Salicylic acid (SA) and Benzoic acid (BA)

1. 1 g of the sample accurately weighed is extracted with three 10 ml portions of isopropyl alcohol at 90°C and cooled. Combined organic extract is extracted with four 10 ml portions of 1 N sodium hydroxide and combined alkaline extract is diluted with water to get a concentration of 20 mcg/ml of salicylic acid. Measure the extinction at 298 nm which corresponds only to salicylic acid.
2. Calculate total acids (BA and SA) by the UV spectrophotometric method described in method 4 of this formulation. By subtracting the contents of salicylic acid obtained by the method 1 above, we can find out the contents of benzoic acid in the sample under analysis.

Total acids

Accurately weigh the sample, add 30 ml of 50% v/v neutral alcohol, warm gently to melt the ointment base and titrate when still warm with 0.1 N sodium hydroxide using phenolphthalein solution as indicator. After determining the end point, add 2 to 3 ml of the 0.1 N sodium hydroxide and reserve this solution for the determination of salicylic acid.

Calculations

$$\text{Volume of 0.1 N sodium hydroxide used in titration } (V) = \frac{\text{Titre value} \times \text{Normality of sodium hydroxide}}{0.1}$$

ml of 0.1 N sodium hydroxide equivalent to total acid in 1 g of the sample = V/a where a is weight (g) of the sample taken for analysis.

Salicylic acid

Cool and filter the titrated solution obtained in the assay for total acids through Whatman filter paper No. 1. Wash the filter paper with several small portions of water and add washing to the main filtrate. Collect the filtrate in a 150 ml beaker and evaporate the filtrate in order to completely remove alcohol present in the solution. Transfer this solution to a 250 volumetric flask with the aid of small portion of water and make up the volume. Transfer 50 ml of this solution to an iodine flask and exactly add 25 ml of 0.1 N bromine solution, 5 ml of hydrochloric acid and immediately insert the stopper. Shake the flask for 30 minutes, add quickly 5 ml of potassium iodide solution (1 in 5). Shake thoroughly, remove the stopper and rinse it and the neck of the flask with little water, so that the washings flow into the flask. Add 1 ml of chloroform, shake the mixture well and titrate the liberated iodine with 0.1 N sodium thiosulphate using solution of starch as indicator, to be added when the end point is almost near. Run a blank side by side.

Note

Bromination of salicylic acid proceeds extremely rapidly. Due to blocked phenolic function, the aromatic in aspirin is insufficiently reactive for electrophilic attack by bromine. Aspirin also does not form complex with ferric chloride for these reasons.

Calculations

1. Salicylic acid (mg)/g of the sample (B) $= \dfrac{(A-a)\times 2.3\times 250}{w\times 50}$

   where A = ml of 0.1 N bromine added; a = ml of 0.1 N sodium thiosulphate required to titrate the excess bromine; w = weight (g) of the sample taken for analysis.
2. Benzoic acid : Volume (ml) of 0.1 N sodium hydroxide equivalent to the salicylic acid present in 1 g of the sample (v) = $B/13.81$
   where B = mg of salicylic acid present in 1 g of the sample found by the method for salicylic acid.
   Volume (ml) of 0.1 N sodium hydroxide equivalent to benzoic acid present in 1 g of sample (C) = ($V - v$); where V is the volume (ml) of 0.1 N sodium hydroxide equivalent to total acids.

METHOD 2

(a) Weigh accurately the sample equivalent to 25 mg of salicylic acid and add 100 ml of hot water (75°C) and 2 drops of phenolphthalein solution. Then, add enough 0.1 N sodium hydroxide so that the mixture is light pink. Heat to 85°C and add more sodium hydroxide to get clear pink colour. Cool the solution and dilute to 250 ml with distilled water. Filter, reject first few ml of the filtrate. Take 15 ml of this solution, add 5 ml of ferric nitrate solution (0.1% in 1%

nitric acid) and dilute to 50 ml and read the pink colour at 525 nm. Compare with the standard solution processed by the above method. This method gives the amount of salicylic acid (% w/v) present in the sample.

(b) Suspend the sample accurately weighed in 200 ml of alcohol and estimate the total acid (salicylic acid and benzoic acid) as per method given under total acids. Subtract the volume of 0.1 N sodium hydroxide equivalent to the amount of salicylic acid to calculate the contents of benzoic acid as per method given above.

METHOD 3

In this method, iso-absorption point for the two compounds is determined using standard solutions of salicylic acid (40 mcg/ml) and benzoic acid (40 mcg/ml) in 0.5 N sodium hydroxide. Record the UV spectra of both the standard solutions separately on the same graph to get iso-absorption point and maxima for salicylic acid.

Iso-absorption point = 267 nm
Absorption maxima for salicylic acid = 299 nm

	Absorption value at		
	299 nm	267 nm	Ratio 299/267
Salicylic acid (40 mcg/ml)	0.930	0.190	4.94 (Q_1)
Benzoic acid (40 mcg/ml)	0.00	0.190	0.00 (Q_2)
Standard mixture (40 mcg/ml of each acid)	0.940	0.380	2.47 (Q_M)

Absorptivity (g/lit) at 267 nm = 4.75 (A)

$$C_1 \text{ [amount (g) of salicylic acid/L]} = \frac{Q_M - Q_2}{Q_1 - Q_2} \times \frac{a}{A} \quad \ldots(1)$$

$$C_2 \text{ [amount (g) of benzoic acid/L]} = \frac{Q_M - Q_2}{Q_2 - Q_1} \times \frac{a}{A} \quad \ldots(2)$$

where a = absorption of the mixture at iso-absorption point, A = absorptivity.

Typical laboratory analysis

A formulation contains 7% w/w salicylic acid, 3% w/w benzoic acid, 5% boric acid and 0.5% w/w thymol.

Procedure

Take sample accurately weighed (0.71 g), add 20 ml of ether and suspend the contents by slight warming. Extract the ether layer with four 10 ml portions of 0.5 N sodium hydroxide. Shake the combined alkaline extract with 10 ml of ether, reject ether layer and adjust the alkaline layer to 50 ml. Dilute 2 ml of this solution to 50 ml with 0.5 N sodium hydroxide and read at 267 nm and 299 nm.

Absorption of the mixture at 267 nm = 0.27 ...(a)
Absorption of the mixture at 299 nm = 0.92

$$\text{Value for } Q_M = \frac{0.92}{0.27} = 3.40$$

Substitute the standard values and the values obtained for the sample in analogous equations, 1 and 2 described above.

$Q_1 = 4.92$
$Q_2 = 0.00$
$Q_M = 3.40$
Absorptivity (A) = 4.75

$$\text{Amount of salicylic acid (g \%)} = \frac{Q_M - Q_2}{Q_1 - Q_2} \times \frac{a}{A}$$

$$= 0.0394 \text{ g/L}$$

$$= \frac{0.0394 \times 50 \times 50}{0.71 \times 2 \times 10} = 7.2\% \text{ w/w}$$

$$\text{Claim} = 7.0\% \text{ w/w}$$

$$\text{Amount of benzoic acid (g \%)} = \frac{Q_M - Q_2}{Q_2 - Q_1} \times \frac{a}{A}$$

$$= \frac{4.92 - 3.40}{0.00 - 4.92} \times \frac{0.27}{4.75}$$

= 1.5 3.92 0.27 4.75 = 0.0176 g/L
= 0.0176 50 50 0.71 2 10 = 3.0% w/w
Claim = 3.0% w/w

METHOD 4

Total acids (BA and SA)

This iso-absorption method can be applied efficiently for determination of total acids. By taking the values obtained for Q_M in the above formulation, the total acids can easily be calculated.

$$\text{Total acids (g/L)} = \frac{a}{A} = \frac{0.27}{4.75}$$

$$= 0.057 \text{ g/L}$$

$$\text{Total acids (g \%)} = \frac{0.057 \times 50 \times 50}{0.71 \times 2 \times 10}$$

$$= 10.2\% \text{ w/w}$$

Claim for total acid = 10% w/w (7% + 3%)

Total volatile contents

Weigh the sample accurately and follow the method 1 or 2 as described under formulation 4 of chapter on rubefacient.

Thymol

Follow the method 1 for determination of thymol as described under formulation of the chapter on rubefacients.

Menthol

Follow the method described in formulation of the chapter on rubefacients.

Note

Carry out the distillation of volatile material as described in formulation 4 of the chapter on rubefacients under method 1 for estimation of total volatile contents and use the distillate for estimation of menthol and thymol. Since salicylic acid and benzoic acid present in the formulation are volatile, the contents should be suspended in 1 N sodium hydroxide before subjecting to distillation.

ESTIMATION

Identification of Camphor

Two derivative formulations i.e. 2,4-dinitrophenylhydrazone and the oxime are the most suitable reactions for analytical purpose, the former being used commonly based on reaction with carbonyl (C=O) function of the molecule.

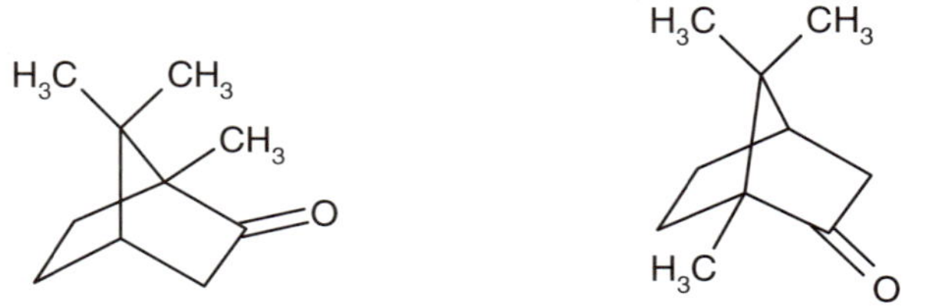

L-form **d-form**

Camphor

(a)

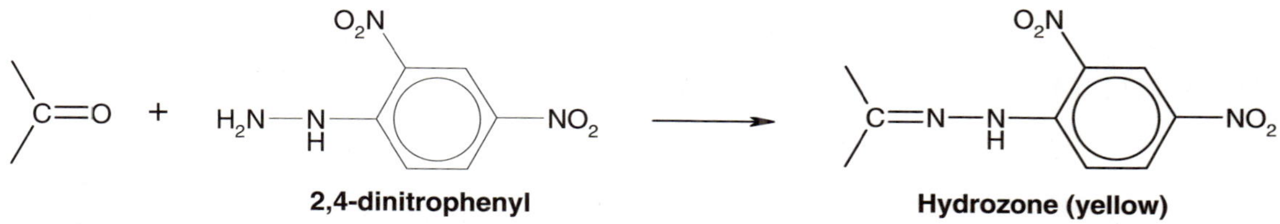

(b)

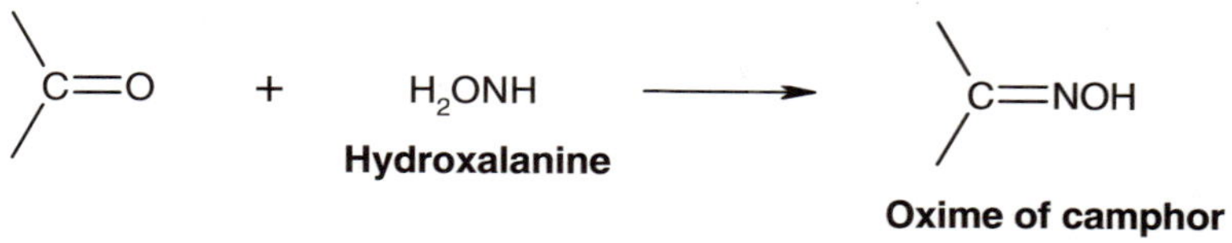

Note

Both oximes and phenylhydrazone are crystalline compounds and are used primarily for identification test; can be developed for quantitative work as well.

Other reagent used for hydrazone is phenylhydrazone. One can use semicarbazide to get semicarbazone.

Reference

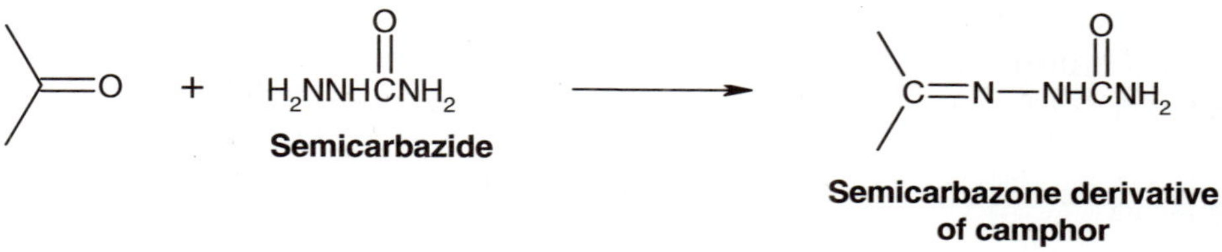

1. Organic Chemistry by Norman L. Allinger et al., Worth Publishers Inc., 1971, pp. 210, 482.
2. Pharmaceutical Chemistry (Vol. 2) by H.J. Roth, p. 135.

A UV spectrophotometric method of estimation has also been proposed (λ_{max} 289 nm—methanol).

Formulation 6

Salicylic acid, Benzoic acid, Boric acid, Soft paraffin base

ESTIMATION

METHOD 1

Benzoic acid and Salicylic acid

Procedure

Extract the sample with five 40 ml portions of ether (retain the residue for determination of boric acid). Evaporate the ether layer on water-bath at low temperature. Add about 20 ml of alcohol, while nearing complete evaporation and titrate the alcoholic extract with 0.1 N sodium hydroxide using phenolphthalein as indicator. Each ml of 0.1 N sodium hydroxide is equivalent to 0.01301 g of combined salicylic acid/benzoic acid (total acids).

Boric acid

The residue reserved for boric acid in the above method is suspended in 50 ml mixture of water-glycerin (1 : 1) by slight warming. The contents are titrated with 0.1 N sodium hydroxide using phenolphthalein as indicator. Each ml of sodium hydroxide is equivalent to 0.006183 g of boric acid. From the volume of 0.1 N sodium hydroxide consumed in the titration, the total amount of boric acid is calculated. Determine the contents of salicylic acid by bromination as described in the formulation 4 of this chapter. Deduct the amount of salicylic acid thus determined from the total acids to get the amount of benzoic acid in the formulation.

Note

For extraction, chloroform can be used.

Boric acid behaves as a very weak monobasic acid.

$$\underset{\text{Boric acid}}{H_3BO_3} \rightleftharpoons H^+ + \underset{\text{Metaborate ion}}{BO_2^-} + H_2O$$

The metaborate ion is strongly basic and forces the above reaction backward, thus titration with sodium hydroxide is not practicable. However, when glycerine is added, it forms a slightly dissociated complex with metaborate ion preventing the backward reaction and thus titration with NaOH becomes possible.

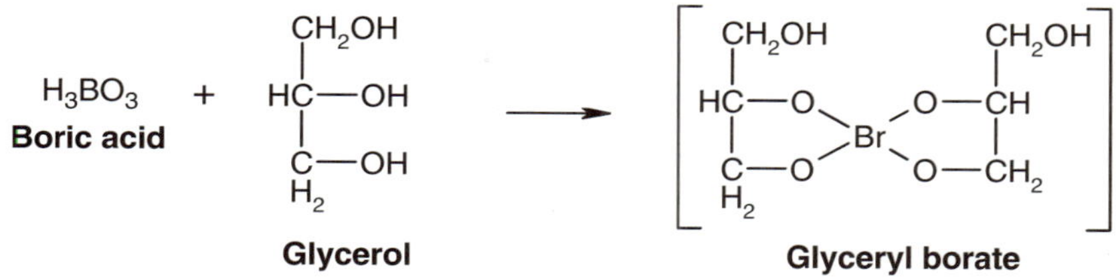

METHOD 2

(a) Take 10 g of the sample accurately weighed and suspend in 40 ml of ethyl alcohol by slight warming. Add 20 ml of water and warm for complete suspension. Make up the volume to 100 ml with distilled water. Take 50 ml of the solution and titrate with 0.1 N sodium hydroxide using phenolphthalein solution as indicator. Calculate the amount of combined salicylic acid/benzoic acid (total acids) from the volume of 0.1 N sodium hydroxide consumed in above titration as explained in method 1 above.

(b) As soon as the above titration for total acids is complete, add 25 ml of glycerin and continue titration to pink end point. From the amount of sodium hydroxide consumed in the second titration, boric acid contents are calculated as discussed above.

(c) The remaining portion of the sample solution is appropriately diluted with 0.1 N sodium hydroxide to get a solution of 20 mcg/ml of salicylic acid and measure the extinction at about 298 nm, specific for salicylic acid (see method under formulation 4 of this chapter). Benzoic acid does not absorb at 298 nm.

METHOD 3

Take sample accurately weighed, suspend in ether by slight warming and extract with fine 20 ml portions of 0.1 N sodium hydroxide. Shake the combined alkaline extract with 5 ml of ether. Adjust the alkaline layer to get concentration of 10 mcg/ml of salicylic acid. Carry out the quantitative determination of salicylic acid and benzoic acid by iso-absorption method as described in formulation 4 of this chapter. Boric acid does not interfere.

Boric acid

The ether layer obtained under method 3 above is evaporated and suspended in 50 ml of water-glycerin mixture (1 : 1) by slight warming. Carry out the titration and calculation as per method 1 discussed above.

Formulation 7

Salicylic acid, Benzoic acid, Resorcinol

Combined (Salicylic acid and Benzoic acid) acids—Total acids

Take 25 ml of water in a separator and volume of the sample equivalent to 175 mg of salicylic acid. Add 30 ml of petroleum ether (40-60°C), shake well and run the aqueous solution to another separator. Wash petroleum ether with 10 ml of water. Mix the aqueous layers and extract with four 25 ml portions of solvent ether. Wash each ether extract with same 10 ml of water and make up the volume to 100 ml with solvent ether. Evaporate 25 ml of ether extract below 40°C, cool and dissolve the residue in 20 ml of alcohol, warm the alcohol if necessary. Cool and titrate with 0.1 N sodium hydroxide using phenol red as indicator. Each ml of 0.1 N sodium hydroxide is equivalent to 0.01381 g of salicylic acid and 0.01221 g of benzoic acid. After finding out the contents of salicylic acid, salicylic acid should be deducted from combined acids to know the amount of benzoic acid present in the sample taken for analysis.

Salicylic acid

The aqueous solution obtained above is made alkaline and filtered. The filtrate is acidified with hydrochloric acid extracted with four 25 ml portions of chloroform. The combined chloroform layer is extracted with five 20 ml portions of saturated solution of sodium bicarbonate, washing each extract with the same 20 ml of ether. Acidify the bicarbonate extract with hydrochloric acid and extract with four 25 ml portions of solvent ether. Combine ether layer and make up to 100 ml. Evaporate 25 ml of the ether extract and take up the residue in 5 ml of 0.5 N sodium hydroxide and carry out the bromination method described in formulation 4 of this chapter. Each ml of 0.1 N bromine is equivalent to 0.002302 g of salicylic acid.

Resorcinol

METHOD 1

Take sample accurately weighed equivalent to 20 mg of resorcinol and evaporate to about 2 ml. Transfer into a separator, wash the beaker two times with 5 ml of water and extract with 25 ml of chloroform. Run the aqueous layer to another separator. Wash the chloroform layer with 10 ml of water and mix washing with the aqueous layer and make up the volume to 100 ml with water. To 25 ml, add 50 ml of 0.1 N bromine, 10 ml of hydrochloric acid and shake vigorously. Allow to stand for 15 minutes, then add 10 ml of potassium iodide solution. Shake vigorously and titrate with 0.1 N sodium thiosulphate using towards end starch mucilage as indicator. Each ml of 0.1 N bromine is equivalent to 0.001835 g of resorcinol. Run blank side by side. Salicylic acid and benzoic acid remain in chloroform layer.

Probable Reaction Mechanism

This involves bromination of polyphenol. Excess bromine is allowed to react with iodide which is oxidized to iodate (IO_3^-) and finally liberated I_2 is titrated with sodium thiosulphate.

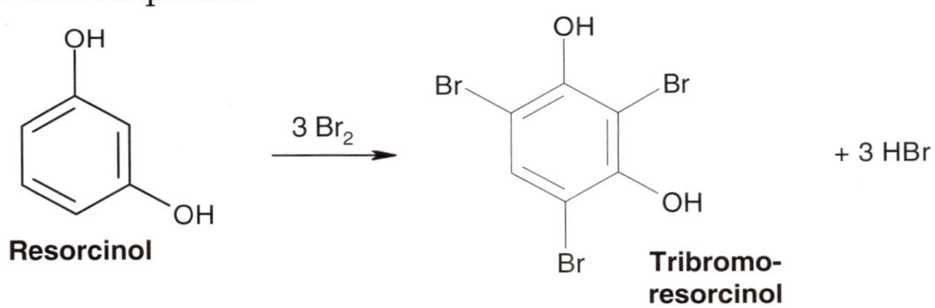

$$2\,KI + Br_2 \longrightarrow I_2 + KBr$$

$$I_2 + 2Na_2S_2O_3 \longrightarrow 2NaI + Na_2S_4O_6$$

METHOD 2

Reagents

1. About 0.12% w/v solution of iodine in chloroform. The standardization of this reagent is not necessary.
2. Acetate buffer, pH 5.7.
3. 1% w/v solution of starch.
4. 0.5% w/v solution of potassium iodide in water.
5. 0.001 and 0.01 N sodium thiosulphate solution. This may be standardized against potassium iodate solution of similar normality.
6. The bromine water, saturated.

Standard solution

1 mg/ml solution of resorcinol in water. The solution may be diluted as required.

Sample solution

The sample may be dissolved/extracted with water and diluted appropriately to get a concentration of 1 mg/ml.

Procedure

(a) **Titrimetric method:** In a 100 ml separating funnel, place a suitable volume of the sample representing 500 mcg of the resorcinol. Add 10 ml buffer solution, pH 5.7 and 10 ml of iodine solution. Shake exactly for 1 minute and separate the organic layer. Remove the last traces of iodine from aqueous layer by extraction with 10 ml of chloroform. Transfer quantitatively the aqueous phase into conical flask. Add 2 ml of bromine water, shake for 3 minutes and destroy excess of bromine with 1 ml of formic acid. Add about 2.5 g of potassium iodide and titrate the liberated iodine with 0.01 N sodium thiosulphate solution using starch as indicator. Run a blank determination. If the sample under estimation contains less than 500 mcg of the compound, preferably use 0.001 N sodium thiosulphate solution. Each ml of 0.01 sodium thiosulphate solution is equal to 61.17 mcg of resorcinol.

(b) **Spectrophotometric method:** Carry out the extraction procedure as described under titrimetric method with about 100 mcg of resorcinol. Transfer the iodide formed into 50 ml volumetric flask, add 1 ml of 0.5 N sulphuric acid and 0.5 ml of bromine water. Shake for 2 minutes, add 1 ml of formic acid, shake for 2 minutes and add 2 ml of potassium iodide solution, 2 ml of starch solution and dilute with water. Measure the extinction of blue solution at 600 nm against reagent blank and calculate the results.

Note

1. Iodination time should not be allowed to exceed one minute as excessive time gives higher results.
2. pH higher than 5.7 usually gives higher results.
3. Phenol, salicylic acid, hydroquinone and cresol do not interfere even when present 25 folds.

(a) This method involves iodination of the compound in buffered medium. The resulting iodide is oxidized with bromine to give iodate and finally iodine which is titrated with sodium thiosulphate.

(b) Instead of titrating the liberated iodine, blue colour is developed by adding starch solution and absorbance of blue colour measured at 600 nm.

Probable Reaction Mechanism

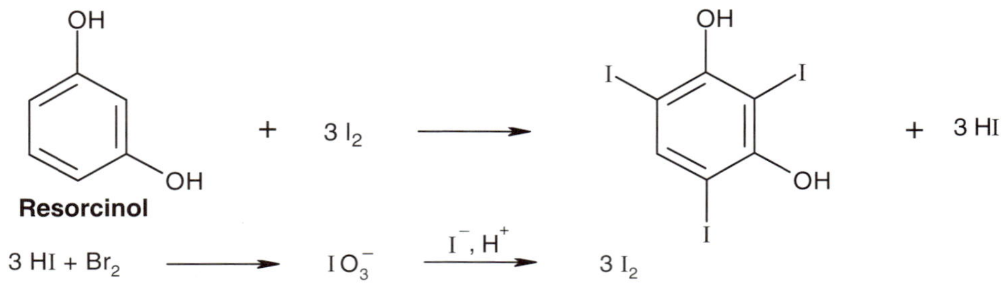

Reference

Darwish Amin & S.T. Sulaiman, *Analyst*, **109**, 739-741, 1984.

METHOD 3

Reagents

1. 1 M sodium hydroxide solution.
2. 0.04% p-aminophenol (PAP) solution in methanol.

Sample and standard solutions

10 µg/ml of resorcinol in water.

Procedure

To 2 ml of each sample and standard solutions add 2 ml of sodium hydroxide solution and 1.4 ml of 'PAP' reagent, adjust the volume to 10 ml and measure the absorbance at 585 nm against reagent blank.

Probable Reaction Mechanism

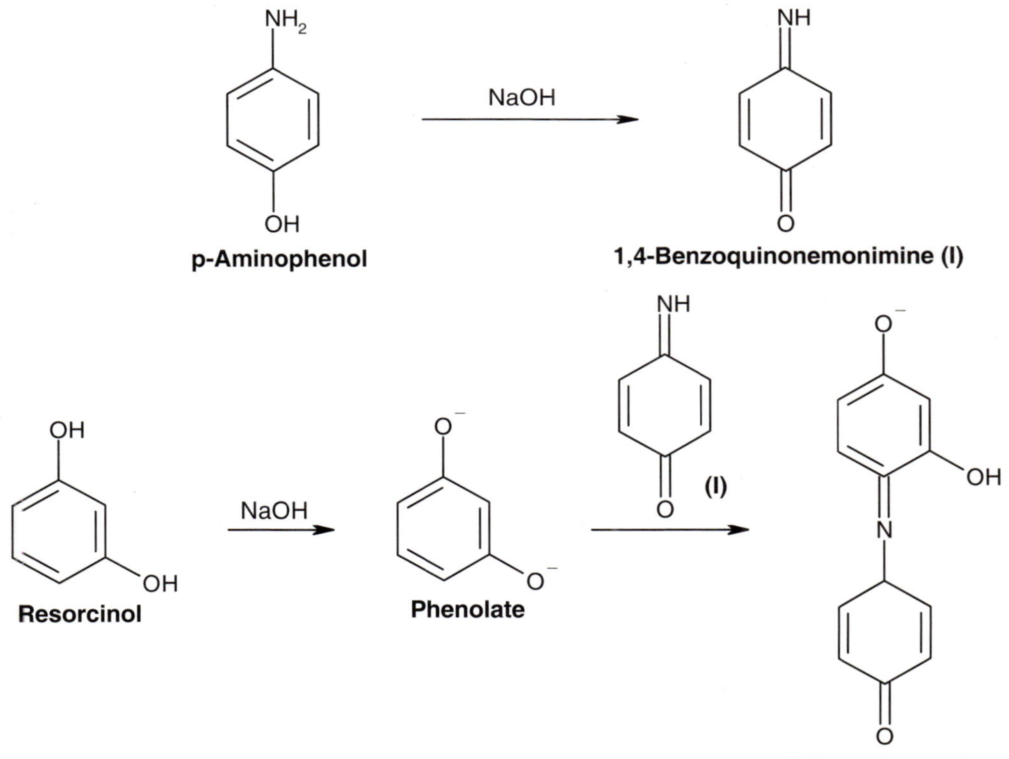

Coloured complex
(λ_{max} 585 nm)

Reference

R.T. Sane & C.H. Thombare, *J. Ind. Chem. Soc.*, **Vol. LVII**, 349, 1980.

Another titrimetric method has been reported by Amin & Bashir (1984). This method is based on the reaction of the compound with excess bromine to form tribromoaryl hypobromite.

Procedure

Sample equivalent to 0.5 mg of resorcinol taken in separating funnel, add 10 ml of water, 1.5 ml of saturated bromine water, stopper the funnel, shake the flask for 2 min. Destroy excess bromine by shaking with 1 ml of formic acid for 1 min. Add 1 ml of 1% potassium iodide solution (5%), shake for 2 min, extracted the liberated iodine with 3 × 10 ml of chloroform, combine the chloroform layers and reduce the iodine to iodide by shaking with 10 ml water containing 1 ml of 1% sodium sulphite solution. Transfer the aqueous layer containing iodide to 50 ml conical flask, add 2 ml of bromine water, shake for 3 min, add 2 ml of formic acid to remove excess of bromine, add about 0.5 g of KI and titrate the liberated iodine with 0.01 M sodium thiosulphate solution using starch as indicator. For low concentration, use of 0.001 M thiosulphate solution is suggested. Each ml of 0.01 N sodium thiosulphate solution is equivalent to 0.046 mg of resorcinol.

Probable Reaction Mechanism

Resorcinol readily undergoes bromination giving tribromo derivative and with large excess of bromine, substitution goes further to form tribromophenyl hypobromite. Both —OH groups in resorcinol undergo substitution.

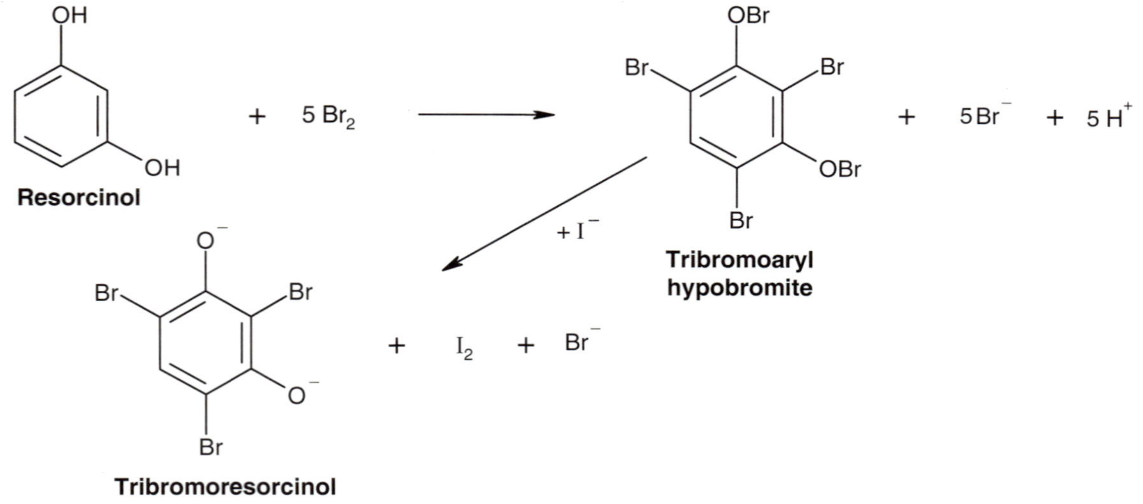

Note

Bromination of the compound is very fast and is complete within 1-2 min. Reduction of the tribromophenyl hypobromite to tribromophenol can be achieved with 0.5-1 ml of KI solution (5%). Large excess of KI hindres extraction of iodine with chloroform due to formation of tri-iodide. Complete liberation of iodine requires 1-2 min.

Reference

D. Amin & W.A. Bashir, *Talanta*, **31(4)**, 283-284, 1984.

Formulation 8

Salicylic acid, Benzoic acid, Ichthammol, Triamcinolone acetonide

ESTIMATION

Salicylic acid

Follow the method described in formulation 4 of this chapter.

Benzoic acid

Follow the method described in formulation 4 of this chapter for estimation of salicylic acid and benzoic acid as total acids by titrating with 0.1 N sodium hydroxide. Then deduct the volume of 0.1 N sodium hydroxide required for salicylic acid contents as estimated above taking each ml of 0.1 N sodium hydroxide as equivalent to 0.01381 g of salicylic acid. Excess volume of sodium hydroxide consumed will be due to benzoic acid. The contents of benzoic acid in the formulation can then be calculated by taking factor of 0.01221 g of benzoic acid.

Triamcinolone acetonide

Follow the method described in the chapter on topical antifungal preparations under fluocinolone acetonide.

Note

Separation by preparative thin layer chromatography using dichloromethane-diethyl ether-methanol (77 + 15 + 8%) as mobile phase, elution of separated spot with methanol as subsequent colour development with tetrazolium blue has seen found to give higher results.

Ichthammol

The method is based on estimation of organically combined sulphur contents. Accurately weighed quantity of sample taken in crucible is mixed with 1 g of analysing sodium carbonate, add 2-3 ml of chloroform and heat gently on water-bath with constant stirring till no smell of chloroform. Add 2 g of cupric nitrate and heat on a gas burner. Cool and place the crucible in a 500 or 1000 ml beaker. Add drop by drop 20 ml of concentrated hydrochloric acid. After the reaction has stopped, add 100 ml of water and boil for 15-20 minutes for copper oxide to dissolve. Filter and heat the filtrate gently for about 15 minutes. Add 20 ml of barium chloride solution (20%) and set aside for complete precipitation. Filter through fine filter paper to collect the precipitates. Ignite the precipitate at 800°C till constant weight. Each g of the residue so obtained is equivalent to 0.1374 g of combined sulphur.

Formulation 9

Salicylic acid, Lactic acid

ESTIMATION

METHOD 1

Salicylic acid and Lactic acid (total acids)

Weigh accurately about 0.5 g of the sample containing about 170 mg of total acids, add 30 ml of water and shake for 5-10 min. Add 25 ml of 0.1 N sodium hydroxide and allow to stand at room temperature in a stoppered flask for 30 min (this is sufficient for complete hydrolysis of lactic anhydride to lactic acid usually present in lactic acid and subsequent neutralization with sodium hydroxide). Titrate the excess alkali with 0.1 N hydrochloric acid using phenolphthalein as indicator.

Record the volume of 0.1 N sodium hydroxide consumed by both the acids—X ml.

Salicylic acid

Follow the method described in formulation of this chapter. Alternatively, extract in sample with 0.1 N sodium hydroxide and dilute to get final solution of 10 mcg/ml. Measure the absorption of both sample and standard solution (10 mcg/ml) at 298 nm and calculate the amount of salicylic acid present in the sample. Lactic acid does not absorb at 298 nm. From the amount of salicylic acid so determined, calculate the equivalent volume of 0.1 N sodium hydroxide (13.80 mg of salicylic acid represents 1 ml of 0.1 N sodium hydroxide—Y ml.

Lactic acid

Determine the volume of 0.1 N alkali consumed by lactic acid (X – Y) and calculate the contents of lactic acid in the sample. Each ml of 0.1 N sodium hydroxide consumed for estimation of lactic acid is equivalent to 9.008 mg of lactic acid.

METHOD 2

Reagent

0.1% w/v solution of ferric chloride: To 100 mg of ferric chloride, add 5 ml of methanol and dilute to 100 ml with water, prepare fresh.

Standard solution

100 mcg/ml of lactic acid and salicylic acid in water.

Sample solution

Extract accurately weighed quantity of the sample with slightly warm water to get final concentration of 100 mcg/ml in respect of both the acids.

Procedure

To 10 ml each of sample and standard solutions, add 1 ml of ferric chloride reagent and immediately measure the absorption at 390 nm (lactic acid) and at 530 nm (salicylic acid) against reagent blank.

Typical laboratory analysis

Weight of lactic acid taken for standard solution = 0.1 g
Weight of salicylic acid taken for standard solution = 0.1230 g

	Absorption value	
	530 nm	390 nm
Sample	0.452	0.232
Standard	0.585	0.223

$$\text{Salicylic acid (\%)} = \frac{0.452}{0.585} \times d_f \times \frac{0.1230}{100} \times \frac{0.9575 \times 100}{16.7}$$

$$= 107\% \text{ of claim } (16.7\%)$$

$$\text{Lactic acid (\%)} = \frac{0.232}{0.223} \times d_f \times \frac{0.1}{100} \times \frac{0.9575 \times 100}{16.7}$$

$$= 103.46\% \text{ of claim } (16.7\%)$$

(0.9575 is the weight/ml)

Note

Lactic acid has practically no absorption at 530 nm, whereas salicylic acid does not absorb at 390 nm; both wavelengths being λ_{max} of each compound, hence no mutual interference.

Probable Reaction Mechanism

Reaction of salicylic acid with $FeCl_3$ cannot be explained only due to phenolic function and due to presence of neighbouring carbonyl group.

Salicylic acid

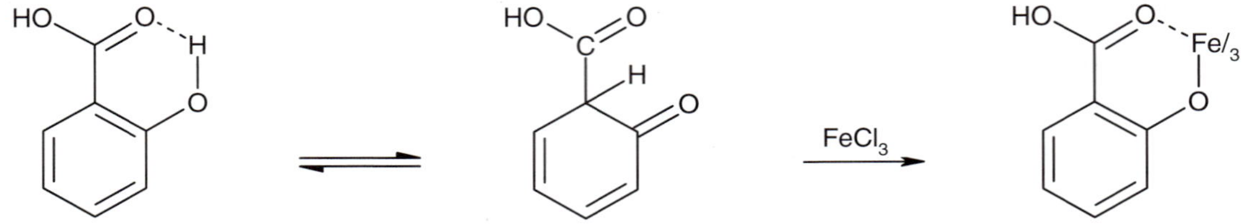

Salicylic acid **Salicylic acid** **Salicylic acid - Fe(3) complex**
(λ_{max} 530 nm)

Another possible structure of complex is:

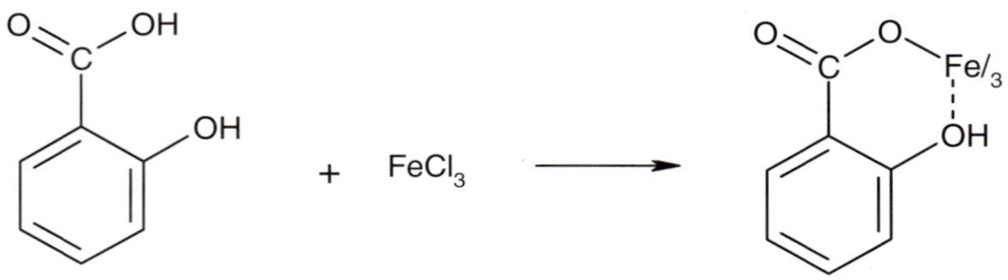

Salicylic acid - Fe(3) complex
(λ_{max} 530 nm)

Lactic acid

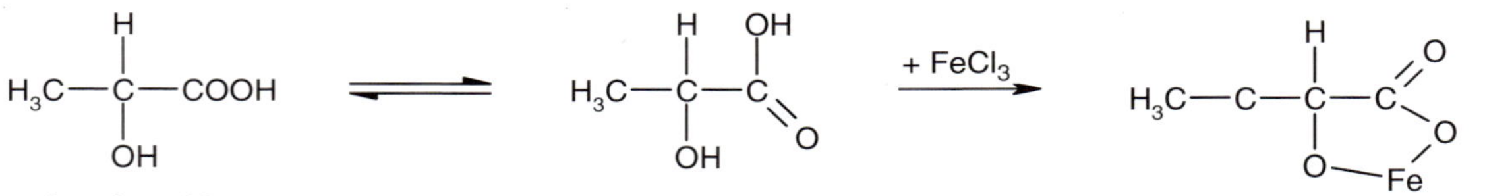

Lactic acid **Lactic acid - Fe(3) complex**
(λ_{max} 390 nm)

Note

Lactic acid on mild oxidation yields pyruvic acid. Pyruvic acid can react with 2,4-dinitrophenyl hydrazine to give hydrazone.

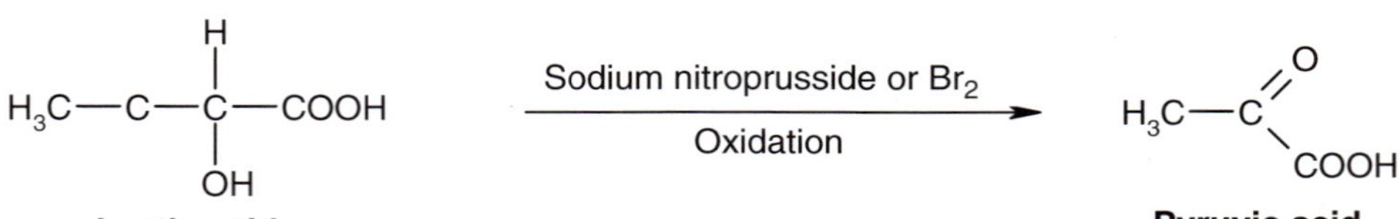

Lactic acid **Pyruvic acid**

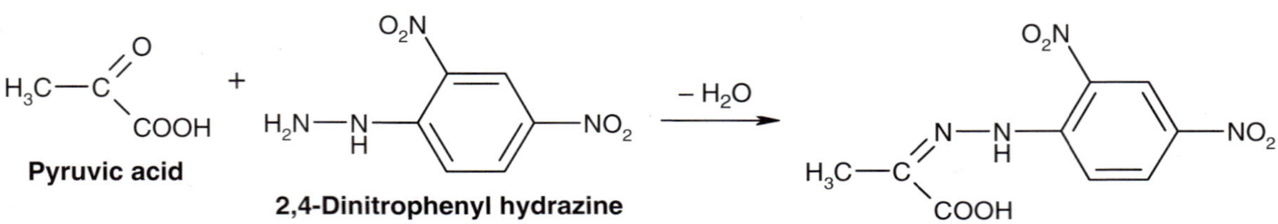

Pyruvic acid **2,4-Dinitrophenyl hydrazine** **Yellow-coloured hydrazone derivative**

Reference

Pharmaceutical Chemistry (Vol. 2) by H.J. Roth, p. 160.

METHOD 3 (Salicylic acid)

Reagents

1. 1% w/v copper acetate solution in water.
2. Sodium acetate buffer, pH 5.5.

Standard/sample solution

10 mg/ml in 0.1 M NaOH.

Procedure

To 1 ml of sample/standard solution add 1 ml of copper acetate solution and 1 ml of buffer solution, dilute to 10 ml with water and measure the absorbance at 730 nm against reagent blank.

Note

This method is suitable for estimation of salicylic acid in the presence of sulphur, ZnO. However, benzoic acid will interfere.

Explanatory Note

Here the phenolic oxygen containing lone pair of electrons can readily coordinate with Cu(2) resulting in the formation of coordinate bond. Oxygen attached to C==O group may not readily donate electrons as C==O group is an electron withdrawing group, hence phenolic oxygen will form covalent (→) bond with Cu(2) as shown below.

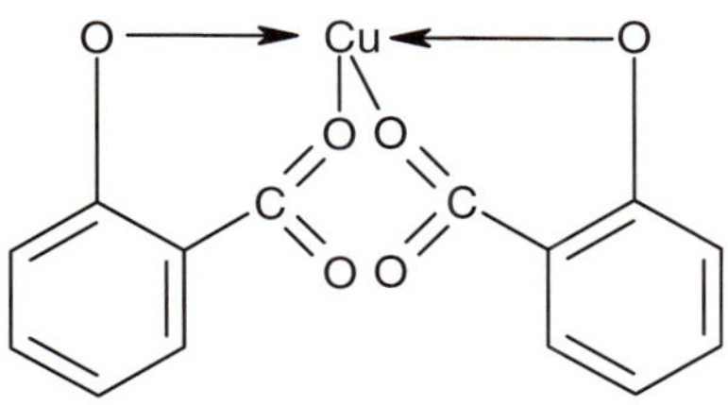

Salicylic acid - copper complex
(λ_{max} 730 nm)

Note

Ampicillin, amoxycillin, calcium pantothenate and α-amino acids form similar chelates with Cu(2).

Reference

Utpal Saha & Kalyan Baksi, *Analyst*, **110**, 739-741, 1985.

Salicylic acid, because of the presence of phenolic —OH function, can couple with Gibbs reagent in alkaline medium. The reagent acts as oxidizing agent and attacks free para position to the phenolic —OH as shown below.

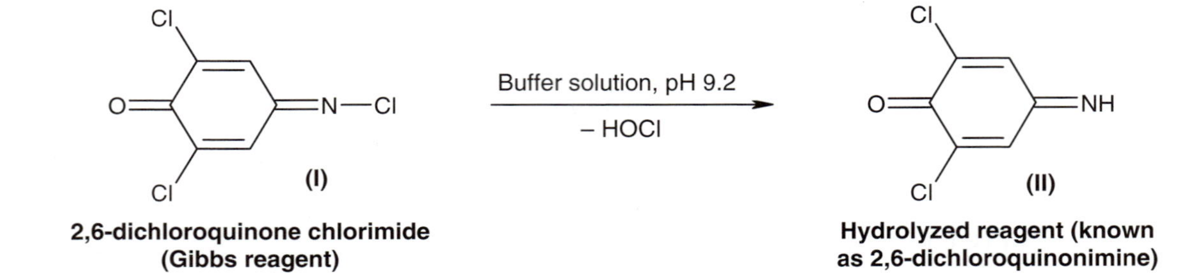

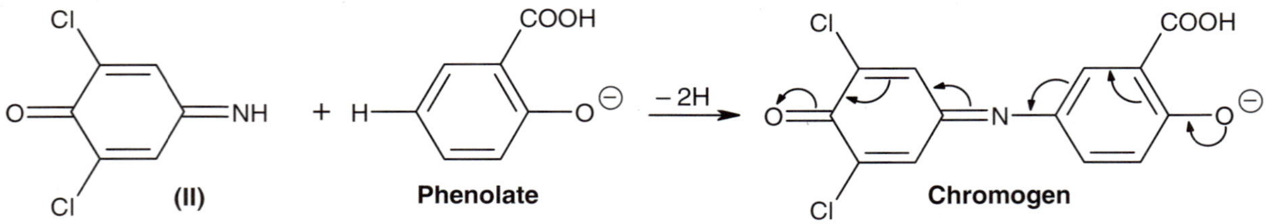

Because of the presence of phenolic —OH group, the compound undergoes nitrosation reaction and the product so formed is stabilized by chelating with Hg(II).

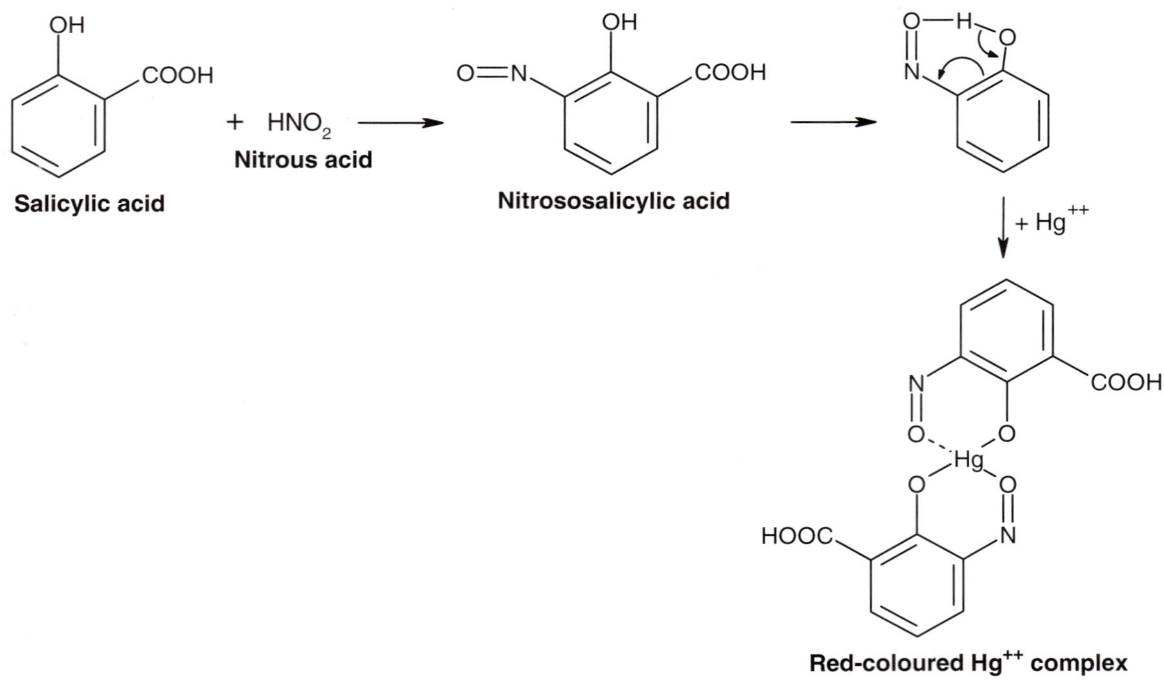

Formulation 10

Dithranol, Salicylic acid

ESTIMATION

Salicylic acid

Reagents

1. Phosphate solution: 5% w/v solution of sodium phosphate in water.
2. 5% w/v solution of potassium iodide in water.

Procedure

Weigh accurately sample (ointment) equivalent to 50 mg of salicylic acid, disperse in chloroform and extract with phosphate solution (3 ´ 20 ml). Collect the aqueous layer. Wash the chloroform layer further with water (2 ´ 20 ml) and add the washings to the main aqueous layer (combined aqueous layer may be warmed to remove dissolved chloroform). Transfer the entire aqueous solution to iodine flask, make it slightly acidic (hydrochloric acid), add 30 ml of 0.1 N bromine and 10 ml of concentrated hydrochloric acid. Shake intermittently during 45 min, add 10 ml of potassium iodide solution and titrate with 0.1 N sodium thiosulphate using starch as indicator. Carry out the blank titration without the sample. Each ml of 0.1 N bromine is equivalent to 0.0023 g of salicylic acid.

This method involves bromination of salicylic acid. Bromination causes displacement of carboxyl group with the formation of corresponding 2,4,6-tri substituted bromophenol. The excess of bromine acting as oxidizing agent liberates iodine from potassium iodide which is titrated with sodium thiosulphate.

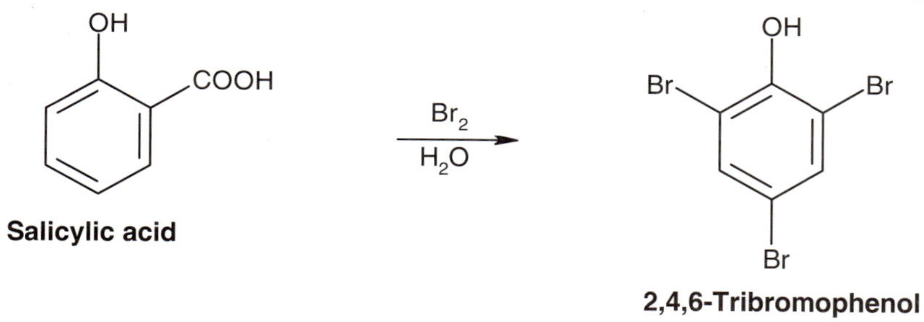

Probable reaction mechanism for displacement of carboxylic group by Br^-

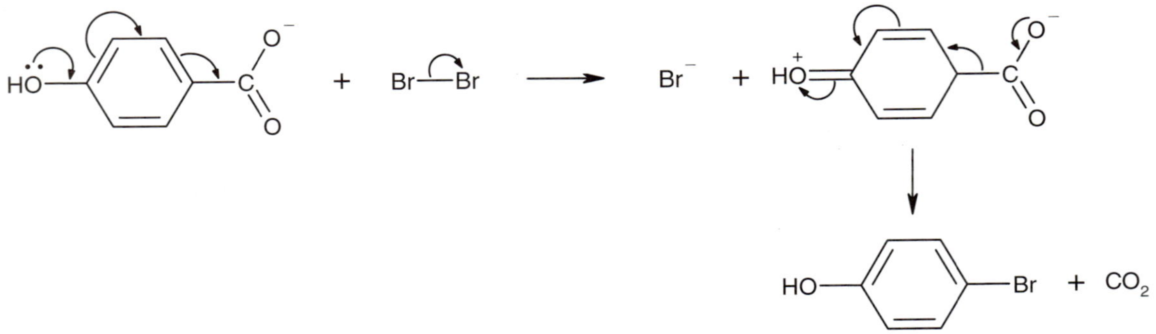

Note

A titrimetric method is reported using sodium methoxide as titrant and DMF as solvent. This method is suitable for titration of phenols and some phenolic acids such as salicylic acid. It was observed that brilliant orange was found suitable indicator for neutralization point of both —COOH and phenolic —OH groups whereas tilan yellow for that of —COOH group. By using different indicators one can determine total —COOH and —OH moiety or only carboxylic (COOH moiety). The compound having —COOH and —OH groups ortho to each other consume only one equivalent of the titrant per mole probably due to intramolecular hydrogen bonding, whereas ortho and p-hydroxy benzoic acid consume two equivalents of titrant as there is no intramolecular hydrogen bonding. For simultaneous determination of —COOH and —OH in phenolic acid in one run was not possible as titrating first using tilan yellow as indicator and then adding brilliant yellow after the first end-point as brilliant yellow formed deep red compound with tilan yellow. Hence two separate titrations are to be carried out for determining total —OH to COOH or only —COOH groups.

Reference

S.S.M. Hassan & T.M.Z. Zaki, *Talanta*, **22**, 863-847, 1975.

Since p-position to the phenolic —OH is unoccupied, Emerson reaction is feasible for analytical purpose.

Dithranol

Standard solution

30 mcg/ml of dithranol in glacial acetic acid.

Sample solution

To accurately weighed quantity of the sample equivalent to 15 mg of the substance, add 20-30 ml of glacial acetic acid, warm in water-bath for 5 min with stirring. Cool and make up the volume to 50 ml. Filter and dilute 5 mg of the filtrate to 50 ml with glacial acetic acid.

Procedure

To 5 ml each of sample and standard solutions, add 1 ml of sodium nitrite solution (5%), keep in boiling water-bath for 2 min, cool and dilute to 25 ml with glacial acetic acid. Measure the absorbance of both the solutions of 460 nm against reagent blank within 10 min. Calculate the results by comparison.

Note

1. Maximum colour intensity is observed within 2 min of heating, it tends to fade if heating is continued.
2. One may be confronted with formation of turbidity on addition of sodium nitrite solution; the solution is clear on dilution.

In acidic medium it forms nitroso derivative ortho to phenolic function which has λ_{max} 460 nm.

Probable Reaction Mechanism

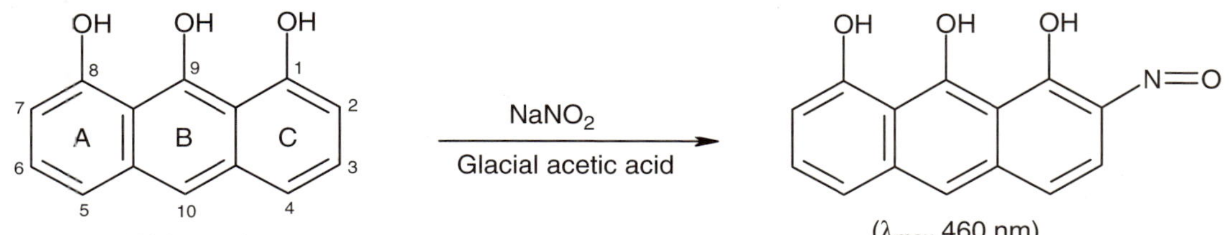

Dithranol

(λ_{max} 460 nm)

In sodium hydroxide, yellow colour of the compound is changed to red with fluorescence due to intramolecular hydrogen bridge.

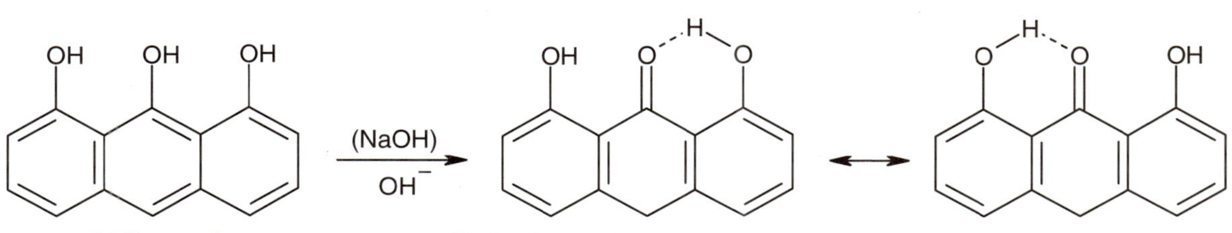

(Yellow-red) Red colour with green fluorescence

Reference

Pharmaceutical Chemistry (Vol. 2) by H.J. Roth, pp. 93-94.

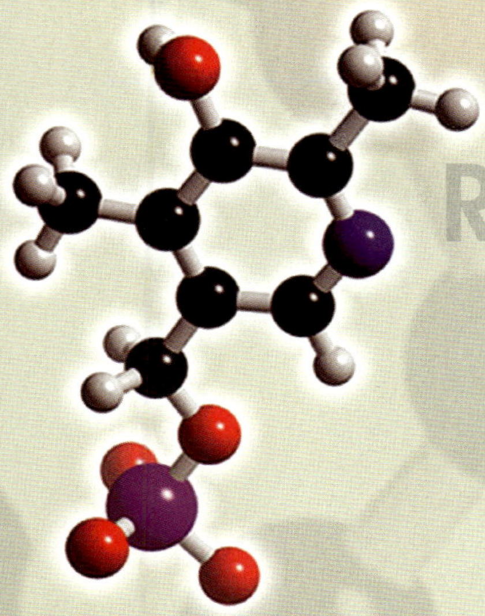

Reaction Mechanism

18

Miscellaneous (Vitamins, Minerals and Digestive Enzyme Preparations)

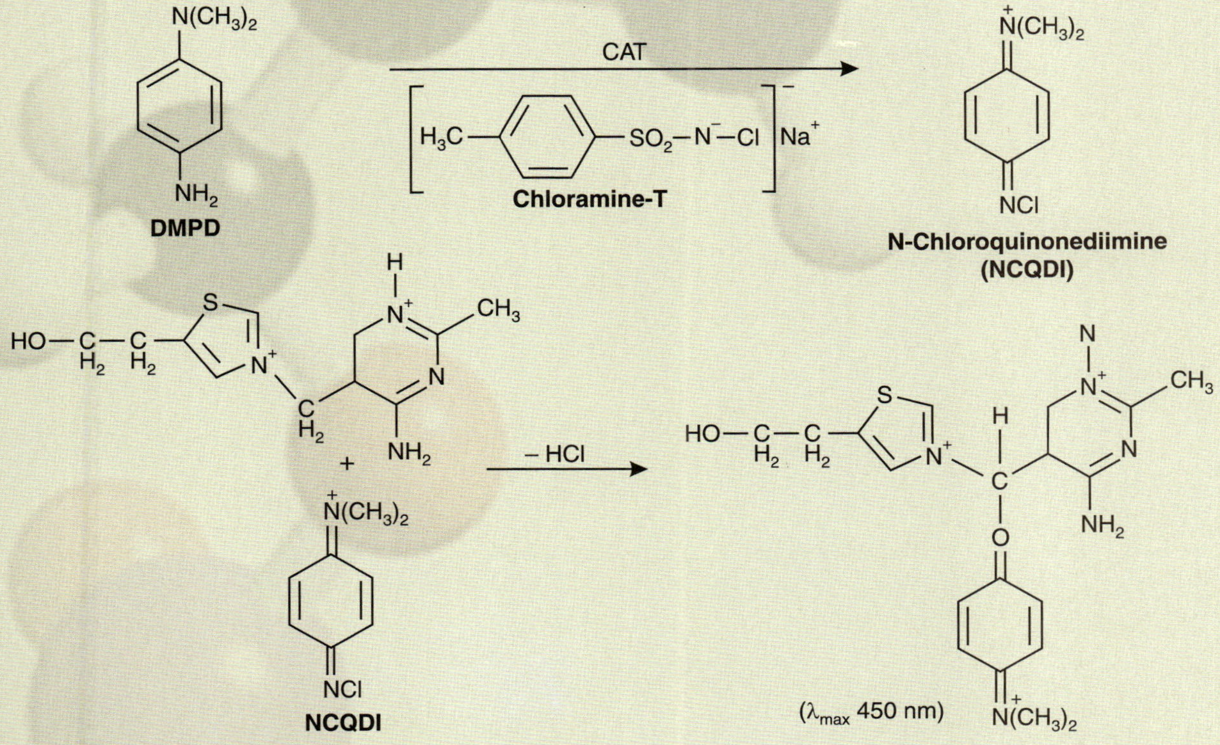

Formulation 1

Thiamine hydrochloride (Vitamin B_1)

METHOD 1

Reagents

1. 0.04% w/v solution of p-aminophenol in ethyl alcohol.
2. 0.1 M ammonium hydroxide solution.

Standard solution

Dissolve 100 mg of thiamine hydrochloride (previously dried at 100°C) in distilled water to produce 100 ml. Dilute this solution suitably with water to give a concentration of 20 mcg/ml.

Sample solution

Dissolve and dilute suitably with water to give a concentration of 20 mcg/ml. In case of tablets having coloured coating, remove the colour by rubbing with cotton wetted with water or organic solvent.

Procedure

To 3 ml of sample and standard solutions add 3 ml of 0.1 M ammonium hydroxide solution and 0.5 ml of p-aminophenol reagent. Wait for 5 minutes and extract the coloured complex with 10 ml of chloroform. Measure the absorption of organic layer at about 430 nm against reagent blank. The contents of thiamine are calculated by comparison. The method obeys Beer's law in the concentration range of 3-12 mcg/ml in final solution.

The following compounds do not interfere in the above method. The figures in brackets indicate the number of folds excess the compounds can be tolerated.

- Pyridoxine (5)
- Niacinamide (20)
- Riboflavin (1)
- Vitamin B_{12} (0.05)
- Ascorbic acid (2)

- Folic acid (1)
- Menadione (15)
- Calcium glycerophosphate (25)
- Magnesium glycerophosphate (5)
- Dried yeast (10)
- Calcium pantothenate (1)
- Ferrous sulphate (100)
- Sodium glycerophosphate (75)
- Potassium glycerophosphate (50)

If the preparations contain high percentage of minerals, they form hydroxides and get precipitated in ammoniacal medium. It is therefore necessary to centrifuge the alkaline solution before proceeding with addition of the reagent and colour development.

Precautions

1. p-aminophenol should be freshly sublimed or freshly prepared.
2. The reagent should be prepared every day.
3. Concentration of the reagent should not be more than 0.04%, otherwise the reagent blank is very high, sometime even the solution turns black.
4. Reagent blank and sample blank should be prepared simultaneously.
5. When ascorbic acid is present in the formulation, a slightly longer time is required (10 min) to get the full intensity of the colour.
6. When ascorbic acid is present in the formulation, add 6-7 ml of 0.1 M ammonium hydroxide instead of usual 3 ml.

If ascorbic acid is present in the formulation, the following treatment is also suggested before following method 1 above.

To 10 mg of vitamin B_1 add 5 ml of hydrochloric acid and 200 ml of water. Warm to dissolve, cool and dilute to 250 ml with water (40 mcg/ml). To 25 ml of this solution, add 10 ml of 1 N sodium hydroxide, mix and add 200 mg of manganese dioxide. Heat on water-bath for 30 minutes with frequent agitation, cool and dilute to 50 ml with water and filter. Take 3 ml of the filtrate and follow method 1 as described above.

The reaction mechanism as proposed by the author is as under:

Probable Reaction Mechanism

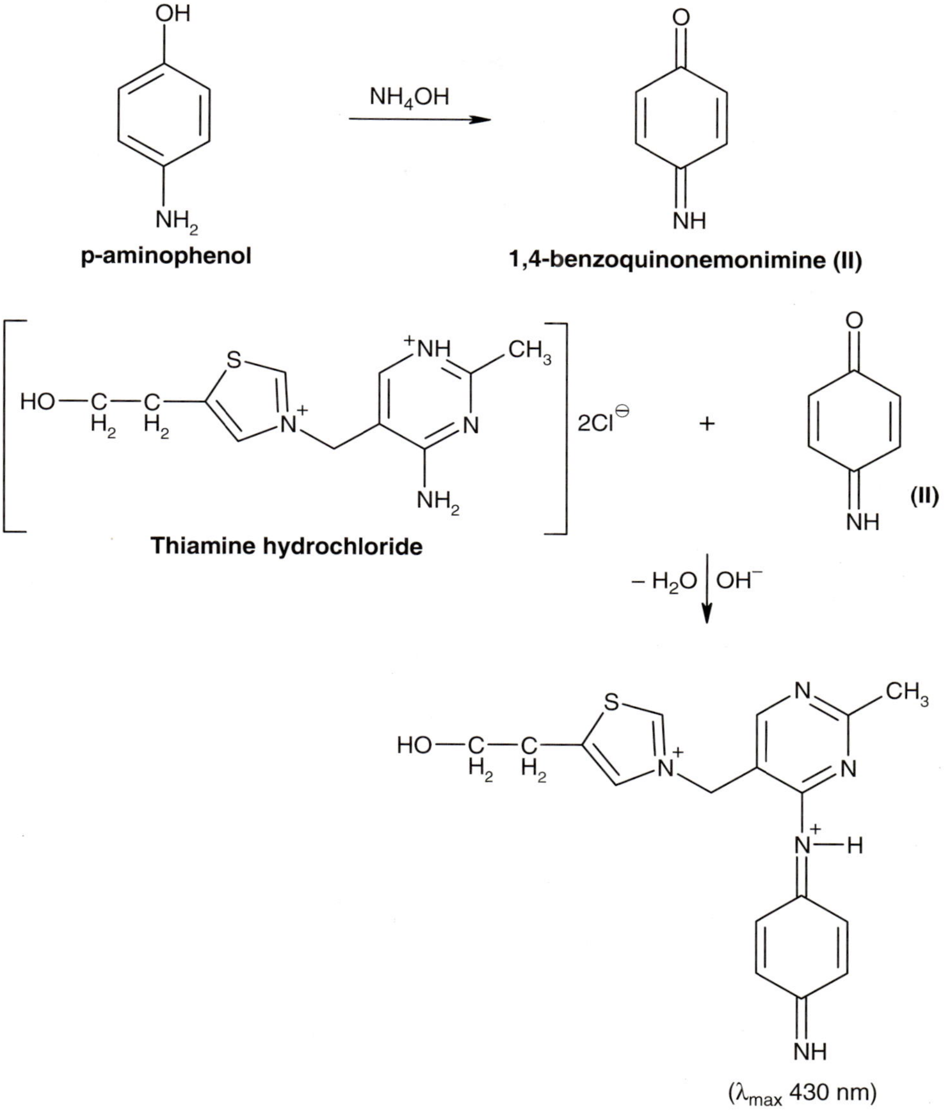

p-aminophenol; 1,4-benzoquinonemonimine (II); Thiamine hydrochloride; (λ_{max} 430 nm)

Reference

R.T. Sane & U.A. Ghorpade, *Acta Vitaminol. Enzymol.*, **5(1)**, 29-34, 1988.

An alternative reaction is described by Roth. In alkaline medium (about pH 9) position 2′ of the thiazole ring is attacked by —OH ion resulting in the formation of mercaptal-like structure finally yielding thiol form. Then p-aminophenol reacts with carbonyl group of the formyl structure to give Schiff's base.

Probable Reaction Mechanism

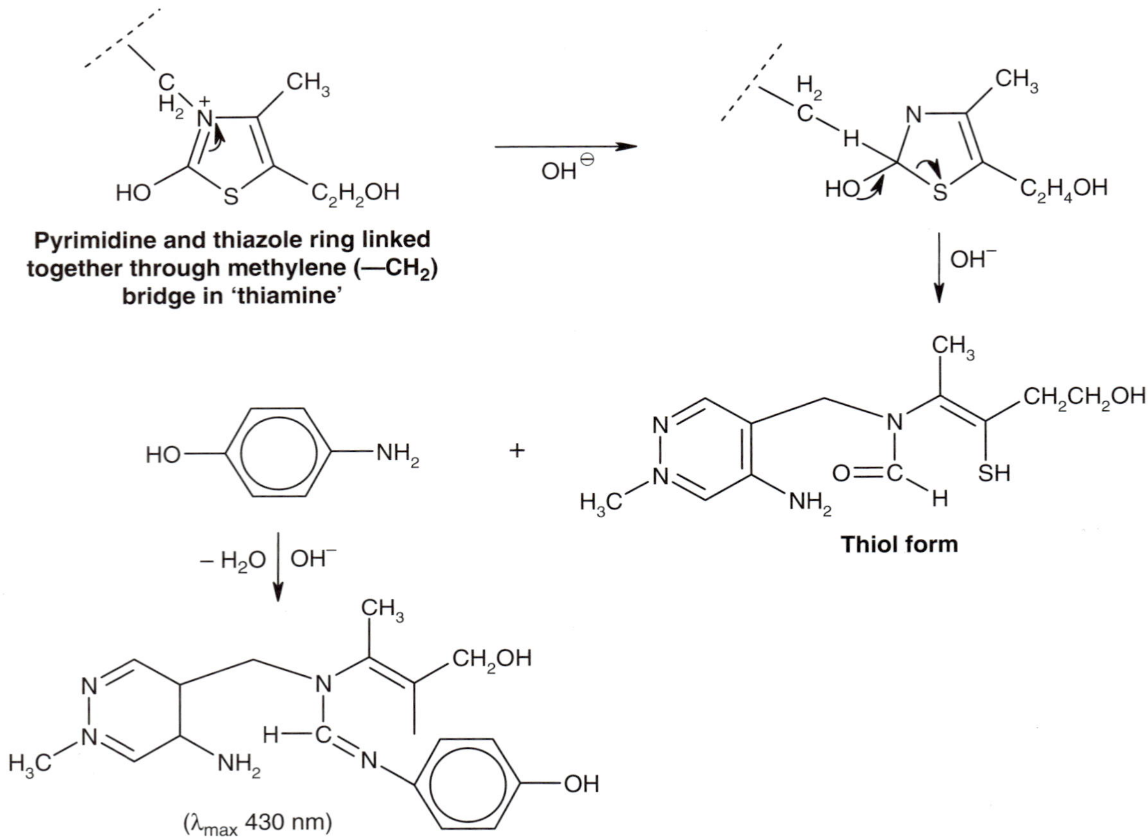

Reference

1. R.T. Sane, U.M. Vaidya & K.D. Deodhar, *Ind. J. Pharm. Sci.*, **40(2)**, 72-73, 1970.
2. Pharmaceutical Chemistry (Vol. 2) by H.J. Roth, p. 547.

METHOD 2

A spectrophotometric method was described by Sane et al. (1985).

Reagents

1. Ammonia solution (25%).
2. 0.1% w/v solution of metol (p-methylaminophenol sulphate).
3. Chloroform.

Sample/standard solution

20 µg/ml of thiamine hydrochloride or mononitrate in water.

Procedure

To 2 ml each of sample and standard solutions add 0.5 ml of metol solution and 1 ml of ammonia solution, keep for 7 min with frequent stirring, dilute to 10 ml with water and measure the absorbance of the solution at 420 nm against reagent blank. The developed colour can also be extracted into chloroform for spectrophotometric measurements. Since p-aminophenol is easily oxidizable, metol is preferred as a reagent.

Note

Most of the water-soluble and fat-soluble vitamins do not interfere.

Probable Reaction Mechanism

The following reaction was proposed by the authors:

A complex formation occurs between p-methylaminophenol and thiamine hydrochloride. The structure of the proposed complex formed is as shown below:

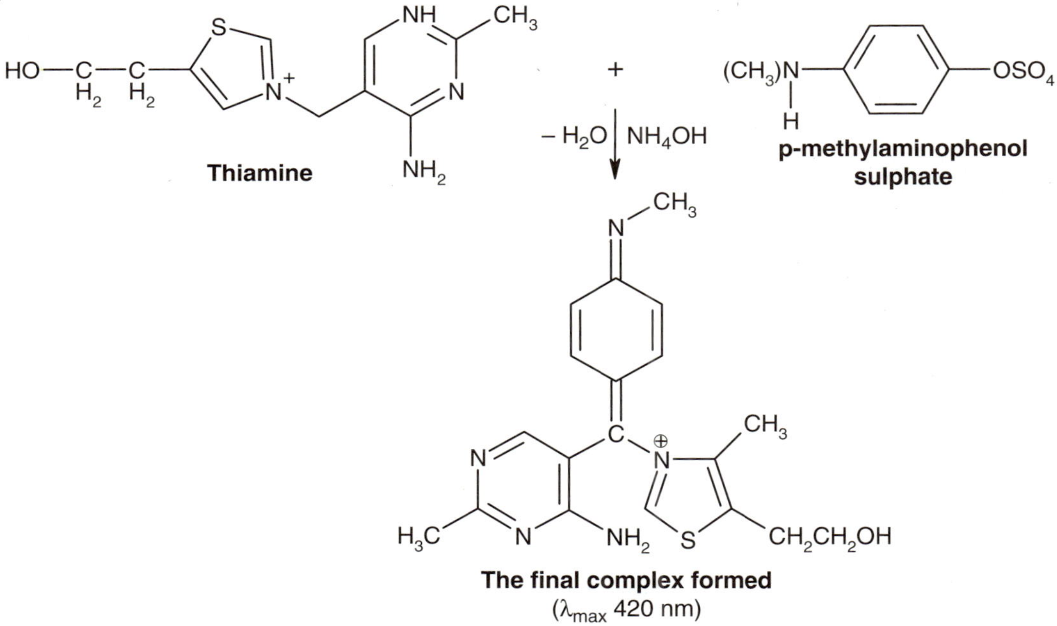

Note

Vitamins B_2, B_6, C, A, D and E, niacinamide, calcium pantothenate, folic acid and biotin do not interfere.

Reference

R.T. Sane, Vipul J. Doshi, Swati Jukar, Sanjay K. Doshi, Satish V. Sawant & Ulhas R. Pandit, *J. Assoc. Off. Anal. Chem.* (*JAOAC*), **68(1)**, 83-85, 1985.

METHOD 3

A spectrophotometric method has been reported by Viswanath et al. (1986) for the estimation of thiamine hydrochloride.

Reagents

1. 0.1 M and 1 M hydrochloric acid.
2. 5% solution of sodium nitrite in water.
3. 0.2 M solution of sodium hydroxide.
4. Diazotized phenylhydrazine-4-sulphonic acid sodium salt.

Sample and standard solutions

Weigh sample/standard equivalent to 10 mg, suspend in 50 mg of 0.1 M hydrochloric acid and heat on water-bath for 30 min, cool, dilute to 100 ml with water (100 μg/ml).

Procedure

To 2 ml of diazotized phenylhydrazine add 5 ml of alcohol and 5 ml each of sample/standard solution, keep aside for 10 min and then dilute to 50 ml with 0.2 M sodium hydroxide solution and measure the absorbance of the resulting solution at 490 nm against reagent blank.

Probable Reaction Mechanism

Heating of thiamine hydrochloride for 30 min in a water-bath by addition of 0.1 M HCl causes acid hydrolysis of thiamine resulting in the formation of hydroxymethylene-substituted pyrimidine and thiazole derivative as shown below.

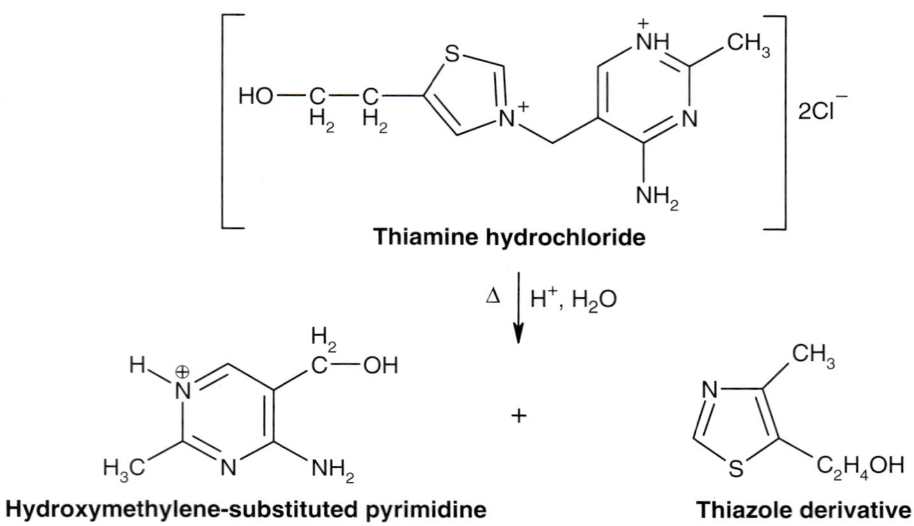

Coupling occurs between diazotized phenylhydrazine and amino group of hydroxymethylene-substituted pyrimidine resulting in the formation of diazo amine compound.

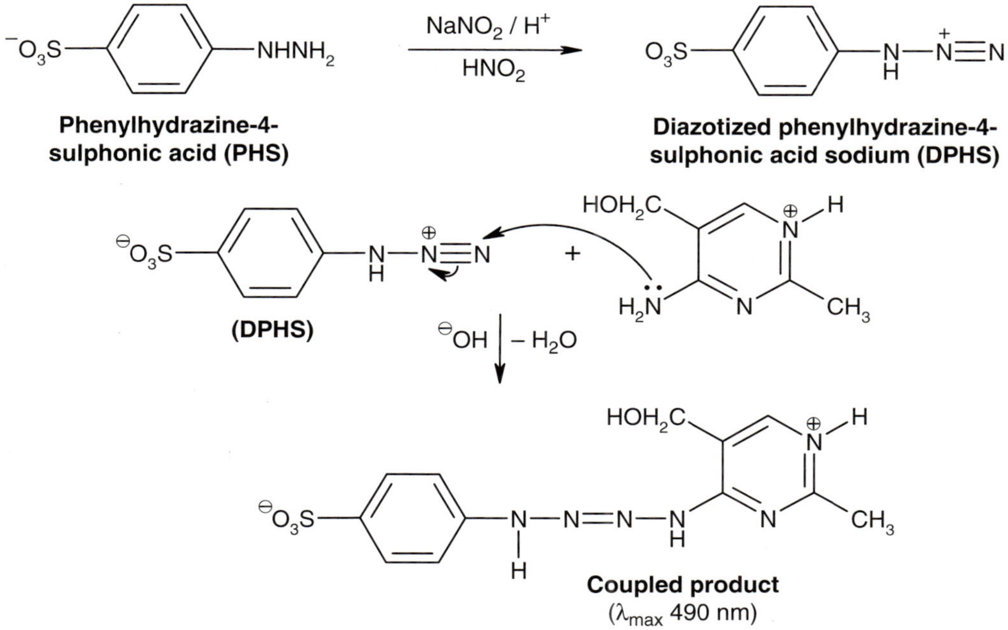

Note

The method using diazotized sulphanilic acid as coupling reagent has been described. Orange-red chromogen has λ_{max} 455 nm.

Reference

A. Rajasekaran & B. Jayakar, *Eastern Pharmacist*, pp. 121-122, May 1997.

Another method based on coupling with p-acetylphenyl diazonium salt was described by Mickelsen O. (1958). As usual coupling occurs between diazotized component and the amino group present in thiamine.

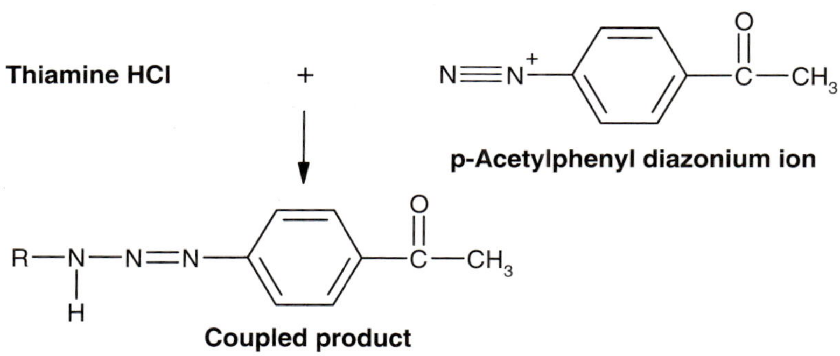

Reference

1. Mickelsen O. & Yamamoto R.S., *Methods Biochemical Analysis*, **6**, 221, 1958.
2. Textbook of Practical Organic Chemistry by Vogel, pp. 946-948.
3. K.K. Viswanath, Rao A. Satya Prasad & M.V. Sivaramakrishnan, *Ind. J. Pharm. Sci.*, May-June 1986, pp. 80-83.

Note

Vitamins B_6 and B_{12} did not interfere; vitamins C and B_2 interfered.

The method is based on alkaline oxidation of thiamine into thiochrome which has fluorescent property and can be used for quantitative estimation. Thiochrome so formed is extractable into isobutyl alcohol.

Probable Reaction Mechanism

Thiazole form of the compound is first changed into close ring which loses one proton to form monoanion which is oxidized into thiochrome; or closed thiazole ring is directly oxidized to thiochrome.

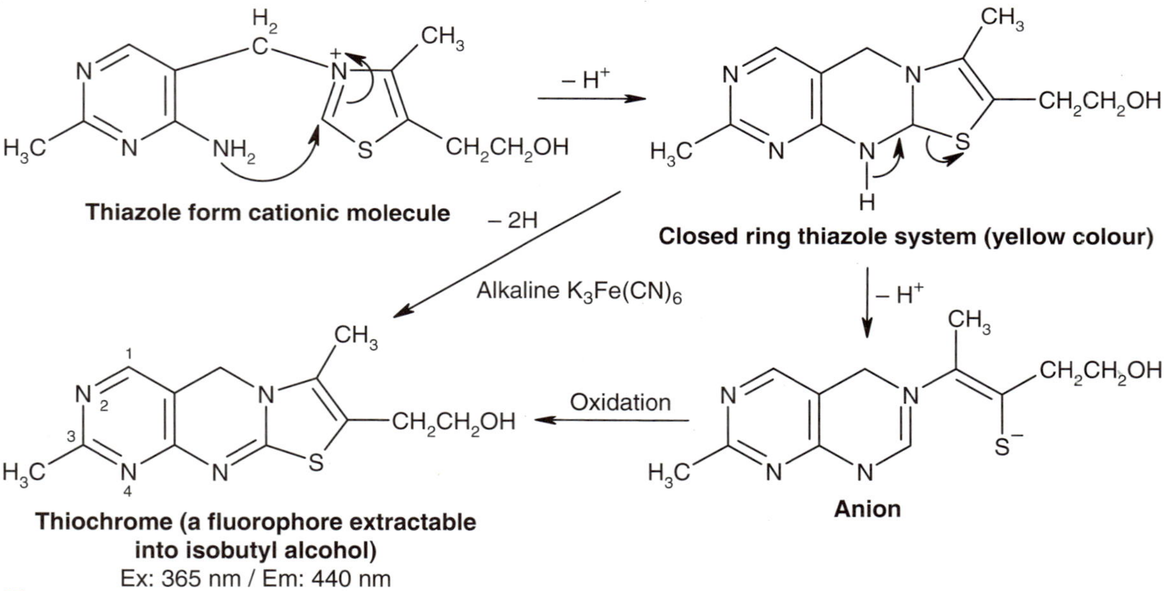

Note

1. Excess $K_3Fe(CN)_6$ destroys thiochrome.
2. Cyanogen bromide or mercuric oxide have been used as oxidizing agents by certain authors.

To make the reaction specific, sodium sulphite can be added. In the presence of sodium sulphite (HSO_3^-) no fluorescence is produced. In weakly acidic solution, sulphite ions are more strongly nucleophilic than water and attack at methylene group (CH_2) to produce irreversible cleavage of the molecule into pyrimidine derivative and thiazole derivative. None of them is fluorescent.

Probable Reaction Mechanism

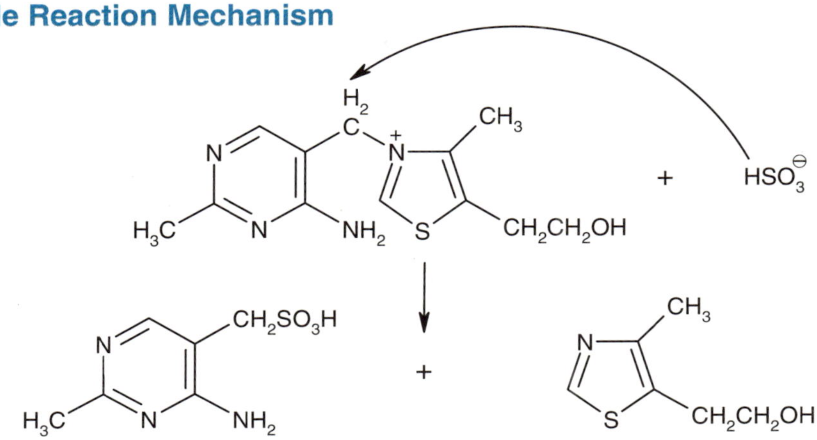

Pyrimidine derivative **Thiazole derivative**

(None of these is fluorescent)

Reference

Pharmaceutical Chemistry (Vol. 2) by H.J. Roth, pp. 548-552.

Preparation of p-aminophenol

To procure p-aminophenol as a white crystalline powder is quite difficult. Para-aminophenol, a raw material for synthesis of paracetamol, is usually available as black crystalline powder. To get the desired grade of purity for use in estimation of vitamin B_1, the commercially available p-aminophenol can be purified by sublimation. However, an easier and cheaper method for its preparation is described which involves the acid-hydrolysis of paracetamol.

Dissolve paracetamol in minimum amount of 4 N hydrochloric acid by slight warming in boiling water-bath (usually for every 1 g of paracetamol, 3-4 ml of 4 N hydrochloric acid is required). Reflux on boiling water-bath under water condenser in a fume cupboard for 30-40 minutes, allow it to cool. Crystals of p-aminophenol separate out. Filter through G_3 sintered funnel under vacuum. Wash the crystals with small amount of water to remove acid. Collect the crystals, dry them between folds of filter paper and store in amber-coloured bottles. Prepare fresh stock when crystals develop more than slightly brown colour. The compound is stable for about 2 months if stored under proper conditions.

Note

When stored under toluene, it remains stable and colourless for a longer period.

METHOD 4

The method is suitable in the presence of vitamins B_6 and B_{12}.

Standard solution

(a) 16 mcg/ml thiamine hydrochloride in 0.1 N sulphuric acid.
(b) 16 mcg/ml thiamine hydrochloride in 0.01 N sodium hydroxide.

Sample solution

Extract the sample with water and then 2 equal volumes are diluted separately with 0.1 N sulphuric acid and 0.01 N sodium hydroxide to get a concentration of 16 mcg/ml.

The absorbance of the acid solution is measured at 265 nm using alkaline solution in the reference cell. The method obeys Beer's law in the concentration range of 8 to 56 mcg/ml.

METHOD 5

This method is based on simultaneous spectrophotometric determination of thiamine (B_1) and pyridoxine (B_6) in the presence of vitamin B_{12} using iso-absorption point method. Record the spectra of standard solutions of vitamin B_1 (20 mcg/ml) and vitamin B_6 (20 mcg/ml) in 0.1 N hydrochloric acid. The solutions exhibit iso-absorption point at 276 nm and maximum for vitamin B_6 at 291 nm and for vitamin B_1 at 247 nm.

By applying absorbance ratio method and using two analogous equations, the amount of both the vitamins can be estimated.

$$C_1 = \frac{Q_0 - Q_2}{Q_1 - Q_2} \times \frac{A_1}{a_1} \qquad \text{...(1)}$$

$$C_2 = \frac{Q_0 - Q_1}{Q_2 - Q_1} \times \frac{A_1}{a_1} \qquad \text{...(2)}$$

where

C_1 = concentration (g/L) of thiamine hydrochloride in the sample;
C_2 = concentration (g/L)of pyridoxine hydrochloride in the sample;
Q_0 = ratio of absorbance value of unknown binary mixture at two wavelengths (291 : 276);
Q_1 = ratio of absorbance values of thiamine hydrochloride (20 mcg/ml) at two wavelengths (291 : 276);
Q_2 = ratio of absorbance values of pyridoxine hydrochloride (20 mcg/ml) at two wavelengths (291 : 276);
A_1 = absorbance values of the sample at iso-absorption point (276 nm);
a_1 = absorptivity of components at iso-absorption point (276 nm).

Absorptivity (a_1) at 276 nm	21
Q_1 (Vitamin B_6) (291 : 276)	2.0
Q_2 (Vitamin B_1) (291 : 276)	0.119
Q_0 (Sample) (291 : 276)	to be determined

Note

1. The values of Q_1, Q_2 and a_1 as noted above are mean of 5 determinations on standard solutions of both vitamins (20 mcg/ml).
2. These values are likely to differ from laboratory to laboratory. Hence these values are required to be determined on the available instrument and placed in record for future use.

Several market preparations (tablets and injections) containing three vitamins were analysed. Lignocaine, common preservatives and excipients do not interfere. Analgin present in one of the formulations along with three vitamins interfere in this method.

Working example

Each ml of the formulation is labelled to contain:

Vitamin B_1	50 mg
Vitamin B_6	25 mg
Vitamin B_{12}	500 mcg
Lignocaine	1% w/v

1 ml of the above formulation was diluted to 100 ml with 0.1 N hydrochloric acid and 2 ml was subsequently diluted to 100 ml with 0.1 N hydrochloric acid. Absorbance of the resultant solution was measured at 276 and 291 nm and absorbance ratio of the mixture calculated.

Q_2 (vitamin B_6) = 2.00
Q_1 (vitamin B_1) = 0.110
Absorbance of the mixture at 291 nm = 0.265
Absorbance of the mixture at 276 nm = 0.395

$$Q_0 = \frac{0.265}{0.395} = 0.670$$

Absorptivity at 276 nm = 21

Calculations

$$\text{Amount of vitamin B}_1\text{ (mg/ml)} = \frac{Q_0 - Q_2}{Q_1 - Q_2} \times \frac{A_{276}}{21} = \frac{0.67 - 2.00}{0.119 - 2.00} \times \frac{0.395}{21}$$

$$= 13.30 \times \text{dilution factor}$$

$$= 13.30\left(\frac{100}{1} \times \frac{100}{2}\right) \times \frac{1}{1000}$$

$$= 66.5 \text{ mg}$$

$$\text{Claim} = 50 \text{ mg}$$

Usually 20% overages of the vitamins are added.

$$\text{Amount of vitamin } B_2 \text{ (mg/ml)} = \frac{Q_0 - Q_1}{Q_2 - Q_1} \times \frac{0.395}{21} = \frac{0.67 - 0.119}{1.881} \times \frac{0.395}{21}$$

$$= \frac{0.55}{1.881} \times \frac{0.395}{1}\left(\frac{100}{1} \times \frac{100}{2}\right) \times \frac{1}{1000}$$

$$= 27.5 \text{ mg}$$

$$\text{Claim} = 25.0 \text{ mg}$$

The method was tried on several formulations with satisfactory results.

METHOD 6

This is based on the formation of coloured ion-pair complex between vitamin B_1 and alizarin-violet-3B in the aqueous phase of pH 4.5, which is extractable into chloroform.

Reagents

1. Potassium acid phthalate–sodium hydroxide buffer, pH 4.5.
2. 0.2% w/v solution of alizarin-violet-3B (CI No. 60725).

Standard solution

200 mcg/ml of pure thiamine hydrochloride in water.

Sample solution

Different solid and liquid formulations are either diluted or extracted with water to get a concentration of 200 mcg/ml.

Procedure

To 0.5 ml of the sample and standard solutions add 2 ml of dye solution, 6 ml of buffer solution and water to get 10 ml. Add 25 ml of chloroform. Shake for 2 minutes, separate chloroform layer and measure its absorbance at about 575 nm against reagent blank. Vitamins and other ingredients usually present along with vitamin B_1 do not interfere, even when they are present 15 folds excess.

Choline chloride, panthenol, pantothenyl alcohol, riboflavine, nicotinic acid, nicotinamide, ascorbic acid, folic acid, pyridoxine, vitamin B_{12}, sodium chloride, glucose, sucrose, gelatin, urea and lignocaine do not interfere.

METHOD 7

Reagents

1. 0.05% w/v solution of p-N,N-dimethylphenylenediamine dihydrochloride (DMPD).
2. 0.1% w/v solution of chloramine-T.
3. Glycine–sodium hydroxide buffer, pH 8.5-10.

Standard solution

500 mcg/ml of thiamine hydrochloride in water.

Sample solution

(a) Tablets: Powdered sample material equivalent to 50 mg of vitamin B_1 is dissolved in water, filtered and diluted to 100 ml with water (500 mcg/ml).

(b) Syrups, liquids and injections: An appropriate aliquot of the composite sample is diluted with water to produce 500 mcg/ml.

Procedure

To 2 ml of the sample and standard solutions add 10 ml of buffer solution, 2 ml of 'DMPD' solution and 2 ml of chloramine-T solution. Keep aside for 5 minutes and dilute to 25 ml with buffer solution. Measure the absorbance of the coloured complex at about 450 nm against reagent blank. The method obeys Beer's law over a concentration range of 10-80 mcg/ml. The coloured complex is stable for at least 5 hours. Water soluble vitamins and choline chloride do not interfere in this method.

Probable Reaction Mechanism

Chloramine-T first oxidizes DMPD to N-chloroquinonediimine (NCQDI) and subsequent coupling of NCQDI at methylene group of the molecule.

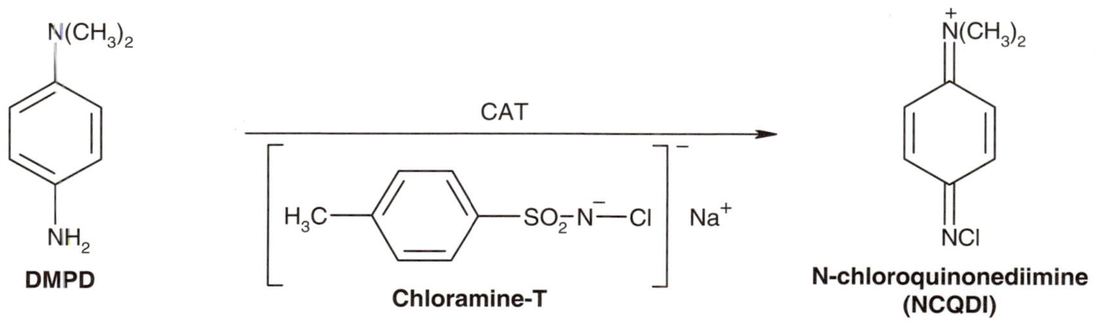

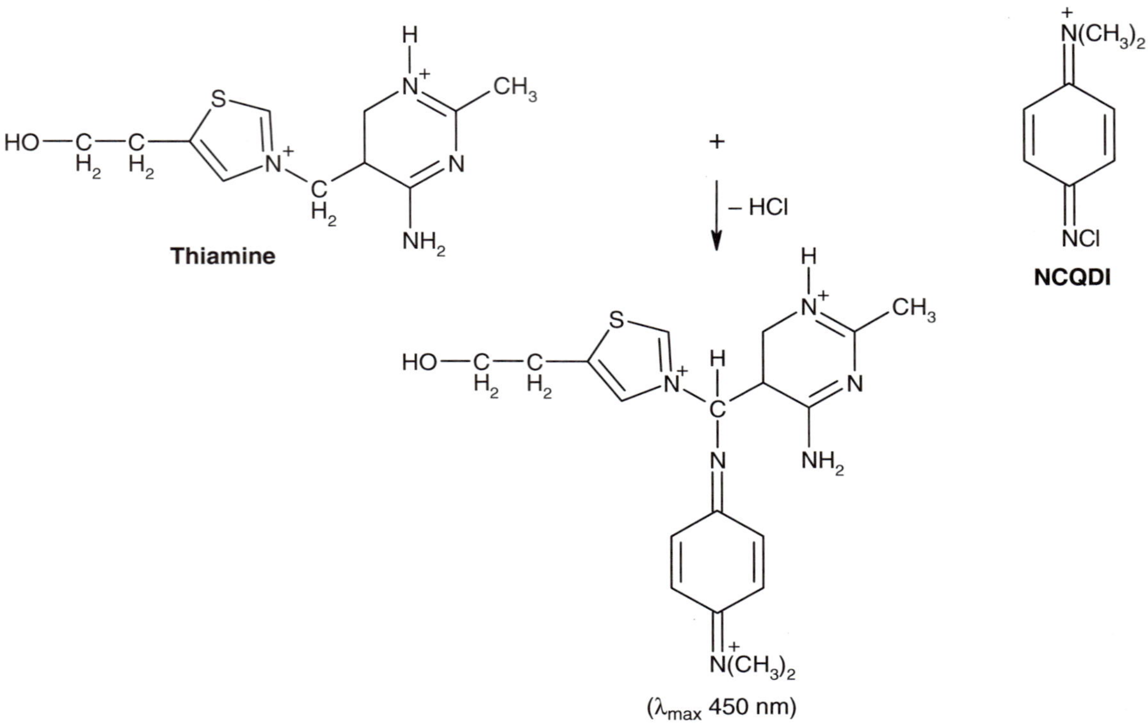

METHOD 8

Reagents

1. Bromothymol blue solution: 62.44 mg of the dye is dissolved in chloroform to make 250 ml.
2. Buffer solution, pH 6.6: To 50 ml of 0.2 M potassium hydrogen phosphate add appropriate volume of 0.2 M sodium hydroxide and dilute to 20 ml with water.

Standard solution

Stock solution of thiamine hydrochloride or thiamine mononitrate is prepared in water. Working standards may be prepared freshly in phosphate buffer, pH 6.6 (20 mcg/ml).

Sample solution

Appropriate quantity of the sample is extracted or diluted with buffer of get concentration of 40 mcg/ml.

Procedure

To 10 ml each of sample and standard solutions add 10 ml of dye. Shake vigorously and separate chloroform layer. The aqueous layer is further extracted with three 10 ml portions of chloroform. Combine the chloroform layer and make up to 50 ml. Centrifuge and measure the absorbance of clear solution at about 420 nm. Calculate the results by comparison.

Note

1. The method obeys Beer's law in the concentration range of 5-20 mcg/ml.
2. Decomposition products of thiamine and other vitamins likely to be present do not interfere.
3. In liquid formulations, if alcohol is present it should be removed by gently heating the sample before assay as alcohol will interfere in assay.

Reference

V.D. Gupta et al., *J. Pharm. Sci.*, **57**, 112, 1968.

METHOD 9

Reagents

1. 4.5% w/v solution of sodium nitrite in water.
2. Phenol buffer: 0.85 ml of phenol diluted to 100 ml with methanol.
3. 1% w/v solution of thymol blue in methanol (indicator).
4. Sodium bicarbonate–sodium hydroxide solution: 2.88 g of sodium bicarbonate and 2.0 g of sodium hydroxide are dissolved in water to produce 100 ml.
5. 2 N sodium hydroxide.
6. 0.635% w/v solution of 4-aminoacetophenone in 0.1 N hydrochloric acid.
7. Diazotizing reagent: To 1.66 ml of 4-aminoacetophenone solution add 1.66 ml of sodium nitrite solution. Wait for 15 min and dilute to 10 ml with sodium nitrite solution.

Standard solution

100 mcg/ml of thiamine mononitrate/hydrochloride in water.

Sample solution

Extract accurately weighed quantity of powdered sample with water to get solution of 100 mcg/ml in respect of thiamine mononitrate/hydrochloride.

Procedure

To 5 ml each of sample and standard solutions add 30 ml of buffer solution, 0.9 ml of indicator, 0.9 ml of 2 N sodium hydroxide, 75 ml of sodium bicarbonate–sodium hydroxide solution and 7.5 ml of diazotizing reagent. Then add 25 ml of xylene or toluene and shake vigorously for 10 min. Allow the layers to separate and measure absorbance of xylene layer at about 550 nm against blank prepared by using water instead of sample/standard.

Note

1. If the sample is not coloured, extraction with xylene is not necessary; the solution after reaction with diazotized reagent may be diluted with isopropyl alcohol for measurement at 550 nm.
2. Common water soluble vitamins and iron do not interfere.

Probable Reaction Mechanism

Thiamine reacts with diazotized reagent to give purple-red complex (λ_{max} 550 nm).

$$NaNO_2 + HCl \longrightarrow NaCl + HNO_2$$

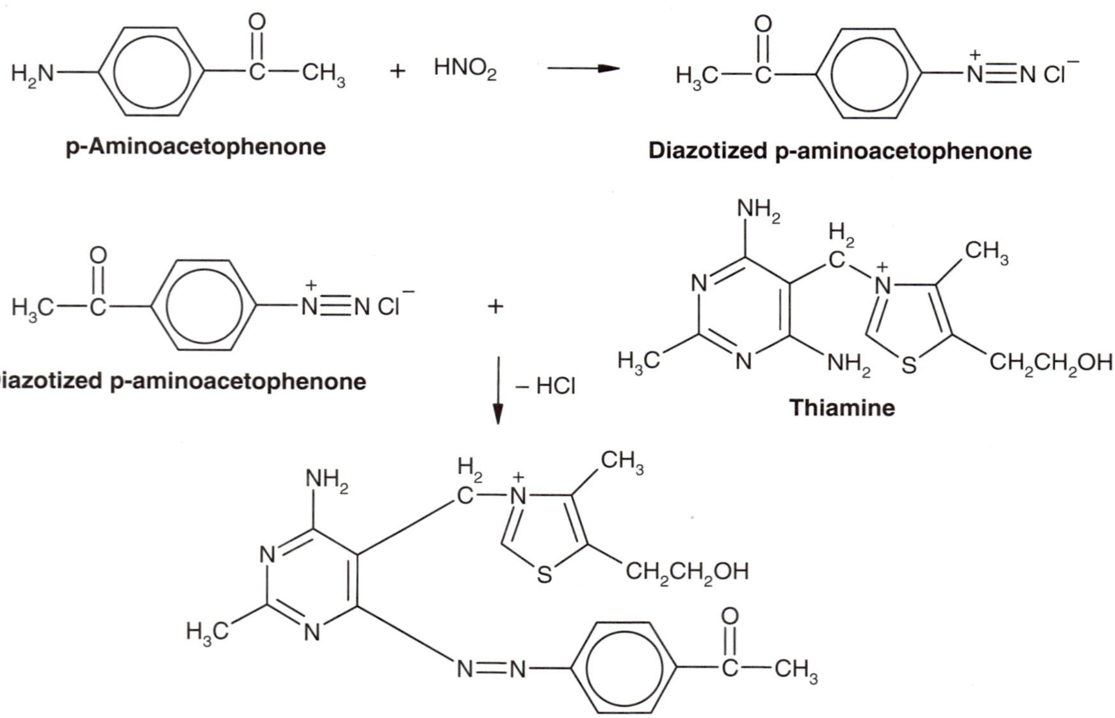

Purple-red complex
(λ_{max} 550 nm)

Reference

M.E. Auerbach, *J. Am. Pharm. Assoc.*, **29**, 313, 1940.

Note

Diazotized phenylhydrazine-1-sulphonic acid sodium salt gives similar reaction as explained earlier.

METHOD 10

Nirmal Chandar & Balasubramanian have described a spectrophotometric method for the estimation of thiamine.

Reagents

1. 0.05 M and 0.1 M solution of sodium hydroxide.
2. 2 mg/ml solution of zinc acetate in water.
3. 0.02% solution of potassium dichromate in water.
4. 1.5% solution of N,N-diethyl-p-phenylenediamine in cold mixture of sulphuric acid - water (15 : 65 v/v).

Sample and standard solutions

50 μg/ml of thiamine hydrochloride in water.

Procedure

To 0.5 ml each of sample and standard solutions add 5 ml of 0.05 M sodium hydroxide solution and 1 ml of zinc solution. Heat in a boiling water-bath for 45 min, cool, add 1 ml of amine reagent and 2 ml of dichromate solution, dilute to 25 ml with water and measure the absorbance of the solution at 670 nm against reagent blank.

Probable Reaction Mechanism as proposed by the authors

This method is based on the ability of Zn^{++} salt to form zinc sulphide on heating with an alkaline solution of thiamine. The zinc sulphide so formed is changed to hydrogen sulphide on acidification which reacts with the amine reagent to give a stable ethylene blue dye (λ_{max} 670 nm). Zinc (II) in the presence of alkali and heating causes quantitative desulphurisation of thiamine leading to the formation of H_2S.

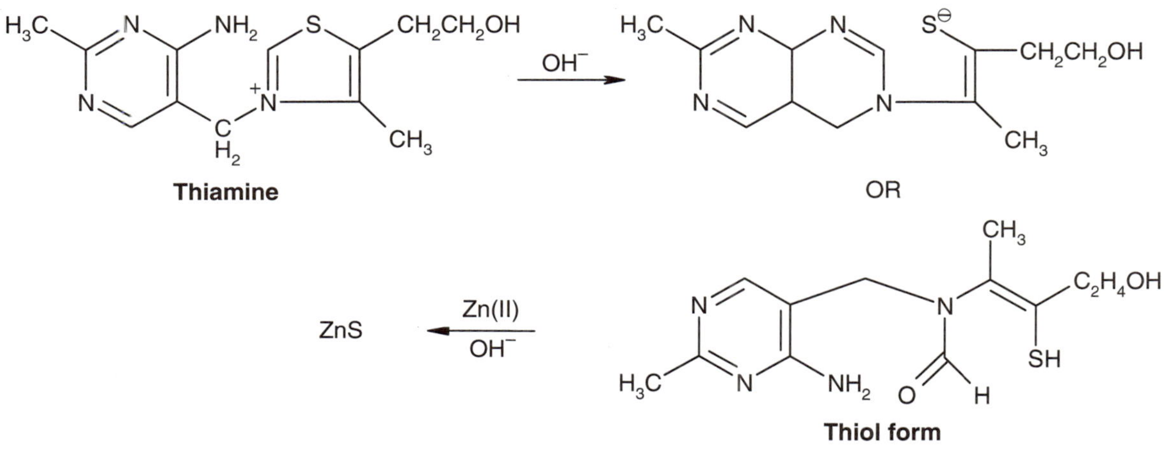

$$ZnS + H^+ \longrightarrow H_2S$$

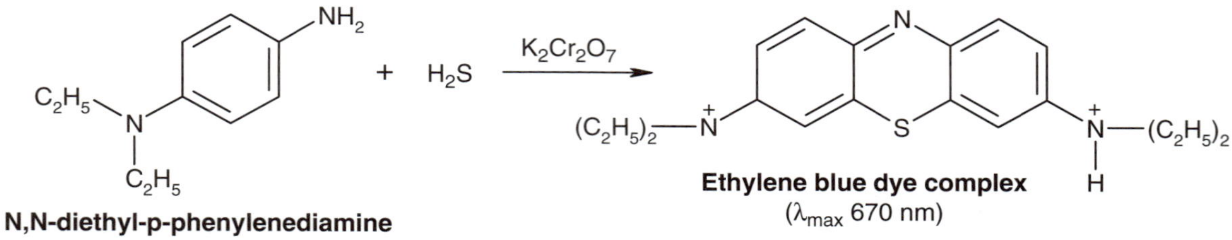

Reference

V. Nirmal Chandar & N. Balasubramanian, *Indian Drugs*, **26(5)**, 233-237, 1989.

In acidic medium, methylene group between two heterocyclic molecules is nucleophilically degraded (hydrolysis) to give pyrimidine derivative and thiazole derivative.

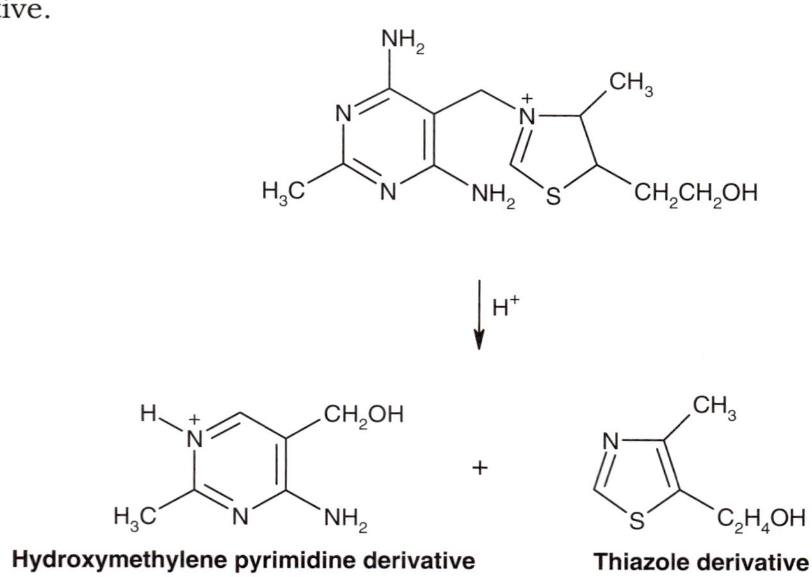

Pyrimidine derivative can be used for quantitative estimation as NH_2 group can be diazotized and coupled with NED.

A spectrophotometric method based on colour reaction with 2,6-dichloro-p-benzoquinone-4-chlorimine (DDQ) in the presence of methanolic hydrobromic acid (HBr) was applied to thiamine propyldisulphide and thiamine disulphide. 'DDQ' — Gibbs' reagent is well-known chromogen reagent for phenolic compounds.

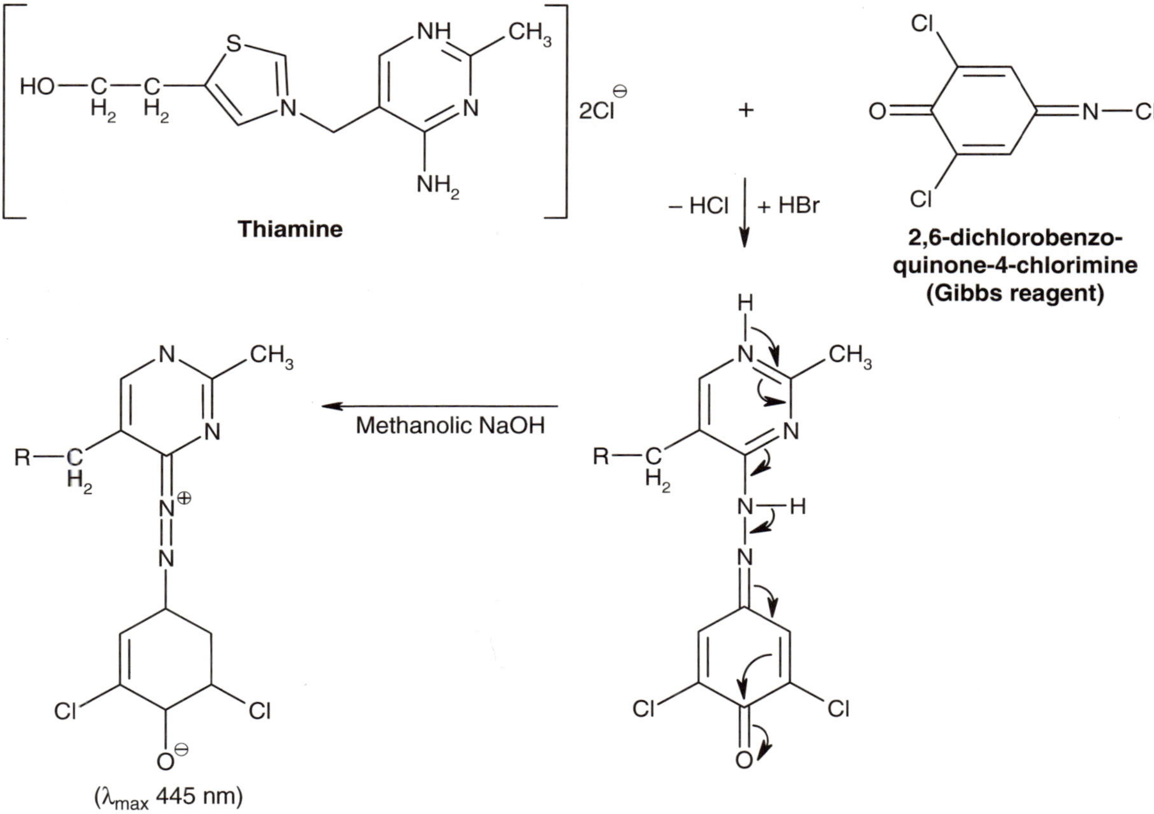

Note

This method is suitable for thiamine disulphide and thiamine propyldisulphide.

Reference

M.V. Sivarama Krishnan, S.N. Mahajan & G. Rama Rao, Analyst, **101**, 601-610, 1976.

General reaction for phenolic drugs involves oxidative coupling with N,N-dimethyl-p-phenylene diammonium dihydrochloride (DMPD). The reaction is carried out in the presence of oxidizing agent [$K_3Fe(CN)_6$] in slight alkaline medium ($NaHCO_3$). The coupling forms highly coloured indaniline dyes extractable into chloroform. In case of para-substituted phenolic drugs, the substituent facilitates formation of quinoidal form of phenol undergoing indaniline coupling with the displacement of para substituent. In general, the drugs reported to undergo this coupling are ICHQ, DIHQ, amoxycillin, dithranol, oxymetazoline, resorcinol, phenylephrine hydrochloride, pyridoxine, thymol, paracetamol, vitamin E, terbutaline, salbutamol sulphate and triamcinolone.

Probable Reaction Mechanism

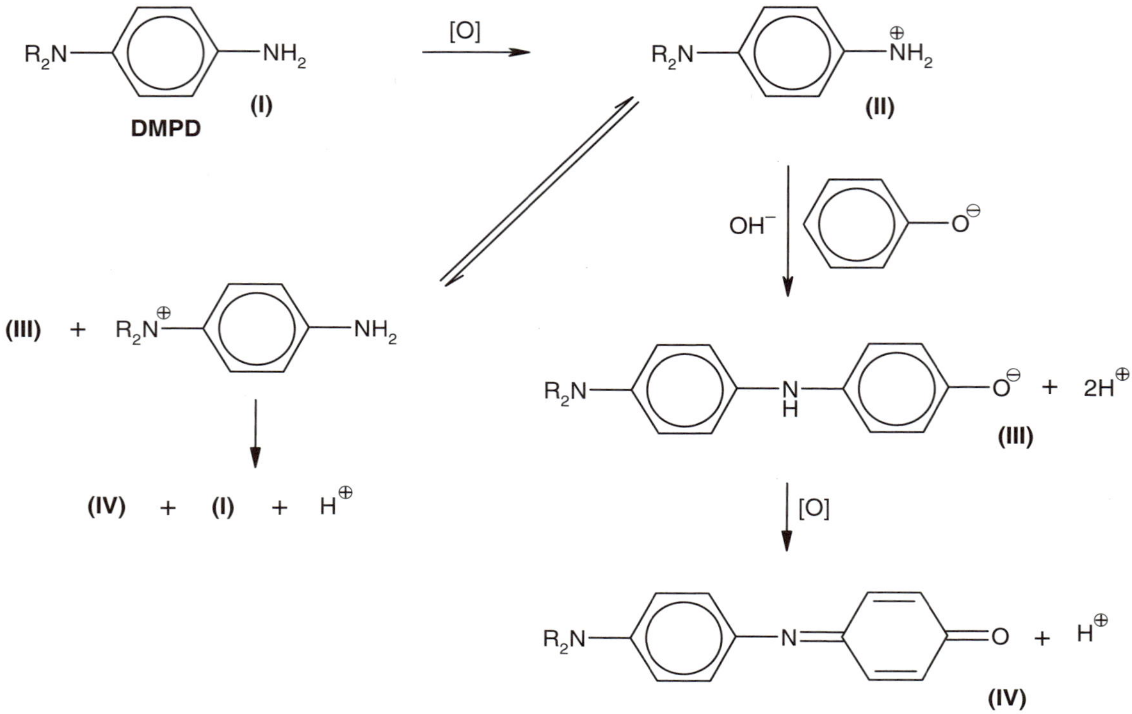

Reference

R.T. Sane, R.S. Samani, S.V. Desai, M.L. Kubal, V.G. Nayak & A.D. Nadkarni, *Indian Drugs*, **22(11)**, 592-596, 1985.

Gupta & Jain described a fluorimetric method using phosphomolybdic acid as fluorogenic reagent in alkaline medium.

To appropriate quantity of the sample/standard, 2 ml of phosphomolybdic solution (0.1%) was added followed by 5 ml of sodium hydroxide solution (0.4%) and the resulting solution was subjected to fluorescence measurements (Exc: 370 nm; Em: 400 nm).

Reference

M.K. Gupta, C.L. Jain & J. Kasliwal, *Indian Drugs*, **29(8)**, 372-374, 1992.

A spectrophotometric method based on fluorescence quenching effect of thiamine on hemoglobin-catalyzed reaction of H_2O_2 with L-lysine is reported by Yahong Chen et al. (2011). Fluorescence quenching (decrease in fluorescence) effect of thiamine is directly related to its concentration.

Probable Reaction Mechanism

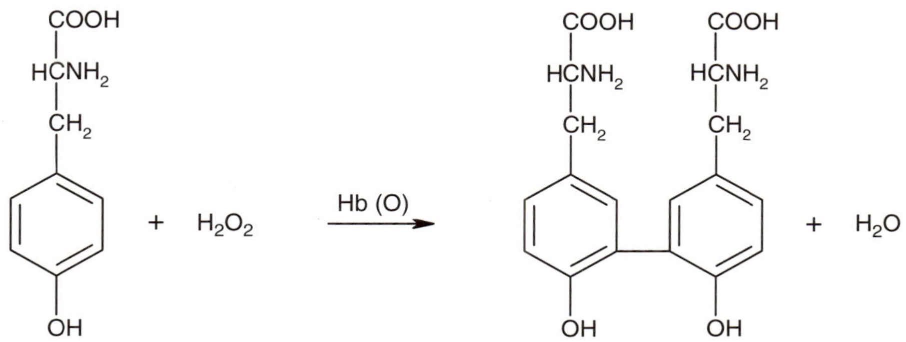

L-Tyrosine Fluorescence dimer

Reference

Yahong Chen, Jianfu Zhang, Fengshou Tian & Yinghua Zhang, *Asian J. Chem.*, **23(5)**, 2169-2171, 2011.

Formulation 2

Riboflavine (Vitamin B_2)

METHOD 1

Reagents

1. 0.1% w/v solution of methyldopa in 0.1 N hydrochloric acid.
2. 0.4% w/v solution of ortho-aminophenol in alcohol.
3. 0.1 M, 1 M and 4 M ammonium hydroxide solution.

Standard solution

Prepared by dissolving in distilled water 50 mg of the compound previously dried for 2 hours at 105°C. To this add 1 ml of 0.1 N sodium hydroxide to clear the solution, followed by 1 ml of glacial acetic acid to preserve the solution. The volume is made to 250 ml with distilled water to give 200 mcg/ml of riboflavine. Ten ml of the stock solution is further diluted with water to 100 ml to give 20 mcg/ml.

Sample solution

The sample solution is prepared by dissolving and diluting the sample with water to give a concentration of 20 mcg/ml. The colour coating in the case of tablets is removed by rubbing the tablet with cotton wetted with water and/or organic solvent.

Procedure

(a) **Methyldopa:** In clean, dry 10 ml graduated test tubes, 3 ml of standard solution and 3 ml of sample solution are taken separately. 5 ml of 0.4 M ammonia and 0.5 ml of the reagent are added and diluted to the mark with water. Absorbance is measured at 445 nm against reagent blank after about 10 minutes and results calculated by comparison.

(b) **Ortho-aminophenol:** In 10 ml graduated test tubes, 3 ml of standard solution and 3 ml of sample solution are taken. Add 1.5 ml of reagent, 2 ml of 4 M ammonia and dilute to the mark with water. Absorbance is measured at about 440 nm against a reagent blank after about 10 minutes and results calculated by comparison.

Probable Reaction Mechanism (Methyldopa)

Amino group of methyldopa reacts with carbonyl group at C-4 of riboflavin.

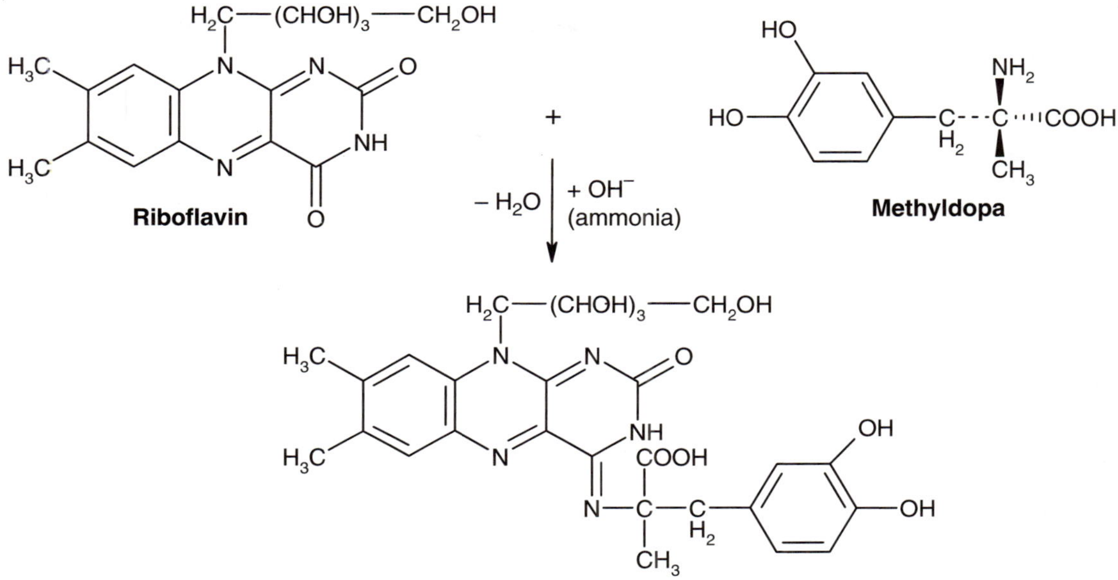

Condensed product
(λ_{max} 445 nm)

Probable Reaction Mechanism (o-Aminophenol)

It is similar to the reaction with methyldopa.

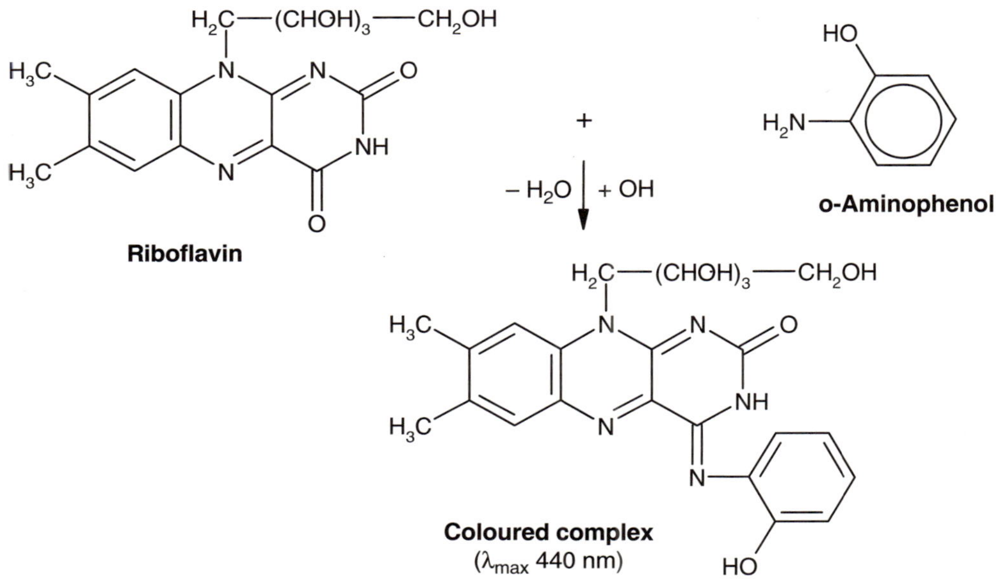

Coloured complex
(λ_{max} 440 nm)

The following compounds do not interfere up to the minimum folds indicated in brackets. Thiamine (8), Niacinamide (2), Pyridoxine (5), Calcium pantothenate (3), Ascorbic acid (33), Calcium glycerophosphate (65), Magnesium oxide (15), Manganese sulphate (1), Phosphorus (6), Copper sulphate (1), Zinc sulphate (0.5), Vitamin B_{12} (0.004), Folic acid (1), Calcium phosphate (25), Manganese glycerophosphate (8).

Reference

R.T. Sane & U.M. Vaidya, *J. Ind. Chem. Soc.*, **56**, 308-309, 1979.

Riboflavin, lactoflavin and vitamin B_2 are synonyms. Neutral riboflavin solution in UV radiation exhibits yellow-green fluorescence with λ_{max} 223 nm, 267 nm, 373 nm and 445 nm, the last being responsible for yellow colour of the substance. Fluorescence being pH dependant, in strong acid and strong alkali or reducing agent, the compound does not fluoresce, so anion and cation do not fluoresce i.e. acid or alkali or reducing agent shall quench fluorescence of the compound.

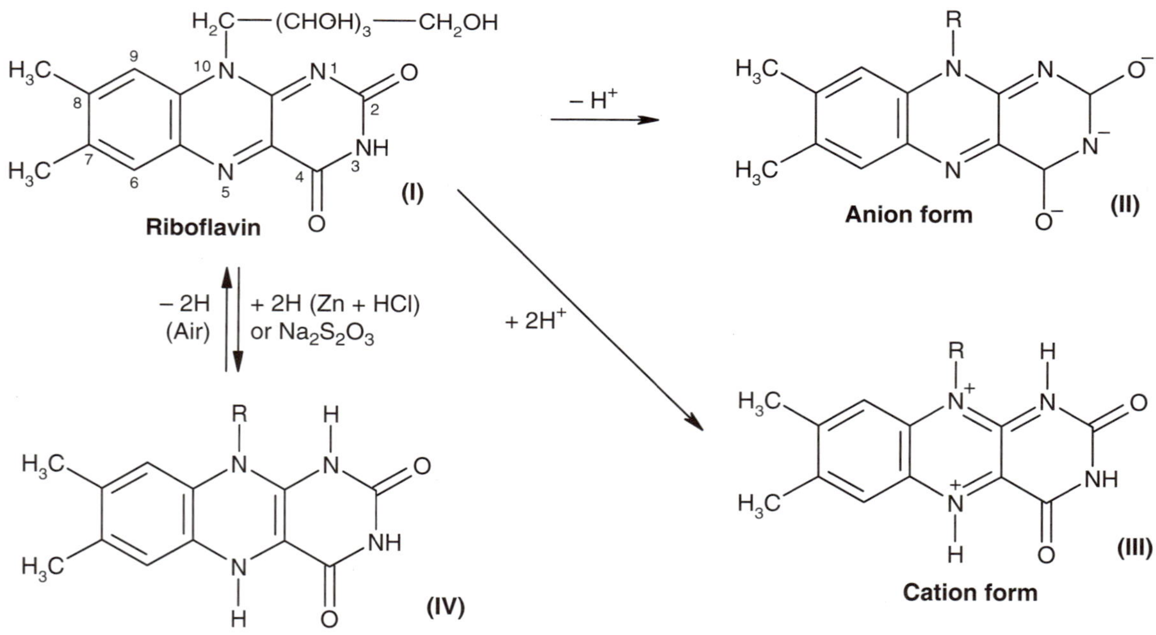

Dihydroriboflavin
(Nitrogen at positions 1 and 5 gets hydrogenated. Compounds II, III and IV do not fluoresce.)

Reference

Pharmaceutical Chemistry (Vol. 2) by H.J. Roth, p. 656.

In alkaline medium, hydroxide ion attacks at position 10a and the product formed is urea which can form the basis for quantitative estimation of the drug.

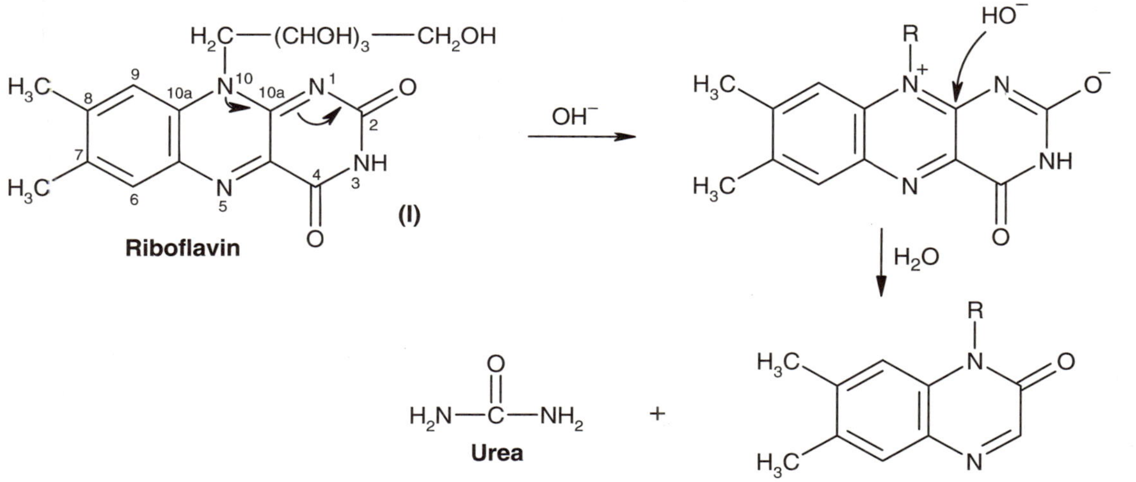

METHOD 2

In preparations containing diastase, papain, pepsin, vitamin B_1, vitamin B_6, niacinamide and choline dihydrogen citrate the following method gives reliable results.

Standard solution

To 100 mg of accurately weighed pure vitamin B_2 add 2 ml of glacial acetic acid and dilute to 500 ml with water and treat as under sample solution.

Sample solution

Weigh accurately sample equivalent to 200 mcg of vitamin B_2, add 0.2 ml of 5 N sodium hydroxide and 0.5 ml of glacial acetic acid. Heat on boiling water-bath, cool and extract with 20 ml of n-butanol shaking vigorously. Allow the layers to separate and measure extinction of alcoholic layer at 445 nm. Treat the standard similarly and calculate the results by comparison.

METHOD 3

This method is based on chromatographic separation over a column of talc, followed by colorimetric measurements. Talc is one of the weakest adsorbents, but has sufficient adsorption affinity for riboflavine, whereas other constituents pass freely.

Reagents

1. Talc, purified, IP.

2. Dioxane: Its absorbance at 267, 374 and 445 nm (usual wavelength used for measurements of vitamin B_2) should not exceed 0.03.
3. 0.01 N hydrochloric acid.
4. 10% v/v and 20% v/v dioxane in 0.01 N hydrochloric acid.
5. Glass column: 200 mm × 10 mm (i.d.).

Talc: Although the mesh size of the talc is not very critical but to maintain a reasonable flow rate, finer particles have to be removed. About 50-75 g of talc is suspended in 500-700 ml of water, shake and allow to settle for about 2 min. Decant off unsettled portion and repeat the process till supernatant liquid is almost free from fine particles. After this treatment, the talc is found to have size of 25-50 micron.

Procedure

The aqueous slurry of the talc is poured into the column to get 8-10 cm working bed. The column is repeatedly washed with water till washings are colourless. The sample equivalent to 50 mcg of vitamin B_2 contained in about 5-10 ml of water is poured on the top of the column and is allowed to be adsorbed. Then wash the column with 0.01 N hydrochloric acid, followed by 10% dioxan in order to elute other constituents adsorbed on talc column. Washings are continued till the eluate is colourless. Finally elute the yellow-coloured band of riboflavin with 20% dioxan. The absorbance of yellow solution is measured at 445 nm (to maintain a flow rate of 80-100 drops per minute, the use of slight suction may be required). The above column chromatographic separation has been tried on several liquid samples containing various vitamin B group, glycerophosphates, liver extract, caffeine, panthenol etc. successfully. It is possible to eluate the entire band of riboflavine in about 3-4 ml of solvent and the method gives excellent results with recovery of more than 95%.

The above method has also been tried on yeast tablets with satisfactory results.

Note

Change the receiver when yellow band of vitamin B_2 is near the tip of the column.

METHOD 4

Reagents

1. 0.1 N sodium hydroxide.
2. Phosphate buffer (1 M), pH 6.0.
3. Glacial acetic acid.
4. 2% w/v solution of potassium permanganate.
5. Hydrogen peroxide (30%).

Standard solution

150 mcg/ml of riboflavin in 0.1 N hydrochloric acid.

Sample solution

Weigh accurately a quantity of the sample equivalent to 15 mg of riboflavin, extract with acid to make 100 ml.

Procedure

To 2 ml each of sample and standard solutions add 1 drop of phenolphthalein solution and neutralize with 0.1 N sodium hydroxide. Add 10 ml of buffer solution followed by 2 ml of acetic acid, 1 ml of potassium permanganate solution. Allow to stand for 2 minutes, neutralize pink colour with 1 ml of hydrogen peroxide. Shake vigorously and dilute to 25 ml with water.

Measure the absorption of both the solutions at about 445 nm and calculate the results by comparison.

Note

The method is applicable to most of the vitamin combinations and gives good results.

METHOD 5

Reagents

1. Acetate buffer, pH 4.0: Prepared by mixing 10 ml of glacial acetic acid and 30 ml of 1 N sodium hydroxide.
2. 1% w/v solution of potassium permanganate in water.
3. Hydrogen peroxide 30%.
4. Concentrated sulphuric acid.

Procedure

Accurately weighed quantity of the powdered sample equivalent to 1 mg of riboflavin was extracted with 1 ml of concentrated sulphuric acid. Add 30 ml of acetate buffer (pH 4) and keep in water-bath for 30 min, cool and filter. Add potassium permanganate solution till pink colour persists for 30 seconds. Add hydrogen peroxide to remove the excess colour and finally dilute to 100 ml with buffer solution. Measure the extinction at 444 nm using acetyl buffer pH 4 as blank (prepared by adding 20 mg of sodium dihydrogen sulphide to 5 ml of above solution and measuring the extinction at 444 nm within 5 seconds). Calculate the results taking 323 as value of A 1%, 1 cm at maximum, i.e., 444 nm.

Note

1. Initial with sulphuric acid removes all the impurities.
2. Various ingredients of multivitamin formulations including minerals (iron, calcium, manganese, phosphorus, magnesium) did not interfere.

METHOD 6

Reagents

1. 1 N sodium hydroxide.
2. Glacial acetic acid.
3. 5% sodium dithionate solution.

Standard solution

Weigh accurately 100 ml of riboflavin, add 30 ml of 1 N sodium hydroxide and 5 ml of glacial acetic acid. Heat on boiling water-bath and dilute to 100 ml with water. 5 ml of this solution is finally diluted to 500 ml with water (10 mcg/ml).

Sample solution

Sample equivalent to 1 mg of riboflavin is suspended in 3 ml of 1 N sodium hydroxide and 5 ml of glacial acetic acid; solution is effected by heating on water-bath. Dilute to 100 ml with water (10 μg/ml).

Procedure

To 5 ml of sample and standard solutions add 0.5 ml of sodium dithionate solution, allow to stand for 1 min and measure the absorbance at 445 nm. Then aerate the solution by shaking for 1 min and again measure the absorbance at 445 nm. The difference between the two readings is used for calculation of riboflavin contents.

Explanatory Note

On addition of reducing agent like (zinc + HCl) or sodium dithionate, the yellow colour of the compound disappears and dihydroriboflavin (leucoriboflavin) is formed which is devoid of fluorescence property and has no absorption at 445 nm. On aeration, the fluorescence property is restored due to re-oxidation to riboflavin. This is reversible alteration of the molecule.

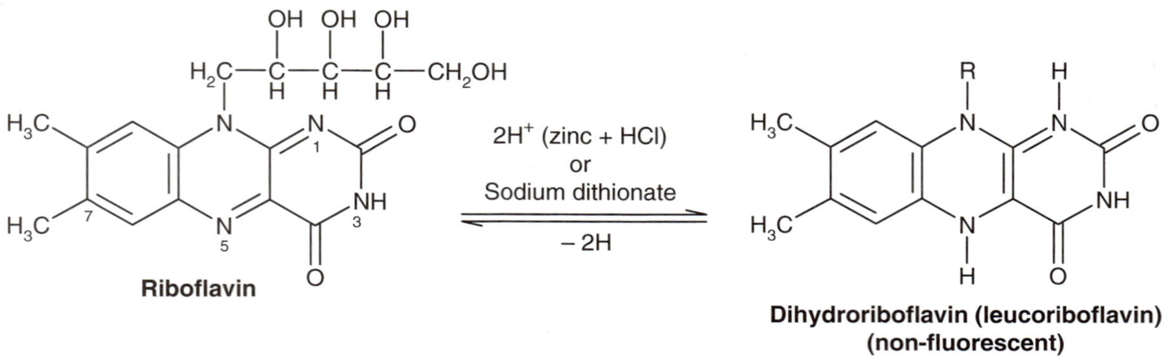

METHOD 7

This method is based on oxidation of riboflavin with periodate. Due to presence of —CH(OH)CH_2OH group in the side chain, one mole of formaldehyde is produced during periodate oxidation and the resulting formaldehyde reacts with chromotropic acid to produce complex with absorption maxima at about 570 nm. However, the chromotropic acid reagent being very corrosive this method is no more popular. Further, vitamin C or any other substance having —CH(OH)CH_2OH grouping will interfere.

Reagents

1. Chromotropic acid solution: Dissolve 1 g in 100 ml of water and mix with 450 ml of 24 N sulphuric acid.
2. 0.1 M sodium periodate solution in water.
3. 5% solution of sodium metabisulphite in water.

Sample and standard solutions

Initially the sample is suspended in water, brought into solution by adding minimum quantity of 0.1 M NaOH drop by drop, adjusted to pH 7.0 with 0.1 M HCl and dilute to volume.

Procedure

To 2 ml each of sample and standard solutions add 0.5 ml of sodium periodate solution, keep in dark for 30 min at room temperature. Then add 0.5 ml of sodium metabisulphite solution to remove excess iodate/periodate. 1 ml of the resulting solution is mixed with 5 ml of chromotropic acid solution in a glass-stoppered test tube, heat at 100°C for 30 min, cool, add 0.5 ml of half saturated solution of thiourea to remove background colour. Mix the contents and measure the absorbance of resulting purple-coloured solution at 570 nm. For reaction mechanism between HCHO and chromotropic acid, refer to details under analgin.

Probable Reaction Mechanism

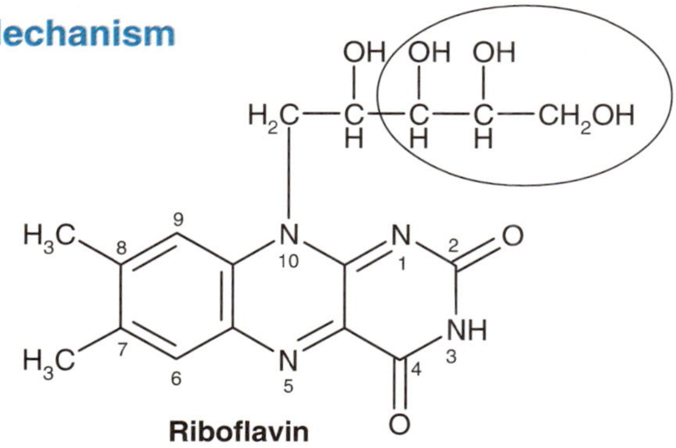

Riboflavin

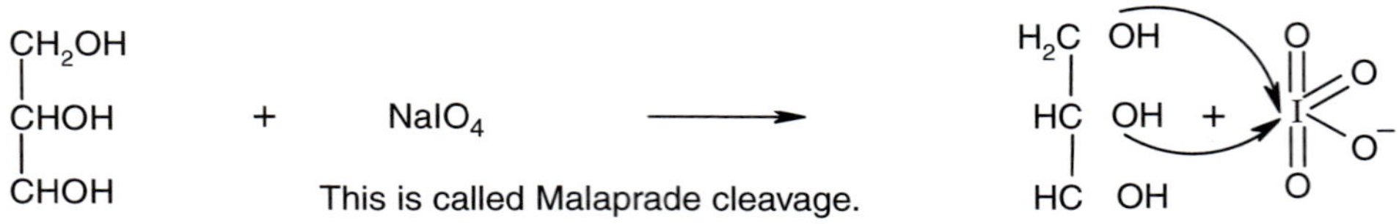

Formaldehyde is produced from ribityl component of the molecule.

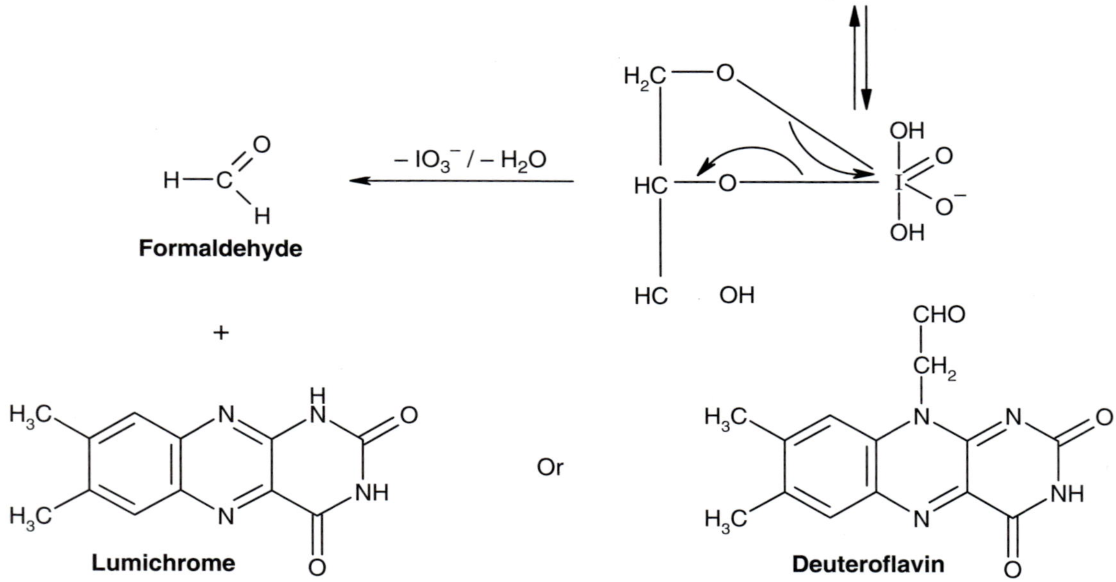

HCHO reacts with chromotropic acid to give complex (λ_{max} 570 nm).

Note

1. Only 1 mole equivalent of formaldehyde is produced by periodate oxidation of the compound.
2. Sodium metabisulphite is added to remove interference due to iodate and periodate.
3. The method is not suitable if vitamin C is present in the formulation as vitamin C also yields formaldehyde on periodate oxidation.

Reference

E.V Rao & M.N. Narayanan, *Ind. J. Pharm.*, **30**, 70, 1968.

Formulation 3

Pyridoxine hydrochloride (Vitamin B_6)

METHOD 1

The method is suitable for estimation of vitamin B_6 in the presence of vitamins B_1 and B_{12}.

Prepare solution of 10 mcg/ml of the vitamin in acidic and alkaline solutions. For details, see method 2 for vitamin B_1. Read absorbance of alkaline solution at 300 nm and 310 nm using acidic solution in reference cell. The difference between the absorbance of alkaline solution at 300 nm and 310 nm is linear to the concentration of B_6 in the range of 4-28 mcg/ml.

METHOD 2

Refer to method 3 for estimation of vitamin B_1 which is based on simultaneous spectrophotometric determination of both vitamins B_1 and B_6.

METHOD 3

Reagents

1. Buffer solution, pH 7.0: Dissolve 11.876 g of disodium hydrogen phosphate, monohydrate in sufficient distilled water to produce 1000 ml (solution A). Dissolve 9.078 g of potassium dihydrogen phosphate in sufficient distilled water to produce 1000 ml (solution B). Transfer 1000 ml of the solution A to a beaker and add sufficient quantity of solution B to get a pH of 7.0 as measured with a glass electrode (about 500 ml of the solution B is usually needed).
2. 0.1% w/v diethyl-p-phenylenediamine solution: Dissolve 100 mg of diethyl-p-phenylenediamine sulphate (p-aminoaniline diethyl sulphate) in sufficient distilled water to produce 100 ml. Prepare fresh for every estimation. This solution is sensitive to light.
3. 1% w/v potassium ferricyanide solution in water, prepare fresh.
4. 5% w/v boric acid solution in water.
5. 1 N hydrochloric acid.
6. 1 N sodium hydroxide.

Pyridoxine standard solution

Dissolve 100 mg of pure pyridoxine hydrochloride in 1000 ml of 0.1 N hydrochloric acid. This stock solution can be stored in the refrigerator for 1 to 2 months. Shortly before use, pipette 5 ml of the stock solution (pre-warmed to 25°C) into a 100 ml volumetric flask and dilute to volume with distilled water. Each ml of this standard solution contains 5 mcg of pyridoxine hydrochloride.

Sample solution

The sample solution should have a pH of 7.0 and contains approximately 5 mcg of pyridoxine hydrochloride per ml.

(a) Solid preparations: Finely powder the sample and weigh accurately a quantity equivalent to about 1 mg of pyridoxine hydrochloride into a 150 ml beaker. Add 80 ml of distilled water and 10 ml of 1 N hydrochloric acid. Heat on a steam-bath for 10 minutes, agitating occasionally. Cool to room temperature and adjust the pH to 7.0 with 1 N sodium hydroxide, using glass electrode. Transfer quantitatively to a 200 ml volumetric flask with distilled water and dilute to volume. This is the sample solution containing approximately 5 mcg of pyridoxine hydrochloride per ml.

(b) Liquid preparations: Transfer sample equivalent to about 1 mg of pyridoxine hydrochloride to a 150 ml beaker. Add 80 ml of distilled water and adjust the pH to 7.0 with 1 N sodium hydroxide or 1 N hydrochloric acid, using glass electrodes. Transfer quantitatively to a 200 ml volumetric flask with distilled water and dilute to volume. This is the sample solution containing approximately 5 mcg of pyridoxine per ml.

Procedure

Pipette into seven glass-stoppered centrifuge tubes (capacity about 35 ml) the following reagents:

	A1 (ml)	A2 (ml)	A3 (ml)	B1 (ml)	B2 (ml)	B3 (ml)	Blank (ml)
Distilled water	—	—	—	—	—	—	2
Sample solution	—	—	—	2	2	2	—
Pyridoxine standard solution	2	2	2	—	—	—	—
Buffer solution, pH 7.0	10	10	10	10	10	10	10
Chloroform	10	10	10	10	10	10	10
Diethyl-p-phenylene-diamine solution (DEPPDA)	1	1	1	1	1	1	1

Proceed successively with each of these mixtures as follows: Rapidly add 1 ml of potassium ferricyanide solution and immediately mix by shaking for 30 seconds (delayed mixing yields low assay values). Centrifuge the seven tubes for 5 minutes in order to separate the layers. Pipette 4-5 ml of the clear blue chloroform layer each of sample and standard preparations into a dry 1 cm cell and measure the absorption at 605 nm against chloroform layer of the blank preparation and calculate the results by taking average extinction of three samples and three standard solutions.

Probable Reaction Mechanism

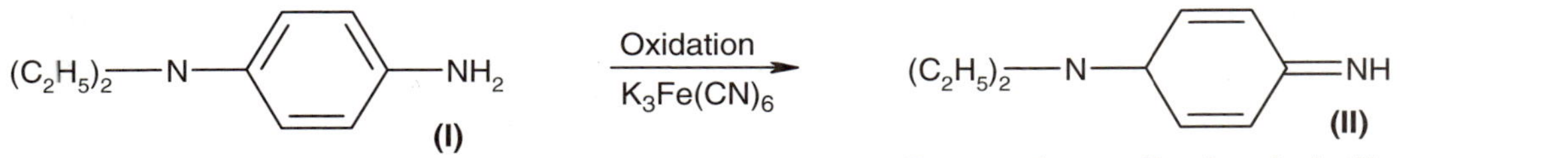

DEPPDA **Benzoquinone diamine derivative**

Benzoquinone reacts with the drug at para or ortho positions to phenolic —OH as phenolic —OH is both ortho and para-directing. As both ortho and para positions are rich in electrons and hence attack of electron-deficient reagent occurs at these positions. As ortho is occupied, the reaction shall take place at p-position.

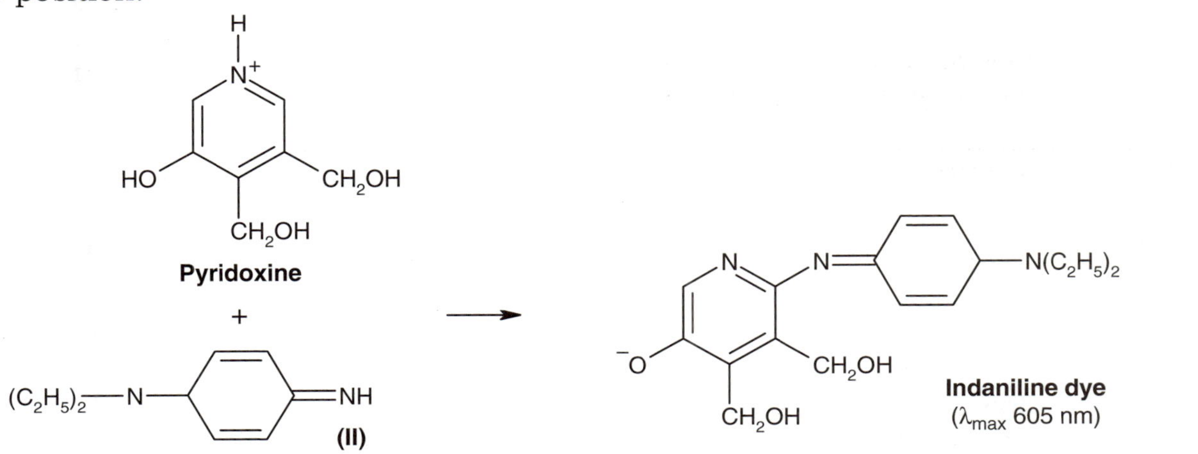

Role of boric acid is same as under method 4.

Phenolic drugs involving oxidative coupling with DMPPDA yield indaniline dyes which can be extracted into chloroform or benzene. Several p-substituted phenolic drugs, where the substituents withdraw electrons or facilitate the formation of quinoidal form of phenol, undergo the indaniline coupling with the displacement of p-substituents. If the para position is free, direct coupling shall take place.

General reaction mechanism of DMPPDA and phenolic drugs

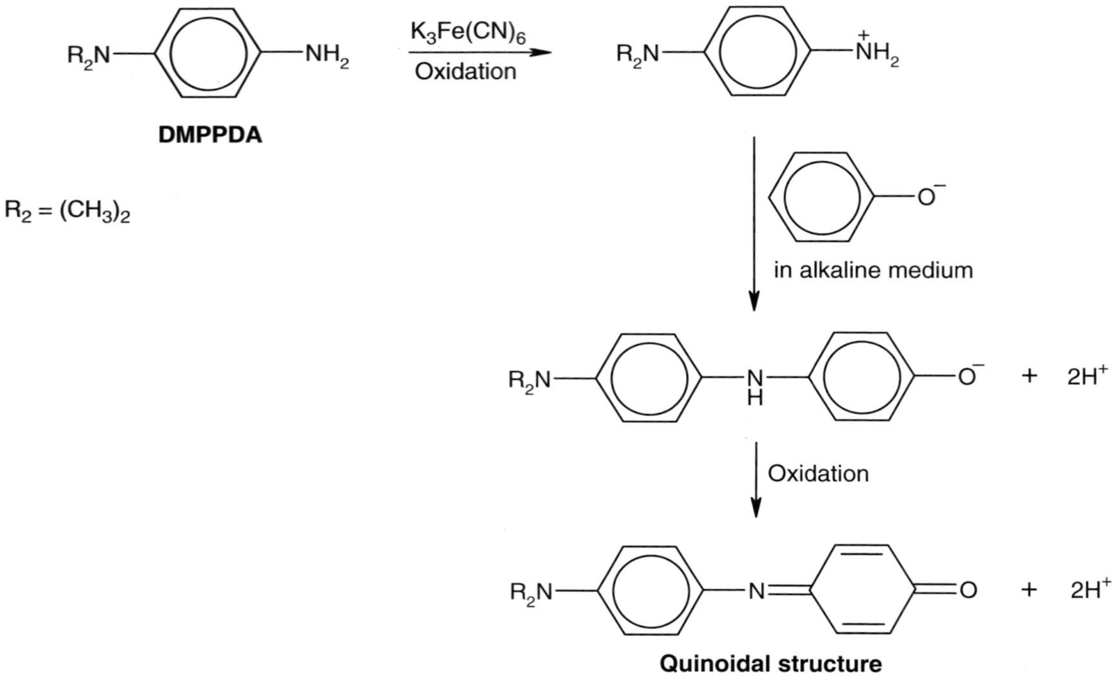

The following drugs are reported to couple with DMPPDA under reported conditions to give individual dyes with varying λ_{max}.

Compound	λ_{max} (nm)
Iodochlorhydroxyquinoline	630
Amoxycillin	596
Dibromohydroxyquinoline	620
Chlorothymol	590
Dithranol	610
Pyridoxine hydrochloride	605
Isoxsuprine hydrochloride	590
Oxymetazoline hydrochloride	490
Resorcinol	580
Nylidrin hydrochloride	596
Phenylephrine hydrochloride	600
Thymol	585
Thiamine hydrochloride	450
Oxedrine tartrate	596

Reference

R.T. Sane, R.S. Samant, S.V. Desai, M.L. Kubal, V.G. Nayak & A.D. Nadkarni, *Indian Drugs*, **22(11)**, 592, 1985.

Note

Interference due to presence of foreign substances which are soluble in chloroform and which exhibit some absorption at 605 nm can be eliminated by following method: Shake 5 ml of chloroform layers of the sample preparations and of the blank preparation for one minute with 5 ml of boric acid solution and centrifuge. Measure the extinctions of the chloroform layers again as described above and subtract their mean value from the average extinction of the original determinations. If the chloroform solution in the cells shows some haze or turbidity, this can be eliminated by slight mixing with a thin glass rod.

Natural source of vitamin B_6 contains all the three forms (I, II, II), however, only pyridoxine, the most stable of the three, is used in pharmaceutical preparations. This method is based on indophenol test, the general reaction for phenolic compounds which are unsubstituted in para position to phenolic hydroxyl group. This reaction involves coupling of pyridoxine with 2,6-dichloroquinone chlorimide (Gibbs' reagent) in buffer solution to produce blue colour (λ_{max} 650 nm). This test has been made more specific by adding boric acid as pyridoxine reacts with boric acid to form a complex which no longer reacts with chloroimide reagent. Thus, by the addition of boric acid one can differentiate pyridoxine from other phenolic substances and also from pyridoxamine and pyridoxal. These two forms of vitamin B_6 do not react with boric acid as they do not possess hydroxymethylene group at C-4. The boron chelate formed spontaneously blocks the phenolic hydroxyl group so that the para position is not activated for electrophilic attack and the reaction does not take place; thus interference due to other phenolic compounds is eliminated. Further addition of boric acid increases the specificity of the method.

Probable Reaction Mechanism

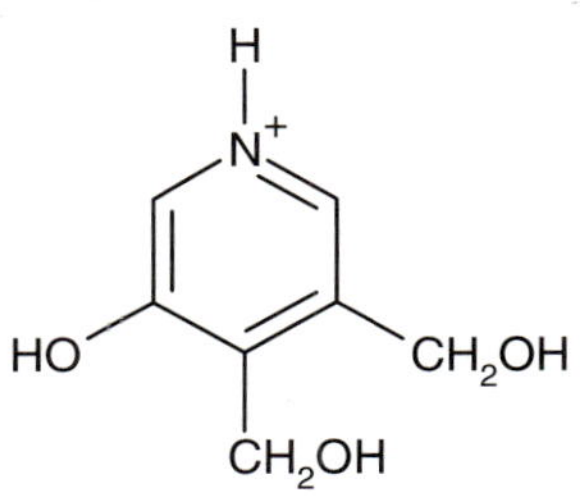

(I)
Pyridoxine

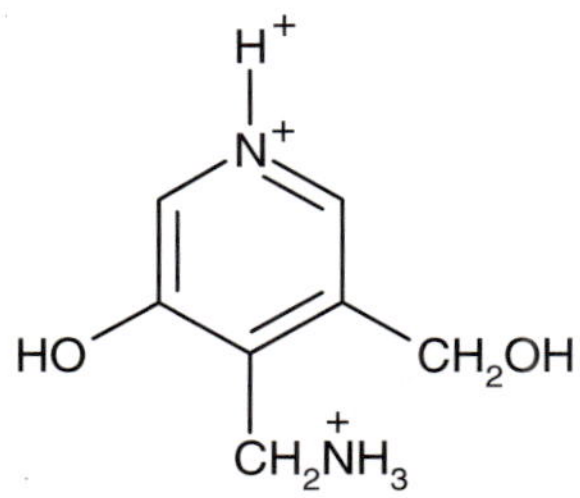

(II)
Pyridoxamine

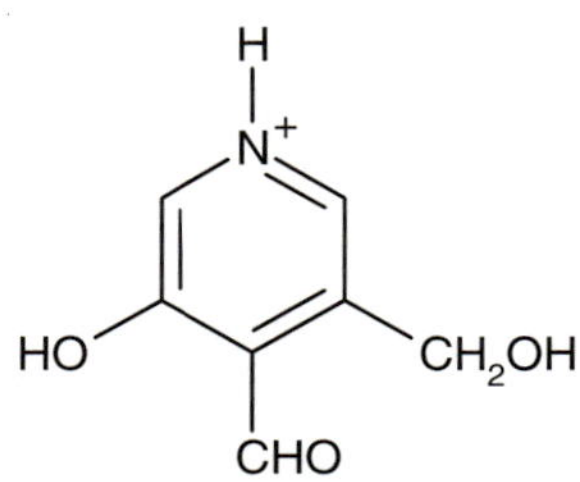

(III)
Pyridoxal

METHOD 4

Reagents

1. 20% w/v solution of sodium acetate in water.
2. 5% w/v solution of boric acid in water.
3. 1 N sodium hydroxide in water.
4. Chlorimide reagent (Gibbs reagent): Dissolve 20 mg of 2,6-dichloroquinone chlorimide in 50 ml of isopropyl alcohol. Store in refrigerator.
5. Ammonia–ammonium chloride buffer: Dissolve 8 g of ammonium chloride in 5 ml of water, add 8 ml of strong ammonia solution, dilute to 50 ml with water.

Standard solution

(a) Stock solution: 200 mcg/ml of pyridoxine hydrochloride in 0.1 N hydrochloric acid.
(b) Dilute solution: Dilute 5 ml of solution to 100 ml with water (10 mcg/ml).
(c) Working standard: Dilute 10 ml of dilute solution to 50 ml with isopropyl alcohol.

Sample solution

Weigh accurately powdered sample equivalent to 2.5 mg of pyridoxine, add 5 ml of hydrochloric acid and 100 ml of water. Digest in boiling water-bath for 45 min, cool and adjust to 250 ml with water. Filter, and to 10 ml of the filtrate add 4 ml of 1 N sodium hydroxide and make up the volume to 50 ml with isopropyl alcohol. Shake well and filter.

Procedure

To 2.5 ml each of sample and standard solutions, taken separately in 2 test tubes each, add the following in succession:

	Sample		Standard	
	(A) ml	(B) ml	(A) ml	(B) ml
Ammonium chloride buffer	1	1	1	1
Sodium acetate	1	1	1	1
Water	1	—	1	—
Boric acid	—	1	—	1

Shake well. Add 1 ml of chlorimide reagent to the respective blanks of sample and standard marked (B) and adjust the instrument to 100% transmittance at 650 nm exactly 1 min after addition of the reagent. Then add 1 ml of the chlorimide reagent to the sample and standard (marked A) and absorbances are measured at maximum at about 650 nm.

Note

As there is small progressive change within blank, the readings for sample and standard should also be taken exactly one minute after addition of the reagent and no further adjustment of the instrument should be made with the blank.

1 mole of boric acid reacts with 2 moles of pyridoxane to give a compound which no longer reacts with chlorimide reagent, hence serves as blank and also increases the sensitivity of the method. Other analogues of vitamin B_6 such as pyridoxamine and pyridoxal do not react with boric acid as they do not possess hydroxymethylene group (CH_2OH) at position 4.

Probable Reaction Mechanism

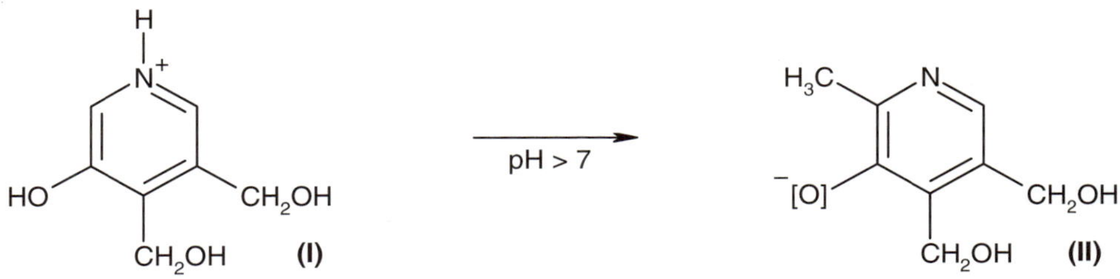

Pyridoxine **Phenolate ion**

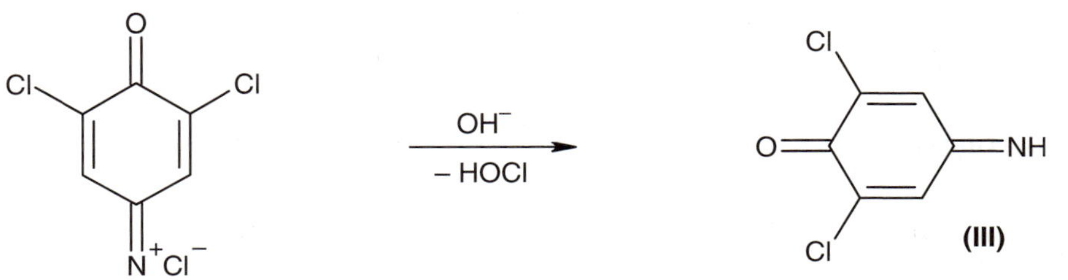

2,6-dichloroquinone-4-chlorimide (DCQ) (Gibbs' reagent) **2,6-dichloroquinonimine**

It is 2,6-dichloroquinonimine which is rapidly produced from DCQ in alkaline aqueous solution which ultimately reacts with pyridoxine.

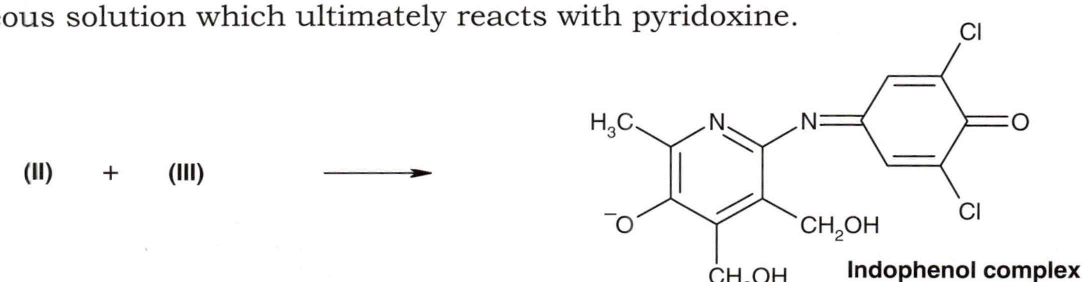

Indophenol complex
(λ_{max} 650 nm)

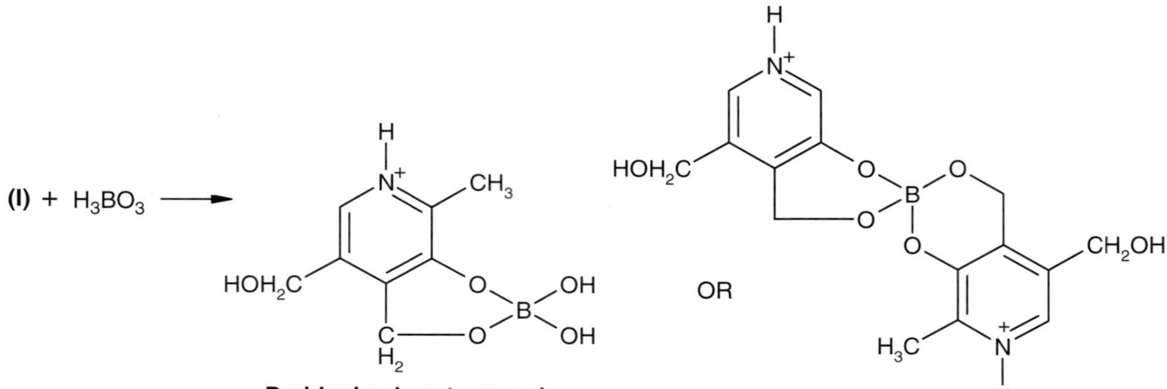

Pyridoxine borate complex

Reference

1. M.K. Gupta & C.L. Jain, *Indian Drugs*, **28(6)**, 275-277, 1991.
2. Assay of Vitamins in Pharmaceutical Preparations by M.H. Hashmi, p. 195, 1973.
3. Pharmaceutical Chemistry (Vol. 2) by H.J. Roth, p. 533.

METHOD 5

Reagents

1. 0.05% solution of p-nitroaniline: Dissolve 0.05 g of p-nitroaniline in 5 ml of methanol and dilute to 100 ml with 0.033 M orthophosphoric acid.
2. 0.1% w/v solution of sodium nitrite in water.
3. Phosphate buffer, pH 8.0: Adjust the pH of 0.5 M solution of disodium hydrogen phosphate to 8.0 with sodium hydroxide or orthophosphoric acid.
4. Acetate buffer, pH 4.25: Prepare 5% solution of sodium acetate and adjust the pH to 4.25 with acetic acid.
5. Mercury acetate solution: Dissolve 0.1589 g of mercury (II) acetate in acetate buffer of pH 4.25.
6. 0.2% solution of sodium carbonate in water.

Standard solution

10 mcg/ml of pyridoxine hydrochloride in water.

Sample solution

Weigh accurately powdered sample equivalent to 10 mg of the substance and extract with water to produce 100 ml. Further dilutions are done with water to get solution of 10 mcg/ml. For oily preparations, suspend the sample in water and extract with petroleum ether (40-60°) and use aqueous layer for analysis.

Procedure

Take 10 ml each of sample and standard solutions, add 2.5 ml of phosphate buffer (pH 8.0). In separate test tube mix 20 ml of p-nitroaniline solution and 20 ml of sodium nitrite solution. Add 2.5 ml of this solution to 10 ml each of sample and standard solutions followed by 5 ml of mercury (II) acetate solution. Make up the volume to 25 ml and measure the absorbance at 530 nm against reagent blank.

Explanatory Note

Diazotized p-nitroaniline couples with pyridoxine at position para to phenolic hydroxide in phosphate buffer. The complex in turn reacts with Hg^{++} in acetate buffer to give azo dye (λ_{max} 530 nm).

Probable Reaction Mechanism as proposed by the authors

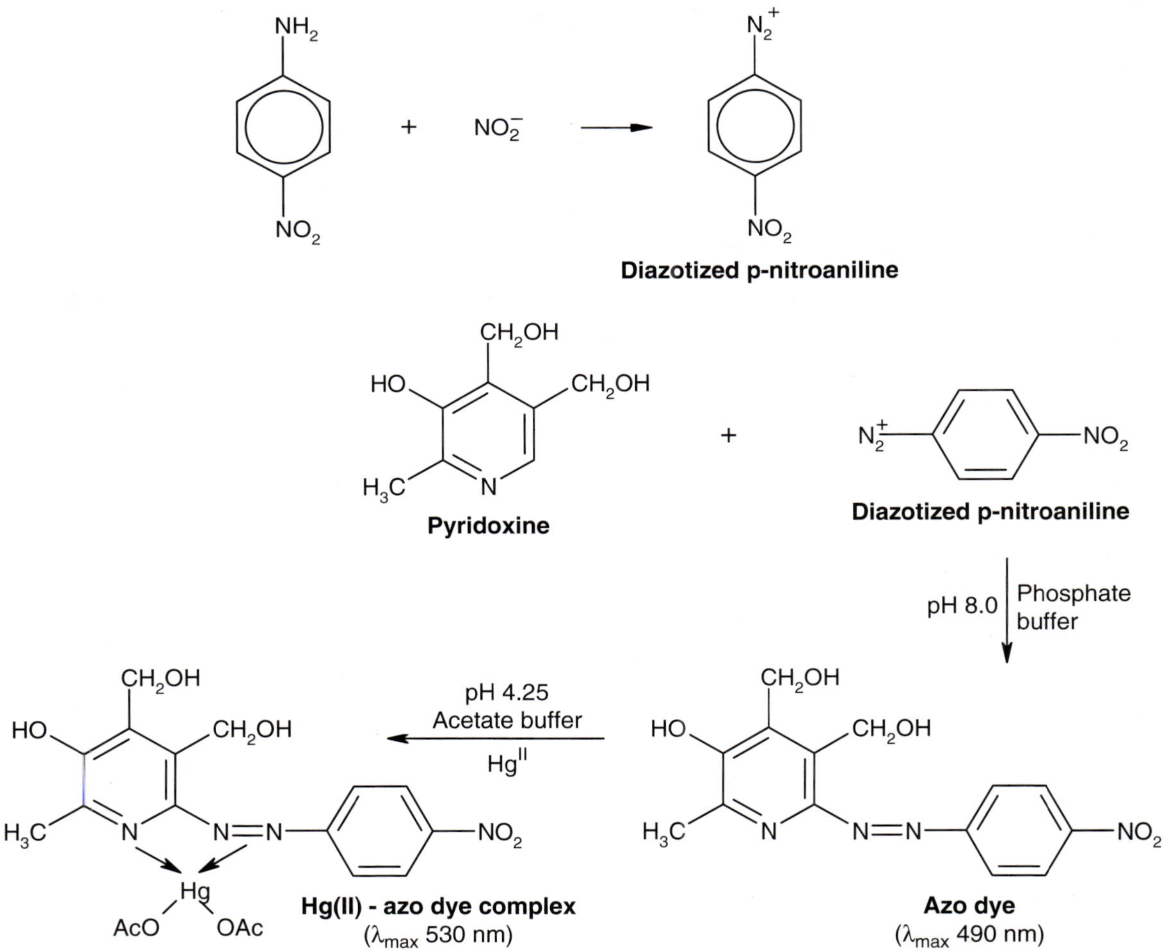

Note

1. Since the colour of the azo dye was stable for only 10 min, the colour was stabilized by complexing with Hg(II). The developed colour was stable for 24 hr. Further formation of Hg(II) complex resulted in bathochromic (490 → 530 nm) shift and hyperchromic effect (2-fold).
2. Vitamins B_1, B_2, nicotinic acid, folic acid, vitamin C and fat-soluble vitamins did not interfere.

Reference

V. Nirmal Chandar & N. Bala Subramanian, *Analyst*, **113**, 1097-1099, 1988.

Alternatively, unreacted p-nitrodiazonium ion can couple with 'NED' to give p-NA-NED azo dye (λ_{max} 545 nm).

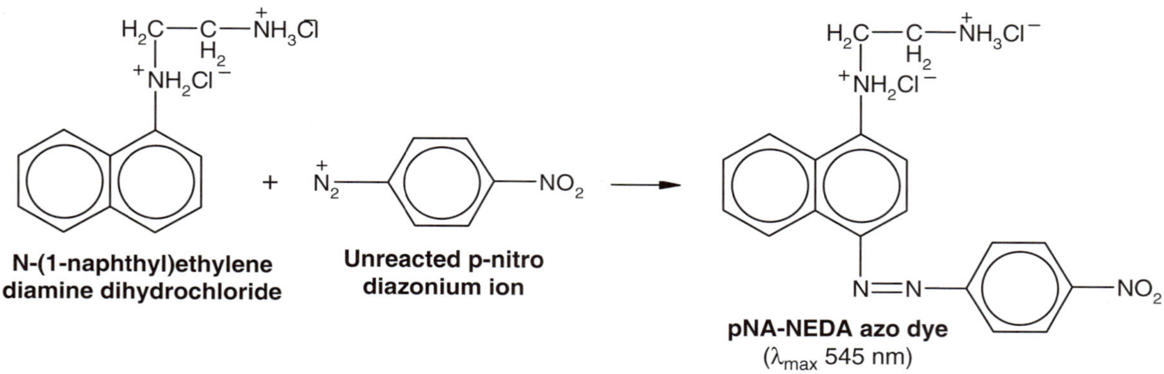

Diazotized aniline gives better results.

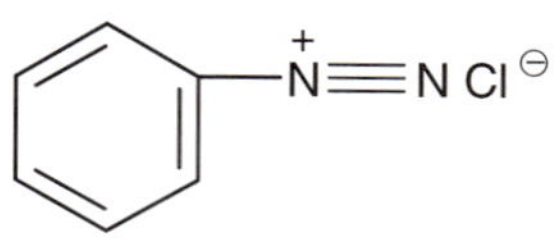

Benzene diazonium chloride

It is a cation. So active electrophilic can attack other electron-rich aromatic ring. Electrophilic attack by terminal nitrogen atom of diazonium salt forms a C–N bond to an electron-rich aromatic ring to produce a coloured azo compound.

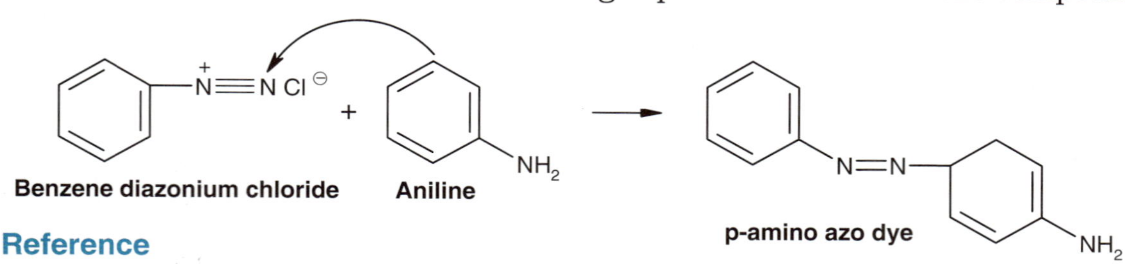

Reference

Organic Chemistry by Fox, p. 554.

METHOD 6

A spectrophotometric method involving coupling of diazotized sulphanilic acid and dapsone with the drug has been described by Sane et al. After diazotization reaction is complete, sodium carbonate solution is added to stabilize the diazonium salt and to take care of excess nitrous acid.

Reagents

1. Sulphanilamide.
2. Dapsone.
3. Acid mixture: Mix 86 ml of trichloroacetic acid with 20 ml of sulphuric acid and 94 ml of water under cold conditions.
4. 0.1% w/v aqueous solution of sodium nitrite.
5. 4% sodium carbonate solution.

Sample and standard solutions

250 μg/ml of pyridoxine in water.

Procedure

To doazotized sulphanilamide and dapsone add 0.5 ml each of sample and standard solutions and 3 ml of sodium carbonate solution, allow to stand for 3 min and measure the absorbance at 440 nm (sulphanilamide) and 465 nm (dapsone) against reagent blank.

Probable reaction mechanism proposed by the authors based on infrared and NMR studies

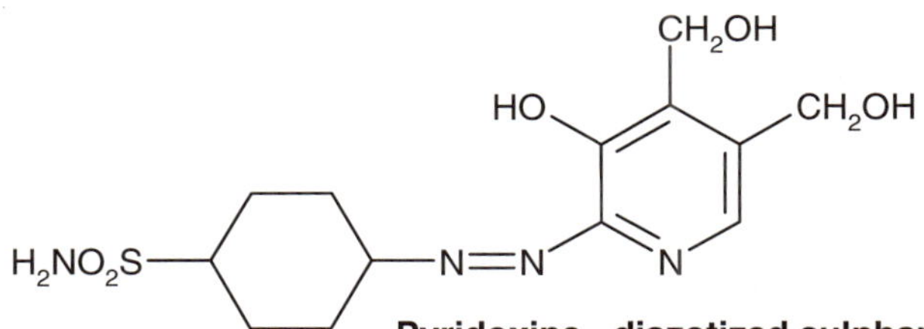

Pyridoxine - diazotized sulphanilamide complex
(λ_{max} 440 nm)

Note

Substitution can take place at para position as well.

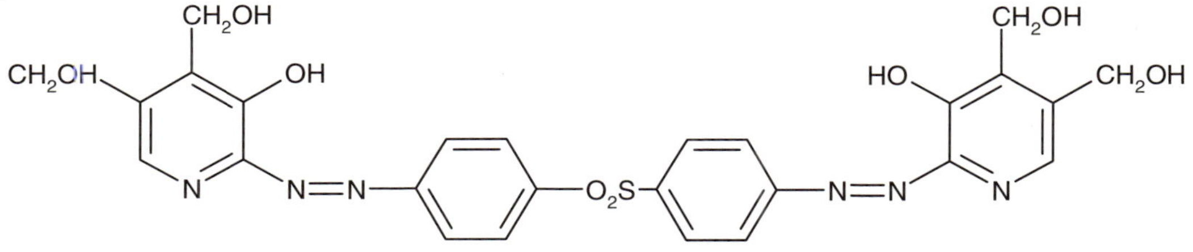

Pyridoxine - diazotized dapsone complex
(λ_{max} 485 nm)

Note

Since para position to phenolic —OH is free, these substitution reactions should take place at that position. This is similar to the reaction with diazotized p-nitroaniline method.

Note

Vitamins B_1 and B_{12} do not interfere.

Reference

R.T. Sane, V.J. Doshi & S.K. Doshi, *J. Assoc. Off. Anal. Chem.*, **66(1)**, 158-160, 1983.

METHOD 7

A spectrophotometric method based on modification of the method described by Snell & Snell (1961) has been reported by G. Ramana Rao et al. (1979). The method involves coupling of diazotized phenylhydrazine-4-sulphonic acid (DPHS) giving a stable yellow-coloured product (λ_{max} 430 nm).

Procedure

To 5 ml of the 'DPHS' solution add 2 ml of alcohol, allow to stand for 5 min and then add 2 ml of aliquot of sample and standard solutions and make up the volume to 25 ml with 0.1 M sodium carbonate solution, shake and allow to stand for 10 min and then measure the absorbance at 430 nm against reagent blank.

Note

1. The colour was stable for 4 hr.
2. Vitamins B_1 and B_{12} do not interfere.

Probable Reaction Mechanism

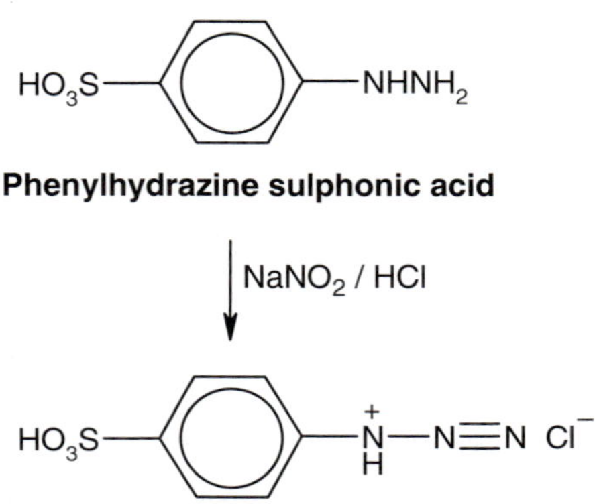

Diazotized phenylhydrazine sulphonic acid (DPHS)

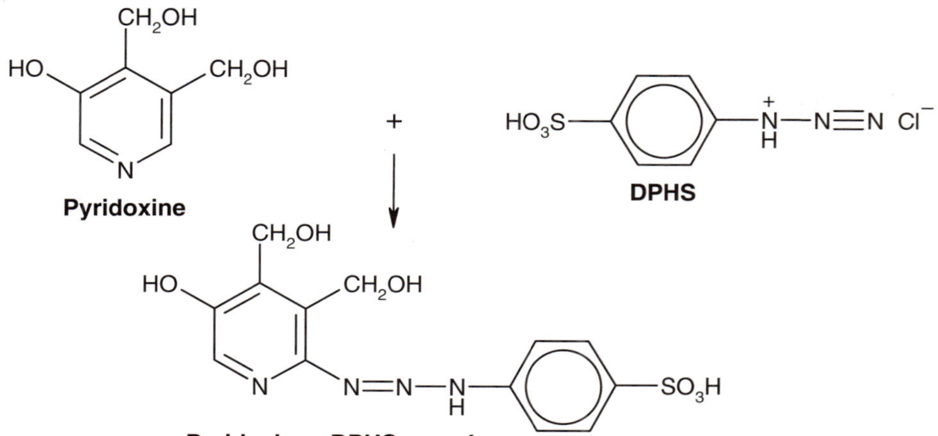

Pyridoxine - DPHS complex
(λ_{max} 430 nm)

Reference

1. Colorimetric Method of Analysis (Vol. 3) by F.D. Snell & C.T. Snell, 1961, p. 102.
2. G. Ramana Rao, M.V. Sivaramakrishna, Geeta Kanjilal & C.M.R. Srivastava, *Ind. J. Pharm. Sci.*, **41(5)**, 203-205, 1979.

METHOD 8

Reagents

1. 1% w/v solution of cerric ammonium sulphate in 0.7 M sulphuric acid.
2. 0.2% w/v solution of 3-methylbenzothiazolin-2-one-hydrazine (MBTH).

Standard solution

200 μg/ml in water.

Sample solution

Appropriate quantity of the sample extracted with water to get 200 μg/ml solution.

Procedure

To 2 ml each of sample and standard solutions add 3 ml of MBTH reagent, shake for 2 min and then add 3 ml of cerric ammonium sulphate solution, dilute to 10 ml with water and measure the absorbance at 620 nm against reagent blank.

Probable Reaction Mechanism

This is oxidative coupling of the reagent with compound having phenolic function. MBTH on oxidation loses two electrons and one proton forming a electrophilic intermediate, being the active coupling species. This undergoes electrophilic substitution at p-position to phenolic —OH group, thus forming a coloured product (λ_{max} 620 nm).

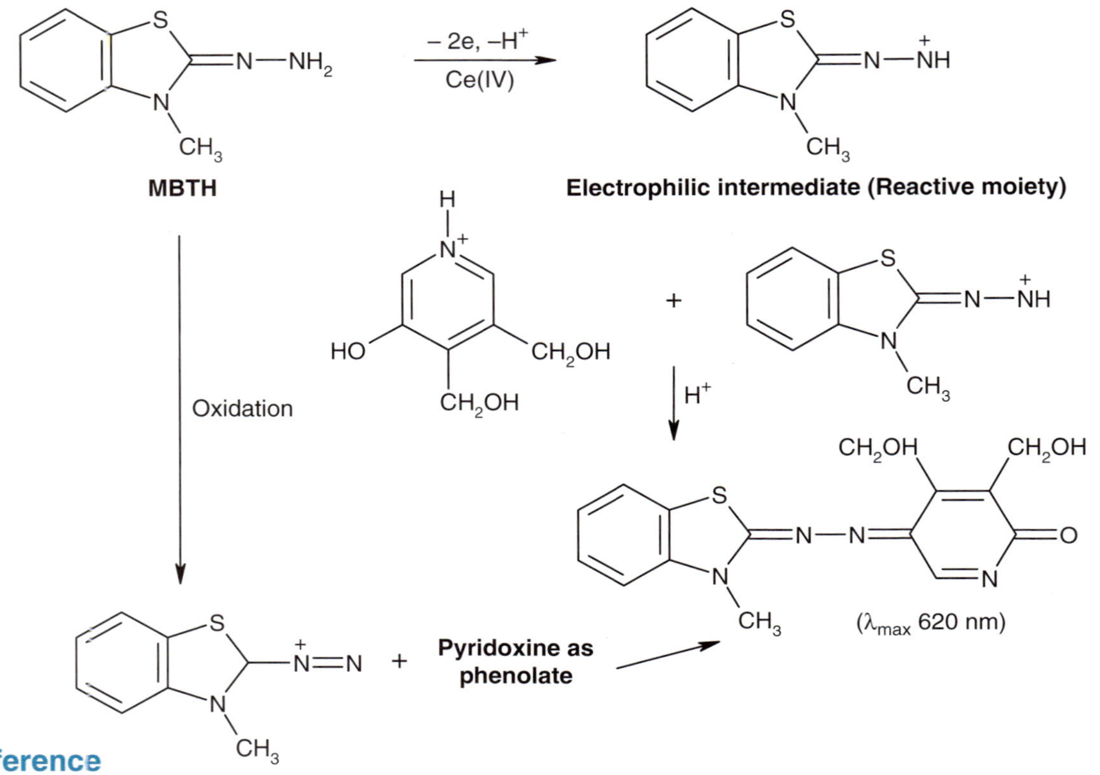

Reference

M. Narayana Reddy, Siva Prasad Rao & D. Gowri Sankar, *Indian Drugs*, **33(4)**, 569-570, 1996.

METHOD 9

Reagents

1. 1% sodium carbonate solution in water.
2. 0.4% w/v solution of 4-aminoantipyrin (AAP) in water.
3. 1% solution of ammonium persulphate in water.

Standard solution

50 μg/ml of pyridoxine hydrochloride in water.

Sample solution

Appropriate quantity of the powdered sample suspended in water, filtered and adjusted with water to get 50 μg/ml of the sample. If ascorbic acid is present, treat the sample with lead acetate, adjust the pH to 7.6 with ammonia, filter and remove excess lead as carbonate, filter and use the filtrate for the estimation of pyridoxine. To remove any interference due to pyridoxal and pyridoxamine, to one portion of the sample add 1 ml of boric acid (1%), adjust pH to 7.0 with sodium carbonate, add 1 ml of additional sodium carbonate solution and carry out the procedure as under.

Procedure

To 2.5 ml each of sample and standard solutions add 1 ml of sodium carbonate solution followed by 1 ml each of 'AAP' and ammonium persulphate solution. Dilute to 10 ml with water and after 20 min measure the absorbance of the solution at 420 nm against reagent blank.

Probable Reaction Mechanism

The method is based on oxidative coupling of pyridoxine with 4-aminoantipyrin in the presence of ammonium persulphate (oxidizing agent in alkaline medium) at para position to the phenolic group.

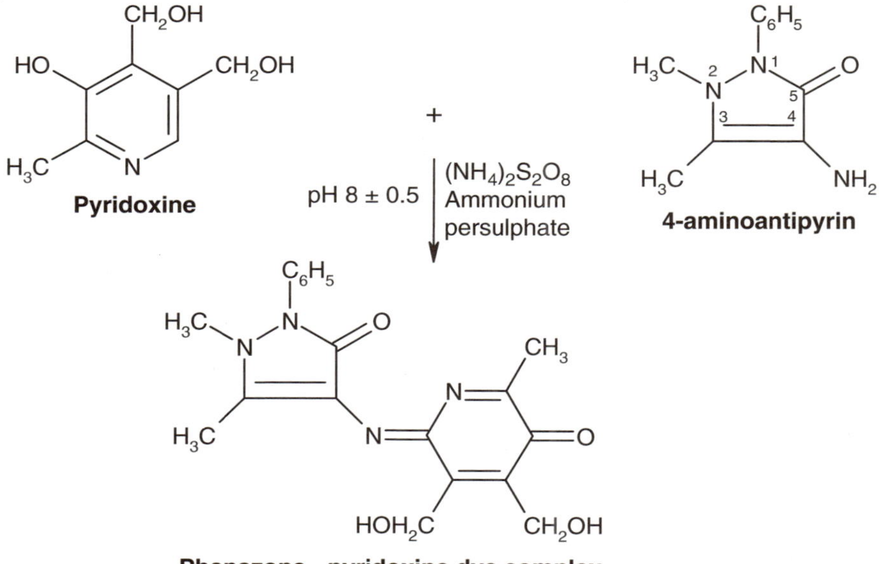

Phenazone - pyridoxine dye complex
(λ_{max} 420 nm)

Note

The reaction is similar to the one described with 'MBTH'.

Reference

V. Nirmal Chandar, Rajganesh Viswanathan & N. Balasubramanian, *Analyst*, **112(5)**, 653-655, 1987.

METHOD 10

Reagents

1. 10% ferric nitrate solution in 5% nitric acid.
2. 0.02 M 1,10-phenanthroline in water.

Sample and standard solutions

200 μg/ml in water.

Procedure

To 2 ml each of sample and standard solutions add 0.5 ml of ferric nitrate and 3 ml of phenanthroline reagent, set aside for 10 min and dilute to 10 ml with water. Measure the absorbance at 510 nm against reagent blank and calculate the results.

Probable Reaction Mechanism

Fe(3) oxidizes pyridoxine and itself gets reduced to Fe(2) which couples with tertiary nitrogen of the phenanthroline moiety. Hydroxylic group in pyridoxine gets oxidized to yield dicarboxylic derivative.

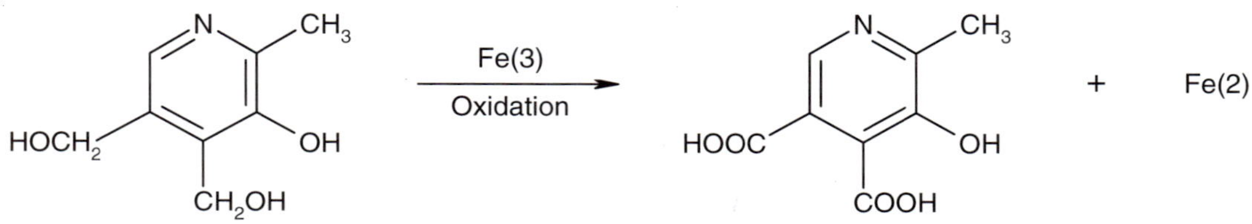

Pyridoxine **Dicarboxylic acid derivative**

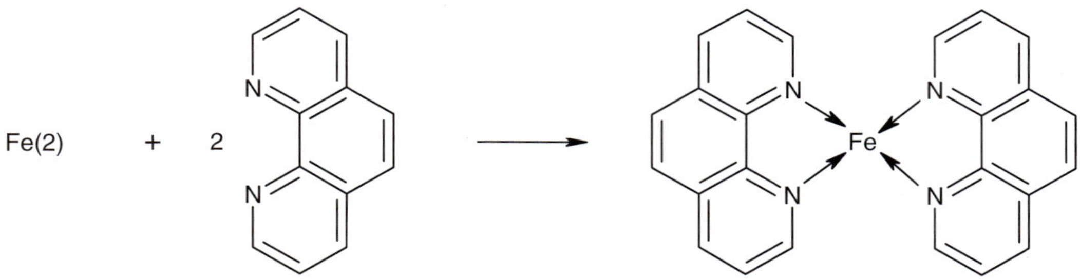

1,10-phenanthroline **Ferrous - phenanthroline complex**
(λ_{max} 510 nm)

Reference

B.S. Kuchekar, S.V. Thakkar, M.R. Hiren, P.P. Chothe & D.B. Shinde, *Ind. J. Pharm. Sci.*, **64(2)**, 158-160, 2002.

Other possibility of oxidation of the compound by ferric chloride, as explained below, leads to the formation of a brown-coloured compound (λ_{max} 480 nm).

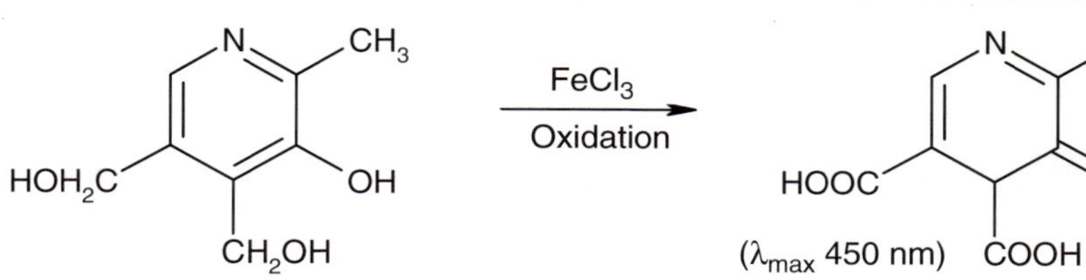

Siegel & Blake (1962) had reported a spectrophotometric method for the estimation of pyridoxal in the presence of pyridoxamine and pyridoxine based on reaction of aldehyde (—CHO) group with acetone in alkaline medium producing a yellow-coloured product.

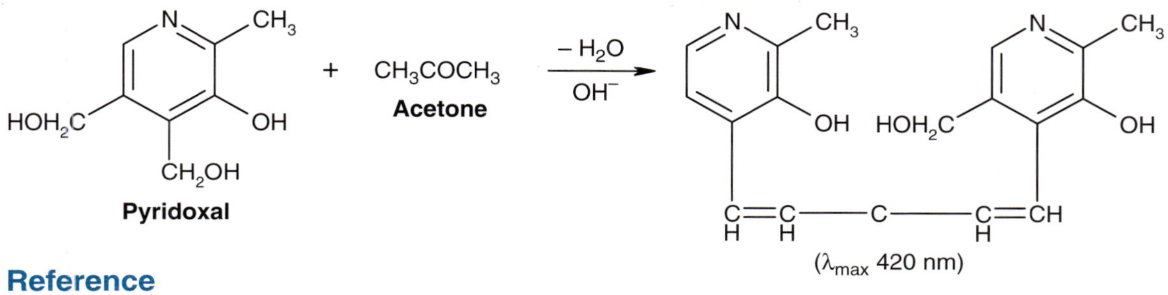

Reference

F.P. Siegel & M.I. Blake, *Anal. Chem.*, **34**, 397, 1962.

The dicarboxylic acid derivative formed after oxidation, as under method 1, on heating is converted to anhydride which on reaction with resorcinol yields a fluorescent derivative which can form the basis of an analytical method.

Probable Reaction Mechanism

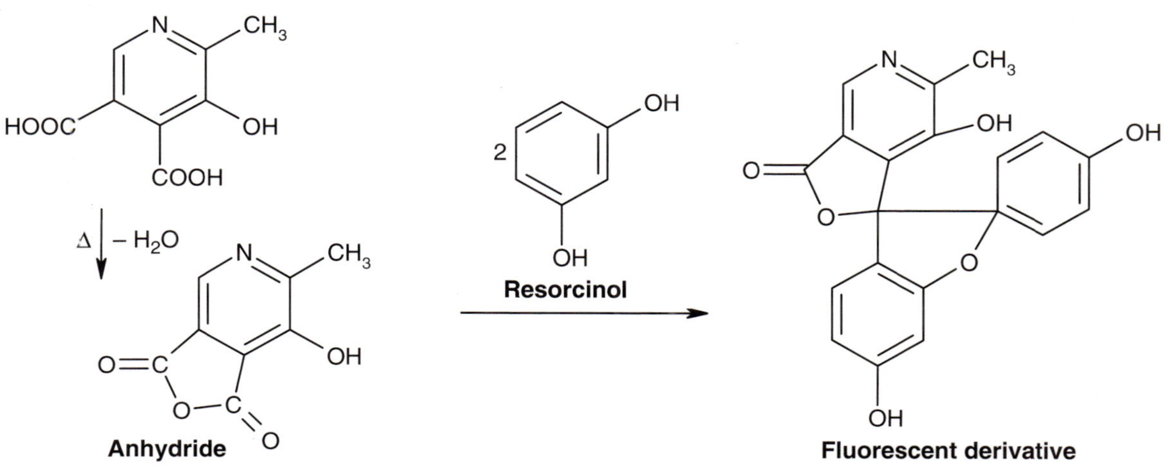

Reference

Pharmaceutical Chemistry (Vol. 2) by H.J. Roth, p. 535.

Formulation 4

Nicotinamide / Niacinamide

Ammonia distillation method when applied to nicotinamide in combination with B-complex vitamins or liver extract usually gives high results owing to the interference of volatile, titrable bases formed by the action of sodium hydroxide on the other constituents of the formulation during distillation.

A well-tried thin-layer chromatographic method is reported here for the convenience of those analysts who are well conversant with this procedure and facilities are available in their laboratories.

METHOD 1

Material and reagents

1. Glass plates (20 × 20 cm) coated with silica gel GF-254 (0.25 mm).
2. Solvents: (a) Water; (b) Ethanol–chloroform (25 : 60 v/v).
3. 0.1 N Hydrochloric acid.

Sample preparation

A. Concentrate the sample on water-bath to remove alcohol (if present) and water. Extract the semi-solid mass with dry ether. Evaporate the ether layer and take the residue in methanol for application to TLC plates.

B. To the solid mass obtained under A above, add ethanol and leave in refrigerator overnight. Decant off the supernatant liquid and adjust the volume to get concentration of 1 mg/ml of nicotinamide for application. This step ensures removal of sugars.

C. Extract the tablets, capsules directly with methyl alcohol to get 1 mg/ml concentration.

Procedure

Apply, by means of a microlitre pipette, solution obtained under A, B or C above, equivalent to 100 mcg in the form of a streak about 6 cm long, evaporating the solvent after each application with the help of hot air. Allow the plate to cool and develop the plate using solvent (a) or (b) as the case may be and allow the solvent front to travel upto 10-12 cm. Remove the plate, dry and examine under short UV

(254 nm) to locate the band of nicotinamide with the help of spot of a reference standard. Scrap off the silica gel corresponding to nicotinamide and transfer to 10 ml volumetric flask. Extract with 0.1 N hydrochloric acid by shaking for 2 minutes and adjust the volume. Centrifuge or filter and measure the extinction at about 261 nm. Calculate the results by using 454 as value of E 1%, 1 cm.

Blank: Scrap off silica gel GF 254 from the plate equivalent to the area used for samples and extract with 0.1 N hydrochloric acid in similar way.

METHOD 2

Reagents

1. Sulphanilic acid buffered solution: To 2.5 g sulphanilic acid, add 15 ml water and 2 ml dilute ammonia solution. Mix, add with stirring more dilute ammonia solution if necessary to dissolve the substance, adjust pH of the solution to 4.5 with dilute ammonia.
2. 10% w/v solution of cyanogen bromide in water.
3. Dilute ammonia solution: Dilute 2 ml strong ammonia solution to 100 ml with water.

Standard solution

100 mcg/ml of nicotinamide in water.

Sample solution

Weigh powdered sample accurately equivalent to 10 mg of the substance, suspend in water to make 100 ml, stir and filter.

Procedure

To 2 ml each of sample and standard solutions, add 2 ml of sulphanilic acid buffered solution, 5 ml water, shake well and add 2 ml of cyanogen bromide solution. Measure the extinction of both sample and standard solutions at 450 nm after 2 min against reagent blank and calculate the contents of nicotinamide by comparison.

Probable Reaction Mechanism

$$Br_2 + KCN \longrightarrow Br{-}C{\equiv}N + KBr$$

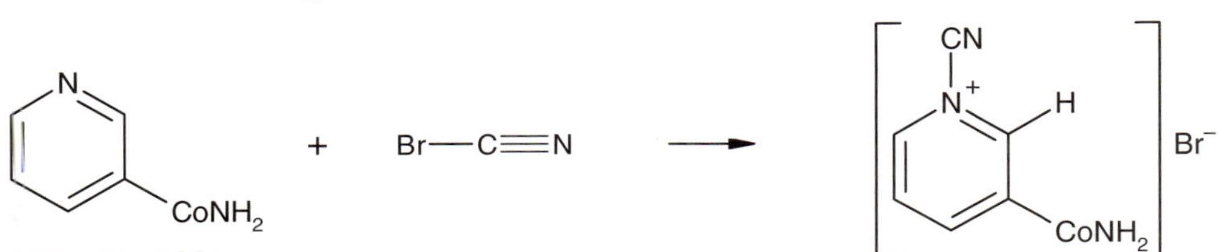

Nicotinamide

N-Cyanopyridinium bromide derivative

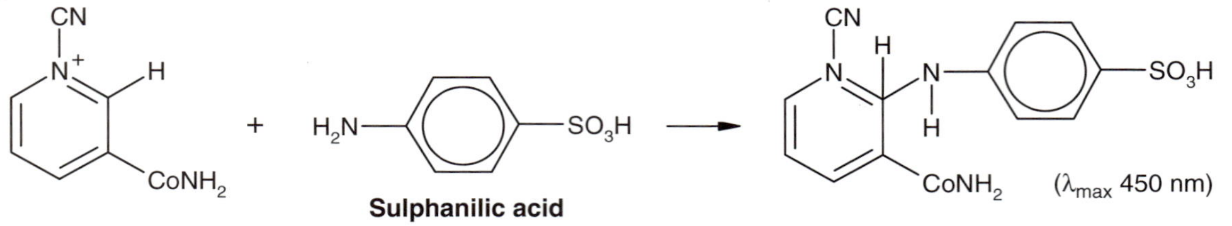

An important analytical method was proposed by J.S. Estere-Romero et al. (1995). The method involves the use of sodium dodecyl sulphate (SDS), an anionic surface acting agent giving micellar medium. The micellar medium inhibits undesirable reactions (hydrolysis and photolysis), stabilization of the reaction intermediates and increases the reaction rate.

Procedure

To 5 ml of 0.2 M sodium acetate buffer pH 5, add 5 ml of 0.5 M SDS and 2.5 ml of sample/standard solutions, followed by 5 ml of cyanogen bromide solution. After 10 min (time required for complete hydrolysis of the sample/standard), add 0.4 ml of 0.6 M arylamine solution, allow to stand for 15 min and measure the absorbance at 440 nm.

Note

Spectrophotometric method for estimation of organic compounds has been improved by use of such micellar media such as coupling of diazotized arylamine with NED, coupling of phenols with diazotized 4-aminoantipyrin.

Probable Reaction Mechanism

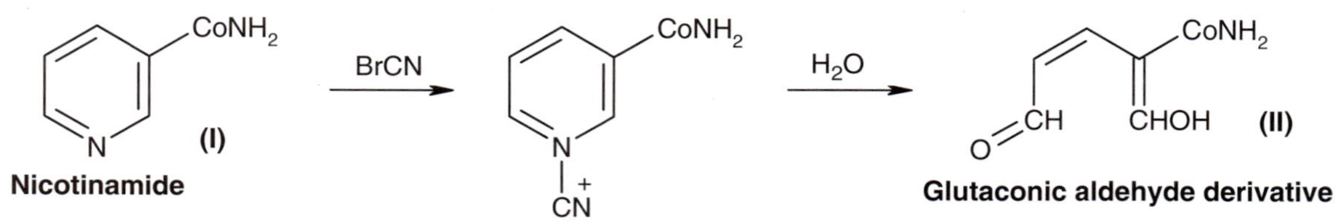

Allow to stand for 10 min to complete the hydrolysis to glutaconic aldehyde derivative.

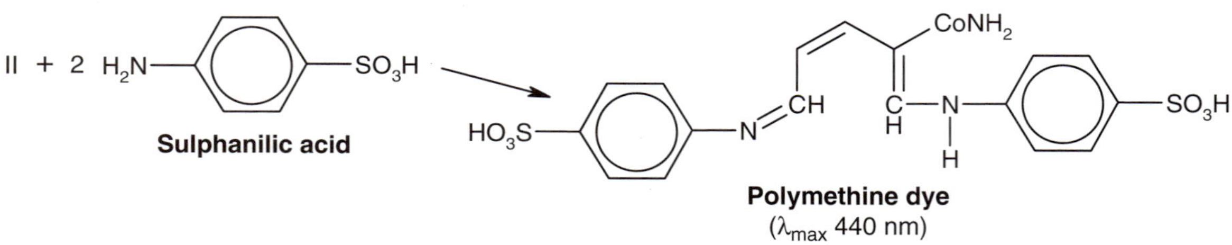

This is based on König reaction (W.J. König, *J. Prakt. Chem.*, **19**, 70, 1904).

Reference

J.S. Estere-Romero, Ll. Monferrer-Pons, G. Remis-Romos & M.C. Garcia-Alvarez-Cogue, *Talanta*, **42(5)**, 737-745, 1995.

Nudelman et al. (1976) have described a spectrophotometric method based on reaction of nicotinamide with 1-chloro-2,4-dinitrobenzene. The reaction proceeds via nucleophilic attack at C-1 of the reagent giving 2,4-dinitrophenyl pyridinium chloride. This compound when treated with sodium hydroxide develops violet colour (λ_{max} 540 nm).

Probable Reaction Mechanism

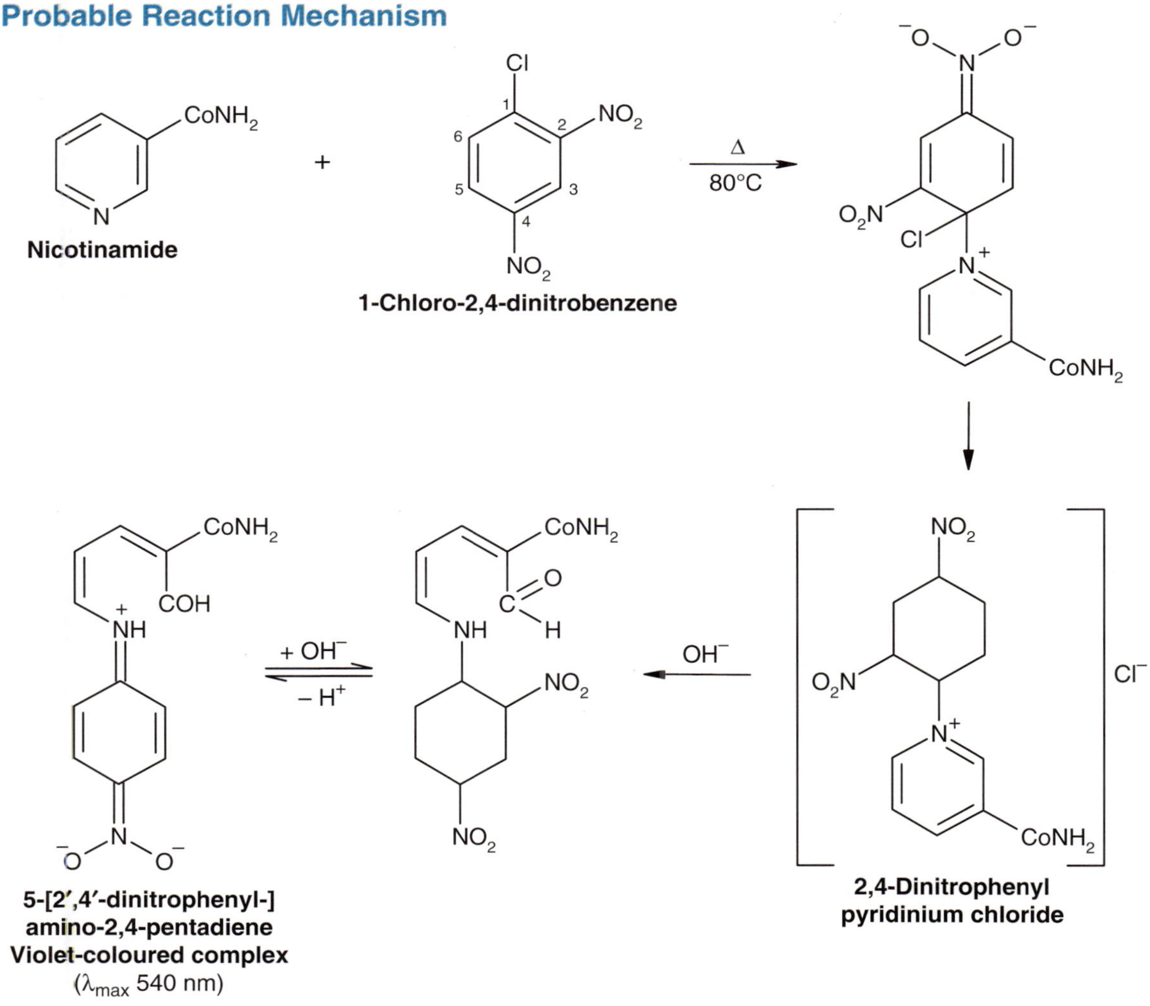

The above reaction mechanism is similar to the one proposed by König with cyanogen bromide (CNBr).

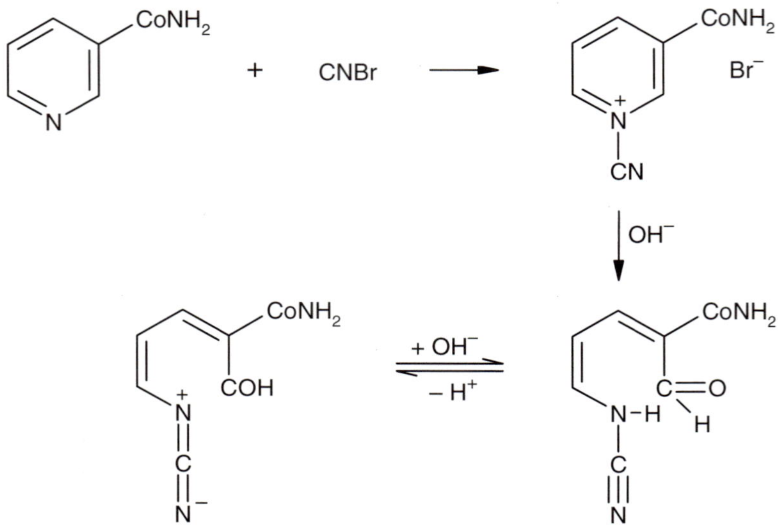

Reference

1. N. Sbarbati Nudelman & O. Nudelman, *J. Pharm. Sci.*, **65(1)**, 65-67, 1976.
2. Thin-Layer Chromatography – Reagents and Detection Methods (Vol. 1b) by Jork, Funk et al. , p. 127.

Formulation 5

Vitamin B_{12} / Cyanocobalamine

ESTIMATION

The method is based on isolating vitamin B_{12} by passing through a column of weekly acidic ion-exchange resin. There is no loss of vitamin in this process. Since vitamin B_{12} is eluted as a narrow band, enrichment of the solution also occurs. This is followed by spectrophotometric measurements for quantitative determination.

Reagents

1. Ion-exchange resin CG-50 (type-II) or XE-97.
2. 1 N sodium hydroxide.
3. 0.1 N and 1 N hydrochloric acid.
4. Tetrahydrofuran–hydrochloric acid: 60 ml of tetrahydrofuran, 10 ml of 1 N hydrochloric acid and 30 ml of water are mixed.
5. Dioxane–hydrochloric acid mixture: 60 ml of freshly distilled dioxane is mixed with 10 ml of 1 N hydrochloric acid and 30 ml of water.
6. Buffer solution, pH 4: 65 g of sodium citrate and 60 g of citric acid are dissolved in water to produce 1000 ml. The solution is adjusted to pH 4 with sodium hydroxide or citric acid.
7. 10% w/v solution of ferric chloride in water.
8. 1% w/v solution of potassium ferricyanide in water.
9. 5% w/v solution of potassium cyanide in water.
10. 50% w/v solution of p-chlorophenol in carbon tetrachloride.
11. Aqueous acetone, 85% v/v.

Glass column

2 cm (i.d.) × 20 cm fitted with glass stopcock and a sintered glass disc of zero porosity.

Activation of ion-exchanger

The resin is shaken with water and mixture allowed to stand for at least 2 hours. The turbid supernatant liquid is decanted and resin is again shaken with water. After 10 minutes, it is again decanted and the process is repeated till supernatant liquid is practically clear. After the last portion is decanted, 1 N sodium hydroxide solution is added and is allowed to act on the resin for 1 hour, and then poured off. The resin is washed with water till washings are neutral to litmus. The water is decanted and the resin is kept under buffer solution of pH 4 for 1 hour. The material is now ready for use.

Preparation of ion-exchange column

Sufficient resin suspension is poured into the column having a plug of glass wool on the sintered disc to give a column height of about 10 cm on setting. The liquid is drained off and buffer is further added. The tube is closed and tilted to mix the resin with the solution and then column is allowed to settle slowly. Wash the column with buffer till the pH of the eluate is 4.0. Cover the top of the column with glass wool and drain the solvent to level of 1 cm above the glass wool.

Assay

The sample containing at least 100 mcg of vitamin B_{12} is accurately weighed and suspended in 50-80 ml of water. This solution is passed through the prepared column. After the entire sample solution is passed through the column, wash the column with 100 ml of 0.1 N hydrochloric acid. Collect two 5 ml aliquots of the eluate in two separate test tubes. In one tube, add few drops of ferric chloride solution, brown colour should be absent (confirms removal of vitamin B_6); to the other tube, add 5 ml of 2 N sodium hydroxide, 10 ml of potassium ferricyanide solution and 5 ml of isobutyl alcohol, shake, alcoholic layer exhibits no fluorescence (confirms removal of vitamin B_1). When the washing of the column is complete, it is eluted with dioxane–hydrochloric acid mixture and the enriched red colour is collected in 5 ml volumetric flask until the dripping liquid is colourless. Adjust the volume with dioxane–hydrochloric acid mixture, filter and measure the extinction at 548 nm and 361 nm against water as blank. The absorbance ratio at 361 and 548 nm should be between 3.0 and 3.5.

Note

1. The same column can be used several times on the same day but after every use it should be washed with buffer solution, pH 4, and it may be ensured that the washing has pH 4 before using the column again.
2. After the experiment is complete, the resin is removed into a clean beaker and washed with water till the washing is practically neutral. Add 1 N hydrochloric acid and keep it for at least 1 hour. Decant the supernatant liquid and wash the resin with water till washings are neutral. Preserve the resin in water. This material can again be used for estimation of vitamin B_{12}.

Total Vitamin B_{12}

To estimate total vitamin B_{12} contents as cyanocobalamin in liver extract or in vitamin B_{12} solution, which may contain aquo- or hydroxycobalamin, the cobalamins are first converted into cyanocobalamin by treating with potassium cyanide. The sample solution containing about 100-150 mcg of vitamin B_{12} is treated with 2 ml of potassium cyanide solution and the pH is adjusted to between 4 and 6 with citric acid (make use of pH meter as indicator paper imparts its colour to the solution which may get eluted by the solvent). Keep the solution in fume hood for 15-20 minutes; the solution is then poured onto the prepared ion-exchange column.

Assay of vitamin B_{12} in tablets and capsules

The tablets and capsules containing equivalent to 100 mcg of vitamin B_{12} are powdered and suspended in 30-35 ml of water. The solution is then treated with potassium cyanide and chromatographed as above.

Assay of vitamin B_{12} in feeding stuff

The extraction and potassium cyanide treatment is done as above. After addition of potassium cyanide, the mixture is heated on water-bath for about 30 minutes. Potassium cyanide treatment not only converts B_{12} to 'cyano' form but also liberates the vitamin from proteins.

Assay of vitamin B_{12} in very dilute solutions

Very low levels of vitamin B_{12} are usually encountered in the form of drop or syrups for oral use. Because of their relatively high viscosity, filtration through column is difficult. In such cases, the vitamin can be enriched by extraction with chlorophenol before proceeding with ion-exchange separation. Such samples are diluted with water and then treated with 2 drops of potassium cyanide.

The above solution is extracted with three 10 ml portions of chlorophenol solution. To the combined extract add 10 ml of carbon tetrachloride and 20 ml of n-butanol. The resulting mixture is shaken with two 5 ml portions of water. The aqueous layer is used for ion-exchange separation.

Note

1. While carrying out the estimation of vitamin B_{12} in foodstuff, it is recommended that after the column has been washed with 0.1 N hydrochloric acid the column should be treated with 50-100 ml of aqueous acetone before proceeding with elution by dioxane–hydrochloric acid mixture.
2. Allowances for losses in extraction with p-chlorophenol should be made in calculations. Usually 5-10% of vitamin is lost in above purification procedure.

Thin-layer chromatography

Aquocobalamin and cyanocobalamin can be differentiated by TLC using silica gel G coated plates. 20 μl of the sample containing about 5-10 mcg of the vitamin are applied on the plate which is developed with 1 : 1 mixture of methanol–water. The cyanocobalamin has Rf value of about 0.5, whereas aquocobalamin remains almost at the starting point.

Eluting mixtures

It has been seen that after the column has been washed, reddish colour of adsorbed vitamin B_{12} is mainly confined to upper part of the column. If the washing has been complete, there should be no other foreign coloration on the exchanger.

(a) **Dioxane–hydrochloric acid mixture:** This is used when the vitamin B_{12} left on the upper part of the column has characteristic colour, no other brownish substances being observed on the column. This is the case with simple pharmaceutical preparations containing sufficiently large amount of vitamin B_{12}.

(b) **Tetrahydrofuran–hydrochloric acid mixture:** Elution with this solvent is essential while analysing the vitamin in feeding stuff. In the analysis of some pharmaceutical specialities, certain brown colour material cannot be removed in spite of repeated washings. These substances behave like vitamin B_{12} and get eluted with the vitamin. In such cases purification by chlorophenol extraction is advisable after chromatography.

Time required

If the determination cannot be completed in a single day, it can be interrupted before elution of the vitamin if the column is filled with 0.1 N hydrochloric acid (acetone, if used, must be completely displaced with hydrochloric acid).

The solution of vitamin B_{12} in hydrochloric acid is stable until the following day. It is not stable in solutions containing dioxane or tetrahydrofuran.

Formulation 6

Ascorbic acid (Vitamin C)

ESTIMATION

METHOD 1

Reagents

1. 10% v/v sulphuric acid in water.
2. 10% w/v solution of ammonium molybdate in water.

Standard solution

100 mcg/ml of ascorbic acid in water.

Sample solution

Dilute or extract the sample with water to get 100 mcg/ml concentration.

Procedure

To 2 ml of the sample and standard solutions add 2 ml of sulphuric acid and 4 ml of ammonium molybdate solution. Keep at room temperature for 60 minutes and dilute with water to 25 ml. Measure the absorbance of both the sample and standard solutions at maximum at about 650 nm against reagent blank. The method obeys Beer's law in the concentration range of 2-10 mcg/ml. Since the colour starts fading after 1 hour, so reading must be taken within this period.

Note

1. This method has been tried on different liquid and solid formulations containing water and fat soluble vitamins, rutin, cysteine, reducing sugars and different iron salts and found to give reliable results.
2. Analgin, if present in the formulations, was found to interfere in this method.
3. The method is based on reduction of molybdate by ascorbic acid to yield molybdenum blue.

Reference

Assay of Vitamins in Pharmaceutical Preparations by M.H. Hashmi, p. 310, 1973.

METHOD 2

Reagents

1. 0.01 M chloramine-T reagent: Solution prepared by dissolving 2.81 g of sodium N-chloro-4-toluene sulphonamide, trihydrate in 1000 ml of water. The solution can be standardized iodometrically.
2. 0.025 M sodium tetrathionate solution: This solution is prepared freshly by titrating 100 ml of 0.1 M sodium thiosulphate with 0.05 M iodine to the first appearance of iodine colour which is bleached by dropwise addition of 0.01 M sodium thiosulphate. This solution is stored in amber-coloured bottle.
3. 1% w/v solution of 2-furfuraldehyde.
4. 0.01% w/v solution of methyl red in alcohol.

Procedure

A. Accurately weighed quantity of powdered tablets/capsules is stirred with 30 ml of water containing 1 ml of glacial acetic acid. After 15 minutes, the residual solid is filtered and washed with water. To the filtrate (test solution) add (a) 0.5 g of potassium iodide, 1 ml of 0.5% w/v starch solution and 2 ml of 0.1 N sulphuric acid, or (b) 0.5 g of potassium bromide, 2-3 drops of methyl red and 2 ml of 1 N sulphuric acid and the resultant solution is titrated with 0.01 M chloramine-T to the appearance of a blue colour of starch–iodine or to the sharp bleaching of the red colour of methyl red.

B. If the preparation contains sulphite along with vitamin C, then to the 10 ml of test solution as obtained under method A add 5 ml of furfuraldehyde solution and allow to stand for 15 minutes. The mixture is diluted to 20 ml, then mixed with 0.5 g of potassium iodide, 1 ml of 0.5% w/v starch solution and 2 ml of 0.1 N sulphuric acid. Vitamin C is then titrated with 0.01 M chloramine-T to the appearance of a blue colour. Each ml of 0.01 M chloramine-T is equivalent to 0.8806 mg of vitamin C.

Note

1. Vitamins B_1, B_2, B_6, B_{12}, folic acid, calcium pantothenate, nicotinamide, ferrous fumarate and acetylsalicylic acid do not interfere in this method.
2. The method is based on oxidation of ascorbic acid to dehydroascorbic acid. Although titration with iodine, an oxidizing agent, had been approved in USP but use of chloramine-T as oxidizing agent is preferred over iodine as end point is sharp.

Reference

S.K. Ganguly, *Ind. J. Pharm.*, **10**, 3, 1948.

Ascorbic acid is selectively oxidized by N-bromosuccinimide before other reducing substances that may be present in the formulation such as vitamins B_1, B_2, glucose, lactose and starch which do not interfere.

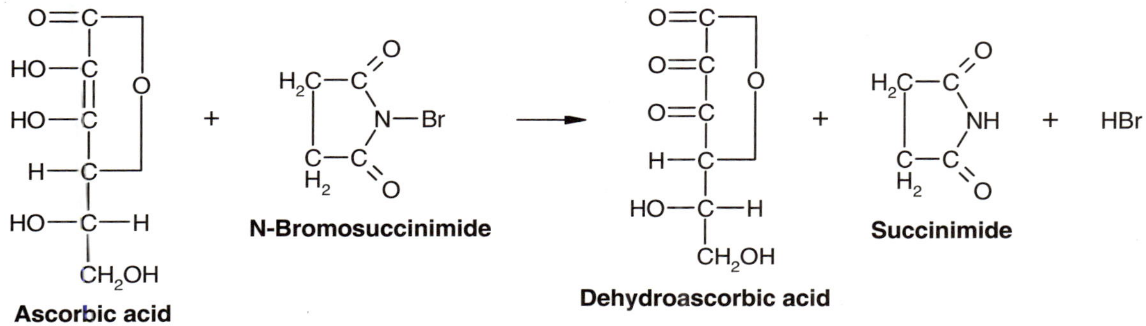

Reference

M.Z. Barakal et al., *Anal. Chem.*, **27**, 536, 1955.

Another method based on reducing property of ascorbic acid was reported by M.Z. Barakal et al. (1955) involving reduction of 1,2-naphthoquinone-4 sulphonic acid sodium.

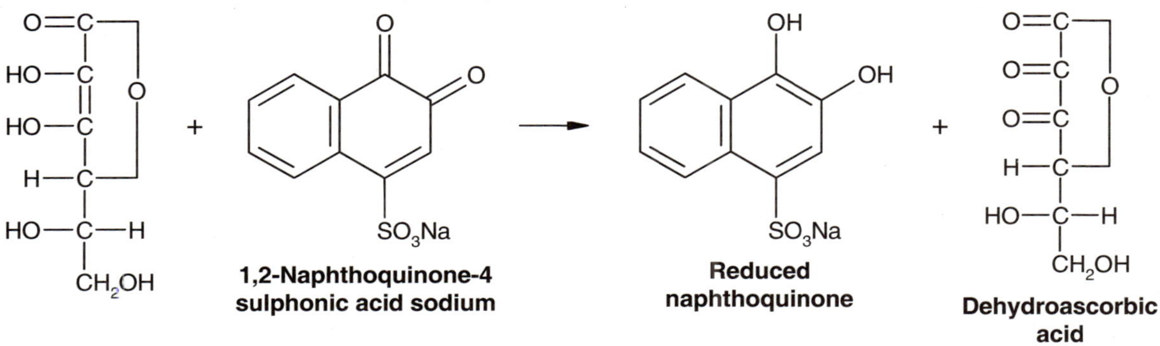

Reference

M.Z. Barakal et al., *Analyst*, **80**, 828, 1955.

Dehydroascorbic acid obtained on oxidation of ascorbic acid gives fluorescent compound on reaction with o-phenylene diamine as explained below.

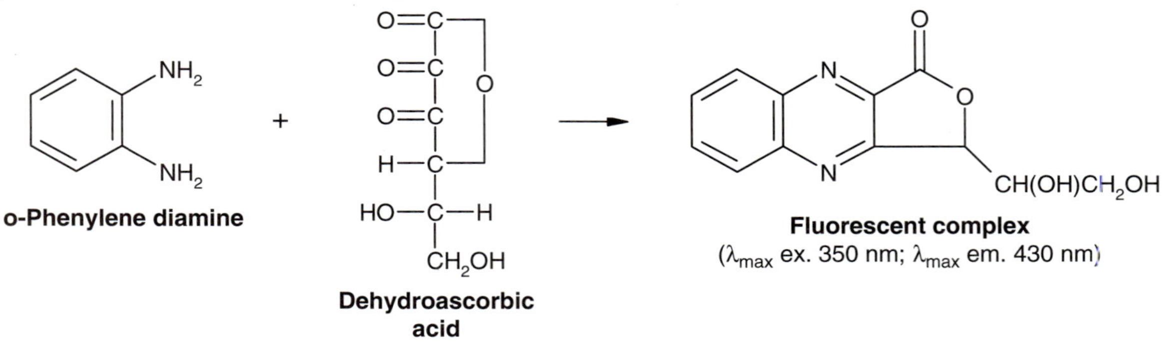

Reference

Assay of Vitamins in Pharmaceutical Preparations by M.H. Hashmi, p. 301, 1973.

Formulation 7

Folic acid

ESTIMATION

METHOD 1

This method is based on the reaction of folic acid with formaldehyde to yield a coloured product having absorption maximum at 360 nm.

Reagents

1. 0.01 N sodium hydroxide.
2. 1 M sulphuric acid.

Standard solution

100 mcg/ml of folic acid in 0.01 N sodium hydroxide.

Sample solution

Weigh a quantity of powdered tablets accurately equivalent to 5 mg of folic acid and extract with 25 ml of 0.01 N sodium hydroxide by shaking for 15 minutes, filter and dilute to 50 ml with water.

Procedure

To 10 ml each of sample and standard solutions add 13 ml of 1 M sulphuric acid and 3 ml of formaldehyde solution. Close the tube with rubber stopper in which a hypodermic needle has been inserted. Heat on a boiling water-bath for 1 hour, cool and dilute to 25 ml with water. Measure the absorbance of sample and standard solutions at maximum at about 360 nm against a reagent blank prepared by adding 13 ml of 1 M sulphuric acid to 10 ml of sample solution and diluting to 25 ml with water.

METHOD 2

This method is based on reductive cleavage of folic acid to 2,4,5-triamino-6-hydroxypyrimidine which gives colour with ninhydrin.

Reagents

1. 3% w/v solution of ninhydrin in 2-methoxy ethanol, to be freshly prepared.
2. Zinc dust.

Standard solution

1 mg/ml of folic acid in 0.1 N sodium hydroxide. It is stable for 4 days if stored in dark under toluene.

Sample solution

Extract accurately weighed quantity of powdered material equivalent to 20 mg of folic acid with 0.1 N sodium hydroxide to produce 1 mg/ml.

Procedure

To 10 ml each of sample and standard solutions add 10 ml of water and 20 ml of 4 N hydrochloric acid and 2 g of zinc dust. Maintain at 35°C ± 0.5°C for 45 minutes, filter and dilute to 100 ml with water. To 1 ml of the above solutions (sample and standard) add 10 ml of isopropyl alcohol, 2 ml of ninhydrin solution and dilute to 25 ml with isopropyl alcohol. Keep at room temperature and after 10 minutes, but not later than 30 minutes after addition of ninhydrin reagent, measure the absorbance of both the solutions at about 550 nm and calculate the results.

Probable Reaction Mechanism

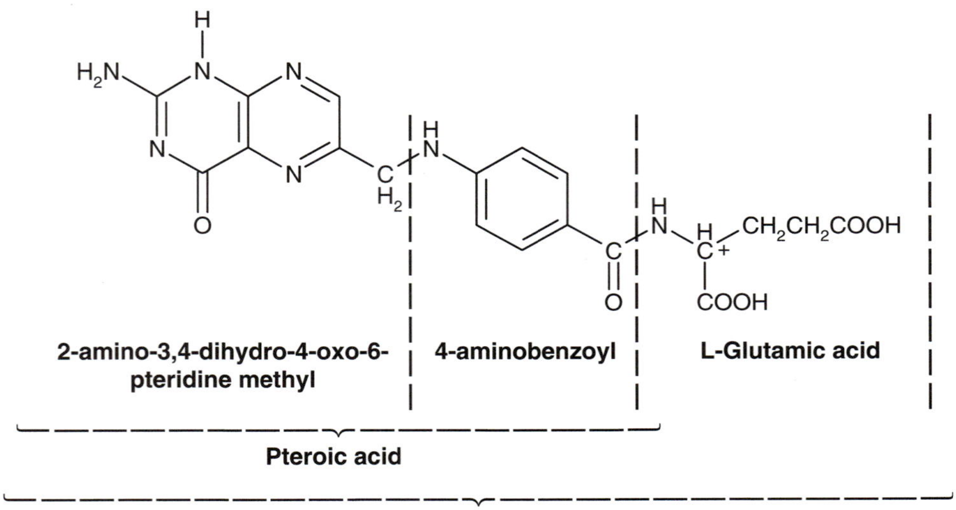

Folic acid (1)

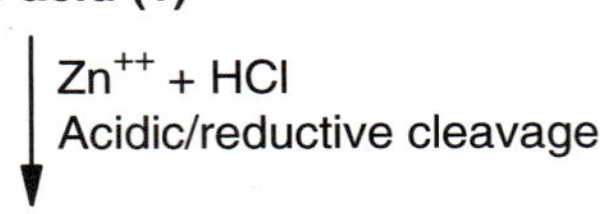

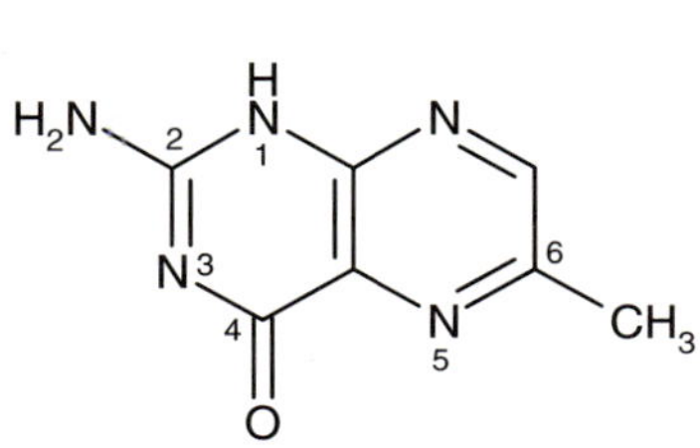

6-methylpteridine (2)

+

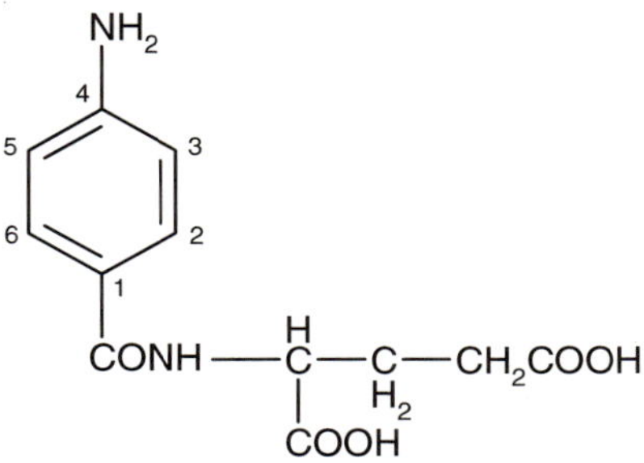

4-aminobenzoylglutamic acid (3)

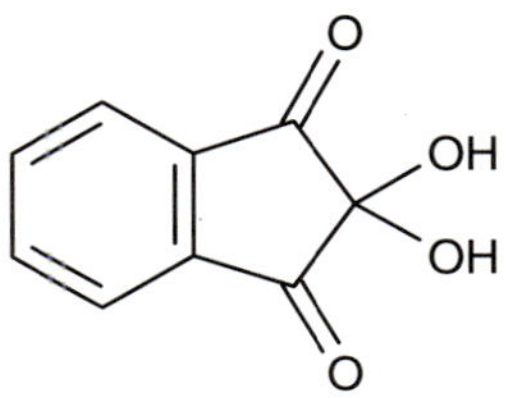

Ninhydrin

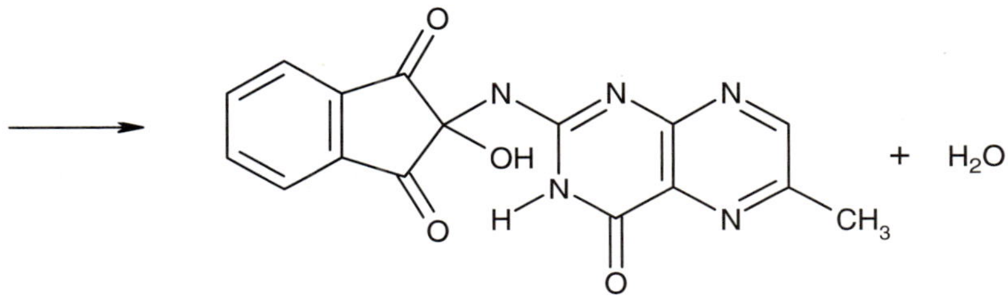

Coloured complex
(λ_{max} 550 nm)

Note

1. Vitamins B_1, B_6, vitamin C, ferrous sulphate and ferrous gluconate do not interfere.
2. Vitamin B_2 interferes and leads to low assay value.
3. If niacin is also present in the formulation, measure the colour exactly after 10 minutes after addition of ninhydrin.
4. The method obeys Beer's law in the range of 4.5-45 mcg/ml.

Alternatively, the following reaction mechanism is also possible.

Folic acid is reduced to 2,4,5-triamino-6-hydroxypyrimidine with Zn and HCl i.e. reductive cleavage.

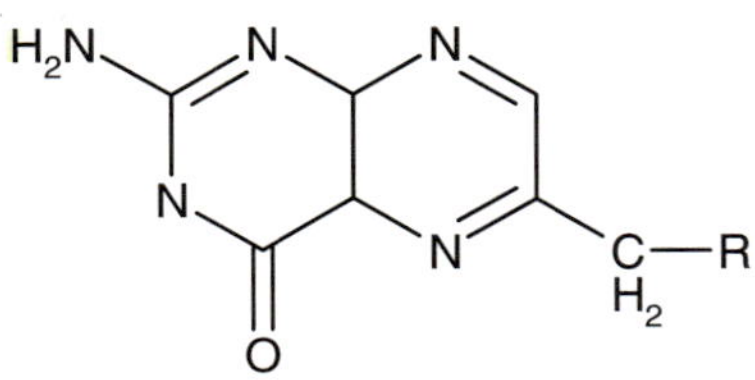

Folic acid

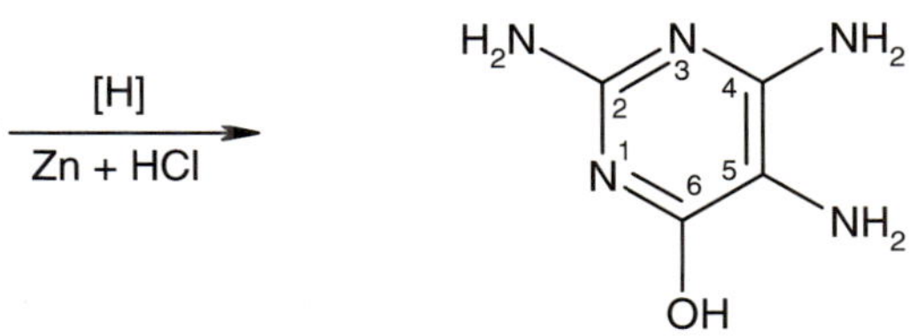

2,4,5-triamino-6-hydroxypyrimidine (TAPH)

Now the amino group at the 5th position of 2,4,5-triamino-6-hydroxypyrimidine will react with ninhydrin resulting in the formation of the product.

The amino group at the 5th position can react due to the presence of phenolic —OH group at position 6. This phenolic group at position 6 can undergo tautomerism and can give rise to structure as follows:

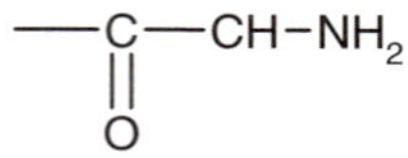

This makes hydrogen at amino group more acidic because of the electron withdrawing capacity of carbonyl group. Thus, the reaction between amino group at position 5 and ninhydrin occurs.

Probable Reaction Mechanism

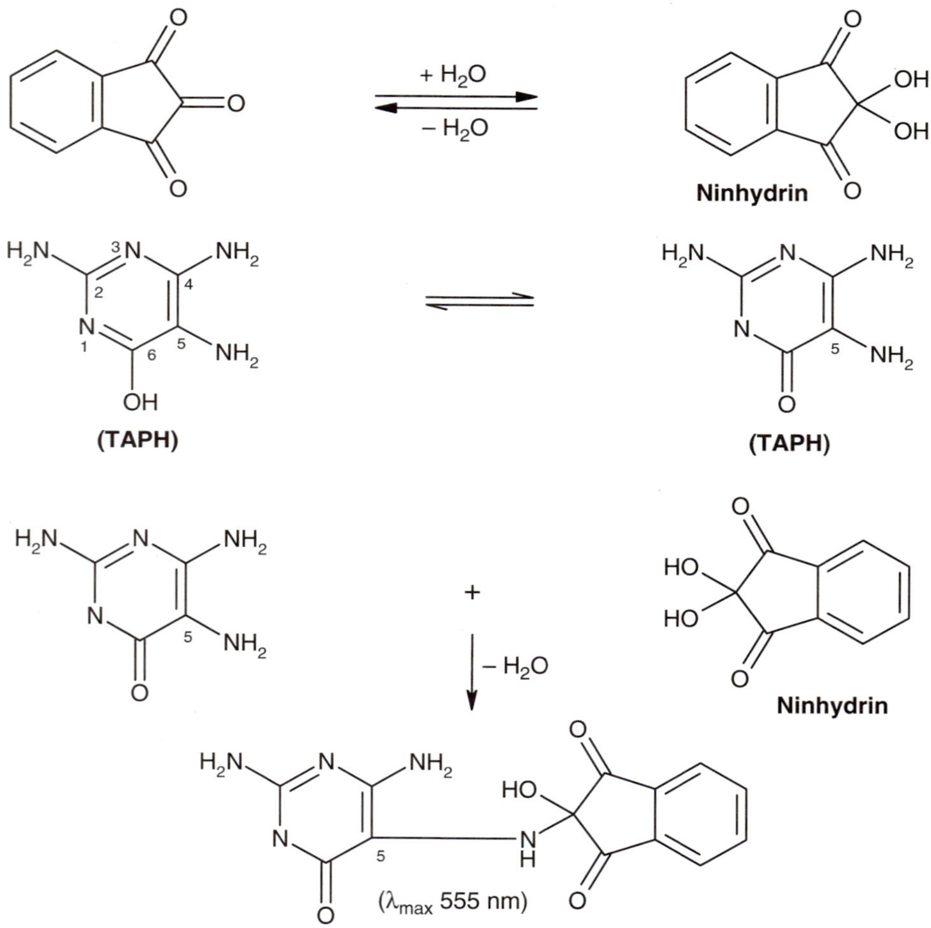

Reference

G. Ramana Rao, Surinder N. Mahajan, Geeta Kanjilal & Katta R. Mohan, *J. AOAC*, **60(3)**, 531-535, 1977.

All the three amino groups can react with ninhydrin resulting in the formation of a product.

Probable Reaction Mechanism

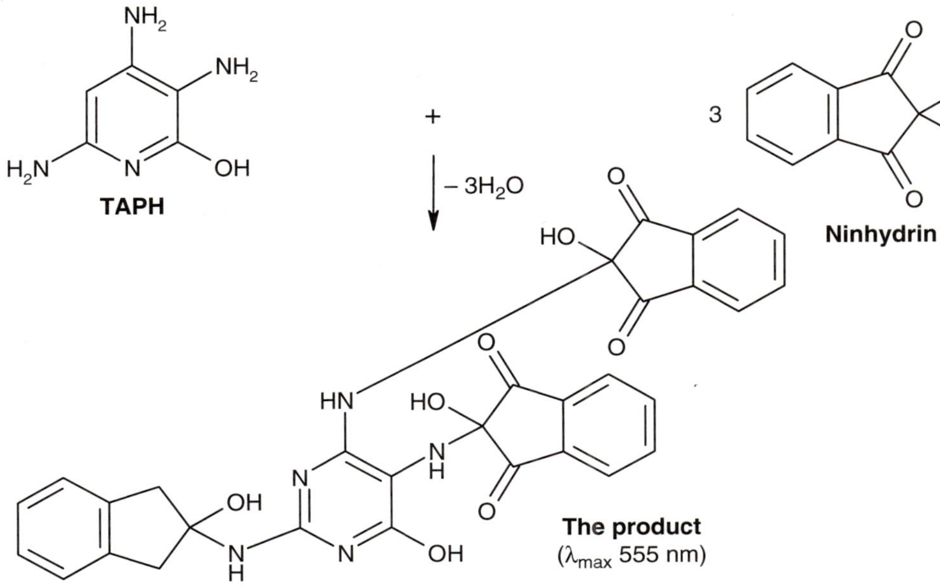

The product
(λ_{max} 555 nm)

Reference

K. Rama Mohan, Geeta Kanjilal, S.N. Mahajan & G. Ramana Rao, *Curr. Sci.*, **45(4)**, 154, 1976.

METHOD 3

This method works well for preparations containing iron and vitamin B_{12}.

Reagents

1. 0.3% w/v solution of 1,2-naphthoquinone-4-sulphonic acid (sodium salt).
2. 0.1 M and 0.2 M potassium hydroxide.
3. Zinc dust.
4. 0.2 M potassium hydrogen phthalate solution.
5. 3% w/v solution of calcium lactate in water.
6. 8% w/v solution of trisodium phosphate in water.
7. Buffer solution, pH 5.0: 500 ml of 0.2 M potassium hydrogen phthalate solution is mixed with 238.5 ml of 0.2 M potassium hydroxide and diluted to 2000 ml with freshly boiled and cooled water. Adjust the pH to 5, if necessary with 0.1 M potassium hydroxide or 0.2 M potassium hydrogen phthalate solution.
8. Lactophosphate buffer: Mix equal volumes of calcium lactate and trisodium phosphate solutions.

Standard solution

150 mg of pure folic acid is dissolved in 0.1 N sodium hydroxide to produce 100 ml (150 mcg/ml).

Sample solution

Accurately weighed quantity of the powdered material is extracted with 0.1 N sodium hydroxide to produce 150 mcg/ml concentration.

Note

If tablets contain iron then weigh material equivalent to 25 mg of folic acid and add 250 ml of lactophosphate buffer and heat at 50° in water-bath. Shake the flask thoroughly and allow to stand for 1 hr. Black precipitates separate out. Filter, reject first 20 ml of the filtrate and use the remaining for estimation.

Procedure

To 20 ml of sample and standard solutions add 2 g of zinc dust, shake for 20 minutes, filter and adjust to 100 ml with water. Protect the filtrate from light. To 5 ml of the filtrate add 2 ml of naphthoquinone reagent and adjust to 50 ml with pH 5.0 buffer and measure the absorbance at about 485 nm. Ascorbic acid, if present, will interfere.

In acidic solution folic acid exists as partial amidine structure. The primary aromatic amino group of the amidine structure undergoes Michael addition with 1,2-naphthoquinone-4-sulphonic acid eliminating HSO_3^- radical.

Probable Reaction Mechanism

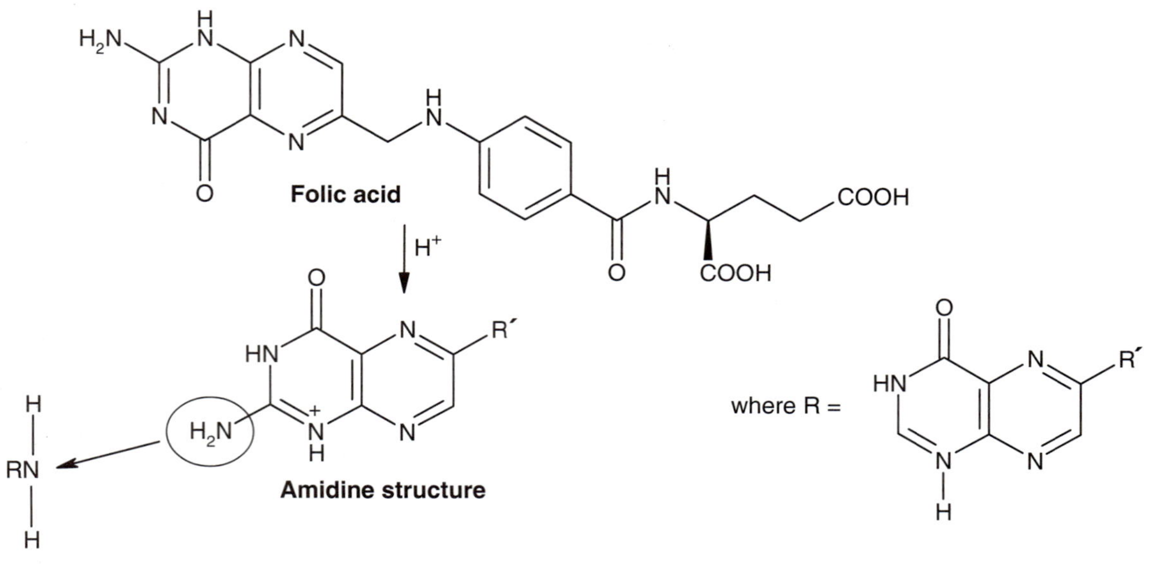

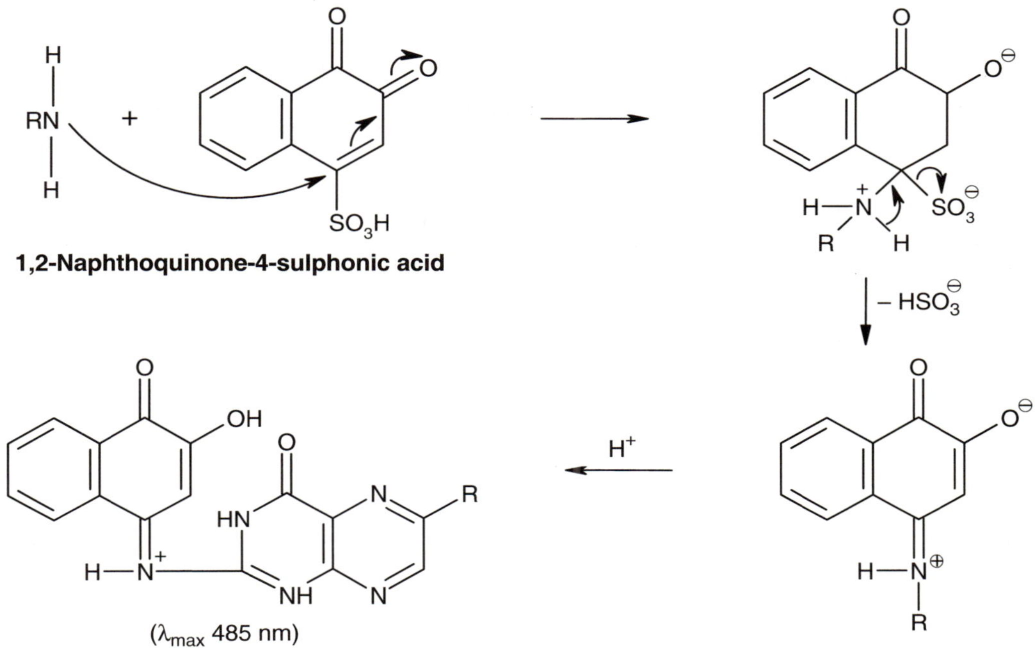

Reference

Pharmaceutical Chemistry (Vol. 2) by H.J. Roth, p. 379.

METHOD 4

Reagents

1. 4 N hydrochloric acid.
2. 0.1% w/v solution of sodium nitrite in water.
3. 0.5% w/v ammonium sulphamate in water.
4. 0.1% w/v solution of N-(1-naphthyl)-ethylenediamine dihydrochloride (NED) in water.
5. 5% w/v solution of sodium edetate in water.

Procedure

Weigh or measure accurately aliquot of the sample equivalent to 5 mg of folic acid and dilute to 100 ml with water. To 10 ml of the above solution, add 5 ml of edetate solution and 10 ml of 4 N hydrochloric acid. Dilute to 100 ml with water. This is called unreduced solution (URS).

To about 75 ml of 'URS' solution add 1 g of zinc dust, shake for 10 minutes and filter. This is called reduced solution (RS).

To each of two test tubes marked 'RT' and 'RB' add 2 ml of reduced solution. In another two test tubes marked 'URT' and 'URB' add 2 ml of unreduced solution. Store all the tubes in ice-bath (15°C), add 0.5 ml of 4 N hydrochloric acid to each tube. Add 1 ml of sodium nitrite solution to tubes marked 'RT' and 'URT' and keep in ice-bath for 2 minutes. Take out of ice-bath and add 1 ml of ammonium sulphamate solution, keep at room temperature for 3 minutes, add 1 ml of 'NED' solution to each tube and allow to stand for 10 minutes and finally adjust the volume of each tube to 10 ml with water. Measure the absorbance at about 550 nm. The calculations are based on the net absorbance due to reduced molecule of folic acid. Treat the standard solution of folic acid similarly and calculate the contents of folic acid by comparison.

Explanatory Note

4-aminobenzoyl glutamic acid formed as a result of reductive splitting of folic acid (method 2) is diazotized and coupled with β-naphthol or NED to give purple colour (λ_{max} 550 nm).

Probable Reaction Mechanism

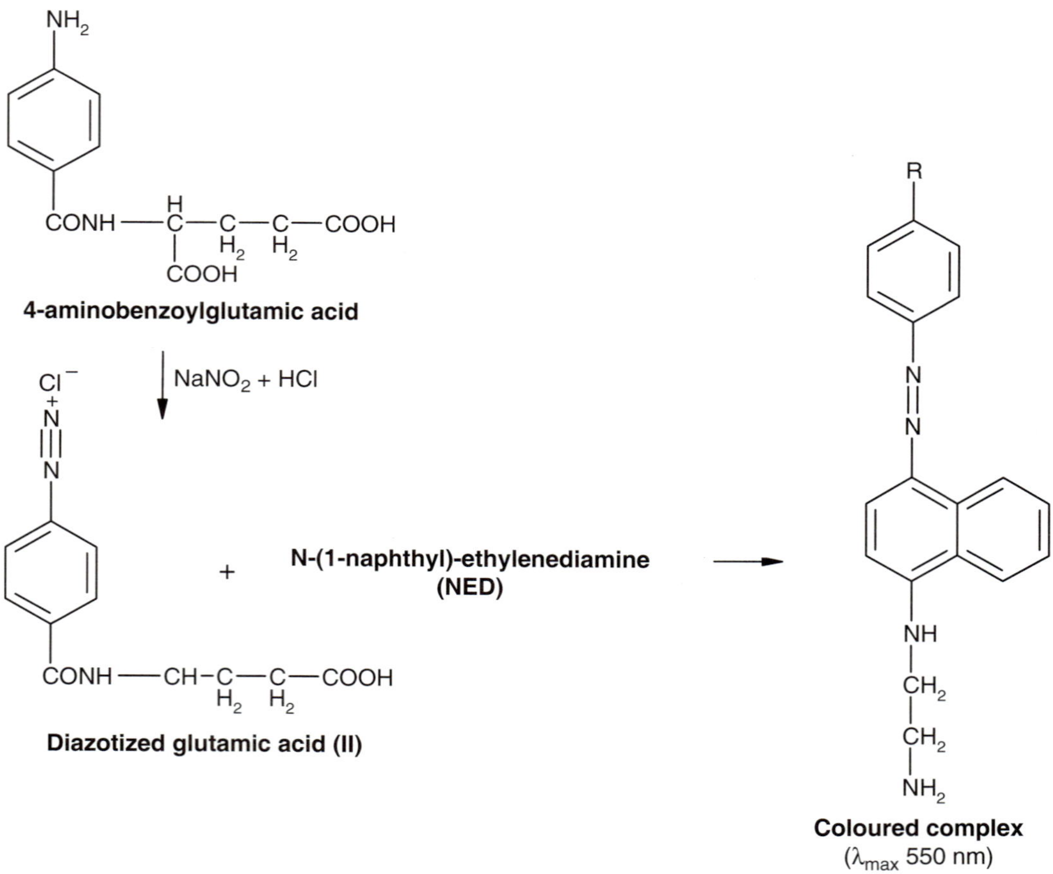

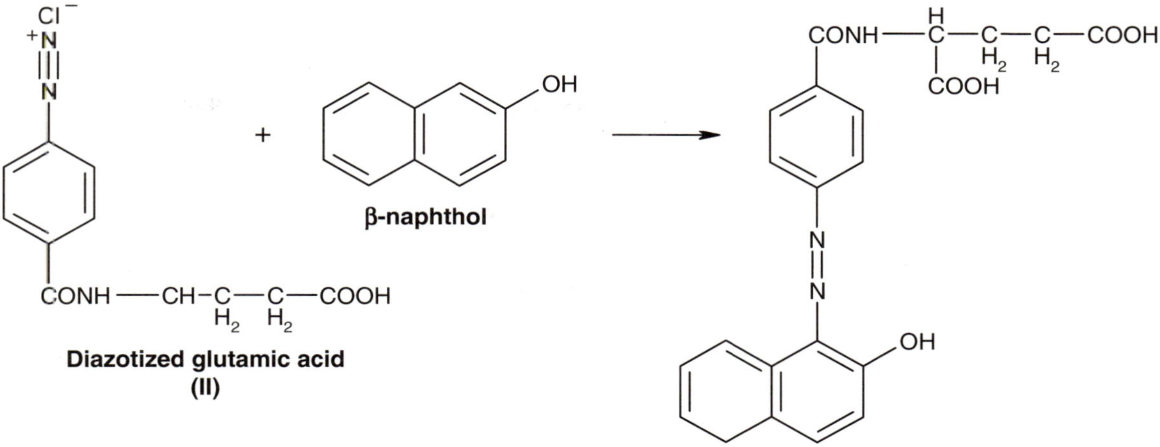

Diazotized glutamic acid (II)

Red-coloured complex
(λ_{max} 490 nm)

Oxidative splitting of folic acid produces a carboxylic acid which is highly fluorescent and can be used for fluorimetric assay of the compound.

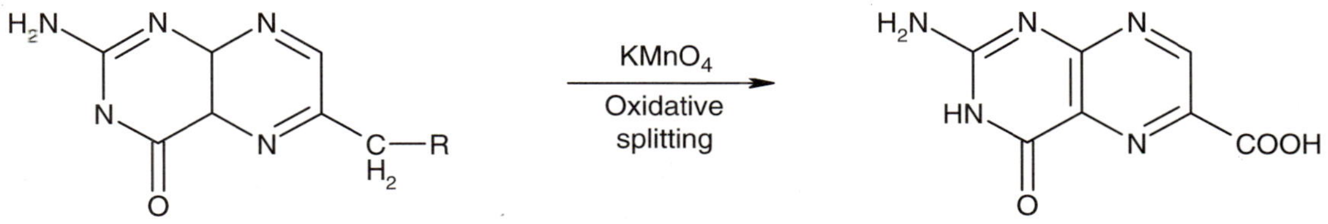

Fluorescent moiety

Reference

Pharmaceutical Chemistry (Vol. 2) by H.J. Roth, p. 650.

Folic acid in alkaline medium forms complex with several divalent cations. The general formula with cation (Cu^{++}) is as under:

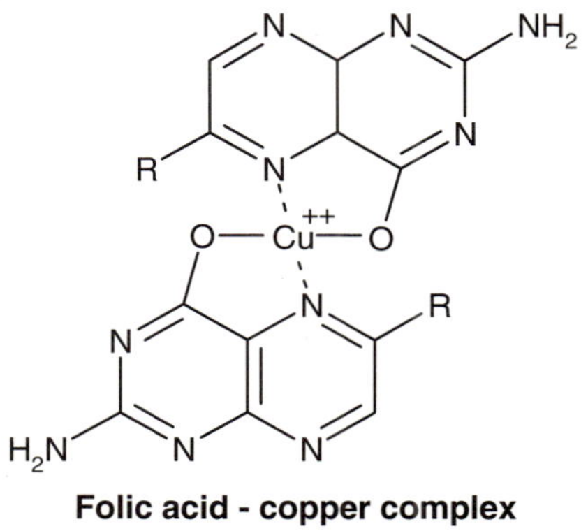

Folic acid - copper complex

METHOD 5

Reagents

1. 0.1% w/v solution of sodium nitrite in water.
2. 0.5% w/v solution of ammonium sulphamate in water.
3. 0.1% w/v solution of phloroglucinol in water.
4. 15% w/v solution of sodium hypochlorite in water.
5. 6% w/v solution of phenol in water.
6. 0.1% w/v solution of p-dimethylaminocinnamaldehyde (PDCA) in alcohol.
7. 4 N hydrochloric acid.
8. 2 N sodium hydroxide.

Procedure for reduction of folic acid

Weigh accurately either pure compound or the formulation equivalent to 100 mg of folic acid. Add 10 ml of 4 N hydrochloric acid and 1.2 g of zinc dust. Allow to stand for 1 hour at room temperature and filter through a plug of cotton wool. Wash the residue with three 5 ml portions of alcohol and adjust the total filtrate to 100 ml with alcohol.

Procedure

(a) To an aliquot of reduced folic acid solution equivalent to 100 mcg add 0.5 ml of p-dimethylaminocinnamaldehyde solution, 2 ml of 4 N hydrochloric acid and dilute to 10 ml with alcohol. Measure the absorbance of the purple colour at 520 nm after 2 minutes. The results are calculated by comparison with the standard. The method obeys Beer's law in the concentration range of 2.5-20 mcg/ml.

(b) To an aliquot of reduced folic acid solution equivalent to 200 mcg add 5 ml of 4 N hydrochloric acid and 5 ml of sodium nitrite solution. Wait for 5 minutes and add successively 5 ml of ammonium sulphamate solution, 5 ml of phloroglucinol solution and dilute to 50 ml with water. Measure the absorbance of the orange-red coloured complex at 450 nm against reagent blank and calculate the results by comparison with the standard. The method obeys Beer's law in the concentration range of 0.5-5 mcg/ml.

(c) To an aliquot of reduced folic acid solution equivalent to 1.5 mg add 2 ml of 2 N sodium hydroxide, 2 ml of phenol solution, 1 ml of sodium hypochlorite solution and dilute to 10 ml. After 10 minutes measure the absorbance of greenish-blue complex at 610 nm against reagent blank. Compute the results by comparison with the standard. The method obeys Beer's law in the concentration range of 25-175 mcg/ml.

Vitamins and excipients commonly present in formulation do not interfere in above method.

Probable Reaction Mechanism

Method 5 (a)

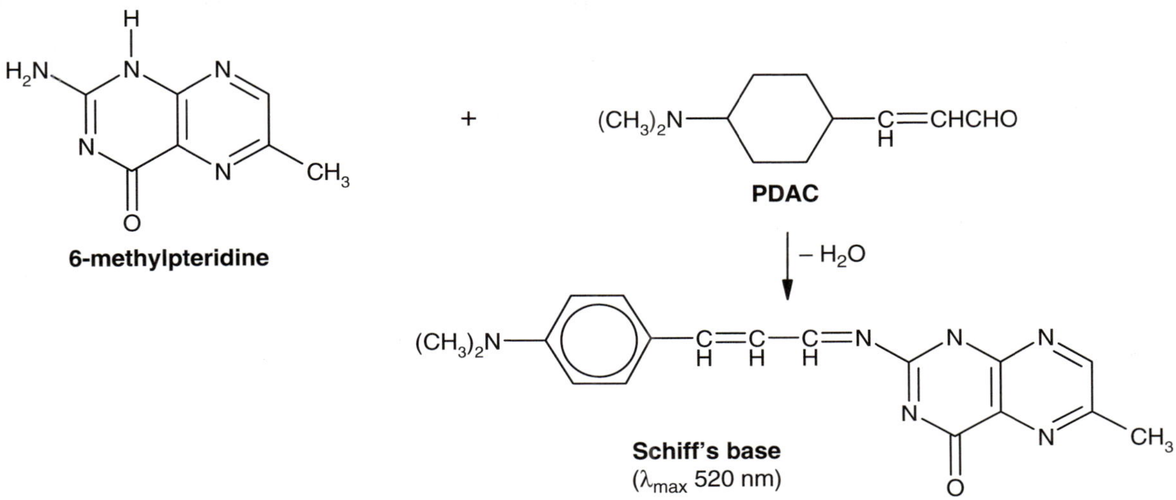

Method 5 (b)

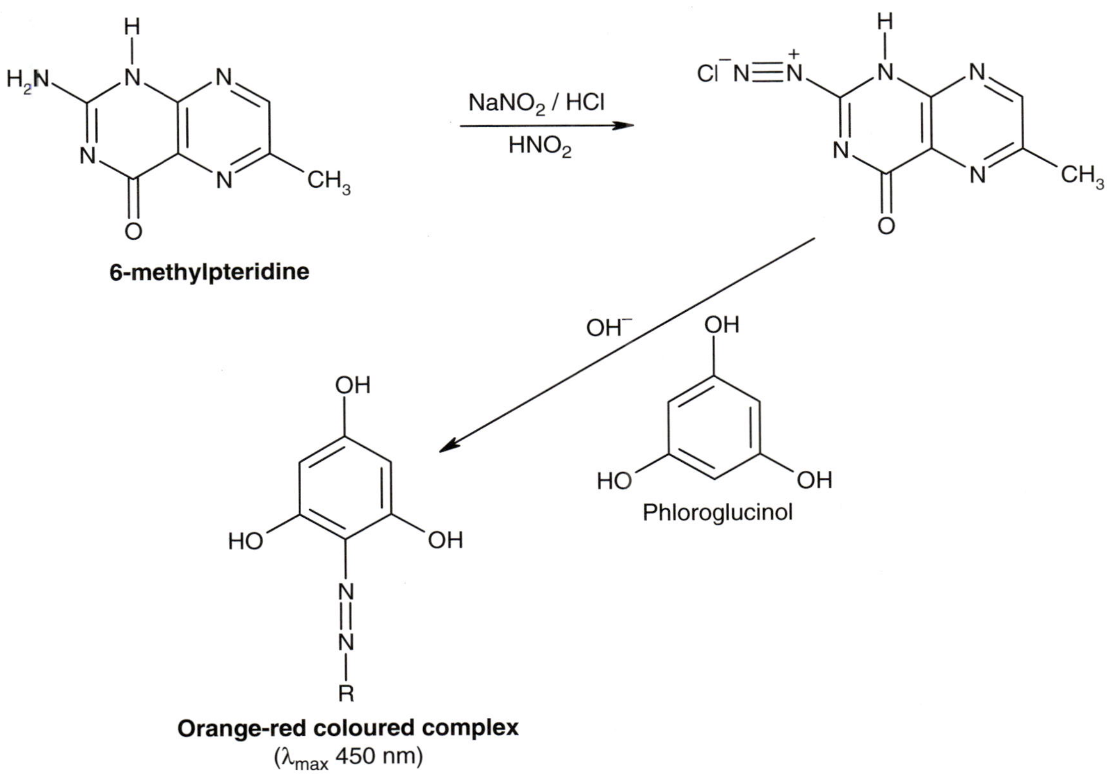

Method 5 (c)

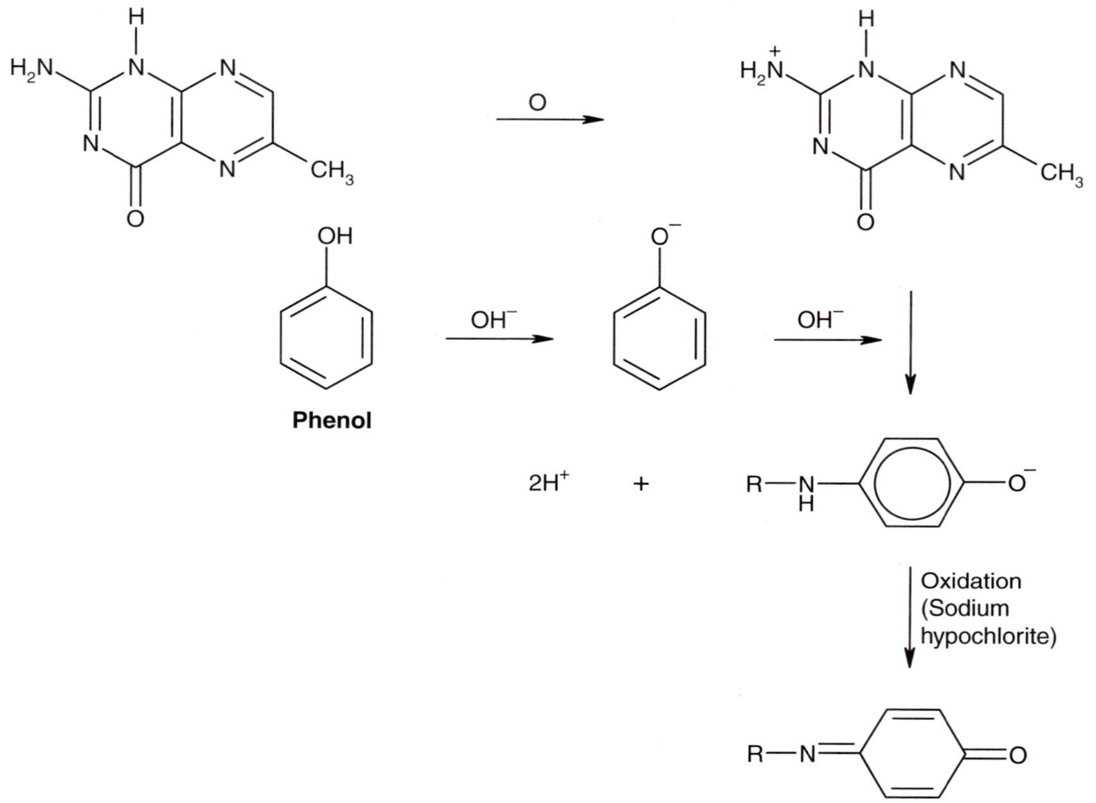

Indaniline dye complex
(λ_{max} 610 nm)

For detailed reaction mechanism, see under thiamine hydrochloride.

Formulation 8

Calcium pantothenate, Panthenol

ESTIMATION

Removal of interferences by solvent extraction

Purification of panthenol

To the sample equivalent to 5-10 mg of panthenol in water add 7 g of ammonium sulphate. Shake for 5-10 min, add 20 ml of benzyl alcohol and again shake mechanically for 10-15 min. Centrifuge to separate the layer. To 10 ml of benzyl alcohol layer (upper) add 10 ml of toluene and 20 ml of water, shake for 15 min and centrifuge. The lower aqueous layer will contain panthenol which can be used for any of the methods described below. (In the presence of ammonium sulphate, the compound is extracted with benzyl alcohol layer and re-extracted with aqueous layer with the use to toluene.)

Purification of calcium pantothenate

To 10 ml of aqueous solution of the sample containing 3-5 mg of calcium pantothenate add 13 g of sodium dihydrogen phosphate, shake vigorously for 15 min, add 20 ml of benzyl alcohol. Shake for 15 min, centrifuge to separate the layer. To 15 ml of organic layer (upper) add 10 ml of toluene and 12 ml of boric acid solution (5%). Shake for 15 min and centrifuge. The lower boric acid layer containing calcium pantothenate is appropriately diluted.

Removal of decomposition product, β-alanine

A. Prepare slurry with 5 g of the bile and pour over filtration funnel. Pass 5 ml of the sample solution obtained above through the slurry and let it drain. Wash the slurry with two 5 ml portions of water to complete the elution. Talc, being weak adsorbent, is capsule of retaining amino acid and riboflavin, but calcium pantothenate is not adsorbed.

B. Suspend prepared florisil in water and add to the glass column (250 mm × 12 mm, i.d., fitted with G_2 sintered disc) under suction. Pass the solutions of the sample and standard as obtained above through column and elute with water.

Prepared florisil

50-100 g of the florisil is taken in beaker and covered with sufficient volume of solvent (glacial acetic acid–pyridine–water; 02 : 20 : 78 v/v). Boil gently for several minutes and allow to settle. Remove the supernatant liquid and repeat the washing process twice. Finally wash it with hot water till there is no perceptible smell of pyridine. Florisil thus treated is dried at 110 ± 10°C and stored in close container to be used for preparatory column for purification of sample.

METHOD 1

This method is based on hydrolytic cleavage of the substance in acid medium with the formation of pantoyl lactone. The lactone reacts with hydroxylamine in alkaline medium to form hydroxamic acid of pantoyl lactone. Hydroxamic acid derivative so produced yields a purple-coloured complex on acidification in the presence of ferric chloride.

Reagents

1. 1% w/v solution of ferric chloride in water.
2. Hydroxylamine–sodium hydroxide reagent: Prepared by dissolving 7.5 g of hydroxylamine hydrochloride in 100 ml of 1 N sodium hydroxide. Prepare the solution fresh.

Standard solution

1.5 mg/ml of calcium pantothenate or panthenol in water.

Sample solution

After purification, as discussed above, appropriate dilution with water to get solution of 1.5 mg/ml.

Hydrolysis

To 5 ml each of the sample and standard solutions add 3 ml of 1 N hydrochloric acid. Cap the flask loosely and heat the mixture for 5 hrs at 69 ± 1°C for effecting the hydrolysis. Cool to room temperature and to each of the hydrolysed solutions add 2 ml of hydroxylamine reagent, followed by 5 ml of 1 N sodium hydroxide. Allow to stand for 5 min, adjust the pH to 2.7 ± 0.1 (pH meter) with 1 N hydrochloric acid and make up the volume to 50 ml with water.

Procedure

To 5 ml of hydrolysed solutions each of the sample and standard add 1 ml of ferric chloride solution, mix and tap the tubes against table top to remove air bubbles and measure the absorbance of purple colour so developed at about 500 nm against blank and calculate the results by comparison.

Blank: Prepared by heating 5 ml each of the sample and standard solutions in the same manner except hydrolysis procedure in acid medium. Blank so prepared will eliminate interference due to any pre-formed pantoyl lactone.

Note

1. Pantoyl lactone has melting point of 92°C; some decomposition might occur at temperature higher than 70°C.
2. pH 2.7 is critical as excess of hydrochloric acid results in marked decrease in colour intensity.
3. As alkaline medium is necessary for formation of hydroxamic acid of pantoyl lactone, there is possibility of formation of some pantoic acid. It is therefore advisable that after addition of sodium hydroxide the solution should be brought to pH 2.7 immediately after 5 min; longer exposure to alkali gives lower assay values.

Probable Reaction Mechanism

Panthenol and calcium pantothenate undergo hydrolytic cleavage in acid medium leading to the formation of pantoyl lactone and β-alanol or β-alanine. Pantoyl lactone reacts with hydroxylamine in alkaline medium to form hydroxamic acid of pantonyl lactone. On acidification and in the presence of Fe(III) chloride it yields purple-coloured complex (λ_{max} 500 nm).

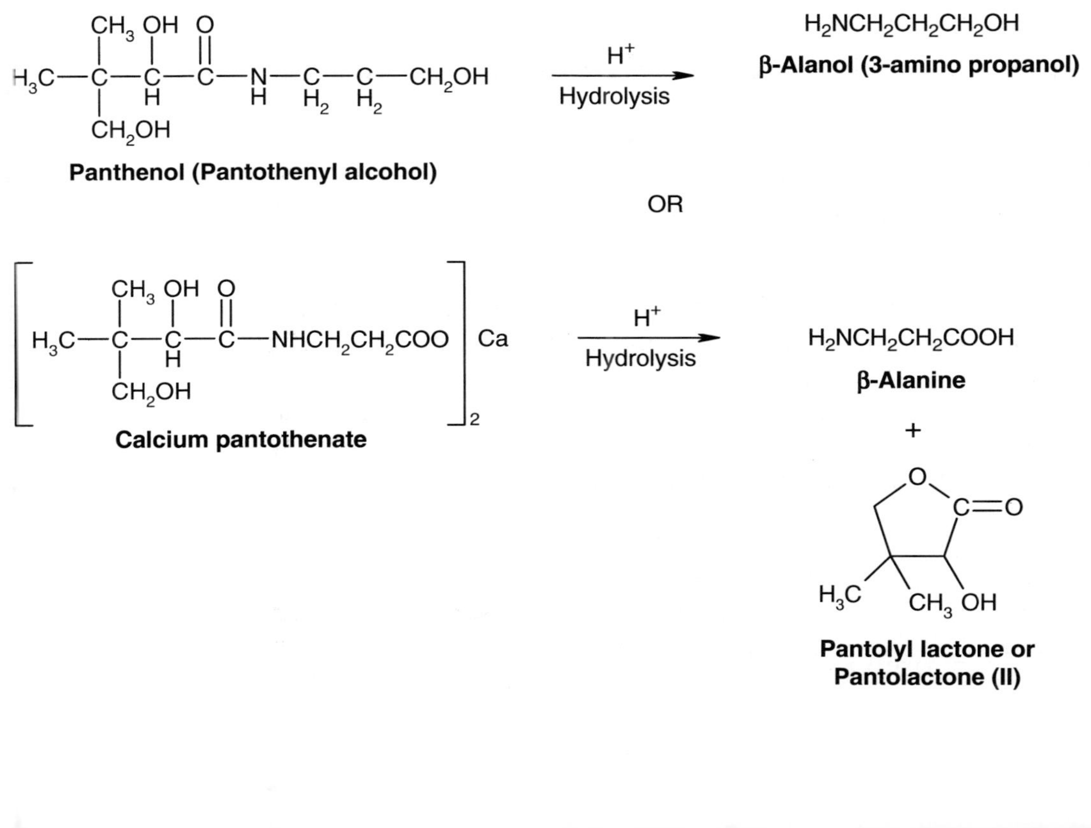

Note

Ease of dissociation of amide group can be attributed to the neighbouring group effect of the end position hydroxyl group.

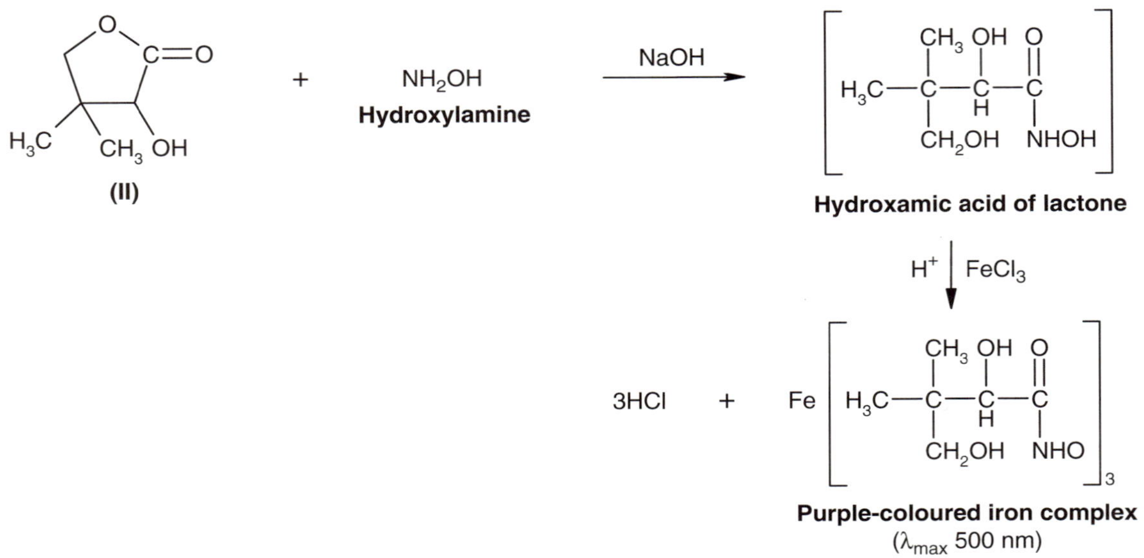

Reference

E.G. Wollish & Morton Schmall, Anal. Chem., **22**, 1033-39, 1950.

METHOD 2

This method involves alkaline hydrolysis of panthenol or calcium pantothenate and β-alanol or β-alanine so formed reacts with naphthoquinone reagent to give brownish-yellow coloured complex having absorption maxima at 465 nm.

Hydrolysis: To aliquots of the sample and standard containing 2-5 mg of the substance in 40 ml of water as purified by the method described above add 3 ml of 2.5 N sodium hydroxide solution and heat in boiling water-bath for 1 hr to ensure complete cleavage of the molecule, cool, adjust the volume to 50 ml with water.

Reagents

1. 0.04 M formaldehyde prepared by diluting 3 ml of 40% formaldehyde to 1000 ml with water.
2. Acidic formaldehyde: 0.3 N hydrochloric acid in 0.04 M formaldehyde.
3. 0.05 M sodium thiosulphate in water.
4. 0.5% w/v solution of 1,2-naphthoquinone-4-sulphamate, sodium salt in water; prepare fresh.

Procedure

5 ml each of hydrolysed sample and standard solutions are adjusted to pH 9.3 with 0.1 N sulphuric acid. Add 1 ml of naphthoquinone reagent and heat for 10 min in boiling water-bath, cool to room temperature, add 1 ml of acidic formaldehyde followed by 1 ml of thiosulphate solution. Allow to stand at room temperature for 10 min and dilute to 25 ml with methanol. Measure the absorbance of both sample and standard solutions at 465 nm against respective blanks prepared with hydrolysed sample without naphthoquinone reagent.

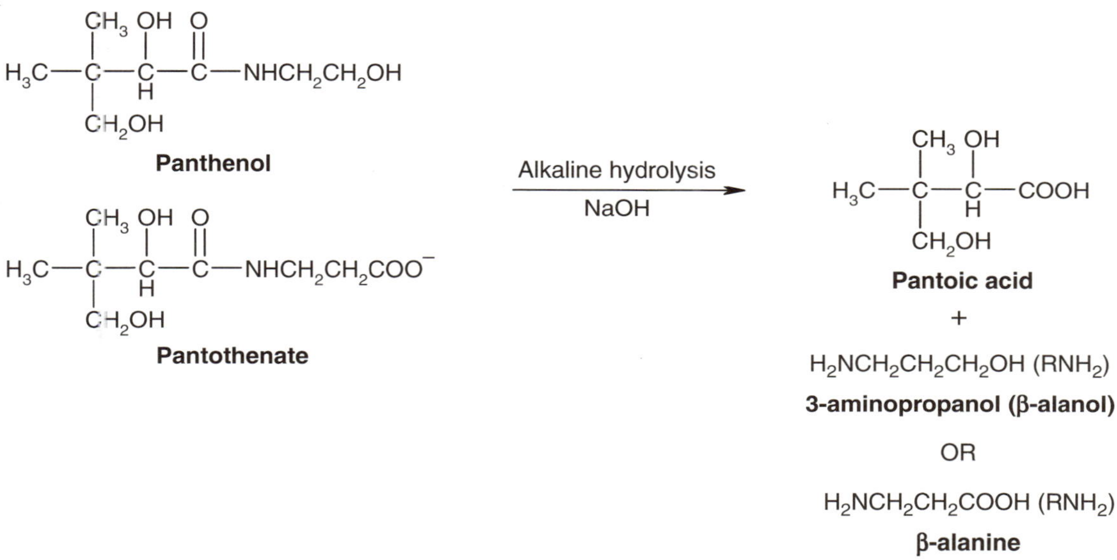

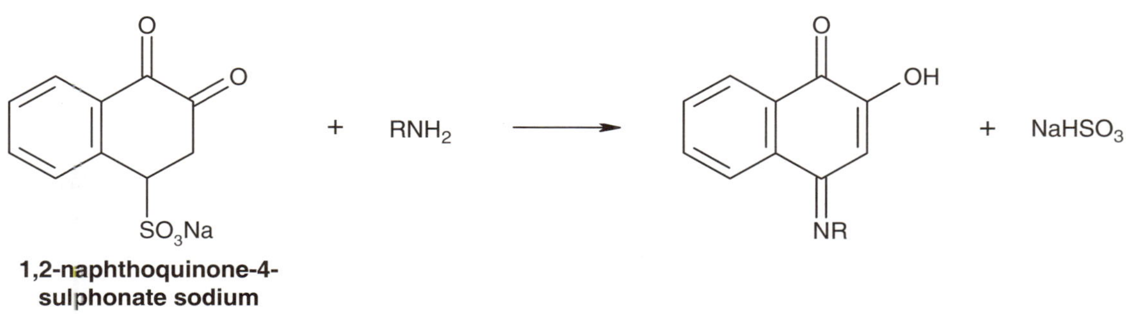

R = CH_2CH_2COOH or $CH_2CH_2CH_2OH$

Brownish yellow colour

(λ_{max} 465 nm)

Reference

M. Schmall & E.G. Wollish, *Anal. Chem.*, **29(10)**, 1509-1513, 1957.

In alkaline medium it forms Cu^{++} complex, indicative of β-alanine structure. β-alanine can also be determined by formol titration.

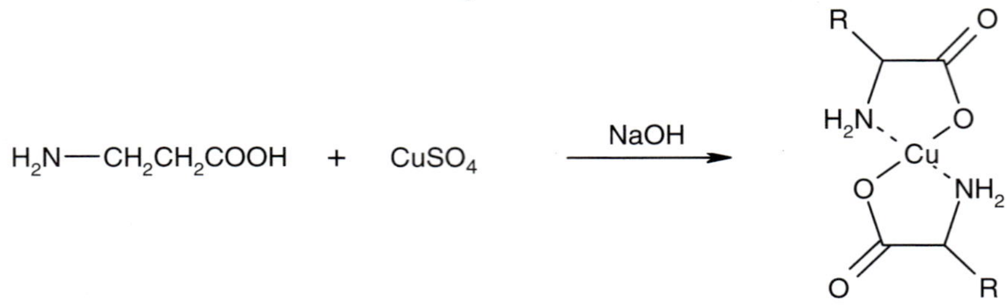

Violet-blue copper complex

Note

Calcium pantothenate can also form copper complex as under:

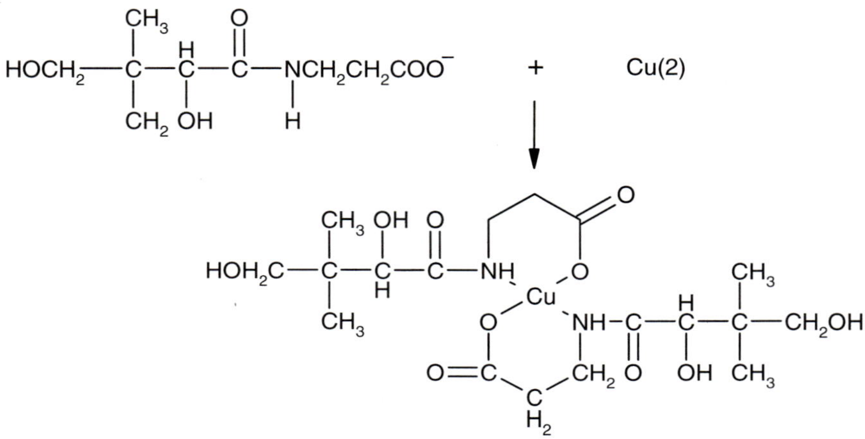

Cu(2) - pantothenate complex

METHOD 3

Reagents

1. 0.2 M citrate buffer, pH 5: Dissolve 21 g of citric acid in 200 ml of 1 N sodium hydroxide and dilute to 500 ml with water. Check pH 5.0 ± 0.1.
2. 0.2% w/v solution of stannous chloride dihyride in citrate buffer.
3. 2% w/v solution of ninhydrin in methanol.
4. Ninhydrin–stannous chloride reagent: Mix equal volumes of reagents 2 and 3.

Procedure

After alkaline hydrolysis, the solution is made distinctly acidic with 1 N sulphuric acid. Add 50 ml of methanol and dilute to 100 ml with water. To 2 ml aliquot of the above solution add 1 ml of citrate buffer and 1 ml of ninhydrin reagent. Heat in water-bath at 95-100°C for 5 min, cool and adjust to 10 ml with 60%

methanol. The absorbance of both sample and standard solutions is measured at about 570 nm against reagent blank and results calculated by comparison.

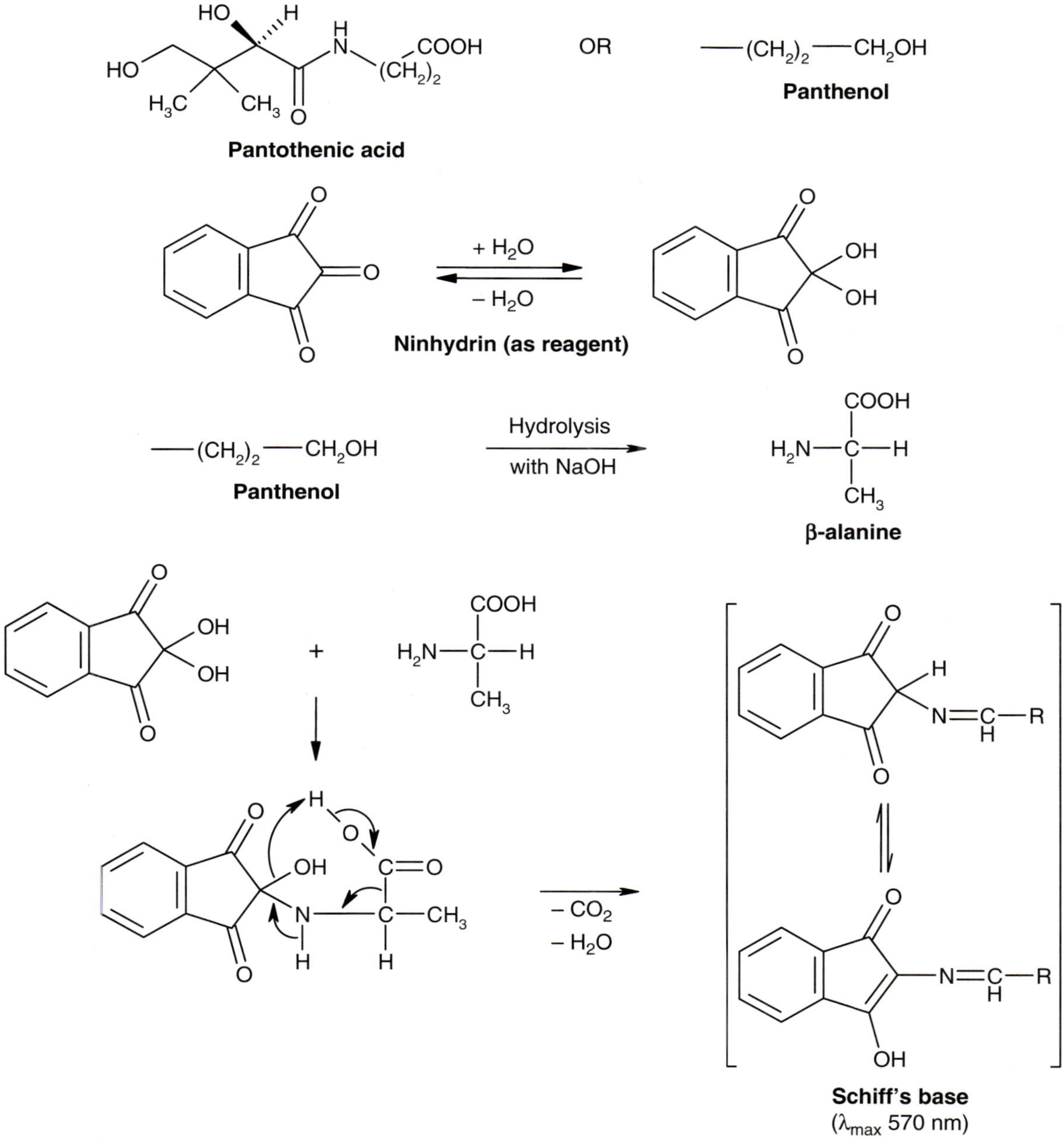

Reference

Mohamed S. Karawya, Mohamed G. Ghourab & Esther N. Ibrahim, *J. of the AOAC*, **57(6)**, 1357-1359, 1974.

METHOD 4

Reagents

1. Zinc metal, granules.
2. Talc (purified).
3. Benzyl alcohol.
4. Sodium acid phosphate.
5. 0.5% w/v solution of ninhydrin in absolute alcohol.
6. Pyridine cyanide reagent: Dilute 2 ml of 0.065% freshly prepared aqueous solution of potassium cyanide to 100 ml with ammonia-free pyridine.
7. 5% w/v solution of boric acid in water.
8. 50% w/v solution of sodium hydroxide in water.

Standard solution

Dissolve 100 mg of the substance in water, add 2-3 drops of hydrochloric acid and dilute with water to 100 ml (1 mg/ml).

Sample solution

(a) Tablets/capsules: Weigh accurately a quantity of the sample equivalent to 0.5 mg of calcium pantothenate and dissolve in 5 ml of water containing 1-2 drops of hydrochloric acid. Filter, wash the residue with water to produce 25 ml (solution A). Prepare slurry with 5 g of the talc and pour in funnel. Pass 5 ml of the solution A and let it drain. Wash the slurry with two 5 ml portions of water. Add 0.2 ml of sodium hydroxide solution to the liquid, concentrate to 2 ml on hot plate (sample solution).

(b) Dried yeast: Weigh 2.5 g of yeast, macerate with 25 ml of water for 12 hr and centrifuge. Wash the precipitates with water. Filter and transfer to a separating funnel, add 7 g of sodium acid phosphate and 20 ml of benzyl alcohol. Shake for 15 minutes and let the layers separate. Transfer the organic layer to another separating funnel, add 12.5 ml of toluene and 12.5 ml of boric acid solution. Shake for 15 minutes, filter and dilute the filtrate to 25 ml with boric acid solution. Transfer 10 ml of this solution to the top of talc slurry and continue as under tablets/capsules beginning with the words "let it drain".

Procedure

To sample and standard solutions equivalent to 100 mcg of the compound add 1 ml of hydrochloric acid and 50 mg of zinc granules. Heat on water-bath (90°C) until zinc dissolves completely (5 min). Make solution alkaline (phenolphthalein) with 50% sodium hydroxide solution. Filter the precipitated zinc hydroxide. Wash the precipitates twice with 2 ml water, add washing to the filtrate. Make filtrate slightly acidic to phenolphthalein with 0.1 N hydrochloric acid, add 0.5 ml of pyridine–cyanide reagent and 0.5 ml of ninhydrin reagent. Heat on water-bath (85-90°C) for 10 minutes, cool to room temperature and dilute with water to 25 ml. Measure the absorbance of the colour at maximum at about 570 nm and compute the results by comparison.

The method obeys Beer's law in the concentration range of 2-15 mcg/ml in respect of final volume.

Probable Reaction Mechanism

Reaction of pantothenate with Zn and HCl results in the cleavage and hydrogenation resulting in the formation of an aldehyde and β-alanine.

Step 1:

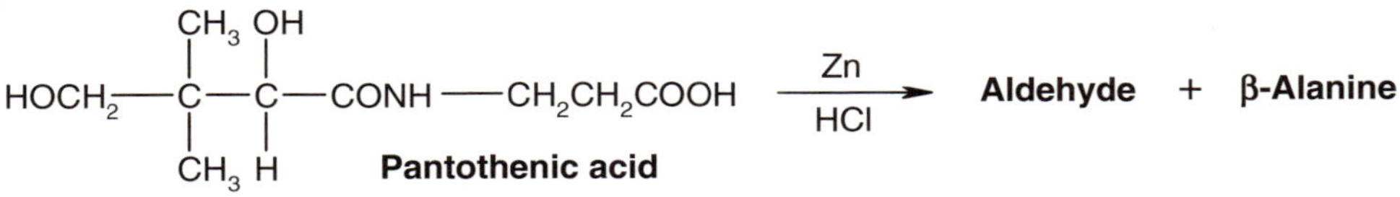

Pantothenic acid

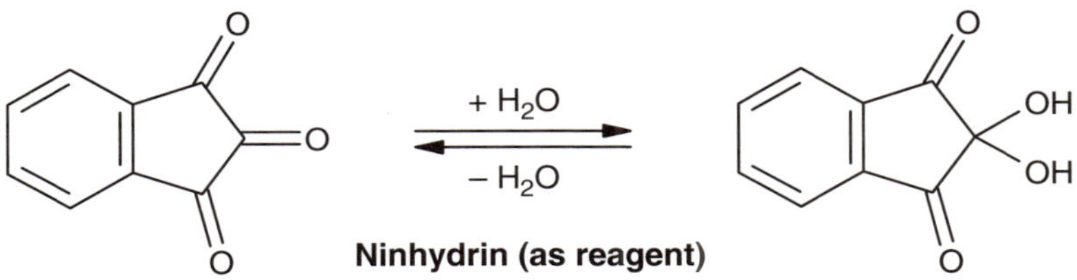

Ninhydrin (as reagent)

β-Alanine being an amino acid reacts with ninhydrin resulting in the formation of a violet-coloured complex.

The Schiff's base as formed in this method undergoes hydrolysis to give 2-amino-1,3-indane dione.

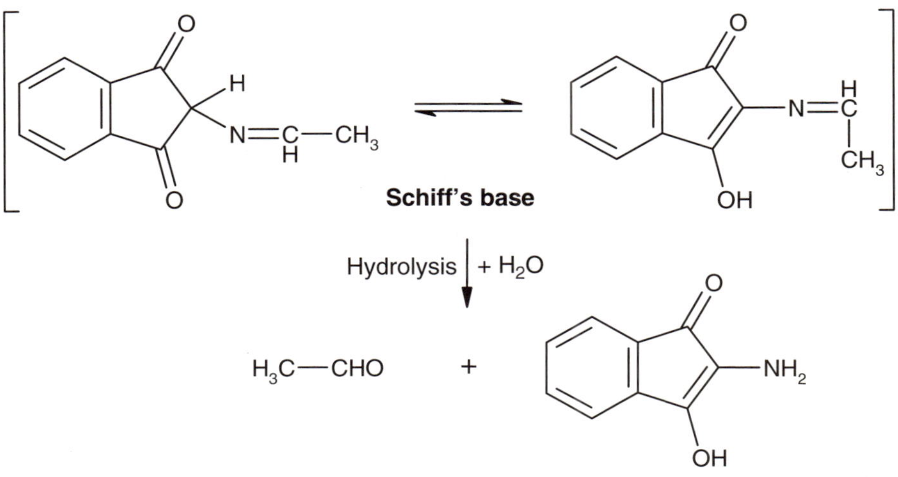

2-amino-1,3-indane dione (A)

Hydrolysis of 2-amino-1,3-indane dione (A) results in the formation of 2-hydroxyindane-1,3-dione (B).

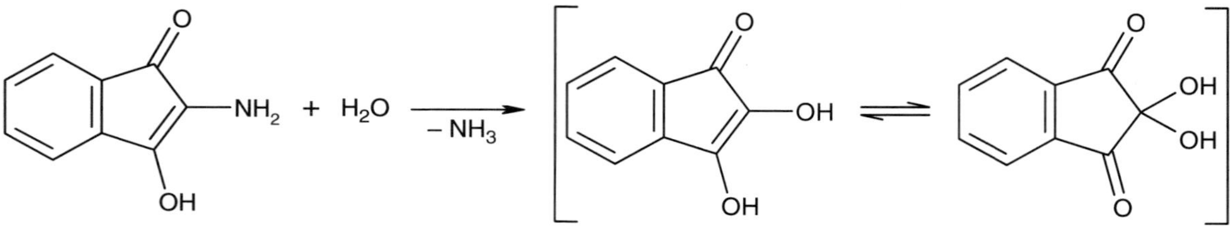

2-amino-1,3-indane dione **2-hydroxyindane-1,3-dione (B)**

Now 2-amino-1,3-indane dione being a reducing agent reduces ninhydrin and oxidises itself to 2-iminoindane-1,3-dione (C).

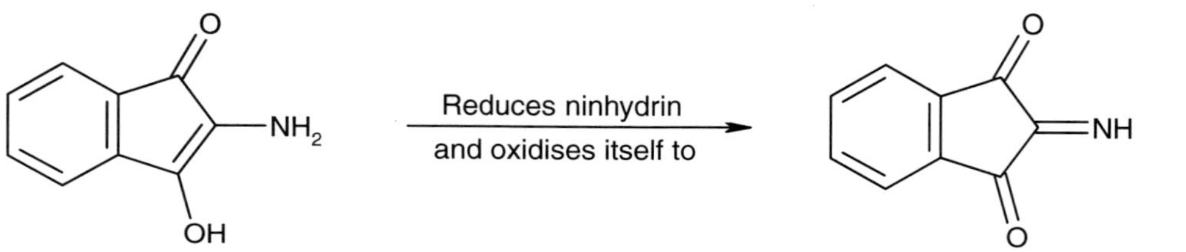

2-amino-1,3-indane dione **2-iminoindane-1,3-dione (C)**

In the next step, condensation reaction occurs between (B) and (C) resulting in the formation of azaoxonol which is an anion and can be represented by three mesomeric forms.

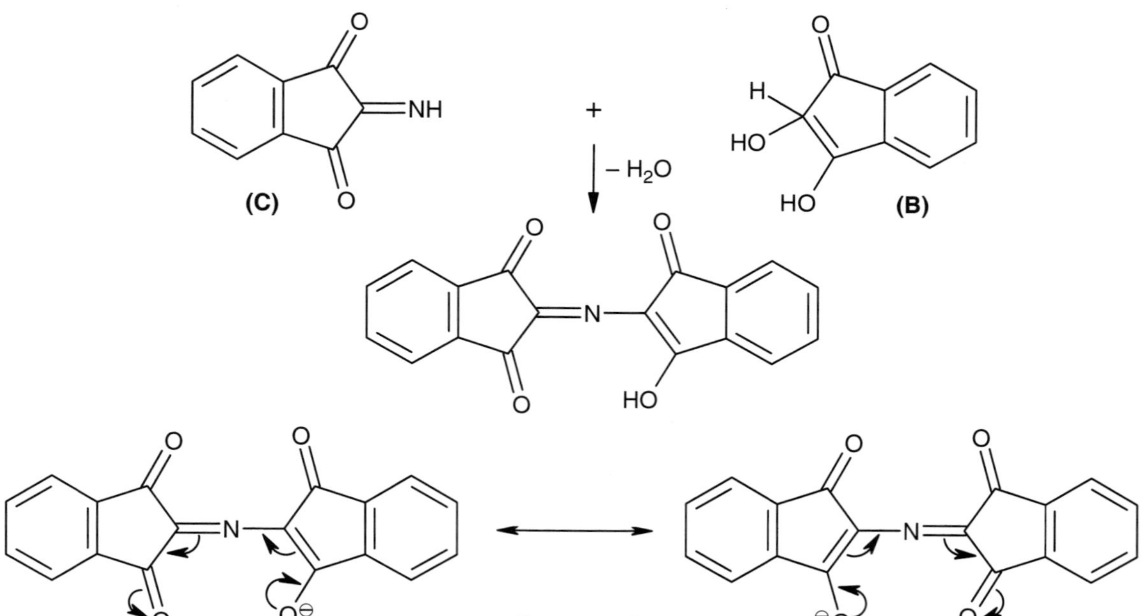

Azaoxonol

Note

Interference due to nicotinamide is removed by alkali treatment and treatment with talc removes amino acids and riboflavin. The retention of amino acids on talc can be successfully used for isolation of calcium pantothenate from β-alanine which is present as its decomposition product.

The following types of column are used for extraction and purification of the compound:

Reagents and material

1. Glass column: A glass column 25 cm × 1.2 cm (i.d.) is used.
2. Acetic acid–pyridine mixture: 2 parts v/v acetic acid and 20 parts v/v pyridine are mixed with water to produce 100 ml.
3. Florisil: About 50-100 g of florosil is taken in beaker and covered with sufficient volume of acetic acid–pyridine mixture, boiled gently for several minutes and allowed to settle. The supernatant liquid is decanted and washing is repeated thrice with cold water, followed by final washing with hot distilled water to remove acetic acid–pyridine. Florisil thus obtained is dried at 100-120°C and is stored in closed container for preparation of the column.

Preparation of column

Suspend 4 g of treated florisil in water and add to the column under gentle suction. Wash the column with 50 ml of distilled water before use.

Standard solution

1 mg/ml of calcium pantothenate in water.

Sample solution

The sample is appropriately diluted with water to get 1 mg/ml.

Procedure

Sample and standard solutions equivalent to 10 mg of calcium pantothenate are passed through the column and the column is eluted with water to collect 50 ml of the eluate. The contents of panthenol/calcium pantothenate are determined by method 1 or by reaction with naphthoquinone reagent as described above.

On hydrolysis, β-alanine and pantoic acid are produced. Pantoic acid, on treatment with $KMNO_4$, is oxidized to an aldehyde which reacts with phenylhydrazine to give coloured hydrazone.

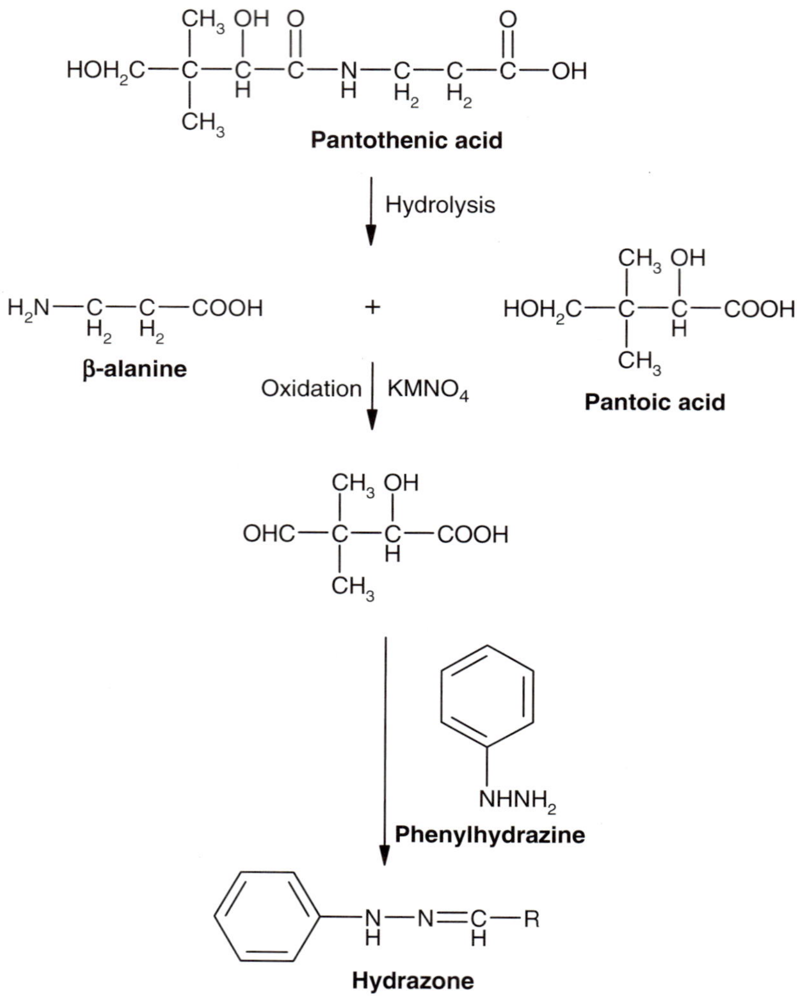

Reference

Assay of Vitamins in Pharmaceutical Preparations by M.H. Hashmi, p. 136, 1973.

Formulation 9

Ergocalciferol (Vitamin D_2) and Cholecalciferol (Vitamin D_3)

METHOD 1

This method is based on the measurement of salmon-pink colour as a result of interaction of vitamin D with antimony trichloride in chloroform. The absorbance of pink colour is measured at 500 nm. Prior to the colour development, vitamin D is separated chromatographically from vitamin A.

This is a well tried method being used in several National Drug Control Laboratories.

Reagents and materials

1. Silica gel GF_{254}.
2. Fuller's earth (fine powder): Dry 100 g of Fuller's earth at 110°C for 4 hours. Add 7 to 8 ml of water, mix by shaking vigorously and store it in a tight stoppered bottle.
3. Chloroform: Wash chloroform with water and store over anhydrous sodium sulphate overnight. Distil and collect at 60°C. Only this chloroform should be used throughout experiment; prepare fresh.
4. Ether petroleum (40-60°C).
5. Anaesthetic ether (peroxide-free).
6. Butylated hydroxytoluene.
7. Chloroform–acetic anhydride (1 : 1 v/v), inhibitor.
8. TLC plates (20 × 20 cm), coated with silica gel GF_{254} (0.5 mm thick).
9. Chromatographic column: 2.5 cm (i.d.) and about 20 cm long fitted with sintered glass support of G_2 porosity, a stop cock and a funnel on top.
10. Antimony trichloride stock solution: Rapidly weigh and powder 110 g of pure, crystalline antimony trichloride in a mortar and transfer to 1000 ml Erlenmeyer flask. Immediately add 500 ml of chloroform and dissolve by warming gently in a water-bath at 60°C, agitating the flask occasionally. Filter through a folded filter paper into a 1000 ml glass bottle with a ground stopper. Add 10 ml of acetic anhydride, mix well and allow to stand overnight in the closed bottle. Stored in the dark; this clear and almost colourless stock solution is stable for several weeks.

11. Antimony trichloride reagent: On the day of use, mix cautiously 49 volumes of the stock solution with 1 volume of acetyl chloride using a glass bottle with a ground stopper. Allow to stand for one hour before use. This reagent must be prepared fresh every day.
12. Chromatographic chamber (vapour-saturated chamber): Line the chromatographic chamber with filter paper. Pour into the chamber sufficient of mobile phase to saturate the filter paper and to form a layer 1.5 cm deep. Close the chamber and allow to stand for 1 hr at room temperature.
13. Mobile phase:
    (i) Petroleum ether : Chloroform (7 : 3 v/v).
    (ii) Benzene : Ether : Cyclohexane (2 : 1 : 1 v/v).
    (iii) Cyclohexane : Ether (1 : 1 v/v).
    (iv) Cyclohexane : Ethyl acetate (3 : 1 v/v).

Note

All mobile phases contain 0.01% w/v of butylated hydroxytoluene.

Vitamin D standard solution

Weigh accurately about 100 mg of vitamin D_2 (ergocalciferol) or vitamin D_3 (cholecalciferol), reference standard, 40 miu/g, or an equivalent product into a 100 ml volumetric flask, dissolve and dilute to volume with chloroform. Dilute 5 ml of 100 ml with chloroform.

Thin layer chromatography and elution of vitamin D

Spot quantitatively standard and sample solutions containing at least 2000 I.U. on two halves of a 20 × 20 cm TLC plate as a streak in minimum time. The streaks should be about 2.5 cm from lower edge and not less than 2 cm from the sides of plate. Transfer the plate to chromatographic chamber and allow the mobile phase-I to ascend 10 cm. Take out the plate and allow the solvent to evaporate but not completely from the plate. Place the plate in second chromatographic chamber and allow the mobile phase-II to ascend 10 cm. Take out the plate and allow the solvent to evaporate but not completely. Expose the plate to shortwave ultraviolet lamp and mark the D_2 bands with a pointer using minimum of time. Scrape the D_2 band corresponding to sample and standard preparations separately on butter paper.

Add 3 g of Fuller's earth to the glass column. Transfer the scraped bands corresponding to vitamin D_2 on different columns and elute with about 80 ml of chloroform. Evaporate chloroform in smaller lots in 50 to 100 ml round-bottom flasks to dryness under reduced pressure at 40°C taking precaution to evaporate last few ml at room temperature under nitrogen. Dissolve the residue immediately in chloroform.

Colour development

Pipette into dry cells the quantities of reagents and solutions as specified below:

	A_1	A_2	A_3	A_4	B_1	B_2	B_3	B_4	Blank	
									I	II
Sample	—	—	—	—	1.0	1.0	1.0	1.0	—	—
Standard eluate	2	2	2	2	—	—	—	—	—	—
Chloroform	—	—	—	—	1	1	—	—	2	1
Inhibitor	—	—	—	—	—	—	1	1	—	1

Proceed successively with each of these mixtures as follows: Add rapidly 3 ml of antimony trichloride reagent directly into the cell and mix briefly. After 10 to 20 seconds measure the extinction of the orange to dirty blue solution at 500 nm directly in the cells using a suitable spectrophotometer.

Before each reading calibrate the instrument for 100% transmission with the corresponding blank solution (blank 1 for samples without inhibitor; blank 2 for samples with inhibitor). If there is at least 10 ml of the extract solution, carry out the colour development four times with and without the addition of inhibitor to get an average value.

Calculation

$$\text{Vitamin D (IU/ml) of the extract solution} = \frac{E_B \times C \times 2}{E_A}$$

where

E_B = average extinction of B_1 and B_2 (without inhibitor) minus average extinction of B_3 and B_4 (with inhibitor);

E_A = average extinction of A_1, A_2, A_3 and A_4;

C = I.U. of vitamin D contained in 1 ml of the vitamin D standard solution (approximately 1000 I.U.).

Note

Vitamin D solutions are unstable. In particular, they are sensitive to light. All operations must be undertaken in the absence of actinic light. If the form of vitamin D present in the sample is unknown, use vitamin D_2 standard in the determination. For thin layer chromatography, at least 1000 I.U. of vitamin D are required. If the preparation to be tested has sufficient contents of vitamin D, 4000 I.U. should be chromatographed, if possible.

Sample solution (in the presence of vitamin A)

(a) **Solids:** Take an aliquot of powdered tablets or capsules containing 2000 to 4000 I.U. of vitamin D_2/D_3 into a stout walled test tube, add 5 ml of 2% v/v ammonia (pre-warmed to 60°C), flush with nitrogen and heat in a water-bath at 60°C stirring occasionally with a glass-rod. Care must be taken that the powder is thoroughly moistened and no particles remain adhering to the wall of the test tube. After about 10 minutes, transfer contents quantitatively to a separating funnel with the aid of 10 ml of water and sufficient ethanol. Extract with three 50 ml portions of petroleum ether (40-60°C). Evaporate the combined ether extracts in smaller lots in 50-100 ml ground-glass standard joint round-bottom flask to dryness under reduced pressure at 40°C taking precautions to evaporate the last few ml at room temperature. Continue the evaporation till the petroleum ether is completely expelled out. Then, add immediately sufficient quantity of chloroform but not less than 2 ml to attain the concentration of 1000 I.U. of vitamin D_2 or D_3 per ml.

(b) **Syrups:** Take an aliquot of the sample containing not less than 2000 I.U. of vitamin D_3 into a separating funnel. If sample is a thick syrupy preparation, add sufficient water to get a relatively less viscous consistency. Add enough ethanol to get ethanol concentration of 30 to 35 per cent in the mixture. Extract with three portions each of 50 ml of petroleum ether (40-60°C). Continue ether extracts and wash with water. Filter ether extracts through 35 to 40 g of anhydrous sodium sulphate in a conical flask and wash anhydrous sodium sulphate with sufficient petroleum ether. Evaporate the combined ether extracts in smaller lots in 50-100 ml of standard joint round-bottom flask to dryness under reduced pressure at 40°C taking precautions to evaporate the last few drops at room temperature. Add immediately sufficient chloroform but not less than 2 ml to get a concentration of 1000 I.U. of vitamin D_3 per ml.

(c) **Tablets containing calcium salts and isoniazid:** Soxhlate an aliquot of powdered tablets equivalent to 3000 to 5000 I.U. of vitamin D_2 or D_3 with sufficient petroleum ether (40-60°C) for 2 hours. Evaporate petroleum ether extract to about 5 ml. Add small portion of chloroform and continue evaporation till it is free from ether smell. Care should be taken to see that the solution does not evaporate completely to dryness. If needed, further small portion of chloroform may be added. Transfer chloroform solution quantitatively to 25 ml volumetric flask. Wash the sides of the container with small portions of chloroform and transfer the washings to the volumetric flask and dilute the solution up to the mark with chloroform.

(d) **Colloidal calcium with vitamins D_2 and D_3 and colloidal calcium with vitamin B_{12} and vitamins D_2 and D_3 injections:** Reflux an aliquot of the sample containing 3000 to 5000 I.U. of vitamin D_3 in 250 ml standard joint flask with 3 ml of 100 per cent w/v potassium hydroxide solution, 30 ml of alcohol and 0.1 g hydroquinone for 30 minutes. Cool and extract with three 70 ml portions of anaesthetic ether. Combine ether extracts and wash with 20 ml of 0.05 N potassium hydroxide solution, followed by 20 ml portions of water till the water wash is neutral to phenolphthalein solution. Filter through 35 to 40 g of anhydrous sodium sulphate in a conical flask and wash anhydrous sodium sulphate by filtering 50 ml of anaesthetic ether. Combine ether portions and evaporate on a water-bath to about 5 ml. Add small portion of chloroform and continue the evaporation till it is free from ether smell. Care should be taken to see that the solution does not evaporate completely. If needed, further small portion of chloroform may be added. Transfer chloroform solution quantitatively to 25 ml of volumetric flask. Wash the sides of the conical flask with small portion of chloroform, transferring it to same volumetric flask and make the solution to volume.

Antimony trichloride ($SbCl_3$) forms coloured π-complex with double bond system.

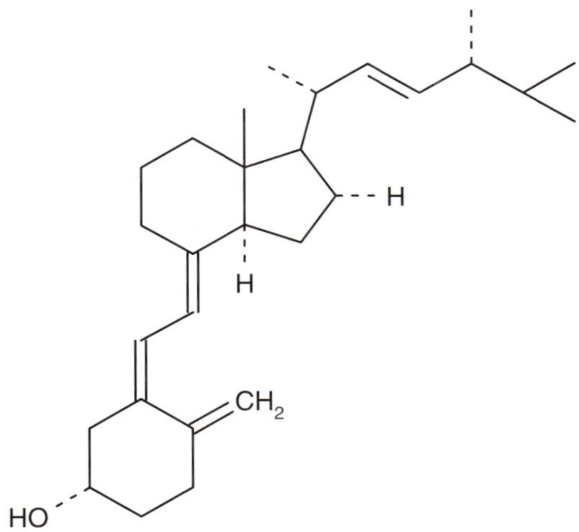

Ergocalciferol (vitamin D_2)

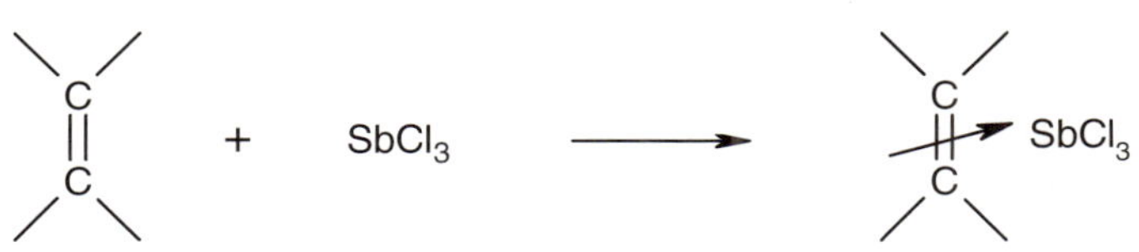

METHOD 2

The antimony (III) chloride method for determination of vitamin D_2/D_3 as described earlier suffers from certain disadvantages:

1. The reagent is extremely corrosive.
2. The reagent absorbs moisture from the atmosphere, thus forming oxychlorides and leaving a film of antimony oxychloride on the absorption cells.
3. Colour produced in unstable, non-specific and its intensity varies from batch to batch of the reagent and from day to day.

After the vitamin D_2/D_3 has been separated by TLC, it is subjected to the following method.

Reagents

1. Absolute methanol.
2. 1% v/v solution of anisaldehyde in methanol.
3. 10% v/v sulphuric acid in methanol.

Standard solution of vitamin D_2/D_3

20 mcg/ml of vitamin D_2/D_3 reference substance in methanol.

Sample solution

Proceed as described under method 1 except that at the end the residue is taken up in methanol instead of chloroform.

Procedure

To 2 ml of sample and standard solutions add 0.6 ml of anisaldehyde reagents and 1.25 ml of sulphuric acid (added dropwise with constant agitation). Allow the mixture to stand for 1 minute and then dilute to 25 ml with 10% v/v sulphuric acid. Measure the absorbance of greenish-blue colour in both the solutions at 685 nm against reagent blank treated similarly and calculate the results by comparison. The colour is stable for 35 minutes and the method obeys Beer's law over a range of 0.1 to 0.5 mg of vitamin D_2/D_3.

Formulation 10

Rutin

METHOD 1

Reagents

1. 0.1 M aluminium chloride: 24.1 g of aluminium chloride is dissolved in water to produce 100 ml.
2. 1 M potassium acetate: 24.5 g of potassium acetate is dissolved in water to produce 250 ml.

Standard solution

Weigh accurately 10 mg of pure rutin, dissolve and make up the volume to 100 ml with ethyl alcohol. 10 ml of the resulting solution is diluted to 100 ml with ethyl alcohol.

Sample solution

Remove the colour of the tablet with water and powder in a mortar. Wash the powder with 25 ml solvent ether and keep for some time. Decant ether layer and repeat the above step five times. Dry pestle mortar in the oven to remove traces of ether. Add about 40 ml of hot absolute alcohol to the pestle mortar and mix thoroughly. Transfer quantitatively into a 100 ml centrifuge tube with the aid of absolute alcohol. The volume should not exceed 60 ml. To this add about 3-4 g of Fuller's earth and mix thoroughly. Centrifuge the solution and filter supernatant solution into a 100 ml volumetric flask. Wash the filter paper thoroughly with absolute alcohol and make up to volume with it. Mix well and designate it as sample solution.

Procedure

Take 2 ml each of sample and standard solutions and add 3 ml of aluminium chloride solution, 5 ml of potassium acetate solution and 1 ml of 1 N hydrochloric acid. Mix well and keep at room temperature for 15 minutes. Prepare respective blanks and measure the absorbance at 433 nm against blanks. Deduce the results by comparison.

Probable Reaction Mechanism

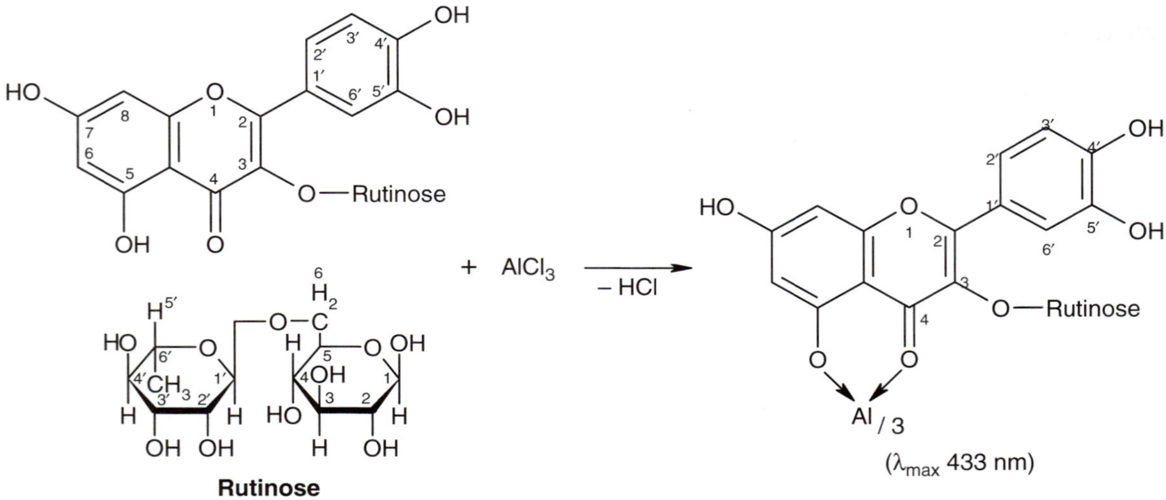

Rutin (vitamin P)

Note

Rutin alone has λ_{max} 259, 266 & 363 nm; this bathochromic shift on addition of Al^{+++} (327 → 433 nm) is indicative of 5 —OH free.

When rutin is treated with sodium acetate and boric acid we get boric acid complex between 3′,4′ —OH along with bathochromic shift from 363 to 387 nm, indicative of 3′,4′ —OH being free. On addition of sodium acetate we get bathochromic shift from 259 to 271 nm i.e. 7 —OH free. On treatment with NaOH the bathochromic effect from 363 to 415 nm is indicative of 4 —OH free.

Probable Reaction Mechanism

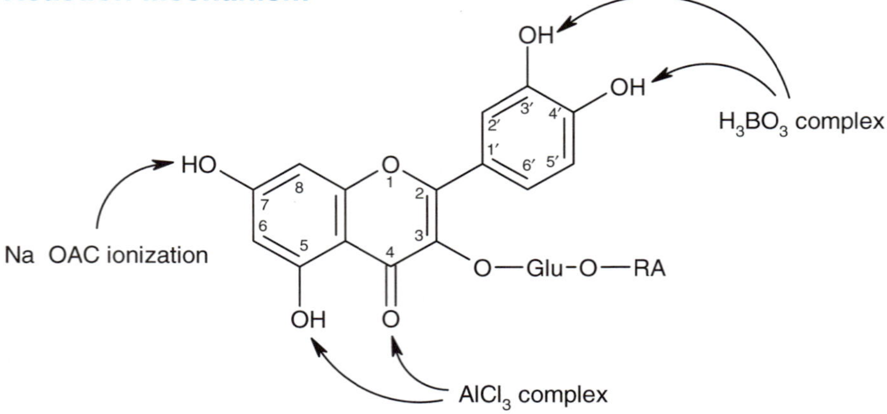

Rutin - $AlCl_3$ and H_3BO_3 complex

Diazotized p-aminobenzoic acid ($NaNO_2 + H_2SO_4$) couples with the compound at C-6, i.e., ortho to C-5 —OH group to give a coloured product which is stabilized with NaOH having λ_{max} 420 nm.

Probable Reaction Mechanism

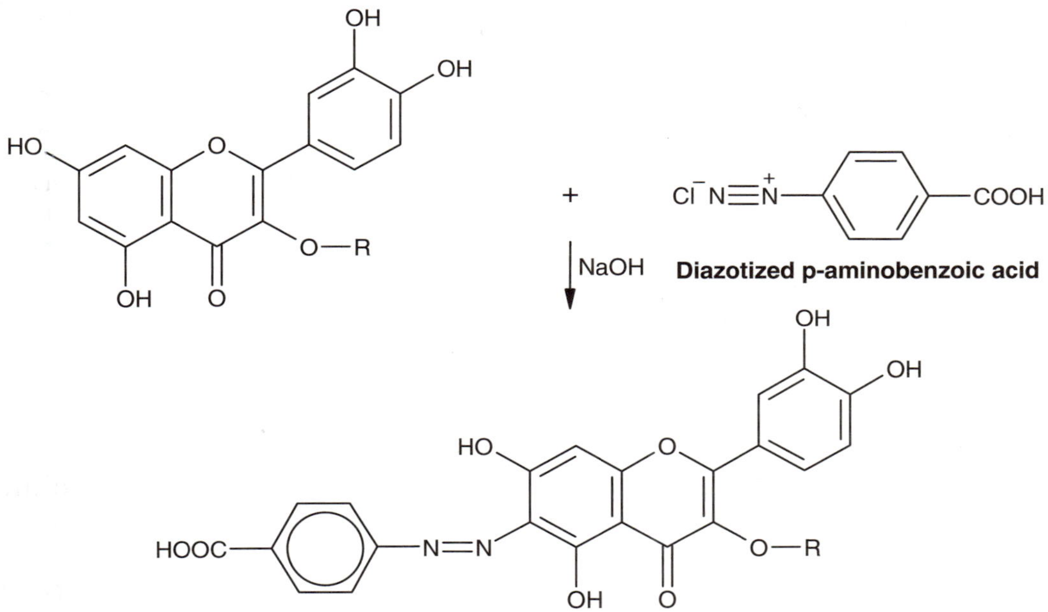

Coloured product
(λ_{max} 420 nm)

Reference

Analytical Profile of Drug Substances (Vol. 12) by Klaus Florey, p. 663.

METHOD 2

Standard solution

1 mg/ml of rutin in ethyl alcohol.

Sample solution

Accurately weighed quantity of the powdered tablets equivalent to 25 mg of rutin is shaken with hot ethanol, cooled and adjusted to 25 ml.

Procedure

To 1 ml of the sample and standard solutions add 1 ml of hydrochloric acid and 100 mg of pure magnesium powder. Cool the flask under running tap water and adjust the volume to 10 ml with ethanol. The colour of the resultant solution is measured at about 520 nm against reagent blank.

Probable Reaction Mechanism

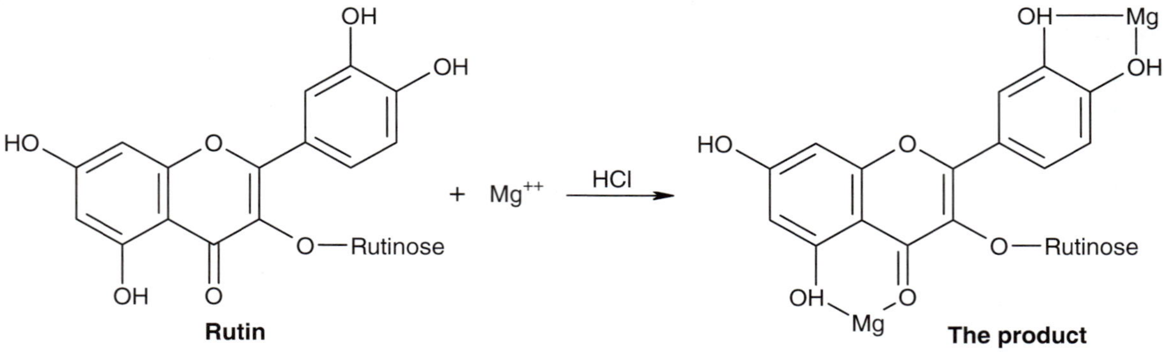

The product
(λ_{max} 520 nm)

Reference

P.K. Sengupta & R. Chanda, *Eastern Pharmacist*, p. 113, June 1980.

METHOD 3

Standard solution

1 mg/ml of rutin in isopropyl alcohol. An appropriate aliquot of the above solution is further diluted with isopropyl alcohol to get 20 mcg/ml concentration.

Sample solution

The sample is extracted with isopropyl alcohol to get a concentration of 20 mcg/ml.

Procedure

The extinction of both sample and standard solutions is measured at 363 nm, the absorption maxima for rutin and results are calculated using 285 as the $E^{1\%}_{1\ cm}$.

Formulation 11

Ascorbic acid, Menadione, Ferrous gluconate, Calcium lactate, Citrus bioflavonoid compound

ESTIMATION

Ascorbic acid

METHOD 1

Reagents

1. Dilute sulphuric acid.
2. 0.1 N iodine.
3. Starch solution.

Procedure

Dissolve the accurately weighed sample equivalent to 150 mg of ascorbic acid in 25 ml of dilute sulphuric acid and add 60 ml of water. Titrate with 0.1 N iodine using starch solution as indicator. Each ml of 0.1 N iodine is equivalent to 0.008806 g of ascorbic acid.

Iodine oxidizes ascorbic acid to dehydroascorbic acid and excess iodine reacts with indicator to give blue colour.

Probable Reaction Mechanism

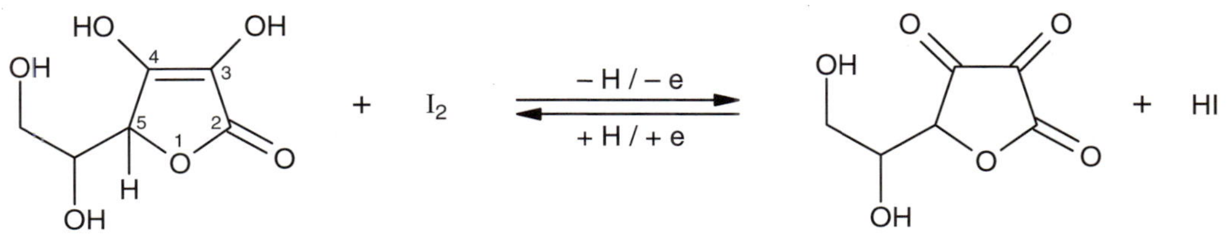

Ascorbic acid

Dehydroascorbic acid

Note

The acidity of ascorbic acid is due to presence of —OH group at C-4.

The compound forms coloured complex with Cu(2) (λ_{max} 540 nm).

Probable Reaction Mechanism

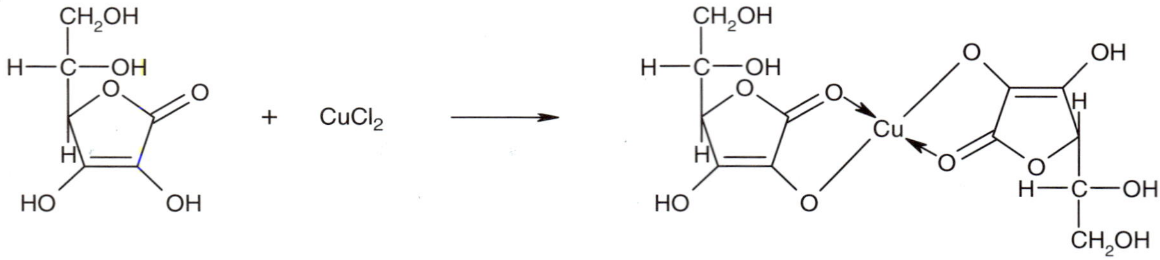

On treatment with HCl, ascorbic acid is quantatively converted into furfuraldehyde. Furfuraldehyde so formed reacts with o-toulidine in acetic acid medium resulting in the formation of the product.

Probable reaction mechanism as proposed by the authors

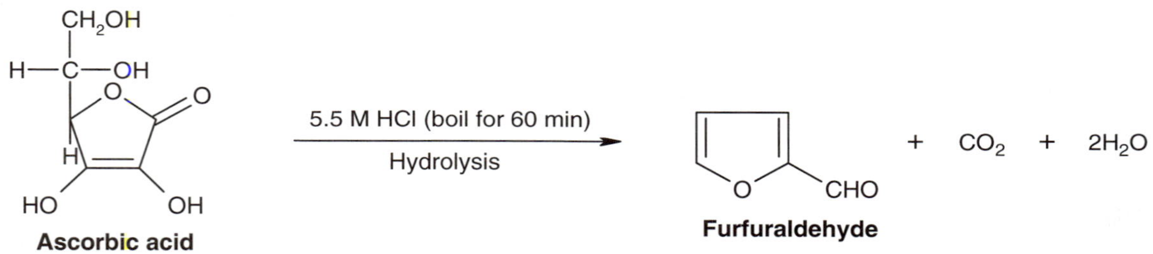

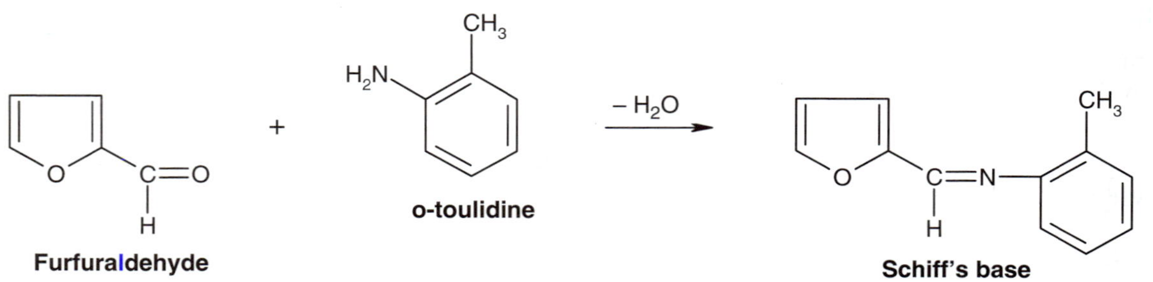

Under the reaction condition employed, the five-membered furan ring of formaldehyde opens up resulting in another molecule of o-toulidine reacting with furfuraldehyde (opened ring) and forming the product.

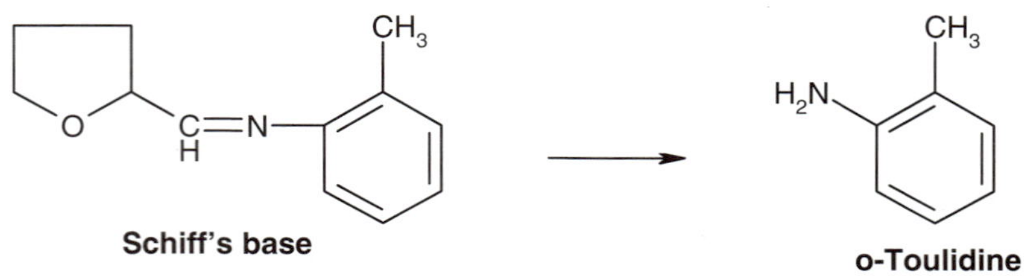

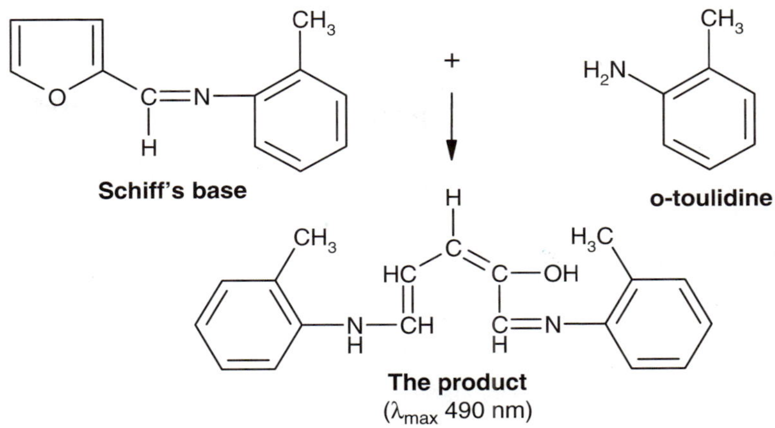

Note

1. During acidic hydrolysis, 5 ml of xylene is added. Xylene prevents loss of ascorbic acid due to steam volatility and also acts as collector. After hydrolysis, xylene layer containing furfural is diluted with acetic acid (glacial) and subjected to colour development.
2. Vitamins B_1, B_2 and B_6 do not interfere.

Reference

V. Nirmal Chandar, Elizabeth K. John & N. Balasubramanian, *Indian Drugs*, **25(7)**, 309, 1988.

METHOD 2

Balasubramanian et al. have described an analytical method based on oxidation by iodate in acidic medium in the presence of chloride ion.

Reagents

1. 0.04% solution of potassium iodate in water.
2. 0.5 M sulphuric acid.
3. 6% w/v solution of sodium chloride.
4. 0.01% solution of dye (2′,7′-dichlorofluoroscein) in 1 M sodium hydroxide.
5. 1 M sodium hydroxide.
6. Monochloroacetic acid reagent: Dissolve 19 g of monochloroacetic acid in 30 ml of water, add 8 g of sodium hydroxide, dilute to 100 ml with water; pH of the reagent is about 4.35.

Standard solution

100 μg/ml of ascorbic acid in water.

Sample solution

Appropriate quantity of the sample suspended in water and processed to get 100 μg/ml.

Procedure

Take 5 ml of iodate solution and 1 ml of sodium chloride, mix, make acidic by adding 1 ml of 0.5 M sulphuric acid. Then add 3 ml of dye and 2 ml of sample or standard solution. Allow to stand for 5 min and then to each flask add 2.5 ml of chloroacetic acid reagent, dilute to 25 ml with water, measure the absorbance at 525 nm against reagent blank.

Probable Reaction Mechanism

Firstly, IO_3 is reduced by ascorbic acid to iodine (I_2). Liberated iodine is further oxidized by excess iodate and stabilized as ICl_2 in the presence of NaCl. Stabilized species (ICl_2) acts as iodinating agent to iodinate the dye (ICl_2 is a superior iodinating agent than I_2). Iodinated complex is coloured (λ_{max} 525 nm).

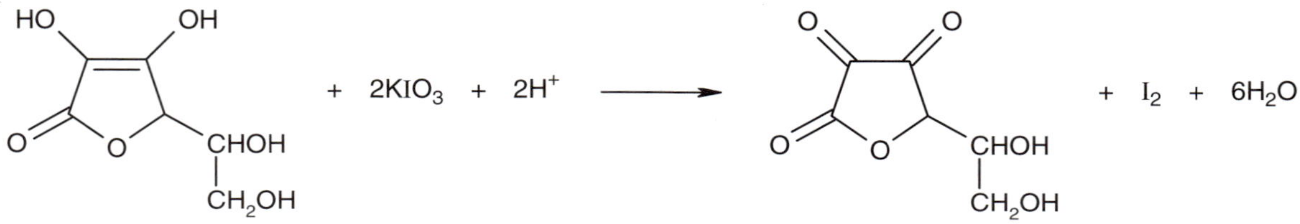

Dehydroascorbic acid

$$2I_2 + KIO_3 + 6H^+ \; 5Cl^- \,(NaCl) \longrightarrow 5ICl + 3H_2O$$

$$5ICl + 5Cl^- \longrightarrow 5ICl_2^-$$

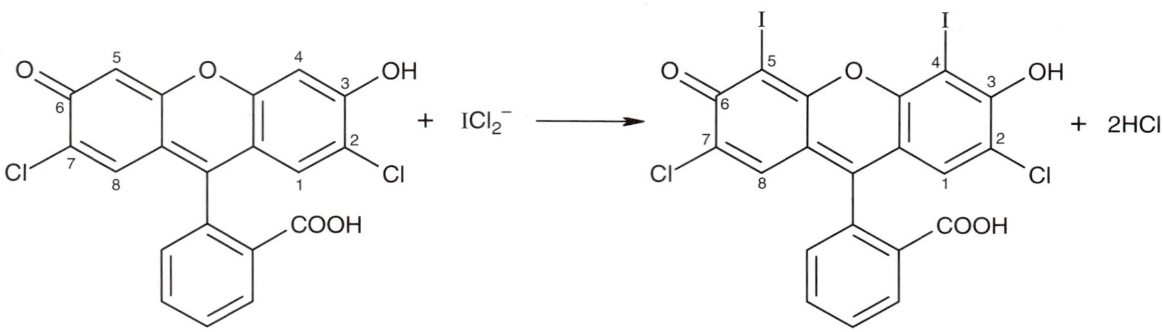

2′,7′-dichlorofluorescein **2′,7′-dichloro-4′,5′-diiodofluorescein** (λ_{max} 525 nm)

Note

Nicotinic acid, vitamin B_6 (5000 μg), riboflavin (100 μg), folic acid (25 μg), thiamine (1500 μg), Co^{+2}, Mg^{+2}, Fe^{+2}, Zn^{+2}, Cu^{+2} (4000 μg) do not interfere.

Reference

N. Balasubramanian, S. Usha & K. Srividya, *Indian Drugs*, **32(2)**, 78-83, 1985.

Citrus bioflavonoid compound (CFC)

This method is based on estimation of hespiridin contents.

Reagents

1. Methanol AR.
2. 0.04% w/v solution of copper sulphate in water.
3. 0.1 N hydrochloric acid.

Standard solution

Heat 150 mg of 'CFC' standard in 50 ml of methanol, cool and make up to 100 ml with methanol.

Sample solution

Heat the sample equivalent to 150 mg of 'CFC' in 50 ml of methanol, cool, make up to 100 ml with methanol and filter.

Procedure

To 5 ml each of the standard and sample solutions add 1 ml of copper sulphate solution, 1 ml of 0.1 N hydrochloric acid and dilute to 100 ml with methanol. Measure the extinction of the resulting solutions at the maximum at about 283 nm and deduce the results by comparison.

Probable Reaction Mechanism

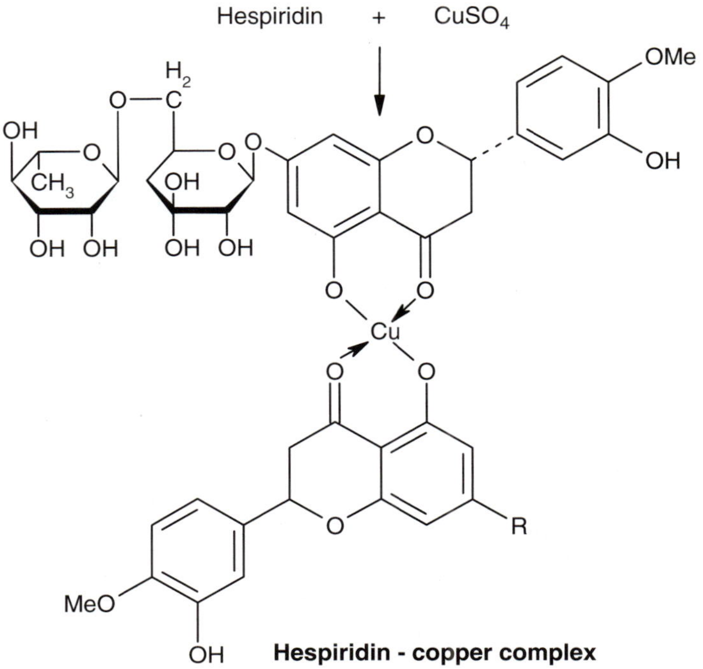

Hespiridin - copper complex

Calcium lactate

Reagents

1. Ammonia–ammonium chloride buffer solution.
2. 0.05 M EDTA solution.
3. 10% w/v solution of potassium cyanide.
4. Solochrome black T solution.

Procedure

Dissolve an accurately weighed sample equivalent to 150 mg of calcium lactate in about 100 ml of water, add 2 ml of potassium cyanide solution and 5 ml of buffer. Titrate the above solution with 0.05 M EDTA solution using solochrome black T solution as indicator. Each ml of 0.05 M EDTA solution is equivalent to 0.01542 g of calcium lactate.

Alternatively estimate (Ca^{++}) by flame photometric method described in formulation 34 of the chapter on alimentary drugs.

Ferrous gluconate

Reagents

1. Nitric acid.
2. Hydrochloric acid.
3. Dilute sulphuric acid.
4. 10% w/v solution of ammonium thiocyanate.

Standard solution

40 mcg/ml solution of Fe^{++} (as ferrous sulphate).

Sample solution

To accurately weighed sample equivalent to 50 mg of ferrous gluconate add 1 ml of nitric acid and 5 ml of hydrochloric acid. Heat on water-bath till there are no fumes of nitrous acid. Dilute to 250 ml with water and filter.

Procedure

To 2 ml each of the sample and standard solutions add 5 ml of ammonium thiocyanate solution, dilute to 25 ml with dilute sulphuric acid. Measure the absorption of the sample and standard solutions at about 520 nm and deduce the results by comparison.

Note

The method is based on formation of coloured complex with NH_4SCN (λ_{max} 520 nm).

In acidic medium, gluconic acid is formed which is spontaneously converted to gluconic acid lactone forming iron chelate of hydroxamic acid.

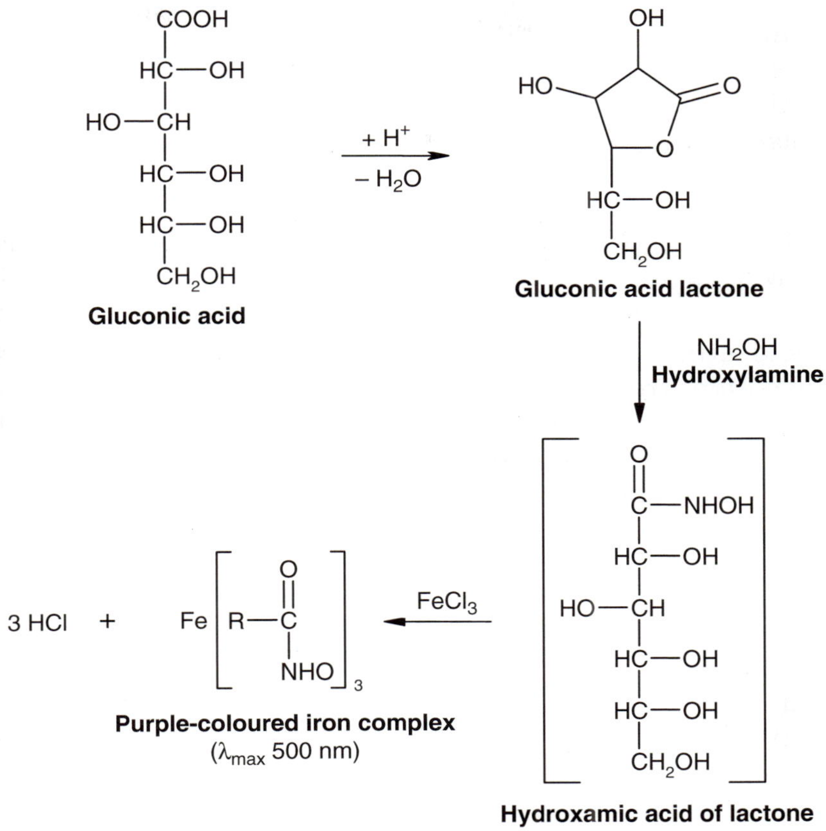

Note

Gluconic acid portion of the molecule, i.e., polyols shall undergo Malaprade cleavage forming formic acid which can be used for quantitative method.

Menadione

METHOD 1

Reagents

1. Chloroform.
2. 0.2% w/v solution of 2,4-dinitrophenyl hydrazine in hydrochloric acid–alcohol (1 : 5 v/v) mixture.
3. Ammonia–alcohol (1 : 1) mixture.

Standard solution

5 mcg/ml solution of menadione in chloroform.

Sample solution

Suspend an accurately weighed sample equivalent to 300 mcg in 5 ml of water and extract with three 10 ml portions of chloroform, make up to 50 ml with chloroform and filter.

Procedure

To 5 ml each of standard and sample solutions add 2 ml of 2,4-dinitrophenyl hydrazine solution. Heat on water-bath to almost dryness, add 15 ml of ammonia–alcohol mixture and dilute to 50 ml with alcohol. Measure the extinction of the standard and sample solutions at about 635 nm and deduce the results by comparison.

Menadione in acid–ethanolic solution condenses with 2,4-dinitrophenylhydrazine and subsequent treatment with ethanolic ammonia produces green colour. For attack on ninhydrin in this acid catalysed carbonyl reaction, there are two conceivable positions C-1 and C-4; since there is electron-repelling CH_3 group at C-2, so increased electron density at C-1, so less electrophilic attraction at C-1 than C-4, so hydrazine attacks at C-4. Hydrazone so formed is deprotonated by the addition of ethanolic ammonia giving dark blue-coloured compound (λ_{max} 635 nm).

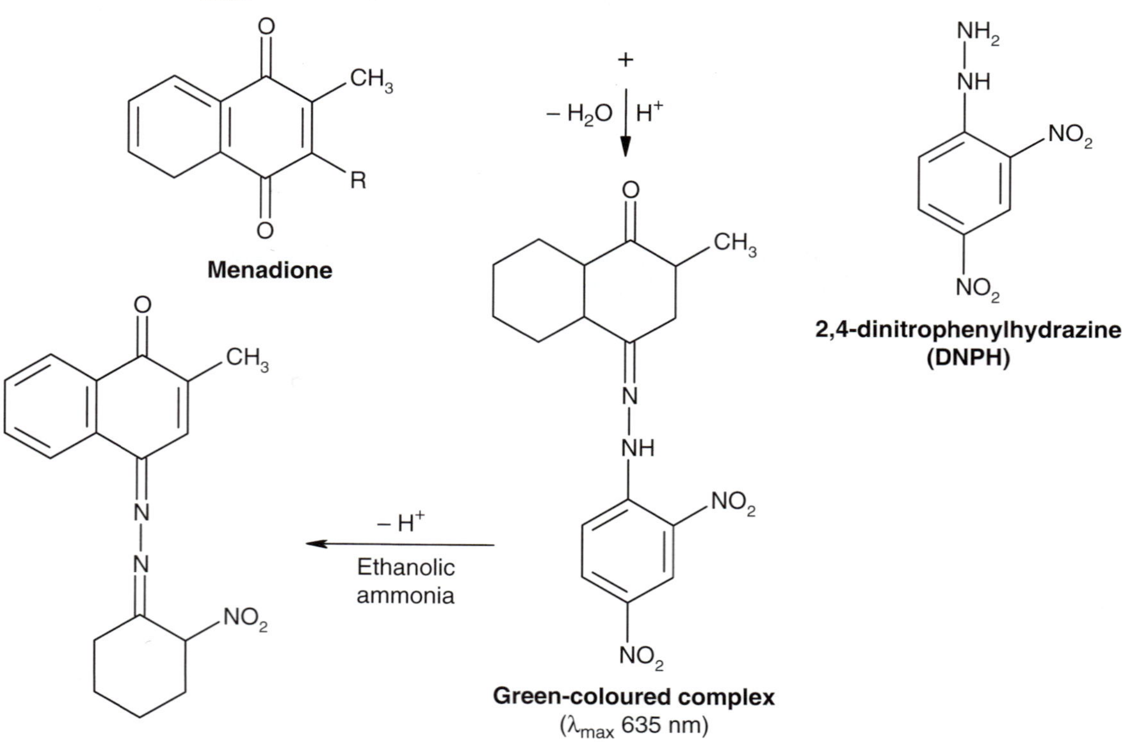

R = **H (K_3)**

R = 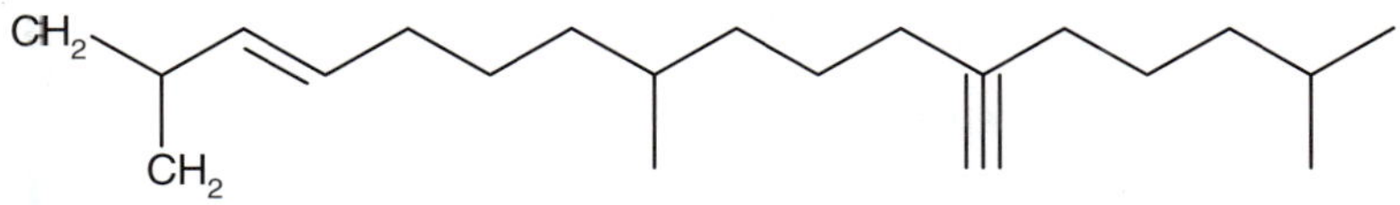

Phytyl radical (K_1)

Menadione, a quinone, can be reduced to hydroquinol with zinc and hydrochloric acid, and hydroquinol so formed can be estimated by ceriometric titration; compound gets reoxidized to quinone (menadione).

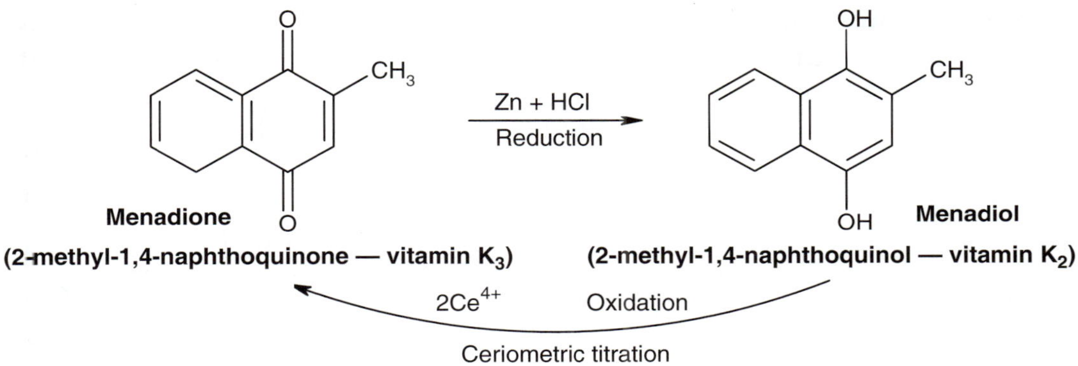

Sane et al. have reported the estimation of vitamin K_4 based on reaction with p-aminophenol forming indophenol dye in alkaline medium (sodium hydroxide) with λ_{max} 630 nm.

Probable Reaction Mechanism

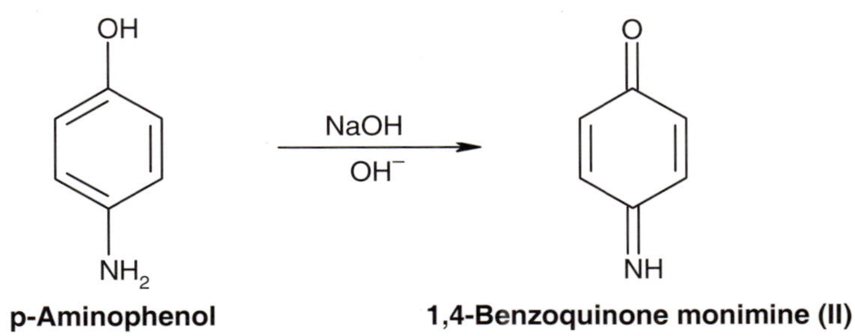

The coupling takes place at ortho position to position 4 —OH giving indophenol dye.

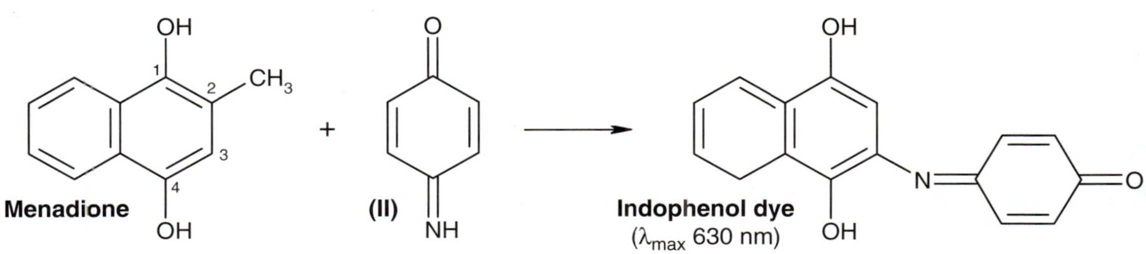

Reference

R.T. Sane & A.Y. Sathe, *J. of University of Bombay*, Science (Vol. L), No. 77, 1981.

The drug forms complex with p-phenylene diamine dihydrochloride on alkaline oxidation by coupling at ortho position to phenolic —OH group present in the ring.

Probable Reaction Mechanism

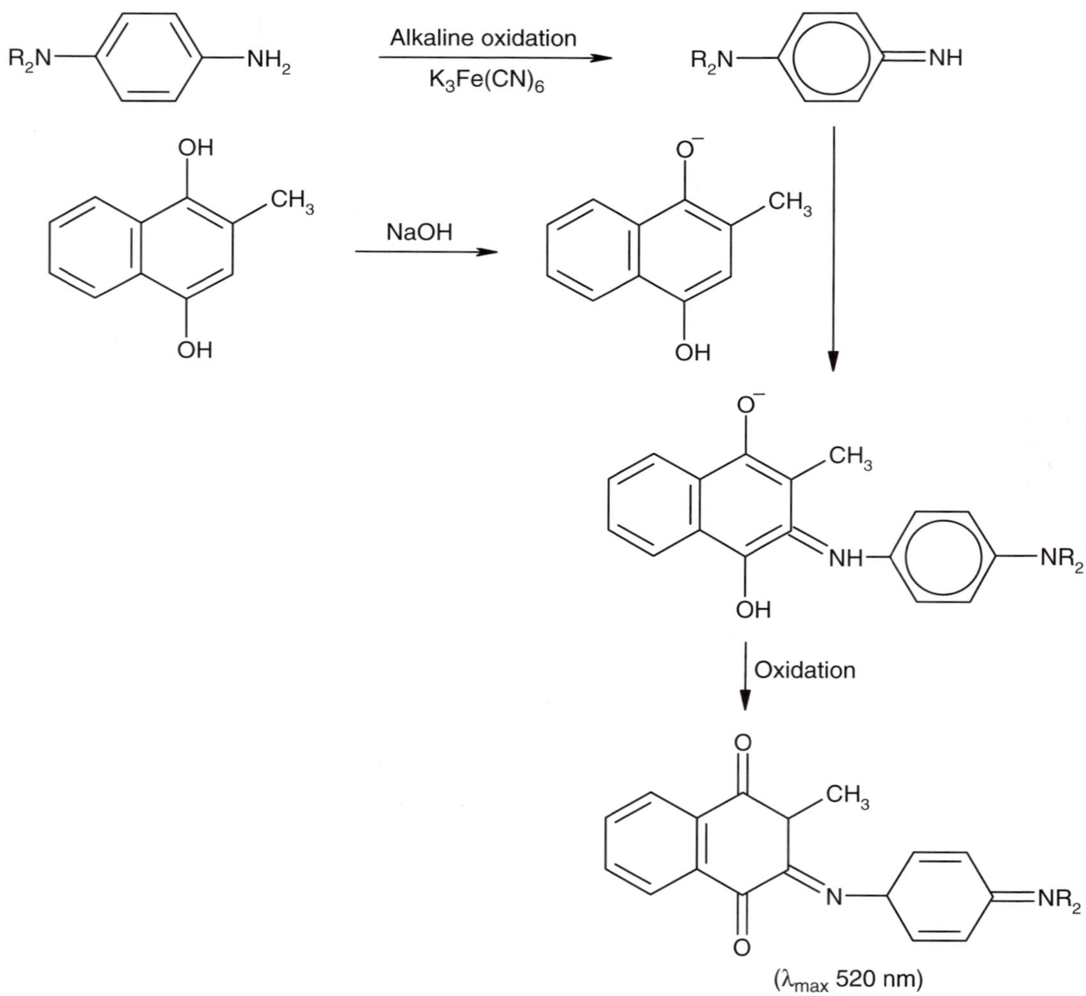

Reference

R.T. Sane, V.J. Doshi, S.R. Jukar, S.K. Joshi & S.V. Sawant, *Indian Drugs*, **21(1)**, 30-31, 1983.

METHOD 2

Reagents

1. 5 M sodium hydroxide solution.
2. 0.5% w/v solution of 3-methyl-2-benzothiazolinone (MBTH) hydrazone hydrochloride in water.
3. 0.2% resorcinol solution in methanol.
4. Conc. sulphuric acid.

Standard solution

(a) Standard solution of menadione (1 mg/ml) prepared in methanol.
(b) Standard solution of menadione sodium bisulphite (MSB) (1 mg/ml) prepared in water.

Further dilutions made with methanol or water to get 200 μg/ml.

Sample solution

Powdered sample equivalent to 100 mg of menadione suspended in water, shake, filter and dilute appropriately. For injection, sample was diluted with methanol.

Procedure

(a) To 2.5 ml each of sample and standard solutions add 5 ml of "MBTH" reagent and 2 ml of 5 M NaOH, set aside for 5 min, dilute to 25 ml with water and measure the absorbance at 625 nm against reagent blank and calculate the results.
(b) To 2 ml each of sample and standard solutions add 2 ml of methanol, 1 ml of resorcinol solution followed by 5 ml of conc. sulphuric acid, set aside for 5 min, cool and dilute to 25 ml with water and measure the absorbance of red-coloured product at 520 nm against reagent blank and calculate the results by comparison.

Probable Reaction Mechanism

In method (a), menadione and MSB form diazo complex with MBTH in alkaline medium. This readily loses a molecule of nitrogen to form coupled blue product; whereas in method (b), oxygen atom of menadione and MSB gets protonated in the presence of concentrated sulphuric acid to form carbo cation which may undergo electrophilic addition with electron-rich resorcinol to form a product with the loss of water to form red-coloured complex (λ_{max} 520 nm).

Method A

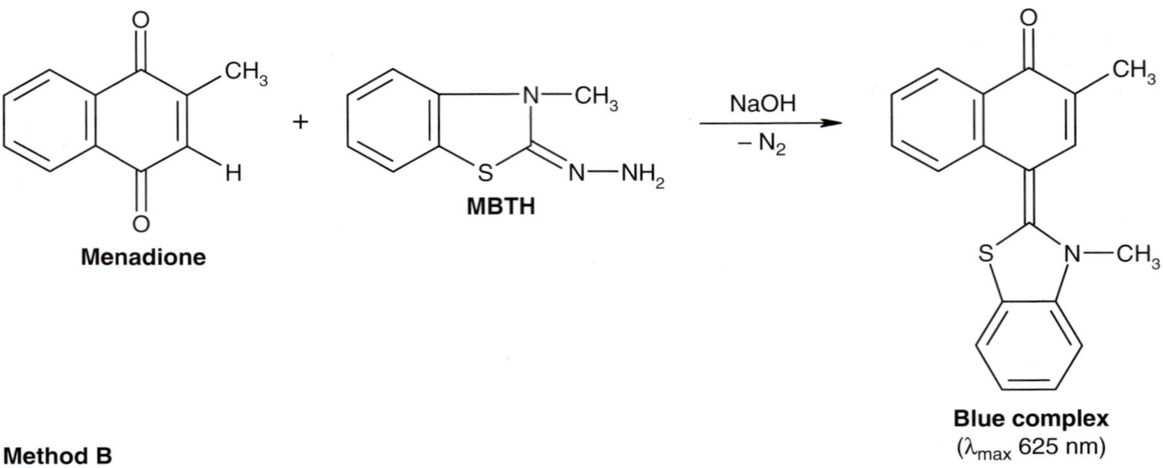

Method B

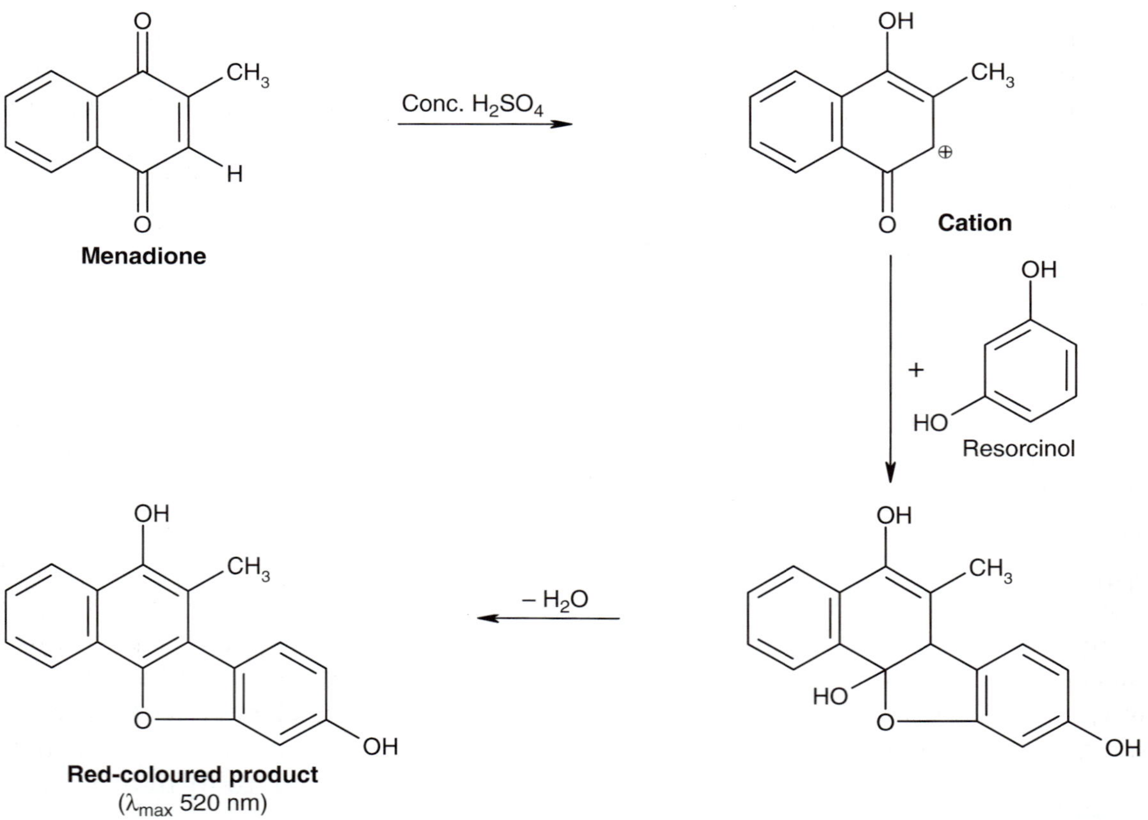

Reference

P. Nagaraja, R.A. Vasantha & H.S. Yathiraju, *J. Pharm. Biomed. Anal.*, **28**, 161-168, 2002.

Formulation 12

Inositol, N-Hydroxymethyl nicotinamide, Vitamin B_{12}

ESTIMATION

Inositol

Reagents

1. Borate buffer: Dissolve 4 mg of boric acid in 200 ml of water and adjust the pH to 8.0 with 1 N sodium hydroxide solution.
2. Potassium periodate solution: Weigh about 120 mg of potassium periodate and dissolve in water to produce 100 ml.
3. 2% w/v solution of potassium iodide in water, prepare fresh.
4. 1 N sodium hydroxide.

Standard solution

20 mcg/ml of inositol in water.

Sample preparation

Weigh accurately powdered sample equivalent to 100 mg of the substance and dissolve in water to produce 100 ml. Shake, filter and dilute 5 ml of the filtrate to 250 ml with water (20 mcg/ml).

Procedure

Transfer 10 ml each of standard and sample solutions to two different tubes, add 10 ml of water and 2 ml of potassium periodate solution. Shake and keep at 50°C for 2 hrs and cool. Take 2 ml each of the above solutions, add 15 ml of borate buffer and 8 ml of potassium iodide solution. Shake and dilute to 50 ml with borate buffer. Measure the extinction of both the solutions after 5 minutes at 352 nm and calculate the results.

Probable Reaction Mechanism

The compound undergoes Malaprade cleavage by sodium metaperiodate. The excess reagent reacts with KI to give iodine, the final solution having λ_{max} 352 nm.

$$\underset{\substack{\textbf{Inositol} \\ \textbf{(Hexahydroxycyclohexane)}}}{C_6H_6O_6} + NaIO_4 \longrightarrow -CHO + NaIO_3$$

$$NaIO_4 + KI \xrightarrow{\text{Alkaline medium}} NaIO_3 + I_2 + KOH$$

Iodine is responsible for λ_{max} 352 nm.

N-hydroxymethyl nicotinamide (pyridine-3 carboxylic acid hydroxymethylamide)

Reagent

Citrate buffer: 0.2 N solution of sodium acid citrate is prepared in boiled water, cooled and adjusted to pH 6. Alternatively, 25 g of citric acid is dissolved in 75 ml of water and pH adjusted to 6 with 40% w/v sodium hydroxide solution.

Standard solution

Dissolve about 50 mg of pure compound in water to produce 100 ml (500 mcg/ml).

Sample solution

Shake an accurately weighed portion of the sample equivalent to 100 mg of the substance with 70 ml of water for 20-25 min. Dilute to 200 ml and filter.

Procedure

To 5 ml each of sample and standard solutions add 10 ml of citrate buffer, pH 6, and dilute to 100 ml with water. Measure the extinction of both the solutions at 262 nm and deduce the results by comparison.

Vitamin B_{12}

Weigh accurately powdered material equivalent to 200 mcg of vitamin B_{12} and add 50 ml of distilled water. Shake and add 30 g of ammonium sulphate and 100 ml of isobutyl alcohol. Shake well and collect the separated isobutyl alcohol layer. Shake the alcoholic layer with 5 ml of water and use aqueous layer for estimation by ion-exchange method described under general assay methods for vitamin B_{12}.

Formulation 13

Cyproheptadine hydrochloride, Lysine monohydrochloride, Dried Yeast

ESTIMATION

Cyproheptadine hydrochloride

METHOD 1

Reagents

1. Methanol (anhydrous).
2. Acetic anhydride.
3. Citric acid (monohydrate).
4. Citric acid–acetic anhydride reagent: Dissolve 2 g of citric acid (monohydrate) in 5 ml of methanol (anhydrous) and dilute to 100 ml with acetic anhydride.

Standard solution

100 mcg/ml of cyproheptadine hydrochloride in chloroform.

Sample solution

Weigh accurately a quantity of the sample equivalent to 10 mg of the substance, extract with four 20 ml portions of chloroform, filter through sintered funnel. Wash the residue with chloroform and make up the volume to 100 ml (100 mcg/ml). Retain the residue for estimation of lysine monohydrochloride.

Procedure

Evaporate 1 ml each of sample and standard solutions to dryness, add 1 ml of citric acid reagent and immerse in water-bath for 30 min. Cool and dilute to 10 ml with acetic anhydride. Measure the absorption of both the solutions at about 570 nm against reagent blank and calculate the results by comparison.

Explanatory Note

On heating the substance with citric acid–acetic anhydride, a red-violet colour is produced. Citric acid reacts with acetic anhydride to give acetyl citric acid γ-anhydride which yields red colour with pyridine or piperidine derivative.

METHOD 2

Alternatively, it can be estimated as under:

Reagents

1. Acetone.
2. Hydrochloric acid.
3. Modified Dragendorff's reagent.

Procedure

To both sample and standard solutions add Dragendorff's reagent, stir for 15 min, filter the precipitates through G_4 sintered funnel, dissolve the precipitates in acetone and measure the absorbance of the resulting solution at 470 nm for quantitative analysis.

Probable Reaction Mechanism

Iodine present in the reagent attacks at double bond of the ring B as under:

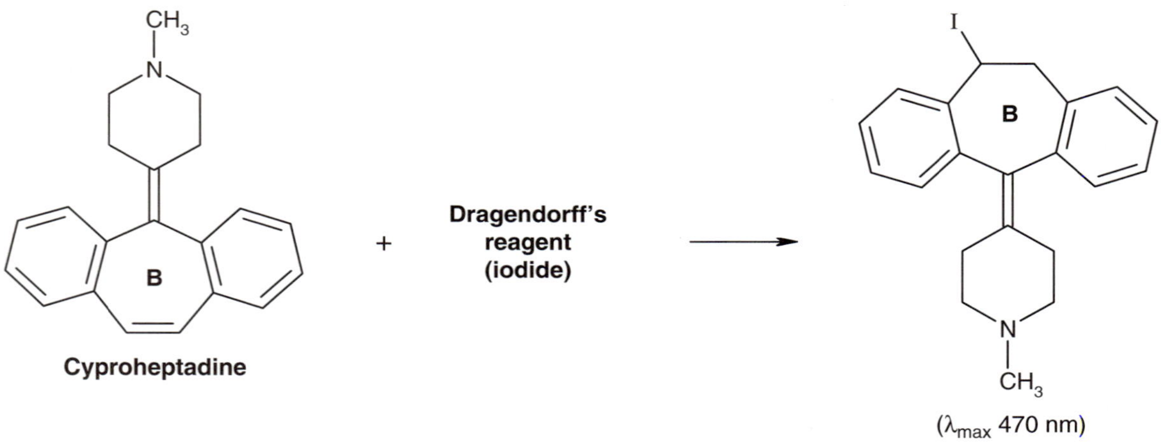

The drug forms ion-pair complex with bromocresol. The complex is extractable into chloroform for quantitative evaluation (λ_{max} 410 nm).

Reference

Adamski, S., Ind. *J. Pharm. Sci.*, **63(3)**, 111, 1981.

A spectrophotometric method based on precipitation of the drug as reinckate (ammonium reinckate) in acidic medium and subsequently dissolving the precipitates in acetone and subjected to spectrophotometric analysis (λ_{max} 525 nm).

Reference

Indian Drugs, 505-506, Sept. 1982.

Lysine monohydrochloride

METHOD 1

Reagents

1. 0.1% w/v solution of copper sulphate in methanol.
2. 0.5% w/v solution of ninhydrin in methanol–pyridine mixture.
3. Methanol–pyridine mixture (1 : 1) v/v.

Standard solution

50 mcg/ml of lysine monohydrochloride in water.

Sample solution

Extract the accurately weighed quantity of the sample with water to get a concentration of 50 mcg/ml of the substance.

Procedure

To 2 ml each of the sample and standard solutions add 5 ml of ninhydrin solution. Keep in water-bath for 10 min, cool and dilute to 25 ml with copper sulphate solution. Measure the absorption of both the solutions at about 530 nm against reagent blank. Calculate the results by comparison.

Alternatively, dissolve the residue retained in estimation of cyproheptadine in water to get a concentration of 100 mcg/ml of lysine monohydrochloride and follow the above method.

METHOD 2

Reagents

1. 0.2% w/v solution of ninhydrin in ethyl alcohol.
2. 50% w/v solution of copper nitrate in water. Dilute 0.5 ml to 100 ml with water just before use.
3. 10% v/v n-propanol in water.
4. TLC plates (glass), 20 × 20 cm, coated with silica gel G (0.25 mm). After coating, the plates are allowed to dry in air overnight (do not activate in the oven).
5. Mobile phase: n-propanol : water : glacial acetic acid (7 : 3 : 1) v/v.

Standard solution

(a) Stock solution: 1 mg/ml of lysine monohydrochloride in aqueous propanol.
(b) Working standard: Dilute stock solution appropriately to get 200 mcg/ml. To be prepared freshly on the day of use.

Sample solution

Extract the sample with 10% n-propanol to get a concentration of 200 mcg/ml.

Procedure

Line the chromatographic chamber with filter paper on 3 sides. Spot 100 µl each of sample and standard solutions as streaks. Dry and develop the plate up to a distance of 10 cm. Remove and dry in oven at 90°C for 10 min. Cool and spray evenly with ninhydrin reagent. Again heat in oven at 90°C for 30 min. The coloured spots (Rf 0.45) corresponding to sample and standard are scraped and transferred quantitatively to stoppered centrifuge tube. Add 10 ml of dilute copper nitrate solution, shake vigorously and centrifuge to get clear solution. Measure the absorption of both the solutions at about 520 nm using dilute copper nitrate solution as blank. Calculate the results by comparison.

One of the amino groups present in lysine condenses with ninhydrin and the product formed gives copper complex, thus colour of ninhydrin is stabilized.

Probable Reaction Mechanism (Methods 1 & 2)

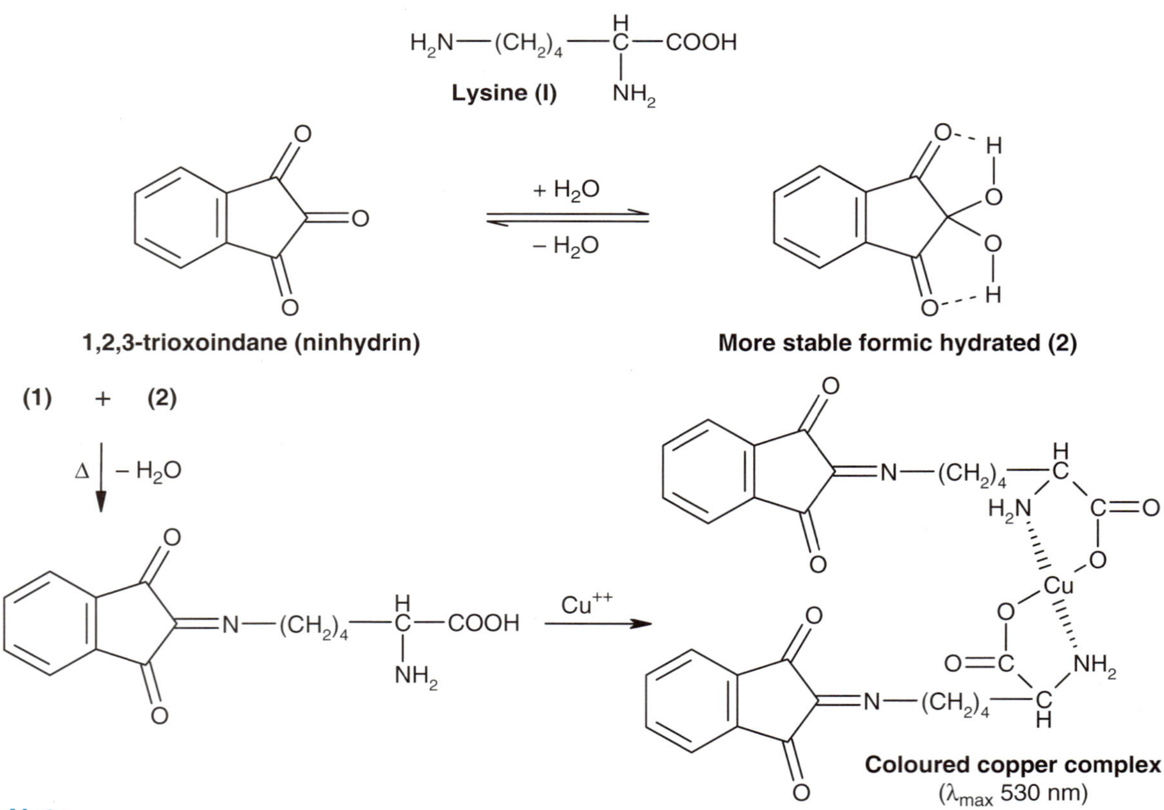

Note

Other divalent metal cations (Co^{2+} and Zn^{2+}) can be substituted for stabilization of ninhydrin colour.

METHOD 3

Evaporate appropriate volume of the sample equivalent to 100 mg of lysine monohydrochloride. Dissolve the residue with the aid of 0.5 ml of water and 50 ml glacial acetic acid. Add 10 ml of mercuric acetate solution and carry out the non-aqueous titration with 0.1 N perchloric acid using crystal violet or naphtholbenzein as indicator. Each ml of 0.1 N perchloric acid is equivalent to 9.133 mg of lysine monohydrochloride. This method gives good results in formulations containing ferrous gluconate, folic acid and pyridoxine.

METHOD 4

Lysine undergoes "Nash reaction" i.e. reaction of primary aliphatic amino group with HCHO and acetylacetone. This reaction is answered by glutamic acid as well.

Reagent

Formaldehyde - acetylacetone reagent (FAA): Mix 15 ml of formaldehyde (37%) with 7.8 ml of acetylacetone, dilute to 100 ml with acetate buffer, pH 4.7.

Procedure

To 2 ml each of sample and standard solutions (1 mg/ml), add 5 ml of 'FAA' reagent, heat in boiling water-bath for 20 min, cool and dilute to 25 ml with water and measure the absorbance at 425 nm against reagent blank.

Probable Reaction Mechanism

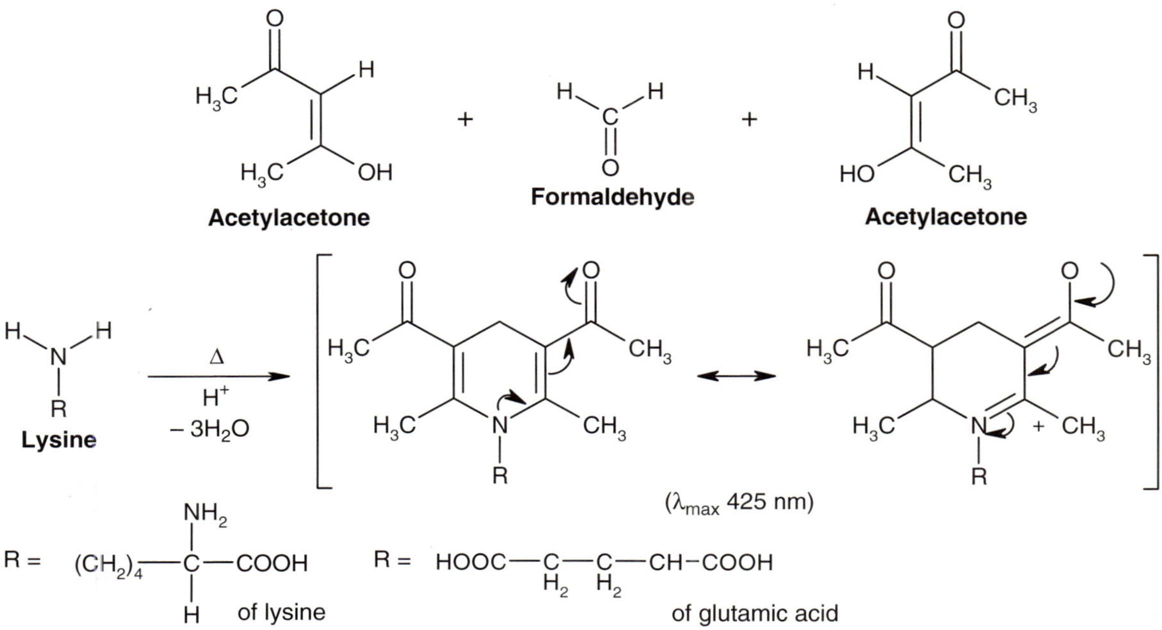

Reference

S.A. Shah, R.S. Shah, M.B. Devani, C.J. Shishoo & K.P. Soni, *Ind. J. Pharm. Sci.*, **54(5)**, 201-203, 1992.

METHOD 5

Paper chromatographic separation and estimation of lysine in the presence of methionine

This method is extremely useful for preparations containing lysine and methionine in combination and gives excellent results.

Support material: Whatman No. 1 paper.

Amount to be applied: 100 mcg (100 µl) in 70% v/v alcohol.

Mobile phase: N-propanol : Water : Benzyl alcohol
3 : 1 : 1 v/v

Spray reagent: 0.3% w/v solution of ninhydrin in ethyl alcohol.

Detection method: After spray the paper is heated at 105°C for 10-15 min. Lysine, which remains near the line of application, appears as violet spot.

Elution and estimation: The area in the paper representing the colour of lysine is cut and reduced to small pieces. Extract with 70% alcohol to produce 25 ml. Measure the absorbance at 560 nm. Subject the standard also to similar treatment for comparison.

Note

Methionine moves near to the front line and can be estimated based on colour reaction with ninhydrin.

METHOD 6

Sample equivalent to 75 mg of the compound is taken and to this add 300 ml of water. The solution is neutralized to phenolphthalein. Add 25 ml of neutralized formaldehyde and titrate with 0.1 N sodium hydroxide. Each ml of 0.1 N sodium hydroxide is equivalent to 0.0182 g of lysine monohydrochloride. Perform sample blank without formaldehyde.

Note

1. Syrupy preparations are likely to contain acidic substances. It is, therefore, desirable that the sample should be neutralized to phenolphthalein before the addition of formaldehyde. The volume of 0.1 N sodium hydroxide consumed after addition of formaldehyde is related to lysine contents.
2. Although certain laboratories have reported to have used this method in liquid formulations it has been found that the volume of 0.1 N sodium hydroxide consumed in formol titration is not in stoichiometric ratio; hence this method is not preferred.

Explanatory Note

In aqueous solution amino acid exists as "Zwitterion" in which protonation of amino group and ionization of carboxyl group both are present. Schiff et al. found that the presence of formaldehyde permitted titration of amino acids as acid as it forms imine which is very much weaker base than is the amine.

Probable Reaction Mechanism

There are several ways that reaction with formaldehyde can be depicted.

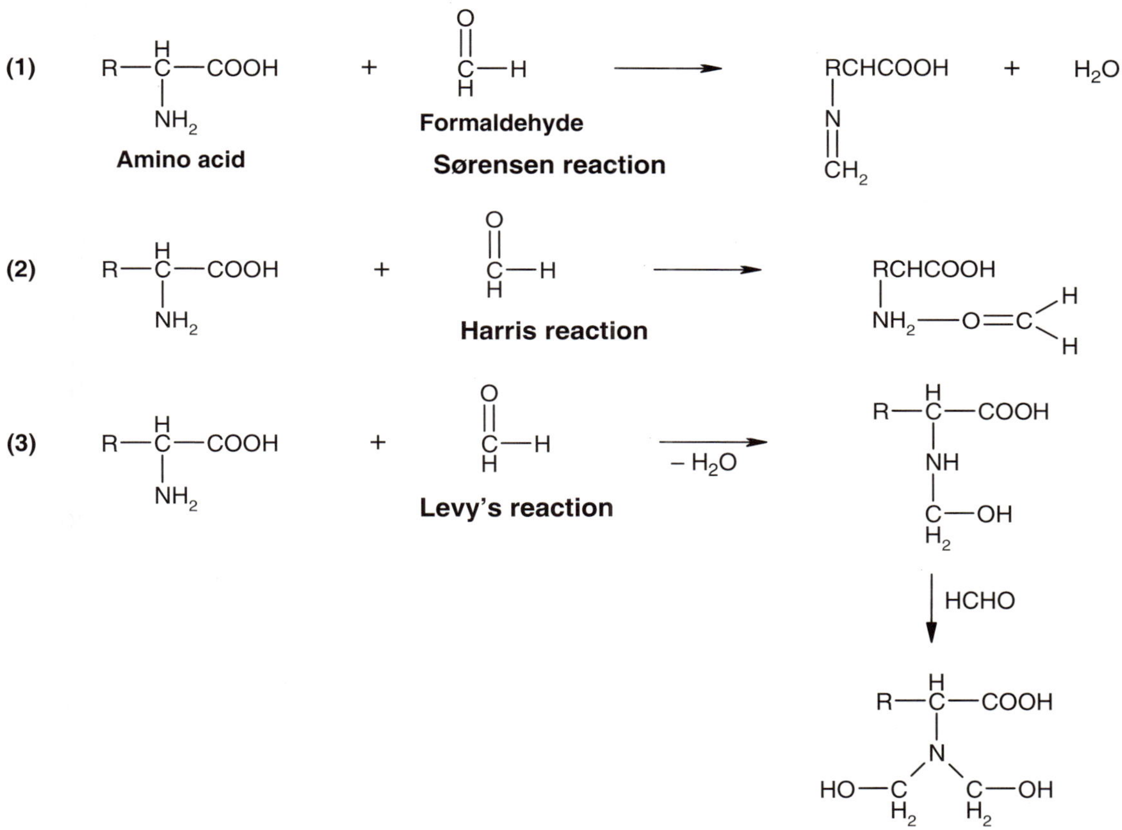

Reaction of α-amino group with formaldehyde destroys its Zwitterion relationship to carboxyl group. Carboxyl group then exhibits usual properties of an acid which can be titrated with NaOH. This is commonly called formol titration. This principle applies for titration of ammonium salts in the presence of formaldehyde.

$$H_3\overset{+}{N}RCOO^{-} + OH \rightleftharpoons H_2NRCOO^{-} + H_2O$$

Lysine reacts with diazotized 4-nitroaniline to produce a triazene structure which has intense red colour (λ_{max} 510 nm).

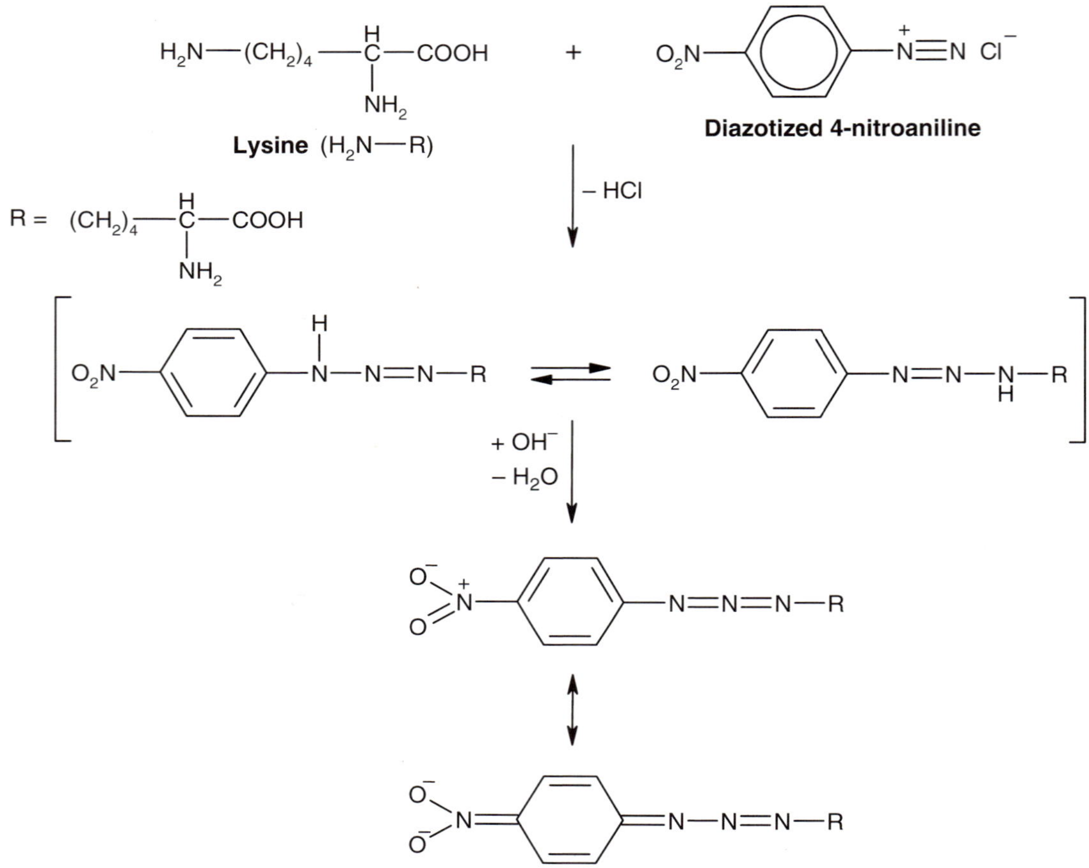

Stabilized anion
(λ_{max} 510 nm)

Reference

Pharmaceutical Chemistry (Vol. 2) by H.J. Roth, 1991, p. 220.

The amino group present in the molecule reacts with Sanger's reagent (2,4-dinitrofluorobenzene (DNFB)). Aromatic moiety in the reagent is activated and is attacked by the amino group leading to the formation of a coloured product.

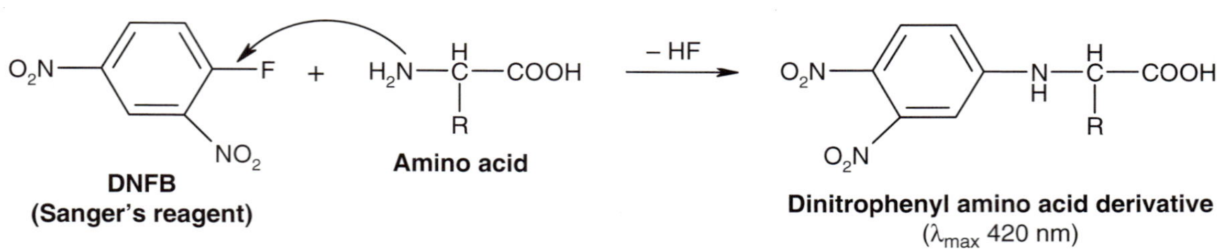

The reaction is carried out in slightly alkaline medium. 'DNFB' has the tendency to hydrolyse in slightly alkaline medium to dinitrophenolate which is coloured (λ_{max} 368 nm). This colour shall interfere in assay of lysine. At the end of reaction, acidify the medium, colourless compound is formed which does not interfere.

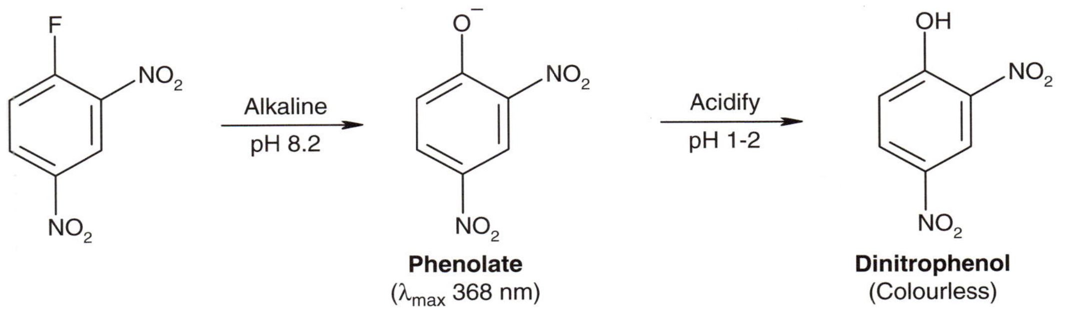

Dried yeast

The yeast is usually analysed for various vitamins preferably for B_1 and B_2 and calcium pantothenate.

Riboflavin (vitamin B_2)

METHOD 1

Reagents

1. 2% w/v solution of potassium permanganate in water.
2. Hydrogen peroxide (30%) solution.
3. Glacial acetic acid.
4. Phosphate buffer, pH 6.0.

Standard solution

30 mcg/ml of riboflavin in phosphate buffer.

Sample solution

Take appropriate quantity of the sample. Add 60-70 ml of phosphate buffer, pH 6.0, boil under reflux for 30 min, cool and adjust to 100 ml with buffer. Final solutions in buffer should contain 30 mcg/ml of riboflavin.

Procedure

To 10 ml of the standard and sample solutions add 2 ml of glacial acetic acid and 1 ml of potassium permanganate solution. Keep for 2 min, add 1 ml of hydrogen peroxide, shake vigorously and dilute to 25 ml with water. Measure the absorption of both the solutions at about 445 nm and calculate the results by comparison.

METHOD 2

Chromatographic separation through a column of talc gives satisfactory results. For details, refer to the method 3 for estimation of riboflavin under formulation 2 of this chapter.

Dried yeast may be analysed for calcium pantothenate contents. Carry out the estimated by method 1 described in formulation 8 of this chapter.

Formulation 14

Cyproheptadine hydrochloride, Lysine monohydrochloride, Dried Yeast, Tricholine citrate

ESTIMATION

Cyproheptadine hydrochloride

METHOD 1

Reagent

Citric acid–acetic anhydride reagent: Dissolve 2 g of citric acid (monohydrate) in 5 ml of methanol (anhydrous) and dilute to 100 ml with acetic anhydride.

Standard solution

100 mcg/ml of cyproheptadine hydrochloride in chloroform.

Sample solution

Weigh accurately a quantity of the sample equivalent to 10 mg of the substance, extract with four 20 ml portions of chloroform, filter through sintered funnel. Wash the residue with chloroform and make up the volume to 100 ml (100 mcg/ml). Retain the residue for estimation of lysine monohydrochloride.

Procedure

Evaporate 1 ml each of sample and standard solutions to dryness, add 1 ml of citric acid reagent and immerse in water-bath for 30 min. Cool and dilute to 10 ml with acetic anhydride. Measure the absorption of both the solutions at about 570 nm against reagent blank and calculate the results by comparison.

Alternatively, the residue is dissolved in methanol to produce 100 ml, filtered and extinction measured at maximum at about 286 nm and contents of cyproheptadine hydrochloride calculate by taking 355 as value of A 1%, 1 cm.

METHOD 2

To accurately weighed quantity of sample (syrup), add 20 ml of sodium bicarbonate solution (0.1%) and extract with iso-octane (2×25 ml). Wash the combined iso-octane layer with 50 ml of sodium bicarbonate solution, discard the aqueous layer. Iso-octane layer is extracted with 0.1 N sulphuric acid (3 × 25 ml). The acidic layer is combined and diluted to 100 ml. Filter and measure the extinction at maximum at about 286 nm using 0.1 N sulphuric acid as blank. Calculate the contents of cyproheptadine hydrochloride taking 355 as value of A 1%, 1 cm.

The drug forms ion-pair complex with bromocresol green; complex extracted into methylene chloride (λ_{max} 410 nm); extracted back into 0.1 M sodium hydroxide (λ_{max} 615 nm). It also forms complex with tropeolin OOO in pH 1.0 buffer (λ_{max} 485 nm).

Reference

1. BP, 1973, p.139.
2. Y.A. Beltagy, A. Issa & S.M. Riola, Pharmazie.

Lysine monohydrochloride

METHOD 1

Reagents

1. 0.1% w/v solution of copper sulphate in methanol.
2. 0.5% w/v solution of ninhydrin in methanol–pyridine mixture.
3. Methanol–pyridine mixture (1 : 1) v/v.

Standard solution

50 mcg/ml of lysine monohydrochloride in water.

Sample solution

Extract the accurately weighed quantity of the sample with water to get a concentration of 50 mcg/ml of the substance.

Procedure

To 2 ml each of the sample and standard solutions add 5 ml of ninhydrin solution. Keep in water-bath for 10 min, cool and dilute to 25 ml with copper sulphate solution. Measure the absorption of both the solutions at about 530 nm against reagent blank. Calculate the results by comparison.

Alternatively, dissolve the residue retained in estimation of cyproheptadine in water to get a concentration of 50 mcg/ml of lysine monohydrochloride and follow the above method.

A method based on precipitation of compound as reineckate using ammonium reineckate $NH_4[Cr(NH_3)_2(SCN)_3]$ as precipitating reagent and subsequently dissolving the insoluble precipitate in acetone for spectrophotometric estimation (λ_{max} 525 nm).

Reference

J. Emmanuel & T.V. Yegyanarayanan, *Indian Drugs*, **19**, 505-507, 1982.

METHOD 2

Reagents

1. 0.2% w/v solution of ninhydrin in ethyl alcohol.
2. 50% w/v solution of copper nitrate in water. Dilute 0.5 ml to 100 ml with water just before use.
3. 10% v/v n-propanol in water.
4. TLC plates (glass) 20 × 20 cm, coated with silica gel G (0.25 mm). After coating the plates are allowed to dry in air overnight (do not activate in the oven).
5. Mobile phase: n-propanol–water–glacial acetic acid (7 : 3 : 1) v/v.

Standard solution

(a) Stock solution: 1 mg/ml of lysine monohydrochloride in aqueous propanol.
(b) Working standard: Dilute stock solution appropriately to get 200 mcg/ml. To be prepared freshly on the day of use.

Sample solution

Extract the sample with 10% n-propanol to get a concentration of 200 mcg/ml.

Procedure

Line the chromatographic chamber with filter paper on 3 sides. Spot 100 ml each of sample and standard solutions as streaks. Dry and develop the plate up to a distance of 10 cm. Remove and dry in oven at 90°C for 10 min. Cool and spray evenly with ninhydrin reagent. Again heat in oven at 90°C for 30 min. The coloured spots (Rf 0.45) corresponding to sample and standard are scraped and transferred quantitatively to stoppered centrifuge tube. Add 10 ml of dilute copper nitrate solution, shake vigorously and centrifuge to get clear solution. Measure the absorption of both the solutions at about 520 nm using dilute copper nitrate solution as blank. Calculate the results by comparison.

For reaction mechanism, see under formulation 13 of this chapter.

Dried yeast

Estimate the nitrogen contents and calculate the amount of protein. The yeast can also be analysed for various vitamins preferably for B_1 and B_2 and calcium pantothenate.

Riboflavin (Vitamin B_2)

METHOD 1

Reagents

1. 2% w/v solution of potassium permanganate in water.
2. Hydrogen peroxide (30%) solution.
3. Glacial acetic acid.
4. Phosphate buffer, pH 6.0.

Standard solution

30 mcg/ml of riboflavin in phosphate buffer.

Sample solution

Take appropriate quantity of the sample. Add 60-70 ml of phosphate buffer, pH 6.0, boil under reflux for 30 min, cool and adjust to 100 ml with buffer. Final solutions in buffer should contain 30 mcg/ml of riboflavin.

Procedure

To 10 ml of the standard and sample solutions add 2 ml of glacial acetic acid and 1 ml of potassium permanganate solution. Keep for 2 min, add 1 ml of hydrogen peroxide, shake vigorously and dilute to 25 ml with water. Measure the absorption of both the solutions at about 445 nm and calculate the results by comparison.

METHOD 2

Chromatographic separation through a column of talc gives satisfactory results. For details, refer to the method for estimation of riboflavin under formulation 2 of this chapter.

Tricholine citrate

To the sodium bicarbonate layer obtained during estimation of cyproheptadine hydrochloride add 10 ml of freshly prepared ammonium reineckate. The precipitates are dried at 105°C, weighed and multiplied by 0.397 to give the weight of tricholine citrate present in the volume of the sample taken for analysis. For further details refer to formulation 13 of this chapter.

Formulation 15

Ascorbic acid, Ferrous gluconate, Calcium lactate, Rutin, Adrenochrome monosemicarbazone, Menadione sodium bisulphite, Methyl hespiridin

ESTIMATION

For estimation of ascorbic acid, calcium lactate and ferrous gluconate follow the method described under formulation 6 of this chapter.

Rutin

Reagents

1. 0.1 M aluminium chloride: Weigh and dissolve 2.41 g of aluminium chloride in water to produce 100 ml.
2. 1 M potassium acetate: 9.81 g in water to produce 100 ml.
3. 1 N hydrochloric acid.

Standard solution

100 mcg/ml of rutin in alcohol.

Preparation of sample

Accurately weigh powdered sample equivalent to 10 mg of rutin, add 80 ml of ethyl alcohol. Heat on water-bath to boil, cool to room temperature, make up to 100 ml with ethyl alcohol.

Procedure

Carry out the colour development as follows:

	Standard	Standard blank	Sample	Sample blank
Prepared solutions	2 ml	2 ml	2 ml	2 ml
Aluminium chloride reagent	3 ml	—	3 ml	—
Potassium acetate solution	5 ml	5 ml	5 ml	5 ml
1 N hydrochloric acid	1 ml	1 ml	1 ml	1 ml
Distilled water	—	3 ml	—	3 ml

Allow to stand at room temperature for about 20 minutes, make up to 25 ml. Measure the absorbance of the sample against sample blank and standard against standard blank at about 420 nm. Calculate the results by comparison.

For reaction mechanism, see formulation 10 of this chapter.

Menadione sodium bisulphite (MSB)

METHOD

Weigh the powdered sample accurately equivalent to 60 mg of MSB, add 25 ml of water and 2-3 pellets of sodium hydroxide and saturate with sodium chloride. Shake and extract with three 50 ml portions of chloroform. Combine all the chloroform extracts, pass through anhydrous sodium sulphate, wash the sodium sulphate layer with additional 20 ml of chloroform. Evaporate combined chloroform layer to dryness.

Treat the residue by any one of the following two methods for estimation.

(a) Dissolve the residue in 10 ml of glacial acetic acid followed by 10 ml of dilute hydrochloric acid. Add 3 g of zinc dust and the flask is shaken. Allow the flask to stand in the dark with intermittent shaking (every 10 minutes) for one hour. Filter the solution through cotton plug wetted with water. Wash the reduction flask with three 10 ml portions of water (CO_2-free). To the combined filtrate add 2-3 drops of orthophenanthroline solution and titrate with 0.02 N cerric ammonium sulphate or cerric sulphide. Each ml of 0.02 N cerric ammonium sulphate is equivalent to 3.03 mg of menadione sodium bisulphite.

OR

(b) Dissolve the residue obtained after evaporation of chloroform layer in 10 ml of glacial acetic acid. Add 5 ml of 10% w/v solution of sodium potassium tartrate and 4 g of anhydrous sodium carbonate. Immediately titrate with 0.2 N titanous chloride using few drops of 0.1% solution of indigo carmine as indicator. Each ml of 0.2 N titanous chloride is equivalent to 3.03 mg of menadione sodium bisulphite.

Adrenochrome monosemicarbazone (AMS)

Reagents

1. 0.5% w/v solution of sodium nitrite in water.
2. 0.5% v/v hydrochloric acid.
3. 13.25% w/v solution of sodium carbonate in water.

Standard solution

Weigh the analyte mixture as prepared under preparative TLC accurately equivalent to 2 mg of AMS. Add 80 ml of water, shake continuously for 2 hours and centrifuge. Transfer the supernatant liquid to 100 ml volumetric flask, wash the residue with 2 × 5 ml water, centrifuge again, transfer clear liquid to volumetric flask and make up to 100 ml with water (20 mcg/ml in respect of AMS).

Sample solution

Weigh the powdered sample accurately equivalent to about 2 mg of AMS and extract with 80 ml of water, proceed further as described under standard preparation.

Procedure

To 2 ml each of standard and sample solutions add 2 ml each of 0.5% hydrochloric acid and of 0.5% sodium nitrite solution. Shake gently till colourless. Then add 3 ml of sodium carbonate solution and 3 ml of water. Measure the absorbance of both sample and standard solutions at about 430 nm using mixture of 2 ml each of water, 0.5% hydrochloric acid, 0.5% sodium nitrite, 3 ml of sodium carbonate and 3 ml of water as blank.

Probable Reaction Mechanism

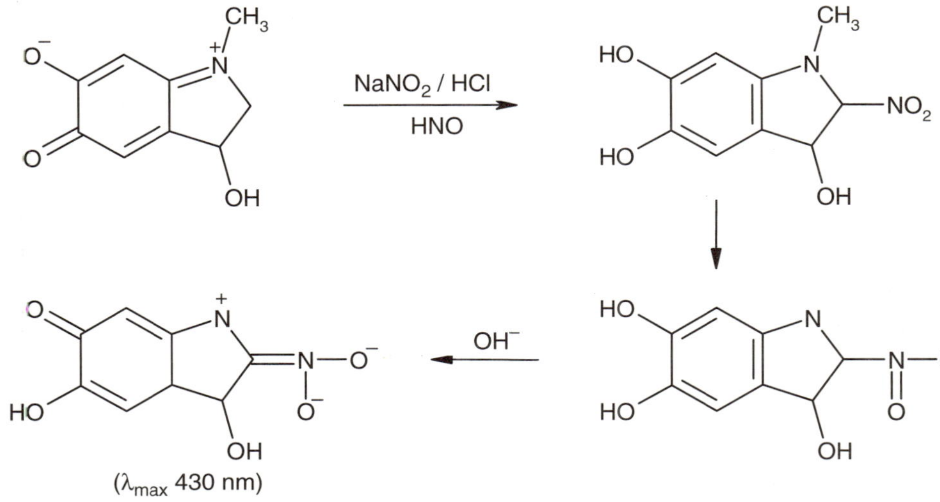

Note

Na_2CO_3 neutralizes excess of HNO_2, thus removing interference due to HNO_2 and also it stabilizes the nitro derivative.

Adrenochrome monosemicarbazone (AMS) and Methyl hespiridin (MH) by preparative TLC

Absorbent layer: Silica gel GF_{254}
TLC plates: Precoated plates, 20 × 20 cm (0.2 mm thickness)
Solvent system: Ethyl acetate–formic acid (85%)–acetic acid–water (100 : 11 : 11 : 27) v/v
Volume used: 200 ml
Chamber saturation: Chamber lined on three sides with filter paper and saturated for 60 minutes.
Preparation of analyte mixture: The pure samples of various ingredients as present in the tablet (adrenochrome monosemicarbazone, methyl hespiridin, ascorbic acid, rutin, menadione bisulphite representing 10 tablets = 10 mg of AMS) were weighed and mixed.

(The analyte mixture stored in air-tight amber-coloured bottle may be used for further analysis of sample.)

Preparation of standard solution

Analyte mixture was weighed accurately and shaken with methanol to produce 5 ml (200 mcg/ml of AMS).

Preparation of sample solution

Weigh accurately powdered sample equivalent to 1 mg of AMS. Add sufficient methanol to produce 5 ml. Shake vigorously for 10-15 minutes, centrifuge and use clear supernatant liquid for spotting.

Procedure

Apply 100 μl (0.1 ml) each of sample and standard solutions as bands (about 7.5 cm long) with the help of graduated microcapillary and current of air, drying after each application. Dry the plate and transfer to pre-saturated developing chamber. Develop the plate to a distance of about 15-17 cm. Remove the plate and allow the solvent to evaporate. Examine the plate under visible light for (AMS) and UV (for methyl hespiridin) to locate the compounds. Scrap the relevant portions representing sample and standard separately. MH gives three bands; all the three bands are scraped and the material mixed together for analysis.

Adrenochrome monosemicarbazone

Extract the scraped material of both sample and standard separately with methanol to produce 5 ml. Filter and measure the absorbance of clear filtrates of both sample and standard solutions at 444 nm and calculate the results by comparison.

Note

On basification, adrenochrome is converted to adrenolutin which is slightly fluorescent.

Probable Reaction Mechanism

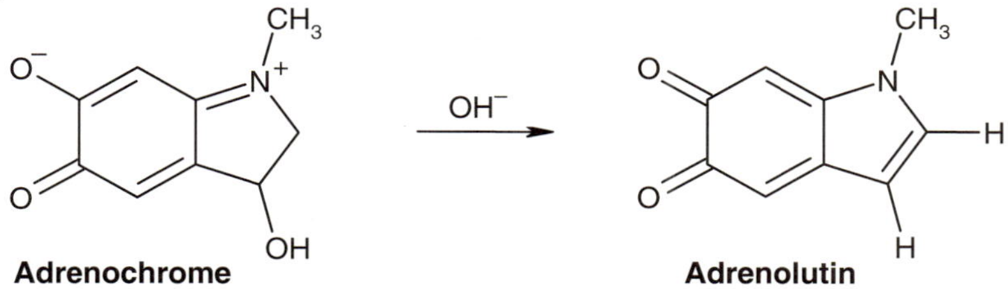

Adrenochrome   Adrenolutin

Reference

Pharmaceutical Chemistry (Vol. 2) by H.J. Roth, p. 389.

Methyl hespiridin

Extract the combined scraped material of three bands of both sample and standard with methanol to produce 100 ml, filter and measure the extinction of both sample and standard solutions at maxima at about 283 nm.

Blank: Scrap the silica gel of similar area from similarly developed plate, extract with 5 ml of methanol, filter and use as blank.

Note

See method involving formation of copper complex under citrus bioflanoid compounds (CFC) in formulation 11 of this chapter.

Formulation 16

Ferrous fumarate/Ferrous gluconate, Folic acid, Calcium phosphate dibasic, Ascorbic acid, Vitamin B_{12}

ESTIMATION

Ferrous fumarate/Ferrous gluconate

METHOD 1

Reagents

1. 1 N sodium hydroxide.
2. 0.1 N cerric ammonium sulphate.
3. Ortho-phenanthroline solution (indicator).
4. Concentrated sulphuric acid.

Procedure

Transfer accurately weighed quantity of the sample equivalent to 300 mg of ferrous fumarate. Add 200 ml of water and 20 ml of 1 N sodium hydroxide. Mix, filter and transfer the precipitates (iron hydroxide) quantitatively to filter paper with the aid of water. Wash the precipitates with water till the filtrate is almost colourless (use the filtrate for estimation of folic acid). Pierce the filter paper with a glass rod and wash the precipitates to a 250 ml conical flask with the aid of water. Add slowly through sides with stirring concentrated sulphuric acid till the precipitates just dissolve, add 2-5 ml more of sulphuric acid. Add about 1 g of zinc dust, plug the flask loosely with cotton and allow it to stand at room temperature for 30 min. Filter, wash the flask and residue with small volume of water and filter. Titrate the combined filtrate and washings with 0.1 N cerric ammonium sulphate using orthophenanthroline solution as indicator. Each ml of 0.1 N cerric ammonium sulphate is equivalent to 0.017167 g of ferrous fumarate or 0.02061 g of ferrous gluconate.

Note

The method is based on oxidation of iron by Ce^{4+} using o-phenanthroline as indicator.

METHOD 2

Reagents

1. Nitric acid.
2. Hydrochloric acid.
3. Dilute sulphuric acid.
4. 10% w/v solution of ammonium thiocyanate in water.

Standard solution

40 mcg/ml of Fe^{++} (as ferrous sulphate).

Sample solution

To accurately weighed quantity of the sample equivalent to 50 mg of ferrous fumarate or gluconate add 1 ml of nitric acid and 5 ml of hydrochloric acid. Heat on a water-bath till there are no fumes of nitrous acid. Dilute to 250 ml and filter.

Procedure

To 2 ml each of sample and standard solutions add 5 ml of ammonium thiocyanate solution, dilute to 25 ml with dilute sulphuric acid. Measure the absorption of both the solutions at about 520 nm against reagent blank. Calculate the results by comparison.

Probable Reaction Mechanism

On heating the sample/standard with HNO_3 and HCl, Fe^{2+} is oxidized to Fe^{3+} which then reacts with NH_4SCN to give reddish colour (λ_{max} 520 nm).

$$Fe^{3+} + NH_4SCN \longrightarrow \underset{(\lambda_{max}\ 520\ nm)}{FeNH_4(SCN)_3}$$

METHOD 3

Reagents

1. Acetate buffer, pH 4.7: To 2.9 ml of acetic acid (glacial) add 6.805 g of sodium acetate and dilute to 1000 ml with water. Adjust the pH to 4.7 with sodium acetate solution or with glacial acetic acid as required.
2. 5% w/v solution of sodium metabisulphite in water.
3. 3% w/v solution of 2,2′-bipyridyl in water.
4. 10% v/v sulphuric acid in water.

Standard solution

To 50 mg of ferrous fumarate accurately weighed add 20 ml of 10% sulphuric acid, heat on water-bath for about 30 min, shake, cool and dilute to 100 ml with water. Dilute 2.5 ml of the resulting solution to 50 ml with water.

Sample solution

Weigh accurately quantity of the sample equivalent to 50 mg of the substance and proceed for sample preparation as under standard solution.

Procedure

To 5 ml each of sample and standard solutions add 5 ml of buffer solution and 2.5 ml of sodium metabisulphite solution. Allow to stand at room temperature for 15 min, add 2.5 ml of bipyridyl solution, shake and adjust to 25 ml with water. Measure the absorbance of both sample and standard solutions at about 510 nm against reagent blank and calculate the results by comparison.

Probable Reaction Mechanism

This method is based on reaction of Fe^{2+} with 2,2′-bispyridine. On heating with sulphuric acid the component breaks into iron (2+) and corresponding acid. Fe^{2+} complexes with 2,2′-bispyridine to give coloured product (λ_{max} 510 nm).

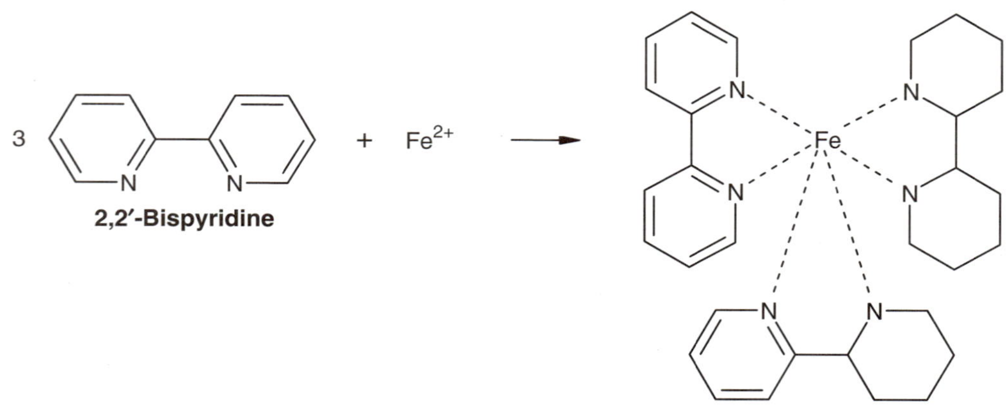

Iron - bispyridine complex
(λ_{max} 510 nm)

Two nitrogen atoms in 2,2′-bispyridine have one unshared pair of electrons which can be shared by Fe^{2+}.

Reference

Thin-Layer Chromatography: Reagents and Detection Methods by H. Jork et al., Vol. 1(a), p. 217.

Ascorbic acid

Follow the method described in formulation 6 of this chapter.

Folic acid

Follow the method 3 described under formulation 7 of this chapter.

Note

Precipitation of iron with alkali results in low recovery of folic acid as it gets trapped in creamy precipitates of iron hydroxide. Standard solution should also be treated similarly after addition of appropriate amount of ferrous fumarate.

Vitamin B_{12}

Follow microbiological method. However in such formulations initial extraction should be done with 25% alcohol to enhance the solubility of vitamin, thus complete extraction. Stock solution may be diluted with buffer or water as necessary.

Calcium phosphate, dibasic

Reagent

Vanadate–ammonium molybdate solution: To 20 g of ammonium molybdate and 1 g of ammonium vanadate add about 500 ml of water and warm. Add 140 ml of concentrated nitric acid to dissolve, dilute to 1000 ml with water.

Standard solution

200 mcg/ml of calcium phosphate (dibasic) in 1 N hydrochloric acid.

Sample solution

Weigh sample accurately equivalent to 100 mg of the substance, add 50-60 ml of 1 N hydrochloric acid, warm on water-bath for 30 min to dissolve the substance. Make the volume to 100 ml with the acid and further dilute appropriately with 1 N hydrochloric acid to get 200 mcg/ml.

Procedure

To 5 ml of sample and standard solutions add 5 ml of vanadate molybdate solution, mix, allow to stand for 10 min, and measure the absorbance at about 450 nm against reagent blank. Deduce the results by comparison.

Formulation 17

Haemoglobin, Alcohol

Such liquid preparations contain about 5-7% v/v of alcohol and are quite viscous.

Estimation

Haemoglobin

Take sample equivalent to about 3 g of haemoglobin, heat in a crucible on a burner to char the sample completely. Cool and moisten with 1 ml of concentrated sulphuric acid and again heat till all fumes are expelled out. Transfer the contents to furnace and heat at 450-500°C till ashing is complete. Cool, moisten with little water, add about 20 ml of concentrated hydrochloric acid, warm on water-bath till ash dissolves. Transfer the extract to 250 ml conical flask with the aid of water. Now add strong ammonia solution drop by drop till slight brown precipitate appears in solution (the pH at this stage is about 4). Add about 0.25 g of salicylic acid, warm on water-bath at about 60°C and titrate the hot solution with 0.05 M edetate, end-point being change of deep violet colour (colour of iron salicylate) to bright yellow, indicating the complete titration of iron. Each ml of 0.05 M edetate is equivalent to 0.8502 g of haemoglobin.

Alcohol

Reagents

1. 10% w/v solution of potassium iodide in water.
2. 0.1 N sodium thiosulphate.
3. Nitrochromium reagent.

Procedure

Take 25 g of the sample, add 300 ml of water and distil to collect 100 ml. Dilute 10 ml of the distillate to 50 ml with water.

To 10 ml of the resultant solution add 10 ml of nitrochromium reagent. Keep at room temperature for 30 minutes, then add 100 ml of water and 10 ml of potassium iodide solution. After 5 minutes titrate the liberated iodine with 0.1 N sodium thiosulphate, the end-point is from yellow (colour of iodine) to pale green (colour of chromium salt).

$$\text{Alcohol \% w/v} = \frac{A \times 1.448 \times \text{density}}{\text{weight (g) of the sample}}$$

'*A*' is the net volume (ml) of 0.1 N sodium thiosulphate consumed in the titration.

Probable Reaction Mechanism

Alcohol is oxidized to aldehyde by chromium (VI) reagent. Excess reagent reacts with KI to give iodine which is titrated with sodium thiosulphate.

$$3CH_3CH_3OH + 3Cr_2O_7^{2-} + 8H^+ \xrightarrow{\text{Oxidation}} 2Cr^{3+} + 3CH_3CHO + 7H_2O$$

$$Cr_2O_7^{2-} + 6KI + H^+ \longrightarrow 2Cr^{3+} + 3I_2 + 7H_2O$$

$$I_2 + Na_2S_2O_3 \longrightarrow 2NaI + \underset{\textbf{Sodium tetrathiosulphate}}{Na_2S_4O_6}$$

Formulation 18

Ergometrine maleate, Adrenochrome monosemicarbazone, Rutin, Dicalcium phosphate, Menadione sodium bisulphite

ESTIMATION

Rutin, Adrenochrome monosemicarbazone and Menadione sodium bisulphite

Follow the method described in formulation 15 of this chapter.

Dicalcium phosphate

Follow the method described in formulation 16 of this chapter.

Ergometrine maleate

Reagents

1. 1% w/v solution of p-dimethylaminobenzaldehyde (PDAB) in hydrochloric acid (Ehrlich's reagent).
2. Brine solution.

Standard solution

20 mcg/ml of the substance in tartaric acid.

Sample solution

Weigh accurately quantity of powdered sample equivalent to 4 mg of substance, suspend in 15 ml of brine solution and make alkaline with ammonia. Extract with 5 × 25 ml portions of diethyl ether (anaesthetic). Wash the combined ether extract with 3 × 5 ml portions of brine and reject the brine layer. Extract the ether layer with tartaric acid to get final concentration of 20 mcg/ml.

Procedure

To 5 ml each of sample and standard solutions add 10 ml of PDAB solution and measure the absorbance of both the solutions at 550 nm against reagent blank and calculate the results by comparison.

The method is based on reaction with Ehrlich's reagent. This involves electrophilic substitution at C-2 of the indole, followed by elimination of water to form coloured complex (λ_{max} 550 nm).

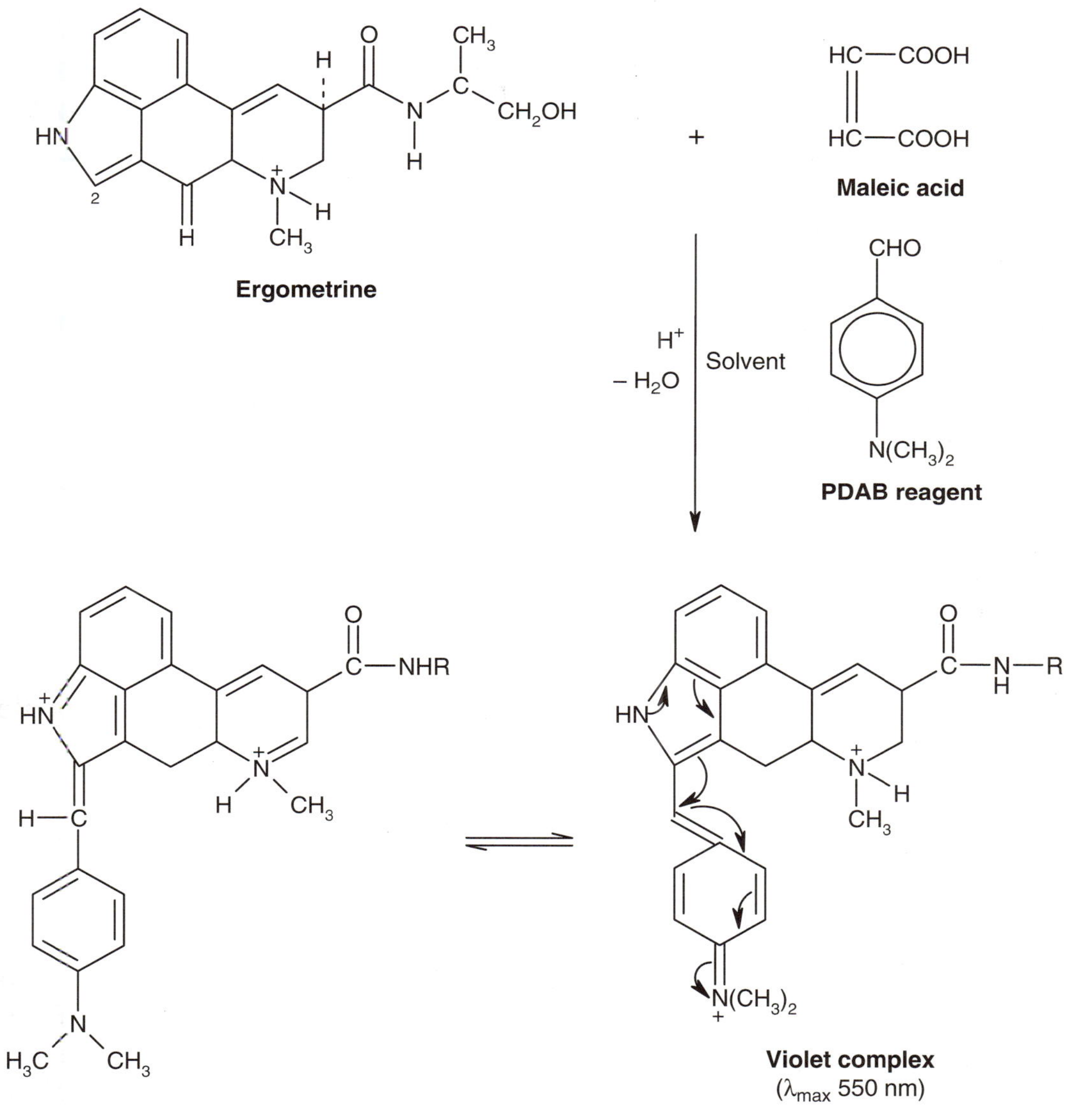

Reference

H. York et al., Thin Layer Chromatography: Reagents and Detection Methods, Vol. 1b, pp. 245 & 253.

Formulation 19

Cyproheptadine hydrochloride, L-Lysine hydrochloride, Peptone

ESTIMATION

Cyproheptadine hydrochloride

Follow the method 2 described in formulation 13 of this chapter.

L-Lysine hydrochloride

Follow the colorimetric method described in formulation 13 of this chapter.

Peptone

Digest the sample with sulphuric acid, basify and carry out ammonia distillation by Kjeldahl method. From the total nitrogen subtract the amount of nitrogen equivalent to both the other ingredients.

$$\text{Peptone (mg/ml)} = [N_T - (N_C + N_2)] \times 6.7843$$

where

N_T (total nitrogen) = $T_R \times N \times 35.025$

$N_C = a \times 0.399$

$N_L = b \times 0.1534$

a = contents of cyproheptadine determined in 5 ml of the sample

b = contents of L-lysine determined in 5 ml of the sample

T_R = Titre value (blank) – Titre value (back titration)

Formulation 20

Haemoglobin, Ferric ammonium citrate, Folic acid, Cyanocobalamin

ESTIMATION

Haemoglobin

This method is based on oxidation of haemoglobin into methaemoglobin and subsequent conversion to cyanmethaemoglobin which is coloured.

METHOD 1

Reagent

Ferricyanide–cyanide reagent: Dissolve 0.2 g of potassium ferricyanide, 0.05 g of potassium cyanide and 0.14 g of potassium and phosphate in water to produce 1000 ml; pH should be between 7.0 and 7.4 (adjacent if necessary).

Transfer accurately measured quantity of the sample equivalent to 200 mg of haemoglobin to 250 ml volumetric flask, add about 100 ml of water, shake well and add 10 ml of ferricyanide–cyanide reagent and dilute to 250 ml with water. Allow to stand for 10 min, filter and measure the absorbance of the solution at 540 nm against blank and calculate the results. If solution is hazy it may be centrifuged.

$$\text{Haemoglobin (g)}/15\text{ ml} = \frac{A_U}{11} \times \frac{16114.5}{1000} \times \frac{200}{1000} \times \frac{15}{10} \times \frac{\text{S.G.}}{1}$$

where A_U = absorbance of the sample
11 = factor of A 1%, 1 cm
S.G. = specific gravity of the preparation

Alternatively, use standard haemoglobin for comparison.

METHOD 2

Take sample equivalent to about 3 g of haemoglobin, heat in a crucible on a burner to char the sample completely. Cool and moisten with 1 ml of concentrated sulphuric acid and again heat till all fumes are expelled out.

Transfer the contents to furnace and heat at 450-500°C till ashing is complete. Cool, moisten with little water, add about 20 ml of concentrated hydrochloric acid, warm on water-bath till ash dissolves. Transfer the extract to 250 ml conical flask with the aid of water. Now add strong ammonia solution drop by drop till slight brown precipitate appears in solution (the pH at this stage is about 4). Add about 0.25 g of salicylic acid, warm on water-bath at about 60°C and titrate the hot solution with 0.05 M disodium edetate, end point being change of deep violet colour (colour of iron salicylate) to bright yellow, indicating complete titration of iron. Each ml of 0.05 M disodium edetate is equivalent to 0.8502 g of haemoglobin.

Note

Haemoglobin contains 0.34% of elemental iron.

METHOD 3

Weigh sample equivalent to 500 mg of the substance and transfer to Kjeldahl flask, add 1 g of copper sulphate and 10 g of sodium sulphate. Add 20 ml of sulphuric acid. Heat until solution is clear blue (this will ensure conversion of nitrogen into ammonium sulphate). Cool, add water and 100 ml of 40% sodium hydroxide. Collect the distillate with 50 ml of 0.1 N sulphuric acid. Titrate excess of the acid with 0.1 N sodium hydroxide using methyl red as indicator (*A* ml). Perform the blank (*B* ml). Each ml of 0.1 N sulphuric acid is equivalent to 1.4 mg of nitrogen.

From the total nitrogen (mg), calculate the content of haemoglobin.

$$\text{Glycerrinated haemoglobin} = \frac{B \times A \times N \times 1.4 \times 6.38 \times W \times 100}{0.1 \times W_1 \times 35}$$

where B = blank reading

A = volume consumed by the sample

N = normality of sodium hydroxide

W = average fill of the capsule

W_1 = weight of the sample taken for analysis

Ferric ammonium citrate (FAC)

METHOD 1

Reagents

1. 20% w/v solution of citric acid.
2. Strong ammonia solution.
3. 80% thioglycollic acid.

4. Concentrated hydrochloric acid.
5. Strong ammonia solution.

Standard solution

To accurately weighed sample equivalent to 200 mg of ferric ammonium citrate add 10 ml of concentrated hydrochloric acid and dilute to 100 ml with water. Further dilute 5 ml to 100 ml with water.

Sample solution

To appropriate quantity of the sample add 10 ml of concentrated hydrochloric acid and then dilute with water.

Procedure

To 10 ml each of sample and standard solutions add 2 ml of citric acid solution, 0.1 ml of thioglycollic acid and 5 ml of strong ammonia, dilute to 25 ml with water. Measure the absorbance of both the solutions at 525 nm against reagent blank. This will give total quantity (mg) of iron in the sample.

Note

100 mg of ferric ammonium citrate contains 21.5 mg of elemental iron.

METHOD 2

Digest accurately weighed quantity of the sample with 4-5 ml of concentrated hydrochloric acid. Transfer to 250 ml flask with the help of water. Add 15 ml of potassium iodide solution (10% w/v). Keep in the dark for 5 min and titrate the liberated iodine with 0.1 N sodium thiosulphate using starch paste as indicator, added near the end of titration. Each ml of 0.1 N sodium thiosulphate is equivalent to 5.585 mg of iron. Calculate the contents of FAC in the sample considering each 100 mg of FAC equivalent to 21.5 mg of iron.

Folic acid

Follow the methods described in this chapter.

Cyanocobalamin

Follow the microbiological method.

Formulation 21

Thiamine hydrochloride, Riboflavin, Nicotinamide, Pyridoxine hydrochloride, Folic acid, Calcium pantothenate, Ascorbic acid, Zinc sulphate, Vitamin B_{12}, Glutamic acid, Lactobacillus sporogenes, Sodium selenite, Copper sulphate, Manganese sulphate

ESTIMATION

Ascorbic acid

Accurately weighed quantity of powdered sample equivalent to 150 mg of ascorbic acid is diluted in 300 ml of water and 20 ml of dilute sulphuric acid and titrated with 0.1 N cerric ammonium sulphate using ferric sulphate as indicator. Each ml of 0.1 N cerric ammonium sulphate is equivalent to 8.8806 mg of ascorbic acid.

Zinc sulphate

Follow the method described in formulation 18 of this chapter which is based on titration with EDTA.

Selenium (Sodium selenite)

To 5 ml of 1 mmol solution of sodium selenite add 10 ml of dilute hydrochloric acid and 5 ml of potassium iodide (10%), shake for 2 min, add 10 ml of water and 2 ml of chloroform. Mixture was titrated with 1 mmol (0.176%) of l-ascorbic acid using starch as indicator.

$$\text{Selenium } (\mu g) = V \times C \times \frac{\text{Atomic weight of selenium}}{\text{Molecular weight of ascorbic acid} \times 2}$$

$$= V \times C \times \frac{78.96}{176 \times 2}$$

$$= V \times C \times 0.23$$

where V = volume of standard ascorbic acid
C = concentration (mg or mu g/ml) of l-ascorbic acid

1 ml of 0.004 N ascorbic acid ≡ 78.96 μg of selenium
1 ml of 0.1 N ascorbic acid ≡ 4.325 mg of sodium selenite

Copper sulphate

Accurately weighed quantity of the sample equivalent to 1.25 mg of copper sulphate is ignited at 450°C, add 5 ml of hydrochloric acid and evaporate to dryness, add 2.5 ml of nitric acid and evaporate. Extract the residue with three 5 ml portions of hot hydrochloric acid, combine the acid extract and dilute to 25 ml with water.

To 1 ml of this solution add 10 ml of edetate–citrate solution, 0.1 ml of thymol blue solution and sufficient dilute ammonia solution to produce green to blue-green colour. Add 10 ml sodium diethyldithiocarbamate solution and extract the yellow colour with four 5 ml portions of carbon tetrachloride. Combine the organic extracts and dilute to 20 ml with carbon tetrachloride. Measure the absorption at maxima at about 435 nm. Use standard solution of copper sulphate for comparison.

Manganese sulphate

METHOD 1

To 2 ml of the solution obtained during estimation of copper sulphate add 2.5 ml of dilute sulphuric acid, evaporate to dryness. To the residue add 3 ml of phosphoric acid, 6 ml of water and 0.5 g of sodium periodate and dissolve by aid of heat. Heat in a water-bath for 30 min, cool, dilute to 10 ml with water. Measure the absorption of the resulting solution at the maximum at about 526 nm. The result can be calculated from a standard curve prepared by diluting 1, 2, 3, 4, 5 ml of 0.005% w/v solution of potassium permanganate to 10 ml with water. Each mg of potassium permanganate is equivalent to 1.4114 mg of $MnSO_4 \cdot 4H_2O$.

METHOD 2

Reagents

1. 0.002% w/v solution of rhodamine B.
2. 0.015 N solution of potassium periodate.
3. 0.5 M solution of sodium fluoride.
4. 0.025% w/v solution of 1,10-phenanthroline in 10% alcohol.
5. 0.5 M acetic acid–sodium acetate buffer (pH 3.8).

Standard solution

0.1 mcg/ml of manganese (Mn^{++}).

Sample solution

Containing equivalent to 0.1 mcg/ml of manganese (Mn^{++}).

Procedure

To 0.4 ml of rhodamine B solution add 1.6 ml of mixture of 1,10-phenanthroline, potassium iodate, sodium fluoride and buffer solution (1 + 1 + 1 + 7). Then add 0.2 ml each of sample and standard solutions, adjust the volume to 4 ml with water. Heat at 60°C for 8.5 min, cool quickly to terminate the reaction. Measure the absorbance of sample and standard solutions against reagent blank. Oxidation of rhodamine B by potassium periodate in acidic medium results in decoloration of the dye. This oxidation reaction is accelerated by 1,10-phenanthroline and minute quantity of manganese. The decrease in colour intensity is proportional to the amount of manganese. Other elements such as Co, Ni, Cu^{++}, chromium (III), Zn, Fe^{+++}, Fe^{++}, Ca^{++}, Mg^{++}, Al^{+++} have insignificant interference.

Glutamic acid

Reagents

1. 0.5% w/v solution of ninhydrin in methanol.
2. 1% w/v solution of copper sulphate in water.
3. Pyridine.
4. Methanol.

Standard solution

60 mcg/ml of glutamic acid in water.

Sample solution

Accurately weighed quantity of sample is extracted with water (treat with charcoal if colour is present).

Procedure

To 5 ml each of sample and standard solutions add 5 ml of ninhydrin solution and 5 ml of pyridine and heat in water-bath for 15 min. Cool, add 1 ml of copper sulphate solution and dilute to 50 ml with methanol. Measure the absorbance of both the solutions at 500 nm against reagent blank and calculate the contents of glutamic acid by comparison.

Note

For detailed reaction mechanism, see under lysine as described in this chapter.

Lactobacillus sporogenes

Determine the viable spore count and lactic acid producing capacity.

Formulation 22

Microcrystalline hydroxyapatite (Calcium orthophosphate), L-lysine monohydrochloride, Zinc sulphate

ESTIMATION

Phosphate

Reagents

1. Ammonium molybdate reagent: Introduce drop by drop 13.9 ml of concentrated sulphuric acid in 80 ml of ice-cooled water, cool and add 3.3 g of ammonium molybdate, dissolve and dilute to 100 ml with water, filter before use.
2. 2 N sulphuric acid.
3. Nitric acid.
4. Ammonia solution.
5. Reducing reagent: Dissolve 3 g of ferrous sulphate in 10 ml of water, add 5 ml of 2 N sulphuric acid, dilute to 100 ml with water and filter. Reducing solution should always be freshly prepared.

Standard solution

Weigh accurately 50-60 mg of sodium or potassium acid phosphate and dissolve in water to produce 100 ml. Dilute further 10 ml of this solution to 100 ml with distilled water.

Sample solution

Take sample equivalent to 20 mg of phosphorus, evaporate to dryness on steam-bath in a silica dish and ignite the contents to almost white ash. Cool, weigh and calculate the concentration of the ash. Dissolve the ash in a mixture of 15 ml water and 10 ml nitric acid. Boil for 3-5 min, cool, neutralize the solution with ammonia solution. Then, acidify with 2 N sulphuric acid and add 35 ml of 2 N sulphuric acid in excess. Transfer to 250 ml volumetric flask, rinse silica dish with water, add the washings to volumetric flask and dilute to 250 ml with water. 20 ml of the resultant solution is further diluted to 100 ml (sample solution).

Procedure

To 5 ml each of sample and standard solutions add 2 ml of ammonium molybdate reagent and then 2 ml of reducing agent. Shake well and measure the absorbance of both the solutions at about 660 nm after 10 minutes against reagent blank.

Note

This method was experimentally checked on number of formulations and found to give excellent results. The method is simpler than official methods. Commonly used glycerophosphate can be estimated by this method for phosphate contents.

Zinc sulphate

Weigh accurately sample equivalent to 100 mg of zinc sulphate and dissolve in 100 ml of water. Filter and add 5 ml of strong ammonia–ammonium chloride solution and 0.1 ml of eriochrome black-T solution and titrate with 0.05 M EDTA until deep blue colour. Each ml of 0.05 M EDTA is equivalent to 14.38 mg of zinc sulphate.

Lysine monohydrochloride

Follow the method described in formulation 14 of this chapter.

Calcium (Ca^{++})

Weigh sample accurately equivalent to 100 ml of calcium (Ca^{++}), dissolve in dilute hydrochloric acid to make 100 ml. To 25 ml of this solution add 25 ml of ammonium oxalate solution (saturated) and heat on water-bath for 1 hr. Filter through 42 Whatman filter paper. Wash the precipitates with hot water till precipitates are free from oxalate ions. Dissolve the precipitates along with filter paper in warm dilute sulphuric acid and titrate while still warm with 0.1 N potassium permanganate until faint pink colour persists for 15 seconds. Each ml of 0.1 N potassium permanganate is equivalent to 2.004 mg of calcium (Ca^{++}).

Formulation 23

Microcrystalline hydroxyapatite (Calcium orthophosphate), Zinc sulphate, Ferrous fumarate, Folic acid, Vitamin B_{12}

ESTIMATION

Phosphate of calcium

Follow the method described in formulation 22 of this chapter.

Zinc sulphate

Follow the method described in formulation 22 of this chapter.

Ferrous fumarate

Weigh accurately sample equivalent to 1.5 g of ferrous fumarate and dissolve in 15 ml of dilute sulphuric acid with the aid of gentle heat. Cool, add 50 ml of water, filter and titrate the whole filtrate with 0.1 N cerric ammonium sulphate using ferrous sulphate as indicator. Each ml of 0.1 N cerric ammonium sulphate is equivalent to 16.99 mg of ferrous fumarate.

Folic acid

Follow the general method described for folic acid in this chapter.

Vitamin B_{12}

Follow the microbiological method as per I.P. or the method described in this chapter under vitamin B_{12}.

Formulation 24

Melatonin, Pyridoxine hydrochloride

ESTIMATION

Melatonin

Reagents

1. 0.01% w/v solution of cerric ammonium sulphate (CAS).
2. 0.1 M sulphuric acid.
3. 0.3% w/v solution of 3-methylbenzothiazole-2-one-hydrazone (MBTH).
4. 10% w/v solution of ferric nitrite in 5% nitric acid.
5. 0.02 M 1,10-phenanthroline solution in water.

Standard solution

60 μg/ml of melatonin in water.

Sample solution

Powdered sample equivalent to 6 mg of melatonin suspended in 75 ml of water, shake, make up the volume to 100 ml with water, filter and use the aliquot for assay.

Procedure

To 2 ml of sample and standard solutions add 3.5 ml of 'CAS' solution and 1.5 ml of MBTH reagent, heat in boiling water-bath for 5 min, cool, dilute to 10 ml with water and measure the absorbance at 530 nm against reagent blank. The method obeys Beer's law in the range of 1.5-15 μg/ml.

Probable Reaction Mechanism

The method involves oxidative coupling reaction of the drug with MBTH in the presence of 'CAS' producing reddish-coloured chromogen (λ_{max} 530 nm).

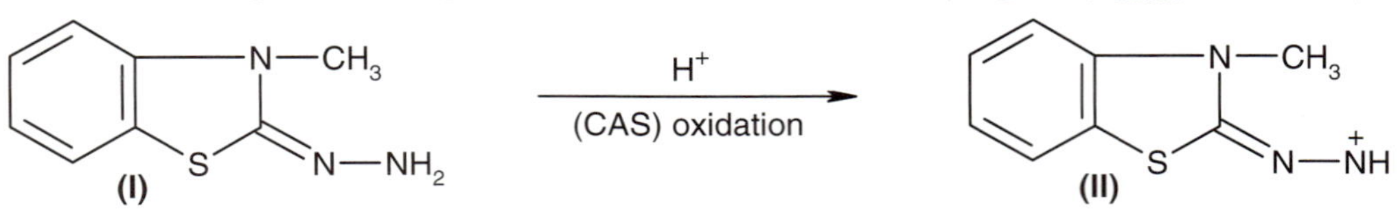

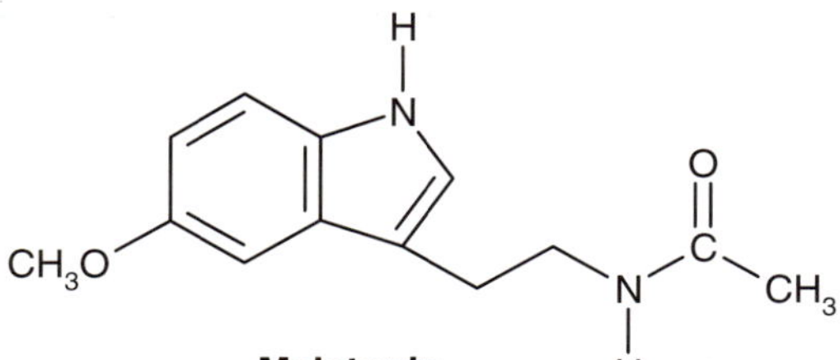

Melatonin

i.e.

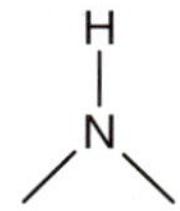

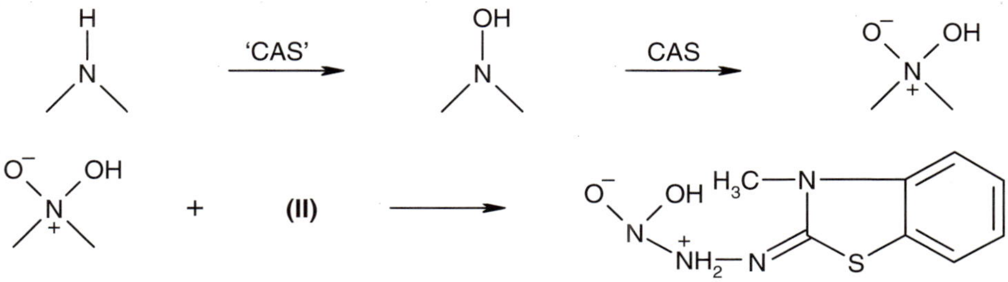

Reddish-coloured chromogen
(λ_{max} 530 nm)

Reference

B.S. Kuchekar et al., *Ind. J. Pharm. Sci.*, March-April 2002, pp. 158-160.

Pyridoxine

For details refer to method under pyridoxine hydrochloride. This method is based on oxidation of phenolic —OH by Fe(III) chloride and getting reduced to Fe(II) which complexes with 1,10-phenanthroline yielding reddish-brown coloured product (λ_{max} 510 nm).

The author has proposed the following structure for Fe(II) - phenanthroline complex.

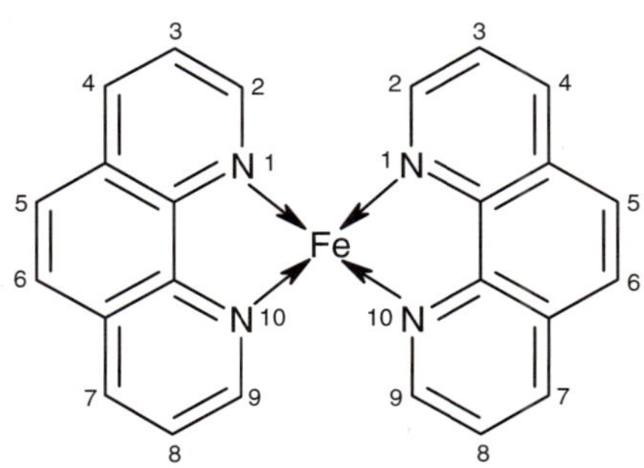

Fe(II) - phenanthroline complex
(λ_{max} 510 nm)

Formulation 25

Ethamsylate, Tranexamic acid

ESTIMATION

Ethamsylate

METHOD 1

Standard preparation

Weigh 50 mg of ethamsylate working standard in a 250 ml volumetric flask. Dissolve using water and make up to volume with water, dilute 10 ml to 50 ml with water.

Sample preparation

Weigh 50 mg equivalent of ethamsylate powdered tablets in a 250 ml volumetric flask. Dissolve using water and make up to volume with water, filter, dilute 10 ml of the above solution to 50 ml with water. Measure the absorbance of standard and sample at 301 nm using water as blank.

METHOD 2

Reagents

1. 3% w/v solution of sodium nitrite in water.
2. 1 M hydrochloric acid.
3. 1% w/v solution of copper acetate.

Sample and standard solutions

100 µg/ml in water.

Procedure

To 2 ml each of sample and standard solutions add 2 ml of sodium nitrite solution, mix, add 2 ml of copper acetate solution and 3 ml of hydrochloric acid, heat in boiling water-bath for 25 min, cool and measure the absorbance at 525 nm against reagent blank.

Probable Reaction Mechanism

$$NaNO_2 + HCl \longrightarrow HNO_2 + NaCl$$

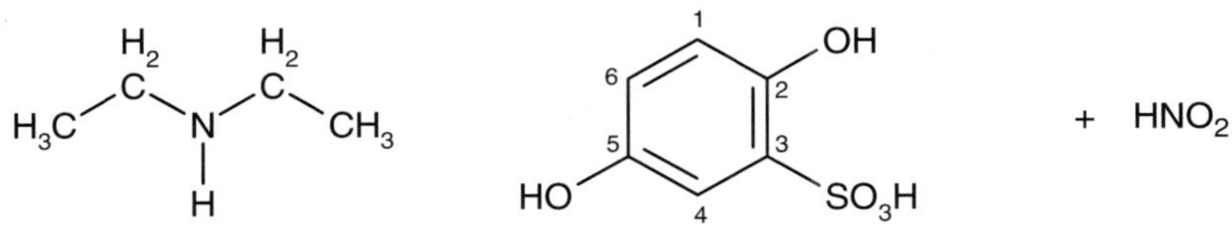

N-ethylethanamine **2,5-dihydroxybenzene sulphonic acid**

Ethamsylate

Phenolic —OH being ortho-directing, we first get ortho nitroso derivative.

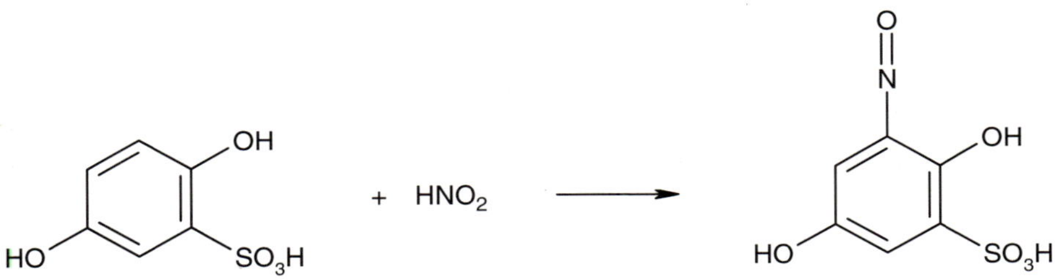

Partial structure of ethamsylate

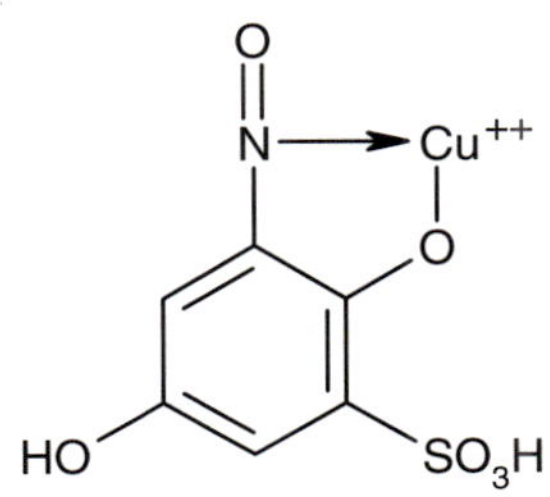

Copper - nitroso complex
(λ_{max} 525 nm)

In order to increase the sensitivity of the nitrosation reaction, the method was extended to chelating power of the nitroso derivative. Nitroso-phenol is capable of forming chelates with Cu(2) - Co(2) ions as the chelating agent contains phenolic —OH group (a group with an easily replacable proton) ortho to the nitroso (N==O) group. Nitroso group offers a lone pair of electrons to the Cu^{++} ions thus forming a coloured chelate.

Note

This reaction mechanism is analogous to the one described for paracetamol by S.F. Belal et al. (*Analyst*, 104, 919-927, 1979).

METHOD 3

Reagents

1. 0.1 M ferric chloride solution.
2. 0.02% potassium ferricyanide.

Sample and standard solutions

100 µg/ml.

Procedure

To 2 ml each of sample and standard solutions add 0.5 ml each of ferric chloride solution and potassium ferricyanide solution, keep for 5 min for reaction to complete and then dilute to 10 ml with water. Measure the absorbance at 750 nm against reagent blank.

Probable Reaction Mechanism

Fe^{+++} oxidizes the phenolic —OH to quinone and some Fe^{+++} gets reduced to Fe(II) which reacts with ferricyanide to produce Prussian blue or Turnbull's blue (λ_{max} 750 nm). This reagent, iron(III) chloride - potassium hexacyanoferrate (III), is called Barton's reagent.

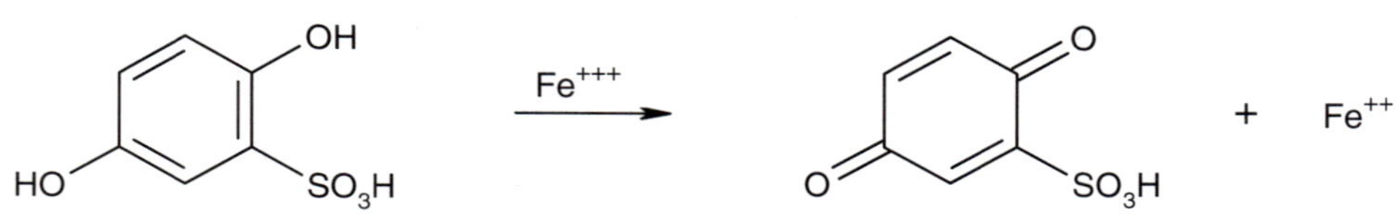

Partial structure of ethamsylate

METHOD 4

Reagents

1. 5% ferric nitrate solution in 5% nitric acid.
2. 0.02 M 1,10-phenanthroline in 1% hydrochloric acid.

Sample and standard solutions

100 µg/ml in water.

Procedure

To 2 ml each of sample and standard solutions add 0.5 ml of ferric(III) nitrate solution and 1.5 ml of phenanthroline reagent, keep for 5 min for reaction to complete and then measure the absorbance at 435 nm against reagent blank.

Probable Reaction Mechanism

Fe(III) oxidizes the drug and gets reduced to Fe(II). (For oxidation reaction by Fe(III), see method 3.) Then Fe(II) forms complex with phenanthroline to give coloured complex (λ_{max} 435 nm).

$$Fe^{+++} \longrightarrow Fe^{++}$$

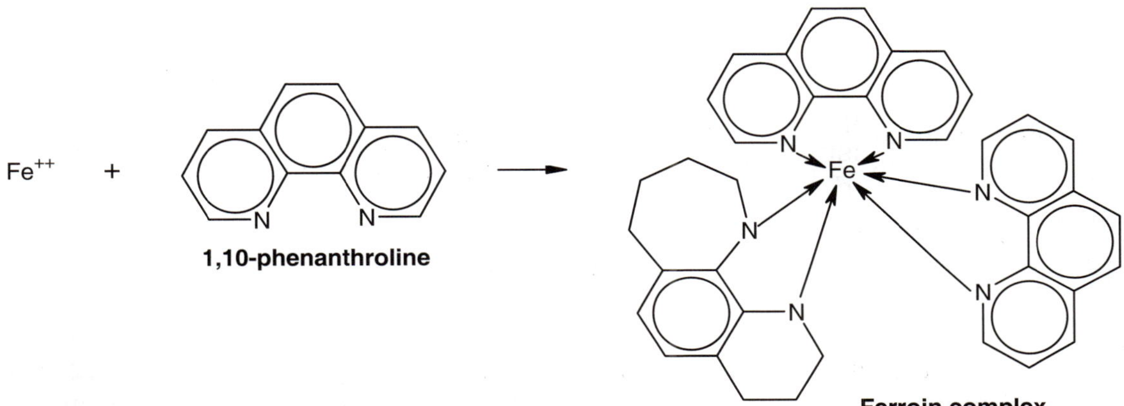

Ferroin complex
(λ_{max} 435 nm)

Reference (Methods 3 & 4)

K. Chitra, K. Sujatha, Iman Rabia Ahmed, K. Shalini, B. Lakshmi Priya & Sharon S. Varghese, *Ind. J. Pharm. Sci.*, **67(1)**, 98-100, 2005.

Reference

B.S. Kuchekar, V.S. Randive, A.P. Chaudhari & S.S. Bhise, *Ind. J. Pharm. Sci.*, **65(2)**, 184-186, 2003.

Tranexamic acid

METHOD 1

Weigh 250 mg equivalent of tranexamic acid in a conical flask, add 50 ml of acetic acid previously neutralized and titrate with 0.1 M perchloric acid using crystal violet solution as indicator. Each ml of 0.1 M perchloric acid is equivalent to 15.72 mg of tranexamic acid.

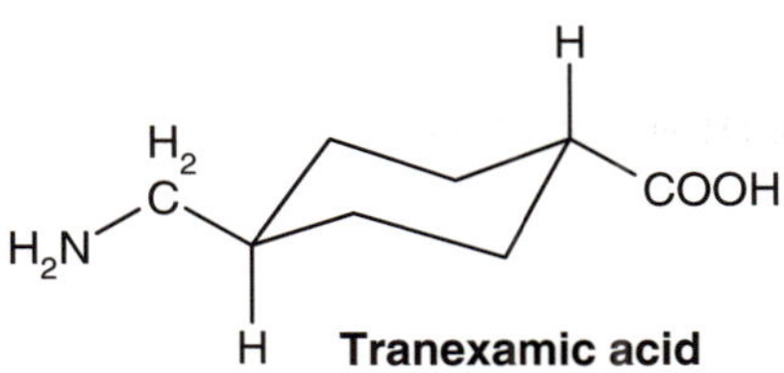

Tranexamic acid

METHOD 2

Since the drug has both amino group and carboxylic (—COOH) group [trans-4-(aminomethyl)cyclohexane carboxylic acid] it can be estimated by formol titration similar to amino acids which involve addition of neutral formaldehyde and then titrating with 0.1 M sodium hydroxide (phenolphthalein). The method is based on formol titration.

METHOD 3

Reagents

1. Saturated solution of chloranil in ethanol.
2. 0.05 M sodium tetraborate solution in water (pH 9.0).

Standard and sample solutions

100 μg/ml of tranexamic acid in water.

Procedure

To 2.5 ml each of sample and standard solutions add 10 ml of chloranil solution and 2 ml of pH 9.0 borate buffer, mix and dilute to 50 ml with water. Allow to stand at room temperature for 40 min and then measure the absorbance at 346 nm against reagent blank.

Probable Reaction Mechanism

The authors have suggested that reaction involvs (1 : 1) charge-transfer (C-T) complex formation as suggested earlier between amino acids and chloranil.

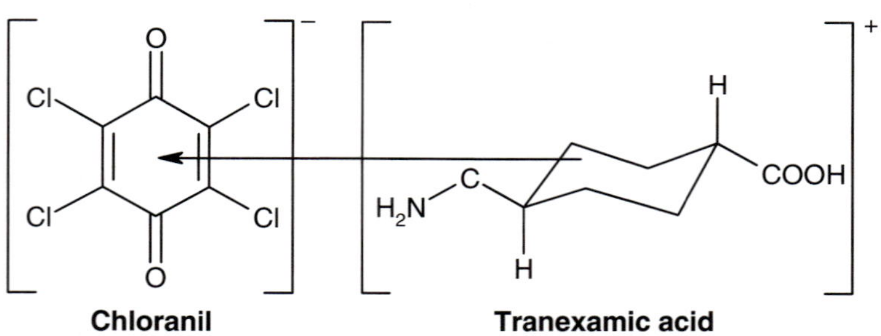

Charge-transfer (C-T) complex
(λ_{max} 346 nm)

Reference

Abdel-Aziz M. Wahbi, Essam A. Lotfi & Hanan Y. Aboul-Enein, *Talanta*, **31(1)**, 77-78, 1984.

METHOD 4

K. Chitra et al. (2004) have described a spectrophotometric method based on condensation of the drug with 'PDAB' in acidic medium yielding a yellow-coloured Schiff's base.

Procedure

To 0.5 ml each of sample and standard solutions (100 μg/ml in water) add 5 ml of 1% PDAB solution and 5% sulphuric acid, keep for 5 min and dilute to 10 ml with water. Measure the absorbance at 410 nm against reagent blank.

Probable Reaction Mechanism

The amino group present in the drug condenses with 'PDAB' to yield Schiff's base.

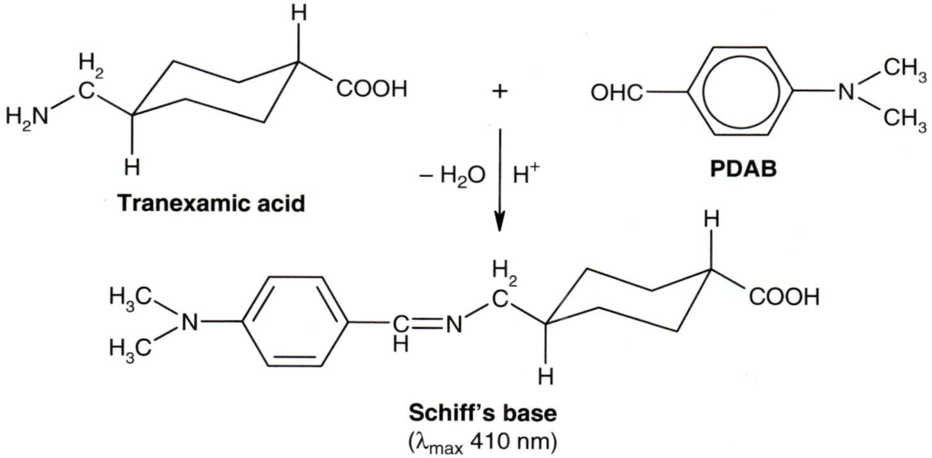

Reference

K. Chitra, K. Sujata, Iman Rabia Ahmed, K. Shalini & B. Lakshmi Priya, *Ind. J. Pharm. Sci.*, **66(6)**, 836-839, 2004.

Formulation 26

Starch Digesting Enzymes

The starch digesting enzymes are being used by pharmaceutical manufacturers in their digestive preparations. Depending on the mode of action, starch digesting enzymes, biochemically known as amylases, are fundamentally of two types:

(a) Dextrinogenic
(b) Saccharogenic.

The first type of enzymes, dextrinogenic, degrade starch only up to a stage of dextrins and not below it, the end product being dextrins. The second type of enzymes, saccharogenic, degrade starch right down to reducing sugars, the end product being predominantly maltose. These saccharogenic enzymes are mainly useful for digestive aid formulations.

Diastase from *Aspergillus oryzae* contains primarily α-amylase which is known to liquefy starch paste by reducing viscosity. In order to arrive at some meaningful idea of the comparative activity of enzymes, it is necessary that a standard way of expression is used. This is all the more important considering that there is proliferation of the ways of this expression.

Amylases are of animal or plant origin. Animal amylases are termed as α-amylases, whereas plant amylases are termed as β-amylases; pancreatin contains α-amylases.

For α-amylases of bacterial origin, a buffer of pH 6.0 and for α-amylases of fungal origin, acetate buffer of pH 5.3 is used for estimation of diastase activity. For β-amylases, buffer solution of pH 5.6 may be used.

Note

It is absolutely essential that the type of diastase added in the formulation is correctly indicated on the label to enable the analyst to use buffer of appropriate pH.

Number of methods are available for measurement of starch-digesting capacity of amylases, the important among them are:

1. Starch–iodine coloration method.
2. Estimation making use of fall in viscosity of starch solution.
3. Estimation of reducing sugars formed by the enzymic action on starch.

ESTIMATION

Diastase activity

METHOD 1

The method determines the diastase activity in term of starch hydrolysed to a stage when it gives no blue colour with iodine.

Reagents

1. Freshly prepared normal saline solution (0.9%), pH 5.0. Use dilute acetic acid to adjust the pH.
2. Soluble starch having about 15% moisture content. BDH grade starch is most suitable.
3. Buffer solution, pH 5.0 (0.1 N sodium acetate): Weigh accurately 2.05 g of sodium acetate, dissolve in sufficient quantity of water and make the volume to 250 ml. When 5.9 ml of 0.1 N acetic acid is mixed with 14 ml of 0.1 sodium acetate, solution will attain pH 5.0.
4. Iodine solution, 0.1 N (stock solution): Weigh accurately 1.276 g of iodine and dissolve in 15 ml of water containing 4 g of potassium iodide and make the volume to 100 ml. Standardise this solution to get a solution of exactly 0.1 N.
5. Iodine solution, 0.02 N: Dilute 20 ml of the stock solution (0.1 N) with 80 ml of water to obtain 0.02 N iodine solution. Prepare 0.02 N iodine solution just before use, and use 1 drop of this solution per tube.
6. 10 N hydrochloric acid, to arrest the enzymatic reaction.
7. Substrate: Weigh 200 mg of soluble starch accurately (on dry weight basis) and transfer into 200 ml measuring flask with little quantity of water. Boil the suspension till it gets into solution, constantly shaking the flask while boiling. Cool under tap water, add 5.9 ml of 0.1 N acetic acid, 14 ml of 0.1 N sodium acetate and finally make the volume to 200 ml with normal saline, pH 5.0. Dispense this solution in 5 ml aliquot to each tube. Thus each tube contains 5 mg of soluble starch.

Dilution of sample (enzyme dilution): All dilutions are to be made with normal saline, pH 5.0. The sample is diluted so that the final solution contains 200 mcg/ml of 1 in 50 enzyme. This solution is used as test enzyme solution in graded amounts of 0.1 ml to 1.0 ml per tube.

Procedure

Dispense substrate (starch solution) and saline solution as shown in the following table, and pre-incubate the tubes for 5 min in a water-bath at 37°C (± 0.5°C). Then, add graded amount of diluted enzyme solution, shake to mix well and incubate for one hour at 37°C. At the end of incubation period stop the enzyme action by adding 5 drops of 10 N hydrochloric acid. Shake the tube well after adding hydrochloric acid. Add to each tube 1 drop of 0.02 N iodine and shake well. Note the change of colour in the tubes. With increasing concentration of enzyme, there will be fall in the intensity of the colour from light purple, red to colourless. The tube showing no colour on the addition of iodine is to be taken as the end point. It is assumed that amount of enzyme present in the tube showing no colour on the addition of iodine solution has fully digested the quantity of starch present, viz. 5 mg.

	Tube No.										
	1	2	3	4	5	6	7	8	9	10	11
Substrate, starch solution (ml) 1 mg/ml	5.0	5.0	5.0	5.0	5.0	5.0	5.0	5.0	5.0	5.0	5.0
Saline, pH 0.5 (ml)	0.9	0.8	0.7	0.6	0.5	0.4	0.3	0.2	0.1	0.0	1.0
Diluted enzyme solution (ml) 200 mcg/ml	0.1	0.2	0.3	0.4	0.5	0.6	0.7	0.8	0.9	1.0	0.0

Calculations

Each tube contains 5 mg of starch. At the end of incubation period, stop the reaction and add solution of iodine. Let us assume that tube No. 5 shows no colour with iodine. Thus 100 mcg of enzyme digests 5 mg of starch in one hour.

$$\text{Diastase activity} = \frac{5 \times 1000}{100} = \frac{5000}{100} = 50 \text{ units (1 in 50)}$$

Claimed = 50 (1 in 50), i.e., the ratio = 1 : 50

Note

The starch–iodine complex has a change of colour from blue → violet purple → reddish-brown → colourless, depending upon the degradation of starch to lower molecular weight products; dextrin showing reddish-brown colour. This test only ensures that the starch is degraded to below the stage of dextrins, but this does not necessarily mean that starch is digested to the stage of reducing sugars, maltoses.

METHOD 2

Undigested starch reacts with iodine to give blue colour having absorption maximum at about 610 nm.

Reagents

1. Soluble starch (BDH) solution, substrate: Boil 80 ml of water and into this pour 1 g of starch previously suspended in 5 ml of water, stir till a clear solution is obtained. Cool and dilute to 100 ml with water.

2. Phthalate buffer (0.2 M), pH 5.4.
3. 0.5 M solution of sodium chloride.
4. Stock solution of iodine, 0.1 N: To be prepared as described under method 1 above.
5. 0.01 N iodine solution: Dilute 10 ml of the stock solution to 100 ml with water.
6. 2 N hydrochloric acid.

Standard enzyme solution

Weigh accurately standard diastase of known enzymatic activity and dilute with water to produce concentration similar to the sample.

Sample solution

Take appropriately weighed or measured aliquot of the sample equivalent to 50 mg of diastase (1 in 400) and extract or dilute with water to produce 100 ml.

Procedure

Take two tubes of 50 ml each. To each add 10 ml of substrate, 6 ml of buffer solution, pH 5.4, and 2 ml of sodium chloride solution, mixing after each addition. Place them in water-bath maintained at 40°C ± 0.5°C. Add 1 ml of sample and 1 ml of water to the sample and blank tubes and note the starting point. Shake the tubes and keep in water-bath (40°C) for 15 minutes. Then, add 1 ml of 2 N hydrochloric acid to arrest the reaction. Transfer contents of both the tubes to 100 ml volumetric flask and dilute to 90 ml with water. Then, add accurately 1 ml of 0.01 N iodine and make up the volume with water. Dilute 5 ml of the digested mixtures (sample and blank) further to 25 ml with water and measure the absorbance of blue colour of sample and blank solutions at about 610 nm. Calculate the activity; amount (g) of starch digested by the enzyme. Repeat the procedure with the standard enzyme solution.

Amount (g) of starch digested by enzyme present in each tablet =

$$= \frac{A_s - A_u}{A_s} \times C \times \frac{\text{Average weight of tablets}}{\text{Weight of the sample (g) taken}} \times d_f$$

where

A_s = absorbance of blank;
A_u = absorbance of sample;
C = quantity of starch used as substrate for digestion (0.1 g);
d_f = dilution factor.

METHOD 3

By this method, liquefying power of the enzyme is determined. Two methods are proposed to determine this activity.

Method (a): This is based on the measurement of outflow time of liquefied starch. The outflow time decreases with the fall in viscosity of the substrate.

Reagents

1. Potato starch, BDH grade.
2. Sodium chloride.
3. 1 N sodium hydroxide.
4. Acetate buffer solution: Mix 16.4 g of anhydrous sodium acetate and make up the volume to 500 ml with water.
5. Starch solution, substrate: Weigh 25 g of potato starch (BDH) and make a paste with 50 ml of water in a 150 ml beaker. In a 1000 ml beaker having a 500 ml mark, dissolve 2 g of sodium chloride in 450 ml water and heat this to boiling. Add the above starch suspension to the boiling water in 1000 ml beaker with continuous stirring and transfer any residue of starch suspension with minimum quantity of water. Note the time when boiling commences throughout the entire mass and continue boiling for 5 minutes. Remove the source of heat, cool, add 5 ml of acetate buffer solution. Mix thoroughly by pouring and make up the volume to 500 ml with water.

Procedure

Set a thermostatically controlled water-bath at a temperature of 40 ± 1°C. Take five 150 ml beakers, each with a stirring rod, and to each of the beakers add 100 ml of starch solution. Mark three beakers as A_1, A_2, A_3 and other two beakers as B_1, B_2. Put the beakers containing the starch solution in the water-bath and allow them to attain the temperature of the bath (40°C). When the starch solution inside the beakers has attained the temperature of 40 ± 1°C, add 0.25 ml of the sample to each of the three beakers marked A_1, A_2, A_3. At the same time, add 0.25 ml of water to each of two beakers marked B_1, B_2. Immediately after addition, stir thoroughly the solution in the beaker for one minute and allow them to remain in the bath for 10 minutes after addition of the sample. Take out the beakers and while stirring add 1 ml of 1 N sodium hydroxide solution to each of the beakers and stir for 30 seconds more. Allow 2-3 minutes time interval between operation of successive beakers for proper manipulation of the experiment.

Allow the contents of the beaker to cool to room temperature. Measure the outflow time with the help of a 100 ml pipette and record the time taken by each of three samples marked A_1, A_2, A_3 and take mean of three readings. Also measure the time taken by the solutions in B_1, B_2 and take mean. Express the liquefying power by the mean time taken by the sample against the mean time taken by the blank solution.

Method (b): In this method, liquefying power is estimated by fuchsin colour test.

Reagents

1. Starch suspension: 10 g of potato starch (moisture-free basis) is suspended in 10 ml of 0.1 M acetate buffer solution, pH 6.0, and made to 100 ml with distilled water.
2. Fuchsin solution: 0.2 g of fuchsin is dissolved in 1.5 ml alcohol and made to 200 ml with distilled water.

Enzyme solution

The enzyme preparation is mixed with an appropriate amount of distilled water, allowed to stand for 30 minutes at 30°C with occasional shaking and filtered.

Procedure

10 ml of starch suspension is placed in each of ten test tubes. Add 0.1, 0.2, ..., 1.0 ml of the enzyme solution and 0.9, 0.8, ..., 0.0 ml of distilled water to each of these test tubes respectively (the final content of each tube should be (11 ml). These test tubes are heated at successive time intervals in a boiling water-bath with vigorous shaking to keep starch suspension homogeneous. As soon as the content is gelatinised, the test tube is transferred to a water-bath kept at 40°C and incubated for 10 minutes exactly. Then, the tube is heated in a boiling water-bath for 5-7 minutes to destroy amylase and cooled in a water-bath at 20°C for 3 minutes. To each tube add 1 ml fuchsin solution. The tube is stoppered, turned upside down gently twice, and the colour distribution is observed. Among the tubes whose contents are uniformly coloured, the one to which has been added the least amount of test enzyme solution is picked up. The activity of unknown enzyme in the sample is calculated by comparing with the standard.

Formulation 27

Pepsin

ESTIMATION

Proteolytic activity of pepsin

METHOD 1

Reagents

1. Acidified water: Dilute 65 ml of 1 N hydrochloric acid to 1000 ml with distilled water.
2. Coagulated egg albumin: Hen's eggs, preferably of countryside, 5-10 days old are selected. Boil the eggs for 5 minutes, cool to room temperature, separate the white. At once, rub through sieve No. 44, rejecting first portion that passes through the sieve.

Note

1. Fresh eggs give erratic results.
2. Eggs are generally boiled for 5 minutes and allowed to cool to room temperature. Prolonged heating is not desirable as it produces hard coagulation.
3. Stored egg-white should have final moisture content of 80-85%.

Sample solution

Dilute accurately measured aliquot of the sample with acidified normal saline to produce approximately 0.5 mg of the pepsin per ml. If the sample is in powder form, triturate with acidified normal saline and dilute with the same solvent to contain about 0.5 mg of pepsin per ml.

Procedure

Triturate 12.5 g or 15 g of freshly prepared coagulated egg albumin, depending upon the activity of pepsin i.e. 1 in 2500 or 1 in 3000, in a small mortar with 50 ml of acidified water until reduced to uniform paste. Transfer to a 250 ml flask, rinse the mortar with 60 ml of acidified water and add the rinsing to the contents of the flask. Immerse the flask in a water-bath maintained at 50-52°C, its contents being on a lower level than water in the bath. When the contents of the flask have attained the temperature of the bath, add 10 ml of assay preparation and dilute the contents of the flask to 125 ml with acidified water. Cover the flask with butter paper and digest for 4 hrs, shaking at interval of fifteen minutes. Centrifuge the contents of the flask and pour out the greater portion of the clear liquid. Wash remainder into a 10 ml graduated cylinder and allow to stand for 30 minutes. Measure the volume of the undissolved albumin residue.

Note

1. One can either repeat the experiment using different amounts of albumin (7.5 g to 15.0 g) or different volume of assay preparations (6-10 ml) and find out the minimum amount of assay preparation for which residue left after digestion is not more than 2 ml.
2. Diluted enzyme solution should be used within 1 hr of preparation. Care should be taken that while diluting the enzyme sample it is not shaken vigorously as it may result in the detachment of the enzyme.
3. Sodium chloride stabilizes the enzyme.

Working example

Suppose a flask containing 15 g of egg albumin and 8 ml of sample solution (0.5 mg/ml) leaves 1.8 ml of sedimentation, the pepsin activity is 4 mg of pepsin I.P. digests 15 g of egg albumin. However, as per claim (1 in 3000), it should digest 12 g of egg albumin.

Amount of pepsin present in 8 ml aliquot of the sample $= \frac{15}{12} \times 4 = 5$ mg.

Net content (mg) of pepsin (1 in 3000) = 5 × dilution factor.

METHOD 2

Reagents

1. 0.1 N sodium hydroxide.
2. 1 N sodium hydroxide.
3. 1 N hydrochloric acid.
4. 20% w/v solution of sodium sulphate in water.
5. Acidic sodium chloride solution: 1% solution of sodium chloride in 0.065 N hydrochloric acid.
6. Formaldehyde.

7. 5% casein solution, substrate: Triturate 50 g of casein with little water, then add 50 ml of 1 N sodium hydroxide and dilute to 1000 ml with water. Heat on boiling water-bath for 30 minutes, cool and again adjust the volume to 1000 ml. Filter through glass wool.

Enzyme solution

The sample of enzyme solution is prepared in acidified sodium chloride solution and pH of the substrate is adjusted to 2 to 2.8.

METHOD

To 100 ml of casein solution add 12 ml of 1 N hydrochloride acid and known quantity of pepsin. Mix and incubate for 1 h at 40°C ± 0.5°C. Then, add sufficient sodium sulphate solution to produce 400 ml. Filter to remove undigested casein. To 100 ml of the filtrate add 10 ml of neutralized (phenolphthalein) formaldehyde and titrate with 0.1 N sodium hydroxide using undigested casein as blank. Prepare the standard curve for volume of 0.1 N sodium hydroxide required in titration against the concentration of pepsin taken for the test. Pepsin concentrations varying from 5-100 mg are usually employed for this purpose. The sample is subjected to above method and amount of pepsin in the sample calculated from the standard curve.

This is based on formol titration as applicable for the estimation of amino acids.

Note

Papain, if present, interferes in this test. In such cases, pepsin is assayed by egg albumin method and papain by casein digestion method at pH 7 at which pepsin will not interfere as it gets inactivated at higher pH.

Formulation 28

Papain

ESTIMATION

Proteolytic activity of papain

METHOD 1

Reagents

1. Solution of cysteine hydrochloride: Dissolve 0.5 g of cysteine hydrochloride, accurately weighed, in 10 ml of water, adjust to pH 7.0 with solution of sodium hydroxide. It should be freshly prepared.
2. Solution of casein, substrate: Dissolve 4.0 g of purified casein (Hammerstan grade) accurately weighed by shaking with 90 ml of water. Adjust to pH 7.0 with 1 N sodium hydroxide and dilute to 100 ml with water.

Sample preparation

Transfer sample equivalent to 1 tablet into a stoppered flask containing 50 ml of 30% v/v glycerine in water (previously maintained at 37°C). Shake for 3 minutes only and keep aside for about 30 minutes to settle down the undissolved material. Transfer the supernatant into a centrifuge tube and centrifuge for about 40 minutes or more (if necessary) to separate charcoal. Now take out exactly 25 ml of the supernatant into a 100 ml volumetric flask, add 10 ml of cysteine hydrochloride solution and dilute to 100 ml with water (solution A).

Sample blank preparation

Transfer 25 ml of solution (A) to a 150 ml conical flask. Boil for 5 minutes, cool and transfer to 25 ml volumetric flask, rinse with water and dilute to volume with water.

Procedure

To two 250 ml conical flasks add 10 ml of water, 15 ml of casein solution and keep at 60°C for 15 minutes. Add to one of the flasks, labelled as SA, 25 ml of sample solution; and to the other flask, labelled as SB, add 25 ml sample blank solution. Keep the flasks at 60°C over water-bath for 30 min. Stir both flasks (SA and SB) at regular intervals of 5 min. After 30 min, remove the flasks and cool immediately to room temperature. Add 10 ml of formaldehyde solution previously neutralized (by 0.1 M NaOH) solution using phenolphthalein indicator. Titrate sample solution SA and sample blank SB to a pH of 8.3 using 0.02 M sodium hydroxide solution. The difference between the two titrations is not less than 4.5 ml of 0.1 M sodium hydroxide.

Calculation

Each ml of 0.02 M NaOH = 1.1112 mg of papain

$$\text{Papain} = \frac{(\text{SA} - \text{SB}) \times M \times 50 \times 100 \times AW \times 1.1112}{0.02 \times W \times 25 \times 25}$$

where

SA = Volume of 0.02 M sodium hydroxide consumed for sample
SB = Volume of 0.02 M sodium hydroxide consumed for sample blank
M = Exact molarity of 0.02 M sodium hydroxide
AW = Average weight of tablet in mg
W = Weight of sample taken in mg

Note

1. Ordinary grade of casein does not give satisfactory results.
2. It has been experienced that boiling of liquid sample solution for 3 min is often not adequate to destroy completely the enzyme due to buffering property of the sample and lower pH (3.5–5.5) as papain is highly stable in buffered medium. Longer heating time may be required while handling oral liquid samples.
3. In liquid dosage forms, the pH is normally maintained between 3.0–6.0 and on boiling at 100°C for 3 min to destroy the enzyme there is further variation in pH. These changes in pH, if not taken care of, can lead to erroneous results. It is, therefore, required that pH should be adjusted prior to incubation. After addition of enzyme solution (boiled or as such) to the substrate, pH should be rapidly adjusted to 7.0 before taken for incubation (60°C) in a thermostatically controlled water-bath. After incubation, carry out the formol titration.

Reference

N.M. Ranga Raju, K.M. Raghu & G.A. Vinolia, *Indian Drugs*, **25(8)**, 345-346, 1988.

METHOD 2

Reagents

1. Buffer solution, pH 7.6.
   (a) Weigh 11.41 g of potassium phosphate diabasic and make up to 500 ml with distilled water.
   (b) Weigh 6.804 g of potassium phosphate monobasic and make up to 500 ml with distilled water. Adjust solution (a) to pH 7.6 with solution (b).
2. Casein solution, substrate: Dissolve 1 g of casein in pH 7.6 buffer solution and make up to 100 ml with the same buffer.
3. 5% w/v trichloroacetic acid in water.

Standard preparation

Weigh 50 mg of standard papain, add 5 ml of 0.1 N hydrochloric acid and make up to 100 ml with water. Take 100 ml, add 1 ml of 0.1 N hydrochloric acid and make up to 100 ml with water.

Sample preparation

Take sample powder equivalent to 25 mg of papain. Add 10 ml of distilled water, followed by 5 ml of 0.1 N hydrochloric acid, make up to 100 ml with distilled water and filter. Pipette 20 ml, add 1 ml of 0.1 N hydrochloric acid and make up to 100 ml with distilled water.

Procedure

Take 1 ml of the sample solution in one test tube and 1 ml of the standard solution in two test tubes, one of which serves as a blank. Add to all test tubes 1 ml of buffer solution, pH 7.6, and then, add 2 ml of casein solution except in blank. Add 6 ml of trichloroacetic acid in blank only and maintain all the tubes at 37°C for 20 minutes. Then, add 6 ml of trichloroacetic acid to the sample and the standard. Keep for one hour at room temperature, filter and measure the extinction at 280 nm of both sample and standard solutions against blank and calculate the results by comparison. This method is based on spectrophotometric measurement of amino acid - tyrosine released as a result of proteolytic action of papain on casein, the protein.

Note

Trichloroacetic acid, in addition to removing the substrate (casein) by precipitation, also acts as denaturing agent which causes drastic irreversible changes in papain structure and activity.

Formulation 29

Pepsin, Papain, Diastase, Choline dihydrogen citrate, Tricholine citrate, Methionine

ESTIMATION

Pepsin

Follow method 1 described for pepsin using appropriate aliquots of egg albumin and enzyme preparations.

Papain

Use casein as substrate in pH 7.0 buffer and determine the contents of papain by formol titration method. For details, refer to method 1 for determination of proteolytic activity of papain in this chapter.

Diastase

Follow method 1 described under determination of diastase activity. This method determines diastase activity in term of starch hydrolysed to a stage when it gives no blue colour with iodine. Calculate the diastase activity as per example explained under method 1 for estimation of diastase activity.

Note

Type of diastase (fungal or bacterial) must be indicated on the label to enable the analyst to use buffer of correct pH. Refer to formulation 1 of this chapter.

Choline dihydrogen citrate

Wash solution

Prepared by diluting 2 ml of saturated aqueous ammonium reineckate solution to 1000 ml with water.

Procedure

Transfer an accurately weighed portion of the sample equivalent to 100 mg of choline dihydrogen citrate to a beaker and dissolve in 40 ml of water. Filter and to the filtrate add carefully 10 ml of freshly prepared saturated reineckate solution from a pipette, allowing it to run down the side of the beaker so that it forms a layer under the sample solution without producing turbulence. Mix by rotating the beaker gently and allow to stand in a refrigerator for one hour. Filter, collect the precipitates in 30 ml low form sintered glass crucible of medium porosity using gentle suction. Rinse the beaker with three 10 ml portions of wash solution previously cooled to 5°C and pass through the crucible containing the precipitates. Remove most of the water by suction, then dry in an oven at 105°C for an hour. Cool in desiccator and weigh as choline reineckate. The weight of the choline reineckate multiplied by 0.6988 gives the weight of choline dihydrogen citrate.

In case of tricholine citrate, each g of the residue (as reineckate) is equivalent to 0.4114 g of tricholine citrate:

$$0.6988 \times \frac{295.29}{501.63} = 0.4114\,\text{g}$$

295.29 = Mol. wt. of choline dihydrogen citrate
422.51 = Mol. wt. of choline reineckate
501.63 = Mol. wt. of tricholine citrate

Methionine

Reagents

1. Bentonite.
2. 10% w/v solution of sodium nitroprusside in water or iodine solution.
3. 20% v/v hydrochloric acid.
4. 1% w/v solution of glycine in water.

Standard solution

1 mg/ml of methionine, in water.

Sample solution

Weigh accurately a quantity of powdered sample equivalent to 50 mg of methionine. Add 50 ml of water, 1 g of bentonite, 0.5 g of sodium chloride, shake for 15 minutes and dilute to 100 ml with water.

Procedure

To accurately measured volume of sample and standard solutions, representing 2 mg of methionine, add water to produce 6 ml. Add 1 ml of 5 N sodium hydroxide, 1 ml of glycine solution and 0.5 ml of sodium nitroprusside solution. Shake for 15-20 seconds and keep on water-bath (40°C) for 10 minutes. Cool and add 2 ml of hydrochloric acid. Shake well and measure the extinction of both the sample and standard solutions at about 530 nm against reagent blank and calculate the results by comparison.

Note

The sample can be subjected to paper chromatography or thin layer chromatography. For details regarding chromatographic separation and colour development, refer to the method described for estimation of lysine monohydrochloride in formulation 10 of the chapter on vitamins and minerals.

Explanatory Note

On gentle heating of alkaline solution of the substance with sodium nitroprusside, cooling and addition of hydrochloric acid gives red colour. This involves oxidation of methionine with sodium nitroprusside.

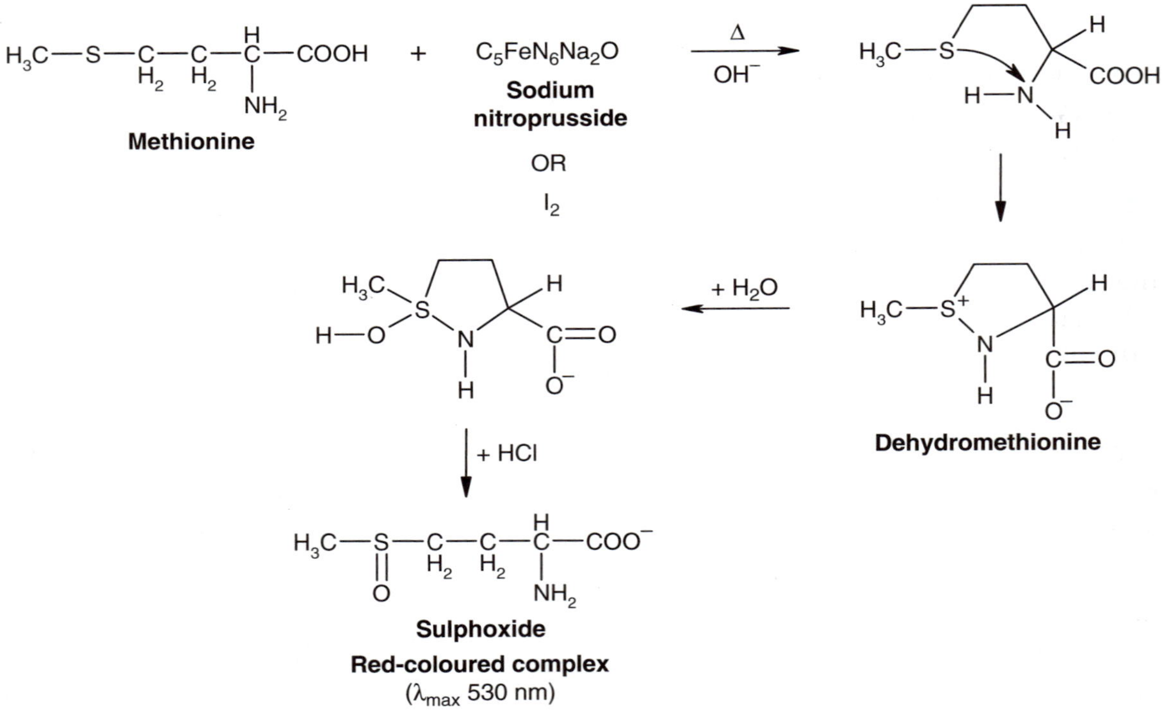

Note

Bromine or sodium periodate have been used as oxidizing agents. With bromine, sulphoxide or sulphone 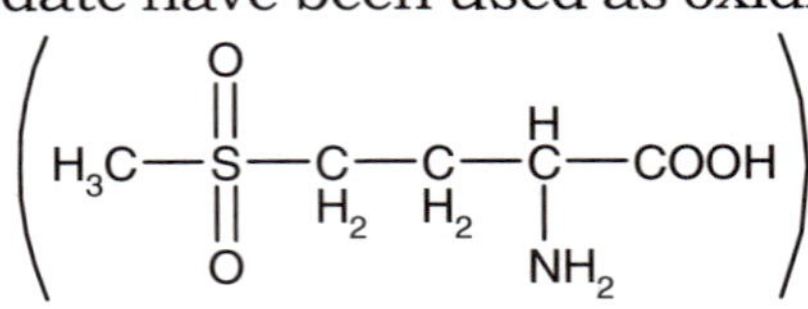 are formed.

Formulation 30

Papain, Fungal diastase, Iodochlorhydroxyquinoline, Diphenhydramine hydrochloride, Methyl polysiloxane, Thiamine hydrochloride, Riboflavine, Nicotinamide

ESTIMATION

Iodochlorhydroxyquinoline (ICHQ)

METHOD 1

Reagents

1. 5% w/v solution of sodium nitrite in water.
2. Glacial acetic acid.
3. Dilute ammonium hydroxide solution.

Standard solution

Weigh accurately 100 mg of pure 'ICHQ' and dissolve it in 50 ml of glacial acetic acid. Warm on water-bath for 3-4 minutes, cool and make up to 100 ml with glacial acetic acid. Filter, rejecting first few ml of the filtrate. Dilute further appropriately with glacial acetic acid to get a concentration of 100 mcg/ml.

Sample solution

Transfer sample equivalent to 100 mg of 'ICHQ', add 50 ml of glacial acetic acid. Warm on water-bath for 3-4 minutes shaking intermittently to dissolve, cool and make up the volume to 1000 ml with glacial acetic acid. Dilute further to get 100 mcg/ml concentration.

Procedure

To 2 ml of the sample and standard solutions, taken in two separate test tubes, add 2 ml of sodium nitrite solution. Shake and allow to stand at room temperature for 10 minutes. Add 10 ml of dilute ammonia solution and shake. Measure the extinction of both the solutions at maxima at about 450 nm against reagent blank prepared by using 2 ml of water instead of sample solution. Calculate the results by comparison.

METHOD 2

Follow the method described in the chapter on antidiarrhoeals.

Diphenhydramine hydrochloride

Reagents

1. Citrate - phosphate buffer: 17.65 ml of 0.2 M citric acid and 82.35 ml of 0.2 M disodium phosphate are mixed together to give pH 7.0 buffer (adjust pH to 7.0 either with 0.2 M citric acid or 0.2 M disodium phosphate).
2. Buffered dye solution: 50 ml of 0.2% w/v matanil yellow is mixed with 50 ml of buffer solution, pH 7.0, and extracted with chloroform till no more dye is extracted in chloroform (this treatment reduces the blank reading considerably).
3. Dilute acetic acid.

Standard solution

Weigh accurately 200 mg of diphenhydramine hydrochloride, add 10 ml of acetic acid and about 50 ml of water. Digest for some time in water-bath, cool and dilute to 100 ml with water. 10 ml of the resulting solution is diluted to 1000 ml with acetic acid.

Sample solution

Weigh accurately a quantity of powdered tablets equivalent to 20 mg of the substance, add 10 ml of acetic acid, 25 ml of water and digest for 30 minutes in water-bath. Cool and dilute to 100 ml with water. Filter through filter paper.

Procedure

Take 1 ml each of sample and standard solutions, add 15 ml of water and 3 ml of buffered dye solution. Shake to mix and extract with three 25 ml portions of chloroform. Combine chloroform extracts and swirl gently with 10 ml of water. Allow the two layers to separate, reject aqueous layer and then extract chloroform layer with dilute hydrochloric acid. Dilute the acid layer to 200 ml with dilute acid and measure the absorbance of both the solutions at 405 nm against reagent blank prepared without substance and calculate the results.

Fungal diastase

Follow method 1 described under estimation of diastase activity in this chapter.

Methyl polysiloxane (MPS)

Amount of 'MPS' can be estimated making use of its defoaming activity. Use 0.2% w/v aqueous solution of sodium lauryl sulphate to generate the foam. For details of the procedure, refer to formulation 2 of the chapter on antacids.

Riboflavine

Follow method 2 described under general assay methods for riboflavine.

Thiamine hydrochloride

Follow method 2 described under general assay method for thiamine hydrochloride.

Nicotinamide

Reagents

1. 4% w/v solution of aniline in ethyl alcohol.
2. Cyanogen bromide solution.
3. Buffer solution: To 196 ml of water add 33 ml of ethyl alcohol and 1 ml of 1 N sodium hydroxide, mix well.

Standard solution

Weigh accurately 25 mg of nicotinamide, add 50 ml of 6 N hydrochloric acid. Digest on boiling water-bath for 40 minutes, cool and adjust to 100 ml with water. To 10 ml of the resulting solution add about 70-80 ml of water, adjust the pH to 7.0 and dilute to 100 ml with water.

Sample solution

Weigh powdered tablets accurately equivalent to 25 mg of the compound, digest and treat as under standard solution.

Procedure

Take 2 ml of sample and standard solutions, add 5 ml of buffer solution, 1 ml of aniline solution and 6 ml of cyanogen bromide solution. Shake well and measure the absorbance of both the solutions at 420 nm against reagent blank.

Papain

Follow method 1 described under estimation of proteolytic activity of papain in this chapter.

Formulation 31

Pancreatin, Bromelain, Ox-bile

ESTIMATION

Pancreatin

Estimate the proteolytic, lipolytic and amylolytic activities of pancreatin as per methods described in standard pharmacopoeias, i.e., I.P., B.P., U.S.P.

Bromelain

Unit of enzyme activity is defined as that quantity of enzyme which under the test conditions as described below releases the amount of compounds which react positively with Folin–ciocalteaus–phenol reagent which correspond to 1 μm of tyrosine in depth of colour.

Reagents

1. Folin–ciocalteaus–phenol reagents: 100 g of sodium tungstate, 25 g of sodium molybdate and 50 ml of phosphoric acid (85%) are refluxed with 800 ml of water for 3 hrs. This reagent is quite stable and sensitive.
2. Haemoglobin, substrate.
3. Sodium chloride.
4. 0.5 N sodium hydroxide.
5. 1 N sodium hydroxide.
6. 0.2 N hydrochloric acid.
7. 1 N hydrochloric acid.
8. 5% w/v trichloroacetic acid solution in water.
9. L-tyrosine.
10. Boric acid solution: 4.12 g of boric acid and 0.195 g of sodium chloride are dissolved in water by slight warming and adjusted with water to 100 ml.
11. Folin–ciocalteaus (FC) solution: Mix 1 part of the reagent with 2 parts of water. Prepare fresh as and when required.

12. Solution of haemoglobin, substrate: Suspend 2 g of haemoglobin in 150 ml beaker with 25 ml of water, add 36 g of urea and 80 ml of 1 N sodium hydroxide. Stir for 50-60 minutes, add 15 ml of boric acid solution and adjust the pH to 6.0 with 1 N hydrochloric acid. Make up the volume to 100 ml with water.
13. Buffer solution, pH 4.0: Dissolve 22.6 g of diammonium hydrogen citrate in 900 ml of water, adjust the pH to 4.0 with 1 N hydrochloric acid and dilute to 1000 ml with water, mix well.
14. Buffer solution, pH 6.0: Dissolve 22.6 g of diammonium hydrogen citrate in 900 ml of water, adjust the pH to 6.0 with 1 N hydrochloric acid and dilute to 1000 ml with water.

Tyrosine standard solution

Weigh accurately 18.12 mg of L-tyrosine and dilute to 100 ml with 0.2 N hydrochloric acid. 0.5 ml of the resulting solution is further diluted to 25 ml with 0.2 N hydrochloric acid.

Tyrosine standard curve

Take 1, 2, 3, 4, 5 ml of tyrosine standard solution in separate tubes, adjust to 5 ml where necessary with 0.2 N hydrochloric acid. To each tube add 10 ml of 0.5 N sodium hydroxide, mix and add 3 ml of Folin–ciocalteaus solution and mix. Measure the absorbance of different solutions at maximum at about 750 nm against reagent blank. Plot the graph of absorbance against quantities of tyrosine. Above quantities of tyrosine correspond to 0.2 to 1 μm of L-tyrosine.

Sample solution

Bromelain coating is usually done over the protective cellulose acetate coating. Therefore pancreatin which is present in lower coating of the tablet will not interfere in this assay. Take whole tablet equivalent to 750 units of bromelain, add 50 ml of buffer solution, pH 4.0 and stir for 10-15 minutes. Care should be taken not to damage inner layer while extracting bromelain. 5 ml of above suspension is diluted to 50 ml with buffer solution, pH 6.0.

Procedure

Add 1 ml of sample solution to 5 ml of the substrate [previously maintained at 35°C (± 0.5°C) for 15 minutes]. Incubate exactly for 10 minutes and then add 10 ml of trichloroacetic acid. After 20 minutes, filter, and to 5 ml of the filtrate add 10 ml of 0.5 N sodium hydroxide and 3 ml of Folin's solution. After 5 minutes measure the absorbance of the sample solution at 750 nm against blank, prepared by adding 1 ml of sample solution after addition of 10 ml of trichloroacetic acid. Calculate the amount of bromelain from the standard curve.

Calculation

Units/tablet: $E \times 3.2 \times d_f$

From the absorbance of sample (E), calculate the μm of tyrosine from the standard curve.

3.2 = ratio value (16 : 5)

Total digesting volume comes to 16 ml (1 + 5 + 10) and out of this 5 ml is taken for colour development.

Bile constituents (Cholic acid)

The main constituent is sodium desoxycholate which is estimated as cholic acid.

Reagents

1. 60% v/v acetic acid.
2. Solution of furfural (1 in 100): Measure 1 ml of freshly distilled furfural and make to 100 ml with water. This solution is prepared fresh every time.
3. Dilute sulphuric acid: Mix cautiously 50 ml of sulphuric acid with 65 ml of water and cool.

Standard cholic acid solution

Dissolve 25 mg of cholic acid, accurately weighed in 10 ml of 60% acetic acid, and make up the volume to 50 ml with acetic acid (0.5 mg/ml).

Sample solution

Weigh accurately about 700 mg of finely powdered tablets and suspend them in 20 ml of alcohol. Shake well and make the volume to 50 ml with alcohol. Shake again for about 10 minutes and filter. This solution should contain about 0.5 mg/ml of cholic acid.

Procedure

Pipette exactly 1 ml each of standard and sample solutions into two test tubes. To each tube add exactly 1 ml of furfural solution and place the tubes at once in an ice-bath for 5 minutes. Then, add to each tube exactly 18 ml of dilute sulphuric acid. Thoroughly mix the contents of the tubes and place them in water-bath maintained at 70°C for 10 minutes. At the end of this period, place the tube immediately in ice water for 2 minutes and determine the absorbance of each solution at about 650 nm. A blank is taken by omitting the addition of furfural. Calculate the results by comparison.

Cholic acid has two functional groups of analytical interest. First is carboxyl (—COOH) group present in the acid molecule in the side chain at C-17. Second are the hydroxy (—OH) groups present at C-3, 7 & 12. The acid group can be titrated with potassium hydroxide using thymol blue as indicator.

The above procedure is based on the work of Irwin et al. (1944) which is the modification of classical Pattenkofer reaction. This involves addition of aldehyde group present in the reagent to the alcoholic (—OH) group of the molecule in acidic medium. The acid acts as catalyst in the formation of hemiacetal. Hemiacetal being highly unstable and in the presence of the ? acid reacts with one more mole of the drug to form acetal (λ_{max} 650 nm).

Probable Reaction Mechanism

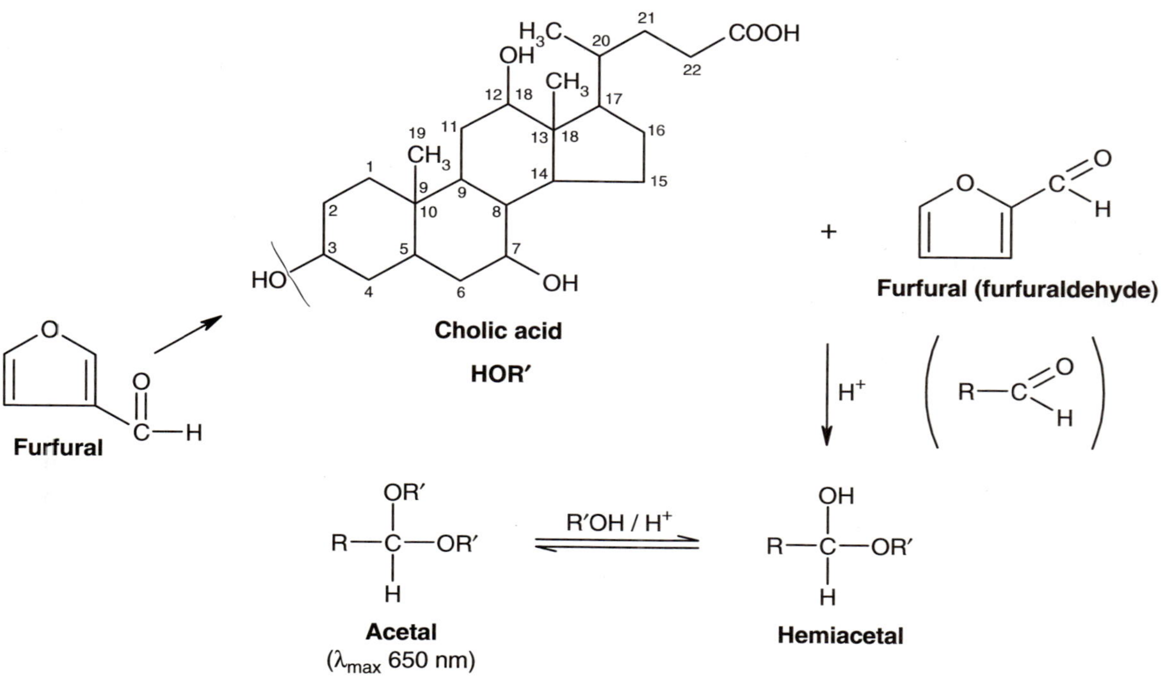

Reference

1. J.L. Irwin, C.G. Johnston & J. Kopala, *J. Biol. Chem.*, **153**, 439, 1944.
2. Pharmaceutical Analysis by Higuchi et al., 1997, p. 116.
3. Organic Chemistry (Vol. 1), 6th ed. by I.L. Finar, p. 222.
4. Organic Chemistry by Norman L. Allinger, 1971, Worth Publishers, Inc., p. 476.

Formulation 32

L-ornithine-L-aspartate, Pancreatin

ESTIMATION

Pancreatin

Follow the method described in formulation 31 of this chapter for proteolytic, amylolytic and lipolytic activities.

L-ornithine-L-aspartate

METHOD 1

This method is based on post-derivatisation preparative thin layer chromatography.

Standard solution (30 mg/ml)

Dissolve 300 mg of L-ornithine-L-aspartate working standard in water sufficient to produce 10 ml.

Sample solution

Weigh 20 tablets and take powder equivalent to 300 mg of L-ornithine-L-aspartate and shake vigorously with 10 ml of water for about 15 minutes and centrifuge. Use supernatant as sample solution.

Stationary phase

Silica gel $60F_{254}$ pre-coated on aluminium back.

Mobile phase

h-butanol : glacial acetic acid : water (50 : 25 : 25) v/v

Derivatising agent

1% ninhydrin solution in acetone.

Development, derivatisation and elution procedure

Saturate the chamber with mobile phase for 20 minutes. Wash the silica gel plate in methanol and activate it. Apply 100 ml of standard and sample solutions in the form of a band. Run the plate up to 150 mm and air dry. Spray ninhydrin solution and heat it for 10 minutes at 110°C. Violet purple spots (two) appear on the plate for L-ornithine-L-aspartate. Cut out both the bands carefully for standard and sample separately. (In sample some extra spot appears for pancreatin, so take care while cutting the bands for sample.) Extract both the bands with 5 ml of methanol and centrifuge for 10 minutes. Prepare the blank in similar manner using silica gel from the same plate. Measure the absorbance of both sample and standard solutions at about 595 nm against reagent blank and calculate the results by comparison.

Note

The above sample was also analysed by HPTLC using the same mobile phase. L-ornithine and L-aspartate could be estimated separately. The spot with lower Rf value corresponds to ornithine.

METHOD 2

Procedure

Weigh accurately a quantity of powdered tablets equivalent to 70 mg of L-ornithine-L-aspartate into a dry 250 ml conical flask and dissolve it in 5 ml of anhydrous formic acid. Add about 50 ml of previously neutralised glacial acetic acid and titrate against 0.1 M perchloric acid using crystal violet as indicator. Each ml of 0.1 M HClO4 is equivalent to 8.84 mg.
Calculation

$$\frac{\text{Titration value} \times 8.84 \times \text{Normality of } 0.1\,\text{M}\, HClO_4 \times \text{Av. wt.}}{\text{Weight of test taken} \times 0.1}$$

METHOD 3

Reagents

1. 5% w/v solution of copper sulphate.
2. 0.5% ninhydrin solution in 1 : 1 mixture of methanol–pyridine.

Sample and standard solutions

50 µg/ml of the substance in water.

Procedure

Take 2 ml each of standard and test solutions for CD in a 25 ml volumetric flask. Add 5 ml of reagent and heat on boiling water-bath for 5 min. Cool and make the final volume to 25 ml in methanol containing 2 drops of 5% copper sulphate solution. Measure the absorbance of the solutions at 525 nm against reagent blank.

Note

This method is based on general reaction of amino acids with ninhydrin followed by coupling with Cu^{++} as Cu^{++} stabilizes the colour.

Formulation 33

Cellulase and Hemicellulase

Cellulases are group of enzymes that catalyse the degradation of cellulose to glucose.

Determination of Cellulase and Hemicellulase activity

METHOD 1

Cellulases and hemicellulases split hydrated cellulose. The reducing groups released by this process are determined iodometrically.

Reagents

1. Cellulose suspension, substrate: Moisten 50 g of thin picked cellulose with 450 ml of concentrated hydrochloric acid in a 5 litre flask and keep for 3 hours under frequent swirling. Dilute the mass with 2.5 litres of water, shake well and let hydrated cellulose to settle. Remove the supernatant solution as completely as possible and suspend the sediment again in 2.5 litres of water. Repeat this procedure till the supernatant liquid is free of chloride ions. Transfer the precipitate to a suction filter and suspend the residue homogeneously in 500 ml of water. Then determine the content of cellulose in this suspension by drying 5 ml to constant weight at 105°C. Dilute the rest of the suspension with water so that 10 ml of the cellulose substrate suspension contains 320 mg of hydrated cellulose.
2. Buffer solution (0.04 M), pH 4.5: Dissolve 2.4 ml of glacial acetic acid and 5.44 g of crystalline sodium acetate, trihydrate, in water and make up to 1000 ml with water. Check pH.
3. Starch solution: Dissolve 1.0 g of soluble starch (BDH) in 100 ml of water and heat the mixture under swirling just to boiling.
4. 0.02 N iodine solution.
5. 0.02 N sodium hydroxide solution.
6. 0.02 N sodium thiosulphate solution.
7. Dilute sulphuric acid.

Enzyme suspension

Suspend the finely powdered sample homogeneously in 100 ml of water and use 5 ml of the previously well stirred suspension for the test.

Procedure

A blank value is necessary for every test. The blank test distinguishes itself from the analysis test by the fact that immediately after addition of the enzyme suspension, the enzymes are inactivated by boiling the whole mixture for a few minutes.

Scheme of the reactions

Solutions	*Sample*	*Blank*
Cellulose substrate suspension	10.0 ml	10.0 ml
Buffer solution, pH 4.5	4.0 ml	4.0 ml
Enzyme suspension	5.0 ml	5.0 ml

Immediately after addition of the enzyme suspension, boil the blank only for 5 minutes and then incubate both the blank and the sample for 8 hours in a thermostatic water-bath at 30°C ± 0.5°C. Cool and proceed with addition of other reagents to each tube as below:

0.02 N iodine solution	20.0 ml	20.0 ml
0.02 N sodium hydroxide	40.0 ml	40.0 ml
(To be added slowly with swirling)		

After 15 minutes, proceed with the addition of other reagents as given below:

Dilute sulphuric acid (3 N)	10.0 ml	10.0 ml
Starch solution	2.0 ml	2.0 ml

Titrate both sample and the blank with 0.02 N sodium thiosulphate from a microburette till the blue colour disappears. Record the volume (ml) of 0.02 N sodium thiosulphate used for sample (a) and blank (b).

Calculation

The unit is defined as the amount of enzyme which splits, during 8 hours at a pH of 4.5 and temperature of 30°C, amount of hydrated cellulose (320 mg) present in 20 ml at a rate which is equivalent to an increase of iodine consumption of 2 ml of 0.02 N iodine solution. Then calculate the activity as follows:

$$\text{Grassmann units} = \frac{(b-a)\times F \times \text{Average weight of the tablet}}{2\times 60}$$

where F is the normality factor of the 0.02 N sodium thiosulphate solution.

Note

Carboxymethyl cellulose - Na has been used as substrate and glucose, the final product, estimated.

METHOD 2

Reagents

1. 1 N hydrochloric acid.
2. 0.1 N iodine solution.
3. 0.1 N sodium thiosulphate.
4. 0.1 N sodium hydroxide.
5. 0.5 N sodium chloride solution.
6. 20% v/v sulphuric acid.
7. 1% solution of soluble starch: 1 g of soluble starch is stirred in 20 ml of water and poured into boiling water, boiled for 2 min and made up to 100 ml.
8. Phosphate buffer, pH 5.3: Prepared by mixing 21.5 ml of 0.1 N disodium hydrogen phosphate dihydrite and 978.5 g of potassium dihydrogen phosphate.
9. Enzyme solution: To 300 mg of mass (after removal of coating, if any) add 9 ml of water and shake for about 30 min, separate the undissolved portion by centrifuging at high speed and use the supernatant solution for assay.

Procedure

In a 250 ml iodine flask add 25 ml of (7) and 10 ml of buffer solution (8) and 1 ml of (5). Keep in a thermostatic water-bath at 37°C for 15 min, and then add 3 ml of enzyme solution. After exactly 2 hrs, stop the enzyme reaction by addition of 2 ml of (1) and then 15 ml of iodine solution (2) and then 45 ml of (4) is added slowly and drop by drop while shaking. After 15 min, the entire reaction mixture as obtained above is acidified with 5 ml of (6) and excess iodine is titrated with thiosulphate (3) using 1 ml of solution (7) as indicator.

Blank: Blank titration is performed as main titration except 2 ml of (1) is added before the addition of enzyme solution.

Results

Difference between the sample and the blank titration should not be less than 2 ml of 0.1 N iodine for each 30 mg of tablet mass.

Note

We may use 1% solution of lichenin (stir 1 g of lichenin with 20 ml of water, pour into boiling water, boil for 1-2 min and make up to 100 ml with water) instead of soluble starch as substrate.

Formulation 34

Serratiopeptidase, Paracetamol

Estimation

Serratiopeptidase

Reagents

1. Sodium borate–hydrochloric acid buffer, pH 9.0: Prepared by dissolving 19.0 g of disodium tetraborate (borax) in 900 ml of water, adjust the pH to 9.0 with 1 M hydrochloric acid, dilute to 1000 ml with water.
2. Trichloroacetic acid (TCA) solution prepared by dissolving 18 g of TCA, 30 g of sodium acetate and 20 ml of glacial acetic acid in water to produce 1000 ml.
3. 0.2 M hydrochloric acid.
4. Folin's reagent: Mix 1 ml of the Folin's reagent with 2 ml of water just before use.
5. 5% v/v solution of ammonium sulphate in water.

Casein solution (substrate)

Dissolve 1.2 g of casein (Hammerstein grade) in 100 ml of borate buffer of pH 9.0 by keeping in boiling water-bath for 1-2 min to make the solution clear, filter through cotton plug and dilute to 200 ml with buffer.

Standard solution (tyrosine)

Dissolve 80 mg of tryptosine in ammonium sulphate solution to produce 50 ml. Further dilute 1 ml to 100 ml with borate buffer, pH 9.0.

Test solution

Sample equivalent to 50 mg of the enzyme is dry extracted with anhydrous acetone, filtered through G_4 sintered funnel. The residue left on the funnel is extracted with 3 × 15 ammonium sulpahte solution, final volume made up to 50 ml. Further dilute 1 ml to 200 ml with pH 9.0 borate buffer.

Procedure

Sample: To 1 ml of test enzyme solution add 5 ml of casein solution, maintain at 37°C for 20 min, then add 5 ml of TCA solution and again keep at 37°C for 30 min, filter and use 2 ml of the filtrate for further treatment.

Blank: To 5 ml of casein solution add 5 ml of TCA solution and then proceed as under sample solution, filter.

To 2 ml each of sample, blank (as obtained above) and standard, add 5 ml of sodium carbonate solution (6%) and 1 ml of diluted Folin's reagent. Incubate at 37°C for 30 min, cool and measure the absorbance of blank, test and standard solutions using distilled water as blank.

Calculations

$$\text{Serratiopeptidase (units/mg)} = \frac{A_1 - A_2}{A_3 - A_4} \times 176 \times \frac{1}{20} \times 200$$

Conversion coefficient of enzyme reaction mixture = 176

$$\text{Total volume of enzyme mixture} \times \frac{32}{2} = 176$$

$$11(1 + 5 + 5) \times \frac{32}{2} = 176$$

20 = Reaction time in min
200 = Dilution factor
A_1 = Absorbance of the test solution
A_2 = Absorbance of the blank
A_3 = Absorbance of the standard solution
A_4 = Absorbance of 0.2 N HCl
32 = Content of tyrosine in 2 ml of the standard solution taken for assay

$$\text{Potency of tablets} = \frac{\text{Activity obtained}}{\text{Activity declared on label}} \times 100$$

Precautions

1. Enzyme sample should be assayed within 15 min of its preparation.
2. Tyrosine used for determination of moisture content should not be used for assay.
3. Folin's reagent should be diluted less than 5 minutes before addition into the assay.
4. Tablets of the enzyme should be crushed to a fine powder (100 mesh) for the purpose of extraction.

Probable Reaction Mechanism

This method is based on proteolytic activity of the enzyme liberating amino acids. The Folin's reagent used for colour development is specific for phenolic compounds. Out of the common amino acids liberated as a result of protein (casein) hydrolysis (such as glycine, alanine, valine, methionine, tryptophan, lysine, arginine, asparagine, tyrosine and cysteine), tyrosine is the only amino acid with phenolic function in its structure. The main component of the reagent molybdenum(VI) is a strong oxidizing agent.

Initially, phosphoric acid (H_3PO_4), comparatively stronger acid, can replace weaker acids (H_2MoO_4 and H_2WO_4) from their salts forming sodium phosphate (Na_3PO_4) and corresponding acid. Lithium sulphate is added to maintain ionic nature i.e. $MoO_3 \cdot H_2O \rightarrow H_2MoO_4$ and $WO_3 \cdot H_2O \rightarrow H_2WO_4$ so that oxo-anions are made to behave as Lewis acid or anion base.

ortho-molybdic acid   ortho-tungstic acid

In the presence of ortho-molybdic acid, ortho-tungstic acid tyrosine is ionized easily and the acid reacts with phenolic anion to give blue colour (λ_{max} 650 nm). This reaction is analogous to the reaction of $FeCl_3$ with phenol.

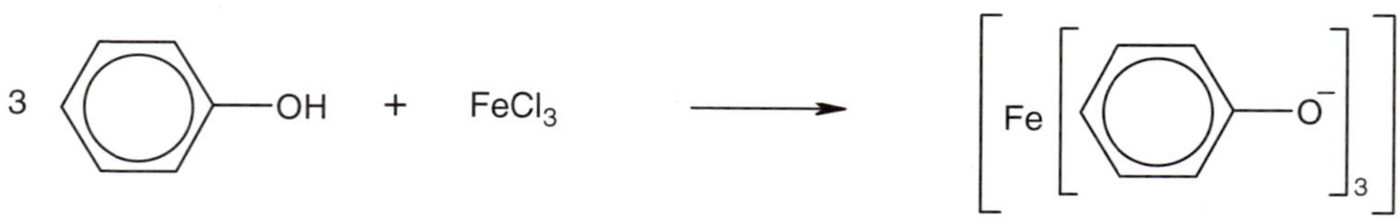

Violet colour

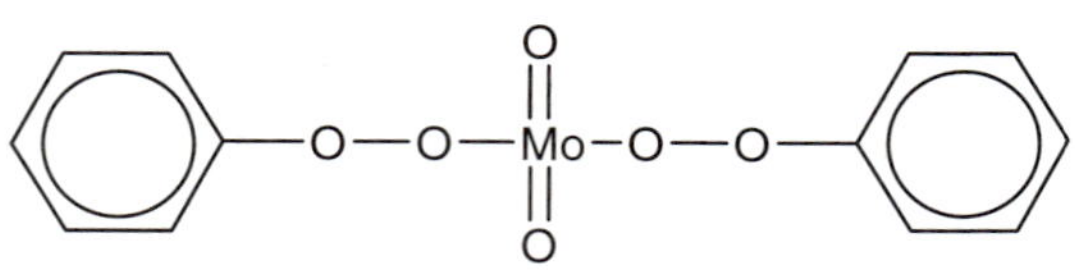

Blue colour
(λ_{max} 650 nm)

Alternatively, phosphomolybdate oxidizes phenolic (—OH) moiety of the amino acid (tyrosine) liberated as a result of enzymatic hydrolysis of caseine and itself (Mo (VI)) gets reduced to Mo (IV) which forms blue-grey mixed oxide with remaining Mo (VI).

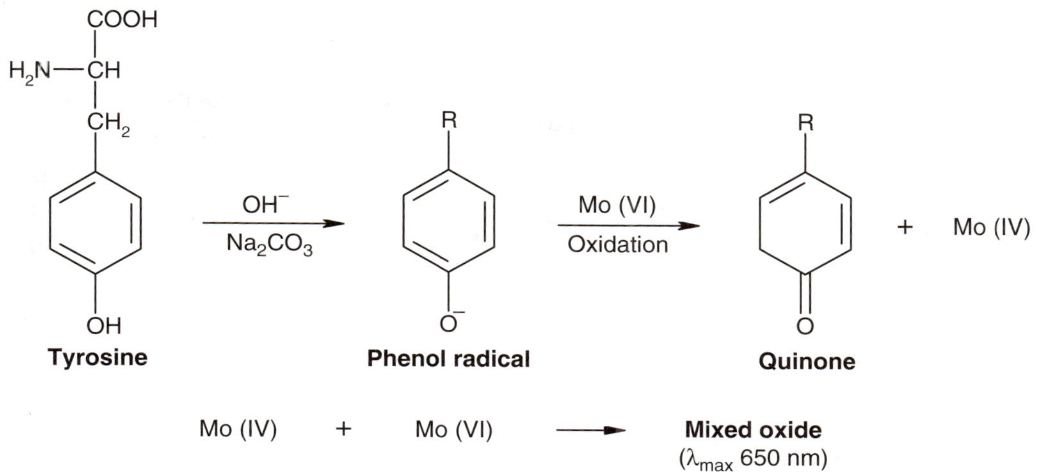

The phenolic (—OH) function of tyrosine present in hydrolysate can be estimated by Pauly's reaction. Diazotized 4-nitroaniline shall couple at ortho position to phenolic group, para being occupied in tyrosine.

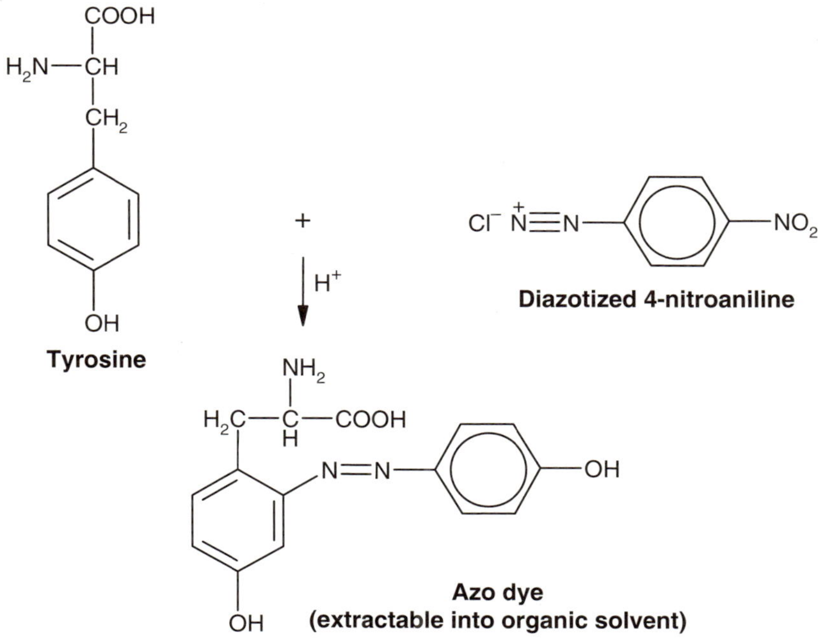

Note

Usually diazotized sulphanilic acid is used as coupling reagent in Pauly reaction, but diazotized nitroaniline is preferred as the azo dye form can be extracted into organic solvent. Tyrosine, because of its phenolic function, shall react with Gibbs' reagent and MBTH reagent for quantitative analysis.

Reference

Pharmaceutical Chemistry (Vol. 2) by H.J. Roth, pp. 210, 519, 599.

After removing paracetamol, after acetone extraction, the enzyme can be analysed by reaction with ninhydrin by heating in a boiling water-bath leading to formation of a coloured product with two maxima, i.e., 440 nm and 566 nm. Actual analysis was carried out in the laboratory and λ_{max} 440 nm was found to give reproducible result.

Note

1. As such there is significant interference from paracetamol, hence to be removed.
2. Acetone was the most appropriate solvent for removal of paracetamol.

Reference

F.A. Mehta et al., Abstract No. F 40, 559th IPC, 2007.

Paracetamol

Powdered sample equivalent to 50 mg of paracetamol is suspended in 0.1 M hydrochloric acid, shake, filter and dilute the filtrate suitably and measure the extinction of the resulting solution at 246 nm and calculate the results by using E 1%, 1 cm value of the drug.

Note

The enzyme did not interfere.

Drug Index

X

Z